Diabetes Mellitus

A Fundamental and Clinical Text

Diabetes Mellitus

A Fundamental and Clinical Text

Edited by

Derek LeRoith, MD, PhD

Section Chief, Diabetes Branch
National Institute of Diabetes, Digestive, and Kidney Diseases
National Institutes of Health
Bethesda, Maryland

Simeon I. Taylor, MD, PhD

Branch Chief, Diabetes Branch
National Institute of Diabetes, Digestive, and Kidney Diseases
National Institutes of Health
Bethesda, Maryland

Jerrold M. Olefsky, MD

Professor of Medicine
University of California Medical School
San Diego, California;
Veterans Administration Medical Center
La Jolla, California

With 176 additional contributors

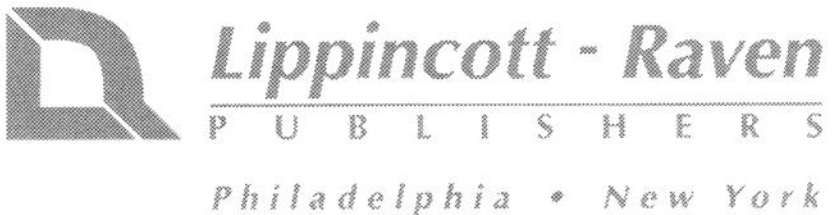

Lippincott - Raven
PUBLISHERS
Philadelphia • New York

Acquisitions Editor: Lisa McAllister
Developmental Editor: Melissa James
Production Editor: Virginia Barishek
Production Manager: Janet Greenwood
Production: P. M. Gordon Associates
Cover Designer: Robert Freese Design
Compositor: Compset, Inc.
Printer/Binder: Quebecor, Kingsport
Color Separator: Fidelity Color
Color Insert Printer: Sheridan Press

Library of Congress Cataloging-in-Publication Data

Diabetes mellitus / [edited by] Derek LeRoith, Simeon I. Taylor, Jerrold M. Olefsky ; with 176 additional contributors.
p. cm.
Includes bibliographical references and index.
ISBN 0-397-51456-5
1. Diabetes—Pathophysiology. 2. Diabetes—Molecular aspects. I. LeRoith, Derek, 1945– . II. Taylor, Simeon I. III. Olefsky, Jerrold M.
[DNLM: 1. Diabetes Mellitus. WK 810 D536 1996]
RC660.D4544 1996
616.4′62—dc20
DNLM/DLC
for Library of Congress 96-10271
CIP

The material contained in this volume was submitted as previously unpublished material, except in the instances in which credit has been given to the source from which some of the illustrative material was derived.

Great care has been taken to maintain the accuracy of the information contained in the volume. However, neither Lippincott–Raven Publishers nor the editors can be held responsible for errors or for any consequences arising from the use of the information herein.

The authors and publishers have exerted every effort to ensure that drug selection and dosage set forth in this text are in accord with current recommendations and practice at the time of publication. However, in view of ongoing research, changes in government regulations, and the constant flow of information relating to drug therapy and drug reactions, the reader is urged to check the package insert for each drug for any change in indications and dosage and for added warnings and precautions. This is particularly important when the recommended agent is a new or infrequently employed drug.

Materials appearing in this book prepared by individuals as part of their official duties as U.S. Government employees are not covered by the above-mentioned copyright.

9 8 7 6 5 4 3 2 1

Contributors

E. Dale Abel, MB, BS, DPhil
The Harvard Thorndike Research Laboratory
Department of Medicine
Beth Israel Hospital
Boston, Massachusetts

Domenico Accili, MD
Visiting Scientist
Diabetes Branch
National Institutes of Health
Bethesda, Maryland

John M. Amatruda, MD
Professor of Medicine, Adjunct
Section of Endocrinology
Yale University School of Medicine;
Director of Metabolic Disorders Research
Bayer Research Center;
Medical Staff
Yale–New Haven Hospital
New Haven, Connecticut

Robert C. Anderson, PhD
Senior Associate Director, Medicinal Chemistry
Sandoz Research Institute
East Hanover, New Jersey

Tammy Antonucci, PhD
Parke-Davis Pharmaceutical Research Division
Ann Arbor, Michigan

Plamen Atanasov, PhD
Research Professor
Department of Chemical and Nuclear Engineering
University of New Mexico School of Engineering
Albuquerque, New Mexico

Illani J. Atwater, PhD
Researcher
National Institute of Diabetes, Digestive, and Kidney Diseases
Laboratory of Cell Biology and Genetics
National Institutes of Health
Bethesda, Maryland

Joseph Avruch, MD
Professor of Medicine
Harvard Medical School
Chief, Diabetes Unit
Massachusetts General Hospital
Boston, Massachusetts

Pina L. Balducci-Silano, PhD
Postdoctoral Associate
Department of Pathology and Laboratory Medicine
University of Florida
Gainesville, Florida

Andrew B. Becker, MD, PhD
Mendel Group Inc.
Redwood City, California

Henning Beck-Nielsen, MD, PhD, DSc
Professor of Medicine
Clinical Research Institute
Odense University;
Chief Physician
Odense University Hospital
Odense, Denmark

Christine A. Beebe, MS, RD, CDE
Director of Saint James Health and Wellness Center
Chicago Heights, Illinois

Per A. Belfrage, MD, PhD
Professor
Medical and Physiological Chemistry
Faculty of Medicine
Lund University
Lund, Sweden

Peter H. Bennett, MB, FRCP, FFCM
Chief, Phoenix Epidemiology and Clinical Research Branch
National Institute of Diabetes, Digestive, and Kidney Diseases
Phoenix, Arizona

Michael Berelowitz, MB, ChB, FCP(SA)
Professor of Medicine, Physiology and Biophysics
Director, Division of Endocrinology and Metabolism
SUNY at Stoney Brook
Stoney Brook, New York

Vicky Blakesley, MD
Clinical Associate
Diabetes Branch
National Institute of Diabetes, Digestive, and Kidney Diseases
National Institutes of Health
Bethesda, Maryland

Clifton Bogardus, MD
Chief, Clinical Diabetes and Nutrition Section
National Institute of Diabetes, Digestive, and Kidney Diseases
National Institutes of Health
Phoenix, Arizona

Susan Bonner-Weir, PhD
Associate Professor of Medicine
Harvard Medical School;
Senior Investigator
Joslin Diabetes Center
Boston, Massachusetts

Kenneth L. Brayman, MD, PhD
Assistant Professor of Surgery
Director of the Pancreas and Human Islet Transplant Program
University of Pennsylvania Medical Center
Philadelphia, Pennsylvania

Michael Brownlee, MD
Anita and Jack Saltz Professor of Diabetes Research
Co-Director, Diabetes Research Center
Albert Einstein College of Medicine
New York, New York

John D. Brunzell, MD
Department of Medicine
University of Washington
Seattle, Washington

Thomas A. Buchanan, MD
University of Southern California School of Medicine;
LAC and USC Medical Center
Los Angeles, California

Peter C. Butler, MD
Endocrine Research Unit
Mayo Medical Center
Rochester, Minnesota

Maria M. Byrne, MD
Section of Endocrinology
The University of Chicago
The University of Chicago Hospitals
Chicago, Illinois

Michael G. Carlson, MD
Assistant Professor of Medicine
Division of Diabetes and Metabolism
Vanderbilt University School of Medicine
Vanderbilt University Medical Center
Nashville, Tennessee

Jose F. Caro MD
Magee Professor of Medicine
Chairman of the Department
Jefferson Medical College
Thomas Jefferson University;
Attending Physician
Thomas Jefferson University Hospital
Philadelphia, Pennsylvania

Alan Chait, MD
Professor of Medicine
Department of Medicine
Division of Metabolism, Endocrinology, and Nutrition
University of Washington
Seattle, Washington

Bentley Cheatham, PhD
Instructor in Medicine
Harvard Medical School;
Research Associate
Elliott P. Joslin Research Laboratory
Section on Cellular and Molecular Physiology
Joslin Diabetes Center
Boston, Massachusetts

Alan D. Cherrington, PhD
Professor
Department of Molecular Physiology and Biophysics
Vanderbilt University School of Medicine
Nashville, Tennessee

Lawrence B. Colen, MD
Associate Professor
Plastic and Reconstructive Surgery
Eastern Virginia Medical School
Norfolk, Virginia

Richard J. Comi, MD
Associate Professor of Medicine
Dartmouth Medical School;
Staff Endocrinologist/Diabetologist
Dartmouth–Hitchcock Medical Center
Lebanon, New Hampshire

Ellen L. Connor, MD
Fellow, Endocrinology
Department of Pediatrics
Shands Teaching Hospital
Gainesville, Florida

Philip E. Cryer, MD
Professor of Medicine
Director, Division of Endocrinology, Diabetes, and Metabolism
Washington University School of Medicine;
Director, General Clinical Research Center
Barnes Hospital
St. Louis, Missouri

Michael P. Czech, PhD
Professor
Department of Biochemistry and Molecular Biology
Director of the Program in Molecular Medicine
University of Massachusetts Medical Center
Worcester, Massachusetts

Erik J. Dasbach, PhD
Senior Research Fellow
Merck Research Laboratories
Blue Bell, Pennsylvania

Eva Degerman, MD, PhD
Department of Medical Chemistry
University of Lund
Lund, Sweden

Alison S. Depto, PhD
Assistant Professor
Diabetes Institute
Department of Internal Medicine
Neuropathy Study Group of the Diabetes Institute
Norfolk, Virginia

George Dimitriadis, MD, DPhil
Associate Professor of Medicine
Athens University Medical School,
Athens, Greece

Li Ding, PhD
Post-Doctoral Fellow
Department of Molecular Pharmacology
Stanford Medical Center
Stanford, California

Boris Draznin, MD, PhD
Professor and Vice Chairman
Department of Medicine
University of Colorado Health Sciences Center;
Chief, Endocrine Section
Veterans Administration Medical Center
Denver, Colorado

Richard C. Eastman
Director
Division of Diabetes, Endocrinology, and Metabolic Diseases
National Institute of Diabetes, Digestive, and Kidney Diseases
National Institutes of Health
Bethesda, Maryland

Steven V. Edelman, MD
Associate Professor of Medicine
Division of Diabetes and Metabolism
University of California San Diego;
Veterans Administration Medical Center
San Diego, California

Shimon Efrat, MD
Associate Professor
Department of Molecular Pharmacology
Albert Einstein College of Medicine
Bronx, New York

George S. Eisenbarth, MD, PhD
Professor of Medicine, Pediatrics and Immunology
University of Colorado School of Medicine;
Executive Director
Barbara Davis Center for Childhood Diabetes
University of Colorado Health Sciences Center
Denver, Colorado

Elizabeth D. Ennis, MD
Clinical Assistant Professor of Medicine
University of Alabama;
Assistant Director of Internal Medicine Education
Baptist Health Systems
Birmingham, Alabama

James L. Erwin, PhD
Department of Biochemistry and Molecular Biology
University of Massachusetts Medical Center
Worcester, Massachusetts

Susan J. Faas, PhD
Division of Immunogenetics
Department of Pediatrics
Rangos Research Center;
Children's Hospital of Pittsburgh
University of Pittsburgh School of Medicine
Pittsburgh, Pennsylvania

Stefan S. Fajans, MD
Professor Emeritus (Active) of Internal Medicine
University of Michigan Medical School
University of Michigan Hospitals
Ann Arbor, Michigan

Alberto Falorni, MD
Research Associate
Department of Molecular Medicine
Karolinska Institute
Stockholm, Sweden

Robert V. Farese, MD
Associate Chief of Staff for Research and Development
Professor and Director
Division of Endocrinology/Metabolism
J.A. Haley Veterans Administration Hospital
University of South Florida
Tampa, Florida

Ele Ferrannini, MD
Professor of Internal Medicine
University of Pisa School of Medicine;
Chief, Metabolism Unit
CNR Institute of Clinical Physiology
Pisa, Italy

Fred T. Fiedorek, Jr, MD
Assistant Professor
Department of Medicine
Curriculum in Genetics and Molecular Biology
University of North Carolina
Chapel Hill, North Carolina

Paul J. Flakoll, PhD
Assistant Professor
Departments of Surgery and Biochemistry
Vanderbilt University Medical Center
Nashville, Tennessee

Norman Fleischer, MD
Professor of Medicine
Director of Endocrinology and the Diabetes Research Center
Albert Einstein College of Medicine
Bronx, New York

Jeffrey S. Flier, MD
Professor of Medicine
Harvard Medical School;
Chief, Division of Endocrinology
Beth Israel Hospital
Boston, Massachusetts

James F. Foley, PhD
Executive Director Metabolic Diseases Department
Sandoz Research Institute
East Hanover, New Jersey

Saul Genuth, MD
Professor of Medicine
Case Western Reserve University;
Chief of Endocrinology
Mt. Sinai Medical Center of Cleveland
Cleveland, Ohio

Michael German, MD
Department of Medicine
Hormone Research Institute
University of California at San Francisco
San Francisco, California

Eugene How Go, MD
Fellow, Division of Endocrinology and Metabolism
SUNY at Stoney Brook
Stoney Brook, New York

Barry J. Goldstein, MD, PhD
Director, Division of Endocrinology and Metabolism Diseases
Associate Professor of Medicine
Department of Medicine
Jefferson Medical College
Thomas Jefferson University
Thomas Jefferson Hospital
Philadelphia, Pennsylvania

Daryl K. Granner, MD
Professor and Chairman
Department of Molecular Physiology and Biophysics
Vanderbilt University School of Medicine
Nashville, Tennessee

Carla J. Greenbaum, MD
Assistant Professor
Department of Medicine
Division of Endocrinology, Metabolism, and Nutrition
University of Washington
Veterans Administration Medical Center
University of Washington Medical Center
Seattle, Washington

Douglas A. Greene, MD
Professor of Internal Medicine
Chief, Division of Endocrinology and Metabolism
Director, Michigan Diabetes Research and Training Center
University of Michigan Medical Center
Ann Arbor, Michigan

Dale L. Greiner, PhD
Professor of Medicine
University of Massachusetts Medical School
Worcester, Massachusetts

Gerold M. Grodsky, PhD
Professor Emeritus (Active) of Biochemistry, Biophysics, and Medicine
University of California San Francisco
San Francisco, California

Angelika C. Gruessner, MS, PhD
Assistant Professor
Surgical Sciences
University of Minnesota Hospital
Minneapolis, Minnesota

Rainer W.G. Gruessner, MD, PhD
Associate Professor of Surgery
University of Minnesota;
University of Minnesota Hospital
Minneapolis, Minnesota

Joel F. Habener, MD
Professor of Medicine
Harvard Medical School;
Chief, Laboratory of Molecular Endocrinology
Massachusetts General Hospital;
Investigator
Howard Hughes Medical Institute
Boston, Massachusetts

Jeffrey B. Halter, MD
Professor of Internal Medicine
Chief, Division of Geriatric Medicine
Director, Geriatrics Center
Medical Director
Institute of Gerontology
University of Michigan;
Veterans Administration Medical Center
Ann Arbor, Michigan

Hans-Peter Hammes, MD
Associate Professor
Third Medical Department
Internal Medicine
Justus-Liebig University
Giessen, Germany

Barbara C. Hansen, PhD
Director, Obesity and Diabetes Research Center
Professor
Department of Physiology
University of Maryland at Baltimore
School of Medicine
Baltimore, Maryland

MAUREEN I. HARRIS, PHD, MPH
Director, National Diabetes Data Group
National Institute of Diabetes, Digestive, and Kidney Diseases
National Intitutes of Health
Bethesda, Maryland

LEONARD C. HARRISON, MD, DSC, FRACP, FRCPA
Professor
Director, Burnet Clinical Research Unit
Walter and Eliza Hall Institute of Medical Research
Royal Melbourne Hospital
University of Melbourne
Victoria, Australia

ROBERT HENRY, MD
Associate Professor of Medicine
Department of Endocrinology and Metabolism
Veterans Administration Medical Center
San Diego, California

WILLIAM H. HERMAN, MD, MPH
Chief, Epidemiology and Statistics Branch
Division of Diabetes Translation
Center for Disease Control and Prevention
Atlanta, Georgia

MICHAEL A. HILL, PHD
Department of Physiology
Eastern Virginia Medical School
Norfolk, Virginia

MARIE T. HOLLAND, MD
Assistant Professor of Neurology
Eastern Virginia Medical School
Sentara-Norfolk General Hospital
Norfolk, Virginia

EDWARD S. HORTON, MD
Professor of Medicine
Harvard Medical School;
Medical Director
Joslin Diabetes Center;
Director, Endocrinology and Metabolism
New England Deaconess Hospital
Boston, Massachusetts

GÖKHAN S. HOTAMISLIGIL, MD, PHD
Research Fellow in Cell Biology
Dana-Farber Cancer Institute
Harvard Medical School
Boston, Massachusetts

OLE HOTHER-NIELSEN, MD
Consultant Physician
Department of Medical Endocrinology
Odense University Hospital
Odense, Denmark

BARBARA V. HOWARD, PHD
Research Professor of Medicine
University of Maryland
George Washington University;
President
Medlantic Research Institute
Washington, DC

JONATHAN C. JAVITT, MD
Associate Professor of Ophthalmology
Director, Glaucoma Service
Georgetown University Medical Center;
Director
Worten Center for Eye Care Research
Washington, DC

ALEXANDRA L. JENKINS, BSC, RD
Research Associate
Department of Nutritional Sciences
Faculty of Medicine
University of Toronto;
Clinical Nutrition and Risk Factor Modification Center
St. Michael's Hospital
Toronto, Ontario, Canada

DAVID J.A. JENKINS, MD, PHD, DSC
Professor
Departments of Nutritional Sciences and Medicine
Faculty of Medicine
University of Toronto;
Director, Clinical Nutrition and Risk Factor Modification Center
St. Michael's Hospital
Toronto, Ontario, Canada

ZHEN Y. JIANG, MD, PHD
Research Fellow
Harvard Medical School
Joslin Diabetes Center
Brigham and Women's Hospital
Boston, Massachusetts

JOHN H. JOHNSON, PHD
Department of Internal Medicine
University of Texas
Southwestern Medical School
Veterans Administration Medical Center
Dallas, Texas

TAKASHI KADOWAKI, MD
Assistant Professor
Third Department of Internal Medicine
Faculty of Medicine
University of Tokyo
Tokyo, Japan

BARBARA B. KAHN, MD
Associate Professor of Medicine
Harvard Medical School;
Chief of the Diabetes Unit
Beth Israel Hospital
Boston, Massachusetts

C. Ronald Kahn, MD
Mary K. Iacocca Professor of Medicine
Harvard Medical School;
Director
Elliott P. Joslin Research Laboratory
Joslin Diabetes Center
Boston, Massachusetts

Thomas W.H. Kay, PhD, MBBS, FRACP, FRCPA
First Assistant
Burnet Clinical Research Unit
Walter and Eliza Hall Institute of Medical Research;
Immunologist
Royal Melbourne Hospital
Victoria, Australia

David M. Kendall, MD
Diabetes Center
Division of Diabetes, Endocrinology, and Metabolism
Department of Medicine
University of Minnesota Medical School
Minneapolis, Minnesota

Giulia Kennedy, MD
Millennium Pharmaceutical Inc.
Cambridge, Massachusetts

Norma S. Kenyon, PhD
Research Assistant Professor
Diabetes Research Institute
University of Miami School of Medicine
Miami, Florida

Anjaneyulu Kowluru, PhD
Senior Scientist
Section of Endocrinology
Department of Medicine
University of Wisconsin-Madison;
William S. Middleton Memorial Veterans Hospital
Madison, Wisconsin

Robert A. Kreisberg, MD
Clinical Professor of Medicine
University of Alabama
Director of Internal Medicine Education
Baptist Health Systems
Birmingham, Alabama

Jack L. Leahy, MD
Acting Chief
Division of Endocrinology, Diabetes, Metabolism, and Molecular Medicine
Associate Professor of Medicine
New England Medicine
Tufts University School of Medicine
Boston, Massachusetts

Åke Lernmark, PhD
Professor of Medicine
R.H. Williams Laboratory
University of Washington
Seattle, Washington

Derek LeRoith, MD, PhD
Section Chief, Diabetes Branch
National Institute of Diabetes, Digestive, and Kidney Diseases
National Institutes of Health
Bethesda, Maryland

Marie Joselie Leroy, PhD
Inserm Maternite Baudeloqove
Paris, France

Susan Lightman, MB, BS, FRCP, FRCOphth, PhD
Professor of Clinical Ophthalmology
Consultant Ophthalmologist
Moorfields Eye Hospital
London, England

Francis J. Liuzzi, PhD
Associate Professor
Department of Anatomy and Neurobiology
Director, Molecular Neurobiology Laboratory
Eastern Virginia Medical School
Norfolk, Virginia

Dean H. Lockwood, MD
Vice President for Clinical Research
Warner-Lambert/Parke-Davis
Ann Arbor, Michigan

Constantine Londos, DDS, PhD
Chief, Membrane Regulation Section
Laboratory of Cellular and Developmental Biology
National Institute of Diabetes, Digestive, and Kidney Diseases
National Institutes of Health
Bethesda, Maryland

Philip Luthert, MB, BS, BSc, MRCP, MRCPath
Professor of Ophthalmology
Institute of Ophthalmology
London, England

Noel K. Maclaren, MD
Professor and Chairman
Department of Pathology and Laboratory Medicine
Shands Teaching Hospital
Gainesville, Florida

Vincent C. Manganiello, MD, PhD
Chief, Section of Biochemical Physiology
Pulmonary-Critical Care Medicine
National Heart, Lung, and Blood Institute
National Institutes of Health
Bethesda, Maryland

Jennifer B. Marks, MD
Associate Professor of Clinical Medicine
University of Miami School of Medicine
Jackson Memorial Hospital
Miami, Florida

PAT MCNITT, RN
Clinical Research
Diabetes Research Institute
Eastern Virginia Medical School
Norfolk, Virginia

DAVID MEARS, PHD
National Institute of Diabetes, Digestive, and Kidney Diseases
Laboratory of Cell Biology and Genetics
National Institutes of health
Bethesda, Maryland

STEWART A. METZ, MD
Professor of Medicine
Section of Endocrinology
Department of Medicine
University of Wisconsin-Madison
William S. Middleton Memorial Veterans Hospital
Madison, Wisconsin

ZVONKO MILICEVIC, MD
Department of Internal Medicine
The Diabetes Institute
Eastern Virginia Medical School
Norfolk, Virginia

DANIEL H. MINTZ, MD
Mary Lou Held Professor of Medicine and Scientific Director
Diabetes Research Institute
University of Miami School of Medicine
Jackson Memorial Hospital
Miami, Florida

MENACHEM MIODOVNIK, MD
Professor of Obstetrics and Gynecology
Professor of Pediatrics
University of Cincinnati College of Medicine
University of Cincinnati Hospital
Cincinnati, Ohio

DAVID E. MOLLER, MD
Assistant Professor of Medicine
Harvard Medical School
Beth Israel Hospital
Boston, Massachusetts

JOHN P. MORDES, MD
Professor of Medicine
University of Massachusetts Medical School;
Physician
University of Massachusetts Medical Center
Worcester, Massachusetts

JERRY L. NADLER, MD
Director, Department of Diabetes, Endocrinology, and Metabolism
City of Hope National Medical Center
Duarte, California;
Adjunct Associate Professor of Medicine
University of Southern California
Los Angeles, California

DAVID M. NATHAN, MD
Associate Professor of Medicine
Harvard Medical School;
Director, Diabetes Research Center and Diabetes Clinic
Director, General Clinical Research Center
Massachusetts General Hospital
Boston, Massachusetts

CHRISTOPHER B. NEWGARD, PHD
Gifford O. Touchstone, Jr. and Randolph G. Touchstone Professor in Diabetes Research
Department of Biochemistry and Internal Medicine
The University of Texas Southwestern Medical Center at Dallas
Dallas, Texas

PAULINE G. NEWLON, PHD
Associate Director
Office of Research
Department of Medicine
Eastern Virginia Medical School
Norfolk, Virginia

ERIC A. NEWSHOLME, MA, PHD, DSC
Reader in Cellular Nutrition
Oxford University
Oxford, England

ROGER D. NOLAN, PHD
Departments of Biochemistry and Internal Medicine
The Diabetes Institutes
Eastern Virginia Medical School
Norfolk, Virginia

RICHARD M. O'BRIEN, MD
Department of Molecular Physiology and Biophysics
Vanderbilt University School of Medicine
Nashville, Tennessee

NIALL M. O'MEARA, MD
Section of Endocrinology
The University of Chicago
The University of Chicago Hospitals
Chicago, Illinois

JERRY P. PALMER, MD
Professor of Medicine
University of Washington;
Chief, Endocrinology and Metabolism
Veterans Administration Medical Center
Seattle, Washington

GARY L. PITTENGER, PHD
Assistant Professor
Department of Internal Medicine, Anatomy, and Neurobiology
Eastern Virginia Medical School
Norfolk, Virginia

Vincent Poitout, DVM, PhD
Diabetes Center
Division of Diabetes, Endocrinology, and Metabolism
Department of Medicine
University of Minnesota Medical School
Minneapolis, Minnesota

Kenneth S. Polonsky, MD
Professor of Medicine
Chief, Section of Endocrinology
The University of Chicago
The University of Chicago Hospitals
Chicago, Illinois

Alexander Rabinovitch, MD
Professor of Medicine and Immunology
Department of Medicine
University of Alberta
Edmonton, Alberta, Canada

Daniel J. Rader, MD
Director, Lipid Referral Center
Assistant Professor
Department of Medicine
Division of Medical Genetics
University of Pennsylvania Medical Center
Hospital of the University of Pennsylvania
Philadelphia, Pennsylvania

Steven E. Raper, MD
Associate Professor
Department of Surgery
University of Pennsylvania Medical Center
Hospital of the University of Pennsylvania
Philadelphia, Pennsylvania

Robert E. Ratner, MD
Associate Professor of Medicine
Division of Endocrinology
George Washington University
School of Medicine;
Director
Medlantic Clinical Research Center
Medlantic Research Institute
Washington, DC

Gerald M. Reaven, MD
Professor of Medicine
Head, Division of Endocrinology and Metabolism
Stanford University School of Medicine;
Director, Geriatric Research, Education, and Clinical Center
Veterans Administration Medical Center
Palo Alto, California

J. Bruce Redmon, MD
Diabetes Center
Division of Diabetes, Endocrinology, and Metabolism
Department of Medicine
University of Minnesota Medical School
Minneapolis, Minnesota

Jane E-B. Reusch, MD
Associate Professor of Medicine
University of Colorado Health Sciences Center;
Research Associate
Veterans Administration Medical Center
Denver, Colorado

Christopher J. Rhodes, PhD
Assistant Professor of Medicine (Biochemistry)
Harvard Medical School;
Investigator
Research Division
Joslin Diabetes Center
Boston, Massachusetts

Steven S. Rich, PhD
Professor of Public Health Sciences, Epidemiology and Neurology
Bowman Gray School of Medicine
Winston-Salem, North Carolina

Camillo Ricordi, MD
Professor of Surgery
Chief, Division of Cellular Transplantation
Co-Director, Diabetes Research Institute
University of Miami School of Medicine
Miami, Florida

Peter J. Roach, PhD
Professor of Biochemistry and Molecular Biology
Department of Biochemistry and Molecular Biology
Indiana University School of Medicine
Indianapolis, Indiana

R. Paul Robertson, MD
Professor of Medicine
Director, Division of Diabetes, Endocrinology, and Metabolism
University of Minnesota Medical School
University of Minnesota Hospital and Clinics
Minneapolis, Minnesota

Edouard Rojas, PhD
National Institute of Diabetes, Digestive, and Kidney Diseases
Laboratory of Cell Biology and Genetics
National Institutes of Health
Bethesda, Maryland

Barak M. Rosenn, MD
University of Cincinnati College of Medicine
University of Cincinnati
Cincinnati, Ohio

Luciano Rossetti, MD
Associate Professor of Medicine
Department of Medicine
Albert Einstein College of Medicine
Bronx, New York

Aldo A. Rossini, MD
Professor of Medicine
University of Massachusetts Medical School;
Physician
University of Massachusetts Medical Center
Worcester, Massachusetts

Richard A. Roth, PhD
Associate Professor
Department of Molecular Pharmacology
Stanford University School of Medicine
Stanford, California

Alan R. Saltiel
Warner-Lambert/Parke-Davis
Ann Arbor, Michigan

David S. Schade, MD
Professor of Medicine
University of New Mexico School of Medicine
Albuquerque, New Mexico

Elizabeth R. Seaquist, MD
Diabetes Center
Division of Diabetes, Endocrinology, and Metabolism
Department of Medicine
University of Minnesota Medical School
Minneapolis, Minnesota

Peter R. Shepherd, PhD
The Harvard Thorndike Research Laboratory
Department of Medicine
Beth Israel Hospital
Boston, Massachusetts

Alan R. Shuldiner, MD
Associate Professor of Medicine
Johns Hopkins University School of Medicine
Baltimore, Maryland

Kristi D. Silver, MD
Johns Hopkins University School of Medicine
Baltimore, Maryland

Alexander V. Skurat, PhD
Assistant Scientist
Assistant Professor
Department of Biochemistry and Molecular Biology
Indiana University School of Medicine
Indianapolis, Indiana

Jay S. Skyler, MD
Professor of Medicine, Pediatrics, and Psychology
University of Miami School of Medicine
Miami, Florida

Mark W. Sleeman, PhD
Department of Biochemistry and Molecular Biology
University of Massachusetts Medical Center
Worcester, Massachusetts

Bruce M. Spiegelman, PhD
Professor of Cell Biology
Dana Farber Institute
Harvard Medical School
Boston, Massachusetts

Kevin B. Stansberry, BS
Clinical Research
Diabetes Research Institute
Eastern Virginia Medical School
Norfolk, Virginia

Michael P. Stern, MD
Professor of Medicine
Chief, Clinical Epidemiology
University of Texas Health Sciences Center at San Antonio
San Antonio, Texas

Naftali Stern, MD
Associate Professor of Medicine
Sackler Faculty of Medicine
Tel Aviv University;
Director, Institute of Endocrinology
Tel Aviv-Sourasky Medical Center
Tel Aviv, Israel

Martin J. Stevens, MD
Assistant Professor
Department of Internal Medicine
Division of Endocrinology and Metabolism
University of Michigan Medical Center
Ann Arbor, Michigan

Jeppe Sturis, MD
Section of Endocrinology
The University of Chicago
The University of Chicago Hospitals
Chicago, Illinois

David E.R. Sutherland, MD, PhD
Professor of Surgery
University of Minnesota Hospitals
Minneapolis, Minnesota

Masato Taira, MD, PhD
Second Department of Internal Medicine
Chiba University School of Medicine
Chiba, Japan

Simeon I. Taylor, MD, PhD
Branch Chief, Diabetes Branch
National Institute of Diabetes, Digestive, and Kidney Diseases
National Intitutes of Health
Bethesda, Maryland

Hamish M.A. Towler, MB, ChB, BMedBiol, MRCP, FRCSE, FRCOphth
Lecturer in Clinical Ophthalmology
Institute of Ophthalmology
London, England

Roberto Trevisan, MD, PhD
Endocrinology
University of Padua;
Senior Registrar
Policlinico Universitario di Padova
Padua, Italy

Massimo Trucco, MD
Hillman Professor of Pediatric Immunology
Division of Immunogenetics
Department of Pediatrics
Children's Hospital of Pittsburgh
University of Pittsburgh School of Medicine
Pittsburgh, Pennsylvania

Michael L. Tuck, MD
Professor of Medicine
University of California Los Angeles
Los Angeles, California;
Chief, Endocrinology-Metabolism
UCLA San Fernando Valley Medical Program
Sepulveda, California

Charles F. Verge, MB, BS, FRACP
Barbara Davis Center for Childhood Diabetes
University of Colorado Health Sciences Center
Denver, Colorado

GianCarlo Viberti, MD, FRCP
Professor of Diabetes and Metabolic Medicine
Head, Unit for Metabolic Medicine
Division of Medicine
United Medical and Dental Schools
University of London;
Honorary Consultant Physician
Guy's and St. Thomas' Hospital Trust
London, England

Aaron I. Vinik, MBBch, PhD
Professor of Internal Medicine, Anatomy, and Neurobiology
Director, Diabetes Research Institute
Eastern Virginia Medical School
Norfolk, Virginia

Timothy F. Walseth, PhD
Diabetes Center
Division of Diabetes, Endocrinology, and Metabolism
Department of Medicine
University of Minnesota Medical School
Minneapolis, Minnesota

Gordon C. Weir, MD
Professor of Medicine
Harvard Medical School;
Head, Section of Islet Transplantation and Cell Biology
Joslin Diabetes Center
Boston, Massachusetts

Randall Whitcomb
Warner-Lambert/Parke-Davis
Ann Arbor, Michigan

Morris F. White, PhD
Associate Professor of Biological Chemistry
Department of Medicine
Harvard Medical School;
Investigator
Joslin Diabetes Center
Boston, Massachusetts

Ebtisam S. Wilkins, PhD
Professor of Chemical and Nuclear Engineering
University of New Mexico
Albuquerque, New Mexico

James M. Wilson, MD, PhD
Director, Institute for Human Gene Therapy
John Herr Musser Professor and Chair
Department of Molecular and Cellular Engineering;
Professor of Medicine
Chief, Division of Medicinal Genetics
University of Pennsylvania Medical Center
Hospital of the University of Pennsylvania
Philadelphia, Pennsylvania

Lori Winer, MD
Assistant Physician
Department of Diabetes, Endocrinology, and Metabolism
City of Hope Medical Center
Duarte, California

Ji-Won Yoon, PhD
Professor and Director
Julia McFarlane Diabetes Research Centre
Department of Microbiology and Infectious Diseases
Faculty of Medicine
University of Calgary
Calgary, Alberta, Canada

Hui-Jian Zhang, MD
Diabetes Center
Division of Diabetes, Endocrinology and Metabolism
Department of Medicine
University of Minnesota Medical School
Minneapolis, Minnesota

Preface

There are a number of excellent textbooks on diabetes mellitus available to the practicing physician. They cover most aspects of diabetes from a practical standpoint. However, we, the editors, were particularly struck by the lack of in-depth information on the basic molecular and cellular aspects of diabetes in these textbooks. Thus, we felt the need to assemble a volume that encompasses the many exciting advances in basic molecular and cellular components of diabetes as well as new therapeutic modalities. This textbook represents the culmination of this work.

The book is divided into ten parts; each part is divided into chapters authored by experts in that particular field. The text begins with a discussion of the basic pathophysiology of insulin secretion and insulin action. Insulin secretion is a tightly regulated phenomenon and the multiple influences, in addition to the well-known effects, of glucose are only now being unraveled. These newly discovered pathways are described in detail in this section.

The molecular details of the signaling pathways which mediate the various biologic effects of insulin are rapidly coming into focus, with new information emerging on a regular basis. One of the challenges in this field is to understand which sets of signaling molecules mediate the various diverse actions of insulin and how the specificity for the signaling pathways is manifested. These aspects are discussed in detail to provide the reader a current understanding of this emerging field.

In recent years, there have been major advances in our understanding of the autoimmune mechanisms which cause the destruction of islet cells. Furthermore, progress is being made to identify genes which may predispose individuals to such autoimmune destruction. In addition to the major histocompatibility locus method, positional cloning has been used to begin to identify other type I "diabetes genes." This section is immediately followed by a discussion of therapeutics, with particular attention paid to innovative and novel approaches to preventing diabetes and its complications.

The etiology of type II diabetes is similarly complex. We now understand that most patients destined to develop NIDDM manifest insulin resistance in the early pre-diabetic state. This leads to compensatory hyperinsulinemia, but, after a variable period of years, the beta cells no longer maintain this hyperinsulinemic state. Consequently, insulin secretion declines and the hyperglycemic NIDDM state ensues. This is a heterogenous syndrome with genetic and acquired factors combining to cause the final pathophysiologic state.

The application of modern methods of molecular genetics has begun to shed light on the genetic basis of type II diabetes mellitus. For example, mutations have been identified in several candidate genes in uncommon forms of type II diabetes. Additionally, efforts are underway to apply the positional cloning strategies useful in identifying type I "diabetes genes" to also identify type II "diabetes genes." And remarkable progress has been made in identifying genes that predispose individuals to the development of obesity using animal models of "diabesity" (e.g., the mouse obese gene). Finally, the large, recent U.S. clinical trial on the prevention of type II diabetes and the advent of a new class of insulin-sensitizing drugs promise to affect the treatment of millions of patients with diabetes.

The underlying mechanisms involved in the changes which occur during pregnancy as well as the effects of these changes on the mother and the offspring are still poorly understood. Similarly, the devastating complications of diabetes will only be significantly reduced once a better understanding of pathogenesis and pathophysiology is achieved.

The pace of the field of diabetology has been rapid in recent years. Not only have there been major advances in established areas of investigation, but entirely new areas of inquiry have evolved. For this text, we have striven to collect chapters by experts in the field to cover both the known etiologic factors involved in atherosclerosis, such as hyperinsulinemia, hypertension, and hyperlipidemia, as well as less well-known factors, such as free radicals, growth factors, glycation products, and autoimmunity. We have attempted to provide sufficient basic and clinical information to satisfy inquiry about either of these facets. The structure of the chapters (multiple, short reviews on each topic accompanied by extensive reference lists) was chosen to help our readers derive maximum information within a limited period while providing a tremendous resource for delving deeper into each subject by utilizing the up-to-date references. We sincerely hope that our approach in this fundamental and clinical textbook will provide a better understanding of the basic mechanisms involved in diabetes and, consequently, a more rational, effective approach to therapy.

This book represents the efforts of a great many individuals. We are indebted to our families for their patience and forbearance during the writing and editing of this textbook. Also, we owe a debt of appreciation to our contributing authors for their excellent scholarship and also for their willingness to share in this project and make it successful. Without their energy, this book could not have been possible and we thank them. Finally, we wish to express our gratitude to the staff at Lippincott–Raven Publishers for their assistance and understanding during the months of assembling the chapters.

Derek LeRoith, MD, PhD
Simeon I. Taylor, MD, PhD
Jerrold M. Olefsky, MD

Contents

Part I
Insulin Secretion 1

Part II
Insulin Action 119

Part III
Definition/Classification 249

Part IV
Type I Diabetes 261

Part V
Type I Diabetes: Therapeutics 371

Part VI
Type II Diabetes 453

PART I

Insulin Secretion

Diabetes Mellitus, edited by Derek LeRoith, Simeon I. Taylor, and Jerrold M. Olefsky. Lippincott–Raven Publishers, Philadelphia © 1996.

CHAPTER 1

Insulin Secretion in Humans: Physiologic Regulation and Alterations in Disease States

MARIA M. BYRNE, JEPPE STURIS, NIALL M. O'MEARA, AND KENNETH S. POLONSKY

Methods to Quantitate β-Cell Function

The development of the insulin radioimmunoassay was the first major advance in our attempt to understand in vivo β-cell function,[1] and it has remained the standard method used to evaluate β-cell secretory activity.[2,3] The measurement of peripheral insulin has significant limitations. Fifty to 60% of the insulin produced by the pancreas is extracted by the liver and does not reach the systemic circulation.[4,5] The standard radioimmunoassay for the measurement of insulin concentrations is also limited by its inability to distinguish between endogenous and exogenous insulin. The problem is further compounded when subjects taking exogenous insulin develop anti-insulin antibodies, because these antibodies interfere with the insulin radioimmunoassay. In addition, the polyclonal anti-insulin antibodies used to measure insulin have a high degree of cross-reactivity with proinsulin and the proinsulin conversion intermediates.[6]

Within the islet cells, proinsulin is cleaved into one molecule of insulin and one molecule of C-peptide. Insulin is subsequently released into the circulation at concentrations equimolar to those of C-peptide. Small amounts of intact proinsulin and proinsulin conversion intermediates are also released. These proinsulin-related peptides constitute 20% of total circulating insulin-like immunoreactivity, although their contribution to insulin's biologic activity is considerably less.[6] It has been estimated that the biologic potency of proinsulin is only 10% of that of insulin,[7,8] whereas the potency of split proinsulin is intermediate between that of proinsulin and insulin.[9,10] Their low concentration in serum, however, ensures that under normal physiologic conditions, their in vivo effects are negligible. In subjects with non–insulin-dependent diabetes mellitus (NIDDM) and even impaired glucose tolerance, however, there is a disproportionate increase in pro-insulin-related peptides to approximately 30% of the total immunoreactive insulin in the serum.

In contrast to insulin and proinsulin, C-peptide does not appear to be metabolically active.[11,12] It is considered to be a good marker of insulin secretion because of its equimolar secretion with insulin, negligible hepatic extraction,[5,13,14] and constant peripheral clearance at different plasma concentrations and in the presence of alterations in plasma glucose concentrations.[15,16] It is excreted exclusively by the kidney, and its plasma half-life of approximately 30 minutes contrasts sharply with the short plasma half-life (approximately 4 minutes) of insulin.[17] C-peptide assays are now widely available in which the relative molar cross-reactivity of proinsulin and proinsulin conversion products compared to C-peptide is approximately 10%, and therefore negligible.

The use of plasma C-peptide levels as an index of β-cell function is dependent on the critical assumption that the mean clearance rates of C-peptide are constant over the range of C-peptide levels observed under normal physiologic conditions. This assumption has been shown to be valid in both dogs and humans[5,18]; using this approach, insulin secretion rates can be derived from plasma C-peptide concentrations under steady-state conditions.[18] Under non–steady-state conditions (e.g., after a glucose infusion), because of its long plasma half-life, peripheral plasma C-peptide levels do not change in proportion to the changing insulin secretory rate[18,19]; under such circumstances, insulin secretion rates are best calculated by the use of the two-compartmental model initially proposed by Eaton and coworkers.[20] This approach involves nonlinear least-squares regression analysis of C-peptide decay curves to derive model parameters in individual subjects. The kinetic parameters of C-peptide are sufficiently reproducible that it is also possible to derive accurate estimates of the insulin secretion rate with the use of standard literature parameters.[21] Once the fractional rate constants and distribution volume are known, peripheral C-peptide concentrations can be analyzed mathematically and the corresponding secretion rates derived. With the use of this methodology, estimates of the secretion rate of insulin in human subjects have been reported to be 98 ± 3% of the actual rate as it is increasing and 100 ± 2% as it is decreasing.[18] Therefore, under steady-state conditions, whole plasma C-peptide levels provide an accurate index of the insulin secretory rate; under non–steady-state conditions, β-cell secretion rates of insulin can be more accurately and most easily derived from mathematical analysis of peripheral C-peptide concentrations using a two-compartmental model. In interpreting the validity of experimental results evaluating insulin secretion in vivo, the limitations of the method used to assess β-cell function should always be taken into account.

The Normal Insulin Secretory Profile

Dose-Response Relationship Between Glucose and Insulin Secretion

The in vivo dose-response curve that describes the relationship between insulin secretion and glucose in humans is sigmoidal in shape.[22–24] In vivo studies utilizing a low-dose graded glucose infusion have shown that in normal-weight, nondiabetic subjects, β-cell responses to glucose can be modified by a number of physiologic factors, including low-dose glucose infusion, fasting, and refeeding. As illustrated in Figure 1-1, after an overnight fast, the dose-response relationship between glucose and insulin secretion is linear at glucose levels below 15 mM. If dose-response curves between glucose and insulin secretion are constructed before and after an exogenous infusion of glucose for 42 hours, changes in the sensitivity of the β-cell to glucose can be demonstrated. Glucose administration primes β-cell responses to the same glucose stimulus, resulting in a shift in the dose-response curve to the left, with a 52% increase in insulin secretion rates over the 5–9 mM glucose concentration range. After a 72-hour fast, however, the glucose insulin secretion dose-response curve is shifted to the right, with a 32% reduction in insulin secretion (see Fig. 1-1). This reduction in β-cell responsiveness to glucose is reversed by refeeding.[25]

This priming effect of glucose to increase the sensitivity of the β-cell to a subsequently administered glucose stimulus[26–28] also has been observed in humans, in the isolated rat pancreas, and in isolated rat islets. Flax et al.[29] demonstrated that in response to 2 days of basal hyperglycemia (6.0 mM), both basal and stimulated

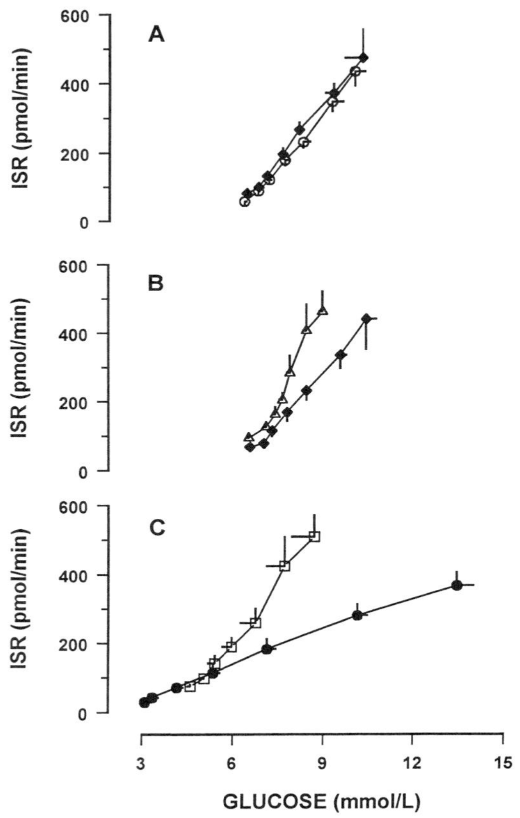

Figure 1-1. Relationship between average glucose concentrations and ISR during graded IV glucose infusion study. Lowest glucose levels and ISR were measured under basal conditions, and subsequent levels were obtained during glucose infusion rates of 1, 2, 3, 4, 6, and 8 mg/kg/min. *A,* ◆ = Data from the initial study; ○ = data from the repeat study. *B,* ◆ = Data from the initial study; △ = data from postglucose infusion study. *C,* ● = Data from the fasting study; □ = data from the refeeding study. (Redrawn with permission from Byrne MM, Sturis J, Polonsky KS. Insulin secretion and clearance during low-dose graded glucose infusion. Am J Physiol 1995;268:E21.)

β-cell responses to glucose were enhanced. Leahy et al.[30] demonstrated that 48 hours of mild hyperglycemia in rats (i.e., an increase in glucose of 1 mM) potentiated glucose-induced insulin secretion. Exposure to very high doses of glucose for prolonged periods, however, may actually induce defects in insulin secretion.[31]

The mechanism whereby changes in β-cell sensitivity to glucose are mediated has been studied in vitro and has been suggested to result from upregulation of the enzyme glucokinase. Changes in β-cell sensitivity to glucose correlate with alterations in the levels and activity of glucokinase in vitro.[27,32] Unlike liver glucokinase, expression of islet glucokinase appears to regulated by serum glucose levels. The activity of glucokinase in the islet plays a crucial role in glucose-induced insulin secretion.[33] It has also been postulated that the glucose transporter GLUT-2 may be important in glucose-stimulated insulin secretion. Alterations in β-cell GLUT-2 expression occur in animals with glucose infusion. Hyperglycemic clamping in Wistar rats for 5 days (glucose 200 ± 50 mg/dL) increased GLUT-2 mRNA by 46%.[34]

Studies in laboratory animals have indicated that the β-cell sensitivity to glucose is reduced in the fasting state.[35] Efendic et al.[36] showed that 24-hour starvation in rats reduced the magnitudes of the early and the late insulin-secretion phases to a similar extent.[36] In fact, they noted that the insulin response of "fasted" rats is similar to that of mildly diabetic subjects. It has been suggested that the reduction in glucokinase that occurs with fasting may be responsible for the associated reduction in insulin secretion. In studies of insulin release in pancreatic islets during fasting and refeeding, glucokinase activity decreased 31% after a 72-hour fast. After 48 hours of refeeding, glucokinase activity was higher than in islets from control rats who had been fed.[37]

Postprandial Responses and Circadian Variations in Secretion

It has been estimated that 50% of the total amount of insulin secreted by the pancreas during a 24-hour period represents basal secretion, and the remainder is secreted in response to meals. The β-cell response to a particular stimulus appears in part to be dependent on the clock time at which the stimulus is administered. The administration of three standard meals at different clock times demonstrates that maximum postprandial responses are observed consistently after breakfast.[38–40] Similar results were those found when oral glucose tolerance tests were performed at different times of the day.[41–43] Maximum insulin secretory responses were observed in the morning, with lower responses occurring in the afternoon and evening. These diurnal variations were found to be present after IV glucose tolerance tests (IVGTTs) and during a prolonged 24-hour glucose infusion study, during which the nocturnal rise in glucose concentration was not accompanied by a similar increase in the insulin secretory rate.[44] It has been postulated that these circadian differences may reflect a diminished responsiveness of the β-cell to glucose in the afternoon and evening.[43]

Oscillatory Insulin Secretion

In vivo studies of β-cell secretory function have demonstrated that insulin is released in a pulsatile fashion. Rapid oscillations occur every 8–15 minutes,[45–48] which are superimposed on slower (ultradian) oscillations that occur at a periodicity of 80–150 minutes[39,44,49–51] (Fig. 1-2). These rapid oscillations have been observed in a variety of species in addition to humans, including monkeys,[45,52] baboons, and dogs.[53,54] Their presence also has been noted in a number of in vitro experiments[55–58] and in subjects who have undergone pancreas transplantation[59,60]; accordingly, neural factors are unlikely to be responsible for their generation. These pulses could be a reflection of the activity of an intrinsic pancreatic pacemaker.[61] Because the periodicity of these oscillations is more rapid in vitro[56,58] and after transplantation,[60] however, it appears that neural factors modulate the activity of the pacemaker which generates these oscillations.

The rapid oscillations of insulin are of small amplitude in the systemic circulation, averaging between 0.4 and 3.2 μU/mL in several published human studies.[46–48,62] Because these values are very close to the limits of sensitivity of most standard insulin radioimmunoassays, the characterization of these oscillations is subject to considerable pitfalls, not the least of which being the need to differentiate between true oscillations of small amplitude and random assay noise. This latter problem can in part be overcome by increasing the accuracy of laboratory estimations through the use of frequent measurements (six to eight) at each sampling time point in contrast to the standard practice of relying solely on duplicate measurements.[51] In addition, we have recently shown that the detection and characterization of these pulses in the systemic circulation is greatly facilitated by the application of several different analytic approaches to each pulsatile or oscillatory profile obtained in an individual subject.[51]

The low amplitude of the rapid oscillations in the systemic circulation contrasts sharply with observations in the portal vein, where pulse amplitudes of 20–40 μU/mL have been recorded in dogs.[54,55] Although the physiologic importance of these low-ampli-

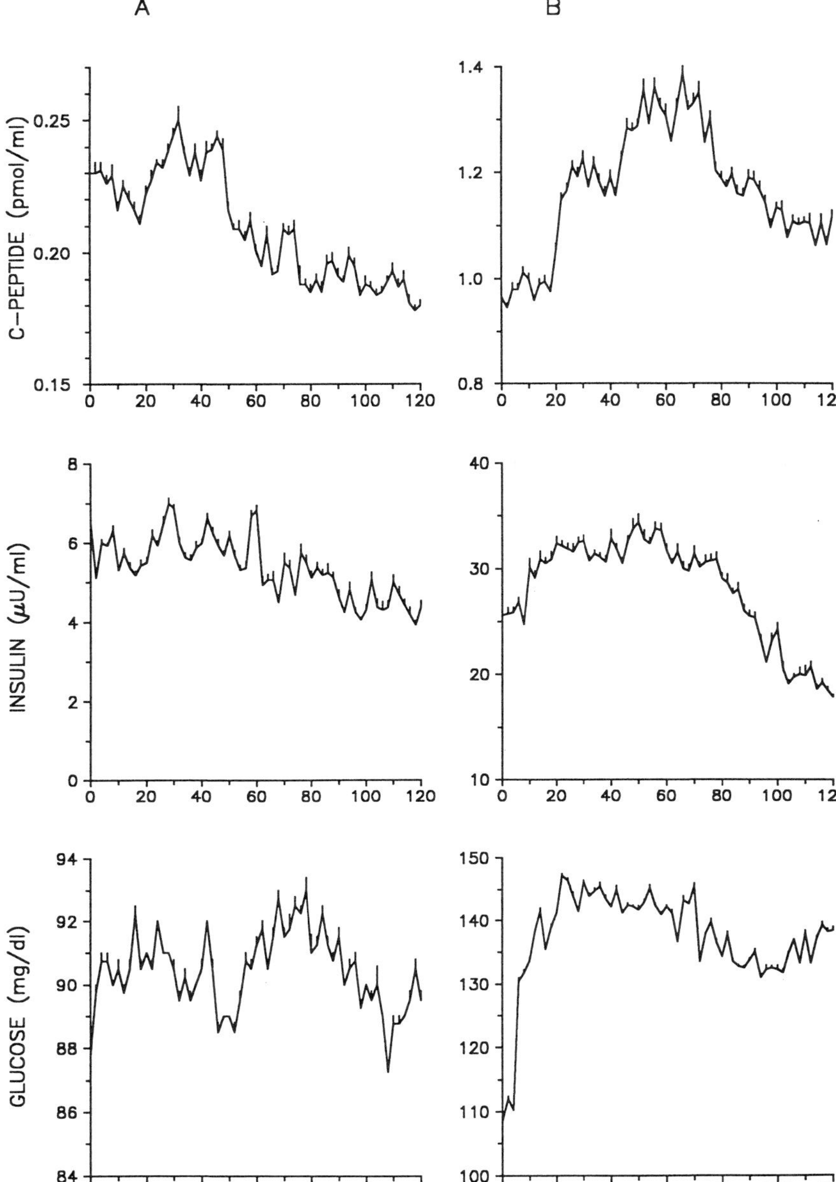

Figure 1-2. Profiles in one subject of glucose, insulin, and C-peptide during basal conditions (*A*) and during constant glucose infusion (*B*). All sample measurements (4 for glucose and 16 for insulin and C peptide) were averaged before profiles were plotted. (Reproduced with permission from O'Meara NM, Sturis J, Blackman JD, et al. Analytical problems in detecting rapid insulin secretory pulses in normal humans. Am J Physiol 1993;264:E231.)

tude rapid pulses in the periphery is unclear, they are likely to be of physiologic importance in the portal vein. It is possible that the liver responds more readily to insulin delivered in a pulsatile fashion than to insulin delivered at a constant rate.[63–65]

In contrast to the rapid oscillations, the slower (ultradian) oscillations are of much larger amplitude in the peripheral circulation. They are present under basal conditions, but are amplified postprandially[39,66] and have been observed in subjects receiving IV glucose,[44,50] suggesting that they are not generated by intermittent absorption of nutrients from the gut. Furthermore, they do not appear to be related to fluctuations in glucagon or cortisol levels[50] and are not regulated by neural factors because these oscillations are also present in recipients of successful pancreas transplants.[59,67] Many of these ultradian insulin and C-peptide pulses are synchronous with pulses of similar oscillatory period in glucose,[39,44,66] raising the possibility that these oscillations are a product of the insulin-glucose feedback mechanism. Ultradian oscillations are self-sustained during constant glucose infusion at various rates, they are increased in amplitude after stimulation of insulin secretion without change in frequency, and there is a slight temporal advance of the glucose versus the insulin oscillation. These findings suggest that the ultradian oscillations may be entirely accounted for by the major dynamic characteristics of the insulin-glucose feedback system, with no need to postulate the existence of an intrapancreatic pacemaker.[68] In support of this hypothesis, Sturis et al.[69] demonstrated that when glucose is administered in an oscillatory pattern, ultradian oscillations in plasma glucose and insulin secretion are generated that are 100% concordant with the oscillatory period of the exogenous glucose infusion. This close relationship between the ultradian oscillations in insulin secretion and similar oscillations in plasma glucose was further exemplified in a series of dose-response studies where the largest amplitude oscillations in insulin secretion were observed in those subjects exhibiting the largest-amplitude glucose oscillations, which in turn were directly related to the infusion dose of glucose.[70] It has recently been shown that in normal humans, insulin is more effective in reducing plasma glucose levels when administered intravenously as a 120-minute oscillation than when delivered at a constant rate.[71] These results indicate that the ultradian oscillations have functional significance.

Alterations of Insulin Secretion

Obesity

Subjects who are obese are insulin resistant and hyperinsulinemic.[72–75] Insulin hypersecretion has been observed in both animal models and obese humans. Increased β-cell mass or islet hypertrophy, or both, have been reported.[76,77] Although decreased insulin clearance has been demonstrated in obese subjects,[78] most evidence suggests that the elevated insulin levels in this population subgroup represent a compensatory adaptive response of the β-cell to the accompanying insulin resistance. Increased insulin secretory rates, both basally and after meals, have been demonstrated in obese subjects and correlate strongly with body mass index.[79] As in normal subjects, basal insulin secretion accounts for 50% of the total daily insulin production, and the increased secretion of insulin in obese subjects is not associated with any alteration in the proinsulin:insulin molar ratio.[80] In a recent study of juvenile obesity, the sequence of metabolic dysfunction began with an abnormal pattern of postprandial hyperinsulinemia caused by β-cell dysfunction. This defect was then followed by permanent hyperinsulinemia and insulin resistance. These defects worsened with the duration of obesity.[81] These results are consistent with animal studies in which experimental lesions of the ventromedial hypothalamus caused hyperinsulinemia in response to oral glucose or meals before the animals accumulated excess weight.[82,83]

Oscillatory insulin secretion is also preserved in obese subjects. Small-amplitude rapid oscillations in secretion occurring every 10–12 minutes[47] and slower oscillations of larger amplitude occurring every 1-1/2–2 hours[39,79] have been demonstrated, the latter once again being tightly coupled to oscillations of similar period in plasma glucose.[84] A recent study of women with abdominal obesity demonstrated blunted ultradian secretory pulse amplitudes, a phenomenon also observed in overtly NIDDM subjects. This suggests that in abdominal obesity, the increase in pancreatic insulin output is limited and the secretory pulsatilities aberrant, suggesting a defect in the insulin secretory process.[85]

Aging

In the general population, glucose tolerance declines with age in unaffected as well as affected subjects. Peripheral insulin resistance, impaired glucose tolerance, and hyperinsulinemia are metabolic changes observed with aging.[86–88] Physical inactivity and obesity appear to be important factors in causing the reduction in insulin sensitivity in the elderly population.[89,90] On completion of exercise training programs, elderly subjects demonstrated marked improvements in insulin sensitivity from baseline,[90] which was associated with a corresponding reduction in β-cell secretory responses to glucose.

Insulin secretion has been shown to be reduced in elderly rats, but studies of elderly human subjects have yielded conflicting results: Diminished, normal, and increased insulin secretory activity all have been reported.[86,91–93] This discrepancy in results among these studies may have resulted in part from the fact that young and elderly subjects were not always studied at comparable levels of insulin and glucose sensitivity. In a study by Gumbiner et al.,[94] ten elderly subjects demonstrated basal hyperinsulinemia and enhanced insulin secretory responses to meals. When glucose levels were matched during hyperglycemic clamping, however, the insulin secretory response, although normal in absolute terms, was disproportionately low in the elderly patients, especially when viewed in relation to the degree of insulin resistance associated with aging. These findings were recently confirmed by Kahn et al.,[95] who demonstrated that insulin secretory responses to glucose and arginine in an elderly group of subjects were significantly lower than in the weight-matched younger group. Thus, although elderly subjects have enhanced insulin-secretion rates due to insulin resistance, the β-cell secretory responses still are inappropriately low for the level of insulin sensitivity. Diminished insulin clearance does not appear to be a contributory factor to the observed hyperinsulinemia in this population subgroup.[93,94] A recent study has demonstrated decreased amplitude of ultradian oscillations in insulin secretion as a result of aging.[96] In recent preliminary studies performed in elderly subjects, the ability of glucose to entrain the ultradian insulin secretory oscillations also has been suggested to be impaired, suggesting the presence of a β-cell defect in the elderly.[97]

Diabetes Mellitus

Insulin-Dependent (Type I) Diabetes Mellitus

Patients with type I diabetes mellitus are insulin deficient and have practically no β-cell response to glucose and nonglucose stimuli.[98] The initial period after diagnosis, however, often is associated with an improvement in glucose tolerance to the point where normoglycemia can be maintained for a self-limiting duration in some patients in the absence of any definitive therapy.[99] This ''honeymoon period'' is associated with improvement in the C-peptide and insulin responses to glucose.[3,100,101] Although β-cell secretory capacity is improved during this period, it is still less than that observed in normal subjects. In addition to this quantitative defect, a qualitative defect is also present, as manifested in serum by an increased molar ratio of proinsulin to C-peptide.[102,103] Thus during the honeymoon period, the pancreas in addition to secreting less insulin also releases the contents of immature β-cell granules into the circulation. The subsequent and inevitable deterioration in glycemia control heralding the end of the honeymoon period is preceded by a gradual reduction in the secretory capacity of the β-cell.[3] The assessment of β-cell function in patients with recently diagnosed type I diabetes mellitus may be of clinical relevance in view of the evidence suggesting that the degree of residual β-cell function at this stage may be an important prognostic indicator of which patients are most likely to benefit from a period of immunosuppression.

The β-cell secretory responses during the period before the onset of type 1 diabetes mellitus are also of interest. Studies of normoglycemic islet cell antibody–positive monozygotic twins whose co-twins were already insulinopenic, have demonstrated a progressive diminution in the first-phase insulin response to glucose for a number of years before the development of overt type 1 diabetes mellitus.[104] A study by Bingley et al.[62] demonstrated that the rapid oscillations lose their regularity in islet cell antibody–positive nondiabetic subjects. A recent study of β-cell function in a person who developed type I diabetes over a 13-month period while under observation, showed that despite lower absolute secretory rates, ultradian oscillations in insulin secretion persisted in the period before and immediately after the onset of type I diabetes, but they were less tightly coupled to glucose than in nondiabetic subjects.[105] Hence, an abnormal pattern of insulin secretion was present when the subject's fasting glucose and glycosylated hemoglobin levels were still normal. During this ''early'' diabetic phase, the β-cell response to other secretagogues including arginine, tolbutamide, and glucagon is also impaired, but to a much smaller extent.[106] In the future, the early identification of β-cell dysfunction in persons at high risk for developing type I diabetes mellitus may be of therapeutic value in preventing the onset of the disease in this group. Intensive therapy with insulin early in the course of type I diabetes has been found to preserve β-cell function, and when less toxic immunosuppressive agents become available, early immunosuppression may be a viable therapeutic option.

Insulin Secretion in Classic Non–Insulin-Dependent (Type II) Diabetes Mellitus

Patients with type II diabetes are often hyperinsulinemic, but the degree of hyperinsulinemia is inappropriately low for the prevailing glucose concentrations. Nevertheless, many of these patients have sufficient β-cell reserve to maintain a euglycemic state during dietary restriction with or without an oral agent. Type II diabetes is recognized to arise from a combination of insulin resistance and impaired β-cell function. In Pima Indians[107] and Mexican-Americans,[108] insulin resistance is the first identifiable defect, whereas in white populations β-cell deficiency appears to be more marked at an early stage in the development of diabetes.[109,110] Once overt diabetes has occurred subjects have hyperglycemia, insulin resistance and impaired insulin responses. The β-cell defect in patients with NIDDM is characterized by an absent first-phase insulin and C-peptide response to an IV glucose load and a reduced second-phase response,[98,111] delayed and blunted secretory responses to mixed meals, increased concentrations of proinsulin and proinsulin-breakdown intermediates, and alterations in the ultradian oscillations and rapid pulses of insulin secretion. Although in vitro studies using the isolated perfused pancreas have emphasized the importance of hyperglycemia in mediating these changes,[112,113] the abnormal first-phase response to IV glucose persists in patients whose diabetic control has been greatly improved,[98,114] thus supporting the hypothesis that patients with type II diabetes may have an intrinsic defect in the β-cell. Furthermore, when subjects develop mild impaired glucose tolerance, first phase insulin secretion is blunted.[115] An attenuated insulin response to oral glucose has been observed in normoglycemic co-twins of patients with type II diabetes,[109,110] a group at very high risk for NIDDM and who can legitimately be classified as being "prediabetic." This pattern of insulin secretion during the so-called prediabetic phase is also seen in subjects with impaired glucose tolerance who later develop NIDDM,[116–119] and in normoglycemic obese subjects with a recent history of gestational diabetes[120–123]; this later group is also at high risk for developing NIDDM in the future.[124] β-cell abnormalities may therefore precede the development of overt NIDDM by many years.

Many studies in recent years have examined the effects of type II diabetes on levels of proinsulin in serum. These studies have consistently demonstrated elevated levels of proinsulin in association with increases in the molar ratio of proinsulin to insulin,[123,125,126] suggesting that the β-cells of patients with type II diabetes release an excess of immature secretory granules into the circulation. The amount of proinsulin produced in these patients appears to be related to the degree of glycemic control rather than the duration of diabetes. In one series, proinsulin levels contributed nearly 50% of the total insulin immunoreactivity in patients with type II diabetes who had marked hyperglycemia.[126] Because conventional assays of levels of immunoreactive insulin also measure proinsulin, it is possible that hyperinsulinemia reported in patients with type II diabetes represents to some degree the combined contributions of insulin and proinsulin rather than hyperinsulinemia alone.[127,128] In a recent study a sensitive insulin assay was used that did not cross-react with proinsulin, and the results showed that insulin levels in both obese and nonobese subjects with type II diabetes were lower than in weight-matched controls.[127] The patients with diabetes in this series had elevated circulating proinsulin levels and 32-33 split proinsulin (a proinsulin conversion intermediate molecule). When insulin levels in this study population were measured with a conventional insulin assay, the differences between diabetic patients and controls were less apparent. Proinsulin levels also have been measured in subjects with impaired glucose tolerance, and conflicting results have been obtained: Both elevated and normal levels of proinsulin have been reported.[126,129]

Abnormalities in the temporal pattern of insulin secretion also have been demonstrated in patients with type II diabetes.[130] In normal subjects, equal amounts of insulin are secreted basally and postprandially in a 24-hour period. Subjects with NIDDM secrete a greater proportion of their daily insulin under basal conditions.[131] There is reduction in the amplitude of the secretory pulses of insulin, rather than the number of pulses occurring after meals. In a recent study utilizing a 28-hour oscillatory glucose infusion with the amplitude of the oscillations being 33% above and below the mean infusion rate and their respective periods being 144 minutes (slow oscillatory infusion) or 96 minutes (rapid oscillatory infusion), we demonstrated that the tight temporal coupling between glucose and insulin secretion rate (ISR) in the nondiabetic controls was impaired in the impaired glucose tolerance (IGT) and NIDDM groups as demonstrated by pulse analysis, cross-correlation analysis, and spectral analysis.[84] Figure 1-3 demonstrates the glucose, insulin, and ISR responses to a slow oscillatory infusion (i.e., with a period of 144 minutes in a control subject [Fig. 1-3*C*], one subject with impaired glucose tolerance [Fig. 1-3*B*], and one subject with NIDDM [Fig. 1-3*A*]. The absolute amplitude of the ISR pulses progressively declined with the transition from obesity to IGT to NIDDM, and the absolute amplitude of the ISR oscillations failed to increase appropriately with increasing absolute amplitude of the glucose oscillations in the IGT and NIDDM subjects compared to the control group. This study demonstrates that the insulin-glucose feedback mechanism, which plays an important role in the regulation and generation of the ultradian oscillations in nondiabetic subjects, is disrupted in NIDDM, even in conditions where glucose tolerance is only minimally impaired. The resultant uncoupling of the normally tight relationship between glucose and ISR pulses is reflected in (1) a reduction in the spectral power of the ultradian oscillations of insulin secretion when oscillatory glucose is administered, and (2) a discrepancy between the dominant period of the spectra of insulin secretion and glucose. The dissociation between the oscillations in glucose and insulin becomes more severe with the progression from IGT to NIDDM. Whether the abnormal secretory oscillations play a pathogenetic role in the progression to overt diabetes or whether they are merely reflective of underlying defects in the β-cell and peripheral tissues remains to be determined. Similar findings are observed in subjects with NIDDM studied under fasting conditions.[70]

The rapid insulin pulses that occur every 8–15 minutes superimposed on the ultradian oscillations are also disrupted in NIDDM.[132] The cycles are shorter and more irregular than those observed in normal subjects. O'Rahilly et al.[133] observed similar findings in a group of first-degree relatives of patients with NIDDM who had only mild glucose intolerance, indicating that abnormalities in oscillatory activity may be an early manifestation of β-cell dysfunction in NIDDM.

Insulin Secretion in Maturity-Onset Diabetes of the Young

It has been determined recently that maturity-onset diabetes of the young (MODY), a form of NIDDM with early age of onset <25 years and autosomal dominant inheritance, may result from the presence of the diabetes susceptibility gene on chromosome 20q12 in the region of the adenosine deaminase gene in the RW pedigree,[134] or from mutations in the glycolytic enzyme glucokinase gene (*GCK*).[135–137]

Froguel and coworkers[138] recently found that MODY was linked to glucokinase in a number of French families. They described this form of diabetes as being characterized by mild fasting hyperglycemia (i.e., glucose levels >6.1 mM), which is evident in childhood. Heterozygous mutations in the *GCK* gene were subsequently identified. The enzyme glucokinase is the first rate-limiting step in glucose metabolism by the β-cell and has been postulated to represent the glucose sensor.[33] We have recently performed detailed studies of subjects with *GCK* mutations to gain a further

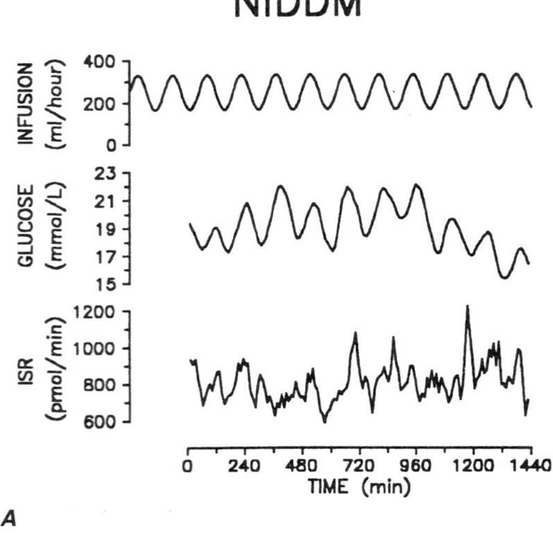

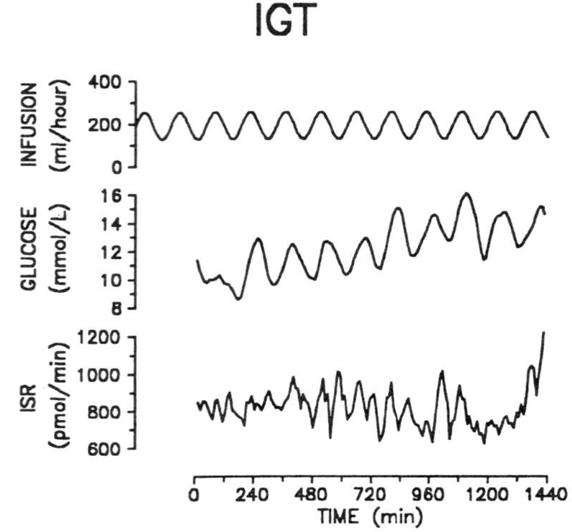

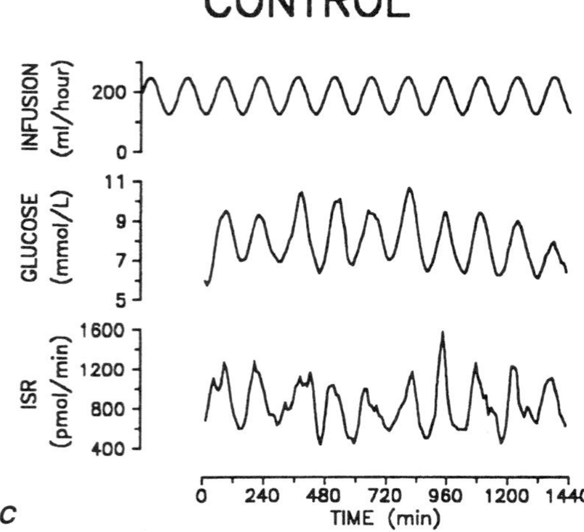

FIGURE 1-3. Profiles of the glucose infusion rate, glucose concentrations, and the ISRs, during a slow oscillatory infusion (period of 144 minutes) in one subject with NIDDM (*A*), one subject with IGT (*B*), and one control subject (*C*). (Redrawn with permission from O'Meara NM, Sturis J, Van Cauter E, Polonsky KS. Lack of control by glucose of ultradian insulin secretory oscillations in impaired glucose tolerance and in non–insulin-dependent diabetes mellitus. J Clin Invest 1993;92:262.)

understanding of the in vivo regulation of insulin secretion in this condition as well as the pathophysiology of the glucose intolerance that is found in these patients.[139]

Insulin secretory responses were evaluated over a 24-hour period while subjects consumed a weight-maintenance diet consisting of three meals. Subjects with *GCK* mutations had fasting glucose concentrations of ≈7.0 mM and peak postprandial levels of ≈10 mM. These levels are significantly less than those seen in subjects with classic NIDDM and higher than controls (Fig. 1-4). The 24-hour ISRs were not significantly different from controls, and the delayed and blunted insulin secretory responses to meals characteristic of classic NIDDM were not seen.[131] First-phase insulin secretory responses during IVGTTs were normal in subjects with *GCK* mutations, in contrast to classic NIDDM and subjects with IGT where first-phase insulin secretion is markedly blunted or absent.

To test the ability of the β-cell to sense and respond to small increments in plasma glucose concentrations, we used a low-dose glucose infusion protocol. Figure 1-5 shows the dose-response curves in subjects with *GCK* mutations and controls before and after a 42-hour glucose infusion. In normal subjects the relationship between glucose and ISR was linear in the physiologic range (i.e., 5–9 mM). The β-cell was most sensitive to glucose levels of 5.5–6.0 mM. In contrast, in subjects with *GCK* mutations, the relationship between glucose and ISR was not linear because the β-cell was poorly responsive to glucose within the normal fasting range. The point of maximal responsiveness was increased to 6.5–7.5 mM. The dose-response curve was shifted to the right in these patients, and a comparison of ISRs at different glucose levels demonstrated that the presence of a mutation in this enzyme was associated globally with a 60% reduction in insulin secretion.

The responsiveness of the β-cell to glucose in subjects with *GCK* mutations was improved after the administration of low doses of glucose for 42-hours. After the glucose infusion, the glucose-ISR dose-response curve was shifted to the left, with the insulin secretory responses at each glucose concentration increasing by 45%. We assume that this increase in insulin responsiveness results from increased levels of glucokinase activity in the β-cell, as has been previously described in vitro.[27,32] Using computer modeling,[140] we also investigated whether the magnitude of the observed decrease in insulin secretion was to be expected based on the known in vitro activities of the mutant forms of *GCK* present in the subjects.[141] We found that in two subjects who had a mutation that led to a relatively mild impairment of enzymatic activity, the reduction in insulin secretion was entirely predicted by the model. In subjects who had a mutation that led to more severe impairment of *GCK* activity, the insulin secretory response was greater than

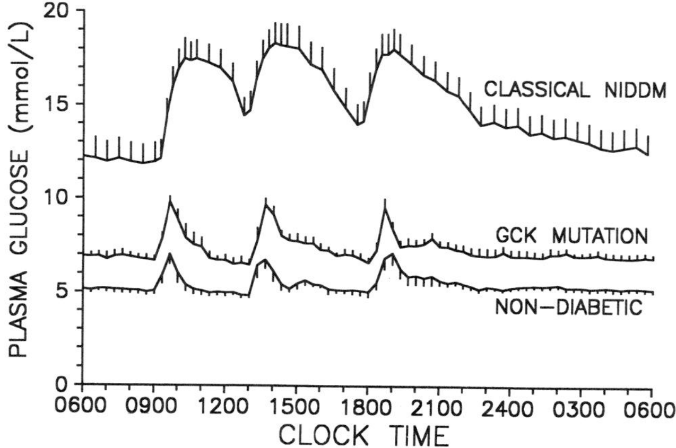

FIGURE 1-4. Mean 24-hour profiles of glucose and insulin secretion in controls, subjects with *GCK* mutations, and subjects with classic NIDDM. Breakfast, lunch, and dinner were presented at 0900, 1300, and 1800 hours, respectively.

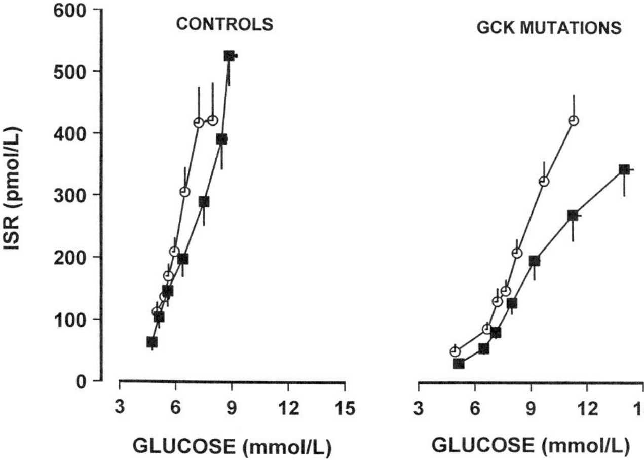

FIGURE 1-5. Relationship between average glucose concentrations and ISRs during the graded IV glucose infusion studies. (■) = after an overnight fast (baseline) study; (○) = after a 42-hour glucose infusion (postglucose) at a rate of 4–6 mg/kg/min. (Redrawn with permission from Byrne MM, Sturis J, Clément K, et al. Insulin secretory abnormalities in subjects with hyperglycemia due to glucokinase mutations. J Clin Invest 1994;93:1120.)

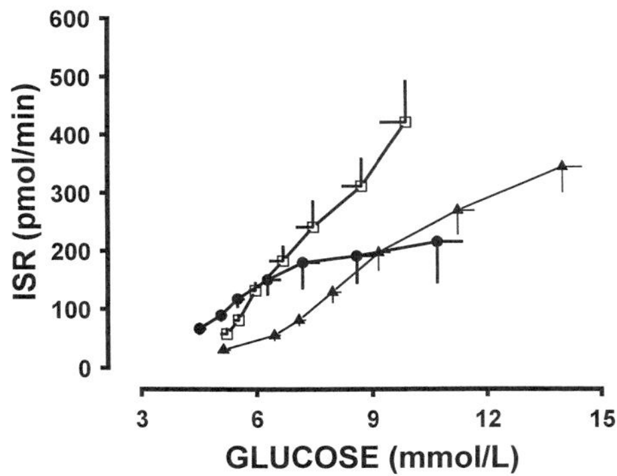

FIGURE 1-6. Relationship between average glucose concentrations and ISRs during the graded glucose infusion studies in the 10 marker-positive (●) and 6 marker-negative subjects (□) from the RW family and in 6 subjects with *GCK* mutations (▲). (Redrawn with permission from Byrne MM, Sturis J, Fajans SS, et al. Altered insulin secretory responses to glucose in subjects with a mutation in the *MODY1* gene on chromosome 20. Diabetes 1995;in press.)

predicted by the model, indicating the presence of compensatory mechanisms operating in vivo in these subjects.[140]

During a 12-hour oscillatory glucose infusion, the average amplitude of the ultradian oscillations in ISR tended to be lower in subjects with *GCK* mutations. In contrast to controls, where the oscillatory glucose infusion resulted in entrainment of plasma glucose and insulin secretion, the glucose and ISR patterns exhibited reduced entrainment in the subjects with *GCK* mutations.[139] This lack of entrainment of ISR is consistent with previous data in patients with classic NIDDM or IGT.[84]

A large Michigan kindred to the RW family has been assembled recently.[142] In this family, MODY is linked to the presence of an at-risk allele at the *MODY1* locus on chromosome 20.[134] Subjects who are marker-positive usually develop diabetes before the age of 25 years. Previous studies have shown that nondiabetic subjects from this family who have inherited the at-risk allele at the *MODY1* locus (i.e., are marker-positive) but who still have completely normal plasma glucose concentrations have normal first-phase insulin responses to IV glucose and do not demonstrate insulin resistance. Compared to nondiabetic marker-negative subjects from the same family, however, significant alterations in insulin secretory responses to prolonged glucose infusion were demonstrated, including decreased mean plasma C-peptide levels, decreased ISR, and reduced absolute amplitude of ultradian insulin secretory oscillations.[142]

Dose-response relationships between glucose and ISRs have been established in 6 marker-negative subjects and 10 marker-positive subjects. The dose-response relationship was normal in the marker-negative group. The marker-positive group had normal insulin secretion until the plasma glucose reached 7 mM and then the curve was shifted downward and to the right (i.e., glucose concentrations >7 mM did not enhance insulin secretion). Figure 1-6 shows the dose-response curves in the marker-positive and marker-negative subjects of the RW family and in the subjects with *GCK* mutations. *GCK* mutations resulted in an impaired ISR at lower glucose levels, but the ISR increased as glucose levels continued to rise. In contrast, marker-positive subjects of the RW family secreted normal amounts of insulin at lower glucose levels and were unable to increase the ISR at higher glucose levels.[143] The priming effect of a 42-hour glucose infusion was lost in 9 of 10 marker-positive subjects.

The defect in the RW family appears to be a primary insulin secretory defect, which is demonstrable in subjects with normal glucose tolerance. We believe that the *MODY1* gene either functions in the regulation of glucose-induced insulin secretion at a cellular level distal to glucokinase or is involved in a process regulating β-cell mass.

References

1. Yalow RS, Berson SA. Immunoassay of endogenous plasma insulin in man. J Clin Invest 1960;39:1157
2. Cerasi E, Luft R. Insulin response to glucose infusion in diabetic and nondiabetic monozygotic twin pairs: Genetic control of insulin response. Acta Endocrinol 1967;55:330
3. Weber B. Glucose-stimulated insulin secretion during "remission" of juvenile diabetes. Diabetologia 1972;8:189
4. Polonsky KS, Jaspan J, Emmanouel D, et al. Differences in hepatic and renal extraction of insulin and glucagon in the dog: Evidence for saturability of insulin metabolism. Acta Endocrinol 1983;102:420
5. Polonsky KS, Jaspan J, Pugh W, et al. Metabolism of C-peptide in the dog: In vivo demonstration of the absence of hepatic extraction. J Clin Invest 1983;72:1114
6. Melani FA, Rubenstein AH, Steiner DF. Human serum proinsulin. J Clin Invest 1970;49:497
7. Bergenstal RM, Cohen RM, Lever E, et al. The metabolic effects of biosynthetic human proinsulin in individuals with type I diabetes. J Clin Endocrinol Metab 1984;58:973
8. Revers RR, Henry R, Schmeiser L, et al. The effects of biosynthetic human proinsulin on carbohydrate metabolism. Diabetes 1984;33:762
9. Peavy DE, Brunner MR, Duckworth WC, et al. Receptor binding and biological potency of several split forms (conversion intermediates) of human proinsulin: Studies in cultured IM-9 lymphocytes and in vivo and in vitro in rats. J Biol Chem 1985;260:13989
10. Gruppuso PA, Frank BH, Schwartz R. Binding of proinsulin and proinsulin conversion intermediates to human placental insulin-like growth factor 1 receptors. J Clin Endocrinol Metab 1988;67:194
11. Polonsky KS, Rubenstein AH. C-peptide as a measure of the secretion and hepatic extraction of insulin: Pitfalls and limitations. Diabetes 1984;33:486
12. Wojcikowski C, Blackman J, Ostrega D, et al. Lack of effect of high-dose biosynthetic human C-peptide on pancreatic hormone release in normal subjects. Metabolism 1990;39:827
13. Polonsky KS, Pugh W, Jaspan JB, et al. C-peptide and insulin secretion: Relationship between peripheral concentrations of C-peptide and insulin and their secretion rates in the dog. J Clin Invest 1984;74:1821
14. Bratusch-Marrain PR, Waldhausl WK, Gasic S, Hofer A. Hepatic disposal of biosynthetic human insulin and porcine proinsulin in humans. Metabolism 1984;33:151

15. Licinio-Paixao J, Polonsky KS, Given BD, et al. Ingestion of a mixed meal does not affect the metabolic clearance rate of biosynthetic human C-peptide. J Clin Endocrinol Metab 1986;63:401
16. Gumbiner B, Polonsky KS, Beltz WF, et al. Effects of weight loss and reduced hyperglycemia on the kinetics of insulin secretion in obese non-insulin dependent diabetes mellitus. J Clin Endocrinol Metab 1990;70:1594
17. Faber OK, Hagen C, Binder C, et al. Kinetics of human connecting peptide in normal and diabetic subjects. J Clin Invest 1978;62:197
18. Polonsky KS, Licinio-Paixao J, Given BD, et al. Use of biosynthetic human C-peptide in the measurement of insulin secretion rates in normal volunteers and type I diabetic patients. J Clin Invest 1986;77:98
19. Shapiro ET, Tillil H, Rubenstein AH, Polonsky KS. Peripheral insulin parallels changes in insulin secretion more closely than C-peptide after bolus intravenous glucose administration. J Clin Endocrinol Metab 1988;67:1094
20. Eaton RP, Allen RC, Shade DS, et al. Prehepatic insulin production in man: Kinetic analysis using peripheral connecting peptide behavior. J Clin Endocrinol Metab 1980;51:520
21. VanCauter E, Mestrez F, Sturis J, Polonsky KS. Estimation of insulin secretion rates from C-peptide levels: Comparison of individual and standard kinetic parameters for C-peptide clearance. Diabetes 1992;41:368
22. Grodsky GM. Threshold distribution hypothesis for packet storage of insulin and its mathematical modeling. J Clin Invest 1972;51:2047
23. Karam JH, Grodsky GM, Ching KN, et al. "Staircase" glucose stimulation of insulin secretion in obesity: Measure of beta cell sensitivity and capacity. Diabetes 1974;23:763
24. Turner RC, Harris E, Ounsted E, Ponsford C. Two abnormalities of glucose-induced insulin secretion: Dose-response characteristics and insulin sensitivity. Acta Endocrinol 1976;92:148
25. Byrne MM, Sturis J, Polonsky KS. Insulin secretion and clearance during low-dose graded glucose infusion. Am J Physiol 1995;268:E21
26. Brelje TC, Sorenson RL. Nutrient and hormonal regulation of the threshold for glucose-stimulated insulin secretion in isolated rat pancreas. Endocrinology 1988;123:1582
27. Liang Y, Najafi H, Smith RM, et al. Concordant glucose induction of glucokinase, glucose usage, and glucose-stimulated insulin release in pancreatic islets maintained in organ culture. Diabetes 1992;41:792
28. Ward WK, Halter JB, Beard JC, Porte D. Adaptation of B and A cell function during prolonged glucose infusion in human subjects. Am J Physiol 1984; 246:E405
29. Flax H, Matthews DR, Levy JC, et al. No glucotoxicity after 53 hours of 6.0 mmol/L hyperglycemia in normal man. Diabetologia 1991;34:570
30. Leahy JL, Bonner-Weir S, Weir GC. B-cell dysfunction induced by chronic hyperglycemia. Diabetes Care 1992;15:442
31. Leahy JL, Cooper HE, Deal DA, Weir GC. Chronic hyperglycemia is associated with impaired glucose influence on insulin secretion. J Clin Invest 1986;77:908
32. Meglasson MD, Matschinsky FM. Pancreatic islet glucose metabolism and regulation of insulin secretion. Diabetes Metab Rev 1986;2:163
33. Matchinsky FM. Glucokinase as glucose sensor and metabolic signal generator in pancreatic beta-cells and hepatocytes. Diabetes 1990;39:647
34. Chen L, Alam T, Johnson JH, et al. Regulation of B-cell glucose transporter gene expression. Proc Natl Acad Sci USA 1990;87:4088
35. Zawalich WS, Dye ES, Pagliara AS, et al. Starvation diabetes in the rat: Onset, recovery, and specificity of reduced responsiveness of pancreatic β-cells. Endocrinology 1979;104:1344
36. Efendic S, Cerasi E, Luft R, Gladnikoff G. Potentiation of glucose-induced insulin release by glucose in the isolated pancreas of fed and fasted rats. Diabetes 1976;25:949
37. Burch PT, Trus MD, Berner DK, Leontire A, et al. Adaptation of glycolytic enzymes: Glucose use and insulin release in rat pancreatic islets during fasting and refeeding. Diabetes 1981;30:923
38. Malherbe C, DeGasparo M, DeHertogh R, et al. Circadian variations of blood sugar and plasma insulin levels in man. Diabetologia 1969;5:397
39. Polonsky KS, Given BD, VanCauter E. Twenty-four-hour profiles and pulsatile patterns of insulin secretion in normal and obese subjects. J Clin Invest 1988;81:442
40. Tasaka Y, Sekine M, Wakatssuki M, et al. Levels of pancreatic glucagon, insulin and glucose during twenty-four hours of the day in normal subjects. Horm Metab Res 1975;7:205
41. Jarrett RJ, Baker IA, Keen H, et al. Diurnal variation in oral glucose tolerance: Blood sugar and plasma insulin levels morning, afternoon and evening. Br Med J 1972;1:199
42. Carroll KF, Nestel PJ. Diurnal variation in glucose tolerance and in insulin secretion in man. Diabetes 1973;22:333
43. Alparicio NJ, Puchulu FE, Gadliardino JJ, et al. Circadian variation of the blood glucose, plasma insulin and human growth hormone levels in response to an oral glucose load in normal subjects. Diabetes 1974;23:132
44. Van Cauter E, Desir D, Decoster C, et al. Nocturnal decrease in glucose tolerance during constant glucose infusion. J Clin Endocrinol Metab 1989;69: 604
45. Goodner CJ, Walike BC, Koerker DJ, et al. Insulin, glucagon and glucose exhibit synchronous sustained oscillations in fasting monkeys. Science 1977; 195:177
46. Lang DA, Matthews DR, Peto J, Turner RC. Cyclic oscillations of basal plasma glucose and insulin concentrations in human beings. N Engl J Med 1979;301:1023
47. Hansen BC, Jen KC, Pek SB, Wolfe RA. Rapid oscillations in plasma insulin, glucagon and glucose in obese and normal weight humans. J Clin Endocrinol Metab 1982;54:785
48. Matthews DR, Lang DA, Burnett MA, Turner RC. Control of pulsatile insulin secretion in man. Diabetologia 1983;2:231
49. Simon C, Brandenberger G, Follenius M. Ultradian oscillations of plasma glucose, insulin and C-peptide in man during continuous enteral nutrition. J Clin Endocrinol Metab 1987;64:669
50. Shapiro ET, Tillil H, Polonsky KS, et al. Oscillations in insulin secretion during constant glucose infusion in normal man: Relationship to changes in plasma glucose. J Clin Endocrinol Metab 1988;67:307
51. O'Meara NM, Sturis J, Blackman JD, et al. Analytical problems in detecting rapid insulin secretory pulses in normal humans. Am J Physiol 1993;264: E231
52. Koerker DJ, Goodner CJ, Hansen BW, et al. Synchronous sustained oscillations of C-peptide and insulin in the plasma of fasting monkeys. Endocrinology 1978;102:1649
53. Goodner CJ, Koerker DJ, Weigle DS, et al. Decreased insulin and glucose pulse amplitude accompanying B-cell deficiency induced by streptozotocin in baboons. Diabetes 1989;38:925
54. Jaspan JB, Lever E, Polonsky KS, et al. In vivo pulsatility of pancreatic islet peptides. Am J Physiol 1986;251:E215
55. Matthews DR, Hermansen K, Connolly AA, et al. Greater in vivo than in vitro pulsatility of insulin secretion with synchronized insulin and somatostatin secretory pulses. Endocrinology 1987;120:2272
56. Goodner CJ, Koerker DJ, Stagner JI, et al. In vitro pancreatic hormonal pulses are less regular and more frequent than in vivo. Am J Physiol 1991;260:E422
57. Stagner JI, Samols E, Weir GC. Sustained oscillations of insulin, glucagon and somatostatin from the isolated canine pancreas during exposure to a constant glucose concentration. J Clin Invest 1980;65:939
58. Safarik RH, Joy RM, Curry DL. Episodic release of insulin by rat pancreas: Effects of CNS and state of satiety. Am J Physiol 1988;254:E384
59. Sonnenberg GE, Hoffmann RG, Johnson CP, et al. Low and high frequency insulin secretion pulses in normal subjects and pancreas recipients: Role of extrinsic innervation. J Clin Invest 1992;90:545
60. O'Meara NM, Sturis J, Blackman JD, et al. Oscillatory insulin secretion following pancreas transplantation. Diabetes 1993;42:855
61. Bergstrom RW, Fujimoto WY, Teller DC, et al. Oscillatory insulin secretion in perfused isolated rat islets. Am J Physiol 1989;257:E479
62. Bingley PJ, Matthews DR, Williams AJK, et al. Loss of regular oscillatory insulin secretion in islet cell antibody positive non-diabetic subjects. Diabetologia 1992;35:32
63. Matthews DR, Naylor BA, Jones RG, et al. Pulsatile insulin has greater hypoglycemic effect than continuous delivery. Diabetes 1983;32:617
64. Bratusch-Marrain PR, Komjati M, Waldhausl W. Efficacy of pulsatile versus continuous insulin administration on hepatic glucose production and glucose utilization in type I diabetic humans. Diabetes 1986;35:922
65. Ward GM, Walters JM, Aitken PM, et al. Effects of prolonged pulsatile hyperinsulinemia in humans: Enhancement of insulin sensitivity. Diabetes 1990;39:501
66. Simon C. Brandenberger G, Follenius M. Postprandial oscillations of plasma glucose, insulin and C-peptide in man. Diabetologia 1987;30:769
67. Blackman JD, Polonsky KS, Jaspan JB, et al. Insulin secretory profiles and C-peptide clearance kinetics at 6 months and 2 years after kidney-pancreas transplantation. Diabetes 1992;41:1346
68. Sturis J, Polonsky KS, Mosekilde E, Van Cauter E. Computer model for mechanisms underlying ultradian oscillations of insulin and glucose. Am J Physiol 1991;260:E801
69. Sturis J, Van Cauter E, Blackman JD, Polonsky KS. Entrainment of pulsatile insulin secretion by oscillatory glucose infusion. J Clin Invest 1991;87:439
70. Sturis J, O'Meara NM, Shapiro ET, et al. Differential effects of glucose stimulation upon rapid pulses and ultradian oscillations of insulin secretion. J Clin Endocrinol Metab 1993;76:895
71. Sturis J, Scheen AJ, Leproult R, et al. 24-hour glucose profiles during continuous or oscillatory insulin infusion: Demonstration of the functional significance of ultradian insulin oscillations. J Clin Invest 1995;95:1464
72. Olefsky JM, Faquhar JW, Reaven GM. Reappraisal of the role of insulin in hypertriglyceridemia. Am J Med 1974;57:551
73. Kissebah AH, Vydelingum N, Murray R, et al. Relation of body fat distribution to metabolic complications of obesity. J Clin Endocrinol Metab 1982; 54:254
74. Peiris AN, Mueller RA, Smith GA, et al. Splanchnic insulin metabolism in obesity: Influence of body fat distribution. J Clin Invest 1986;78:1648
75. Savage PJ, Flock EV, Mako ME, et al. C-peptide and insulin in Pima Indians and Caucasians: Constant fractional hepatic extraction over a wide range of insulin concentrations and in obesity. J Clin Endocrinol Metab 1979;48:594
76. Ogilive RF. The islets of Langerhans in 19 cases of obesity. J Pathol 1933; 37:473
77. Mahler RJ. The pathogenesis of pancreatic islet cell hyperplasia and insulin insensitivity in obesity. Adv Metab Disord 1974;7:213
78. Rossell R, Gomis R, Casamitjana R, et al. Reduced hepatic insulin extraction in obesity: Relationship with plasma insulin levels. J Clin Endocrinol Metab 1983;56:608
79. Polonsky KS, Given BD, Hirsch L, et al. Quantitative study of insulin secretion and clearance in normal and obese subjects. J Clin Invest 1988;81:435
80. Shiraishi I, Iwamoto Y, Kuzuya T, et al. Hyperinsulinemia in obesity is not accompanied by an increase in serum proinsulin/insulin molar ratio in groups

of human subjects with and without glucose intolerance. Diabetologia 1991; 34:737
81. Le Stunff C, Bougneres P. Early changes in postprandial insulin secretion, not in insulin sensitivity, characterize juvenile obesity. Diabetes 1994;43:696
82. Hales CN, Kennedy GC. Plasma glucose, nonesterified fatty acids and insulin concentrations in hypothalamic-hyperphagic rats. Biochem J 1964;90:620
83. Bernardis LL, Frohman LA. Effect of hypothalamic lesions at different loci on development of hyperinsulinemia and obesity in the weaning rat. J Comp Neurol 1971;141:107
84. O'Meara NM, Sturis J, Van Cauter E, Polonsky KS. Lack of control by glucose of ultradian insulin secretory oscillations in impaired glucose tolerance and in non–insulin-dependent diabetes mellitus. J Clin Invest 1993; 92:262
85. Sonnenberg GE, Hoffman RG, Mueller RA, Kissebah AH. Splanchnic insulin dynamics and secretion pulsatilities in abdominal obesity. Diabetes 1994; 43:468
86. DeFronzo RA. Glucose intolerance and aging: Evidence for tissue insensitivity to insulin. Diabetes 1979;28:1095
87. Davidson MB. The effect of aging on carbohydrate metabolism: A review of the English literature and a practical approach to the diagnosis of diabetes mellitus in the elderly. Metabolism 1979;28:688
88. Fink RI, Kolterman OG, Olefsky JM. The physiological significance of glucose intolerance of aging. J Gerontol 1984;39:273
89. Tonino RP. Effects of physiological training on the insulin resistance of aging. Am J Physiol 1989;256:E352
90. Kahn SE, Larson VG, Beard JC. Effect of exercise on insulin action, glucose intolerance and insulin secretion in aging. Am J Physiol 1990;258:E937
91. Dudl RJ, Ensinck JW. Insulin and glucagon relationships during aging in man. Metabolism 1977;26:33
92. Crockford PM, Herbeck RJ, Williams RH. Influence of age on intravenous glucose tolerance and serum immunoreactive insulin. Lancet 1966;1:465
93. Chen M, Bergman RN, Pacini G, Porte D Jr. Pathogenesis of age-related glucose intolerance in man: Insulin resistance and decreased β-cell function. J Clin Endocrinol Metab 1985;60:13
94. Gumbiner B, Polonsky KS, Beltz WF, et al. Effects of aging on insulin secretion. Diabetes 1989;38:1549
95. Kahn SE, Larson VG, Schwartz RS. Exercise training delineates the importance of B-cell dysfunction to the glucose intolerance of human aging. J Clin Endocrinol Metab 1992;74:1336
96. Scheen AJ, Sturis J, Polonsky KS, Van Cauter E. Alterations in the ultradian oscillations of insulin secretion and plasma glucose in aging. Diabetologia: in press
97. Ortiz J, Sturis J, Smith M, et al. Glucose control of ultradian insulin secretory oscillations is impaired in elderly humans. Diabetes 1994;43(suppl 1): 246A
98. Pfeifer MA, Halter JB, Porte D Jr. Insulin secretion in diabetes mellitus. Am J Med 1981;70:579
99. Carlstrom S, Ingemanson CA. Juvenile diabetes with long-standing remission. Diabetologia 1967;3:465
100. Johansen K, Ørskov H. Plasma insulin during remission in juvenile diabetes mellitus. Br Med J 1969;1:676
101. Block MB, Rosenfield RL, Mako ME, et al. Sequential changes in beta-cell function in insulin-treated diabetic patients assessed by C-peptide immunoreactivity. N Engl J Med 1973;288:1144
102. Heding LG, Ludvigsson J, Kasperska-Czyzykowa T. β-cell secretion in non-insulin and insulin-dependent-diabetics. Acta Med Scand 1981;656(suppl):5
103. Snorgaard O, Hartling SG, Binder C. Proinsulin and C-peptide at onset and during 12 months cyclosporin treatment of type I (insulin-dependent diabetes mellitus. Diabetologia 1990;33:36
104. Srikanta S, Ganda OP, Jackson RA, et al. Type I diabetes mellitus in monozygotic twins: Chronic progressive beta cell dysfunction. Ann Intern Med 1983;99:320
105. O'Meara NM, Sturis J, Herold KC, et al. Alterations in the patterns of insulin secretion before and after diagnosis of IDDM. Diabetes Care 1995;18:in press
106. Ganda OP, Srikanta S, Brink SJ, et al. Differential sensitivity to β-cell secretagogues in "early" type I diabetes mellitus. Diabetes 1984;33:516
107. Bogardus C. Insulin resistance in the pathogenesis of NIDDM in Pima Indians. Diabetes Care 1993;16:228
108. Gulli G, Ferrannini E, Stern M, et al. The metabolic profile of NIDDM is fully established in glucose-tolerant offspring of two Mexican-American NIDDM parents. Diabetes 1992;41:1575
109. Barnett AH, Sphlopoulos AJ, Pyke DA, et al. Metabolic studies in unaffected co-twins of non–insulin-dependent diabetes. Br Med J 1981;282:1656
110. Vaag A, Henriksen JE, Madsbad S, et al. Insulin secretion, insulin action, and hepatic glucose production in identical twins discordant for non–insulin-dependent diabetes mellitus. J Clin Invest 1995;95:690
111. Ward WK, Boliano DC, McNight B, et al. Diminished β-cell secretory capacity in patients with non–insulin-dependent diabetes mellitus. J Clin Invest 1984;74:1318
112. Leahy JL, Bonner-Weir S, Weir GC. Minimal chronic hyperglycemia is a critical determinant of imparied insulin secretion after an incomplete pancreatectomy. J Clin Invest 1988;81:1407
113. Leahy JL, Weir GC. Evolution of abnormal insulin secretory responses during 48-h in vivo hyperglycemia. Diabetes 1988;37:217
114. Garvey WT, Olefsky JM, Griffin J, et al. The effect of insulin treatment on insulin secretion and insulin action in type II diabetes mellitus. Diabetes 1985;34:222
115. O'Rahilly SP, Nugent Z, Rudenski AS, et al. Beta-cell dysfunction rather than insulin insensitivity is the primary defect in familial type 2 diabetics. Lancet 1986;11:360
116. Kosaka K, Hagura R, Kuzuya T. Insulin responses in equivocal and definite diabetes with special reference to subjects who had mild glucose intolerance but later developed definite diabetes. Diabetes 1977;26:944
117. Kadowaki T, Miyake Y, Hagura R, et al. Risk factors for worsening to diabetes in subjects with impaired glucose tolerance. Diabetologia 1984;26:44
118. Efendic S, Luft R, Wajngot A. Aspects of the pathogenesis of type 2 diabetes. Endocrine Rev 1984;5:395
119. Mitrakou A, Kelley D, Mokan M, et al. Role of suppression of glucose production and diminished early insulin release in impaired glucose tolerance. N Engl J Med 1992;326:22
120. Ward WK, Johnston CLW, Beard JC, et al. Insulin resistance and impaired insulin secretion in subjects with histories of gestational diabetes. Diabetes 1985;34:861
121. Byrne MM, Sturis J, O'Meara NM, Polonsky KS. Insulin secretion in insulin resistant women with a history of gestational diabetes. Metabolism 1995; 44:1067
122. Ryan EA, Imes S, Liu D, et al. Defects in insulin secretion and action in women with a history of gestational diabetes. Diabetes 1995;44:506
123. Ward WK, LaCava EC, Paquette TL, et al. Disproportionate elevation of immunoreactive proinsulin in type 2 (non–insulin-dependent) diabetes mellitus and in experimental insulin resistance. Diabetologia 1987;30:698
124. O'Sullivan JB. Body weight and subsequent diabetes mellitus. JAMA 1982;248:949
125. Duckworth WC, Kitabchi AE, Heinemann M. Direct measurement of plasma proinsulin in normal and diabetic subjects. Am J Med 1972;53:418
126. Saad M, Kahn SE, Nelson RG, et al. Disproportionately elevated proinsulin in Pima Indians with non-insulin dependent diabetes mellitus. J Clin Endocrinol Metab 1990;70:1247
127. Temple RC, Carrington CA, Luzio SD, et al. Insulin deficiency in non–insulin-depedent diabetes. Lancet 1989;1:293
128. Temple RC, Clark PMS, Nagi DK, et al. Radioimmunoassay may overestimate insulin in non–insulin-dependent diabetics. Clin Endocrinol 1990;32: 689
129. Yoshioka N, Kuzuya T, Matsuda A, et al. Serum proinsulin levels at fasting and after oral glucose load in patients with type 2 (non–insulin-dependent) diabetes mellitus. Diabetologia 1988;31:355
130. Sturis J, Polonsky KS, Shapiro ET, et al. Abnormalities in the ultradian oscillations of insulin secretion and glucose levels in type 2 (non–insulin-dependent) diabetic patients. Diabetologia 1992;35:681
131. Polonsky KS, Given BD, Hirsch LJ, et al. Abnormal patterns of insulin secretion in non-insulin dependent diabetes mellitus. N Engl J Med 1988; 318:1231
132. Lang DA, Matthews DR, Burnett M, et al. Brief irregular oscillations of basal plasma insulin and glucose concentrations in diabetic man. Diabetes 1981;30:435
133. O'Rahilly S, Turner RC, Matthews DR. Impaired pulsatile secretion of insulin in relatives of patients with non–insulin-dependent diabetes. N Engl J Med 1988;318:1225
134. Bell GI, Xiang KS, Newman MV, et al. Gene for non–insulin-dependent diabetes mellitus (maturity-onset diabetes of the young subtype) is linked to DNA polymorphism on human chromosome 20q. Proc Natl Acad Sci USA 1991;88:1484
135. Froguel P, Vaxillaire M, Sun F, et al. Close linkage of glucokinase locus on chromosome 7p to early-onset non–insulin-dependent diabetes mellitus. Nature 1992;356:162
136. Vionnet N, Stoffel M, Takeda J, et al. Nonsense mutation in the glucokinase gene causes early-onset non–insulin-dependent diabetes mellitus. Nature 1992; 356:721
137. Hattersley AT, Turner RC, Permutt MA, et al. Linkage of type 2 diabetes to the glucokinase gene. Lancet 1992;339:1307
138. Froguel P, Zouali H, Vionnet N, et al. Familial hyperglycemia due to mutations in glucokinase. N Engl J Med 1992;328:697
139. Byrne MM, Sturis J, Clément K, et al. Insulin secretory abnormalities in subjects with hyperglycemia due to glucokinase mutations. J Clin Invest 1994;93:1120
140. Sturis J, Kurland IJ, Byrne MM, et al. Compensation in pancreatic β-cell function in subjects with glucokinase mutations. Diabetes 1994;43:718
141. Gidh-Jain M, Takeda J, Xu LZ, et al. Glucokinase mutations associated with non–insulin-dependent (type II) diabetes mellitus have decreased enzymatic activity: Implications for structure/function relationships. Proc Natl Acad Sci USA 1993;90:1932
142. Herman WH, Fajans SS, Ortiz FJ, et al. Abnormal insulin secretion, not insulin resistance, is the genetic or primary defect of MODY in the RW pedigree. Diabetes 1994;43:40. Published erratum appears in Diabetes 1994; 43:1171
143. Byrne MM, Sturis J, Fajans SS, et al. Altered insulin secretory responses to glucose in subjects with a mutation in the MODY 1 gene on chromosome 20. Diabetes 1995;44:699

Diabetes Mellitus, edited by Derek LeRoith, Simeon I. Taylor, and Jerrold M. Olefsky. Lippincott–Raven Publishers, Philadelphia © 1996.

Chapter 2
Kinetics of Insulin Secretion: Current Implications

Gerold M. Grodsky

Glucose and other secretagogues affect insulin release by acting on multiple ionic and metabolic mechanisms. These mechanisms not only overlap and interrelate, but they change in quantitative significance with time and concurrent or prior exposure to stimulators and inhibitors. Although current knowledge remains limited, in this chapter we will attempt to correlate these metabolic events with the kinetics of insulin secretion. Phenomena to be considered include the following: (1) multiphasic release, (2) rate sensitivity, (3) time-dependent potentiation (memory), (4) "delayed" insulin secretion in non–insulin-dependent diabetes mellitus (NIDDM), and (5) oscillatory release. Finally, some emphasis is made on the abilities of the β-cell to adapt (or counter-regulate) after chronic stimulation, and in special circumstances, to release hormone constitutively.

Multiphasic Insulin Secretion: Kinetics

β-Cells are sensitive to the rate of change as well as the actual concentration of a secretagogue.[1–3] Characteristics of insulin release in response to a rapid-onset stimulation by glucose are as follows (Fig. 2-1)[4]:

1. Initial response is a transient, rapid rise in release (first phase), which terminates in 5–10 minutes.
2. This is followed by a progressively increasing second phase in which glucose continually amplifies its own signal.* The phases have identical dose sensitivities to glucose,[8] indicating that the same initial steps in glucose metabolism are required for both.
3. When glucose is rapidly reduced to a lower, but still stimulating concentration, negative rate sensitivity is reflected by a transient negative spike of insulin secretion.
4. If the pancreas or islets are exposed to elevated glucose levels for periods of more than 15 minutes, they become primed or potentiated so that, after a brief rest period, their response to the same stimulus is greater than seen initially. This memory component can persist for more than 1 hour and is referred to as priming or *time-dependent potentiation* (TDP).[3,8–10]

Inhibition of protein synthesis does not affect the first phase and has only a small effect on second-phase secretion[1] for up to 3 hours (Grodsky, GM, and Bolaffi, J., 1994). Thus, the acute kinetics of insulin secretion reflects changes in the release of preformed, stored insulin rather than changes in insulin production.

As shown in Figure 2-2, if the pancreas or islets are further stimulated by glucose beyond 1–3 hours, insulin release spontaneously declines to a low level, which can be maintained for up to 48 hours (third phase).[11–14] The reduced third-phase secretion is not caused by depletion of total insulin content[12,13] and is therefore related to signals affecting secretion.

*Second-phase release, prominent in humans and rats, is relatively low and flat for most strains of mice.[5–7]

Both the first and second phases of insulin secretion are demonstrable in humans when glucose is given as a rapid, continuous IV stimulation.[15] Because first-phase release is more pronounced with a fast rate of change in glucose concentration, it is not obvious when glucose is given as a slow, gradual increase, as after a glucose meal. It does result, however, in higher insulin levels than would have occurred otherwise, and its importance to maintain glucose homeostasis is recognized. For example: (1) rapid first-phase release of insulin is necessary for normal regulation of hepatic glucose output[16]; (2) closed-loop insulin infusion devices require algorithms for fast insulin release proportional to the rate of change of glucose concentration in order to prime target tissues and to prevent overinsulinization and a subsequent delayed hypoglycemia[17]; and (3) impaired first-phase release predicts impending development of insulin-dependent diabetes mellitus (IDDM) and is an early feature of impaired β-cell function in non–insulin-dependent diabetes mellitus (NIDDM).[18–20]

Quantitative Relationship of Insulinogenesis to Secretion

Although, as noted above, stimulation of phasic insulin secretion during a period of several hours is relatively independent of insulinogenesis, it is obvious that insulin synthesis is required as the ultimate source of hormone for release. Production and regulation of insulin mRNA and insulin synthesis is discussed in detail elsewhere (see Chapter 3 by M. German) and is beyond the scope

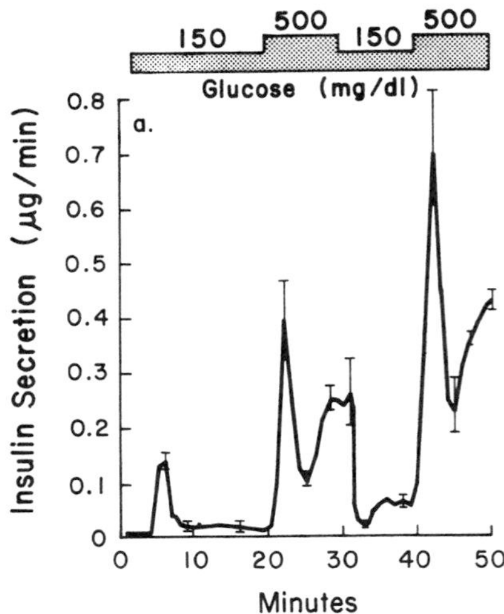

Figure 2-1. Characteristic insulin secretion from the in vitro perfused pancreas of the rat in response to steps in glucose concentration. (Reproduced with permission from Gold G, Grodsky GM. Kinetic aspects of compartmental storage and secretion of insulin and zinc. Experientia 1984;40:1105.)

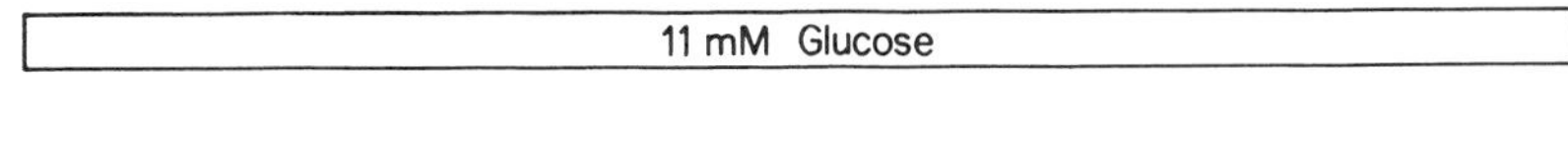

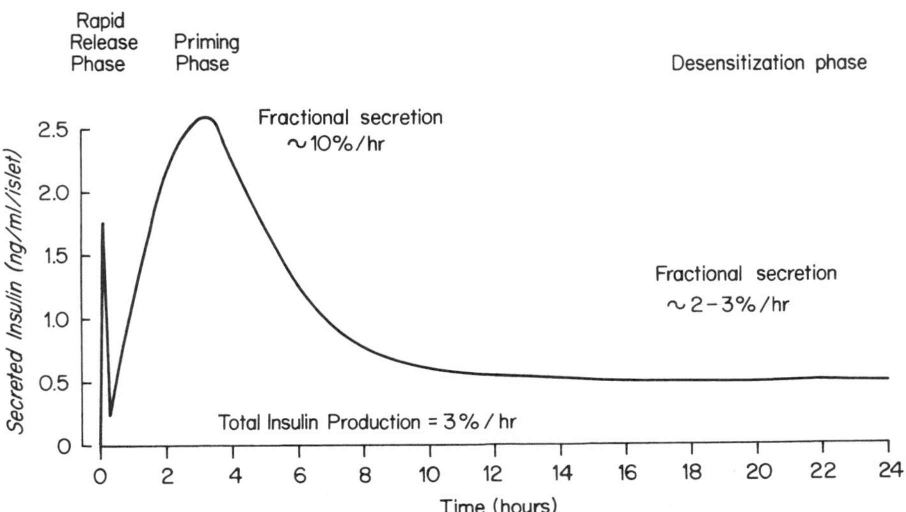

Figure 2-2. Schematic of the characteristic three phases of insulin secretion during continuous stimulation of islets with glucose (11 mM). (Reproduced with permission from Grodsky GM. A new phase of insulin secretion: How will it contribute to our understanding of β-cell function? Diabetes 1989; 38:673.)

of this review. In brief, glucose increases—or stabilizes—insulin mRNA during a 24-hour period, but the changes are slow and of small magnitude.[21] Glucose also increases the rate of synthesis of proinsulin at the translational level by several orders of magnitude within minutes.[22–23] Despite this demonstrated increase in the rate of insulin synthesis by glucose, the actual amounts of insulin synthesized in relationship to release are unclear. In recent 24-hour islet programmed-perifusion experiments, the *amount* of insulin synthesis (measured as a change in the net recovery in islets and media) was only one-third of secretion during peak second-phase release, but was sufficient to partially replace secreted hormone during the third phase.[13] These studies provide quantitative support for previous observations that elevated glucose in vivo results in net degranulation and depleted insulin content, an indication that release exceeds insulinogenesis, whereas under conditions where secretion is low, pancreatic β-cells are replenished back to their normal steady-state insulin content.

Model of Insulin Secretion

Mathematic models do not specifically identify the processes that drive multiphasic insulin secretion, but they help in their ultimate identification by defining the quantitative and temporal characteristics that the processes must express. Figure 2-3 depicts a two-

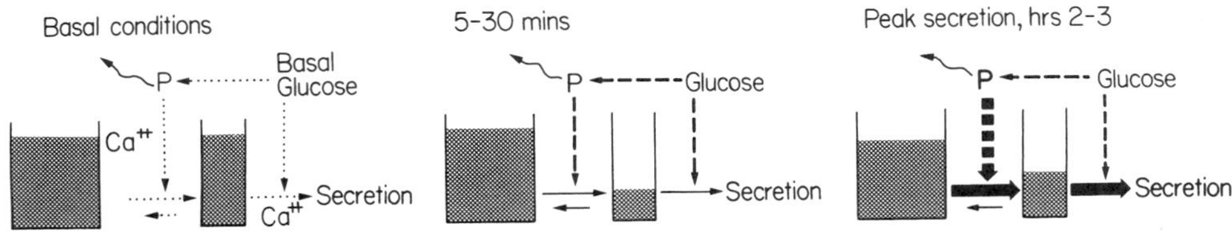

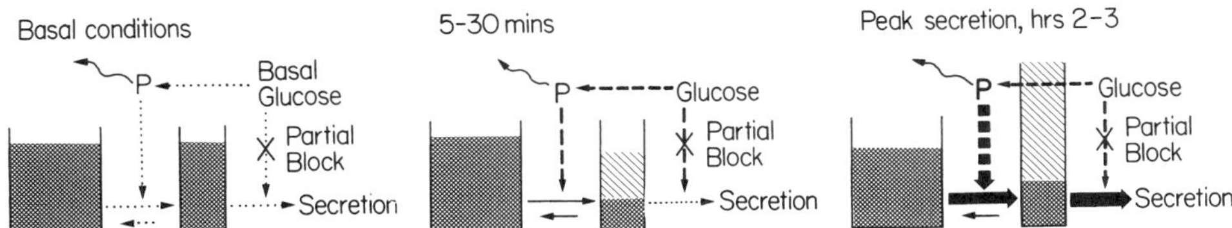

Figure 2-3. Two-compartmental model of insulin secretion. (For mathematical and quantitative development, see refs. 3 and 8). ***A,*** Glucose stimulates first-phase release by rapidly depleting insulin (or a metabolic signal similarly depleted during secretion). Glucose also stimulates a potentiating signal, P, that accumulates gradually and drives the increasing second phase secretion. ***B,*** Results when a partial, but constant, defect for release from the small compartment is introduced. Response to glucose is initially inhibited. With time, P causes a compensating increased content in the small compartment; release is now regulated solely by P and is normal. (Reproduced with permission from Grodsky GM. An update on implications of phasic insulin secretion. In: Flatt PR, Lenzen S, eds. Insulin secretion and pancreatic B-cell research: 1994;421–430.)

compartmental model, shown previously[3,8] to reproduce the first and second phases of insulin secretion from the perfused pancreas when stimulated by glucose added in various patterns and concentrations. In this model, the two compartments may consist of insulin, but also may represent secretion signals that are depleted and produced as indicated. A sudden increase in glucose causes first-phase insulin release and rate sensitivity by depleting the smaller labile compartment. Because progressively higher concentrations of glucose cause first-phase secretion of greater magnitude but with identical transient kinetics, it was required that the small compartment not be homogeneous, but that it consist of storage components with different threshold sensitivities to glucose.[8] These release their contents in an all-or-nothing fashion when their thresholds are exceeded by the ambient glucose.[8] Kinetic analysis of insulin secretion, therefore, predicted the subsequent observation that β-cells from a single islet, or insulin storage granules in a single β-cell[24–28] differ in their sensitivity to glucose. A negative feedback or exitor-inhibitor concept can alternatively be invoked to describe transient first-phase release.[3]

The second phase is produced by a potentiating factor (P), which in response to constant glucose, gradually increases. In contrast to first-phase release, P is not depleted during insulin secretion, but is degraded by independent processes with a determined half-time of 20–60 minutes. These characteristics of P metabolism create the memory (priming) or TDP in the β-cell.[8–10] Thus, after a prior stimulation, both insulin release and synthesis of P stops. Residual P, however, although is decreases slowly, continues to cause supernormal accumulation of insulin or signal into the small compartment; restimulation by glucose produces the time-dependent hyperinsulin secretion.

Inherent in the model are the following additional concepts: (1) both phases require functioning of the small compartment, and (2) with increasing time, the metabolic parameters generating the P provide the major signals for late insulin secretion.

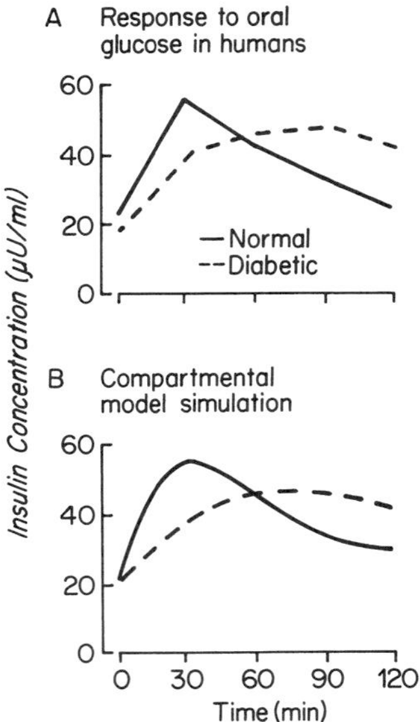

Figure 2-4. Quantitative simulation by the two-compartmental model of "delayed" hyperinsulin release in mild NIDDM. ***A,*** Experimental pattern of insulin secretion during oral glucose tolerance in subjects with mild NIDDM. (Reproduced with permission from Hales CN, Greenwood FC, Mitchell FL, Strauss WT. Blood-glucose, plasma-insulin and growth hormone concentrations of individuals with minor abnormalities of glucose tolerance. Diabetologia 1968;4:73.) ***B,*** Simulated insulin secretion using a whole body computer model incorporating the two-compartmental concept for β-cell function (see Fig. 2-3*A*). Simulations assumed a 60% inhibition of release from the small compartment and unchanged production and effectiveness of P for second phase release (see Fig. 2-3*B*). A 75% inhibition of peripheral glucose utilization was also incorporated to produce the characteristic mild hyperglycemia (refer to ref. 20). The whole-body model was developed in collaboration with H. Landahl and M. O'Connor.

Phasic Insulin Release in Clinical Diabetes

Figure 2-4 illustrates the classic "delayed" insulin release followed by hyperinsulin secretion typical for the mild NIDDM diabetic given an oral glucose tolerance test.[20] An almost identical curve is produced by the compartmental model if a partial, but constant, defect in first-phase release is incorporated while the production and action of potentiator, P, is kept normal. In the model, the defect in release causes a transient reduction in the rise of insulin secretion. In time, insulin (or signal) in the small compartment increases to a higher than normal compensating level, and secretion now is regulated solely by P, which is normal. Thus, delayed hyperinsulin secretion is the mathematic resultant of a constant defect in factors regulating first-phase release. Insulin resistance and hyperinsulinism occur in NIDDM, but model analysis emphasizes the hazards of defining hyperinsulinism on the basis of late insulin levels during an oral glucose tolerance test. After 30 minutes, insulin levels can be higher than normal whether caused by a hyperinsulin state, or in contrast, by a defect in insulin release.

Metabolic Factors Regulating Insulin Release

Although it has long been established that products of glucose metabolism mediate insulin secretion,[29,30] the target mechanisms or pathways on which they act are numerous, complex, and highly interrelated (Fig. 2-5) (reviewed in [31,32]). How these mechanisms temporally affect phasic insulin secretion is poorly understood.

Ion Flux

As one of its actions, glucose inhibits ATP-sensitive K^+ channels (presumably through its stimulation of ATP production), thereby causing membrane depolarization; depolarization activates the L-type voltage-dependent Ca^{++} channels resulting in Ca^{++} entry and an increase in cytosolic Ca^{++} ($Ca^{++}[i]$).[33–38] Because extracellular Ca^{++} production[31,39] and energy production[40,41] are required for stimulation of all phases of insulin secretion by conventional secretagogues, it often is implied that the complete action of glucose is to cause depolarization and Ca^{++} influx. Early studies, have showed, however,[1,42,43] that this sole action was insufficient to cause glucose-stimulated biphasic insulin release; continuous tolbutamide or K^+ cause depolarization and Ca^{++} entry by inhibiting the ATP-dependent K^+ channel via a tolbutamide-binding protein, or by directly depolarizing the cell, respectively. In the absence of glucose, however, these agents primarily stimulate first-phase secretion (Fig. 2-6). That the predominant effect of ion flux is on first-phase release was further supported by the demonstration that diazoxide, an activator of the K^+ channel, preferentially inhibits this phase.[43]

More recent experiments have confirmed that glucose acts on phasic insulin secretion by mechanisms in addition to its effect on Ca^{++} influx.[44,45] Thus, in the combined presence of diazoxide and high K^+, used to inhibit the K^+ channel while permitting depolarization and Ca^{++} uptake, glucose still had a large additive effect on secretion—primarily to cause second-phase release. Therefore, although Ca^{++} entry is required for both phases of insulin release,

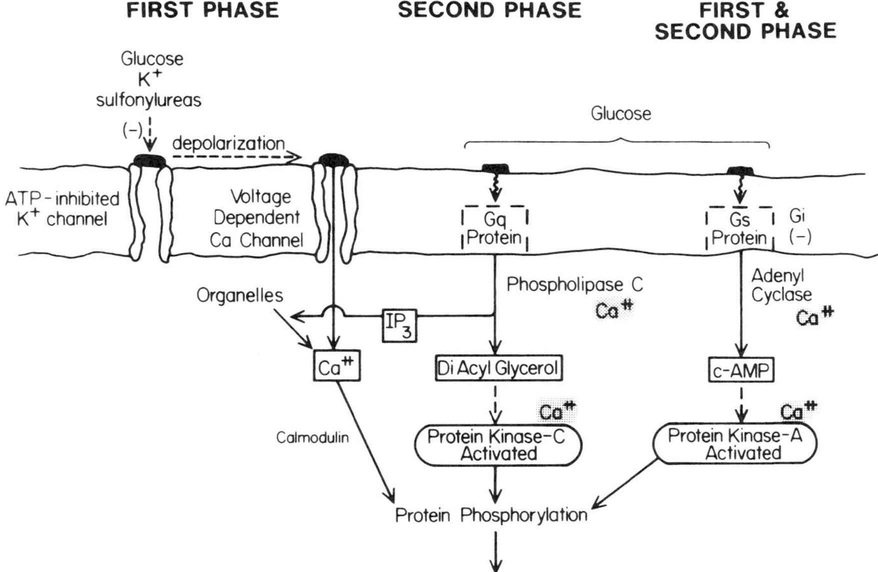

Figure 2-5. Metabolic functions in the β-cell and the phases of insulin secretion that they regulate.

it is insufficient to explain the diphasic stimulation of insulin release by glucose.

In the compartmental model (see Fig. 2-3), Ca^{++}(i) is depicted as regulating total insulin secretion by mediating signals at the small compartment. The Ca^{++} requirement for the second phase is at the level of the effectiveness of P, subsequent to its production (experimentally, production of time-dependent potentiation (and, therefore, P) does not require Ca^{++}).[9]

cAMP

Glucose stimulates adenyl cyclase and cAMP levels that mediate protein kinase A activity and phosphorylation of intracellular proteins[31,46] (see Fig. 2-5). Although an increase in cAMP alone elicits only a small nonphasic insulin release (Fig. 2-7),[46,47] it enhances both phases in the presence of glucose, K^+, or tolbutamide. An effect on first-phase release is consistent with observations that cAMP facilitates ion flux and Ca^{++} uptake into the β-cell.[48,49] By acting on additional mechanisms,[50] it amplifies both phases of secretion. In the model (Fig. 2-3), cAMP activates both release from the small compartment and production of P.

Because many gastrointestinal hormones (e.g., glucagon-like peptide, GLP), whose levels increase with meals, act primarily on adenyl cyclase in the β-cell, production of cAMP is a major regulating event for insulin secretion in vivo (reviewed in [50]).

Phosphoinositol Metabolism

Activation of phospholipase C results in phosphoinositol hydrolysis, causing production of both diacylglycerol and inositol phosphates. Diacylglycerol phosphate, in turn, activates protein kinase C and phosphorylation of protein substrates different from those

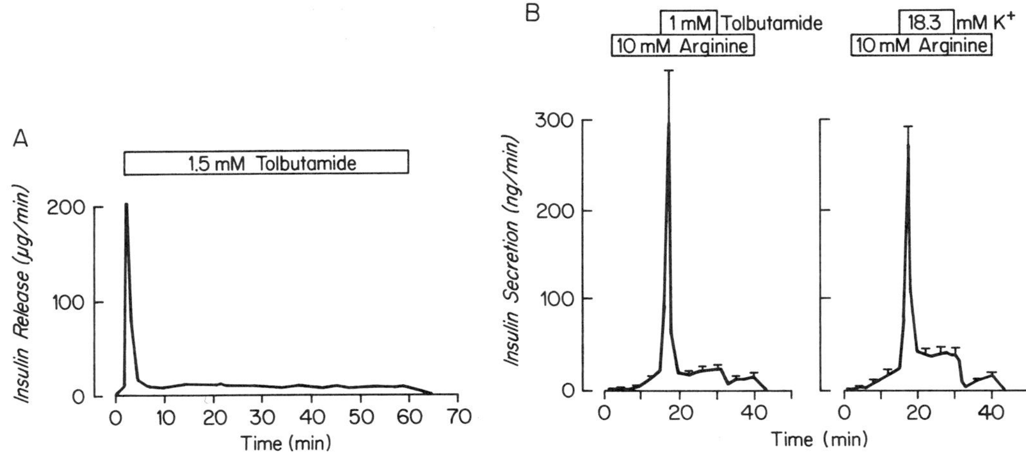

Figure 2-6. Effect of tolbutamide or K^+ on phasic insulin secretion from the isolated perfused pancreas of the rat. ***A,*** Reproduced with permission from Curry DL, Bennett LL, Grodsky GM. Dynamics of insulin secretion by the perfused rat pancreas. Endocrinology 1968;83:572. ***B,*** Reproduced with permission from Grodsky GM, Epstein GH, Fanska R, Karam JH. Pancreatic action of the sulfonylureas. FASEB 1977;36:2714.

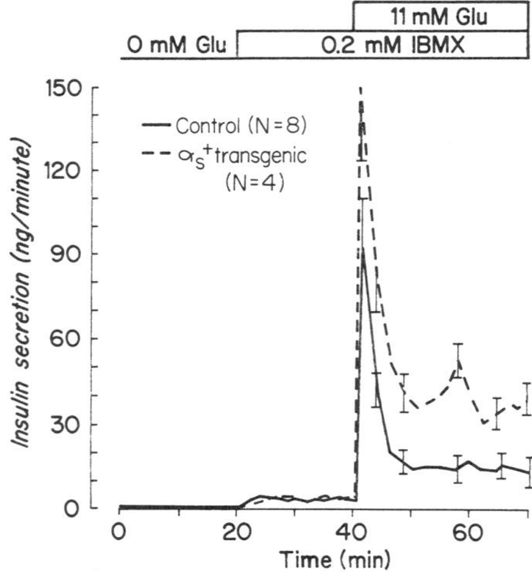

Figure 2-7. Insulin secretion from the isolated perfused pancreas of control normal mice and transgenic mice expressing constitutively active mutant α_s subunit of G_s (refer to ref. 46). Transgenics, stimulated with glucose + IBMX, hypersecrete both phases of insulin secretion. When stimulated with glucose alone, responses from transgenic pancreas are normal (data not shown). (Modified with permission from Ma YH, Landis CA, Wang J, et al. Over-expression of β-cell G-protein α_s in transgenic mice causes down-regulated hyperinsulin secretion. Endocrinology 1993;42(suppl 1):558.)

phosphorylated by cAMP (see Fig. 2-5). The role of this pathway in insulin secretion is still controversial. Though probable that stimulation of this pathway by cholinergic agents enhances insulin secretion, it is debated if glucose acts directly at this level.[31,51–56] Alternatively, glucose may increase diacyl glycerol directly from the trioses generated during its metabolism.

Nevertheless, current evidence indicates that the phosphoinositol pathway is an important positive contributor to the regulation of second-phase insulin secretion. For example: (1) phosphoinositol metabolism and protein kinase C translocation to the plasma membrane increase concurrently with the kinetics of second-phase secretion; and (2) stimulators (e.g., phorbol esters) or inhibitors (e.g., staurosporine) of protein kinase C are particularly effective on second-phase secretion (reviewed in [53]).

Other pathways that may affect insulin secretion, but whose role on phasic release is unclear, include those generating arachidonic acid,[31] cADP ribose,[57] nitric oxide,[58] malonyl CoA,[59] long-chain fatty acyl CoA,[60,61] and glycogen.[62] Additionally, the glycerol P shuttle that provides glucose-generated reducing equivalents to the mitochondria may be a sensitive step in the insulin secretory process.[63]

Ubiquitous Role of Ca^{++} on Phasic Secretion

Defining the role of the various metabolic pathways in the first and second phases of insulin secretion is complicated because cytosolic Ca^{++} itself modulates all these pathways at various steps (see Fig. 2-5). In turn, Ca^{++} influx is directly affected by cAMP or protein kinase C,[48,56] and inositol phosphates produced in the phosphoinositol pathway can mobilize stored intracellular Ca^{++} from the endoplasmic reticulum.

The penultimate signal for second-phase secretion may not be Ca^{++}(i) modulated protein phosphorylation as indicated in Fig. 2-5, but cytosolic Ca^{++} itself. During glucose stimulation, cytosolic Ca^{++} can be diphasic, sometimes paralleling that of biphasic insulin secretion.[64,65] Thus, it is unclear if the late rise in Ca^{++}(i) drives second-phase as well as first-phase secretion or if it acts on second phase as a secondary modulator of the metabolic pathways. Resolution of these alternate possibilities may require illucidation of newly discovered Ca^{++} channels that can mobilize intracellular Ca^{++} from the ER,[66] or are activated by ER calcium levels ([67], see Chapter 9).

Furthermore, nearly all considerations of the role of Ca^{++} for insulin secretion have focused on its regulation of signal pathways (see Fig. 2-5). However, numerous Ca^{++}-dependent membrane fusion proteins involved in vesicular transport and exocytosis (e.g., small G-proteins, annexins, syntaxins, soluble *N*-ethylmaleimide–sensitive attachment proteins [SNAPs]) are being identified.[68] It is apparent that a direct permissive effect of Ca^{++} on the β-cell secretory process itself is important and adds to the complexity.

Oscillations of Insulin Secretion

Although usually measured as relatively smooth secretion curves, insulin release, when stimulated with glucose and other secretagogues actually oscillates with a reproducible frequency. These oscillations are presumed important to prevent downregulation of insulin receptors in vivo, and therefore to maximize insulin action. "Slow" oscillations have a frequency of 10–15 minutes in vivo.[69,70] The process is inherent to the β-cell because oscillations (of somewhat greater frequency) are found with isolated β-cells.[71] Secretagogue increases cause an increase in amplitude, and therefore total insulin release, with no change in the oscillatory frequencies. Recent studies have shown a temporal correlation between oscillations of insulin secretion and oscillations in cytosolic Ca^{++}, suggesting that Ca^{++} flux is the driving force.[65,72,73] The possibility that both first-phase and oscillatory insulin secretion are related phenomena may explain why both are suppressed as early defects in the mild type II diabetic.[20,74]

The causes for these oscillations of Ca^{++}(i) and insulin release are unclear. Glucose, in addition to its positive effects on Ca^{++}(i) as a result of increasing uptake of extracellular Ca^{++} can also deplete Ca^{++}(i) by transferring cytosolic Ca^{++} to storage organelles,[75] a feed-back situation that could favor oscillations. Alternatively, oscillations could arise from elevated Ca^{++}(i) depleting itself by activating K^+ channels in the membrane[76] or from changes in a newly described, ER calcium-regulated ion channel (Calcium Releasing Activating Current Channel, CRAC[67]; see Chapter 9). A second type of Ca^{++}(i) oscillation has a greater frequency (2–3/min) but a small amplitude. These oscillations, superimposed on the slow ones, correspond to bursts of action potentials.[73,77]

A third type of oscillation of insulin secretion (ultradian) is observed only in vivo and is impaired in subjects with NIDDM.[78] Pulses are of low frequency (2–3 hours). Ultradian oscillations are not inherent to the β-cell, but result from "entrainment" driven by oscillating blood glucose.

Regulation and Counter-Regulation of β-Cell Function

The β-cell is affected by long-term chronic exposure to various agents, which can result in downregulation or compensatory upregulation of phasic insulin release.

Third-Phase Insulin Secretion: Relationship to Desensitization

Details of desensitization of β-cell function by chronic hyperglycemia in vivo are presented elsewhere (see Chapter 10 by J. Leahy; reviewed in [79]). In vitro, chronic exposure of the perfused pancreas or normal islets to glucose for 1–3 hours results in spontaneous decreased secretion (third phase) (see Fig. 2-2).[11,14] Although third-phase release may not duplicate all of the phenomena related to glucose-induced desensitization generated in vivo, it can provide insights into some of the characteristics involved. Both insulin synthesis (discussed above) and conversion of proinsulin to insulin are stimulated by glucose.[80–82] Neither of these glucose-regulated events, however, are downregulated during third-phase secretion,[80] suggesting that inhibition is not caused by a general impairment of glucose metabolism or insulin production, but is at the level of signals regulating the release process. This is further suggested by observations that third-phase release occurs with nonglucose secretagogues.[9]

Reports of a change in Ca^{++} flux during glucose-induced desensitization in vitro are inconsistent. In the same 24-hour perifusion conditions illustrated in Figure 2-2, however, Ca^{++} uptake either basally or stimulated by glucose was unchanged.[83] Hence, it is unlikely that suppressed Ca^{++} flux is solely responsible for the low insulin secretion of the third phase. In fact, excess Ca^{2+}(i) caused by chronic glucose may contribute to the desensitization process.[84]

An increase in cAMP produced by isobutylmethylxanthine (IBMX) or forskolin enhances the total amount of insulin release in all phases, but does not delay or prevent the spontaneous onset of the third phase,[11] indicating that cAMP depletion is not responsible.

As shown in Figure 2-5, insulin secretion is amplified by the phosphoinositol pathway, particularly in the second phase. Phosphoinositol metabolism and the functional activity of protein kinase C decline during third-phase insulin secretion, or with desensitization produced in vivo in hyperglycemic animal models,[53] suggesting an important role for this process in both phenomena.

As noted above, downregulation of insulin secretion in vitro during the third phase is not caused by decreased insulin storage.[13] However, apparent desensitization resulting from prolonged hyperglycemia in vivo may in part, reflect depleted insulin stores.[79,85] Recently, an improvement of acute stimulated insulin release was demonstrated when hyperglycemic animals were chronically treated with the β-cell inhibitor diazoxide.[86,87] Although this improved function was ascribed to reduction of the hyperinsulinemia per se, it was mathematically proportional to the increased insulin content produced during inhibition of insulin release by the diazoxide. Therefore, any evaluation of downregulation during chronic stimulation must carefully dissociate alterations in secretory mechanisms from a simple prior depletion of β-cell content.

One caveat in relating insulin secretion to total insulin content is that not all stored insulin is equally available for release. Insulin is stored in compartments within the β-cell that differ in their biochemical or geographic availability (e.g., proinsulin and insulin still in ER and golgi, insulin in labile granules proximal to the plasma membrane,[24] or "old" insulin destined for degradation and not available for secretion[88]). Additionally, heterogeneity can be caused by differences in the sensitivity of individual β-cells to stimulators of both synthesis and secretion.[25–28]

Counter-Regulation of Inhibition

After chronic exposure, β-cells can become desensitized both to inhibitors as well as to stimulating agents.[11,83] Verapamil inhibits the L-type Ca^{2+} channel and is therefore a highly effective inhibitor of insulin secretion. In 24-hour islet perifusion experiments, inhibition by verapamil of glucose-stimulated insulin secretion is dramatic during the first 2–3 hours of exposure. After 20 hours, however, inhibition is no longer detectable; if verapamil is added for the first time at 20 hours, the inhibitor is fully active. Similar neutralization of the inhibitory effect of somatostatin is also demonstrable. Because both of these inhibitory agents act on ion flux, it is possible that K^+ and or Ca^{++} channels can compensate for the effects of inhibitors within a few hours.

Phase-Dependent Effects of Agents

Because different mechanisms control each phase of insulin secretion (see Fig. 2-5), the effect of an agent depends highly on the underlying phase occurring when the agent is added.[89] For example, 3,4,5-trimethoxybenzoic acid 8-(dimethylamine)octyl ester, (TMB) and tetracane have inhibitory effects if added during second-phase insulin secretion or during time-dependent potentiation (both are conditions in which potentiator, P [see Fig. 2-3] is the predominating factor regulating secretion). In contrast, when these agents are added during the third phase, they are potent stimulators.[89] Based on the assumptions previously discussed, these agents could act by blocking the phosphoinositol path because they inhibit insulin secretion during the second phase, when this pathway predominates as the effective signal for insulin release. Positive stimulation, occurring during third-phase secretion when the contribution of phosphoinositol metabolism is reduced, can result from uncovering these agents' known ability to increase Ca^{++}(i) (see Fig. 2-5). These results emphasize that the kinetic state of the β-cell must be considered when evaluating effects of agents on insulin secretion. As a practical application, secretion results obtained with fresh islet cell preparations (in the first and second phases) should be distinguished carefully from those obtained with islets cultured with glucose (in the third phase).

Positive Compensation

Although chronic exposure to glucose downregulates or desensitizes β-cell function, more extensive exposure to glucose (>24 hours) can cause a compensatory partial recovery of the secretory process. This is characterized by a shift in the glucose sensitivity curve for insulin secretion to the left and a corresponding increase in glucokinase mRNA, protein, and activity.[90–92] Thus, there can be compensatory increases in insulin secretion despite coexisting desensitization. Possibly, an inability to make these compensations could contribute to the impaired insulin secretion of NIDDM.

Indirect Counter-Regulation

Counter-regulation of β-cell function may occur in sites modifying a regulatory pathway, but not necessarily located directly in it. A mutant, α_s^+ subunit of the Gs protein (which increases adenyl cyclase production) has been expressed in a constitutively active form in the β-cells of transgenic mice.[47] In this case, overproduction of cAMP and hyperinsulin secretion were normalized by a compensatory increase in cAMP catabolism.

Constitutive (Unregulated) Insulin Release

In the normal β-cell, release is tightly regulated, approximately 99% of the insulin being secreted by the secretagogue-induced, Ca^{++}-dependent, pathway.[27,93] The β-cell, however, is capable of constitutive release of newly synthesized hormone, which (1) is rapid (within minutes), (2) is rich in proinsulin and proinsulin-split products, and (3) does not require Ca^{++} (reviewed in [94]). Constitutive release of (pro)insulin has been observed previously only from transformed cells or from isolated islets of transgenic mice.[95] Recently, a unique constitutive release from the intact pancreas of transgenic mice expressing mutant, monomeric insulin was observed.[96] The mouse pancreas responded normally to Ca^{++} plus secretagogues, indicating a relatively intact regulated secretory system; however, in contrast to normal mice, the hormone was secreted constitutively and nonphasically in the absence of Ca^{++} (Fig. 2-8). In this model, Ca^{++} was actually a rapid inhibitory

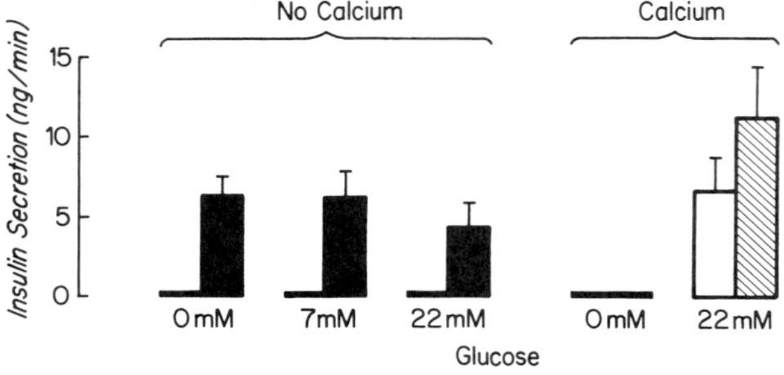

Figure 2-8. Insulin release (measured by insulin radioimmunoassay [IRI]) in the presence and absence of calcium from the isolated perfused pancreas of normal control mice and transgenic mice expressing B9,B27 mutant proinsulin. The B9,B27 mutant hormone is restricted to its monomeric state, but can form aggregates and crystals with high calcium. In the absence of calcium (no calcium + EGTA), transgenics spontaneously release large amounts of "insulin" measured as IRI, which may include proinsulin, proinsulin-split products, and some fully processed insulin itself (refer to [92]); solid bars (right). In contrast, the normal pancreas does not secrete without calcium; solid bars (left). With calcium, normal (open bar) and transgenic pancreata (hatched bar) respond with typical glucose-regulated release.

signal (Fig. 2-9); glucose and arginine were mild inhibitors. Thus, constitutive release of proinsulin required both expression of a monomeric form of insulin and the absence of extracellular Ca^{++}, two conditions that reduce aggregation during the sorting process. These results support the hypothesis that aggregation of proteins favor sorting to regulatory release, whereas reduced aggregation results in nonphasic constitutive secretion.[94] It is to be established whether any or a part of the elevated proinsulin and proinsulin-split products that occur in NIDDM result from impaired sorting and a shift to constitutive release. At the least, such studies demonstrate that under special circumstances, a nearly complete reversal of kinetic insulin secretion (i.e., inhibition by secretagogues and enhancement by Ca^{++}-deprivation) can occur.

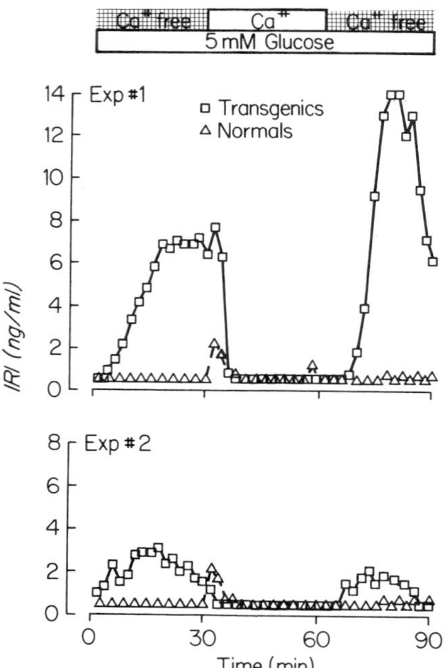

Figure 2-9. Acute effect of extracellular calcium on constitutive IRI release from the isolated perfused pancreas of transgenic mice expressing B9,B27 mutant proinsulin (see legend for Fig. 2-8 and [96] for additional details).

Summary

The three phases of insulin release occurring during constant stimulation reflect the changing and overlapping contributions of different ionic and metabolic signals. The quantitative characteristics required for these signals to produce phasic insulin secretion is described by the classic two-compartmental model. First-phase release is caused by emptying of a small compartment (containing insulin or a signal similarly depleted); the second and third phases result from a progressive rise and then fall in signals, causing provision via a putative potentiator, P. Time-dependent potentiation (memory) is generated by the residual levels of this same P. The "delayed" high insulin levels characteristic of mild NIDDM during a glucose tolerance test can be produced in the model by introducing a constant defect in release from the terminal small compartment while allowing signals for provision to remain normal.

First-phase release is particularly under ionic control; agents stimulating only β-cell depolarization and Ca^{++} uptake (in the absence of glucose) predominantly produce this phase. Glucose stimulates ion flux and first-phase release, but in addition, causes second-phase release mediated by the cAMP, phosphoinositol, and other pathways. Ca^{++} can modulate all these pathways and is involved in the terminal exocytotic process itself. Thus Ca^{++} has an ubiquitous, but not exclusive, role in regulating phasic insulin secretion. Oscillations of insulin secretion also are driven by cytosolic Ca^{++}, which itself oscillates by unknown causes.

Stimulatory or inhibitory effects of agents on the function of the β-cell can vary, depending on the phase of insulin secretion occurring when they are administered.

New evidence is accumulating that the β-cell counter-regulates when overexposed to stimulators (and inhibitors) in an attempt to reestablish normal homeostasis. The spontaneous reduction in insulin secretion (third phase) during prolonged high glucose may represent one form of counter-regulation similar to the glucose-induced desensitization occurring in NIDDM. Finally, constitutive or unregulated nonphasic release of (pro)insulin has been demonstrated from the intact pancreas of transgenic mice expressing a mutant, nonaggregating form of insulin. It is not yet established whether constitutive insulin secretion plays any role in the hyper-(pro)insulinism of NIDDM.

References

1. Curry DL, Bennett LL, Grodsky GM. Dynamics of insulin secretion by the perfused rat pancreas. Endocrinology 1968;83:572
2. O'Connor MDL, Landahl HD, Grodsky GM. Role of rate of change as a signal for insulin release. Endocrinology 1977;101:85
3. O'Connor MDL, Landahl H, Grodsky GM. Comparison of storage- and signal-limited models of pancreatic insulin secretion. Am J Physiol 1980;238:R378
4. Gold G, Grodsky GM. Kinetic aspects of compartmental storage and secretion of insulin and zinc. Experientia 1984;40:1105
5. Ma YH, Wang J, Rodd GG, Bolaffi JL, Grodsky GM. Differences in insulin secretion between the rat and mouse: Role of cAMP. Eur J Endocrinol 1995;132/3:370–376
6. Lenzen S. Insulin secretion by isolated perfused rat and mouse pancreas. Am J Physiol 1979;236:E391
7. Grodsky GM, Ma YH, Cullen B, Sarvetnick N. Effect on insulin production, sorting, and secretion by MHC class II gene expression in the pancreatic beta cell of transgenic mice. Endocrinology 1992;131:933
8. Grodsky GM. Threshold distribution hypothesis for packet storage of insulin and its mathematical modeling. J Clin Invest 1972;51:2047
9. Nesher R, Praiss M, Cerasi E. Immediate and time-dependent effects of glucose on insulin release: Differential calcium requirement. Acta Endocrinol 1988;117:409
10. Grill V. Time and dose dependencies for priming effect of glucose on insulin secretion. Am J Physiol 1981;240:E24

11. Bolaffi JL, Rodd G, Ma Y, Grodsky GM. Effect of glucagon or somatostatin on desensitized insulin secretion. Endocrinology 1990;126:1750
12. Grodsky GM. A new phase of insulin secretion: How will it contribute to our understanding of β-cell function? Diabetes 1989;38:673
13. Bolaffi JL, Bruno L, Heldt A, Grodsky GM. Characteristics of desensitization of insulin secretion in fully in vitro systems. Endocrinology 1988;122:1801
14. Bolaffi JL, Heldt A, Lewis LD, Grodsky GM. The third phase of in vitro insulin secretion: Evidence for glucose insensitivity. Diabetes 1986;35:370
15. Ward WK, Beard JC, Porte D Jr. Clinical aspects of islet β-cell function in non–insulin-dependent diabetes mellitus. Diabetes Metab Rev 1986;2:297
16. Luzi L, DeFronzo RA. Effect of loss of first-phase insulin secretion on hepatic glucose production and tissue glucose disposal in man. Am J Physiol 1989;257:E241
17. Albisser AM, Leibel BS, Ewart TG, Dividovac Z, Botz CK, Zingg W. An artificial endocrine pancreas. Diabetes 1974;23:389
18. Simpson RG, Benedetti A, Grodsky GM, Karam JH, Forsham PH. Early phase of insulin release. Diabetes 1968;17:684
19. Cerasi E, Luft R, Efendic S. Decreased sensitivity of the pancreatic beta cells to glucose in prediabetic and diabetic subjects: A glucose dose-response study. Diabetes 1972;21:224
20. Hales CN, Greenwood FC, Mitchell FL, Strauss WT. Blood-glucose, plasma-insulin and growth hormone concentrations of individuals with minor abnormalities of glucose tolerance. Diabetologia 1968;4:73
21. Welsh M, Nielsen DA, MacKrell AJ, Steiner DF. Control of insulin gene expression in pancreatic B-cells and in an insulin producing cell line: RIN-5F cells. II. Regulation of insulin mRNA stability. J Biol Chem 1985;260:13590
22. Nagamatsu S, Bolaffi JL, Grodsky GM. Direct effects of glucose on proinsulin synthesis and processing during desensitization. Endocrinology 1987;120:1225
23. Itoh N, Okamoto H. Translocation control of proinsulin synthesis by glucose. Nature 1980;283:100
24. Bokvist K, Eliasson L, Ammala C, Renstrom E, Rorsman P. Co-Localization of L-type Ca^{2++} channels and insulin-containing secretory granules and its significance for the initiation of exocytosis in mouse pancreatic B cells. EMBO 1995;14:50
25. Salomon D, Meda P. Heterogeneity and contact-dependent regulation of hormone secretion by individual B cells. Exp Cell Res 1986;162:507
26. Pipeleers DG. Heterogeneity in pancreatic β-cell population. Diabetes 1992; 41:777
27. Gold G, Landahl HD, Gishizky ML, Grodsky GM. Heterogeneity and compartmental properties of insulin storage and secretion in rat islets. J Clin Invest 1982;69:554
28. Halban P. Differential rates of release of newly synthesized and of stored insulin from pancreatic islets. Endocrinology 1982;110:1183
29. Grodsky GM, Batts AA, Bennett LL, Vcella C, McWilliams NB, Smith DF. Effects of carbohydrates on secretion of insulin from isolated rat pancreas. Am J Physiol 1963;205:638
30. Coore HG, Randle PJ. Regulation of insulin secretion studied with pieces of rabbit pancreas incubated in vitro. Biochem J 1964;93:66
31. Prentki M, Matschinsky FM. Ca^{++}, cAMP, and phospholipid-derived messengers in coupling mechanisms of insulin secretion. Physiol Rev 1987;67:1185
32. Ostenson C-G, Khan A, Abdel-Halim SM, et al. Abnormal insulin secretion and glucose metabolism in pancreatic islets from the spontaneous diabetic GK rat. Diabetologia 1993;36:3
33. Ammala C, Eliasson L, Bokvist K, et al. Exocytosis elicited by action potentials and voltage-clamp calcium currents in individual mouse pancreatic B-cells. J Physiol 1993;472:665
34. Ashcroft FM, Rorsman P. Electrophysiology of the pancreatic β-cell. Prog Biophys Molec Biol 1989;54:87
35. Santos RM, Rosario LM, Nadel A, Garcia-Sancho J, Soria B, Valdeolmillos M. Widespread synchronous $[Ca^{2+}]_i$ oscillations due to bursting electrical activity in single pancreatic islets. Pfugers Archiv 1991;418:417
36. Henquin JC, Meissner HP. Significance of ionic fluxes and changes in membrane potential for stimulus-secretion coupling in pancreatic B-cells. Experientia 1984;40:1043
37. Rosario LM, Atwater I, Scott AM. Pulsatile insulin release and electrical activity from single ob/ob mouse islets of Langerhans. Adv Exper Med Biol 1987;211:413
38. Boyd AE 3d, Rajan AS, Baines KL. Regulation of insulin release by calcium. In: Draznin B, Melmed S, LeRoith D, eds. Molecular and Cellular Biology of Diabetes Mellitus. New York, NY: Alan R Liss;1989;93–105
39. Grodsky GM, Bennett LL. Cation requirements for insulin secretion in the isolated perfused pancreas. Diabetes 1966;15:910
40. Ashcroft SJH, Weerasinghe LCC, Randle PJ. Interrelationship of islet metabolism, adenosine triphosphate content and insulin release. Biochem J 1973; 132:223
41. Misler S, Barnett DW, Gillis KD, Pressel DM. Electrophysiology of stimulus-secretion coupling in human β-cells. Diabetes 1992;41:1221
42. Grodsky GM, Epstein GH, Fanska R, Karam JH. Pancreatic action of the sulfonylureas. FASEB 1977;36:2714
43. Levin SR, Charles MA, O'Connor M, Grodsky GM. Use of diphenylhydantoin and diazoxide to investigate insulin secretory mechanisms. Am J Physiol 1975;229:49
44. Sato Y, Aizawa T, Komatsu M, Okada N, Yamada T. Dual functional role of membrane depolarization/Ca^{++} influx in rat pancreatic B-cell. Diabetes 1992;41:438
45. Gembal M, Detimary P, Gilon P, Gao Z-Y, Henquin JC. Mechanisms by which glucose can control insulin release independently from its action on adenosine triphosphate-sensitive K^+ channels in mouse β cells. J Clin Invest 1993;91:871
46. Charles MA, Fanska R, Schmid FG, Forsham PH, Grodsky GM. Adenosine 3′,5′-monophosphate in pancreatic islets: Glucose-induced insulin release. Science 1973;179:569
47. Ma YH, Landis CA, Wang J, et al. Over-expression of β-cell G-protein α_s in transgenic mice causes down-regulated hyperinsulin secretion. Endocrinology 1993;42(suppl 1):558
48. Henquin JC, Meissner HP. The ionic, electrical, and secretory effects of endogenous cyclic adenosine monophosphate in mouse pancreatic β-cells: Studies with forskolin. Endocrinology 1984;115:1125
49. Rajan AS, Hill RS, Boyd III AE. Effect of rise in cAMP levels on Ca^{++} influx through voltage-dependent Ca^{++} channels in HIT cells. Diabetes 1989;38:874
50. Rasmussen H, Zawalich KS, Ganesan S, Calle R, Zawalich WS. Physiology and pathophysiology of insulin secretion. Diabetes Care 1990;13:655
51. Kelley GG, Zawalich KC, Zawalich WS. Calcium and a mitochondrial signal interact to stimulate phosphoinositide hydrolysis and insulin secretion in rat islets. Endocrinology 1994;134:1648
52. Gao Z-Y, Gilon P, Henquin J-C. The role of protein kinase-C in signal transduction through vasopressin and acetylcholine receptors in pancreatic B-cells from normal mouse. Endocrinology 1994;135:191
53. Ganesan S, Calle R, Zawalich K, Smallwood JI, Zawalich WS, Rasmussen H. Glucose-induced translocation of protein kinase C in rat pancreatic islets. Proc Natl Acad Sci 1990;87:9893
54. Laychock SG. Identification and metabolism of polyphosphoinositides in isolated islets of Langerhans. Biochem J 1983;216:101
55. McDaniel BA, Easom RA, Hughes JH, McDaniel ML, Turk J. Secretagogue-induced diacylglycerol accumulation in isolated pancreatic islets. Mass spectrometric characterization of the fatty acyl content indicates multiple mechanisms of generation. Biochemistry 1989;28:429
56. Biden TJ, Peter-Riesch B, Schlegel W, Wollheim CB. Ca^{2+}-mediated generation of inositol 1,4,5-triphosphate and inositol 1,3,4,5-tetrakisphosphate in pancreatic islets. J Biol Chem 1987;262:3567
57. Takasawa S, Nata K, Yonekura H, Okamoto H. Cyclic ADP-ribose in insulin secretion from pancreatic B cells. Science 1993;259:370
58. Jones PM, Persaud SJ, Bjaaland T, Pearson JD, Howell SL. Nitric oxide is not involved in the initiation of insulin secretion from rat islets of Langerhans. Diabetologia 1992;35:1020
59. Corkey BE, Glennon MC, Chen KC, Denney JT, Matschinsky FM, Prentki M. A role for malonyl-CoA in glucose-stimulated insulin secretion from clonal pancreatic β-cell. J Biol Chem 1989;264:21608
60. Prentki M, Vischer S, Glennon MC, Regazzi R, Denney JT, Corkey BE. Malonyl-CoA and long chain acyl-CoA esters as metabolic coupling factors in nutrient-induced insulin secretion. J Biol Chem 1992;267:5802
61. Warnotte C, Gilon P, Henquin M, Henquin J-C. Mechanisms of the stimulation of insulin release by saturated fatty acids. Diabetes 1994;43:703
62. Lundquist I, Panagiotidis G. The relationship of islet amyloglucosidase activity and glucose-induced insulin secretion. Pancreas 1992;7:352
63. Sener A, Malaisse WJ. Hexose metabolism in pancreatic islets: Ca^{2+}-dependent activation of the glycerol phosphate shuttle by nutrient secretagogues. J Biol Chem 1992;267:13251
64. Rojas E, Carroll PB, Ricordi C, et al. Control of cytosolic free calcium in cultured human pancreatic B-cells occurs by external calcium-dependent mechanisms. Endocrinology 1994;134:1771
65. Bergsten P, Grapengiesser E, Gylfe E, Tengholm A, Hellman B. Synchronous oscillations of cytoplasmic Ca^{2+} and insulin release in glucose-stimulated pancreatic islets. J Biol Chem 1994;269:1
66. Worley JF, McIntyre MS, Spencer RJ, Mertz RJ, Roe MW, Dukes ID. Endoplasmic reticulum calcium store regulates membrane potential in mouse islet B cells. J Biol Chem 1994;269:14359
67. Bertram R, Smolen P, Sherman A, Mears D, Atwater A, Martin F. A role for calcium release-activated current (CRAC) in cholinergic modulation of electrical activity in pancreatic B-cells. Biophysical J 1995;68:2323
68. Bean AJ, Zang X, Hokfelt T. Peptide secretion: What do we know? FASEB 1994;8:630
69. Goodner CJ, Walike BC, Koerker DJ, et al. Insulin, glucagon and glucose exhibits synchronous sustained oscillations in fasting monkeys. Science 1977;195:177
70. Lang DA, Matthews DR, Peto PJ, Turner RC. Cyclic oscillations of basal plasma glucose and insulin concentrations in human beings. N Engl J Med 1979;301:1023
71. Grapengiesser E, Gylfe E, Hellman B. Glucose-induced oscillations of cytoplasmic Ca^{2+} in the pancreatic β-cell. Biochem Biophys Res Commun 1988;151:1299
72. Bergstrom RW, Fujimoto WY, Teller DC, De Haen C. Oscillatory insulin secretion in perifused isolated rat islets. Am J Physiol 1989;257:E479
73. Rosario LM, Atwater I, Scott AM. Pulsatile insulin release and electrical activity from single ob/ob-mouse islets. In: Atwater I, Rojas E, Soria B, eds. Biophysics of the Pancreatic β-Cell. New York, NY: Plenum Press;1986:413
74. O'Rahilly S, Turner RC, Matthews DR. Impaired pulsatile secretion of insulin in relatives of patients with non–insulin-dependent diabetes. N Engl J Med 1988;318:1225
75. Hellman B, Gylfe E. Calcium and the control of insulin secretion. In: Cheung WY, ed. Calcium and Cell Function. Orlando, Fla: Academic Press;1986:6:253
76. Atwater I, Dawson CM, Ribalet B, Rajas E. Potassium permeability activated by intracellular calcium ion concentration in the pancreatic β-cell. J Physiol 1979;288:575

77. Santos RM, Rosario LM, Nadal A, Garcia-Sancho J, Soria B, Valdeolmillos M. Widespread synchronous $[Ca^{2+}]_i$ oscillations due to bursting electrical activity in single pancreatic islets. Pfugers Arch 1991;418:417
78. Sturis J, Van Cauter E, Blackman JD, Polonsky KS. Entrainment of pulsatile insulin secretion by oscillatory glucose infusion. J Clin Invest 1991;87:439
79. Robertson RP, Olson LK, Zhang H-J. Differentiating glucose toxicity from glucose desensitization: A new message from the insulin gene. Diabetes 1994;43:1085
80. Nagamatsu S, Grodsky GM. Glucose regulated proinsulin processing in isolated islets from rat pancreas. Diabetes 1988;37:1426
81. Alcaron C, Lincoln B, Rhodes CJ. The biosynthesis of the subtilisin-related proprotein convertase PC3, but not that of the PC2 convertase, is regulated by glucose in parallel to proinsulin biosynthesis in rat pancreatic islets. J Biol Chem 1993;268:4276
82. Gishizky ML, Grodsky GM. Differential kinetics of rat insulin I and II processing in rat islets of Langerhans. FEBS Lett 1987;223:227
83. Bolaffi JL, Rodd GG, Ma YH, Bright D, Grodsky GM. The role of Ca^{++}-related events in glucose-stimulated desensitization of insulin secretion. Endocrinology 1991;129:2131
84. Thams P, Hansen SE, Capito K, Hedeskov J. Role of glucose metabolism and phosphoinositide hydrolysis in glucose-induced sensitization/desensitization of insulin secretion from mouse pancreatic islets. Acta Physiol Scand 1995;154:65
85. Leahy JL, Bumbalo LM, Chen C. Diazoxide causes recovery of B-cell glucose responsiveness in 90% pancreatectomized diabetic rats. Diabetes 1994;43:173
86. Sako Y, Grill VE. Coupling of β-cell desensitization by hyperglycemia to excessive stimulation and circulating insulin in glucose-infused rats. Diabetes 1990;39:1580
87. Sako Y, Grill VE. Diazoxide infusion at excess but not at basal hyperglycemia enhances β-cell sensitivity to glucose in vitro in neonatally streptozotocin-diabetic rats. Metabolism 1992;41:738
88. Halban PA, Wollheim CB. Intracellular degradation of insulin stored by rat pancreatic islets in vitro: An alternative pathway for homeostasis of pancreatic insulin content. J Biol Chem 1980;255:6003
89. Bolaffi JL, Rodd GG, Ma YH, Grodsky GM. Opposite, phase-dependent effects of TMB or tetracaine on islet function during three phases of glucose-stimulated insulin secretion. Endocrinology 1993;132:2325
90. Purrello F, Buscema M, Rabuazzo AM, et al. Glucose modulated glucose transporter affinity, glucokinase activity, and secretory response in rat pancreatic β-cells. Diabetes 1993;42:199
91. Liang Y, Najafi H, Matschinsky FM. Glucose at physiological levels induces glucokinase, glucose usage and insulin secretion in cultured pancreatic islets. Diabetes 1991;40(suppl 1):705
92. Timmers KI, Powell AM, Voyles NR, Solomon D, Wilkins SD, Bhathena S, Recant L. Multiple alternations in insulin response to glucose in islets from 48-h glucose-infused nondiabetic rats. Diabetes 1990;39:1436
93. Rhodes CJ, Halban PA. Newly synthesized proinsulin/insulin and stored insulin are released from pancreatic β cells predominantly via a regulated, rather than a constitutive, pathway. J Cell Biol 1987;105:145
94. Halban PA, Irminger JC. Sorting and processing of secretory proteins. Biochem J 1994;299:1
95. Carroll RC, Hammer RE, Chan SJ, Swift HH, Rubenstein AH, Steiner DF. A mutant human proinsulin is secreted from islets of Langerhans in increased amounts via an unregulated pathway. Proc Natl Acad Sci USA 1988;85:8943
96. Ma YH, Lores P, Wang J, Jami J, Grodsky GM. Spontaneous hormone release in transgenic mice expressing monomeric insulin. Endocrinology 1995;xx:2622

Diabetes Mellitus, edited by Derek LeRoith, Simeon I. Taylor, and Jerrold M. Olefsky. Lippincott–Raven Publishers, Philadelphia © 1996.

CHAPTER 3
Insulin Gene Regulation

GIULIA C. KENNEDY AND MICHAEL GERMAN

Insulin is among the best studied of the polypeptide hormones, having been the first protein for which the complete amino acid sequence was determined as well as the first hormone to be molecularly cloned. Insulin is released into the circulation by pancreatic β-cells in response to rising blood glucose levels. Insulin binds to specific receptors present on cell surfaces, and this binding signals the uptake of nutrients, storage of energy, and growth. A fall in insulin levels in response to low blood glucose results in the release of this stored energy and synthesis of glucose by the liver. Lack of insulin secretion or impaired insulin action leads to the metabolic derangement characteristic of diabetes mellitus.

The human insulin gene (*INS*) is located on chromosome 11p15.5, between the tyrosine hydroxylase (*TH*) and insulin-like growth factor-2 (*IGF2*) genes (Fig. 3-1).[1] The *INS* gene contains three exons and two introns, and the final spliced mRNA transcript is 446 bp in length, and codes for the preproinsulin peptide.

Insulin mRNA is first detected in the primordial gut of the mouse on embryonic day nine (E9), a full 3 days before the morphologic development of the pancreatic lobules.[2] Transcription of *INS* appears to be the restricting step for insulin synthesis and secretion because non–β-cells can produce—and even process, package, and secrete insulin—as long as they are engineered to transcribe exogenously introduced insulin by recombinant DNA technology.[3] Such "artificial β-cells" could become an important source of insulin for patients with insulin-dependent diabetes mellitus (IDDM).

Insulin Gene Promoter

Transcription of the *INS* gene depends on more than just the transcribed sequences of the gene. Transcription is regulated at least in part by the untranscribed sequences immediately upstream (5′ flanking sequences) of the transcription start site: the insulin promoter (see Fig. 3-1). The insulin promoter consists of all of the 5′ flanking DNA necessary for appropriate initiation of transcription. The exact 5′ end of the promoter is ill-defined, but it is known that sequences at least 4 Kb upstream contribute to regulation of transcription.[4,5]

The insulin promoter can function as an independent unit. When isolated from the remainder of the gene and linked to a reporter gene, such as the bacterial gene for chloramphenicol acetyltransferase (CAT), the promoter directs the correct transcription start site for RNA polymerase and drives expression of the heterologous gene.[6,7]

Like the intact gene, the promoter functions in a distinctly cell type–specific fashion. In both cultured cells[6–11] and transgenic animals,[12] the promoter limits expression of linked genes to the β-cells, with at least a 40-fold lower expression even in closely related α-cells[13,14] (M. German and J. Wang, unpublished data, 1995).

What allows the insulin promoter to distinguish β-cells from other cells? The sequence of the insulin promoter must encode a regulatory signal that only the β-cells can read correctly. This code is formed by a series of sequence elements along the promoter that

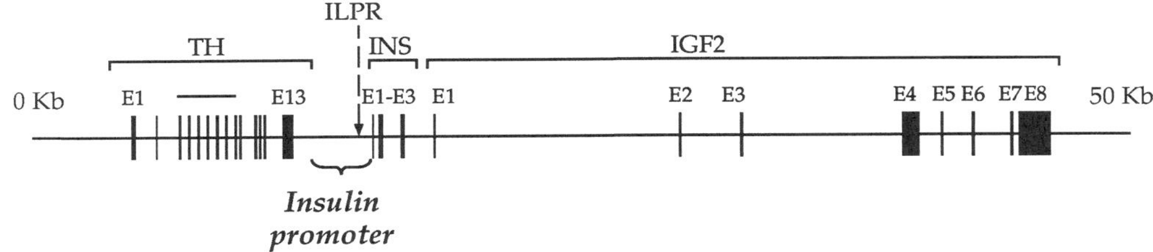

Figure 3-1. The *INS* gene and surrounding loci on chromosome 11.

act as recognition sites for DNA binding proteins. The names for these promoter sequence elements have been simplified recently; the new and old names are outlined in Figure 3-2.[15] Proteins found in the β-cell nucleus bind to these sites and form a unique DNA-protein complex that activates transcription. Other cell types do not contain the same set of nuclear proteins and therefore cannot form the unique β-cell complex and cannot activate transcription. Some of the promoter sequence elements and their cognate binding proteins have been identified (Fig. 3-3) and we are starting to learn how these pieces fit together and activate transcription.

E-Box Elements

The proximal rat insulin I promoter contains two identical eight-base pair sequence elements, E1 and E2. Mutation of either of these elements causes a 90% loss of promoter activity in insulinoma cells, and mutation of both ablates all promoter activity.[16] Although the E2 element is poorly conserved, the E1 element is absolutely conserved in all of the known mammalian insulin promoters[15,17]; its importance has also been demonstrated in the rat insulin II[10,18] and human insulin promoters[19] (H. Odagiri, J. Wang, and M. German, 1995). These elements contain the core sequence CANNTG, a common promoter sequence found in critical sequence elements called *E-boxes* in a number of other genes.[20]

β-Cell nuclei contain several protein complexes that bind to the insulin E-boxes.[19,21–25] One complex (which appears to be a set of several very similar complexes) is not present in most other cells, although similar or identical complexes are found in α-cell[13,14,21,26] and pituitary cell nuclei.[21] These complexes contain three similar proteins: Pan1, Pan2, and HEB.[21,24,27–29] Pan1 and 2 (also termed E41/E12 [human][30] or A1 [mouse][31]) are differential RNA splicing products of the same gene, *E2A*.[32] The Pan proteins and HEB belong to a family of DNA-binding proteins that share a common amino acid sequence motif: a basic domain adjacent to a helix-loop-helix structure (bHLH).

The bHLH proteins bind to DNA as dimers. The HLH region is required for dimerization and DNA binding; the basic domain is required for DNA binding. Although the bHLH proteins can form dimers with two identical partners (homodimers), in most cells the DNA-binding forms are heterodimers. Heterodimerization explains an apparent inconsistency: Both the Pan proteins and HEB are found in all cells, but in β-cells they are present in the β-cell–specific E-box–binding complex. We assume, therefore, that these ubiquitously expressed bHLH proteins preferentially heterodimerize with a set of bHLH proteins that are selectively expressed in β-cells.

One potential β-cell bHLH partner, the INSAF protein, has been described.[33] A partial cDNA for human INSAF has been cloned and sequenced. Although larger than the predicted size for β-cell bHLH partners,[34] INSAF is expressed in α- and β-cells and binds to Pan1 in vitro.[33] Based on the presence of multiple E-box–binding complexes in β-cells, however, INSAF may not be the only β-cell–specific bHLH partner.

A Elements

The A elements are a group of short adenosine/thymidine-rich sequences found on either side of E1, and immediately downstream of E2. An additional A site, A5, is found upstream of E2 in *INS* (see Fig. 3-2). Mutation of the A3 element (H. Odagiri, J. Wang, and M. German, unpublished data, 1995)[35] (or A3+A4 in the rat insulin I gene[16,36]) causes a marked loss of promoter activity, but

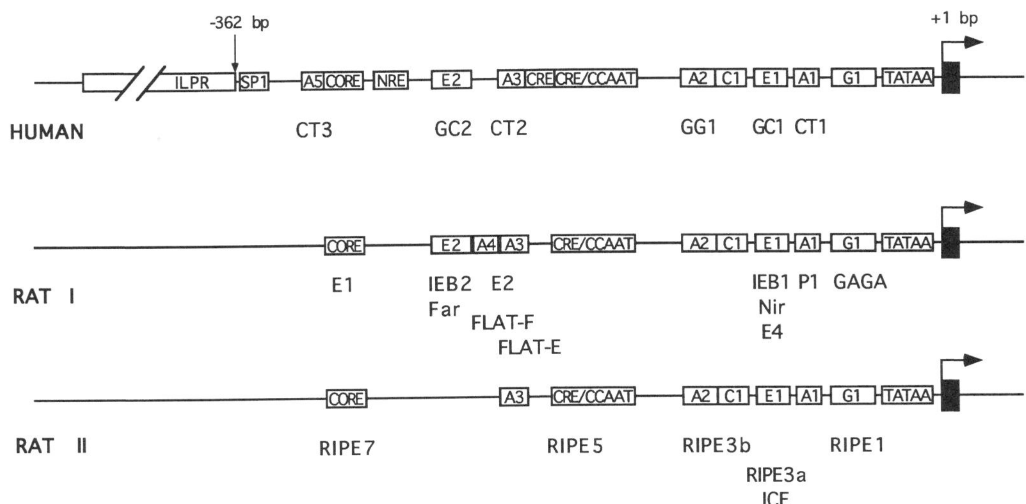

Figure 3-2. Insulin promoter sequence elements. The new names are in boxes; the old names are shown below each gene.

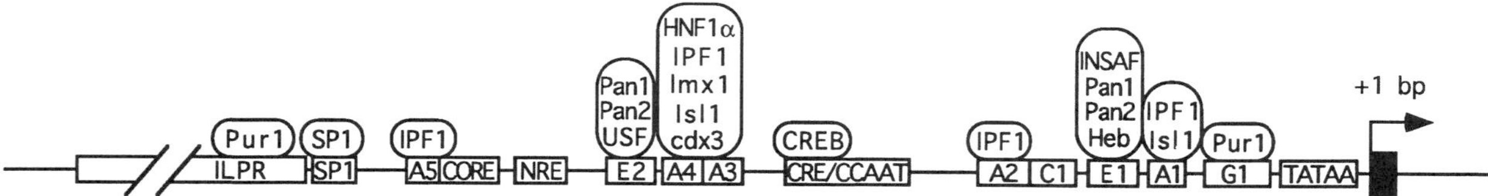

FIGURE 3-3. A composite insulin promoter with known sequence elements and binding factors. The boxes represent characterized sequence elements. The cloned binding proteins are circled above the promoter.

mutation or deletion of the other A elements causes little or no loss of activity.[16,18,36] Similar sequences have been recognized in transcriptionally important elements in other β-cell and islet genes, including β-cell–specific glucokinase,[37,38] islet amyloid polypeptide,[37] glucagon,[39] and somatostatin.[40,41]

A elements have in common the core sequence TAAT. β-Cell nuclei contain several different protein complexes that bind the A elements,[13,26,37,42,43] and cDNAs encoding a number of these proteins have been isolated.[44–50] All of the binding proteins share a common sequence of 61 amino acids, the *homeodomain,* which forms a helix-turn-helix structure that binds to DNA. Homeodomain proteins have been identified in a growing number of species and appear to be common to all eukaryotic organisms. Expressed in a variety of cell types, homeodomain proteins play determining roles in development, differentiation, and gene transcription.

Four of the β-cell homeodomain proteins, isl-1,[44] lmx-1.1,[45] lmx-1.2 (A. Rudnick and M. German, unpublished data, 1995), and lmx-2,[46] share an additional feature: a pair of cysteine-rich regions, termed *LIM domains,* that coordinate zinc atoms.[51] LIM domains have been implicated in protein-protein interactions[52,53] and also may regulate DNA binding by the homeodomain.[54] Although not ubiquitously expressed, isl-1 and lmx-2 are expressed in a variety of different cell types,[46,55–57] while lmx-1.1 and lmx-1.2 appear to be more limited in distribution[45] (A. Rudnick, H. Odagiri, and M. German, unpublished data, 1995).

IPF1,[48] also called STF1[50] and IDX1,[49] is a recently described homeodomain protein that is expressed in the duodenum and pancreas. During development, all or most of the pancreatic cells express IPF1, but with maturation, expression of IPF1 becomes largely limited to the β-cells and duodenum, with occasional expression in non–β islet cells and duct cells.[48,58] IPF1 can activate portions of the insulin promoter in non–β-cells[35,48,50] and binds to all of the A sites in the human and rat insulin I promoters (H. Odagiri and M. German, unpublished data). Interestingly, mice that are homozygous for a targeted disruption of the *IPF1* gene lack a pancreas and die shortly after birth, demonstrating that *IPF1* is required for pancreatic development.[59] The role of *IPF1* in differentiation of the β-cell, however, remains unknown.

Several other cDNAs encoding homeodomain proteins have been cloned from β-cells. Two of these, the cad-related protein cdx3[45] and the POU-homeodomain protein HNF1α,[47] can activate the insulin promoter in non–β-cells. The relative contributions of the various homeodomain proteins to insulin gene expression are unknown.

The C1 Element

Between the A2 and E1 elements lies a well-conserved, cytosine-rich sequence, the C1 element. Mutation of this element in the context of the rat insulin II promoter causes a dramatic loss of activity.[18,24,60,61] A unique β-cell nuclear complex binds to this site.[24] This complex has not been found in any other cell types tested, even in the closely related α-cells[14] (H. Odagiri and M. German, unpublished data, 1995).

The G Elements

Many genes contain purine-rich stretches immediately upstream of the transcription start site. These regions of DNA, often called *GAGA boxes,* are thought to play key roles in transcription.[62] The insulin promoter contains a conserved GAGA box, the G1 element, at positions −40 to −57, which has been shown by mutational analysis to be critical for insulin transcription in primary cultures of fetal rat islets,[63] and to a lesser extent, in the hamster-insulinoma cell line (*HIT*).[16] The rat insulin I G1 element was shown to bind several proteins in vitro; subsequently a transcription factor, Pur-1, was isolated by expression cloning and was found to bind to the insulin GAGA box.[64,65] Pur-1 contains six zinc fingers (DNA-binding motifs similar to those found in steroid hormone receptors), and is a potent activator of transcription from the insulin promoter.[64] Pur-1 also binds to the rat insulin II G1 element and a similar GAGA box in the islet amyloid polypeptide promoter, as well as to the purine-rich insulin-linked polymorphic region[66] (see below).

Other Sequence Elements

Upstream of the E1 element, between −279 and −258 bp in the human insulin promoter, lies the *negative regulatory element,* a sequence that has been shown to inhibit insulin promoter function in a β-cell tumor line.[19] This sequence also inhibited transcription when linked to a heterologous promoter and transfected into either β-cell or non–β-cell tumor lines.[19] Walker et al.,[6] however, found no effect upon removal of the negative regulatory element from the insulin promoter, and we have noted that the negative regulatory element region actually functions as a potent transcriptional activator in primary cultures of rat β-cells (H. Odagiri, J. Wang, M. Sander, and M. German, unpublished data, 1995). It appears that the function of the negative regulatory element may depend on the exact construction of the test plasmid or on the cell line used.

Four additional elements in the insulin promoter have been recognized based on their similarity to characterized elements from other genes. The Sp1 element in the human insulin promoter is a consensus binding site for the ubiquitous transcription factor Sp1, although the importance of Sp1 for function of this element is uncertain.[67] The overlapping CCAAT element and *cAMP regulatory element* (CRE) are well conserved in mammalian insulin promoters. The insulin promoter CRE binds to CRE binding factor (CREB) produced in vitro, but in β-cell nuclei CREB binds only weakly to the insulin promoter,[68] and cAMP is only a modest activator of insulin gene transcription.[36,68–70] The core element (also previously called E1[71]) has a similar sequence to the SV40 core element. Mutation or deletion of this region reduces activity in the rat insulin I promoter,[16,36] and the core element binds a β-cell nuclear complex of limited tissue distribution.[23,26,71]

Synergistic Activation

The insulin promoter should not be viewed as a simple series of binding sites, each binding a protein that independently adds to the activity of the promoter. Instead, the sequence elements with their cognate binding factors interact to activate transcription synergistically. As a result, in the β-cell nucleus, the insulin promoter forms a large DNA-protein complex whose function is dependent on all of its parts. Removal or substitution of any of the individual parts of this complex incapacitates the entire promoter. This complexity results in exquisite cell specificity. The nuclei of closely related cell types such as α-cells have most of the transcription factors that bind to the insulin promoter in β-cells. Without the complete set, however, the insulin promoter is not active in these cells.

To understand how this synergy works, we have used the example of the E and A elements. In the insulin promoter, these elements are always juxtaposed. We found that a small minienhancer that included the rat insulin I E2 and A3/A4 elements functions as a potent, β-cell–specific transcriptional activator.[37,72] However if either the E1 or the A3/A4 elements are removed by deletion or mutation, the minienhancer becomes inactive.[37] This synergy results from specific interactions between the proteins that bind at these elements. The E2A3/A4 minienhancer does not function in the fibroblast cell line BHK21, and addition of plasmids expressing high levels of Pan1 (which binds to E2) or lmx1.1 (which binds to A3 and A4) results in little or no activation. Expression of both proteins together, however, activates minienhancer-driven transcription approximately 1000 fold (Fig. 3-4).

The capacity for synergistic activation extends to other elements in the promoter. We have tested the various E-A combinations in the human promoter and found that all but the E2-A3 combination are synergistic (H. Odagiri, J. Wang, and M. German, unpublished data, 1995). The human E2 site is poorly conserved,[15,17] and it binds the Pan proteins weakly at best,[13,19] which may explain its inability to synergize with the A3 site. In the rat insulin II gene, the E1 element interacts synergistically with the adjacent C1 element,[24,60,61] although the possibility that the activity observed could result from E1 interaction with A2 has not been rigorously excluded.

Metabolic Regulation of the Insulin Promoter

β-Cells tightly control the rate of insulin synthesis and secretion in response to the feeding state of the organism, using the circulating glucose concentration as a gauge of nutritional status. Glucose causes a rise in insulin mRNA levels in cultured β-cells because of the combined effects of increased insulin gene transcription and decreased insulin mRNA degradation.[73,74] The effect of glucose on transcription in the β-cell is selective for the insulin gene and is due at least in part to activation of the insulin promoter.[69]

Glucose stimulates insulin gene transcription indirectly through the end products of its catabolism.[63] The rate-limiting step for glycolysis in β-cells is phosphorylation of glucose to glucose-6-phosphate. When the rate of glucose phosphorylation is increased by the expression of high levels of hexokinase I in β-cells, glycolysis is accelerated and the insulin promoter is activated.[63] The intermediates of glycolysis are required for this response.[63]

Mapping the sequence elements responsible for glucose activation of the insulin promoter has proved confusing. Both the rat

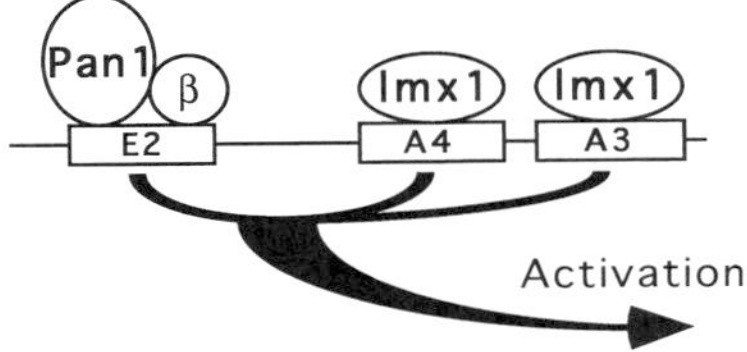

Figure 3-4. Synergistic activation of the rat insulin I E2A4/A3 minienhancer in β-cells. β represents the selectively expressed heterodimer partner found in β-cells.

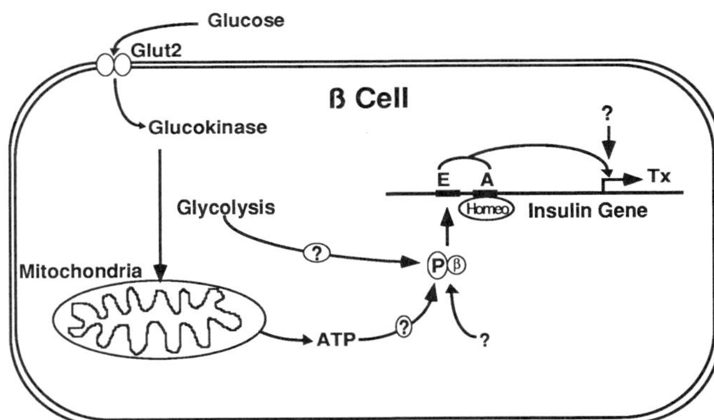

Figure 3-5. One pathway for glucose regulation of insulin gene expression. P represents Pan1 or Pan2, and β represents the selectively expressed heterodimer partner found in β-cells. Question marks indicate unknown steps in the pathway or probable intersection with other pathways.

insulin I E2A4/A3 minienhancer[69,75] and the rat insulin II C1E1 minienhancers[58] respond to glucose. Further mapping has implicated the E2,[36] A4/A3,[75] and C1[58] elements. These differences may be a result of the type of β-cells used in the studies or the exact experimental design; however, the multiplicity of metabolic regulatory elements demonstrates that, like cell type-specific transcription, glucose regulation also results from the combined interaction of several elements.[36]

We have found that the Pan-containing complexes that bind the E elements increase in response to glucose.[36] Furthermore, overexpression of Pan1 or truncated Pan1 ablates the glucose response by the E-A minienhancers.[36] We have concluded from these results that glucose catabolism by the β-cell results in the activation of the Pan-β-cell–bHLH complex. This complex then binds the E elements and synergizes with the A element–binding factors to activate insulin gene transcription (Fig. 3-5).

The Insulin-Linked Polymorphic Region

The insulin-linked polymorphic region (ILPR) (also called the insulin variable number of tandem repeats [VNTR]) was originally detected when the first two cloned human insulin genes were found to have different restriction fragment lengths due to an insertion or deletion of DNA in the 5′ flanking region of the gene.[76] The ILPR is a highly polymorphic repetitive DNA element (minisatellite) that is unique for several reasons: (1) it has been found only in primates, suggesting that it is a recent evolutionary acquisition; (2) it is found as a single copy in the human genome, in contrast to other widely dispersed repetitive elements; (3) it adopts unusual higher-order structures in vitro; (4) its location in the promoter of the insulin gene suggests that it might be involved in gene regulation; and (5) it probably encodes a locus for IDDM susceptibility. In the decade after its discovery, the ILPR has been the subject of numerous investigations aimed toward elucidating its function.

Length and Sequence Polymorphisms

The initial observation of a length polymorphism in the 5′ flanking DNA of the human insulin gene prompted Bell and coworkers to examine this region in other subjects.[77] The nature of the restriction fragment lengths was found to be an insertion located approximately 500 bp from the transcription start site.[77] Furthermore, the sizes of the insertions vary from subject to subject, falling into three general classes: short (class I), medium (class II), and long (class III). Approximately 60% of the subjects studied possess two different sizes of insertions (i.e., are heterozygous at this locus), making the ILPR a highly polymorphic region (hence the derivation of its name). Shortly thereafter, nucleotide sequencing of the insertion site revealed that the ILPR is composed of 14 bp sequences repeated in tandem.[78] The two original insulin alleles that were sequenced contain 34 and 45 copies, respectively, of the 14 bp sequence (both are class I alleles). Since then, the nucleotide sequences of two more ILPR alleles have been determined, one with 139 repeats (class III)[79] and the other with 81 repeats (class II).[80]

In addition to length heterogeneity of the ILPR, nucleotide sequence analysis of the various alleles showed that there are minor sequence variations in the 14 bp repeats[78] (Table 3-1). The most common repeat has the sequence ACAGGGGTGTGGGG; and a total of 14 different variants of this sequence (lettered a–n), most of which reflect one or two nucleotide substitutions, have now been described.[78–80] Each of the ILPR alleles differs not only in the number of total repeats, but in the type and arrangement of the repeats. Furthermore, not all of the repeats are present in any one ILPR. For instance, the class II ILPR isolated and sequenced by Rotwein and coworkers[80] lacks repeats e, h, and k, while containing three repeats l, m, and n, which are absent from the other three ILPR alleles.

Role of the Insulin-Linked Polymorphic Region in Insulin Gene Regulation

From the time of its discovery to the present, numerous laboratories have studied the ILPR in an attempt to elucidate its function. Because of its location in the 5′ flanking region of the *INS,* it was hypothesized that the ILPR might affect insulin transcription. This hypothesis was tested by deleting the ILPR from the human insulin promoter and testing its activity in vitro. Walker et al.[6] using one of the original insulin genes containing a short (class I) ILPR, showed that deletion of the ILPR resulted in the loss of only 20% of total transcriptional activity, when assayed by transient transfection into the insulinoma cell line HIT. They concluded that the ILPR did not significantly affect insulin gene transcription. At the time these experiments were performed, no long (class III) ILPR alleles had been molecularly cloned or sequenced, and it was therefore not known whether insulin promoters containing different classes of ILPR have the same effect on transcription.

Recently the role of the ILPR in transcription has been reexamined by the testing of insulin promoter constructs containing a long (class III) ILPR allele.[66] It was found that a long ILPR is associated with higher transcriptional activity than a short ILPR, when tested in fetal rat islets and HIT cells.[66] Thus, contrary to previous models of insulin promoter action, these results show that the ILPR can contribute significantly to overall transcription rates in vitro. Furthermore, these experiments show that two naturally occurring human ILPR alleles differ in their transcriptional activities in vitro, raising the possibility that additional ILPR alleles might have varying amounts of transcriptional activity.

Like the other promoter elements, the ILPR probably affects transcription by binding to proteins that interact with the basal transcriptional machinery. It has been shown recently that the transcription factor gene *Pur-1* binds to the ILPR and can activate transcription of a downstream reporter gene.[66] Each of the polymorphic repeats was tested individually for binding and transcriptional activation by *Pur-1,* and a wide range in activity among the repeats was found, despite seemingly minor variations in nucleotide sequence. For instance, the most common polymorphic repeat "a" has the highest binding affinity for *Pur-1,* whereas repeat "g" binds poorly to *Pur-1;* other repeats fall between these two extremes. Thus, in addition to the overall length of the ILPR, the sequence and arrangements of the repeats could also influence overall transcription rates.[66]

Higher-Order Structure of the Insulin-Linked Polymorphic Region

The ILPR exhibits unusual structural properties both in vivo and in vitro. For example, it shows distinct patterns of nuclease hypersensitivity; the purine-rich strand is a poor substrate for *Taq* polymerase, which is consistent with the presence of a secondary structure.[81–83] Electron microscopic analysis reveals that one strand of the ILPR exists primarily as a looped-out single strand, the other strand adopting a shorter, more compressed configuration.[81] The ILPR repeats are unusually guanine-rich, and thus resemble telomeric sequences, which readily form quadruplex structures in vitro through guanine-guanine (Hoogsteen) basepairing.[84] Studies using chimeric oligonucleotides indicate that sequences contained within the ILPR can form four-stranded structures under high NaCl concentrations.[85] Under single-stranded conditions, the most common polymorphic repeat (ACAGGGGTGTGGGG) can snap back on itself to form intramolecular hairpin structures and, at higher DNA concentrations, intermolecular interactions through guanine-guanine basepairs (G. Kennedy and W. Rutter, unpublished observations, 1994).

The significance of these DNA structures is unclear, nor is it known whether the ILPR adopts these configurations as it exists in *INS* in vivo. The structure of the ILPR in vivo could have an impact on its ability to enhance transcription. Almost certainly, the nuclear proteins that bind the ILPR will differ depending on its structure. Independent of proteins binding at the ILPR, the structure of the ILPR could also affect transcription by altering the conformation and protein-binding characteristics of the remainder of the promoter, or by influencing RNA polymerase directly.

Genetic Studies

At the time the ILPR was discovered, minisatellite DNA was just beginning to emerge as a powerful tool for genetic mapping. In fact, the ILPR was the second highly polymorphic locus discovered in the human genome, and the first linked to a known gene. Its polymorphic nature and its location in the 5′ flanking region of *INS* has made it possible to use the ILPR as a genetic marker to distinguish maternal and paternal insulin alleles in a given meiosis. This distinction is central to all genetic mapping efforts; more specifically, it allows one to test the hypothesis that an altered *INS* gene or closely linked locus is associated with genetic susceptibility to diabetes. Numerous early studies examined possible associations between different classes of the ILPR and diabetes. A population association study found a significantly higher number of class I (short) ILPR alleles in patients with IDDM.[86] Subsequent family linkage studies analyzing affected sibling pairs, however, were unable to demonstrate linkage of ILPR alleles to IDDM[87–90]; this has been attributed to the high prevalence of the disease-associated allele (i.e., the short ILPR) in the general population.[91] By restricting their analysis to offspring with heterozygous parents, Julier et al.[92] found significant linkage to a 19 Kb region spanning the *INS/IGF2* loci, which includes the ILPR. This linkage was even more significant when transmission to HLA-DR4-positive subjects was examined, suggesting an interaction between these two loci. The linkage between IDDM and the ILPR has been confirmed by several groups using different ethnic populations,[91,93,94] although these studies found no association between HLA-DR haplotypes and the ILPR polymorphisms.

The molecular mechanisms underlying ILPR association with IDDM are unclear. Although it has been shown recently that the ILPR is transcriptionally active and that there are differences in activity between two naturally occurring ILPR alleles,[66] it is not known whether transcription by the ILPR per se is involved in genetic susceptibility to IDDM, or whether another feature of the ILPR is implicated. Furthermore, the ILPR may indirectly affect other genes in addition to *INS*. The ILPR could modify transcription

Table 3-1. Polymorphic Repeats in Four ILPR Alleles

Repeat Designation	Nucleotide Sequence*				ILPR Allele Number			
					λHI-1	λHI-2	λHI-3	λHI4
a	ACA	GGGG	TGT	GGGG	15	24	81	46
b	ACA	GGGG	TCCT	GGGG	7	7	7	9
c	ACA	GGGG	TCT	GGGG	5	6	20	6
d	ACA	GGGG	TCC	GGGG	2	1	7	3
e	ATA	GGGG	TGT	GGGG	1	0	10	0
f	ACA	GGGG	TCCC	GGGG	1	5	10	10
g	ACA	GGGG	TCT	GAGG	1	0	0	1
h	ACA	GGGG	TGT	GGGC	1	0	0	0
i	ACA	GGG	TCCT	GGGG	1	1	1	1
j	ACA	GGGG	TGT	GAGG	0	1	2	1
k	ATA	GGGG	TGT	GTGG	0	0	1	0
l	ACA	GGGG	TCCG	GGGG	0	0	0	2
m	ACA	GGGG	TCCC	GGGT	0	0	0	1
n	ACA	GGGG	TCG	TAGG	0	0	0	1
	Total number of repeats				34	45	139	81

*The sequence is shown for each of the variant repeats found in the known ILPRs. The number of copies of each repeat is shown for four alleles: λHI-1,[78] λHI-2,[78] λHI-3,[79] and λHI-4.[80]
ILPR = insulin-linked polymorphic region.

of either of the two closely linked genes on human chromosome 11, *TH* and *IGF2,* or a distant gene that could affect some aspect of β-cell function or the immune response. Thus, despite the genetic linkage data, which strongly suggests that the ILPR encodes genetic susceptibility to IDDM, and the recent data showing that the ILPR does in fact possess transcriptional activity, there has been no experimental evidence to tie these two observations together.

The finding that polymorphisms in the *INS* promoter that affect transcription are also linked to IDDM demonstrates the importance of investigating the role of *INS* regulation and β-cell–specific gene expression in diabetes. The regulators of these processes (e.g., the transcription factor genes such as *Pur-1, IPF1,* and *lmx-1*) should be considered candidates for genetic studies of diabetes.

Acknowledgments

The work from our laboratory was supported by grant R01 DK-21344 (W.J. Rutter) from the National Institutes of Health, a Juvenile Diabetes Foundation fellowship (G.K.), and a Juvenile Diabetes Foundation career development award (M.G.).

References

1. Owerbach D, Bell GI, Rutter WJ, Shows TB. The insulin gene is located on chromosome 11 in humans. Nature 1980;286:82
2. Gittes G, Rutter WJ. Onset of cell-specific gene expression in the developing mouse pancreas. Proc Natl Acad Sci USA 1992;89:1128
3. Moore HPH, Walker MD, Lee F, Kelly RB. Expressing a human proinsulin cDNA in a mouse ACTH-secreting cell: Intracellular storage, proteolytic processing and secretion of stimulation. Cell 1983;35:531
4. Laimins L, Holmgren-Konig M, Khoury G. Transcriptional "silencer" element in rat repetitive sequences associated with the rat insulin 1 gene locus. Proc Natl Acad Sci USA 1986;83:3151
5. Fromont-Racine M, Bucchini D, Madsen O, et al. Effect of 5′-flanking sequence deletions on expression of the human insulin gene in transgenic mice. Mol Endocrinol 1990;4:669
6. Walker MD, Edlund T, Boulet AM, Rutter WJ. Cell-specific expression controlled by the 5′ flanking regions of the insulin and chymotrypsin genes. Nature 1983a;306:557
7. Edlund T, Walker MD, Barr PJ, Rutter WJ. Cell-specific expression of the rat insulin gene: Evidence for the role of two distinct 5′ flanking sequences. Science 1985;230:912
8. Nir U, Walker MD, Rutter WJ. Regulation of rat insulin 1 gene expression: Evidence for negative regulation in nonpancreatic cells. Proc Natl Acad Sci USA 1986;83:3180
9. Takeda J, Ishii S, Seino Y, et al. Negative regulation of human insulin gene expression by the 5′-flanking region in non-pancreatic cells. FEBS Lett 1989;247:41
10. Whelan J, Poon D, Weil PA, Stein R. Pancreatic β-cell-type-specific expression of the rat insulin II gene is controlled by positive and negative cellular transcription elements. Mol Cell Biol 1989;9:3253
11. Cordle SR, Whelan J, Henderson E, et al. Insulin gene expression in nonexpressing cells appears to be regulated by multiple distinct negative-acting control elements. Mol Cell Biol 1991b;11:2881
12. Hanahan D. Heritable formation of pancreatic β-cell tumors in transgenic mice expressing recombinant insulin/simian virus 40 oncogenes. Nature 1985;315:115
13. Clark AR, Petersen HV, Read ML, et al. Human insulin gene enhancer-binding proteins in pancreatic α and β cell lines. FEBS Lett 1993a;329:139
14. Robinson GLWG, Peshavaria M, Henderson E, et al. Expression of the trans-active factors that simulate insulin control element-mediated activity appear to precede insulin gene transcription. J Biol Chem 1994;269:2452
15. German M. Insulin gene structure and regulation. In Draznin B, LeRoith D, eds. Molecular Biology of Diabetes. Totowa, NJ: Humana Press; 1994:91–117
16. Karlsson O, Edlund T, Moss JB, et al. A mutational analysis of the insulin gene transcription control region: Expression in β-cells is dependent on two related sequences within the enhancer. Proc Natl Acad Sci USA 1987;84:8819
17. Steiner DF, Chan SJ, Welsh JM, Kwok SCM. Structure and evolution of the insulin gene. Ann Rev Genet 1985;19:463
18. Crowe DT, Tsai M-J. Mutagenesis of the rat insulin II 5′-flanking region defines sequences important for expression in HIT cells. Mol Cell Biol 1989;9:1784
19. Boam D, Clark A, Docherty K. Positive and negative regulation of the insulin gene by multiple *trans*-acting factors. J Biol Chem 1990;265:8285
20. Ephrussi A, Church G, Tonegawa S, Gilbert W. B lineage-specific interactions of an immunoglobulin enhancer with cellular factors in vivo. Science 1985;227:134
21. Aronheim A, Ohlsson H, Park CW, et al. Distribution and characterization of helix-loop-helix enhancer-binding proteins from pancreatic β-cells and lymphocytes. Nucleic Acids Res 1991;19:3893
22. Moss LG, Moss JB, Rutter WJ. Systematic binding analysis of the insulin gene transcription control region: Insulin and immunoglobulin enhancers utilize similar transactivators. Mol Cell Biol 1988;8:2620
23. Ohlsson H, Karlson O, Edlund T. A β-cell-specific protein binds to the two major regulatory sequences of the insulin enhancer. Proc Natl Acad Sci 1988;85:4228
24. Sheih S, Tsai M. Cell-specific and ubiquitous factors are responsible for the enhancer activity of the rat insulin II gene. J Biol Chem 1991;266:16708
25. Read ML, Clark AR, Docherty K. The helix-loop-helix transcription factor USF (upstream stimulating factor) binds to a regulatory sequence of the human insulin gene enhancer. Biochem J 1993;295:233
26. Ohlsson H, Thor S, Edlund T. Novel insulin promoter- and enhancer-binding proteins that discriminate between pancreatic α- and β-cells. Mol Endocrinol 1991b;5:897
27. German MS, Blanar MA, Nelson C, et al. Two related helix-loop-helix proteins participate in separate cell-specific complexes that bind to the insulin enhancer. Mol Endocrinol 1991;5:292
28. Cordle SR, Henderson E, Masuoka H, et al. Pancreatic β-cell-type–specific transcription of the insulin gene is mediated by basic helix-loop-helix DNA-binding proteins. Mol Cell Biol 1991;11:1734
29. Peyton M, Moss LG, Tsai M-J. Two distinct class A helix-loop-helix transcription factors, E2A and BETA1, form separate DNA binding complexes on the insulin gene E box. J Biol Chem 1994;269:25936

30. Murre C, McCaw PS, Baltimore D. A new DNA binding and dimerization motif in immunoglobulin enhancer binding, daughterless, MyoD, and *myc* proteins. Cell 1989;56:777
31. Walker MD, Park CW, Rosen A, Aronheim A. A cDNA from a mouse pancreatic β-cell encoding a putative transcription factor of the insulin gene. Nucleic Acids Res 1990;18:1159
32. Sun XH, Baltimore D. An inhibitory domain of E12 transcription factor prevents DNA binding in E12 homodimers but not in E12 heterodimers. Cell 1991;64:459
33. Robinson GLWG, Cordle SR, Henderson E, et al. Isolation and characterization of a novel transcription factor that binds to and activates insulin control element-mediated expression. Mol Cell Biol 1994;14:6704
34. Park CW, Walker MD. Subunit structure of cell-specific E box-binding proteins analyzed by quantitation of electrophoretic mobility shift. J Biol Chem 1992;267:15642
35. Petersen HV, Serup P, Leonard J, et al. Transcriptional regulation of the human insulin gene is dependent on the homeodomain protein STF1/IPF1 acting through the CT boxes. Prox Natl Acad Sci USA 1994;91:10465
36. German M, Wang J. The insulin gene contains multiple transcriptional elements that respond to glucose. Mol Cell Biol 1994;14:4067
37. German MS, Moss LG, Wang J, Rutter WJ. The insulin and islet amyloid polypeptide genes contain similar cell-specific promoter elements that bind identical β-cell nuclear complexes. Mol Cell Biol 1992;12:1777
38. Shelton KD, Franklin AJ, Khoor A, et al. Multiple elements in the upstream glucokinase promoter contribute to transcription in insulinoma cells. Mol Cell Biol 1992;12:4578
39. Philippe J, Drucker DJ, Knepel W, et al. Alpha-cell–specific expression of the glucagon gene is conferred to the glucagon promoter element by the interactions of DNA-binding proteins. Mol Cell Biol 1988;8:4877
40. Leonard J, Serup P, Gonzalez G, et al. The LIM family transcription factor Isl-1 requires cAMP response element binding protein to promote somatostatin expression in pancreatic islet cells. Proc Natl Acad Sci USA 1992;89:6247
41. Vallejo M, Miller C, Habener JF. Somatostatin gene transcription regulated by a bipartite pancreatic islet D-cell specific enhancer coupled synergistically to a cAMP response element. J Biol Chem 1992;267:12868
42. Boam DSW, Docherty K. A tissue-specific nuclear factor binds to multiple sites in the human insulin-gene enhancer. Biochem J 1989;264:233
43. Scott V, Clark AR, Hutton JC, Docherty K. Two proteins act as the IUF1 insulin gene enhancer binding factor. FEBS Lett 1991;290:27
44. Karlsson O, Thor S, Norberg T, et al. Insulin gene enhancer binding protein isl-1 is a member of a novel class of proteins containing both a homeo- and a cys-his domain. Nature 1990;344:879
45. German MS, Wang J, Chadwick RB, Rutter WJ. Synergistic activation of the insulin gene by a LIM-homeodomain protein and a basic helix-loop-helix protein: Building a functional insulin minienhancer complex. Genes Dev 1992b;6:2165
46. Rudnick A, Ling T, Odagiri H, et al. β-Cells express numerous unique homeodomain proteins. Endocrine Society 76th Annual Meeting 1994;741 (Abstract). Washington, D.C.
47. Emens LA, Landers DW, Moss LG. Hepatocyte nuclear factor 1α is expressed in a hamster insulinoma line and transactivates the rat insulin I gene. Proc Natl Acad Sci USA 1992;89:7300
48. Ohlsson H, Karlsson K, Edlund T. IPF1, a homeodomain-containing transactivator of the insulin gene. EMBO J 1993;12:4251
49. Miller CP, McGehee RE, Habener JF. IDX-1: A new homeodomain transcription factor expressed in rat pancreatic islets and duodenum that transactivates the somatostatin gene. EMBO J 1994;13:1145
50. Leonard J, Peers B, Johnson T, et al. Characterization of somatostatin transactivating factor-1, a novel homeobox factor that stimulates somatostatin expression in pancreatic islet cells. Mol Endocrinol 1993;7:1275
51. Archer VEV, Breton J, Sanchez-Garcia I, et al. Cysteine-rich LIM domains of LIM-homeodomain and LIM-only proteins contain zinc but not iron. Proc Natl Acad Sci USA 1994;91:316
52. Schmeichel KL, Beckerle MC. The LIM domain is a modular protein-binding interface. Cell 1994;79:211
53. Valge-Archer VE, Osada H, Warren AJ, et al. The LIM protein RBTN2 and the basic helix-loop-helix protein TAL1 are present in a complex in erythroid cells. Proc Natl Acad Sci USA 1994;91:8617
54. Sanchez-Garcia I, Osada H, Forster A, Rabbitts TH. The cysteine-rich LIM domains inhibit DNA binding by the associated homeodomain in isl-1. EMBO J 1993;12:4243
55. Dong J, Asa SL, Drucker DJ. Islet cell and extrapancreatic expression of the LIM domain homeobox gene isl-1. Mol Endocrinol 1991;5:1633
56. Thor S, Ericson J, Brannstrom T, Edlund T. The homeodomain LIM protein isl-I is expressed in subsets of neurons and endocrine cells in the adult rat. Neuron 1991a;7:1
57. Barnes JD, Crosby JL, Jones CM, et al. Embryonic expression of Lim-1, the mouse homolog of Xenopus XLim-1, suggests a role in lateral mesoderm differentiation and neurogenesis. Dev Biol 1994;161:168
58. Peshavaria M, Gamer L, Henderson E, et al. XIHbox 8, an endoderm-specific Xenopus homeodomain protein, is closely related to a mammalian insulin gene transcription factor. Mol Endocrinol 1994;8:806
59. Jonsson J, Carlsson L, Edlund T, Edlund H. Insulin-promoter-factor 1 is required for pancreas development in mice. Nature 1994;371:606
60. Hwung Y, Gu Y, Tsai M. Cooperativity of sequence elements mediates tissue specificity of the rat insulin II gene. Mol Cell Biol 1990;10:1784
61. Sharma A, Stein R. Glucose-induced transcription of the insulin gene is mediated by factors required for beta-cell-type specific expression. Mol Cell Biol 1994;14:871
62. Kerrigan LA, Croston GE, Lira LM, Kadonaga JT. Sequence-specific transcriptional antirepression of the Drosophila Kruppel gene by the GAGA factor. J Biol Chem 1991;266:574
63. German M. Glucose sensing in pancreatic islet beta cells: The key role of glucokinase and the glycolytic intermediates. Proc Natl Acad Sci USA 1993;90:1781
64. Kennedy GC, Rutter WJ. Pur-1, a zinc-finger protein that binds to purine-rich sequences, transactivates an insulin promoter in heterologous cells. Proc Natl Acad Sci USA 1992;89:11498
65. Kennedy GC, Rutter WJ. Characterization of a cDNA encoding the insulin gene GAGA-binding factor, Pur-1. Biochem Soc Trans 1993;21:178
66. Kennedy GC, German MS, Rutter WJ. The minisatellite in the diabetes susceptibility locus IDDM2 regulates insulin transcription. Nat Genet 1995;9: 293–298
67. Docherty K. The regulation of insulin gene expression. Diabet Med 1992c; 9:792
68. Oetjen E, Diedrich T, Eggers A, et al. Distinct properties of the cAMP-responsive element of the rat insulin I gene. J Biol Chem 1994;269:27036
69. German MS, Moss LG, Rutter WJ. Regulation of insulin gene expression by glucose and calcium in transfected primary islet cultures. J Biol Chem 1990;265:22063
70. Philippe J, Missotten M. Functional characterization of a cAMP-responsive element of the rat insulin I gene. J Biol Chem 1990;265:1465
71. Ohlsson H, Edlund T. Sequence-specific interactions of nuclear factors with the insulin gene enhancer. Cell 1986;45:35.
72. Karlsson O, Walker MD, Rutter WJ, Edlund T. Individual protein-binding domains of the insulin gene enhancer positively activate β-cell-specific transcription. Mol Cell Biol 1989;9:823
73. Nielsen DA, Welsh M, Casadaban MJ, Steiner DF. Control of insulin gene expression in pancreatic β-cells and in an insulin-producing cell line, RIN-5F cells I. Effects of glucose and cyclic AMP on the transcription of insulin mRNA. J Biol Chem 1985;260:13585
74. Welsh M, Nielsen DA, MacKrell AJ, Steiner DF. Control of insulin gene expression in pancreatic β-cells and in an insulin-producing cell line, RIN-5F cells II. Regulation of insulin mRNA stability. J Biol Chem 1985;260:13590
75. Melloul D, Ben-Neriah Y, Cerasi E. Glucose modulates the binding of an islet-specific factor to a conserved sequence within the rat I and the human insulin promoters. Proc Natl Acad Sci USA 1993;90:3865
76. Bell GI, Pictet R, Rutter WJ. Analysis of the regions flanking the human insulin gene and sequence of an Alu family member. Nucleic Acids Res 1980;8:4091
77. Bell GI, Karam JH, Rutter WJ. Polymorphic DNA region adjacent to the 5′ end of the human insulin gene. Proc Natl Acad Sci USA 1981;78:5759
78. Bell GI, Selby M, Rutter WJ. The highly polymorphic region near the human insulin gene is composed of simple tandemly repeating sequences. Nature 1982;295:31
79. Owerbach D, Aagaard L. Analysis of a 1963-bp polymorphic region flanking the human insulin gene. Gene 1984;32:475
80. Rotwein P, Yokoyama S, Didier DK, Chirgwin JM. Genetic analysis of the hypervariable region flanking the human insulin gene. Am J Hum Genet 1986;39:291
81. Hammond-Kosack MCU, Dobrinski B, Lurz R, et al. The human insulin gene linked polymorphic region exhibits an altered DNA structure. Nucleic Acids Res 1992;20:231
82. Hammond-Kosack MCU, Kilpatrick MW, Docherty K. Analysis of DNA structure in the human insulin gene-linked polymorphic region *in vivo*. J Mol Endocrinol 1992;9:221
83. Hammond-Kosack MCU, Kilpatrick MW, Docherty K. The human insulin gene-linked polymorphic region adopts a G-quartet structure in chromatin assembled *in vitro*. J Mol Endocrinol 1993;10:121
84. Henderson E, Hardin CC, Walk SK, et al. Telomeric DNA oligonucleotides form novel intramolecular structures containing guanine-guanine base pairs. Cell 1987;51:899
85. Hammond-Kosack MCU, Docherty K. A consensus repeat sequence from the human insulin gene linked polymorphic region adopts multiple quadriplex DNA structures in vitro. FEBS Lett 1992;301:79
86. Bell GI, Horita S, Karam JH. A polymorphic locus near the human insulin gene is associated with insulin-dependent diabetes mellitus. Diabetes 1984;33:176
87. Hitman GA, Tarn AC, Winter RM, et al. Type 1 (insulin-dependent) diabetes and a highly variable locus close to the insulin gene on chromosome 11. Diabetologia 1985;28:218
88. Ferns GA. DNA polymorphic haplotypes on the short arm of chromosome 11 and the inheritance of type I diabetes mellitus. J Med Genet 1986;23:210
89. Cox NJ, Baker L, Spielman RS. Insulin gene-sharing in sib pairs with insulin-dependent mellitus: No evidence for linkage. Am J Hum Genet 1988;42:167
90. Cox NJ. Restriction fragment polymorphisms of the HLA-DR, HLA-DQ and insulin gene regions in IDDM: The GAW5 data. Genet Epidemiol 1989;6:21
91. Lucassen AM, Julier C, Beressi J-P, et al. Susceptibility to insulin dependent diabetes mellitus maps to a 4.1 kb segment of DNA spanning the insulin gene and associated VNTR. Nat Genet 1993;4:305
92. Julier C, Hyer RN, Davies J, et al. Insulin-IGF2 region on chromosome 11p encodes a gene implicated in HLA-DR4-dependent diabetes susceptibility. Nature 1991;354:155
93. Bain SC, Prins JB, Hearne CM, et al. Insulin gene region-encoded susceptibility to type I diabetes is not restricted to HLA-DR4-positive individuals. Nat Genet 1992;2:212
94. van der Auwera BJ, Heimberg H, Schrevens AF, et al. 5′ insulin gene polymorphism confers risk to IDDM independently of HLA class II susceptibility. Diabetes 1993;42:851

Diabetes Mellitus, edited by Derek LeRoith, Simeon I. Taylor, and Jerrold M. Olefsky. Lippincott–Raven Publishers, Philadelphia © 1996.

CHAPTER 4

Processing of the Insulin Molecule

CHRISTOPHER J. RHODES

The pancreatic β-cell's primary function is the production, storage, and regulated secretion of insulin. Under normal circumstances, the β-cell maintains a condition where there is always a readily available pool of insulin that can be rapidly secreted in response to a stimulus, such as a rise in blood glucose. Any increase in insulin release is compensated for by a corresponding increase in insulin biosynthesis, so that β-cell insulin stores are constantly maintained. Thus, a biosynthesis and processing of the insulin molecule along the β-cell's secretory pathway is a highly regulated and dynamic process.

The Insulin Molecule

Biologically active human insulin consists of two polypeptide chains,[1] the A-chain (21 amino acids) and B-chain (30 amino acids), joined by two interchain disulfide-linked bridges at A-Cys^7/B-Cys^7 and A-Cys^{20}/B-Cys^{19}. There is also an intrachain disulfide bridge between A-Cys^6/A-Cys^{11}. Insulin structure is highly conserved in higher vertebrate evolution,[2] showing several regions of invariability including (1) the position of cysteines that form the disulfide bridges, (2) the N- and C-terminal regions of the A-chain, and (3) hydrophobic residues at the C-terminus of the B-chain.[1,3] At an acidic pH in the presence of Zn^{++}, insulin forms a hexameric crystal unit, which consists of three insulin dimers arranged around an axis of two Zn^{++} atoms interacting with B-His^{10} of the insulin molecules.[1,4,5] Each insulin dimer is held together by hydrogen bonding between amino acids B^{24}-B^{26} of the two insulin B-chains, forming an antiparallel β-sheet structure.[1] Intramolecular insulin structure appears stable because the conformation of monomeric insulin is similar to that of its associated forms in solution.[6]

Insulin is initially synthesized, however, as the precursor molecule prepoinsulin,[7,8] which is composed of a 24-amino-acid N-terminal hydrophobic signal peptide, followed by the insulin B-chain, an Arg-Arg sequence, 31 amino acids of the connecting peptide (C-peptide or proregion), a Lys-Arg sequence, and then the insulin A-chain (Fig. 4-1). The signal peptide of preproinsulin is structurally typical of a newly synthesized protein that is to enter the secretory pathway of eukaryotic cells.[3,9] The signal peptide facilitates translocation of preproinsulin from the cytoplasm (where biosynthesis is initiated) across the rough endoplasmic reticulum (RER) membrane[10] (see below). Removal of the preproinsulin signal peptide occurs cotranslationally as the newly synthesized peptide is translocated into the lumen of the RER, thus generating the proinsulin precursor molecule. The C-peptide moiety of proinsulin is thought to aid correct structural alignment and disulfide linkage of the insulin A- and B-chains.[11,12] Proinsulin is able to form dimers, which in the presence of Zn^{++} hexamers are similar to that of insulin,[13,14] but has <5% of insulin's biologic activity.[1,15] The C-peptide region of proinsulin varies in length between higher vertebrates from 26 (bovine) to 38 (goose fish) amino acid residues, and it has considerably more sequence variation compared to the A- and B-chain regions.[16] C-peptide itself encodes little secondary structure, so that the three-dimensional structure of proinsulin

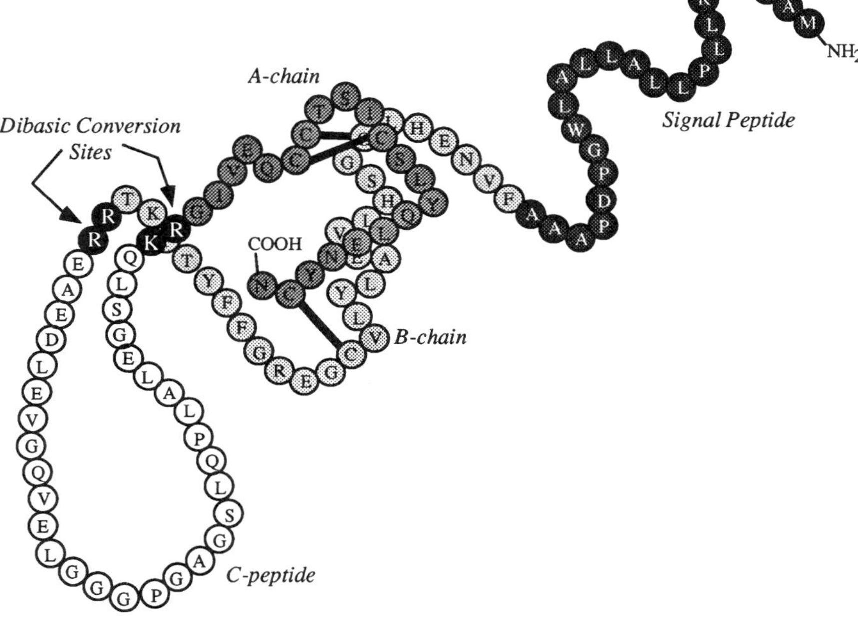

FIGURE 4-1. The human preproinsulin molecule. The signal peptide, B-chain, C-peptide, and A-chain domains of preproinsulin are indicated, as are the two dibasic conversion sites.

closely resembles that of insulin.[17,18] The flexibility of C-peptide, however, indicates that it may interact with the surface of the insulin A- and B-chains, perhaps accounting for reduced biologic activity of proinsulin. The two dibasic sites on proinsulin that border the C-peptide region (which are essential for the proteolytic conversion of proinsulin to insulin[1,3,19] [see below]) are very close to each other on the outer surface of the molecule.[17] A degree of stable structure has been indicted at the C-peptide–A-chain junction (named the "CA-knuckle"), which in intact proinsulin may be a determinant affecting accessibility of the endopeptidase that specifically cleaves at this site[17,19,20] (see below).

Insulin Biosynthesis

Translation and Translocation

The final product of insulin gene transcription is preproinsulin mRNA, which is transported from the nucleus into the β-cell cytosol (as described in Chapter 6). A simplified outline of the individual steps in the translation of preproinsulin mRNA is illustrated in Figure 4-2. Preproinsulin mRNA translation is initiated by promoting the binding of free 40S and 60S ribosomal subunits, and methionyl-tRNA to the AUG start codon, to form an 80S translation initiation complex in the β-cell cytosol. The assembly of such a translation initiation complex in β-cells would be tightly controlled by a family of proteins known as eukaryotic initiation factors (eIFs).[21–23] Translation of preproinsulin mRNA to preproinsulin protein then proceeds in an elongation phase. Translational elongation involves a repetitive cycle of codon-directed addition of specific aminoacyl-tRNAs to the ribosomal-preproinsulin mRNA translation complex that is catalyzed by proteins known as eukaryotic elongation factors (eEFs).[21,23] The codon sequence on preproinsulin mRNA dictates the order of aminoacyl-tRNA addition; then peptide bonds are formed between the amino acids brought in a series to the translation complex, so that the correct amino acid sequence of newly synthesized preproinsulin begins to emerge. More than one ribosomal complex can bind to a single preproinsulin mRNA at a time to form polysomes, in which a series of ribosomes follow each other along the mRNA template to synthesize many preproinsulin copies from a single mRNA.

As elongation proceeds, the ribosomal-preproinsulin mRNA translation complex is transported to the RER and newly synthesized preproinsulin translocated across the RER membrane into the RER lumen (Fig. 4-3). This process is assisted by the action of certain protein factors outlined in Figure 4-3. The appearing nascent signal peptide sequence is likely chaperoned early on (fewer than 30 amino acids) by a nascent-polypeptide–associated protein complex.[24] This complex sits over a channel in the larger ribosomal subunit and is thought to prevent the nascent signal peptide sequence from inappropriate folding, or improper interaction with other chaperon proteins.[24] As the peptide sequence extends (i.e., to >50 amino acids), there is interaction of preproinsulin signal peptide with the 54-kD subunit of the signal recognition particle (SRP), an 11S ribonucleoprotein complex.[25–27] Transfer of newly synthesized preproinsulin from the cytosol to the RER membrane occurs cotranslationally, and it is mediated by SRP.[25,26,28] Association of the SRP/newly forming signal peptide/preproinsulin mRNA ribosomal complex with the RER membrane is facilitated via an interaction of the SRP with an integral RER membrane SRP-receptor or docking protein,[29] which occurs when 70–80 amino acids of preproinsulin have been polymerized.[25] In addition, attachment of the ribosome to the RER membrane is facilitated by another RER integral membrane protein, the ribosomal receptor of 180 kD.[30] When SRP binds to the SRP receptor, SRP dissociates from both the signal peptide and the ribosome.[31] The 54-kD subunit of SRP is a guanine triphosphate (GTP)–binding protein with intrinsic GTPase activity, and when GTP is hydrolyzed, SRP is released from its receptor to the cytosol.[31] The preproinsulin signal peptide is then shifted to another RER integral membrane protein, the signal sequence receptor,[32] which has been proposed to be part of a protein translocation pore.[33] As newly synthesized preproinsulin is translocated into the intralumenal space of the RER, an RER membrane—associated signal peptidase removes the signal peptide to yield proinsulin.[34] Preproinsulin peptide chain elongation is completed at a stop codon (UAG for human preproinsulin[8]); then a GTP-binding protein releasing factor induces release of the newly synthesized peptide from the ribosomal complex concomitant with releasing factor GTP hydrolysis[21] and disassembly of the translational machinery. The efficient termination action of releasing factor allows the recycling of ribosomes for another round of translation.

Effectors of Proinsulin Biosynthesis

The rate of proinsulin biosynthesis is controlled by many factors, including nutrients, neurotransmitters, hormones, and protein kinase activities.[35,36] A list of some effectors of insulin biosynthesis reported in the literature is presented in Table 4-1, but glucose is the most physiologically relevant regulator of proinsulin biosynthesis. The metabolism of glucose is necessary to generate intracellular signals to stimulate proinsulin biosynthesis,[37] as indicated by inhibition of glucose-induced biosynthesis in the presence of mannoheptulose, which blocks metabolism by inhibiting glucokinase-induced phosphorylation of glucose to glucose-6-phosphate.[38–41] The threshold concentration of glucose required to stimulate insulin secretion is 4–6 mM; however, that required to stimulate proinsulin biosynthesis is only 2–4 mM.[40–43] A maximum rate of proinsulin biosynthesis is reached at a glucose concentration of 10–12 mM.[38,40,41] Increased proinsulin biosynthesis within an islet population of β-cells may be mediated by a glucose dose-dependent increased recruitment of β-cells into a higher proinsulin biosynthetic rate.[44,45] The response of the proinsulin biosynthetic machinery to a rise in glucose concentration is rapid,[40,41,46,47] and for short-term stimulation

FIGURE 4-2. Translation of preproinsulin mRNA. A simplistic outline of the individual steps for the initiation and early elongation phases of human preproinsulin mRNA are illustrated (for detailed view of eukaryotic protein translation refer to refs. 21–23. Essentially, the initiation phase involves binding of the 40S ribosomal subunits and initiator met-tRNA to the 5′-cap region of preproinsulin mRNA. The mRNA is then "scanned" in the 5′–3′ direction to the AUG start codon with which met-tRNA associates, and then the 60S ribosomal subunit is attached to form the 80S initiation complex. Formation of the preproinsulin mRNA 80S initiation complex is catalyzed by a large number of cytosolic protein initiation factors (eIFs) (refer to refs. 21–23). The elongation phase of translation involves continued codon scanning of the 80S ribosomal complex along the preproinsulin mRNA template (in a 5′–3′ direction). Aminoacyl tRNAs bring the appropriate amino acid as dictated by the codon order on the mRNA template. Peptide bond formation occurs between the evolving amino acid at the 80S ribosomal complex, and gradually a nascent preproinsulin peptide sequence emerges. The potential sites of glucose regulation on preproinsulin mRNA translation are indicated. ▶

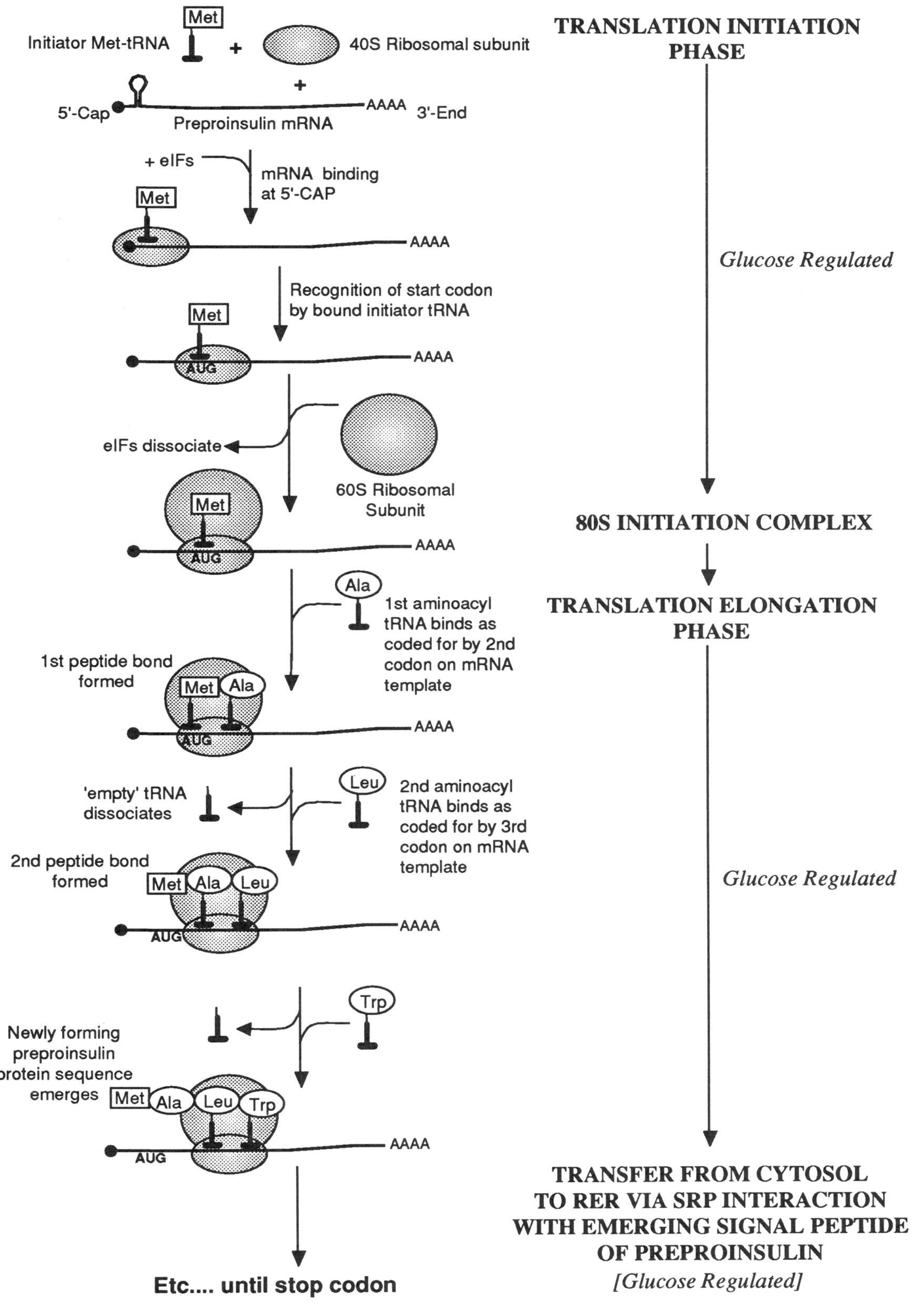

Met
Initiator Met-tRNA
+
40S Ribosomal subunit
+
5'-Cap
AAAA
3'-End
Preproinsulin mRNA
+ eIFs
mRNA binding at 5'-CAP
Met
AAAA
Recognition of start codon by bound initiator tRNA
Met
AUG
AAAA
eIFs dissociate
60S Ribosomal Subunit
Met
AUG
AAAA
Ala
1st aminoacyl tRNA binds as coded for by 2nd codon on mRNA template
1st peptide bond formed
Met
Ala
AUG
AAAA
'empty' tRNA dissociates
Leu
2nd aminoacyl tRNA binds as coded for by 3rd codon on mRNA template
2nd peptide bond formed
Met
Ala
Leu
AUG
AAAA
Trp
Newly forming preproinsulin protein sequence emerges
Met
Ala
Leu
Trp
AUG
AAAA
Etc.... until stop codon
TRANSLATION INITIATION PHASE
Glucose Regulated
80S INITIATION COMPLEX
TRANSLATION ELONGATION PHASE
Glucose Regulated
TRANSFER FROM CYTOSOL TO RER VIA SRP INTERACTION WITH EMERGING SIGNAL PEPTIDE OF PREPROINSULIN
[Glucose Regulated]

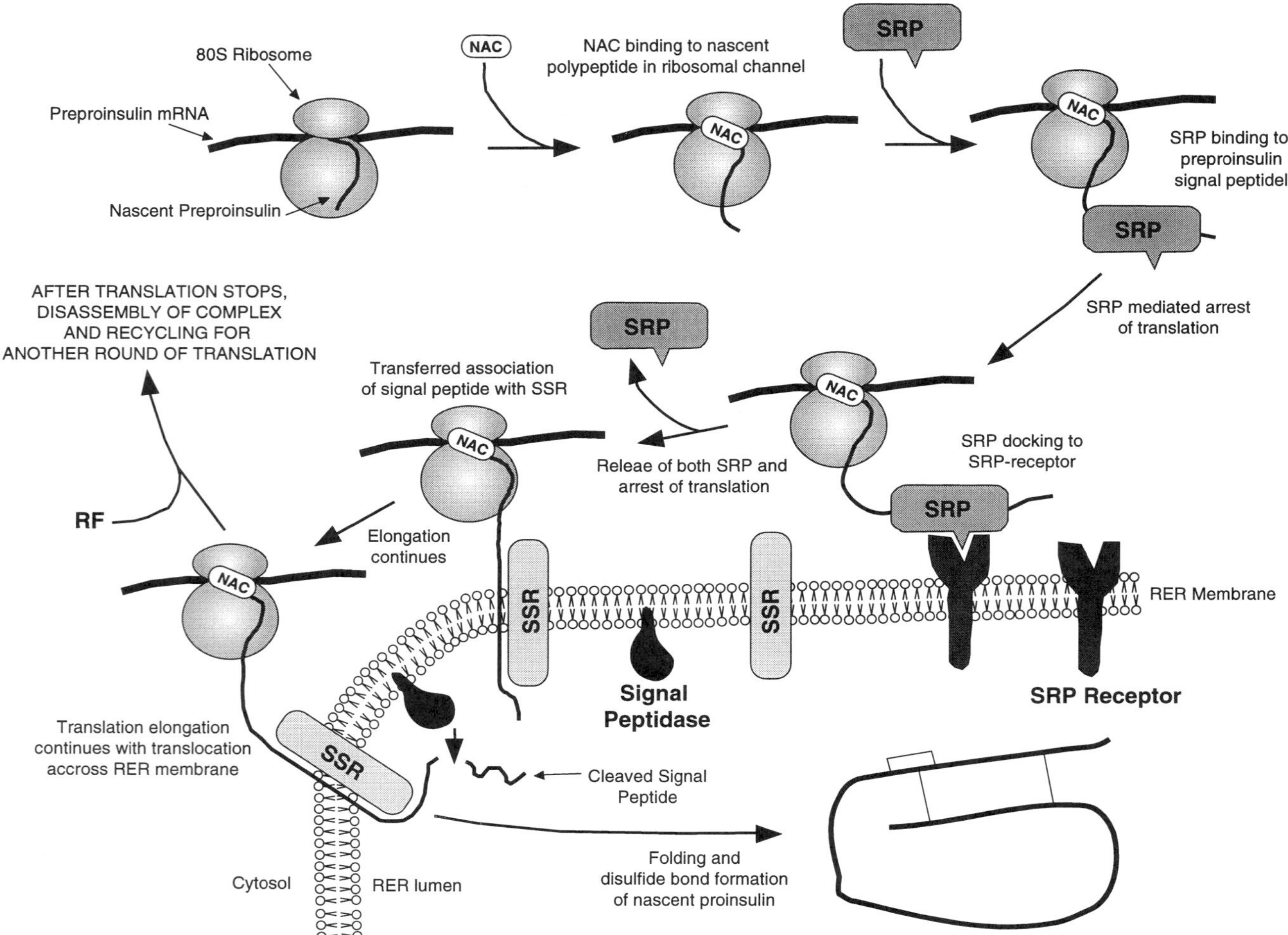

Figure 4-3. Translocation of preproinsulin across the endoplasmic reticulum. The translation of preproinsulin mRNA begins in the β-cell cytoplasm. The first few amino acids of the nascent signal peptide associate with a nascent-polypeptide–associated protein complex (NAC). With further peptide elongation, there is interaction with the signal recognition particle (SRP) which transiently halts translation. This allows the binding of the preproinsulin mRNA translation complex to the rough endoplasmic reticulum (RER) membrane via docking of SRP with the SRP-receptor. SRP is then released and the nascent signal peptide transferred to the signal sequence receptor (SSR) in the RER membrane. Translation then resumes, and the elongating preproinsulin peptide chain translocates across the membrane into the RER lumen. As this translocation occurs, the signal peptidase (associated with the lumenal side of the RER membrane) removes the signal peptide and proinsulin correctly forms in the RER lumen. Once the stop codon is reached, translation terminates and releasing factor (RF) dissociates the translation complex so that it can recycle for another round of protein synthesis.

(<2 hours) it appears to be entirely mediated at the translational level.[48,49] Significant glucose-induced proinsulin biosynthesis can be observed 20 minutes after introduction of a glucose stimulus, reaching a maximum rate (often as much as a 30–40-fold increase) by 60 minutes.[40,41,47] Once the stimulus is removed, the ''off-rate'' of proinsulin biosynthesis is relatively slow, taking more than 1 hour to return a basal rate.[47] For longer glucose stimulation periods (e.g., >4 hours, starvation, and non–insulin-dependent diabetes mellitus), there is an additional degree of transcriptional regulation[86,87,90–93] and an increase in mRNA stability[94] that would contribute to the control of proinsulin biosynthesis. Nevertheless, under normal physiologic circumstances, the fine control of proinsulin biosynthesis is predominantly mediated at the translational level.[36,40] Remarkably, the β-cell's translational response to glucose appears to be relatively specific for proinsulin biosynthesis[38] (as well as a small subset of other β-cell proteins[3]). For the vast majority of β-cell proteins, biosynthesis is unaffected by glucose at the translational level.

Stimulus-Coupling Mechanism for Proinsulin Biosynthesis

Unlike that for glucose-induced insulin secretion,[95,96] information concerning the signal transduction pathway for glucose-stimulated proinsulin biosynthesis is sadly lacking. Glucose metabolism is required,[37,38] but the secondary signals emitted from an increased rate of glycolytic flux that activate the proinsulin translational machinery are unknown. Nevertheless, several lines of experi-

TABLE 4-1. Effects of Various Agents on Proinsulin Biosynthesis

Effector	Stimulator (+) or Inhibitor (−)	Remarks	References
Nutrients			
Glucose	+	Primary physiologic stimulus	38, 42, 46, 50–52
Mannose	+	Similar to glucose stimulation	38, 50
Mannoheptulose	−	Inhibits glucose stimulation	38, 39
Fructose	No effect	May potentiate glucose stimulation	38, 42
Xylitol	No effect		37, 42
Ribose	+/−	Conflicting reports in literature	42, 53
Galactose	No effect		42, 50
N-acetylglucosamine	+		38, 54
Other sugars	No effect	Including sucrose, sorbitol, 2-deoxyglucose and 3-methylglucose	37
Leucine	+		55
α-Ketoisocaproate	+		55
Dihydroxyacetone	+		38
Glyceraldehyde	+	Concentration dependent	56
Inosine	+		38, 53
Guanosine	+		53
Adenosine	+		57
Ketone bodies	+		58
Fatty acids	−	Long-term fatty acid exposure	59
Arginine	−	Not a specific effect	60, 61
Hormonal			
Growth hormone	+		62, 63
Epinephrine	−	Inhibits glucose stimulation	64
Glucagon	+	Potentiates glucose stimulation	65
GLP-1(7-37)	+	In the presence of glucose	66
Somatostatin	No effect		67
IAPP	No effect		68, 69
Pancreastatin	No effect		70
Interferon	No effect	Inhibits at very high concentrations	71, 72
Interleukin-1	+/−	Concentration dependent	73–75
Pharmacologic			
Sulfonylureas	No effect	Some reports show slight inhibition	3, 52, 76
cAMP	+	Potentiates glucose stimulation	42, 43, 64, 65, 77, 78
Phorbol esters	+	Potentiates glucose stimulation	79
Physiologic			
Pregnancy	+		80, 81
Obesity	+	Gold-thioglucose–induced obesity	82
Starvation	−		80, 83
Aging	−		84
Hyperglycemic models			
NIDDM	−		85, 86
Glucose infusion	+		87–89

GLP-1 = glucagon-like peptide-1; IAPP = Islet amyloid polypeptide; NIDDM = non–insulin-dependent diabetes mellitus.

mental evidence suggest that the stimulus-coupling pathway for glucose-regulated insulin release is quite different from that of glucose-regulated biosynthesis:

1. The glucose threshold concentration required to stimulate proinsulin biosynthesis is lower than that required for insulin release.[42,43]
2. Regulated proinsulin biosynthesis does not require extracellular Ca^{++}, whereas it is an essential requirement for insulin release.[95,97]
3. Sulphonylureas are very effective at inducing insulin release, but they appear to have little effect on proinsulin biosynthesis.[3,52,76]
4. Somatostatin inhibits insulin release, but not proinsulin biosynthesis.[67]
5. Mg^{++} appears to be a requirement of proinsulin biosynthesis, but not necessarily insulin release.[78]
6. Diazoxide inhibits insulin release,[96] but not proinsulin biosynthesis.[78]
7. Inhibitors of Ca^{++} calmodulin (CaM) kinase activity (e.g., trifluoperazine) inhibit insulin release,[98,99] but they have no effect on proinsulin biosynthesis.[100]

Analogous to general protein synthesis translation, proinsulin biosynthesis has a dependence for GTP, which likely resides in the GTP requirement of the action of the 54 kD subunit of SRP,[101] or eIF2.[21–23] Finally, there is some limited evidence that the activities of both protein kinase A and C might be involved in modulating glucose-induced proinsulin biosynthesis,[42,43,64,65,77–79] but the molecular mechanism behind this has yet to be defined.

Translational Regulation of Proinsulin Biosynthesis

Inhibition of insulin gene transcription with actinomycin-D does not affect short-term glucose-stimulated proinsulin biosynthesis.[40,41,102] Furthermore, short-term glucose stimulation of pancreatic islets does not alter the total amount of preproinsulin mRNA in a β-cell,[48,49,103] even though proinsulin biosynthesis is raised more than 10–20 fold.[38] Thus, the rapid response to glucose of stimulated proinsulin biosynthesis uses translational regulation of preexisting preproinsulin mRNA.[1,3] Translational control of proinsulin biosynthesis has been implicated at the level of initiation, SRP–SRP-receptor interaction, and elongation. Although total preproinsulin mRNA does not change, there is a redistribution of it in the β-cell when proinsulin biosynthesis is induced.[48,49,104] Upon glucose stimulation, there is a transfer of preproinsulin mRNA from a cytosolic pool to polysomes associated with the RER.[48,49] This suggests that glucose increases the initiation rate of translation as well as the transfer of initiated preproinsulin mRNA free in the cytosol to membrane-bound polysomes (i.e., the major site of preproinsulin mRNA translation). The initiation phase of translation is usually the rate-limiting step in protein synthesis, and thus is implicated as the major point of control in the mechanism.[22,23] Cell-free translation of preproinsulin mRNA has demonstrated a significant degree of translational control at the level of initiation[105,106] and may be mediated, in part, by the phosphorylation state of eIFs.[22,107] Glucose does not, however, affect the phosphorylation state of eIF2α, eIF3 p120, or eIF4e in isolated rat islets.[108] Nevertheless, it is possible that glucose could instigate a change in the phosphorylation state of other eIFs in the β-cell or the binding of certain protein factors to untranslated regions of preproinsulin mRNA,[108,109] but this remains to be demonstrated.

Glucose also induces an increased rate of SRP-mediated transfer of the SRP/newly forming signal peptide/preproinsulin mRNA/80S ribosomal complex from the cytoplasm to the RER. In vitro translation in islet homogenates has suggested that a contribution to translation control of preproinsulin biosynthesis may be mediated by an increased rate of SRP–SRP-receptor interaction.[49] The mechanism of leucine-stimulated proinsulin biosynthesis[55] is similar to that of glucose preproinsulin mRNA translation.[104] cAMP does not, however, affect SRP–SRP-receptor interaction, but only translation initiation.[104] This raises the possibility that protein kinase A phosphorylates an eIF or related protein factor involved in specific translation of preproinsulin mRNA.

Translational control of proinsulin biosynthesis also has been observed at the elongation phase[49]; however, this effect can only be observed at glucose concentrations <5 mM.[49] No effect on the translational elongation rate of preproinsulin biosynthesis has been observed in the more physiologic glucose concentration range above 5 mM.[106] It has been shown that CaM kinase III is able to phosphorylate elongation factor 2 (EF2) in pancreatic islets,[110] but it is unclear whether this could modulate the rate of preproinsulin mRNA translation, especially when generic inhibitors of CaM kinase activity do not affect glucose-regulated proinsulin biosynthesis.[100] Nevertheless, further investigations of effects on elongation at glucose concentrations <5 mM could provide some insight into the general control of the translational machinery in pancreatic β-cells.

As with all eukaryotic cells, several thousand proteins are likely to be synthesized at any given moment in the β-cell;[21–23] however, glucose stimulates the biosynthesis of only an exclusive subset of β-cell proteins (approximately 50 proteins plus some isoforms of these in all[111]). Thus, translational regulation of proinsulin biosynthesis is a relatively specific mechanism.[38,102] Regulatory effects at the levels of initiation, SRP–SRP-receptor interaction (for β-cell secretory pathway proteins), and elongation in translation may affect general β-cell protein biosynthesis. It is more likely therefore that the specific nature of translational control of proinsulin biosynthesis resides in the 5′-untranslated regions (UTRs) or 3′-UTRs, or both, of glucose-regulated mRNAs. It is possible that the UTRs of glucose-regulated mRNAs contain common structural elements that allow preferential recognition of the β-cell translational machinery under glucose stimulation. Translational regulation directed toward secondary structures in 5′-UTRs has been proposed to adjust accessibility of the translation initiation machinery to the 5′ cap of mRNAs.[22] For preproinsulin mRNAs, a predicted "stem-loop" mRNA secondary structure in the 5′-UTR is conserved across species and has been proposed to be involved in the translational control mechanism.[108,109] A similar stem-loop structure in ferritin mRNA has been shown to be key to the specific translational regulation of ferritin biosynthesis by iron.[112] In future studies, it will be key to (1) identify β-cell cytosolic proteins that specifically bind to the 5′-UTRs of glucose-regulated mRNAs as either repressors or activators of translation[107] and (2) to demonstrate that these are involved in translational control.

Translational Regulation of Other β-Cell Protein Biosynthesis

Proinsulin in only one of a small subset of β-cell proteins (50–100 in all[3,111]) whose biosynthesis is regulated by glucose at the translational level. Other glucose-regulated proteins include a common secretory granule matrix protein, chromogranin A (CgA)[40]; a secretory granule membrane glycoprotein, SGM-110[113]; and the proinsulin processing endopeptidase, PC3.[41] The glucose regulation of these β-cell proteins' biosynthesis does not appear to be uncoupled from that of proinsulin.[40,41,113] Thus, the translational control mechanism for CgA, SGM-110, and PC3 biosynthesis is likely common to that of proinsulin. Two-dimensional electrophoresis analysis of isolated islets has revealed that the majority of glucose-regulated proteins are constituents of insulin secretory granules (also named β-granules)[111]; however, not all secretory granule proteins have their biosynthesis regulated. Glucose does not appear to regulate the biosynthesis of the other proinsulin conversion enzymes, PC2,[41] or carboxypeptidase-H (CP-H)[40] in normal rat isolated islets. Both PC2 and CP-H are cotranslationally inserted into the RER lumen along with newly synthesized preproinsulin, CgA, SGM-110, and PC3.[40,41,113] This suggests that alleviation of SRP-mediated arrest may be an adaptive mechanism in translational control rather than a specific one, in order to cater to increased protein translation of newly synthesized secretory pathway proteins.[3,49] Furthermore, the biosynthesis of a small number of β-cell cytosolic proteins (which are synthesized on free polysomes in the cytosol as opposed to RER polysomes) also appear to be translationally regulated by glucose,[111] thus implying translational control at the level of initiation rather than SRP–SRP-receptor interactions.[3]

Proinsulin Folding in the Endoplasmic Reticulum

Translocation of a newly synthesized proinsulin into the RER lumen marks its entrance into the β-cell's secretory pathway.[114–116] The compartments of the β-cell secretory pathway are outlined in Figure 4-4. Here, proinsulin undergoes a folding process so that the disulfide linkage between the A- and B-chains of insulin are correctly aligned. This process is likely catalyzed by a disulfide isomerase enzyme activity[117,118] and a molecular chaperon BiP,[119] both of which are located in the RER of eukaryotic cells.[10,118,119] BiP (a member of the heat-shock protein family[120]) is thought to bind transiently to newly synthesized, incompletely folded proteins to prevent nonspecific aggregation.[10,119] BiP permanently binds to

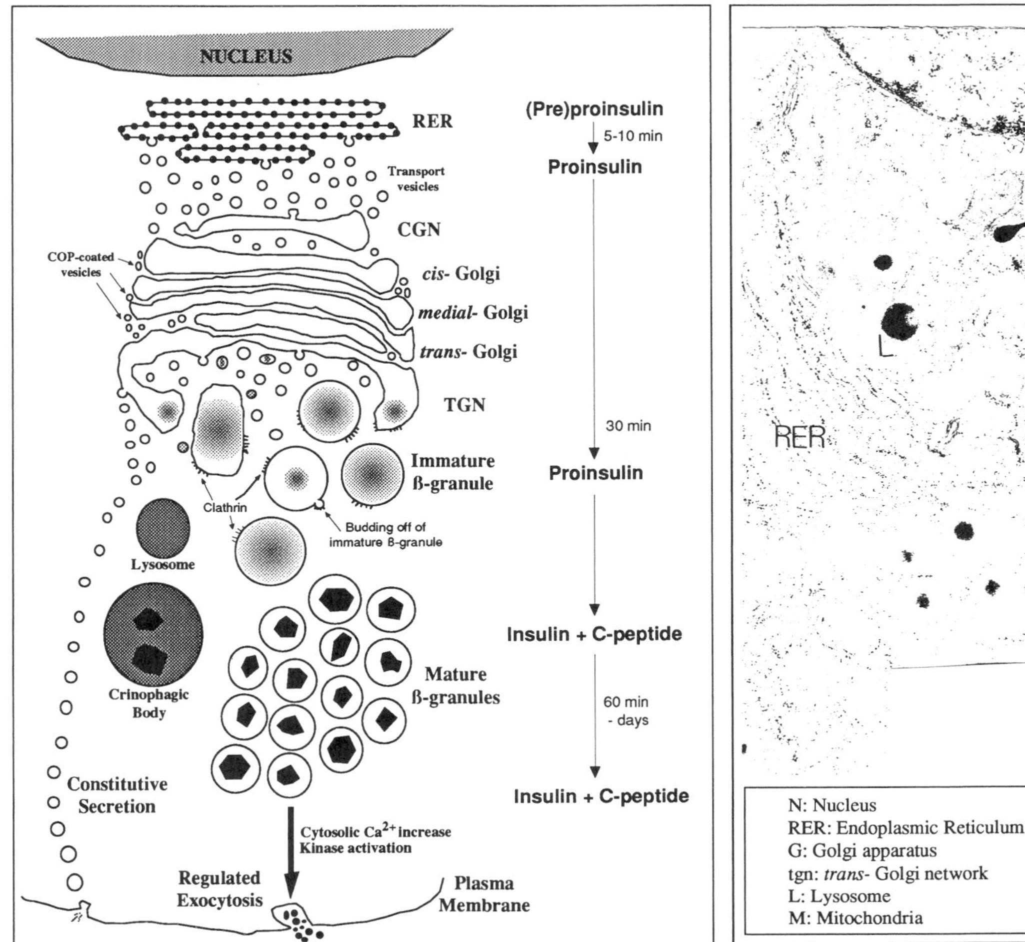

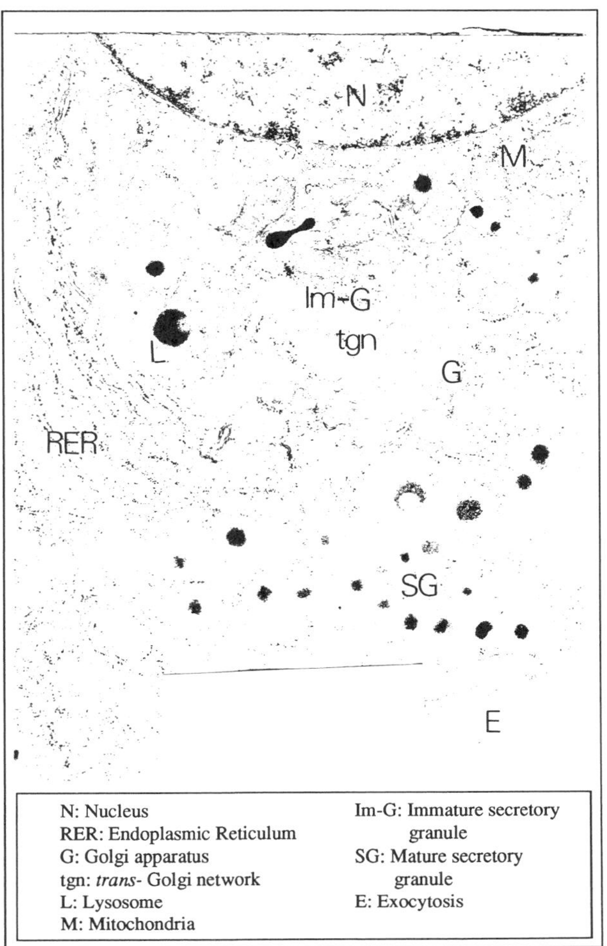

Figure 4-4. The β-cell's secretory pathway. The left panel shows a diagram of the β-cell secretory pathways. The right panel shows an electron micrograph (×24,200) of rat insulinoma tissue; key organelles of the secretory pathway are labeled. The timing of passage of newly synthesized proinsulin through the β-cell secretory pathway is also indicated (where time zero is the start of translation). Newly synthesized proinsulin in the rough endoplasmic reticulum (RER) is transferred to the *cis*-Golgi network (CGN), through the Golgi apparatus, to the *trans*-Golgi network (TGN) where immature β-granules form. The TGN is the sorting point of β-granule, lysosomal, and constitutively secreted proteins. A post-TGN editing mechanism (refer to refs. 174–176) is indicated as a budding off of the clathrin-coated region of an immature β-granule. Proinsulin is targeted to the β-granule compartment, where it undergoes proteolytic conversion to insulin and C-peptide. Mature β-granules are then held in an intracellular storage compartment awaiting a signal to stimulate transport to, and then fusion with, the plasma membrane for exocytosis.

incorrectly folded proteins, blocking their further progress along the secretory pathway and marking their rapid degradation within the RER.[119,120] The cleaved signal peptide of preproinsulin is also rapidly degraded in the RER.[34] The majority of proteins that enter into the secretory pathway at the RER are *N*-glycosylated,[121,122] but the primary structure of proinsulin does not contain an *N*-glycosylation consensus sequence (Asn-X-Ser or Asn-X-Thr, where X is any amino acid except proline[121,122]) and remains unglycosylated.

Correctly folded proinsulin, once past the RER's internal quality-control system,[123] can then be delivered to the *cis*-Golgi apparatus from the RER in transport vesicles in an ATP-dependent process.[124] The RER to *cis*-Golgi transport mechanism also requires the integrity of the β-cell's microfilament/microtubular network,[125] cytosolic Ca^{++},[126] GTP hydrolysis,[126,127] possible protein phosphorylation,[128] and certain cytosolic protein factors including *N*-ethylmaleimide-sensitive fusion protein NSF,[129] ADP-ribosylation factor (ARF),[130] heterotrimeric G-proteins,[127] and the Ras-related GTP-binding proteins, Rab1 and Rab2.[126,131,132] Generally, export from the RER is facilitated via a bulk flow mechanism.[115] When a protein's export from the RER is slower than the rate of bulk flow, however, it is thought to reflect a longer time period required for folding of that protein, hence a delay on leaving the RER.[133] An example of such retardation in the β-cell is the proinsulin-processing endopeptidase PC2, whose passage along the secretory pathway is slower than that of proinsulin.[134,135] It has been proposed recently that PC2 folding is assisted by a novel chaperon, 7B2, that may account for its slow exit from the RER.[136,137]

Resident RER proteins are sorted away from other newly synthesized secretory pathway proteins in that they possess a C-terminal sequence Lys-Asp-Glu-Leu (KDEL) that signals their RER retention.[119] Putative KDEL receptors have been proposed[138–140] that appear to be located in a ''salvage'' compartment or *cis*-Golgi network.[115] It appears that RER-resident proteins are retrieved in this network and then returned to the RER.[115] Proinsulin does not contain a KDEL signal, so it proceeds along the β-cell secretory pathway onto the *cis*-Golgi apparatus.

Vesicular Transport Through the Golgi Apparatus

The Golgi apparatus is the major intracellular site for post-translational modifications of secretory pathway proteins, including *N*-glycosylation modifications, *O*-glycosylation, glycosaminoglycan addition, mannose-6-phosphate addition for lysosomal proteins (this being a signal for sorting to lysosomes[141]), sulfation, and perhaps some lipid attachment.[141,142] None of these modifications, however, apply to the proinsulin molecule, which as no such post-translational additions. Trafficking of proinsulin from the stacks of *cis*- via the *medial*- to the *trans*-Golgi apparatus is mediated by vesicular transport.[115,122,141,143–145] Transport between Golgi stacks is mediated by coated (but not clathrin-coated) vesicles.[115] The coat consists of a protein complex of cytosolic coatmer proteins (α-, β-, ∂-, and γ-) in stoichiometric amounts, and ARF.[115] Before fusion of a transport vesicle with a Golgi-stack target membrane, the coat is lost in a GTP-[146,147] and possibly an ATP-dependent mechanism.[115] Intercisternal transport between Golgi stacks also requires cytosolic factors, including *N*-ethylmaleimide sensitive factor (NSF),[147] Rab6 and ARF GTP-binding proteins,[115,126,132,148] SNAPs (soluble NSF-attachment proteins),[149,150] and fatty acyl coenzyme-A.[151] Transport through the Golgi apparatus results in newly synthesized proinsulin accumulating in clathrin-coated regions of the *trans*-Golgi network (TGN),[152] which are the sites of secretory granule biogenesis.

Secretory Granule Biogenesis

In the TGN, proinsulin is targeted to the regulated secretory pathway.[153–155] This involves sorting of proinsulin, and other proteins designated for the secretory granule compartment, away from plasma-membrane proteins, secretory proteins destined to the constitutive pathway,[153–155] and proteins targeted to lysosomes.[156,157] The specific sorting of lysosomal proteins is relatively well defined. It is mediated by a mannose-6-phosphate modification to lysosomal protein glycosylation and their interaction via a mannose-6-phosphate receptor in the TGN membrane.[156,157] Delivery of secretory and plasma membrane proteins to the constitutive pathway is thought to be facilitated by a default bulk flow mechanism, where no specific sorting signal or mechanism is required.[153,154,158] Although an active area of cell biology research, the actual mechanism of protein sorting to the regulated secretory pathway has not yet been defined clearly. It is believed, however, to involve a positive dominant signal[159,160] and is likely to be either some sort of receptor-mediated process[161] or a mechanism of selective aggregation of secretory granule proteins[162,163] in limited regions of the TGN.[3,153,154,163] It has been postulated that secretory granule proteins possess some kind of sorting signal (analogous to the KDEL sequence for RER retention[119] or mannose-6-phosphate for lysosomal sorting[156]), but such a consensus sequence for specific sorting to the regulated secretory pathway in secretory granule proteins has not yet been identified. It has been indicated, however, that some degree of structural integrity of certain secretory granule proteins is required for efficient sorting to a secretory granule compartment, because disruption of disulfide-linked bonds in chromogranin B was found in one study to result in its mistargeting to the constitutive secretory pathway.[164] Some hormone-specific binding proteins have been found in the TGN that have been proposed to be ''receptors'' for sorting to the regulated secretory pathway,[161] but whether these proteins are in fact chaperon molecules that enhance the selective aggregation of proteins destined for the secretory granule has not been ruled out.[3,154] Presently, the *aggregation hypothesis* is favored (though certainly not proven),[154,163] which proposes that common physicochemical properties of secretory granule proteins make them prone for a possible Ca^{++}-dependent aggregation in the mildly acidic pH internal environment of the TGN.[135,154,162,165] Sorting by aggregation is likely to be a complex mechanism, however, considering that 50–100 β-granule proteins,[111,166] must be coordinately delivered to the site of secretory granule biogenesis. It is unlikely that the sorting of secretory granule proteins is simply a consequence of their being in the vicinity as proinsulin (the major secretory granule component) condenses in the TGN, especially considering that certain proteins clearly are efficiently sorted to the granule compartment in parallel to proinsulin.[87,166,167]

Examination of secretory granule biogenesis in ''cell-free'' model systems has identified acidic pH 6.5,[165] Ca^{++} concentration,[165] ATP,[162] and GTP-hydrolysis[168] as necessary components of this sorting mechanism.[3,154] Both small GTP-binding proteins[169] and heterotrimeric G-proteins[170] have been identified in secretory granule formation and budding off of the TGN. Secretory granule biogenesis occurs in limited clathrin-coated regions of the TGN,[152] but constitutive vesicle formation does not require clathrin.[3,171] Clathrin has been shown to be required for the mannose-6-phosphate receptor–mediated lysosomal pathway and selective endocytosis,[172] but its precise role in secretory granule formation remains unclear.[154] Experiments in clathrin-deficient yeast, however, have indicated that clathrin is not an essential component of vesicular traffic along the biosynthetic secretory pathway.[173] Rather, it may be involved in a scavenger receptor mechanism that retrieves TGN-membrane proteins and missorted lysosomal proteins after a newly formed immature secretory granule has budded off of the TGN.[163,173] In support of this *post-TGN editing/recycling hypothesis,* small clathrin-coated vesicles have been observed budding off of newly formed secretory granules in anterior pituitary cells[174] and pancreatic β-cells (see Fig. 4-4). Furthermore, it has been shown in pancreatic β-cells that retrieval of lysosomal enzymes away from condensed secretory granule contents occurs in a post-TGN immature secretory granule compartment.[135,175] This post-TGN editing mechanism most likely accounts for a minor degree of ''constitutive-like'' proinsulin secretion observed in normal isolated pancreatic islets.[154,176]

Whatever the mechanism, sorting of proinsulin to the regulated secretory pathway is a highly efficient process, with >99% of newly synthesized proinsulin being delivered to a secretory granule compartment.[177] Processing of proinsulin to insulin does not appear to be required for sorting to secretory granules because >99% of newly synthesized proinsulin released in normal pancreatic islets is secreted via the regulated secretory pathway.[177] Moreover, mutant proinsulins with the C-peptide domain either deleted, altered, or reduced were sorted correctly to secretory granules even though they were not efficiently processed to mature insulin.[16,178,179] In contrast, a single mutation in the insulin B-chain moiety of proinsulin, His^{10} to Asp^{10}, significantly disrupted both proinsulin processing and sorting to secretory granules.[180,181] The B10 His is involved in the formation of proinsulin and insulin hexamers in associated with Zn^{++}.[1] Thus, it is probable that sorting signal information is present in the secondary or tertiary structure of the proinsulin molecule in the presence of Zn^{++}, and further suggests aggregation of proinsulin molecules in the TGN as being important for targeting to a secretory granule compartment.

Once an immature partially clathrin-coated β-granule has budded off of the TGN, it undergoes a maturation process.[152] The immature secretory granule is the intracellular compartment where the vast majority of proinsulin-to-insulin conversion takes place (see below).[152,182–184] Maturation of secretory granules involves proinsulin conversion, progressive intragranular acidification, loss of the clathrin-coated regions, and formation of hexameric insulin crystals.[3,152,154] Acidification is mediated by a proton-pump ATPase present in β-granule membranes[185] that provides the correct intragranular pH (pH 5.0–5.5) for proinsulin processing to proceed,[152,182–184] and optimal insulin crystal formation around insulin's isoelectric point (pKi 5.3).[1,3] Clathrin can be removed from coated vesicles by a cytosolic ATP-dependent uncoating protein.[186] It is not known, however, whether this uncoating protein can remove the partial clathrin-coat from immature β-granules directly, or whether these coat regions are removed during the clathrin coated-vesicle budding from newly formed granules in a post-TGN editing/recycling mechanism (described above).[174–176]

Proinsulin Conversion

The major site for processing of the proinsulin precursor molecule to biologically active insulin is the immature granule compartment of the β-cell.[182,184,187] Proinsulin conversion proceeds in this compartment as part of the secretory granule maturation process previously discussed.

The Proinsulin Processing Enzymes

There are two dibasic sites on the human proinsulin molecule: Arg[31], Arg[32] and Lys[64], Arg[65] (see Fig. 4-1). These signal limited proteolytic processing of proinsulin to excise the C-peptide moiety and to generate insulin with its A- and B-chains correctly aligned.[1,3,19] This post-translational proteolytic maturation of a precursor molecule is common to many peptide hormones and neurotransmitters,[188–190] as well as some constitutively secreted plasma membrane and viral proteins.[154,191–193] Endoproteolytic peptide bond cleavage of proinsulin occurs on the carboxylic side of the Arg[31], Arg[32] or Lys[64], Arg[65], followed by rapid and specific exopeptidic removal of the newly exposed basic amino acids by carboxypeptidase-H (CP-H).[194,195] A scheme of proinsulin conversion is illustrated in Figure 4-5.

A secretory granule Ca^{++}-dependent proinsulin-processing endopeptidase activity with an acidic pH optimum[196] was first discovered about 20 years after that of proinsulin.[197,198] Later this activity was found by anion exchange chromatography actually to consist of two individual endopeptidases.[183] One (type I) cleaved specifically at the Arg[31], Arg[32] site of proinsulin, whereas the other (type II) had a strong preference for the Lys[64], Arg[65] site (see Fig. 4-5).[183] The substrate specificity of these endopeptidase activities was confirmed by the use of active-site–directed inhibitors,[20,199] and by examination of the in vitro processing of proinsulin[200] and proalbumin variants.[201] These two enzyme activities appeared to be related to the bacterial subtilisin-like prohormone processing endopeptidase in *Saccharomyces cerevisiae,* named the Kex2 protease.[191,202–204] The subsequent cloning of Kex2,[205] then provided a means whereby mammalian homologue proprotein endopeptidases could be cloned.[191–193] Among this novel family of mammalian proprotein-specific endopeptidases are two endopeptidases named PC2[206,207] and PC3[208] (also known as PC1[209]) that are specifically expressed in neuroendocrine cell-types.[154,210] It has now been established that PC2 and the type-II proinsulin-processing endopeptidase activity are indeed the same protein.[135,211] Furthermore, PC3 is biochemically[212] and immunologically[213] indistinguishable from the type I proinsulin-processing endopeptidase activity. Cotransfection studies of proinsulin with PC3 and PC2 have additionally reaffirmed these enzymes as the proinsulin processing endopeptidase equivalent to type I and type II activities, respectively.[214]

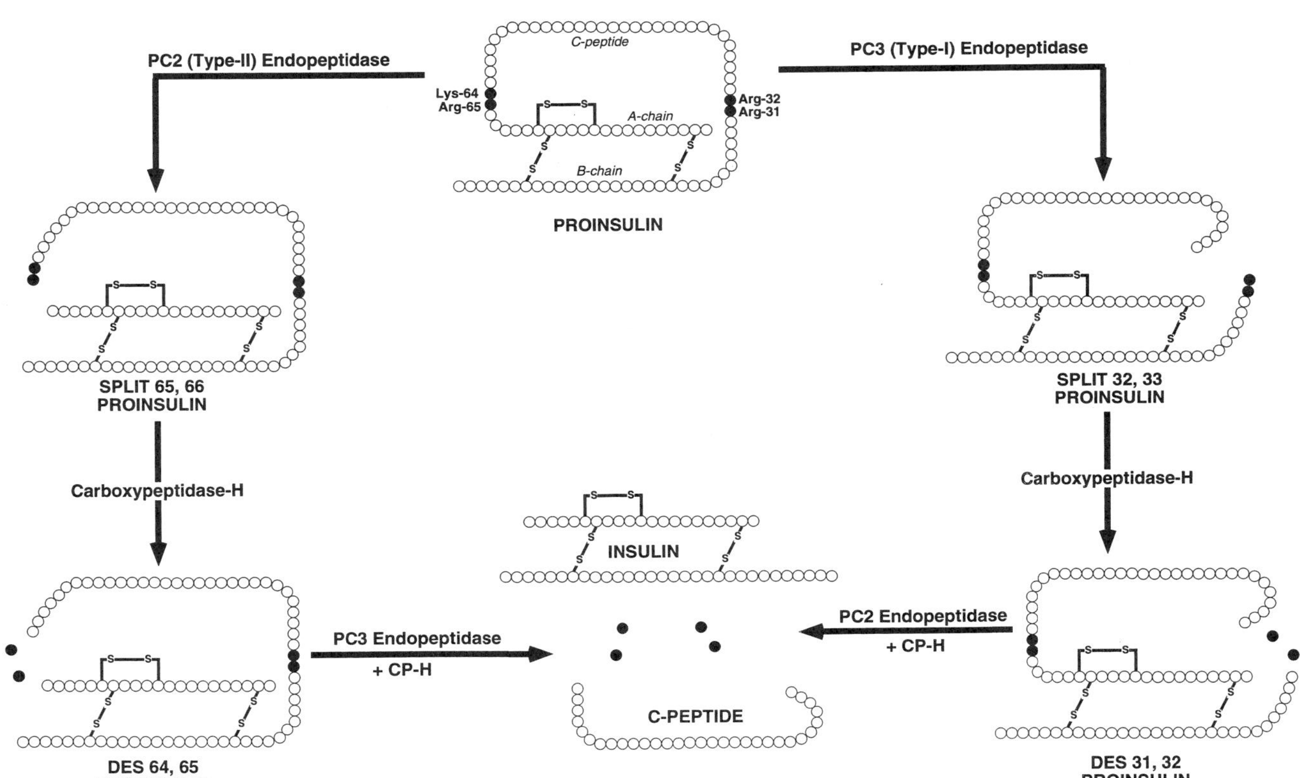

FIGURE 4-5. Proteolytic conversion of proinsulin to insulin and C-peptide.

Structural Requirements and Sequential Processing of Human Proinsulin

As well as the primary sequence of Arg^{31},Arg^{32} and Lys^{64},Arg^{65}, the PC2 and PC3 endopeptidase activities may also require an additional structural feature around these processing sites.[19,135] A basic amino acid at position −4 to the peptide bond cleaved (e.g., Lys^{29} on human proinsulin [see Fig. 4-1]) has been suggested to enhance cleavage at Arg^{31},Arg^{32} by PC3.[214–217] Predicted secondary structures of β-turns and Ω-loops have been implicated to play a role in endopeptidase recognition of a proprotein substrate.[218,219] Indeed for human proinsulin, β-turns before both Arg^{31},Arg^{32} and Lys^{64},Arg^{65} are predicted, as are Ω-loops after these processing sites.[135] Nuclear magnetic resonance (NMR) studies of proinsulin have revealed that the A- and B-chain conformation is similar to that of insulin,[12,17] and that the two dibasic processing sites are in close proximity to each other (4–8 Å) on the outside of the molecule. Thus, the processing sites on proinsulin are readily available for endopeptidase recognition even in a hexameric conformation.[1] In addition, because these two processing sites are neighboring each other, processing at one site might affect conformation at the other site.[17,20,200] A region of ordered structure around the C-peptide/A-chain junction (Lys^{64},Arg^{65}), named the CA-knuckle, has been postulated to influence substrate recognition by PC2.[17] It is thought that the CA-knuckle may represent a structural constraint that prevents PC2 from cleavage at Lys^{64},Arg^{65} in intact proinsulin.[19,20] However, this constraint is alleviated after cleavage at Arg^{31},Arg^{32} by PC3 to generate des 31,32 proinsulin, which is a much preferred substrate of PC2.[20,213] This, in part, has led to the idea that the processing of human proinsulin is sequential, where PC3 cleaves intact proinsulin at Arg^{31},Arg^{32} first to generate des 31,32 proinsulin (after CP-H trimming), which is then processed by PC2 at Lys^{64},Arg^{65} to generate the final products (after CP-H trimming): insulin, C-peptide, and free basic amino acids.[19] This sequential processing hypothesis predicts that because PC2 cleavage of intact proinsulin is very inefficient,[20,213] the product of PC2 cleavage of intact proinsulin (i.e., des 64,65 proinsulin intermediate) would be very low compared to the des 31,32 proinsulin intermediate. This has been supported in isolated human islets studies where des 31,32 proinsulin has been found to be much more abundant as a transient processing intermediate than des 64,65 proinsulin.[220] Furthermore, in the human circulation there are measurable levels of des 31,32 proinsulin, but negligible levels of des 64,65 proinsulin.[221,222] Thus, in humans, the sequential processing of proinsulin via des 31,32 proinsulin is the predominant route, where PC3 cleaves intact proinsulin first, followed by PC2 cleavage of des 31,32 proinsulin. Because PC3 initiates human proinsulin conversion, it is likely to be the key enzyme that regulates proinsulin processing,[19] and this hypothesis is supported in that PC3 is apparently more abundant than PC2 in pancreatic β-cells.[223] However, sequential processing may not be apparent for all mammalian proinsulins. Both rat proinsulin I and II possess an Arg^{62} at position −4 relative to Lys^{64},Arg^{65}, instead of Leu^{62} in human proinsulin.[216] The introduction of an Arg^{-4} renders processing at Lys^{64},Arg^{65} in intact rat proinsulins more efficient and perhaps makes this site available for processing by PC3.[214–217] Furthermore, in rat proinsulin II, the Lys^{-4} relative to the Arg^{31},Arg^{32} site is replaced by Met^{29}, rendering PC3 processing at this site inefficient.[215] Thus, subtle differences in the primary and secondary structure of proinsulins can reveal different processing patterns, although under normal circumstances the predominant final products ($<90\%$) remain insulin and C-peptide.

Regulation of Proinsulin Conversion

PC2 and PC3 are Ca^{++}-dependent enzyme activities with an acidic pH 5–5.5 optimum.[20,183,212,213] The β-granule contains an intraorganellar environment of 1–10 mM free Ca^{++}[224] and acidic pH 5.5,[185] which ideally suits the requirements for optimal endopeptidase and CP-H activities within this organelle.[183,195] This also ensures that insulin is produced mainly in the intracellular β-granule compartment in which it is stored.[19,183] To render PC2 and PC3 fully active for proinsulin processing in a newly formed β-granule, it follows that activation of the proton-pumping ATPase[184,185,225] and Ca^{++}-translocation proteins[226] are key regulatory events. It has been shown that Ca^{++} cannot be taken up or released from isolated β-granules,[227] but it is possible that Ca^{++} is introduced at a point earlier along the secretory pathway (i.e., before the immature β-granule), and sequestered into a newly forming β-granule as part of the proinsulin condensing process in the TGN.[160,162]

The relative abundance of PC2 and PC3 present in a cell can dictate the ''phenotypic processing pattern'' of a peptide prohormone.[228–231] In rat pancreatic islet β-cells, the cellular levels of PC3 are greater than those of PC2, whereas in the islet non–β-cells PC2 is more abundant.[223] It has been proposed that differences in PC2 and PC3 levels in β-cells among different species could contribute to the differing patterns of proinsulin processing observed.[216] Indeed, deficient processing of proinsulin at Arg^{31},Arg^{32} in a β-cell line (INS-1 cells) has been shown to correlate with a low expression of PC3.[232]

The mammalian Kex2-related family of proprotein-specific endopeptidases have homology to bacterial subtilisin and possess a conserved active site domain consisting of a catalytic triad (Asp, His, Ser) and an oxy-anion hole (Asn, except Asp in PC2).[135,192] Bacterial subtilisin has a proregion that enables the molecule to fold correctly, and once folded the proregion is autocatalytically cleaved.[233] Similarly, the related proteases Kex2 and furin also undergo autocatalytic cleavage activation.[234,235] PC2 and PC3 are initially synthesized as proproteins that are subsequently cleaved by limited proteolysis.[41,134] In pancreatic islets PC2 is initially synthesized as a 75-kD glycoprotein which is N-terminally cleaved via 71 and 68 kD intermediates to a mature 64–66-kD β-granule form.[41,134,236,237] A N-terminal proregion of PC3 is rapidly cleaved from a 92–94-kD glycoprotein precursor at an Arg-Lys-Lys-Arg[110] site,[207] and then later processed at its C-terminal region to a 66-kD mature β-granule form.[41,238] The early N-terminal processing PC2 and PC3 precursors is thought to occur in the RER[135,192] and the later C-terminal processing of PC3 in the TGN/immature granule compartment.[41,135] It has yet to demonstrated, however, whether proteolysis of PC2 and PC3 is an autocatalytic or activation process, or both.[135,192,233] Nevertheless, similarities to bacterial subtilisin, Kex2 and furin, suggest this is a potential control of PC2 and PC3 activities in the β-cell.[135]

Passage of newly synthesized proinsulin, PC3 and CP-H, appears to be relatively similar along the β-cell secretory pathway, although PC3 and CP-H might exit the RER slightly earlier than proinsulin.[135] In contrast, PC2 appears to be held up in the RER for 5–10 times longer.[134,135] PC2 has been shown to interact with a chaperon protein, 7B2,[137] which specifically inhibits PC2 activity.[136] A transient interaction between PC2 and 7B2 might be an influence on proinsulin processing regulation.

Proinsulin biosynthesis can be stimulated by glucose at both translational and transcriptional levels.[49,93,94] This places an increased demand on the proinsulin conversion mechanism in β-cells, but it seems that proinsulin conversion is adaptable to changes in glucose.[239] The biosynthesis of PC3 is stimulated in parallel with that of proinsulin at a translational level.[41] In contrast, the biosynthesis of PC2[41] and CP-H[40] are not glucose-regulated. Given that PC3 initiates the majority of sequential processing of proinsulin conversion in human β-cells,[19] the coordinate glucose regulation of PC3 with its proinsulin substrate at the biosynthetic level ensures that proinsulin conversion proceeds efficiently and is adaptable to varying glucose concentrations.[177] It remains to be shown whether the proinsulin convertase genes are coordinately transcriptionally regulated with the preproinsulin gene by long-term exposure to glucose.[91,240,241] This is a distinct possibility, especially considering that it has been shown that PC2 and PC3 mRNAs are coordinately regulated with proopiomelanocortin mRNA in pituitary cells.[242]

The β-Granule Storage Pool and Insulin Degradation

Mature β-granules containing insulin in crystalline form and soluble C-peptide are kept in an intracellular storage pool awaiting an intracellular signal to trigger their transport to the plasma membrane for exocytosis. Such a storage pool and regulated release of a major hormone product is typical of a regulated secretory pathway found in neuroendocrine cells.[116,153] Insulin is almost entirely released (>99%) from β-cells via a regulated secretory pathway.[177] The insulin content of pancreatic β-cells stays remarkably constant under normal circumstances, there being a balance maintained among insulin secretion, (pro)insulin biosynthesis, and intracellular insulin degradation.[243,244] This ensures that there is always a readily available and rapidly releasable pool of insulin.[36] The half-life of a β-granule is several days, and if it is not marked for exocytosis it is eventually degraded within the β-cells by fusion with lysosomes, a process known as *crinophagy*.[152,243,244] During a high demand for insulin release, insulin degradation is downregulated; when there is a low rate of insulin release, degradation increases.[243–245] The regulatory mechanism behind crinophagy in β-cells is not known. The degradation of insulin is rather slow, which is thought to be due to the high stability of the insulin crystal in the β-cell lysosomal compartment.[246,247] Nevertheless, intracellular degradation of insulin is irreversible and marks the final stage of processing of the insulin molecule, that is, if a β-granule does not undergo exocytosis. The final step is this latter case would be secretion of insulin from the β-cell.

Transport of Secretory Granules to the Plasma Membrane

Experimental evidence suggests that transport of β-granules to the plasma membrane is enhanced via a β-granule interaction with the β-cell cytoskeletal framework of microtubules and microfilaments.[125,248–251] Microtubules are not essential for secretory granule transport, but they are required to guide the specific direction of granule movement.[251] This could well be important considering that β-cells are polarized.[252,253] It is not clear whether β-granules in the storage pool are already attached to β-cell microtubules or whether there is a specific mechanism of attachment when β-granule transport to the plasma membrane is required. Preferential release of newly synthesized insulin[177,254,255] suggests that newly formed β-granules are more likely to be transported to the plasma membrane than those in a storage pool, perhaps because of a prior attachment to microtubules.[177] β-Granule movement along microtubules is likely driven by microtubule-associated proteins and motors (e.g., kinesin and dynein[251,256–259]; kinesin has been identified in β-cells[260]). Besides evoking exocytosis, the stimulation of insulin release must involve increased recruitment of β-granules to the plasma membrane. In this light, glucose has been shown to increase tubulin polymerization in pancreatic islets,[261] and microtubule stability can be affected by Ca^{++}, GTP, and protein kinase phosphorylation.[258]

The role of microfilaments in β-granule transport to the β-cell plasma membrane is not particularly clear, but they are thought to provide a proportion of motive force for β-granule transport.[125,262,263] This could be mediated by myosin light-chain kinase activity found in β-cells,[264,265] which promotes association between myosin- and actin-containing microfilaments.[125] The microfilament network occurs in bundles just beneath and parallel to the plasma membrane of the β-cell, forming a "cell-web."[263] This may actually block access of β-granules to fuse with the plasma membrane for exocytosis. The β-cell may therefore be analogous to the chromaffin cell, where there is limited disassembly of actin filaments just before exocytosis, instigated by sciderin and ATP.[266]

Exocytosis

The pancreatic β-cell is a typical endocrine cell in the sense that its primary secretory product, insulin, is predominately secreted via a regulated secretory pathway.[153,177,267] In accordance with this process,[116,153] insulin is stored in the β-cell's secretory granule compartment in the resting state; it is not released from the β-cell unless there is a specific signal that stimulates exocytosis.[152,177] Stimulation of insulin exocytosis is generally thought to be instigated by intracellular secondary signals,[153] the most prominent of which is a rise in cytosolic Ca^{++}.[95,96] A rise in $[Ca^{++}]i$, however, is not likely to be the only regulator of β-cell exocytosis.[268] G-proteins[269–272] and protein kinase activities[98,273–276] also have been identified as contributing to the triggering of insulin exocytosis. There are likely to be several stages of regulated insulin exocytosis, including: (1) "priming" a β-granule for exocytosis, (2) "docking" a secretory granule to a site on the plasma membrane, (3) "fusing" the secretory granule and plasma membranes, and (4) "expelling" secretory granule contents into the extracellular space. Unfortunately, the molecular mechanism of insulin exocytosis in β-cells is essentially unknown, but it is likely to be analogous to that of related neuroendocrine cells, in which the mechanism is thought to be controlled by interactions among various secretory granule, cytosolic, and plasma membrane proteins.[169,271,277–279]

References

1. Steiner DF, Bell GI, Tager HS. Chemistry and biosynthesis of pancreatic protein hormones. In: DeGroot LG, ed. Endocrinology. 2nd ed. Philadelphia, Pa: WB Saunders 1990;1263–1289
2. Steiner DF, Chan SJ, Welsh JM, Kwok SC. Structure and evolution of the insulin gene. Ann Rev Genet 1985;19:463
3. Bailyes EM, Guest PC, Hutton JC. Insulin synthesis. In: Ashcroft FM, Ashcroft SJH, eds. Insulin: Molecular Biology to Pathology. Oxford, UK: Oxford University Press;1992:64–92
4. Blundell TL, Dodson GG, Dodson E, et al. X-ray analysis and the structure of insulin. Recent Prog Horm Res 1971;27:1
5. Chothia C, Lesk AM, Dodson GG, Hodgkin DC. Transmission of conformational change in insulin. Nature 1983;302:500
6. Hefford MA, Oka G, Kaplan H. Structure function relationships in the free insulin monomer. Biochem J 1986;237:663
7. Chan SJ, Keim P, Steiner DF. Cell free synthesis of rat preproinsulins: Characterization and partial amino acid sequence determination. Proc Natl Acad Sci USA 1976;73:1964
8. Bell GI, Pictet RL, Rutter WJ, et al. Sequence of the insulin gene. Nature 1980;284:26
9. Briggs MS, Gierasch LM. Molecular mechanisms of protein secretion: The role of the signal sequence. Adv Protein Chem 1986;38:109
10. Pfeffer SR, Rothman JE. Biosynthetic protein transport and sorting by the endoplasmic reticulum and Golgi. Ann Rev Biochem 1987;56:829
11. Steiner DF. On the role of the proinsulin C-peptide. Diabetes 1978; 27(suppl 1):145
12. Snell CR, Smythe DG. Proinsulin: A proposed three-dimensional structure. J Biol Chem 1975;250:6291
13. Steiner DF. Cocrystallization of proinsulin and insulin. Nature 1973;243:528
14. Frank BH, Veros AJ. Interaction of zinc with proinsulin. Biochem Biophys Res Commun 1970;38:284
15. Galloway JA, Hooper SA, Spradlin CT, et al. Biosynthetic human proinsulin: Review of chemistry, in vitro and in vivo receptor binding, animal and human pharmacology studies, and clinical trial experience. Diabetes Care 1992;15:666
16. Gross DJ, Villa-Komaroff L, Kahn CR, et al. Deletion of a highly conserved tetrapeptide sequence of the proinsulin connecting peptide (C-peptide) inhibits proinsulin to insulin conversion by transfected pituitary corticotroph (AtT20) cells. J Biol Chem 1989;264:21486
17. Weiss MA, Frank BH, Khait I, et al. NMR and photo-CIDNP of human proinsulin and prohormone processing intermediates with application to endoprotease recognition. Biochemistry 1990;29:8389
18. Derewenda U, Derewenda Z, Dodson GG, et al. Molecular structure of insulin: The insulin monomer and its assembly. Br Med Bull 1989;45:4

19. Rhodes CJ, Alarcón C. What β-cell defect could lead to hyperproinsulinemia in NIDDM: Some clues from recent advances made in understanding the proinsulin conversion mechanism. Diabetes 1994;43:511
20. Rhodes CJ, Lincoln B, Shoelson SE. Preferential cleavage of des 31,32 proinsulin over intact proinsulin by the insulin secretory granule type-II endopeptidase: Implications for a favored route for prohormone processing. J Biol Chem 1992;267:22719
21. Merrick WC. Mechanism and regulation of eukaryotic protein synthesis. Microbiol Rev 1992;56:291
22. Clemens MJ. Regulatory mechanisms in translational control. Curr Op in Cell Biol 1989;1:1160
23. Hershey JWB. Translational control in mammalian cells. Ann Rev Biochem 1991;60:717
24. Wiedmann B, Sakai H, Davis TA, Wiedmann M. A protein complex required for signal-sequence-specific sorting and translocation. Nature 1994;370:434
25. Eskridge EM, Shields D. Cell-free processing and segregation of insulin precursors. J Biol Chem 1983;258:11487
26. Okun MM, Eskridge EM, Shields D. Truncations of a secretory protein define minimum lengths required for binding to signal recognition particle and translocation across the endoplasmic reticulum membrane. J Biol Chem 1990;265:7478
27. Wolin SL, Walter P. Discrete nascent chain lengths are required for the insertion of presecretory proteins into microsomal membranes. J Cell Biol 1993;121:1211
28. Siegel V, Walter P. Functional dissection of the signal recognition particle. Trends Biochem Sci 1988;13:314
29. Meyer DI, Krause E, Dobberstein B. Secretory protein translocation across membranes—the role of the 'docking protein.' Nature 1982;297:647
30. Savitz AJ, Meyer DI. Identification of a ribosome receptor in the rough endoplasmic reticulum. Nature 1990;346:540
31. Miller JD, Wilhelm H, Gierasch L, et al: GTP binding and hydrolysis by the signal recognition particle during initiation of protein translocation. Nature 1993;366:351
32. Wiedmann M, Kurzchalia TV, Hartman E, Rapoport TA. A signal sequence receptor in the endoplasmic reticulum membrane. Nature 1987;328:830
33. Gorlich D, Prehn E, Hartman E, et al. The signal sequence receptor has a second subunit and is part of a translocation complex in the endoplasmic reticulum as probed by bifunctional reagents. J Cell Biol 1990;111:2283
34. Lively MO. Signal peptidases in protein biosynthesis and intracellular transport. Curr Opin Cell Biol 1989;1:1188
35. Campbell IC, Hellqvist LNB, Taylor KW. Insulin biosynthesis and its regulation. Clin Sci 1982;62:449
36. Shoelson SE, Halban PA. Insulin biosynthesis and chemistry. In: Kahn CR, Weir GC, eds. Joslin's Diabetes Mellitus. 13th ed. Malvern, Pa: Lea & Febiger;1994:29–55
37. Ashcroft SJH. Glucoreceptor mechanisms and the control of insulin release and biosynthesis. Diabetologia 1980;18:5
38. Ashcroft SJH, Bunce J, Lowry M, et al. The effect of sugars on (pro)insulin biosynthesis. Biochem J 1978;174:517
39. Lin BJ, Haist RE. Insulin biosynthesis: Effects of carbohydrates and related compounds. Can J Physiol Pharmacol 1969;47:791
40. Guest PG, Rhodes CJ, Hutton JC. Regulation of the biosynthesis of insulin secretory granule proteins: Co-ordinate translational control is exerted on some but not all granule matrix constituents. Biochem J 1989;257:431
41. Alarcón C, Lincoln B, Rhodes CJ. The biosynthesis of the subtilisin-related proprotein convertase PC3, but not that of the PC2 convertase, is regulated by glucose in parallel to proinsulin biosynthesis in rat pancreatic islets. J Biol Chem 1993;268:4276
42. Pipeleers DG, Michael M, Malaisse WJ. The stimulus coupling of glucose-induced insulin release. XIV. Glucose-regulation of insular biosynthetic activity. Endocrinology 1973;93:1001
43. Maldonato A, Renold AE, Sharp GWG, Cerasi E. Glucose-induced proinsulin biosynthesis: Role of islet cAMP. Diabetes 1977;26:538
44. Schuit FC, In't Veld PA, Pipeleers DG. Glucose stimulates proinsulin biosynthesis by a dose-dependent recruitment of pancreatic β-cells. Proc Natl Acad Sci USA 1988;85:3865
45. Kiekens R, In't Veld PA, Mahler T, et al. Differences in glucose recognition by individual rat pancreatic β-cells are associated with differences in glucose-induced biosynthesis activity. J Clin Invest 1992;89:115
46. Steiner DF, Kemmler W, Clark JL, et al. The biosynthesis of insulin. In: Greep RO, Astwood EB, eds. Handbook of Physiology, Section 7. Washington, DC: American Physiological Society;1972:175–198
47. Kaelin D, Renold AE, Sharp GWG. Glucose-stimulated proinsulin biosynthesis: Rates of turn off after cessation of the stimulus. Diabetologia 1978;14:329
48. Itoh N, Okamoto H. Translational control of proinsulin synthesis by glucose. Nature 1980;283:100
49. Welsh M, Scherberg N, Gilmore R, Steiner DF. Translational control of insulin biosynthesis: Evidence for regulation of elongation, initiation and signal-recognition-particle–mediated translational arrest by glucose. Biochem J 1986;235:459
50. Parry DG, Taylor KW. The effects of sugars on incorporation of [^{3}H]leucine into insulins. Biochem J 1966;100:2
51. Howell SL, Taylor KW. Effects of glucose concentration on incorporation of [^{3}H]leucine into insulin using isolated mammalian islets of Langerhans. Biochim Biophys Acta 1966;130:517
52. Morris GE, Korner A. The effect of glucose on insulin biosynthesis by isolated islets of Langerhans of the rat. Biochim Biophys Acta 1970;208:404
53. Jain K, Logothetopoulos J. Stimulation of proinsulin biosynthesis by purine-ribonucleosides and D-ribose. Endocrinol 1977;100:923
54. Ashcroft SJH, Crossley JR, Crossley PC. The effect of N-acetylglucosamines on the biosynthesis and secretion of insulin in the rat. Biochem J 1976;154:701
55. Andersson A. Stimulation of insulin biosynthesis in isolated mouse islets by L-leucine, 2-aminobornane-2 carboxylic acid and α-keto-isocaproic acid. Biochim Biophys Act 1976;437:345
56. Jain K, Logothetopoulos J, Zucker P. The effects of D- and L-glyceraldehyde on glucose oxidation, insulin secretion and insulin biosynthesis by pancreatic islets of the rat. Biochim Biophys Acta 1975;399:384
57. Andersson A. Opposite effects of starvation on oxidation of [^{14}C]adenosine and adenosine-induced insulin release by mouse pancreatic islets. Biochem J 1978;176:619
58. Malaisse WJ, Lebrun P, Yaylali B, et al. Ketone bodies and islet function: ^{45}Ca handling, insulin synthesis, and release. Am J Physiol 1990;259:E117
59. Zhou YP, Grill VE. Long-term exposure of rat pancreatic islets to fatty acids inhibits glucose-induced insulin secretion and biosynthesis through a glucose fatty acid cycle. J Clin Invest 1994;93:870
60. Patzelt C. Differential inhibitory action of cationic amino acids on protein synthesis in rat pancreatic islets. Diabetologia 1988;31:241
61. Lin BJ. An apparent inhibition of insulin biosynthesis resulting from inhibition of transport of neutral amino acids by arginine. Diabetologia 1977;13:77
62. Whittaker PG, Taylor KW. Direct effects of rat growth hormone on rat islets of Langerhans in tissue culture. Diabetologia 1980;18:323
63. Billestrup N, Moldrup A, Serup P, et al. Introduction of exogenous growth hormone receptors augments growth hormone-responsive insulin biosynthesis in rat insulinoma cells. Proc Natl Acad Sci USA 1990;87:7210
64. Malaisse WJ, Pipeleers DG, Levy J. The stimulus-secretion coupling of glucose-induced insulin release. XVI. A glucose-like and calcium-independent effect of cAMP. Biochim Biophys Acta 1974;362:121
65. Schatz H, Maier V, Hinz M, et al. Stimulation of [^{3}H]leucine incorporation into proinsulin and insulin fraction of isolated pancreatic mouse islets in the presence of glucagon, theophylline and cAMP. Diabetes 1973;22:433
66. Fehmann HC, Habener JF. Insulinotropic hormone glucagon-like peptide-I(7-37) stimulation of proinsulin gene expression and proinsulin biosynthesis in insulinoma beta TC-1 cells. Endocrinology 1992;130:159
67. Olsson SE, Anderson A, Petersson B, Hellerström C. Effects of somatostatin on the biosynthesis and release of insulin from isolated pancreatic islets. Diabete Metab 1976;2:199
68. Nagamatsu S, Carroll RJ, Grodsky GM, Steiner DF. Lack of islet amyloid polypeptide regulation of insulin biosynthesis or secretion in normal rat islets. Diabetes 1990;39:871
69. Nagamatsu S, Nishi M, Steiner DF. Effects of islet amyloid polypeptide (IAPP) on insulin biosynthesis or secretion in rat islets and mouse β-TC3 cells. Biosynthesis of IAPP in mouse β-TC3 cells. Diabetes Res Clin Pract 1992;15:49
70. Ostenson CG, Sandler S, Efendic S. Effects of pancreastatin on secretion and biosynthesis of insulin and glucose oxidation of isolated rat pancreatic islets. Pancreas 1989;4:441
71. Rhodes CJ, Taylor KW. Effect of lymphoblastoid interferon in isolated pancreatic islets. Diabetologia 1984;27:601
72. Rhodes CJ, Taylor KW. The effect of interferon and double stranded RNA on β-cell function on mouse islets of Langerhans. Biochem J 1985;228:87
73. Sandler S, Andersson A, Hellerström C. Inhibitory effects of interleukin-1 on insulin secretion, insulin biosynthesis and oxidative metabolism of isolated rat pancreatic islets. Endocrinology 1987;121:1424
74. Spinas GA, Hansen BS, Linde S, et al. Interleukin-1 dose-dependently affects the biosynthesis of (pro)insulin in isolated rat islets of Langerhans. Diabetologia 1987;30:474
75. Hansen BS, Nielsen JH, Linde S, et al. Effect of interleukin-1 on the biosynthesis of proinsulin and insulin in isolated rat pancreatic islets. Biomed Biochim Acta 1988;47:305
76. Levy J, Malaisse WJ. The stimulus-secretion coupling of glucose-induced insulin release- XVII. Effects of sulfonylureas and diazoxide on insular biosynthetic activity. Biochem Pharmacol 1975;24:235
77. Tanese T, Lazarus NR, Devrim S, Recant L. Synthesis and release of proinsulin and insulin by isolated rat islets of Langerhans. J Clin Invest 1970;49:1394
78. Lin BJ, Haist RE. Effects of some modifiers of insulin secretion and insulin biosynthesis. Endocrinology 1973;92:735
79. Gwilliam DJ, Jones PM, Persaud SJ, Howell SL. The role of protein kinase C in insulin biosynthesis. Acta Diabetol 1993;30:99
80. Bone AJ, Taylor KW. Metabolic adaptation to pregnancy shown by increased biosynthesis of insulin in islets of Langerhans from pregnant rats. Nature 1976;262:501
81. Bone AJ, Taylor KW. Alterations in regulation of insulin biosynthesis in pregnancy and starvation studies in isolated rat islets of Langerhans. Biochem J 1977;166:501
82. Caterson ID, Taylor KW. Islet cell function in gold-thioglucose-induced obesity in mice. Diabetologia 1982;23:119
83. Tjioe TO, Bouman PR. Effect of fasting on the incorporation of [^{3}H]-L-phenylalanine into proinsulin-insulin and total protein in isolated rat pancreatic islets. Horm Metab Res 1976;8:261
84. Wang SY, Halban PA, Rowe JW. Effects of aging on insulin synthesis and secretion: Differential effects on preproinsulin messenger RNA levels, proinsulin biosynthesis, and secretion of newly made and preformed insulin in the rat. J Clin Invest 1988;81:176

85. Portha B. Decreased glucose-induced insulin release and biosynthesis by islets of rats with non–insulin-dependent diabetes: Effect of tissue culture. Endocrinology 1985;115:1735
86. Permutt MA, Kakita K, Malinas P, et al. An in vivo analysis of pancreatic protein and insulin biosynthesis in a rat model for non-insulin dependent diabetes. J Clin Invest 1984;73:1344
87. Alarcón C, Leahy JL, Schuppin GT, Rhodes CJ. Hyperproinsulinemia in a glucose-infusion rat model of non insulin dependent diabetes mellitus is a symptom of increased secretory demand rather than a defect in the proinsulin conversion mechanism. J Clin Invest 1995;95:1032
88. Heinze E, Hagele U, Fussganger RD, Pfeiffer EF. Insulin biosynthesis and release in isolated islets from hyperglycemic male rats. Horm Metab Res 1980;12:190
89. Zucker P, Logothetopoulos J. Persisting enhanced proinsulin-insulin and protein biosynthesis (^{3}H-incorporation) by pancreatic islets of the rat after glucose exposure. Diabetes 1975;24:194
90. Brunstedt J, Chan SJ. Direct effect of glucose on the preproinsulin mRNA level in isolated pancreatic islets. Biochem Biophys Res Commun 1982; 106:1383
91. Giddings SJ, Chirgwin J, Permutt MA. Effects of glucose on proinsulin mRNA in rats in vivo. Diabetes 1982;31:624
92. Giddings SJ, Chirgwin J, Permutt MA. The effects of fasting and feeding on preproinsulin mRNA in rats. J Clin Invest 1981;67:952
93. Nielsen DA, Welsh M, Casadaban MJ, Steiner DF. Control of insulin gene expression in pancreatic β-cells and in an insulin producing cell line, RIN-5F cells. 1. Effects of glucose and cAMP on the transcription of insulin mRNA. J Biol Chem 1985;260:13586
94. Welsh M, Nielsen DA, MacKrell AJ, Steiner DF. Control of insulin gene expression in pancreatic β-cells and in an insulin producing cell line, RIN-5F cells. 2. Regulation of insulin mRNA stability. J Biol Chem 1985;260:13590
95. Prentki M, Matchinsky FM. Ca^{++}, cAMP, and phospholipid-derived messengers in coupling mechanisms of insulin secretion. Physiol Rev 1987;67:1185
96. Ashcroft FM, Ashcroft SJH. Mechanism of insulin secretion. In: Ashcroft FM, Ashcroft SJH, eds. Insulin: Molecular Biology to Pathology. Oxford, UK: Oxford University Press;1992:97–150
97. Pipeleers DG, Marichal M, Malaisse WJ. The stimulus coupling of glucose-induced insulin release. XV. Participation of cations in the recognition of glucose by the B-cell. Endocrinology 1973;93:1012
98. Wenham RM, Landt M, Easom RA. Glucose activates the multifunctional Ca^{2+}/calmodulin-dependent protein kinase II in isolated rat pancreatic islets. J Biol Chem 1994;269:4947
99. Ammala C, Eliaason L, Bokvist K, et al. Exocytosis elicited by action potentials and voltage-clamp calcium currents in individual mouse pancreatic B-cells. J Physiol 1993;472:665
100. Gagliardino JJ, Harrison DE, Christie MR, et al. Evidence for the participation of calmodulin in stimulus-secretion coupling in the pancreatic β-cell. Biochem J 1980;192:919
101. Welsh N, Oberg C, Welsh M. GTP-binding proteins may stimulate insulin biosynthesis in rat pancreatic islets by enhancing the signal-recognition-particle–dependent translocation of the insulin mRNA poly-/monosome complex to the endoplasmic reticulum. Biochem J 1991;275:23
102. Permutt MA, Kipnis DM. 1. Insulin biosynthesis: On the mechanism of glucose stimulation. J Biol Chem 1972;247:1194
103. Itoh N, Ohshima Y, Nose K, Okamoto H. Glucose stimulates proinsulin synthesis in pancreatic islets without a concomitant increase in proinsulin mRNA synthesis. Biochem Int 1982;4:315
104. Welsh N, Welsh M, Steiner DF, Hellerström C. Mechanisms of leucine- and theophylline-stimulated insulin biosynthesis in isolated rat pancreatic islets. Biochem J 1987;246:245
105. Lomedico PT, Saunders GF. Cell-free modulation of proinsulin synthesis. Science 1977;198:620
106. Permutt MA. Effect of glucose on initiation and elongation rate in isolated pancreatic islets. J Biol Chem 1974;248:2738
107. Kozak M. Regulation of translation in eukaryotic systems. Ann Rev Cell Biol 1992;8:197
108. Rhodes CJ. The unique regulation of proinsulin biosynthesis. J Cell Biochem 1994;Abstract(Suppl 18A):125
109. Knight SW, Docherty K. RNA-protein interactions in the 5′-untranslated region of preproinsulin mRNA. J Mol Endocrinol 1992;8:225
110. Hughes SJ, Smith H, Ashcroft SJH. Characterization of Ca^{2+} calmodulin-dependent protein kinase in rat pancreatic islets. Biochem J 1993;289:795
111. Guest PC, Bailyes EM, Rutherford NG, Hutton JC. Insulin secretory granule biogenesis: Co-ordinate regulation of the biosynthesis of the majority of constituent proteins. Biochem J 1991;274:73
112. Klausner RD, Rouault TA, Harford JB. Regulating the fate of mRNA: The control of cellular iron metabolism. Cell 1993;72:19
113. Grimaldi KA, Siddle K, Hutton JC. Biosynthesis of insulin granule membrane proteins: Control by glucose. Biochem J 1987;245:567
114. Palade G. Intracellular aspects of the process of protein synthesis. Science 1975;189:347
115. Rothman JE, Orci L. Molecular dissection of the secretory pathway. Nature 1992;355:409
116. Kelly RB. Pathways of protein secretion in eukaryotes. Science 1985;230:25
117. Tang J-G, Wang C-C, Tsou C-L. Formation of native insulin from scrambled molecules by disulfide isomerase. Biochem J 1988;255:451
118. Freedman RB. Native disulfide bond formation in protein biosynthesis: Evidence for the role of protein disulfide isomerase. Trends Biochem Sci 1984;9:438
119. Pelham HRB. Control of protein export from the endoplasmic reticulum. Ann Rev Cell Biol 1989;5:1
120. Georgopoulos C, Welch WJ. Role of the major heat shock proteins as molecular chaperons. Ann Rev Cell Biol 1993;9:601
121. Kornfeld R, Kornfeld S. Assembly of asparagine-linked oligosaccharides. Ann Rev Biochem 1985;54:631
122. Hirschberg CB, Snider MD. Topography of glycosylation in the rough endoplasmic reticulum and Golgi apparatus. Ann Rev Biochem 1987;56:63
123. Hurtley SM, Helenius A. Protein oligomerization in the endoplasmic reticulum. Ann Rev Cell Biol 1989;5:277
124. Howell SL. Role of ATP in the intracellular translocation and insulin in the rat pancreatic β-cell [Letter]. Nature New Biol 1972;235:85
125. Howell SL. The mechanism of insulin secretion. Diabetologia 1984;26:319
126. Balch WE. Small GTP-binding proteins in vesicular transport. Trends Biochem Sci 1990;15:473
127. Schwaninger R, Plutner H, Bokoch GM, Balch WE. Multiple GTP-binding proteins regulate vesicular transport from the ER to Golgi membranes. J Cell Biol 1992;119:1077
128. Davidson HW, McGowan CH, Balch WE. Evidence for the regulation of exocytic transport by protein phosphorylation. J Cell Biol 1992;116:1343
129. Beckers CJM, Block MR, Glick BS, et al. Vesicular transport between the endoplasmic reticulum and the Golgi stack requires the NEM-sensitive fusion protein. Nature 1989;339:397
130. Balch WE, Kahn RA, Schwaninger R. ADP-ribosylation factor is required for vesicular trafficking between the endoplasmic reticulum and the cis-Golgi compartment. J Biol Chem 1992;267:13053
131. Tisdale EJ, Bourne JR, Khosravi-Far R, et al. GTP-binding mutants of Rab1 and Rab2 are potent inhibitors of vesicular transport from the endoplasmic reticulum to the Golgi complex. J Cell Biol 1992;119:749
132. Zerial M, Stenmark H. Rab GTPases in vesicular transport. Curr Opin Cell Biol 1993;5:613
133. Lodish HF, Kong N. Perturbation of cellular calcium blocks exit of secretory proteins from the rough endoplasmic reticulum. J Biol Chem 1990;265:10893
134. Guest PC, Arden SD, Bennett DL, et al. The post-translational processing and intracellular sorting of PC2 in the islets of Langerhans. J Biol Chem 1992;267:22401
135. Hutton JC. Insulin secretory granule biogenesis and the proinsulin-processing endopeptidases. Diabetologia 1994;37(suppl 2):S48
136. Martens GJM, Braks JAM, Eib DW, et al. The neuroendocrine polypeptide 7B2 is an endogenous inhibitor of prohormone convertase PC2. Proc Natl Acad Sci USA 1994;91:5784
137. Braks JAM, Martens GJM. 7B2 is a neuroendocrine chaperone that transiently interacts with prohormone convertase PC2 in the secretory pathway. Cell 1994;78:263
138. Lewis MJ, Pelham HRB. A human homologue of the yeast HDEL receptor. Nature 1990;348:162
139. Semenza JC, Hardwick KG, Dean N, Pelham HRB. ERD2, a yeast gene required for the receptor-mediated retrieval of luminal ER proteins from the secretory pathway. Cell 1990;61:1349
140. Vaux D, Tooze J, Fuller S. Identification by anti-idiotypic antibodies of an intracellular membrane protein that recognizes a mammalian endoplasmic reticulum retention signal. Nature 1990;345:495
141. Farquhar MG. Progress in unraveling pathways of Golgi traffic. Ann Rev Cell Biol 1985;1:447
142. Olofsson SO, Bjursell G, Bostrom K, et al. Apolipoprotein B: Structure, biosynthesis and role in the lipoprotein assembly process. Atherosclerosis 1987;68:1
143. Rothman JE. The compartmental organization of the Golgi apparatus. Sci Am September 1985;74
144. Rothman JE. The Golgi apparatus: Two organelles in tandem. Science 1981;213:1212
145. Balch WE. Biochemistry of interorganelle transport: A new frontier in enzymology emerges from versatile in vitro model systems. J Biol Chem 1989;264:16965
146. Melançon P, Glick BS, Malhotra V, et al. Involvement of GTP binding "G" proteins in transport through the Golgi stack. Cell 1987;51:1053
147. Orci L, Malhotra V, Amherdt M, et al. Dissection of a single round of vesicular transport: Sequential intermediates for intercisternal movement of the Golgi stack. Cell 1989;56:357
148. Goud B, Zahraoui A, Tavitian A, Saraste J. Small GTP binding protein associated with Golgi cisternae. Nature 1990;345:553
149. Clary DO, Griff IC, Rothman JE. SNAPs: a family of NSF attachment proteins involved in intracellular membrane fusion in animals and yeast. Cell 1990;61:709
150. Söllner T, Whiteheart SW, Brunner M, et al. SNAP receptors implicated in vesicle targeting and fusion. Nature 1993;362:318
151. Glick BS, Rothman JE. Possible role for fatty acyl-coenzyme A in intracellular protein transport. Nature 1987;326:309
152. Orci L. The insulin factory: A tour of the plant surroundings and a visit to the assembly line. Diabetologia 1985;28:528
153. Burgess TL, Kelly RB. Constitutive and regulated secretion of proteins. Ann Rev Cell Biol 1987;3:243

154. Halban PA, Irminger J-C. Sorting and processing of secretory proteins. Biochem J 1994;299:1
155. Griffiths G, Simons K. The trans Golgi network: Sorting at the exit site of the Golgi complex. Science 1986;234:438
156. Griffiths G, Hoflack B, Simons K, et al. The mannose 6-phosphate receptor and the biogenesis of lysosomes. Cell 1988;52:329
157. Kornfeld S, Mellman I. The biogenesis of lysosomes. Ann Rev Cell Biol 1989;5:483
158. Wieland FT, Gleason ML, Serafini TA, Rothman JE. The rate of bulk flow from the endoplasmic reticulum to the cell surface. Cell 1987;50:289
159. Moore H-PH, Kelly RB. Rerouting of a secretory protein by fusion with growth hormone sequence. Nature 1986;321:443
160. Rosa P, Weiss U, Pepperkok R, et al. An antibody against secretogranin 1 (chromogranin B) is packaged into secretory granules. J Cell Biol 1989;109:17
161. Chung K-N, Walter P, Aponte GW, Moore H-PH. Molecular sorting in the secretory pathway. Science 1989;243:192
162. Tooze SA, Huttner WB. Cell free protein sorting to the regulated and constitutive secretory pathways. Cell 1990;60:837
163. Huttner WB, Bauerfeind R. Biogenesis of constitutive secretory vesicles, secretory granules and synaptic vesicles. Curr Opin Cell Biol 1993;5:628
164. Chanat E, Weiss U, Huttner WB, Tooze SA. Reduction of the disulfide bond of chromogranin B (secretogranin I) in the trans-Golgi network causes its missorting to the constitutive secretory pathways. EMBO J 1993;12:2159
165. Gerdes H-H, Rosa P, Phillips E, et al. The primary structure of human secretogranin II, a widespread tyrosine-sulfated secretory granule protein that exhibits low pH and calcium-induced aggregation. J Biol Chem 1989;264:12009
166. Sopwith AM, Hales CN, Hutton JC, Pancreatic β-cells secrete a range of novel peptides besides insulin. Biochim Biophys Acta 1984;803:342
167. Guest PG, Pipeleers D, Rossier J, et al. Co-secretion of carboxypeptidase-H and insulin from isolated rat islets of Langerhans. Biochem J 1989;264:503
168. Tooze SA, Weiss U, Huttner WB. Requirement for GTP hydrolysis in the formation of secretory granules. Nature 1990;347:207
169. Nuoffer C, Balch WE. GTPases: Multifunctional molecular switches regulating vesicular traffic. Ann Rev Biochem 1994;63:949
170. Barr FA, Leyte A, Mollner S, et al. Trimeric G-proteins of the trans-Golgi network are involved in the formation of constitutive secretory vesicles and immature secretory granules. FEBS Lett 1991;294:239
171. Fine RE. Vesicles without clathrin: Intermediates in bulk flow exocytosis. Cell 1989;58:609
172. Pearse BMF, Robinson MS. Clathrin, adapters and sorting. Ann Rev Cell Biol 1990;6:151
173. Payne GS, Shekman R, Clathrin: A role in the intracellular retention of a Golgi membrane protein. Science 1989;245:1358
174. Tooze J, Tooze SA. Clathrin coated vesicular transport of secretory proteins during the formation of ACTH-containing secretory granules in AtT-20 cells. J Cell Biol 1986;103:839
175. Kuliawat R, Arvan P. Distinct molecular mechanisms for protein sorting within immature secretory granules of pancreatic β-cells. J Cell Biol 1994; 126:77
176. Kuliawat R, Arvan P. Protein targeting via the "constitutive-like" pathway in isolated pancreatic islets: Passive sorting in the immature granule. J Cell Biol 1992;118:521
177. Rhodes CJ, Halban PA. Newly-synthesized proinsulin/insulin and stored insulin are released from pancreatic B-cells via a regulated, rather than a constitutive pathway. J Cell Biol 1987;105:145
178. Powell SK, Orci L, Moore H-PH. Efficient targeting to storage granules of human proinsulins with altered propeptide domains. J Cell Biol 1988;106:1843
179. Taylor NA, Docherty K. Sequence requirements for processing of proinsulin in transfected mouse pituitary AtT20 cells. Biochem J 1992;286:619
180. Carroll RJ, Hammer RE, Chan SJ, et al. A mutant human proinsulin is secreted from islets of Langerhans in increased amounts via an unregulated pathway. Proc Natl Acad Sci USA 1988;85:8943
181. Gross DJ, Halban PA, Kahn CR, et al. Partial diversion of a mutant proinsulin (B10 aspartic acid) from the regulated to the constitutive secretory pathway in transfected AtT-20 cells. Proc Natl Acad Sci USA 1989;86:4107
182. Kemmler W, Steiner DF. Conversion of proinsulin to insulin in a subcellular fraction from rat islets. Biochem Biophys Res Commun 1970;41:1223
183. Davidson HW, Rhodes CJ, Hutton JC. Intraorganellar Ca and pH control proinsulin cleavage in the pancreatic β-cell via two site-specific endopeptidases. Nature 1988;333:93
184. Rhodes CJ, Lucas CA, Mutkoski RL, et al. Stimulation by ATP of proinsulin to insulin conversion in isolated rat pancreatic islet secretory granules: Association with ATP-dependent proton pump. J Biol Chem 1987;262:10712
185. Hutton JC. The internal pH and membrane potential of the insulin secretory granule. Biochem J 1982;204:171
186. Chappell TG, Konforti BB, Schmid SL, Rothman JE. The ATPase core of a clathrin uncoating protein. J Biol Chem 1987;262:746
187. Orci L, Ravazzola M, Storch M-J, et al. Proteolytic maturation of insulin is a post-Golgi event which occurs in acidifying clathrin-coated secretory vesicles. Cell 1987;49:865
188. Docherty KD, Steiner DF. Post-translational proteolysis in polypeptide hormone biosynthesis. Ann Rev Physiol 1982;44:625
189. Loh YP, Brownstein MJ, Gainer H. Proteolysis in neuropeptide processing and other neural functions. Ann Rev Neurosci 1984;7:189
190. Douglass J, Civelli O, Herbert E. Polyprotein gene expression: Generation of diversity of neuroendocrine peptides. Ann Rev Biochem 1984;53:665
191. Hutton JC. Subtilisin-like proteinases involved in the activation of proproteins of the secretory pathway of eukaryotic cells. Curr Opin Cell Biol 1991;2:1131
192. Steiner DF, Smeekens SP, Ohagi S, Chan SJ. The new enzymology of precursor processing endopeptidases. J Biol Chem 1992;267:23435
193. Lindberg I. The new eukaryotic precursor processing proteinases. Mol Endocrinol 1991;5:1361
194. Docherty KD, Hutton JC. Carboxypeptidase activity in the insulin secretory granule. FEBS Lett 1983;162:137
195. Davidson HW, Hutton JC. The insulin secretory granule carboxypeptidase-H: purification and demonstration of involvement in proinsulin processing. Biochem J 1987;245:575
196. Davidson HW, Peshavaria M, Hutton JC. Proteolytic conversion of proinsulin into insulin: Identification of a Ca^{++}-dependent acidic endopeptidase in isolated insulin secretory granules. Biochem J 1987;246:279
197. Steiner DF, Oyer PE. The biosynthesis of insulin and probable precursor of insulin by a human islet cell adenoma. Proc Natl Acad Sci USA 1967;57:473
198. Steiner DF, Cunningham D, Spigelman L, Aten B. Insulin biosynthesis: Evidence for a precursor. Science 1967;157:697
199. Rhodes CJ, Zumbrunn A, Bailyes EM, et al. The inhibition of proinsulin-processing endopeptidase activities by active-site-directed peptides. Biochem J 1989;258:305
200. Docherty KD, Rhodes CJ, Taylor NA, et al. Proinsulin endopeptidase substrate specificities defined by site-directed mutagenesis of proinsulin. J Biol Chem 1989;264:18335
201. Rhodes CJ, Brennan SO, Hutton JC. Proalbumin to albumin conversion by a proinsulin processing endopeptidase of insulin secretory granules. J Biol Chem 1989;264:14240
202. Fuller RS, Sterne RE, Thorner J. Enzymes required for yeast prohormone processing. Ann Rev Physiol 1988;50:345
203. Fuller RS, Brake A, Thorner J. Yeast prohormone processing enzyme (KEX2 gene product) is a Ca^{++}-dependent serine protease. Proc Natl Acad Sci USA 1989;86:1434
204. Julius D, Brake A, Blair L, et al. Isolation of the putative structural gene for the lysine-arginine cleaving endopeptidase for processing yeast prepro-a-factor. Cell 1984;37:1075
205. Mizuno K, Nakamura T, Oshima T, et al. Yeast KEX2 genes encodes an endopeptidase homologous to subtilisin-like proteases. Biochem Biophys Res Commun 1988;156:246
206. Smeekens SP, Steiner DF. Identification of a human insulinoma cDNA encoding a novel mammalian protein structurally related to the yeast dibasic processing KEX2. J Biol Chem 1990;265:2997
207. Seidah NG, Gaspar L, Mion P, et al. cDNA sequence of two distinct pituitary proteins homologous to Kex2 and furin gene products: Tissue-specific mRNAs encoding candidates for pro-hormone processing proteinases. DNA Cell Biol 1990;9:415
208. Smeekens SP, Avruch AS, LaMendola J, et al. Identification of a cDNA encoding a second putative prohormone convertase related to PC2 in AtT20 cells and islets of Langerhans. Proc Natl Acad Sci USA 1991;88:340
209. Seidah NG, Marcinkiewicz M, Benjannet S, et al. Cloning and primary sequence of a mouse candidate prohormone convertase PC1 homologous to PC2, Furin, and Kex2: Distinct chromosomal localization and messenger RNA distribution in brain and pituitary compared to PC2. Mol Endocrinol 1991;5:111
210. Seidah NG, Benjajjet S, Day R, Chrétien M. mPC1 and mPC2 are distinct pro-hormone processing proteinases. J Cell Biochem 1991; Abstract(suppl 15G):136
211. Bennett DL, Bailyes EM, Nielson E, et al. Identification of the type-II proinsulin processing endopeptidase as PC2, a member of the eukaryotic subtilisin family. J Biol Chem 1992;267:15229
212. Bailyes EM, Shennan KIJ, Seal AJ, et al. A member of the eukaryotic subtilisin family (PC3) has the enzymic properties of the type-I proinsulin-converting endopeptidase. Biochem J 1992;285:391
213. Bailyes EM, Bennett DL, Hutton JC. Proprotein-processing endopeptidases of the insulin secretory granule. Enzyme 1991;45:301
214. Smeekens SP, Montag AG, Thomas G, et al. Proinsulin processing by the subtilisin-related proprotein convertases furin, PC2 and PC3. Proc Natl Acad Sci USA 1992;89:8822
215. Sizonenko SV, Halban PA. Differential rates of conversion of rat proinsulins I and II. Biochem J 1991;278:621
216. Halban PA. Proinsulin processing in the regulated and the constitutive secretory pathway. Diabetologia 1994;37(suppl 2):S65
217. Zhou Y, Lindberg I. Purification and characterization of the prohormone convertase PC1 (PC3). J Biol Chem 1993;268:5615
218. Rholam M, Cohen P, Brakch N, et al. Evidence for β-turn structure in model peptides reproducing pro-ocytocin/neurophysin proteolytic processing site. Biochem Biophys Res Commun 1990;168:1066
219. Bek E, Berry R. Prohormone cleavage sites are associated with omega loops. Biochemistry 1990;29:178
220. Sizonenko S, Irminger J-C, Buhler L, et al. Kinetics of proinsulin conversion in human islets. Diabetes 1993;42:933
221. Sobey WJ, Beer SF, Carrington CA, et al. Sensitive and specific two-site immunoradiometric assays for human insulin, proinsulin, 65-66 and 32-33 split proinsulins. Biochem J 1989;260:535
222. Temple RC, Carrington CA, Luzio SD, et al. Insulin deficiency in non–insulin-dependent diabetes. Lancet February 1989;293

223. Neerman-Arbez M, Cirulli V, Halban PA. Levels of the conversion endoproteases PC1 (PC3) and PC2 distinguish between insulin-producing pancreatic beta cells and non-beta cells. Biochem J 1994;300:57
224. Hutton JC, Penn EJ, Peshavaria M. Low molecular weight constituents of isolated insulin secretory granules. Bivalent cations, adenine nucleotides and inorganic phosphate. Biochem J 1983;210:297
225. Orci L, Ravazzola M, Amherdt M, et al. Conversion of proinsulin to insulin occurs coordinately with acidification of maturing secretory granules. J Cell Biol 1986;103:2273
226. Formby B, Capito K, Egeberg J, Hedeskov CJ. Ca-activated ATPase activity in subcellular fractions of mouse pancreatic islets. Am J Physiol 1976;230:441
227. Rhodes CJ, Dawson AP, Hutton JC. Secretory granule Ca and the proteolytic conversion of prohormones. In Reid E, Cook GMW, Luzio P, eds. Biochemical Approaches to Cellular Calcium. Methodological Surveys in Biochemistry and Analysis, Volume 19. The Royal Society of Chemistry, London UK 1988:281–288
228. Benjannet S, Rondeau N, Day R, et al. PC1 and PC2 are pro-protein convertases capable of cleaving POMC at distinct pairs of basic residues. Proc Natl Acad Sci USA 1991;88:3564
229. Benjannet S, Reudelhuber T, Mercure C, et al. Proprotein conversion is determined by a multiplicity of factors including convertase processing, substrate specificity, and intracellular environment: Cell type-specific processing of human prorenin by the convertase PC1. J Biol Chem 1992;267:11417
230. Thomas L, Leduc R, Thorne BA, et al. Kex2-like endoproteases PC2 and PC3 accurately cleave a model prohormone in mammalian cells: Evidence for a common core of neuroendocrine processing enzymes. Proc Natl Acad Sci USA 1991;88:5297
231. Rhodes CJ, Thorne BA, Lincoln B, et al. Processing or proopiomelanocortin by insulin secretory granule proinsulin processing endopeptidases. J Biol Chem 1993;268:4267
232. Neerman-Arbez M, Sizonenko SV, Halban PA. Slow cleavage at the proinsulin B-chain/connecting peptide junction associated with low levels of endoprotease PC1/3 in transformed β-cells. J Biol Chem 1993;268:16098
233. Takagi H, Matsuzawa H, Ohta T, et al. Studies on the structure and function of subtilisin E by protein engineering. Ann N Y Acad Sci 1992;672:52
234. Wilcox CA, Fuller RS. Posttranslational processing of the prohormone-cleaving Kex2 protease in the *Saccharomyces cerevisiae* secretory pathway. J Cell Biol 1991;115:297
235. Rehemtulla A, Dorner A, Kaufman RJ. Regulation of PACE/furin processing: Requirement for a post-endoplasmic reticulum compartment and autoproteolytic activation. Proc Natl Acad Sci USA 1992;89:8235
236. Shennan KIJ, Smeekens SP, Steiner DF, Docherty K. Characterization of PC2, a mammalian Kex2 homologue, following expression of the cDNA in microinjected Xenopus oocytes. FEBS Lett 1991;284:277
237. Shennan KIJ, Seal AJ, Smeekens SP, et al. Site-directed mutagenesis and expression of PC2 in microinjected Xenopus oocytes. J Biol Chem 1991; 266;24011
238. Vindrola O, Lindberg I. Biosynthesis of the prohormone convertase mPC1 in AtT-20 cells. Mol Endocrinol 1992;6:1088
239. Nagamatsu S, Bolaffi JL, Grodsky GM. Direct effects of glucose on proinsulin synthesis and processing during desensitization. Endocrinology 1987;120:1225
240. Permutt MA, Chirgwin J, Giddings S, et al. Insulin biosynthesis and diabetes mellitus. Clin Biochem 1981;14:230
241. German MS, Moss LG, Rutter WJ. Regulation of gene expression by glucose and calcium in transfected primary islet cultures. J Biol Chem 1990;265:22063
242. Birch NP, Tracer HL, Hakes DJ, Loh YP. Coordinate regulation of mRNA levels of pro-opiomelanocortin and the candidate processing enzymes PC2 and PC3, but not furin, in rat pituitary intermediate lobe. Biochem Biophys Res Commun 1991;179:1311
243. Halban PA, Wollheim CB. Intracellular degradation of insulin stores by rat pancreatic islets in vitro. J Biol Chem 1980;255:6003
244. Halban PA, Renold AE. Influence of glucose of insulin handling by rat islets in culture: A reflection of integrated changes in insulin biosynthesis, release and intracellular degradation. Diabetes 1983;32:254
245. Schnell AH, Swenne I, Borg LAH. Lysosomes and pancreatic islet function: A quantitative estimation of crinophagy in the mouse pancreatic β-cell. Cell Tiss Res 1988;252:9
246. Rhodes CJ, Halban PA. The intracellular handling of insulin related peptides in isolated pancreatic islets: Evidence for differential rates of degradation of insulin and C-peptide. Biochem J 1988;251:23
247. Halban PA, Mutkoski R, Dodson G, Orci L. Resistance of the insulin crystal to lysosomal proteases: Implications for pancreatic B-cell crinophagy. Diabetologia 1987;30:348
248. Lacy PE, Howell SL, Young DA, Fink CJ. New hypothesis of insulin secretion. Nature 1968;219:1177
249. Lacy PE, Walker MM, Fink CJ. Perifusion of isolated islets in vitro: Participation of the microtubular system in the phasic mechanism of insulin release. Diabetes 1972;21:987
250. Malaisse WJ, Malaisse-Legae F, Van Obberghen E, et al. Role of microtubules in the phasic pattern of insulin release. Ann N Y Acad Sci 1975;253:630
251. Kelly RB. Microtubules, membrane traffic and cell organization. Cell 1990; 61:5
252. Bonner-Weir S. Morphological evidence for pancreatic polarity of β-cell within islets of Langerhans. Diabetes 1988;37:616
253. Lombardi T, Montesano R, Wohlwend AL, et al. Evidence for the polarization of plasma membrane domains in pancreatic endocrine cells. Nature 1985; 313:694
254. Howell SL, Taylor KW. The secretion of newly synthesized insulin in vitro. Biochem J 1967;102:922
255. Halban PA. Differential rates of release of newly synthesized and of stored insulin from pancreatic islets. Endocrinology 1982;110:1183
256. Cleveland DW. Microtubule MAPping. Cell 1990;60:701
257. Vale RD, Goldstein LSB. One motor, many tails: An expanding repertoire of force-generating enzymes. Cell 1990;60:883
258. Gelfand VI, Bershadsky AD. Microtubule dynamics: Mechanism, regulation and function. Ann Rev Cell Biol 1991;7:93
259. Porter ME, Johnson KA. Dynein structure and function. Ann Rev Cell Biol 1989;5:119
260. Balczon R, Overstreet KA, Zinkowski RP, et al. The identification, purification, and characterization of a pancreatic β-cell form of the microtubule adenosine triphosphatase kinesin. Endocrinology 1992;131:331
261. Montague W, Howell SL, Green IC. Insulin release and the microtubular system in islets of Langerhans. Biochem J 1975;148:237
262. Wang JL, Easom RA, Hughes JH, McDaniel ML. Evidence for a role of microfilaments in insulin release from purified β-cells. Biochem Biophys Res Commun 1990;171:424
263. Orci L, Gabbay KH, Malaisse WJ. Pancreatic β-cell web: Its possible role in insulin secretion. Science 1972;175:1128
264. Penn EJ, Brocklehurst KW, Sopwith AM, et al. Ca^{++}-calmodulin dependent myosin light-chain phosphorylating activity in insulin secreting tissues. FEBS Lett 1982;139:4
265. MacDonald MJ, Kawluru A. Calcium-calmodulin myosin phosphorylation in pancreatic islets. Diabetes 1982;31:566
266. Vitale ML, Rodriquez Del Castillo A, Tchakarov L, Trifaró JM. Cortical filamentous actin dissembly and sciderin redistribution during chromaffin cell stimulation precede exocytosis, a phenomenon not exhibited by gelsolin. J Cell Biol 1991;113:1057
267. Halban PA. Proinsulin trafficking and processing in the pancreatic β-cell. Trends in Endocrinology and Metabolism 1990;May:261
268. Gembal M, Gilon P, Henquin J-C. Evidence that glucose can control insulin release independently from its action on ATP-sensitive K^+ channels in mouse β-cells. J Clin Invest 1992;89:1288
269. Vallar L, Biden TJ, Wollheim CB. Guanine nucleotides induce Ca^{++}-independent insulin secretion from permeabilized RINm5F cells. J Biol Chem 1987;262:5049
270. Li G, Regazzi R, Balch WE, Wollheim CB. Stimulation of insulin release with permeabilized HIT-T15 cells by a synthetic peptide corresponding to the effector domain of the small GTP-binding protein Rab3. FEBS Lett 1993;327:145
271. Olszewski S, Deeney JT, Schuppin GT, et al. Rab3A effector domain peptides induce insulin exocytosis via a specific interaction with a cytosolic protein doublet. J Biol Chem 1994;269:27987
272. Baffy G, Yang L, Wolf BA, Williamson JR. G-protein specificity in signaling pathways that mobilize calcium in insulin secreting beta-TC3 cells. Diabetes 1993;42:1878
273. Ashcroft SJH. Protein phosphorylation and beta cell function. Diabetologia 1994;37(suppl 2):S21
274. Howell SL, Jones PM, Persaud SJ. Regulation of insulin secretion: The role of second messengers. Diabetologia 1994;37(suppl 2):S30
275. Sorenson RL, Brelje TC, Roth C. Effect of tyrosine kinase inhibitors on islets of Langerhans: Evidence for tyrosine kinases in the regulation of insulin secretion. Endocrinology 1994;134:1975
276. Ratcliff H, Jones PM. Effects of okadaic acid on insulin secretion from rat islets of Langerhans. Biochim Biophys Acta 1993;1175:188
277. Bennett MK, Scheller RH. The molecular machinery for secretion is conserved from yeast to neurons. Proc Natl Acad Sci USA 1993;90:2559
278. Kelly RB. Storage and release of neurotransmitters. Neuron 1993;10:43
279. Bennett MK, Scheller RH. A molecular description of synaptic vesicle membrane trafficking. Ann Rev Biochem 1994;63:63

Diabetes Mellitus, edited by Derek LeRoith, Simeon I. Taylor, and Jerrold M. Olefsky. Lippincott–Raven Publishers, Philadelphia © 1996.

Chapter 5

The Role of Glucose Transport and Phosphorylation in Glucose-Stimulated Insulin Secretion

John H. Johnson and Christopher B. Newgard

A General Biochemical Overview of Glucose-Stimulated Insulin Secretion

Glucose homeostasis is maintained in normal animals by the reciprocal regulation of insulin secretion by β-cells and glucagon secretion by α-cells of the islets of Langerhans. The mechanisms by which changes in blood glucose are recognized by these cells have been the subject of intensive investigation for many years. In this chapter, we will focus on the role of glucose transport and phosphorylation in dictating the dose dependence and magnitude of the glucose-stimulated insulin secretion response.

Early work on how β-cells recognize and respond to changes in blood glucose evolved into a debate over the "glucose-receptor" versus the "fuel" hypotheses.[1–3] The former model holds that glucose binds to a β-cell receptor that triggers insulin release via unidentified second messengers, whereas the latter model argues that the metabolism of glucose itself produces the key coupling factor or factors. Over time, the bulk of evidence has accumulated in favor of the requirement of a metabolic signal (or signals) for the initiation of the cascade resulting in insulin secretion.[1,3] Major support for the now favored fuel hypothesis comes from the fact that both glucose uptake and metabolism are required to support insulin secretion. Nonmetabolizable analogs of glucose are incapable of evoking insulin secretion, and inhibitors of glucose metabolism blunt the insulin secretory response.[1,3] The curves used to demonstrate the glucose concentration dependence of insulin release and glycolytic rate are virtually superimposable,[1] but it is still possible that metabolism alone is not sufficient for insulin secretion. The finding that there are insulin secretory response differences, but no glucose metabolism differences, in cell lines transfected with different isoforms of the glucose transporter suggests that combined events including, but not limited to, glucose metabolism are at work.[4]

The exact metabolic signals triggering the insulin secretory cascade have not yet been identified, although several candidates have been suggested. Recent work has focused on the mitochondrial glycerol phosphate shuttle[5,6] and the malate-aspartate shuttle[6] as important contributors of reduced nicotinamide adenine dinucleotide (NADH) for mitochondrial ATP formation during β-cell glucose oxidation. A primary role for flavin adenine dinucleotide–linked mitochondrial glycerol phosphate dehydrogenase in generating reducing power for ATP production is suggested by the fact that glyceraldehyde is a potent insulin secretagogue, whereas pyruvate is not. Changes in the β-cell ATP:ADP ratio brought about by glucose metabolism are thought to inhibit the ATP-sensitive K^+ channel, which results in membrane depolarization and activation of voltage-sensitive L-type Ca^{++} channels. Glucose usage has been shown to close K^+ channels[7] and to stimulate Ca^{++} entry into β-cells.[8] Further, agents that inhibit L-type Ca^{++} channel flux into β-cells inhibit glucose-stimulated insulin secretion,[8,9] and the α_1 subunit containing the voltage sensor and Ca^{++} pore is downregulated in response to glucose infusion in vivo.[10] Although the K_{ATP} and Ca^{++} channel activities are clearly regulated by glucose in β-cells, the sugar has little effect on islet cell ATP:ADP ratios.[11] Thus, the mechanisms by which nucleotide signal ion channel activity remain to be elucidated, although one intriguing possibility is that nucleotide concentration changes may be occurring in a localized setting. A variety of other metabolic events, such as changes in mitochondrial metabolites, phospholipid turnover, and fatty acid oxidation, are influenced by glucose flux and may be important in glucose-induced insulin secretion.[8,9,12]

Exocytosis of insulin secretory vesicles in response to ion fluxes is believed to be modulated by one or more protein kinase activities. The Ca^{++} calmodulin class of protein kinases is thought to associate with cytoskeletal elements of the β-cell and is a potential participant in the final membrane fusion events.[13] Also, protein kinase C has been shown to be translocated from the cytosol to the plasma membrane in a manner that is dependent on β-cell glucose metabolism.[14] In one study, glucose was found to increase the phosphorylation of the protein kinase C substrate myristolated alanine-rich protein C kinase substrate (MARCKS), resulting in its dissociation from cytoskeletal elements.[15] Further, protein kinase C activation by diacylglycerol could provide a link between insulin secretion and phospholipid metabolism in response to glucose.[9] Thus, the protein kinases may play a modulatory role in insulin secretion by controlling the interactions of secretory vesicles with cytoskeletal elements. The foregoing concepts are summarized in schematic form in Figure 5-1.

The Role of GLUT-2 and Glucokinase in the Regulation of Glucose-Induced Insulin Secretion

Insulin secretion in response to increases in blood glucose levels requires both transport and metabolism of glucose because nonmetabolizable analogs of glucose are clearly transported but do not stimulate insulin release.[1] In mammalian cells, the first two steps of metabolism are transport and phosphorylation, carried out by a family of facilitated glucose transport proteins and glucose phosphorylating enzymes, respectively, which differ in their tissue distribution and catalytic activities.[1,16] In the β-cell, these are represented by GLUT-2 and glucokinase, whose activities change throughout the range of blood glucose concentrations.

Under normal conditions, GLUT-2–mediated transport activity greatly exceeds the rate of glucose utilization, and therefore glucokinase has been postulated to be the point at which glucose utilization in β-cells is controlled.[1,17] This model is supported by the fact that glucokinase activity in β-cells is substantially lower than other potentially regulatory enzymes (e.g., phosphofructokinase, pyruvate kinase[1,18]). Furthermore, the glucose concentration dependence of glucokinase is virtually identical to glucose metabo-

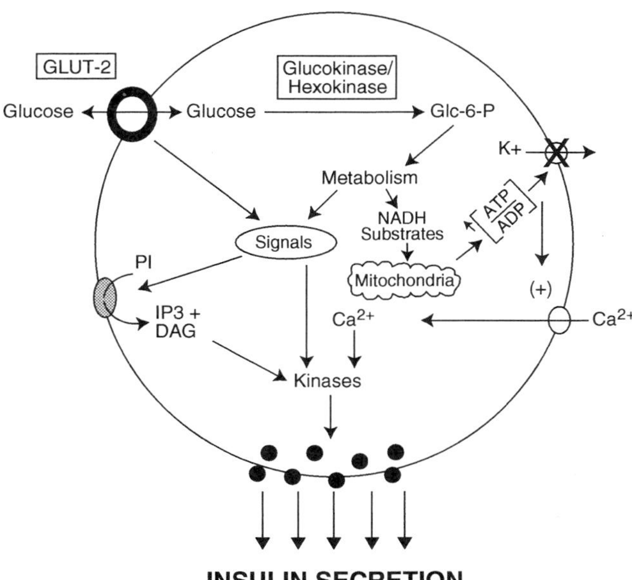

Figure 5-1. Schematic summary of biochemical events in the glucose-stimulated insulin secretion pathway. See text for details.

lism in islets,[1] and inhibitors of glucokinase activity (e.g., alloxan, mannoheptulose, glucoseamine) also inhibit glucose-stimulated insulin secretion.[1,3,19–21]

The hexokinase family consists of four members (I–IV). Hexokinases I–III have apparent affinities for glucose in the 10–100 μM range and have molecular weights of approximately 100 kd. In contrast, glucokinase (or hexokinase IV) has an apparent K_m for glucose of about 8 mM, a molecular weight of about 50 kd, and shows a sigmoidal dependence on glucose concentration with a Hill coefficient of 1.5.[22] Glucose-6-phosphate is a potent allosteric inhibitor of hexokinases I–III, but has little effect on glucokinase.[23] Glucokinase has a discrete tissue distribution and is found in liver, β-cells of the islets, gastrointestinal cells, and anterior pituitary cells.[24–28] It is noteworthy that each of these tissues may play a role in mammalian glucose homeostasis. Glucokinase is encoded by a single gene in rodents and humans.[24–27,29–31] The glucokinase protein expressed in islets and pituitary cells is identical to that found in liver except for the N-terminal sequence of 15 amino acids.[25–27] Alternative splicing of unique segments encoded by different exonic regions produce liver and islet/pituitary isoforms of glucokinase in rats, and similar isoforms plus a second liver type in humans (see Fig. 2 for comparison of the N-terminal sequences). The physiologic significance of the different isoforms is at present unclear, although it has been suggested that the highly charged nature of the additional amino acids in the β-cell protein may allow it to interact with other cellular proteins or structures.[26]

The kinetic properties of glucokinase and its tissue distribution has long suggested a regulatory role for the enzyme in β-cell glucose metabolism.[1,32] Islets contain both low and high K_m hexokinase activities.[1] Given that GLUT-2 maintains glucose concentrations close to equilibrium across the β-cell membrane under steady-state conditions, levels of glucose-6-phosphate within the β-cell may curtail low-K_m hexokinase activity, following glucokinase to play the primary regulatory role.[18,33]

Recent molecular and genetic studies provide strong support for an essential role of glucokinase in glucose sensing. Families with an autosomal dominant form of non–insulin-dependent diabetes (NIDDM) termed maturity-onset diabetes of the young (MODY) have been shown to have at least 28 different mutations in the glucokinase gene, many of which have been shown to result in altered activity of the enzyme (see Chapters 1 and 27).[34–37] Using the sequences of glucokinase, the activity alterations associated with mutations found in MODY patients, and inferences based on the X-ray crystallographic structure of yeast hexokinase, Pilkis et al.[38] presented a structural model of glucokinase. In this model, the MODY mutations affecting enzyme activity fall for the most part within the postulated glucose binding cleft. Conservative mutations appear to have modest effects on glucokinase function, whereas replacement of amino acids with residues incapable of interacting with the glucose molecule or disrupting the secondary protein structure around the binding cleft results in severe impairment of glucokinase function.[36,37] Interestingly, in this model two of the polymorphisms that have been identified in β-cell glucokinase are not predicted to affect its function, and this has been confirmed in one instance.[36,37] All MODY patients with glucokinase mutations studied to date are heterozygotes, with one normal and one affected allele. The threshold for glucose-stimulated insulin secretion is higher in MODY patients, and the total amount of insulin released is less than in normal patients.[39,40] The severity of these defects is generally correlated with the function of the mutant allele, as revealed by expression of the mutant genes in bacteria and kinetic analysis of the purified proteins.[36,37]

```
                            (-)   (-)   (+)         (+)         (-)               (+)   (+)   (-)   (+)
Human Islet     Met   Len   Asp   Asp   Arg   Ala   Arg   Met   Glu   Ala   Ala   Lys   Lys   Glu   Lys   Val

                 |     |     |     |     |     |     |     |     |     |           |     |     |     |     |
                            (-)   (-)   (+)         (+)         (-)               (+)   (+)   (-)   (+)
Rat Islet       Met   Len   Asp   Asp   Arg   Ala   Arg   Met   Glu   Ala   Thu   Lys   Lys   Glu   Lys   Val

                 |                 |                 |                 |                                   |
                                  (-)               (+)
Rat Liver       Met   Ala   Met   Asp   Thr   Thr   Arg   Cys   Gly   Ala   Trp   Leu   Leu   Thr   Leu   Val

                 |     |     |     |           |     |                 |     |           |     |     |     |
                                  (-)               (+)
Human Liver2    Met   Ala   Met   Asp   Val   Thr   Arg   Ser   Trp   Ala   Trp   Thr   Leu   Thr   Leu   Val
                                                                                     \/
                             |                       |     |     |                   Ala                  |
                                        (+)         (+)                                                   |
Human Liver1                Met   Pro   Arg   Pro   Arg   Ser   Trp   Leu   Pro   Tvp   Asn   Ser   Tvp   Val
                                                                                     \/
                                                                                     Pro
```

Figure 5-2. Alignment of the N-terminal sequences of human and rat glucokinase isoforms. Note the near-exact sequence identity of rat and human islet glucokinase sequences, compared with the lesser homology between the rat liver and the two human liver forms of the enzyme. Data taken from references 25–27 and 29–31.

The effect of altered β-cell glucokinase activity also has been studied in transgenic mice, in which a glucokinase-specific "ribozyme" was used to decrease the expression of the enzyme by 70%.[41] Although the animals remained normoglycemic, pancreas perfusion studies revealed a change in the glucose response threshold and a reduction in total insulin release similar to that described in MODY patients. The molecular and genetic studies thus clearly provide evidence for a rate-limiting role for glucokinase, and show that decreasing the normal complement of enzyme activity has detrimental effects on glucose responsiveness. Interestingly, the glucose transport capacity and activities of distal glycolytic steps such as phosphofructokinase exceed glucokinase activity by one order of magnitude or more,[1,18,42] suggesting that overexpression of the latter enzyme may cause a significantly enhanced secretory response. The actual consequences of overexpression of glucose phosphorylating enzymes in islets are discussed below.

The precise role of GLUT-2 in the glucose-sensing pathway is more difficult to define. It has been appreciated for some time that glucose is rapidly taken up and is in near equilibrium across the cell membrane of islet cells.[1,42] This has been shown to be largely a property of β-cell glucose handling because purified α-cells are much slower in equilibrating intracellular and extracellular concentrations of glucose.[43] GLUT-2 belongs to a family of facilitated diffusion glucose transporters and is unique in that it has a high capacity for transport and a low affinity for glucose.[16,44,45] The other members of the family have K_ms for glucose in the 1–3 mM range and would be expected to be operating at or near their maximum velocities under normal blood glucose conditions, whereas GLUT-2 has a K_m of 17 mM and would respond to changes in blood glucose concentrations by dramatically increasing its activity.[44,45] This would ensure that β-cells and other cells expressing GLUT-2 could readily discriminate between changes in blood glucose and thus respond appropriately. These characteristics make the relationship of GLUT-2 to other members of the glucose transporter family similar to the relationship of glucokinase to the hexokinases. Also, GLUT-2 and glucokinase have very similar tissue distributions and are found in tissues that are critically important in the maintenance of normal glucose homeostasis.[26,28,44] Unlike glucokinase, the GLUT-2 primary sequence is identical in all tissues examined within a species. There is a small (3000-kd) difference in molecular weight between liver and β-cell proteins, which is due probably to a difference in the glycosylation of the molecule.[44] Thorens and coworkers[46] have shown that >95% of GLUT-2 expression is at the cell surface of β-cells, that the protein does not recycle into intracellular vesicles, and that expression of the transporter occurs with a half-time of approximately 7 hours.

Alignment of the primary sequences of the entire family of facilitated diffusion glucose transporters reveals that they are related proteins. There is remarkable conservation of the transmembrane segments of these proteins, whereas extramembranous regions such as the N- and C-termini, the large extracellular loop between membrane spanning regions 1 and 2, and the large intracellular loop between membrane spanning segments 6 and 7 are much less conserved (see reference 16 for review). Substitution of the C-terminal segment of GLUT-1 with the corresponding region of GLUT-2 produced a chimeric transporter with a K_m that was significantly greater than that of native GLUT-1 when the two molecules were expressed in COS cells.[47] Native GLUT-2 was expressed only at very low levels in these experiments, so it remains to be determined whether other structural elements are also required for full GLUT-2–like activity.

Finally, GLUT-2 expression appears to be regulatable in vivo. In one study, hyperinsulinemic clamping resulted in a sharp decrease in GLUT-2 mRNA levels in islets and a commensurate decrease in glucose transport capacity.[48] Various iatrogenic agents producing diabetes in animals, such as dexamethasone and streptozotocin, have similar effects on GLUT-2 expression. Interestingly, there appears to be tissue specificity to this regulation (discussed below). Future work on structure/function relationships will be important because there is evidence from some experimental systems that the effects of GLUT-2 on glucose sensing are not necessarily linked to changes in glycolytic flux (see below).

Lessons from Animal Models

A great deal has been learned about the glucose-stimulated insulin secretory pathway from the study of animal models of both insulin-dependent diabetes mellitus (IDDM) and NIDDM. Although these two disease forms have different etiologies, they share the common feature of a progressive decline in glucose-stimulated insulin secretion during the preovert phases of the disease until, at onset, there is no glucose-stimulated insulin secretion while the insulin secretory response to nonglucose secretagogues remains intact. In the BB/Wor rat, a rodent model of IDDM, a progressive loss of glucose-stimulated insulin secretion has been documented to be accompanied by a large reduction in the ability of islet cells to transport glucose.[50] In the first 24 hours of diabetes, islet glucose transport rates were reduced by >90%, and it was proposed that this loss of transport might play a role in the loss of glucose responsiveness.[50] Subsequent work showed that as these animals progressed to having IDDM, the β-cells of the islets progressively lost glucose responsiveness as well as GLUT-2 at their cell surface.[51] On the first day of diabetes, only 45% of the surviving β-cells expressed immunodetectable GLUT-2. Coupled with the loss of β-cell mass, this reduction in expression of GLUT-2 could account for the loss of glucose recognition by the remaining cells.[50,51]

In contrast to the autoimmune destruction of β-cells in IDDM, the NIDDM form of diabetes is associated with the loss of sensitivity of peripheral tissues to insulin as well as a deterioration of regulated insulin secretion despite an apparently normal complement of β-cells in the islet. Because insulin resistance is a common feature of obesity and because only a fraction of subjects with obesity-related insulin resistance develop diabetes, it follows that insulin resistance may be required but is not sufficient for the development of NIDDM. Additionally, loss of glucose sensitivity appears to play a role and, as in IDDM, β-cells from humans or experimental animals with NIDDM-like syndromes fail to secrete insulin in response to a glucose challenge at the onset of disease.[52–55]

The expression of β-cell GLUT-2 has been studied in a variety of genetic and pharmacologic models of NIDDM. The male Zucker diabetic rat (ZDF/DRT-fa) is an obese, diabetic animal with associated insulin resistance.[56] The male rat becomes diabetic with a frequency of virtually 100% within 6–8 weeks, whereas the female rat is obese and insulin resistant but does not develop NIDDM. Temporal studies of this genetic model have shown that glucose-stimulated insulin secretion progressively declines until, at the onset of NIDDM, there is no response to glucose while the response to arginine remains completely intact.[54] These pancreata also show a decline in GLUT-2 expression until, at onset, the protein is detectable in only 60% of the β-cells.[54] This decline continues until the transporter ultimately becomes undetectable.[57] The correlation of the loss of GLUT-2 and the loss of glucose-stimulated insulin secretion was $r = 0.98$, and 3-*O*-methyl glucose transport rates of these islet cells were reduced by 80% at 15 mM concentrations.[54]

Feeding the glycosidase inhibitor, acarbose, prevented the development of hyperglycemia in these animals but was not found to prevent the downregulation of expression of β-cell GLUT-2.[57] Furthermore, hyperglycemic infusion[48] or incubation of islets at high glucose concentrations[57] increased GLUT-2 expression. These results are consistent with recent findings showing that the GLUT-2 promoter/enhancer is activated by glucose in INS-1 cells.[58] Thus, hyperglycemia per se could not have been responsible for GLUT-2 downregulation. Although insulin infusion downregulates GLUT-2 in normal animals,[48] it is doubtful that this can explain the reduced GLUT-2 expression in Zucker diabetic fatty rats, considering that the obese female rat is as hyperinsulinemic as the male rat but does not become diabetic and retains β-cell GLUT-2.[54,57] Although correlations do not prove a cause-and-effect relationship, the dramatic loss of transport function in conjunction with protein expression suggests that GLUT-2 regulation could play a role in β-cell dysfunction in the Zucker diabetic rat.

The Zucker rat model is not unique in this regard. Similar observations have now been documented in the db/db mouse,[59] the GK rat,[55,60] the dexamethasone-treated Wistar and Zucker fatty female rat,[61] and the streptozotocin-treated rat.[62] Decreased GLUT-2 protein is partially accounted for by decreased GLUT-2 mRNA in the Zucker rat[54] and db/db mouse.[59] It is important to note that although GLUT-2 expression is downregulated in β-cells in every model of NIDDM or IDDM studied to date, no effects on liver GLUT-2 expression have been observed, suggesting that the GLUT-2 gene is differentially regulated in liver and islet cells.

Glucocorticoid-induced diabetes occurs in normal rats with a frequency similar to that seen in humans.[61] In this model, all animals show some degree of hyperinsulinemia, but only 16% become diabetic. The diabetic animals show loss of glucose-stimulated insulin secretion at onset of diabetes and reduced β-cell GLUT-2 expression. The animals that do not become diabetic show GLUT-2 expression on 100% of their β-cells and mount a normal secretory response to a glucose challenge.[61] In contrast to other models, however, the dexamethasone-induced diabetes model has mRNA levels for GLUT-2 that are increased relative to controls, suggesting a post-transcriptional mechanism for downregulation.[61] Table 5-1 summarizes changes in glucose-stimulated insulin secretion, GLUT-2 expression, and glucose uptake in all of the models that we have discussed in this chapter.

What are the factors involved in this downregulation? An elegant set of experiments was performed by Thorens et al.[59] suggesting that the factors are external and may even be humoral in origin. In these experiments, islets from diabetic db/db mice were transplanted under the kidney capsule of normal mice, resulting in restoration of GLUT-2 expression. Conversely, transplantation of islets from normal animals into diabetic db/db mice or animals rendered diabetic by streptozotocin injection resulted in the downregulation of expression of the protein.[59] These data strongly suggest the importance of environmental factors in GLUT-2 expression. Insulin clearly is eliminated as a candidate factor because down-regulation of GLUT-2 occurred in both insulin-deficient and hyperinsulinemic forms of diabetes. Based on work cited above, in which experimentally induced hyperglycemia caused an increase rather than a decrease in GLUT-2 expression, it also seems unlikely that glucose per se is responsible for the effects. Recent work of Unger[63] implicates circulating fatty acids as a potential modulator of the glucose-stimulated insulin secretion response: When cultured for 7 days in the presence of 2 mM free fatty acids, cultured islets exhibited basal hyperinsulinemia and an attenuated response to stimulatory glucose levels. The role of lipids in downregulation of GLUT-2 in transplantation models remains to be investigated.

Lessons from Insulinoma Cell Lines

Insulinoma cell lines have long been used for studies of glucose-induced insulin secretion. Such lines are easy to manipulate but often exhibit glucose responses that are quite different from those of normal islets. For example, the RINm5F cell line is unresponsive to glucose,[64] whereas the MIN6, INS-1, and βTC-6 cell lines respond to glucose at concentrations similar to those eliciting responses in pancreatic β-cells.[65–67] Interestingly, unresponsive lines exhibit absent or low GLUT-2 or glucokinase expression, whereas the glucose-responsive lines retain expression of both proteins.

The RIN 1046-38 cell line secretes insulin in response to a glucose challenge, but the response is maximal at 0.5 mM glucose. These cells progressively lose their ability to respond to glucose with passage in culture until at about passage 35 they become unresponsive.[68,69] Analysis of GLUT-2 and glucokinase expression in these cells reveals substantial levels of both gene products at low passage numbers, and a decline in both paralleling the loss of glucose sensitivity.[69] As will be shown later, the restoration of GLUT-2 expression at critical times during the passage-dependent loss of glucose sensing in RIN 1046-38 cells results in restoration of their glucose-sensing capacity.

A number of insulinoma cell lines have been established from tumors of transgenic animals wherein expression of the SV40 large T-antigen is directed by the insulin promoter/enhancer. Early lines produced by this method (e.g., βTC-1, βTC-3) secreted insulin in response to subphysiologic glucose concentrations and expressed low levels of GLUT-2 and high levels of GLUT-1.[70,71] The shift to the left of the dose-response curve in these cells has been correlated with a leftward shift in the glucose utilization curve, and thus the secretory profiles are consistent with a shift to both low K_m transport and metabolism.[71] Newer lines generated using the same strategy secrete insulin at or near normal physiologic glucose concentrations. Miyazaki et al.[65] reported on two lines, designated MIN6 and MIN7, that have different phenotypes and different insulin secretory profiles despite being generated with the identical insulin promoter–SV40 large T-antigen construct. The MIN6 line showed a 10-fold increase in insulin secretion when glucose concentrations were raised from 5 to 25 mM, whereas the MIN7 line was found to be unresponsive to glucose. The MIN6 line was found to express high levels of GLUT-2 and low levels of GLUT-1, whereas the MIN7 line expressed GLUT-1 and virtually no GLUT-2.[65] Thus, in these and other cell lines, the expression of GLUT-2 appears to be important for the maintenance of the glucose-induced secretory response at any level. Work by Efrat et al. has resulted in the establishment of the βTC-6 and βTC-7 cell lines, which secrete insulin in response to glucose in a manner similar to β-cells.[67] These cells retain GLUT-2 expression, but also retain glucokinase:hexokinase ratios that are similar to those of the β-cell. In one study,[67] passaging these cells in culture resulted in a

Table 5-1. Glucose-Stimulated Insulin Secretion, Glucose Uptake and GLUT-2 Expression in Animal Models of Diabetes

Model	Insulin Secretion	Glucose Uptake	GLUT-2 Expression	References
BB/Wor rat	D	D	D	50, 51
ZDF rat	D	D	D	54, 57
GK rat	D	D	D	55, 60
db/db mouse	D	ND	D	59
neonatal				
streptozotocin rat	D	ND	D	62
dexamethasone rat	D	D	D*	61

*In the case of GLUT-2 expression in the dexamethasone-injected rat, GLUT-2 protein levels were decreased while mRNA was increased. D = decreased; I = increased; ND = not determined.

leftward shift in the glucose dose-response curve with no apparent change in the expression of GLUT-2 and GLUT-1. Glucokinase activity rose twofold in these cells but hexokinase activity rose sixfold, resulting in a shift toward low K_m glucose utilization. The increased hexokinase-mediated phosphorylation of glucose was proposed to be the basis of the leftward shift in glucose-induced insulin secretion in these cells by increasing the levels of intermediates for secretion signaling at low glucose concentrations.

Efrat et al.[70] reported that soft agar cloning of single cells from the βTC6 cell line resulted in the establishment of a line that retains glucose responsiveness at physiologic glucose concentrations through at least 55 passages (greater than 1 year). This line, designated βTC6-F7, expresses high levels of glucokinase and GLUT-2, low levels of hexokinase activity, and does not express detectable GLUT-1. The conclusions reached by these authors is that these types of insulinomas represent a heterogeneous population of cells with respect to the glucose-response phenotype, and that the less differentiated cells in the population have a selective advantage in culture over the more differentiated cells. These results also suggest that it is possible for the specialized proteins of the glucose-sensing apparatus to remain functional in a transformed, proliferating cell line.[72]

For most insulinoma lines, the bulk of evidence suggests that although GLUT-2 may be an essential enabling factor for glucose responsiveness, the critical step for determining the concentration threshold of the response is glucose phosphorylation, and more specifically, the glucokinase:hexokinase ratio (see the following section of this chapter). One exception to this may be the hamster insulinoma cell line HIT, which responds to glucose at subphysiologic glucose concentrations and expresses low levels of GLUT-2. Culturing these cells in different concentrations of glucose changes the levels of GLUT-2 mRNA (and presumably protein) and results in roughly proportional changes in the magnitude of the insulin secretory response, suggesting that glucose transport rather than phosphorylation is limiting in these cells.[73]

Lessons from Engineered Cell Lines

To assess more directly the relative contributions of glucose transport and phosphorylation in the glucose-induced insulin secretory pathway, we and others have been using molecular techniques to alter the level of expression of these molecules in insulin-secreting cell lines. Two types of cells have been used for these studies. AtT-20ins cells are derived from corticotropin-secreting cells of the anterior pituitary, and they are stably transfected with the human insulin cDNA driven by a viral promoter.[74] Other studies have been performed with RIN 1046-38 or MIN insulinoma cell lines.

The AtT-20ins cell line completely lacks the ability to secrete insulin in response to a glucose challenge although it constitutively expresses the β-cell form of glucokinase.[27] These cells express low levels of glucokinase enzymatic activity, consistent with their expression of a mixture of normal and cryptically deleted glucokinase transcripts.[27,75] Expression of these deleted products in bacteria confirmed that they do not encode for functional protein.[75,76] Unlike the liver and β-cell, AtT-20ins cells do not express GLUT-2, but instead contain low levels of GLUT-1.[27]

Stable transfection of AtT-20ins cells with the GLUT-2 cDNA driven by the cytomegalovirus promoter/enhancer resulted in isolation of clones with levels of GLUT-2 mRNA and protein similar to the normal islet.[77] Further, the kinetic constants derived for 3-*O*-methyl glucose transport in these lines were essentially indistinguishable from those measured in dispersed islet cell preparations. GLUT-2 expression conferred a clear glucose-induced insulin secretory response, albeit with maximal responsiveness at 10–50 μM, well below the threshold for stimulation of normal β-cells.[77] In perifusion studies, GLUT-2 expressing AtT-20ins cells responded to glucose within 2 minutes of exposure to glucose and in some cases showed a biphasic secretory response reminiscent of islets.[4] To rule out the possibility that increased glucose flux across the cell could be the important determinant of glucose sensitivity, two types of experiments were performed. The first experiment showed that nonmetabolizable analogs of glucose could not stimulate insulin secretion in these cells. The results of the second experiment were even more important: Overexpression of GLUT-1 in these cells was shown to be ineffective in conferring glucose sensitivity despite raising transport rates by more than one order of magnitude.[4] Surprisingly, overexpression of either GLUT-1 or GLUT-2 had no significant effect on glucose utilization compared to untransfected cells.[4] These results with GLUT-1–overexpressing cells do not prove the lack of a requirement for a threshold level of glucose transport because their capacity for glucose uptake (V_{max}) was still only one-third that of the GLUT-2 lines. Nevertheless, the fact that glucose utilization rates were similar in these lines suggests that a structural element of GLUT-2 that is distinct from GLUT-1 may be important in glucose signaling.[4]

Because the RIN 1046-38 cell line is a β-cell–derived tumor line that loses GLUT-2 and glucokinase in parallel with glucose responsiveness during continuous passage in culture, similar strategies were employed with these cells.[69] Transfection of GLUT-2 into intermediate-passage cells (35 passages) resulted in a restoration of glucose recognition, whereas transfection of GLUT-2 into high-passage cells (90 passages) did not restore glucose responsiveness. These results suggest that other essential components of the glucose-sensing apparatus are lost with continuous culture. The presence of GLUT-2 in these cells may have delayed, but did not prevent the loss of these components, because growth of intermediate-passage, glucose-responsive GLUT-2–transfected cells for an additional 30 passages resulted in diminished glucose responsiveness.[69]

Interestingly, GLUT-2 transfection of intermediate-passage RIN 1046-38 cells, but not AtT-20ins cells, resulted in a fourfold increase in glucokinase enzymatic activity that was at least partially accounted for by an increase in immunodetectable glucokinase protein.[69] The increase in glucokinase was not observed in GLUT-2–transfected high-passage cells. Despite the increase in high K_m glucokinase activity, GLUT-2–transfected intermediate-passage RIN cells still exhibited a maximal insulin secretory response at subphysiologic levels of glucose.[69] This was likely due to the fact that hexokinase activity was approximately four times greater in these cells than in normal islets. To test this hypothesis, GLUT-2–transfected, intermediate passage RIN cells were preincubated with 2-deoxyglucose and challenged with glucose. The rationale for this experiment was that the accumulation of 2-deoxyglucose 6-phosphate would accumulate and inhibit hexokinase but not glucokinase. Pretreatment of the cells with 2-deoxyglucose resulted in a shift of the dose-response curve for glucose from a maximal stimulatory concentration of 50 μM to 5 mM, a change of two orders of magnitude.[69] Although this is still clearly lower than the stimulatory threshold of normal β-cells, these data provide encouragement for the development of molecular strategies that might permanently modulate the glucokinase:hexokinase activity ratio. Consistent with demonstrating a major role for this parameter in dictating the threshold for glucose responsiveness in insulinoma cells, Ishihara and colleagues[78] showed that overexpression of hexokinase I in MIN6 cells resulted in a sharp leftward shift in the threshold for activation of insulin release and glucose usage, whereas overexpression of GLUT-1 had no effect on glucose dose response.

Lessons from Gene Transfer Studies in Normal Islets

As discussed earlier, recent molecular and genetic studies have clearly demonstrated the consequences of reduced expression of glucokinase in normal islet β-cells.[34–37,39–41] We and other researchers have used molecular techniques to investigate the metabolic and secretory consequences of increasing the glucose phosphorylating capacity, and also have determined whether any such effects are dependent on the hexokinase isoform expressed. German[79] demonstrated that overexpression of hexokinase I in fetal islets resulted in a sharp reduction in the concentration threshold for glucose activation of a cotransfected insulin promoter/chloramphenicol acetyl transferase plasmid.[79] Similarly, Epstein and coworkers[80] showed that overexpression of low K_m yeast hexokinase in β-cells of transgenic mice resulted in a leftward-shifted glucose-stimulated insulin secretion response and an increase in total insulin output. Finally, Becker et al.[81,82] developed the recombinant adenovirus system for efficient delivery of metabolic regulatory genes to isolated islets. A virus containing the *Escherichia coli* β-galactosidase gene (AdCMV-βGAL)[83] has been used to demonstrate gene transfer to islet cells with an average efficiency of approximately 70%,[82] slightly lower than observed by us in isolated hepatocytes (86%)[84] or insulinoma cells (100%)[69] but considerably better than the 10–20% generally observed with more traditional physical methods such as electroporation or Ca_2PO_4 coprecipitation. Importantly, untreated and AdCMV-βGAL–treated islets responded identically to stimulation with glucose or glucose plus arginine.[82]

Treatment of freshly isolated rat islets with a recombinant virus containing the hexokinase I cDNA (AdCMV-HKI) results in an 8-fold increase in total glucose phosphorylation.[82] Overexpression of hexokinase in this manner resulted in a doubling of insulin secretion from islets perifused at a nonstimulatory glucose concentration (3 mM), but did not alter the increment of response to stimulatory glucose (20 mM) or stimulatory glucose + 30 mM arginine relative to untreated or AdCMV-βGAL–treated islets. Overexpression of hexokinase I in islets also caused a 2.5–4 fold increase in 5-^{3}H glucose usage and lactate production at 3 mM glucose relative to the control groups.

More recently Becker, et al. have studied the effects of glucokinase overexpression by preparing recombinant viruses containing the cDNAs encoding either the liver or islet isoforms of the enzyme.[86] Treatment of islets with either virus resulted in increases in total glucose phosphorylating activity in crude extracts of up to 20-fold relative to untreated or AdCMV-βGAL treated islets. In contrast to the clear metabolic and secretory effects of low Km hexokinase I overexpression, adenovirus-mediated delivery of either isoform of glucokinase resulted in no change in 5-^{3}H glucose usage or lactate production relative to control islets. Furthermore, glucokinase overexpression enhanced insulin secretion in response to stimulatory glucose or glucose + arginine by only 36–53% relative to control islets. In contrast to the lack of metabolic impact of overexpressed glucokinase in islets, a clear metabolic effect can be demonstrated when glucokinase activity is increased in the kidney cell line CV-1[86] or in hepatoma cells.[87] That this result cannot be ascribed to the glucokinase regulatory protein that inhibits the enzyme in a hexose-phosphate regulated manner in liver is indicated by the very low levels of regulatory protein mRNA and activity in islet extracts.[86,88] These data provide evidence for functional partitioning of glucokinase and hexokinase, and suggest that glucokinase must interact with factors found in limiting concentration in the islet cell in order to become activated and engage in metabolic signalling. Whether this functional partitioning is related to the known capacity of hexokinase, but not glucokinase to associate with islet mitochondria[82,86] remains to be determined.

Summary

Advances in our understanding of the early biochemical events involved in glucose-stimulated insulin secretion have been gained in recent years through genetic analyses of humans with MODY, and molecular, physiologic and biochemical studies of animal models of diabetes and insulin-secreting cell lines. Although many of the details of this process remain to be elucidated, several conclusions can be drawn from these studies with respect to the contribution of the proteins involved in the first steps of glucose recognition. The glucokinase:hexokinase ratio appears to be the major determinant of the threshold for activation of glucose-stimulated insulin release in cell lines and islet β-cells. The role of the glucose transport step is less clear, although it appears that some GLUT-2 expression is required for glucose responsiveness, and that this requirement may be independent of any metabolic effects exerted by this transporter. Areas for future study include mechanistic aspects of the interrelationship between expression of GLUT-2 and glucokinase, as well as further studies on manipulation of the activities of glucose transporters and glucose phosphorylating enzymes in isolated islets, cell lines, and transgenic animals.

Acknowledgments

Research was supported by United States Public Health Service grants DK42582 and DK46492, as well as a Merit Review from the Department of Veterans Affairs.

References

1. Meglasson MD, Matschinsky FM. Pancreatic islet glucose metabolism and regulation of insulin secretion. Diabetes Metab Rev 1986;2:163
2. Landgraf R, Kotler-Brajburg J, Matschinsky FM. Kinetics of insulin from the perfused rat pancreas caused by glucose, glucoseamine and galactose. Proc Natl Acad Sci USA 1971;68:546
3. Ashcroft SJH. Metabolic controls of insulin release. In: Cooperstein SJ, Watkins D, eds. The Islets of Langerhans. London: Academic Press; 1981:117–148
4. Hughes SD, Quaade C, Johnson JH, et al. Transfection of AtT-20ins cells with GLUT 2 but not GLUT 1 confers glucose-stimulated insulin secretion: Relationship to glucose metabolism. J Biol Chem 1993;268:15205
5. Dukes ID, McIntyre MS, Mertz RJ, et al. Dependence on NADH produced during glycolysis for β-cell signaling. J Biol Chem 1994;269:10979
6. MacDonald MJ. Elusive proximal signals of β-cells for insulin secretion. Diabetes 1990;29:1461
7. Ashcroft FM, Harrison DE, Ashcroft SJH. Glucose induces closure of single potassium channels in isolated rat pancreatic islets. Nature 1984;312:446
8. Prentki M, Matschinsky FM. Ca^{2+}, cAMP and phospholipid-derived messengers in coupling mechanisms of insulin secretion. Physiol Rev 1987;67:1185
9. Turk J, Wolf BA, McDaniel ML. The role of phospholipid-derived mediators including arachodonic acid, its metabolites, and inositoltriphosphophate and of intracellular Ca^{2+} in glucose-induced insulin secretion in pancreatic islets. Prog Lipid Res 1987;26:125
10. Boyd AE III. The role of ion channels in insulin secretion. J Cell Biochem 1992;48:234
11. Ghosh A, Ronner P, Cheong E, et al. The role of ATP and free ADP in metabolic coupling during fuel-stimulated insulin release from islet β-cells in the isolated perfused pancreas. J Biol Chem 1991;266:22887
12. Newgard CB, McGarry JD. Metabolic coupling factors in pancreatic beta-cell signal transduction. Ann Rev Biochem 1995;64:689–719
13. Ashcroft SJH, Hughes SJ. Protein phosphorylation in the regulation of insulin secretion and biosynthesis. Biochem Soc Trans 1990;18:116
14. Ganesan S, Calle R, Zawalich K, et al. Immunocytochemical location of a-protein kinase C in rat pancreatic β-cells during glucose-induced insulin secretion. J Cell Biol 1992;119:313
15. Calle R, Ganesan S, Smallwood JI, Rasmussen H. Glucose-induced phosphorylation of myristolated alanine-rich C kinase substrate (MARCKS) in isolated rat pancreatic islets. J Biol Chem 1992;267:18723
16. Bell GI, Kayano T, Buse JB, et al. Molecular biology of mammalian glucose transporters. Diabetes Care 1990;13:198
17. Hellman B, Lernmark A, Sehlin J, Taljedal I-B. Effects of phlorizin on metabolism and function of pancreatic β-cells. Metabolism 1972;21:60
18. Trus MD, Zawalich WS, Burch PT, et al. Regulation of glucose metabolism in pancreatic islets. Diabetes 1981;30:911
19. Meglasson MD, Burch PT, Berner DK, et al. Identification of glucokinase as an alloxan-sensitive glucose sensor of the pancreatic β-cell. Diabetes 1986;35:1163
20. Coore HG, Randle PJ. Inhibition of glucose phosphorylation by mannoheptulose. Biochem J 1964;91:56
21. Balkan B, Dunning BE. Glucoseamine inhibits glucokinase in vitro and produces glucose-specific impairment of in vivo insulin secretion in rats. Diabetes 1994;43:1173
22. Meglasson MD, Matschinsky FM. New perspectives on pancreatic islet glucokinase. Am J Physiol 1984;246:E1

23. Wilson JE. Regulation of mammalian hexokinase activity. In: Beitner R, ed. Regulation of Carbohydrate Metabolism. Boca Raton, Fla: CRC Press; 1984:45–85
24. Iynedjian PB, Pilot P-R, Nouspikel T, et al. Differential expression and regulation of the glucokinase gene in liver and islets: Implications for control of glucose homeostasis. Proc Natl Acad Sci USA 1989;86:7838
25. Magnuson MA, Shelton KD. An alternate promoter in the glucokinase gene is active in the pancreatic β-cell. J Biol Chem 1989;264:15936
26. Newgard CB, Quaade C, Hughes SD, Milburn JL. Glucokinase and glucose transporter expression in liver and islets: Implications for control of glucose homeostasis. Biochem Soc Trans 1990;18:851
27. Hughes SD, Quaade C, Milburn JL, et al. Expression of normal and novel glucokinase mRNAs in anterior pituitary and islet cells. J Biol Chem 1991; 266:4921
28. Jetton TL, Liang Y, Pettefer CC, et al. Analysis of upstream glucokinase promoter activity in transgenic mice and identification of glucokinase in rare neuroendocrine cells in the brain and gut. J Biol Chem 1994;269:3641
29. Tanizawa Y, Koranyi LI, Welling CM, Permutt MA. Human liver glucokinase gene: Cloning and sequence determination of two alternatively spliced cDNAs. Proc Natl Acad Sci USA 1991;88:7294
30. Koranyi LI, Tanizawa Y, Welling CM, et al. Human islet glucokinase gene: Isolation and sequence analysis of a full-length cDNA. Diabetes 1992;41:807
31. Stoffel M, Frougel P, Takeda J, et al. Human glucokinase gene: Isolation, characterization, and identification of two missense mutations linked to early-onset noninsulin-dependent (type 2) diabetes mellitus. Proc Natl Acad Sci USA 1992;89:7698
32. Coore HG, Randle PJ. Regulation of insulin secretion studied with pieces of rabbit pancreas incubated in vitro. Biochem J 1964;93:66
33. Giroix M-H, Sener A, Pipeleers DG, Malaisse WJ. Hexose metabolism in pancreatic islets: Inhibition of hexokinase. Biochem J 1984;223:447
34. Frougel P, Vaxillaire M, Sun F, et al. Close linkage of glucokinase locus on chromosome 7p to early-onset noninsulin-dependent diabetes mellitus. Nature 1992;356:162
35. Vionnet N, Stoffel M, Taqkeda J, et al. Nonsense mutation in the glucokinase gene causes early-onset noninsulin-dependent diabetes mellitus. Nature 1992;356:721
36. Gidh-Jain M, Takeda J, Xu LZ, et al. Glucokinase mutations associated with noninsulin-dependent (type 2) diabetes mellitus have decreased enzymatic activity: Implications for structure/function relationships. Proc Natl Acad Sci USA 1993;90:1932
37. Takeda J, Gidh-Jain M, Xu LZ, et al. Structure/function studies of human β-cell glucokinase. J Biol Chem 1993;268:15200
38. Pilkis SJ, Weber IT, Harrison RW, Bell GI. Glucokinase: Structural analysis of a protein involved in susceptibility to diabetes. J Biol Chem 1994;269:21925
39. Vehlo G, Frougel P, Clement K, et al. Primary pancreatic beta-cell secretory defect caused by mutations in glucokinase gene in kindreds of maturity onset diabetes of the young. Lancet 1992;340:444
40. Byrne MM, Sturis J, Clemment K, et al. Insulin secretory abnormalities in subjects with hyperglycemia due to glucokinase mutations. J Clin Invest 1994;93:1120
41. Efrat S, Leiser M, Wu Y-J, et al. Ribozyme-mediated attenuation of pancreatic β-cell glucokinase expression in transgenic mice results in impaired glucose-induced insulin secretion. Proc Natl Acad Sci USA 1994;91:2051
42. Matschinsky FM, Ellerman JE. Metabolism of glucose in the islets of Langerhans. J Biol Chem 1968;243:2730
43. Gorus FK, Malaisse WJ, Pipeleers DG. Differences in glucose handling by pancreatic α- and β-cells. J Biol Chem 1984;259:1196
44. Thorens B, Sarkar HK, Kaback HR, Lodish HF. Cloning and functional expression in bacteria of a novel glucose transporter in liver, intestine, kidney and beta-pancreatic islet cells. Cell 1988;55:281
45. Johnson JH, Newgard CB, Milburn JL, et al. The high K_m glucose transporter of islets of Langerhans is functionally similar to the low affinity transporter of liver and has an identical primary sequence. J Biol Chem 1990;265:6548
46. Thorens B, Gerard N, Deriaz N. GLUT 2 expression and intracellular transport via the constitutive pathway in pancreatic β-cells and insulinoma: Evidence for a block in trans-Golgi network exit by brefeldin A. J Cell Biol 1993;123:1687
47. Katagiri H, Asano T, Ishihara H, et al. Replacement of intracellular C-terminal domain of GLUT 1 glucose transporter with that of GLUT increases V_{max} and K_m of transport activity. J Biol Chem 1992;267:22550
48. Chen L, Alam T, Johnson JH, et al. Regulation of β-cell glucose transporter gene expression. Proc Natl Acad Sci USA 1990;87:4088
49. Unger RH. Diabetic hyperglycemia: Link to impaired glucose transport in pancreatic β-cells. Science 1991;251:1200
50. Tominaga M, Komiya I, Johnson JH, et al. Loss of insulin response to glucose but not arginine during the development of autoimmune diabetes in the BB/Wor rat: Relationship to islet volume and glucose transport rate. Proc Natl Acad Sci USA 1986;83:9749
51. Orci L, Unger RH, Ravazzola M, et al. Reduced β-cell glucose transporter in new-onset diabetic BB rats. J Clin Invest 1990;86:1615
52. Cerasi E, Luft R. Decreased sensitivity of pancreatic beta cells to glucose in prediabetic and diabetic subjects. Diabetes 1971;21:224
53. Pfeifer MA, Halter JB, Porte D. Insulin secretion in diabetes mellitus. Am J Med 1981;70:579
54. Johnson JH, Ogawa A, Chen L, et al. Underexpression of β-cell high K_m glucose transporter in noninsulin-dependent diabetes. Science 1990;250: 546
55. Portha B, Serradas D, Bailbe K-I, et al. β-cell insensitivity to glucose in the GK rat, a spontaneous nonobese model for type II diabetes. Diabetes 1991;40: 227
56. Clark JB, Palmer CJ, Shaw WN. The diabetic Zucker fatty rat (41611). Proc Soc Exp Biol Med 1983;173:68
57. Orci L, Ravazzola M, Baetens D, et al. Evidence that downregulation of β-cell glucose transporters in noninsulin-dependent diabetes may be the cause of diabetic hyperglycemia. Proc Natl Acad Sci USA 1990;87:9953
58. Waeber G, Thompson N, Haefliger J-A, Nicod P. Characterization of the murine high Km glucose transporter GLUT2 gene and its transcriptional regulation by glucose in a differentiated insulin-secreting cell line. J Biol Chem 1994;269:26912
59. Thorens B, Wu Y-J, Leahy JL, Weir GC. The loss of GLUT 2 expression by glucose-unresponsive β-cells of db/db mice is reversible and is induced by the diabetic environment. J Clin Invest 1992;90:77
60. Ohneda M, Johnson JH, Inman LI, et al. Glut 2 expression and function in β-cells of the GK rat with NIDDM: Dissociation between reduction in glucose transport and glucose-stimulated insulin secretion. Diabetes 1993;42:1065
61. Ohneda M, Johnson JH, Inman LI, Unger RH. GLUT 2 function in glucose-unresponsive β-cells of dexamethosone-induced diabetes in rats. J Clin Invest 1993;92:1950
62. Thorens B, Weir GC, Leahy JL, et al. Reduced expression of liver/beta cell glucose transporter isoform in glucose-insensitive beta cells of diabetic rats. Proc Natl Acad Sci USA 1990;87:6492
63. Unger RH. Lipotoxicity in the pathogenesis of obesity-dependent NIDDM: Genetic and clinical implications. Diabetes 1995;44:863–870
64. Halban PA, Praz GA, Wollheim CB. Abnormal glucose metabolism accompanies failure of glucose to stimulate insulin release from a pancreatic line (RINm5F). Biochem J 1983;212:439
65. Miyazaki J-I, Araki K, Yamoto E, et al. Establishment of a pancreatic β-cell line that retains glucose-inducible insulin secretion: Special reference to glucose transporter isoforms. Endocrinology 1990;127:126
66. Asafari M, Janjic D, Meda P, et al. Establishment of 2-mercaptoethanol-dependent differentiated insulin-secreting cell lines. Endocrinology 1992; 130:167
67. Efrat S, Leiser M, Surana M, et al. Murine insulinoma cell line with normal glucose-regulated insulin secretion. Diabetes 1993;42:901
68. Clark SA, Burnham BL, Chick WL. Modulation of glucose-induced insulin secretion from a rat clonal β-cell line. Endocrinology 1990;127:2779
69. Ferber S, BeltrandelRio H, Johnson JH, et al. GLUT-2 gene transfer into insulinoma cells confers both low and high affinity glucose-stimulated insulin release: Relationship to glucokinase activity. J Biol Chem 1994;269:11523
70. Efrat S, Linde S, Kofod H, et al. Beta-cell lines derived from transgenic mice expressing a hybrid insulin gene-oncogene. Proc Natl Acad Sci USA 1988;85:9037
71. Whitesell RR, Powers AC, Regen DM, Abumrad NA. Transport and metabolism of glucose in an insulin-secreting cell line, βTC-1. Biochemistry 1991;30:11560
72. Knaak D, Fiore DM, Surana M, et al. Clonal insulinoma cell line that stably maintains correct glucose responsiveness. Diabetes 1994;43:1413
73. Inagaki N, Yasuda K, Inoue G, et al. Glucose regulation of glucose transport activity and glucose transporter mRNA in hamster β-cell line. Diabetes 1992;41:592
74. Moore H-P, Walker MD, Lee F, Kelly RB. Expressing a human proinsulin cDNA in a mouse ACTH-secreting cell: Intracellular storage, proteolytic processing and secretion on stimulation. Cell 1983;35:531
75. Liang Y, Jetton T, Zimmerman EC, et al. Effects of alternate RNA splicing on glucokinase isoform activities in the pancreatic islet, liver, and anterior pituitary. J Biol Chem 1991;266:6999
76. Quaade C, Hughes SD, Coats WS, et al. Analysis of the protein products encoded by variant glucokinase transcripts via expression in bacteria. FEBS Lett 1991;280:47
77. Hughes SD, Johnson JH, Quaade C, Newgard CB. Engineering of glucose-stimulated insulin secretion in non-islet cells. Proc Natl Acad Sci USA 1992;89:688
78. Ishihara H, Asano T, Tsukuda K, et al. Overexpression of hexokinase I but not GLUT 1 glucose transporter alters the concentration dependence of glucose-stimulated insulin secretion in pancreatic beta cells. J Biol Chem 1994; 269:3081
79. German MS. Glucose sensing in pancreatic islet beta cells: The key role for glucokinase and the glycolytic intermediates. Proc Natl Acad Sci USA 1993;90:1781
80. Epstein PN, Boschero AC, Atwater I, et al. Expression of yeast hexokinase in pancreatic β-cells of transgenic mice reduces blood glucose, enhances insulin secretion and decreases diabetes. Proc Natl Acad Sci USA 1992;89:12038
81. Becker TC, Noel RJ, Coats WS, et al. Use of recombinant adenovirus for metabolic engineering of mammalian cells. Methods Cell Biol 1994;43:161
82. Becker TC, BeltrandelRio H, Noel R, et al. Overexpression of hexokinase I in isolated islets of Langerhans by recombinant adenovirus: Enhancement of glucose metabolism and insulin secretion at basal but not stimulatory glucose levels. J Biol Chem 1994;269:21234
83. Herz J, Gerard RD. Adenovirus-mediated transfer of low density lipoprotein receptor gene acutely accelerates cholesterol clearance in normal mice. Proc Natl Acad Sci USA 1993;90:2812

84. Gomez-Foix AM, Coats WS, Baque S, et al. Adenovirus-mediated transfer of the muscle glycogen phosphorylase gene into hepatocytes confers altered regulation of glycogen metabolism. J Biol Chem 1992;267:25129
85. Voss-McCowan ME, Xu B, Epstein PN. Insulin synthesis, secretory competence and glucose utilization are sensitized by transgenic yeast hexokinase. J Biol Chem 1994;269:15814
86. Becker TC, Noel RJ, Johnson JH, et al. Differential effects of overexpressed glucokinase and hexokinase I in isolated islets; evidence for functional segregation of the high and low Km enzymes. J Biol Chem, in press, 1995
87. Valera A, Bosch F. Glucokinase expression in rab hepatoma cells induces glucose uptake and is rate limiting in glucose utilization. Eur J Biochem 1994;222:533–539
88. Malaisse WJ, Malaisse-Lagal F, Davies DR, et al. Regulation of glucokinase by a fructose-1–phosphate-sensitive protein in pancreatic islets. Eur J Biochem 1990;190:539–545

Diabetes Mellitus, edited by Derek LeRoith, Simeon I. Taylor, and Jerrold M. Olefsky. Lippincott–Raven Publishers, Philadelphia © 1996.

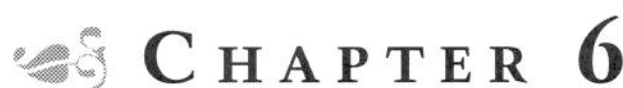

Chapter 6

GTP-Binding Proteins and Regulation of Pancreatic Islet Function: Part I. Heterotrimeric Proteins, Insulin Gene Expression, and Insulin Secretion

R. Paul Robertson, Elizabeth R. Seaquist, Timothy F. Walseth, Hui-Jian Zhang, J. Bruce Redmon, Vincent Poitout, and David M. Kendall

The endocrine pancreas is of paramount importance for regulation of glucose and fatty acid metabolism. The hormonal output of pancreatic islets of Langerhans is regulated by extracellular and intracellular signals, many of which depend on heterotrimeric G-proteins. The islets constitute 2–3% of the total mass of the pancreas, and each islet contains four main cell types: The core of the islet is made up primarily of *beta cells,* which synthesize and secrete insulin; the other three cell types are the *alpha, delta,* and *PP cells,* which synthesize and secrete glucagon, somatostatin, and pancreatic polypeptide (PP) respectively. This chapter emphasizes the β-cell because the vast majority of experiments to study the role of heterotrimeric G-proteins and the islet have been performed with this cell type. Information regarding heterotrimeric G-proteins and the α-cell is just beginning to emerge and is virtually nonexistent for the delta and PP cells.

β-Cells and α-cells continually undergo positive and negative regulation by a large array of fuels, hormones, and autacoids. Glucose is considered the most important stimulant of insulin secretion from the β-cell, but amino acids such as arginine also play important roles as physiologic stimulators of insulin secretion. Most of the prominent inhibitors of insulin secretion are produced within the islet. For example, prostaglandin E_2 (PGE_2) is made within the β-cell itself, somatostatin by δ-cells, and norepinephrine and galanin by nerves supplying the islet, whereas epinephrine travels from the adrenal medulla via the systemic circulation to reach the β-cell. Probably the most important stimulatory signal to the α-cell to release glucagon is *hypoglycemia.* Glucagon provides the body's primary defense against dangerously low circulating glucose levels by virtue of its glycogenolytic effect on the liver. Arginine and epinephrine also stimulate glucagon release, whereas somatostatin and hyperglycemia inhibit it. For the purposes of this chapter it is important to realize that many, but not all, of these stimulators and inhibitors of β- and α-cells have mechanisms of action on secretion that are mediated by heterotrimeric G-proteins.

As a final introductory note, a brief historical perspective on the intense interest in and excitement about heterotrimeric G-proteins by researchers involved in pancreatic islet function may be helpful. Until just little more than a decade ago, knowledge about the mechanisms of actions of endogenous regulators of insulin and glucagon secretion essentially stopped at the cell membrane. It was known that many agonists and antagonists had specific cell membrane receptors. This information was developed through the use of pharmacologic receptor antagonists and radiolabeled ligand binding studies of both whole cells and plasma membrane fragments of cells. Despite our appreciation that cAMP and protein phosphorylation were involved, however, our knowledge about postreceptor events after hormone-receptor binding, or transport of fuels such as glucose, was in its infancy. In the last decade we have witnessed an impressive expansion of knowledge about postreceptor events. Much of this expansion has come from a recognition of the roles that heterotrimeric G-proteins play in regulating the pancreatic islet at the level of both gene expression and hormone exocytosis.

Heterotrimeric G-Proteins

The term *G-protein* is an abbreviation of the phrase guanine nucleotide binding protein. Heterotrimeric G-proteins are so called because they consist of three subunits: the *alpha, beta,* and *gamma subunits.* Heterotrimeric G-proteins are coupled to hundreds of receptors that bind hormones, neurotransmitters, autacoids, and growth factors. Odorant receptors and photo receptors are also examples of G-protein–coupled receptors. Effector molecules that are regulated by G-proteins include adenylyl cyclases, phospholipases, and ion channels.[1–7] Receptors that are coupled to heterotrimeric G-proteins usually contain seven domains that span the plasma membrane of the cell. The amino terminus of the receptor projects into the extracellular space, and the carboxyl terminus projects into the cell's cytosol.

Because the number of ligands and their specific receptors that interact with heterotrimeric G-proteins is at least 10 times greater than the number of G-proteins themselves, it is reasonable to assume that the specificity of the cellular consequences that follow the interaction between the ligand, its receptor, and a G-protein is primarily provided by the ligand-receptor complex. Nonetheless, another level of specificity can be provided by the variety of alpha, beta, and gamma subunits of heterotrimeric G-proteins. Although these numbers still increase with each passing year, it can be stated with a fair degree of accuracy that 20 different alpha subunits, 8 different gamma subunits, and 4 different beta subunits have been described. This variety of subunits is produced by different genes, some of which utilize alternative RNA splicing to generate alternative forms of the subunits. Although it was initially thought that activation of the alpha subunit and subsequent coupling to an effector molecule was primarily responsible for G-protein action, it is now known that G-proteins can also act through the beta-gamma subunit complex.

Myristoylation and isoprenylation appear to be important determinants of subunit function. Myristoylation of alpha subunits appears to be required for binding to membranes or beta-gamma complexes, and gamma subunits appear to require isoprenylation for binding to membranes. Generally speaking, myristoylation of alpha subunits takes place at the amino terminus and isoprenylation of gamma subunits takes place at a cysteine on the carboxyl terminus. Thus, many heterotrimeric G-protein structural variables exist that provide potential regulation of their activity in addition to the specificity inherent in the initial ligand-receptor–G-protein interaction. One should note that little has been published about the cloning or regulation of G-protein genes found in the pancreatic islet.

The consensus mechanism of action for heterotrimeric G-proteins is provided in Figure 6-1. In this example, the initial event is coupling of a hormone to its specific receptor. The hormone-receptor complex in turn associates with a heterotrimeric G-protein that is in a quiescent state at the cell membrane. In this state the alpha subunit is bound to guanosine diphosphate (GDP). Formation of the hormone-receptor–G-protein complex causes the GDP bound by the alpha subunit to be exchanged for guanosine triphosphate (GTP). This exchange destabilizes the heterotrimeric structure of the G-protein, which causes dissociation of the GTP-liganded alpha subunit from the combined beta-gamma subunits. In the example shown in Figure 6-1, it is the GTP-activated alpha subunit that leads to the physiologic effect (i.e., modulation of insulin secretion, rather than the beta-gamma complex), although in some other situations the beta-gamma complex may actively participate in signal transduction. The second half of the cycle begins with deactivation of the alpha subunit which is initiated by its own intrinsic GTPase activity. Consequent to hydrolysis of GTP to GDP, the alpha subunit is free to reassociate with the beta-gamma subunit complex. This reassociation returns the heterotrimeric G-protein to a quiescent state in which it is again available for activation upon binding to a hormone-receptor complex.

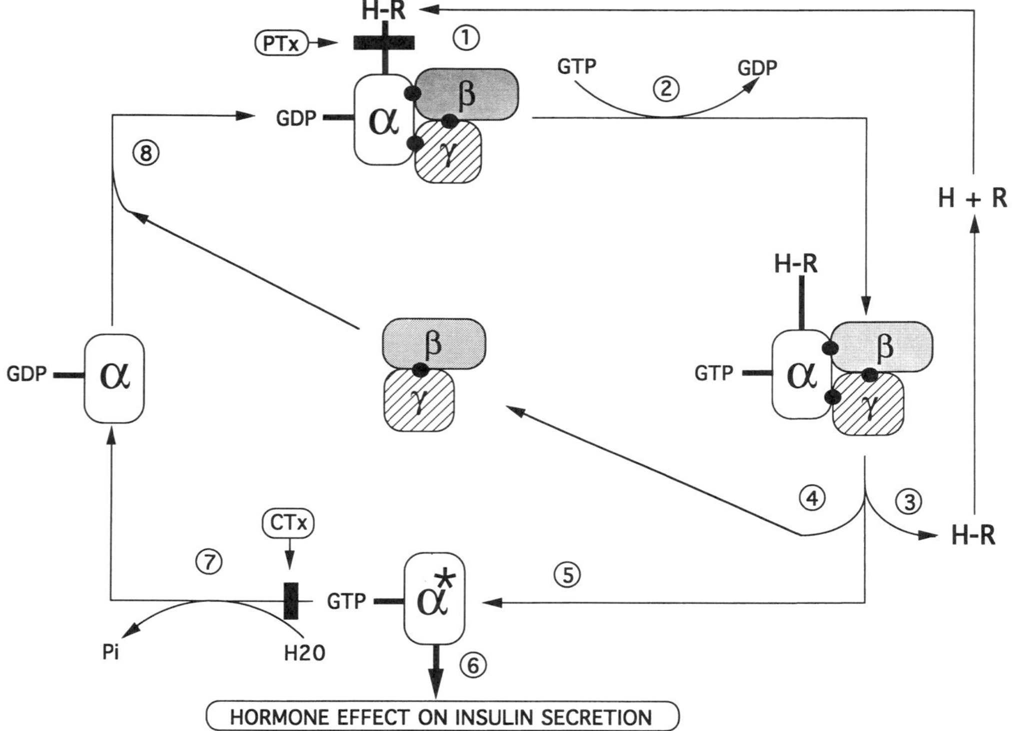

Figure 6-1. Mechanism of action for G proteins. The hormone-receptor complex (H-R) associates with GDP-binding G-protein, which comprises the α, β, and γ-subunits (Step 1). This union promotes exchange of GTP for GDP on α-subunit (Step 2) which forms an unstable complex that quickly dissociates into free H-R complex (Step 3), free β-γ-subunits (Step 4), and activated α-subunit (Step 5). The activated species then influences the activity of various islet effector systems (e.g., adenylyl cyclase, ion channels, phospholipases, and distal sites in exocytosis; Step 6). Activated α-subunit is inactivated by its intrinsic GTPase activity, which hydrolyzes bound GTP to GDP (Step 7) and allows reassociation of α-GDP with the β-γ-subunit (Step 8). This completes the cycle and returns G-protein to its quiescent state. PTx irreversibly ADP-ribosylates G-proteins such as $G_{1\alpha}$ and $G_{o\alpha}$ and prevents interaction of H-R with GDP-binding G-protein at Step 1. CTx irreversibly ADP-ribosylates $G_{s\alpha}$ and $G_{t\alpha}$, blocks intrinsic GTPase activity, and consequently prevents Step 7. (Modified with permission from Robertson RP, Seaquist ER, Walseth TF. G proteins and modulation of insulin secretion. Diabetes 1991;40:1.)

Pertussis toxin (PTx) and *cholera toxin* (CTx) potently influence the activation-deactivation cycle of heterotrimeric G-proteins. Both toxins catalyze the addition of ADP-ribose to alpha subunits. ADP-ribosylation by PTx occurs on cysteine molecules in the carboxy terminus of certain alpha subunits and prevents coupling with the hormone-receptor complex. It thereby wholly or partially prevents the physiologic consequences of hormones that depend on the G-protein involved. ADP-ribosylation by CTx occurs on asparagine molecules on the alpha subunit and inhibits the intrinsic GTPase activity of alpha subunits. This prevents hydrolysis of GTP to form GDP and thereby leads to prolonged and irreversible activation of the subunit. In this case, the cellular consequence brought about by activation of the alpha subunit continues unabatedly.

As will be seen in the final section of this chapter, PTx and CTx are important investigative tools for the study of G-protein regulation of cellular events. These toxins can be used to test hypotheses both in intact animals and in vitro by virtue of their ability to perturb the normal G-protein activation-deactivation cycle. Advantage is also taken of the ADP-ribosylation reaction to detect PTx- and CTx-sensitive substrates chemically and to assess their molecular size in preparations of cellular membranes.

Identification of Heterotrimeric G-Proteins in the Pancreatic Islet and in Islet Cell Lines

Currently, evidence for the existence of 13 heterotrimeric G-protein alpha subunits within the pancreatic islet or in islet cell lines has been reported (Table 6-1). Identification of G-proteins has generally been performed by Western analysis (immunodetection of the protein by a specific antiserum). The first pancreatic islet G-protein identified was $G_{s\alpha}$ (S = stimulatory for adenylyl cyclase), a CTx-sensitive G-protein. Walseth et al.[8] detected two CTx substrates in HIT-T15 cells, an insulin-secreting clonal cell line (Fig. 6-2). These two substrates were 52 and 45 kd in size, respectively. Interestingly, the number of the 45-kd species (but not the 52-kd form) increased in late passages of HIT-T15 cells. The identity of these CTx substrates was established by immunoblots using antisera that were specific for the alpha subunits of G_s. Walseth et al.[8] also examined the biologic activity of the G_s species, using extracts of HIT-T15 cell membranes to reconstitute guanine nucleotide-sensitive adenylyl cyclase in S49 cyc$^-$ cell membranes. These S49 cyc$^-$ cells lack G_s and thus do not form cAMP when stimulated with an adenylyl cyclase agonist. Their data suggested functional differences between the 45- and 52-kd $G_{s\alpha}$-subunits. Extracts of late-passage HIT-T15 cells containing a severalfold abundance of the 45-kd form were much more efficacious than extracts of cells from earlier passages containing equal amounts of the 45- and 52-kd

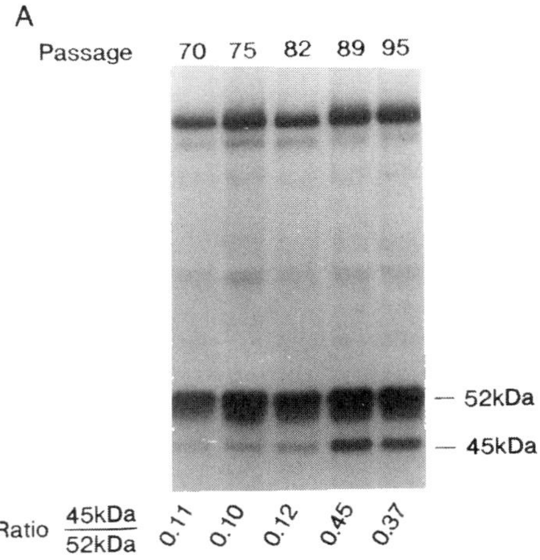

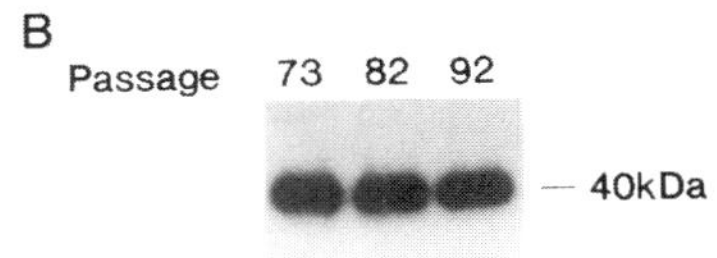

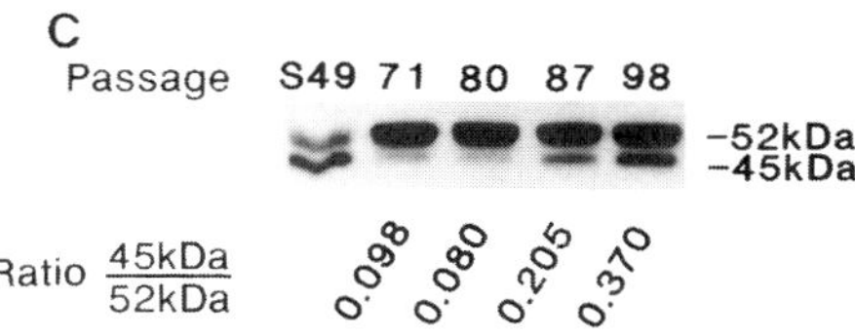

Figure 6-2. Demonstration of two forms of G_s in various passages of HIT-T15 cells. ***A,*** CTx-induced ADP-ribosylation of cell membranes detecting 52-kd and 45-kd substrates. The 45-kd substrate increases with increasing passage. ***B,*** PTx-induced ADP-ribosylation detecting one substrate that does not increase with increasing passage. ***C,*** Identification by Western analysis of the 52-kd and 45-kd substrates has two forms of G_s. (Reproduced with permission from Walseth, Zhang H-J, Olson LK, et al. Increase in G_s and cyclic AMP generation in HIT cells. J Biol Chem 1989;264:21106.)

subunits in terms of stimulating cAMP synthesis. Subsequently, Zigman et al.[9] reported expression of $G_{s\alpha}$-subunit mRNA in pancreatic islets. They used degenerate oligonucleotide primers and reverse transcriptase-polymerase chain reaction to amplify cDNA fragments, which were then subcloned and sequenced. The finding of only one species of G_s-mRNA is consistent with the concept that the two forms of $G_{s\alpha}$-protein detected by Walseth et al.[8] had been synthesized by alternative splicing of G_s-RNA.

All of the other reports identifying heterotrimeric G-proteins in islets or islet cell lines have come from work focused on G-proteins other than G_s (e.g., G_i, where i = inhibitory for adenylyl cyclase; and G_o, where o = other). Hsu et al.[10] screened an HIT-T15 cell cDNA library with a G_o- specific oligodeoxynucleotide probe and isolated six recombinant phages whose inserts encoded two forms of α_o, termed α_{o1} and α_{o2}. After in vitro transcription and translation, the peptide encoded in the α_{o1} and α_{o2} cDNAs could be ADP-ribosylated by PTx in the presence of added beta-gamma dimers. These authors pointed out the close structural similarity of the α_{o1} and α_{o2} proteins and their nucleotide sequences and proposed that α_{o1} and α_{o2} arise from alternative splicing of a single α_o transcript.

Table 6-1. Heterotrimeric G-Proteins Identified in Pancreatic Islets and β-Cell Lines

G-Protein	References (No. of Forms)
$G_{s\alpha 45}$	8, 9
$G_{s\alpha 52}$	8
$G_{i\alpha 1}$	11, 12, 14, 16
$G_{i\alpha 2}$	11, 12, 14, 15, 17
$G_{i\alpha 3}$	12, 14, 17
$G_{o\alpha}$	10 (2), 11 (2), 14 (3), 15 (2), 16 (1), 17 (1)
$G_{\alpha q}$	16
$G_{11\alpha}$	9
$G_{14\alpha}$	9
$G_{z\alpha}$	9
$G_{12\alpha}$	9

Using PTx ADP-ribosylation and immunoblotting, Schmidt et al.[11] and Cormont et al.[12] identified the alpha-subunits in RIN m5F cells. Schmidt et al. reported $G_{i\alpha 1}$, $G_{i\alpha 2}$, $G_{o\alpha 2}$, and another $G_{o\alpha}$-subtype; Cormont et al. found $G_{i\alpha 1}$, $G_{i\alpha 2}$, $G_{i\alpha 3}$, and two forms of $G_{o\alpha}$. Cormont et al. also reported that galanin binding to cell membranes was decreased by an antibody that selectively recognized $G_{i\alpha 1}$ and $G_{i\alpha 2}$. They also reported the absence of effects of other antibodies specifically directed against $G_{i\alpha 3}$ or $G_{\alpha o}$. They concluded that G_{i1} or G_{i2}, or both, interact with the galanin receptor and mediate the effects of galanin, an inhibitor of insulin secretion, in pancreatic β-cells. Their laboratory[13] later reported that $G_{i\alpha 3}$ may also be involved in galanin effects in the islet.

Shortly thereafter in 1992, Seaquist et al.[14] reported studies of PTx-sensitive G-proteins in HIT-T15 cell membranes. They found ADP-ribosylation of six different proteins by PTx: Western analysis with a panel of antisera provided evidence for the presence of $G_{i\alpha 1}$, $G_{i\alpha 2}$, $G_{i\alpha 3}$, and three forms of $G_{o\alpha}$ (Fig. 6-3). The most abundant form was a species of $G_{o\alpha}$, and the second most abundant was $G_{i\alpha 2}$. This differs from the report of Cormont et al.[12] described above, in which the most abundant form in RIN5mF cells was $G_{i\alpha 2}$. In the same year, Berrow et al.[15] reported evidence for $G_{i\alpha 2}$ and two forms of $G_{o\alpha}$ in rat pancreatic islet membranes from experiments using immunoblots.

Heterotrimeric G-protein identification in the β-cell was performed by Baffy et al.[16] through use of a newer glucose-responsive insulin-secreting β-cell line, the BTC-3 cell. Western analysis revealed the presence $G_{i\alpha}$, $G_{o\alpha}$, and $G_{q\alpha}$ with no marked differences in abundance among the three. In contrast, a preliminary report by Poitout et al.[17] using Western analysis and BTC-6 cells identified $G_{i\alpha 2}$, $G_{i\alpha 3}$, and $G_{o\alpha 2}$. Baffy et al.[16] microinjected anti–G-protein antibodies into the cells to inactivate G-proteins and to characterize the consequences on glucose- and carbachol-induced calcium mobilization. Anti–$G_{\alpha q}$-antibodies completely inhibited calcium-mobilization by carbachol but not by glucose. The anti–$G_{\alpha o}$-antibody had a partial effect on glucose-induced calcium mobilization, whereas the anti–$G_{\alpha i}$-antibody had no effect.

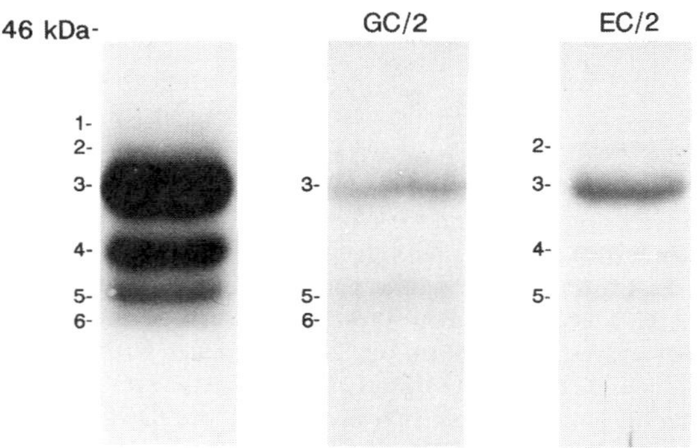

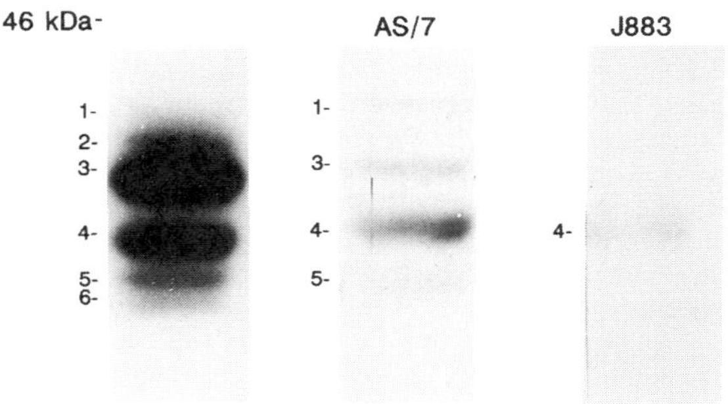

Figure 6-3. Detection of six PTx-sensitive substrates in HIT-T15 cell membranes (top and bottom left). Two different photographic exposures were used to facilitate identification of the PTx-sensitive substrates. Identification by Western analysis of the six PTx-sensitive substrates as $G_{i\alpha 1}$, $G_{i\alpha 2}$, $G_{i\alpha 3}$, and three forms of $G_{o\alpha}$ (center and right top and bottom). (Reproduced with permission from Seaquist ER, Neal AR, Shoger KD, et al. G-proteins and hormonal inhibition of insulin secretion from HIT-T15 cells and isolated rat islets. Diabetes 1992;41:1390.)

Most recently, Zigman et al.[9] used oligodeoxynucleotide primers to detect cDNA fragments in pancreatic islets (as mentioned above). Besides detecting G_s, they also identified six other G_α-subunits: $G_{i1\alpha}$ or $G_{i3\alpha}$, $G_{i2\alpha}$, $G_{11\alpha}$, $G_{14\alpha}$, $G_{z\alpha}$, and $G_{t2\alpha}$. They also demonstrated the presence of $G_{t2\alpha}$-mRNA in a clonal mouse pancreatic α-cell line.

All these reports together indicate there are at least 13 heterotrimeric G-protein alpha subunits in pancreatic islets, pancreatic β-cell lines, and pancreatic α-cell lines. As reflected by the attempts of Schmidt et al.,[11] Cormont et al.,[12] and Baffy et al.,[16] a major immediate investigative challenge is to devise technologies whereby these various G-proteins can be convincingly linked to specific physiologic events after stimulation of β- and α-cells by ligand-receptor complexes.

Heterotrimeric G-Protein Regulation of Islet Gene Expression and Hormone Secretion

Gene Expression

Somatostatin and epinephrine have been known for many years to be inhibitors of insulin secretion. More recently, these hormones have been reported to have complementary effects on insulin gene expression. Zhang et al.[18] first observed this in experiments in which measurements of insulin secretion, insulin content, and insulin mRNA levels were correlated in HIT-T15 cells. They reported that both somatostatin and epinephrine decreased not only insulin secretion, but also insulin content and insulin mRNA levels—all to approximately 50% of control values (Fig. 6-4). Because it was already known that PTx could prevent the inhibitory effects of somatostatin and epinephrine on insulin secretion (see below), these investigators examined whether it could also prevent the inhibitory effects of these hormones on insulin gene expression. They observed that the decrement in insulin mRNA levels caused by somatostatin and epinephrine could be partially prevented by preincubation of HIT-T15 cells with a concentration of PTx sufficient to ADP-ribosylate all available substrates completely. These observations suggested that these two hormones negatively modulate insulin availability through a guanine nucleotide binding protein-mediated step in insulin synthesis *before* insulin enters the exocytotic pathway. They proposed that this mechanism might allow these two hormones to serve as more long-term regulators of insulin availability, as distinct from their shorter term and more readily reversible inhibitory effects on exocytosis.

These studies were later extended by Redmon et al.[19] who studied human insulin gene (*INS*) transcription using a chloramphenicol acetyltransferase reporter gene (*CAT*) driven by the enhancer-promoter region of *INS*. They observed that epinephrine, and to a lesser extent somatostatin, significantly inhibited *INS-CAT* expression (Fig. 6-5). Both somatostatin and epinephrine inhibited *INS-CAT* activity in a concentration-dependent manner that paralleled their inhibition of insulin secretion. The authors concluded that (1) somatostatin and epinephrine reduce HIT-T15 cell insulin mRNA levels in part by inhibiting *INS* transcription and (2) that these hormones were capable of coordinately regulating insulin synthesis and insulin secretion at the levels of *INS* and insulin exocytosis, respectively. More recently, a report by Kendall et al.,[20] involving HIT-T15 cells, which secretes glucagon as well as insulin, indicates that somatostatin also decreases glucagon gene expression. Although the studies by Redmon et al.[19] were the first to report that epinephrine inhibits *INS* transcription, somatostatin had

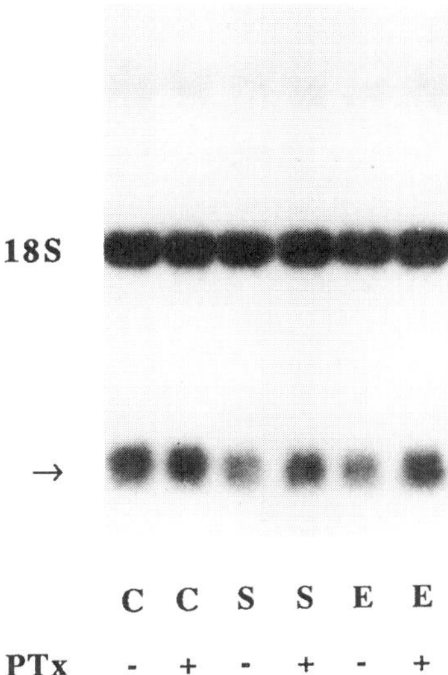

Figure 6-4. Demonstration by Northern analysis that incubation of HIT-T15 cells with somatostatin (S) or epinephrine (E) decreases the level of insulin mRNA compared to control (C) cells. Decrements of insulin mRNA could be prevented by pretreating the cells with PTx. (Reproduced with permission from Zhang H-J, Redmon JB, Andresen JM, Robertson RP. Somatostatin and epinephrine decrease insulin messenger ribonucleic acid in HIT cells through a pertussis toxin–sensitive mechanism. Endocrinology 1991;129:2409.)

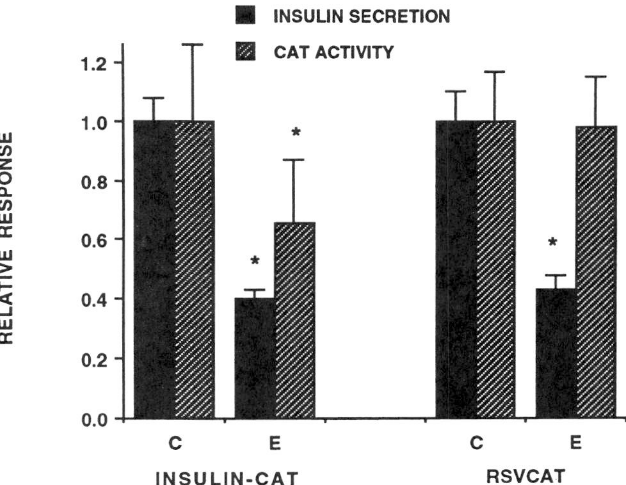

Figure 6-5. The effect of epinephrine on *CAT* activity in HIT-T15 cells transiently transfected with an insulin enhancer-promoter region–driven *CAT* construct. Pretreatment of HIT-T15 cells with epinephrine decreased both insulin secretion and *CAT* activity. No decrease in *CAT* activity was seen in control experiments in which a Rous sarcoma virus–driven *CAT* construct was transfected. (Reproduced with permission from Redmon JB, Towle HC, Robertson RP. Regulation of human insulin gene transcription by glucose, epinephrine, and somatostatin. Diabetes 1994;43: 546.)

been reported previously to affect rat insulin I gene transcription. German et al.[21] observed that somatostatin decreased the activity of a rat insulin I reporter gene transfected into fetal rat islets by 40%. Philippe[22] later confirmed the report of Zhang et al.[18] that somatostatin decreased insulin mRNA levels in HIT-T15 cells. He did not, however, observe effects on *INSCAT* activity, but did observe that somatostatin decreased insulin mRNA half-life. Thus, the reports of Redmon et al.[19] and Philippe[22] together suggest both transcriptional and post-transcriptional effects of somatostatin on the insulin gene.

The mechanism whereby somatostatin inhibits islet gene expression seems likely to involve cAMP response elements of both the *INS* and glucagon genes. The promoter region of the human, rat I and rat II, and mouse *INS* genes contain cAMP response elements that include an eight base pair sequence with close homology. Philippe and Mistotten[23] suggested that an intact cAMP response element is required for full expression of both basal and cAMP-stimulated *INS* expression based on experiments using the rat insulin I promoter region linked to *CAT*. Therefore, because both somatostatin and epinephrine are known to decrease cAMP levels in the islet and β-cell lines, it seems reasonable to maintain that the mechanism for their inhibition of islet gene expression may involve the cAMP response element.

Exocytosis

Evidence for G-protein participation in the post-receptor mechanisms involved in positive and negative regulation of islet hormone secretion by several hormones has been available for two decades. Beginning in 1975, a series of manuscripts[24–32] have been published in which extensive studies, both in vivo in rats and in vitro using isolated islets, have demonstrated that PTx prevented the decrease in cAMP and inhibition of insulin secretion caused by epinephrine and somatostatin. These investigators were the first to demonstrate that PTx ADP-ribosylates an islet protein that mediates hormonally induced inhibition of adenylate cyclase activity.[33] Since these seminal observations by Ui and colleagues, information reported within the past decade substantially added to our appreciation of the extent to which heterotrimeric G-proteins interact with several inhibitors of insulin secretion, namely, PGE_2, epinephrine, somatostatin, and galanin.

Prostaglandin E_2

Among the arachidonic acid metabolites that have been examined, PGE_2 is the most potent inhibitor of insulin secretion. This prostaglandin inhibits glucose-induced insulin secretion in humans, animals, and some pancreatic islet preparations.[34–37] In 1987, Robertson et al.[38] reported that the mechanism of action of PGE_2 in pancreatic islets and in HIT-T15 cells involved a ligand-receptor interaction with a PTx-sensitive substrate. They observed that PGE_2 bound to a specific receptor, decreased cAMP concentrations, and decreased insulin secretion. They also demonstrated that PTx ADP-ribosylated a 40-kd substrate in HIT-T15 cell membranes and that pretreatment of intact HIT-T15 cells partially prevented the inhibitory effects of PGE_2 on glucose-induced insulin secretion. Seaquist et al.[39] extended these observations, using a perifusion system in which phasic glucose-induced insulin secretion was examined. They demonstrated that perifusion of HIT-T15 cells with PGE_2 decreased both first and second phases of glucose-induced insulin release to approximately 50% of control, and that pretreatment with PTx largely prevented PGE_2 inhibition of phasic insulin release (Fig. 6-6). This inhibition of insulin release was completely prevented when PTx was included in the perifusion, suggesting that G-protein heterotrimer reassociation had occurred during the perifusion period in the first set of experiments. Seaquist et al.[39] also observed that cAMP levels were decreased by PGE_2 and that pretreatment with PTx could partially prevent this effect. There was a significant correlation between the inhibition of cAMP levels and the inhibition of glucose-induced insulin release. These findings

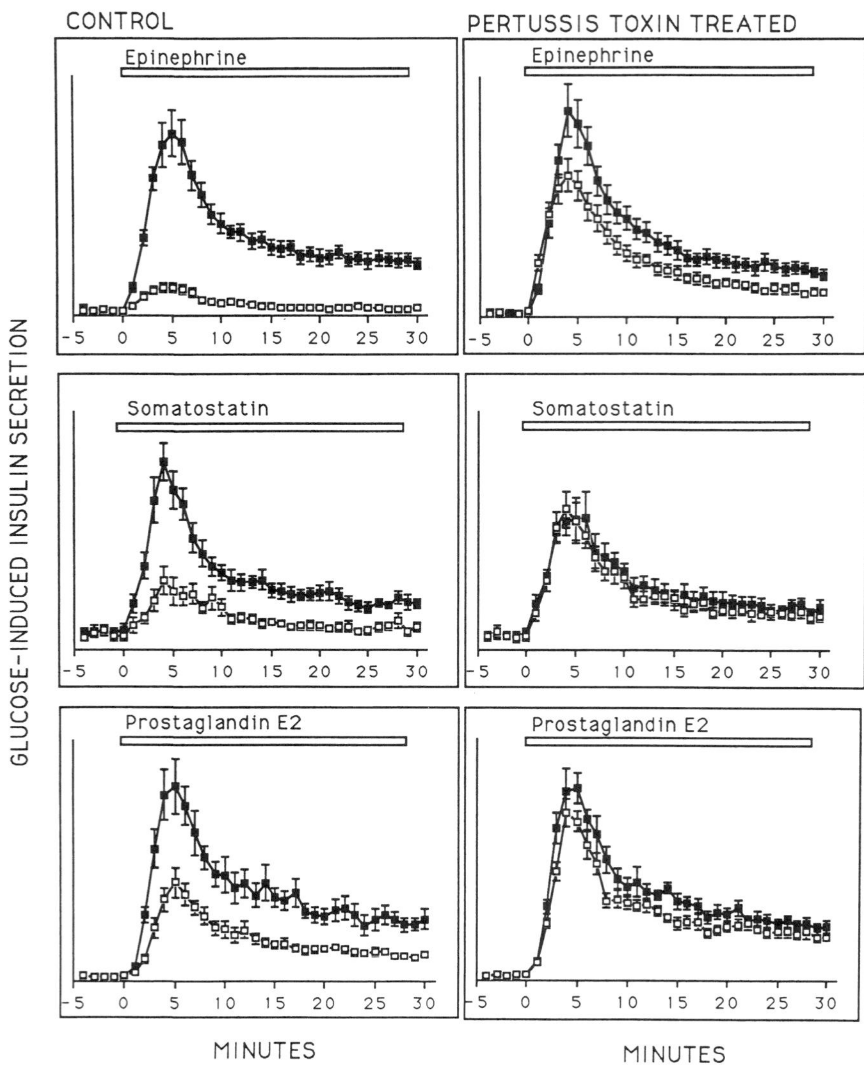

Figure 6-6. The effect of PTx pretreatment of HIT-T15 cells on the ability of epinephrine, somatostatin and PGE_2 to inhibit glucose-induced insulin secretion during perifusion. In all instances, PTx pretreatment partially or wholly prevented the inhibitory effects of these agents. (Reproduced with permission from Robertson RP, Seaquist ER, Walseth TF. G. proteins and modulation of insulin secretion. Diabetes 1991;40:1.)

were consistent with a mechanism involving inhibition of adenylate cyclase activity, presumably mediated by a form of G_i. More recently, Kowluru and Metz[40] have shown that PGE_2 stimulates a GTPase activity in secretory granule-rich fractions of both rat and human islets. This PGE_2 effect was blocked by PTx pretreatment. They concluded that there may be a PGE_2-stimulatable inhibitory G-protein located on the secretory granule that regulates exocytosis.

Epinephrine

Epinephrine was first shown to inhibit insulin secretion in vitro by Coore and Randle[41] in 1964. The mechanism of action for epinephrine was discovered to involve α_2-adrenergic receptors, inhibition of adenylate cyclase, and reduction of intracellular cAMP levels. More recently, Schmidt et al.[11] reported that epinephrine's α-adrenergic property stimulated GTPase activity in RIN m5F cells.[11] Whether or not decreased cAMP levels can explain inhibition of insulin secretion by epinephrine, however, has been the subject of much debate. Ullrich and Wollheim[42] reported that cAMP analogs did not reverse inhibitory effects of epinephrine on insulin secretion in islets and that cAMP levels did not correlate with the rate of insulin secretion in RIN m5F cells. They proposed a model in which α_2-adrenergic receptors coupled to two effector systems: adenylate cyclase and an exocytotic site. Further evidence for a distal site of epinephrine action was provided by Metz,[43] who found no relationship between epinephrine-induced inhibition of insulin secretion and changes in labeled calcium efflux from rat islets. Similar conclusions were reached by Persaud et al.,[44] who confirmed in rat islets an earlier observation by Malaisse et al.[45] that PTx ADP-ribosylated a 41-kd substrate. Persaud et al.[44] questioned whether a decrease in cAMP concentration could explain α_2-adrenergic inhibition of insulin secretion completely because they found that clonidine-induced, but not norepinephrine-induced, inhibition of insulin secretion was associated with a decrease in cellular cAMP levels. Nonetheless, clonidine is known to act through α_2-adrenergic receptors, and PTx treatment was successful in preventing clonidine-induced decrements in cAMP levels and insulin secretion. Thus, the possibility that catecholamines inhibit insulin secretion through adenylate cyclase-dependent and -independent mechanisms was raised once again. Importantly, Persaud et al.[44] found that PTx had no effect on specific binding of yohimbine, a specific α_2-antagonist, to islets. This implies that the effects of PTx are not simply due to a decrease in binding sites for catecholamines and is consistent with the concept that the PTx mechanism of action involves uncoupling of adrenergic receptors from adenylate cyclase.

Rorsman et al.[46] suggested that an alternative site for epinephrine effects on the islet might involve the sulfonylurea-insensitive, low-conductance K^+ channel, which is distinct from the ATP-dependent K^+ channel. Using HIT-T15 cells, Hsu et al.[47] examined the effects of α_2-adrenergic agonists on insulin secretion, rubidium efflux (as a marker for K^+ channel flux), and free intracellular Ca^{++} levels. They observed that epinephrine and clonidine inhibit the increase in Ca^{++} and insulin secretion caused either by K^+ depolarization or stimulation of the voltage-dependent Ca^{++} channel with the agonist Bay K 8644. Pretreatment of cells with PTx abolished the inhibitory effects of epinephrine and clonidine on both Ca^{++} levels and insulin secretion. Hsu et al.[47] suggested that one mechanism by which α_2-adrenergic agonists may inhibit Ca^{++} influx is through a PTx-sensitive G-protein governing the voltage-dependent Ca^{++} channel. In these studies, α_2-adrenergic agonists did not stimulate rubidium efflux from HIT-T15 cells, implying that their mechanism of action did not depend on an ATP-sensitive K^+ channel. Through the whole cell clamp technique, Keahey et al.[48] earlier observed that catecholamines and clonidine directly inhibit HIT-T15 cell Ca^{++} currents.

The theme that epinephrine inhibits glucose-induced insulin secretion by several different mechanisms was further reinforced by Hillaire-Buys et al.,[49] who used the isolated rat pancreas, and by Seaquist et al.,[14] who used isolated islets and HIT-T15 cells. Hillaire-Buys et al. reported PTx-sensitive and -insensitive mechanisms for epinephrine-induced inhibition of insulin secretion, both of which operated through α_2-adrenergic receptors. The data of Seaquist et al.[14] also suggested that epinephrine's effect on the islet may be mediated through multiple G-protein–regulated sites. In contrast to the report by Ullrich and Wollheim,[42] Seaquist et al.[14] demonstrated that a cAMP analog partially prevented the inhibitory effects of epinephrine on insulin secretion in the HIT-T15 cell. These authors also reported that epinephrine inhibited glipizide-induced insulin release noncompetitively through a PTx-sensitive mechanism and that the effects of epinephrine are additive to the inhibitory effects of nickel chloride. Hence, they suggested that epinephrine may act at additional sites distal to the glipizide-binding site on the ATP-sensitive K^+ channel, which could involve ion channels (as suggested by others[46–48]) or more distant exocytotic sites (as suggested by Ullrich and Wollheim[42]).

Somatostatin and Galanin

Less controversy surrounds the mechanisms of action for somatostatin- and galanin-induced inhibition of insulin secretion. Nilsson et al.[50] reported that PTx completely abolished the inhibitory effects of both somatostatin and galanin on glucose-stimulated insulin release from mouse islets. They proposed that both somatostatin and galanin suppress insulin release by a mechanism involving not only repolarization-induced reduction in intracellular Ca^{++}, but also by decreased sensitivity of the secretory machinery to Ca^{++} as well as direct interaction with the exocytotic process. All of these effects were postulated to be mediated by a PTx-sensitive G-protein. Hsu et al.[51] later reported data from whole cell patch-clamp experiments in HIT-T15 cells demonstrating that somatostatin decreased Ca^{++} currents and insulin release, both in the basal state and during depolarization with K^+ and the Ca^{++}-channel agonist, Bay K 8644. They observed that pretreatment of HIT-T15 cells with PTx prevented these effects of somatostatin. Consequently, Hsu et al.[51] concluded that one mechanism by which somatostatin can decrease insulin secretion is by inhibiting PTx-sensitive Ca^{++} influx via voltage-dependent Ca^{++} channels. In their experiments, somatostatin had no significant effects on cAMP levels during stimulation of the cells with Bay K 8644; moreover, it did not activate rubidium efflux, which mitigated against the ATP-sensitive K^+ channel as the site of action for somatostatin.

These conclusions differ from those previously published by Nilsson et al.[50] and DeWeille et al.[52] who favored the ATP-sensitive K^+ channel as the site for somatostatin action. Unlike the work of Hsu et al.,[51] however, the work of Nilsson et al. and DeWeille et al. utilized electrophysiologic techniques, which provide a more direct test of this hypothesis. The studies by Seaquist et al.[14] mentioned earlier reported that PTx completely prevented the inhibitory effects of somatostatin on glucose-induced insulin secretion in HIT-T15 cells and that addition of a cAMP analog partially prevented the inhibitory effect of this hormone. In this study,[14] somatostatin, like epinephrine, inhibited glipizide-induced insulin release noncompetitively through a PTx-sensitive mechanism and was additive to the inhibitory effects of nickel chloride. Most recently, Skoglund et al.[53] and Seaquist et al.[54] reported that galanin and somatostatin, respectively, stimulate PTx-sensitive GTPases in β-cell lines.

Conclusions

The intent of this chapter was to provide information that would allow a full appreciation of the impact that work with heterotrimeric G-proteins in the past decade has made in increasing our understanding of the postreceptor mechanism of action of regulators of pancreatic islet function in gene transcription. Both stimulatory and inhibitory heterotrimeric G-proteins express regulatory influences on pancreatic β-cells at multiple levels, including insulin gene expression and glucose-induced insulin exocytosis. Species of $G_{i\alpha}$ and $G_{o\alpha}$ probably have multiple roles in mediating the effect of multiple inhibitors of insulin secretion, including PGE_2, epinephrine, somatostatin, and galanin. Evidence points toward the existence of multiple sites of action for these inhibitory agents, both at the level of insulin gene expression and throughout the exocytotic pathway. Thus, pancreatic islet cells are exquisitely regulated by numerous mechanisms involving a large array of stimulators and inhibitors of hormone synthesis and secretion, many of which depend on heterotrimeric G-proteins for their mechanisms of action.

Acknowledgments

This work was supported by grants R01 DK38325 (R.P.R.), K08 DK01920 (E.R.S.), K08 DK02134 (J.B.R.), and 5T32 DK 07203 (D.M.K.) from the National Institutes of Health, Bethesda, Md, and by an Albert Renold Fellowship from the European Association for the Study of Diabetes (V.P.).

References

1. Spiegel AM, Downs RW Jr. Guanine nucleotides: Key regulators of hormone receptor-adenylate cyclase interaction. Endocr Rev 1981;2:275
2. Casey PJ, Gilman AG. G protein involvement in receptor-effector coupling. J Biol Chem 1988;263:2577
3. Birnbaumer L, Abramowitz J, Brown AM. Receptor-effector coupling by G proteins. Biochim Biophys Acta 1990;1031:163
4. Robertson RP, Seaquist ER, Walseth TF. G proteins and modulation of insulin secretion. Diabetes 1991;40:1
5. Simon MI, Strathmann MP, Gautam N. Diversity of G proteins in signal transduction. Science 1991;252:802
6. Lefkowitz RJ. The subunit story thickens. Nature 1992;358:372
7. Seaquist ER, Walseth TF, Redmon JB, Robertson RP. G-protein regulation of insulin secretion. J Lab Clin Med 1994;123:338
8. Walseth TF, Zhang H-J, Olson LK, et al. Increase in G_s and cyclic AMP generation in HIT cells. J Biol Chem 1989;264:21106
9. Zigman JM, Westermark GT, LaMendola J, Steiner DF. Expression of cone transducin, $G_z\alpha$, and other G-protein α-subunit messenger ribonucleic acids in pancreatic islets. Endocrinology 1994;135:31
10. Hsu WH, Rudolph U, Sanford J, et al. Molecular cloning of a novel splice variant of the α subunit of the mammalian G_o protein. J Biol Chem 1990; 265:11220
11. Schmidt A, Hescheler J, Offermans S, et al. Involvement of pertussis toxin-sensitive G-proteins in the hormonal inhibition of dihydropyridine-sensitive Ca^{2+} currents in an insulin secreting cell line (RIN 5mF). J Biol Chem 1991;266:18025
12. Cormont M, Marchand-Brustel YL, Van Obberghen E, et al. Identification of G protein α-subunits in RINm5F cells and their selective interaction with galanin receptor. Diabetes 1991;40:1170
13. Gillison SL, Sharp GWG. ADP ribosylation by cholera toxin identifies three G-proteins that are activated by the galanin receptor: Studies with RINm5F cell membranes. Diabetes 1994;43:24

14. Seaquist ER, Neal AR, Shoger KD, et al. G-proteins and hormonal inhibition of insulin secretion from HIT-T15 cells and isolated rat islets. Diabetes 1992;41:1390
15. Berrow NS, Milligan G, Morgan NG. Immunological characterization of the guanine-nucleotide binding proteins G_i and G_o in rat islets of Langerhans. J Mol Endocrinol 1992;8:103
16. Baffy G, Yang L, Wolf BA, Williamson JR. G-protein specificity in signaling pathways that mobilize calcium in insulin-secreting β-TC3 cells. Diabetes 1993;42:1878
17. Poitout V, Stout LE, Armstrong MB, et al. Morphologic and functional characterization of beta-TC6 cells, an insulin-secreting cell line derived from transgenic mice. Diabetes 1995;44:306
18. Zhang H-J, Redmon JB, Andresen JM, Robertson RP. Somatostatin and epinephrine decrease insulin messenger ribonucleic acid in HIT cells through a pertussis toxin-sensitive mechanism. Endocrinology 1991;129:2409
19. Redmon JB, Towle HC, Robertson RP. Regulation of human insulin gene transcription by glucose, epinephrine, and somatostatin. Diabetes 1994;43:546
20. Kendall DM, Olson LK, Poitout V, et al. Somatostatin coordinately regulates pancreatic α cell function via inhibition of both glucagon gene transcription and exocytosis. J Clin Invest 1995;96:2496
21. German MS, Moss LG, Rutter WJ. Regulation of insulin gene expression by glucose and calcium in transfected primary islet cultures. J Biol Chem 1990;265:22063
22. Philippe J. Somatostatin inhibits insulin-gene expression through a posttranscriptional mechanism in a hamster islet cell line. Diabetes 1993;42:244
23. Philippe J, Mistotten M. Functional characterization of a cAMP-responsive element of the rat insulin I gene. J Biol Chem 1990;265:1465
24. Sumi T, Ui M. Potentiation of the adrenergic *beta*-receptor-mediated insulin secretion in pertussis-sensitized rats. Endocrinology 1975;97:352
25. Katada T, Ui M. Perfusion of the pancreas isolated from pertussis-sensitized rats: Potentiation of insulin secretory responses due to β-adrenergic stimulation. Endocrinology 1977;101:1247
26. Katada T, Ui M. Spontaneous recovery from streptozotocin-induced diabetes in rats pretreated with pertussis vaccine or hydrocortisone. Diabetologia 1977;13:521
27. Yajima M, Hosoda K, Kanbayashi Y, et al. Biological properties of islets-activating protein (IAP) purified from the culture medium of *Bordetella pertussis*. J Biochem 1978;83:305
28. Toyota T, Kakizaki M, Kimura K, et al. Islet activating protein (IAP) derived from the culture supernatant fluid of Bordetella pertussis: Effect on spontaneous diabetic rats. Diabetologia 1978;14:319
29. Yajima M, Hosoda K, Kanbayashi Y, et al. Islets-activating protein (IAP) in *Bordetella pertussis* that potentiates insulin secretory responses of rats. J Biochem 1978;83:295
30. Katada T, Ui M. Effect of *in vivo* pretreatment of rats with a new protein purified from *Bordetella pertussis* on *in vitro* secretion of insulin: Role of calcium. Endocrinology 1979;104:1822
31. Katada T, Ui M. Slow interaction of islet-activating protein with pancreatic islets during primary culture to cause reversal of α-adrenergic inhibition of insulin secretion. J Biol Chem 1980;255:9580
32. Katada T, Ui M. Islet-activating protein: A modifier of receptor-mediated regulation of rat islet adenylate cyclase. J Biol Chem 1981;256:8310
33. Ui M, Katada T, Murayama T, et al. Islet-activating protein, pertussis toxin: A specific uncoupler of receptor-mediated inhibition of adenylate cyclase. In: Greengard P, et al., ed. Advances in Cyclic Nucleotide and Protein Phosphorylation Research, Vol. 17. New York, NY: Raven Press;1984:145
34. Robertson RP, Gavareski DJ, Porte D Jr, Bierman EL. Inhibition of *in vivo* insulin secretion by prostaglandin E_1. J Clin Invest 1974;54:310
35. Burr IM, Sharp R. Effects of prostaglandin E_1 and of epinephrine on the dynamics of insulin release *in vitro*. Endocrinology 1974;94:835
36. Robertson RP, Chen M. A role for prostaglandin E in defective insulin secretion and carbohydrate intolerance in diabetes mellitus. J Clin Invest 1977;60:747
37. Metz SA, Robertson RP, Fujimoto WY. Inhibition of prostaglandin E synthesis augments glucose-induced insulin secretion in cultured pancreas. Diabetes 1981;30:551
38. Robertson RP, Tsai P, Little SA, et al. Receptor-mediated adenylate cyclase-coupled mechanism for PGE_2 inhibition of insulin secretion in HIT cells. Diabetes 1987;36:1047
39. Seaquist ER, Walseth TF, Nelson DM, Robertson RP. Pertussis toxin-sensitive G protein mediation of PGE_2 inhibition of cAMP metabolism and phasic glucose-induced insulin secretion in HIT cells. Diabetes 1989;38:1439
40. Kowluru A, Metz SA. Stimulation by prostaglandin E_2 of a high-affinity GTPase in the secretory granules of normal rat and human pancreatic islets. Biochem J 1994;297:399
41. Coore HG, Randle PJ. Regulation of insulin secretion studied with pieces of rabbit pancreas incubated *in vitro*. Biochem J 1964;93:66
42. Ullrich S, Wollheim CB. GTP-dependent inhibition of insulin secretion by epinephrine in permeabilized RINm5F cells. J Biol Chem 1988;263:8615
43. Metz SA. Epinephrine impairs insulin release by a mechanism distal to calcium mobilization: Similarity to lipoxygenase inhibitors. *Diabetes* 1988;37:65
44. Persaud SJ, Jones PM, Howell SL. Effects of *Bordetella pertussis* toxin on catecholamine inhibition of insulin release from intact and electrically permeabilized rat islets. Biochem J 1989;258:669
45. Malaisse WJ, Svoboda M, Dufrane SP, et al. Effect of *Bordetella pertussis* toxin on ADP-ribosylation of membrane proteins, adenylate cyclase activity and insulin release in rat pancreatic islets. Biochem Biophys Res Commun 1984;124:190
46. Rorsman P, Bokvist K, Åmmälä C, et al. Activation by adrenaline of a low-conductance G protein-dependent K^+ channel in mouse pancreatic B cells. Nature 1991;349:77
47. Hsu WH, Xiang H, Rajan AS, Boyd AE III. Activation of α_2-adrenergic receptors decreases Ca^{2+} influx to inhibit insulin secretion in a hamster β-cell line: An action mediated by a guanosine triphosphate-binding protein. Endocrinology 1991;128:958
48. Keahey HH, Boyd III AE, Kunze DL. G protein-dependent modification of calcium currents in clonal pancreatic β-cells. Am J Physiol 1990;257:C1171
49. Hillaire-Buys D, Gross R, Roye M, et al. Adrenergic inhibition of insulin secretion involves pertussis toxin-sensitive and -insensitive mechanisms. Eur J Pharmacol 1992;218:359
50. Nilsson T, Arkhammar P, Rorsman P, Berggren P-O. Suppression of insulin release by galanin and somatostatin is mediated by a G-protein: An effect involving repolarization and reduction in cytoplasmic free Ca^{2+} concentration. J Biol Chem 1989;264:973
51. Hsu WH, Xiang H, Rajan AS, et al. Somatostatin inhibits insulin secretion by a G-protein-mediated decrease in Ca^{2+} entry through voltage-dependent Ca^{2+} channels in the beta cell. J Biol Chem 1991;266:837
52. DeWeille JR, Schmid-Antomarchi H, Fosset M, Lazdunski M. Regulation of ATP-sensitive K^+ channels in insulinoma cells: Activation by somatostatin and protein kinase C and the role of cAMP. Proc Natl Acad Sci USA 1989;86:2971
53. Skoglund G, Bliss CR, Sharp GWG. Galanin-stimulated high-affinity GTPase activity in plasma membranes from RIN m5F cells. Diabetes 1993;42:74
54. Seaquist ER, Armstrong MB, Gettys TW, Walseth TF. Somatostatin selectively couples to $G_{o\alpha}$ in HIT-T15 cells, a clonal line of glucose-responsive pancreatic beta cells. Diabetes 1995;44:85

Diabetes Mellitus, edited by Derek LeRoith, Simeon I. Taylor, and Jerrold M. Olefsky. Lippincott–Raven Publishers, Philadelphia © 1996.

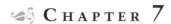

CHAPTER 7

GTP-Binding Proteins in the Regulation of Pancreatic β-Cell Function: Part II. Putative Roles for Low-Molecular-Weight Proteins

STEWART A. METZ AND ANJANEYULU KOWLURU

Overview of GTP-Binding Proteins (GBPs)

Protein trafficking plays a number of important roles in secretory cells. Peptide-secreting endocrine cells require signaling systems that target nascent proteins for translocation into the lumen of the endoplasmic reticulum (ER), and then direct these proteins in the early secretory pathway along the ER to the Golgi; there, in turn, they must be packaged into secretory granules (or vesicles) and somehow be "addressed" for the late (constitutive or regulated) pathways of secretion. After this targeting, secretory granules must be directed to and marginate at the plasma membrane, where they fuse and release their contents under the influence of appropriate secretagogues.

It is widely believed that GTP-binding proteins (GBPs) play central roles as "molecular switches" in such cellular protein traffic, probably in association with (and even complexed to) one or more proteins of the secretory granule or plasma membrane. This group of proteins may include phospholipases, protein kinases, and synaptic vesicle or plasma membrane proteins (e.g., synaptotagmin, syntaxin, 25-kd synaptosomal-associated protein, *N*-ethylmaleimide-sensitive fusion protein (NSF), synaptobrevin). Many of these proteins share common structural motifs (C2 domains). Such domains identify them as Ca^{++}- and phospholipid-binding proteins[1] and possibly Ca^{++} "sensors," especially since some of them may associate with Ca^{++} channels.[2] Together with GBPs, these proteins may serve as docking or fusion proteins, mediating the shuttling of secretory products between various cellular compartments (e.g., secretory granule and plasma membrane) followed by fusion between carrier and recipient membranes. Several biologically active lipids (such as arachidonic acid, lysophospholipids, or phosphatidic acid) are fusigenic under appropriate conditions; therefore, it is possible that phospholipases constitute one class of target or effector molecules for activated GBPs.* Indeed, GBPs activate phospholipase C in insulin-secreting cells[5] and have been shown to have a similar effect on phospholipases A_2 and D in other cells.[6]

Other potential effector targets of GBPs include Ca^{++} or K^+ channels, adenylate cyclases, protein kinases, and elements of the secretory granule and cytoskeleton. Subunits of G_i or G_o, or both, may modulate protein trafficking from the ER to the Golgi, and thence to secretory vesicles or granules.[7] There is evidence of specific linkage of the alpha subunit of one heterotrimeric GBP, G_i, to the inhibition of adenylate cyclase (see Chapter 6 by Robertson) or the modulation of Ca^{++} or K^+ channels,[8] or both. The alpha subunits of G_o species have been linked to inhibition of plasmalemmal Ca^{++} channels,[9] whereas G_q or G_{11}, and perhaps ADP-ribosylation factor (ARF)[10], rho, or ras, are GBPs coupled to phospholipase activation (see footnote denoted by an asterisk [*]). Some analogous evidence exists in studies of insulin-secreting cells (Table 7-1; see Chapter 6).[5,11–14] It is important to note, however, that a particular α subunit may be linked to more than one effector. Furthermore, the activation of an α subunit requires its dissociation from the βγ dimer; βγ subunits can themselves modulate the activity of various effector systems[15] including, potentially, those *not* altered by the respective α subunit. Thus, considerable opportunity for "cross-talk" exists.

This chapter focuses only on relatively *late* steps in regulated, exocytotic insulin secretion as well as selected aspects of the potential role(s) therein of the low-molecular-weight (monomeric) GBPs, emphasizing their identity, post-translational modifications, and activation. (Similar aspects of the heterotrimeric, higher molecular weight GBPs are discussed by Robertson in Chapter 6.) It should be noted, however, that this distinction is somewhat artificial, considering that some recent studies have suggested that important functional relationships may exist between the two classes of GBPs.[16–19] No discussion has been made of the potentially important roles of GBPs in constitutive secretion (which may control, for example, the expression of GLUT-2 on β-cell membranes[20]) or in *early* events in regulated secretion, including the biosynthesis and sorting of secretory products.

Potential Role of Low-Molecular-Weight GBPs in Secretory Processes: Overview

Studies in yeast, and more recent studies in mammalian amine-secreting cells (such as mast cells and adrenal chromaffin cells), have provided precedent for a role of monomeric GBPs in secretory processes. In a pivotal paper, Fernandez and colleagues[21] reported in 1984 that the introduction of a stable GTP analog into mast cells was capable of triggering calcium-*independent* exocytotic secretion. This observation has been confirmed (with minor differences) in many other cell types,[22] including insulin-secreting cells.[5] In more recent studies, introduction of peptides containing the effector domain of one monomeric GBP (e.g., rab 3A) into β-cells has induced insulin release.[23] Such studies are complemented by the use of pharmacologic probes such as mastoparan, a polycationic peptide that directly activates GBPs[24] and also promotes insulin release.[25–29] Because these approaches have elicited insulin release even in permeabilized cells (wherein the levels of many soluble cell messengers can be fixed), it is frequently speculated that one (or more) proteins, referred to as G_E or G_{Ei}, play key roles in

*Some studies purporting to demonstrate the activation of phospholipases by GBPs may require reassessment in view of recent data demonstrating that GBPs can also perturb the degradation or disposal of phospholipid hydrolytic products, including lysophospholipids,[3] diglycerides,[4] and arachidonic acid. Recently, phospholipase inhibitory GBPs have been described.

Table 7-1. Classes of GTP-Binding Proteins

Type	Identification Techniques	Structure	NTP Preferred	Identity in Islets/ β-Cells*	Putative Effector(s)
Heterotrimeric	Immunologic ADP ribosylation (some)	αβγ (holoprotein > 80 kd)	GTPγS	G_o (several) $G_{i(1-3)}$ G_q G_s (2 α subunits) G_{olf} G_{12}, G_{13}, G_z	Adenylate cyclase; K^+ (ATP) channel; insulin gene; phospholipase(s); Ca^{++} channels; traffic from ER → Golgi → secretory granules or vesicles (see text)
Low-molecular-weight (monomeric)	GTP overlay (some) Immunologic ADP ribosylation (some)	Monomeric (20–27 kd) ± regulatory proteins (GDI, GDS, GEP, GAP)	(often) GTP	Cdc42 rhoA rab 3A,3B,3C† rac2 Arf [GDI]	? (? cytoskeleton) ? (? cytoskeleton) Late regulated secretory pathway ? Golgi function and early secretory pathway —
Miscellaneous		Mostly monomeric (49–102 kd)	Both (?)	Signal recognition particle; initiation, elongation, and termination factors; tubulin, etc.	Protein biosynthetic apparatus; cytoskeleton (e.g., ref. 81)

*Data from multiple investigators in Geneva, Minneapolis, Ithaca, Madison, Staffordshire, Uppsala, Philadelphia, Marburg, Boston, Berlin.
†Initial studies indicate that the following genes are detected in human islets: rab 4 and 8A, $G_{s\alpha}$, $G_{i\alpha3}$, ARF_{1-3}, N-*ras* (Takeda J, Yano H, Eng S, Zeng Y, Bell GI, *Hum. Molec. Genet.* 2:1793–1798, 1993). Expression of the rab 3A gene was detected in RIN (but not HIT) cells (Lankat-Buttgereit B, Göke R, Fehmann H-C, Niess C, Göke B, FEBS Lett 312:183–6, 1992). In mouse pancreatic islets, the gene expression of the following α subunits was detected: G_s, G_{i1} or G_{i2}, G_{11}, G_{14}, G_z, and G_t (transducin) (Zigman JM, Westermark GT, LaMendola J, Steiner DF. Endocrinol 135:31–7, 1994).
ER = endoplasmic reticulum; GAP = GTPase-activating protein; GDI = GDP-dissociation inhibitor; GDP = guanosine diphosphate; GDS = GDP-dissociation stimulator; GEP = GTP/GDP exchange protein; NTP = nucleoside triphosphate

the promotion or inhibition, of respectively terminal steps in the exocytotic cascade (Table 7-2, Fig. 7-1).

Such putative proteins could involve representatives of one or both of two major classes of GBPs. The heterotrimeric GBPs are complexes of α, β, and γ subunits and largely reside in the plasma membrane; however, more recent studies have identified such GBPs in intracellular organelles such as secretory granules,[30,31] mitochondria, the Golgi apparatus, and even cytosol in certain circumstances.[32] Heterotrimeric GBPs have been implicated in the inhibitory modulation of exocytotic secretion from nonislet mammalian cells,[33] and clearly are involved in the inhibitory control of insulin release (see Chapter 6; see Fig. 7-1); they might also provide stimulatory signals (see below).[25,27] When heterotrimeric GBPs are activated by occupancy of a surface receptor, guanosine diphosphate (GDP) dissociates from the α subunit, which then binds GTP; this active form ($G_{\alpha\cdot GTP}$) then can interact with various effector systems. Recent studies have suggested that the βγ subunits do not merely fill a passive role in anchoring the α subunit to the membrane, but are themselves capable of interacting with various effector systems,[†15] and therefore may play a direct role both in modulating secretion and in other phenomena such as cellular desensitization.[37] Hydrolysis of GTP by the GTPase activity intrinsic to the heterotrimeric GBPs is an off-signal; therefore, nonhydrolyzable or poorly hydrolyzable analogs of GTP (e.g., GTPγS, GTPβS) or AlF_4^- (fluoroaluminate, which mimics the terminal phosphate of GTP) often are used as probes to activate trimeric GBPs.

In contrast, the large family of low-molecular-weight GBPs exist as monomers. Recent studies (see below), however, indicate that small GBPs can complex with one or more modulatory factors as heterodimers,[31] an interaction that affects both their cellular localization and their activity. Bourne[38] and other investigators have described a cell cycle wherein GTP binding to the monomeric GBPs is associated with their translocation to a membranous compartment (or compartments), where they exert their effects; this is followed by hydrolysis of the GTP, which returns them to the inactive, GDP-liganded form in the cytosol, thereby concluding one cycle. For at least some low-molecular-weight GBPs, the ongoing hydrolysis of GTP is considered necessary to permit repetitive cycles of cell activation[‡]; therefore, it is not surprising that fluoroaluminate does not activate, and GTPγS may even inhibit, low-molecular-weight GBPs.[41] There is some evidence that formation of vesicles requires only GTP binding, whereas their transport involves GTP hydrolysis.[42]

Unlike the heterotrimeric GBPs, many (albeit not all) monomeric GBPs retain the ability to bind radiolabeled GTP after their separation on denaturing (i.e., SDS-PAGE) gels. Specific proteins can then be identified immunologically. These techniques have enabled a variety of low-molecular-weight GBPs to be identified in normal rodent or human pancreatic islets,[30] or in cultured and transformed β-cell lines (Table 7-1). Which of these might act as G_E? Studies using normal islets[25] or transformed β-cells[28] showing

†To complicate issues, β subunits share structural homology with a phospholipase A_2 activating protein[34] and with cellular receptors for protein kinase C.[35] Furthermore, βγ subunits bind to a number of signaling molecules containing pleckstrin domains,[36] including β-adrenergic receptor kinase and, potentially, phospholipase C-γ, GTPase-activating protein, or GTP/GDP exchange protein.[36]

‡Unfortunately, such finds are not invariate because GTPγS may activate some low-molecular-weight GBPs.[19] Furthermore, it may be difficult to interpret the effects of GTPγS when introduced into permeabilized cells. In β-cells, such effects could represent the persistent activation of a trimeric G_E; however, alternatively, they could reflect the freezing (i.e., locking in an activated state) of a monomeric G_{Ei}, which requires GTP hydrolysis to cycle. For example, the observation[39] that GTPγS *prevents* the capacitative entry of extracellular Ca^{++} that follows the emptying of intracellular Ca^{++} stores has been used to infer a *stimulatory* role in that process for monomeric GBPs that hydrolyze GTP. A similar effect of GTPγS on Ca^{++} entry has been described in islet cells.[40]

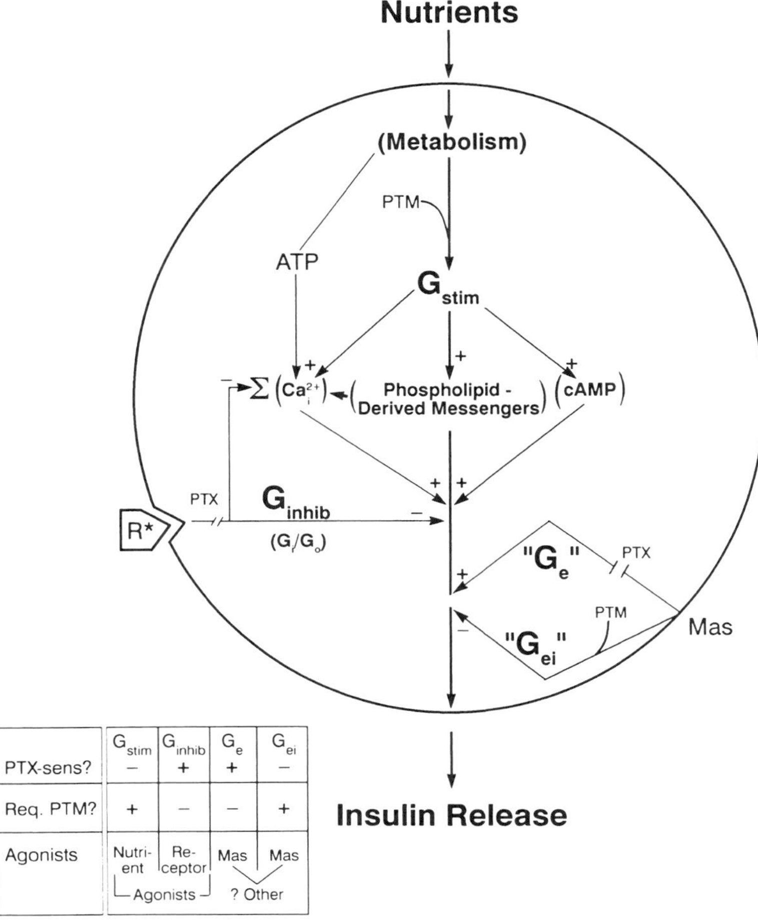

	G_{stim}	G_{inhib}	G_e	G_{ei}
PTX-sens?	−	+	+	−
Req. PTM?	+	−	−	+
Agonists	Nutrient	Receptor	Mas	Mas
	Agonists		? Other	

Figure 7-1. A model, compatible with data in ref. 25 (and A. Kowluru, S. Metz, unpublished data, 1994–1995), suggesting sites of action of GBPs in insulin secretion from normal islets. Nutrients, via their metabolism, appear to modulate one or more stimulatory GBPs (G_{stim}) relatively proximal in the cascade of stimulus-secretion coupling. These may include GBPs which activate phospholipases or generate messengers such as cyclic AMP or intracellular Ca^{++}. The summation (Σ) of effects of these second messengers mediates or accelerates physiologic insulin release (+). (An antecedent rise in intracellular ATP closes K^+ channels [K^+(ATP)] and initiates Ca^{++} influx; this event might also involve a GBP.) At least one G_{stim} requires post-translational modification (PTM), because nutrient-induced secretion is *reduced* by inhibitors of isoprenylation, carboxymethylation or protein acylation. Mastoparan (Mas), a direct activator of GBPs, presumably does *not* promote secretion primarily at this stage because its effects are *resistant* to blockade by PTM inhibitors.

It has been proposed that a stimulatory GBP (G_E) might also mediate *terminal* events in exocytosis. Indeed, mastoparan initiates secretion in a fashion partially sensitive to inhibition by PTx, suggesting the involvement of a stimulatory, heterotrimeric GBP. However, PTx does not block the effect of any *physiologic* agonist, including glucose or Ca^{++}.[5,118] Furthermore, if early metabolic events are bypassed by directly providing more distal signals, such as a phorbol ester, a rise in [Ca^{++}] (via a depolarizing concentration of K^+), or mastoparan, the ensuing insulin release is largely resistant to inhibition by PTM blockers. Thus, there is no unequivocal evidence for a *distal* G_E acting in *physiologic, regulated* secretion. Although the existence of such a protein is not excluded, if it exists, it presumably does not require post-translational modification; alternatively, it is possible that it is sufficiently stable and long-lived that a depletion of its PTM-processed form would not be detectable within the time course of the studies.[25] Another possibility is that mastoparan activates a PTx-sensitive GBP mediating *constitutive* secretion, rather than regulated secretion.

In fact, a dramatic *potentiation* of mastoparan-induced secretion is unmasked by PTM inhibitors such as AFC. This suggests the presence of one or more distally acting, inhibitory GBPs (G_{inhib}). Indeed, because mastoparan activates most or all GBPs, it would be expected to have both inhibitory and stimulatory effects. One G_{inhib} known to be present in islets is activated by receptor (R*) agonists (e.g., epinephrine, prostaglandin E_2, galanin, somatostatin); such agents can alter proximal events such as glucose metabolism and ion channels, but they also inhibit insulin release (at least in part) *distal* to the fuel-activated accumulation of second messengers and in a fashion which is largely sensitive to inhibition by PTx. One G_{inhib} could thus be the heterotrimeric GBPs G_i and/or G_o, or both (see Chapter 6). AFC-induced potentiation of at least some distally acting agonists (phorbol ester, mastoparan), however, is unchanged by prior PTx pretreatment. Furthermore, AFC pretreatment fails to block the inhibitory effects of epinephrine. Therefore, the proteins on which PTx and AFC act appear to differ, suggesting the presence of a second inhibitory GBP acting distally in exocytosis (G_{Ei}). An alternative interpretation for the potentiation of such secretion by AFC, might be that inhibition of the post-translational modifications of the C-terminus of a G_{stim} alters its interaction with inhibitory modulators (e.g., βγ, GDI, GAP), thereby either enhancing its activity directly, or permitting the release of free βγ subunits, which can directly interact with effector systems.

A summary of the experimental findings for this formulation is provided in tabular form in the figure *inset*. (Adapted with permission from Metz SA, Rabaglia ME, Stock JB, Kowluru A. Modulation of insulin secretion from normal rat islets by inhibitors of the post-translational modifications of GTP-binding proteins. Biochem J 1993;295:31. Additional unpublished data from A Kowluru and S Metz, 1993.)

Table 7-2. Evidence for G_E and G_{Ei} in β-Cells

Observation	Cell Type	Effector Systems Excluded	Investigator (reference)
GTPγS stimulates Ca^{++}-independent, GDPβS-sensitive secretion	Permeabilized RINm5F cells	PLC PKA PKC $[Ca^{++}{}_i]$	Vallar et al.[5]
rab3A effector domain potentiates basal-, Ca^{++}-stimulated, and GTPγS-stimulated secretion	Permeabilized HIT cells	$[Ca^{++}{}_i]$	Li et al.[23]
Mastoparan initiates secretion	Permeabilized or intact islets (PTx or GDPβs sensitive) RINm5F (PTx-insensitive)*	$[Ca^{++}{}_i]$ PKA PKC NDPK	Metz et al.,[25] Jones et al.,[26] Kowluru et al.[70] Sharp et al.;[28] Hillaire-Buys et al.,[29] Yokokawa et al.[27]
PGE_2, somatostatin, epinephrine, and galanin inhibit secretion (PTx-sensitive)	Permeabilized and intact HIT cells Islets	(Both at and) distal to cAMP, ion channels, $[Ca^{++}{}_i]$	Robertson, Sharp, Jones, Tamigawa, Ullrich, Metz, Nilsson and colleagues

*In RIN cells, PTx may actually potentiate the effects of mastoparan.[28]
GDP = guanosine diphosphate; GTP = guanosine triphosphate; NDPK = nucleoside diphosphokinase; PGE_2 = prostaglandin E_2; PKA = protein kinase A; PKC = protein kinase C; PLC = phospholipase C; PTx = pertussis toxin.

that mastoparan stimulates insulin release are by themselves of limited help in answering this question, since mastoparan directly activates both high- and low-molecular-weight GBPs. Because mastoparan-induced secretion can be reduced by one-half to two-thirds by prior treatment of normal islets[§] with pertussis toxin (PTx),[25,27] one or more heterotrimeric GBPs might be involved in secretory processes (see Fig. 7-1). Recent data,[25,47,48] however, implicate monomeric GBPs in promoting the insulin secretion induced by physiologic, nutrient secretagogues. Blockade of the function of such GBPs (i.e., by impeding their post-translational modifications; see below) reduces fuel-induced secretion (but not mastoparan-induced secretion) by approximately 50%. It has been suggested[25] that Cdc42 (a 23-kd "monomeric" GBP of the rho family) may be one critical GBP in this regard (Table 7-3). Cdc42 may have a role in budding and polarized cell growth in yeast and, interestingly, localizes to the vicinity of secretory vesicles.[49] The rab 3 family may also be involved[‖] because introduction into islet cells of peptides containing its effector domain promotes secretion.[23] Most frequently implicated is rab 3A, but recent studies[52,53] suggest that rab 3B or 3C could be involved and probably are present in insulin-secreting cells.[31] A third observation that could be interpreted to implicate small GBPs is that an adequate content of GTP in β-cells is a prerequisite for fuel-induced insulin secretion.[54,55] Because most trimeric GBPs have high affinities for GTP (i.e., K_m for GTP in the nanomolar to low micromolar range), they presumably would not be regulated by ambient GTP concentration (which in islet cells is normally 750–1,000 μM). Indeed, even a marked reduction in the GTP content of islet cells impedes neither the inhibition of insulin release induced by epinephrine[54] nor the potentiation of secretion induced by carbachol (S Metz, 1993 unpublished data): The effects of the former are mediated by the trimeric GBPs G_i or G_o, or both (see Chapter 6), and those of the latter are mediated (at least in part) by G_q (a phospholipase-linked GBP).[11] The possibility remains, however, that a monomeric GBP mediates this function of GTP. It is of interest, then, that we have recently described[30] in insulin-secreting cells the presence of a low-affinity, high K_m GTPase. This protein has a K_m (750–800 μM) for GTP such that its function might be impeded by decrements in the ambient GTP concentration in islet cells. The identity of this putative stimulatory GBP has not yet been deduced. It may be relevant, however, that in many other cells as well the concentrations of GTP required to activate intracellular signaling events[55] and secretion[56–58] are also well into the micromolar range, even when poorly hydrolyzable analogs of GTP are used. It remains to be determined whether these findings are attributable to effects of GTP unrelated to GBPs or to the fact that some GBPs, in the milieu of complex membranes, have affinities for GTP that are lower than those calculated in studies of simpler systems (i.e., isolated membranes or pure proteins). Very recent studies[59] also suggest that the local GTP:GDP ratio could modulate the activity of some GBPs.

§In transformed β-cells, in contrast, pertussis toxin (PTx) does not reduce and may *potentiate* mastoparan-induced secretion.[28] This is one of several examples of differences between normal and transformed/cultured β-cells.[30,44] Nonetheless, if this finding in RIN cells indicates that mastoparan also can activate a GBP *inhibitory* to secretion, it confirms the presence of such an inhibitory GBP in intact islets, which has been deduced by other means[25] (see Fig. 7-1). GBPs inhibiting not only ion fluxes and adenylate cyclases, but also phospholipases,[45] are well described. Note also that insulin release stimulated by GTPγS is resistant to PTx in RINm5F cells.[5] This result may not exclude the possibility, however, that at least one G_E is a PTx-sensitive, trimeric GBP, considering that direct, receptor-*independent* activation of such GBPs by GTPγS may not always be prevented by PTx.[46]

‖Very recent studies suggest, however, that rab 3A might serve an inhibitory role in granule/vesicle fusion.[50,51]

Regulation and Targeting of GTP-Binding Proteins: General Aspects

Knowledge of the regulation of GTP-binding proteins is still evolving (Table 7-4), and the field has reached a bewildering level of complexity. The presence of a divalent cation, especially Mg^{++}, is required for most functions of GBPs at several different regulatory sites; however, *changes* in the intracellular concentrations of divalent cations probably are not regulatory for GBPs. One major site of regulation is the "off rate" for the inactive guanine nucleotide GDP. In the case of trimeric GBPs, this event is activated by the binding of extracellular ligands to receptors that are coupled to GBPs. In the case of the major physiologic islet agonists (i.e., nutrients), however, there is no extracellular ligand, a situation that necessitates the search for soluble, intracellular mediators of GTP binding. One class of these may be biologically active lipids (see below); nitric oxide might be another such diffusible activator of GBP.[60]

The activation of monomeric GBPs can be facilitated (or dampened) by a family of proteins that interact directly with them and alter their ability to bind or hydrolyze GTP, as well as to

Table 7-3. Data* Implicating Cdc42 in Fuel-Induced Insulin Release

I. A. Cdc42 is present in rat islets, human islets, and insulin-secreting, pure β-cells (HIT or RIN), based on immunologic evidence.
   B. Each of these insulin-secreting cells has endogenous methyl transferase activity that can mediate guanine nucleotide–specific carboxyl methylation of endogenous as well as exogenous pure Cdc42. Glucose stimulates the carboxyl methylation specifically of Cdc42.
   C. Incubation of homogenates of insulin-secreting cells with GTPγS and S-adenosyl methionine results in an increase in the translocation of Cdc42 from the soluble to the membrane fraction.

II. Inhibition of prenylcysteine carboxyl methylation by AFC correlates with a concomitant reduction of nutrient-induced phospholipase C activation and insulin release from normal islets. An analog of AFC that does not inhibit carboxyl methylation in islets also does not alter phospholipase activity on secretion. Based on immunoprecipitation experiments, most AFC-sensitive carboxyl methylation is attributable to Cdc42.

III. In transformed β-cells, lovastatin reduces the prenylation of Cdc42 (and rab 3A), and thereby impedes its complexing with GDI. This, in turn, leads to its redistribution from membranes to cytosol, effects not seen with some other low-molecular-weight GBPs (rho or ARF). Concomitantly, lovastatin impedes insulin release.†

*Data from refs. 25, 31, 48, and 108.
†The effects of nutrients are blocked in intact islets, whereas in transformed β-cells, only the effects of certain receptor agonists (arginine vasopressin, bombesin) are blocked.

interact with membranes and effectors. These factors sometimes are referred to as GTP/GDP exchange proteins (GEPs) or GDP-dissociation stimulators (GDSs) when they stimulate GDP release and thereby facilitate GTP binding; they are called GDP-dissociation inhibitors (GDIs) when they inhibit GDP release. Others (e.g., GTPase-activating proteins [GAPs]) promote the hydrolysis of GTP once it is bound, thereby terminating the activation. Of these peptide factors, only the presence of GDI has been well documented thus far in insulin-secreting cells.[31,47] Recently, in a reconstituted system using islet subcellular fractions, we observed the presence of a putative GEP in pancreatic islets, which was stimulated by insulinotropic lipids, such as arachidonic acid, lyso-PC, or phosphatidic acid.[61] An interesting property of GDIs is that, by binding to and masking the prenylated and carboxyl methylated C-terminal domains of GBPs (see the following section) they decrease the affinity of the GBP for the membranous compartment.[31] GDIs thereby can actually extract GBPs into the soluble compartment, where presumably they are poised for a new round of binding and activation when exposed to a suitably potent GEP.[62] It is possible that one or more of these regulatory factors is the site of control of islet GBPs by biologically active lipids (see below).[63,64] Regulatory proteins such as GDIs, GDSs, and GAPs have been described only for the monomeric GBPs; however, recent descriptions[36,65] of proteins that bind to the βγ complex of certain trimeric GBPs suggest that similar peptide interactions and heterodimerization of high-molecular-weight GBPs might exist. It is interesting that the βγ complex of the latter acts as a membrane anchor for the α subunit and promotes return to the αβγ (trimeric) form; therefore, it facilitates inactivation of G_α by sequestering it, thus playing a role somewhat analogous to GDI action on low-molecular-weight GBPs. The analogy is furthered by the fact that both βγ and GDI (or GAP) also may have direct or indirect effector functions (e.g., GAP itself, like βγ, may act ''downstream'' of its GBP to modulate effector function).[66] Additionally, GDIs may possibly prevent the dissociation or hydrolysis, or both, of any bound GTP as well[67]; therefore, it might prolong the ''half-life'' of a GBP in its *active* form, thereby acting under certain circumstances as a *potentiator* of GBP function by competing with GAP. Conversely, some effector

Table 7-4. Potential Regulatory Sites for GTP-Binding Proteins

Step Regulated	Regulatory Event or Regulator
GTP/GDP exchange (Mg^{++}-dependent)	Agonist binding to receptors (trimeric GBPs)
	GDI/GDS/GEP (monomeric GBPs)
	Lipid mediators
	Phosphotransfer mechanisms
	[GTP] or GTP:GDP ratio
GTPase	Intrinsic activity (trimeric GBPs)
	GAP, GDI (monomeric GBPs)
	Lipid mediators
	Effector molecules
	Toxins (e.g., PTx or cholera acting on some trimeric GBPs)
Rapid and reversible post-translational modifications	Carboxyl methylation
	Acylation (with palmitate, ? arachidonate)
	Phosphorylation
Steps required for function, but not involved in acute regulation	Divalent cations (Mg^{++})
	Myristoylation
	Isoprenylation
	Ribosylation (e.g., PTx, cholera or botulinum toxins; some modify trimeric GBPs, and some modify small GBPs)

GAP = GTPase-activating protein; GBPs = GTP-binding proteins; GDI = GDP-dissociation inhibitor; GDP = guanosine diphosphate; GDS = GDP-dissociation stimulator; GEP = GTP/GDP exchange protein; GTP = guanosine triphosphate; PTx = pertussis toxin.

systems for GBPs (e.g., phospholipase C, cyclic guanosine monophosphate [cGMP] phosphodiesterase, tyrosine kinase) have been shown recently to have GAP-like or GDI-like activity[68,69]—that is, they modulate GTP hydrolysis and might thereby provide a physiologic feedback loop or desensitizing effect on GBP action. These possibilities remain unexplored in islet cells.

Regulation of GTP-Binding Proteins in Insulin-Secreting Cells

The effects of receptor occupancy or nucleotide exchange factors can be mimicked pharmacologically by application of any of a series of polycationic probes, including the prototype mastoparan, and other similar drugs such as compound 48/80, melittin, and polymyxin. These are not ideal probes, however, because they can induce a number of nonspecific, membrane-active effects; therefore, a suitable control should be studied in tandem.[70] One such control is mastoparan-17, a structurally similar drug but one that lacks the ability to activate GBPs.[24] Because mastoparan can activate most if not all classes of GBPs, its net effect may reflect the summation of its effects on multiple stimulatory and inhibitory GBPs. Indeed, whereas mastoparan-induced insulin secretion is blunted by PTx (see Table 7-2), it is potentiated by blockade of the post-translational modification of small GBPs,[25] suggesting that at least one G_E-like protein, and at least one G_{Ei}-like protein, are simultaneously activated by mastoparan (see Fig. 7-1). It should be noted, however, that mastoparan-induced secretion is resistant to ATP depletion, diazoxide, removal of extracellular Ca^{++}, or epinephrine[26] (S. Metz and M. Rabaglia, 1993, unpublished observations); therefore, it might conceivably represent promotion of *constitutive*-type secretion, rather than a model for GBP-mediated *regulated* secretion.

Recently, novel mechanisms for activating GBPs have been described in normal islets and in β-cells.[71,72] Both involve formation of a transient high-energy phosphate intermediate of the ''transmitter'' molecule; this protein can then transfer its phosphate (via a classic ''ping-pong'' mechanism) to GDP, either liganded to an inactive GBP (the ''receiver'' module) or to GDP free in the soluble fraction, thereby converting them to their active form (Table 7-5). The phosphorylated amino acid on the transmitter is probably histidine, based on criteria summarized in Table 7-6. In cytosol, nucleoside diphosphokinase (NDPK) subserves the role of transmitter molecule; in the membranous fraction of islets, the β subunit of the trimeric GBPs serves this role.[72¶] This transmitter-receiver tandem[73] is analogous to the phosphohistidine relay systems that transduce a number of sensory functions in bacteria.[74,75] There is some evidence, albeit controverted,[76] that NDPK may be directly coupled to certain GBPs[77] as well as to phospholipases[78]; if so, NDPK action could either directly phosphorylate GDP on GBPs or channel the free GTP that it forms in the cytosol directly to the guanine nucleotide–binding domain of GBPs, or both. In these systems, the formation of GTP, generated via the action of NDPK, utilizes ATP as substrate. This raises the possibility that GTP, or the local GTP:GDP ratio, may be the proximate mediator of some (but probably not all) of the effects of ATP in exocytotic secretion.[56,57,80] For example, we have observed (M. Meredith and S. Metz, 1994, unpublished data) that virtually any maneuver that elevates or decreases islet content of ATP (or the ATP:ADP ratio) is accompanied by parallel changes in the content of GTP (and the GTP:GDP ratio) and uridine triphosphate (UTP), both of which are phosphate donors used by NDPK to regenerate ATP. We have been able to dissociate the effects of guanine and adenine nucleotides in only one condition: The provision of mycophenolic acid reduces GTP and the GTP:GDP ratio in islets but does not change the ATP:ADP ratio. Under these conditions, insulin secretion is reduced; therefore, GTP may indeed have primacy over ATP under some conditions. It is worth noting that the GTP:GDP ratio in islet cells is between 3 and 5 (M. Meredith and S. Metz, 1994, unpublished data). As pointed out by Welsh et al.,[81] this is lower than the ratio found in some other cells and suggests that small changes in the phosphorylation potential of guanine nucleotides, perhaps mediated by receptor-*in*dependent activation of NDPK, could alter the on-rate of GTP for GBPs (cf. ref. 77 re. receptor-independent activation of atrial K^+ channels by NDPK-induced local changes in GTP/GDP ratio). Evidence that GBP function may be modulated by the ambient GTP:GDP ratio has been summarized.[59,79]

¶Interestingly, we (A. Kowluru and S. Metz, 1994, unpublished data) have noted considerable sequence homology in the active regions of NDPK and of the β-subunit, suggesting that they might represent examples from a family of related phosphorelay molecules having functional similarities also to succinyl CoA synthetase in mitochondria. These phosphorelay systems are reminiscent of those involved in bacterial sensory transduction systems,[73,74] where the ''transmitter'' molecule relays its high-energy phosphate from a histidine residue, but often to an aspartate residue on the ''receiver'' protein (rather than to GDP). Interestingly in bacteria, the signals activating this phosphorelay system (e.g., glutamine or α-ketoglutarate, phosphate, osmolarity[74]) often are not peptides, suggesting by analogy that nutrient metabolites perhaps could activate such a system in islets.

Table 7-5. Summary of Transmitter and Receiver Molecules in Islets

Characteristics	Transmitters	
	G_β	NDPK
Primary localization	Membrane	Cytosol
Metal ion requirement	Magnesium = manganese > calcium	Magnesium = manganese > calcium
Receiver molecule	$G_{\alpha\text{-GDP}}$ or GDP	Any NDP
High-energy phosphointermediate	36–37 kd	18–20 kd
Phosphoamino acid	Histidine	Histidine
Undergoes autophosphorylation?	No	Yes
Positive modulators	Arachidonate (biphasic), spermine	Arachidonate, linoleate, oleate
Inhibitors	UDP, heparin, diethylpyrocarbonate	UDP, zinc, -SH- modifying reagents, diethylpyrocarbonate

GDP = guanosine diphosphate; NDP = nucleoside diphosphate; NDPK = nucleoside diphosphokinase; SH = sulfhydryl; UDP = uridine diphosphate.

Table 7-6. Classes of Phosphoamino Acids

Amino Acid Residue	Chemical Class	Sensitivity to: Acid	Base	Diethylpyrocarbonate
Ser, Threo	O-p (alcoholic O-monoester)	−	+	−
Tyr, (Cys)	O-p (phenolic O-monoester)	−	−	(rare)
	S-p (thioester)	−	−	−
His (Lyr,Arg)	N-p (phosphoramidate)	+	−	+*
Asp, Glu	Acyl-p (carboxylate acid anhydride)	+	+	− (?)

*Forms ethoxycarbonyl derivative (*N*-carbethoxy-histidine).

One problem with this formulation is that concentrations of NTPs in islets are always far above the concentrations required for near-maximal NDPK activity: If NDPK were always activated, a futile shuttling of phosphates between various nucleoside diphosphates (NDPs) would result. Therefore, NDPK presumably has an as yet unidentified acute regulatory mechanism (assuming that it serves more than a ''housekeeping'' role). One logical candidate might be the phosphorylation potential of cellular nucleotides (i.e., nucleoside triphosphate (NTP):NDP ratio). We have also found that NDPK can be stimulated by arachidonic acid.[82] Because glucose increases the intraislet content of arachidonic acid (see below), this could be one mechanism by which non–receptor-mediated agonists (such as nutrients) might activate GBPs (Table 7-7; see below). Mastoparan also appears to activate NDPK. In this case, however, the effect can be mimicked by analogs of mastoparan that do not activate GBPs or promote insulin release[70]; this action of mastoparan appears to represent the nonspecific ability of such cationic drugs to fulfill the requirement of NDPK for multivalent cations.[70]

Low-molecular-weight GBPs (as well as subunits of heterotrimeric GBPs) also may be regulated at several sites involving their post-translational modifications (see Table 7-4; Table 7-8).[25] The first such modification (prenylation) involves incorporation of a 15- or 20-carbon moiety (itself derived from mevalonic acid) to a cysteine residue on the carboxyl-terminus of the GBP. In many cases, this is followed by proteolytic removal of several terminal amino acids (up to a maximum of three). A proteolytic enzyme (70 kd) of microsomal origin subserving this function has been purified recently from pig brain; a similar protease has been purified from rat brain with properties akin to classic thiol-dependent carboxypeptidases.[83,84] Often, a carboxyl methylation step then modifies the newly exposed terminal cysteine (to distinguish among types of protein carboxyl methylation, see Table 7-9). In some cases, the covalent addition of a long chain fatty acid, typically palmitate,[#] completes the cascade. Degtyarev et al.[85] demonstrated that receptor activation increased the acylation of $G_{S\alpha}$, suggesting a physiologic regulation of GBPs by acylation. Furthermore, other recent evidence suggests that other fatty acids (e.g., arachidonate) also can be incorporated covalently into GBP subunits.[86] This is important in the context of pancreatic islets because of all the fatty acids, arachidonic acid is the most potent insulin secretagogue.[87]

Because the prenylation of GBPs occurs shortly after their synthesis and because the ''half-lives'' of prenylated proteins are rather long, this is not likely to be an acute regulatory step. However, prenylation is in many cases necessary (albeit not sufficient by itself), to increase the hydrophobic nature of the GBP in order to allow it to intercalate into the relevant membrane compartment. Indeed, blockade of isoprenoid synthesis using lovastatin (an inhibitor of mevalonic acid synthesis) results in the accumulation of GBPs in the cytosolic fraction of islet cells.[25,31,48] Subsequent modifications render the protein even more hydrophobic and anchor the GBP to the membrane. It is likely that the carboxyl methylation of GBPs or their acylation, or both, occurs over a sufficiently acute time period to be regulatory. Tan and Rando[88] described the presence

[#]In addition to acute acylation steps that usually involve palmitic acid, certain GBPs (e.g., ARF, α subunit of heterotrimeric GBPs) are stably and cotranslationally modified by myristoylation, which increases their affinity for key membrane compartments.

Table 7-7. Effects* of Biologically Active Lipids on Functional Properties of GTP-Binding Proteins and Related Proteins in Insulin-Secreting Cells

Lipid(s)	Target Protein(s)	Effects on Target Protein(s)	Effects on Insulin Release
AA, lyso-PC, PA, linoleate, oleate	GTPase	Inhibitory†	↑
Lyso-PC, PA	GTP binding	Stimulatory†	↑
AA, lyso-PC, PA	GDP/GTP exchange	Stimulatory†	↑
AA, linoleate, oleate	NDPK activity	Stimulatory†	↑
AA	β-subunit phosphorylation	Biphasic	↑
Prostaglandin E_2	GTPase	Stimulatory	↓

*Based on refs. 61, 113, and A Kowluru and S Metz (1993, unpublished data). This table comprises only a portion of a growing body of evidence on the effects of lipid messengers on GBP function. Based on recent experimental evidence in other systems, additional effects of AA in insulin-secreting cells might include its ability to do the following: (1) translocate GBPs from the soluble to the membrane fraction,[115] analogous to GTPγS-dependent stimulation of translocation of CDC42 as well as the effects of AA described in neutrophils[63,116]; (2) inhibit GTPase-activating protein activity[64]; (3) acylate low-molecular-weight GBPs and α subunits of trimeric GBPs[86]; and (4) potentiate the effects of GTP in membrane fusion.[117]

†These effects on stimulation of GTP formation, GTP-binding, and GDP/GTP exchange, with a simultaneous inhibition of GTPase activity, would facilitate putative GBPs to achieve (and remain in) the GTP-liganded (active) configuration required for effector regulation.

AA = arachidonic acid; GDP = guanosine diphosphate; GTP = guanosine triphosphate; Lyso-PC = lysophosphatidylcholine; NDPK = nucleoside diphosphokinase; PA = phosphatidic acid.

Table 7-8. Post-Translational Modifications of Low-Molecular-Weight GTP-Binding and Related Proteins in Insulin-Secreting Cells: Their Role(s) in Nutrient-Induced Insulin Secretion

Modification	Precursors Used	Proteins Modified	Inhibitors Used	Effect of Inhibitors on Insulin Secretion	Known Stimulators	Additional Comments	Refs.
Isoprenylation	[14C] mevalonic acid	5 (21–27 kDa)	Lovastatin, perillic acid	Inhibitory	—	Inhibition of insulin release was reversed by mevalonic acid Lovastatin treatment resulted in accumulation of GBPs in cytosol	25, 31, 48
Carboxyl methylation	[3H] methionine *or* [3H]S-adenosyl methionine	2 (21–23) kDa	AFC	Inhibitory	GTP or GTPγS	Identified as Cdc42 and rap1	*, 108
		1 (<10 kDa)	AFC				
		1 (36–38 kDa; AFC-insensitive)	—		?	Tentatively identified as γ subunit of GBP ? Protein phosphatase 2A	
Acylation	Not determined	Not determined	Cerulenin	Inhibitory	—	—	25
Phosphorylation	[32P] ATP *or*	2 (18–20 kDa)	DEPC, UDP	Not tested	—	Identified as subunits of NDPK	*, 71
	[32P] GTP	1 (36–37 kDa)	DEPC, UDP, heparin		Polyamines	Identified as β subunits of heterotrimeric GBPs	72

*A. Kowluru and S. Metz, 1993–1994, unpublished data.
AFC = *N*-acetyl-S-*trans,trans*-farnesyl-L-cysteine; DEPC = diethylpyrocarbonate; GBP = GTP-binding protein; GTP = guanosine triphosphate; NDPK = nucleoside diphosphokinase; UDP = uridine diphosphate.

in bovine rod outer segments of a methyl esterase activity selective for isoprenylated cysteine residues. This may be a regulatory enzyme for the interconversion of methylated to nonmethylated GBPs. Indeed, evidence has been provided that blockade of the carboxyl methylation of certain islet low-molecular-weight GBPs, using specific inhibitors such as *N*-acetyl-S-*trans,trans*,farnesyl-L-cysteine (AFC), may impede nutrient-induced insulin secretion (see Tables 7-3 and 7-8).[25] Receptor stimulation may also acutely stimulate the palmitoylation[89] or depalmitoylation[90] of GBPs, or both. Phosphorylation by classic protein kinases is another post-translational modification that may be regulatory for certain GBPs. For example, phosphorylation may modulate GBPs directly, or they may modify their modulatory proteins (e.g., GAPs).[91,92]

Modifications of GBPs that promote their adherence to biologically relevant membranes by increasing hydrophobicity cannot fully explain the selectivity within the cell in the actions of each GBP. The protein must also be addressed (i.e., targeted) to a *particular,* appropriate cellular compartment. Therefore, it is likely that individual membranes contain acceptor or recognition proteins. Each intracellular organelle probably has its own group of GBPs (and docking/fusion proteins[93]) required for the trafficking of proteins to or from that compartment. Very little is yet known about such acceptors. However, rab 3 has been shown in neuronal cells to bind to a protein (rabphilin) that is suitably situated for it to act as an acceptor or effector protein,[94] or both; however it has not been possible thus far to demonstrate rabphilin in β cells. As indicated above, it is likely that such GBPs also interact with other regulatory proteins, especially calcium- and phospholipid-binding proteins; indeed, rabphilin-3A also has a C2 domain. Additionally, each subcellular compartment may have specific "receptors" for the binding proteins of GBPs (e.g., GDIs) or for proteins that dissociate the two,[95,96] permitting translocation to that particular organelle followed by GTP binding and activation. Alternatively, the "hypervariable domains" of GBPs near their C-terminus may contain targeting motifs.[97] Such possibilities remain to be explored in endocrine cells.

An additional area that merits investigation is the subacute or chronic regulation of GBP function at the level of gene transcription or translation.[9,51,98] Changes in gene expression may provide a long-term mechanism to upregulate or downregulate the function of certain GBPs. It is possible that such gene effects are involved in the differences between normal cells and transformed or cultured cell lines, particularly after prolonged passage.[99] Antisense "knock-out" experiments using islet cells are needed to complement studies involving the overexpression of GBPs, in order to deduce the physiologic function of GBPs. Indeed, such studies have strengthened the putative role of rab 3 (in this case, rab 3B) in secretion from pituitary cells[52] and have helped clarify the effector systems linked to various trimeric GBPs.[9] Homologous recombination experiments have been used[100] to suggest that rab 3A is necessary for recruitment of synaptic vesicles, but not for exocytosis itself, at least in hippocampal pyramidal cells. G_s and ras have been overexpressed in insulin-secreting cell lines with some interesting results[101–103]; however, such studies (as well as those in which effector domains of GBPs are introduced into permeabilized islet cells) must be interpreted with extreme caution. For example, introduced (or overexpressed) GBPs might compete somewhat nonspecifically for endogenous nucleotides as well as for the various (stimulatory or inhibitory) regulatory factors described above.[66] Therefore, it is difficult to determine whether the observed effects of overexpressed or exogenously provided proteins are direct and physiologic, or whether they merely reflect competition for various binding molecules, effector proteins, or substrates. Indeed, a recent study[104] involving various structural analogs of the effector domain of a rab protein reached the conclusion that the stimulatory effect may not reflect a specific function of rab 3. Effects on secretion also are not restricted to GBPs of the rab family; other GBPs, such as ARF[105] and the α subunit of G_{i3},[106] inhibited or stimulated secretion, respectively, when introduced into permeabilized cells or neutralized with antisera. Such studies again raise questions about the specificity of the effects seen with rab 3A (which has a mastoparan-like, amphipathic α-helical structure[17,107]) or at least suggest that GBPs exert controls at multiple levels of the secretory process. Another caveat in studies involving the permeabilization of islet cells is that low-molecular-weight, modulatory factors may leak from such cells; this effect may perturb the function of the residual endogenous (or exogenously provided) proteins. Fernandez et al., and Söllner, Rothman and colleagues,[93] have been proponents of

Table 7-9. Classes of Protein Carboxymethyl* Transferases

Amino Acid Residues	Function	GTPγS-Stimulated? (Usual Subcellular Localization)	AFC-Inhibited?	Product Base-Labile?
L-glutamyl	Chemotactic bacteria	? (Soluble)	−	+ (?)
Aspartyl, isoaspartyl	Protein repair (?)	Usually − (Soluble)	−	Extreme†
Terminal prenyl-cysteine (α-carboxyl)	*ras*-like proteins; γ subunits of GBPs	+ (some cases) (usually membrane-bound)	+	+
Leucyl	Regulation of protein phosphatase 2A activity	? (Soluble)	−	+

*Excludes *N*-methylation, such as calmodulin.
†Does not survive Laemmli conditions.
AFC = *N*-acetyl-S-*trans,trans*-farnesyl-L-cysteine; GBPs = GTP-binding proteins; GTP = guanosine triphosphate.

the concept of the exocytotic "scaffold" or *vesicle fusion apparatus*. These investigators believe that for exocytosis to occur a *series* of proteins, including (but not limited to) GBPs and their effector or recognition proteins, needs to be present in the correct configuration both on the secretory granule membrane and on the plasma membrane. This concept suggests that studies of the effect of GBPs in isolation from these other proteins may yield an incomplete picture.

Selected Aspects of GTP-Binding Proteins in Insulin-Secreting Cells

Isoprenylation

Several low-molecular-weight GBPs have been shown to undergo isoprenylation in pancreatic islets (see Table 7-8).[4,25,31] Besides these, γ subunits of heterotrimeric GBPs have been shown to undergo isoprenylation; however, in pancreatic islets, such data are not yet available. Emerging evidence indicates that blocking the production of mevalonic acid, the precursor for isoprene groups, by using drugs such as lovastatin (a blocker of hydroxymethylglutaryl-CoA-reductase), induces the selective accumulation of nonprenylated proteins in the soluble fractions,[25,31,48] which is analogous to findings in yeast mutants lacking a prenylation consensus site.[49] After lovastatin exposure, the ability of fuels to stimulate insulin secretion is significantly impaired in normal islets.[25] Moreover, provision of exogenous mevalonic acid reverses lovastatin's effects.[25] Interestingly, secretion potentiated by bombesin or arginine vasopressin, but not that induced by nutrients alone, is impaired by lovastatin in transformed β-cells.[48] No identification of the isoprenylated proteins has been carried out in insulin-secreting cells thus far.

Proteolysis

A protease selectively removes the C-terminal three amino acid residues of GBPs, thus exposing the carboxylate anion of the prenylated cysteine for subsequent methylation. This has been the least studied post-translational modification of GBPs and is unstudied in islets. Inferentially, such a protease must be present in insulin-secreting cells, considering that the islet GBP identified as Cdc42 by immunochemical methods (21–23 kd) undergoes carboxyl methylation.[108] Cdc42 is a GBP with a consensus sequence of CAAX (where C = cysteine, A = aliphatic amino acid, and X = any amino acid); proteolysis of the terminal three amino acids must take place in order for Cdc42 to undergo carboxyl methylation (see below).

Carboxyl Methylation

Carboxyl methylation involves the transfer of methyl groups from a methyl donor (S-adenosyl methionine) to the carboxylate anion of prenylated cysteine catalyzed by prenyl-cysteine methyl transferases (see Table 7-9). Recent studies[25,108] have, indeed, identified this GBP modification in pancreatic islets; further, a particulate prenylcysteine methyltransferase has been identified in β cells (G Li, A Kowluru, S Metz, 1995, submitted). One such candidate protein is Cdc42; this is a calcium-binding protein of the rho family involved in cytoskeletal organization, cell polarity, and budding of secretory vesicles in yeast. Based on immunofluorescence data, Ziman et al.[49] have implicated a role for Cdc42 at the site of secretory vesicle-plasma membrane fusion. Using rat islets, human islets, and pure β-cells (HIT or RIN), we have demonstrated that Cdc42 undergoes a guanine nucleotide–dependent carboxyl methylation.[108] This guanine nucleotide–dependent modification may promote a tight membrane association after the translocation of Cdc42 from cytosol to the particulate fraction.[108] Furthermore, it may promote the ability of GBPs to activate phospholipase C in β cells, since inhibition of prenylcysteine carboxyl methylation reduces the latter (J Vadekakelam, S Metz, 1995, submitted). Additionally, glucose itself promotes the methylation of Cdc42 (and rap1) in β cells (A Kowluru, S Metz, 1995, submitted). Additional details of the carboxyl methylation of this Cdc42 protein and its putative role in insulin secretion are summarized in Tables 7-3 and 7-8 and in Figure 7-1.

Besides Cdc42 and rap1, at least two other proteins (one <10 kd, in membranes; the other 36–38 kd, primarily cytosolic) undergo carboxyl methylation in islets.[25,108] Based on comigration with a purified γ subunit and its inhibitability by AFC, the smaller protein was tentatively identified as the γ subunit of heterotrimeric GBPs. Several studies have suggested that carboxyl methylation of the γ-subunit is critical in order for it to form a stable αβγ trimer. Based on molecular weight and its cytosolic distribution, the 36–38 kd carboxyl methylated protein may represent a subunit of protein phosphatase 2A. Recent studies by Lee and Stock[109] demonstrated that protein phosphatase 2A is carboxyl methylated by a 40-kd carboxyl methyl transferase that seems to differ from prenylcysteine methyl transferases (see Table 7-9) in three ways: (1) it carboxyl methylates a C-terminal leucyl residue, as opposed to

C-terminal cysteine; (2) it is insensitive to guanine nucleotides; and (3) it is not inhibited by AFC.

Acylation

In nonendocrine cells, α subunits of high-molecular-weight GBPs recently have been shown to be able to incorporate labeled palmitic acid[110] or arachidonic acid[86] in thioester linkage. The concentrations of arachidonic acid required to subserve acylation functions are similar to those found in glucose-stimulated pancreatic islets.[111] To our knowledge, no direct demonstration of the acylation of GBPs has yet been demonstrated in insulin-secreting cells. Recent studies from our laboratory,[25] however, have provided indirect evidence that acylation reactions play a role in glucose-induced insulin secretion. Cerulenin, an inhibitor of such acylation, was shown to cause a significant (>60%) inhibition of glucose-induced insulin secretion. It is unclear whether cerulenin inhibits the acylation of GBPs selectively; other proteins involved in secretion (e.g., 25-kd synaptosomal-associated protein) may also be acylated.[112]

Effects of Biologically Active Lipids

Arachidonate and other biologically active lipids that stimulate or inhibit insulin release have a number of effects on GBPs in islet subcellular fractions that would be expected to potentiate the activation of stimulatory or inhibitory GBPs, respectively (see Table 7-7).[30,113] Although the physiologic importance of these effects requires more study, GBPs may serve as one locus wherein phospholipase activation culminates in insulin secretion.[114]

Conclusions

Although much has been learned about GBPs in insulin-secreting cells, the extant studies are, by and large, descriptive. Studies of the regulation and physiologic effects of GBPs are limited. It is difficult to define such roles, since the selective perturbation of the activity of a single GBP in intact cells (i.e., those able to secrete in response to physiologic stimuli) is not easily achieved. Molecular biologic studies involving mutational analysis and gene "knock-out" will doubtless help in this regard, and are likely to reveal the regulation of β cell function by GBPs at multiple levels in the cell.

Acknowledgments

Research of the authors was supported by the Veterans Administration, the National Institutes of Health (grant DK 37312), and the Juvenile Diabetes Foundation.

References

1. Davletov BA, Südhof TC. A single C_2 domain from synaptotagmin I is sufficient for high affinity Ca^{++}/phospholipid binding. J Biol Chem 1993;268:26386
2. Lévêque C, El Far O, Martin-Moutot N, et al. Purification of the N-type calcium channel associated with syntaxin and synaptotagmin. J Biol Chem 1994;269:6306
3. Metz SA, Dunlop M. Sodium fluoride unmasks the accumulation of lysophosphatidylcholine in intact pancreatic islet cells. Biochem Biophys Res Commun 1990;167:61
4. Bursten SL, Harris WE, Bomsztyk K, Lovett D. Interleukin-1 rapidly stimulates lysophosphatidate acyltransferase and phosphatidate phosphohydrolase activities in human mesangial cells. J Biol Chem 1991;266:20732
5. Vallar L, Biden TJ, Wollheim CB. Guanine nucleotides induce Ca^{++}-independent insulin secretion from permeabilized RINm5F cells. J Biol Chem 1987;262:5049
6. Cockcroft S. G-protein-regulated phospholipases C, D, and A_2-mediated signalling in neutrophils. Biochem Biophys Acta 1992;1113:135
7. Leyte A, Barr FA, Kehlenbach RH, Huttner WB. Multiple trimeric G-proteins on the trans-Golgi network exert stimulatory and inhibitory effects on secretory vesicle formation. EMBO J 1992;11:4795
8. Yatani A, Mattera R, Codina J, et al. The G protein-gated atrial K^+ channel is stimulated by three distinct G_i α-subunits. Nature 1988;336:680
9. Kleuss C, Hescheler J, Ewel C, et al. Assignment of G-protein subtypes to specific receptors inducing inhibition of calcium currents. Nature 1991;353:43
10. Cockcroft S, Thomas GMH, Fensome A, et al. Phospholipase D: A downstream effector of ARF in granulocytes. Science 1994;263:523
11. Baffy G, Yang L, Wolf BA, Williamson JR. G-protein specificity in signaling pathways that mobilize calcium in insulin-secreting β-TC3 cells. Diabetes 1993;42:1878
12. Schmidt A, Hescheler J, Offermanns S, et al. Involvement of pertussis toxin-sensitive G-proteins in the hormonal inhibition of dihydropyridine-sensitive Ca^{++} currents in an insulin-secreting cell line (RINm5F). J Biol Chem 1991;266:18025
13. Hsu WH, Xiang H, Rajan AS, et al. Somatostatin inhibits insulin secretion by a G-protein-mediated decrease in Ca^{++} entry through voltage-dependent Ca^{++} channels in the beta cell. J Biol Chem 1991;266:837
14. Richardson SB, Laya T, Gibson M, et al. Somatostatin inhibits vasopressin-stimulated phosphoinositide hydrolysis and influx of extracellular calcium in clonal hamster β (HIT) cells. Biochem J 1992;288:847
15. Clapham DE, Neer EJ. New roles for G-protein βγ-dimers in transmembrane signalling. Nature 1993;365:403
16. Evans T, Brown ML, Fraser ED, Northup JK. Purification of the major GTP-binding proteins from human placental membranes. J Biol Chem 1986; 261:7052
17. Law GJ, Northrop AJ, Mason WT. rab3-Peptide stimulates exocytosis from mast cells via a pertussis toxin-sensitive mechanism. FEBS Lett 1993;333:56
18. Crespo P, Xu N, Simonds WF, Gutkind JS. Ras-dependent activation of MAP kinase pathway mediated by G-protein βγ subunits. Nature 1994;369:418
19. Barbieri MA, Li G, Colombo MI, Stahl PD. Rab5, an early acting endosomal GTPase, supports *in vitro* endosome fusion without GTP hydrolysis. J Biol Chem 1994;269:18720
20. Thorens B, Gérard N, Dériaz N. GLUT2 surface expression and intracellular transport via the constitutive pathway in pancreatic β cells and insulinoma: Evidence for a block in trans-Golgi network exit by Brefeldin A. J Cell Biol 1993;123:1687
21. Fernandez JM, Neher E, Gomperts BD. Capacitance measurements reveal stepwise fusion events in degranulating mast cells. Nature 1984;312:453
22. Gomperts BD. G_E: A GTP-binding protein mediating exocytosis. Ann Rev Physiol 1990;52:591
23. Li G, Regazzi R, Balch WE, Wollheim CB. Stimulation of insulin release from permeabilized HIT-T15 cells by a synthetic peptide corresponding to the effector domain of the small GTP-binding protein rab3. FEBS Lett 1993;327:145
24. Higashijima T, Burnier J, Ross EM. Regulation of G_i and G_o by mastoparan, related amphophilic peptides, and hydrophobic amines. J Biol Chem 1990; 265:14176
25. Metz SA, Rabaglia ME, Stock JB, Kowluru A. Modulation of insulin secretion from normal rat islets by inhibitors of the post-translational modifications of GTP-binding proteins. Biochem J 1993;295:31
26. Jones PM, Mann FM, Persaud SJ, Wheeler-Jones CPD. Mastoparan stimulates insulin secretion from pancreatic β-cells by effects at a late stage in the secretory pathway. Mol Cell Endocrinol 1993;94:97
27. Yokokawa N, Komatsu M, Takeda T, et al. Mastoparan, a wasp venom, stimulates insulin release by pancreatic islets through pertussis toxin sensitive GTP-binding protein. Biochem Biophys Res Commun 1989;158:712
28. Komatsu M, McDermott AM, Gillison SL, Sharp GWG. Mastoparan stimulates exocytosis at a Ca^{++}-independent late site in stimulus-secretion coupling. J Biol Chem 1993;268:23297
29. Hillaire-Buys D, Mousli M, Landry Y, et al. Insulin releasing effects of mastoparan and amphophilic substance P receptor antagonists on RINm5F insulinoma cells. Mol Cell Biochem 1992;109:133
30. Kowluru A, Rabaglia ME, Muse KE, Metz SA. Subcellular localization and kinetic characterization of guanine nucleotide binding proteins in normal rat and human pancreatic islets and transformed β cells. Biochim Biophys Acta 1994;1222:348
31. Regazzi R, Vallar L, Ullrich S, et al. Characterization of small-molecular-mass guanine-nucleotide-binding regulatory proteins in insulin-secreting cells and PC12 cells. Eur J Biochem 1992;208:729
32. Muntz KH, Sternweis PC, Gilman AG, Mumby SM. Influence of γ subunit prenylation on association of guanine nucleotide-binding regulatory proteins with membranes. Mol Biol Cell 1992;3:49
33. Vitale N, Mukai H, Rouot B, et al. Exocytosis in chromaffin cells. J Biol Chem 1993;268:14715
34. Peitsch MC, Borner C, Tschop J. Sequence similarity of phospholipase A_2 activating protein and the G protein β-subunits: A new concept of effector protein activation in signal transduction? Trends Biochem Sci 1993;18:292
35. Ron D, Chen C-H, Caldwell J, et al. Cloning of an intracellular receptor for protein kinase C: A homolog of the β subunit of G proteins. Proc Natl Acad Sci USA 1994;91:839
36. Touhara K, Inglese J, Pitcher JA, et al. Binding of G protein βγ-subunits to pleckstrin homology domains. J Biol Chem 1994;269:10217

37. Pitcher JA, Inglese J, Higgins JB, et al. Role of $\beta\gamma$ subunits of G proteins in targeting the β-adrenergic receptor kinase to membrane-bound receptors. Science 1992;257:1264
38. Bourne HR. Do GTPases direct membrane traffic in secretion? Cell 1988; 53:669
39. Putney JW Jr, Bird GStJ. The signal for capacitative calcium entry. Cell 1993;75:199
40. Ämmälä C, Berggren P-O, Bokvist K, Rorsman P. Inhibition of L-type calcium channels by internal GTP[γS] in mouse pancreatic β cells. Pflugers Arch 1992;420:72
41. Kahn RA. Fluoride is not an activator of smaller (20-25 kDa) GTP-binding proteins. J Biol Chem 1991;266:15595
42. Oka T, Nakano A. Inhibition of GTP hydrolysis by Sarlp causes accumulation of vesicles that are a functional intermediate of the ER-to-Golgi transport in yeast. J Cell Biol 1994;124:425
43. Göke R, Göke B. Analysis of low molecular mass GTP-binding proteins in insulinoma-derived RINm5F cells by two-dimensional gel electrophoresis. Horm Metab Res 1991;23:304
44. Kowluru A, Metz SA. GTP and its binding proteins in the regulation Part I of insulin exocytosis. In: Draznin B, LeRoith D, eds. Molecular Biology of Diabetes. Totowa, NJ: The Humana Press;1994:249–283
45. Watkins DC, Moxham CM, Morris AJ, Malbon CC. Suppression of $G_{i\alpha 2}$ enhances phospholipase C signalling. Biochem J 1994;299:593
46. Cantiello HF, Pantenaude CR, Ausiello DA. G protein subunit, α_i-3, activates a pertussis toxin-sensitive Na^+ channel from the epithelial cell line, A6. J Biol Chem 1989;264:20867
47. Regazzi R, Kikuchi A, Takai Y, Wollheim CB. The small GTP-binding proteins in the cytosol of insulin-secreting cells are complexed to GDP dissociation inhibitor proteins. J Biol Chem 1992;267:17512
48. Li G, Regazzi R, Roche E, Wollheim CB. Blockade of mevalonate production by lovastatin attenuates bombesin and vasopressin potentiation of nutrient-induced insulin secretion in HIT-T15 cells. Biochem J 1993;289:379
49. Ziman M, Preuss D, Mulholland J, et al. Subcellular localization of CDC42p, a *Saccharomyces cerevisiae* GTP-binding protein involved in the control of cell polarity. Mol Biol Cell 1993;4:1307
50. Holz RW, Brondyk WH, Senter RA, et al. Evidence for the involvement Rab3A in Ca^{++}-dependent exocytosis from adrenal chromaffin cells. J Biol Chem 1994;269:10229
51. Johannes L, Lledo P-M, Roa M, et al. The GTPase *Rab*3a negatively controls calcium-dependent exocytosis in neuroendocrine cells. EMBO J 1994; 13:2029
52. Liedo P-M, Vernier P, Vincent J-D, et al. Inhibition of Rab3B expression attenuates Ca^{++}-dependent exocytosis in rat anterior pituitary cells. Nature 1993;364:540
53. Fischer von Mollar G, Stahl B, Khokhlatchev A, et al. Rab3C is a synaptic vesicle protein that dissociates from synaptic vesicles after stimulation of exocytosis. J Biol Chem 1994;269:10971
54. Metz SA, Rabaglia ME, Pintar TJ. Selective inhibitors of GTP synthesis impede exocytotic insulin release from intact rat islets. J Biol Chem 1992;267:12517
55. Metz SA, Meredith M, Kowluru A. Purine nucleotide metabolism and GTP-binding proteins in the pancreatic β-cell. In: Flatt P, Lenzen S, eds. Insulin Secretion and Pancreatic B-cell Research. London: Smith-Gordon Press; 1994:277–286
56. Wagner PD, Vu N-D. Thiophosphorylation causes Ca^{++}-independent norepinephrine secretion from permeabilized PC12 cells. J Biol Chem 1989; 264:19614
57. Lillie THW, Gomperts BD. Kinetic characterization of guanine-nucleotide-induced exocytosis from permeabilized rat mast cells. Biochem J 1993; 290:389
58. Koffer A. Calcium-induced secretion from permeabilized rat mast cells: Requirements for guanine nucleotides. Biochim Biophys Acta 1993;1176:231
59. Haney SA, Broach JR. Cdc25p, the guanine nucleotide exchange factors for the Ras proteins of *Saccharomyces cerevisiae*, promotes exchange by stabilizing Ras in a nucleotide-free state. J Biol Chem 1994;269:16541
60. Lander HM, Sehajpal PK, Novogrodsky A. Nitric oxide signaling: A possible role for G proteins. J Immunol 1993;151:7182
61. Kowluru A, Metz SA. Regulation of guanine-nucleotide binding proteins in islet subcellular fractions by phospholipase-derived lipid mediators of insulin secretion. Biochim Biophys Acta 1994;1222:360
62. Novick P, Brennwald P. Friends and family: The role of the Rab GTPases in vesicular traffic. Cell 1993;75:597
63. Chuang T-H, Bohl BP, Bokoch GM. Biologically active lipids are regulators of Rac·GDI complexation. J Biol Chem 1993;268:26206
64. Tsai M-H, Lu C-L, Wei F-S, Stacey DW. The effect of GTPase activating protein upon Ras is inhibited by mitogenically responsive lipids. Science 1989;243:522
65. Reig JA, Yu L, Klein DC. Pineal transduction: Adrenergic → cyclic AMP-dependent phosphorylation of cytoplasmic 33-kDa protein (MEKA) which binds $\beta\gamma$-complex of transducin. J Biol Chem 1990;265:5816
66. Yatani A, Quilliam LA, Brown AM, Bokoch GM. Rap1a antagonizes the ability of Ras and Ras-Gap to inhibit muscarinic K^+ channels. J Biol Chem 1990;266:22222
67. Hart JM, Maru Y, Leonard D, et al. A GDP dissociation inhibitor that serves as a GTPase inhibitor for the Ras-like protein CDC42Hs. Science 1992;258:812
68. Manser E, Leung T, Salihuddin H, et al. A brain serine/threonine protein kinase activated by Cdc42 and Rac1. Nature 1994;367:40
69. Pagès F, Deterre P, Pfister C. Enhancement by phosphodiesterase subunits of the rate of GTP hydrolysis by transducin in bovine retinal rods. J Biol Chem 1993;268:26358
70. Kowluru A, Seavey SE, Rabaglia ME, Metz SA. The stimulatory effects of mastoparan on pancreatic islet nucleoside diphosphokinase activity: Dissociation from insulin secretion. Biochem Pharmacol 1995;49:263
71. Kowluru A, Metz SA. Characterization of nucleoside diphosphokinase activity in human and rodent pancreatic β cells. Biochemistry 1994;33:12495
72. Kowluru A, Seavey SE, Rhodes CJ, Metz SA. A novel regulatory mechanism for Trimeric GTP-binding proteins in the membrane and secretory granule fractions of human and rodent β cells. Biochem J, in press, 1995
73. Kofoid EC, Parkinson JS. Transmitter and receiver modules in bacterial signaling proteins. Proc Natl Acad Sci U S A 1988;85:4981
74. Alex LA, Simon MI. Protein histidine kinases and signal transduction in prokaryotes and eukaryotes. Trends Genet 1994;10:133
75. Stock JB, Ninfa AJ, Stock AM. Protein phosphorylation and regulation of adaptive responses in bacteria. Microbiol Rev 1989;53:450
76. Kikkawa S, Takahashi K, Takahashi K-i, et al. Conversion of GDP into GTP by nucleoside diphosphate kinase on the GTP-binding proteins. J Biol Chem 1990;265:21536
77. Heidbüchel H, Callewaert G, Vereecke J, Carmelier E. Acetylcholine-mediated K^+ channel activity in guinea-pig atrial cells is supported by nucleoside diphosphate kinase. Pflugers Arch 1993;422:316
78. Fan X-T, Sherwood JL, Haslam RJ. Stimulation of phospholipase D in rabbit platelet membranes by nucleoside triphosphates and by phosphocreatine: Roles of membrane-bound GDP, nucleoside diphosphate kinase and creatine kinase. Biochem J 1994;299:701
79. Kimura N. Role of nucleoside diphosphate kinase in G-protein action. In: Dickey BF, Birnbaumer L, eds. Handbook of Environmental Pharmacology, Vol. 108/II. Berlin: Springer-Verlag;1993:485–498
80. Koffer A, Churcher Y. Calcium and GTP-γ-S as single effectors of secretion from permeabilized rat mats cells: Requirements for ATP. Biochim Biophys Acta 1993;1176:222
81. Welsh N, Öberg C, Welsh M. GTP-binding proteins may stimulate insulin biosynthesis in rat pancreatic islets by enhancing the signal-recognition-particle-dependent translocation of the insulin mRNA poly-/mono-some complex to the endoplasmic reticulum. Biochem J 1991;275:23
82. Kowluru A, Metz SA. Transmitter and receiver molecules in pancreatic beta cells: Two novel mechanisms to regulate GTP binding proteins? Clin Res 1994;42:334A
83. Akopyan TN, Couedel Y, Beaumont A, et al. Cleavage of farnesylated COOH-terminal heptapeptide of mouse N-ras by brain microsomal membranes: Evidence for carboxypeptidase which specifically removes the COOH-terminal methionine. Biochem Biophys Res Commun 1992;187:1336
84. Akopyan TN, Couedel Y, Orlowski M, et al. Proteolytic processing of farnesylated peptides: Assay and partial purification from pig brain membranes of an endopeptidase which has the characteristics of E.C. 3.4.24.15. Biochem Biophys Res Commun 1994;198:787
85. Degtyarev MY, Spiegel AM, Jones TLZ. Increased palmitoylation of the G_s protein α subunit after activation of the β-adrenergic receptor or cholera toxin. J Biol Chem 1993;268:23769
86. Hallak H, Muszbek L, Laposata M, et al: Covalent binding of arachidonate to G protein α subunits of human platelets. J Biol Chem 1994;269:4713
87. Metz SA. Exogenous arachidonic acid promotes insulin release from intact or permeabilized rat islets by dual mechanisms: Putative activation of Ca^{++} mobilization and protein kinase C. Diabetes 1988;37:1453
88. Tan EW, Rando R. Identification of isoprenylated cysteine methyl ester hydrolase activity in bovine rod outer segment membranes. Biochemistry 1992;31:5572
89. Mumby SM, Kleuss C, Gilman AG. Receptor regulation of G-protein palmitoylation. Proc Natl Acad Sci U S A 1994;91:2800
90. Wedegaertner PB, Bourne HR. Activation and depalmitoylation of $G_{S\alpha}$. Cell 1994;77:1063
91. Itoh T. Kaibuchi K, Sasaki T, Takai Y. The *smg* GDS-induced activation of *smg* p21 is initiated by cyclic AMP-dependent protein kinase-catalyzed phosphorylation of *smg* p21. Biochem Biophys Res Commun 1991;177:1319
92. Manser E, Leung T, Salihuddin H, et al. A non-receptor tyrosine kinase that inhibits the GTPase activity of $p21^{cdc42}$. Nature 1993;363:364
93. Söllner T, Whiteheart SW, Brunner M, et al. SNAP receptors implicated in vesicle targeting and fusion. Nature 1993;362:318
94. Shirataki H, Kaibuchi K, Sakoda T, et al. Rabphilin-3A, a putative target protein for *smg* p25A/*rab*3A p25 small GTP-binding protein related to synaptotagmin. Mol Cell Biol 1993;13:2061
95. Dirac-Svejstrup AB, Soldati T, Shapiro AD, Pfeffer SR. Rab-GDI presents functional rab9 to the intracellular transport machinery and contributes selectivity to rab9 membrane recruitment. J Biol Chem 1994;269:15427
96. Novick P, Garrett MD. No exchange without receipt. Nature 1994;369:18
97. Chavrier P, Gorvel J-P, Stelzer E, et al. Hypervariable C-terminal domain of rab proteins acts as a targeting signal. Nature 1991;353:769
98. Goetzl EJ, Shames RS, Yang J, et al. Inhibition of human HL-60 cell responses to chemotactic factors by antisense messenger RNA depletion of G proteins. J Biol Chem 1994;269:809
99. Walseth TF, Zhang H-J, Olson LK, et al. Increase in G_s and cyclic AMP generation in HIT cells. J Biol Chem 1989;264:21106
100. Geppert M, Bolshakov VY, Siegelbaum SA, et al. The role of rab3A in neurotransmitter release. Nature 1994;369:493

101. Efrat S, Fleischer N, Hanahan D. Diabetes induced in male transgenic mice by expression of human H-*ras* oncoprotein in pancreatic β cells. Mol Cell Biol 1990;10:1779
102. Ma YH, Landis C, Tchao N, et al. Constitutively active stimulatory G-protein α_s in β-cells of transgenic mice causes counterregulation of the increased adenosine 3′,5′-monophosphate and insulin secretion. Endocrinology 1994; 134:42
103. Berggren P-O, Hallberg A, Welsh N, et al. Transfection of insulin-producing cells with a transforming c-Ha-*ras* oncogene stimulates phospholipase C activity. Biochem J 1989;259:701
104. MacLean CM, Law GJ, Edwardson JM. Stimulation of exocytotic membrane fusion by modified peptides of the rab3 effector domain: Re-evaluation of the role of rab3 in regulated exocytosis. Biochem J 1993;294:325
105. Morgan A, Burgoyne RD. A synthetic peptide of the N-terminus of ADP-ribosylation factor (ARF) inhibits regulated exocytosis in adrenal chromaffin cells. FEBS Lett 1993;329:121.
106. Aridor M, Rajmilevich G, Beaven MA, Sagi-Eisenberg R. Activation of exocytosis by the heterotrimeric G protein G_{i3}. Science 1993;262:1569
107. Law GJ, Northrup AJ. Synthetic peptides to mimic the role of GTP binding proteins in membrane traffic and fusion. Ann N Y Acad Sci 1994;710:196
108. Kowluru A, Seavey SE, Rabaglia ME, Metz SA. GTP stimulates methylation and translocation of CDC42 in rodent and human islets: A required step in insulin exocytosis. Diabet Metab 1994;20:169
109. Lee J, Stock J. Protein phosphatase 2A catalytic subunit is methyl-esterified at its carboxyl terminus by a novel methyltransferase. J Biol Chem 1993;268:19192
110. Linder ME, Middleton P, Hepler JR, et al. Lipid modifications of G proteins: α Subunits are palmitoylated. Proc Natl Acad Sci U S A 1993;90:3675
111. Wolf BA, Pasquale SM, Turk J. Free fatty acid accumulation in secretagogue-stimulated pancreatic islets and effects of arachidonate on depolarization-induced insulin secretion. Biochemistry 1991;30:6372
112. Hess DT, Slater TM, Wilson MC, Pate Skene JH. The 25 kDa synaptosomal-associated protein SNAP-25 is the major methionine-rich polypeptide in rapid axonal transport and a major substrate for palmitoylation in adult CNS. J Neurosci 1992;12:4634
113. Kowluru A, Metz SA. Stimulation by prostaglandin E_2 of a high-affinity GTPase in the secretory granules of normal rat and human pancreatic islets. Biochem J 1994;297:399
114. Metz SA. The pancreatic islet as Rubik's cube: Is phospholipid hydrolysis a piece of the puzzle? Diabetes 1991;40:1565
115. Sawai T, Asada M, Nunoi H, et al. Combination of arachidonic acid and guanosine 5′-0-(3-thiotriphosphate) induces translocation of *rac* p21s to membrane and activation of NADPH oxidase in a cell-free system. Biochem Biophys Res Commun 1993;195:264
116. McPhail LC, Qualliotine-Mann D, Agwu DE, McCall DE. Phospholipases and activation of the NADPH oxidase. Eur J Haematol 1993;51:294
117. Paiement J, Lavoie C, Gavino GR, Gavino VC. Modulation of GTP-dependent fusion by linoleic and arachidonic acid in derivatives of rough endoplasmic reticulum from rat liver. Biochim Biophys Acta 1994;1190:199
118. Ullrich S, Wollheim CB. GTP-dependent inhibition of insulin secretion by epinephrine in permeabilized RINm5F cells. J Biol Chem 1988;263: 8615

Diabetes Mellitus, edited by Derek LeRoith, Simeon I. Taylor, and Jerrold M. Olefsky. Lippincott–Raven Publishers, Philadelphia © 1996.

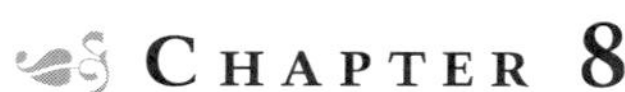

CHAPTER 8

Insulinotropic Glucagon-Like Peptides

JOEL F. HABENER

During the transition from the fasting to fed states, and vice versa, major alterations occur in the activities of enzymes and other factors involved in the metabolism of nutrients in the liver, muscle, and adipose tissue. To a large extent, the modulation of these changes in cellular metabolism is mediated by hormones such as insulin, glucagon, and somatostatin emanating from the endocrine pancreas (the islets of Langerhans). The secretion of islet hormones in response to the ingestion of oral nutrients is regulated not only by blood levels of nutrients (glucose, amino acids, fatty acids) absorbed from the gastrointestinal tract, but also by peptide hormones known as *incretins,* secreted from specialized enteroendocrine cells that reside in the intestines.[1–3] An important aspect in the hormonal control of nutrient metabolism is the contribution of the intestinally derived incretins that in turn modulate the hormonal output of the endocrine pancreas, constituting the enteroinsular axis controlling nutrient homeostasis. Although the concept of the incretin effect was described more than six decades ago,[4] the identification of the actual substance or substances that comprise the incretin components of the enteroinsular axis remained elusive until the discoveries of the structures of gastric inhibitory polypeptide (GIP) in 1981,[5] and of glucagon-like peptide (GLP) in 1982.[6] It now appears that GLP-1, a split product of proglucagon in the intestines, and GIP are the major relevant insulinotropic incretins.[7]

The Incretin Effect

The incretin effect is defined as the observation that intestinally derived factors released in response to oral glucose augment glucose-stimulated insulin secretion.[2] The as yet then unidentified intestinal factors that stimulate the secretions of the endocrine pancreas were termed *incretins,* as opposed to *excretins,* which are hormones such as secretin that stimulate secretions from the exocrine pancreas. The incretins comprise the hormonal components of the *enteroinsular axis,* a term coined by Unger and Eisentraut[8] to describe the neural, hormonal, and nutrient regulation of the pancreatic islets by the intestine in response to the oral ingestion of nutrients. In later studies, researchers demonstrated the incretin effect by showing that an orally administered glucose load was much more effective at releasing insulin and C-peptide than an "isoglycemic" glucose load given intravenously to mimic the rise in blood glucose levels produced by the oral glucose (Fig. 8-1).[9] Further, it was observed that the incretin effect is attenuated in subjects with non–insulin-dependent (type II) diabetes mellitus (NIDDM).[9] In 1935, Heller[10] showed that extracts prepared from the duodenum dampened postprandial hyperglycemia. These early observations were followed 35 years later by the isolation from

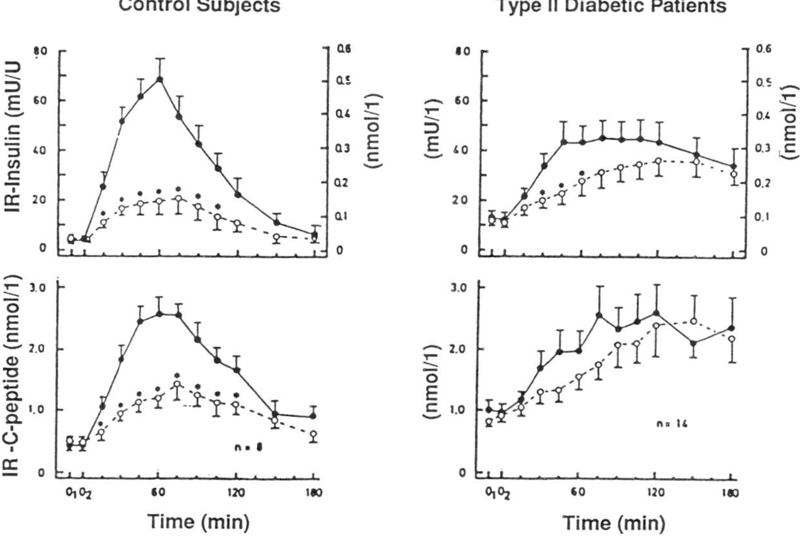

FIGURE 8-1. Reduced incretin effect in NIDDM. Measurements of plasma insulin (top panels) and plasma C-peptide (lower panels) after oral glucose tolerance tests (solid symbols) and during "isoglycemic" IV glucose infusions (open symbols) in metabolically healthy subjects (left panels) and NIDDM patients (right panels). The incretin effect of augmentation of insulin and C-peptide stimulation by an oral glucose load compared to an equivalent amount of glucose infused intravenously is blunted in the NIDDM subjects. (Modified with permission from Nauck M, Stöckman F, Ebert R, Creutzfeld W. Reduced incretin effect in type 2 (non–insulin-dependent) diabetes. Diabetologia 1986; 29:46.)

extracts of pig intestines of the first incretin,[11] *gastric inhibitory polypeptide* (GIP), so named because as an unidentified component in porcine duodenal extracts it inhibited gastric motility and acid secretion.[12,13] The correct amino acid sequence of GIP was determined in 1981 by Jöurnvall et al.[5] Subsequently, GIP was found to stimulate insulin secretion directly in a glucose-dependent manner,[14,15] and it was proposed that the term "gastric inhibitory polypeptide" be changed to "glucose-dependent insulinotropic polypeptide."[16] GIP, however, did not account for the entire intestinal incretin activity, in as much as immunoneutralization of GIP in animals in vivo and in extracts in vitro administered to animals and to human subjects led to the conclusions that GIP could only account for 20% of the incretin effect.[17] Thus, the search continued to identify additional incretins.

Glucagon-Like Peptide-1(7-37)/(7-36)Amides: Newly Discovered Potent Incretins

The search for intestinal incretins in addition to GIP was rewarded unexpectedly in 1982, 10 years after the isolation of GIP from extracts of intestines, by a finding arising from the experimental approach of "reverse genetics."[6] The cloning of the cDNAs encoding the proglucagon of the anglerfish,[6] followed by cloning of the mammalian proglucagon cDNAs[18,19] and genes[20,21] predicted the encodement of two new glucagon-related peptides in addition to glucagon in the proglucagon prohormone. GLP-1 has proved to be a potent glucose-dependent insulinotropic peptide distinct from GIP. It is important to realize that proglucagon (the prohormonal precursor for GLP-1) and proGIP (the prohormone for GIP) are encoded by distinct genes.[22] The combination of the two hormones GIP and GLP-1, however, appears to constitute most if not all of the relevant hormonal component of the incretin effect.[7] Additional perspectives on the GLPs are given in several reviews.[3,23–26]

Alternative Post-Translational Processing of Proglucagon in Intestines and Pancreas

The proglucagon expressed in the α-cells of the endocrine pancreas and in the enteroendocrine L-cells of the intestine arises from the transcription of a single gene and the translation of identical mRNAs in these two tissues. Biologic diversity in the expression of the proglucagon gene occurs at the level of a remarkably tissue-specific alternative post-translational processing, resulting in the formation of the bioactive peptide glucagon in the pancreas and the reciprocal insulin-stimulating GLPs in the intestine[27] (Fig. 8-2). The glucagon and GLP sequences in intestine and pancreas, respectively, are retained as unprocessed proglucagon fragments: *enteroglucagon* (glicentin) in the intestine and *major proglucagon fragment* in the pancreas. It is notable that the alternative processing of the identical proglucagon in the intestine and pancreas gave rise to peptides whose physiologic functions are opposed. GLP-1 is an anabolic hormone that facilitates stimulation of insulin secretion and glucose uptake during feeding, whereas glucagon is a most important catabolic hormone that acts during periods of fasting to break down glycogen and to increase glucose output by the liver, skeletal muscle, and adipose tissue (see ahead to Fig. 8-4).

The proteolytic cleavages of the GLP-1s from the proglucagon in the intestine are part of a complicated process. At least four isopeptides result from the processing: two peptides of 37 and 36 amino acids, GLP-1(1-37) and GLP-1(1-36)amide; and two amino-terminally truncated isopeptides, GLP-1(7-37) and GLP-1(7-36) amide.[23–26] Only the two truncated GLP-1s have insulinotropic activities.[28,29] Thus far, no biologic activities have been found either for the amino-terminally extended forms of GLP-1 or for GLP-2, also liberated from proglucagon in the intestine with high efficiency. Both isopeptides of GLP-1, GLP-1(7-37) and GLP-1(7-36) amide, have identical insulinotropic potencies in all systems in which they have been studied so far,[3] including humans.[30] Thus, the two isopeptides appear to be interchangeable and are heretofore referred to collectively as GLP-1.

Stimulatory Actions of Glucagon-Like Peptide-1 on Hormone Secretion from Pancreatic Endocrine Cells

Glucagon-like peptide-1 is a potent direct stimulator of insulin and somatostatin secretion from β- and δ-cells, respectively, and suppresses glucagon secretion from α-cells, either directly or indirectly, by the paracrine suppressive actions of insulin.[31] In the perfused rat pancreas, one of the most sensitive experimental models for assaying the effectiveness of secretagogues for the stimulation of insulin secretion, GLP-1 releases insulin at concentrations as low as 5 pM.[27] In this experimental system, GLP-1 is approximately 100 times more potent than glucagon in releasing insulin[32] (Fig. 8-3*A*). Although glucagon has been proposed to be important

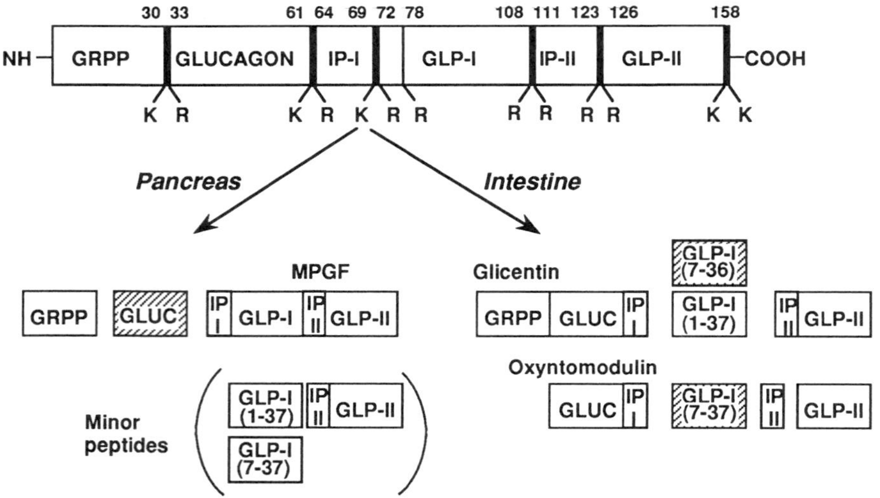

Figure 8-2. Alternative post-translational processing of proglucagon in the pancreas and intestines. The basic amino acids arginine (R) and lysine (K) are sites for enzymatic cleavages by prohormone convertases in the α-cells of the pancreatic islets and the L-cells of the intestine. The major recognized bioactive peptides formed by cleavages (shaded) are glucagon in the pancreas and the two isoforms of GLP-1 in the intestines. (Reproduced with permission from Fehmann H-C, Habener JF. Insulinotropic glucagon-like peptide-1(7-37)–(7-36)amide: A new incretin hormone. Trends Endocrinol Metab 1992;3:158.)

GLP-1

His - **Ala** - **Glu** - *Gly* - *Thr* - *Phe* - *Thr* - *Ser* - *Asp* - **Val** -

Ser - **Ser** - *Tyr* - *Leu* - **Glu** - **Gly** - **Gln** - **Ala** - *Ala* - **Lys** -

Glu - *Phe* - **Ile** - **Ala** - *Trp* - *Leu* - **Val** - **Lys** - **Gly** - **Arg** - *Gly*

NH_2

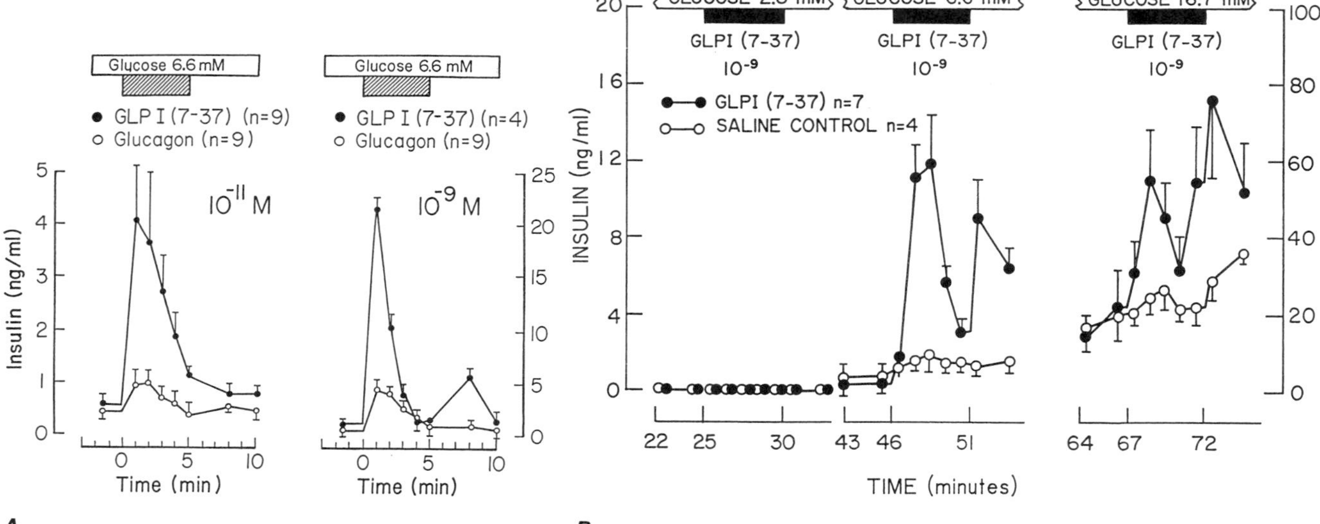

Figure 8-3. *A*, Effects of different concentrations of synthetic GLP-1(7-37) and glucagon on insulin secretion from the perfused rat pancreas. GLP-1(7-37) (●: n = 9 for 10^{-11} M; n = 4 for 10^{-9} M) and synthetic glucagon (○: n = 9). Background perusate contains 6.6 mM glucose. *B*, Glucose dependency of effect of 10^{-9} M GLP-1(7-37) (●: n = 7) on insulin from isolated perfused rat pancreas. Insulin responses at 2.8 and 6.6 mM glucose determined by scale at left; those at 16.7 mM determined by scale at right (○, saline control: n = 4). (Reproduced with permission from Weir GC, Mojsov S, Hendrick GK, Habener JF. Glucagon-like peptide I(7-37) actions on endocrine pancreas. Diabetes 1989;38:338.)

in the augmentation of glucose-stimulated insulin secretion, it remains uncertain whether this effect is mediated by specific glucagon receptors that reside on β-cells. As discussed below, glucagon is a proven weak full agonist on GLP-1 receptors (100-fold weaker [K_d 100 nM] than GLP-1 [K_d 1 nM]), raising the possibility that the stimulation of insulin secretion by glucagon at supraphysiologic concentrations represents a pharmacologic cross-binding of glucagon to the GLP-1 receptor. GLP-1 also appears to be a more potent incretin than GIP, as shown in the perfused rat pancreas and during glucose-clamp studies in human subjects, in whom GLP-1 is at least three times more potent than GIP on a molar basis in stimulating insulin secretion.[33] However, the relative rise in GIP levels after an oral glucose load is greater than that of GLP-1 and may therefore contribute substantially to the incretin effect.[34] The existence of specific distinct receptors for GIP appears to be established by the cloning of the GIP receptor from islet cell cDNA.[35] Whether specific glucagon receptors are expressed in β-cells remains to be determined.

The actions of GLP-1 to stimulate insulin secretion from β-cells depend directly on the glucose concentrations. The effectiveness of GLP-1 as an insulin secretagogue increases as the glucose levels rise and is attenuated as glucose levels fall[31] (Fig. 8-3*B*). In human subjects, all insulin-releasing actions of GLP-1 are lost when blood glucose levels fall to 60 mg/dL (reference no. 36; and Habener JF, McManus K, Nathan DM, unpublished data, 1995). This important property of GLP-1, as well as other incretins such as GIP, to autoregulate the potencies of their actions on augmenting insulin secretion in step with ambient glucose concentrations is a protective measure against hypoglycemia. A cellular mechanism in β-cells to explain this interdependence between glucose and GLP-1 actions involves a synergetic cross-talk between the glycolysis (glucose metabolism) and cAMP signaling pathways (see below). This mutual interdependence between glucose metabolism and GLP-1 actions on β-cells is referred to as the *glucose competence concept* (i.e., glucose is required for β-cells to respond to GLP-1, and GLP-1 [or other incretins] is required to render β-cells competent to respond to glucose.[37]

In addition to its insulin-releasing actions on β-cells, GLP-1 also stimulates somatostatin secretion from δ-cells,[38,39] and suppresses glucagon secretion from α-cells.[39–43] The actions of GLP-1 on δ-cells, as on β-cells, are mediated directly through specific receptors for GLP-1 (see below). However, the actions of GLP-1 on α-cells may or may not depend on receptor interactions with GLP-1. They may be manifested by an indirect effect secondary to the intraislet paracrine suppression of glucagon secretion by insulin.[31] Receptors for GLP-1, however, may also reside on the α-cells that produce glucagon.[44]

The effects of GLP-1 on somatostatin and insulin secretion appear to play an important role in the physiology of insulin secretion and action (Fig. 8-4). Somatostatin suppresses insulin secretion, at least in part, by a paracrine mechanism. The stimulation of somatostatin release by GLP-1 may provide a short-loop negative feedback on insulin secretion.[38] As an anti-insulin hormone, glucagon antagonizes the actions of insulin—particularly on hepatic glucose production, which is stimulated by glucagon and suppressed by insulin. Thus GLP-1, via its actions to stimulate insulin secretion during feeding, acts not only peripherally to enhance uptake of glucose, but also locally within the islets by paracrine mechanisms to suppress glucagon secretion, thereby further enhancing insulin actions by diminishing glucagon-mediated hepatic glucose output.

This paracrine mechanism of regulation within the islets is important in modulating the balance between insulin and glucagon levels during the fasting versus feeding states. In fully manifested NIDDM, in contrast to the earlier stages of impaired glucose tolerance in which blood insulin levels are relatively high, the decreased insulin secretion by β-cells characteristic of NIDDM impairs the paracrine suppression of glucagon mediated by insulin (see below). Ensuing hyperglucagonemia exacerbates the hyperglycemia caused by insulin resistance of peripheral tissues and diminished glucose responsivity of β-cells by stimulating hepatic glucose output.

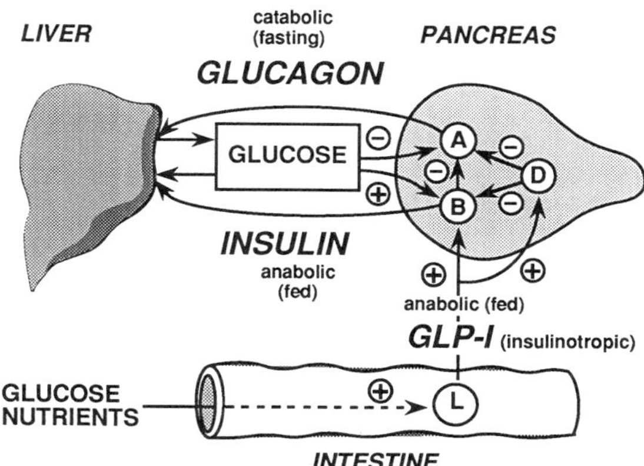

FIGURE 8-4. Model depicting the proposed physiologic actions of GLP-1. Nutrients in the intestinal lumen (glucose, food) stimulate the release of GLP-1, which augments glucose-stimulated insulin and somatostatin secretion and suppresses glucagon secretion, either indirectly via paracrine actions of insulin or through GLP-1 receptors on α-cells. Insulin is an anabolic hormone that stimulates glucose uptake by liver, muscle, and fat during feeding. Glucagon is a catabolic hormone that stimulates glucose production in these organs during fasting. Thus, alternative proteolytic processing of proglucagon produces GLP-1 in the intestines during feeding and glucagon in the pancreas during fasting. (Reproduced with permission from Fehmann H-C, Habener JF. Insulinotropic glucagon-like peptide-1(7-37)-(7-36)amide: A new incretin hormone. Trends Endocrinol Metab 1992;3:158.)

Mechanisms of Action of Glucagon-Like Peptide-1

Soon after GLP-1 was discovered to be a potent glucose-dependent insulin secretagogue, it was found that the peptide bound to high-affinity sites on β-cells (K_d = 1 nM) and stimulated the formation of cAMP in insulinoma cell lines.[45] These findings predicted the likelihood that the hormone acts through specific receptors located on the surface of β-cells that are coupled to the stimulatory G-protein (G_s).

Receptors

In one study, direct screening of a recombinant rat islet cDNA library with ^{125}I-labeled GLP-1 provided a recombinant cDNA encoding the GLP-1 receptor (GLP-1R).[46] The receptor is a member of the seven-membrane–spanning, G-protein–coupled family of receptors. By sequence similarities, GLP-1R falls into a new subclass of receptors that includes glucagon,[47] vasoactive intestinal peptide,[48] secretin,[49] GIP,[50] pituitary adenylyl cyclase activating peptide (PACAP),[51] growth hormone-releasing hormone,[52] calcitonin,[53] and parathyroid hormone.[54] Ligand-binding analyses of the recombinant receptors expressed in and assembled on the surface of β-cells or heterologous cells show that the selectivity for the binding of GLP-1 is approximately 1 nM, whereas all of the other peptides of the glucagon superfamily bind poorly or not at all with the exception of glucagon, which is a weak, full agonist with a binding affinity 100–1,000-fold less (0.1 to 1.0 μM) than that of GLP-1.[46] The amino-terminally truncated form of exendin (exendin 9-39), a peptide related in structure to GLP-1 and the other glucagon-related peptides, is a potent antagonist of GLP-1.[55] Although exendin is not a pure antagonist of GLP-1, the ratio of antagonist to agonist activities is greater than 100 (K_i = 1 nM, K_a = 100 nM).

At present, it is uncertain whether glucagon receptors are expressed on β-cells. Suprapharmacologic concentrations (10 nM or greater) of glucagon are required to bind to and activate GLP-1 receptors and to stimulate cAMP formation.[45,46] The cloned rat hepatic glucagon receptor expressed in Cos GS-1 cell membranes has a K_d for glucagon of 5–10 mM and appears not to bind GLP-1 (K_d > 1 μM).[56]

The matter of the relative ligand specificities of GLP-1 and glucagon for their respective receptors is far from clear. In Cos-7 cells transfected with and expressing the recombinant human hepatic glucagon receptor, GLP-1 binds with a K_d of approximately 100 nM.[57] Moreover, relatively high affinity (1 nM) sites that bind GLP-1 have been demonstrated in adipocytes,[58] skeletal muscle,[59] brain,[60] stomach,[61] and hepatocyte membranes.[62] RNA assays (reverse transcription polymerase chain reaction and RNase protection assays) detect relatively low levels of mRNAs for the *GLP1R* gene in brain, kidney, heart, fat, skeletal muscle, liver, and intestine.[63,64] As discussed further below, binding of GLP-1 to these tissues correlates with the stimulation of biologic activities (e.g., lipogenesis, glycogenesis).

The *GLP1R* gene is highly expressed in lung,[65] stomach,[61] and pancreatic islets.[64] Notably, the lung *GLP1R* binds both GLP-1, vasoactive intestinal peptide, and peptide methionine isoleucine (PMI) with equivalent affinities of approximately 1 nM, resulting in the stimulation of mucous secretion and of smooth muscle contraction.[65] The amidated isopeptide GLP-1(7-36)amide has been reported to inhibit gastric motility and acid secretion.[66]

One potential mechanism for the alteration of *GLP1R* conformation or structure is by alternative exon-splicing at the level of nuclear processing of RNA encoding the *GLP1R*. A somewhat unusual feature of *GLP1R* and the other genes of this family of receptors is the large number of exons (12–16). Alternative splicing of exons in the glucagon, growth hormone-releasing hormone, and PACAP receptors has been demonstrated. In the PACAP-receptor RNA, two small exons designated HIP and HOP are alternatively spliced within the third cytoplasmic loop and thereby change the signal transduction coupling from cAMP (G_s) to phosphoinositol turnover (G_q).[51] The structure of the *GLP1R* is not yet known, but is likely to consist of numerous exonic sequences as well. Thus far, the coupling of *GLP1R* to cellular signaling appears to be restricted to the cAMP pathway. Stimulation of phosphoinositol turnover induced by *GLP1R* transfected and expressed in the COS-7 cell line has been reported, but may be a consequence of artifactual recruitment of G_q by the greatly overexpressed numbers of receptors.[67]

The GLP-1R is susceptible to rapid, reversible homologous desensitization in β-cells (Fig. 8-5).[68] Addition of 100 mM GLP-1 to HIT cells for 5 minutes attenuates insulin secretion and cAMP formation in response to a 10-mM stimulatory dose of GLP-1. Return of receptor responsivity occurs during a "ligand washout" recovery period of 10–20 minutes. This apparent propensity of *GLP1R* to undergo reversible desensitization is an important consideration in the development of GLP-1 as a potential therapy for NIDDM (see below).

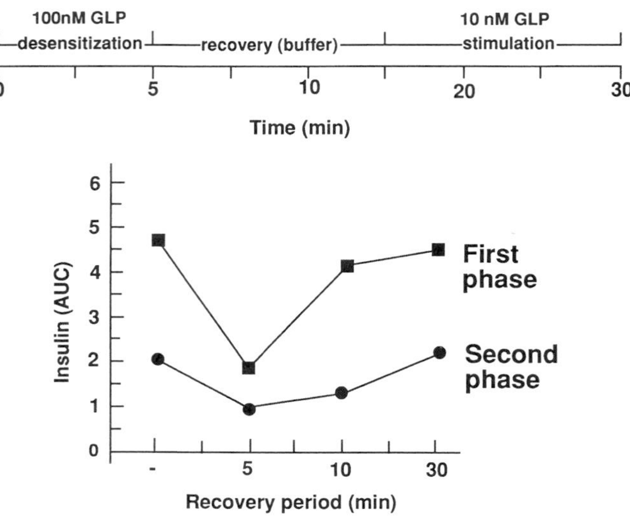

Figure 8-5. Rapid and reversible homologous desensitization of the GLP-1 receptor on hamster insulinoma (HIT-T15) cells. Shown are the integrated insulin secretory responses to 10 nM GLP-1 (7-37) after a 5-minute periperfusion with 100 mM GLP-1(7-37) and a washout period of 5, 10, and 30 minutes. ■ = first phase (1–10 minutes); ● = second phase (11–30 minutes) of insulin secretion. (Reproduced with permission from Fehmann H-C, Habener JF. Homologous desensitization of the insulinotropic glucagon-like peptide-I(7-37) receptor on insulinoma (HIT-T15) cells. Endocrinology 1991;128:2880.)

Stimulation of Insulin Gene Transcription and Insulin Production

In addition to stimulating glucose-dependent insulin secretion, GLP-1 stimulates transcription of the insulin gene proinsulin mRNA levels, insulin biosynthesis, and accumulation of cellular stores of insulin.[69] These unique insulinotropic actions of GLP-1 contrast markedly with the actions of the sulfonylurea class of oral hypoglycemic drugs that stimulate the secretion, but not the production, of insulin.[70] The reason for these differences in the actions of GLP-1 and the sulfonylurea drugs appears to be that GLP-1, unlike sulfonylureas, stimulates the formation of cAMP. The cAMP signaling pathway stimulates transcription of the insulin gene by activating the DNA-binding transcription cAMP response element (CRE)-binding factor[71] that binds to a key CRE located in the promoter of the insulin gene, thereby enhancing the efficiency of the gene's transcription (Fig. 8-6). The effects of cAMP are mediated through the activation of cAMP-dependent protein kinase A (PKA), an enzyme that phosphorylates the CREB bound to the CRE in the promoter of the insulin gene. This circumstance couples the protein-DNA complex consisting of CREB bound to the CRE into the basal RNA polymerase II transcriptional machinery, resulting in enhancement of insulin gene transcription.

Activation of Ion Channels

Studies of ion channels in β-cells have elucidated a mechanism by which elevated glucose levels result in the secretion of insulin.[72,73] Insulin secretion requires the influx of Ca^{++} from the extracellular fluid into the cell, a process that triggers *exocytosis:* fusion of secretory granules with the plasma membrane, lysis of the granules, and release of insulin into the extracellular fluid or blood stream (Fig. 8-7). The influx of Ca^{++} depends largely on the opening of voltage-sensitive calcium channels (Ca-VS), whose activation (opening) depends in turn on the voltage potential between the inside and outside of the cell controlled by the ATP-sensitive potassium channels (K-ATP). This inwardly rectifying K^+ channel appears to be the important target for glucose and cAMP signaling, as determined by electrophysiologic studies using whole-cell patch clamp and excised patch studies, in which the electrical potential of the cell and activities of single channels located on

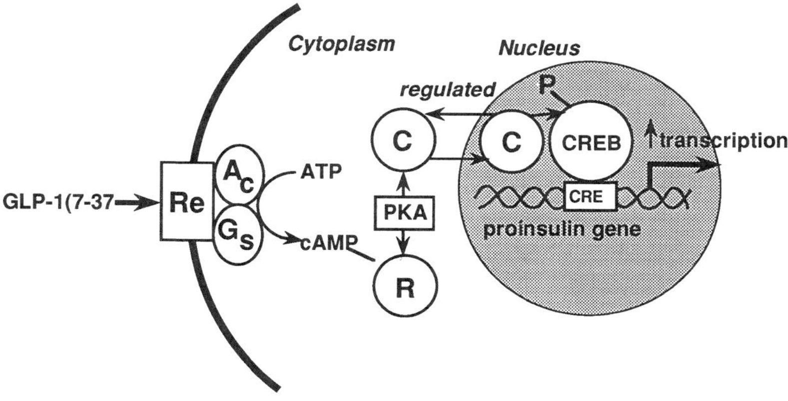

Figure 8-6. Insulinotropic actions of GLP-1 on β-cells mediated by activation of the cAMP signaling pathway. The binding of GLP-1 to its receptor activates adenylyl cyclase, resulting in the formation of cAMP, which activates the cAMP-dependent phosphorylase, protein kinase A (PKA). PKA phosphorylates and therefore activates the nuclear transcriptional activator protein CREB bound to the CRE located in the promoter of the *INS* gene. This cascade of signaling results in a stimulation of transcription of *INS* and increased insulin biosynthesis to replete stores of insulin secreted in response to nutrients (glucose) and incretins (GLP-1).

the plasma membrane are recorded.[37,72,73] The K-ATP of β-cells is also believed to be the receptor for the actions of the sulfonylurea drugs.[70,72]

The sequence of events in the activation of the secretory responses of β-cells is as follows (see Fig. 8-7). In conditions of normoglycemia and the absence of activation of the cAMP signaling pathway, K-ATP on β-cells are open, resulting in a resting potential of −70 to −60 mV, due to the concentration gradient of

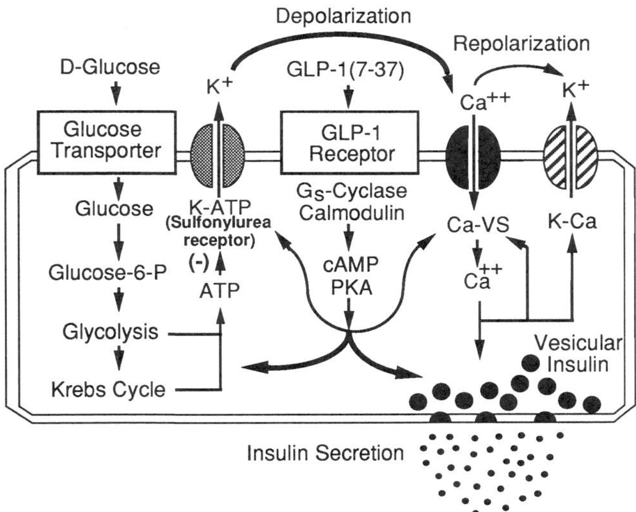

Figure 8-7. Model of the proposed ion channels and signal transduction pathways in a pancreatic β-cell involved in the mechanisms of insulin secretion in response to glucose and GLP-1. The key elements of the model are the requirement of dual inputs of (1) the glucose-glycolysis signaling pathway, and (2) the GLP-1/receptor-mediated cAMP protein kinase A (PKA) signaling pathways to effect closure of ATP-sensitive potassium channels (K-ATP). The closure of these channels results in a rise in the resting potential (depolarization) of the β-cell, leading to opening of voltage-sensitive calcium channels (Ca-VS). The influx of Ca^{++} through the open-end Ca-VS triggers vesicular insulin secretion by the process of exocytosis. Repolarization of the β-cell is achieved by the opening of calcium-sensitive potassium channels (K-Ca). It is believed that the GLP-1 receptor is coupled to a stimulatory G-protein (G_s) and a calcium-calmodulin–sensitive adenylyl cyclase. (Reproduced with permission from Holz GG IV, Habener JF. Signal transduction crosstalk in the endocrine system: Pancreatic β-cells and the glucose competence concept. Trends Biochem Sci 1992;17:388.)

K^+ between the inside (130 mM) and outside (4–5 mM) of the cell. An elevation in glucose levels in the extracellular fluid results in the transport of glucose into the β-cell via the type 2 glucose transporter (GLUT-2), glycolysis, and an increase in the intracellular ATP : ADP ratio. The binding of ATP to K-ATP concomitant with phosphorylation of K-ATP closes the channel, resulting in depolarization of the β-cell. When the potential of the β-cell reaches 30–40 mV, the Ca-VS opens, leading to an influx of Ca^{++} and resultant secretion of insulin. The increase in intracellular Ca^{++} then activates (opens) voltage sensitive potassium channels (K-VS), thereby restoring the resting potential to −70 to −60 mV. This cycle of depolarization, insulin secretion, and repolarization of β-cells occurs in an oscillatory manner with a periodicity of 10–15 minutes, as long as the glucose and cAMP signaling pathways are maintained.

Glucagon-Like Peptide-1 and the Glucose Competence Concept

Single, isolated β-cells appear not to respond to a glucose signal alone, but rather require the simultaneous activation of a second signaling pathway, such as the cAMP-dependent pathway.[37,74,75] This requirement for a cross-talk between glucose-glycolysis–mediated and cAMP-dependent signaling stimulated by GLP-1 is referred to as the glucose competence concept.[37,75] As alluded to above, the closure of K-ATP channels is hypothesized to be an important component of the mechanism involved in the depolarization of the β-cell and consequent insulin secretion (see Fig. 8-7). To close the K-ATP channels, this model of β-cell activation requires the dual input of the ATP signal generated by a glucose-sensing signal consisting of glucose transport and glycolysis, and the cAMP signal produced by the activation of the GLP-1 receptor when bound by GLP-1 to close the K-ATP channels. It is believed, although not definitely proved at this time, that mechanistically both the binding of ATP to K-ATP and the phosphorylation of K-ATP by cAMP-dependent PKA are necessary to effect closure of the channels, resulting in depolarization and the opening of Ca-VS channels. Thus, insulin secretion is stimulated during a meal by the simultaneously occurring rises of both glucose and GLP-1 in the blood perfusing the β-cells. GLP-1 is only one of *several* proposed candidate incretins produced by the intestines in response to oral nutrients that may activate cAMP or other signaling pathways required for glucose to stimulate insulin secretion and production. Evidence has been presented, however, that the combined release of both GLP-1 and GIP during meals may account for most, if not all, of the physiologically relevant incretin effect.[7]

Radioimmunoassays

Sensitive radioimmunoassays for the detection of GLP-1 have been developed, and others are under development. The background of some assays may be artifactually elevated because of the secretion by the pancreas of the major proglucagon fragment in which GLP-1 is retained in an incomplete form with a prolonged clearance time. Thus assay values for circulating levels of GLP-1 reported in the literature are variable because of the problems of cross-reactivities with long-lived proglucagon fragments and possible cross-reactivities with other peptide hormones related to GLP-1 in their amino acid sequences.

For circulating levels of GLP-1 in normal human subjects, however, assays that appear to be relatively specific for the detection of the biologically active isopeptides GLP-1(7-37) and GLP-1 (7-36)amide[74] can provide concensus values. In response to a 400-kcal meal in six nondiabetic subjects, peak levels (90 minutes) of GLP-1(7-37) rose from 6 pM (fasting) to 10 pM; levels of GLP-1 (7-36)amide rose from 7 pM fasting to 41pM[76] (Fig. 8-8). These values for the two GLP-1 isopeptides reflect the ratio of their concentrations measured in extracts of human distal small intestine: GLP-1(7-37), 7 pmol/g tissue; GLP-1(7-36)amide, 28 pmol/g tissue.[76]

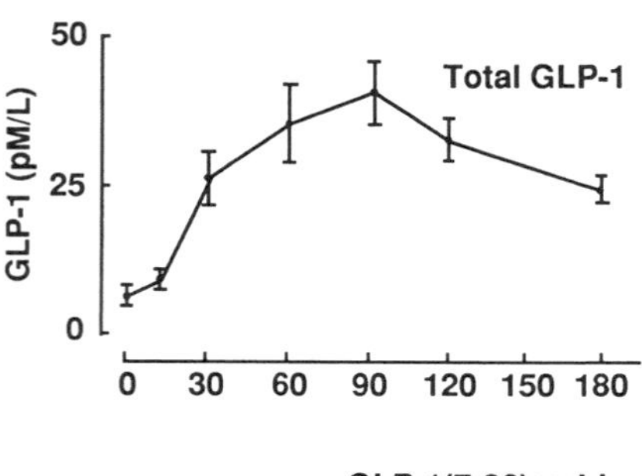

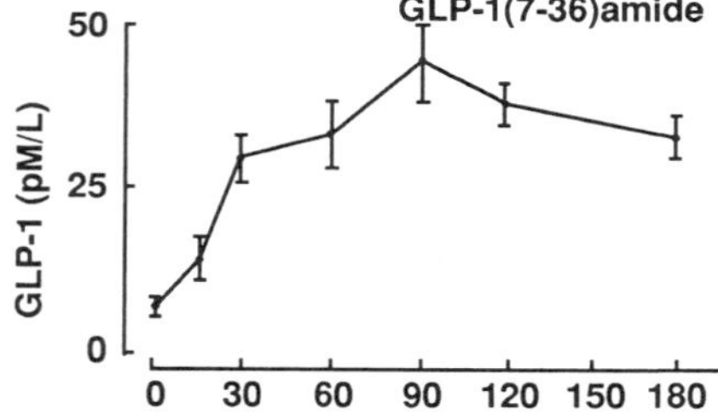

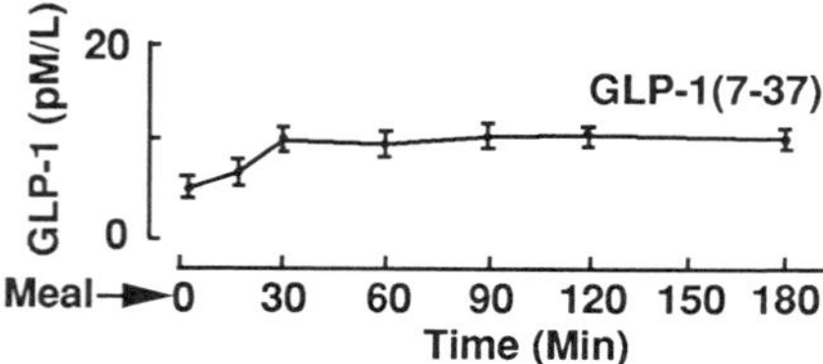

Figure 8-8. Secretory responses of GLP-1 isopeptides GLP-1(7-37) and GLP-1(7-36)amide to a meal in six nondiabetic subjects. Radioimmunoassays are relatively specific for detection of the differences in the COOH-termini of the two isopeptides. Approximately 80% of the total GLP-1 consists of the GLP-1(7-36)amide. (Reproduced with permission from Ørskov C, Rabenhøj L, Wettergren A, et al. Tissue and plasma concentrations of amidated and glycine-extended glucagon-like peptide I in humans. Diabetes 1994;43:535.)

Intestinal Secretion of Glucagon-Like Peptide-1

In the enteroendocrine L-cells of the intestine, GLP-1 is expressed from the same gene from which it is expressed in the pancreas. As noted earlier, however, the post-translational processing of proglucagon in the intestine and pancreas differ markedly: The predominant bioactive peptides secreted from the intestine are the GLPs, not glucagon as in the pancreas. During the intestinal processing of proglucagon, the glucagon peptide remains part of an incompletely processed fragment of proglucagon, known as *glicentin* (or enteroglucagon).

The L-cells that produce GLP-1 are located predominantly in the distal small intestine (ileum) and colon in contrast to the cells that secrete GIP, which is expressed in the more proximal regions of the small intestine.[25] Both GLP-1 and glicentin are cosecreted from the intestinal L-cells in response to the ingestion of nutrients: glucose, protein, and fat. Oral glucose alone is an effective stimulator of GLP-1 secretion as well as protein and fat potentiate secretion. As discussed above, the two isoforms of GLP-1, the glycine-extended GLP-1(7-37) and the amidated GLP-1(7-36)amide, are cosecreted at a ratio of approximately 1 : 4 (see Fig. 8-8), reflecting the composition of the GLP-1 stored in the intestine.[76,77]

The secretion of GLP-1 in response to meals is probably mediated to a large extent by neuroenteric reflexes. Elevations of GLP-1 in the circulation are seen 15–30 minutes after a subject begins to ingest a meal (see Fig. 8-8); luminal nutrients would not be expected to reach the distal ileum, where the L-cells that produce GLP-1 reside, within that 15–30 minute period. Thus, it appears that the initial early stimulation of GLP-1 is due to neural, or perhaps hormonal, influences and that the prolonged phase of elevated levels (90–180 minutes) reflects a direct stimulation of L-cells by luminal nutrients. Such dual pathways for the stimulation of GLP-1 secretion may be important in regulating glucose-dependent secretion of insulin.

The hypersecretion of GLP-1 has been described in at least two situations: *postgastrectomy dumping syndrome* and diabetes mellitus.[25,78] Apparently, gastrectomy or partial gastrectomy results in (1) an exaggerated neuroenteric stimulation of GLP-1 secretion, or (2) a very rapid transit time for nutrients into the small intestine, or both. The hypersecretion of GLP-1 in the dumping syndrome is substantial—fivefold to sixfold elevated above normal.[79] Elevations in blood levels of GLP-1 in patients with NIDDM are less pronounced than they are in patients with dumping syndrome; basal levels and levels stimulated by oral glucose are reported as 1.5–2 fold above those of nondiabetic subjects.[78] Because the differences in GLP-1 levels between diabetic and nondiabetic subjects are small and radioimmunoassay technology is still under development, it is uncertain whether or not elevated GLP-1 levels correlate with diabetes.

Metabolism

The clearance of GLP-1 peptides from the circulation is quite rapid. The half-time of disappearance of both GLP-1(7-37) and GLP-1(7-36)amide in human subjects is 8–10 minutes.[80] The metabolic clearance rate for both peptides is 12–15 mL/min/kg.[80] In comparison, the clearance time for both the larger proglucagon fragment glicentin (containing glucagon) and the major proglucagon fragment (containing GLP-1) is approximately 30 minutes. The kidney appears to be an important organ involved in the clearance of GLP-1 from the circulation; glucagon is cleared by both kidney and liver.[81] Both GLP-1 and GIP, as well as growth-hormone releasing hormone are rapidly inactivated in the circulation via cleavage of the amino terminal two amino acids by a dipeptidyl protease.[82] The biologic activities of many of the peptides in the glucagon superfamily are dependent on the amino terminal histidine or tyrosine with the free alpha amino group available. Either removal of the histidine or tyrosine or extension of the amino-terminus by additional peptide sequence extensions markedly impairs the biologic activities of the glucagon-related peptides.[83]

Potential Role of Glucagon-Like Peptide-1 in Diabetes Mellitus

Because a major role of GLP-1 and GIP is to augment glucose-stimulated insulin release, the possibility arises that an impairment or alteration in the production, secretion, or actions of GLP-1 (or GIP) may contribute to or even be a cause of the blunted insulin secretory dynamics of, or the diminished sensitivity of peripheral tissues to, the actions of insulin, or both possibilities. Of the two prevalent forms of diabetes mellitus, insulin-dependent (type I) diabetes mellitus (IDDM) and maturity-onset NIDDM, the latter disease may be more likely to have a role in defective regulation of GLP-1. Unlike IDDM, in which the β-cells are destroyed, the β-cells of patients with NIDDM are intact and are capable of secreting insulin, albeit with abnormal secretory dynamics resulting in insufficient insulin levels to counteract the hyperglycemia characteristic of diabetes. In the early stages of the development of diabetes before hyperglycemia is manifested, the β-cells hypersecrete insulin to maintain normoglycemia (normal glucose tolerance to oral glucose).[84] As the resistance of peripheral tissues (e.g., skeletal muscle, fat) to the actions of insulin increases, the production of insulin by the β-cells can no longer compensate and postprandial hyperglycemia (impaired glucose tolerance) ensues, which then worsens and progresses to fasting hyperglycemia (diabetes).[84] Such a decompensation of the capacity of the β-cell to produce insulin during the development of NIDDM may be aggravated by, or even caused by, a loss of effectiveness of the GLP-1 incretin hormone. Decreased secretion of GLP-1, increased metabolism, or diminished sensitivity of the β-cells to GLP-1 could be responsible for the loss of effectiveness. It is known that in patients with NIDDM, the incretin effect to augment insulin secretion is reduced

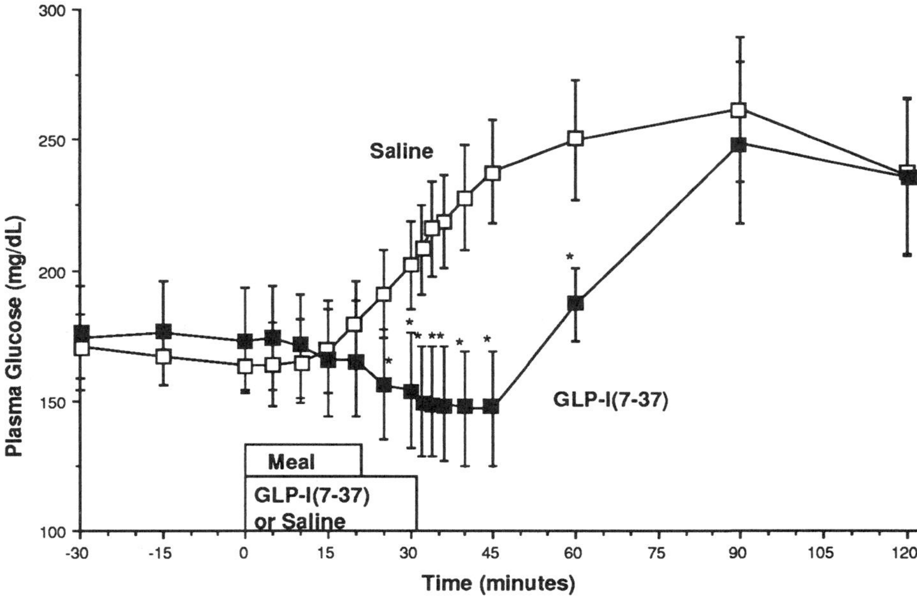

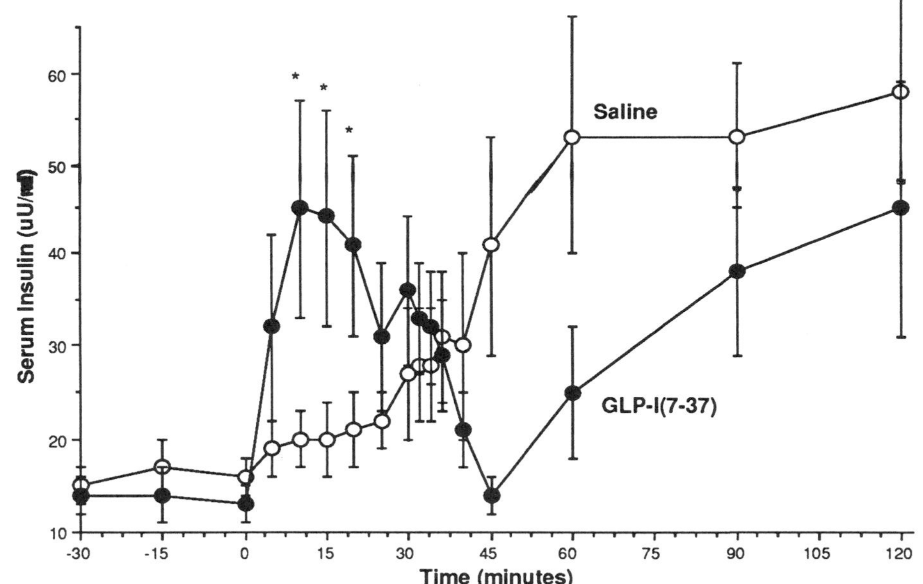

FIGURE 8-9. GLP-1(7-37) administered to diabetic subjects stimulates insulin secretion and lowers blood glucose levels in response to meals. GLP-1 (■, ●: 5 ng/kg/min) and saline (□, ○) infusion in five NIDDM subjects were concurrent with the ingestion of a standard test meal. *$P < 0.05$ GLP-1(7-37) versus placebo. (Reproduced with permission from Nathan DM, Schrieber E, Fogel H, et al. Insulinotropic action of glucagon-like peptide-1(7-37) in diabetic and nondiabetic subjects. Diabetes Care 1992; 15:270.)

or lost.[9,85] This loss appears to occur in the face of enhanced secretion of the incretin hormones GLP-1 and GIP,[13,79] suggesting that the elevated levels of the incretins may in some way desensitize their action on their respective receptors. Perhaps the hypothetical desensitization occurs by way of a partial uncoupling of the receptor from the stimulatory G-protein that activates adenylyl cyclase in the cAMP-mediated signaling pathway. Even a slight impairment in receptor coupling to cAMP formation may be envisioned to impair phosphorylation of the K-ATP channel and thereby to reduce the probability of K-ATP closure (see Fig. 8-7). The result of this chain of events would be a lessening of the incretin effect in augmenting the glucose-stimulated secretion of insulin.

With the recent reports of GLP-1 binding sites on adipocytes[58,63,86,87] and receptor mRNA in skeletal muscle and adipose tissues of rats,[63] it is possible that a partial desensitization of the GLP-1 receptor on these tissues may contribute to the insulin resistance of diabetes apart from the desensitization of the receptor on β-cells. The concept of GLP-1 receptor desensitization and its relevance to diabetes requires that the desensitization be incomplete. Otherwise, as discussed below, the administration of GLP-1 to patients with NIDDM would not be expected to enhance insulin secretion therapeutically, as it appears to do.

Desensitization of the GLP-1 receptor on β-cells in patients with NIDDM may also influence glucagon secretion. Either the diminished insulin secretion resulting from reduced insulinotropic actions of GLP-1 on β-cells or the desensitization of GLP-1 receptors on α-cells, or both, would reduce suppressive effects on α-cells, resulting in excessive secretion of glucagon. Clearly, the actions of excessive glucagon antagonize those of insulin in the target tissues, liver, muscle, and fat, thus worsening the diabetic condition. It is not known whether GLP-1 receptors on the δ-cells that secrete somatostatin undergo desensitization. If they did desensitize, however, the decrease in the suppressive effect of somatostatin on insulin secretion predictably would be diminished, thereby serving to restore insulin secretion. If the GLP-1 receptor on δ-cells were not desensitized, however, the inhibition of insulin secretion would be enhanced.

Potential Use of Glucagon-Like Peptide-1 in the Treatment of Diabetes

In view of the findings described above, GLP-1 offers several potential therapeutic advantages over current modes of therapy for NIDDM. Stimulation of endogenous insulin from the pancreas, which results in the delivery of insulin directly to the liver and other insulin-responsive organs via the combined portal and system circulation, is much preferred to the systemic delivery of insulin administered subcutaneously. Unlike the sulfonylurea drugs, which stimulate insulin secretion but not biosynthesis and have the potential disadvantage of exhausting β-cell supplies of insulin, GLP-1 stimulates both insulin secretion and production. Further, because the sulfonylurea drugs are believed to act directly on the K-ATP channels to pharmacologically close the channels, the extent of closure is not regulated by means other than adjustments of the administered dose. For example, the potency of sulfonylurea actions is not modulated by the ambient glucose concentrations, as is the case for GLP-1. As discussed above, the relative potency of GLP-1 in modulating the closure of K-ATP channels is directly related to the concentration of glucose. Thus, sulfonylurea drugs continue to act in conditions of low blood glucose, potentially leading to the severe effects of hypoglycemia. In contrast, the actions of GLP-1 are abrogated as blood glucose levels fall into the low-normal range, and this circumstance guards against the occurrence of hypoglycemia.

Preliminary studies of the potential efficacy of GLP-1 as a means of controlling hyperglycemia in patients with NIDDM are promising. The administration of GLP-1 to patients with NIDDM during meals effectively restores the early phase of insulin secretion characteristically absent in NIDDM (Fig. 8-9) and consequently attenuates the excessive prandial rise in blood glucose levels.[88,89] Further, in studies in which the blood glucose concentrations of patients with diabetes were controlled by a closed-loop insulin infusion system (artificial pancreas), GLP-1 was shown to have an antidiabetogenic effect. In patients with NIDDM, GLP-1 reduced the mean calculated isoglycemic meal-related insulin requirement by eightfold, so that the plasma free insulin was decreased despite the stimulation of insulin release.[90] Remarkably, in insulin-deficient patients with IDDM, GLP-1 administration significantly increased glucose utilization, suggesting that GLP-1 improved the insulin sensitivity of extrapancreatic tissues.[90] In addition, administration of GLP-1 to patients with mild NIDDM was insulinotropic, whereas GIP was not, indicating that in contrast to GIP the incretin activity of GLP-1 is preserved.[33,34]

Summary

The proglucagon gene is expressed in both the endocrine pancreas and the intestine. Alternative post-translational processing of proglucagon results specifically in the formation of glucagon in the pancreas and two glucagon-like peptides (GLPs) in the intestine. One of the GLPs, GLP-1, is a potent insulinotropic hormone, released from the intestine in response to oral nutrients, and is one of the most potent incretin hormones recognized to augment glucose-stimulated insulin secretion (see Fig. 8-4). Administration of GLP-1 during meals to patients with NIDDM restores the absent or blunted first phase of insulin secretion and lowers plasma glucose levels. Unlike the sulfonylurea drugs that can cause hypoglycemia and possibly β-cell exhaustion of insulin stores, the insulinotropic actions of GLP-1 depend entirely on extracellular glucose concentrations: At plasma glucose levels of 60 mg/dL and below, all actions of GLP-1 are lost. Further, GLP-1 stimulates the production as well as secretion of insulin. Experimental evidence provides potential explanations for these apparently unique properties of GLP-1. The mechanism of action of GLP-1 involves binding to a cAMP-coupled receptor on β-cells that, in concert with increased levels of ATP generated by glucose metabolism (glycolysis), modulates ATP-sensitive K^+ channels that in turn regulate Ca^{++} entry into the cell and resultant insulin secretion by Ca^{++}-dependent mechanisms of exocytosis. Thus, the simultaneous and synergetic activation of both cAMP and biosynthesis is enhanced by cAMP-induced stimulation of proinsulin gene transcription mediated by interactions of cAMP-dependent transcription factor CREB with CREs resident in the promoter of the insulin gene. Moreover, it appears that a substantial degree of the glucose-lowering actions of GLP-1 may occur by mechanisms independent of the direct actions of insulin, possibly mediated by (1) GLP-1-responsive receptors tentatively identified on skeletal muscle and adipose tissue, or (2) inhibition of glucagon release by insulin (or by GLP-1), or both, resulting in decreased hepatic glucose output. The unique mechanisms of action of GLP-1 provide potential advantages over the sulfonylureas as a treatment for NIDDM. Unlike the sulfonylurea drugs, GLP-1 stimulates the production as well as secretion of insulin, and its actions on β-cells are regulated by plasma glucose concentrations. Therefore, hypoglycemia is not anticipated to be an untoward side effect of GLP-1 administration.

Acknowledgments

Joel F. Habener is an investigator with the Howard Hughes Medical Institute. Appreciation is extended to Scott Heller, Ph.D., and Tim Kieffer, Ph.D., for helpful comments and to T. Budde, B.A., for help in preparation of the manuscript. The studies were supported in part by USPHS grant DK30834.

References

1. Creutzfeldt W, Ebert R. New developments in the incretin concept. Diabetologia 1985;28:565
2. Ebert R, Creutzfeldt W. Gastrointestinal peptides and insulin secretion. In: Diabetes/Metabolism Reviews. New York, NY: John Wiley & Sons; 1987; 3:1–26
3. Habener JF. The incretin notion and its relevance to diabetes. Endocrinol Metab Clin North Am 1993;22:775
4. Zunz E, La Barre J. Contributions à l'étude des variations physiologiques de la sécrétion interne du pancreas: Relation entre les sécrétions externe et interne du pancreas. Arch Int Physiol Biochim Biophys 1929;31:20
5. Jöurnvall H, Carlquist M, Kwauk S, et al. Amino acid sequence and heterogeneity of gastric inhibitory polypeptide (GIP). FEBS Lett 1981;123:205
6. Lund PK, Goodman RH, Montminy MR, et al. Anglerfish islet pre-proglucagon II. J Biol Chem 1982;158:3280
7. Nauck M, Baftels E, Ørskov C, et al. Insulinotropic effects of a combination of human synthetic GIP and GLP-1 (7-36 amide) at physiological plasma glucose in man. Diabetologia 1991;34(suppl 2):A14
8. Unger RH, Eisentraut AH. Entero-insular axis. Arch Intern Med 1979;123:261
9. Nauck M, Stöckmann F, Ebert R, Creutzfeldt W. Reduced incretin effect in type 2 (non-insulin-dependent) diabetes. Diabetologia 1986;29:46
10. Heller H. Über das insulinotrope Hormon der darmschleimhaut (Duodenin). Naunyn Schmiedebergs Arch Pharmacol 1935;147:127
11. Brown JC, Mutt V, Pederson RA. Further purification of a polypeptide demonstrating enterogastrone activity. J Physiol Lond 1970;209:57
12. Brown JC, Pederson RA. A multiparameter study on the action of preparations containing cholecystokinin-pancreozymin. Scand J Gastroenterol 1970;5:537
13. Krarup T. Immunoreactive gastric inhibitory polypeptide. Endocr Rev 1988; 9:122
14. Pederson RA, Brown JC. The insulinotropic action of gastric inhibitory polypeptide in the perfused isolated rat pancreas. Endocrinology 1976;99:780
15. Andersen DK, Elahi D, Brown JC, et al. Oral glucose augmentation of insulin secretion: Interactions of gastric inhibitory polypeptide with ambient glucose and insulin levels. J Clin Invest 1978;62:152
16. Brown JC, Pederson RA. GI hormones and insulin secretion. In: Proc 5th International Congress on Endocrinology, Hamburg, Vol. 2. Amsterdam: Excerpta Medica;1977:568
17. Ebert R, Creutzfeldt W. Influence of gastric inhibitory polypeptide antiserum on glucose-induced insulin secretion in rats. Endocrinology 1982;111:1601
18. Heinrich G, Gros P, Lund PK, et al. Preproglucagon messenger RNA: Nucleotide and encoded amino acid sequences of the rat pancreatic cDNA. Endocrinology 1984;115:2176
19. Lopez LC, Frazier ML, Su CJ, et al. Mammalian pancreatic preproglucagon contains three glucagon-related peptides. Proc Natl Acad Sci U S A 1983; 80:5485
20. Bell GI, Sanchez-Pescador R, Laybourn PJ, Najarian RC. Exon duplication and divergence in the human preproglucagon gene. Nature 1983;304:368
21. Heinrich G, Gros P, Habener JF. Glucagon gene sequence—four of six exons encode separate functional domains of rat pre-proglucagon. J Biol Chem 1984;259:14082
22. Takeda J, Seino Y, Tanaka K-I, et al. Sequence of an intestinal cDNA encoding human gastric inhibitory polypeptide precursor. Proc Natl Acad Sci U S A 1987;84:7005
23. Fehmann H-C, Habener JF. Insulinotropic glucagon-like peptide-1(7-37)-(7-36)amide: A new incretin hormone. Trends Endocrinol Metab 1992;3:158
24. Fehmann H-C, Göke R, Göke B. Glucagon-like peptide-1(7-37)/(7-36)amide is a new incretin. Mol Cell Endocrinol 1992;85:C39
25. Ørskov C. Glucagon-like peptide-1, a new hormone of the entero-insular axis. Diabetologia 1992;35:701
26. Thorens B, Waeber G. Glucagon-like peptide-1 and the control of insulin secretion in the normal state and in NIDDM. Diabetes 1993;42:1219
27. Mojsov S, Heinrich G, Wilson IB, et al. Preproglucagon gene expression in pancreas and intestine diversifies at the level of post-translational processing. J Biol Chem 1986;261:11880
28. Mojsov S, Weir GC, Habener JF. Insulinotropin: Glucagon-like peptide-I (7-37) co-encoded in the glucagon gene is a potent stimulator of insulin release in the perfused rat pancreas. J Clin Invest 1987;79:616
29. Holst JJ, Ørskov C, Nielsen V, Schwartz TW. Truncated glucagon-like peptide-I, an insulin-releasing hormone from the distal gut. FEBS Lett 1987;211:169
30. Ørskov C, Wettergren A, Holst JJ. Biological effects and metabolic rates of GLP-1 7-36 amide and GLP-1 7-37 in healthy subjects are indistinguishable. Diabetes 1993;42:658
31. Stagner JI, Samols E. The vascular order of islet cellular perfusion in the human pancreas. Diabetes 1992;41:93
32. Weir GC, Mojsov S, Hendrick GK, Habener JF. Glucagon-like peptide I (7-37) actions on endocrine pancreas. Diabetes 1989;38:338
33. Elahi D, McAloon-Dyke M, Fukagawa NK, et al. The insulinotropic actions of glucose-dependent insulinotropic polypeptide (GIP) and glucagon-like peptide-1(7-37) in normal and diabetic subjects. Regul Pept 1994;51:63
34. Nauck MA, Bartels E, Ørskov C, et al. Additive insulinotropic effects of exogenous synthetic human gastric inhibitory polypeptide and glucagon-like peptide-1-(7-36)amide infused at near-physiological insulinotropic hormone and glucose concentrations. J Clin Endocrinol Metab 1993;76:912
35. Usdin TB, Mezey É, Button DC, et al. Gastric inhibitory polypeptide receptor, a member of the secretin-vasoactive intestinal peptide receptor family, is widely distributed in peripheral organs and the brain. Endocrinology 1993;133:2861
36. Nauck M, Heimesaat MM, Ørskov C, et al. Normalization of fasting hyperglycaemia by exogenous glucagon-like peptide 1 (7-36) in type 2 (non-insulin-dependent) diabetic patients. Diabetologia 1993;36:741
37. Holz GG IV, Habener JF. Signal transduction crosstalk in the endocrine system: Pancreatic β-cells and the glucose competence concept. Trends Biochem Sci 1992;17:388
38. Fehmann HC, Habener JF. Functional receptors for the insulinotropic hormone glucagon-like peptide-1(7-37) on a somatostatin secreting cell line. FEBS Lett 1991;279:335
39. d'Alessio DA, Fujimoto WY, Ensinck JW. Effects of glucagonlike peptide I-(7-36) on release of insulin, glucagon, and somatostatin by rat pancreatic islet cell monolayer cultures. Diabetes 1989;38:1534
40. Kawai K, Suzuki S, Ohashi S, et al. Comparison of the effects of glucagon-like peptide-1-(1-37) and -(7-37) and glucagon on islet hormone release from isolated perfused canine and rat pancreases. Endocrinol 1989;124:1768
41. Komatsu R, Matsuyama T, Namba M, et al. Glucagonostatic and insulinotropic action of glucagonlike peptide 1-(7-36)-amide. Diabetes 1989;38:902
42. Ørskov C, Holst JJ, Nielsen OV. Effect of truncated glucagon-like peptide-1 [proglucagon-(78-107)amide] on endocrine secretion from pig pancreas, antrum, and non-antral stomach. Endocrinology 1988;123:2009
43. Suzuki S, Kawai K, Ohashi S, et al. Comparison of the effects of various C-terminal and N-terminal fragment peptides of glucagon-like peptide-1 on insulin and glucagon release from the isolated perfused rat pancreas. Endocrinology 1989;125:3109
44. Ørskov C, Poulsen SS. Glucagonlike peptide-1-(7-36)-amide receptors only in islets of Langerhans: Autoradiographic survey of extracerebral tissues in rats. Diabetes 1991;40:1292
45. Drucker DJ, Philippe J, Mojsov S, et al. Glucagon-like peptide I stimulates insulin gene expression and increases cyclic AMP levels in a rat islet cell line. Proc Natl Acad Sci U S A 1987;84:3434
46. Thorens B. Expression cloning of the pancreatic β cell receptor for the gluco-incretin hormone glucagon-like peptide 1. Proc Natl Acad Sci U S A 1992; 89:8641
47. Jelinek LJ, Lok S, Rosenberg GB, et al. Expression cloning and signaling properties of the rat glucagon receptor. Science 1993;259:1614
48. Ishihara T, Shigemoto R, Mori K, et al. Functional expression and tissue distribution of a novel receptor for vasoactive intestinal peptide. Neuron 1992;8:811
49. Ishihara T, Nakamura S, Kaziro Y, et al. Molecular cloning and expression of a cDNA encoding the secretin receptor. EMBO J 1991;10:1635
50. Usdin TB, Mezey E, Button DC, et al. Gastric inhibitory polypeptide receptor, a member of the secretin-vasoactive intestinal peptide receptor family, is widely distributed in peripheral organs and the brain. Endocrinology 1993;133:2861
51. Spengler D, Waeber C, Pantaloni C, et al. Differential signal transduction by five splice variants of the PACAP receptor. Nature 1993;365:170
52. Mayo KE. Molecular cloning and expression of a pituitary-specific receptor for growth hormone-releasing hormone. Mol Endocrinol 1992;6:1734
53. Lin HY, Harris TL, Flannery MS, et al. Expression cloning of an adenylate cyclase-coupled calcitonin receptor. Science 1991;254:1022.
54. Jüppner H, Abou-Samra AB, Freeman M, et al. A G protein-linked receptor for parathyroid hormone and parathyroid hormone-related peptide. Science 1991;254:1024
55. Göke R, Fehmann H-C, Linn T, et al. Exendin-4 is a high potency agonist and truncated exendin-(9-39)-amide an antagonist at the glucagon-like peptide 1 (7-36)-amide receptor of insulin-secreting β-cells. J Biol Chem 1993;268: 19650
56. Svoboda M, Ciccarelli E, Tastenoy M, et al. A cDNA construct allowing the expression of rat hepatic glucagon receptors. Biochem Biophys Res Commun 1993;192:135
57. MacNeil DJ, Occi JL, Hey PJ, et al. Cloning and expression of a human glucagon receptor. Biochem Biophys Res Commun 1994;198:328
58. Valverde I, Merida E, Delgado E, et al. Presence and characterization of glucagon-like peptide-1(7-36)amide receptors in solubilized membranes of rat adipose tissue. Endocrinology 1993;132:75
59. Villanueva-Penacarrillo ML, Alcantara AI, Clemente F, et al. Potent glycogenic effect of GLP-1(7-36)amide in rat skeletal muscle. Diabetologia 1994;37: 1163
60. Kanse SM, Kreymann B, Ghatei MA, Bloom SR. Identification and characterization of glucagon-like peptide-1 7-36amide-binding sites in the rat brain and lung. FEBS Lett 1988;241:209
61. Uttenthal LO, Blazquez E. Characterization of high-affinity receptors for truncated glucagon-like peptide-1 in rat gastric glands. FEBS Lett 1990;262:139
62. Valverde I, Morales M, Clemente F. Glucagon-like peptide 1: A potent glycogenic hormone. FEBS Lett 1994;349:313
63. Egan JM, Montrose-Rafizadeh C, Wang Y, et al. Glucagon-like peptide-1 (7-36)amide (GLP-1) enhances insulin-stimulated glucose metabolism in 3T3-L1 adipocytes: One of several potential extrapancreatic sites of GLP-1 action. Endocrinology 1994;135:2070
64. Campos RV, Lee YC, Drucker DJ. Divergent tissue-specific and developmental expression of receptors for glucagon and glucagon-like peptide-1 in the mouse. Endocrinology 1994;134:2156
65. Richter G, Göke R, Göke B, et al. Characterization of receptors for glucagon-like peptide-1(7-36)amide on rat lung membranes. FEBS Lett 1990;267:78

66. Hansen AB, Gespach CP, Rosselin GE, Holst JJ. Effect of truncated glucagon-like peptide-1 on cAMP in rat gastric glands and HGT-1 human gastric cancer cells. FEBS Lett 1988;236:119
67. Wheeler MB, Lu M, Dillon JS, et al. Functional expression of the rat glucagon-like peptide-I (GLP-I) receptor, evidence for coupling to both adenylyl cyclase and phospholipase C. Endocrinology 1993;133:57
68. Fehmann HC, Habener JF. Homologous desensitization of the insulinotropic glucagon-like peptide-I(7-37) receptor on insulinoma (HIT-T15) cells. Endocrinology 1991;128:2880
69. Fehmann HC, Habener JF. Insulinotropic hormone glucagon-like peptide-I (7-37) stimulation of proinsulin gene expression and proinsulin biosynthesis in βTC-1 insulinoma cells. Endocrinology 1992;130:159
70. Gerich JE. Oral hypoglycemic agents. In: Oates JA, Wood AJJ, eds. Medical Intelligence: Drug Therapy 1989;321:1231–1245
71. Meyer TE, Habener JF. Cyclic AMP response element binding protein CREB and related transcription-activating DNA-binding proteins. Endocrinol Rev 1993;14:269
72. Rajan AS, Aguilar-Bryan L, Nelson DA, et al. Ion channels and insulin secretion. Diabetes Care 1990;13:340
73. Prentki M, Matschinsky FM. Ca^{2+}, cAMP, and phospholipid-derived messengers in coupling mechanisms of insulin secretion. Physiol Rev 1987;67:1185
74. Pipeleers D. The biosociology of pancreatic B cells. Diabetologia 1987;30:277
75. Holz GG, Kühtreiber WM, Habener JF. Pancreatic beta-cells rendered glucose-competent by the insulinotropic hormone glucagon-like peptide-1(7-37). Nature 1993;361:362
76. Ørskov C, Rabenhøj L, Wettergren A, et al. Tissue and plasma concentrations of amidated and glycine-extended glucagon-like peptide I in humans. Diabetes 1994;43:535
77. Mojsov S, Kopczynski M, Habener JF. Both amidated and nonamidated forms of glucagon-like peptide I are synthesized in the rat intestine and the pancreas. J Biol Chem 1990;265:8001
78. Ørskov C, Jeppesen J, Madsbad S, Holst JJ. Proglucagon products in plasma of noninsulin-dependent diabetics and nondiabetic controls in the fasting state and after oral glucose and intravenous arginine. J Clin Invest 1991;87:415
79. Miholic J, Ørskov C, Holst JJ, et al. Emptying of the gastric substitute, glucagon-like peptide-1 (GLP-1), and reactive hypoglycemia after total gastrectomy. Dig Dis Sci 1991;36:1361
80. Schjoldager BTG, Mortensen PE, Christiansen J, et al. GLP-1 (glucagon-like peptide 1) and truncated GLP-1, fragments of human proglucagon, inhibit gastric acid secretion in humans. Dig Dis Sci 1989;34:703
81. Ruiz-Grande C, Alarcón C, Alcántara A, Valverde I. Renal catabolism of truncated glucagon-like peptide 1. Horm Metab Res 1993;25:612
82. Kieffer TJ, McIntosh CHS, Pederson RA. Degradation of glucose-dependent insulinotropic polypeptide and truncated glucagon-like peptide 1 in vitro and in vivo by dipeptidyl peptidose IV. Endocrinology 1995;136:3585
83. Mojsov S. Structural requirements for biological activity of glucagon-like peptide-I. Int J Pept Protein Res 1992;40:333
84. Beck-Nielsen H, Groop LC. Metabolic and genetic characterization of prediabetic states: Sequence of events leading to non-insulin-dependent diabetes mellitus. J Clin Invest 1994;94:1714
85. Creutzfeldt W, Ebert R, Nauck M, Stöckmann F. Disturbances of the entero-insular axis. Scand J Gastroenterol Suppl 1983;83:111
86. Ruiz-Grande C, Alarcon C, Merida E, Valverde I. Lipolytic action of glucagon-like peptides in isolated rat adipocytes. Peptides 1992;13:13
87. Oben J, Morgan L, Fletcher J, et al. Effect of the entero-pancreatic hormones, gastric inhibitory polypeptide and glucagon-like polypeptide-1(7-36)amide, on fatty acid synthesis in explants of rat adipose tissue. J Endocrinol 1991;130:267
88. Nathan DM, Schreiber E, Fogel H, et al. Insulinotropic action of glucagon-like peptide-I(7-37) in diabetic and non-diabetic subjects. Diabetes Care 1992;15:270
89. Nauck MA, Kleine N, Ørskov C, et al. Normalization of fasting hyperglycaemia by exogenous GLP-1(7-36)amide in type 2-diabetic patients. Diabetologia 1993;36:741
90. Gutniak M, Ørskov C, Holst JJ, et al. Antidiabetogenic effect of glucagon-like peptide-1 (7-36)amide in normal subjects and patients with diabetes mellitus. New Engl J Med 1992;326:1316

Diabetes Mellitus, edited by Derek LeRoith, Simeon I. Taylor, and Jerrold M. Olefsky. Lippincott–Raven Publishers, Philadelphia © 1996.

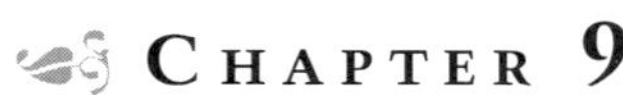

Chapter 9

Electrophysiology of the Pancreatic β-Cell

Illani Atwater, David Mears, and Eduardo Rojas

Pancreatic β-cells constitute 70–80% of the cell population of the islet of Langerhans and play a central role in the maintenance of glucose homeostasis by secreting insulin in response to elevated plasma glucose levels (Fig. 9-1). Defects in β-cell glucose responsiveness lead to severe metabolic disorders, such as those associated with type II diabetes mellitus. The biophysical mechanisms underlying the ability of the β-cell to sense and respond to glucose, as well as the modulation of insulin output by various physiologic and pharmacologic stimuli, has been the subject of intense research effort for more than 25 years. This effort has led to the clear understanding that a key step in stimulus-secretion coupling is the production of a characteristic pattern of β-cell membrane electrical activity subsequent to metabolic processing of glucose and other nutrient secretagogues. Furthermore, the actions of many modulators of insulin secretion, such as muscarinic agonists and drugs used in the treatment of insulin secretory disorders, also involve alteration of the β-cell membrane potential. Therefore, knowledge of the cellular and molecular processes involved in the generation and control of β-cell electrical activity is fundamental to developing a complete picture of glucose homeostasis in the physiologic state as well as the pathogenesis of type II diabetes mellitus.

β-Cell electrical activity results from and is affected by temporal changes in the permeability of the cell membrane to various ions, particularly K^+ and Ca^{++}. Ion permeability is controlled by membrane proteins known as ion channels, which govern the movement of charge across the plasmalemma. The unique assortment of ion channels in the β-cell membrane and the regulation of their activity by various metabolic intermediates, second messengers, and the membrane potential itself allows the coupling of intracellular events (i.e., metabolism of glucose) to membrane events (i.e., flow of ionic currents). These ionic currents trigger the exocytosis of insulin from the cell, making β-cell electrical activity a crucial link between the signal (elevated glucose) and the response (insulin secretion). This chapter focuses on the cellular and molecular basis of β-cell electrophysiology. The first section describes the characteristic glucose-induced electrical activity and its relationship to insulin secretion. The ionic mechanisms underlying the electrical activity and the modulatory effects of various

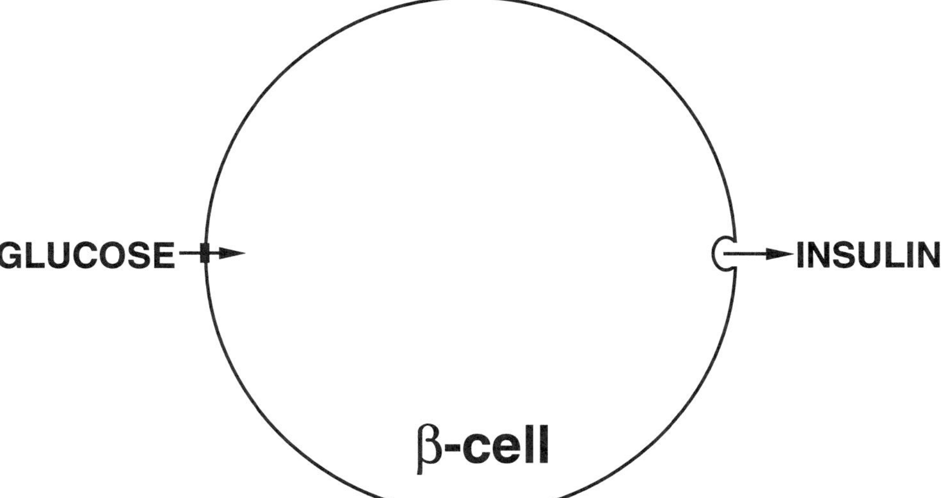

Figure 9-1. Glucose stimulates insulin secretion from the pancreatic β-cell.

physiologic and pharmacologic stimuli are then discussed. Finally, the role of intercellular communication within the islet of Langerhans, which seems to be a requirement for proper β-cell electrical and secretory responsiveness to glucose, is addressed. By adding details to the minimal β-cell model in Figure 9-1, we demonstrate that β-cell function is mediated by complex interactions between extracellular, intracellular, intercellular, and membrane events that link stimulus to response.

Glucose-Induced Electrical Activity

The mouse islet of Langerhans has been the preparation of choice for the majority of studies involving β-cell membrane potential.[1] The common procedure is to dissect a single islet of Langerhans by hand from the mouse pancreas and place it in a sample chamber, where it is continuously perifused with a bicarbonate-buffered Krebs solution at 37°C. High-resistance, saline-filled microelectrodes are used to impale and record membrane potential from a

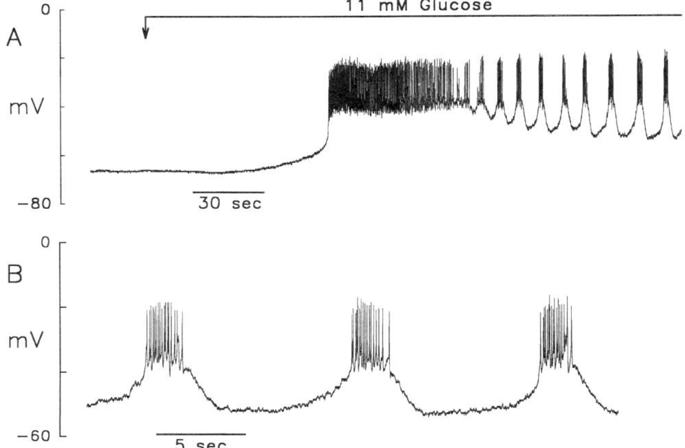

Figure 9-2. Glucose-induced electrical activity in the mouse β-cell. ***A,*** Biphasic pattern of glucose-induced electrical activity recorded from a β-cell in an intact mouse islet. ***B,*** The last three bursts in ***A*** are shown on an expanded time scale. Action potentials, or spikes, arise from the depolarized phase of the slow oscillations in membrane potential.

single β-cell within the islet. This technique allows the study of electrical activity with the β-cell in its native environment, under conditions that are as close to physiologic as can be achieved in vitro.[2,3]

In the absence of glucose, the β-cell membrane potential is constant at a hyperpolarized level, usually between −65 and −70 mV. Addition of glucose at concentrations of up to 7 mM results in a gradual depolarization of the membrane to a new steady-state level, with no apparent electrical activity. Higher concentrations of the sugar (Fig. 9-2*A*) cause the membrane to depolarize to threshold (ca. −50 mV) and initiate a periodic electrical activity known as *bursting*.[4,5] Bursting consists of oscillations in membrane potential between the *active phase,* during which action potentials arise from a depolarized plateau potential (ca. −35 mV), and the *silent phase,* with the membrane remaining quiescent at a level just below threshold. Figure 9-2*B* shows the bursts on an expanded time scale. The active phase spikes are typically 10–20 mV in magnitude, and during the silent phase the membrane slowly depolarizes until threshold is reached, initiating the next cycle.[6] This oscillatory pattern of electrical activity can be maintained for hours in the presence of constant, stimulatory glucose concentrations. Note also in Figure 9-2*A* that the β-cell electrical response to glucose is biphasic. The first phase is similar to a sustained active phase, which can last from 45 seconds to several minutes, and gradually gives way to the steady-state bursting described previously. The steady-state behavior has received the bulk of attention in the literature in terms of elucidating the mechanisms underlying glucose-induced electrical activity, and will be the focus of most of the discussion in this chapter. As discussed below, however, there is one recent theory that the depletion of calcium from intracellular stores may activate an ion channel that can account for the presence of the first phase (CRAC model).[7]

Figure 9-3 shows the effect on steady-state electrical activity of changes in glucose concentration within the stimulatory range.[8] Increasing the glucose concentration lengthens the active phase and shortens the silent phase, with little or no change in the absolute potential levels.[4] Thus, higher glucose concentrations lead to increased spike frequency by increasing the relative time during which action potentials are being fired (referred to as the relative duration of active phase, or plateau fraction). Spiking becomes continuous at higher glucose levels (> 22 mM), although the frequency of the spikes continues to rise with glucose concentration until approximately 27 mM. Although the data is far less comprehensive, there is evidence that β-cells in the rat and human pancreas exhibit similar membrane potential responsiveness to glucose.[9,10]

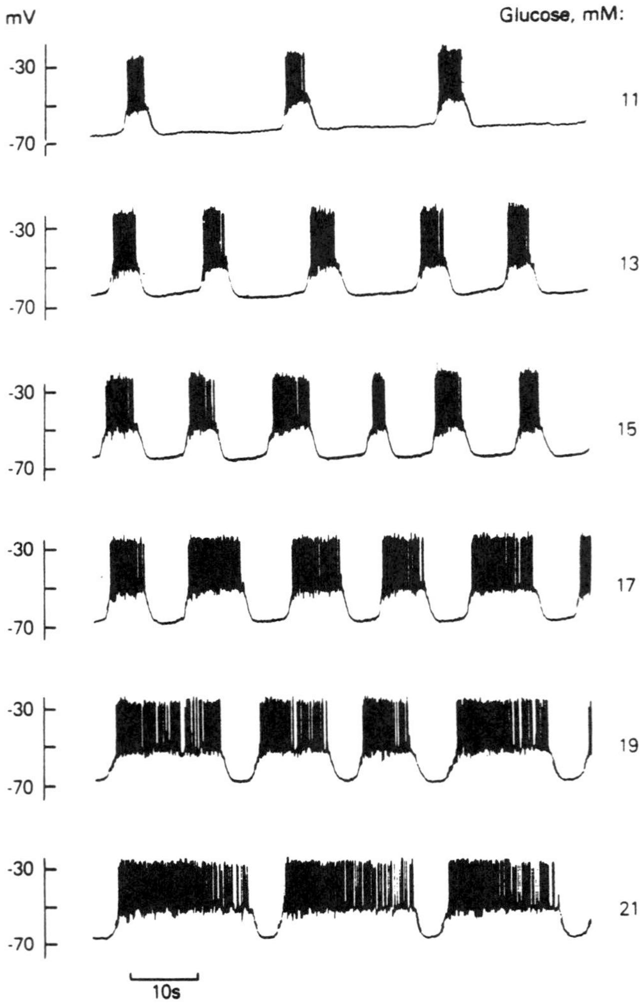

FIGURE 9-3. Modulation in the burst pattern of electrical activity by graded concentrations of glucose. Steady-state glucose concentrations are given over each trace. (Reproduced with permission from Atwater I, Carroll P, Li MX. Electrophysiology of the pancreatic B-cell. In: Draznin B, Melmed S, LeRoith D, eds. Molecular and Cellular Biology of Diabetes Mellitus. New York, NY: Alan R. Liss;1989:49–68.)

Relationship Between Electrical Activity and Insulin Release

The observations that many physiologic and pharmacologic agents that alter insulin secretion also modify β-cell electrical activity led to the hypothesis that the two phenomena are causally related.[5,11,12] In general, electrical activity is enhanced by stimulators and suppressed by inhibitors of insulin secretion. The effects of several such agents are described below.

Pharmacologic Agents

Glyburide and tolbutamide, sulfonylurea drugs that have been used for years as oral hypoglycemic agents, are potent stimulators of insulin secretion and induce electrical activity in β-cells similar to that observed in high glucose concentrations (Fig. 9-4*A*).[5,12] Diazoxide is a related compound that blocks insulin secretion and is used to treat nesideoblastosis and insulinomas (diseases associ-

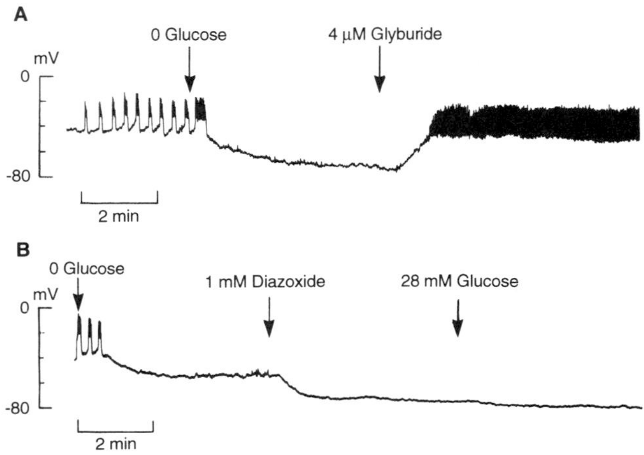

FIGURE 9-4. Effects of sulphonylureas on β-cell membrane potential. ***A,*** Electrical activity induced by 4 μM glyburide in the absence of glucose. Compare continuous spike activity to burst pattern in 11 mM glucose shown at the beginning of the trace. ***B,*** Removal of glucose (at beginning of the trace) induces hyperpolarization. When 1 mM diazoxide is added, the cell hyperpolarizes further. Readdition of glucose, at concentrations of up to 28 mM, in the presence of diazoxide does not elicit an electrical response (P. Carroll and I. Atwater, unpublished data, 1991).

ated with oversecretion of insulin). Figure 9-4*B* shows that diazoxide hyperpolarizes the β-cell and inhibits glucose-induced electrical activity.[13] Nifedipine, a dihydropyridine antagonist of L-type voltage-dependent Ca^{++} channels, also blocks insulin release and electrical activity,[8,14] which may account for the hyperglycemia that often accompanies the use of this drug in the treatment of hypertension.

Physiologic Agents

Acetylcholine (ACh), released during parasympathetic stimulation, enhances glucose-induced insulin release from the islet of Langerhans.[15] Electrophysiologic studies[16,17] revealed that this effect is accompanied by characteristic changes in β-cell electrical activity. When ACh is added to a medium containing 11 mM glucose (Fig. 9-5*A*), the cells depolarize to a level at or slightly above the plateau potential, and the electrical activity changes to a pattern of very high frequency bursts with little or no hyperpolarization during the short, silent phases. The enhancement of electrical activity by ACh involves interaction of the neurotransmitter with M_1 and M_3 subtype muscarinic receptors,[18,19] and hence the bursting pattern shown in Figure 9-5*A* has been termed "muscarinic bursting."[7]

Forskolin and glucagon (produced by the α-cells of the islet) elevate intracellular levels of cAMP and enhance glucose-induced insulin secretion.[20] Like ACh, these substances depolarize the silent phase and increase both the frequency and plateau fraction of glucose-induced bursts (Fig. 5*B*).[21] The same effect is seen when the islet is exposed to membrane-permeant analogs of cAMP. Although sulfonylurea drugs can stimulate electrical activity and insulin secretion in the absence of glucose, ACh, glucagon, and cAMP analogs are potentiators of β-cell activity because they increase the electrical and secretory response to stimulatory glucose concentrations, but have little effect by themselves.[22] Finally, somatostatin, a hormone secreted by islet δ-cells, is a physiologic inhibitor of insulin secretion[23] that also suppresses electrical activity.[24] The mechanism of action of several physiologic stimuli on islet electrical activity are discussed in later sections.

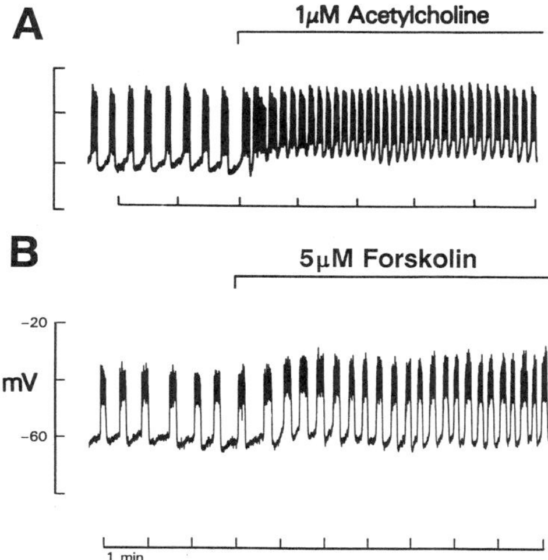

Figure 9-5. Effects of ACh and cAMP on β-cell electrical activity. *A,* "Muscarinic bursts" induced by 1 μM ACh in the presence of 11 mM glucose. Higher concentrations of ACh first induce a transient hyperpolarized phase, followed by fast bursts similar to those shown here. *B,* Forskolin (an activator of adenylate cyclase) induces muscarinic-like bursts in the presence of 11 mM glucose with high frequency and a depolarized silent phase (R.M. Santos and E. Rojas, unpublished data, 1989).

Simultaneous Measurements

Insulin secretion from single, large perifused mouse islets of Langerhans has been measured simultaneously with electrical activity from a single cell within the islet.[25] Figure 9-6 shows that the electrical activity induced by 22 mM glucose is accompanied by elevated secretory activity.[26] The curves of steady-state insulin release rate and electrical activity versus glucose concentration (Fig. 9-7) have similar slopes,[26] although the curve for electrical activity is shifted slightly to the left compared to that for secretion. Figure 9-8 shows the temporal course of spike frequency and insulin release from a single islet. Electrical activity appears slightly earlier than insulin secretion at the onset of glucose stimulation, and insulin release continues for several minutes after membrane hyperpolarization after glucose removal.[8] Figure 9-9 demonstrates that insulin release coincides with the active phase of electrical activity.[27] As discussed in detail below, because the active phase corresponds to a period of increased Ca^{++} permeability[4,28] and extracellular Ca^{++} is a requirement for insulin secretion,[29] the theory was adopted that electrical activity is coupled to insulin secretion via Ca^{++} influx. Fura-2 fluorescence measurements of cytosolic Ca^{++} (Fig. 9-10) have since confirmed that glucose induces intracellular Ca^{++} accumulations that are also in phase with electrical activity and insulin release.[30,31] Thus, although the details may be intricate, the basic picture of stimulus-secretion coupling in the β-cell can be formulated as follows: stimulatory glucose concentrations induce electrical activity, which elevates the intracellular Ca^{++} level, which in turn acts on the secretory machinery of the cell to stimulate insulin release.

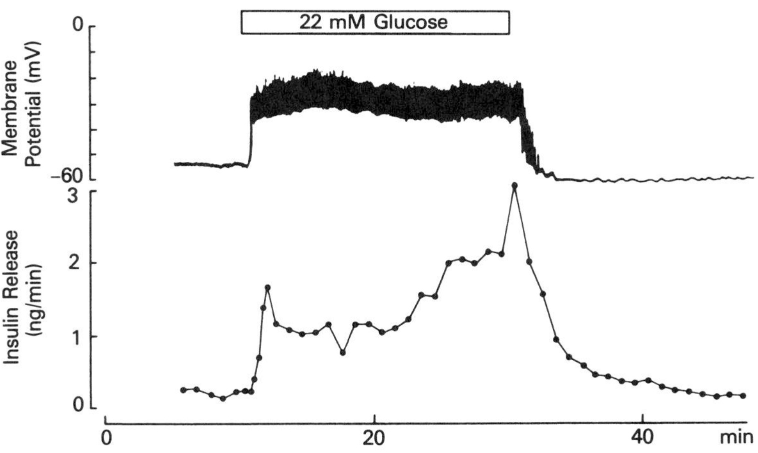

Figure 9-6. Electrical activity recorded from a β-cell and insulin secretion from the whole mouse islet in response to glucose. Insulin release rate from the entire islet (bottom trace) was determined by sampling aliquots of perfusate simultaneously with the measurement of electrical activity from a cell within the islet (top trace) and later by assaying the samples for insulin content. The period of elevated electrical activity was accompanied by increased insulin secretion. (Reproduced with permission from Atwater I, Goncalves A, Herchuelz A, et al. Cooling dissociates glucose-induced insulin release from electrical activity and cation fluxes in rodent pancreatic islets. J Physiol (London) 1984;348:615.)

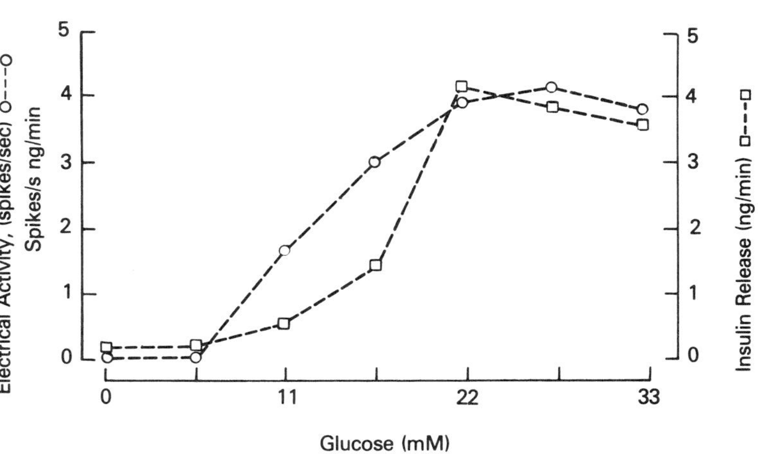

Figure 9-7. Steady-state insulin release rate from a single, microdissected mouse islet and steady-state spike frequency measured simultaneously from a β-cell within the same islet as a function of glucose concentration. At each concentration, the insulin release rate (□) and spike frequency (○) were determined by averaging over the last three minutes of a 20-minute exposure. Insulin secretion from individual islets is variable in amplitude, depending on the size of the islet, whereas electrical activity is fairly constant between cells from different islets. In six individual islets studied, electrical activity showed a significant shift toward lower glucose concentrations compared with insulin release. (Reproduced with permission from Scott AM, Atwater I, Rojas E. A method for the simultaneous measurement of insulin release and B-cell membrane potential in single mouse islets of Langerhans. Diabetologia 1981;21:470.)

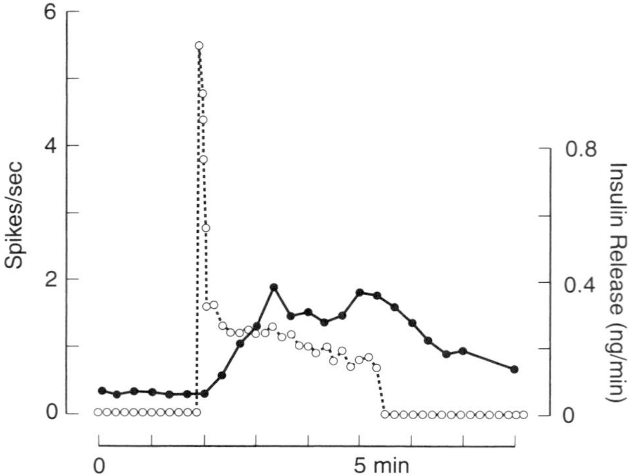

Figure 9-8. Temporal course of spike frequency and insulin release during exposure to 11 mM glucose. (Samples were collected simultaneously, as in Figs. 9-6 and 9-7.) Electrical activity appeared 20 seconds before detectable changes in secretion, and insulin release remained elevated several minutes longer than electrical activity after the stimulus was removed. Diffusion of insulin from the extracellular space of the perifused islet occurred in approximately 20 seconds. There was always a significant delay in the appearance of action potentials after the application of glucose (nearly 2 minutes in this experiment); insulin secretion was never detected before the appearance of electrical activity. (Reproduced with permission from Atwater I, Carroll P, Li MX. Electrophysiology of the pancreatic B-cell. In: Draznin B, Melmed S, LeRoith D, eds. Molecular and Cellular Biology of Diabetes Mellitus. New York, NY: Alan R. Liss;1989:49–68.)

The elevated Ca^{++} resulting from glucose-induced electrical activity initiates a complex sequence of events leading to insulin secretion, but a detailed description of the process is beyond the scope of this chapter. We wish to point out, however, that the steps linking elevated Ca^{++} to secretion are also subject to physiologic regulation, such that insulin release can be modulated independent of electrical activity, and in some cases the two phenomena can be completely dissociated. Reduction of perifusate temperature to 27°C abolishes insulin secretion (Fig. 9-11*A*) while electrical activity continues unchanged at all glucose concentrations (Fig. 9-11*B*).[26] Also, sympathetic agonists such as adrenaline and noradrenaline prevent insulin secretion,[15] but inhibit electrical activity only transiently.[32] In these cases, secretion is being blocked at some step distal to the generation of electrical activity, such that the increased Ca^{++} is unable to trigger exocytosis. Insulin secretion also can be enhanced without simultaneous enhancement of electrical activity. Figure 9-12*A* shows that glucose does not significantly change spike frequency in the presence of glyburide, yet under these conditions the rate of insulin secretion increases in a dose-dependent manner with glucose concentration (Fig. 12*B*).[8] Similarly, insulin secretion in response to depolarization-induced Ca^{++} influx is enhanced by activation of protein kinase A and C, with only small changes in the amount of Ca^{++} entering the cell.[33] These findings indicate that phosphorylation (and possibly other glucose-stimulated processes) play a role in sensitizing the secretory machinery to the elevated Ca^{++} brought about by bursting. Finally, it is important to realize that elevated intracellular Ca^{++} alone is not sufficient to stimulate secretion. Figure 9-13 shows that in the absence of glucose, ACh (which stimulates release of Ca^{++} from intracellular stores) elevates intracellular Ca^{++} similarly to a maximal glucose challenge,[34] yet ACh does not induce secretion in the absence of glucose.[35] Because there have been no cases described in which insulin secretion is stimulated in the absence of β-cell depolarization and Ca^{++} influx, generation of electrical activity therefore is considered crucial to stimulus-secretion coupling under normal conditions. The remainder of this chapter is devoted to discussion of the mechanisms by which elevated glucose and other stimuli produce or alter β-cell electrical activity.

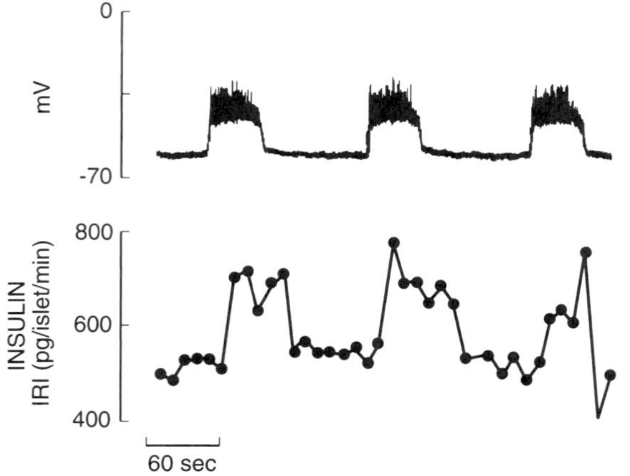

Figure 9-9. Bursts of insulin secretion occur in phase with bursts of electrical activity. Electrical activity of a single β-cell (top trace) and insulin release from the entire islet (IRI) (bottom trace) during steady-state exposure to 16.7 mM glucose. Extracellular Ca^{++} was increased in order to increase the separation between the bursts and thus improve the time resolution of the insulin collections. (Reproduced with permission from Rosario LM, Atwater I, Scott AM. Pulsatile insulin release and electrical activity from single *ob/ob* mouse islets of Langerhans. Adv Exp Med Biol 1985; 211:413.)

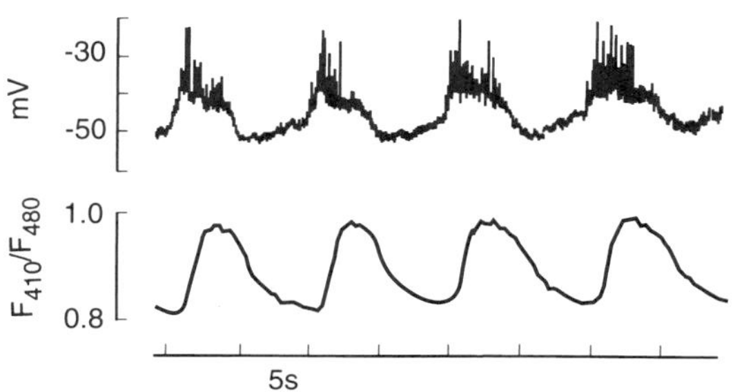

Figure 9-10. Cyclic changes in intracellular Ca^{++} occur in phase with bursts of electrical activity. Membrane potential from a single β-cell (upper trace) and intracellular Ca^{++} concentration measured from an islet loaded with fura-2 (bottom trace) during steady-state exposure to 11 mM glucose. An increase in F410/F480 indicates Ca^{++} increase. Cytoplasmic calcium increases during the active phase. (Reproduced with permission from Santos RM, Rosario LM, Nadel A, et al. Widespread synchronous $[Ca^{++}]_i$ oscillations due to bursting electrical activity in single pancreatic islets. Pflugers Arch 1991;418:417.)

Role of Metabolism

Three lines of evidence demonstrate the dependence of glucose-induced electrical activity on metabolism of the hexose:

1. When metabolic uncouplers such as sodium azide and 2,4-dinitrophenol[11] are added to a medium containing 11 mM glucose, the cells hyperpolarize and both electrical activity and insulin secretion cease.

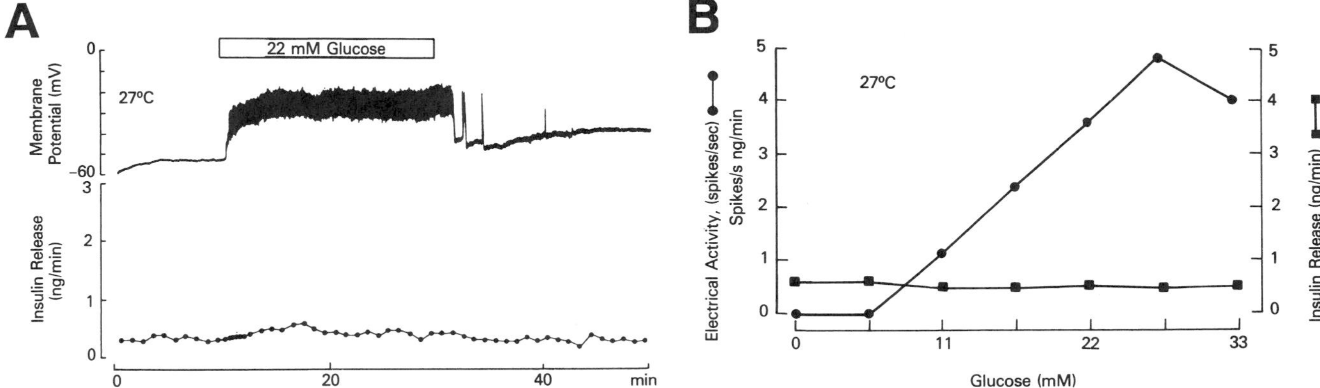

Figure 9-11. Dissociation of electrical activity from insulin secretion by cooling. *A,* At 27°C, electrical activity occurs in 22 mM glucose without a simultaneous increase in insulin release rate (compare to Fig. 9-6). *B,* Dose-response curves of steady-state insulin release and electrical activity versus glucose concentration show that the dissociation at 27°C occurs at all concentrations of glucose (compared to Fig. 9-7). (Reproduced with permission from Atwater I, Goncalves A, Herchuelz A, et al. Cooling dissociates glucose-induced insulin release from electrical activity and cation fluxes in rodent pancreatic islets. J Physiol (London) 1984;348:615.)

2. Nonmetabolizable glucose derivatives such as 2-deoxyglucose are unable to elicit electrical or secretory responses from β-cells,[12] and they antagonize the effects of glucose on β-cell membrane potential.[36]
3. The glycolytic intermediate glyceraldehyde[12] and nonglucose metabolic substrates such as leucine[37] and α-ketoisocaproate[38] induce electrical activity and insulin secretion in pancreatic β-cells.

These observations show that glucose sensing by the β-cell does not involve a specific membrane receptor for the sugar. Rather, as shown in Figure 9-14, the glucose signal is coupled to electrical activity (and hence Ca^{++} influx and insulin secretion) through the interactions of metabolic intermediates with the ion channels of the β-cell membrane. This process is discussed in detail in the following section.

Ionic Events in the β-Cell

Initially, the ionic constituents of β-cell electrical activity were examined using isotope fluxes, membrane resistance measurements, and by observing the effects of ion substitutions and pharmacologic blockers of specific ion channels on membrane potential.

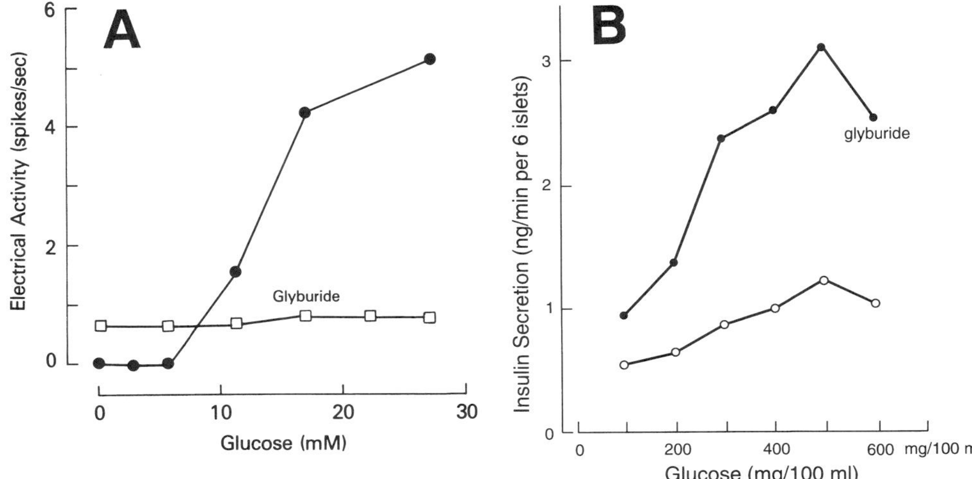

Figure 9-12. Enhancement of secretion by glucose in the presence of glyburide without significant increases in spike frequency. *A,* Steady-state electrical activity (spikes per second averaged over 3 minutes) versus glucose concentration recorded from a single β-cell in the presence (□) and absence (●) of 4 μM glyburide. (Reproduced with permission from Atwater I, Carroll P, Li MX. Electrophysiology of the pancreatic B-cell. In: Draznin B, Melmed S, LeRoith D, eds. Molecular and Cellular Biology of Diabetes Mellitus. New York, NY: Alan R. Liss;1989:49–68.) *B,* Insulin secretion rate from perifused mouse islet versus glucose concentration in the presence (●) and absence (○) of glyburide (11 mM glucose = 200 mg/100 mL). (P. Carroll and I. Atwater, unpublished observations, 1991.)

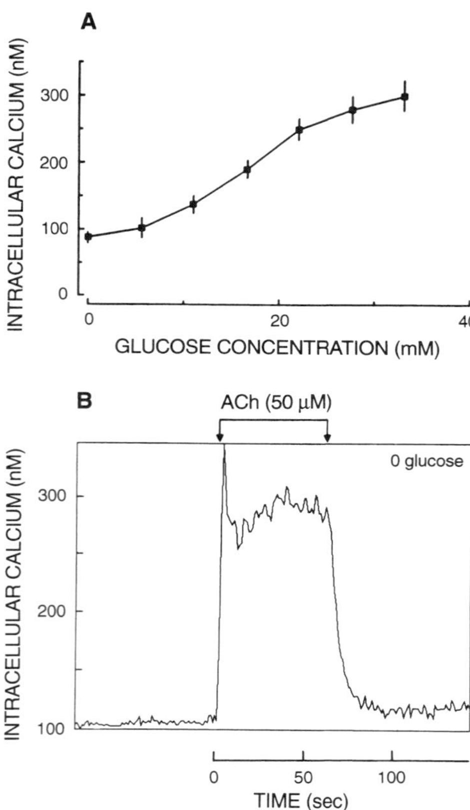

Figure 9-13. Glucose and ACh induced increases in cytoplasmic calcium concentration. ***A,*** Steady-state intracellular Ca^{++} level versus glucose concentration for isolated human β-cells. ***B,*** Elevation of intracellular Ca^{++} in an isolated human β-cell stimulated by 50 μM ACh in the absence of glucose. Ca^{++} was measured by indo-1 fluorescence ratio method. (Reproduced with permission from Rojas E, Carroll PB, Ricordi C, et al. Control of cytosolic free calcium in cultured human pancreatic β-cells occurs by external calcium-dependent and independent mechanisms. Endocrinology 1994;134:1771.)

The properties of some ion channels were determined by statistical analysis of voltage noise measurements. These studies quantified changes in ion permeability under different conditions as well as at different phases of steady-state electrical activity. The application of the patch-clamp technique to the study of β-cell electrophysiology allowed the identification of many of the ion channels resident in the β-cell membrane and the characterization of currents carried by these proteins at the single-channel and whole-cell level. Together, these studies have provided a wealth of information concerning the interactions between metabolically regulated, voltage-regulated, and receptor-operated ion channels that mediate β-cell glucose sensing.

Metabolically Regulated Ion Channels

ATP-Regulated Potassium Channels

The resting β-cell membrane potential in the absence of glucose (ca. −70 mV) is close to the reversal potential for K^+. Thus it is not surprising that under resting conditions, ion substitutions revealed that the membrane K^+ permeability dominates over that of other ions.[2,39,40] Figure 9-15 shows that membrane depolarization brought about by glucose in the subthreshold range reflects a decrease in the ratio of K^+ permeability relative to other ions. Unlike many other excitable cells, however, the reduction in permeability ratio results from a decrease in the K^+ permeability rather than an increase in permeability to other cations (Na^+ or Ca^{++}). The two lines of evidence supporting this idea are that glucose reduces the efflux of $^{42}K^+$ from isolated islets of Langerhans (Fig. 9-16),[41,42] and membrane resistance increases upon addition of glucose (Fig. 9-17).[2,8] Therefore the glucose sensitivity of the β-cell membrane potential in this range of concentrations of the sugar is mediated by a glucose-sensitive K^+ permeability.

Electrophysiologic recordings from cell-attached patches revealed the presence of a K^+ channel in the β-cell membrane that is blocked when the cell is exposed to glucose (Fig. 9-18*A*).[43] Studies using excised patches (Fig. 9-18*B*) showed that the channel is inhibited by ATP on the intracellular side (K_M 10 μM, complete block 1 mM), and so the channel became known as the K_{ATP} channel.[44] This channel belongs to a family of ATP-regulated K^+ channels that were first identified in cardiac myocytes and since have been found in a variety of cells. The presence of the K_{ATP} channel in the β-cell membrane led to the hypothesis that an increase in ATP (or more likely, the ATP : ADP ratio), by inhibiting the K_{ATP} channel, links glucose metabolism to β-cell depolarization.

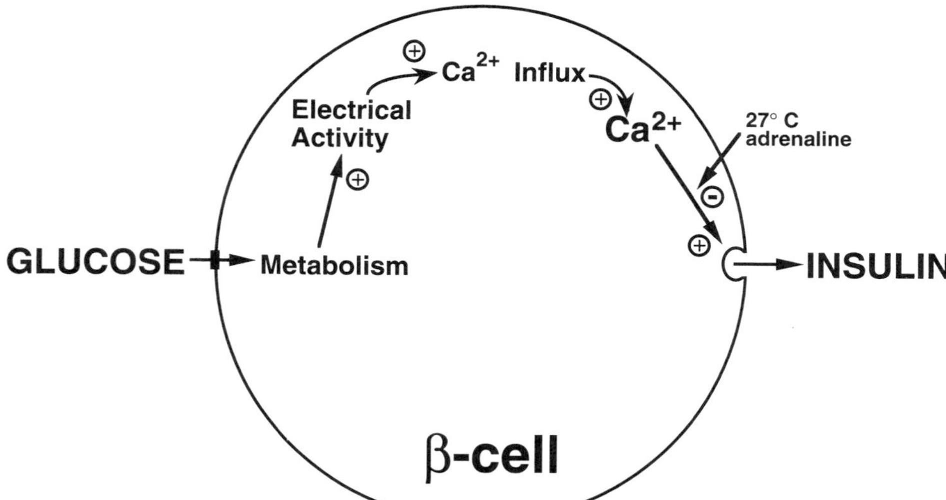

Figure 9-14. Basic events involved in glucose-induced insulin secretion from the β-cell. Glucose is transported into the β-cell and its metabolism induces (⊕) electrical activity that stimulates (⊕) Ca^{++} influx, which in turn increases (⊕) cytoplasmic Ca^{++} concentration and triggers (⊕) insulin secretion. Lowering temperature or adding adrenaline inhibits (⊖) insulin secretion, dissociating the rise in intracellular Ca^{++} from the exocytotic process.

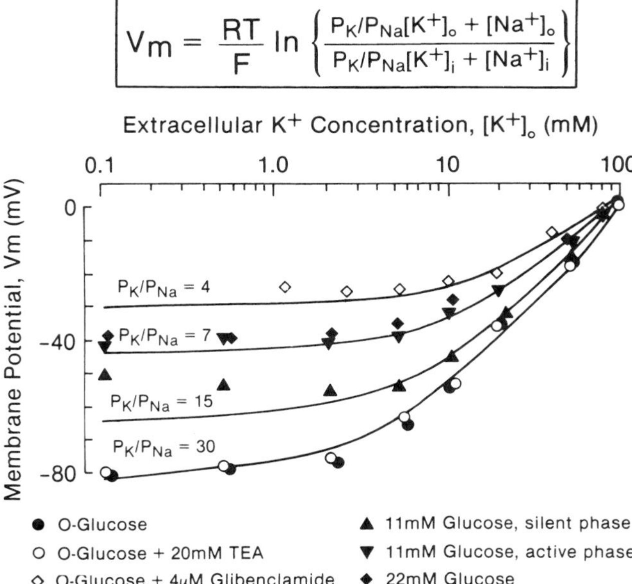

FIGURE 9-15. Beta cell membrane potential (from intact, perifused mouse islet) as a function of extracellular K^+ concentration under various conditions. Solid curves represent predictions of the Goldman-Hodgkin-Katz equation, shown at top, for membrane potential. The permeability ratios (P_K:P_{Na}) are indicated over each curve. The permeability ratio decreases as a function of glucose concentration and is lower during the active phase than during the silent phase at the same glucose level. Without glucose, the ratio is reduced by glyburide but not TEA. (Reproduced with permission from Atwater I, Carroll P, Li MX. Electrophysiology of the pancreatic B-cell. In: Draznin B, Melmed S, LeRoith D, eds. Molecular and Cellular Biology of Diabetes Mellitus. New York, NY: Alan R. Liss;1989:49–68.)

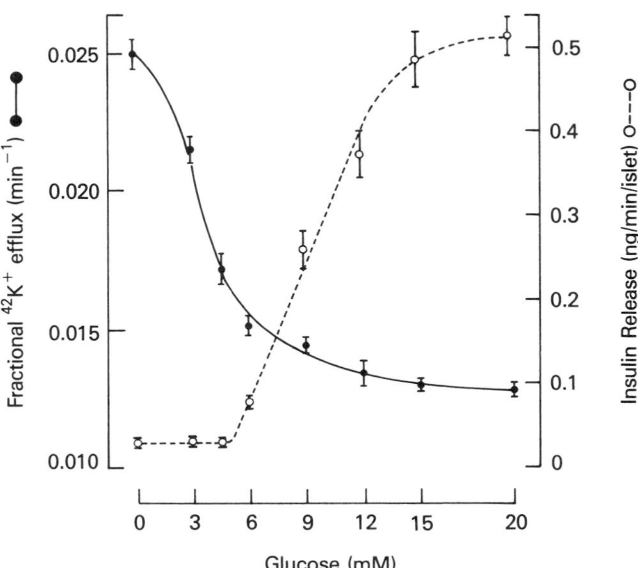

FIGURE 9-16. Insulin secretion and $^{42}K^+$ efflux from collagenase-isolated rat islets of Langerhans. Islets were loaded with $^{42}K^+$ and the efflux of the tracer measured as a function of glucose concentration (solid line). Increases in glucose concentration from 0 to 12 mM reduced the rate of $^{42}K^+$ efflux, indicating a reduction of K^+ permeability by glucose. Increasing glucose from 6 to 15 mM increased the rate of insulin secretion (dashed line) (compare with Fig. 9-7). (Reproduced with permission from Henquin JC. D-glucose inhibits potassium efflux from pancreatic islet cells. Nature 1978;271:271.)

The properties of the K_{ATP} channel are discussed below and are reviewed in detail elsewhere.[45]

In cell-attached patches with no glucose present, the K_{ATP} channel opens in bursts separated by longer closed periods (see Fig. 9-18*A*, inset), whereas openings of other K^+ channels at the hyperpolarized resting potential are rare. The single-channel conductance is 50–80 picosiemens, and in excised patches, both the open probability and conductance are relatively insensitive to the transmembrane potential. The channel exhibits a marked inward rectification in cell-attached patches when high K^+ is present in the patch pipette (illustrated below in Fig. 24). When physiologic K^+ levels are used,[46] the conductance decreases and the current-voltage curve becomes linear. Addition of glucose inhibits the channel in cell-attached patches by reducing the open probability without changing the single-channel conductance. As shown in Figure 9-18*A*, the channel is almost completely inhibited by glucose concentrations as low as 3 mM.[43] This would seem to preclude a role for the channel in determining the K^+ permeability of the cell at higher glucose levels. Also, the channel in excised patches is inhibited by ATP concentrations that are much lower than the millimolar levels observed in intact β-cells (see Fig. 9-18*B*).[44] Finally, the K_{ATP} channel is inhibited by bicarbonate buffer, implying that the activity of the channel under physiologic conditions is even less than that observed under patch-clamp conditions.[47]

Despite these discrepancies, the K_{ATP} channel appears to control the resting potential and to constitute the major metabolically regulated K^+ conductance of the β-cell. Evidence indicates that the ATP sensitivity of the channel may be reduced in the intact β-cell such that single-channel studies underestimate the ATP concentration required for maximal inhibition.[48] Chloride may play a

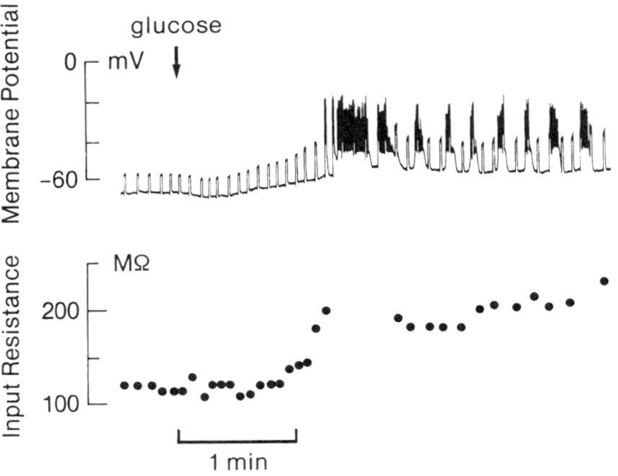

FIGURE 9-17. Addition of glucose increases β-cell input resistance. Input resistance (lower trace) of a β-cell within the intact mouse islet was measured by injecting current through the recording electrode (using a bridge amplifier to compensate for electrode resistance) during measurement of membrane potential (top trace). Resistance was calculated by dividing the magnitude of the voltage deflections on the membrane potential record by the size of the current pulse. The increase in input resistance after addition of glucose indicates reduced overall membrane permeability. (Reproduced with permission from Atwater I, Carroll P, Li MX. Electrophysiology of the pancreatic B-cell. In: Draznin B, Melmed S, LeRoith D, eds. Molecular and Cellular Biology of Diabetes Mellitus. New York, NY: Alan R. Liss;1989:49–68.)

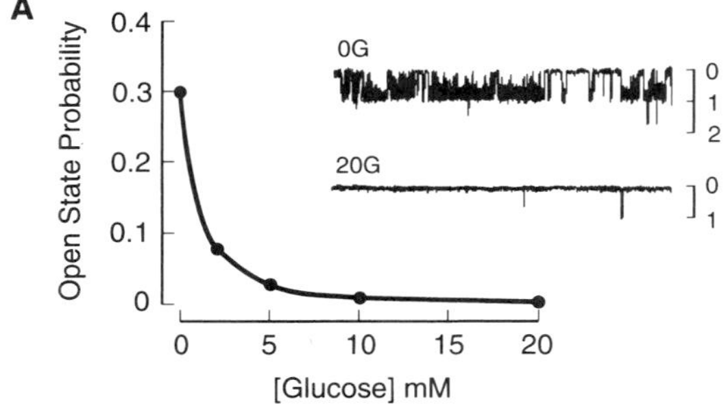

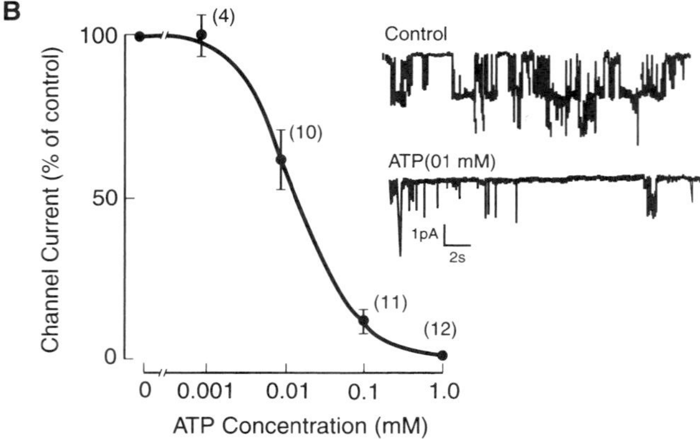

Figure 9-18. Properties of K_{ATP} channel activity. ***A,*** K_{ATP} channel open probability versus glucose concentration in cell-attached patch recordings from isolated rat β-cells. Insert shows inhibition of channel activity by glucose. (Reproduced with permission from Ashcroft FM, Harrison DE, Ashcroft SJH. Glucose induces closure of single potassium channels in isolated rat pancreatic β-cells. Nature 1984;312:446.) ***B,*** K_{ATP} channel open probability versus ATP concentration in recordings from an excised patch of membrane from fetal rat β-cells. Insert shows block of K_{ATP} channel current by ATP on the intracellular side of excised membrane patches. (Reproduced with permission from Cook DL, Hales CN. Intracellular ATP directly blocks K^+-channels in pancreatic B-cells. Nature 1984;311:269.)

role in this phenomenon, since K_{ATP} channels in excised patches appear to be more active when the Cl^- concentration on the intracellular side is lowered to cytoplasmic levels.[49] Furthermore, the density of channels in the cell may be high enough (10^3–10^4 per cell) that even when the channels are 90–99% inactivated, enough K_{ATP} permeability remains to control the membrane potential and to provide additional glucose sensitivity.[48]

Perhaps the most compelling evidence that the K_{ATP} channel dominates the resting K^+ permeability and is the target for metabolite-induced depolarization of the β-cell is the action of sulfonylureas on the channel. Glyburide and tolbutamide specifically reduce the open probability of the K_{ATP} channel[50] and induce β-cell depolarization, whereas diazoxide activates the channel[51] and antagonizes the depolarizing effect of glucose. Figure 9-19 illustrates the decrease and increase, respectively, of the efflux of $^{86}Rb^+$ (a tracer used to follow K^+ fluxes) in response to tolbutamide and diazoxide.[52] Thus the K_{ATP} channel mediates the glucose-induced depolarization of the β-cell and is also the target for clinically useful alterations of potential and secretion by pharmacologic agents.

The role of the K_{ATP} channel in modulating electrical activity at higher glucose concentrations is uncertain. Oscillatory K_{ATP} conductance is unlikely to be responsible for the cyclic nature of β-cell electrical activity because the channel does not activate periodically during glucose-induced bursting, and intracellular ATP levels do not appear to oscillate with a time course similar to the bursts. Further block of the K_{ATP} channel at stimulatory glucose concentrations may increase the plateau fraction by providing an additional depolarizing effect that must be overcome by whatever cyclic hyperpolarizing influence drives the cell into the silent phase. The observation that intracellular ATP is constant at glucose concentrations above approximately 5 mM argues strongly against this hypothesis.

Recently, a gene identified by scanning a human pancreatic cDNA library with a probe spanning the M1 to M2 region of a guanosine nucleotide–binding protein (G-protein)–gated K^+ channel was cloned and expressed in Xenopus oocytes and mammalian CHO cells.[53] The transfected cells possess a membrane K^+ conductance that is blocked by intracellular ATP and enhanced by diazoxide in whole-cell recordings. This K^+ channel gene may code for the β-cell K_{ATP} channel, although the exact localization of the functional gene to β-cells rather than the abundant acinar cells of the pancreas has not yet been reported. The cloning of other K^+ channels, particularly a K_{ATP} channel from rat kidney,[54] may prove useful in predicting conserved regions in the β-cell K_{ATP} channel. From sequence analysis of such channels, it seems likely that the pore-forming region of the β-cell K_{ATP} channel should be similar to those studied in the Shaker family of channels, and intuition predicts the presence of nucleotide-binding regions. The kidney K_{ATP} channel does not appear to have a sulfonylurea binding domain, which is consistent with the idea that the sulfonylurea receptor may be a distinct entity that is closely associated with the K_{ATP} channel.[55] Given its role in glucose sensing, the complete characterization of the molecular properties of the K_{ATP} channel promises to provide important insights into β-cell function in the normal and pathologic state.

Glucose-Activated Calcium Channels

Human pancreatic β-cells express a small Ca^{++} channel that is activated by glucose metabolism.[10] Cell-attached recordings were made at hyperpolarized membrane potentials with high Ca^{++}, tetramethylammonium (TMA), and tetraethylammonium (TEA) in the pipette to block K^+-channel activity. Figure 9-20*A* shows that under such conditions, inward channel openings are rare at the onset of glucose stimulation. Forty seconds after addition of glucose to the medium (Fig. 9-20*B*) there is a rapid increase in the frequency of channel opening events. The openings continue simultaneous with glucose-induced action potentials (Fig. 9-20*C*). The same channel is activated by α ketoisocaproate (KIC) and stimulation of the channel by glucose is antagonized in the presence of mannoheptulose, indicating that the channel (referred to as the Ca_G channel) is activated subsequent to glucose metabolism. Figure 9-20*E* illustrates that the Ca_G channel has a voltage-independent unitary conductance of 4.9 picosiemens. The Ca_G channel may play some role in membrane depolarization at subthreshold glucose levels. Furthermore, the voltage-independent nature of the channel suggests that it could mediate a background Ca^{++} flux throughout the burst cycle. Such a background current may be responsible for the modulation of burst duration over the range of stimulatory glucose concentrations.

Voltage-Regulated Ion Channels

Calcium Channels

β-Cell action potentials resemble Ca^{++} action potentials observed in other tissues. Spikes can be generated by depolarization of the membrane to about −40 mV with elevated extracellular K^+ or current injections, and they can be suppressed by removal of Ca^{++} from the medium or addition of Ca^{++}-channel blockers such as cobalt, cadmium, or nifedipine. Also consistent with increased Ca^{++} permeability during the active phase are decreased membrane

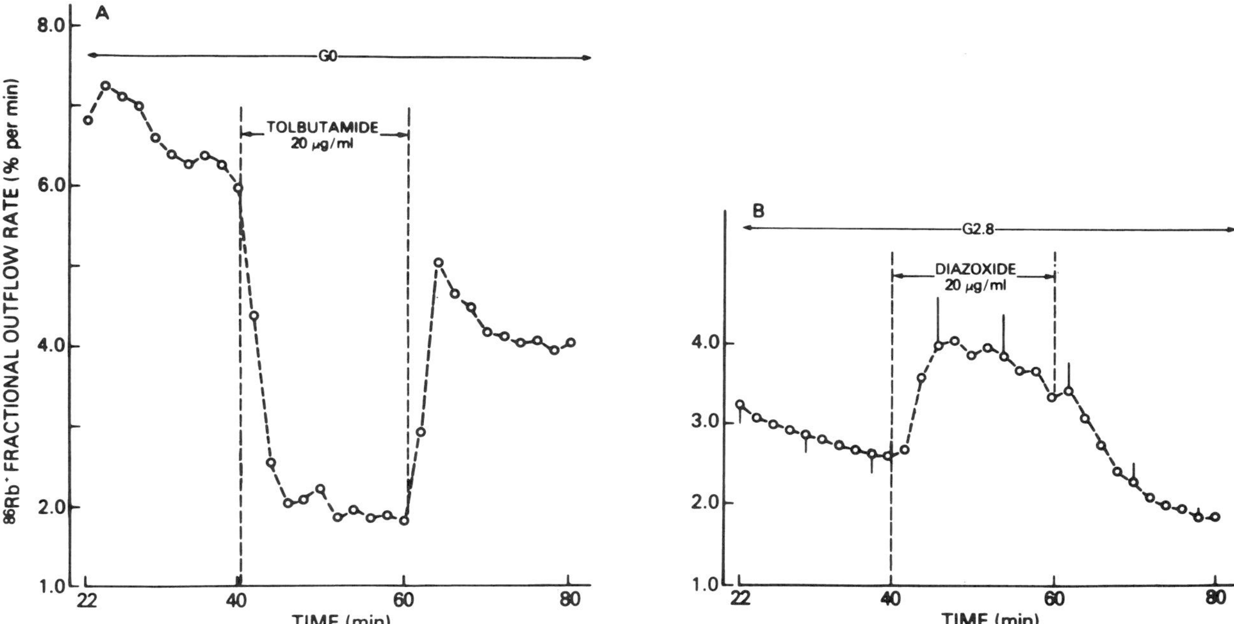

Figure 9-19. K^+ permeability is decreased by tolbutamide and increased by diazoxide. Collagenase isolated rat islets were loaded with $^{86}Rb^+$, a tracer for K^+ fluxes, and the efflux was measured in response to tolbutamide (*A*) and diazoxide (*B*) at the glucose concentrations indicated. (Reproduced with permission from Boschero AC, Tombaccini D, Carneiro EM, Atwater IJ. Differences in K^+ permeability between cultured adult and neonatal rat islets of Langerhans in response to glucose, tolbutamide, diazoxide, and theophylline. Pancreas 1993;8:44.)

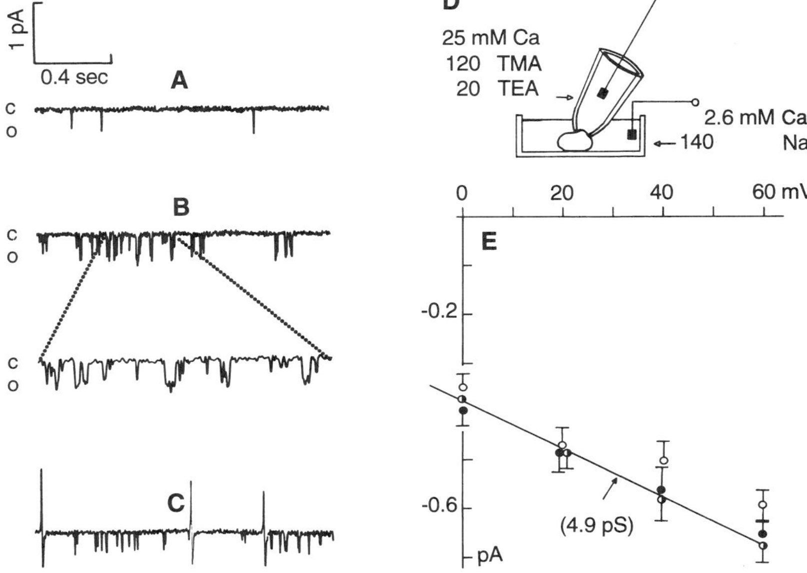

Figure 9-20. Inward channel opening events recorded from a cell-attached patch on a human pancreatic β-cell. The cell was part of a cluster of cells dissociated from collagenase isolated islets. *A,* Record was made 20 seconds after addition of 11 mM glucose. *B, C,* Records were made 40 seconds and 4 minutes, respectively, after record *A*. Inset under *B* illustrates single channel activity on an expanded time scale. *D,* Pipette solution was held at +20 mV with respect to the bath solution. *E,* Current-voltage relationship and unitary conductance for the channel activated by glucose. Potential on abscissa is that of the pipette solution with respect to the bath. (Reproduced with permission from Rojas E, Hilgado J, Carroll PB, Atwater I. A new class of calcium channels activated by glucose in human pancreatic β-cells. FEBS Lett 1990;261:265.)

resistance,[2] accumulation of intracellular Ca^{++} (see Fig. 9-10),[30] and depletion of Ca^{++} in the extracellular space (shown later in Fig. 9-32*B*)[56] during this portion of the cycle. The important role of Ca^{++} fluxes in insulin release suggests that modulation of Ca^{++}-channel activity may be an important mechanism for the alteration of secretion by various signals.

Initial characterization of β-cell Ca^{++} channels was carried out by voltage noise analysis subsequent to elevation of the membrane potential with KCl. Figure 9-21*A,B* shows the transient spiking and elevated voltage noise induced by high KCl. The spikes are blocked by extracellular cobalt, indicating that they are due to the activation of Ca^{++} channels. The amplitude of voltage fluctuations (Fig. 21*C*) revealed the unitary conductance of the channel to be about 5 picosiemens in 2.5 mM external Ca^{++}, and power spectrum analysis (Fig. 21*D*) of the voltage noise indicated an average channel open time at −22 mV of about 43 milliseconds.[57] In accord with this finding, patch-clamp studies later revealed the presence of a voltage-activated Ca^{++} channel in the mouse β-cell with conductance of 2–3 picosiemens after adjusting for the effect of high barium concentrations in the patch pipette, which are used to increase channel conductance.[58] Whole-cell Ca^{++} currents recorded from mouse β-cells activate at potentials positive to −50 mV, reach peak amplitude near +10 mV, and exhibit Ca^{++}-dependent inactivation. The dihydropyridines nifedipine and nitrendipine reduce the amplitude of whole-cell and ensemble currents, as well as the open probability in single-channel recordings, whereas Bay K 8644 increases the peak currents without altering the voltage dependence.[36,59,60] There is also evidence for slow voltage-dependent inactivation of the Ca^{++} current, with a time constant of several seconds.[61] These properties are characteristic of the L-type voltage-gated Ca^{++} channel (Ca_{Vm}), which has been identified in a variety of excitable cells.

Unlike those of the mouse, rat β-cells appear to possess both L-type and T-type voltage-gated Ca^{++} channels.[62] Whole-cell and

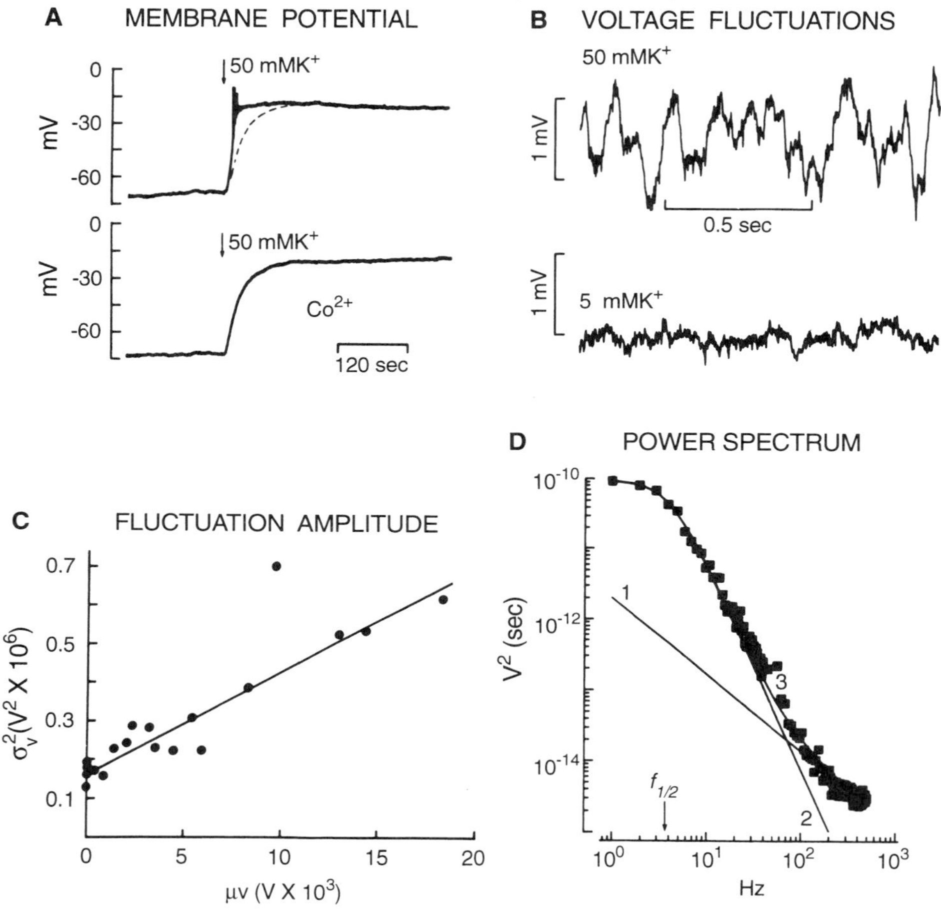

FIGURE 9-21. Noise analysis of voltage fluctuations to measure single Ca^{++} channel properties. ***A,*** Effect of 50 mM K^+ on membrane potential recorded from β-cells in the intact mouse islet in the absence (top) and presence (bottom) of 2 mM cobalt. No glucose was present in either trace. ***B,*** Segments of the recordings from ***A*** shown on expanded amplitude and time bases to demonstrate the voltage noise levels at 5 and 50 mM K^+. ***C,*** Variance (mean square value of amplitude of voltage fluctuations) graphed in relation to the deviation of membrane potential from expected voltage changes (see dashed line in ***A***). These measurements were used to calculate a single channel conductance of 5 picosiemens. ***D,*** Voltage fluctuation frequency distribution (at −22 mV) after Fourier Transform. Corner frequency of 3.7 Hz (indicated by arrow) describes average channel open time of 43 milliseconds for this membrane potential. (Reproduced with permission from Atwater I, Dawson CM, Eddleston GT, Rojas E. Voltage noise measurements across the pancreatic β-cell membrane: Calcium channel characteristics. J Physiol 1981;314:195.)

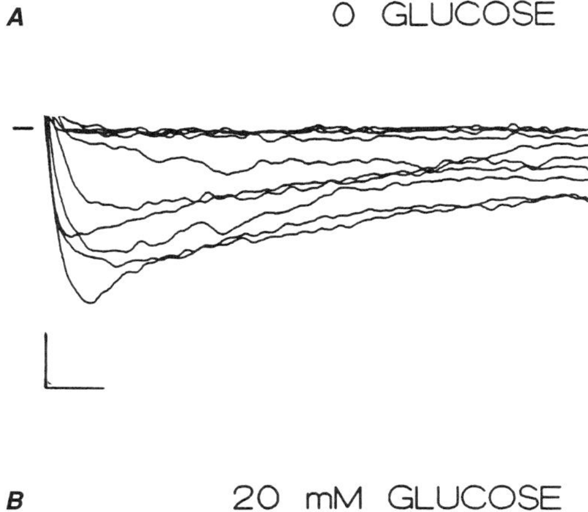

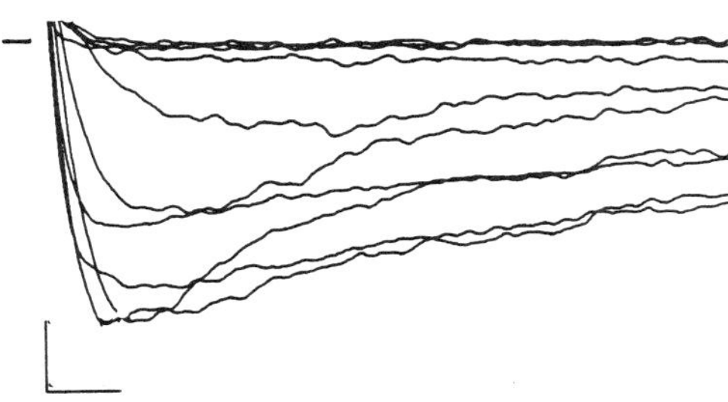

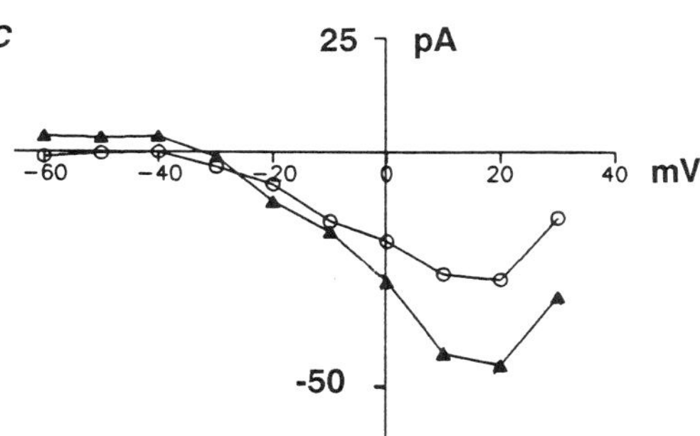

Figure 9-22. Effect of glucose on calcium currents. Inward whole-cell currents in response to depolarizing voltage pulses, recorded from an isolated rat β-cell in the absence (***A***) and presence (***B***) of glucose. Calibrations: vertical, 20 pA; horizontal, 20 milliseconds. Membrane patch was permeabilized with nystatin to preserve the intracellular milieu. Bottom trace (***C***) shows steady-state current-voltage (I-V) relation of the inward current with (▲) and without (○) glucose. Peak current occurs at a potential of approximately +20 mV and is almost doubled in the presence of glucose. (Reproduced with permission from Atwater I, Kukuljan M, Pérez-Armendariz EM. Molecular biology of the ion channels in the pancreatic β-cell. In: Draznin B, LeRoith D, eds. Molecular Biology of Diabetes, Part I. Totowa, NJ: Humana Press;1994:303–331.)

ensemble currents from rat β-cells possess a rapidly inactivating component that disappears when the holding potential is raised to −40 mV. This channel may carry a substantial portion of the Ca^{++} current in rat β-cells, but its absence from the mouse β-cell indicates that the channel is not necessary for glucose-induced bursting.

Although membrane potential is the main determinant of the activity of L-type Ca^{++} channels, the kinetics also can be modulated by a variety of other factors, some of which may play a role in the alteration of electrical activity by different stimuli. Figure 9-22 shows that glucose metabolism increases the whole-cell current through L-type Ca^{++} channels,[36] although this modulation may be too slow to account for the rapid change in electrical activity brought about by glucose.[63] cAMP-dependent phosphorylation antagonizes the inactivation of these channels, but the resulting increase in intracellular Ca^{++} is not large enough to account for the magnitude of the elevation in secretion.[64] L-type channels are affected by interactions with G-proteins in other tissues, and it is tempting to hypothesize that changes in electrical activity and intracellular Ca^{++} levels owing to stimulation by various hormones and neurotransmitters may be mediated by similar interactions.

Delayed-Rectifier Potassium Channels

Whole-cell voltage-clamp recordings from mouse pancreatic β-cells (isolated[59] or in situ[46]) revealed the presence of an outward, voltage-activated current carried by K^+.[59] Families of current traces in response to voltage pulses of increasing height are shown in Figure 9-23*A,B,D,E* for various recording conditions.[46] In each case, the current activates slowly at potentials positive to −30 mV (time constant approximately 20 milliseconds) and is sustained for the duration of the depolarizing pulse. These properties are characteristic of the family of ion channels known as *delayed rectifier potassium channels* (K_{dr}), which are present in many excitable cells. The K_{dr} current is active at depolarized membrane potentials, indicating a role for these channels in repolarization of the action potentials during the active phase. Thus, the increased action potential height and duration in the presence of 2 mM TEA may result from blocking of K_{dr} channels, although TEA also inhibits other voltage-gated K^+ channels. The I-V curves in Figure 9-23*C,F* illustrate important differences in the properties of the voltage-activated outward current based on recording conditions. The currents recorded from single rat β-cells under ideal patch-clamp conditions (cultured cells, room temperature, Hepes buffer) (see Fig. 9-23*A,B*) are larger than those recorded from mouse β-cells in situ under physiologic conditions (37°C, bicarbonate buffer) (see Fig. 9-23*D,E*). This difference may reflect an increase in β-cell size during culture; alternatively, the formation of tight junctions between adjacent β-cells in situ may sequester a significant portion of the membrane area, making β-cells within the islet effectively smaller. Furthermore, the voltage-dependent outward current in mouse β-cells in situ is enhanced by glucose (see Fig. 9-23*F*),[46] but the identification of the affected channels, the mechanism of stimulation, and the physiologic role of the enhanced current has not yet been addressed.

Calcium-Activated Potassium Channels

Early studies of the effects of Ca^{++} on membrane potential and resistance suggested the presence of a Ca^{++}- and voltage-activated K^+ permeability in the β-cell membrane. To date, three Ca^{++}-activated K^+ (K_{Ca}) channels have been identified with the patch-clamp technique. The first of these channels, the "maxi" K_{Ca} channel, is common to many tissues. Figure 9-24 shows the channel to have a large conductance (200 picosiemens) with 140 mM K^+ in the pipette, compared to the K_{ATP} channel with a conductance of 55 picosiemens for inward and 34 picosiemens for outward-going currents.[8] Ca^{++} increases the open probability of the channel by shifting the activation curve to more negative potentials.[65] Although the open probability of the channel in cell-attached patches is inhibited by glucose when the cells have been flooded with Ca^{++}

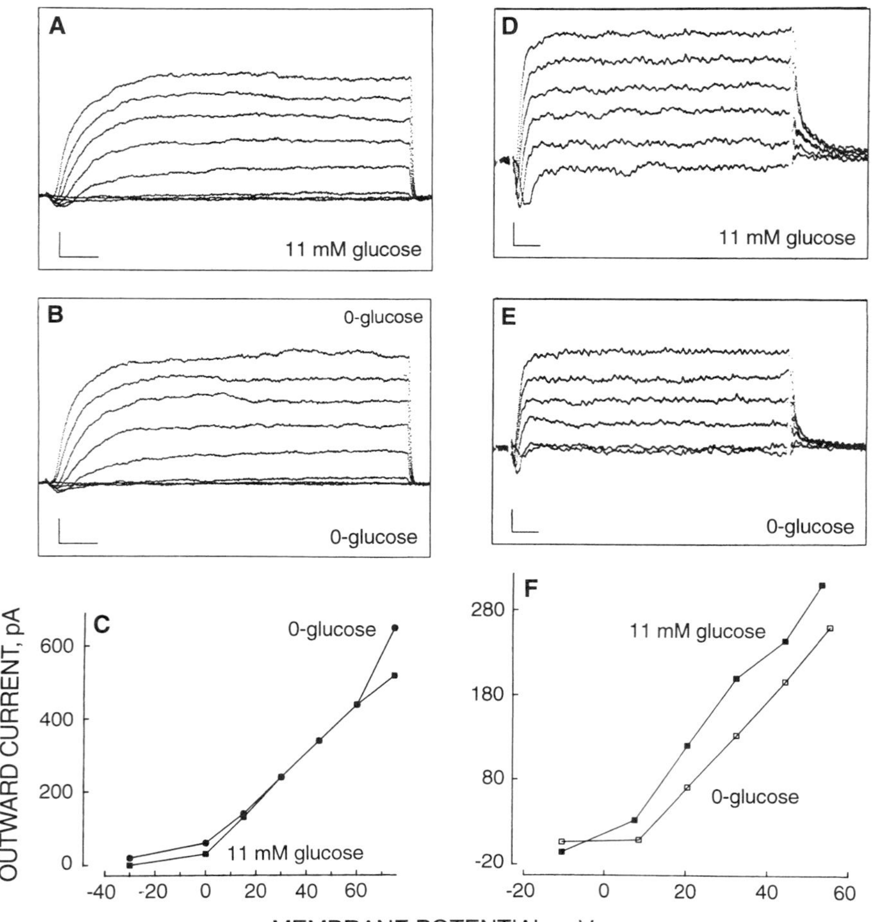

Figure 9-23. Comparison between isolated single-cell and in situ single-cell voltage-clamp currents. Whole-cell currents in response to depolarizing voltage pulses recorded from isolated, cultured rat β-cells at room temperature, with (**A**) and without (**B**) 11 mM glucose. Membrane patches were permeabilized with nystatin; bath solution was without bicarbonate and was buffered with Hepes solution. Linear currents were removed from the record by adding the response of four hyperpolarizing pulses of size P/4 to the response to the depolarizing pulse of size P. I-V relation of the steady-state outward current is plotted in (**C**) with (■) and without (●) glucose. Whole-cell currents were recorded from a mouse β-cell in situ with (**D**) and without (**E**) 11 mM glucose at 37°C, with physiologic Krebs solution as the perifusate. Voltage-clamp was achieved with an intracellular microelectrode. I-V relation (**F**) with (■) and without (●) glucose. (Reproduced with permission from Rojas E, Stokes CL, Mears D, Atwater I. Single microelectrode voltage clamp measurements of pancreatic β-cell membrane ionic currents *in situ*. J Membr Biol 1995;143:65.)

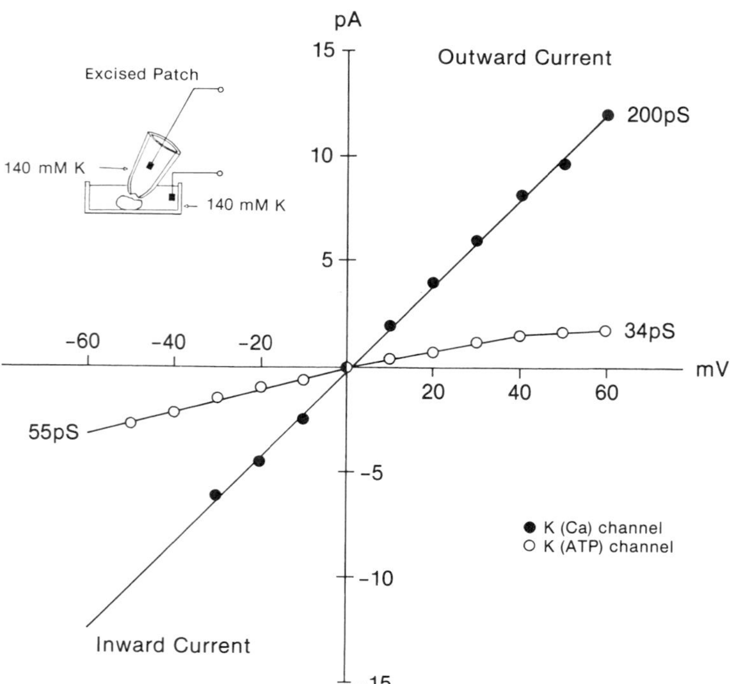

Figure 9-24. I-V relationship of K_{Ca} and K_{ATP} channels. Channel activity was recorded from excised patches of rat β-cell membrane with symmetric KCl solutions in the bath and pipette. Single channel conductance (in picosiemens) is as indicated. (Reproduced with permission from Atwater I, Carroll P, Li MX. Electrophysiology of the pancreatic B-cell. In: Draznin B, Melmed S, LeRoith D, eds. Molecular and Cellular Biology of Diabetes Mellitus. New York, NY: Alan R. Liss;1989:49–68.)

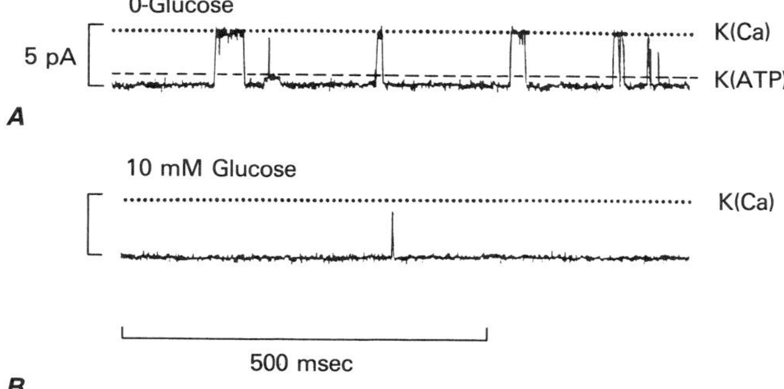

Figure 9-25. Cell attached patch recording from a rat β-cell in high K^+ concentration. ***A,*** In the absence of glucose but presence of 140 mM K^+, a condition that increases cytoplasmic Ca^{++} concentration, both K_{ATP} and K_{Ca} channel activity are present. ***B,*** Ten minutes after addition of 10 mM glucose, the frequency of opening of both channels is reduced. Pipette holding potential 0 mV, solutions (in mM): pipette 135 NaCl, 5 KCl, 2.6 $CaCl_2$, 10 Hepes, pH 7.4; bath 140 KCl, 2.6 $CaCl_2$, 10 Hepes, pH 7.4. (Reproduced with permission from Atwater I, Carroll P, Li MX. Electrophysiology of the pancreatic B-cell. In: Draznin B, Melmed S, LeRoith D, eds. Molecular and Cellular Biology of Diabetes Mellitus. New York, NY: Alan R. Liss;1989:49–68.)

(Fig. 9-25),[8] the role of the maxi K_{Ca} channel in β-cell electrical activity remains elusive. At physiologic intracellular Ca^{++} levels, maxi K_{Ca} channels can be activated only by depolarization to positive potentials, conditions that are never achieved during glucose-induced bursting. Furthermore, charybdotoxin, a potent and sensitive inhibitor of the maxi K_{Ca} channel is without effect on the essential features of glucose-induced bursting.[66] Thus the theory that periodic activation/inactivation of the maxi K_{Ca} channel (driven by periodic changes in intracellular Ca^{++} concentration as in Fig. 9-10) controls the oscillatory β-cell electrical activity has been dismissed. Maxi K_{Ca} channels may play a more important role in electrical activity during modulation of bursting by various agonists rather than under glucose stimulation.

The apamine-sensitive K_{Ca} channel, which is involved in oscillatory electrical activity in cells such as pituitary gonadotropes, does not appear to be important in β-cell electrophysiology because apamine does not modulate glucose-induced electrical activity.[67] Recently a K^+ current activated by inositol triphosphate (IP_3)-induced release of Ca^{++} from intracellular stores was described in mouse pancreatic β-cells. Although the channel responsible for this effect has not been identified directly in single-channel recordings, it was proposed that the channel controls the cycle of electrical activity by opening and closing in response to oscillations in stored Ca^{++}.[68] The bursts described in the study[68] were significantly different from the usual glucose-induced bursts, and thus this hypothesis requires further experimental verification.

Three of the channels discussed to this point (i.e., K_{ATP}, Ca_{Vm}, K_{dr}) are sufficient to provide glucose-induced β-cell depolarization as well as Ca^{++}-dependent action potentials (Fig. 9-26). The others have been proposed to be involved in modulation of the burst pattern by glucose. The following section describes receptor-activated ion channels, which are important in the modulation of β-cell electrical activity by hormones and neurotransmitters.

Receptor-Activated Ion Channels

Calcium-Release–Activated Ion Channels

Depletion of Ca^{++} from intracellular stores (most importantly the endoplasmic reticulum) stimulates an inward Ca^{++} current in a variety of nonexcitable cells.[69,70] The current seems to be activated by a diffusible messenger, *calcium influx factor* (CIF), that is released from the calcium-depleted organelle(s) and interacts with ion channels directly or through other second messengers.[71] The *calcium-release–activated current* (CRAC) plays a role in the refilling of calcium stores and is a crucial part of Ca^{++} signaling in nonexcitable cells. Recent evidence indicates that communication between intracellular organelles and the plasmalemma also exists in pancreatic β-cells.[72] Figure 9-27 shows the effect on β-cell electrical activity of thapsigargin, a drug that passively empties intracellular calcium stores by blocking Ca^{++} uptake by the sarco endoplasmic reticulum calcium ATPase, or Ca^{++} pump.[7] Exposure to thapsigargin in the presence of 11 mM glucose results in a

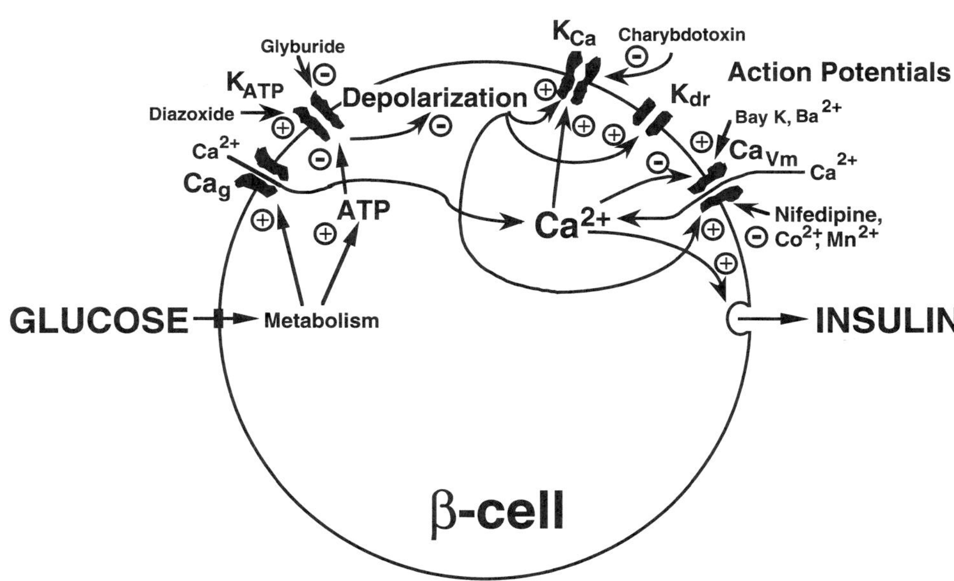

Figure 9-26. Model of stimulus-secretion coupling in the β-cell showing interactions between metabolically and voltage-regulated ion channels responsible for glucose-induced electrical activity. Metabolically regulated channels, Ca_g (⊕) and K_{ATP} (⊖), mediate β-cell membrane depolarization, thereby activating (⊕) voltage-regulated channels, K_{ca}, K_{dr}, Ca_{Vm}, that give rise to the action potentials. Elevations of intracellular Ca^{++}, subsequent to influx through Ca^{++} channels, Ca_g and Ca_{Vm}, open K_{Ca} channels (⊕), close Ca_{Vm} channels (⊖), and trigger (⊕) insulin secretion. Some pharmacologic agents that act directly on β-cell membrane ion channels are indicated.

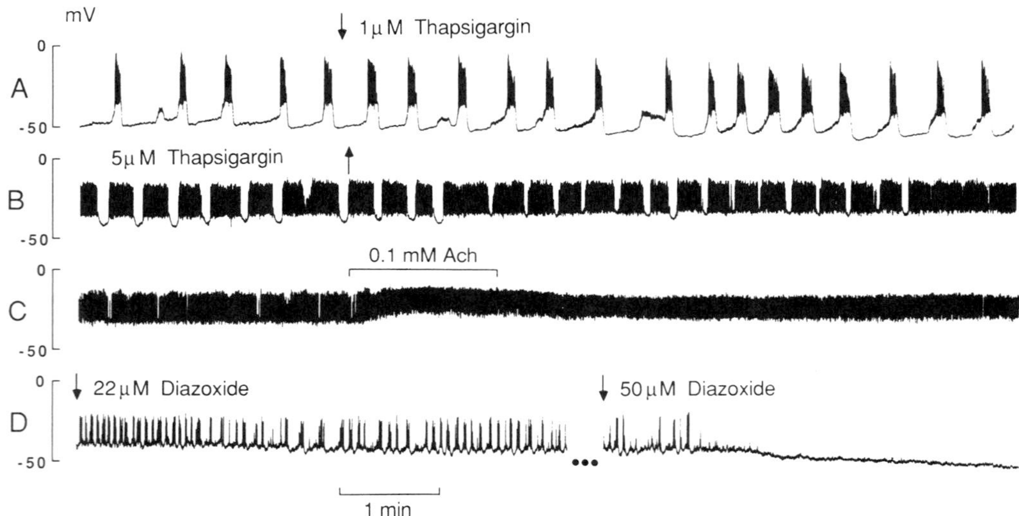

FIGURE **9-27.** Effect of thapsigargin (Tg) on mouse β-cell electrical activity. ***A,*** Addition of 1 μM thapsigargin to the perifusate had little immediate effect on the burst pattern. In the 32 minutes between the top two traces, the Tg concentration was progressively increased to 5 μM, and the silent phase began to depolarize slowly (compare with Fig. 9-5*A,B*). ***B,*** Shortly after removal of Tg, electrical activity changed to a pattern of almost continuous spiking, illustrating the irreversible nature of Tg. ***C,*** The spiking became completely continuous after a brief pulse with 0.1 mM ACh. ***D,*** Titration of diazoxide into the medium restored a muscarinic burst pattern (left side), and further increase in diazoxide concentration (right side) as well as removal of glucose (not shown) hyperpolarized the cell. (Reproduced with permission from Bertram R, Smolen P, Sherman A, et al. A role for calcium release activated current (CRAC) in cholinergic modulation of insulin secretion. Biophys J 1995;68:2323.)

gradual (in 30–60 minutes) depolarization of the silent phase and an increase in plateau fraction (Fig. 9-27*A,B*). After a 90-second exposure to ACh to complete store emptying, the cell spikes continuously (Fig. 9-27*C*), indicating that store depletion is accompanied by a depolarizing current. Furthermore, when diazoxide is added to the medium (Fig. 9-27*D*), a muscarinic burst pattern similar to that observed in the presence of ACh (Fig. 9-6) resulted. Because muscarinic agonists stimulate release of Ca^{++} from intracellular stores, these observations suggest that the effect of muscarinic agonists on β-cell electrical activity may be mediated by calcium store depletion and activation of CRAC.

Results of a theoretic study in which CRAC was added to a mathematic model of the β-cell support this hypothesis (Fig. 9-28).[7] In the model, glucose stimulates uptake of Ca^{++} into intracellular stores, and hence CRAC plays little role in steady-state bursting (bursts in this model are driven by slow inactivation of Ca^{++} channels during the active phase). Application of a muscarinic agonist (simulated by release of stored calcium, shown in Fig. 9-28*C*), however, activates the CRAC current and the cell enters muscarinic bursting (Fig. 9-28*A*). Note that the simulated increase in cytoplasmic Ca^{++} concentration subsequent to calcium store emptying (Fig. 9-28*B*) is similar to the experimental results illustrated previously (see Fig. 9-13). Interestingly, the fast burst pattern after store depletion is driven by periodic activation of K_{Ca} channels in the model, which become more active as a result of the large increase in intracellular Ca^{++}. Thus, in addition to being capable of replicating experimental data, the model suggests a role for the K_{Ca} channel in agonist-stimulated modulation of electrical activity and secretion. The similar effects of ACh and forskolin on electrical activity in the presence of glucose (see Fig. 9-5*A,B*), suggests that the effect of cAMP on membrane potential also may involve activation of CRAC. The recent demonstration that forskolin stimulates release of stored calcium in isolated rat β-cells[73] supports this hypothesis.

The CRAC model is also uniquely able to replicate the long first phase of electrical activity in response to a step increase in glucose concentration (see Fig. 9-2). Figure 9-29*A* illustrates the predicted effects of a step change in glucose concentration; here, the model described above is used, but with the CRAC current removed. The first burst is no longer than steady-state bursts. When CRAC is added to the model,[7] the depolarizing current is active in the absence of glucose, because intracellular calcium stores are depleted (Fig. 9-29*F*) owing to the low cytoplasmic Ca^{++} levels (Fig. 9-29*E*), which depend on membrane potential (Fig. 9-29*D*). The depolarizing effect of CRAC, however, is not able to overcome the dominant hyperpolarizing influence of the open K_{ATP} channels under these conditions, and the cell remains silent. When glucose is added, the K_{ATP} channel closes, but CRAC remains active until Ca^{++} is sequestered. The combined effect of CRAC and blocked K_{ATP} channels produces a long period of continuous activity (Figure 9-29*D*). Only after Ca^{++} uptake has occurred (Fig. 9-29*F*) does the depolarizing CRAC current inactivate, allowing the cell to enter steady-state bursting. The ability of the CRAC model to reproduce both muscarinic alteration of electrical activity and the biphasic response to glucose suggests that communication between subcellular organelles and the plasma membrane plays an important role in β-cell function.

Direct identification of an ion channel activated by calcium depletion has not yet been reported. In contrast to nonexcitable cells, however, CRAC in β-cells does not appear to be carried by Ca^{++} alone. Depletion of extracellular Ca^{++} in whole-cell recordings from β-cells activates an inward current that must be

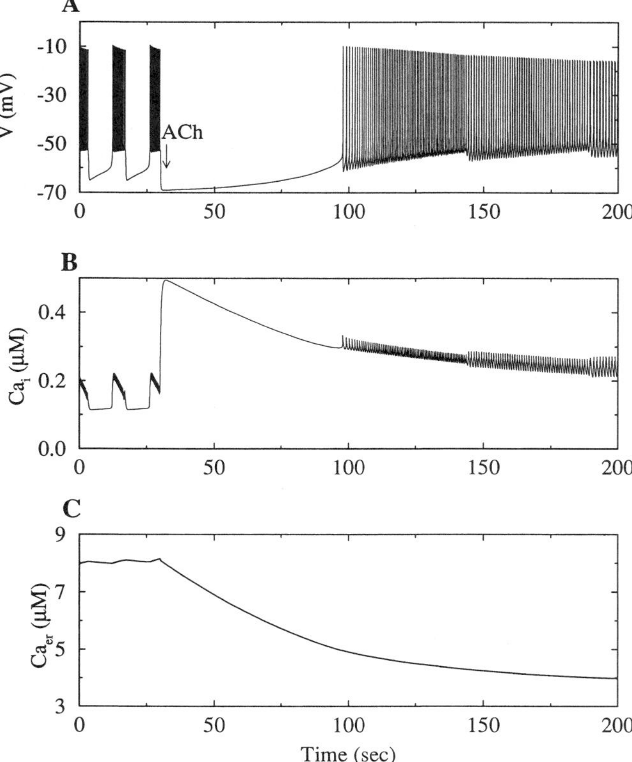

FIGURE 9-28. Mathematic model stimulating effects of acetylcholine (ACh) on β-cell electrical activity. Membrane potential (***A***), cytoplasmic Ca^{++} concentration (***B***), and endoplasmic reticulum (ER) calcium concentration (***C***) predicted by a mathematic model of the β-cell incorporating CRAC. Addition of ACh (***A,*** *arrow*) causes emptying of ER Ca^{++} stores (***C***), increases cytosolic Ca^{++} levels (***B***) (compare to Fig. 9-13*B*), and produces muscarinic bursts (***A***) (compare to Fig. 9-5). (Reproduced with permission from Bertram R, Smolen P, Sherman A, et al. A role for calcium release activated current (CRAC) in cholinergic modulation of insulin secretion. Biophys J 1995;68:2323.)

carried by Na^+,[72] and stimulation of β-cells with muscarinic agonists results in Na^+ uptake.[35,74] In HIT-T15 cells, thapsigargin induces Mn^{++} influx[75]; hence, it appears that the CRAC channel in β-cells may be a nonspecific cation channel.

Adrenergic-Activated Potassium Channels

The α_2-adrenergic agonist clonidine (5 μM) mimics the hyperpolarizing effect of adrenaline on β-cell membrane potential in the presence of glucose. The hyperpolarization is observed in the presence of glyburide or TEA, indicating that K_{ATP}, K_{dr}, and K_{Ca} channels are not involved in the effect. Whole-cell recordings showed that clonidine activates a small outward current carried by K^+, and noise analysis of the current record indicated the channel conductance to be approximately 0.6 picosiemens.[76] Adrenergic stimulation of this channel may involve G-protein interactions because clonidine and adrenaline have no effect on membrane potential after pretreatment of the β-cell with pertussis toxin. As mentioned earlier, adrenaline inhibits glucose-stimulated electrical activity only transiently, and therefore must also act on at least one other step in the stimulus-secretion coupling cascade. The transient nature of adrenergic inhibition of electrical activity may reflect transient activation of the G-protein–coupled K^+ channel (K_{adr}), or a counteracting depolarizing current may be activated more slowly. The mechanisms of receptor-mediated modulation of β-cell electrical activity are summarized schematically in Figure 9-30.

Control of Burst Duration

The mechanism responsible for the oscillatory nature of β-cell electrical activity and the exquisite glucose sensitivity of burst duration (see Fig. 9-3) remains an enigma. In mathematic models, bursting is driven by feedback of a slow process such as ion accumulation or channel inactivation on a fast process (spike generation).[77] The slow variable accumulates during the active phase and exerts a hyperpolarizing influence on the membrane potential, which eventually forces the cell into the silent phase. During the quiescent period, the feedback variable is removed and the cell depolarizes to the next active phase. Note that the hyperpolarizing effect of the feedback variable may actually result from inactivation of a depolarizing current. Glucose can increase plateau fraction by (1) reducing the rate of accumulation of the feedback variable; (2) desensitizing the target ion channels to the feedback variable; or (3) by activating additional depolarizing currents such that the feedback variable must reach higher levels in order to bring the cell into the silent phase. Intracellular calcium accumulation has been a favorite candidate for the slow feedback variable, either via a direct effect on ion channels or by affecting the production of other cellular messengers. Elevation of extracellular calcium shortens active phase duration, increases the length of the silent phase, and shifts the continuous spiking in the presence of high glucose back to a burst pattern.[78,79] Furthermore, after intracellular Ca^{++} is elevated in 11 mM glucose by transient exposure to high KCl, the cell hyperpolarizes and bursts are inhibited for several minutes.[80] The various models in which Ca^{++} acts on a particular ion channel (e.g., K_{Ca}, K_{ATP}, Ca_{Vm}) to produce oscillations, however, have not held up to experimental verification. Fluorescence imaging experiments indicate that the intracellular Ca^{++} concentration rises rapidly at the start of the active phase (see Fig. 9-10),[30] suggesting that Ca^{++} accumulation may not be a slow process at all. Slow voltage-dependent inactivation of L-type Ca^{++} channels as a method of controlling oscillations remains a viable theory,[81] although this may be owing more to a lack of experimental evidence against the idea than to solid evidence supporting it. A role for oscillations in stored calcium (via CRAC or K_{Ca} channels) in controlling bursting awaits experimental verification.

The bistable nature of β-cell electrical activity may result from the combined depolarizing and hyperpolarizing interactions of a number of ion channels. An important point in this discussion is that characterization of the ionic currents in the β-cell are carried out under ideal patch-clamp conditions (single cells, room temperature, Hepes buffer), often with rat β-cells, whereas bursting is reliably seen only in the intact mouse islet under physiologic conditions. Figure 9-23 shows how experimental conditions can dramatically affect the character of cell currents. Thus the inability to reconcile well-defined bursting with current ion channel data may be related to differences in experimental conditions in which the two phenomena are studied.

Importance of Cell-to-Cell Coupling in Glucose Sensing

The characteristic glucose-induced bursting recorded from β-cells in microdissected islets may require communication among at least a small group of cells. In current- and voltage-clamp studies at 25°C, single β-cells usually exhibit spontaneous, disorganized action potentials or remain silent in the presence of glucose,[9,59,66]

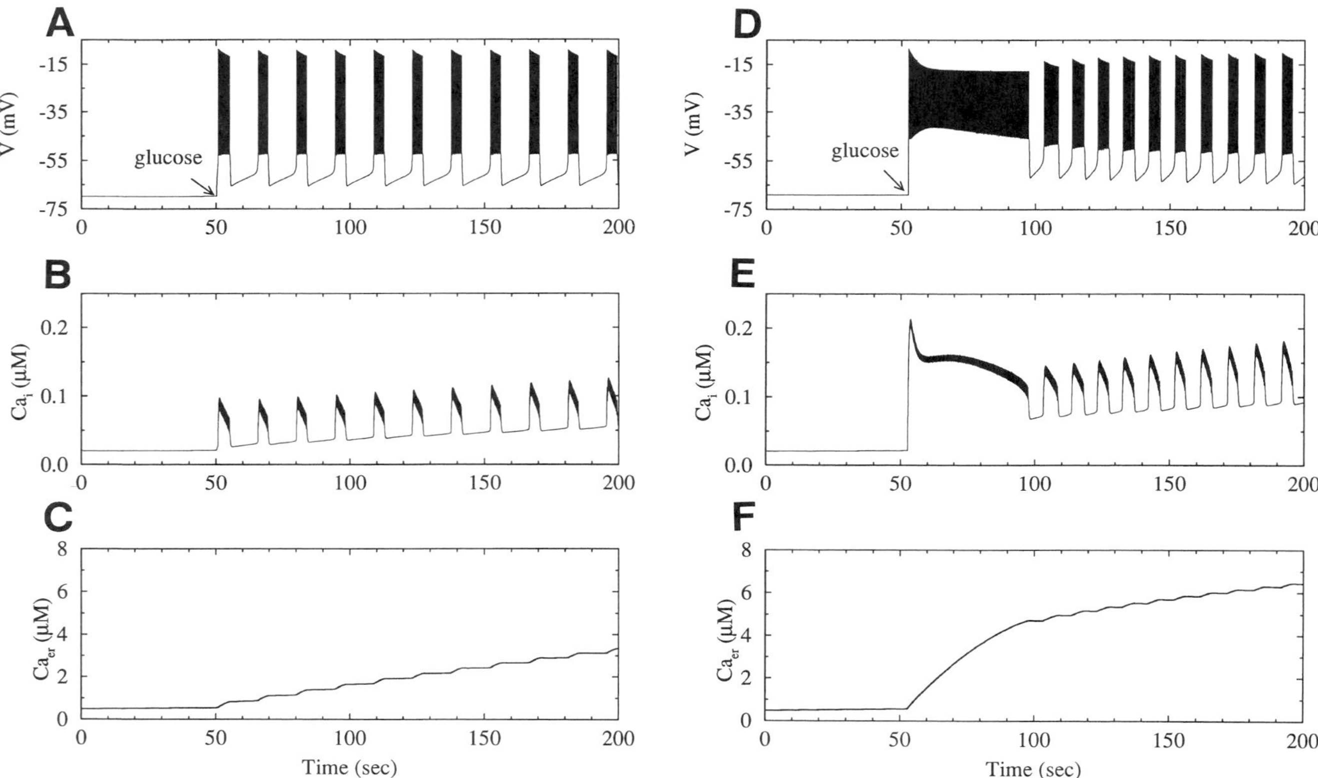

FIGURE 9-29. Mathematic models simulating effects of a sudden increase in glucose concentration on β-cell activity. Changes in electrical activity (*A*) and in intracellular Ca^{++} (*B*) and endoplasmic reticulum calcium (*C*) concentration in response to a step increase in glucose concentration, simulated using the model of Figure 9-28 with CRAC removed. The response is monophasic. (R. Bertram and A. Sherman, unpublished observations, 1995). CRAC included in the model of changes in electrical activity (*D*) and in intracellular (*E*) and endoplasmic reticulum (*F*) concentration in response to the same step increase in glucose concentration. Electrical activity and intracellular calcium traces are biphasic (compare to Fig. 9-2*A*). (Reproduced with permission from Bertram R, Smolen P, Sherman A, et al. A role for calcium release activated current (CRAC) in cholinergic modulation of insulin secretion. Biophys J 1995;68:2323.)

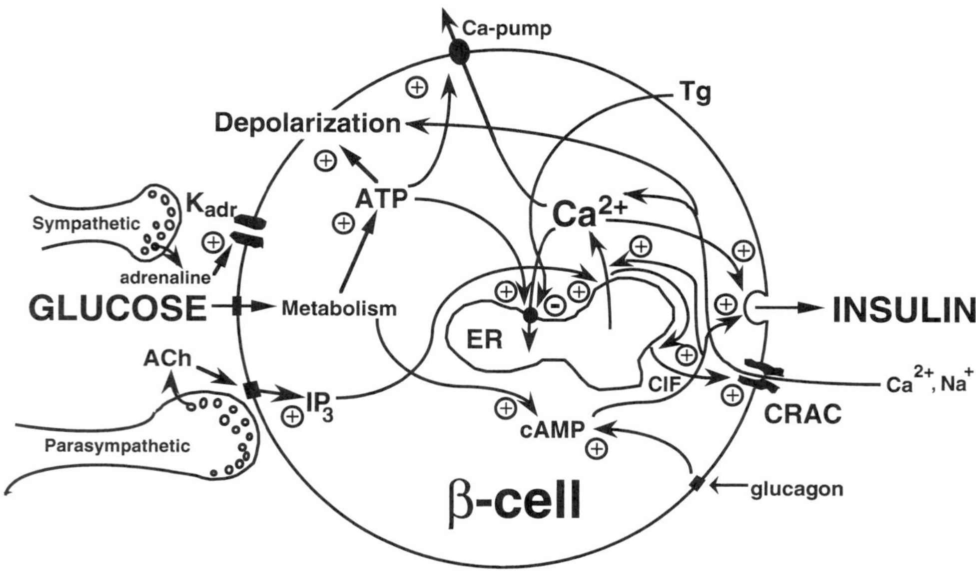

FIGURE 9-30. Model of the β-cell showing mechanisms of receptor-mediated changes in electrical activity and cytoplasmic Ca^{++} concentration. Muscarinic stimuli (ACh) activate CRAC current subsequent to IP_3-dependent depletion of calcium from the endoplasmic reticulum (ER), and adrenaline activates (transiently) a K^+ conductance (Kadr). cAMP, produced in response to glucose metabolism or glucagon, may also induce ER Ca^{++} release as well as affecting insulin secretion directly. Intracellular Ca^{++} released from ER is removed from the cytosol by Ca ATPases in the ER and cell membrane (Ca pump).

whereas clusters 50–100 μm in diameter show regular bursts.[10,59] Similarly, isolated cells release proportionately less insulin when faced with a glucose challenge than those in whole islets.[82,83] There is one report of bursts with large spikes and long periods in a single cell at 30°C[84]; however, temperature is not likely to be the sole cause of the vastly different results reported for single-cell and whole-islet electrical and secretory behavior. The group reporting bursts in single cells[84] confirms that such observations are rare. Electrical activity in intact islets shifts toward higher plateau fractions as temperature is lowered, with continuous spiking occurring near room temperature,[26] but the effect is often transient. Furthermore, even at 37°C, only a small percentage of isolated β-cells show intracellular Ca^{++} oscillations characteristic of bursting islets.[34,85] Thus, although individual β-cells are endowed with the necessary ion channels for glucose sensing, the ability to produce an exquisitely sensitive response to the sugar may be a property of the entire islet.

Gap Junctions in the Islet

Gap junctions are aggregations of large, intercellular channels that allow the passage of ions and small molecules between the cytoplasm of adjacent cells. Both cells of a communicating pair contribute a hexomer of protein subunits (connexins) to each gap junction channel, or *connexon*. At least 12 different isoforms of the connexin family of proteins have been identified, and expression of connexins is tissue-specific.[86] Like ion channels in the nonjunctional membrane, connexons are subject to regulation by various physiologic and pharmacologic signals, and many gap junctions are also sensitive to the transjunctional or transmembrane potential, or both. Furthermore, the extent of intercellular communication within a tissue can be modulated on a long-term basis by stimuli that affect the expression of gap-junction proteins. The strong influence that cell-to-cell coupling appears to have on islet function motivates the investigation of the structural and functional properties of gap junctions in the endocrine pancreas.

Within the islet of Langerhans, β-cells are connected to each other and to the other endocrine cell types (the glucagon-secreting α-cells and the somatostatin-secreting δ-cells) by gap junctions.[87,88] Morphologically, the gap junctions consist of small polygonal or linear arrays of connexons occurring on about 30% of the cell interfaces.[89] Immunolabeling of rat islet sections and Western blots of crude islet membrane preparations with antibodies against the various connexin types has revealed connexin 43 as the major gap junction protein in islets.[86,90,91] Gap junction plaques in β-cells are much smaller than those in other cells expressing connexin 43, having only 10–25 particles per plaque and occupying less than 1 μm^2 (less than 0.5%) of the cell membrane area.[92,93] Given the rather small size of gap junctions in the islet, it seems possible that these cells may also express other connexin isoforms, but at levels that cannot be detected with current techniques.

Extent of Coupling in the Islet

In the presence of glucose, the islet appears to act as a functional syncytium. Figure 9-31 shows simultaneous intracellular recordings of electrical activity from two β-cells within the same islet.[8] Closely adjacent cells (electrode separations of <20 μm) are almost completely synchronous, even at the level of the action potentials; at longer separations, the spike records are less synchronous, and phase lags of 1–2 seconds can occur.[94–96] However, at a given time, the frequency of bursts is identical even across an entire islet (separations of up to 400 μm).[96] Synchronous electrical activity suggests that ion fluxes and secretion also should be synchronous, given the causal relationship between these phenomena. Thus, as discussed previously, secretion of insulin from an entire islet is pulsatile and in phase with bursts of a single β-cell therein (see Fig. 9-9).[27] Furthermore, studies with ion sensitive electrodes (Fig. 9-32) showed that the influx of Ca^{++} during the depolarization of the action potentials and the efflux of K^+ during repolarization results in Ca^{++} depletion and K^+ accumulation in the limited extracellular space of the islet during the active phase.[56] Finally,

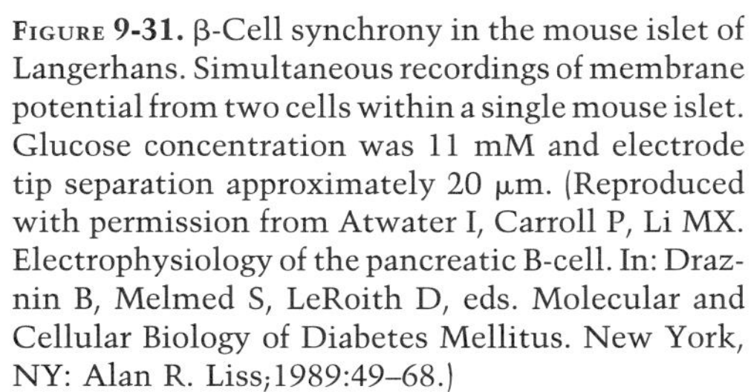

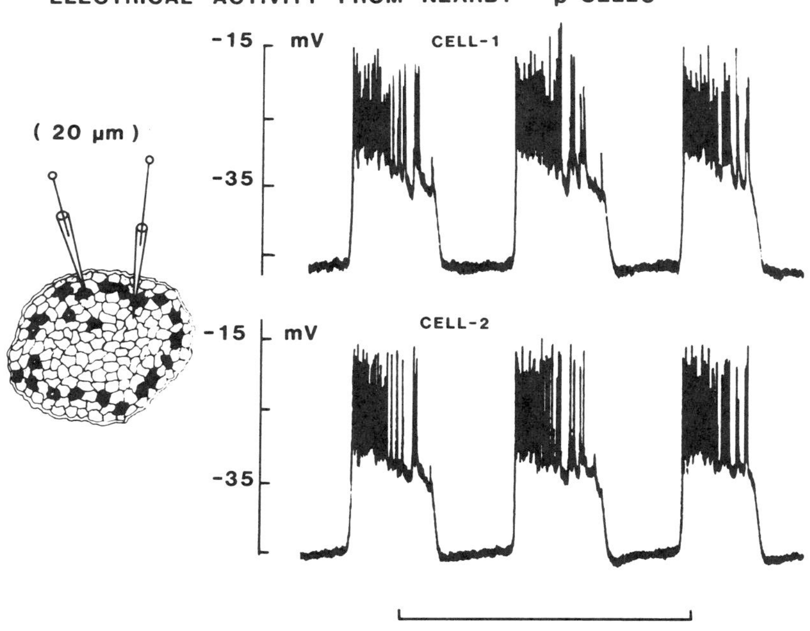

Figure 9-31. β-Cell synchrony in the mouse islet of Langerhans. Simultaneous recordings of membrane potential from two cells within a single mouse islet. Glucose concentration was 11 mM and electrode tip separation approximately 20 μm. (Reproduced with permission from Atwater I, Carroll P, Li MX. Electrophysiology of the pancreatic B-cell. In: Draznin B, Melmed S, LeRoith D, eds. Molecular and Cellular Biology of Diabetes Mellitus. New York, NY: Alan R. Liss;1989:49–68.)

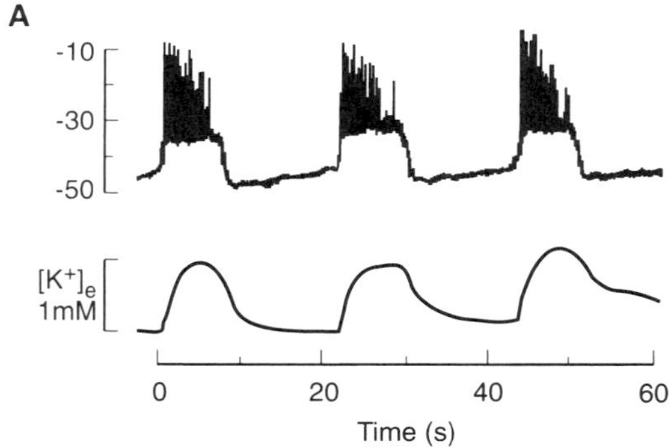

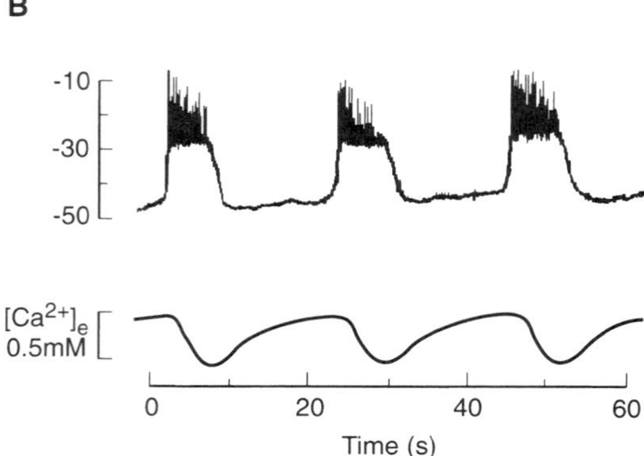

Figure 9-32. Extracellular ion concentrations oscillate in synchrony with β-cell electrical activity. ***A,*** Simultaneous recordings of membrane potential (top) from a β-cell within a mouse islet of Langerhans and K^+ concentration (bottom) measured by placing a K^+-sensitive electrode into the intercellular (i.e., extracellular) space within the same islet. K^+ accumulations occur during the active phase. ***B,*** Same as ***A,*** with K^+ electrode replaced with a Ca^{++}-sensitive electrode. The active phase is also associated with Ca^{++} depletion from the intercellular space within the islet. (Reproduced with permission from Pérez-Armendariz E, Atwater I. Glucose-evoked changes in $[K^+]$ and $[Ca^{++}]$ in the intercellular spaces of the mouse islet of Langerhans. In: Atwater I, Rojas E, Soria B, eds. Biophysics of the Pancreatic β-Cell. New York, NY: Plenum Press;1986:31–51.)

glucose-induced oscillations in intracellular Ca^{++}, detected with fluorescent dyes, are synchronous at different regions of the islet[97] and are also in phase with the electrical activity of a single cell (see Fig. 9-10).[30] Taken together, these findings show that β-cells within an islet act in concert when responding to glucose, and suggest the possibility of extensive cell-to-cell communication.

Most studies of direct communication between islet cells have focused on quantifying the size of coupled domains. In apparent contrast to the widespread synchrony of islet activity, intracellularly injected fluorescent tracers spread to only two to six cells in the cultured rat and microdissected mouse islet.[98–102] Figure 9-33*A* shows the limited spread of Lucifer yellow dye after injection into a single β-cell of the microdissected mouse islet. Sectioning the islet and staining alternate slices with rhodamine-labeled anti-insulin revealed that the dye was present in four cells (Fig. 9-33*B*), all of which were β-cells (Fig. 9-33*C*). Transfer of the dye sometimes occurs between β-cells and the other endocrine cell types within the islet.[99,103] In some cases, although glucose-induced electrical activity can be recorded,[100] the dye does not spread to any neighboring cells, and unlabeled cells are often found within a communicating territory.[101,104] Electrical coupling measured by current injection also exists over a very limited range within the islet of Langerhans. Figure 9-34 illustrates that in the presence of glucose, current injected into one cell via an intercellular electrode causes a voltage deflection in a second cell only if the distance between the cells is <35 μm (three to four cell diameters).[95,96]

There have been several attempts to quantify the magnitude of the electrical conductance of β-cell gap junctions. β-Cells from freshly dispersed mouse islets show a high incidence of coupling (67%), with a mean junctional conductance of 215 picosiemens.[105] This result is in reasonable agreement with the 130-picosiemens value calculated by analyzing the decay of current between two electrodes in a single mouse islet.[95] In another study, only 16% of rat β-cell pairs were coupled.[102] By clamping the voltage of a single β-cell in a bursting islet, electrical coupling in mouse islets can be studied under physiologic conditions.[106] Glucose-induced bursts in surrounding cells drive oscillatory current into the clamped cell, and dividing the magnitude of the current bursts by that of the voltage bursts yields the parallel conductance between the impaled cell and adjacent, bursting β-cells. Figure 9-34 shows that the coupling conductance distribution within the islet is bimodal. The two conductance peaks (2.5 and 3.5 nanosiemens, respectively) may reflect differences in extent of coupling based on location within the islet, which have been suggested by dye coupling[99] and morphologic studies.[89] Using the results of one cell-pair study (67% coupled, 215-picosiemens mean conductance[105]), adjusting for changes in conductance owing to temperature differences,[106] and assuming each β-cell has 12 neighbors, one could predict an average parallel conductance of approximately 2.2 nanosiemens. This value is in reasonable agreement with the lower conductance peak shown in Figure 9-35. The presence of the higher conductance peak suggests that electrical coupling, at least in some locations of the islet, is more extensive than previously predicted.

The available evidence indicates that β-cells are organized into small domains that are dye and electrically coupled, in apparent discrepancy with the widespread synchrony in activity. The coupled domains may be noncommunicating and synchronized by accumulations of K^+ in the extracellular space,[56,107] or there may be a quantitative drop in permeability at the edge of the junctions such that they are electrically coupled, but below the sensitivity of the tracer techniques.

Role of Coupling in Bursting

Two hypotheses have been set forth to explain the difference in electrical behavior between isolated β-cells and those within large clusters or whole islets. The first, known as the *channel-sharing hypothesis,* states that large, stochastic current fluctuations owing to the opening of high conductance K^+ channels (K_{Ca}) would disrupt any organized electrical activity in single cells. Current sharing among cells via gap junctions would reduce the effect of stochastic noise, allowing the cluster to burst in synchrony.[108] Mathematic models incorporating groups of cells and stochastic channel openings have supported this idea (Fig. 9-36), with bursting emerging for clusters of sufficient size.[109,110] Interestingly, when the cells in the model were coupled by physiologic rather than infinite gap-junction conductances, longer burst periods and higher intracellular Ca^{++} oscillations (and presumably increased insulin release) were obtained.[111]

Because mathematic models of single cells support bursting only within a very restricted range of parameter values, a model was developed that takes into account the properties of individual cells (Figs. 9-37 and 9-38). In this model, called the *heterogeneity hypothesis,*[112] individual cell parameters, including cell size, channel conductances, metabolic rate, Ca^{++} removal rate and gap-junction conductance are varied within experimentally determined

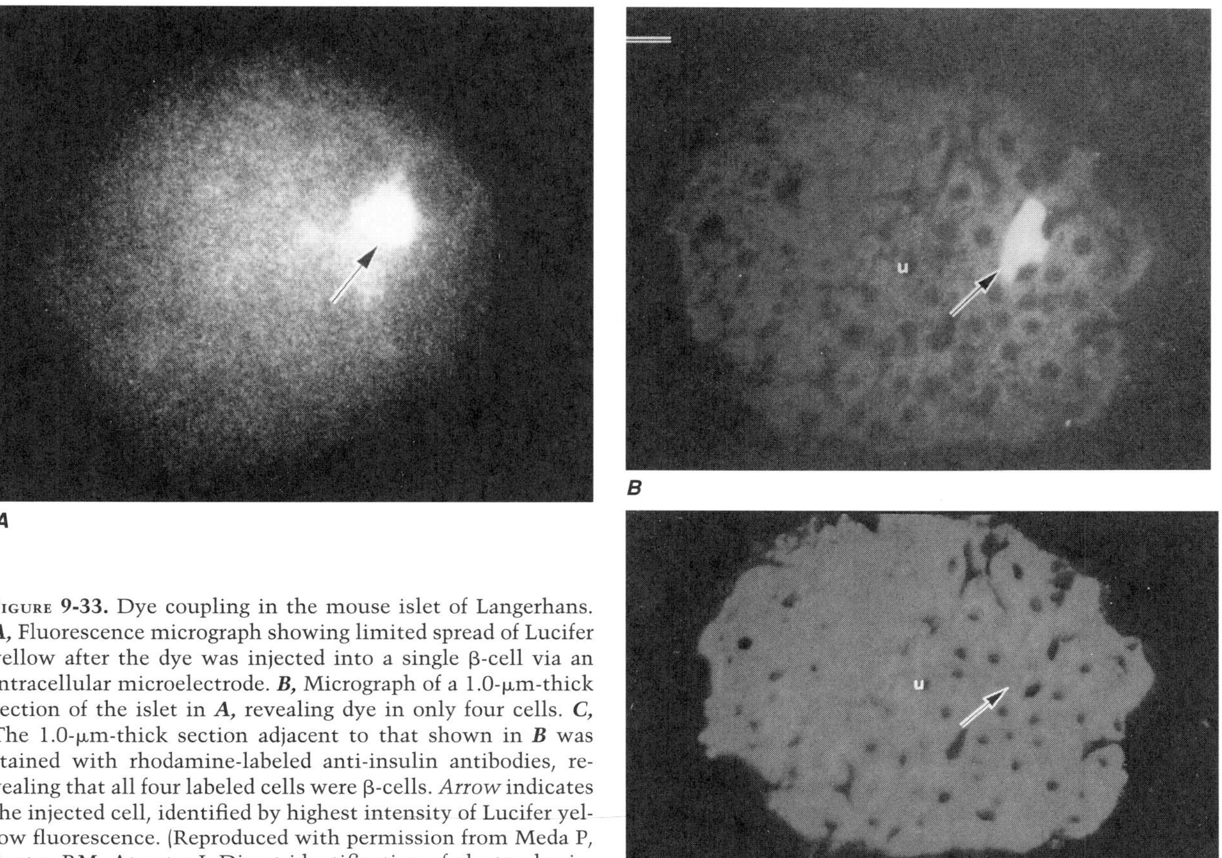

Figure 9-33. Dye coupling in the mouse islet of Langerhans. ***A,*** Fluorescence micrograph showing limited spread of Lucifer yellow after the dye was injected into a single β-cell via an intracellular microelectrode. ***B,*** Micrograph of a 1.0-μm-thick section of the islet in ***A***, revealing dye in only four cells. ***C,*** The 1.0-μm-thick section adjacent to that shown in ***B*** was stained with rhodamine-labeled anti-insulin antibodies, revealing that all four labeled cells were β-cells. *Arrow* indicates the injected cell, identified by highest intensity of Lucifer yellow fluorescence. (Reproduced with permission from Meda P, Santos RM, Atwater I. Direct identification of electrophysiologically monitored cells within intact mouse islets of Langerhans. Diabetes 1986;35:232.)

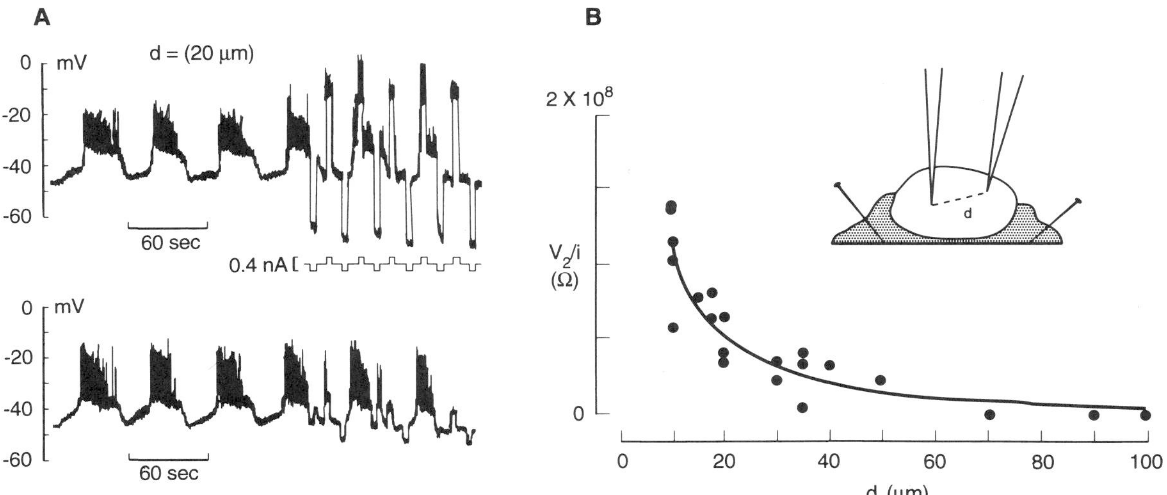

Figure 9-34. Electrical coupling in the mouse islet of Langerhans. ***A,*** Simultaneous membrane potential recordings from two β-cells within the same islet. In 11 mM glucose, current injections into one cell elicited voltage deflections in the other cell when the electrode separation was approximately 20 μm. ***B,*** Plot of interelectrode resistance (voltage response in passive cell divided by size of current pulse) as a function of electrode-tip separation (see inset). Electrical coupling could not be detected in control islets when the separation was greater than 50 μm, or approximately five cells. (Reproduced with permission from Eddlestone GT, Goncalves A, Bangham JA, Rojas E. Electrical coupling between cells in islets of Langerhans from mouse. J Membr Biol 1984;77:1.)

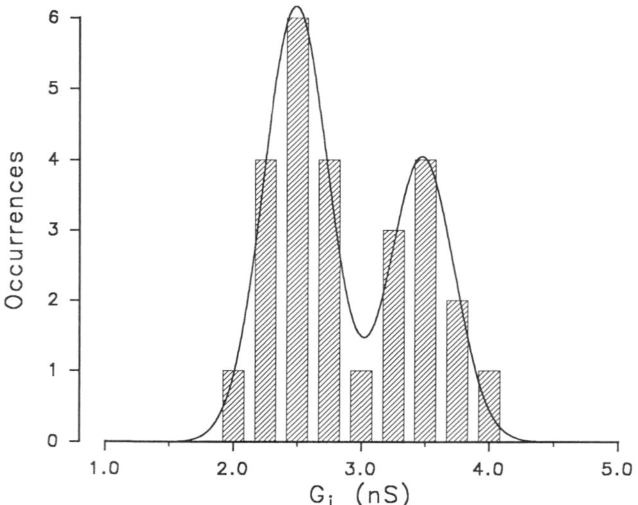

Figure 9-35. Coupling conductance between cells within the islet. Parallel gap-junction conductance between a β-cell and surrounding, active β-cells was measured by clamping the potential of a β-cell within the intact mouse islet. Histogram of coupling conductance from 26 cells in 24 different islets was bimodal. Solid curves are best fit to the data, using a sum of Gaussian distributions with peaks at 2.5 +/− 0.25 nanosiemens and 3.5 +/ − 0.25 nanosiemens. (Reproduced with permission from Mears D, Sheppard NF Jr, Atwater I, Rojas E. Magnitude and modulation of pancreatic β-cell gap junction electrical conductance *in situ*. J Membr Biol 1995;146:163.)

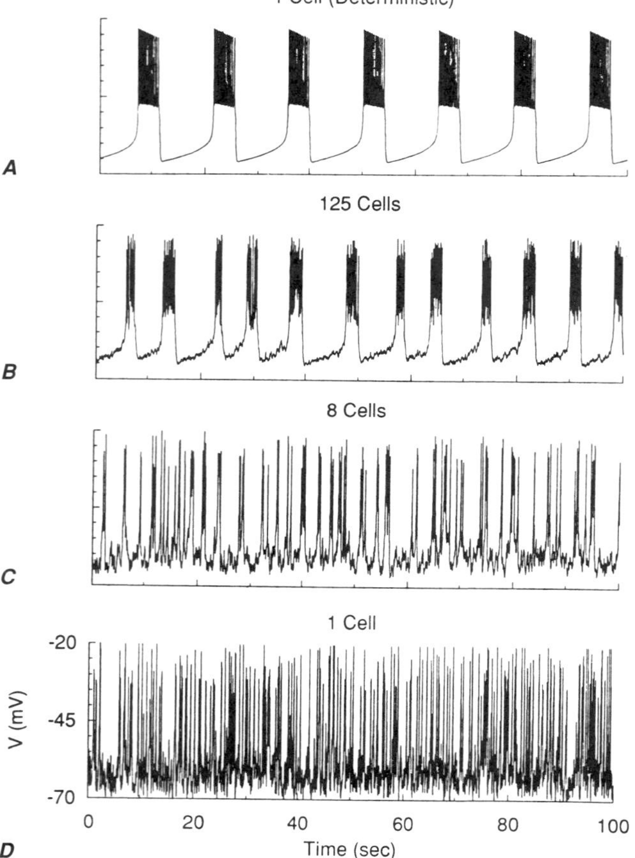

Figure 9-36. The channel-sharing hypothesis for bursting in cell clusters. A mathematic model shows how β-cell coupling can induce the burst pattern when single cells only spike. Glucose-induced bursts simulated by a mathematic model of a single β-cell with no channel noise (***A***). When channel noise is added to the model (by defining the K-Ca channel conductance with a Markov process), the burst pattern progressively gives way to random spiking as the cell cluster size decreases from 125 (***B***) to 8 (***C***) to 1 (***D***) cell. Gap-junction conductances are infinite for the cell clusters (i.e. they behave as a single, large cell). (Figure redrawn from Sherman A, Rinzel J. Model for synchronization of pancreatic β-cells by gap junction coupling. Biophys J 1991;59:547.)

or physiologically reasonable ranges. The result is that most cells have parameters that lie outside the bursting regime, even when the population means are kept within strict limits (Fig. 9-38*B*). Single cells burst only rarely (Fig. 9-37*B*), the majority of cells remaining silent (Fig. 9-37*A*) or spiking continuously (Fig. 9-37*C*) in response to glucose. When coupled by gap junctions with physiologic conductances, the clusters burst (Fig. 37*D*,*E*,*F*).[112] An interesting prediction of the model is that the average intracellular Ca^{++} level (hence rate of secretion) for a group of uncoupled, heterogeneous cells will be a weak, linear function of glucose concentration (Fig. 9-38*A*, open circles). When the same cells are coupled by gap junctions, the dose-response curve becomes sigmoidal, with a

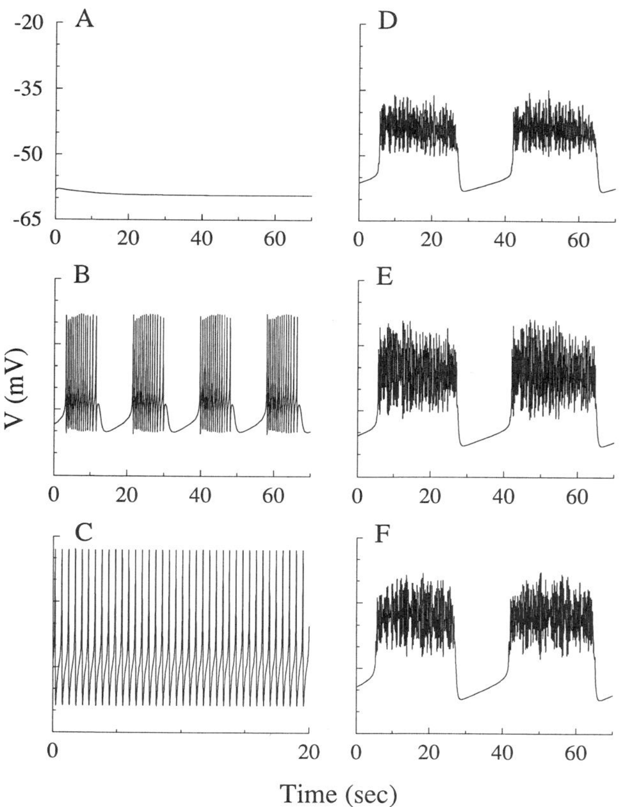

FIGURE 9-37. Mathematic model showing how coupling between heterogenous cells can induce bursting. When parameter values in a β-cell model (including cell size, channel conductances, Ca^{++} removal rate, metabolic rate, etc.) are distributed among the cells, individual cells may remain silent (*A*), burst (*B*), or spike continuously (*C*) in the presence of glucose. When the exact same cells in *A,B,C* are coupled within a cluster of β-cells (125 cells all together), they burst synchronously (*D,E,F*). The predicted variability in action-potential height from cell to cell within a coupled cluster is observed experimentally. (Reproduced with permission from Smolen P, Rinzel J, Sherman A. Why pancreatic islets burst but single β cells do not. Biophys J 1993;64:1668.)

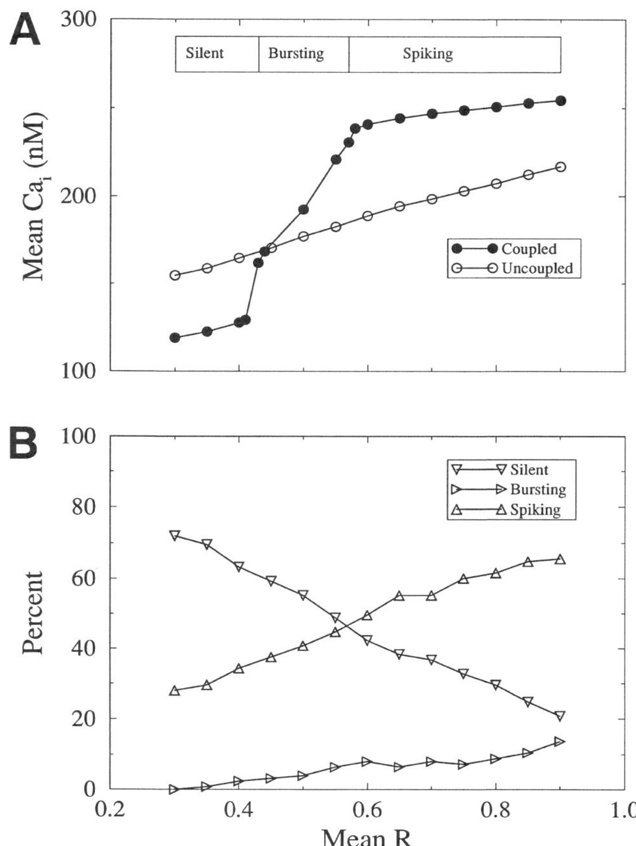

FIGURE 9-38. Mathematic model indicating that coupling may be involved in glucose sensing. *A*, From the model depicted in Figure 9-37, a theoretic prediction of average intercellular calcium level for 125 heterogeneous, uncoupled β-cells as a function of glucose concentration (simulated by a parameter [R] representing metabolic rate) is shown (○). Average intracellular calcium versus glucose level for the same 125 cells coupled by gap junctions with physiologic conductance is also shown (●). Inset in *A* illustrates the predicted electrical activity for the cells in the coupled cluster. The linear response shifts to sigmoidal when the cells are coupled (compare with measured Ca^{++} signals shown in Fig. 9-13*A*). *B*, Percentage of the 125 cells in *A* that, when uncoupled, exhibit continuous spiking or bursting, or are silent, as a function of glucose concentration. The model predicts that only a small percentage of single, isolated cells will burst at a given glucose concentration; this is consistent with experimental observation. (Reproduced with permission from Smolen P, Rinzel J, Sherman A. Why pancreatic islets burst but single β cells do not. Biophys J 1993;64:1668.)

clear threshold for activity (Fig. 9-38*A*, filled circles). Thus the two models (channel sharing and heterogeneity) provide insights into the mechanisms by which intercellular communication can shape glucose responsiveness. The relative importance of each phenomenon, heterogeneity and stochastic noise, awaits experimental determination.

Modulation of Coupling

Gap junction coupling among β-cells is altered by a variety of physiologic and pharmacologic stimuli that also affect islet secretory activity, glucose being the most studied. Long-term exposure to glucose increases the number, but not the size, of gap junctions in freeze-fracture replicas of isolated rat islets,[92] as well as the extent of dye and metabolically coupled domains.[98,99] Short (<10-minute) glucose exposures alter the configuration of gap junctions without changing the number of connexons present.[93] Also, removal of glucose from the perifusion medium causes a rapid cessation of electrical coupling as detected by dual intracellular impalements.[95]

Table 9-1 summarizes the effects of various other stimuli on intercellular communication within the islet.[112–118] Rapid changes in coupling probably reflect direct- or second-messenger–mediated effects on gap-junction channel gating, whereas the change in intercellular communication after a long exposure to some stimuli may result from an alteration in connexin expression. The important information to be gained from Table 9-1 is that coupling is *enhanced* by substances that stimulate or potentiate insulin secretion and *blocked* by inhibitors of secretion. The coupling changes brought about by these stimuli may play a role in the altered secretory activity or simply may be a consequence of the latter. Nevertheless, the strong correlation between changes in intercellular communication and secretory activity, along with the differing behavior between whole islets and isolated cells, hints strongly that the two phenomena are causally related.

TABLE 9-1. Modulation of Cell-to-Cell Coupling in the Islet of Langerhans*

Stimulus	Gap Junction Morphology: Number	Gap Junction Morphology: Size	Gap Junction Morphology: Change Config.	Dye Spread	Electrical Coupling
Glucose	↑ [92,113]	–[92]	↑* [93]	↑ [98,99]	↑* [95]
Glyburide	↑ [92,114]	↑ [92,114]		↑ [101,114]	↑ [96,102]
cAMP	↑ [115]	↑ [115]	↑ [115]	↑ [100]	↑*[21,106]–*[105]
TEA		↑ [116]			
Prolactin				↑ [117]	
A23187				↑* [100]	
Somatostatin				↓ [100]	
Heptanol				↓* [118]	↓* [102,105]

*Arrows pointing upward indicate enhanced coupling; and downward arrows show inhibited coupling. Horizontal lines represent no effect on intercellular communication, and blank squares indicate no result reported. The asterisk indicates a rapid effect (observed within minutes of application of the stimulus).

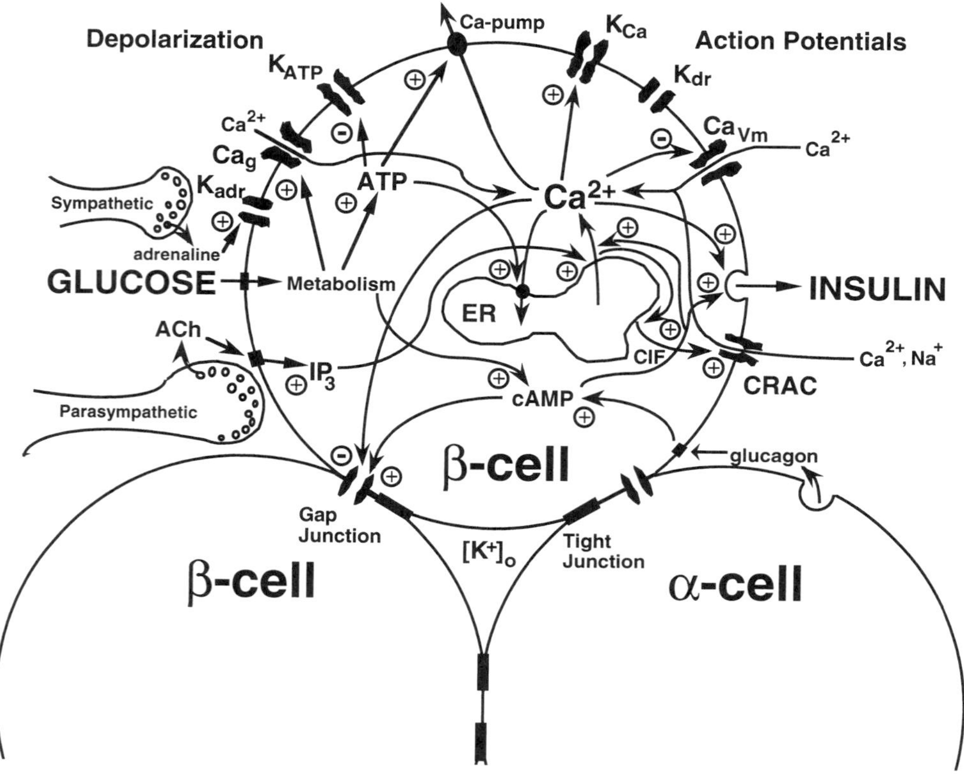

FIGURE 9-39. Composite model of the β-cell, showing the complex physiologic interactions involved in stimulus-secretion coupling. Figure identifies processes related to metabolism, action potential generation, intracellular calcium, cAMP, muscarinic stimulation, adrenergic stimulation, and cell-to-cell coupling.

Conclusions

Glucose-induced insulin secretion is critically dependent on the production of β-cell electrical activity, which results in the intracellular Ca^{++} accumulations necessary to promote exocytosis. Figure 9-39 illustrates the complexity of the interactions among extracellular stimuli (physiologic and pharmacologic signals), intracellular processes (metabolism and second-messenger generation), and membrane events (ionic current flow) that are involved in the generation of β-cell electrical activity. Together, these interactions form an exquisitely sensitive cellular glucose sensor that can be further regulated in times of physiologic need. Although most of the major players involved in the transduction of the glucose signal to electrical events have been identified, questions remain as to which channels are involved in controlling and modulating burst duration, the mechanisms of ion channel regulation at the molecular level, and the role of defects in electrical responsiveness in the pathogenesis of insulin secretory disorders. The application of powerful molecular biologic techniques, such as gene knockout and gene transfer, to the study of β-cell ion channels should answer many of these questions.

Acknowledgments

The authors thank Dr. Patricia Carroll, Dr. Rosa Santos, Dr. Arthur Sherman, and Dr. Richard Bertram for providing figures and sharing unpublished observations. Research was supported in part by a Presidential Young Investigator Award, National Science Foundation, (ECS-9058419) to Dr. Norman F. Sheppard, Jr., from the Department of Biomedical Engineering, Johns Hopkins University, Baltimore, MD, and The Greenwall Foundation, New York, NY. (D.M.).

References

1. Henquin JC, Meissner, HP. Significance of ionic fluxes and changes in membrane potential for stimulus-secretion coupling in pancreatic B-cells. Experientia 1984;40:1043
2. Atwater I, Ribalet B, Rojas E. Cyclic changes in potential and resistance of the β-cell membrane induced by glucose in islets of Langerhans from mouse. J Physiol 1978;278:117
3. Meissner HP. Membrane potential measurements in pancreatic β cells with intracellular microelectrodes. Methods Enzymol 1990;192:235
4. Meissner HP, Schmeltz H. Membrane potential of beta-cells in pancreatic islets. Pflugers Arch 1974;351:195
5. Meissner HP, Atwater I. The kinetics of electrical activity of beta cells in response to a 'square wave' stimulation with glucose or glibenclamide. Horm Metab Res 1976;8:11
6. Atwater I, Beigelman PM. Dynamic characteristics of electrical activity in pancreatic β-Cells. J Physiol (Paris) 1976;72:769
7. Bertram R, Smolen P, Sherman A, et al. A role for calcium release-activated current (CRAC) in cholinergic modulation of electrical activity in pancreatic β-cells. Biophys J 1995;68:2323
8. Atwater I, Carroll P, Li MX. Electrophysiology of the pancreatic B-cell. In: Draznin B, Melmed S, LeRoith D, eds. Molecular and Cellular Biology of Diabetes Mellitus. New York, NY: Alan R. Liss;1989:49–68
9. Falke LC, Gillis KD, Pressel DM, Misler S. Perforated patch recording allows long-term monitoring of metabolite-induced electrical activity and voltage-dependent Ca^{++} currents in pancreatic B cells. FEBS Lett 1989;251:167
10. Rojas E, Hidalgo J, Carroll PB, Atwater I. A new class of calcium channels activated by glucose in human pancreatic β-cells. FEBS Lett 1990;261:265
11. Dean PM, Matthews EK. Glucose-induced electrical activity in pancreatic islet cells. J Physiol 1970;210:255
12. Dean PM, Matthews EK, Sakamoto Y. Pancreatic islet cells: Effects of monosaccharides, glycolytic intermediates and metabolic inhibitors on membrane potential and electrical activity. J Physiol (Lond.) 1975;246:459
13. Henquin JC, Meissner HP. Opposite effects of tolbutamide and diazoxide on $^{86}Rb^{+}$ fluxes and membrane potential in pancreatic β-cells. Biochem Pharmacol 1982;31:1407
14. Malaisse WJ, Boschero AC. Calcium antagonists and islet function. XI. Effect of nifedipine. Horm Res 1977;8:203
15. Wollheim CB, Sharp GWG. Regulation of insulin release by calcium. Physiol Rev 1981;61:914
16. Gagerman E, Idahl LA, Meissner HP, Täljedal IB. Insulin release, cGMP, cAMP, and membrane potential in acetylcholine-stimulated islets. Am J Physiol 1978;4:E493
17. Santos RM, Rojas E. Muscarinic receptor modulation of glucose-induced electrical activity in mouse pancreatic β-cells. FEBS Lett 1989;249:411
18. Rojas E, Santos RM, Atwater I. Role of membrane receptors in stimulus-secretion coupling. In: Hidalgo C, Bacigalupo J, Jaimovich E, Vergara J, eds. Transduction in Biological Systems. New York, NY: Plenum Press; 1990:101–122
19. Boschero AC, Szpak-Glasman M, Carneiro EM, et al. Oxotremorin-m potentiation of glucose-induced insulin release from rat islets involves M_3 muscarinic receptors. Am J Physiol 1995;268:E336
20. Sharp GWG. The adenylate cyclase-cyclic AMP system in islets of Langerhans and its role in the control of insulin release. Diabetologia 1979;16:287
21. Santos RM, Rojas E. Evidence for modulation of cell-to-cell electrical coupling by cAMP in mouse islets of Langerhans. FEBS Lett 1987;220:342
22. Prentki M, Matschinsky FM. Coupling mechanisms in insulin secretion. Physiol Rev 1987;67:1185
23. Efendic S, Luft R, Grill V. Effect of somatostatin on glucose induced insulin release in isolated perfused rat pancreas and isolated rat pancreatic islets. FEBS Lett 1974;42:169
24. Pace CS, Tarvin JT. Somatostatin: Mechanism of action in pancreatic islet beta-cells. Diabetes 1981;30:836
25. Scott AM, Atwater I, Rojas E. A method for the simultaneous measurement of insulin release and B cell membrane potential in single mouse islets of Langerhans. Diabetologia 1981;21:470
26. Atwater I, Goncalves A, Herchuelz A, et al. Cooling dissociates glucose-induced insulin release from electrical activity and cation fluxes in rodent pancreatic islets. J Physiol 1984;348:615
27. Rosario LM, Atwater I, Scott AM. Pulsatile insulin release and electrical activity from single *ob/ob* mouse islets of Langerhans. Adv Exp Med Biol 1985;211:413
28. Dean PM, Matthews EK. Electrical activity in pancreatic islet cells: Effect of ions. J Physiol 1970;210:265
29. Curry DL, Bennett LL, Grodsky GM. Dynamics of insulin secretion by the perfused rat pancreas. Endocrinology 1968;83:572
30. Santos RM, Rosario LM, Nadel A, et al. Widespread synchronous $[Ca^{++}]_i$ oscillations due to bursting electrical activity in single pancreatic islets. Pflugers Arch 1991;418:417
31. Gilon P, Shepherd RM, Henquin JC. Oscillations of secretion driven by oscillations of cytoplasmic Ca^{++} as evidenced in single pancreatic islets. J Biol Chem 1993;268:22265
32. Santana de Sa S, Ferrer R, Rojas E, Atwater I. Effects of adrenaline and noradrenaline on glucose-induced electrical activity of mouse pancreatic β-cell. Q J Physiol 1983;68:247
33. Ämmälä C, Eliasson L, Bokvist K, et al. Activation of protein kinases and inhibition of protein phosphotases play a central role in the regulation of exocytosis in mouse pancreatic β cells. Proc Natl Acad Sci U S A 1994; 91:4343
34. Rojas E, Carroll PB, Ricordi C, et al. Control of cytosolic free calcium in cultured human pancreatic β-cells occurs by external calcium-dependent and independent mechanisms. Endocrinology 1994;134:1771
35. Henquin JC, Garcia MC, Bozem M, et al. Muscarinic control of pancreatic β cell function involves sodium-dependent depolarization and calcium influx. Endocrinology 1988;122:2134
36. Atwater I, Kukuljan M, Pérez-Armendariz EM. Molecular biology of the ion channels in the pancreatic β-cell. In: Draznin B, LeRoith D, eds. Molecular Biology of Diabetes, Part I. Totowa, NJ: Humana Press;1994:303–331
37. Dean PM, Matthews EK. Electrical activity in pancreatic islet cells. Nature 1968;219:389
38. Hutton JC, Sener A, Herchuelz A, et al. Similarities in the stimulus-secretion coupling mechanisms of glucose and 2-keto acid-induced insulin release. Endocrinology 1980;106:203
39. Atwater I. Control mechanisms for glucose-induced changes in the membrane potential of mouse pancreatic B-cell. Cienc Biol (Portugal) 1980;5:299
40. Ferrer R, Atwater I, Omer EM, et al. Electrophysiological evidence for inhibition of potassium permeability in pancreatic β-cells by glibenclamide. Q J Exp Physiol 1984;69:831
41. Sehlin J, Täljedal IB. Glucose-induced decrease in Rb^{+} permeability in pancreatic β-cells. Nature 1975;253:635
42. Henquin JC. D-glucose inhibits potassium efflux from pancreatic islet cells. Nature 1978;271:271
43. Ashcroft FM, Harrison DE, Ashcroft SJH. Glucose induces closure of single potassium channels in isolated rat pancreatic β-cells. Nature 1984;312:446
44. Cook DL, Hales CN. Intracellular ATP directly blocks K^{+}-channels in pancreatic B-cells. Nature 1984;311:269
45. Ashcroft FM. Adenosine-triphosphate sensitive K^{+}-channels. Ann Rev Neurosci 1988;11:97
46. Rojas E, Stokes CL, Mears D, Atwater I. Single microelectrode voltage clamp measurements of pancreatic β-cell membrane ionic currents *in situ*. J Membr Biol 1995;143:65
47. Carroll PB, Li MX, Rojas E, Atwater I. The ATP-sensitive potassium channel in pancreatic B-cells is inhibited by physiological bicarbonate buffer. FEBS Lett 1988;234:208
48. Schmid-Antomarchi H, de Weille J, Fosset M, Lazdunski M. The receptor for antidiabetic sulphonylureas controls the activity of the ATP-modulated K^{+} channel in insulin-secreting cells. J Biol Chem 1987;262:15840
49. Takano M, Ashcroft FM. Effects of internal chloride on ATP-sensitive K-channels in mouse pancreatic β-cells. Pflugers Arch 1994;428:194
50. Sturgess NC, Ashford MLJ, Cook DL, Hales CN. The sulphonylurea receptor may be an ATP-sensitive potassium channel. Lancet 1985;8453:474
51. Trube G, Rorsman P, Ohno-Shosaku T. Opposite effects of tolbutamide and diazoxide on the ATP-dependent K^{+}-channel in pancreatic β-cells. Pflugers Arch 1986;407:493
52. Boschero AC, Tombaccini D, Carneiro EM, Atwater IJ. Differences in K^{+} permeability between cultured adult and neonatal rat islets of Langerhans in response to glucose, tolbutamide, diazoxide, and theophylline. Pancreas 1993;8:44
53. Chan KW, Sui J, Ladias JAA, Logothetis DE. Cloning and functional expression of human pancreatic and brain ATP-sensitive potassium channels. Biophys J 1995;68:A353
54. Ho K, Nichols CG, Lederer WJ, et al. Cloning and expression of an inwardly-rectifying ATP-regulated potassium channel. Nature 1993;362:31
55. Ashcroft SJH, Ashcroft FM. The sulphonylurea receptor. Biochem Biophys Acta 1992;1175:45
56. Pérez-Armendariz E, Atwater I. Glucose-evoked changes in $[K^{+}]$ and $[Ca^{++}]$ in the intercellular spaces of the mouse islet of Langerhans. In: Atwater I, Rojas E, Soria B, eds. Biophysics of the Pancreatic β-Cell. New York, NY: Plenum Press;1986:31–51
57. Atwater I, Dawson CM, Eddlestone GT, Rojas E. Voltage noise measurements across the pancreatic β-cell membrane: Calcium channel characteristics. J Physiol 1981;314:195
58. Rorsman P, Ashcroft FM, Trube G. Single Ca channel currents in mouse pancreatic β-cells. Pflugers Arch 1988;412:597
59. Rorsman P, Trube G. Calcium and delayed potassium currents in mouse pancreatic β-cells under voltage-clamp conditions. J Physiol (Lond.) 1986; 374:531
60. Plant TD. Properties and calcium-dependent inactivation of calcium currents in cultured mouse pancreatic B-cells. J Physiol 1988;404:731
61. Satin LS, Cook DL. Calcium current inactivation in insulin-secreting cells is mediated by calcium influx and membrane depolarization. Pflugers Arch 1989;414:1
62. Satin LS, Cook DL. Evidence for two calcium currents in insulin-secreting cells. Pflugers Arch 1988;411:401
63. Ashcroft FA, Rorsman P. Electrophysiology of the pancreatic β-cell. Prog Biophys Mol Biol 1989;54:87
64. Ämmälä C, Ashcroft FM, Rorsman P. Calcium-independent potentiation of insulin release by cyclic AMP in single β-cells. Nature 1993;363:356
65. Cook DL, Ikeuchi M, Fujimoto WY. Lowering of pH_i inhibits Ca^{++}-activated K^{+}-channels in pancreatic β-cells. Nature 1984;311:269
66. Kukulijan M, Goncalves AA, Atwater I. Charybdotoxin-sensitive K(Ca) chan-

nel is not involved in glucose-induced electrical activity in pancreatic β-cells. J Membr Biol 1991;119:187
67. Lebrun P, Atwater I, Claret M, et al. Resistance to apamin of the Ca^{++}-activated K^+ permeability in pancreatic B-cells. FEBS Lett 1983;161:41
68. Ämmälä C, Bokvist K, Larsson O, et al. Demonstration of a novel apamin-insensitive calcium-activated K^+ channel in mouse pancreatic β cells. Pflugers Arch 1993;422:443
69. Takemura H, Hughes AR, Thastrup O, Putney JJW. Activation of calcium entry by the tumor promoter thapsigargin in parotid acinar cells. J Biol Chem 1989;264:12266
70. Putney JW. Capacitive calcium entry revisited. Cell Calcium 1990;11:611
71. Randriamampita C, Tsien RY. Emptying of intracellular Ca^{++} stores releases a novel small messenger that stimulates Ca^{++} influx. Nature 1993;364:809
72. Worley III JF, McIntyre B, Spencer B, et al. Endoplasmic reticulum calcium store regulates membrane potential in mouse islet β-cells. J Biol Chem 1994;269:14359
73. Xu L, Stokes CL. Regulation of intracellular Ca^{++} by cAMP in the pancreatic β-cell. Biophys J 1995;68:A394
74. Gilon P, Henquin JC. Activation of muscarinic receptors increases the concentration of free Na^+ in mouse pancreatic B-cells. FEBS Lett 1993;315:353
75. Leech CA, Holtz IV GG, Habener JF. Voltage-independent calcium channels mediate slow oscillations of cytosolic calcium that are glucose dependent in pancreatic β-cells. Endocrinology 1994;135:365
76. Rorsman P, Bokvist K, Ämmälä C, et al. Activation by adrenaline of a low-conductance G protein-dependent K^+ channel in mouse pancreatic β-cells. Nature 1991;349:77
77. Sherman A. Theoretical aspects of synchronized bursting in β-cells. In: Huizinga JD, ed. Pacemaker Activity and Intercellular Communication. Boca Raton, Fla: CRC Press;1995:323–337
78. Ribalet B, Beigelman PM. Cyclic variation of K^+ conductance in pancreatic β-cells: Ca^{++} and voltage dependence. Am J Physiol 1979;237:C137
79. Meissner HP, Preissler M, Henquin JC. Possible ionic mechanisms of electrical activity induced by glucose and tolbutamide in pancreatic β-cells. In: Waldhausl WK, ed. Diabetes 1979. Amsterdam: Excerpta Medica; 1980:166–171
80. Dawson CM, Atwater I, Rojas E. The response of pancreatic β-cell membrane potential to potassium-induced calcium influx in the presence of glucose. Q J Exp Physiol 1984;69:819
81. Smolen P, Keizer J. Slow voltage inactivation of Ca^{++} currents and bursting mechanisms for the mouse pancreatic beta-cell. J Membr Biol 1992;127:9
82. Halban PA, Wollheim CB, Blondel B, et al. The possible importance of contact between pancreatic islet cells for the control of insulin release. Endocrinology 1982;111:86
83. Pipeleers D, in't Veld P, Maes E, Van De Winkel M. Glucose-induced insulin release depends on functional cooperation between islet cells. Proc Natl Acad Sci U S A 1982;79:7322
84. Smith PA, Ashcroft FM, Rorsman P. Simultaneous recordings of glucose dependent electrical activity and ATP-regulated K^+-currents in isolated mouse pancreatic β-cells. FEBS Lett 1990;261:187
85. Grapengiesser E, Gylfe E, Hellman B. Ca^{++} oscillations in pancreatic β-cells exposed to leucine and arginine. Acta Physiol Scand 1989;136:113
86. Perez-Armendariz EM, Atwater I, Bennett MVL. Mechanisms for fast intercellular communication within a single islet of Langerhans. In: Huizinga JD, ed. Pacemaker Activity and Intercellular Communication. Boca Raton, Fla: CRC Press;1995:305–321
87. Orci L, Unger RH, Renold AE. Structural coupling between pancreatic islet cells. Experientia 1973;29:1015
88. Orci L, Malaisse-Lagae F, Ravazzola M, et al. A morphological basis for intracellular communication between A- and B-cells in the endocrine pancreas. J Clin Invest 1975;56:1066
89. Meda P, Denef J-F, Perrelet A, Orci L. Non-random distribution of gap junctions between pancreatic β-cells. Am J Physiol 1980;238:C114
90. Meda P, Chanson M, Pepper M, et al. *In vivo* modulation of connexin 43 gene expression and junctional coupling of pancreatic B-cells. Exp Cell Res 1991;192:469
91. Meda P, Pepper MS, Traub O, et al. Differential expression of gap junction connexins in endocrine and exocrine glands. Endocrinology 1993;133:2371
92. Meda P, Perrelet A, Orci L. Increase of gap junctions between pancreatic B-cells during stimulation of insulin secretion. J Cell Biol 1979;82:441
93. in't Veld PA, Pipeleers DG, Gepts W. Glucose alters configuration of gap junctions between pancreatic islet cells. Am J Physiol 1986;251:C191
94. Meissner HP. Electrophysiological evidence for coupling between β cells of pancreatic islets. Nature 1976;262:502
95. Eddlestone GT, Goncalves A, Bangham JA, Rojas E. Electrical coupling between cells in islets of Langerhans from mouse. J Membr Biol 1984;77:1
96. Meda P, Atwater I, Goncalves A, et al. The topography of electrical synchrony among β-cells in the mouse islet of Langerhans. Q J Exp Physiol 1984;69:719
97. Valdeolmillos M, Nadal A, Soria B, Garcia-Sancho J. Fluorescence digital image analysis of glucose-induced $[Ca^{++}]_i$ oscillations in mouse pancreatic islets of Langerhans. Diabetes 1993;42:1210
98. Kohen E, Kohen C, Thorell B. Intercellular communication in pancreatic islet monolayer cultures: A microfluorometric study. Science 1979;204:862
99. Michaels RL, Sheridan JD. Islets of Langerhans: Dye coupling among immunocytochemically distinct cell types. Science 1981;214:801
100. Kohen E, Kohen C, Rabinovitch A. Cell-to-cell communication in rat pancreatic islet monolayer cultures is modulated by agents affecting islet-cell secretory activity. Diabetes 1983;32:95
101. Meda P, Santos RM, Atwater I. Direct identification of electrophysiologically monitored cells within intact mouse islets of Langerhans. Diabetes 1986;35:232
102. Meda P. Junctional coupling modulation by secretagogues in two-cell pancreatic systems. In Peracchia C, ed. Biophysics of Gap Junction Channels. Boca Raton, Fla: CRC Press;1991:191–208
103. Meda P, Perrelet A, Orci L. Endocrine cell interactions in the islets of Langerhans. In: Pitts JD, Finbow ME, eds. The Functional Integration of Cells in Animal Tissues. London: Cambridge University Press;1982:195
104. Meda P. Gap junctional coupling and secretion in endocrine and exocrine pancreas. In: Sperelakis N, Cole WC, eds. Cell Interactions and Gap Junctions. Boca Raton, Fla: CRC Press;1989:59–83
105. Pérez-Armendariz M, Roy C, Spray DC, Bennett MVL. Biophysical properties of gap junctions between freshly dispersed pairs of mouse pancreatic beta cells. Biophys J 1991;59:76
106. Mears D, Sheppard NF Jr, Atwater I, Rojas E. Magnitude and modulation of pancreatic β-cell gap junction electrical conductance *in situ*. J Membr Biol 1995;146:163
107. Stokes CL, Rinzel J. Diffusion of extracellular K^+ can synchronize bursting oscillations in a model islet of Langerhans. Biophys J 1993;65:597
108. Atwater I, Rosario L, Rojas E. Properties of the Ca-activated K^+ channel in pancreatic β-cells. Cell Calcium 1983;4:451
109. Chay TR, Kang HS. Role of single-channel stochastic noise on bursting clusters of pancreatic β-cells. Biophys J 1988;54:427
110. Sherman A, Rinzel J, Keizer J. Emergence of organized bursting in clusters of pancreatic B-cells by channel sharing. Biophys J 1988;54:411
111. Sherman A, Rinzel J. Model for synchronization of pancreatic B-cells by gap junction coupling. Biophys J 1991;59:547
112. Smolen P, Rinzel J, Sherman A. Why pancreatic islets burst but single β cells do not. Biophys J 1993;64:1668
113. Meda P, Halban P, Perrelet A, et al. Gap junction development is correlated with insulin content in the pancreatic B-cell. Science 1980;209:1026
114. Meda P, Michaels RL, Halban PA, et al. In vivo modulation of gap junctions and dye coupling between B-cells of the intact pancreatic islet. Diabetes 1983;32:858
115. in't Veld P, Schuit F, Pipeleers D. Gap junctions between pancreatic B-cells are modulated by cyclic AMP. Eur J Cell Biol 1985;36:269
116. Sheppard MS, Meda P. Tetraethylammonium modifies gap junctions between pancreatic β-cells. Am J Physiol 1981;240:C116
117. Michaels RL, Sorenson RL, Parsons JA, Sheridan JD. Prolactin enhances cell-to-cell communication among β-cells in pancreatic islets. Diabetes 1987;36:1098
118. Meda P, Bosco D, Chanson M, et al. Rapid and reversible secretion changes during uncoupling of rat insulin-producing cells. J Clin Invest 1990;86:759

Diabetes Mellitus, edited by Derek LeRoith, Simeon I. Taylor, and Jerrold M. Olefsky. Lippincott–Raven Publishers, Philadelphia © 1996.

Chapter 10

Detrimental Effects of Chronic Hyperglycemia on the Pancreatic β-Cell

Jack L. Leahy

Introduction

The plasma glucose level acting through a negative feedback loop regulates insulin secretion directly and modulates insulin output from the large number of hormones, nutrients, and neurotransmitters that stimulate insulin secretion (''nonglucose secretagogues'').[1] Key to each of these systems is their high sensitivity, so that small degrees of hypo- or hyperglycemia result in altered insulin release. Over a slightly longer time frame, the biosynthesis of proinsulin, also one of the enzymes used in proinsulin to insulin conversion, is glucose-regulated. More chronically, the β-cell replication rate is glucose-responsive. Thus, the plasma glucose level regulates insulin secretion at multiple sites. Moreover, an exquisitely sensitive, coordinated regulation of insulin synthesis and secretion has for many years been the basis for our understanding of the glucose homeostasis system—how β-cells minimize or prevent abnormal levels of glycemia through adaptive changes in insulin output.

Beginning 15 years ago, a new element was added with the discovery that long-term hyperglycemia is paradoxically harmful to this adaptive system, an idea with important ramifications for human diabetes.[2,3] Best known is the impaired glucostimulatory effect on insulin secretion; the term *glucose toxicity* was coined in reference to this defect. There is also evidence (although less definitive) for defects in nonglucose–mediated insulin secretion, proinsulin biosynthesis, and the β-cell growth rate. Our belief is that glucose toxicity will eventually be recognized as encompassing multiple defects in β-cell glucoregulation, with the current evidence suggesting multiple rather than a single molecular cause.

Interest in this subject stems from non–insulin-dependent diabetes mellitus (NIDDM), in which substantial numbers of β-cells exist in a hyperglycemic environment. Numerous studies have shown partial to full recovery of glucose-stimulated insulin secretion after intensive treatment of the hyperglycemia,[2] reinforcing the notion that identifying the molecular basis for the β-cell glucose unresponsiveness may provide new therapeutic targets for this disease. Important in this area of research is the recognition that few data have come from humans. Many problems exist for measuring the insulin secretion rate in humans, including variable hepatic clearance, complicated oscillatory patterns of secretion, and variable plasma levels of the biologically inactive precursors of insulin (proinsulin and the conversion intermediates) that cross-react in most insulin assays. Also, experimental hyperglycemia is difficult if not impossible to cause in humans. Finally, the nonavailability of pancreas biopsies is a major impediment that has resulted in virtually no molecular or biochemical information about the insulin secretion defects found in persons with NIDDM. Instead, practically all of the information has come from rodent models with experimental or spontaneous hyperglycemia. On the positive side, the β-cell dysfunction seen in diabetic rodents resembles (often closely) that seen in diabetic humans. On the negative side, enough differences exist in the β-cell dysfunction that there is an ongoing debate regarding the relevance of the animal results to humans. This chapter summarizes what we do and do not know about the detrimental effects of chronic hyperglycemia on the β-cell. A number of reviews on selected aspects of this subject have appeared within the last few years.[2–8]

Ninety Percent Pancreatectomy Rat Model

Numerous hyperglycemic rodent models are in use, and a comprehensive review is beyond the scope of this chapter. However, great consistency across the various models has been observed. This chapter focuses on the one used most extensively in our laboratory, the 90% pancreatectomy rat. Our longstanding interest stems from the many advantages of this model for studies of β-cell function. Most prominent of these is that the β-cells (remaining 10% of the pancreas) are known to be normal. As such, functional changes are directly attributable to the hyperglycemia without the uncertainties that occur with β-cell toxin–induced hyperglycemia and spontaneous diabetes. Also, these rats are only mildly hyperglycemic, with normal to slightly subnormal plasma insulin levels.[9] They gain weight normally and are metabolically stable without the need for special diets or hypoglycemic therapies that might affect the β-cell. Another benefit is that this model has been used in most areas of research in this field, making it possible to construct a relatively comprehensive overview of β-cell (dys)function in these rats. Finally, although it is not pertinent to this review, these rats develop insulin resistance,[10] providing a phenotype of insulin secretion and sensitivity that closely resembles that of NIDDM. As such, a reasonable assumption is that this rat can provide important clues to the metabolic abnormalities that occur in human diabetes.

The surgical technique was adapted by Bonner-Weir from the method of Foglia.[9] The pancreas of 5-week-old rats is gently abraded away from the blood vessels with cotton applicators except for the triangular portion bordered by the common bile duct and the duodenum. Postoperatively, they are fed standard rat chow and tap water ad libitum and gain weight normally. In 4–7 days, basal nonfasting blood glucose values rise 1–2 mM, remaining at this level indefinitely, although a deterioration in glucose tolerance 14 weeks after the surgery has been reported coincident with a fall in proinsulin biosynthesis.[11] Some investigators have reported higher levels of glycemia after a 90% pancreatectomy, which probably represents differences in surgical technique and how much of the pancreas remains. Critical for understanding β-cell function in this model is the recognition that substantial islet and exocrine regeneration follows the 90% pancreatectomy, being evident within 3 days and peaking 7 days after surgery.[12] At 8 weeks, the β-cell mass has grown to 42% of age-matched sham-operated rats, a fourfold increase from the original 10%.[9] As such, when viewing insulin secretion in this model (or in any diabetic rodent model) a critical aspect is the fractional β-cell mass.

Impaired Insulin Secretion

The best-known effect of chronic hyperglycemia on the β-cell is to impair glucose-stimulated insulin secretion. This subject is simplified by knowing the terminology. Figure 10-1 shows insulin secretion measured by the in vitro perfused pancreas in normal rats over a glucose range of 0–27.7 mM (broken line). The relationship between glucose concentration and insulin secretion is sigmoidal: insulin output rises most sharply over the physiologic plasma glucose range (showing how small changes in glycemia alter plasma insulin levels) with the half-maximal response (ED_{50}) at 12–15 mM glucose and the maximum near 25 mM glucose. *Glucose sensitivity* (often termed "set-point for secretion") is defined by the ED_{50} value and is reflected at the lower end of the glucose range. *Glucose responsiveness* refers to the maximal insulin response. A common term in this field, *glucose unresponsiveness,* is a near total loss of the glucose stimulatory effect as defined by a markedly reduced insulin output at the high end of the glucose range. It is important to recognize that glucose sensitivity cannot be assessed under these circumstances because of the flatness of the curve.

Also shown is insulin output in the presence of the amino acid arginine (solid line). The shape of the curve is virtually identical to that of glucose alone, with a similar ED_{50} value. The maximal response is threefold higher than with glucose alone, showing the marked insulinotropic effect of arginine. In contrast, note the absence of the secretagogue effect at low glucose levels. This dependence of the insulin stimulatory effect of most nonglucose stimuli on the background glucose level is called *glucose potentiation.*[1] *Defective glucose potentiation* is practically defined as a lowered insulin response to a nonglucose agent that has been administered at a near maximal glucose concentration.

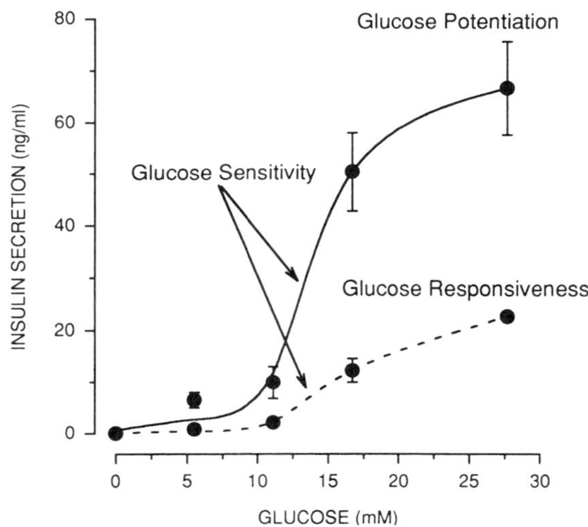

Figure 10-1. Glucose regulation of insulin secretion in the presence (*solid line*) or absence (*broken line*) of 10 mM arginine. Insulin responses to varying levels of glucose were studied in normal rats with the in vitro perfused pancreas. Each point represents the mean effluent insulin concentration from a separate group of rats (n = 3–4).

Selective Glucose Unresponsiveness

Normally, a rise in the plasma glucose level elicits a rapid, biphasic increase in insulin secretion, reflecting direct glucostimulation. Chronic hyperglycemia causes a near total disappearance of this response, an effect first noted in persons with NIDDM given intravenous glucose.[13,14] In contrast, nonglucose stimuli are said to be relatively unaffected, resulting in the term *selective glucose unresponsiveness.* Literally hundreds of studies in vivo in humans and animals and in vitro in diabetic rodents using the perfused pancreas technique have made this observation, although slight differences are found between humans and rodents: only the first phase of glucose-induced insulin secretion is lost in humans, whereas in diabetic rodents, both phases are affected. A typical example from the 90% pancreatectomy rat is shown in Figure 10-2. Insulin output in response to 300 mg/dL glucose (16.7 mM) is virtually absent as opposed to the normal-looking insulin response to the amino acid arginine.

A number of facts have provided seemingly irrefutable evidence for hyperglycemia as the cause of the β-cell glucose unresponsiveness. First, hyperglycemia in both humans and animals, whether it is experimental or spontaneous, is always associated

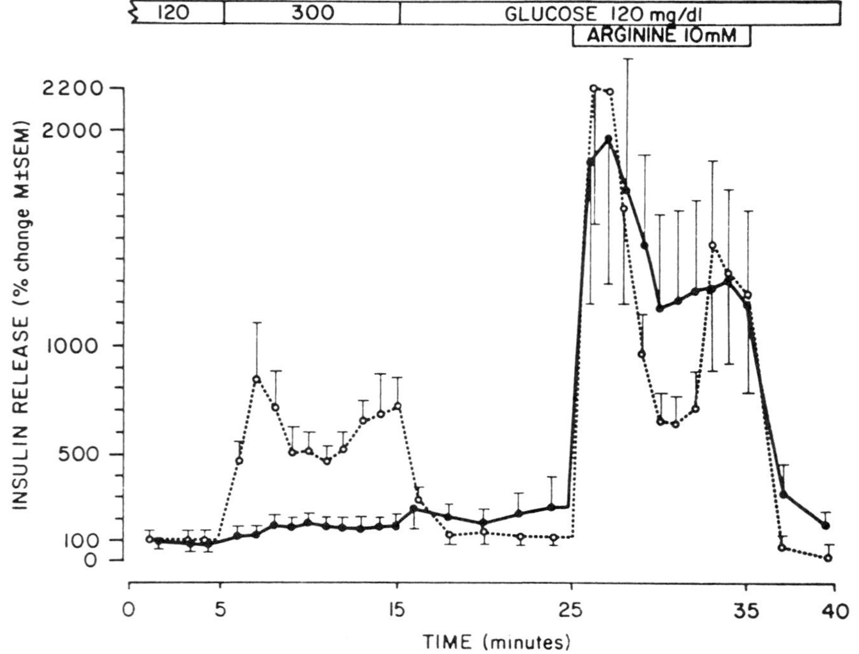

Figure 10-2. Impaired glucose-induced insulin secretion in 90% pancreatectomy rats 8–11 weeks after surgery (*solid line*; n = 9). Data were obtained with the in vitro perfused pancreas. Note there is a brisk response to arginine in these rats, whereas glucose is without effect; this is the classic picture of selective glucose unresponsiveness. Sham-operated control rats (*dashed line*; n = 7) show clear responses to both secretagogues. (Reproduced with permission from Bonner-Weir S, Trent DF, Weir GC. Partial pancreatectomy in the rat and subsequent deficit in glucose-induced insulin release. J Clin Invest 1983;71:1544.)

with this defect. We do not know of even a single contradictory example. Moreover, cross-sectional data in NIDDM have shown that the defect appears after the onset of hyperglycemia.[15] Second, a period of near normalization of blood glucose levels in diabetic humans and animals causes recovery of glucose-induced insulin secretion, establishing the dependence of the defect on hyperglycemia plus its reversibility.[16–18] The rapidity of this reversal effect has been surprising. In 90% pancreatectomy rats that have been hyperglycemic for several weeks, a 6-hour infusion of insulin is sufficient to restore a fourfold rise in insulin output to a high glucose level (16.7 mM).[19] Even more remarkable, Grill showed that perfusing the pancreas of diabetic rats in vitro for 40 minutes with a buffer devoid of glucose causes recovery of glucose-induced insulin secretion,[20] a fact confirmed by many groups in every diabetic model that has been tested. Such rapid recovery is of more than passing interest. Many of the mechanisms described further on that have been postulated for the glucose unresponsiveness are based on reduced cellular levels of a β-cell protein. Rapid recovery is incompatible with this kind of mechanism, since resynthesis cannot occur that fast. However, careful examination of this finding uncovered that only part (the first phase) of glucose-induced insulin secretion recovers with this approach, invalidating this conclusion.[3,21] As such, the recovery time for glucose-induced insulin secretion under optimal conditions is an unanswered question.

Third and most convincing are the results of Rossetti and colleagues showing recovery of glucose-induced insulin secretion in 90% pancreatectomy rats with phloridzin.[22] Phloridzin inhibits renal tubular reabsorption of glucose, restoring normoglycemia through accelerated glycosuria. Of key importance is that plasma insulin levels are unaffected, making phloridzin a specific glucose-lowering agent. The normalization of β-cell glucose responsiveness with phloridzin confirms hyperglycemia as the cause of the secretory defect.

Thus, it is well accepted that chronic hyperglycemia impairs the glucostimulatory effect on insulin secretion. Virtually unrecognized, however, is the converse—that insulin output may not be suppressed appropriately during hypoglycemia—which has important ramifications for NIDDM. This idea has been validated in diabetic rats.[23] Whether the same is true in NIDDM in humans has received surprisingly little attention.

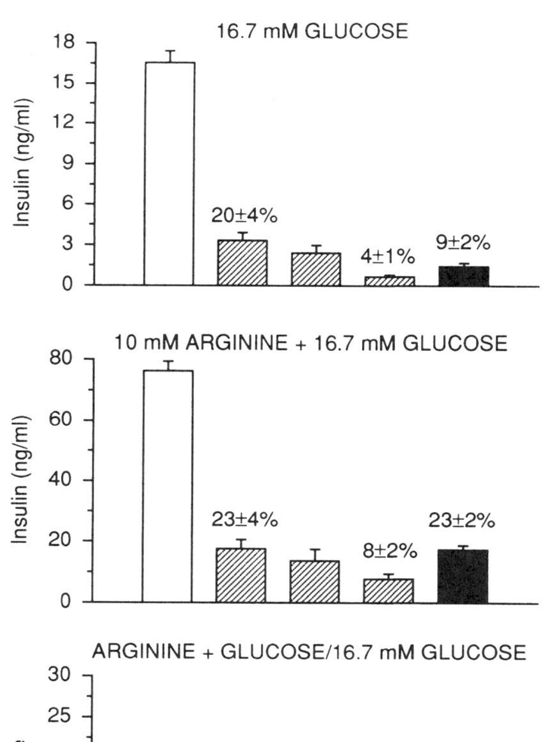

FIGURE 10-3. Natural history of insulin secretion following a 90% pancreatectomy in rats. Insulin secretion in response to 16.7 mM glucose and 16.7 mM glucose/10 mM arginine was assessed with the in vitro perfused pancreas at weekly intervals after a 90% pancreatectomy. The percentage values above the bars are fractional output calculated from the results of the sham-operated control rats (*open bars*). Note the fall in both insulin responses at 3 weeks after surgery, showing the onset of defective glucose responsiveness and glucose potentiation. A 5-day treatment period with diazoxide partially blocked the fall in glucose-induced insulin secretion and normalized that to glucose/arginine (*solid bars*). Data obtained from references 24 and 31.

Other Insulin Secretion Defects

The author and coworkers studied the natural history of insulin secretory responses following a 90% pancreatectomy, looking for insulin secretion defects that precede the glucose unresponsiveness.[24] At 1 week after surgery, insulin responses to 16.7 mM glucose and 16.7 mM glucose/arginine were both normal when adjusted for the lowered mass of β-cells, indicating unimpaired glucose responsiveness and glucose potentiation (Fig. 10-3 shows both to be 20% of normal, which is in keeping with the 90% pancreatectomy). However, the β-cell glucose sensitivity was increased as reflected in lowered ED_{50} values for insulin secretion in response to glucose (5.7 mM glucose versus 16.5 mM glucose in controls) and potentiation of the arginine response (3.5 mM glucose versus 14.8 mM glucose in controls) (Fig. 10-4). This β-cell hypersensitivity to glucose in combination with their hyperglycemia (10.6 ± 0.7 mM versus 8.1 mM in controls, $p<0.001$) caused the β-cells to function near 100% of secretory capacity versus the normal 10–20%. "Left-shifted curves" for glucose-induced insulin secretion and glucose potentiation of nonglucose stimuli have been reported in other diabetic models,[21,25–28] including BB rats, which develop typical autoimmune diabetes.[29] We made the same observation in nondiabetic insulin-resistant[30] and partially pancreatectomized rats.[24] Based on these findings, we view the altered glucose set-point to be an adaptive response that β-cells undergo when faced with an increased demand for insulin output (it magnifies the upregulated insulin secretion). Moreover, as detailed later, the glucose hypersensitivity is an early, necessary step in our model for the mechanism of the glucose unresponsiveness.

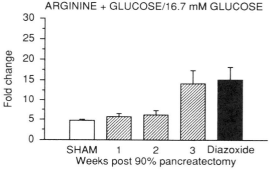

Two weeks after surgery, insulin responses to 16.7 mM glucose and 16.7 mM glucose/arginine were still intact (see Fig. 10-3). However, by 3 weeks the glucose unresponsiveness described above was present, shown by the insulin response to 16.7 mmol glucose falling to 4% of controls (an 80% decrease from 1 week after surgery). Nonglucose stimuli are generally thought to be unaffected by chronic hyperglycemia, and an unexpected finding was that the high glucose/arginine response also fell.[31] The cause was not a loss of β-cells; rather the β-cell mass of the remnant increased during this period because of regeneration.[9,12] Subsequent investigation showed similarly reduced insulin responses at 16.7 mM glucose for the incretin glucagon-like peptide 1 (GLP-1) and the sulfonylurea tolbutamide (Y. A. Hosokawa and J. L. Leahy, unpublished data, 1995), suggesting a global defect in glucose

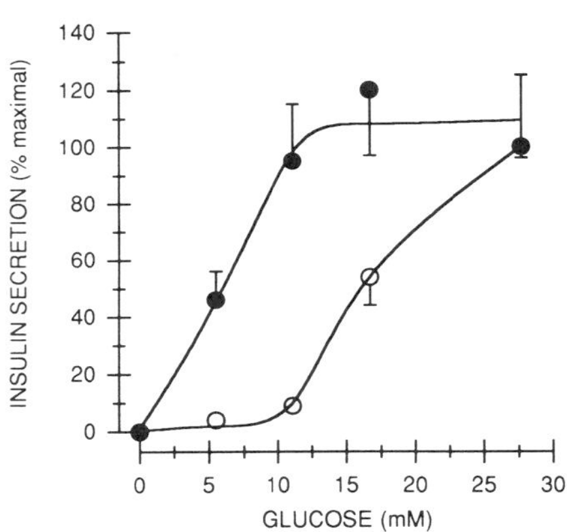

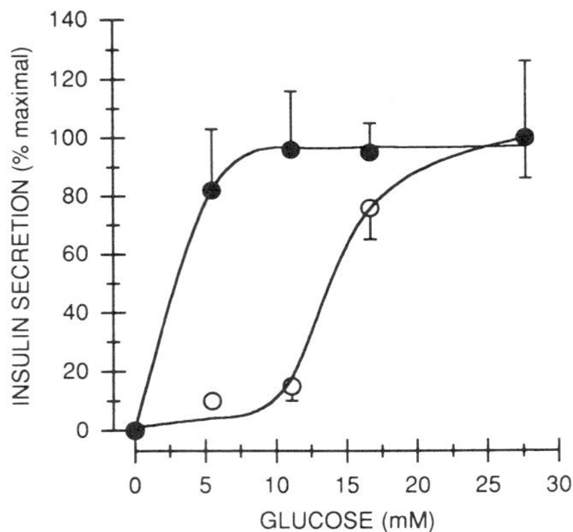

Figure 10-4. Increased β-cell sensitivity to glucose in 90% pancreatectomy rats. Insulin secretion was assessed by the in vitro perfused pancreas in rats 1 week after 90% pancreatectomy (●) or sham-operated control rats (○). Perfusion protocol: 15-minute infusion of 5.5, 11.1, 16.7, or 27.7 mM glucose (*left panel*) followed by another 15 minutes at the same glucose level with the addition of 10 mM arginine (*right panel*). Each point represents the mean effluent insulin concentration from a separate group of rats (n = 3–4). Note that at the usual plasma glucose levels of these rats (10.6 mM glucose in 90% pancreatectomy rats and 8.1 mM glucose in controls), the 90% pancreatectomy β-cells functioned near 100% of secretory capacity versus the normal 10–20%. (Reproduced with permission from Leahy JL, Bumbalo LM, Chen C. Beta-cell hypersensitivity for glucose precedes loss of glucose-induced insulin secretion in 90% pancreatectomized rats. Diabetologia 1993;36:1238.)

potentiation. The presumed cause is hyperglycemia, based on our finding that insulin therapy doubled the insulin secretion to 16.7 mM glucose/arginine in 90% pancreatectomy rats,[19] plus the studies with diazoxide and fasting described below. Additional support would also seem to be the extensive literature showing the same defect in NIDDM.[1,32]

Despite the seemingly clear-cut results in the 90% pancreatectomy rat, hyperglycemia causing defective glucose potentiation is a new concept that requires additional investigation. An important issue is whether hyperglycemia is the cause of the potentiation defect in NIDDM. That question is unanswered because of the dearth of information as to whether intensive blood glucose control reverses this defect in humans. A frequently cited argument against any relationship is finding the same defect in human leukocyte antigen–identical nondiabetic siblings of persons with insulin–dependent diabetes mellitus.[33] Also unanswered is the question of the absence of obviously lowered high glucose/nonglucose insulin responses in some diabetic models.[34,35] Clarification of these issues is important. As shown by the steepness and magnitude of the arginine curve in Figure 10-1, glucose potentiation of nonglucose–mediated insulin secretion is a powerful mechanism for adaptive hyperinsulinemia that far surpasses glucose alone. In theory, intact glucose potentiation would make the impact of the hyperglycemia-induced defect in glucostimulation on overall insulin secretion virtually nil. Instead, the implication of our studies is that "glucose toxicity" is more extensive than previously appreciated, thwarting both adaptive mechanisms for upregulation of insulin secretion.

Reversal Studies

Some of the most valuable tools for investigating hyperglycemia and β-cell function have been hypoglycemic therapies. Numerous studies of NIDDM with diet, sulfonylureas, and insulin have shown partial or complete recovery of glucose-induced insulin secretion.[1,2,16,17] We and others made the same observation using insulin and phloridzin in diabetic rodents.[18,19,22,34] The mechanism of the glucose unresponsiveness is generally assumed to be a direct inhibitory effect of the high glucose level on some critical step in β-cell glucose metabolism, or a second messenger. Also compatible with the experimental findings is that hyperglycemia chronically stimulates insulin secretion, depleting some key substrate, cofactor, nutrient, or other required substance for secretion. This idea is all the more plausible from the data in Figure 10-4 showing that β-cells of 90% pancreatectomy rats function at 90–100% of secretory capacity versus the normal 10–20%. Attempts to differ these two possibilities have been based on inhibitors of insulin secretion, most prominently diazoxide. The theory is that the plasma glucose level is unchanged (or increases) during treatment, allowing a direct effect of hyperglycemia to be differentiated from that caused by overstimulated insulin secretion. Consistent with the latter hypothesis, Sako and Grill reported prevention of the impaired glucose-induced insulin secretion in glucose-infused hyperglycemic rats with diazoxide.[36] In vitro studies implicated a raised β-cell insulin content by diazoxide as the mechanism.[37] Glucose-infused rats are markedly hyperinsulinemic, and the relevance of this finding to the more usual situation of normal to subnormal plasma insulin levels with hyperglycemia was unclear. A subsequent study with diazoxide (2 days) in hypoinsulinemic neonatal streptozocin rats failed to find a clear-cut increase in glucose-induced insulin secretion.[38]

We treated 90% pancreatectomy rats with diazoxide for 5 days, followed by a 36-hour "washout" period.[31] As noted above, insulin secretion defects appear between 2 and 3 weeks after 90% pancreatectomy. Diazoxide reduced the defect in glucose-induced insulin secretion by half and normalized the glucose/arginine response (Figs. 10-3 and 10-5). Accompanying the increased insulin secretion was a 50% elevated pancreatic insulin content.

To further investigate the effects of lowered insulin secretion on subsequent secretory responses, rats 4–6 weeks after 90% pancreatectomy and age-matched controls underwent a 40-hour fast followed by pancreas perfusion using a protocol of 16.7 mM glucose and then 16.7 mM glucose/GLP-1[7–37] (Y. A. Hosokawa and

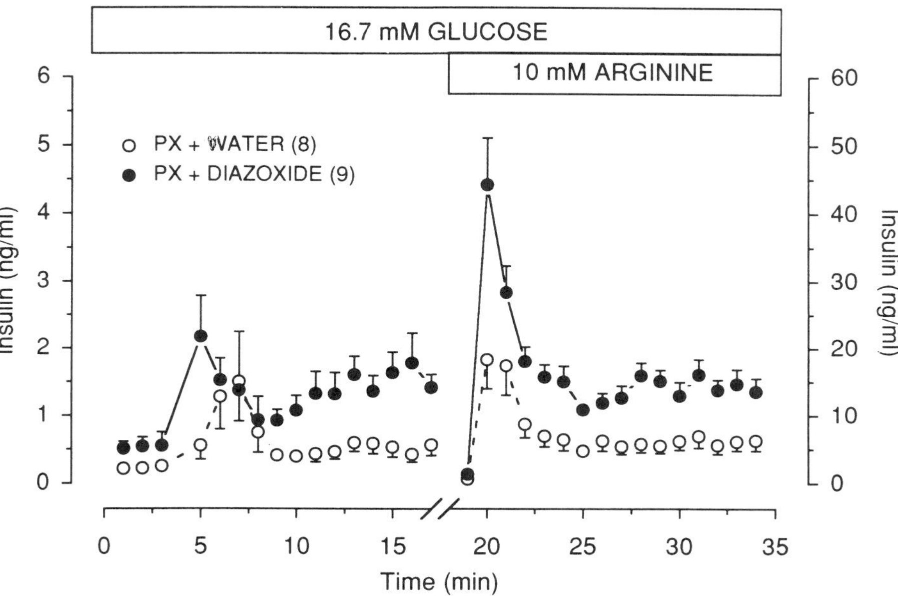

Figure 10-5. Increased insulin secretion in 90% pancreatectomy rats with diazoxide. Diazoxide 30 mg/kg (●-●) or water (○-○) was administered twice daily by gavage tube for 5 days to 90% pancreatectomy rats (Px) that were 3 to 4 weeks after surgery. Insulin secretion was assessed with the in vitro perfused pancreas 36 hours after stopping the diazoxide. Note the separate y axes for insulin responses to 16.7 mM glucose and 16.7 mM glucose/10 mM arginine. (Reproduced with permission from Leahy JL, Bumbalo LM, Chen C. Diazoxide causes recovery of β-cell glucose responsiveness in 90% pancreatectomized diabetic rats. Diabetes 1993; 42:1310.)

J. L. Leahy, unpublished data, 1995). In its role as the primary incretin (incretins are gut peptides released with eating that directly stimulate insulin secretion), GLP-1 is an important physiologic insulin secretagogue. Unfasted 90% pancreatectomy rats had the expected findings: a near total loss of glucose-induced insulin secretion (glucose unresponsiveness), plus insulin output to high glucose/GLP-1 was only 10 ± 2% of the controls, well below the fractional β-cell mass because of regeneration (demonstrating impaired glucose potentiation). Insulin responses normally fall with fasting.[39,40] This effect was noted in the controls (insulin output in response to high glucose levels fell 90%, that to glucose/GLP-1, 60%) in the absence of a change in the pancreatic insulin content. In contrast, in the diabetic rats the insulin response to GLP-1 *rose* threefold, to the level of the control rats, notwithstanding the differences in pancreatic β-cell mass, in association with a tripling of the pancreatic insulin content. This latter result was particularly surprising. When stratified for the reduced β-cell mass, insulin content in the 90% pancreatectomy rats was twice that of the control rats.

Taken together, the diazoxide and fasting studies indicate that maneuvers that reduce insulin secretion and concurrently raise insulin content in 90% pancreatectomy rats result in increased insulin secretory responses, particularly glucose potentiation. These results strongly suggest a causative role for excessive insulin release and/or depleted insulin stores in defective insulin secretion.

Model for Pathogenesis of Hyperglycemia-Induced Insulin Secretion Defects

The model we have developed is based on a cascade of functional changes in β-cells induced by chronic hyperglycemia (Fig. 10-6). First, the glucose sensitivity increases, affecting glucose-induced insulin secretion and glucose potentiation. This results in substantially more insulin output than would be normally expected for mild to moderate hyperglycemia. If normoglycemia is restored, as might occur in the insulin resistance of obesity, the β-cell hypersensitivity to glucose is maintained indefinitely, resulting in the hyperinsulinemia/normoglycemia that clinically defines this state. In contrast, persistent hyperglycemia causes a fall off in insulin output in response to glucose *and* glucose potentiation. The mechanism is speculative, but our data and those of Grill[37] are consistent with lowered pancreatic stores of insulin being the cause of such fall

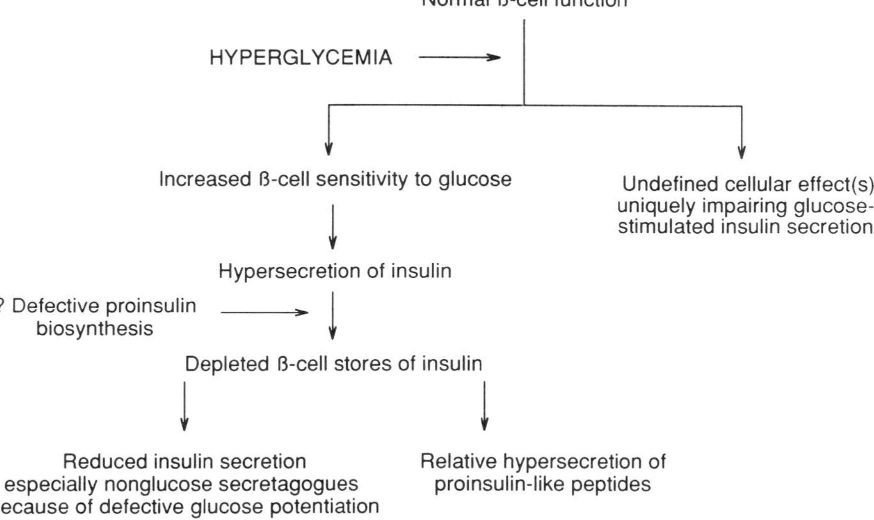

Figure 10-6. Schematic representation of the events that culminate in impaired insulin secretion with chronic hyperglycemia. The sequence is hypothetical and is based on data obtained from animal models, studies conducted in humans, and our own best guesses.

off. Hyperstimulated insulin secretion is clearly an important factor. Whether defective proinsulin biosynthesis also contributes is unclear, since as detailed later the data concerning chronic hyperglycemia leading to reduced insulin synthesis are not definitive. Most important, we view this sequence as explaining only part of the glucose unresponsiveness in terms of glucose-induced insulin secretion (Fig. 10-6), since diazoxide caused only partial recovery of glucose-induced insulin secretion in the 90% pancreatectomy rats.[31] Moreover, as shown in Figure 10-3, the fall in glucose-induced insulin secretion at 3 weeks was proportionately considerably higher than that for high glucose/arginine, causing the fold value for these two measurements to more than double. The increased insulin secretion with diazoxide was not accompanied by any improvement in this measurement, suggesting the presence of two independent defects. We interpret these findings as showing that a combination of defects causes the lost glucostimulatory effect: excessive insulin secretion (diazoxide-responsive element) *and* the "classic" method for glucose toxicity of a direct cellular effect of the high glucose level (diazoxide-unresponsive element). This idea contrasts with that of defective glucose potentiation, which we view as being totally based on overstimulated insulin secretion as reflected in the normalizing of the insulin response to high glucose/arginine by administration of diazoxide.[31]

Mechanism for Direct Cellular Effect of Hyperglycemia on the β-Cell

The last several years have seen the unraveling of the major intracellular steps for glucose-stimulated insulin secretion (Fig. 10-7). Glucose enters the β-cell through a high K_m glucose transporter (GLUT-2), is phosphorylated by glucokinase, and then undergoes glycolysis and oxidation. An offshoot of this process, probably rising ATP/ADP levels, closes the ATP-sensitive K^+ channel, leading to cellular depolarization, opening of the voltage-dependent Ca^{++} channel, and an influx of Ca^{++}. The rise in intracellular Ca^{++}, along with second messengers such as fatty acid metabolites, cAMP, and breakdown of membrane lipids, leads to mobilization of intracellular stores of Ca^{++}, phosphorylation of β-cell proteins, and granule extrusion. Paralleling this information has been extensive investigation of the cellular etiology of why, with chronic hyperglycemia, glucose fails to stimulate insulin secretion. Unfortunately, findings in this area are without consensus. The major problem is the lack of in vitro models that reproduce the profound lack of glucose-induced insulin secretion that is seen in vivo. β-cell biochemical and molecular studies are performed on purified islet tissue so that cellular characteristics can be identified separately from the pancreatic acinar cells. Unfortunately, isolated islets from diabetic rats have been a major disappointment in that glucose-induced insulin secretion is reduced to only a minor extent compared with the in vivo state.[41–43] A typical example is the study by Portha and associates using isolated islets from neonatal streptozocin rats[43]; the fold increase in insulin secretion at 16.7 mmol glucose versus 2.8 mM glucose was 5 in the diabetic islets and 6.6 in control islets. Although statistically different, this minor defect is in marked contrast to the near total absence of glucose-induced insulin secretion in these same rats with the in vitro perfused pancreas.[18] This dichotomy is presumed to reflect the rapid reversibility of this defect. An exception is the spontaneously diabetic GK rat, which is being studied by many groups. GK islets have a profound loss of glucose-induced insulin secretion, which presumably reflects a genetic defect or defects somewhere in the β-cell.[44] An important corollary is that GK islets cannot be expected to teach us much about acquired defects in β-cell function. For models other than the GK rat, this reversal problem has meant that β-cells are studied that *for the most part are without the functional defect*. This fact has not stopped many groups from investigating islets from diabetic rodents and reporting defects at multiple sites. Although seemingly obvious, the minimal nature of the functional defect raises troubling questions about the relevance of the reported biochemical findings. Another limitation of the islet studies is that few have critically measured β-cell mass and β-cell versus non–β-cell proportions in order to exclude functional changes on that basis. Thus, extreme caution must be exercised when reviewing isolated islet studies. An alternate approach is culture of normal islets under conditions of high glucose concentration. Unfortunately, again the secretion defects do not replicate those found in vivo. A short-term exposure to high glucose levels (a few hours) has been reported to cause β-cell glucose desensitization.[45,46] However, the relevance to in vivo secretion defects, which evolve over much longer time periods, is unclear.[47] A potentially interesting model based on a 4–7 day culture period was reported by Xia and Laychock,[48] but additional experience with it is needed. Notwithstanding the limitations of the in vitro models, a number of hypotheses for the β-cell glucose unresponsiveness have been investigated.

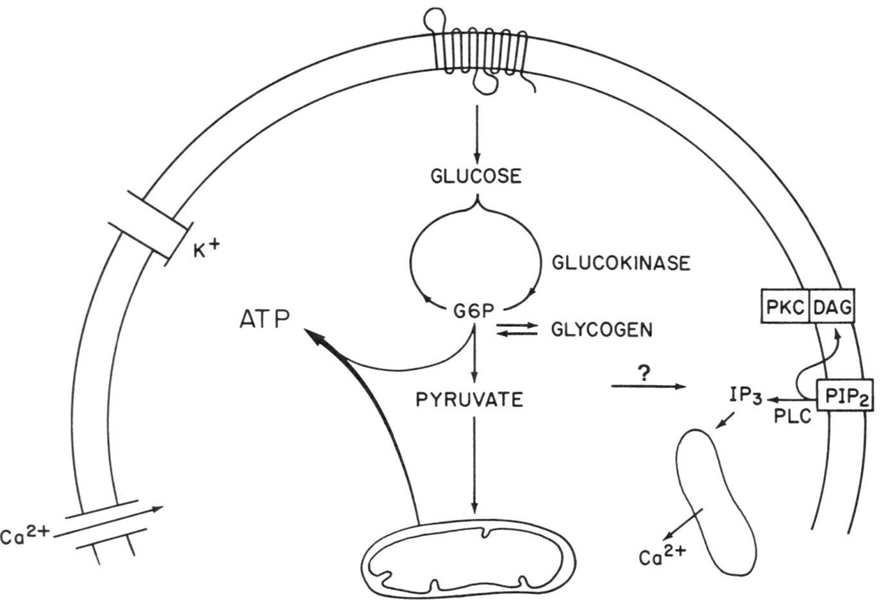

Figure 10-7. Schematic representation of the major intracellular steps that lead to glucose-induced insulin secretion. Glucose enters the β-cell through a high K_m glucose transporter (GLUT-2). It is phosphorylated by glucokinase and then undergoes metabolism and oxidation to CO_2 and H_2O. An offshoot of this process, likely a rising [ATP]/[ADP] ratio, closes the ATP-sensitive K^+ channel leading to cellular depolarization, opening of the voltage-dependent Ca^{++} channel and an influx of Ca^{++}. This rise in intracellular Ca^{++}, along with a variety of second messengers, leads to granule recruitment and extrusion. PKC = phosphokinase C; DAG = diacylglycerol; PLC = phospholipase C; PIP_2 = phosphatidylinositol 4,5-bisphosphate; IP_3 = inositol 1,4,5-triphosphate.

There has been extensive investigation of the possibility that impaired glucose transport into the β-cell causes the lack of glucose responsiveness. The β-cell, like the liver and kidney, contains the high K_m glucose transporter, GLUT-2.[49,50] Every hyperglycemic model investigated to date has a markedly reduced level of GLUT-2 protein in its β-cells, usually with a reduced GLUT-2 messenger RNA level.[51–53] Also, the few studies of glucose transport kinetics have shown equivalent reductions,[54] although some disagreement appeared in a recent study.[55] The key question, and a hotly debated one, is whether reduced glucose transport into the β-cell has an effect on glucose-induced insulin secretion. Its basis is that glucose transport normally far exceeds (as much as 50-fold) glucokinase activity, which is the rate-limiting step for β-cell glucose metabolism.[56] As such, near total reductions in transport are needed for lowered glucose metabolism (and secretion). Consistent with this idea, notwithstanding the reduced GLUT-2 levels in isolated islets from diabetic rodents, most studies have reported normal rates of glucose metabolism. The general consensus is that reduced glucose entry into the β-cell does not cause the defect in glucose-induced insulin secretion. Supporting this idea is a recent report that used normoglycemic transgenic mice with markedly reduced β-cell GLUT-2 levels and found no defect in glucose-stimulated insulin secretion.[57]

A new idea has surfaced: that GLUT-2 levels may influence β-cell glucose responsiveness through a mechanism other than the transport of glucose, that is, some regulatory role of the GLUT-2 protein per se. The evidence is based on transfection studies in which GLUT-2 is overexpressed in cell lines. Functional properties are conferred that seem distinct from the increased glucose transport.[58–60] The role (if any) of this idea in the β-cell glucose unresponsiveness of chronic hyperglycemia awaits delineation of these cellular effects. Although the idea is intriguing, it should not be forgotten that the transgenic studies cited above showed no defect in glucose-induced insulin secretion,[57] plus isolated islets from diabetic rats invariably show minimally impaired glucose-induced insulin secretion despite the markedly reduced GLUT-2 levels.

After transport, the next step in β-cell glucose metabolism is phosphorylation by the high K_m glucose phosphorylation enzyme, glucokinase. Glucokinase is the rate-limiting enzyme in glycolysis. Substantial evidence supports its being the β-cell ''glucose sensor,'' the site where the sensitivity and responsiveness for glucose are determined.[61] The importance of glucokinase has been shown by the recent demonstration that half the cases of maturity onset diabetes of youth are caused by mutations in the glucokinase gene. Given the central role glucokinase plays in regulating glucose-induced insulin secretion, Meglasson and Matschinsky postulated many years ago that an abnormality in glucokinase expression or function causes the insulin secretion defects found with hyperglycemia.[62] This idea became testable only recently. It has now been shown that glucokinase cellular levels and activities are normal to raised in several diabetic rodent models, presumably excluding glucokinase as the site of the defect.[55,63]

An area of active investigation has been mitochondrial defects. Mitochondrial signals play a key role in glucose-induced insulin secretion, as shown by the profound suppression that occurs with inhibitors of mitochondrial function. Unlike in isolated islets, the marked suppression of glucose-induced insulin secretion seen in vivo is found when pancreases of diabetic rats undergo in vitro perfusion (see Fig. 10-2). With this approach, data consistent with a mitochondrial defect have been reported.[64] The focus of much of the investigation has been the *glycerol phosphate shuttle,* which is an important link between glycolysis in the cytosol and glucose oxidation in the mitochondria.[65] During glycolysis, fructose-1,6-bisphosphate is converted to glyceraldehyde-3-phosphate and dihydroxyacetone phosphate (DHAP). Glyceraldehyde-3-phosphate proceeds through glycolysis. DHAP is converted to glyceraldehyde-3-phosphate by an isomerase enzyme and also proceeds through glycolysis. Alternatively, a second pathway is the glycerol phosphate shuttle, whereby DHAP is converted to glycerol-3-phosphate, with the reduced form of nicotinamide-adenine dinucleotide (NADH) being converted to NAD^+ in the process. The mitochondrial enzyme flavin adenine dinucleotide (FAD)-dependent glycerol-3-phosphate dehydrogenase reoxidizes glycerol-3-phosphate to glyceraldehyde-3-phosphate, with generation of $FADH_2$ from FAD. The net result is that hydrogen ions are shuttled into the mitochondria, where they enter the respiratory chain for generation of ATP.[65] This reaction is believed to be a critical step in glucose-induced insulin secretion, in part because the activity of the FAD-dependent glycerol-3-phosphate dehydrogenase is 40–70-fold higher in islets compared to in other tissues.[66] Malaisse has reported defective FAD-dependent glycerol-3-phosphate dehydrogenase activity in islets from multiple diabetic models[67,68] as opposed to other mitochondrial enzymes, which are generally unaffected. The cause of the enzyme defect is unclear. However, the gene for the FAD-dependent glycerol-3-phosphate dehydrogenase enzyme was recently cloned,[69] and studies of the cellular level of the protein and gene expression should appear soon. The significance of this finding, especially its role in the β-cell unresponsiveness to glucose, is also unclear. The literature almost entirely consists of comparisons of enzyme activity in islets from diabetic and control animals. Any attempts to correlate the enzyme defect and secretory dysfunction, such as determining if their times of onset in any diabetic model are the same or dissimilar, are lacking. Alternatively, an obvious question is whether the increased glucose-induced insulin secretion that follows a period of euglycemia is paralleled by an increase in the enzyme activity. Finally, it should not be forgotten that the studies showing reduced activity of this enzyme are performed in islets which, for the most part (except for in GK rats), show rather modest suppression of glucose-induced insulin secretion.

A number of other hypotheses have been suggested for the β-cell glucose unresponsiveness, including defective ATP-sensitive channel activity,[70,71] reduced expression of voltage-dependent calcium channels,[72] defective hydrolysis of membrane inositol phospholipids,[73] overaccumulation of glycogen,[74] cycling of glucose-6-phosphate back to glucose because of increased glucose-6-phosphatase activity,[75,76] and altered Na^+-K^+-ATPase activity coupled with reduced myoinositol uptake.[48]

Thus, our understanding of the molecular basis for defective glucose-induced insulin secretion is plagued by too many hypothesis, with the major stumbling block being inadequate in vitro systems. Regardless, we are undergoing an explosion of information about the physiology and molecular biology of insulin secretion, with important offshoots being new probes, reagents, antibodies, and techniques. It is hoped that the solution to this important question is around the corner, leading to new therapies for NIDDM targeted at specific cellular defects in the β-cell.

Hyperproinsulinemia

A longstanding observation in NIDDM is proportionately raised blood levels of insulin precursors (proinsulin and the conversion intermediates) relative to insulin.[2,77,78] The presumed cause is a relative hypersecretion of these peptides, with several kinds of information implicating hyperglycemia in the pathogenesis. The same observation has been made in diabetes from cystic fibrosis.[79] Cross-sectional data in NIDDM are consistent with the increased proinsulin/insulin ratio occurring after the onset of the hyperglycemia.[80,81] States of increased insulin secretion without hyperglycemia, such as in obesity, have a normal to reduced proinsulin : insulin ratio.[81,82] Finally, most studies have found partial to full normalization of the proinsulin : insulin ratio in NIDDM with hypoglycemic therapies.[83] Two hypotheses have been proposed to explain how hyperglycemia causes a hypersecretion of the proinsulin-like peptides.[84,85] The first is based on intact proinsulin processing machinery: The idea is that a sustained secretory demand from the hyperglycemia shortens the transit time from granule packaging to release, resulting in incomplete peptide processing. The second hypothesis postulates impaired processing machinery.

To investigate these issues, we measured the proinsulin : insulin ratio in pancreas extracts and portal vein samples (obtained during in vitro pancreas perfusion) of 90% pancreatectomy rats.[86] The method entailed separation of the insulins and proinsulin-like peptides (conversion intermediates eluted in the proinsulin peak) by high-pressure liquid chromatography (Fig. 10-8), followed by quantification of the peaks by insulin radioimmunoassay (RIA). The nonavailability of purified proinsulin standards (a problem general to the field) prevented absolute measures of proinsulin; it could only be measured relative to insulin, which was validated by showing parallel dilution curves in the insulin RIA for the insulin and proinsulin peaks. There was an increased abundance of the proinsulin-like peptides relative to insulin in both the pancreas (15.6 ± 1.4% versus 8.3 ± 1.4%, $p<0.01$) and the portal vein samples (10.3 ± 3.0% versus 3.0 ± 0.6%, $p<0.006$) of the diabetic rats.[86] Finding the same defect in diabetic rats as in NIDDM supported the notion of a common cause, that is, hyperglycemia. Moreover, the underlying defect appeared to be storage of material enriched in proinsulin-like peptides.

The pathophysiology of the increased pancreas ratio of proinsulin/insulin was next explored with the intent to determine, based on the hypotheses above, whether hyperglycemia per se or a hyperstimulated insulin secretion is the key pathogenic factor.[87] The model was 48-hour glucose-infused rats. This model has the advantage that different levels of glycemia can be attained, depending on the amount of glucose infused. Rats were infused with 20% glucose (euglycemia with a threefold increased plasma insulin), 30% glucose (plasma glucose raised 2 mM), 35% glucose (plasma glucose raised 5 mM), and 50% glucose (plasma glucose raised 13 mM). The pancreas percentage of proinsulin was increased in the hyperglycemic rats (30%, 35%, 50% glucose) but not in the normoglycemic hyperinsulinemic group (20%). The cause of the increase was a fall in the insulin content, not an increase in proinsulin content as might be expected with defective proinsulin processing (Fig. 10-9). Instead, the data were more consistent with the first hypothesis that hyperstimulated insulin secretion causes release of granules before peptide processing is complete. This idea was confirmed by coinfusing diazoxide (an inhibitor of insulin secretion) into 35% glucose-infused rats. Not surprisingly, the rats were more hyperglycemic. Regardless, the insulin content did not fall and the percent of proinsulin remained normal,[87] clearly showing that a hyperstimulation of insulin secretion was the cause and not a direct cellular effect of hyperglycemia. Additional evidence was obtained by infusing normal rats for 3 days with large amounts of tolbutamide (plus glucose to keep them euglycemic). Tolbutamide stimulates insulin secretion in the absence of promoting biosynthesis.[88] Pancreatic insulin content fell by 50%, raising the pancreatic percentage of proinsulin in the absence of hyperglycemia.[87] Thus, the enriched pancreatic stores of proinsulin-like peptides in diabetic rats are secondary to hyperstimulated insulin secretion. Similar conclusions were recently reached in diabetic sand rats using an overnight fast to reduce insulin secretion.[89]

In collaboration with Dr. Chris Rhodes at the Joslin Diabetes Center, we next investigated whether the proinsulin processing machinery is altered in isolated islets from 50% glucose-induced rats.[90] First, the cellular levels of the processing enzymes PC2, PC3, and carboxypeptidase H were measured by Western blot test. To our surprise, the levels of all the enzymes were reduced. However, the cause was not defective biosynthesis. Rather, the result reflected depletion of granule proteins (including insulin) because of a high secretory rate, as shown by the finding of high levels of the enzymes and proinsulin in the media. The absence of any defect in proinsulin processing was confirmed using pulse

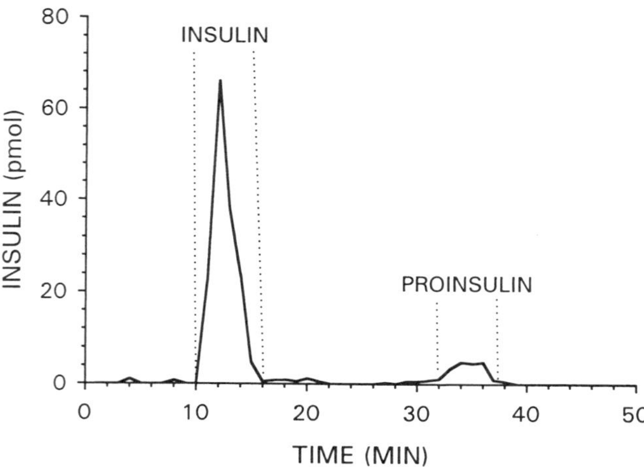

FIGURE 10-8. High-pressure liquid chromatography profile of a pancreas extract from a normal rat. The pancreas underwent extraction and insulin/proinsulin precipitation followed by separation of the insulins and proinsulins by high-pressure liquid chromatography. Fractions were analyzed by insulin radioimmunoassay. (Reproduced with permission from Leahy JL. Increased proinsulin/insulin ratio in pancreas extracts of hyperglycemic rats. Diabetes 1993;42:22.)

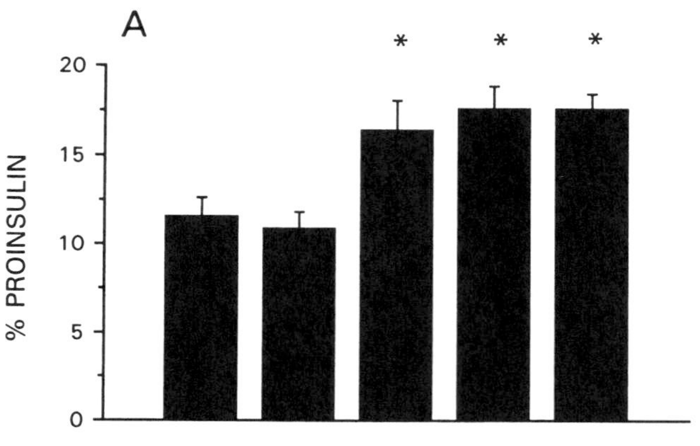

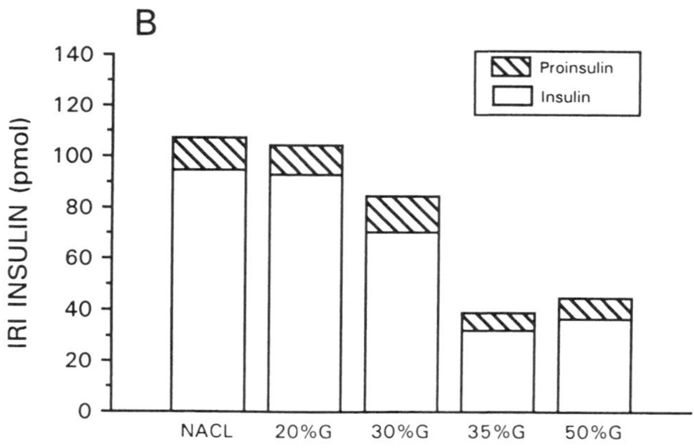

FIGURE 10-9. Relative proportion of proinsulin in pancreas extracts from 48-hour glucose-infused rats. Pancreases underwent extraction, insulin/proinsulin precipitation, and high pressure liquid chromatography separation of the insulins and proinsulins. Equivalent fractions of the total sample were analyzed in all groups. Immunoreactive insulin (IRI) and proinsulin are the areas under the curve of the different peaks as measured by insulin radioimmunoassay. ***A,*** % proinsulin = IRI proinsulin/(IRI insulin + IRI proinsulin). ***B,*** IRI insulin and proinsulin in chromatography samples. (Reproduced with permission from Leahy JL. Increased proinsulin/insulin ratio in pancreas extracts of hyperglycemic rats. Diabetes 1993;42:22.)

chase labeling methodology: The rates in islets from glucose-infused and saline-infused rats were identical.

Thus, the cause of the raised percentage of proinsulin in stored and secreted material from the diabetic rats is a hypermobilization of granules, leading to a rapid transit time that does not allow complete processing. Our evidence strongly argues *against* a defect in proinsulin processing per se. Of note, this hypersecretion scenario fits perfectly with our model for hyperglycemia-induced insulin secretion defects (see Fig. 10-6).

Impaired Proinsulin Synthesis

We have postulated that the pathogenic element that ties the impaired insulin secretion and hyperproinsulinemia together is a hypermobilization of granules leading to depleted β-cell stores of insulin. It is often stated that chronic hyperglycemia inhibits proinsulin biosynthesis; this would be additive to this idea by further depleting the insulin stores (see Fig. 10-6). Also, it would explain the paradox as to why insulin content and secretory responses are not lowered in euglycemic insulin-resistant states despite the insulin hypersecretion.[30] Unfortunately, the data from diabetic rodents on which the idea of impaired proinsulin biosynthesis is based are more confusing than convincing. Using an in vivo technique, Permutt reported reduced proinsulin biosynthesis and reduced proinsulin mRNA levels in neonatal streptozocin diabetic rats.[91,92] Studies in isolated islets from these rats have been contradictory, with three reporting reduced biosynthesis,[42,43,93] and another an increase.[41] Studies in other diabetic models have not clarified the issue. In 48-hour glucose-infused rats, proinsulin biosynthesis and the proinsulin mRNA level were both increased.[94] In contrast, longer term hyperglycemia has mostly been linked with decreased biosynthesis, such as in 4-week grafted islets taken from hyperglycemic mice.[95] However, insulin treatment failed to reverse this defect, making the etiology unclear, especially given the recent report that chronic hyperglycemia lowers the β-cell mass of grafted islets.[96] One explanation for the varying results could be time-based effects on biosynthesis. Supporting such an idea, Orland reported that 90% pancreatectomy rats undergo a worsening of hyperglycemia and a fall in the insulin content 14 weeks after surgery, which he blamed on a fall in the proinsulin mRNA level.[11] No such effect was noted at 1 or 3 weeks. Rather, a compensatory increase in proinsulin mRNA was noted. Of importance, proinsulin mRNA and insulin content were not different at 1 and 3 weeks after surgery, the time we have identified for the onset of the secretory dysfunction,[30] arguing *against* a role for impaired proinsulin synthesis in the β-cell functional abnormalities in these rats.

Besides the lack of consistent results regarding proinsulin biosynthesis in diabetic models, other factors have complicated interpretation of this literature. Routinely, there is no attempt to define what constitutes "normal" biosynthesis for that degree of hyperglycemia. A high glucose level normally stimulates proinsulin biosynthesis at both the transcriptional and post-transcriptional levels. The cited studies simply compare biosynthesis rates or proinsulin mRNA levels in diabetic and control islets without viewing the data in the context of what is the *expected* biosynthesis for that degree of hyperglycemia, that is, the denominator for the data from the diabetic rats is not defined. Also, the fractional β-cell mass of islets from diabetic rats versus normal rats is rarely known, further confusing the denominator for the measurements. Finally, few studies that have reported reduced biosynthesis have followed up that observation with a treatment protocol to restore normoglycemia, looking for reversal of the defect. In fact, we know of no study in which successful reversal was demonstrated. As such, assigning hyperglycemia as the cause of impaired proinsulin biosynthesis is purely speculative.

Robertson and coworkers have studied potential cellular mechanisms for a hyperglycemia-induced impairment of proinsulin transcription. They used a β-cell line (HIT-T15), which in late passages loses glucose-stimulated insulin secretion in combination with a fall off of proinsulin mRNA level and a reduced insulin content. These cells are usually cultured at the supraphysiologic glucose level of 11.1 mM. Culturing them instead at 0.8 mM glucose prevented all the defects.[97] They identified the cause of the decreased insulin gene transcription with standard culture conditions to be an altered ability of a regulatory protein to interact with the insulin gene promoter.[97] Additional investigation of this finding is needed, in particular its relevance to the in vivo state.

Summary

The last decade has seen remarkable progress in identifying and characterizing the defects in insulin secretion that develop with chronic hyperglycemia. Substantial data have been generated in animal models to support the concept that chronic hyperglycemia makes the β-cells selectively unresponsive to glucose. Efforts are now under way to determine the molecular basis for this defect, although a major stumbling block continues to be the lack of in vitro systems that faithfully reproduce the secretory abnormality. Our studies in 90% pancreatectomy rats have identified a cascade of functional changes that occur when β-cells are exposed to chronic hyperglycemia (see Figs. 10-3, 10-4, and 10-6). First, the glucose sensitivity increases, followed a couple of weeks later by a fall off in glucose-induced insulin secretion and glucose potentiation, with the postulated mechanism being reduced β-cell stores of insulin. Our working model is that the β-cell hypersecretion caused by the raised glucose sensitivity is a key pathogenic factor, being responsible for the fall in insulin stores (the contribution if any of defective proinsulin biosynthesis has not been well worked out) as well as the secretion of proinsulin-enriched material (see Fig. 10-6). Our future studies will be directed at finding ways to increase β-cell levels of stored insulin in diabetic rats, to determine if insulin secretory responses increase in parallel, and to look for reversal of the glucose intolerance. Also postulated by our model is a second β-cell defect(s) that uniquely impairs glucose-induced insulin secretion. Multiple candidate defects have been studied but no single hypothesis stands out as able to explain all the characteristics of the secretory abnormalities. As better in vitro systems become available, we can expect to see an explosion of activity directed at identifying the intracellular abnormalities as well as attempts at designing treatments targeted at specific defects. The long-term goal of this line of investigation is to uncover innovative new therapies for NIDDM.

Acknowledgments

This cited work of the author was sponsored by National Institutes of Health grant DK-38543 plus funding from the Juvenile Diabetes Foundation.

References

1. Porte D Jr. β-cells in type II diabetes mellitus. Diabetes 1991;40:166
2. Leahy JL. Natural history of B-cell dysfunction in NIDDM. Diabetes Care 1990;13:992
3. Leahy JL, Bonner-Weir S, Weir GC. Beta-cell dysfunction induced by chronic hyperglycemia: Current ideas on the mechanism of the impaired glucose-induced insulin secretion. Diabetes Care 1992;15:442
4. Rossetti L, Giaccari A, DeFronzo RA. Glucose toxicity. Diabetes Care 1990;13:610
5. Yki-Järvinen H. Glucose toxicity. Endocr Rev 1992;13:415
6. Östenson CG, Khan A, Efendic S. Impaired glucose-induced insulin secretion: Studies in animal models with spontaneous NIDDM. Adv Exp Med Biol 1993;334:1
7. Flatt PR, Barnett CR, Swanston-Flatt SK. Mechanisms of pancreatic β-cell dysfunction and glucose toxicity in non–insulin-dependent diabetes. Biochem Soc Trans 1994;22:18

8. Robertson RP, Olson LK, Zhang H-J. Differentiating glucose toxicity from glucose desensitization: A message from the insulin gene. Diabetes 1994;43:1085
9. Bonner-Weir S, Trent DF, Weir GC. Partial pancreatectomy in the rat and subsequent defect in glucose-induced insulin release. J Clin Invest 1983; 71:1544
10. Rossetti L, Smith D, Shulman GI, et al. Correction of hyperglycemia with phloridzin normalizes tissue sensitivity to insulin in diabetic rats. J Clin Invest 1987;79:1510
11. Orland MJ, Chyn R, Permutt MA. Modulation of proinsulin messenger RNA after partial pancreatectomy in rats. Relationship to glucose homeostasis. J Clin Invest 1985;75:2047
12. Brockenbrough JS, Weir GC, Bonner-Weir S. Discordance of exocrine and endocrine growth after 90% pancreatectomy in rats. Diabetes 1988;37:232
13. Perley MJ, Kipnis DM. Plasma insulin responses to oral and intravenous glucose: Studies in normal and diabetic subjects. J Clin Invest 1967;46:1954
14. Cerasi E, Luft R. The plasma insulin response to glucose infusion in healthy subjects and in diabetes mellitus. Acta Endocrinol 1967;55:278
15. Brunzell JD, Robertson RP, Lerner RL, et al. Relationships between fasting plasma glucose levels and insulin secretion during intravenous glucose tolerance tests. J Clin Endocrinol Metab 1976;42:222
16. Kosaka K, Kuzuya T, Akanuma Y, Hagura R. Increase in insulin response after treatment of overt maturity-onset diabetes is independent of the mode of treatment. Diabetologia 1980;18:23
17. Vague P, Moulin J-P. The defective glucose sensitivity of the B-cell in noninsulin dependent diabetes: Improvement after twenty hours of normoglycemia. Metabolism 1982;31:139
18. Kergoat M, Bailbe D, Portha B. Insulin treatment improves glucose-induced insulin release in rats with NIDDM induced by streptozocin. Diabetes 1987;36:971
19. Leahy JL, Weir GC. B-cell dysfunction in hyperglycemic rat models. Recovery of glucose-induced insulin secretion with lowering of the ambient glucose level. Diabetologia 1991;34:640
20. Grill V, Westberg M, Östenson C-G. B-cell insensitivity in a rat model of non–insulin-dependent diabetes: Evidence for a rapidly reversible effect of previous hyperglycemia. J Clin Invest 1987;80:664
21. Chen C, Thorens B, Bonner-Weir S, et al. Recovery of glucose-induced insulin secretion in a rat model of NIDDM is not accompanied by return of the B-cell GLUT-2 glucose transporter. Diabetes 1992;41:1320
22. Rossetti L, Shulman GI, Zawalich W, DeFronzo RA. Effect of chronic hyperglycemia on in vivo insulin secretion in partially pancreatectomized rats. J Clin Invest 1987;80:1037
23. Leahy JL, Weir GC. Unresponsiveness to glucose in a streptozocin model of diabetes: Inappropriate insulin and glucagon responses to a reduction of glucose concentration. Diabetes 1985;34:653
24. Leahy JL, Bumbalo LM, Chen C. Beta-cell hypersensitivity for glucose precedes loss of glucose-induced insulin secretion in 90% pancreatectomized rats. Diabetologia 1993;36:1238
25. Timmers KI, Powell AM, Voyles NR, et al. Multiple alterations in insulin responses to glucose in islets from 48-hour glucose-infused nondiabetic rats. Diabetes 1990;39:1436
26. Marynissen G, Leclercq-Meyer V, Sener A, Malaisse WJ. Perturbation of pancreatic islet function in glucose-infused rats. Metabolism 1990;39:87
27. Chen N-G, Tassava TM, Romsos DR. Threshold for glucose-stimulated insulin secretion in pancreatic islets of genetically obese (ob/ob) mice is abnormally low. J Nutr 1993;123:1567
28. Thibault C, Guettet C, Laury MC, et al. In vivo and in vitro increased pancreatic beta-cell sensitivity to glucose in normal rats submitted to a 48-hour hyperglycemic period. Diabetologia 1993;36:589
29. Teruya M, Takei S, Forrest LE, et al. Pancreatic islet function in nondiabetic and diabetic BB rats. Diabetes 1993;42:1310
30. Chen C, Hosokawa H, Bumbalo LM, Leahy JL. Mechanism of compensatory hyperinsulinemia in normoglycemic insulin resistant SHR rats: Augmented enzymatic activity of glucokinase in β-cells. J Clin Invest 1994;94:399
31. Leahy JL, Bumbalo LM, Chen C. Diazoxide causes recovery of β-cell glucose responsiveness in 90% pancreatectomized diabetic rats. Diabetes 1994;43:173
32. Ward WK, Bolgiano DC, McKnight B, et al. Diminished B cell secretory capacity in patients with noninsulin-dependent diabetes mellitus. J Clin Invest 1984;74:1318
33. Johnston C, Raghu P, McCulloch DK, et al. β-cell function and insulin sensitivity in nondiabetic HLA-identical siblings of insulin-dependent diabetes. Diabetes 1987;36:829
34. Leahy JL, Cooper HE, Weir GC. Impaired insulin secretion associated with near normoglycemia: Study in normal rats with 96-hour in vivo glucose infusions. Diabetes 1987;36:459
35. Leahy JL, Bonner-Weir S, Weir GC. Abnormal glucose regulation of insulin secretion in models of reduced β-cell mass. Diabetes 1984;33:667
36. Sako Y, Grill VE. Coupling of β-cell desensitization by hyperglycemia to excessive stimulation and circulating insulin in glucose-infused rats. Diabetes 1990;39:1580
37. Björklund A, Grill V. β-cell insensitivity in vitro: Reversal by diazoxide entails more than one event in stimulus-secretion coupling. Endocrinology 1993; 132:1319
38. Sako Y, Grill VE. Diazoxide infusion at excess but not at basal hyperglycemia enhances β-cell sensitivity to glucose in vitro in neonatally streptozotocin-diabetic rats. Metabolism 1992;41:738
39. Malaisse WJ, Malaisse-Lagae F, Wright PH. Effect of fasting upon insulin secretion in the rat. Am J Physiol 1967;213:843
40. Grey NJ, Goldring S, Kipnis DM. The effect of fasting, diet, and actinomycin D on insulin secretion in the rat. J Clin Invest 1970;49:881
41. Halban PA, Bonner-Weir S, Weir GC. Elevated proinsulin biosynthesis in vitro from a rat model of non–insulin-dependent diabetes mellitus. Diabetes 1983;32:277
42. Portha B. Decreased glucose-induced insulin release and biosynthesis by islets of rats with non–insulin-dependent diabetes: Effects of tissue culture. Endocrinology 1985;117:1735
43. Portha B, Giroix M-H, Serradas P, et al. Insulin production and glucose metabolism in isolated pancreatic islets of rats with NIDDM. Diabetes 1988;37:1226
44. Östenson CG, Khan A, Abdel-Halin SM, et al. Abnormal insulin secretion and glucose metabolism in pancreatic islets from spontaneously diabetic GK rat. Diabetologia 1993;36:3
45. Zawalich WS, Zawalich KC. Phosphoinositide hydrolysis and insulin release from isolated perifused rat islets. Studies with glucose. Diabetes 1988;37:1294
46. Grodsky GM, Bolaffi JL. Desensitization of the insulin-secreting beta cell. J Cell Biochem 1992;48:3
47. Leahy JL, Weir GC. Evolution of abnormal insulin secretory responses during 48-hour in vivo hyperglycemia. Diabetes 1988;37:217
48. Xia M, Laychock SG. Insulin secretion, *myo*-inositol transport, and Na^+-K^+-ATPase in glucose-desensitized rat islets. Diabetes 1993;42:1392
49. Thorens B, Sarkar HK, Kaback HR, Lodish HF. Cloning and functional expression in bacteria of a novel glucose transporter present in liver, intestine, kidney, and β-pancreatic islet cells. Cell 1988;55:281
50. Johnson JH, Newgard CB, Milburn JL, et al. The high K_m glucose transporter of islets of Langerhans is functionally similar to the low affinity transporter of liver and has an identical primary sequence. J Biol Chem 1990;265:6548
51. Thorens B, Weir GC, Leahy JL, et al. Reduced expression of the liver/beta-cell glucose transporter isoform in glucose-insensitive pancreatic beta cells of diabetic rats. Proc Natl Acad Sci USA 1990;87:6492
52. Thorens B, Wu Y-J, Leahy JL, Weir GC. The loss of GLUT-2 expression by glucose-unresponsive β cells of db/db mice is reversible and is induced by the diabetic environment. J Clin Invest 1992;90:77
53. Milburn JL Jr, Ohneda M, Johnson JH, Unger RH. Beta-cell GLUT-2 loss and non–insulin-dependent diabetes mellitus: Current status of the hypothesis. Diabetes Metab Rev 1993;9:231
54. Johnson JH, Ogawa A, Chen L, et al. Underexpression of β cell high K_m glucose transporters in noninsulin-dependent diabetes. Science 1990;250:546
55. Liang Y, Bonner-Weir S, Wu Y-J, et al. In situ glucose uptake and glucokinase activity of pancreatic islets in diabetic and obese rodents. J Clin Invest 1994;93:2473
56. Tal M, Liang Y, Najafi H, et al. Expression and function of GLUT-1 and GLUT-2 glucose transporter isoforms in cells of cultured rat pancreatic islets. J Biol Chem 1992;267:17241
57. Tal M, Wu Y-J, Leiser M, et al. [Val12]-HRAS downregulates GLUT-2 in beta cells of transgenic mice without affecting glucose homeostasis. Proc Natl Acad Sci USA 1992;89:5744
58. Hughes SD, Quaade C, Johnson JH, et al. Transfection of $AtT\text{-}20_{inss}$ cells with GLUT-2 but not GLUT-1 confers glucose-stimulated insulin secretion. J Biol Chem 1993;268:15205
59. Ferber S, Beltrandelrio H, Johnson JH, et al. GLUT-2 gene transfer into insulinoma cells confers both low and high affinity glucose-stimulated insulin release. Relationship to glucokinase activity. J Biol Chem 1994;269:11523
60. Morita H, Yano Y, Niswender KD, et al. Coexpression of glucose transporters and glucokinase in *Xenopus* oocytes indicates that both glucose transport and phosphorylation determine glucose utilization. J Clin Invest 1994;94:1373
61. Matschinsky FM. Glucokinase as glucose sensor and metabolic generator in pancreatic β-cells and hepatocytes. Diabetes 1990;39:647
62. Meglasson MD, Matschinsky FM. New perspectives on pancreatic islet glucokinase. Am J Physiol 1984;246:E1
63. Chen C, Bumbalo LM, Leahy JL. Increased catalytic activity of glucokinase in isolated islets from hyperinsulinemic rats. Diabetes 1994;43:684
64. Grill V, Sako Y, Östenson C-G, Jalkanen P. Multiple abnormalities in insulin responses to nonglucose nutrients in neonatally streptozocin diabetic rats. Endocrinology 1991;128:2195
65. MacDonald MJ. Elusive proximal signals of β-cells for insulin secretion. Diabetes 1990;39:1461
66. MacDonald MJ. High content of mitochondrial glycerol 3-phosphate dehydrogenase in pancreatic islets and its inhibition by diazoxide. J Biol Chem 1981;256:8287
67. Malaisse WJ, Malaisse-Lagae F, Kukel S, et al. Could non–insulin dependent diabetes mellitus be attributed to a deficiency of FAD-linked glycerophosphate dehydrogenase? Biochem Med Metab Biol 1993;50:226
68. Malaisse WJ. Pertubation of islet metabolism and insulin release in NIDDM. Adv Exp Med Biol 1993;334:13
69. Brown LJ, MacDonald MJ, Lehn DA, Moran SM. Sequence of rat mitochondrial glycerol-3-phosphate dehydrogenase cDNA. Evidence for EF-hand calcium-binding domains. J Biol Chem 1994;269:14363
70. Purrello F, Vetri M, Vinci C, et al. Chronic exposure to high glucose and impairment of K^+-channel function in perifused rat pancreatic islets. Diabetes 1990;39:397
71. Tsuura Y, Ishida H, Okamota Y, et al. Impaired glucose sensitivity of ATP-sensitive K^+ channels in pancreatic beta-cells in streptozotocin-induced NIDDM rats. Diabetes 1992;41:861

72. Iwashima Y, Pugh W, Depaoli AM, et al. Expression of calcium channel mRNAs in rat pancreatic islets and down-regulation following glucose infusion. Diabetes 1993;42:948
73. Zawalich WS, Zawalich KC, Shulman GI, Rossetti L. Chronic in vivo hyperglycemia impairs phosphoinositide hydrolysis and insulin release in isolated perifused rat islets. Endocrinology 1990;126:253
74. Malaisse WJ, Marynissen G, Sener A. Possible role of glycogen accumulation in B-cell glucotoxicity. Metabolism 1992;41:814
75. Kahn A, Chandramouli V, Östenson C-G, et al. Evidence for the presence of glucose cycling in pancreatic islets of the ob/ob mouse. J Biol Chem 1989;264:9732
76. Kahn A, Chandramouli V, Östenson C-G, et al. Glucose cycling in islets from healthy and diabetic rats. Diabetes 1990;39:456
77. Mako ME, Starr JI, Rubenstein AH. Circulating proinsulin in patients with maturity onset diabetes. Am J Med 1977;63:865
78. Temple RC, Carrington CA, Luzio SD, et al. Insulin deficiency in non–insulin-dependent diabetes. Lancet 1989;1:293
79. Hartling SG, Garne S, Binder C, et al. Proinsulin, insulin, and C-peptide in cystic fibrosis after an oral glucose tolerance test. Diabetes Res 1988;7:165
80. Yoshioka N, Kuzuya T, Matsuda A, et al. Serum proinsulin levels at fasting and after oral glucose load in patients with type 2 (non–insulin-dependent) diabetes mellitus. Diabetologia 1988;31:355
81. Saad MF, Kahn SE, Nelson RG, et al. Disproportionately elevated proinsulin in Pima Indians with noninsulin-dependent diabetes mellitus. J Clin Endocrinol Metab 1990;70:1247
82. Koivisto VA, Yki-Järvinen H, Hartling SV, Pelkonen R. The effect of exogenous hyperinsulinemia on proinsulin secretion in normal man, obese subjects, and patients with insulinoma. J Clin Endocrinol Metab 1986;63:1117
83. Yoshioka N, Kuzuya T, Matsuda A, Iwamoto Y. Effects of dietary treatment on serum insulin and proinsulin response in newly diagnosed NIDDM. Diabetes 1989;38:262
84. Rhodes CJ, Alarcón C. What beta-cell defect could lead to hyperproinsulinemia in NIDDM? Some clues from recent advances made in understanding the proinsulin-processing mechanism. Diabetes 1994;43:511
85. Porte D Jr, Kahn SE. Hyperproinsulinemia and amyloid in NIDDM: Clues to etiology of islet β-cell dysfunction? Diabetes 1989;38:1333
86. Leahy JL, Halban PA, Weir GC. Relative hypersecretion of proinsulin in rat model of NIDDM. Diabetes 1991;40:985
87. Leahy JL. Increased proinsulin/insulin ratio in pancreas extracts of hyperglycemic rats. Diabetes 1993;42:22
88. Schatz H, Steinie D, Pfeiffer EF. Long-term actions of sulfonylureas on (pro-) insulin biosynthesis and secretion: 1. Lack of effect for a compensatory increase in (pro-)insulin biosynthesis after exposure of isolated pancreatic rat islets to tolbutamide and glibenclamide in vitro. Horm Metab Res 1977;9:457
89. Gadot M, Leibowitz G, Shafrir E, et al. Hyperproinsulinemia and insulin deficiency in the diabetic *Psammomys obesus*. Endocrinology 1994;135:610
90. Alárcon C, Leahy JL, Schuppin GT, et al. Increased secretory demand rather than a defect in the proinsulin conversion mechanism causes hyperproinsulinemia in a glucose-infusion rat model of non–insulin-dependent diabetes mellitus. J Clin Invest 1995;95:1032
91. Permutt MA, Kakita K, Malinas P, et al. An in vivo analysis of pancreatic protein and insulin biosynthesis in a rat model for non–insulin-dependent diabetes. J Clin Invest 1984;73:1344
92. Giddings SJ, Orland MJ, Weir GC, et al. Impaired insulin biosynthetic capacity in a rat model for non–insulin-dependent diabetes. Studies with dexamethasone. Diabetes 1985;34:235
93. Welsh N, Hellerström C. In vitro restoration of insulin production in islets from adult rats treated neonatally with streptozotocin. Endocrinology 1990;126:1842
94. Sako Y, Eizirik D, Grill V. Impact of uncoupling glucose stimulus from secretion on β-cell release and biosynthesis. Am J Physiol 1992;262:E150
95. Korsgren O, Jansson L, Andersson A. Effects of hyperglycemia on function of isolated mouse pancreatic islets transplanted under kidney capsule. Diabetes 1989;38:510
96. Montaña E, Bonner-Weir S, Weir GC. Transplanted beta cell response to increased metabolic demand. Changes in beta cell replication and mass. J Clin Invest 1994;93:1577
97. Robertson RP, Zhang H-J, Pyzdrowski KL, Walseth TF. Preservation of insulin mRNA levels and insulin secretion in HIT cells by avoidance of chronic exposure to high glucose concentrations. J Clin Invest 1992;90:320
98. Olson LK, Redmon JB, Towle HC, Robertson RP. Chronic exposure of HIT cells to high glucose concentrations paradoxically decreases insulin gene transcription and alters binding of insulin gene regulatory protein. J Clin Invest 1993;92:514

Diabetes Mellitus, edited by Derek LeRoith, Simeon I. Taylor, and Jerrold M. Olefsky. Lippincott–Raven Publishers, Philadelphia © 1996.

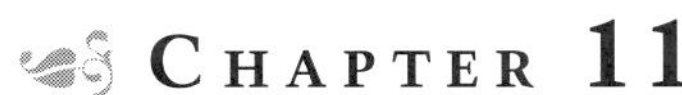

Chapter 11

Islet Amyloid and Its Potential Role in the Pathogenesis of Type II Diabetes Mellitus

Peter C. Butler

Type II diabetes mellitus is characterized by a progressive loss of β-cell function associated with β-cell loss. In their classic text book entitled *The Pathology of Diabetes Mellitus*, published in 1952,[1] Warren and LeCompte recognized the work of earlier investigators who had described deposits of nonspecific material (then referred to as hyaline) in the islets of patients with adult-onset diabetes mellitus. In their book, Warren and LeCompte posed the question: "Is hyalinization of the islands the result of or the cause of diabetes?" In the 40 years since then, it has been demonstrated that the material within the islets is amyloid in nature and consists of a locally expressed protein, islet amyloid polypeptide (IAPP). As a consequence of this information, it is now reasonable to expand the question of Warren and LeCompte into several questions, as follows:

1. What is amyloid?
2. Is islet amyloid really associated with type II diabetes mellitus?
3. What are the normal structure and function of IAPP?
4. Where is IAPP normally expressed, and where in the islet does IAPP-derived amyloid form?
5. Why does IAPP amyloid form in type II diabetes mellitus?
6. Is islet amyloid cytotoxic and of mechanistic significance in the pathogenesis of islet dysfunction?

What Is Amyloid?

Amyloid is an abnormal protein aggregate that possesses the following properties: (1) birefringence under cross-polarizing light with Congo red staining, (2) fibrillar morphology composed of rigid nonbranching fibrils of 75–100 Å in diameter[2] as determined by electron microscopy, and (3) a specific x-ray diffraction pattern.[3] Lansbury reviewed these criteria and pointed out that there is uncertainty as to the molecular basis of amyloid fibrils.[4] However, generally it is assumed that amyloid fibrils are proteins consisting of multiple repeated units of a single constitutive protein in a β-pleated sheet cross-linked configuration.[3] Employing a Fourier Transform Infrared Spectroscopic (FTIR) method, IAPP fibrils have been shown to have a cross β-fibril structure.[4]

Amyloid deposits are thus characterized by both the constitutive protein and the distribution of the amyloid deposits. In some instances, amyloid formation occurs because of a mutation in the relevant protein that results in increased amyloidogenicity.[5] However, in other circumstances, amyloid consists of fibrillar aggregates of a protein with its usual amino acid sequence. These proteins are potentially amyloidogenic in a healthy person, but only under conditions present in some diseases do they become aggregated. Islet amyloid is an example of the latter, since the sequence of the constitutive protein, IAPP, is present in its usual secreted amino acid sequence. These forms of amyloid appear to occur when the protein is expressed (probably usually overexpressed) in cells that are neoplastic (e.g., insulinoma, pituitary tumors, and myeloma) or degenerative (e.g., cerebral cortex in Alzheimer's disease, β-cells in type II diabetes mellitus).

In the case of type II diabetes mellitus, islet amyloid bears some comparison to the focal deposits of amyloid present in the brain of patients with Alzheimer's disease. In both cases, the amyloid deposits are confined to a single tissue (cerebral cortex in Alzheimer's disease and pancreatic islet in type II diabetes mellitus). Both amyloids consist of a normally expressed local protein (β-protein in Alzheimer's disease versus IAPP in the islet). The prevalence of both diseases increases with age, and there is a clear genetic predisposition present in both diseases, although the molecular genetic basis has not yet been identified in either disease. Again, in both diseases the local deposits of amyloid are associated with death and dysfunction of adjacent tissue (brain versus endocrine islet). A vigorous debate as to the mechanism of amyloid formation and its relevance to the pathophysiology of the disease exists for both diseases.

In order to address the potential role of islet amyloid in the pathogenesis of islet dysfunction in type II diabetes mellitus, it is first important to clarify the relationship between islet amyloid and type II diabetes mellitus.

Is Islet Amyloid Really Associated with Type II Diabetes Mellitus?

Study of islet morphology in type II diabetes mellitus has been confounded by several factors. First, islet tissue is dispersed in the exocrine pancreas and is therefore difficult to quantify. Second, in humans the pancreas is usually only available for examination at autopsy, and after death autolysis occurs most rapidly in the pancreas. Finally, autopsy studies are often limited by the availability of clinical data to allow for clinical-pathologic correlations.

It is clearly not possible to perform prospective studies in humans with repeated pancreatic biopsies to determine the relationship between islet amyloid and type II diabetes mellitus. However, similar islet amyloid deposits have been identified in other mammals affected with type II diabetes mellitus (e.g., monkeys,[6] cats,[7]) and also in insulinoma tissue.[8] In patients with type II diabetes mellitus, up to 80% of the β-cell volume may be destroyed, and yet the mean islet area remains comparable in size to that in nondiabetic patients.[9] This observation suggests that the area of the islet occupied by amyloid corresponds to the area formerly occupied by β-cells. The concept that islet amyloid replaces the area occupied by destroyed β-cells is supported by the only available prospective study that reports the progression of islet morphologic abnormalities during the pathogenesis of type II diabetes mellitus in monkeys.[10] Howard, in this remarkable 18-year prospective study, performed sequential pancreatic biopsies and intravenous glucose tolerance tests in monkeys (*Macaca nigra*) as they developed type II diabetes mellitus.[10] The mean area of islet amyloid progressed from 1% in the nondiabetic state to 31% with development of glucose intolerance and 63% with development of type II diabetes mellitus; the area occupied by β-cells declined concurrently. These findings are consistent with a cross-sectional study demonstrating an inverse relationship between the volume of islet amyloid and β-cell volume in obese monkeys developing diabetes mellitus.[11] In humans with NIDDM, the abundance of amyloid in islets shows regional variation in the pancreas that mirrors the regional variation of the abundance of β-cells, that is, most frequent in the tail and least frequent in the polypeptide-rich lobule of the head.[12] However, even within a particular region, the amount of amyloid is highly variable from islet to islet. The reported prevalence of islet amyloid in humans with type II diabetes mellitus varies from 40–100%.[13,14] However, only extracellular deposits of islet amyloid are detectable on light microscopic examination so that an islet in which there is extensive intracellular amyloid may appear as negative for amyloid on light microscopic examination. It is of note that the small amounts of islet amyloid reported in some nondiabetic patients (with increasing prevalence with age[15]) may reflect the fact that these patients died prior to the full clinical development of type II diabetes mellitus.

In conclusion, there appears to be no doubt that islet amyloid is associated with type II diabetes mellitus, and furthermore islet amyloid appears to precede the full development of the disease, leaving open the possibility that it is of mechanistic importance in the pathogenesis of islet dysfunction. The latter warrants careful consideration of the properties of the constitutive protein of islet amyloid.

What Are the Normal Structure and Function of Islet Amyloid Polypeptide?

Structure

Identification of the precursor molecule of islet amyloid was accomplished simultaneously and independently by two groups, from an insulinoma[16] and from pancreatic tissue obtained from patients with type II diabetes mellitus.[17] The resulting protein, IAPP, had a previously undescribed amino acid sequence of 37 amino acids and a theoretical molecular mass of 3850 (Fig. 11-1).[16] The amino acid sequence of IAPP derived from human insulinoma tissue[16] is identical to that present in islet amyloid from patients with NIDDM[18] (and IAPP in healthy humans from cDNA predictions).[19,20]

IAPP structure shows close sequence homology among all species in both the amino terminal (residues 1–19) and the carboxy terminal (residues 30–37) regions.[21,22] In contrast, residues 20–29 show considerable divergence among species (Fig. 11-1). Second-

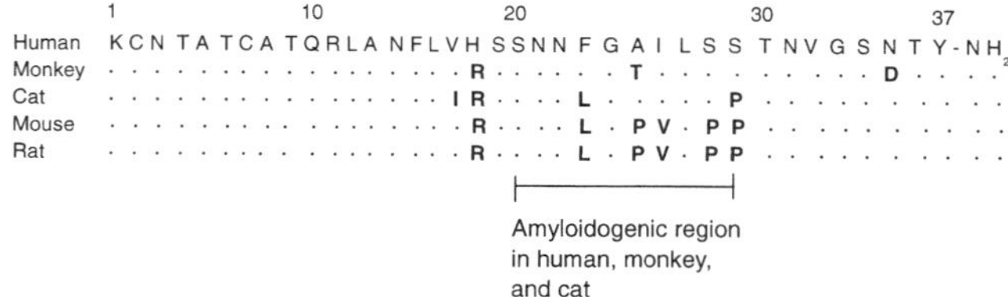

Figure 11-1. Note the considerable species homogeneity in the COOH and NH_2 terminal amino acid sequences among species. However, in the 20–29 amino acid amyloidogenic region of IAPP, species that develop type II diabetes mellitus and islet amyloid (cat, monkey, and human) have close homology, whereas those species that do not develop type II diabetes mellitus (rat and mouse) have a nonamyloidogenic sequence in this region (see references 16–19, 21, 22, 29).

ary structural predictions of amino acids 20–27 in human IAPP indicate a high propensity to form amyloid fibrils.[22] Furthermore, in vitro experiments with synthetic peptides corresponding to the amino acid sequence of human and cat IAPP in the 20–29 region show rapid amyloid formation.[4,22] In contrast, the corresponding synthetic peptides in the rat, guinea pig, and mouse do not form amyloid fibrils.[22] The 25–28 region of human, monkey, and cat IAPP is highly conserved (i.e., Ala-Ile-Leu-Ser [AILS]) and appears to be the most important amyloidogenic sequence (see Fig. 11-1). Thus, substitutions of single amino acids in the 25–28 region of synthetic human IAPP 20–29 significantly reduce or eliminate the amyloidogenicity of these peptides.[22]

In conclusion, IAPP in healthy humans has the necessary properties to form cross β-sheets and hence amyloid. This tendency depends upon a specific amino acid sequence, AILS, in the middle portion of the molecule. Any species that does not have this middle molecular sequence (or a sequence closely related to it) does not spontaneously develop type II diabetes mellitus. This latter theory appears to lend strong support to the possibility that IAPP-derived amyloid does contribute to the pathogenesis of the clinical syndrome of type II diabetes mellitus.

Function

The function of IAPP is controversial. After IAPP was first isolated it was found to inhibit the effects of insulin at pharmacologic concentrations.[23] This led to the speculation that the islet amyloid lesions present in patients with type II diabetes mellitus would be accompanied by high circulating concentrations of this protein, which would contribute to the insulin resistance characteristic of this disease. In fact, it transpired that the circulating concentrations were much lower than those required to cause insulin resistance and that they were no higher in patients with type II diabetes mellitus than in appropriately matched nondiabetic controls.[24]

Although commercial interests have continued to support investigations designed to support the hypothesis that IAPP mediates insulin resistance in patients with type II diabetes mellitus, there are still no data to support this hypothesis. In contrast, there is an increasing body of information to support a regulatory role of IAPP (inhibitory) on insulin secretion.[25] Since IAPP is co-secreted with insulin,[24] it is plausible that the former serves as a brake to rapid increases in insulin secretion after glucose ingestion to reduce the likelihood of subsequent hypoglycemia.

Where Is Islet Amyloid Polypeptide Normally Expressed, and Where in the Islet Does IAPP-Derived Amyloid Form?

Islet amyloid polypeptide immunoreactivity (in healthy humans and most other mammals examined) is almost exclusively located in the pancreatic β-cells.[16,25–27] Also, in situ hybridization studies in the rat showed that IAPP mRNA is predominantly located in β-cells.[28] Ultrastructurally, IAPP immunoreactivity (in humans and cats) is predominantly in β-cell secretory granules.[26,28,29] The co-localization of IAPP and insulin in β-cell secretory granules predicted the subsequent observation that these peptides are co-secreted following appropriate stimuli.[23,30,31,32]

The site of amyloid formation within the islet is more controversial. In islets of patients with established diabetes mellitus, IAPP-derived amyloid is most obviously present in extracellular deposits, frequently adjacent to the capillary endothelium. However abnormal aggregates of IAPP have been noted intracellularly in islet tissue of humans with type II diabetes mellitus.[33] Furthermore, we[34] and others[35] have shown that IAPP-derived amyloid forms intracellularly in human insulinoma tissue. Intracellular formation

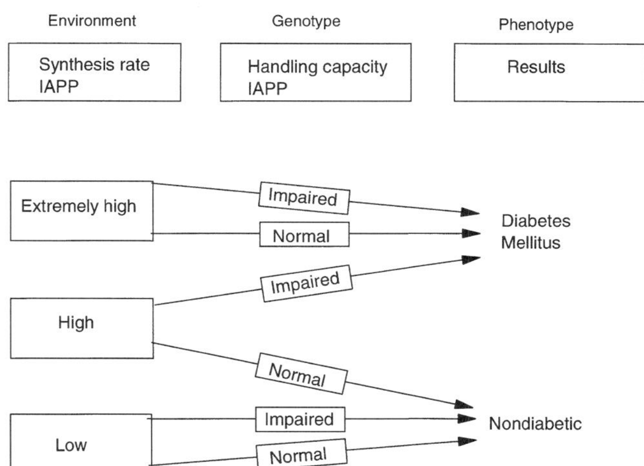

Figure 11-2. A proposed model for islet amyloidogenesis and its role in β-cell destruction. Extremely high rates of IAPP synthesis (e.g., see references 37 and 44) cause intracellular aggregation of IAPP amyloid, β-cell death, and diabetes. At moderately high rates of IAPP synthesis, IAPP forms islet amyloid, leading to diabetes mellitus only under conditions of impaired β-cell capacity to handle IAPP (a potential genotypic variance predisposing to diabetes mellitus). At low rates of IAPP synthesis, this genotypic variance is not sufficient to lead to expression of the diabetes phenotype, and therefore such patients remain nondiabetic.

of IAPP-derived amyloid has also been demonstrated in β-cells of cats with early NIDDM (Fig. 11-2).[36] Furthermore, we have recently shown that IAPP-derived amyloid forms intracellularly in COS cells transiently transfected with the human IAPP gene (Fig. 11-3).[37] Finally, other endocrine-derived amyloid deposits (e.g., growth hormone in growth hormone–secreting pituitary tumors) have also recently been shown to be formed intracellularly.[38]

It therefore seems probable that IAPP amyloid forms within β-cells. Extracellular amyloid may be derived from extrusion of these amyloid fibrils from the cells or from necrosis of the relevant cell (thereby discharging the amyloid to the extracellular environment). Since amyloidogenesis is accelerated by a nidus of amyloid, such extracellular deposits may be the focus for additional amyloid formation from amyloid secreted in a soluble form from adjacent cells.

Why Does Islet Amyloid Polypeptide Form in Type II Diabetes Mellitus?

Since human IAPP forms amyloid fibrils in vitro concentrations of approximately 10^{-9} molar and the concentration of IAPP in the endoplasmic reticulum, Golgi, and secretory granules of healthy human β-cells must far exceed this concentration, it is reasonable to pose the question, Why does human IAPP *not* form amyloid fibrils in the endoplasmic reticulum, Golgi, and secretory granules of all β-cells? It would appear that a mechanism must be present in normal β-cells that prevents the aggregation of IAPP in fibrils.

Important candidates for prevention of IAPP amyloid aggregation would appear to be an acid pH and the presence of chaperone proteins (heat shock proteins). In vitro high concentrations of IAPP can be maintained in solution at very acid pHs. It is thus of interest that the mature insulin secretory vesicle has a pH of approximately 5.[39] Thus, any failure of acidification of the insulin secretory vesicle may predispose to intracellular amyloidogenesis. We have recently reported that patients with cystic fibrosis complicated by diabetes mellitus have a high prevalence of islet amyloid (with intracellular formation).[40] The molecular genetic defect in cystic fibrosis results

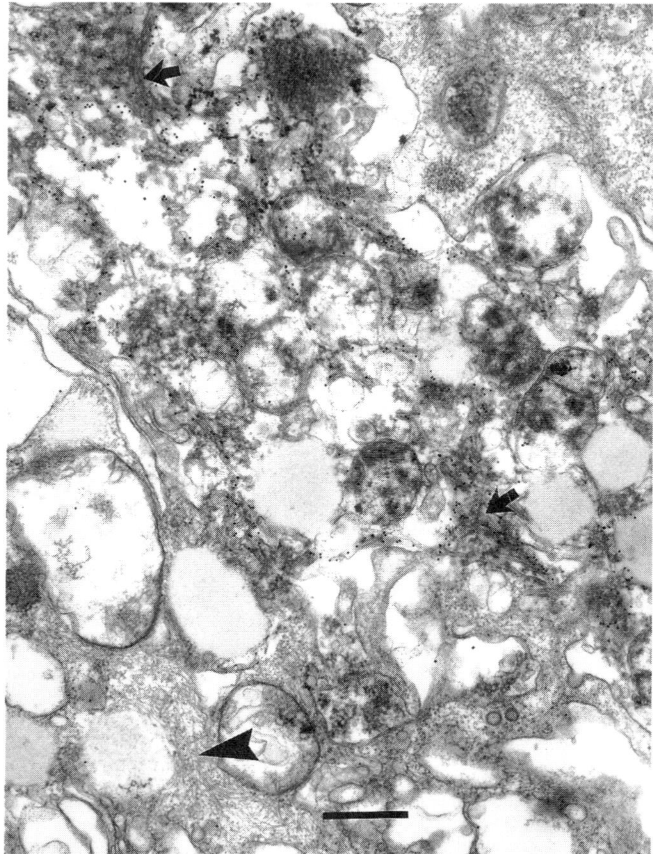

FIGURE 11-3. Electron micrograph of a COS-1 cell 96 hours after transfection with pMT2- human IAPP. Early amyloid formation labeled intensely for IAPP by immunogold is evident. Note the adjacent cytoskeletal filaments (*arrowhead*) that are distinct from the IAPP aggregates (*arrows*) and have no IAPP labeling (bar = 500 nm). (Reproduced with permission from O'Brien TD, Butler PC, Kreutter DK, et al. Human islet amyloid polypeptide expression in COS-1 cells: an *in vitro* model of intracellular amyloidogenesis. Am J Pathol 1995;147:614.)

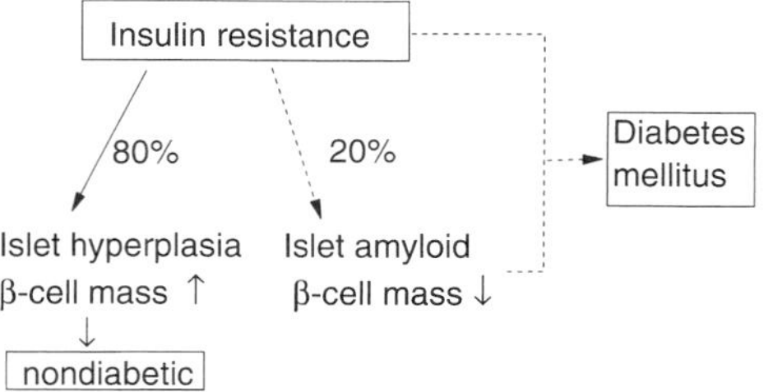

FIGURE 11-4. Epidemiologic data indicate that chronic insulin resistance (fasting hyperinsulinemia) is a major risk factor for expression of type II diabetes genotype. Chronic insulin resistance may be mediated through obesity, multiparity, growth hormone, or glucocorticoid excess. With increasing insulin resistance, there is a progressive increase in rates of IAPP synthesis (see Fig. 11-3). Islets of 80% of people with chronic insulin resistance respond by hyperplasia, and the compensated hyperinsulinemia prevents hyperglycemia. In approximately 20% of the population, chronic insulin resistance results in islet amyloidosis and loss of β-cell mass with the development of diabetes mellitus.

in dysfunction of a chloride channel protein that has been shown to be important in acidification of intracellular vesicles.[41] Therefore, one potential mechanism that might render β-cells vulnerable to intracellular amyloidosis is failure of the insulin secretory vesicles. It remains to be determined if this is a defect that leads to intracellular islet amyloidosis in people with cystic fibrosis.

Chaperone proteins are increasingly recognized as playing an essential role in the appropriate trafficking and folding of nascent proteins within the cell.[42] One key role of chaperone proteins is to prevent insoluble intracellular aggregates of nascent proteins. The latter would be an inevitable occurrence with all proteins with hydrophobic sequences (e.g., those with transmembrane domains), unless chaperone proteins bound to the hydrophobic domains shortly after synthesis and protected these regions from those present in adjacent comparable proteins. There is at least indirect evidence that chaperone proteins play this important role and have a saturable capacity to traffic nascent protein. Thus, cells transfected with highly efficient expression vectors with high rates of synthesis of proteins with hydrophobic sequences frequently are damaged by intracellular aggregates of the relevant protein.

We have previously suggested[43] that the molecular genetic defect in type II diabetes mellitus may at least theoretically result in a decreased capacity of the chaperone protein pathway (e.g., through polymorphisms in the heat shock protein regulatory proteins or the chaperone proteins per se). In the latter circumstance under conditions of increased IAPP synthesis (insulin resistance), free "unprotected" nascent IAPP may become aggregated intracellularly, providing a nidus for subsequent IAPP amyloidogenesis (Fig. 11-3). This latter hypothesis is consistent with the epidemiologic data (Fig. 11-4) that implies that insulin resistance is the environmental factor that leads to expression of the type II diabetes phenotype or the presence of the appropriate genotype.

Thus, although insulin resistance appears to induce type II diabetes mellitus in those genetically predisposed, unless it is extreme,[44] it results in islet hyperplasia and increased insulin secretion, and glycemic control is maintained (Fig. 11-4). Islet hyperplasia in response to insulin resistance might be considered analogous to the parathyroid gland in patients with renal failure and chronically low ionized plasma calcium concentrations in whom the parathyroid gland becomes hyperplastic but does not fail. In contrast, in humans who are genetically predisposed to type II diabetes mellitus, chronic insulin resistance and islet stimulation lead to increased synthesis of IAPP, which is deposited as islet amyloid. If induction of insulin resistance causes intracellular IAPP amyloidogenesis, a key question is whether the intracellular amyloidosis causes the β-cell loss characteristic of type II diabetes mellitus.

Is Islet Amyloid Cytotoxic and of Mechanistic Significance in the Pathogenesis of Islet Dysfunction?

Thus far, two studies have provided evidence that IAPP amyloid may be cytotoxic. When amyloid fibrils derived from IAPP were applied to the cell surface of human and rat islets, they provoked cell death through apoptosis.[45] In a second study, human versus rat IAPP was expressed at a high rate in COS cells to ask the following questions: Does IAPP amyloid form intracellularly, and if so, is it cytotoxic? Cells transfected with the human but not the rat IAPP gene formed intracellular amyloid (see Fig. 11-2), consistent with the observation that human but not rat IAPP is amyloidogenic in vitro[37] (see Fig. 11-1) and that humans but not rats develop type II diabetes mellitus associated with islet amyloid. In the latter experiments, the intracellular IAPP amyloidosis was accompanied by death of the COS cells (although this was not mediated through apoptosis but through necrosis), lending further support to the hypothesis that IAPP amyloidosis is formed intracellularly and is mechanistically important in causing cell death. Based on the observation that extracellular amyloid is cytotoxic,[46] it is possible that extracellular amyloid derived from intracellular sources further contributes to the destruction of adjacent β-cells.

Summary

IAPP-derived amyloid is clearly associated with type II diabetes mellitus. The physical properties of IAPP in humans and other species that develop type II diabetes mellitus are consistent with the tendency of this protein to form amyloid fibrils when present in high concentrations in anything other than a highly acidic environment or bound to other proteins (such as chaperone proteins). Increasing evidence suggests that IAPP amyloidogenesis may originate within β-cells and at least contribute to their destruction. This cytotoxicity may be mediated directly on the cell within which the fibrils are formed or indirectly on adjacent β-cells. The function of IAPP in health remains to be determined, although it appears to inhibit insulin secretion by a paracrine regulatory mechanism. Although many questions remain to be answered, it is becoming increasingly clear that islet amyloid is unlikely to be an innocent bystander in the pathogenesis of type II diabetes mellitus but, in fact, may play a central role.

Acknowledgment

The work of Dr. Peter C. Butler is funded by the United States Public Health Service, DK44341, and the Mayo Foundation.

References

1. Warren S, LeCompte PM. The pancreas in diabetes mellitus. In: The Pathology of Diabetes Mellitus. Philadelphia: Lea & Febiger;1952:31–75
2. Cohen AS, Calkins E. Electron microscopic observations on a fibrous component in amyloid of diverse origins. Nature 1959;183:1202
3. Eanes ED, Glenner GG. X-ray diffraction studies of amyloid filaments. J Histochem Cytochem 1986;16:673
4. Lansbury PT. In pursuit of the molecular structure of amyloid plaque: New technology provides unexpected and critical information. Biochemistry 1992;31:6865
5. Levy E, Carmen MD, Fernandez-Madrid IJ, et al. Mutation of the Alzheimer's disease amyloid gene in hereditary cerebral hemorrhage, Dutch type. Science 1990;248:1124
6. Howard CF Jr. Insular amyloidosis and diabetes in *Macaca nigra*. Diabetes 1978;27:357
7. Johnson KH, Stevens JB. Light and electron microscopic studies of islet amyloid in diabetic cats. Diabetes 1973;22:81
8. O'Brien TD, Hayden DW, O'Leary TP, et al. Canine pancreatic endocrine tumors: Immunohistochemical analysis of the hormone content and amyloid. Vet Pathol 1987;24:308
9. Westermark P, Wilander E. The influence of amyloid deposits on the islet volume in maturity onset diabetes mellitus. Diabetologia 1978;15:417
10. Howard CF. Longitudinal studies on the development of diabetes in individual *Macaca nigra*. Diabetologia 1986;29:301
11. de Koning EJP, Bodkin NL, Hansen BC, Clark A. Diabetes mellitus in *Macaca mulatta* monkeys is characterized by islet amyloidosis and reduction in beta-cell population. Diabetologia 1993;36:378
12. Clark A, Holman RR, Matthews DR, et al. Non-uniform distribution of islet amyloid in the pancreas of maturity onset diabetic patients. Diabetologia 1984;27:527
13. Melato M, Antonutto G, Ferronato E. Amyloidosis of the islets of Langerhans in relation to diabetes mellitus and aging. Beitr Pathol 1977;160:73
14. Narita R, Toshimori H, Nakazato M, et al. Islet amyloid polypeptide (IAPP) and pancreatic islet amyloid deposition in diabetic and non-diabetic patients. Diabetes Res Clin Pract 1992;15:3
15. Maloy AL, Longnecker DS, Greenberg ER. The relation of islet amyloid to the clinical type of diabetes. Hum Pathol 1981;12:917
16. Westermark P, Wernstedt C, Wilander E, et al. Amyloid fibrils in human insulinoma and islets of Langerhans of the diabetic cat are derived from a neuropeptide-like protein also present in normal islet cells. Proc Natl Acad Sci USA 1987;84:3881
17. Cooper GJS, Willis AC, Clark A, et al. Purification and characterization of a peptide from amyloid-rich pancreases of type 2 diabetic patients. Proc Natl Acad Sci USA 1987;84:8628
18. Westermark P, Wernstedt C, Wilander E, Sletten K. A novel peptide in the calcitonin gene related family as an amyloid fibril protein in the endocrine pancreas. Biochem Biophys Res Commun 1986;140:827
19. Nakazato M, Asai J, Miyazato M, et al. Isolation and identification of islet amyloid polypeptide in normal human pancreas. Regul Pept 1990;31:179
20. Nishi M, Bell GI, Steiner DF. Islet amyloid polypeptide (amylin): No evidence of an abnormal precursor sequence in 25 type 2 (non–insulin-dependent) diabetic patients. Diabetologia 1990;33:628
21. Betsholz C, Svensson V, Rorsman F, et al. Islet amyloid polypeptide (IAPP): cDNA cloning and identification of an amyloidogenic region associated with the species-specific occurrence of age-related diabetes mellitus. Exp Cell Res 1989;183:484
22. Westermark P, Engström U, Johnson KH, et al. Islet amyloid polypeptide: Pinpointing amino acid residues linked to amyloid fibril formation. Proc Natl Acad Sci USA 1990;87:5036
23. Leighton B, Cooper GJS. Pancreatic amylin and calcitonin gene related peptide causes resistance to insulin in skeletal muscle in vitro. Nature 1988;335:632
24. Butler PC, Chou J, Carter WB, et al. Effects of meal ingestion on plasma amylin concentrations in NIDDM and nondiabetic humans. Diabetes 1990;39:752
25. Ohsawa H, Kanatsuka A, Yamaguchi T, et al. Islet amyloid polypeptide inhibits glucose-stimulated insulin secretion from isolated rat pancreatic islets. Biochem Biophys Res Commun 1989;160:961
26. Westermark P, Wilander E, Westermark GT, Johnson KH. Islet amyloid polypeptide-like immunoreactivity in the islet B cells of type 2 (non–insulin-dependent) diabetic and non-diabetic individuals. Diabetologia 1987;30:887
27. Johnson KH, O'Brien TD, Hayden DW, et al. Immunolocalization of islet amyloid polypeptide (IAPP) in pancreatic beta cells by means of peroxidase-antiperoxidase (PAP) and protein A-gold techniques. Am J Pathol 1988;130:1
28. Lukinius A, Wilander E, Westermark GT, et al. Co-localization of islet amyloid polypeptide and insulin in the B cell secretory granules of the human pancreatic islets. Diabetologia 1989;32:240
29. Leffert JD, Newgard CB, Okamoto H, et al. Rat amylin: Cloning and tissue specific expression in pancreatic islets. Proc Natl Acad Sci USA 1989;86:3127
30. Clark A, Edwards CA, Ostle LR, et al. Localization of islet amyloid peptide in lipofuscin bodies and secretory granules of human B-cells and in islets of type 2 diabetic subjects. Cell Tissue Res 1989;257:179
31. Hartter E, Svoboda T, Ludvik B, et al. Basal and stimulated plasma levels of pancreatic amylin indicate its co-secretion with insulin in humans. Diabetologia 1991;34:52
32. Mitsukawa T, Takemura J, Asai J, et al. Islet amyloid polypeptide response to glucose, insulin, and somatostatin analogue administration. Diabetes 1990;39:639
33. de Koning EJP, Höppener JWM, Verbeek JS, et al. Human islet amyloid polypeptide accumulates at similar sites in islets of transgenic mice and humans. Diabetes 1994;43:640
34. O'Brien TD, Butler AE, Johnson KH, et al. Islet amyloid polypeptide (IAPP) in human insulinomas: Evidence for intracellular amyloidogenesis. Diabetes 1994;43:329
35. Toshimori H, Narita R, Nakazato M, et al. Islet amyloid polypeptide in insulinoma and in the islet of the pancreas of non-diabetic and diabetic subjects. Virchows Arch A Pathol Anat Histopathol 1991;418:411
36. Yano BL, Hayden DW, Johnson KH. Feline insular amyloid: Ultrastructural evidence for intracellular formation by nonendocrine cells. Lab Invest 1981;45:149
37. O'Brien TD, Butler PC, Kreutter DK, et al. Human islet amyloid polypeptide expression in COS-1 cells: An *in vitro* model of intracellular amyloidogenesis. Am J Pathol 1995;147:609
38. Mori H, Mori S, Saitoh Y, et al. Growth hormone-producing pituitary adenoma with crystal-like amyloid immunohistochemically positive for growth hormone. Cancer 1985;55:96
39. Hutton JC. The internal pH and membrane potential of the insulin-secretory granule. Biochem J 1982;204:171
40. Couce M, O'Brien TD, Moran A, et al. Diabetes mellitus in cystic fibrosis is characterized by islet amyloidosis. J Clin Endocrinol Metab 1996; in press
41. Barasch J, Kiss B, Prince A, et al. Defective acidification of intracellular organelles in cystic fibrosis. Nature 1991;352:70
42. Rothman JE. Polypeptide chain binding proteins: Catalysts of protein folding and related processes in cells. Cell 1989;59:591
43. Butler PC, Eberhardt NL, O'Brien TD. Islet amyloid polypeptide (IAPP) and insulin secretion. In: Draznin B, LeRoith D, eds. Molecular Biology of Diabetes. Totowa, NJ: Humana Press;1994:381–398
44. O'Brien TD, Rizza RA, Carney JA, Butler PC. Islet amyloidosis in a patient with chronic massive insulin resistance due to antiinsulin receptor antibodies. J Clin Endocrinol Metab 1994;79:290
45. Lorenzo A, Razzaboni B, Weir GC, Yankner BA. Pancreatic islet cell toxicity of amylin associated with Type-2 diabetes mellitus. Nature 1994;368:756
46. Molina JM, Cooper GJS, Leighton B, Olefsky JM. Induction of insulin resistance in vivo by amylin and calcitonin gene-related peptide. Diabetes 1990;39:260

Part II

Insulin Action

Diabetes Mellitus, edited by Derek LeRoith, Simeon I. Taylor, and Jerrold M. Olefsky. Lippincott–Raven Publishers, Philadelphia © 1996.

Chapter 12
Physiologic Action of Insulin

Paul Flakoll, Michael G. Carlson, and Alan Cherrington

Introduction

Insulin is commonly felt to be the primary regulator of the blood glucose level. Indeed, an absence of insulin results in an elevated blood glucose concentration, whereas an excess of the hormone results in hypoglycemia. Since both of the above circumstances can be life-threatening, insulin assumes a key role in glucose homeostasis. It is now abundantly clear that insulin also plays a primary role in the control of fat and protein metabolism. Insulin levels increase with food ingestion and fall with food deprivation, thereby providing coordination for the metabolic changes that accompany feeding and fasting. The hormone exerts its effects on muscle, fat, and the liver, tissues primarily concerned with the regulation of fuel metabolism. We will review the effects of insulin on carbohydrate, fat, and protein metabolism in the whole organism.

Insulin and Glucose Metabolism

Insulin and Glucose Production

Insulin is secreted by the β-cells of the pancreas directly into the hepatic portal blood. After an overnight fast in a normal individual, the arterial plasma insulin level can range from 5–15 μU/mL. The level of insulin in the portal vein is approximately threefold greater than its level in arterial plasma, such that the plasma insulin concentration in the liver sinusoids, which contain mixed arterial (20%) and portal (80%) blood, is 15–40 μU/mL. The plasma insulin level falls in response to hypoglycemia, hyperinsulinemia, and in certain circumstances to increased catecholamines. It rises in response to hyperglycemia, amino acids, and nonesterified fatty acids as well as sympathetic and parasympathetic stimulation. As a consequence of these factors, it is not uncommon for the insulin level to decrease by 50% (during exercise or fasting) or to rise by as much as 10-fold (after food ingestion) during the course of a day.

It is now clear that the basal amount of insulin present after an overnight fast exerts a marked inhibitory effect on glucose production. If the insulin level is quickly and selectively reduced to zero (i.e., glucagon is prevented from changing), glucose production doubles in about 30 minutes.[1] This indicates that the basal amounts of insulin seen in blood after an overnight fast produce a half-maximal inhibition of glucose output by the liver. The amount of insulin required to half maximally inhibit the effect of elevated levels of other agonists (e.g., glucagon) on glucose production would of course be greater.

Increments in insulin have long been known to reduce glucose output by the liver.[2] Early studies using tracer methods to explore the effects of insulin on hepatic glucose production, however, overestimated the extent and speed with which the hormone acts. This error was attributable to the presence of a contaminant in the glucose tracer and the use of a less than ideal approach to data analysis. More recent studies using purified tracers and more sophisticated mathematical models have given a more accurate picture of insulin's action on the liver. It now appears that doubling the insulin secretion rate will lead to an inhibition of glucose production by 80%, and, as can be seen in Figure 12-1, a threefold increase in secretion will virtually eliminate glucose production.[3] Further, it is now clear that although insulin's inhibitory action begins quickly (i.e., within a few minutes), it requires as long as 2 hours to be fully manifest.

It has recently been suggested that insulin's action on the liver is secondary to its effects on peripheral tissues.[4–6] Supposedly the hormone inhibits glucose production by decreasing the flow of gluconeogenic precursors and free fatty acids to the liver. Insulin's action in muscle and fat has a slow onset because the hormone must first cross the endothelial barrier to reach the target tissue and exert its effect.[7] This is believed to provide an explanation for the slow time course of insulin's action on the liver. The link between insulin's peripheral action and the liver is still unclear, but data are accumulating to suggest that it relates to the hormone's antilipolytic effect.[8,9]

More recent studies have suggested that the action of insulin on the liver is related both to a direct and an indirect hepatic effect of the hormone.[5] A selective 15 μU/mL increase in the arterial insulin level (brought about in the absence of any change in the portal plasma insulin level or in the arterial or portal plasma glucagon levels) reduced glucose production by 30–40%.[8] A selective increase of 15 μU/mL in the arterial insulin level (brought about in the absence of any change in the portal plasma insulin level or in the arterial or portal plasma glucagon level) also caused a 30–40% fall in glucose production.[8] Since it is clear that any change in insulin secretion would result in a rise in both liver sinusoidal and arterial insulin levels, it is also evident that it would cause both a direct and an indirect inhibition of hepatic glucose production. A doubling of insulin secretion, for instance, would result in a rise in arterial insulin of ≈10 μU/mL, a rise in portal insulin of ≈30 μU/mL, and an increase in liver sinusoidal insulin of 26 μU/mL. The rise in portal insulin (30 μU/mL) would reduce glucose production by ≈60%, whereas the rise in arterial insulin (10 μU/mL) would reduce glucose output by ≈20%. It is thus evident that normally about three-quarters of insulin's effect is attributable to a direct action of the hormone on the liver and about one-quarter is attributable to its indirect actions. When insulin is delivered peripherally, however, as is the case in an individual with diabetes, a 10 μU/mL rise in arterial insulin levels would be associated with a rise in portal insulin of 8 μU/mL, as about 20% of plasma insulin is degraded as blood flows through the gastrointestinal tract. Thus with peripheral insulin administration, approximately half of the hormone's inhibitory action is caused by its peripheral effects. It should also be remembered that under normal circumstances insulin modifies glucose uptake by the α-cell and thus can decrease glucagon secretion.[10] Since glucagon is a very powerful regulator of glucose production, this peripheral action of insulin would also result in decreased glucose production. Insulin thus reduces hepatic glucose output by two indirect mechanisms, one metabolic and one hormonal in nature, as noted in Figure 12-2. If the α-cell response to insulin is considered, it is obvious that when insulin is delivered peripherally its peripheral actions probably explain three-quarters of its effect on the liver.

Glucose production by the liver is attributable both to the breakdown of glycogen and the conversion of gluconeogenic sub-

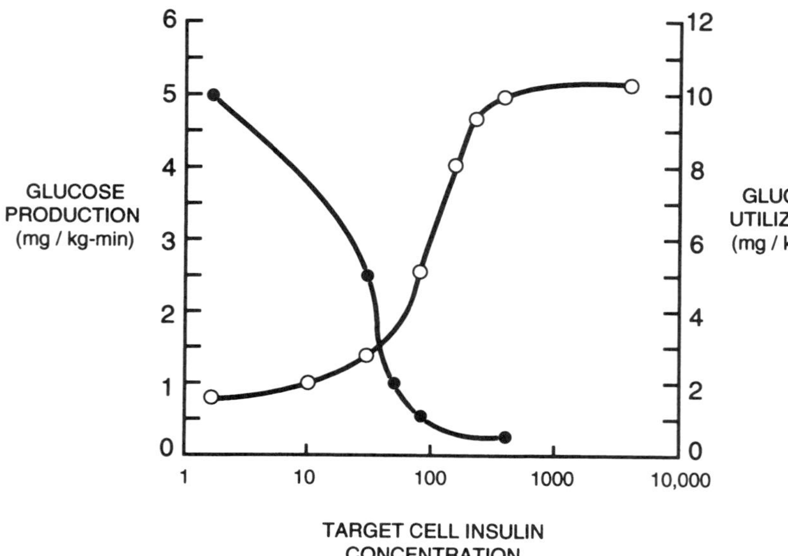

Figure 12-1. Dose-response relationship between the plasma insulin level and glucose production and utilization. Data are taken from references 3, 4, 15, 16, and 20.

strates into glucose. It is important, therefore, to examine insulin's action on both of these processes. Basal amounts of insulin exert a restraining effect on gluconeogenesis.[11] This is clear from glucose production data obtained using a combination of tracer and arteriovenous difference techniques, which showed that gluconeogenic glucose production rose when selective insulin deficiency was produced acutely (i.e., basal glucagon was present). The above methods cannot detect any effect of insulin deficiency on hepatic proteolysis; thus to the extent that proteolysis contributes carbon to gluconeogenesis, the above methods underestimate the inhibitory effect of the hormone. Gluconeogenesis is markedly elevated after prolonged insulin deficiency in the untreated type I diabetic individual.[12,13] This effect seems to result from both an increase in the flow of gluconeogenic precursors to the liver and an increase in their conversion to glucose within the liver (hepatic efficiency).

Increments in insulin secretion as great as fourfold basal, on the other hand, produce little further inhibition of the already low gluconeogenic rate. They do, however, direct some of the gluconeogenically derived glucose into glycogen.[14] The implication of this finding is that small to moderate increments in insulin do not significantly decrease gluconeogenic precursor flow (lactate and amino acids) from muscle to the liver. This has been confirmed by direct observations.[8,15] Increments in insulin do, however, inhibit lipolysis such that glycerol uptake by the liver falls. Since such uptake is only a small contributor to total hepatic gluconeogenic precursor uptake, this has only a limited impact on glucose production. In individuals with obesity or non–insulin-dependent diabetes mellitus (NIDDM), the lipolytic rate can be markedly elevated and as a result the contribution of glycerol to gluconeogenesis would be increased. The more important consequence of insulin's action on fat appears related to the decrease in free fatty acid uptake by the liver, which increases the oxidation rate of glucose within the liver. Small increases in insulin have virtually no effect on the gluconeogenic efficiency of the liver (i.e., the percent of the extracted gluconeogenic precursors that are converted to glucose). Very high levels of insulin, on the other hand, can inhibit hepatic gluconeogenic efficiency,[16] but such levels rarely if ever occur in the course of a normal day.

Basal amounts of insulin inhibit glycogenolysis by about 60% so that selective insulin deficiency increases glycogen breakdown markedly. Unlike gluconeogenesis, glycogenolysis is inhibited by small increments in insulin. In fact, a threefold increase in insulin secretion is enough to completely inhibit glycogenolysis provided that euglycemia is maintained by glucose infusion.

Insulin is clearly a very important regulator of glucose production, but it must be remembered that it acts in concert with glucagon to control the blood glucose level. Glucagon exerts its effect quickly (within minutes), potently stimulating both hepatic glycogenolysis and gluconeogenesis.[3] Basal glucagon is responsible for about two-thirds of glucose production after an overnight fast. A physiologic increase in glucagon has a time-dependent effect on hepatic glucose output, however, so that its effect wanes by almost 50% within 3 hours. The waning is because of a progressive fall in glycogenolysis, the explanation for which is not completely clear. Although glucagon's effect on hepatic gluconeogenic efficiency is sustained, its effect on gluconeogenic glucose production is not because the hormone has little or no effect on muscle or fat and thus fails to increase the supply of gluconeogenic precursors reaching the liver. As a result, once the plasma pool of gluconeogenic precursors is depleted, the reduced substrate supply offsets the enhanced intrahepatic gluconeogenesis and the overall gluconeogenic rate returns to its control value. It should be noted that if fourfold increases in

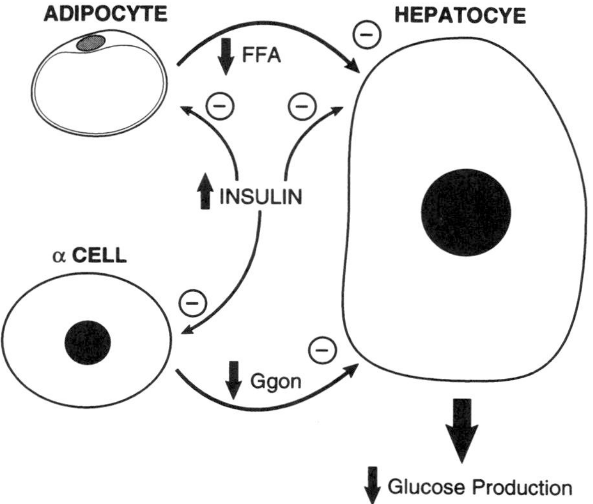

Figure 12-2. Mechanism of insulin's inhibition of glucose production by the liver. Minus sign indicates an inhibitory effect. FFA, free fatty acids.

both insulin and glucagon are brought about together, the inhibitory action of insulin dominates the stimulatory effect of glucagon.[14]

Insulin and Glucose Utilization

Insulin has long been known to increase glucose utilization. It does so by enhancing glucose uptake by the liver, muscle, and fat. In all three tissues it appears to promote the entry of glucose via an effect on the transport-phosphorylation step and to promote the disposition of glucose within the cell through effects on glycogen synthesis and glucose oxidation. The intracellular signals that bring about the above changes are dealt with elsewhere, so we will focus only on the quantitative consequences of insulin action in the whole animal.

After an overnight fast the glucose utilization rate is between 2.0 and 2.5 mg/kg/min. Of that only 25% is insulin-mediated, the rest being glucose uptake by non–insulin-dependent tissues (e.g., nervous system and the formed elements of the blood). Removal of insulin should thus result in only a small fall in glucose utilization. In fact, since a fall in insulin results in a paradoxical increase in plasma glucose, insulin deficiency is usually associated with an increase in glucose utilization.[1] If an index of insulin action is calculated by relating glucose utilization to the prevailing glucose level, however, the impairment induced by insulin removal becomes evident. Examination of any such index shows a decrease in the efficiency of glucose utilization in the absence of insulin.[1]

The ability of increments in insulin to increase glucose utilization has been examined by many investigators using isotope techniques or arteriovenous difference methods or both. Regardless of the technique employed, it is clear that insulin can increase glucose utilization under euglycemic conditions by as much as 25-fold.[14,17–20] Further, a half-maximally effective insulin level would appear to be between 60 and 100 μU/mL. It is of interest to compare insulin's action on glucose production and utilization (see Fig. 12-1). A doubling of insulin secretion will inhibit hepatic glucose output by ≃80% (≃1.5–2.0 mg/kg/min), whereas it will increase glucose utilization by only 20% (≃0.4–0.6 mg/kg/min). On the other hand, the effect of insulin on glucose production is complete when insulin secretion rises threefold, but its effect on glucose utilization does not saturate even with the highest possible physiologic insulin levels. It takes a pharmacologic arterial plasma insulin concentration in excess of 500 μU/mL to saturate glucose uptake under euglycemic conditions. Thus the sensitivity of glucose production to insulin is greater than the sensitivity of glucose utilization to insulin, but the capacity of the glucose utilization response is much greater than the capacity of the glucose production response.

The time course of insulin's action on glucose utilization is, as noted earlier, similar to its time course on glucose production. Both begin to respond in minutes, but the response requires 90–120 minutes to be fully manifest. Bergman and colleagues have provided convincing data indicating that it is the relatively slow movement of insulin across the endothelial barrier and into the interstitial compartment in fat and muscle that explains the slow development of its full effect.[5]

Under euglycemic conditions, physiologic increments in insulin promote the uptake of glucose by muscle, fat, and the liver, but the latter two tissues contribute minimally (<10%) to the increased glucose uptake. Thus muscle is by far the predominant target for insulin action under euglycemic conditions. It should be noted that insulin causes vasodilation in muscle vasculature so that in addition to its direct action on myocytes, it increases the perfusion of muscle. Comparison of the dose-response curves relating glucose uptake by the leg or limb blood flow and the insulin level shows marked similarity (Fig. 12-3). It is difficult to determine the metabolic significance of the flow changes per se, but work by Baron and colleagues suggests that the change in flow contributes in its own right to the overall action of insulin.[20] It is also worth pointing out that although insulin has a direct vasodilatory effect on the vasculature, it also increases sympathetic drive by the central nervous system. Studies in which hyperinsulinemic euglycemic clamps were brought about have clearly shown that insulin increased plasma norepinephrine levels and nerve firing to muscle.[21] Indeed, Davis and coworkers[22] have shown that the brain can respond directly to physiologic changes in the circulating insulin level.

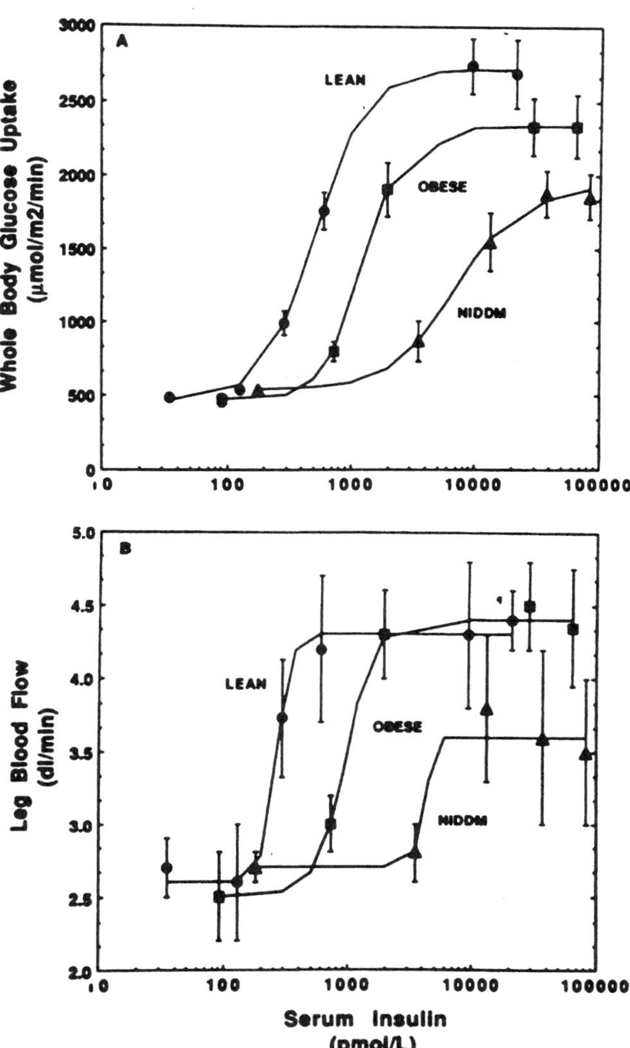

Figure 12-3. Dose-response relationships between the serum insulin level and whole body glucose uptake (*A*), or leg blood flow (*B*) in humans. The data are taken from Baron AD. Hemodynamic actions of insulin. Am J Physiol 1994;267:E187.

It is now clear that insulin also directs the fate of glucose once it enters the muscle cell. Increments in insulin increase both glycogen synthesis and glucose oxidation in muscle, with the effect on the former being predominant. As the plasma insulin level is increased, the effect of the hormone on oxidation changes only slightly, so that the increase in glucose uptake is explained predominantly by an increase in glucose storage. There is also a small increase in the release of glucose carbon in the form of alanine and lactate, again pointing out that increased insulin is not associated with a decreased flux of these gluconeogenic precursors to the liver.[15]

Rarely does insulin rise under euglycemic conditions; thus, the situation seen most commonly is a combination of hyperglycemia and hyperinsulinemia. Hyperglycemia by itself leads to an increase in glucose uptake by muscle as a result of a "mass" effect. As a consequence of this increased glucose uptake, glucose storage and oxidation increase about equally. Addition of a half-maximally effective concentration of insulin under hyperglycemic conditions markedly increases glucose uptake and doubles the increase in glucose oxidation but profoundly increases glucose storage.[15] Thus, extremely high glucose utilization rates (>25 mg/kg/min) can be seen in the presence of very high insulin and very high glucose levels. Although the muscle remains by far the most important repository for glucose under these conditions, some glucose is stored in liver and fat. Surprisingly, however, even with very high levels of insulin and a glucose level twice normal, the liver takes up little glucose when the sugar is infused through a peripheral vein. Net hepatic glucose uptake under such conditions can reach 2 mg/kg/min in the dog[23] and no more than 1.0 mg/kg/min in humans.[24] This raises the question as to the explanation for the marked hepatic glucose uptake (≈5.0 mg/kg/min) seen after oral glucose consumption.[25] It was originally postulated that a gut factor signaled the liver to take up glucose.[24] Studies in which glucose absorption was mimicked by portal glucose infusion, however, showed that portal glucose delivery was also associated with net hepatic glucose uptake of 5.0 mg/kg/min.[23] More recently it has been suggested that when the portal glucose level exceeds the arterial glucose level (such as occurs after glucose ingestion), a response is triggered that changes the distribution of glucose between muscle and liver. This "portal" signal appears to cause a decrease in muscle glucose uptake and an augmentation of liver glucose uptake. The portal signal can increase glucose uptake by the liver in the absence of any change in insulin (for review, see reference 25). It appears that the effects of insulin and the portal signal on the liver are additive.[25] The regulation of hepatic glucose uptake under hyperglycemic conditions is thus only partly dependent on insulin. It should not be forgotten, however, that in the chronic absence of insulin, glucokinase becomes deficient and glucose uptake by the liver ceases whether or not the portal signal is present.[25]

In summary, it is now clear that physiologic levels of insulin have profound effects on glucose production and utilization. Muscle glucose uptake is markedly but somewhat slowly increased in response to increased insulin. Glucose production by the liver, on the other hand, is sensitively decreased by insulin. This effect comes about through both direct and indirect actions of hormone, the latter imparting a slow second phase to the overall response. Insulin is important to the regulation of hepatic glucose uptake under hyperglycemic conditions both in an acute and chronic sense. Clearly, insulin's role in the metabolic adjustment to food intake, food deprivation, and exercise is critical in that in the absence of normal insulin release, normal glucose control is lost.

Insulin and Fat Metabolism

Insulin plays a central role in the regulation of adipose tissue metabolism and in the storage, mobilization, and utilization of adipose tissue triglyceride. The integrated physiologic effects of insulin on lipid metabolism (Table 12-1) facilitate fat storage and inhibit fat mobilization. Through its many metabolic actions, insulin serves to coordinate the availability and utilization of alternative fuels, glucose, and free fatty acids in order to meet the energy demands of the organism throughout the normal cycles of feeding and fasting.

Physiology of Fat Metabolism

Fat is stored in anhydrous form as triglyceride (TG) in the central lipid droplet of adipocytes. Because of its high caloric content (9 kcal/g) and efficient storage form, adipose tissue TG represents the major source of stored fuel available for mobilization when energy requirements are increased (e.g., during exercise) or when glucose availability is reduced (e.g., during fasting). For example, the average adult human weighing 70 kg has approximately 14,000 g of stored adipose tissue TG with an energy equivalent of 126,000 kcal. By comparison, hepatic glycogen stores amount to ~75 g (or 300 kcal) following an overnight fast.[26]

Table 12-1. Insulin Actions on Fat Metabolism

Inhibition of free fatty acid mobilization from adipose tissue
Suppression of adipose tissue lipolysis
Stimulation of intra-adipocyte free fatty acid re-esterification
Inhibition of plasma free fatty acid uptake and oxidation
Suppression of circulating ketone body concentrations
Reduction in supply of free fatty acid substrate to the liver for ketogenesis
Inhibition of intrahepatic ketogenesis
Acceleration of peripheral ketone body clearance and catabolism
Activation of lipoprotein lipase
Increased clearance of TG-rich lipoproteins by peripheral tissues
Stimulation of lipogenesis

Following an overnight fast when blood insulin concentrations are low (~10 μU/mL), fat is mobilized from adipose tissue stores as free fatty acids (Fig. 12-4). The hydrolysis of stored triglyceride (i.e., lipolysis), catalyzed by the adipocyte enzyme, hormone-sensitive lipase, yields free fatty acids and glycerol, the three carbon backbone of triglyceride. The free glycerol is released from the adipocyte and enters the plasma, where its major metabolic fate is extraction by the liver and conversion to glucose (gluconeogenesis).[27] In contrast, whereas most of the free fatty acids generated by lipolysis are released into the plasma, a fraction is immediately re-esterified back to TG without ever leaving the adipose tissue (Fig. 12-4). The glycerol-3-phosphate required for the intra-adipocyte or primary re-esterification of free fatty acids is derived from glycolytic metabolism of glucose within the adipocyte, an insulin-dependent process. Following their release from adipose tissue, plasma free fatty acids circulate complexed with albumin and are available for uptake by tissues such as liver, skeletal muscle, and heart, where they can undergo oxidation or esterification to TG (peripheral or secondary re-esterification). Under postabsorptive conditions, oxidation of free fatty acids provides the bulk of the energy needs of these organs, sparing glucose for use by glucose-requiring tissues such as brain, erythrocytes, and renal medulla.

Following a mixed meal, the rise in blood insulin (to 30–50 μU/mL) levels inhibits adipose tissue lipolysis and restrains free fatty acid mobilization from endogenous fat stores. Exogenous fat from the meal is packaged by the intestine and released as TG-rich chylomicrons. Lipoprotein lipase, an enzyme present on the capillary endothelium in muscle and adipose tissue, hydrolyzes chylomicron-TG with subsequent uptake of the generated fatty acids by muscle or adipose tissue, where they can be oxidized or stored, respectively.[28,29] Meal-stimulated insulin release and the elevated postprandial glucose and insulin levels result in activation of adipose tissue lipoprotein lipase and clearance of TG-rich lipoproteins (mainly chylomicrons). In contrast, the activity of skeletal muscle lipoprotein lipase is inhibited by the postprandial increase in glucose and insulin.[30] The differential effects of insulin on adipose tissue and skeletal muscle lipoprotein lipase activity serve to divert free fatty acids derived from lipoprotein TG away from muscle and to adipose tissue for storage. In states of absolute or relative insulin deficiency such as decompensated insulin-dependent diabetes mellitus or NIDDM, respectively, lipoprotein lipase–mediated clearance of chylomicrons is grossly impaired and can result in profound lipemia and hypertriglyceridemia (TG>1000 mg/dL). Improved diabetes control reverses the defect in lipoprotein lipase activity and reduces serum TG levels.[31]

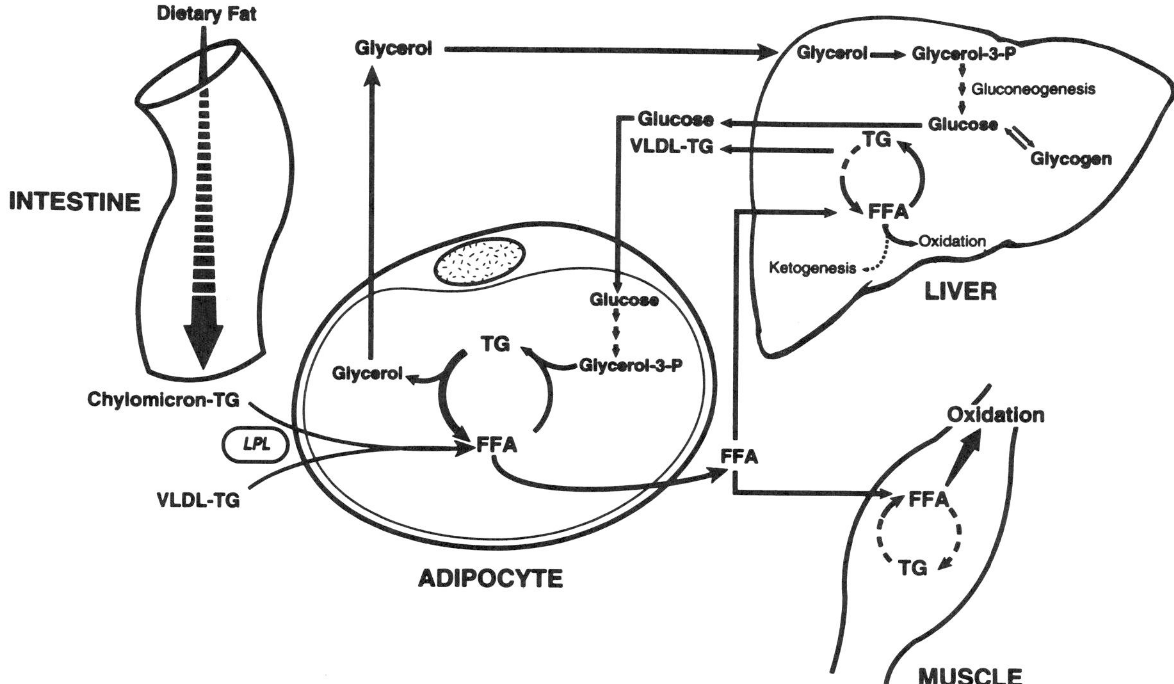

Figure 12-4. Control points in the regulation of fat metabolism. FFA, free fatty acids; VLDL, very low density lipoprotein; LPL, lipoprotein lipase; TG, triglyceride.

Insulin and Free Fatty Acid Availability

Fatty acid mobilization from adipose tissue is exquisitely sensitive to insulin. Among its many metabolic effects, insulin's most potent action is the suppression of adipose tissue lipolysis.[32–34] A rise in plasma insulin concentration of only 5 μU/mL inhibits lipolysis by ~50% from basal levels (Figs. 12-6 and 12-7), whereas a reduction in basal insulin levels results in a marked acceleration of lipolysis. The antilipolytic effect of insulin is mediated through inhibition of hormone-sensitive lipase. Recent work suggests that insulin activates a protein phosphatase that in turn dephosphorylates and inactivates hormone-sensitive lipase.[35] A second mechanism by which insulin inhibits hormone-sensitive lipase involves an insulin-sensitive phosphodiesterase that lowers intracellular cAMP and inhibits the cAMP-dependent protein kinase responsible for phosphorylating and activating hormone-sensitive lipase.[36]

The rate of adipose tissue release of free fatty acids is determined by the net balance between the rate of lipolysis and the rate of intra-adipocyte (or primary) free fatty acid re-esterification (see Fig. 12-4). In addition to its antilipolytic effects, insulin restrains free fatty acid mobilization by stimulating the retention and re-esterification of fatty acids within adipose tissue. As the circulating insulin concentration rises, less free fatty acid is generated by lipolysis, while at the same time a progressively greater fraction of free fatty acid is re-esterified to TG.[32] This stimulation of fractional free fatty acid re-esterification magnifies the degree of suppression of free fatty acid mobilization by insulin in lean healthy humans. The increase in fatty acid esterification induced by insulin is mediated mainly through stimulation of adipocyte glucose uptake and glycolytic metabolism, thereby increasing the availability within the adipocyte of glycerol-3-phosphate for esterification.[37] Insulin may also promote fatty acid activation to fatty acyl CoA and fatty acyl transferase activity.[37]

In obesity, adipose tissue lipolysis is less sensitive to suppression by insulin. However, basal rates of lipolysis corrected for differences in fat mass are not increased in obese nondiabetic humans.[38–40] Rather, the compensatory hyperinsulinemia of obesity is sufficient to overcome the resistance to the antilipolytic effects of insulin. In addition, basal rates of intra-adipocyte free fatty acid re-esterification are increased in obese individuals, and this further limits free fatty acid mobilization.[38] Body fat distribution in obesity also affects the rate of free fatty acid mobilization. Obese individuals with a predominance of intra-abdominal or mesenteric fat (i.e., visceral, upper body, or android obesity) demonstrate excessive rates of free fatty acid mobilization and greater resistance to the antilipolytic effects of insulin when compared to individuals with subcutaneous gluteofemoral adiposity (i.e., lower body or gynecoid obesity).[41,42] The resultant oversupply of free fatty acids to the liver in individuals with visceral obesity can impair hepatic insulin sensitivity and insulin binding and extraction,[43–45] which in turn contributes to the peripheral hyperinsulinemia characteristic of visceral obesity. Furthermore, the increased delivery of free fatty acids to the liver stimulates hepatic gluconeogenesis and net glucose output[46] as well as increased very low density lipoprotein production and hypertriglyceridemia.[47]

Insulin and Free Fatty Acid Disposal

Whole body disposal of circulating free fatty acids occurs by oxidative and nonoxidative (i.e., secondary or peripheral free fatty acid re-esterification) pathways.[32,33,40] Although skeletal muscle, heart, and liver are major sites of free fatty acid oxidation, the re-esterification of circulating free fatty acids occurs predominantly in the liver and is reflected largely by the rate of very low density lipoprotein synthesis.[48] Insulin suppresses both the oxidation and re-esterification of circulating free fatty acids in a dose-dependent manner.[32,33,40] In contrast to the direct hormonal regulation of fatty acid mobilization, rates of uptake and disposal of plasma free fatty acids are largely determined by the circulating free fatty acid concentration. Thus, while insulin decreases tissue uptake and oxidation of free fatty acids, these effects are largely eliminated when free fatty acid availability is maintained experimentally by the intravenous administration of heparin and/or a lipid emulsion to enhance intravascular hydrolysis of circulating TG.[49,50] These studies indicate that the suppression of free fatty acid uptake and oxidation by insulin is predominantly mediated by its potent antilipolytic action and the resultant decrease in free fatty acid availability.

Insulin and Ketone Body Metabolism

Under hypoinsulinemic conditions such as fasting or uncontrolled diabetes, fat mobilization is greatly accelerated and results in an oversupply of free fatty acids to the liver. Under these conditions, the liver synthesizes ketone bodies from the surplus acetyl-CoA produced by the incomplete β-oxidation of long-chain fatty acids. These ketone bodies (acetoacetate, β-hydroxybutyrate, and acetone) are released into the plasma and are taken up and oxidized by extrahepatic tissues, especially skeletal muscle and the heart. During prolonged starvation, the brain is also able to utilize ketone bodies for fuel, thus reducing its obligatory requirement for glucose. The utilization of ketone bodies by extrahepatic tissues is roughly proportional to their concentration in the blood, which in turn is related to the rate of hepatic ketogenesis. At higher concentrations, the ability of extrahepatic tissues to utilize ketone bodies is saturated, such that the accelerated rates of ketonuria and loss of acetone in expired air begin to account for a greater proportion of ketone body disposal.

Insulin potently suppresses circulating ketone body concentrations via three separate mechanisms: (1) inhibition of lipolysis, (2) suppression of intrahepatic ketogenesis, and (3) increased peripheral ketone body clearance. Through its potent antilipolytic effects, insulin restrains free fatty acid mobilization from adipose tissue and decreases the supply of free fatty acids to the liver for ketogenesis. Hepatic fractional extraction of a delivered free fatty acid load does not appear to be affected by insulin.[51] Rather, the decrease in hepatic free fatty acid uptake in response to insulin is mediated solely by the decrease in free fatty acid availability.

Although most of insulin's inhibitory effect on hepatic ketogenesis is accounted for by the decrease in the supply of free fatty acid substrate, physiologic elevations in insulin concentration also exert a direct inhibitory effect on intrahepatic ketogenesis. The direct antiketogenic actions of insulin have been demonstrated in studies in which insulin was administered intravenously to create physiologic hyperinsulinemia while decreases in plasma free fatty acid concentration were prevented. Under these conditions of isolated hyperinsulinemia, rates of hepatic ketogenesis were reduced by ~50% despite no decrease in hepatic free fatty acid uptake.[52] Clinically, this direct inhibitory effect of hyperinsulinemia on hepatic ketogenesis provides one explanation for the resistance to ketosis in obesity and NIDDM despite elevated circulating free fatty acid levels.

Insulin appears to exert its direct inhibitory effect on hepatic ketogenic efficiency by regulating the pathways of intrahepatic free fatty acid metabolism. Following their uptake by the liver, fatty acids may be esterified to TG and secreted in the form of very low density lipoprotein, or they may enter the oxidative pathway (see Fig. 12-4). The entry of long-chain fatty acids into the mitochondria and access to the high capacity enzymes of β-oxidation and ketogenesis are regulated by the outer mitochondrial membrane carrier protein, carnitine acyltransferase I. By inhibiting the activity of carnitine acyltransferase I, insulin suppresses hepatic fatty acid oxidation and ketogenesis and shunts fatty acids into the pathway of TG synthesis.[53] Glucagon counteracts these effects of insulin and appears to be the primary hormone involved in the induction of fatty acid oxidation and ketogenesis in the liver. Thus, intrahepatic ketogenic efficiency is largely determined by the portal concentration ratio of insulin:glucagon.[53,54] The ketogenic capacity of the liver is increased in the fasted state (low insulin:glucagon ratio) and reduced in the fed state (high insulin:glucagon ratio). In addition to the direct hepatic effects of glucagon, physiologic elevations of glucagon such as occur during fasting or exercise may stimulate hepatic ketogenesis indirectly by increasing the supply of free fatty acids to the liver via a direct lipolytic effect of glucagon.[55] This effect however, seems to be limited in magnitude.

Although the major effect of insulin in suppressing circulating ketone body concentrations is mediated through the inhibition of hepatic ketone body production, insulin also influences the rate of ketone body clearance and catabolism by nonhepatic tissues.[56,57] Elevated plasma insulin concentrations result in an increased metabolic clearance rate of ketone bodies. This effect of insulin is mediated both by a direct stimulation of peripheral ketone body disposal and indirectly via the suppression of ketogenesis and lowering of blood ketone body levels. Although total peripheral ketone body uptake increases as circulating ketone body concentrations rise, this increase in uptake by nonhepatic tissues is not linear. In fact, fractional ketone body uptake (i.e., metabolic clearance rate) falls at higher ketone body concentrations.[58] Thus, insulin exerts a direct effect on peripheral tissues and an indirect effect through its suppression of ketogenesis and lowering of ketone body concentrations, which together serve to increase peripheral ketone body clearance and catabolism.

Insulin and Lipogenesis

De novo lipogenesis refers to the biosynthesis of fatty acids from glucose or other substrates. Our understanding of the biochemistry and hormonal regulation of lipogenesis has resulted mostly from in vitro studies in rodents.[59] However, the biologic importance, activity, and tissue distribution of the lipogenic pathways vary greatly among species. Whereas active lipogenesis occurs in liver and adipose tissue in the rat, de novo lipogenesis is an inefficient process in humans; it occurs predominantly in the liver and is of minor significance in human adipose tissue even under conditions of massive carbohydrate overfeeding.[60–62]

The nutritional state of the organism, mediated through changes in circulating insulin concentration, appears to be the major factor determining the rate of lipogenesis. Lipogenesis is high in the fed state and following carbohydrate administration, whereas it is suppressed by fasting, high-fat diets, or insulin deficiency, such as in uncontrolled diabetes. Insulin stimulates de novo lipogenesis from glucose in the liver and adipose tissue by several mechanisms.[59] In adipose tissue, insulin stimulates glucose uptake, thereby increasing the supply of lipogenic substrate. Furthermore, several key enzymes in the lipogenic pathway, including fatty acid synthase and acetyl-CoA carboxylase, are induced by insulin. In addition, the antilipolytic action of insulin reduces free fatty acid availability to the liver and thereby reduces the inhibitory effects of fatty acids on hepatic lipogenesis. Similarly, together the inhibition of lipolysis and the stimulatory effect of insulin on re-esterification of fatty acids in adipose tissue reduce the intra-adipocyte concentration of fatty acyl-CoA, an inhibitor of lipogenesis. Thus, the many actions of insulin serve to increase the biosynthesis of fatty acids for subsequent storage in the form of TG. It should be emphasized, however, that the predominant source of fatty acid substrate for triglyceride synthesis in both adipose tissue and liver comes from circulating free fatty acids derived either from adipose tissue lipolysis or from the intravascular hydrolysis of lipoprotein TG by lipoprotein lipase.

Insulin and Protein Metabolism

A fundamental role for insulin in the regulation of protein metabolism is well established. Throughout history, negative nitrogen balance, lean tissue atrophy, and hyperaminoacidemia have been chronicled as hallmarks to identify uncontrolled diabetes in humans. Findings of additional studies in dogs and rats with experimentally induced diabetes have concurred with these clinical observations, demonstrating increased urinary nitrogen excretion and plasma α-amino nitrogen concentrations.

Although insulin's influence on nitrogen balance and protein accretion has long been recognized, specific mechanisms by which insulin alters protein metabolism have only recently been elucidated (Fig. 12-5). One of these mechanisms is the entry of amino acids into cells, which is regulated via the process of active transport. A second event that contributes to protein homeostasis is proteolysis. The breakdown of proteins into their constitutive amino acids is a perpetual process. Therefore, it is important for the maintenance of body protein that a third event, protein synthesis, also occurs on a continual basis. Amino acids derived from proteolysis as well as from exogenous sources are used to synthesize proteins. These amino acids can also be utilized, however, to form glucose, ketones, urea, and tricarboxylic acid cycle intermediates. Therefore, the interaction of insulin with any of these specific mechanisms could result in alterations in protein accretion.

Insulin and Amino Acid Transport

The movement of amino acids into a cell provides a control site for the regulation of plasma amino acid levels, intracellular amino acid availability, and protein synthesis. Therefore, understanding the control of amino acid transport is fundamental to understanding the regulation of protein metabolism. Intracellular amino acid concentrations are normally greater than corresponding extracellular concentrations. However, this concentration gradient is dependent on the amino acid in question, with glutamine having the largest gradient and branched-chain amino acids the smallest.[63] The maintenance of the gradients requires a number of different transport mechanisms[63,64] (Table 12-2). These systems differ from each other in their specificity for certain amino acids, in how they derive energy for transport, and in their sensitivity to insulin. Furthermore, these transport systems have different activities in various tissues, which have physiologic significance for the movement and disposal of amino acids. For example, while half-maximal transport rates in skeletal muscle occur at much greater than physiologic plasma amino acid concentrations, half-maximal transport across the blood-brain barrier is manifest at physiologic levels.[64-66] Therefore, after ingestion of a protein meal, transport of amino acids into muscle is increased relative to transport into the brain, and muscle acts as a storage depot for excess amino acids.

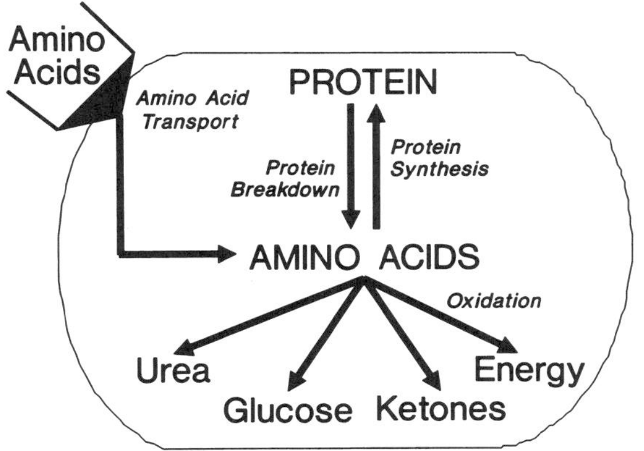

Figure 12-5. General scheme of protein and amino acid metabolism.

Insulin has been implicated in facilitating amino acid transport into hepatocytes, skeletal muscle, and fibroblasts. This potentially explains, in part, the clinical observation that insulin shrinks the plasma pool of amino acids. At least four amino acid transport systems (A, ASC, N^m, and X_c) have been demonstrated to be responsive to insulin. These systems are primarily responsible for the transport of nonessential amino acids. Interestingly, system L, which is responsible for the transport of branched-chain amino acids, is not sensitive to insulin action. Therefore, the influence of insulin on amino acid transport appears to be limited to nonessential amino acids such as alanine, glycine, and glutamine. Furthermore, although insulin's stimulation occurs in a dose-dependent manner, the K_m for insulin's action on system A is approximately 170 μU/mL in hepatocytes[67] and 90 μU/mL in rat skeletal muscle,[66] clearly high physiologic levels. Hence, while in vitro data suggest that the overall action of insulin on amino acid transport involves the stimulation of amino acid movement from extra- to intracellular compartments, the significance of this action in vivo is questionable.

Insulin and Protein Catabolism

The prevailing degree of protein catabolism is important for the maintenance of body protein stores. Proteolytic events control both the quantity of proteins present in a cell and the availability of amino acids within the cellular compartments. Early in vitro studies concluded that insulin decreases proteolysis in skeletal[68-70] and cardiac muscle[68] and in the liver.[71] Furthermore, insulin is known to regulate specific mechanisms of muscle and liver protein breakdown. Although insulin does not act on either cytosolic ATP- or calcium-dependent degradation systems in skeletal muscle, it functions at basal concentrations in muscle by stabilizing lysosomal membranes. In this way it decreases lysosomal uptake and breakdown of cellular constituents.[72] Additionally, basal insulin in muscle decreases free cathepsin D activity, blunting degradation of polyribosomes. Insulin withdrawal enhances muscle lysosome activity and muscle protein catabolism.[73] In the liver, basal insulin diminishes hepatic autophagy by stabilizing lysosomal membranes, decreasing lysosomal uptake of cellular constituents, and reducing lysosomal density.[72] Further increases in insulin above basal levels result in dose-responsive decreases in hepatic proteolysis. Therefore, while sub-basal insulin allows acceleration of both muscle and liver protein catabolism, hyperinsulinemia primarily directs a reduction of liver proteolysis.

Table 12-2. Summary of Amino Acid Transport Systems*

System Type	Amino Acid Specificity	Mechanism
Insulin-Sensitive		
A	Ala, Ser, Gly, Gln, Pro	Na^+ Co-transport
ASC	Ala, Ser, Cys, Gln	Na^+ Co-transport
N^m	Gln, Asp, His	Na^+ Dependent
X^c	Cys, Gln	Substrate coupled
Insulin Sensitivity Undefined		
Y^+	Lys, Arg	Facilitated diffusion
X_{ag}	Asp, Glu	Na^+ Co-transport
Insulin-Insensitive		
L	Leu, Ile, Val	Substrate coupled

*Data are summarized from references 63–67.

A limited number of experiments have examined catabolism of specific tissue proteins in vivo. Breakdown of fixed hepatic proteins is difficult to assess in the whole animal. Although skeletal muscle accounts for only one-fourth of daily total protein turnover, it appears to be the most relevant organ for insulin's mediation of protein metabolism. During insulin deficiency, it has been shown that catabolism of protein is most prevalent in skeletal muscle, with visceral proteins tending to be spared.[72,74] In early studies, Pozefsky and coworkers noted that the normal net loss of amino acids that occurs across the forearm postabsorptively was blunted by local insulin infusion.[75] Furthermore, physiologic hyperinsulinemia diminished skeletal muscle proteolysis assessed by isotopic dilution of phenylalanine across the human forearm.[76] Therefore, while insulin's effects on the catabolism of specific proteins in vivo require further evaluation, it is clear that it plays a significant role in control of skeletal muscle proteolysis.

Clinically, insulin is thought to be anabolic, as insulin treatment is associated with diminished urinary nitrogen loss and restored body mass in diabetic patients.[77] Diabetic patients with negligible plasma insulin concentrations have increased whole body protein breakdown,[78–81] demonstrating a role for basal insulin in suppressing proteolysis. Intensive insulin therapy diminishes proteolysis in insulin-dependent diabetics.[82] Human studies using hyperinsulinemic-euglycemic clamps have shown that physiologic increments in insulin blunt whole body proteolysis in a dose-responsive manner.[83–85] Maximal suppression occurs when protein breakdown is reduced by 40%, suggesting that at least half of the regulation of proteolysis is unresponsive to insulin. It is of interest that maximal and half-maximal suppressive effects in these studies were attained at supraphysiologic insulin levels. Therefore, processes associated with proteolysis in vivo are less sensitive to insulin than those regulating lipolysis or glucose production (Figs. 12-6 and 12-7).

Amino acid availability appears to act with insulin to regulate protein breakdown. During a hyperinsulinemic-euglycemic clamp study, hypoaminoacidemia is prevalent, particularly in the case of essential amino acids. When the fall in plasma amino acids is prevented via exogenous amino acid infusion, insulin suppression of proteolysis is augmented at every insulin dose tested. Furthermore, maintaining amino acid availability enhances responsiveness of proteolysis to insulin but does not change insulin sensitivity.[84] Therefore, this suggests that the interactions of insulin and amino acids are postreceptor or intracellular in nature.

Insulin and Protein Synthesis

Events associated with the synthesis of proteins are also instrumental in the regulation of protein homeostasis and in the utilization of intracellular amino acids. In vitro studies with skeletal and cardiac muscle and liver tissue have suggested that insulin causes an increase in protein synthesis.[86,87] In muscle tissues, insulin is associated with increases in both the number of ribosomes and in their translational efficiency. On the other hand, the stimulation of protein synthesis by insulin in liver tissue may vary, depending upon the specific protein in question. For example, insulin stimulates the synthesis of secretory proteins such as albumin. This increase is facilitated by an elevation in albumin mRNA content as well as in peptide initiation factors. Conversely, insulin reduces the levels of mRNA for proteins involved in gluconeogenesis (e.g., phosphoenolpyruvate carboxykinase[88]).

In direct contrast to in vitro data, however, in vivo studies utilizing hyperinsulinemic-euglycemic clamps have shown a dose-responsive decrease in whole body protein synthesis.[83–85] Half-maximal suppression of protein synthesis occurs at approximately 100 μU/mL. The logic for such disparate results between in vitro and in vivo experiments most likely relates to the availability of amino acids. Although amino acid availability was maintained during in vitro studies, insulin resulted in hypoaminoacidemia during in vivo studies. Therefore, it is difficult to discern the difference between the direct effects of insulin versus the influence of hypoaminoacidemia. Furthermore, it could be postulated that hypoaminoacidemia is the limiting factor for the synthesis of proteins during insulin administration. In studies in which amino acids are infused with insulin to maintain amino acid availability, protein synthetic rates are improved compared to in hypoaminoacidemic conditions. Therefore, it may be postulated that the primary action of insulin is to decrease proteolysis. Furthermore, blunting protein breakdown results in decreased available amino acids, which causes secondary effects such as decreased protein synthesis and amino acid oxidation.

As might be expected, insulin alters the synthesis of different types of proteins in different ways. For example, albumin synthesis is increased while fibrinogen synthesis is decreased when insulin-deficient humans are treated with insulin.[89] Gut and kidney protein synthesis are increased in diabetic rats compared with controls.[72,74] Although data are not conclusive, skeletal muscle protein synthesis

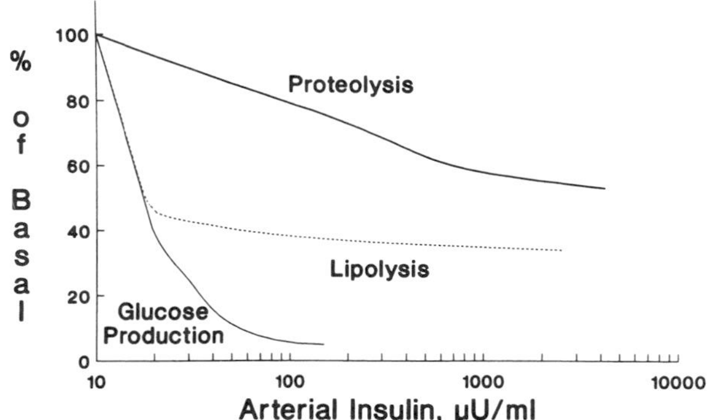

Figure 12-6. Insulin suppression of lipolysis, glucose production, and proteolysis in humans. Data were extracted from references 32, 84, and 101. Values are plotted as percent suppression, which is an estimate of responsiveness.

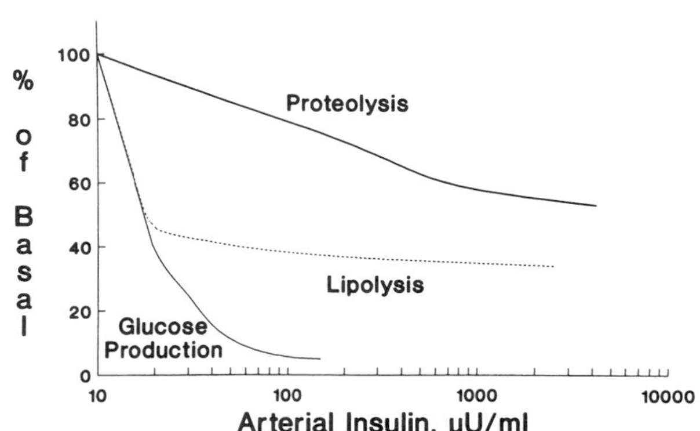

Figure 12-7. Insulin's percent maximal suppression of lipolysis glucose production and proteolysis in humans. Data were extractracted from references 32, 84, and 101. Values are plotted as percent of maximal suppression, which is an estimate of sensitivity.

in vivo does not appear to be dramatically altered with hyperinsulinemia.[76] In view of the limited data regarding the effects of insulin on the synthesis of different proteins, significantly more research is required to allow an integrated view of insulin's interaction with individual proteins and their contributions to overall whole body protein synthesis.

Insulin and Amino Acid Oxidation

Another component of amino acid utilization is amino acid oxidation. Changes in amino acid oxidation could also lead to alterations in protein homeostasis. During prolonged insulin deficiency in type I diabetics, amino acid oxidation is increased.[81] This suggests an important role for basal insulin in the control of amino acid oxidation. Furthermore, during euglycemic-hyperinsulinemic clamp studies, insulin decreases amino acid oxidation in a dose-responsive manner.[84] The levels of insulin at which half-maximal response occurs are very high (~700 μU/mL), diminishing the physiologic relevance of such findings. More significant, however, is the suggestion that amino acid oxidation is highly dependent upon amino acid availability. When plasma amino acid concentrations fall as a result of hyperinsulinemic proteolytic suppression, amino acid oxidation falls. During hyperinsulinemic experiments in which amino acids are maintained, amino acid oxidation is increased.[84] Therefore, insulin's regulation of amino acid oxidation appears to be primarily controlled via regulation of proteolysis and amino acid pool size.

Although many tissues are actively involved in the oxidation of amino acids, skeletal muscle, as the largest insulin-sensitive organ in the body, is particularly important for insulin control of amino acid oxidation. Branched-chain amino acids (BCAAs) make up approximately 60% of the total amino acids taken up by muscle, and insulin promotes their uptake at a greater rate than other amino acids. In the diabetic, skeletal muscle uptake of BCAAs is reduced. These observations are most probably related to insulin's regulation of the BCAA catabolic enzymes (BCAA transaminase and branched-chain ketoacid dehydrogenase), which are more active in muscle than in liver tissue. Therefore, after the ingestion of protein meal, only 15–30% of BCAAs are utilized by the splanchnic bed, with most of the escaping BCAAs being utilized by muscle.[90] Insulin decreases transaminase activity and, therefore, limits leucine conversion to α-ketoisocaproate in skeletal muscle.[91] Insulin's influence on the activity of branched-chain ketoacid dehydrogenase, the rate-limiting enzyme for the catabolism of BCAAs, is mediated by substrate availability. Insulin diminishes leucine oxidation in perfused hindlimbs from fed rats but increases it in perfused hindlimbs from fasted rats.

Leucine is also utilized in adipose tissue. Leucine is a ketogenic amino acid, and therefore its ultimate catabolic fate is carbon dioxide and ketone bodies. It is of interest, therefore, that insulin promotes leucine oxidation and increases the rate of leucine conversion to ketones in adipose tissue.[92] The importance of the use of other amino acids by adipose tissue has not been as well defined.

In the liver, amino acids are utilized for the synthesis of proteins, for direct incorporation into the tricarboxylic acid cycle as sources of energy, and for the de novo synthesis of glucose and ketone bodies. Even at basal concentrations, insulin acts on hepatic amino acid utilization by decreasing gluconeogenesis, thereby making amino acids available for other biochemical processes, such as protein synthesis and oxidation. During insulin withdrawal in diabetic individuals, de novo glucose production from amino acids is enhanced when compared to that in diabetic individuals under insulin therapy.[79]

In summary, insulin, in its role as the primary regulator of protein homeostasis, is active in the control of proteolysis, protein synthesis, amino acid oxidation, and amino acid transport (Fig. 12-8). Insulin's primary function is to decrease proteolysis, which results in decreased amino acid availability. Because of the lack of amino acids, protein synthesis and amino acid oxidation are diminished. The net result of these events yields increased protein deposition, which is amplified in the presence of exogenous amino acids.

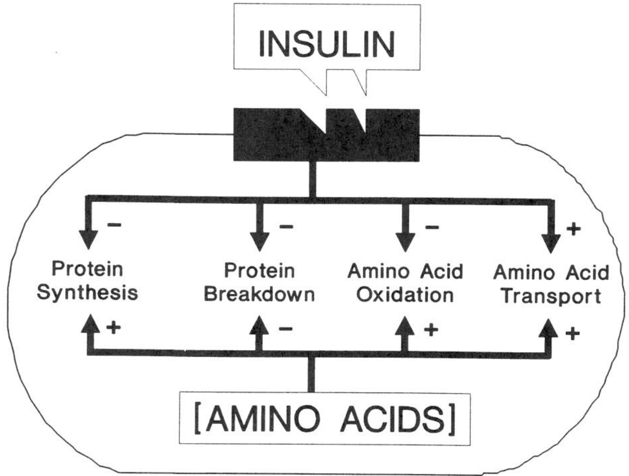

Figure 12-8. Interaction of insulin and amino acids with whole-body protein metabolism.

The Role of Insulin in Daily Metabolic Control

Changes in insulin secretion play a key role in mediating the metabolic responses to circumstances of everyday life, including feeding, food deprivation, and exercise. In response to an ingested carbohydrate load the insulin level can rise as much as 10-fold, glucagon secretion can fall by as much as 50%, and the portal feeding signal is induced. These signals, along with the altered glucose load's reaching the target tissues, result in marked glucose uptake at muscle and liver. The distribution of the ingested glucose is such that about one-third goes to the liver, one-third to muscle, and one-third to non–insulin-sensitive tissues (e.g., central nervous system). Non–insulin-sensitive tissue glucose disposal occurs as a result of the cessation of endogenous glucose production and the continued need of such tissues for glucose. The role of insulin in muscle appears to counter the effect of the portal signal and thereby to ensure adequate glycogen repletion in myocytes. The role of insulin at the liver appears to be to act in concert with the portal signal to ensure optimal glycogen repletion in the hepatocyte. It should be remembered that a physiologic rise in insulin does not modify the gluconeogenic rate appreciably. For this reason, the gluconeogenic pathway remains active during carbohydrate ingestion and about half of the glycogen deposited in the liver comes from gluconeogenically derived carbon (so-called indirect glycogen synthesis) and the other half from circulating glucose (so-called direct glycogen synthesis).

The rise in arterial glucose and insulin concentrations in response to an oral or intravenous carbohydrate load suppresses free fatty acid mobilization and glycerol release from adipose tissue through inhibition of lipolysis and stimulation of fractional free fatty acid re-esterification within adipose tissue. The reduction in availability of free fatty acids contributes to the increased glucose uptake by liver and muscle. In addition, the rise in insulin in response to carbohydrate ingestion produces hypoaminoacidemia and promotes conservation of protein and amino acids in muscle via decreased proteolysis and reduced amino acid oxidation.

The role of insulin in fuel metabolism after mixed meal feeding is less clearly defined but probably is as important as its role after carbohydrate ingestion. When the blood glucose and amino acid levels rise in concert, the insulin level increases much more profoundly than with carbohydrate ingestion alone. Additionally the plasma glucagon level rises instead of falling. As might be expected, the uptake of glucose by the liver is less than is apparent with the ingestion of carbohydrate alone, but amino acid uptake is dramatically enhanced and glycogen synthesis via the indirect pathway is increased so that the glycogen stores can be completely replenished. The precise role of insulin in this outcome remains to be clarified. Following a mixed meal, the increased plasma levels of glucose and insulin potently suppress adipose tissue lipolysis and endogenous free fatty acid availability. Additionally, the activation of adipose tissue lipoprotein lipase by insulin promotes the clearance of circulating chylomicrons and the subsequent storage of meal-derived fatty acids as TG in adipose tissue. The rise in arterial insulin and amino acid levels following a mixed meal stimulates uptake of BCAAs by muscle and accretion of protein via decreased proteolysis and increased protein synthesis.

In response to food deprivation, the plasma glucose level falls. In association with this the plasma insulin level declines and the plasma glucagon level rises. The latter response is at least partly dependent on the degree of hypoglycemia present. The fall in insulin is important to glucose utilization in that it reduces glucose uptake by muscle. In the liver, the fall in insulin and the rise in glucagon act to sustain glucose production. In addition, the above hormonal changes, along with increases in catecholamines, cortisol, and growth hormone during periods of fasting, stimulate lipolysis and proteolysis, thereby providing alternative oxidative fuels in the form of free fatty acids and amino acids. The increased supply of free fatty acids and gluconeogenic substrates reaching the liver contributes to the increase in gluconeogenesis and the maintenance of adequate glucose production in the face of depleted liver glycogen stores. In addition, hepatic ketogenesis is markedly accelerated by the hormonal milieu and the enhanced supply of free fatty acids to the liver. This integrated hormonal and metabolic response to food deprivation limits glucose utilization and provides a number of alternative fuels to meet the energy requirements of the organism during periods of prolonged fasting.

In response to moderate intensity exercise, the blood glucose level declines slightly if at all. There is an increase in glucagon secretion, an increase in catecholamine release, and a decline in plasma insulin secretion, the magnitude of which changes with exercise intensity and duration. The decline in plasma insulin level serves to counter the increase in muscle glucose utilization triggered by exercise per se, thus preventing the occurrence of hypoglycemia. At the liver the decline in insulin acts in concert with the rise in glucagon to ensure that glucose production rises. In this way the energy requirement of the exercising muscle can be met by adequate hepatic glucose production. The coordination of this response is so precise that a 10-fold increase in muscle energy requirement can be satisfied with little or no change in the blood glucose level.

Free fatty acid and glycerol levels rise progressively during low- or moderate-intensity exercise. The increase in free fatty acid mobilization results both from enhanced lipolysis and reduced free fatty acid re-esterification. Free fatty acids provide a significant fraction of the increased energy required during exercise, such that circulating free fatty acids become the major source of oxidative fuel for skeletal muscle during prolonged periods of exercise. Amino acid mobilization also increases during exercise primarily as a result of decreases in protein synthesis and secondarily as a result of increases in protein breakdown. The increased mobilization of amino acids from muscle and of free fatty acids and glycerol from adipose tissue contributes to the enhanced hepatic glucose production and maintenance of a stable blood glucose concentration despite the dramatic exercise-induced increase in glucose utilization.

Effects of Insulin on Growth

Growth is defined as an expansion of body tissues due to both hyperplasia and hypertrophy. During growth, net tissue deposition arises as a result of anabolism's occurring at a faster rate than catabolism. A normal consequence of growth is that priorities between various tissues change throughout development in the typical life cycle. Therefore, growth is a complex event, requiring considerable regulation and control.

Historically, insulin has been classified as an anabolic hormone. Consequently, it is thought to be intrinsically involved in the complex regulation of body growth. Normal insulin function is critical to normal growth. In young diabetics whose disease is poorly controlled, growth is markedly blunted even in the presence of elevated growth hormone levels.[93,94]

Insulin's influence on growth is most likely manifested by its net anabolic effects on protein and lipid metabolism, as described in previous sections. For example, by its inhibition of gluconeogenesis and ketogenesis, insulin allows increased availability of amino acids for synthesis of proteins. Although the classic control of homeostatic variables, such as glucose, lipid, and protein metabolism, is relatively well understood, the control of substrate homeostasis and its interaction with other anabolic and catabolic regulatory processes to produce a net anabolic effect are less clear. Under normal conditions, insulin does not act in isolation but rather its action in combination with other hormones, metabolites, and neural signals influences the net deposition of protein or lipid. Hence, it is appropriate that insulin secretion peaks after a meal, coinciding with the most prominent period of nutrient uptake and storage.

One example of insulin's interaction with other mediators of growth is its stimulation of somatomedin production. Somatomedins, also referred to as insulin-like growth factors (IGF I and II), are polypeptide hormones that mediate the growth-stimulating effects of growth hormone and exhibit insulin-like functions in muscle and adipose tissue. They share structural homologies with insulin and have the ability to bind to the insulin receptor.[95] In both uncontrolled diabetic rats and humans, somatomedin production and plasma concentrations are reduced.[93,96,97] Restoration of normal somatomedin concentrations is accomplished by insulin infusion.

The direct influence of insulin on specific tissues has been well documented. Basic biochemical data support a role for insulin in enlarging adipose stores by increasing lipid uptake and fat deposition. Similar data provide evidence that insulin expands lean tissues via regulation of protein synthetic machinery as well as control of proteolysis. Although alterations in fat and muscle depots are the primary sites responsible for major whole body growth, insulin also alters growth and development of other tissues. For example, King and associates used thymidine incorporation into DNA to demonstrate that insulin promotes growth of cultured human fibroblasts.[98] In utero, insulin also has important growth-promoting abilities. In fact, fetal hyperinsulinemia is a common anomaly associated with pregnancy. Typically, insufficient maternal insulin causes hyperglycemia, which in turn stimulates hyperinsulinemic conditions in the fetus.[99] Repercussions from fetal hyperinsulinemia include elevated birth weights owing to expanded lipid stores and enlarged parenchymal organs.[100]

In summary, it is clear that insulin has a very central role in the regulation of growth. This is best illustrated by observations of diminished growth associated with the insulin insufficiency during diabetes. However, it is also clear that insulin's role is very complex and interactive with many other hormones and substrates. These interactions provide direction for future research.

References

1. Cherrington AD, Lacy WW, Chiasson JL. Effect of glucagon on glucose production during insulin deficiency in the dog. J Clin Invest 1978;62:664

2. Madison LL, Combes B, Adams R, Strickland W. III. The physiological significance of the secretion of insulin into the portal circulation. J Clin Invest 1960;39:507
3. Cherrington AD. The acute regulation of hepatic glucose production. In: Pagliassotti M, Davis S, Cherrington AD, eds. The Role of the Liver in Maintaining Glucose Homeostasis. Austin, Tex: RG Landes Co;1994:19
4. Prager R, Wallace P, Olefsky JM. Direct and indirect effects of insulin to inhibit hepatic glucose output in obese subjects. Diabetes 1987;36:607
5. Ader M, Bergman R. Peripheral effects of insulin dominate suppression of fasting hepatic glucose production. Am J Physiol 1990;258:E1020
6. Giacca A, Fisher SJ, Quing Shi Z, et al. Importance of peripheral insulin levels for insulin-induced suppression of glucose production in depancreatized dogs. J Clin Invest 1992;90:1769
7. Poulin RA, Steil GM, Moore M, et al. Glucose turnover dynamics are more closely related to insulin in hindlimb lymph than in thoracic duct lymph. Diabetes 1994;43:180
8. Sindelar DK, Balcom JH, Chu CA, et al. Comparison of the effects of a selective increase in arterial or portal insulin on hepatic glucose metabolism. Diabetes 1994;3:133A
9. Rebrin K, Steil GM, Getty L, Bergman RN. Free fatty acids as a link in the regulation of hepatic glucose output by peripheral insulin. Diabetes 1995; 44:1038
10. Myers SR, Diamond MP, Adkins-Marshall BA, et al. Effects of small changes in glucagon on glucose production during a euglycemic, hyperinsulinemic clamp. Metabolism 1991;40:66
11. Goldstein RE, Wasserman DH, Lacy DB, et al. The effects of an acute increase in epinephrine and cortisol on carbohydrate metabolism during insulin deficiency. Diabetes 1995;44:672
12. Stevenson R, Williams PE, Cherrington AD. Role of glucagon suppression on gluconeogenesis during insulin treatment of the conscious diabetic dog. Diabetologia 1987;30:782
13. Consoli A, Nurjhan N, Capai F, Gerich J. Predominant role of gluconeogenesis in increased hepatic glucose production in NIDDM. Diabetes 1989;38:550
14. Steiner KE, Williams PE, Lacy WW, Cherrington AD. Effects of insulin on glucagon-stimulated glucose production in the conscious dog. Metabolism 1990;39:1325
15. Mandarino LJ, Consoli A, Jain A, Kelley DE. Differential regulation of intracellular glucose metabolism by glucose and insulin in human muscle. Am J Physiol 1993;265:E898
16. Chiasson JL, Atkinson RL, Cherrington AD, et al. Effects of insulin at two dose levels on gluconeogenesis from alanine in fasting man. Metabolism 1980;29:810
17. McGuinness OP, Friedman A, Cherrington AD. Intraportal hyperinsulinemia decreases insulin-stimulated glucose uptake in the dog. Metabolism 1989; 39:127
18. McGuinness OP, Myers SR, Neal D, Cherrington AD. Chronic hyperinsulinemia decreases insulin action but not insulin sensitivity. Metabolism 1990; 39:931
19. Davis S, McGuinness OP, Cherrington AD. Insulin action in vivo. In: Alberti KGMM, Krall LP, eds. Diabetes Annual IV. New York: Elsevier Science Publishers BV;1990:585
20. Baron AD. Hemodynamic actions of insulin. Am J Physiol 1994;267:E187
21. Lembo G, Napoli R, Capaido B, et al. Abnormal sympathetic overactivity evoked by insulin in the skeletal muscle of patients with essential hypertension. J Clin Invest 1992;90:24
22. Davis SN, Colburn C, Dobbins R, et al. Evidence that the brain of the conscious dog is insulin sensitive. J Clin Invest 1995;95:593
23. Adkins-Marshall BA, Myers SR, Hendrick GK, et al. Interaction between insulin and glucose delivery route in regulation of net hepatic glucose uptake in conscious dogs. Diabetes 1990;39:87
24. DeFronzo RA, Ferrannini E, Hendler R, et al. Influence of hyperinsulinemia, hyperglycemia, and the route of glucose administration on splanchnic glucose exchange. Proc Natl Acad Sci USA 1978;75:5173
25. Pagliassotti MJ, Horton RJ. Hormonal and neural regulation of hepatic glucose uptake. In: Pagliassotti M, Davis S, Cherrington AD, eds. The Role of the Liver in Maintaining Glucose Homeostasis. Austin, Tex: RG Landes Co; 1994:45
26. Cahill GF Jr. Starvation in man. N Engl J Med 1970;282:668
27. Bortz WM, Paul P, Haff AG, Holmes WL. Glycerol turnover and oxidation in man. J Clin Invest 1972;51:1537
28. Eckel RH. Lipoprotein lipase: A multifunctional enzyme relevant to common metabolic diseases. N Engl J Med 1989;320:1060
29. Coppack SW, Frayn KN, Humphreys SM, et al. Effects of insulin on human adipose tissue metabolism in vivo. Clin Sci Lond 1989;77:663
30. Farese RV Jr, Yost TJ, Eckel RH. Tissue-specific regulation of lipoprotein lipase activity by insulin/glucose in normal-weight humans. Metabolism 1991;40:214
31. Simsolo RB, Ong JM, Saffari B, Kern PA. Effect of improved diabetes control on the expression of lipoprotein lipase in human adipose tissue. J Lipid Res 1992;33:89
32. Campbell PJ, Carlson MG, Hill JO, Nurjhan N. Regulation of free fatty acid metabolism by insulin in humans: Role of lipolysis and reesterification. Am J Physiol 1992;263:E1063
33. Bonadonna RC, Groop LC, Zych K, et al. Dose-dependent effect of insulin on plasma free fatty acid turnover and oxidation in humans. Am J Physiol 1990;259:E736
34. Jensen MD, Caruso M, Heiling V, Miles JM. Insulin regulation of lipolysis in nondiabetic and IDDM subjects. Diabetes 1989;38:1595
35. Stralfors P, Bjorgell P, Belfrage P. Hormonal regulation of hormone-sensitive lipase in intact adipocytes: Identification of phosphorylated sites and effects on the phosphorylation by lipolytic hormones and insulin. Proc Natl Acad Sci USA 1984;81:3317
36. Stralfors P, Honnor RC. Insulin-induced dephosphorylation of hormone-sensitive lipase: Correlation with lipolysis and cAMP-dependent protein kinase activity. Eur J Biochem 1989;182:379
37. Vaughan M, Steinberg D. Glyceride biosynthesis, glyceride breakdown, and glycogen breakdown in adipose tissue: Mechanisms and regulation. In: Renold AE, Cahill GF, eds. Handbook of Physiology, Adipose Tissue. Washington, DC: American Physiological Society;1965:24, 239
38. Campbell PJ, Carlson MG, Nurjhan N. Fat metabolism in human obesity. Am J Physiol 1994;266:E600
39. DelPrato S, Enzi G, Vigili de Kreutzenberg S, et al. Insulin regulation of glucose and lipid metabolism in massive obesity. Diabetologia 1990;33:2280
40. Groop LC, Bonadonna RC, Simonson DC, et al. Effect of insulin on oxidative and nonoxidative pathways of free fatty acid metabolism in human obesity. Am J Physiol 1992;263:E79
41. Jensen MD, Haymond MW, Rizza RA, et al. Influence of body fat distribution on free fatty acid metabolism in obesity. J Clin Invest 1989;83:1168
42. Martin ML, Jensen MD. Effects of body fat distribution on regional lipolysis in obesity. J Clin Invest 1991;88:609
43. Peiris AN, Mueller RA, Smith GA, et al. Splanchnic insulin metabolism in obesity. Influence of body fat distribution. J Clin Invest 1986;78:1648
44. Svedberg J, Bjorntorp P, Smith V, Lonnroth P. Free fatty acid inhibition of insulin binding, degradation, and action in isolated rat hepatocytes. Diabetes 1990;39:570
45. Hemmes MMI, Shrago E, Kissebah AH. Receptor and postreceptor effects of free fatty acids on hepatocyte insulin dynamics. Int J Obes 1990;14:831
46. Ferrannini E, Barrett EJ, Bevilacqua S, DeFronzo RA. Effect of fatty acids on glucose production and utilization in man. J Clin Invest 1983;72:1737
47. Kissebah AH, Alfarsi S, Adams PW, Wynn V. Role of insulin resistance in adipose tissue and liver in the pathogenesis of endogenous hypertriglyceridemia in man. Diabetologia 1976;12:563
48. Howard BV, Zech L, Davis M, et al. Studies of very low density lipoprotein metabolism in an obese population with low plasma lipids: Lack of influence of body weight or plasma insulin. J Lipid Res 1980;21:1032
49. Groop LC, Bonadonna RC, Shank M, et al. Role of free fatty acids and insulin in determining free fatty acid and lipid oxidation. J Clin Invest 1991;87:83
50. Capaldo B, Napoli R, Di Marino L, et al. Role of insulin and free fatty acid (FFA) availability on regional FFA kinetics in the human forearm. J Clin Endocrinol Metab 1994;79:879
51. Hagenfeldt L, Wennlung A, Felig P, Wahren J. Turnover and splanchnic metabolism of free fatty acids in hyperthyroid patients. J Clin Invest 1981; 67:1672
52. Keller U, Gerber PPG, Stauffacher W. Fatty acid-independent inhibition of hepatic ketone body production by insulin in man. Am J Physiol 1988; 254:E694
53. McGarry JD, Foster DW. Regulation of hepatic fatty acid oxidation and ketone body production. Annu Rev Biochem 1980;49:395
54. Beylot M, Picard S, Chambrier C, et al. Effect of physiological concentrations of insulin and glucagon on the relationship between nonesterified fatty acids availability and ketone body production in humans. Metabolism 1991; 40:1138
55. Carlson MG, Snead WL, Campbell PJ. Regulation of free fatty acid metabolism by glucagon. J Clin Endocrinol Metab 1993;77:11
56. Sherwin RS, Hendler RG, Felig P. Effect of diabetes mellitus and insulin on the turnover and metabolic response to ketones in man. Diabetes 1976;25:776
57. Keller U, Lustenberger M, Stauffacher W. Effect of insulin on ketone body clearance studied by a ketone body ''clamp'' technique in normal man. Diabetologia 1988;31:24
58. Fery F, Balasse EO. Ketone body production and disposal in diabetic ketosis. A comparison with fasting ketosis. Diabetes 1985;34:326
59. Wakil SJ, Stoops JK, Joshi VC. Fatty acid synthesis and its regulation. Annu Rev Biochem 1983;52:537
60. Acheson KJ, Schutz Y, Bessard T, et al. Glycogen storage capacity and de novo lipogenesis during massive carbohydrate overfeeding in man. Am J Clin Nutr 1988;48:240
61. Hellerstein MK, Christiansen M, Kaempfer S, et al. Measurement of de novo hepatic lipogenesis in humans using stable isotopes. J Clin Invest 1991; 87:1841
62. Hellerstein MK, Neese RA, Schwarz JM. Model for measuring absolute rates of hepatic de novo lipogenesis and reesterification of free fatty acids. Am J Physiol 1993;265:E814
63. Bergstrom J, Furst P, Noree L, Vinnars E. Intracellular free amino acid concentrations in human muscle tissue. J Applied Physiol 1974;36:693
64. Christensen HN. Role of amino acid transport and countertransport in nutrition and metabolism in skeletal muscle. Physiol Rev 1980;70:43
65. Guidotti GC, Gazzola GC. Amino acid transporters: Systematic approach and principles of controls. In: Kilberg M, Haussiger D, eds. Mammalian Amino Acid Transport. New York: Plenum Press;1992:3
66. Tovar AR, Tews JK, Torres N, Harper AE. Neutral amino acid transport into rat skeletal muscle: Competition, adaptative regulation, and effects of insulin. Metabolism 1991;40:410

67. Le Cam A, Freychet P. Effects of insulin on amino acid transport in isolated rat hepatocytes. Diabetologia 1978;15:117
68. Jefferson LS, Rannels DE, Munger BL, Morgan HE. Insulin in the regulation of protein turnover in heart and skeletal muscle. Fed Proc 1974;33:1098
69. Fulks R, Li BJ, Goldberg AL. Effects of insulin, glucose, and amino acids on protein turnover in rat diaphragms. J Biol Chem 1980;250:290
70. Lundholm KS, Edstrom S, Ekman L, et al. Protein degradation in human skeletal muscle tissue: The effect of insulin, leucine, amino acids, and ions. Clin Sci 1981;60:319
71. Mortimore GE, Mondon CE. Inhibition by insulin of valine turnover in the liver. Evidence for a general control of proteolysis. J Biol Chem 1970; 245:2375
72. Kimball SR, Flaim KE, Peavy DE, Jefferson LS. Protein metabolism. In: Ellemberg M, Rifkin M, eds. Diabetes Mellitus, Theory and Practice. New York: Elsevier;1989:41
73. Kettelhut IC, Wing SS, Goldberg AL. Endocrine regulation of protein breakdown in skeletal muscle. Diabetes Metab Rev 1988;4:751
74. McNurlan MA, Garlick PJ. Protein synthesis in liver and small intestine in protein deprivation and diabetes. J Clin Invest 1981;241(Suppl 4):E238
75. Pozefsky T, Felig P, Tobin JC, et al. Amino acids across tissues of the forearm in postabsorptive man. Effects of insulin at two dose levels. J Clin Invest 1969;48:2273
76. Gelfand RA, Baarret EJ. Effect of physiological hyperinsulinemia on skeletal muscle protein synthesis and breakdown in man. J Clin Invest 1987;80:1
77. Atchley DW, Loeb RF, Richards DW, et al. On diabetic acidosis: A detailed study of electrolyte balances following the withdrawal and re-establishment of insulin therapy. J Clin Invest 1933;12:297
78. Nair KS, Garrow JS, Ford C, et al. Effect of poor diabetic control and obesity on whole-body protein metabolism in man. Diabetologia 1983;25:400
79. Rogert JJ, Beaufrere B, Koziet J, et al. Whole-body de novo amino acid synthesis in type 1 (insulin-dependent) diabetes studied with stable isotope-labelled leucine, alanine and glycine. Diabetes 1985;34:67
80. Tessari P, Nosandini R, Trevisan R, et al. Defective suppression by insulin of leucine-carbon appearance and oxidation in type 1, insulin dependent diabetes mellitus: Evidence for insulin resistance involving glucose and amino acid metabolism. J Clin Invest 1986;77:1797
81. Umpleby AM, Boroujerdi MA, Brown PM, et al. The effect of metabolic control on leucine metabolism in type 1 (insulin-dependent) diabetic patients. Diabetologia 1986;29:131
82. Carlson MG, Campbell PJ. Intensive insulin therapy and weight gain in IDDM. Diabetes 1993;42:1700
83. Fukagawa NK, Minaker KL, Rowe JW, et al. Insulin-mediated reduction of whole-body protein breakdown. Dose-responsive effects on leucine metabolism in post-absorptive men. J Clin Invest 1985;76:2306
84. Flakoll PJ, Kulaylat M, Frexes-Steed M, et al. Amino acids augment insulin's suppression of whole body proteolysis. Am J Physiol 1989;257:E839
85. Tessari P, Trevisan R, Inchiostro S, et al. Dose-response curves of the effects of insulin on leucine kinetics in man. Am J Physiol 1986;251:E334
86. Pain WM, Garlick PJ. Effect of streptozotocin diabetes and insulin treatment on the rate of protein synthesis in tissues of the rat *in vivo*. J Biol Chem 1974;249:4510
87. Jefferson LS. The role of insulin in the regulation of protein synthesis. Diabetes 1980;29:487
88. Granner DK, Andreone T, Saski T, Beale E. Inhibition of transcription of the phosphoenolpyruvate carboxylase gene by insulin. Nature 1983;305: 549
89. De Feo P, Gan Gaisano M, Haymond MW. Differential effects of insulin deficiency on albumin and fibrinogen synthesis in humans. J Clin Invest 1991;88:833
90. Bloomgarden ZT, Liljenquist J, Lacy W, Rabin D. Amino-acid disposition by liver and gastrointestinal tract after protein and glucose ingestion. Am J Physiol 1981;241:E90
91. Hutson SM, Cree TC, Harper AE. Regulation of leucine and α-ketoisocaproate metabolism in skeletal muscle. J Biol Chem 1980;255:6286
92. Rosenthal J, Angel A, Farkas J. Metabolic fate of leucine: A significant sterol precursor in adipose tissue and muscle. Am J Physiol 1974;26:411
93. Tamborlane WV, Hintz RL, Bergman M, et al. Insulin-infusion pump treatment of diabetes. Influence of improved metabolic control on plasma somatomedin levels. N Engl J Med 1981;305:303
94. Hayford JT, Danney MM, Hendrix JA, Thompson RG. Integrated concentration of growth hormone in juvenile-onset diabetes. Diabetes 1980;29: 391
95. Megyesi K, Kahn CR, Roth J, et al. Insulin and non-suppressible insulin-like activity (NSILA-S) = evidence for separate plasma membrane receptor sites. Biochem Biophys Res Commun 1974;57:307
96. Phillips LS, Young HS. Nutrition and somatomedin. II. Serum somatomedin activity and cartilage growth activity in streptozotocin-diabetic rats. Diabetes 1976;25:516
97. Miller LL, Schalch DS, Draznin B. Role of the liver in regulating somatomedin activity: Effects of streptozotocin diabetes and starvation on the synthesis and release of insulin-like growth factor and its carrier protein by the isolated perfused rat liver. Endocrinology 1981;108:1265
98. King GL, Kahn CR. Non-parallel evolution of metabolic and growth-promoting functions of insulin. Nature 1982;292:644
99. Pederson J. The Pregnant Diabetic and Her Newborn. Baltimore: Williams & Wilkins;1977
100. Susa JB, McCormick KL, Widness JA, et al. Chronic hyperinsulinemia in the fetal rhesus monkey: Effects on fetal growth and composition. Diabetes 1979;28:1058
101. Rizza RA, Mandarino LJ, Gerich JE. Dose-response characteristics for effects of insulin on production and utilization of glucose in man. Am J Physiol 1981;240:E630

Diabetes Mellitus, edited by Derek LeRoith, Simeon I. Taylor, and Jerrold M. Olefsky. Lippincott–Raven Publishers, Philadelphia © 1996.

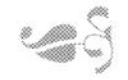

CHAPTER 13

Glucose Counter-regulatory Hormones: Physiology, Pathophysiology, and Relevance to Clinical Hypoglycemia

PHILIP E. CRYER

Introduction

The integrated regulation of systemic glucose balance prevents the devastating consequences of hypoglycemia and hyperglycemia.[1] This remarkable homeostatic feat is accomplished primarily by hormones but also by neurotransmitters and substrate effects, and it reflects the interplay of plasma glucose-lowering and glucose-raising factors. Insulin (see Chapter 12) is the dominant glucose-lowering factor. In contrast, there are redundant glucose-raising (glucose counter-regulatory) factors, including glucagon and epinephrine.[1–4] Given its immediate survival value, the prevention or correction of hypoglycemia must be viewed as the primary physiologic function of the counter-regulatory factors,[1–3] although they affect diverse aspects of intermediary metabolism.[1] Although the counter-regulatory systems may contribute to the pathogenesis of hyperglycemia under some conditions,[6,7] their failure resulting in iatrogenic hypoglycemia is a more important feature of their pathophysiology in diabetes mellitus.[4,5]

Glucose is, by far, the predominant metabolic fuel utilized by the brain.[8] The brain cannot synthesize glucose nor can it store more than a few minutes' supply as glycogen. Therefore, the brain is dependent on a continuous supply of glucose from the circulation. At normal (or elevated) plasma glucose concentrations, the rate of blood-to-brain glucose transport exceeds the rate of brain glucose metabolism. However, as the plasma glucose concentration falls below the physiologic range, blood-to-brain glucose transport becomes limiting to brain glucose metabolism and, thus, survival. Therefore, it is not surprising that physiologic mechanisms that normally very effectively prevent or correct hypoglycemia[1–4] have evolved. Indeed, these are so effective that hypoglycemia is a distinctly uncommon clinical event except in persons who use drugs (such as insulin or sulfonylureas) that lower plasma glucose, particularly in the setting of compromised glucose counter-regulation.[1,4,5]

Iatrogenic hypoglycemia is a major problem for many patients with diabetes mellitus, particularly those with insulin-dependent diabetes mellitus (IDDM).[1,4,5] It is best viewed as the result of the interplay of absolute or relative therapeutic insulin excess and compromised glucose counter-regulation.[4,5]

Physiology

Glucose Counter-regulatory Factors

Potentially important glucose counter-regulatory factors include hormones, neurotransmitters, and substrate effects.[1–4]

Glucagon, secreted from pancreatic α-cells in response to hypoglycemia, raises plasma glucose levels by stimulating hepatic glucose production.[1,6] Both glycogenolysis and gluconeogenesis are increased but the effect of the hormone on glycogenolysis is transient, as is the glycemic response. Epinephrine, an adrenomedullary hormone also secreted in response to hypoglycemia, raises plasma glucose concentrations both by stimulating glucose production and by limiting glucose utilization through complex mechanisms that include both direct and indirect actions and are mediated through both β_2-adrenergic and α_2-adrenergic receptors.[1,4,9,10] Epinephrine stimulates hepatic glycogenolysis and gluconeogenesis and limits glucose utilization in insulin-sensitive tissues such as skeletal muscle through direct (β_2-adrenergic) mechanisms. Because the effect on glucose utilization is sustained, the glycemic response tends to be sustained. Indirect glycemic actions include (β_2-adrenergic) increased lipolysis (which both drives glucose production and limits glucose utilization), glycolysis (which provides precursors for gluconeogenesis such as lactate and alanine), and glucagon secretion and (α_2-adrenergic) limitation of insulin secretion. Limitation of insulin secretion is particularly important; β-adrenergic stimulation alone, as occurs with isoproterenol, increases glucose turnover; however, because it stimulates insulin secretion, it produces only a small increase in plasma glucose concentrations. Nonetheless, there is some increase in insulin secretion as plasma glucose rises in response to epinephrine.[9] That is a critical regulatory event, since it limits the magnitude of the glycemic response to the hormone. When insulin secretion cannot increase, as in patients with IDDM, the glycemic response is exaggerated.[9] This mechanism also undoubtedly underlies the exaggerated hyperglycemic response to other counter-regulatory hormones in IDDM. Whereas glucagon and epinephrine raise glucose levels in minutes, pituitary growth hormone and adrenocortical cortisol do so during a period of hours. Growth hormone and cortisol limit glucose utilization but also support glucose production.[11,12] Many other hormones are released during hypoglycemia.[2]

Potentially important glucose counter-regulatory neurotransmitters include the classic ones, i.e., sympathetic neural norepinephrine and parasympathetic neural acetylcholine. Following sympathetic activation, norepinephrine raises glucose levels through mechanisms similar to those of epinephrine.[1,10] Acetylcholine released from activated parasympathetic neurons decreases hepatic glucose production, an effect demonstrable in humans only in the absence of glucagon release.[13] In addition, it is conceivable that some of the array of neuropeptides released during hypoglycemia might affect glucose metabolism.

Potentially important substrate effects include those of glucose per se, that is, the phenomenon of glucose autoregulation (hepatic glucose production as an inverse function of ambient glucose levels independent of hormonal and neural regulation).[14] In addition, there is an inverse relationship between fatty acid and glucose oxidation.[15]

Glucose Counter-regulation: The Prevention and Correction of Hypoglycemia

Principles. The principles of the physiology of glucose counter-regulation are now known.[1–4] First, the prevention and correction of hypoglycemia involve both dissipation of insulin and activation of glucose counter-regulatory systems. The process is not caused solely by dissipation of insulin. Second, whereas insulin is the dominant glucose-lowering factor, there are redundant glucose counter-regulatory factors. There is a fail-safe system that prevents failure of the counter-regulatory process even when one or perhaps more of the components of the system fail. Third, there is a hierarchy among the counter-regulatory factors; some are more important than others.

The physiology of glucose counter-regulation is outlined in Figure 13-1. Arterialized venous glycemic thresholds for changes in hormone secretion (decreased insulin, increased counter-regulatory hormones) as plasma glucose falls are also shown.[16,17]

Insulin. The first response to falling glucose levels is a decrease in insulin secretion, which occurs with glucose decrements within the physiologic range[3,16] (see Fig. 13-1). There is direct evidence that decreased insulin secretion plays a fundamental role in the correction of hypoglycemia,[18] and it is undoubtedly also important in the prevention of hypoglycemia. Indeed, although there is a body of evidence that regulation of the postabsorptive plasma glucose concentration is accomplished by the interplay of the glucose-lowering action of insulin and the glucose-raising action of glucagon,[6] the possibility that it is generally regulated by changes in insulin secretion alone has been raised.[18] Consistent with the glycemic thresholds demonstrated during decrements in plasma glucose,[16,17] Heller and Cryer[18] found that during recovery from hypoglycemia the counter-regulatory systems disengaged at glucose levels lower than control values when some insulin was provided, and that glucose levels plateaued at levels somewhat below control, postabsorptive levels. That finding suggests that postabsorptive glucose levels are regulated primarily by variations in insulin secretion and that the counter-regulatory factors become relevant only when plasma glucose levels fall just below the physiologic range.

The first evidence that recovery from hypoglycemia is not attributable solely to dissipation of insulin was the finding in a model of hypoglycemia produced by intravenous insulin injection that the changes in glucose kinetics that ultimately restore euglycemia (decrements in insulin-stimulated glucose utilization and increments in insulin-suppressed glucose production) begin while plasma insulin concentrations are still tenfold higher than baseline.[19] Additional evidence is the finding that biologic recovery from hypoglycemia occurs despite approximately twofold peripheral hyperinsulinemia in the absence of calculated portal hypoinsulinemia.[18] Clearly, therefore, additional (glucose counter-regulatory) factors must be involved.

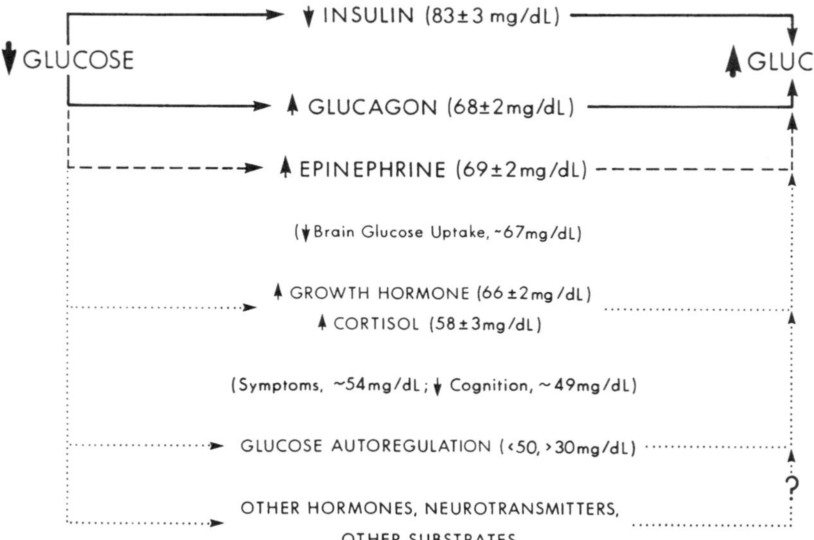

Figure 13-1. Schematic representation of the physiology of glucose counter-regulation. Mean (±SE) arterialized venous glycemic thresholds for the various responses and changes are also shown. These thresholds are from references 16 and 17. (Reproduced with permission from Cryer PE. Glucose counter-regulation: The prevention and correction of hypoglycemia in humans. Am J Physiol 1993;264:E149. Reproduced with the permission of the American Physiological Society.)

Glucagon and Epinephrine. Among the counter-regulatory hormones, glucagon plays a primary role. Recovery from hypoglycemia is impaired by about 40% in the absence of a glucagon secretory response.[20,21] Several counter-regulatory hormones, including glucagon, are released as the plasma glucose falls at glucose levels just below the physiologic range and at glucose levels substantially higher than those required to produce symptoms of hypoglycemia and impair cognitive function[16,17] (see Fig. 13-1). That finding is consistent with but does not prove a role for these hormones in the prevention as well as the correction of hypoglycemia. However, there is considerable direct evidence on this point from studies in the overnight[22] and 3-day[23] fasted states, in the postprandial state,[24] and during physical exercise.[25,26] Under all of these conditions plasma glucose levels fall but then plateau and do not progress to hypoglycemic levels when glucagon secretion is suppressed. Thus, glucagon plays a primary role in both the prevention and correction of hypoglycemia, but additional factors are involved and become critical when glucagon is deficient.

The key additional factor is epinephrine. Neither recovery from hypoglycemia[20,21] nor the prevention of hypoglycemia[22–26] is affected substantially by pharmacologic adrenergic blockade or the epinephrine deficiency state that results from bilateral adrenalectomy. However, hypoglycemia progresses[20,21] or develops[22–26] when both glucagon and epinephrine are deficient and insulin is present. Thus, epinephrine is not normally critical to the correction or prevention of hypoglycemia but it becomes critical when glucagon is deficient.

Other Factors. Clearly, insulin, glucagon, and epinephrine stand high in the hierarchy of redundant glucoregulatory factors (see Fig. 13-1). Both growth hormone and cortisol are demonstrably involved in defense against prolonged hyperinsulinemia and developing hypoglycemia.[11,12,27] However, neither hormone is critical to the correction of hypoglycemia or, at least in adults, to the prevention of hypoglycemia after an overnight fast.[27] Thus, these hormones stand lower in the hierarchy. There is evidence that glucose autoregulation may be operative in humans, although only at very low plasma glucose concentrations.[28,29] In animals there is evidence that additional factors are involved,[30] but their contribution is quantitatively small.[3,30]

Pathophysiology

Syndromes of Compromised Glucose Counter-regulation

Defective Glucose Counter-regulation. The physiology of glucose counter-regulation is seriously deranged in patients with IDDM.[1,4,5] First, as the patient becomes totally insulin-deficient over the first few years of clinical IDDM, the appearance of insulin in the circulation becomes totally unregulated. It is solely a function of passive diffusion from subcutaneous injection sites. As plasma glucose levels fall, insulin levels do not decrease. Second, over approximately the same time frame, the glucagon secretory response to falling glucose levels is lost.[31,32] This is an acquired defect but, because it develops early in the course of IDDM, it is the rule in established IDDM. Interestingly, it is a selective defect. Glucagon secretory responses to other stimuli are largely, if not entirely, intact. Its mechanism is not known but it is tightly linked to and theoretically explainable by absolute insulin deficiency.[33] Thus, glucose counter-regulation is altered fundamentally early in the course of IDDM. Third, after a few more years of IDDM, the epinephrine response to falling glucose levels is reduced.[32,34,35] This, too, is a selective defect. The epinephrine responses to other stimuli remain largely intact. The mechanism of this reduced response is not fully understood but, as discussed shortly, recent antecedent hypoglycemia appears to be one factor. In contrast to the deficient glucagon response, which appears to be absolute, the deficient epinephrine response appears to be a threshold abnormality. An epinephrine response can be elicited but a lower plasma glucose concentration is required.[35] The development of a deficient epinephrine response is a critical pathophysiologic event in a patient with IDDM. When compared with those with deficient glucagon but normal epinephrine responses, patients with combined deficiencies of the glucagon and epinephrine responses to falling plasma glucose concentrations have been shown in prospective studies to be at 25-fold or greater increased risk for the occurrence of severe iatrogenic hypoglycemia[36,37] (Fig. 13-2). Such patients have the syndrome of defective glucose counter-regulation.

Hypoglycemia Unawareness. The syndrome of hypoglycemia unawareness is loss of the warning symptoms of developing hypoglycemia that previously alerted the patient to act (i.e., eat) to prevent its progression to severe hypoglycemia.[4,5,38–44] It is conventional to divide the symptoms of hypoglycemia into two categories, neuroglycopenic and neurogenic (or autonomic) symptoms.[45] Neuroglycopenic symptoms are the direct result of neuronal fuel (glucose) deprivation. They include behavioral changes, confusion, fatigue, seizure, loss of consciousness, and ultimately death. Neurogenic symptoms are the result of the perception of physiologic changes caused by the autonomic nervous system discharge triggered by hypoglycemia. They include adrenergic (catecholamine-mediated) symptoms such as palpitations, tremor, and anxiety and cholinergic (acetylcholine-mediated) symptoms such as sweating, hunger, and paresthesias.[45] The former symptoms are mediated by norepinephrine released from sympathetic postganglionic neurons, the adrenal medullae, or both, and epinephrine released from the adrenal medullae. The latter symptoms are thought to be mediated by acetylcholine released from sympathetic postganglionic neurons, although a contribution from neurotransmitter released from parasympathetic postganglionic neurons cannot be excluded. Because awareness of hypoglycemia is normally largely the result of the perception of neurogenic symptoms,[45] it is reasonable to attribute hypoglycemia unawareness in IDDM largely to loss of these neurogenic symptoms. The mechanism of hypoglycemia unawareness is also not entirely known, but recent antecedent hypoglycemia appears to be a major factor, as discussed farther on. Prospective data indicate that hypoglycemia unawareness substantially increases the risk of severe iatrogenic hypoglycemia in IDDM (Fig. 13-3).[46]

Elevated Glycemic Thresholds During Intensive Therapy. Intensive therapy of IDDM that effectively lowers overall plasma glucose levels results in elevated glycemic thresholds (lower plasma glucose levels required) for symptoms of and counter-regulatory hormone responses to hypoglycemia.[47,48] A critical unresolved issue is whether such therapy does[48,50] or does not[51,52] also produce elevated glycemic thresholds for cognitive dysfunction during hypoglycemia. This question relates directly to the extent to which such elevated glycemic thresholds per se increase the risk of severe hypoglycemia in IDDM. It is well established that effective intensive therapy increases the risk of severe hypoglycemia at least threefold.[53] If glycemic thresholds for symptoms and counter-regulatory hormone responses are elevated but those for cognitive dysfunction are not, the elevated thresholds for the former would likely be responsible for much of the increased risk of hypoglycemia, since cognitive impairment would occur before physiologic and behavioral defenses are activated. Conversely, glycemic thresholds

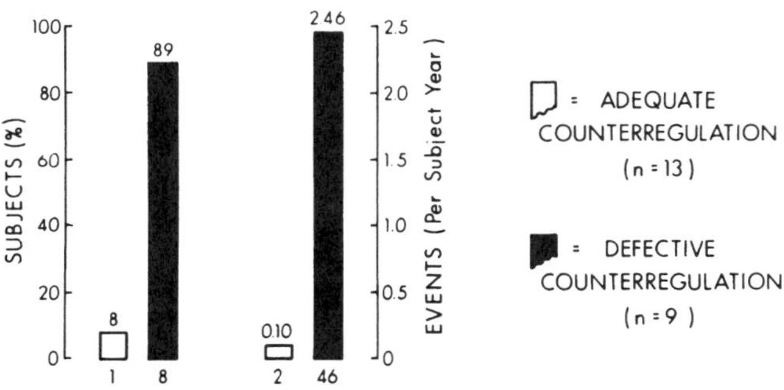

Figure 13-2. Proportion of patients affected and event rates for severe hypoglycemia during intensive therapy of patients with IDDM and adequate (*open columns*) or defective (*closed columns*) glucose counter-regulation. Drawn from data in reference 36.

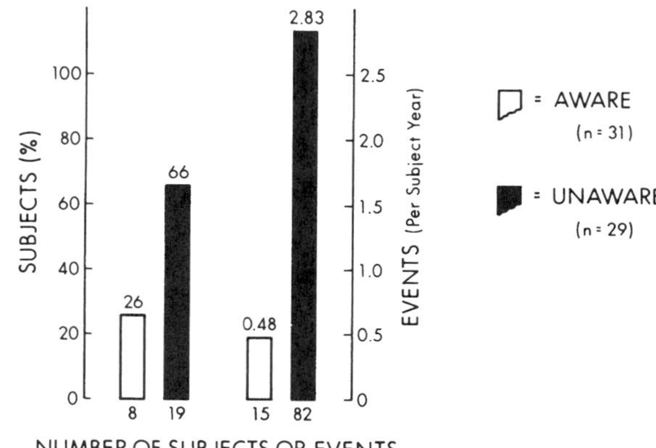

Figure 13-3. Proportion of patients affected and event rates for severe hypoglycemia in patients with IDDM and normal (*open columns*) or reduced (*closed columns*) awareness of hypoglycemia. Drawn from data in reference 46.

for symptoms and counter-regulatory hormone responses are reduced (occur at higher glucose levels) in patients with poorly controlled IDDM.[54] These findings provided the first evidence that glycemic thresholds for at least some responses to hypoglycemia are dynamic rather than static, a concept fundamental to the discussion that follows. Like hypoglycemia unawareness, the mechanism of elevated glycemic thresholds during intensive therapy is not known. Again, recent antecedent hypoglycemia appears to be a major factor.

Hypoglycemia-Associated Autonomic Failure. These three syndromes—defective glucose counter-regulation, hypoglycemia unawareness, and elevated glycemic thresholds during effective intensive therapy—have much in common.[4,35,55] First, they are all associated with a high frequency of severe iatrogenic hypoglycemia. Second, they tend to segregate together clinically. (Parenthetically, they do not segregate together with classic diabetic autonomic neuropathy.[40,41]) Third, they share several pathophysiologic features, including elevated glycemic thresholds for autonomic—adrenomedullary (epinephrine), parasympathetic neural (pancreatic polypeptide), and perhaps sympathetic neural (neurogenic symptoms)—responses to hypoglycemia.[4,35,55] Based on these considerations, it has been suggested that these three syndromes can be conceptualized as examples of hypoglycemia-associated autonomic failure, a functional disorder distinct from classic diabetic autonomic neuropathy.[55]

The pathogenesis of hypoglycemia-associated autonomic failure is not known, need not be the same in all three syndromes and, indeed, could be multifactorial in a given syndrome. We have suggested that recent antecedent iatrogenic hypoglycemia might be one factor in its pathogenesis.[4,35,55] Based largely on our finding that a single episode of afternoon hypoglycemia reduces autonomic and symptomatic responses to hypoglycemia the following morning[56] and conceptually similar findings in other laboratories[57,58] in nondiabetic individuals, we developed the overall hypothesis that in patients with IDDM recent antecedent iatrogenic hypoglycemia is a major cause of hypoglycemia-associated autonomic failure; such failure, by reducing both symptoms of and physiologic defense against developing hypoglycemia, results in recurrent iatrogenic hypoglycemia, thus creating a vicious cycle.[55] As illustrated in Figure 13-4, the hypothesis predicts that episodes of recent antecedent iatrogenic hypoglycemia cause reduced symptomatic responses to (i.e., decreased awareness of) and reduced autonomic responses (including the key epinephrine response) to subsequent falling glucose levels, resulting in recurrent severe iatrogenic hypoglycemia. To date we and others have demonstrated that recent antecedent

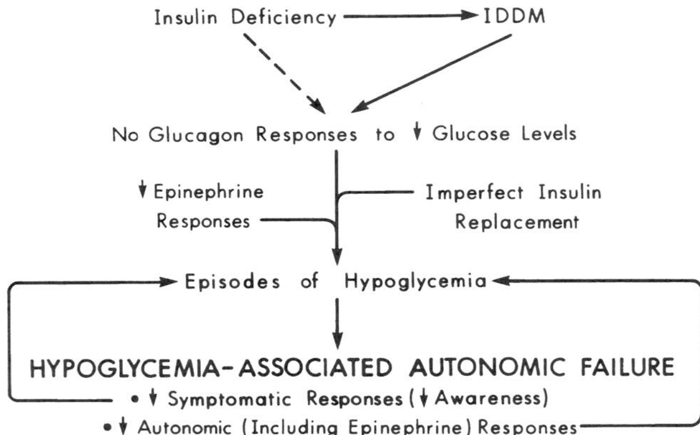

Figure 13-4. Schematic diagram of the hypoglycemia-associated autonomic failure in the IDDM hypothesis. (Modified from Cryer PE. Iatrogenic hypoglycemia as a cause of hypoglycemia-associated autonomic failure in IDDM: A vicious cycle. Diabetes 1992; 41:2550. Reproduced with the permission of the American Diabetes Association.)

hypoglycemia reduces symptomatic and autonomic responses to subsequent hypoglycemia in patients with IDDM,[35,59,60] including those with well-controlled IDDM[61]; impairs glycemic defense against subsequent hyperinsulinemia[35]; is specific for the stimulus of hypoglycemia[61]; and is not attributable to prior autonomic activation per se,[61] all consistent with the overall hypothesis.

To the extent that recent antecedent hypoglycemia is causative of these clinical syndromes, avoidance of iatrogenic hypoglycemia should reverse them. There is now considerable evidence that minimizing the frequency of iatrogenic hypoglycemia reverses the clinical syndrome of hypoglycemia unawareness and the elevated glycemic thresholds for symptoms and autonomic responses associated with effective intensive therapy in patients with IDDM.[62–64] Indeed, hypoglycemia unawareness appears to be completely reversible in that symptomatic responses to hypoglycemia are normalized[62,65] (Fig. 13-5). Although increased but not normalized epinephrine responses have been demonstrated in some studies,[62,63] glucagon responses are affected very little[62] or not at all.[63,64] Thus, although there may be some improvement, the syndrome of defective glucose counter-regulation does not appear to be reversible despite scrupulous avoidance of iatrogenic hypoglycemia. This indicates that factors in addition to recent antecedent hypoglycemia play an important role in the pathogenesis of defective glucose counter-regulation in IDDM.[4,64]

Compromised Glucose Counter-regulation in Non–Insulin-Dependent Diabetes Mellitus

The pathophysiology of glucose counter-regulation has been studied less extensively in non–insulin-dependent diabetes mellitus (NIDDM).[5] Although a key feature of defective glucose counter-regulation—a reduced but not absent glucagon response to hypoglycemia—has been demonstrated in patients with NIDDM,[65] the magnitude of its clinical impact in such patients is not known. On the other hand, hypoglycemia unawareness does occur in NIDDM, and it is reasonable to suspect a role for recent antecedent hypoglycemia in its pathogenesis.

Role in the Pathogenesis of Hyperglycemia

To what extent are the plasma glucose-raising counter-regulatory factors involved in the pathogenesis of hyperglycemia in patients with diabetes mellitus?

A widely held view is that NIDDM is the result of insufficient insulin secretion in the setting of resistance to insulin action. A

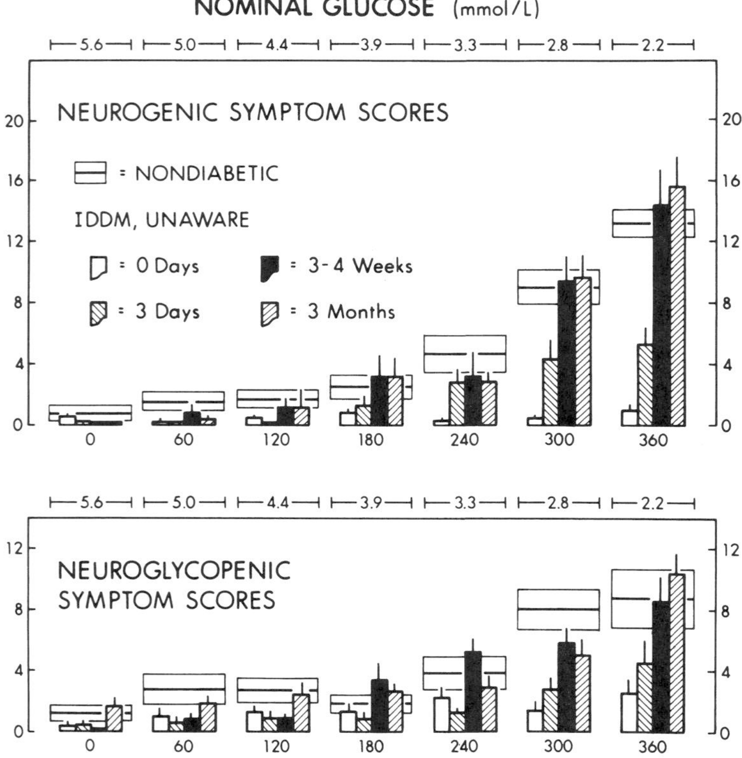

Figure 13-5. Mean (±SE) neurogenic and neuroglycopenic symptom scores during stepped hypoglycemic clamps in patients with IDDM and hypoglycemia unawareness (*columns*) and nondiabetic control subjects (*rectangles*). The initially unaware patients were studied at baseline (*open columns*) and after 3 days (*first set of cross-hatched columns*), 3–4 weeks (*closed columns*), and 3 months (*second set of cross-hatched columns*) of scrupulous avoidance of iatrogenic hypoglycemia. (Reproduced with permission from Dagogo-Jack S, Rattarasarn C, Cryer P. Reversal of hypoglycemia awareness, but not defective glucose counterregulation, in IDDM. Diabetes 1994;43:1426. Reproduced with the permission of the American Diabetes Association.)

substantial body of evidence has been marshalled to support the hypothesis that inappropriately high levels of glucagon secretion contribute to the pathogenesis of insulin resistance, and thus hyperglycemia, in NIDDM.[6]

There is evidence that glucagon[66] but not catecholamines[67] accelerate the development of mild ketoacidosis produced experimentally by insulin withdrawal from patients with IDDM. The levels of these and other glucose-raising factors, including growth hormone and cortisol, are elevated in patients with full-blown diabetic ketoacidosis,[7] and it is conceivable that they contribute to maintenance of the metabolic abnormalities that characterize that disorder. On the other hand, release of glucose-raising hormones caused by psychological ''stress'' does not appear to have a major hyperglycemic effect in patients with IDDM, at least in the short term.[68,69]

Nocturnal growth hormone secretion is the basic cause of the dawn phenomenon—a night-time to morning rise in plasma glucose—in IDDM.[70–72] However, the magnitude of this phenomenon is not great in the clinical setting.[72] An episode of hypoglycemia induces posthypoglycemic insulin resistance mediated initially by catecholamines and later by growth hormone and cortisol.[73–74] Thus, the physiologic basis of the Somogyi hypothesis that hypoglycemia begets hyperglycemia would appear to be sound. However, the magnitude of this effect is not great, and there is now considerable evidence, rhetoric aside, that nocturnal hypoglycemia does not cause clinically important fasting or daytime hyperglycemia in patients with IDDM.[72,75–78] Indeed, for reasons discussed earlier, hypoglycemia begets hypoglycemia rather than hyperglycemia in patients with IDDM.[79]

Clinical Hypoglycemia

Clinical Aspects

The clinical manifestations, classification, frequency, impact, diagnosis, and treatment of iatrogenic hypoglycemia in patients with diabetes mellitus have been reviewed in detail[5] and are not reiterated here.

Hypoglycemia is a major problem for many patients with IDDM and some with NIDDM.[4,5] Indeed, iatrogenic hypoglycemia is the limiting factor in the management of diabetes mellitus.[4] Patients with IDDM receiving conventional therapy suffer an average of one episode of symptomatic hypoglycemia per week and those receiving intensive therapy an average of two such episodes per week. At a minimum, 10% of IDDM patients using conventional therapy and 25% of those using intensive therapy suffer at least one episode of severe, temporarily disabling hypoglycemia, often with seizure or coma, in a given year. It has been estimated from large retrospective series that approximately 4% of deaths of persons with IDDM are the result of hypoglycemia, an alarming iatrogenic mortality rate. Hypoglycemia not only causes recurrent physical morbidity and some mortality; it often causes recurrent or even persistent psychosocial morbidity.

Hypoglycemia is a less frequent problem in drug-treated patients with NIDDM overall.[5] However, its frequency approaches that in IDDM in those who reach the insulin-deficient end of the spectrum of NIDDM.[5] For example, Hepburn and colleagues[80] found the frequency of severe hypoglycemia to be similar in insulin-treated NIDDM patients and in IDDM patients matched for duration of insulin therapy.

Risk Factors for Hypoglycemia

Conventional risk factors for iatrogenic hypoglycemia in IDDM are based on the premise that relative or absolute insulin excess, which must occur from time to time because of the imperfections of all current insulin replacement regimens, is the sole determinant of risk.[4,5] Relative or absolute insulin excess occurs when (1) insulin doses are excessive, ill-timed, or of the wrong type; (2) the influx of exogenous glucose is decreased, as following a missed meal or snack or during an overnight fast; (3) insulin-independent glucose utilization is increased, as during exercise; (4) endogenous glucose production is decreased, as following alcohol ingestion under some conditions; (5) sensitivity to insulin is increased, as during intensive therapy or after exercise or in patients with hypopituitarism or primary adrenocortical insufficiency; and (6) insulin clearance is decreased as with progressive renal insufficiency.

However, the extensive experience of the Diabetes Control and Complications Trial indicates clearly that these conventional risk factors explain only a minority of episodes of severe hypoglycemia in IDDM.[81] Therefore, it is reasonable to view the risk of iatrogenic hypoglycemia as the result of the interplay of relative or absolute insulin excess and compromised glucose counter-regulation. In other words, insulin excess of sufficient magnitude will cause hypoglycemia, but the integrity of the counter-regulatory systems determines whether or not less marked hyperinsulinemia, perhaps more representative of that which occurs in the treatment of IDDM, causes an episode of hypoglycemia. From this perspective issues relevant to hypoglycemia addressed with a given patient should include, in addition to the conventional risk factors, the syndromes of compromised glucose counter-regulation.[4,5]

Acknowledgments

The author acknowledges the substantive input of his several collaborators and postdoctoral fellows to the work from our laboratory summarized here, the skilled assistance of the staff of the Washington University Clinical Research Center and the assistance of our laboratory staff, and the help of Ms. Kay Logsdon in the preparation of this manuscript.

The author's work cited here was supported, in part, by U.S.P.H.S. grants DK27085, DK44235, RR00036, DK20579, and DK07120 and by the American Diabetes Association.

References

1. Cryer PE. Glucose homeostasis and hypoglycemia. In: Wilson JD, Foster DW, eds. Williams Textbook of Endocrinology, 8th ed. Philadelphia: WB Saunders; 1992:1223–1253
2. Cryer PE. Glucose counterregulation: The physiological mechanisms that prevent or correct hypoglycemia. In: Frier BM, Fisher BM, eds. Hypoglycaemia and Diabetes. London: Edward Arnold; 1993:34–55
3. Cryer PE. Glucose counterregulation: The prevention and correction of hypoglycemia in humans. Am J Physiol 1993;264:E149
4. Cryer PE. Hypoglycemia: The limiting factor in the management of IDDM. Diabetes 1994;43:1378
5. Cryer PE, Fisher JN, Shamoon H. Hypoglycemia. Diabetes Care 1994;17:734
6. Unger RH, Orci L. Glucagon secretion, α-cell metabolism, and glucagon action. In: De Groot LJ, ed. Endocrinology, 3rd ed. Philadelphia: WB Saunders; 1995:1337–1353
7. Fleckman AM. Diabetic ketoacidosis. Endocrinol Metab Clin North Am 1993;22:181
8. McCall AL. Effects of glucose deprivation on glucose metabolism in the central nervous system. In: Frier BM, Fisher BM, eds. Hypoglycaemia and Diabetes. London: Edward Arnold; 1993:56–71
9. Berk MA, Clutter WE, Skor D, et al. Enhanced glycemic responsiveness to epinephrine in insulin dependent diabetes mellitus is the result of the inability to secrete insulin. J Clin Invest 1985;75:1842
10. Cryer PE. Catecholamines, pheochromocytoma and diabetes. Diabetes Rev 1993;1:309
11. De Feo P, Perriello G, Torlone E, et al. Demonstration of a role of growth hormone in glucose counterregulation. Am J Physiol 1989;256:E835
12. DeFeo P, Perriello G, Torlone E, et al. Contribution of cortisol to glucose counterregulation in humans. Am J Physiol 1989;257:E35
13. Boyle PJ, Liggett SB, Shah SD, Cryer PE. Direct muscarinic cholinergic inhibition of hepatic glucose production in humans. J Clin Invest 1988;82:445
14. Soskin S, Levine R. Carbohydrate Metabolism, 2nd ed. Chicago: University of Chicago Press; 1952:1–336
15. Randle PJ, Garland PB, Hales CN, Newsholme EA. The glucose-fatty acid

cycle: Its role in insulin sensitivity and the metabolic disturbances of diabetes mellitus. Lancet 1963;i:785
16. Schwartz NS, Clutter WE, Shah SD, Cryer PE. The glycemic thresholds for activation of glucose counterregulatory systems are higher than the threshold for symptoms. J Clin Invest 1987;79:777
17. Mitrakou A, Ryan C, Veneman T, et al. Hierarchy of glycemic thresholds for counterregulatory hormone secretion, symptoms and cerebral dysfunction. Am J Physiol 1991;260:E67
18. Heller SR, Cryer PE. Hypoinsulinemia is not critical to glucose recovery from hypoglycemia in humans. Am J Physiol 1991;261:E41
19. Garber AJ, Cryer PE, Santiago JV, et al. The role of adrenergic mechanisms in the substrate and hormonal response to insulin-induced hypoglycemia in man. J Clin Invest 1976;58:7
20. Gerich J, Davis J, Lorenzi M, et al. Hormonal mechanisms of recovery from insulin-induced hypoglycemia in man. Am J Physiol 1979;236:E380
21. Rizza RA, Cryer PE, Gerich JE. Role of glucagon, catecholamines and growth hormone in human glucose counterregulation. J Clin Invest 1979;64:62
22. Rosen SG, Clutter WE, Berk MA, et al. Epinephrine supports the postabsorptive plasma glucose concentration, and prevents hypoglycemia, when glucagon secretion is deficient in man. J Clin Invest 1984;73:405
23. Boyle PJ, Shah SD, Cryer PE. Insulin, glucagon and catecholamines in the prevention of hypoglycemia during fasting in humans. Am J Physiol 1989; 256:E651
24. Tse TF, Clutter WE, Shah SD, Cryer PE. Mechanisms of postprandial glucose counterregulation in man: Physiologic roles of glucagon and epinephrine vis-a-vis insulin in the prevention of hypoglycemia late after glucose ingestion. J Clin Invest 1983;72:278
25. Hirsch IB, Marker JC, Smith LJ, et al. Insulin and glucagon in the prevention of hypoglycemia during exercise in humans. Am J Physiol 1991;260:E695
26. Marker JC, Hirsch IB, Smith LJ, et al. Catecholamines and the prevention of hypoglycemia during exercise in humans. Am J Physiol 1991;260:E705
27. Boyle PJ, Cryer PE. Growth hormone, cortisol, or both are involved in defense against, but are not critical to recovery from, prolonged hypoglycemia in humans. Am J Physiol 1991;260:E395
28. Bolli GB, DeFeo P, Perriello G, et al. Role of hepatic autoregulation in defense against hypoglycemia in humans. J Clin Invest 1985;75:1623
29. Hansen I, Firth R, Haymond M, et al. The role of autoregulation of hepatic glucose production in man: Response to a physiologic decrement in plasma glucose. Diabetes 1986;35:186
30. Connolly CC, Adkins-Marshall BA, Neal DW, et al. Relationship between decrements in glucose level and metabolic response to hypoglycemia in absence of counterregulatory hormones in the conscious dog. Diabetes 1992;41:1308
31. Gerich J, Langlois M, Noacco C, et al. Lack of glucagon response to hypoglycemia in diabetes: Evidence for an intrinsic pancreatic alpha-cell defect. Science 1973;182:171
32. Bolli G, De Feo P, Compagnucci P, et al. Abnormal glucose counterregulation in insulin-dependent diabetes mellitus: Interaction of anti-insulin antibodies and impaired glucagon and epinephrine secretion. Diabetes 1983;32:134
33. Fukuda M, Tanaka A, Tahara Y, et al. Correlation between minimal secretory capacity of pancreatic β-cells and stability of diabetic control. Diabetes 1988;37:81
34. Hirsch BR, Shamoon H. Defective epinephrine and growth hormone responses in type 1 diabetes are stimulus specific. Diabetes 1987;36:20
35. Dagogo-Jack SE, Craft S, Cryer PE. Hypoglycemia-associated autonomic failure in insulin dependent diabetes mellitus. J Clin Invest 1993;91:819
36. White NH, Skor DA, Cryer PE, et al. Identification of type 1 diabetic patients at increased risk for hypoglycemia during intensive therapy. N Engl J Med 1983;308:485
37. Bolli GB, De Feo P, DeCosmo S, et al. A reliable and reproducible test for adequate glucose counterregulation in type I diabetes mellitus. Diabetes 1984; 33:732
38. Gerich JE, Mokan M, Veneman T, et al. Hypoglycemia unawareness. Endocrine Rev 1991;12:356
39. Cryer PE. Hypoglycemia unawareness in IDDM. Diabetes Care 1993;16:40
40. Hepburn DA, Patrick AW, Eadington DW, et al. Unawareness of hypoglycaemia in insulin-treated diabetic patients: Prevalence and relationship to autonomic neuropathy. Diabetic Med 1990;7:711
41. Ryder REJ, Owens DR, Hayes TM, et al. Unawareness of hypoglycaemia and inadequate glucose counterregulation: No causal relationship with diabetic autonomic neuropathy. Br Med J 1990;301:783
42. Grimaldi A, Bosquet F, Davidoff P, et al. Unawareness of hypoglycemia by insulin-dependent diabetics. Horm Metab Res 1990;22:90
43. Clarke WL, Gonder-Frederick LA, Richards FE, Cryer PE. Multifactorial origin of hypoglycemic symptom unawareness in insulin dependent diabetes mellitus. Diabetes 1991;40:680
44. Hepburn DA, Patrick AW, Brash HM, et al. Hypoglycaemia unawareness in type I diabetes: A lower plasma glucose is required to stimulate sympathoadrenal activation. Diabetic Med 1991;8:934
45. Towler DA, Havlin CE, Craft S, Cryer PE: Mechanisms of awareness of hypoglycemia: Perception of neurogenic (predominantly cholinergic) rather than neuroglycopenic symptoms. Diabetes 1993;42:1791
46. Gold AE, MacLeod KM, Frier BM. Frequency of severe hypoglycemia in patients with type I diabetes with impaired awareness of hypoglycemia. Diabetes Care 1994;17:697
47. Amiel SA, Tamborlane WV, Simonson DC, Sherwin RS: Defective glucose counterregulation after strict control of insulin-dependent diabetes mellitus. N Engl J Med 1987;316:1376
48. Amiel SA, Sherwin RS, Simonson DC, Tamborlane WV. Effect of intensive insulin therapy on glycemic thresholds for counterregulatory hormone release. Diabetes 1988;37:901
49. Ziegler D, Hübinger A, Mühlen H, Gries FA. Effects of previous glycemic control on the onset and magnitude of cognitive dysfunction during hypoglycaemia in type 1 (insulin dependent) diabetic patients. Diabetologia 1992; 35:828
50. Jones TW, McCarthy G, Tamborlane WV, et al. Resistance to neuroglycopenia: An adaptive response during intensive insulin treatment of diabetes (abstract). Diabetes 1991;40:557A
51. Amiel SA, Pottinger RC, Archibald HR, et al. Effect of antecedent glucose control on cerebral function during hypoglycemia. Diabetes Care 1991;14:109
52. Widom B, Simonson DC. Glycemic control and neuropsychologic function during hypoglycemia in patients with insulin-dependent diabetes mellitus. Ann Intern Med 1990;112:904
53. The Diabetes Control and Complications Trial Research Group. The effect of intensive treatment of diabetes on the development and progression of long-term complications in insulin-dependent diabetes mellitus. N Engl J Med 1993;329:977
54. Boyle PJ, Schwartz NS, Shah SD, et al. Plasma glucose concentrations at the onset of hypoglycemic symptoms in patients with poorly controlled diabetes and nondiabetics. N Engl J Med 1988;318:1487
55. Cryer PE. Iatrogenic hypoglycemia as a cause of hypoglycemia-associated autonomic failure in IDDM: A vicious cycle. Diabetes 1992;41:255
56. Heller SR, Cryer PE. Reduced neuroendocrine and symptomatic responses to subsequent hypoglycemia after one episode of hypoglycemia in nondiabetic humans. Diabetes 1991;40:223
57. Davis M, Shamoon H. Counterregulatory adaptation to recurrent hypoglycemia in normal humans. J Clin Endocrinol Metab 1991;73:995
58. Widom B, Simonson DC. Intermittent hypoglycemia impairs glucose counterregulation. Diabetes 1992;41:1597
59. Dans MR, Mellman M, Shamoon H. Further defects in counterregulatory responses induced by recurrent hypoglycemia in type 1 diabetes. Diabetes 1992;41:1335
60. Lingenfelser T, Renn W, Sommerwerck U, et al. Compromised hormonal counterregulation, symptom awareness, and neurophysiological function after recurrent short-term episodes for insulin-induced hypoglycemia in IDDM patients. Diabetes 1993;42:610
61. Rattarasarn C, Dagogo-Jack SE, Zachwieja JJ, Cryer PE. Hypoglycemia-associated autonomic failure in IDDM is specific for the stimulus of hypoglycemia and is not attributable to prior autonomic activation per se. Diabetes 1994; 43:809
62. Fanelli CG, Epifano L, Rambotti AM, et al. Meticulous prevention of hypoglycemia normalizes the glycemic thresholds and magnitude of most neuroendocrine responses to, symptoms of, and cognitive function during hypoglycemia in intensively treated patients with short-term IDDM. Diabetes 1993;42:1683
63. Cranston I, Lomas J, Maran A, et al. Restoration of hypoglycaemia awareness in patients with long duration insulin-dependent diabetes. Lancet 1994;344:283
64. Dagogo-Jack S, Rattarasarn C, Cryer PE. Reversal of hypoglycemia unawareness, but not defective glucose counterregulation, in IDDM. Diabetes 1994;43:1426
65. Bolli GB, Tsalikian E, Haymond MW, et al. Defective glucose counterregulation after subcutaneous insulin in noninsulin dependent diabetes mellitus. J Clin Invest 1984;73:1532
66. Gerich JE, Lorenzi M, Bier DM, et al. Prevention of human diabetic ketoacidosis by somatostatin. N Engl J Med 1975;292:985
67. Beylot M, Sautot G, Dechaud H, et al. Lack of beta-adrenergic role for catecholamines in the development of hyperglycemia and ketonaemia following acute insulin withdrawal in type 1 diabetic patients. Diabete Metab 1985; 11:111
68. Kemmer FW, Bisping R, Steingrüber HG, et al. Psychological stress and metabolic control in patients with type 1 diabetes mellitus. N Engl J Med 1986;314:1078
69. Fernqvist-Forbes E, Linde B. Insulin absorption, glucose homeostasis, and lipolysis in IDDM during mental stress. Diabetes Care 1991;14:1006
70. Campbell PJ, Bolli GB, Cryer PE, Gerich JE. Pathogenesis of the dawn phenomenon in patients with insulin dependent diabetes mellitus: Accelerated glucose production and impaired glucose utilization due to nocturnal surges in growth hormone secretion. N Engl J Med 1985;312:1473
71. Boyle PJ, Avogaro A, Smith L, et al. Absence of the dawn phenomenon and abnormal lipolysis in type 1 (insulin dependent) diabetic patients with chronic growth hormone deficiency. Diabetologia 1992;35:372
72. Cryer PE. Morning hyperglycemia in insulin dependent diabetes mellitus: Insulin lack versus the dawn and Somogyi phenomena. In: Mazzaferri EL, ed. Advances in Endocrinology and Metabolism, vol. 1. Chicago: Year Book Medical Publishers;1990:231–243
73. Atvall S, Eriksson B-M, Fowelin J, et al. Early posthypoglycemic insulin resistance in man is mainly an effect of β-adrenergic stimulation. J Clin Invest 1987;80:437
74. Fowelin J, Attvall S, von Schenck H, et al. Combined effect of growth hormone and cortisol on late posthypoglycemic insulin resistence in humans. Diabetes 1989;38:1357

75. Havlin CE, Cryer PE. Nocturnal hypoglycemia does not result commonly in major morning hyperglycemia in patients with diabetes mellitus. Diabetes Care 1987;10:141
76. Tordjman KM, Havlin CE, Levandoski LA, et al. Failure of nocturnal hypoglycemia to cause fasting hyperglycemia in patients with insulin dependent diabetes mellitus. N Engl J Med 1987;317:1552
77. Perriello G, DeFeo P, Torlone E, et al. The effect of asymptomatic nocturnal hypoglycemia on glycemic control in diabetes mellitus. N Engl J Med 1988;319:1233
78. Hirsch IB, Smith LB, Havlin CE, et al. Failure of nocturnal hypoglycemia to cause daytime hyperglycemia in patients with insulin dependent diabetes mellitus. Diabetes Care 1990;13:133
79. Cryer PE. Hypoglycemia begets hypoglycemia in IDDM. Diabetes 1993; 42:1691
80. Hepburn DA, MacLeod KM, Pell ACH, et al. Frequency and symptoms of hypoglycaemia experienced by patients with type 2 diabetes treated with insulin. Diabetic Med 1993;10:231
81. The Diabetes Control and Complications Trial Research Group. Epidemiology of severe hypoglycemia in the Diabetes Control and Complications Trial. Am J Med 1991;90:450

Diabetes Mellitus, edited by Derek LeRoith, Simeon I. Taylor, and Jerrold M. Olefsky. Lippincott–Raven Publishers, Philadelphia © 1996.

CHAPTER 14
The Biochemistry of Insulin Action

BENTLEY CHEATHAM AND C. RONALD KAHN

Introduction

Insulin's primary physiologic role is the regulation of glucose homeostasis. This involves complex molecular mechanisms that control gluconeogenesis and glucose uptake and metabolism in insulin-sensitive tissues. In normal individuals this scheme is initiated by elevated plasma glucose levels that trigger the secretion of insulin from the β-cells of the pancreas. The resultant increase in circulating levels of insulin inhibits hepatic glucose production and stimulates an increase in glucose uptake and storage in adipose and skeletal muscle, thus bringing glucose levels to normal. In the progression from normal glucose tolerance to type II diabetes, there is a decrease in the ability of tissues to respond to insulin and an inability of the pancreas to produce enough insulin to compensate for the insulin-resistant state, which leads to impaired β-cell function. These two fundamental defects appear to result from the combined effects of both genetic disposition and environmental factors.[1–5]

The effects of insulin on glucose metabolism are immediate, occurring within a few seconds to minutes. More intermediate and long-term effects of insulin on cellular events include regulation of ion and amino acid uptake, protein synthesis and degradation, gene transcription and mRNA turnover, and cellular growth and differentiation.[4,5] To better understand these pathways and thus perhaps the underlying mechanisms of the pathophysiology of insulin resistant states, it is crucial to identify the key molecular components necessary for mediating insulin signaling.

Insulin action can be viewed as occurring at three distinct levels (Fig. 14-1). Level I actions include the initial cell-surface events: insulin binding to its receptor, activation of the insulin receptor tyrosine kinase with subsequent phosphorylation of insulin receptor substrates, and interaction of these substrates with several downstream signaling molecules. Level II actions are composed of a complex set of distinct phosphorylation-dephosphorylation cascades that lead to activation of several key regulatory enzymes involved in cell growth and metabolism. These include Raf-1 kinase, the mitogen-activated protein kinase-kinase (MAPKK, also referred to as MEK), MAPK, and the 70 kd and 90 kd ribosomal S6 kinases. The final biologic effects of insulin make-up level III actions. This involves the movement of insulin-regulated glucose transporters (GLUT-4) from an intracellular pool to the plasma membrane, activation of enzymes involved in glycogen synthesis, lipid synthesis and protein synthesis, and regulation of nuclear events including DNA synthesis and transcription of specific genes. This chapter focuses on describing our current understanding of how these final biologic effects are governed by a complex insulin-regulated network of upstream signaling molecules.

The Insulin Receptor

Following secretion from the β-cells of the pancreas, insulin binds to its specific cell-surface receptor. Almost all mammalian tissues contain insulin receptors, although the numbers vary greatly, with the highest number being present in insulin-sensitive tissues such as liver and adipose (200,000 to 300,000 receptors per cell) and significantly fewer receptors being present in nonclassic target tissues, such as circulating erythrocytes and brain.[4,6] In its native conformation the insulin receptor is a transmembrane glycoprotein composed of two α-subunits (135 kd) and two β-subunits (95 kd) covalently linked through disulfide bonds to form an $\alpha_2\beta_2$ heterotetramer. The α-subunit is entirely extracellular and contains the sites for insulin binding, whereas the β-subunit has a small extracellular portion, a transmembrane domain, and an intracellular insulin-regulated tyrosine protein kinase activity. Both subunits are derived from a single gene via a large proreceptor polypeptide. The proreceptor undergoes glycosylation followed by disulfide bond formation. Final processing occurs in Golgi-derived vesicles where cleavage of the proreceptor occurs at a tetrabasic site located at the junction of the α- and β-subunits (amino acid residues 720–723). This is followed by terminal glycosylation and possible fatty acid acylation.[7–9] The processing of the insulin proreceptor appears to involve a member of the Kex2-related proprotein family of convertases that cleaves the proreceptor at the tetrabasic site.[10]

Since the cloning of the human insulin receptor cDNA, a number of structure and function studies have been performed using in vitro site-directed mutagenesis followed by biochemical and cell biologic analyses of the mutant proteins in transfected cell

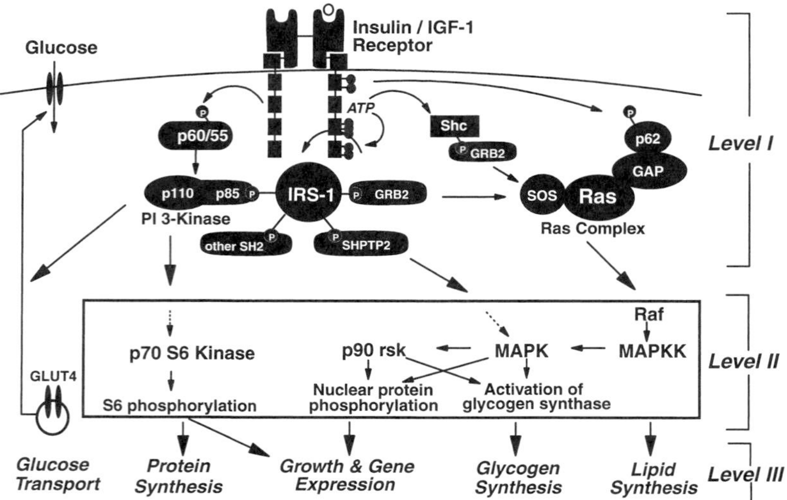

Figure 14-1. The three levels of insulin action. Level I actions include activation of the insulin receptor, phosphorylation of endogenous substrates, and recruitment of signaling molecules. Level II actions involve the activation of complex phosphorylation-dephosphorylation cascades. Level III actions include the final biologic effects of insulin.

culture models. This approach has yielded vital information in understanding the molecular mechanisms of both insulin binding and activation of the tyrosine kinase. Although the detailed structural and functional analysis of the α-subunit is still in the early stages, it is clear that its major role is to suppress the tyrosine kinase activity of the β-subunit. Thus, the insulin receptor behaves as a classic allosteric enzyme in which the binding of insulin to the α-subunit results in a conformational change that releases the inhibitory constraints and allows activation of the tyrosine kinase.[11]

Transmission of the insulin-induced conformational change that signals the β-subunit tyrosine kinase to "turn on" is blocked if the disulfide bond between the α- and β-subunits is disrupted by site-directed mutagenesis, suggesting that covalent interaction between the two subunits is required for communication of the insulin-binding signal.[12,13] In contrast, the inhibitory constraints imposed by the α-subunit that require insulin for disinhibition can also be artificially bypassed. Truncation of the α-subunit by either proteolysis or in vitro site-directed mutagenesis leads to insulin-independent activation of the receptor tyrosine kinase in the absence of insulin.[12] In addition, modifications of the transmembrane domain by site-directed mutagenesis have also resulted in alterations in insulin-stimulated autophosphorylation. These studies showed that the transmembrane domain can tolerate a number of dramatic changes and still be competent for transmitting the conformational change from the extracellular to intracellular domain of the receptor. However, when the transmembrane domain from the *erb*B-2 oncoprotein was substituted for the wild-type transmembrane domain, the mutant insulin receptor displayed maximal levels of autophosphorylation and kinase activity in the absence of insulin, suggesting a role for the transmembrane domain in communicating signals to the intracellular tyrosine kinase, perhaps by promoting ligand-independent receptor oligomerization.[12,14]

What is so important about the insulin receptor tyrosine kinase? A number of studies using mutant insulin receptors that fail to undergo autophosphorylation or are not fully activated show that the kinase activity is imperative for insulin-regulated growth and metabolism.[15] Indeed, some cases of severe insulin resistance are caused by naturally occurring mutations in the insulin receptor that result in impaired kinase activity.[16]

Activation of the tyrosine kinase toward phosphorylation of endogenous substrates is preceded by a complex autophosphorylation cascade involving six or perhaps seven tyrosine residues that are clustered in three regions of the β-subunit.[17,18] The most N-terminal of these regions lies in the juxtamembrane domain and contains Tyr^{960} (and possibly Tyr^{953}); the second region contains three sites of phosphorylation: Tyr^{1146}, Tyr^{1150}, and Tyr^{1151}; the third and more C-terminal region contains Tyr^{1316} and Tyr^{1322}. Each of these regions appears to play a specific role in receptor function. The cluster of Tyr^{1146}, Tyr^{1150}, and Tyr^{1151} has been termed the "regulatory domain," since mutations of these residues either singly or in various combinations result in an impaired kinase activity that is paralleled by a loss in biologic function.[12,19]

The juxtamembrane domain appears to play at least two major roles in receptor function. When Tyr^{960} is deleted or mutated to Phe, these receptors undergo normal kinase activation but fail to phosphorylate endogenous substrates, resulting in an inhibition of signal transmission.[12] In addition, these receptors do not internalize properly.[12,20] It has been suggested that this is because of a disruption of a β-turn structural motif within the Tyr^{960} region. Analysis of secondary structure within the juxtamembrane domain indicates two β-turn motifs[20] at $NPEY^{960}$ and $GPLY^{953}$. Mutations in these regions individually cause a partial reduction in insulin-stimulated receptor internalization, whereas receptors with point mutations at both Tyr^{953} and Tyr^{960} fail to internalize. Thus, this region of the receptor plays two fundamental roles: recognition of substrates and insulin-stimulated receptor endocytosis.

The exact role of the C-terminal sites of phosphorylation is somewhat controversial. Some studies have shown that deletion of the C-terminal 43 amino acids has no effect on kinase activation but results in a decrease in activation of glycogen synthesis. In addition, these receptors display enhanced sensitivity to insulin-stimulated DNA synthesis. However, in a separate study, a similar insulin receptor mutant displayed no alterations in activation of either glycogen synthesis or cell growth.[12] More studies in this region of the receptor are necessary to clarify the role of the C-terminus and its sites of tyrosine phosphorylation in receptor function.

In addition to tyrosine phosphorylation, the insulin receptor undergoes serine and threonine phosphorylation. This is stimulated by a number of agents including cAMP, phorbol esters, and insulin. In contrast to activation by tyrosine phosphorylation, serine phosphorylation has a negative effect on insulin receptor kinase activity.[12] Specific sites of serine-threonine phosphorylation have been identified following insulin or phorbol ester treatment. These include[21,22] Ser^{1293}, Ser^{1294}, and Thr^{1336}. The exact role of these residues in regulating kinase activity or receptor function remains unclear, but it has been suggested that serine phosphorylation plays a role in the decrease in insulin receptor kinase activity observed in non–insulin-dependent diabetes mellitus.[23] It is interesting to note that a serine kinase activity copurifies with the insulin receptor,[21] and more recently some serine kinase activity has been reported to occur by the receptor itself, although the physiologic significance of this activity is unknown.[24]

Phosphorylation of Insulin Receptor Substrate-1 and Signaling Through Interaction with SH2 Domain-Containing Proteins

As described above, level I of insulin action is composed of activation of the insulin receptor kinase followed by subsequent phosphorylation of endogenous substrates. Many advances have been made recently concerning this point in the transmission of the insulin signal.[12,31]

An early hypothesis of insulin action was thought to involve the insulin-stimulated production of second messengers analogous to those where production of small molecules such as cAMP, cGMP, or changes in cellular electrophysiology occurred through fluxes in ion gradients. Indeed, it has been proposed that phosphatidylinositol (PI)-glycans may be insulin-regulated second messengers. This scheme is thought to involve the activation of a specific phospholipase by insulin that acts on a membrane substrate to produce the PI glycan and 1,2-diacylglycerol, which act directly to activate downstream enzymes.[25] Recently, a mutant human erythroleukemia cell line that is incapable of PI glycosylation was shown to be insensitive to insulin stimulation of glycogen synthesis, suggesting a requirement for a PI glycan in insulin action.[26] Insulin has also been shown to alter signaling through heterotrimeric G-proteins. In one study, treatment of plasma membranes from rat liver or adipocytes with insulin inhibited the pertussis toxin–catalyzed ADP ribosylation of G_i.[27] Furthermore, peptides derived from the β-subunit of the insulin receptor have been shown to have a G_i and a G_s-activating function in vitro.[28] In addition, insulin has been shown to induce a conformational change in G_i in the plasma membrane of intact adipocytes.[29] Taken together, these data suggest that there may be communication between the G-protein coupled and insulin signaling pathways.

A more recent hypothesis for insulin action stems from the discovery of proteins with Src homology 2 (SH2) domains that direct noncovalent interactions with specific phosphotyrosine-containing peptide motifs.[30] In this model at least two possibilities exist for downstream signaling by receptor tyrosine kinases; one is exemplified by the receptors for platelet-derived growth factor, epidermal growth factor, and colony-stimulating factor-1, which undergo ligand-stimulated autophosphorylation on multiple tyrosine residues within the intracellular portion of these molecules. These tyrosine phosphorylation sites then provide binding sites for proteins containing SH2 domains such as the phosphatidylinositol-3-kinase (PI-3-kinase), phospholipase Cγ (PLCγ), the Ras GTPase-activating protein, the phosphotyrosine phosphatase SHPTP2, and adapter molecules such as Grb2, nck, and crk. The second model is exemplified by kinases that phosphorylate endogenous substrates; the latter then serve as docking proteins for the SH2 domain containing signaling molecules. The insulin and insulin-like growth factor receptors represent this class. Following activation there is tyrosine phosphorylation of several intracellular substrates. The best characterized of these is a high-molecular-weight protein that was first identified in antiphosphotyrosine immunoprecipitates from insulin-treated hepatoma cells and in livers of intact animals. This protein was termed pp185 and was subsequently partially purified and cloned and renamed insulin receptor substrate-1 (IRS-1).[31,32]

IRS-1 is a cytosolic protein with a predicted molecular weight of 131 kd; however, it migrates on sodium dodecyl sulfate polyacrylamide gels (SDS-PAGE) between 165 and 180 kd, probably as a result of its conformation and high level of serine phosphorylation. IRS-1 is expressed in almost all tissues and is highly conserved among species. Based on its predicted amino acid sequence it contains several notable features, including a potential nucleotide binding site near the N-terminal portion of the molecule, 22 potential tyrosine phosphorylation sites, numerous sites for serine phosphorylation, and a pleckstrin homology domain in the extreme N-terminal domain.[31] This domain of the receptor has recently been shown to be required for efficient interaction-recognition by the insulin receptor, since mutations in this region result in a decrease in IRS-1 phosphorylation and a parallel decrease in signaling capability.[33]

IRS-1 appears to be a relatively specific substrate for the insulin and insulin-like growth factor-1 (IGF-1) receptors, although it has also recently been shown to be a substrate for the interleukin-4 receptor in transfected cell culture models[31,34] and the growth hormone receptor in adipocytes.[35] Of the 22 potential sites for tyrosine phosphorylation, eight have been confirmed by amino acid sequencing of high-pressure liquid chromatography purified proteolytic fragments and include residues 460, 608, 628, 895, 939, 987, 1172, and 1222.[31] Six of these sites reside in peptide motifs with the sequence YMXM or YXXM that are consensus sites for the binding of the SH2 domains of two isoforms of PI-3-kinase, p85α and p85β. IRS-1 has been shown to bind other proteins containing SH2 domains including Grb2, SH-PTP2 (also referred to as Syp, PTP-1D, and PTP-2C), nck, fyn, and perhaps several others that have yet to be identified. The interaction of two of these proteins (the p85 subunit of PI-3-kinase and SH-PTP2) with IRS-1 also appears to be an activation step. Binding of phosphorylated IRS-1 or the respective IRS-1-derived phosphotyrosine-containing peptides to the enzymes in vitro results in an increase in their specific activity.[31]

The binding of a distinct subset of SH2 domain–containing proteins to IRS-1 defines a unique signaling molecule with the potential for a diverse range of downstream effects (Fig. 14-1). Some of the intracellular effects of these proteins have been partially defined, and they do appear to play a role in mediating some insulin actions at both the intermediate stage (level II) and at the level of final biologic effects (level III). In order to discuss the role of IRS-1 in mediating certain aspects of insulin action, a brief description of some of the SH2 domain proteins that associate with IRS-1 follows. Their potential role in insulin signaling is discussed in a later section of this chapter.

PI-3-kinase is a heterodimer composed of an 85 kd regulatory subunit (p85) and a catalytic 110 kd subunit (p110). The p85 subunit contains two SH2 domains and one SH3 domain (a region that directs protein-protein interaction to sites independent of tyrosine phosphorylation. The p85 subunit also displays regions of homology to the break-point cluster region kinase and to the Ras-GTPase-activating protein.[36] Ruderman and coworkers first detected insulin-stimulated PI-3-kinase activity in antiphosphotyrosine immunoprecipitates.[37] Using anti–IRS-1 antibodies, it has since been shown that the majority of the insulin-stimulated PI-3-kinase activity observed in antiphosphotyrosine immunoprecipitates is associated with IRS-1.[31,32] Binding of the p85 subunit to tyrosine phosphorylated IRS-1 or to the consensus phosphopeptides (YMXM or YXXM) is an activation step that results in a 10- to 20-fold increase in PI-3-kinase activity. PI-3-kinase, in turn, phosphorylates PI, PI-4-P, and PI-4,5-P_2 on the D-3 position of the inositol ring to produce PI-3-P, PI-3,4-P_2, and PI-3,4,5-P_3. The exact function of these phospholipids is unclear, but it has been shown that PI-3-kinase activity is required for insulin stimulation of glucose transport and activation of p70 S6 kinase (described below).

Ras is a membrane-associated small GTP-binding protein that plays a key initial role in regulating cell growth and metabolism in a variety of growth factor–regulated signaling systems. The activity of Ras is dependent on its nucleotide-bound state—GTP-bound (active) or GDP-bound (inactive).[38] Guanine nucleotide binding is regulated by specific exchange and releasing factors. mSOS is the guanine nucleotide exchange factor specific for Ras that increases the binding affinity for GTP. Following insulin stimulation, IRS-1 binds Grb2, which associates with mSOS, and this complex results in an increase in the GTP-bound active form of

Ras. Thus, Grb2 acts as a link between IRS-1 and the Ras signaling pathway.[39]

SH-PTP2 is a 70 kd phosphotyrosine phosphatase containing two SH2 domains. It is the homologue of the *Drosophila* corkscrew gene product (csw).[40] SH-PTP2 binds to IRS-1 at Tyr^{1172} following insulin stimulation.[31] Recent data suggest that SH-PTP2 may play a role in the activation of MAPK and in downregulating the insulin signal by dephosphorylation of IRS-1.[41–43]

The Role of IRS-1 in Insulin Action

Although the exact intracellular roles of the individual SH2 proteins that engage IRS-1 are not totally understood, it is clear that IRS-1 and the docking of SH2 domain-containing proteins are necessary components in mediating several downstream insulin effects. These conclusions are based on a series of studies involving a variety of experimental techniques including microinjection of *Xenopus* oocytes, transfected cell culture models, and most recently from transgenic mice that lack the IRS-1 gene.[1,31,44–46]

Insulin and IGF-1 stimulate maturation of primed *Xenopus* oocytes through events requiring tyrosine phosphorylation. Unprimed oocytes do not contain detectable levels of IRS-1 and do not respond to insulin or IGF-1 even though they express IGF-1 receptors. Microinjection of these oocytes with recombinant IRS-1 restores the insulin-IGF-1 maturation response, and this correlates with tyrosine phosphorylation of IRS-1 and the recruitment of PI-3-kinase and Grb2. Formation of either the PI-3-kinase-IRS-1 or the Grb2-IRS-1 complex is effectively blocked when IRS-1 is coinjected along with glutathione S-transferase (GST) fusion proteins containing the SH2 domains of either p85 or Grb2. This results in the blockade of oocyte maturation, providing evidence that the IRS-1 signaling complex is necessary for coupling insulin and IGF-1 receptors with downstream events.[1]

In mammalian cells IRS-1 is also required for insulin-stimulated cell growth. Overexpression of IRS-1 in Chinese hamster ovary cells enhances insulin-stimulated DNA synthesis. In contrast, overexpression of IRS-1 antisense RNA or microinjection of neutralizing antibodies against IRS-1 effectively inhibits the mitogenic effect of insulin, although serum-stimulated growth is unaffected. Furthermore, insulin-stimulated transcriptional activation of a reporter gene construct is also blocked in IRS-1–deficient cells.[31,44,45]

More recently the development of a transgenic mouse that lacks the IRS-1 gene has provided some interesting insight into the impact of IRS-1 signaling in a whole animal model.[46] $IRS\text{-}1^{-/-}$ mice have no detectable IRS-1 protein and as expected display no insulin-stimulated IRS-1 phosphorylation or IRS-1-associated PI-3-kinase activity. Phenotypically, these animals show marked inhibition of intrauterine growth and are 40–50% smaller than their unaffected littermates ($IRS\text{-}1^{+/-}$) at birth (Fig. 14-2). This decreased size is maintained as the mice mature; however, they display no defects in fertility or ability to raise their young. $IRS\text{-}1^{-/-}$ mice are also insulin-IGF-1–resistant, showing an abnormal glucose tolerance (Fig. 14-3*A–E*). Although there is no significant difference between $IRS\text{-}1^{+/+}$ and $IRS\text{-}1^{-/-}$ mice in fasting glucose levels, $IRS\text{-}1^{-/-}$ mice displayed significantly impaired glucose tolerance, increased plasma insulin levels, and a decreased hypoglycemic response to both insulin and IGF-1. In addition, insulin- and IGF-1–stimulated glucose uptake in isolated adipocytes from $IRS\text{-}1^{-/-}$ mice is about 50% that in control mice.

Another interesting observation made in the IRS-1–deficient mice was that although they display no insulin-stimulated PI-3-kinase activity in IRS-1 immunoprecipitates, they still display insulin-stimulated PI-3-kinase activity in antiphosphotyrosine immunoprecipitates. When phosphotyrosine-containing proteins from liver and muscle were analyzed either by direct immunoblotting of total protein or in immunoprecipitates, insulin stimulated the phosphorylation of the insulin receptor in both $IRS\text{-}1^{-/-}$ and controls in a similar manner, whereas as expected IRS-1 was detected only in the control animals. However, antiphosphotyrosine immunoblots of total protein from muscle or liver from $IRS\text{-}1^{-/-}$ mice revealed a band migrating approximately 10 kd higher than the IRS-1 band in control mice (Fig. 14-4). Furthermore, this band was clearly distinct in antiphosphotyrosine immunoblots of anti-p85 immunoprecipitates. This protein band does not cross-react with anti–C-terminal IRS-1 antibody, suggesting that the $IRS\text{-}1^{-/-}$ mice use an alternative substrate of insulin receptor. This protein has been named IRS-2 (Fig. 14-5).

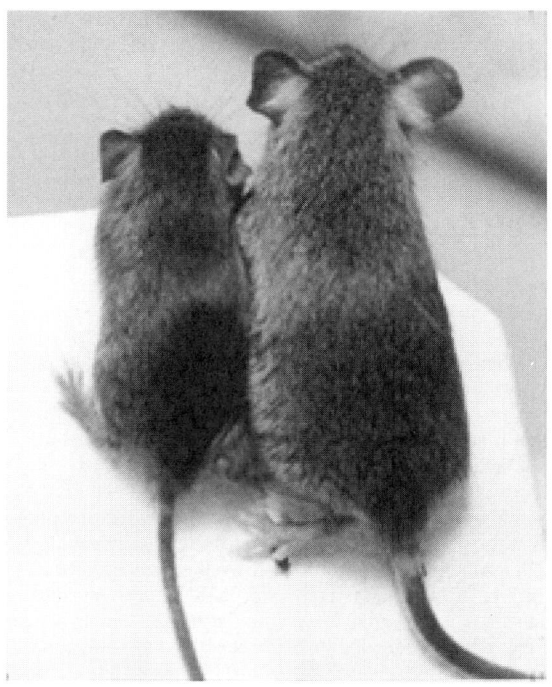

Figure 14-2. IRS-1 knockout mice. Homozygous transgenic mice lacking the IRS-1 gene (*left*) are 40–50% smaller than their heterozygous littermates (*right*).

Alternative high-molecular-weight substrates of the insulin receptor have been suggested to exist. Studies in hepatoma cells indicated that the pp185 band may contain more than one insulin-regulated component.[47] In addition, in myeloid cells overexpressing the insulin receptor, insulin stimulates the tyrosine phosphorylation of a high-molecular-weight protein called 4PS that behaves similarly to IRS-1 in binding of PI-3-kinase but is immunologically distinct from IRS-1. Recently 4PS has been cloned and been shown to be related to IRS-1.[48] Using two different peptide antibodies to 4PS, it is now clear that the IRS-2 in the $IRS^{-/-}$ mice is immunologically related and perhaps identical to 4PS (Patti ME, Kahn CR, et al., J Biol Chem 1995; in press). Additional studies are required to determine the role of these alternate substrates in insulin signaling.

PI-3-Kinase Plays a Diverse Role in Insulin Action

The exact physiologic role of the PI-3-kinase reaction products (PI3-P, PI-3,4-P_2 and PI-3,4,5-P_3) is unknown, but it has been suggested that they may serve as second messengers themselves. They have been implicated in activation of the ζ isoform of protein kinase C (PKC) in vitro, associated with an increase in cellular proliferation, and linked to cytoskeletal rearrangements associated

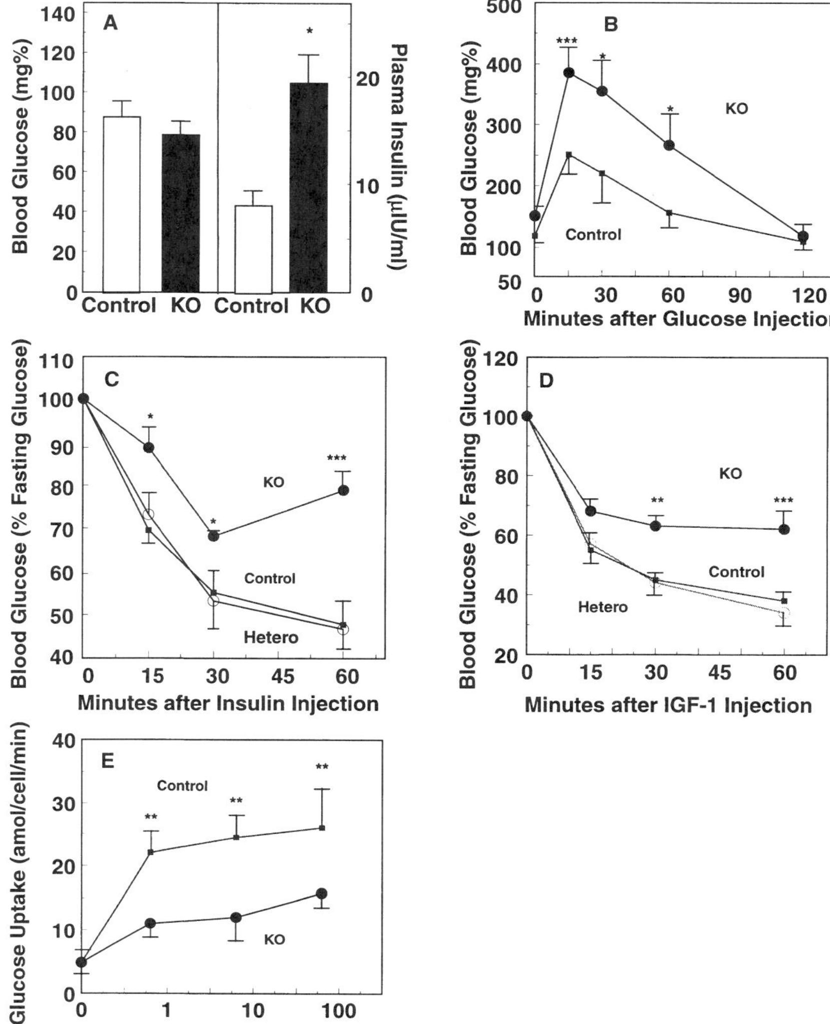

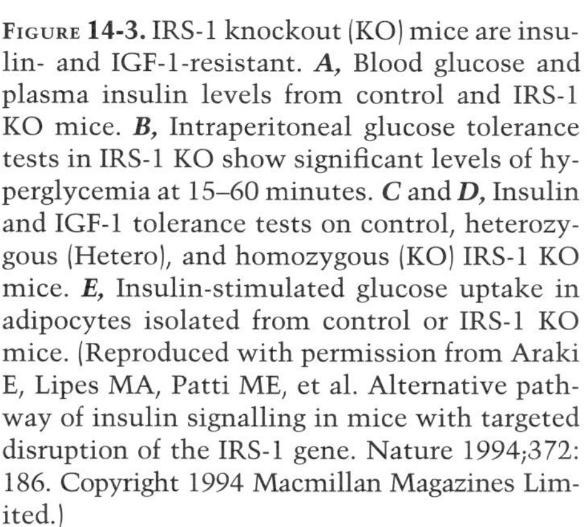
FIGURE 14-3. IRS-1 knockout (KO) mice are insulin- and IGF-1-resistant. *A,* Blood glucose and plasma insulin levels from control and IRS-1 KO mice. *B,* Intraperitoneal glucose tolerance tests in IRS-1 KO show significant levels of hyperglycemia at 15–60 minutes. *C* and *D,* Insulin and IGF-1 tolerance tests on control, heterozygous (Hetero), and homozygous (KO) IRS-1 KO mice. *E,* Insulin-stimulated glucose uptake in adipocytes isolated from control or IRS-1 KO mice. (Reproduced with permission from Araki E, Lipes MA, Patti ME, et al. Alternative pathway of insulin signalling in mice with targeted disruption of the IRS-1 gene. Nature 1994;372:186. Copyright 1994 Macmillan Magazines Limited.)

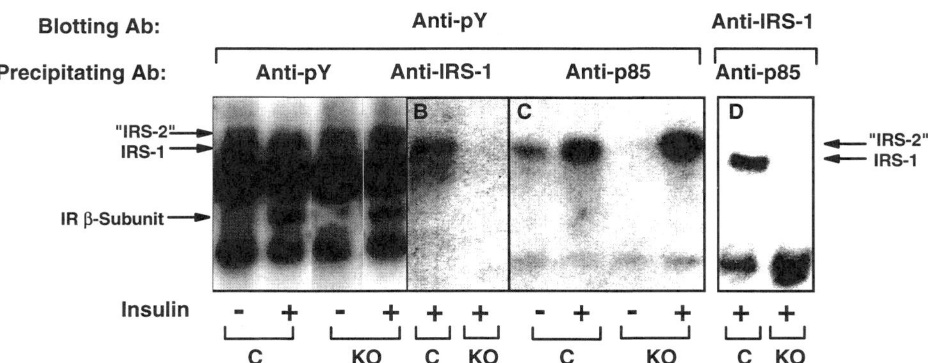

FIGURE 14-4. Insulin-stimulated phosphotyrosine-containing proteins from liver of control (C) or IRS-1 knockout (KO) mice. Proteins were immunoprecipitated followed by immunoblotting with the indicated antibodies. Arrows indicate the tyrosine phosphorylated insulin receptor β-subunit, IRS-1 and IRS-2. The IRS-2 protein is most prominent in anti-p85 immunoprecipitates from IRS-1 KO mice, followed by immunoblotting with antiphosphotyrosine (panel *C*). (Reproduced with permission of Araki E, Lipes MA, Patti ME, et al. Alternative pathway of insulin signalling in mice with targeted disruption of the IRS-1 gene. Nature 1994;372:186. Copyright 1994 Macmillan Magazines Limited.)

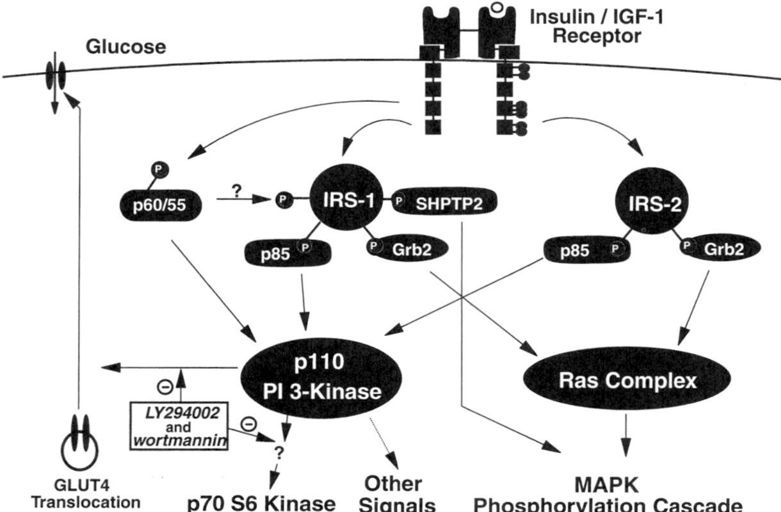

FIGURE 14-5. A potential role for PI-3-kinase in insulin action. Both IRS-1 and IRS-2 bind PI-3-kinase following stimulation with insulin. Inhibition of PI-3 kinase activity with either LY294002 or wortmannin effectively blocks insulin-stimulated GLUT-4 translocation and the activation of p70 S6 kinase.

with actin polymerization. VPS34 is the yeast homologue to the mammalian p110 subunit of PI-3-kinase and is required for proper protein sorting. These data suggest that PI-3-kinase may play a multifunctional role within the cell.[36,49,50]

Inhibitors of PI-3-kinase have recently been used to dissect the role of this enzyme in insulin action.[51–53] Wortmannin and LY294002 are structurally distinct and potent inhibitors of PI-3-kinase. Although treatment of a variety of cell types with either of these compounds does not affect insulin-stimulated receptor phosphorylation or the tyrosine phosphorylation of IRS-1, it does affect certain downstream insulin actions.[51–53]

As noted previously, insulin activates a number of phosphorylation cascades in the intact cell, including the regulation of mitogen-activated protein kinase (MAPK) and members of the ribosomal S6 kinases (p70 S6 kinase and $p90^{rsk}$). These phosphorylation cascades play an important role in coordinating the regulation of kinases and phosphatases involved in protein synthesis and glycogen metabolism. The current hypothesis suggests that insulin-stimulated activation of MAPK and $p90^{rsk}$ is on the same pathway downstream of Ras, whereas the activation of p70 S6 kinase by insulin is unique.[54] p70 S6 kinase is activated by phosphorylation by unknown upstream components. Inhibition of PI-3-kinase with wortmannin or LY294002 effectively blocks the insulin-stimulated phosphorylation-activation of p70 S6 kinase without any effect on insulin-stimulated activation of MAPK or $p90^{rsk}$.[52,55] These data suggest that PI-3-kinase is an upstream component required for mediating the activation of p70 S6 kinase (see Fig. 14-5). Treatment of fibroblasts with the PI-3-kinase inhibitors also blocks insulin- and serum-stimulated DNA synthesis,[52] implying that PI-3-kinase is required for cell cycle progression.

PI-3-kinase activation also appears to be an important component of insulin-stimulated glucose uptake. The majority of facilitative glucose uptake in adipocytes and muscle is carried out by the GLUT-1 and GLUT-4 glucose transporters. Stimulation of glucose uptake by insulin in fat and muscle occurs through the insulin-dependent translocation of vesicles containing the GLUT-4 glucose transporter from an intracellular vesicular pool (where the vesicles are stored under basal conditions) to the plasma membrane; this results in a 10- to 20-fold increase in glucose uptake.[56] The mechanism of this translocation event is unknown; however, several of the proteins (SCAMPs, VAMPs, and small GTP-binding proteins) that are involved in general regulated secretory mechanisms are present in GLUT-4 vesicles[57,58] in addition to some novel proteins that have recently been identified.[59] Pretreatment of adipocytes with either LY294002 or wortmannin inhibits both basal and insulin-stimulated glucose uptake.[52,53] The inhibition of insulin-stimulated glucose uptake results in part from inhibition of GLUT-4 translocation (see Fig. 14-5). Inhibition of p70 S6 kinase with the immunosuppressant rapamycin does not affect glucose uptake,[60] suggesting that p70 S6 kinase is not involved in GLUT-4 trafficking but that PI-3-kinase is upstream at a bifurcation of pathways between p70 S6 kinase activation and GLUT-4 translocation.

Apart from its lipid kinase activity, PI-3-kinase also contains a serine kinase activity that phosphorylates itself on both the 85 kd and 110 kd subunits. The serine phosphorylation of PI-3-kinase results in a three- to sevenfold decrease in activity that can be reversed by treatment with phosphoprotein phosphatase 2A.[61] In vitro reactions using immunoprecipitated PI-3-kinase suggest that IRS-1 may also be a substrate for the serine kinase activity of PI-3-kinase[62]; however, this has not yet been shown in intact cells. Taken together, these data show that PI-3-kinase plays a multifunctional role and is a branch point in insulin signaling, leading to activation of glucose uptake through GLUT-4 translocation, and in regulating upstream components leading to activation of p70 S6 kinase.

Insulin Signaling Through the Ras Pathway

Ras is a 21 kd membrane–associated guanine triphosphate (GTP)-binding protein that is regulated by its cycling between a GTP-bound active form and guanine diphosphate–bound inactive form. Ras is an integral component in regulating signals for cell growth and differentiation for many growth factor signaling pathways. Many advances have been made in understanding the mechanism of Ras signaling through its key role in regulation of a distinct phosphorylation cascade involving at least four different serine kinases.[38]

Following growth factor stimulation there is an increase in the amount of GTP-bound Ras that appears to be governed by the coordinate regulation of GTPase-activating protein (GAP) and the guanine nucleotide exchange factor, mSOS.[39,63] Active Ras then forms a complex with and activates Raf-1 kinase, which in turn phosphorylates and activates MAP kinase-kinase (also known as MAPKK and MEK). MEK phosphorylates and activates MAPK, which then phosphorylates and activates $p90^{rsk}$.[64–67] Active $p90^{rsk}$ is thought to phosphorylate and activate the glycogen-associated protein phosphatase-1 (PP1G), the enzyme that is responsible for dephosphorylation and activation of glycogen synthase. PP1G also dephosphorylates and inactivates phosphorylase kinase.[67] More recently, it has been shown that $p90^{rsk}$ phosphorylates and inactivates the glycogen synthase kinase-3 (GSK-3).[68] Thus, the Ras-MAPK-p90^{rsk} pathway is an extremely important mechanism in mediating insulin signals for both growth and metabolism.

How does insulin initiate this pathway? There are at least two separate and apparently independent signals that couple the active insulin receptor to the Ras-MAPK-p90^{rsk} pathway (see Fig. 14-1). The first of these is binding of the Grb2-mSOS complex to phosphorylated IRS-1. The second involves the insulin-stimulated tyrosine phosphorylation of Shc, which provides a binding site for the SH2 domain of Grb2 and thus leads to the formation of a Shc-Grb2-mSOS complex resulting in activation of Ras.[69]

The potential role for these two different routes into the Ras path is unclear and may vary from cell type to cell type. In normal tissues, such as liver and muscle, IRS-1 phosphorylation appears to be more rapid and prominent than Shc phosphorylation. In some cultured cells the reverse may be true. For example, 32-D myeloid progenitor cells do not contain any detectable IRS-1 and do not respond to insulin as a growth factor. Overexpression of the insulin receptor alone results in a 10-fold increase in insulin-stimulated MAPK activity, presumably via the Shc-Grb2-mSOS pathway. However, introduction of both the insulin receptor and IRS-1 into the cells is required for hormone-sensitive activation of DNA synthesis and also slightly enhances MAPK activation. Likewise, in fibroblasts, microinjection of antibodies against either Shc or IRS-1 blocks the mitogenic response.[31,45,70] Taken together, these data suggest that the insulin receptor can activate the Ras-MAPK pathway through the formation of the Shc-Grb2 complex alone, but activation of DNA synthesis requires IRS-1 and the insulin receptor and possibly Shc as well for a full response.

The formation of the IRS-1-SH-PTP2 complex has also been implicated in regulation of Ras-MAPK activation. Microinjection of fibroblasts with reagents that block activation of SH-PTP2 or its association with IRS-1 inhibited insulin-stimulated cell growth.[41–43] Furthermore, in cells overexpressing a catalytically inactive SH-PTP2 protein, insulin fails to stimulate MAPK activation despite normal tyrosine phosphorylation of IRS-1 and Shc and their association with Grb2.[71] How SH-PTP2 mediates positive insulin-regulated mitogenic signals through the Ras-MAPK pathway is unclear.

Alternative Substrates of the Insulin Receptor

The tyrosine phosphorylation of IRS-1, IRS-2, and Shc is a key step in mediating signals from the insulin receptor. However, there are other potential substrates of the insulin receptor that are less characterized. In some cell lines insulin stimulates tyrosine phosphorylation of a 120-kd protein. This band has been shown to contain two proteins. One is immunologically related to HA4 (an ecto-ATPase) and the second is the focal adhesion kinase (FAK), but their roles in insulin action are unclear.[72,73] In adipocytes that were treated with tyrosine phosphatase inhibitors (vanadate and/or phenylarsine oxide (PAO)), insulin stimulates the phosphorylation of a 15-kd protein that has been identified as the fatty acid binding protein 422 (ap2).[74] Phosphorylation of Ras-GAP has also been detected in PAO-treated cells, and a small fraction of this material is associated with the insulin receptor. However, this interaction is not required for activation of the Ras pathway.[75,76] GAP also associates with two other proteins, p190 and p62. The p190 may couple signals from Ras to the nucleus and regulate gene expression. The p62 is phosphorylated following insulin stimulation; however, its role in insulin action remains to be determined.[76]

Recently, two proteins of 55 and 60 kd have been reported to be tyrosine phosphorylated in response to insulin.[77,78] These proteins are distinct from the GAP-associated p62. It is not yet clear whether p55 and p60 are the same protein, but both associate with PI-3-kinase and cross-react with antibodies against the p85 protein.[78] The role of these proteins in insulin action is unknown, but they represent potential novel regulatory subunits for PI-3-kinase.

Nuclear Actions of Insulin

The regulation of transcription of specific mRNAs by insulin suggests that insulin signals are communicated to the nucleus (Fig. 14-6). A number of insulin-stimulated nuclear phosphoproteins have been observed in several cell types. These include three phosphoproteins ranging from 62 to 66 kd that appear to be immunologically related to the family of nuclear lamins A and C.[79] Nucleolin is an abundant nuclear protein that is involved in rRNA transport and trafficking and is serine phosphorylated in response to subnanomolar concentrations of insulin approximately 2.5-fold; this correlates with an increase in RNA efflux from the nucleus. Phosphorylation of nucleolin may be mediated by casein kinase II, since an inhibitor (5,6-dichlorobenzimidazole-riboside) of casein kinase II blocks insulin-stimulated phosphorylation of nucleolin.[80] Insulin also stimulates the phosphorylation of c-Jun, c-Fos, and several of the Fos-related nuclear transcription factors.[81] Phosphorylation of these proteins has been shown to be mediated by a number of kinases, including GSK-3, MAPK, protein kinase A (PKA), PKC, and casein kinase II. In addition, an increase in tyrosine kinase activity was recently detected in nuclei from insulin-treated cells that is distinct from the insulin receptor.[82] Thus, insulin regulates

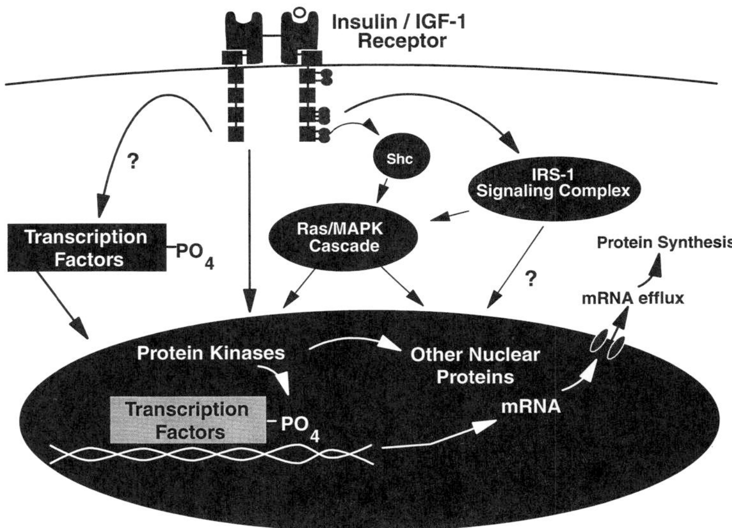

Figure 14-6. Insulin action in the nucleus. Insulin stimulates the phosphorylation of a number of transcription factors, nuclear kinases, and other nuclear proteins including nucleolin, which is involved in RNA transport from the nucleus.

both serine and tyrosine phosphorylation in the nucleus and appears to mediate a number of nuclear-related functions.

Rad: A Potential New Member of the Insulin Signaling Network

Rad is a small Ras-like GTP-binding protein that is overexpressed in muscle from type II diabetic individuals. It was recently cloned using a subtraction library constructed using mRNA isolated from skeletal muscle of normal and type II diabetics.[83] Rad has a predicted molecular weight of ~30 kd (larger than other Ras-like proteins) and contains the five conserved domains (G1–G5) found in Ras-like proteins that are required for nucleotide binding and GTPase activity. Some distinct features of Rad include a proline at position 61 and a glutamic acid at position 108; these correspond to highly conserved glycines (positions 12 and 60) in Ras. Rad does not contain a site for isoprenylation, which is required for membrane localization in other Ras-like molecules.[1,83]

Recently some biochemical characteristics of Rad were described in experiments using a recombinant glutathione S-transferase (GST)-Rad fusion protein.[84] Rad binds guanine nucleotides in a magnesium-dependent manner similar to that of other Ras-like GTP-binding proteins. Rad also possesses a low intrinsic GTPase activity that can be dramatically stimulated by a GAP that appears to be present in all tissues examined thus far, but such stimulating activity is distinct from the p120 Ras-GAP, NF1, p190 Rac-Rho GAP, Rap-GAP, and IQGAP1. Rad is also a substrate for PKA in vitro, and immunoprecipitates of Rad contain a serine-threonine kinase activity that phosphorylates Rad but is distinct from PKA.

A specific function for Rad in insulin signaling is unclear, but the role of Ras in insulin-regulated cell growth and metabolism and the potential roles of Rab4 and Rab3D in insulin-stimulated glucose transport suggest a number of diverse functions for small GTP-binding proteins in insulin signaling. Indeed, in 3T3-L1 adipocytes, overexpression of Rad inhibits insulin-stimulated glucose uptake by approximately 50% (Moyers J, Kahn CR, et al., unpublished data, 1995).

Conclusions and Future Directions

Several of the key regulatory molecules in insulin signal transduction have been identified and appear to play diverse roles in modulating complex phosphorylation cascades that affect downstream growth and metabolic actions. These findings have provided some insight into what was previously considered a ''black box'' where insulin binds and then something happens. Obviously there are still many areas that require further study, such as the characterization of IRS-2 (and perhaps other IRS-1-like molecules), of Rad, the insulin-regulated nuclear kinases, and identification of the specific signaling components in mediating GLUT-4 translocation and glycogen synthesis.

It is apparent that several of the pathways leading from the insulin receptor share signaling components that are common to other signal transduction pathways. For example, insulin, platelet-derived growth factor, and epidermal growth factor each recruit similar SH2 domain–containing proteins into their signal transduction pathways. However, in normal adipocytes only insulin can stimulate glucose uptake and glycogen synthesis, whereas in fibroblasts platelet-derived growth factor and epidermal growth factor are more potent growth factors. How do the various signal transduction pathways utilize these common molecular interactions and yet mediate unique and specific intracellular effects? One obvious difference could simply be in the variable expression of a signaling system's components within a particular cell type. Perhaps another important criterion is the subcellular location of different signaling molecules, where the recruitment of signaling components may have differing effects depending upon the particular intracellular region and its immediate surrounding milieu. Certainly, determining the unique routing of these apparently common signals between the various signaling pathways is imperative to understanding their specific intracellular effects.

References

1. Kahn CR. Insulin action, diabetogenes, and the cause of type II diabetes (Banting Lecture). Diabetes 1994;43:1066
2. Moller DE, Flier JS. Insulin resistance: Mechanisms, syndromes, and implications. N Engl J Med 1991;325:938
3. DeFronzo RA, Bonadonna RC, Ferrannini E. Pathogenesis of NIDDM: A balanced overview. Diabetes Care 1992;15:318
4. Kahn CR, Crettaz M. Insulin receptors and the molecular mechanism of insulin action. Diabetes Metab Rev 1985;1:5
5. Rosen OM. After insulin binds. Science 1987;237:1452
6. Pilch PF, Czech M. The subunit structure of the high affinity insulin receptor. J Biol Chem 1980;255:1722
7. Hedo JA, Simpson IA. Biosynthesis of the insulin receptor in rat adipose cells. Intracellular processing of the Mr-190 000 pro-receptor. Biochem J 1985; 232:71
8. Hedo JA, Gorden P. Biosynthesis of the insulin receptor. Horm Metab Res 1985;17:487
9. Hedo JA, Kahn CR, Hayoshi M, et al. Biosynthesis and glycosylation of the insulin receptor. Evidence for a single polypeptide precursor of the two major subunits. J Biol Chem 1983;258:10020
10. Alarcon C, Cheatham B, Lincoln B, et al. A Kex2-related endopeptidase activity present in rat liver specifically processes the insulin proreceptor. Biochem J 1994;301:257
11. Shoelson SE, White MF, Kahn CR. Tryptic activation of the insulin receptor. J Biol Chem 1988;263:4852
12. Kahn CR, White MF, Shoelson SE, et al. The insulin receptor and its substrate: Molecular determinants of early events in insulin action. Recent Prog Horm Res 1993;48:291
13. Cheatham B, Kahn CR. Cysteine 647 in the insulin receptor is required for normal covalent interaction between alpha- and beta-subunits and signal transduction. J Biol Chem 1992;267:7108
14. Cheatham B, Shoelson SE, Yamada K, et al. Substitution of the erbB-2 oncoprotein transmembrane domain activates the insulin receptor and modulates the action of insulin and insulin-receptor substrate 1. Proc Natl Acad Sci USA 1993;90:7336
15. Ebina Y, Araki E, Taira M, et al. Replacement of lysine residue 1030 in the putative ATP-binding region of the insulin receptor abolishes insulin- and antibody-stimulated glucose uptake and receptor kinase activity. Proc Natl Acad Sci USA 1987;84:704
16. Taylor SI, Cama A, Accili D, et al. Mutations in the insulin receptor gene. Endocr Rev 1992;3:566
17. White MF, Shoelson SE, Keutmann H, Kahn CR. A cascade of tyrosine autophosphorylation in the β-subunit activates the insulin receptor. J Biol Chem 1988;263:2969
18. Feener EP, Backer JM, King GL, et al. Insulin stimulates serine and tyrosine phosphorylation in the juxtamembrane region of the insulin receptor. J Biol Chem 1993;268:11256
19. Wilden PA, Siddel K, Haring E, et al. The role of insulin receptor kinase domain autophosphorylation in receptor-mediated activities. J Biol Chem 1992;267:13719
20. Backer JM, Shoelson SE, Weiss MA, et al. The insulin receptor juxtamembrane region contains two independent tyrosine/beta-turn internalization signals. J Cell Biol 1992;118:831
21. Lewis RE, Wu GP, MacDonald RG, Czech MP. Insulin-sensitive phosphorylation of serine 1293/1294 on the human insulin receptor by a tightly associated serine kinase. J Biol Chem 1990;265:947
22. Lewis RE, Cao L, Perregaux D, Czech MP. Threonine 1336 of the human insulin receptor is a major target for phosphorylation by protein kinase C. Biochemistry 1990;29:1807
23. Thies RS, Molina JM, Ciaraldi TP, et al. Insulin-receptor autophosphorylation and endogenous substrate phosphorylation in human adipocytes from control, obese, and NIDDM subjects. Diabetes 1990;39:250
24. Baltensperger K, Lewis RE, Woon CW, et al. Catalysis of serine and tyrosine autophosphorylation by the human insulin receptor. Proc Natl Acad Sci USA 1992;89:7885
25. Saltiel AR, Fox JA, Sherline P, Cuatrecasas P. Insulin-stimulated hydrolysis of a novel glycolipid generates modulators of cAMP phosphodiesterase. Science 1986;233:967
26. Lazar DF, Knez JJ, Medof ME, et al. Stimulation of glycogen synthesis by insulin in human erythroleukemia cells requires the synthesis of glycosyl-phosphatidylinositol. Proc Natl Acad Sci USA 1994;91:9665
27. Rothenberg PL, Kahn CR. Insulin inhibits pertussis toxin-catalyzed ADP-ribosylation of G-proteins. Evidence for a novel interaction between insulin receptors and G-proteins. J Biol Chem 1988;263:15546

28. Okamoto T, Murayama Y, Hayashi Y, et al. GTP-binding protein-activator sequences in the insulin receptor. FEBS Lett 1993;334:143
29. Record RD, Smith RM, Jarett L. Insulin induces an unmasking of the carboxyl terminus of Gi proteins in rat adipocytes. Exp Cell Res 1993;206:36
30. Moran MF, Koch CA, Anderson D, et al. Src homology region 2 domains direct protein-protein interactions in signal transduction. Proc Natl Acad Sci USA 1990;87:8622
31. White MF, Kahn CR. The insulin signaling system. J Biol Chem 1994;269:1
32. Sun XJ, Rothenberg P, Kahn CR, et al. The structure of the insulin receptor substrate IRS-1 defines a unique signal transduction protein. Nature 1991; 352:73
33. Myers MG Jr, Grammer TC, Brooks J, et al. The pleckstrin homology domain in IRS-1 sensitizes insulin signaling. J Biol Chem 1995;270:11715
34. Wang LM, Keegan AD, Li W, et al. Common elements in IL4 and insulin signaling pathways in factor dependent hematopoietic cells. Proc Natl Acad Sci USA 1993;90:4032
35. Souza SC, Frick GP, Yip R, et al. Growth hormone stimulates tyrosine phosphorylation of insulin receptor substrate-1. J Biol Chem 1994;269:30085
36. Parker PJ, Waterfield MD. Phosphatidylinositol 3-kinase: A novel effector. Cell Growth Differ 1992;3:747
37. Ruderman N, Kapeller R, White MF, Cantley LC. Activation of phosphatidylinositol-3-kinase by insulin. Proc Natl Acad Sci USA 1990;87:1411
38. Hall A. The cellular functions of small GTP-binding proteins. Science 1990;249:635
39. McCormick F. Activators and effectors of ras p21 proteins. Curr Opin Genet Devel 1994;4:71
40. Freeman RM, Plutzky J, Neel BG. Identification of a human src homology 2-containing protein-tyrosine-phosphatase: A putative homolog of *Drosophila* corkscrew. Proc Natl Acad Sci USA 1992;89:11239
41. Xiao S, Roses DW, Sasaoka T, et al. Syp (SH-PTP2) is a positive mediator of growth factor-stimulated mitogenic signal transduction. J Biol Chem 1994;269:21244
42. Milarski KL, Saltiel AR. Expression of catalytically inactive syp phosphatase in 3T3 cells blocks stimulation of mitogen-activated protein kinase by insulin. J Biol Chem 1995;269:21239
43. Yamauchi K, Milarski KL, Saltiel AR, Pessin JE. Protein-tyrosine-phosphatase SHPTP2 is a required positive effector for insulin downstream signaling. Proc Natl Acad Sci USA 1995;92:664
44. Waters SB, Yamauchi K, Pessin JE. Functional expression of insulin receptor substrate-1 (IRS-1) is required for insulin-stimulated mitogenic signaling. J Biol Chem 1993;268:22231
45. Rose DW, Saltiel AR, Majumdar M, et al. Insulin receptor substrate 1 is required for insulin-mediated mitogenic signal transduction. Proc Natl Acad Sci USA 1994;91:797
46. Araki E, Lipes MA, Patti ME, et al. Alternative pathway of insulin signalling in mice with targeted disruption of the IRS-1 gene. Nature 1994;372:186
47. Miralpeix M, Sun XJ, Backer JM, et al. Insulin stimulates tyrosine phosphorylation of multiple high molecular weight substrates in FAO hepatoma cells. Biochemistry 1992;31:9031
48. Sun XJ, Wang LM, Zhang Y, et al. Molecular cloning of 4PS reveals IRS-2: A common element in insulin/IGF-1 and IL4 signaling. Nature 1995; in press
49. Schu PV, Kaoru T, Fry MJ, et al. Phosphatidylinositol 3-kinase encoded by yeast *VPS*34 gene essential for protein sorting. Science 1993;260:88
50. Nakanishi H, Brewer KA, Exton JH. Activation of the zeta isozyme of protein kinase C by phosphatidylinositol 3,4,5-trisphosphate. J Biol Chem 1993;268:13
51. Vlahos CJ, Matter WF, Hui KY, Brown RF. A specific inhibitor of phosphatidylinositol 3-kinase, 2-(4-morpholinyl)-8-phenyl-4H-1benzopyran-4-one (LY294002). J Biochem 1994;269:5241
52. Cheatham B, Vlahos CJ, Cheatham L, et al. Phosphatidylinositol 3-kinase activation is required for insulin stimulation of pp70 S6 kinase, DNA synthesis and glucose transporter translocation. Mol Cell Biol 1994;14:4902
53. Okada T, Kawano Y, Sakakibara T, et al. Essential role of phosphatidylinositol 3-kinase in insulin-induced glucose transport and antilipolysis in rat adipocytes. J Biochem 1994;269:3568
54. Blenis J. Signal transduction via the MAP kinases: Proceed at your own RSK. Proc Natl Acad Sci USA 1993;9089:5889
55. Chung J, Grammer TC, Lemon KP, et al. PDGF- and insulin-dependent pp70S6k activation mediated by phosphatidylinositol-3-OH kinase. Nature 1994;370:71
56. Birnbaum MJ. The insulin-sensitive glucose transporter. Int Rev Cytol 1992; 137:239
57. Laurie SM, Cain CC, Lienhard GE, Castle JD. The glucose transporter gluT4 and secretory carrier membrane proteins (SCAMPs) colocalize in rat adipocytes and partially segregate during insulin stimulation. J Biochem 1993;268: 19110
58. Cormont M, Tanti JF, Zahraoui A, et al. Insulin and okadaic acid induce Rab4 redistribution in adipocytes. J Biol Chem 1993;268:19491
59. Kandror K, Pilch PF. Identification and isolation of glycoproteins that translocate to the cell surface from GLUT4-enriched vesicles in an insulin-dependent fashion. J Biochem 1994;269:138
60. Fingar DC, Hausdorff SF, Blenis J, Birnbaum MJ. Dissociation of pp70 ribosomal protein S6 kinase from insulin-stimulated glucose transport in 3T3-L1 adipocytes. J Biol Chem 1993;268:3005
61. Carpenter CL, Auger KR, Duckworth BC, et al. A tightly associated serine/threonine protein kinase regulates phosphoinositide 3-kinase activity. Mol Cell Biol 1993;13:1657
62. Lam K, Carpenter CL, Ruderman NB, et al. The phosphatidylinositol 3-kinase serine kinase phosphorylates IRS-1-stimulation by insulin and inhibition by wortmannin. J Biol Chem 1994;269:20648
63. Egan SE, Giddings BW, Brooks MW, et al. Association of Sos ras exchange protein with Grb2 is implicated in tyrosine kinase signal transduction and transformation. Nature 1993;363:45
64. Kyriakis JM, App H, Zhang X-F, et al. Raf-1 activates MAP kinase-kinase. Nature 1992;358:417
65. Ahn NG, Seger R, Krebs EG. The mitogen-activated protein kinase activator. Curr Opin Cell Biol 1993;4:992
66. Sturgill TW, Ray LB, Erikson E, Maller JL. Insulin-stimulated MAP-2 kinase phosphorylates and activates ribosomal protein S6 kinase II. Nature 1988; 334:715
67. Dent P, Lavoinne A, Nakielny S, et al. The molecular mechanisms by which insulin stimulates glycogen synthesis in mammalian skeletal muscle. Nature 1990;348:302
68. Eldar-Finkelman H, Seger R, Vandenheede JR, Krebs EG. Inactivation of glycogen synthase kinase-3 by epidermal growth factor is mediated by mitogen-activated protein kinase/p90 ribosomal protein S6 kinase signaling pathway in NIH-3T3 cells. J Biol Chem 1995;270:987
69. Skolnik EY, Lee CH, Batzer A, et al. The SH2/SH3 domain-containing protein GRB2 interacts with tyrosine-phosphorylated IRS-1 and Shc: Implications for insulin control of ras signalling. EMBO J 1993;12:1929
70. Sasaoka T, Rose DW, Jhun BH, et al. Evidence for a functional role of Shc proteins in mitogenic signaling induced by insulin, insulin-like growth factor-1, and epidermal growth factor. J Biol Chem 1994;269:13689
71. Noguchi T, Matozaki T, Horita K, et al. Role of SH-PTP2, a protein-tyrosine phosphatase with Src homology 2 domains, in insulin-stimulated ras activation. Mol Cell Biol 1994;14:6674
72. Lin S-H, Guidotti G. Cloning and expression of a cDNA coding for a rat liver plasma membrane ecto-ATPase. J Biol Chem 1989;264:14408
73. Schaller MD, Borgman CA, Cobb BS, et al. pp125FAK, a structurally distinctive protein-tyrosine kinase associated with focal adhesions. Proc Natl Acad Sci USA 1992;89:5192
74. Hresko RC, Bernier M, Hoffman RD, et al. Identification of phosphorylated 422(aP2) protein as pp15, the 15-kilodalton target of the insulin receptor tyrosine kinase in 3T3-L1 adipocytes. Proc Natl Acad Sci USA 1988;85:8835
75. Pronk GJ, Medema RH, Burgering BMt, et al. Interaction between the p21ras GTPase activating protein and the insulin receptor. J Biol Chem 1993; 267:24058
76. Porras A, Nebreda AR, Benito M, Santos E. Activation of Ras by insulin in 3T3 L1 cells does not involve GTPase-activating protein phosphorylation. J Biol Chem 1992;267:21124
77. Hosomi Y, Shii K, Ogawa W, et al. Characterization of a 60-kilodalton substrate of the insulin receptor kinase. J Biol Chem 1994;269:11498
78. Pons S, Asano T, Glasheen E, et al. The structure and function of $p55^{PIK}$ reveals a new regulatory subunit for the phosphatidylinositol-3 kinase. Mol Cell Biol 1995;15:4453
79. Csermely P, Kahn CR. Insulin induces the phosphorylation of DNA-binding nuclear proteins including lamins in 3T3-F442A cells. Biochemistry 1992; 31:9940
80. Csermely P, Schnaider T, Cheatham B, et al. Insulin induces the phosphorylation of nucleolin: A possible mechanism of insulin-induced RNA efflux from nuclei. J Biol Chem 1993;268:9747
81. Kim S, Kahn CR. Insulin stimulates phosphorylation of c-Jun, c-Fos, and Fos-related proteins in cultured adipocytes. J Biol Chem 1994;269:11887
82. Kim S, Kahn CR. Insulin induces rapid accumulation of insulin receptor and increases tyrosine kinase activity in the nucleus of cultured adipocytes. J Cell Physiol 1993;157:217
83. Reynet C, Kahn CR. Rad: A member of the Ras family overexpressed in muscle of type II diabetic humans. Science 1993;262:1441
84. Zhu J, Reynet C, Caldwell JS, Kahn CR. Characterization of Rad, a new member of Ras/GTPase superfamily, and its regulation by a unique GTPase-activating protein (GAP)-like activity. J Biol Chem 1995;270:4805

Diabetes Mellitus, edited by Derek LeRoith, Simeon I. Taylor, and Jerrold M. Olefsky. Lippincott–Raven Publishers, Philadelphia © 1996.

CHAPTER 15
The Insulin Receptor

JEFFREY S. FLIER

Introduction

The initial step in the diverse regulatory actions of insulin is binding to the insulin receptor, a transmembrane glycoprotein present in the plasma membrane of virtually all vertebrate cells. Since its initial identification as a functional entity in binding studies with radiolabeled insulin over 25 years ago,[1] this protein has been the subject of intense investigation.[2–6] Our understanding of this receptor has progressed through a number of phases, including, in turn, studies of the kinetics of hormone binding and the regulation of receptor expression; evaluation of the role of the receptor in states of altered insulin action; elucidation of the subunit composition and structure of the receptor protein; identification of the receptor as a ligand-activated protein tyrosine kinase; cloning of the receptor cDNA and gene and subsequent structure-function analysis; and, most recently, solving of the crystal structure of the tyrosine kinase domain. The goal of this chapter is to review and summarize our current knowledge regarding this key element in the insulin signaling cascade. The emphasis is on information obtained in the past several years. The related subjects of postreceptor signal transduction and diseases caused by disorders of the insulin receptor, including mutations at this locus, are covered in Chapters 16 and 17.

Expression and Subunit Structure

As determined through binding studies, immunologic techniques, and mRNA expression, insulin receptors are present in virtually all vertebrate cell types. These include the well-known tissues involved in fuel homeostasis, such as liver, muscle, and fat, as well as tissues such as ovarian granulosa cells, renal tubules, and vascular endothelial cells, which play no known role in fuel metabolism. The cellular content of receptors is variable, ranging from less than 100 per erythrocyte to several hundred thousand per adipocyte or hepatocyte.

The insulin receptor cDNA was cloned in 1985.[7,8] The receptor gene maps to the short arm of human chromosome 19.[9] It spans more than 150 Kb, and its 22 exons are transcribed into several mRNA species ranging from 4.2–9.5 Kb in length owing to variation in their 3′-untranslated region.[10] As discussed in detail below, exon 11 is subject to tissue-specific alternative splicing, and forms of the receptor mRNA both with and without the 36 base sequence encoded by this exon exist.[11,12] The abundance of the insulin receptor mRNA is upregulated by differentiation in cultured adipocytes[13] and muscle cell lines.[14] In IM-9 lymphoblasts, exposure to insulin reduces receptor mRNA abundance,[14] and this may be one of several mechanisms accounting for receptor downregulation after chronic exposure to insulin.[15] In these same cells, glucocorticoids increase mRNA levels without altering mRNA half-life,[14] and this may be mediated by an atypical glucocorticoid response element located −345 to −359 bases upstream of the transcription start site. The promoter region of the insulin receptor gene contains no TATA or CAAT boxes and has the characteristics of a housekeeping gene.[9,16] In addition to several SP1 binding sites, two novel nuclear factors have been identified in nuclear extracts of HepG-2 cells that are involved in efficient transcription.[17] With the exception of several cases of extreme insulin resistance in which specific mutations in the receptor gene causing reduced abundance of receptor mRNA have been identified (see Chapter 00), there is as yet no indication that altered receptor mRNA transcription or stability results in the modestly decreased expression of insulin receptors that has frequently been observed in non–insulin-dependent diabetes mellitus or obesity.

Current knowledge of the structure of the insulin receptor has derived from the cDNA sequence and extensive biochemical studies. The physiologically relevant insulin holoreceptor is a heterotetrameric protein composed of two extracellular α-subunits that are each linked to a β-subunit and to each other by disulfide bonds ($\alpha 2\beta 2$) (Fig. 15-1). The disulfide bonds that link the α-subunits (referred to as class I) are thought to be located C-terminal to a cysteine-rich region, via cysteine 435, 468, or 524.[18] Reduction of these bonds produces an α-β heterodimer that binds insulin with reduced affinity.[19] The α-β linkage is via class II disulfide bonds, and cysteine 647 may mediate this linkage.[20] The primary translation product of the insulin receptor is a linear α-β proreceptor sequence. At the N-terminus of the α-subunit there is a deduced signal sequence of 27 hydrophobic amino acids that allows the receptor to enter the endoplasmic reticulum, during which process the signal peptide is cleaved. The proreceptor is further proteolytically processed into distinct α- and β-subunits at a cleavage site consisting of four basic amino acids (Arg-Lys-Arg-Arg), apparently after disulfide linkage of two proreceptor molecules.[21,22]

The mature α-subunit contains either 719 or 731 amino acids (see discussion of alternative splicing farther on) and has a molecular mass of approximately 130 kd on SDS PAGE electrophoresis. (In this chapter, we use the amino acid numbering system for the receptor form that includes the exon 11 sequence that encodes the 12 additional amino acids in the α-subunit.[7]) The α-subunit is entirely extracellular and contains the binding domain for insulin. It also contains a cysteine-rich domain, with 21 cysteine residues being concentrated between amino acids 155 and 312. Similar domains are seen in several other receptors, including the IGF-1, EGF, and LDL receptors. The transmembrane-spanning β-subunit contains 620 amino acids and has an approximate molecular mass of 95 kd. The β-subunit may be viewed as having three overall domains: extracellular, transmembrane, and cytosolic. The cytosolic domain contains the insulin-regulated tyrosine protein kinase activity and has substantial structural homology to other members of the tyrosine protein kinase family.[8] The cytosolic domain of the β-subunit may be viewed as having several subdomains: a juxtamembrane domain, an ATP-binding domain, the trityrosines of the kinase regulatory domain, and a carboxy terminal domain. The functional implications of these domains are discussed below. Both receptor subunits are glycosylated cotranslationally and contain complex N-linked carbohydrate side chains with terminal sialic acid residues.[23,24] These sugar moieties are necessary for normal insulin

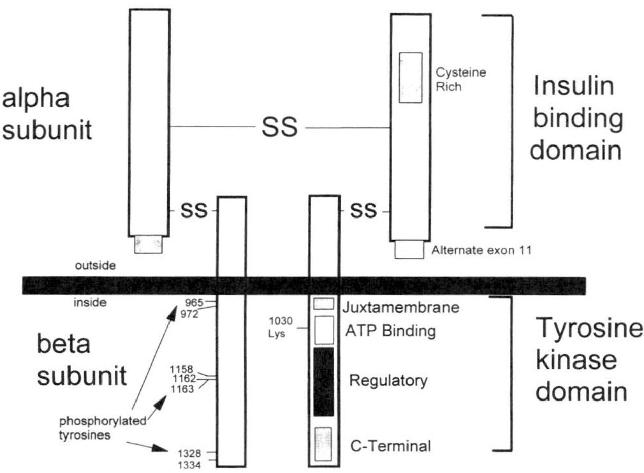

Figure 15-1. The structure of the insulin receptor kinase. See text for details.

binding[25] and they also account for the molecular mass disparity between predicted and observed values. The β-subunit may contain O-linked carbohydrate as well.[24] The mature α2-β2 heterotetramer migrates with a molecular mass of 300–400 kd on SDS-PAGE electrophoresis.

Insulin Receptor Isoforms

Although it is encoded by a single gene, the insulin receptor pre-mRNA transcript undergoes alternative splicing. This produces two isoforms, one with (HIR-B or EX11+) and one without (HIR-A or EX11⁻), the 12 amino acids at the carboxy terminus of the α-subunit, after arg-723, which are encoded by exon 11 (Fig. 15-2). The relative abundance of the two alternatively spliced mRNAs[12] and their encoded proteins[26] is tissue-specific and developmentally regulated. The smaller exon 11− form predominates in hematopoietic cells, the exon 11+ form predominates in the liver, and other tissues such as muscle and adipose cells have both.[12,27] The regulation and conservation of these mRNA splicing events suggest the possibility that the two alternative receptor forms have functionally distinct properties. Although intensive studies have been carried out, the differences that have been found between the two forms have so far been of small magnitude and to some degree controversial. It is agreed that the exon 11− form displays a two- to threefold higher affinity for insulin after expression in cultured cell lines,[28,29] and this form may have accelerated hormone-induced internalization.[29,30] Interestingly, the exon 11− isoform binds IGF-1 with substantially higher affinity than does the exon 11+ form.[29] Whether the two forms differ modestly with respect to kinase activity is unclear,[29,31] and detailed studies of their abilities to activate downstream processes in differentiated cells have not been carried out. Thus, the biologic importance of the two isoforms is not yet clear.

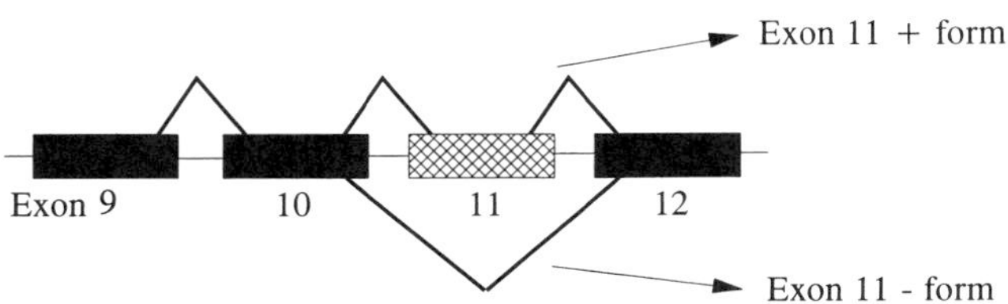

Figure 15-2. Alternative splicing of the insulin receptor gene. The sequence encoded by exon 11 is either included or excluded from the mature mRNA.

Some controversy also exists regarding the status of the alternatively spliced forms of the receptor in disease states. One group reported initially that skeletal muscle of non–insulin-dependent diabetes mellitus (NIDDM) subjects had dramatically increased the fraction of receptor mRNA molecules with the larger, exon 11+ (B) form, compared with controls who had only the smaller, exon 11− (A) species.[32] This was clearly an error in that multiple groups have shown that muscle of nondiabetic individuals as well as those with NIDDM have a predominance of the B form of the mRNA,[26,33] and in one study using an immunologic approach with an antibody specific to the amino acids of exon 11, similar fractions of the two protein isoforms were seen in a small group of subjects.[26] On the other hand, as seen in one recent study, it is possible that a small difference in fractional expression of the B form of the mRNA may exist in muscle from insulin-resistant (90%) versus insulin-sensitive (81%) individuals.[34] Whether such differences, even if paralleled by changes at the level of receptor protein, would have important biologic consequences is unknown at present.

Insulin Binding

The details of insulin binding to its receptor have been studied extensively, beginning with the period when no structural information on the receptor existed and hormone binding was the only receptor attribute available for investigation. A major outcome of such studies was the observation that equilibrium binding isotherms were complex and nonlinear as a result of heterogeneity of sites, negative cooperativity of binding, or a combination of the two.[35] Kinetic experiments in which insulin binding at high concentrations induced a low-affinity state through an increase in the rate of hormone dissociation supported the existence of negative cooperativity of insulin binding.[35,36] New insights derived from structural elucidation of the receptor as a heterotetrameric protein and binding studies with novel insulin analogues have allowed models for insulin binding that incorporate cooperativity to be refined.[36] These models infer the existence of four potential ''contact sites'' for insulin in each α2-β2 holoreceptor, with each a subunit having two distinct classes of sites (Fig. 15-3). According to these models,[36,37] at low ''physiologic'' insulin concentrations one molecule of insulin would bind to both (nonidentical) sites in an asymmetric manner (giving a stoichiometry of 1 for the holoreceptor at ''physiologic conditions''), and the two-site binding would account for the binding's being of high affinity. In the presence of higher (nonphysiologic) levels of insulin, a second molecule of insulin would compete for occupancy of one of the sites, thereby reducing binding affinity and potentially accounting for negative cooperativity. Experimental studies of insulin binding to αβ-heterodimers confirms the prediction that insulin binding to this species occurs as a single class of low-affinity sites.[19,37]

Considerable attention has been focused recently on the structural basis for the insulin binding ''site(s)'' on the receptor. The location of the binding site in the α-subunit was initially inferred from the fact that this subunit is entirely extracellular and is the only subunit ever identified in affinity labeling protocols.[38–40] Two approaches—(1) affinity labeling with insulin followed by isolation of receptor-insulin fragments, and (2) mutagenesis of the receptor, including creation of chimeric insulin/IGF-1 receptors—have been employed to gain further insight into the molecular nature of the hormone-binding site. Establishing the actual contact points will eventually require crystallization of the insulin-receptor complex. Short of that, the above approaches have revealed several features of the binding site interactions. These results, some of which appear to conflict, are not described in detail, but the main conclusions are stated. The dominant binding interactions and a potential ''binding pocket'' appear to involve the first 400–500 amino acids of the α-subunits, including residues N- and C-terminal to the cysteine-

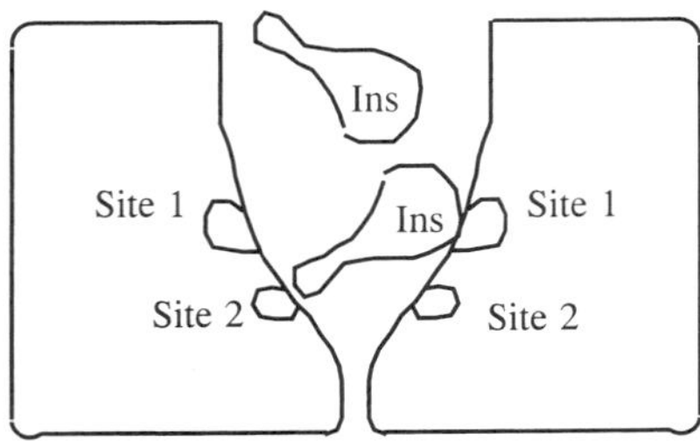

Figure 15-3. A schematic cartoon of the insulin binding sites on the two covalently linked α-subunits in an α2β2 holoreceptor. It is suggested that each insulin molecule has two nonidentical sites that make contact with two nonidentical sites (sites 1 and 2) on the two α-subunits, thus producing a state of high-affinity binding. At high insulin concentrations, a second molecule of insulin can occupy the second site, preventing high affinity (2 site) binding from taking place. This competition for the second site may account for negative cooperativity.

rich region and within this region itself.[41–44] However, since the presence of the 12 amino acids encoded by exon 11 at the C-terminal end of the α-subunit changes binding affinity, this region of the protein has an impact on binding as well. Change in only a single amino acid (Phe 89) abolishes insulin binding.[45] In contrast, replacing amino acids 64–137 of the IGF-1 receptor with corresponding sequences of the insulin receptor confers high-affinity insulin binding, and this is further enhanced by substitution of residues 325–524 of the insulin receptor.[43] It is surprising that IGF-1 binding to this chimera is retained, consistent with the evidence that high-affinity IGF-1 binding, unlike insulin binding to the insulin receptor, is primarily determined by the cysteine-rich region.[44–46]

Insulin Receptor Subunit Interactions

Insulin binding to its receptor rapidly causes receptor autophosphorylation,[47] an event that appears to be critical to both activation of the tyrosine kinase activity toward exogenous substrates and most or all of insulin's actions.[48] The mechanism whereby insulin binding to the α-subunit is transduced to the intracellular β-subunit to cause autophosphorylation is not yet fully understood. There is evidence to suggest that the unoccupied α-subunit in some way actively inhibits the kinase activity of the β-subunit. Thus, the receptor tyrosine kinase is activated by tryptic cleavage and removal of the α-subunit[49] and by a variety of deletion or point mutations in this domain. There have also been attempts to understand the possible role of the single transmembrane domain of the β-subunit in signal transduction. The fact that numerous substitution and deletion mutations introduced into this domain fail to alter receptor processing, binding, kinase activity, or ability to activate downstream pathways[50,51] has suggested a "passive role" for this domain. However, certain substitutions, such as replacing the insulin receptor transmembrane sequence with that of the *neu* oncogene,[51] activate the receptor kinase, suggesting that the status of this domain can influence the conformation of the kinase domain. Several lines of evidence, including the use of "conformation-sensitive" antibodies, directly support the expectation that insulin binding causes conformational changes in the receptor molecule.[52–54] It is likely that the initial conformational change that follows insulin binding will alter the interface between the two α-subunits in a holoreceptor and that this will then change the quaternary structure of the receptor such that the relationship between the two β-subunits is altered, stimulating autophosphorylation. Evidence from the crystal structure of the tyrosine kinase domain[55] related to this point is discussed below.

Receptor Autophosphorylation and Signal Transduction

As mentioned earlier, the insulin receptor is a member of the receptor tyrosine kinase gene family that includes the receptors for EGF and PDGF.[8] It is therefore of interest to draw several distinctions between these receptors and the insulin receptor (and the larger "insulin receptor family," including the IGF-1 receptor and the insulin receptor-related receptor,[56] for which the ligand is not known). Whereas the EGF and PDGF receptors exist as monomers that are induced to form noncovalent dimers as a consequence of ligand binding,[57,58] the insulin receptor exists as a covalent dimer of two αβ-monomers in the unliganded state. This suggests that interactions between β-subunits are important for activation in all members of the tyrosine kinase family, as will be discussed. It is unclear, however, why the molecular strategies employed by the two classes of tyrosine kinase receptors evolved differently. A second difference between these classes of receptors relates to the molecular strategies employed to engage downstream signaling events, discussed in more detail for the insulin receptor in Chapter 16. The EGF and PDGF receptors form relatively stable complexes between specific tyrosine phosphorylated residues in the receptor and downstream mediators via src homology (SH-2) domains in the effector proteins,[57] and an activity of these receptors to tyrosine phosphorylate exogenous substrates is hard to identify. In contrast, the insulin receptor appears not to form such complexes. Instead, the activated receptor tyrosine phosphorylates one or more principal substrates, of which IRS-1 is the best characterized.[59,60] Specific phosphorylated tyrosines on IRS-1 engage downstream mediators, analogous to the sites on the PDGF and EGF receptors proper.[61] Whether the insulin receptor and IRS-1 evolved from a primordial species that contained both elements in a single protein is an open question.

Sites of Tyrosine Autophosphorylation and Functional Domains

Each receptor cytoplasmic domain has 13 tyrosine residues, and considerable effort has been expended in order to map and characterize the importance of the phosphorylation of these sites. Seven of the thirteen tyrosines, occurring in three domains, are phosphorylated in response to insulin binding.[62–65] The most important sites for autophosphorylation and tyrosine kinase activity are the three tyrosines (1158, 1162, and 1163) that lie in the tyrosine kinase catalytic domain. As determined through peptide mapping, phosphorylation of these sites is temporally correlated with 10-–20-fold activation of tyrosine kinase activity.[65,66] Systematic mutagenesis of these residues has led to the conclusion that maximal activation requires triphosphorylation, whereas absence of one or two tyrosines limits activation and capacity to maximally mediate downstream signals in transfected cells.[46,67,68] Like all protein kinases, the insulin receptor has a consensus amino acid sequence encoding an ATP binding domain. This includes a glycine-rich motif (Gly-X-Gly-X-X-Gly) followed by a lysine residue (Lys 1030) that has been shown to be cross-linked with ATP affinity reagents.[69] Substitution of this lysine with other amino acids abolishes autophosphorylation and kinase activity.[70]

An intracellular juxtamembrane domain encoded by exon 16 contains several tyrosines and has been implicated in both signal transduction[71] and internalization of the receptor.[72] In vitro phosphorylation of this region accounts for 15% of the total insulin-stimulated phosphorylation, and this occurs primarily on tyrosine 972.[62] Mutation of this residue does not affect autophosphorylation or exogenous kinase activity but markedly impairs the ability of activated receptor to phosphorylate IRS-1 and mediate downstream events.[71] It is likely, therefore, that this domain participates in substrate recognition.

The role of the insulin receptor C-terminal domain, which extends beyond the tyrosine kinase domain, is unclear. The domain contains two tyrosines (1328 and 1334) that are phosphorylated and account for as much as 40% of the insulin-stimulated phosphorylation.[73,74] In some studies, deletion of the C-terminal 43 amino acids impairs insulin stimulation of glucose transport but augments the stimulation of mitogenesis,[75] suggesting a regulatory effect of this region on postreceptor signaling events. In other studies that used a different fibroblast cell line, no effects of the C-terminal deletion were noted.[76] To resolve this issue, it will probably be necessary to assess receptor function in the differentiated tissues of transgenic mice rather than in fibroblast cell lines in which insulin actions are difficult to quantify. It does appear clear that, unlike receptors for PDGF and EGF, these C-terminal tyrosines in the insulin receptor are not binding sites for signaling proteins via SH-2 domains.

Evidence Against the Obligatory Role of Kinase Activity in Insulin Signaling

Although the evidence favoring an obligatory role of insulin-stimulated kinase activity in the biologic actions of insulin is impressive and in general overwhelming, several observations have been put forward that challenge this view. One report that a site-directed mutant of the receptor with disruption of the ATP binding site and no kinase activity had normal ability to regulate pyruvate dehydrogenase activity[77] is very difficult to understand in the light of all other work. Several studies have used antireceptor monoclonal antibodies to stimulate cells, finding that biologic activities including glucose transport were activated without activation of autophosphorylation or kinase activity.[78] These results have been challenged by others, who ascribe the results to insufficiently sensitive measurement of kinase activity in the prior studies, given that minimal receptor occupancy and activation may be needed to obtain many insulin bioeffects, including glucose transport in adipose cells.[79] Using cells that were overexpressing a particular insulin receptor mutant (at the 1200 position in the kinase domain) that has markedly impaired kinase activity, we observed that insulin's dose-response for stimulation of glycogen synthesis was surprisingly normal.[80] Although this mutant receptor has approximately 3% of the kinase activity of the wild type receptor, the results with glycogen synthesis suggest that downstream signaling can be surprisingly maintained in the face of certain defects in kinase activation.

Serine Phosphorylation

The insulin receptor is phosphorylated on serine and threonine residues in the absence of insulin, and this increases in the presence of phorbol esters,[81] overexpression of protein kinase C isoforms,[82] and activation of cAMP–dependent protein kinase[83] and of insulin itself.[81] One of the sites is serine 1305 or 1306 in the C-terminus[84] and another is in the juxtamembrane region. Serine phosphorylation appears capable of inhibiting insulin signal transduction.[81] The identity of the kinases responsible for the receptor serine phosphorylation is uncertain. It has been reported that the receptor itself may have a low level of intrinsic serine kinase activity,[85] but the significance of this is unknown.

Cis- Versus Trans-phosphorylation in the Activation Process

Since the insulin holoreceptor exists as a covalently linked dimer of two α-β halves, it is important to understand whether the initial act of autophosphorylation and kinase activation occurs as a *cis* process (i.e., self-phosphorylation of each β-subunit) or a *trans* process (i.e., one β-subunit phosphorylating the other). Several lines of evidence, including studies with chimeric receptors in which inactive receptor halves are detectable via a mutation-induced size change,[86] suggest that the initial event is a transphosphorylation. If the half being phosphorylated is inactive as a kinase, this would prevent further ability of the holoreceptor to be activated,[86] and such a mechanism could explain the capacity of kinase defective receptor halves (as can occur in patients with certain receptor mutations) to behave in a dominant negative manner.[87] Although complete phosphorylation of all potentially phosphorylated tyrosines would produce a phosphorylation stoichiometry of 14 (on both α-subunits combined), it is unclear what stoichiometry exists in the intact cell under specific conditions of insulin action. In some in vitro studies, stoichiometries as low as 2 have been reported.[88,89]

Hybrid Insulin Receptor Molecules

It has long been known that insulin and IGF-1 share a spectrum of biologic activities, and that this is in part mediated by affinity of each ligand for the other's primary receptor.[90] It is now also known that subunits of the homologous receptors for insulin and IGF-1 can form hybrid species, in which α-β halves of insulin and IGF-1 receptors exist as covalently linked receptor heterotetramers.[91] The biologic functions, if any, of these hybrid receptors is currently unknown.

Termination of the Insulin Receptor Activated State

The activated state of the insulin receptor kinase is reversed by dephosphorylation of the receptor, mediated by a class of enzymes known as phosphotyrosine phosphatases, or PTPases.[92] These enzymes are divided into two general classes: transmembrane PTPases that appear to be receptors for unknown ligands, with the PTPase existing as the intracellular domain, and a class of smaller, intracellular enzymes, including some that have SH-2 domains.[92] Members of both classes have been shown to have activity against insulin receptor tyrosine-containing peptides,[93,94] but the identity of the actual PTPases that mediate receptor inactivation in relevant target tissues is as yet unknown.

Receptor Internalization and Turnover

Soon after the identification of the insulin receptor through binding studies, it became apparent that the receptor number was subject to regulation, and that insulin itself, through a process described as homologous downregulation or desensitization, was a major regulator of this process.[15] Indeed, both with cultured cells in vitro and in many in vivo models in animals and humans, an inverse relationship between the ambient insulin concentration and the receptor density on the cell surface can be seen. These observations with the downregulation of the insulin receptor by insulin preceded an avalanche of work with other receptor-ligand interactions that explored the mechanism of such regulation and the role of receptor internalization in the process.

It is now known that, in addition to its role as initiator of the insulin signal transduction cascade, the insulin receptor mediates the internalization of insulin.[95,96] When the insulin-receptor complex is internalized via endocytosis, insulin is degraded and the empty receptors are largely recycled to the plasma membrane.[95–97] More prolonged exposure to insulin also increases the rate of receptor degradation, which accounts in large measure for the phenomenon of downregulation.[98,99] Since internalized receptors appear to be active as kinases,[100] it is possible that kinase activity at some intracellular site could play a role in insulin action.

There appear to be at least two functionally distinct pathways for insulin internalization. The first, involving structures called coated pits, requires a functionally competent insulin receptor kinase, triphosphorylation in the regulatory domain of the β-subunit, and two specific tyrosine-containing sequences in the juxtamembrane domain.[101] In some cells, including fibroblastic cell lines frequently used in transfection studies, an additional pathway that is constitutive, nonsaturable, and independent of receptor phosphorylation is seen as a major pathway.[102]

Insights from the Crystal Structure of the Kinase Domain of the Insulin Receptor

The crystal structure of the tyrosine kinase domain of the human insulin receptor was recently determined at 2.1 Å resolution.[55] Although the catalytic domains of several serine kinases have been crystallized and solved, this is the first tyrosine kinase catalytic domain to be examined in this detail. The results appear to provide important new insights into the determinants of substrate preference for tyrosine versus serine as well as a novel autoinhibition mechanism that sheds light on the mechanisms of kinase autophosphorylation and activation.

The region of the receptor that was analyzed is a 306 amino acid fragment of the β-chain of the human receptor, which contains tyrosine kinase activity and the trityrosine autophosphorylation sites (Fig. 15-4). The purified protein (made in a baculovirus expression system) was crystallized in the nontyrosine phosphorylated state. Overall, there is a remarkable degree of structural homology between the insulin receptor and the analogous region of the cAMP–dependent protein kinase, reinforcing the fact that both serine-threonine and tyrosine protein kinases are derived from a common precurser. The catalytic loop conformations of the insulin receptor and cAMP–dependent kinase are very similar despite several sequence differences. Strikingly, the crystal structure reveals that Tyr 1162, a tyrosine that is autophosphorylated upon insulin binding, sits in the active site of the enzyme, seemingly poised for cis-autophosphorylation. The hydroxyl group of the Tyr 1162 phenolyic ring is hydrogen bonded to the carboxylate group of the catalytic base (Asp 1132). In addition, in this state the likely binding pocket for ATP is blocked, so that, in the unphosphorylated form, the Tyr 1162 of each β-subunit sits in that subunit's substrate binding site and also blocks ATP binding, with the result being that the receptor kinase is inactive. This could be viewed as a (cis) autoinhibition mechanism.

It may be predicted that when insulin binds to the α-subunit, the quaternary structure of the β-subunit changes. As a result, the phosphorylation sites (in the trityrosine domain) of one β-chain come within reach of the active site of the other β-chain. When Tyr 1162 disengages, thereby allowing ATP to bind, a transphosphorylation event takes place by causing the Tyr 1162 of the phosphorylated half to disengage from the active site of that segment, which is then predicted to cause that phosphorylated receptor half to become active.

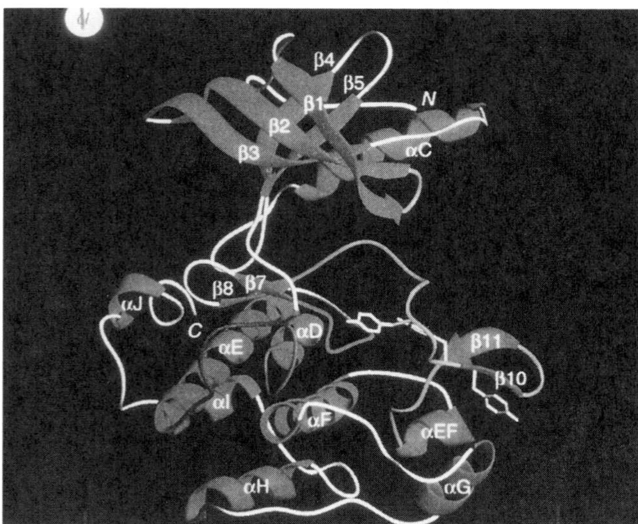

FIGURE 15-4. A ribbon diagram of the structure of the insulin receptor kinase domain (from Val 978 to Lys 1283) as determined through x-ray crystallography. The α helices are shown in red, the β-strands in green, the side chains of tyrosines 1158, 1162, and 1163 in yellow, the nucleotide binding loop is in orange, the catalytic loop is in dark blue, and the activation loop is in violet. The N and C termini are denoted by N and C. An N and a C-terminal lobe with a single connection can be seen.

References

1. Freychet P, Roth J, Neville DM. Insulin receptors in liver: Specific binding of 1251 insulin to the plasma membrane and its relation to insulin bioactivity. Proc Natl Acad Sci USA 1971;68:1833–1837
2. Kahn CR, Roth J. Cell membrane receptors for polypeptide hormones. Application to the study of disease states in mice and men. Am J Clin Pathol 1975;63:656–667
3. Kahn CR, Baird KL, Flier JS, et al. Insulin receptors, receptor antibodies, and the mechanism of insulin action. Recent Prog Horm Res 1981;37:477–538
4. Kahn CR. The molecular mechanism of insulin action. Annu Rev Med 1985;36:429–451
5. Kahn CR, White MF. The insulin receptor and the molecular mechanism of insulin action. J Clin Invest 1988;82:1151–1156
6. Olefsky JM. The insulin receptor: A multifunctional protein. Diabetes 1990;39:1009–1016
7. Ebina Y, Ellis L, Jarnagin K, et al. The human insulin receptor cDNA: The structural basis for hormone-activated transmembrane signalling. Cell 40:747–758
8. Ullrich A, Bell JR, Chen EY, et al. Human insulin receptor and its relationship to the tyrosine kinase family of oncogenes. Nature 1985;313:756–761
9. Seino S, Seino M, Nishi S, Bell GI. Structure of the human insulin receptor gene and characterization of its promoter. Proc Natl Acad Sci USA 1989; 86:114–118
10. Goldstein BJ, Kahn CR. Analysis of mRNA heterogeneity by ribonuclease H mapping: Application to the insulin receptor. Biochem Biophys Res Commun 1989;159:664–669
11. Seino S, Bell GI. Alternatively splicing of human insulin receptor messenger RNA. Biochem Biophys Res Commun 1989;159:312–316
12. Moller DE, Yokota A, Caro JF, Flier JS. Tissue-specific expression of two alternatively spliced insulin receptor mRNA's in man. Mol Endocrinol 1989;3:1263–1269
13. Sibley E, Kastelic T, Kelly TJ, Lane MD. Characterization of the mouse insulin receptor gene promoter. Proc Natl Acad Sci USA 1989;86:9732–9736
14. Mamula PW, McDonald AR, Brunetti A, et al. Regulating insulin-receptor-gene expression by differentiation and hormones. Diab Care 1990;13:288–301
15. Gavin JR 3rd, Roth J, Neville DM Jr, et al. Insulin-dependent regulation of insulin receptor concentrations: A direct demonstration in cell culture. Proc Natl Acad Sci USA 1974;71:84–88
16. Araki E, Shimada F, Uzawa H, Mori M, Ebina Y. Characterization of the promoter region of the human insulin receptor gene. J Biol Chem 1987; 262:16186–16191
17. Lee JK, Tam JWO, Tsai MJ, Tsai SY. Identification of cis- and trans-acting factors regulating the expression of the human insulin receptor gene. J Biol Chem 1992;266:3944–3948
18. Lee J, Pilch PF. The insulin receptor: Structure, function, and signaling. Am J Physiol 1994;266:C319–C334
19. Boni-Schnetzler M, Scott W, Waugh SM, DiBella E, Pilch PF. The insulin

receptor: Structural basis for high affinity ligand binding. J Biol Chem 1987;262:8395–8401
20. Cheatham B, Kahn CR. Cysteine 647 in the insulin receptor is required for normal covalent interaction between α- and β-subunits and signal transduction. J Biol Chem 1992;267:7108–7115
21. Olson TS, Lane MD. Post-translational acquisition of insulin binding activity by the insulin proreceptor. Correlation to recognition by autoimmune antibody. J Biol Chem 1987;6816:6822
22. Salzman A, Wan CF, Rubin CS. Biogenesis, transit, and functional properties of the insulin proreceptor and modified insulin receptors in 3T3-L1 adipocytes. Use of monensin to probe proceptor cleavage and generate altered receptor subunits. Biochemistry 1984;23:6555–6565
23. Hedo JA, Kahn CR, Hayashi M, et al. Biosynthesis and glycosylation of the insulin receptor. Evidence for a single polypeptide precursor of the two major subunits. J Biol Chem 1983;258:10020–10026
24. Herzberg VL, Grigorescu F, Edge AS, et al. Characterization of insulin receptor carbohydrate by comparison of chemical and enzymatic deglycosylation. Biochem Biophys Res Commun 1985;129:789–796
25. Pilch PF, Czech MP. The subunit structure of the high affinity insulin receptor: Evidence for a disulfide-linked receptor complex in fat cell and liver plasma membranes. J Biol Chem 1980;255:1722–1731
26. Benecke H, Flier JS, Moller DE. Alternatively spliced variants of the insulin receptor protein. Expression in normal and diabetic human tissues. J Clin Invest 1992;89:2066–2070
27. Seino S, Bell GI. Alternative splicing of human insulin receptor messenger RNA. Biochem Biophys Res Commun 1989;159:312–316
28. Mosthaf L, Grako K, Dull TJ, et al. Functionally distinct insulin receptors generated by tissue-specific alternative splicing. EMBO J 1990;9:2409–2413
29. Yamaguchi Y, Flier JS, Yokota A, et al. Functional properties of two naturally occurring isoforms of the human insulin receptor in Chinese hamster ovary cells. Endocrinology 1991;129:2058–2066
30. Vogt B, Carrascosa JM, Ermel B. The two isotypes of the human insulin receptor (HIR-A and HIR-B) follow different internalization kinetics. Biochem Biophys Res Commun 1991;177:1013–1018
31. Kellerer M, Lammers R, Ermel B, et al. Distinct α-subunit structures of human insulin receptor A and B variants determine differences in tyrosine kinase activities. Biochemistry 1992;31:4588–4596
32. Mosthaf L, Vogt B, Haring H, Ullrich A. Altered expression of insulin receptor types A and B in the skeletal muscle of non-insulin-dependent diabetes mellitus patients. Proc Natl Acad Sci USA 1991;88:4728–4730
33. Norgren S, Zierath J, Galuska D, et al. Differences in the ratio of RNA encoding two isoforms of the insulin receptor between control and NIDDM patients: The RNA variant with exon 11 predominates in both groups. Diabetes 1993;42:675–681
34. Sell SM, Reese D, Ossowski VM. Insulin-inducible changes in insulin receptor mRNA splice variants. J Biol Chem 1994;49:30769–30772
35. DeMeyts P, Roth J, Neville DM, et al. Insulin interactions with its receptors: Experimental evidence for negative cooperativity. Biochem Biophys Res Commun 1973;55:154–161
36. DeMeyts P, Christoffersen CT, Laturs LJ, et al. Negative cooperativity at the insulin receptor 1973–1993: New insights into the structural basis of site-site interactions. Exp Clin Endocrinol 1993;101:17–19
37. Schaffer L. The high-affinity binding site of the insulin receptor involves both α-subunits. Exp Clin Endocrinol 1993;101:7–9
38. Jacobs S, Hazum E, Schecter Y, Cuatrecasas P. Insulin receptor: Covalent labeling and identification of subunits. Proc Natl Acad Sci USA 1979; 261:4918–4921
39. Pilch PF, Czech MP. Interaction of cross-linking agents with the insulin effector system of isolated fat cells. Covalent linkage of 125I-insulin to a plasma membrane receptor protein of 140,000 daltons. J Biol Chem 1979;254:3375–3381
40. Yip CC, Yeung CWT, Moule ML. Photoaffinity labeling of insulin receptor of rat adipocyte plasma membrane. J Biol Chem 1978;253:1743–1745
41. Kjeldsen T, Andersen AS, Wiberg FC. The ligand specificities of the insulin receptor and the insulin-like growth factor I receptor reside in different regions of a common binding site. Proc Natl Acad Sci USA 1991;4404:4408
42. Gustafson TA, Rutter WJ. The cysteine-rich domains of the insulin and insulin-like growth factor I receptors are primary determinants of hormone binding specificity: Evidence from receptor chimeras. J Biol Chem 1990; 265:18663–18667
43. Schumacher R, Soos MA, Schlessinger J. Signaling-competent receptor chimeras allow mapping of major insulin receptor binding domain determinants. J Biol Chem 1993;268:1087–1094
44. Andersen AS, Kjeldsen T, Wiberg FC, et al. Identification of determinants that confer ligand specificity on the insulin receptor. J Biol Chem 1992; 267:13681–13686
45. DeMeyts P, Gu JL, Shymko RM, et al. Identification of a ligand-binding region of the human insulin receptor encoded by the second exon of the gene. Mol Endocrinol 1990;4:409–416
46. Zhang B, Roth RA. Binding properties of chimeric insulin receptors containing the cysteine-rich domain of either the insulin-like growth factor I receptor or the insulin receptor related receptor. Biochemistry 1991; 30:5113–5117
47. Kasuga MF, Karlsson A, Kahn CR. Insulin stimulates the phosphorylation of the 95,000-dalton subunit of its own receptor. Science Wash DC 1982;215:185–186
48. Rosen OM. After insulin binds. Science 1987;237:1452–1458
49. Shoelson SE, White MF, Kahn CR. Tryptic activation of the insulin receptor. Proteolytic truncation of the α-subunit releases the β-subunit from inhibitory control. J Biol Chem 1988;263:4852–4860
50. Frattali AL, Treadway JL, Pessin JE. Evidence supporting a passive role for the insulin receptor transmembrane domain in insulin-dependent signal transduction. J Biol Chem 1991;266:9829–9834
51. Yamada K, Goncalves E, Kahn CR, Shoelson SE. Substitution of the insulin receptor transmembrane domain with the cnew/erbB2 transmembrane domain constitutively activates the insulin receptor kinase in vitro. J Biol Chem 1992;267:12452–12461
52. Herrera R, Rosen OM. Autophosphorylation of the insulin receptor in vitro. Designation of phosphorylation sites and correlation with receptor kinase activation. J Biol Chem 1986;261:11980–11985
53. Maddux BA, Goldfine ID. Evidence that insulin plus ATP may induce a conformational change in the beta subunit of the insulin receptor without inducing receptor autophosphorylation. J Biol Chem 1991;266:6731–6736
54. Perlman R, Bottaro DP, White MF, Kahn CR. Conformational changes in the α- and β-subunits of the insulin receptor identified by anti-peptide antibodies. J Biol Chem 1989;264:8946–8950
55. Hubbard SR, Wei L, Ellis L, Hendrickson WA. Crystal structure of the tyrosine kinase domain of the human insulin receptor. Nature 1994;372:746–754
56. Shier P, Watt VM. Primary structure of a putative receptor for a ligand of the insulin family. J Biol Chem 1989;264:14605–14608
57. Fantl WJ, Johnson DE, Williams LT. Signalling by receptor tyrosine kinases. Annu Rev Biochem 1993;62:453–481
58. Schlessinger J, Ullrich A. Growth factor signaling by receptor tyrosine kinases. Neuron 1992;9:383–391
59. Myers MG, White MF. The new elements of insulin signaling: Insulin receptor substrate-1 and proteins with SH2 domains. Diabetes 1993;42:643–650
60. Sun XJ, Rothenberg P, Kahn CR, et al. Structure of the insulin receptor substrate IRS-1 defines a unique signal transduction protein. Nature 1991; 352:73–77
61. White MF, Kahn CR. The insulin signaling system. J Biol Chem 1994; 269:1–4
62. Feener EP, Backer JM, King GL, et al. Insulin stimulates serine and tyrosine phosphorylation in the juxtamembrane region of the insulin receptor. J Biol Chem 1993;268:11256–11264
63. Kohanski RA. Insulin receptor autophosphorylation. II. Determination of autophosphorylation sites by chemical sequence analysis and identification of the juxtamembrane sites. Biochemistry 1993;32:5773–5780
64. Tornqvist HE, Pierce MW, Frackelton AR, et al. Identification of insulin receptor tyrosine residues autophosphorylated in vitro. J Biol Chem 1993;262: 10212–10219
65. White MF, Shoelson SE, Keutmann H, Kahn CR. A cascade of tyrosine autophosphorylation in the β-subunit activates the phosphotransferase of the insulin receptor. J Biol Chem 1988;263:2969–2980
66. Lee J, O'Hare T, Pilch PF, Shoelson SE. Insulin receptor autophosphorylation occurs asymmetrically. J Biol Chem 1993;268:4092–4098
67. Wilden PA, Siddle K, Haring E, et al. The role of insulin receptor kinase domain autophosphorylation in receptor-mediated activities. Analysis with insulin and anti-receptor antibodies. J Biol Chem 1992;267:13719–13727
68. Zhang B, Tavare JM, Ellis L, Roth RA. The regulatory role of known tyrosine autophosphorylation sites of the insulin receptor kinase domain. An assessment by replacement with neutral and negatively charged amino acids. J Biol Chem 1991;266:990–996
69. Hanks SK, Quinn AM, Hunter T. The protein kinase family: Conserved features and deduced phylogeny of the catalytic domains. Science 1988; 241:42–52
70. Chou CK, Dull TJ, Russell DS, et al. Human insulin receptors mutated at the ATP-binding site lack protein tyrosine kinase activity and fail to mediate postreceptor effects of insulin. J Biol Chem 1987;262:14663–14667
71. White MF, Livingston JN, Backer JM, et al. Mutation of the insulin receptor at tyrosine 960 inhibits signal transmission but does not affect its tyrosine kinase activity. Cell 1988;54:641–649
72. Rajagopalan M, Neidigh JL, McClain DA. Amino acid sequences Gly-Pro-Leu-Tyr and Asn-Pro-Gly-Tyr in the submembranous domain of the insulin receptor are required for normal endocytosis. J Biol Chem 1991;266:23068–23073
73. Tornqvist HE, Pierce MW, Frackelton AR, et al. Identification of insulin receptor tyrosine residues autophosphorylated in vitro. J Biol Chem 1987;262:10212–10219
74. White MF, Shoelson SE, Keutmann H, Kahn CR. A cascade of tyrosine autophosphorylation in the β-subunit activates the insulin receptor. J Biol Chem 1988;263:2969–2980
75. Thies RS, Ullrich A, McClain DA. Augmented mitogenesis and impaired metabolic signaling mediated by a truncated insulin receptor. J Biol Chem 1989;264:12820–12825
76. Myers MG, Backer JM, Siddle K, White MF. The insulin receptor functions normally in Chinese hamster ovary cells after truncation of the C-terminus. J Biol Chem 1991;266:10616–10623
77. Gottschalk WK. The pathway mediating insulin's effects on pyruvate dehydrogenase bypasses the insulin receptor tyrosine kinase. J Biol Chem 1992;266:8814–8819
78. Hawley DM, Maddux BA, Patel RG, et al. Insulin receptor monoclonal

antibodies that mimic insulin action without activating tyrosine kinase. J Biol Chem 1989;264:2438–2444
79. Steele-Perkins G, Roth RA. Insulin-mimetic anti-insulin receptor monoclonal antibodies stimulate receptor kinase activity in intact cells. J Biol Chem 1990;265:9458–9463
80. Moller DE, Benecke H, Flier JS. Biologic activities of naturally occurring human insulin receptor mutations: Evidence that metabolic effects of insulin can be mediated by a kinase-deficient insulin receptor mutant. J Biol Chem 1991;266:10995–11001
81. Takayama S, White MF, Kahn CR. Phorbol ester-induced serine phosphorylation of the insulin receptor decreases its tyrosine kinase activity. J Biol Chem 1988;263:3440–3447
82. Chin JE, Dickens M, Tavare JM, Roth RA. Overexpression of protein kinase C isoenzymes alpha, beta I, gamma, and epsilon in cells overexpressing the insulin receptor. Effects on receptor phosphorylation and signaling. J Biol Chem 1993;268:6338–6347
83. Stadtmauer L, Rosen OM. Increasing the cAMP content of IM-9 cells alters the phosphorylation state and protein kinase activity of the insulin receptor. J Biol Chem 1986;261:3402–3407
84. Lewis RE, Cao L, Perregaux D, Czech MP. Threonine 1336 of the human insulin receptor is a major target for phosphorylation by protein kinase C. Biochemistry 1990;29:1807–1813
85. Baltensperger KR, Lewis RE, Woon CW, et al. Catalysis of serine and tyrosine autophosphorylation by the human insulin receptor. Proc Natl Acad Sci USA 1992;89:7885–7889
86. Treadway JL, Morrison BD, Soos MA, et al. Transdominant inhibition of tyrosine kinase activity in mutant insulin/insulin-like growth factor I hybrid receptors. Proc Natl Acad Sci USA 1991;88:214–218
87. Moller DE, Yokota A, White MF, et al. A naturally occurring mutation of insulin receptor alanine 1134 impairs tyrosine kinase function and is associated with dominantly inherited insulin resistance. J Biol Chem 1990; 265:14979–14985
88. Argetsinger LS, Shafer JA. The reversible and irreversible autophosphorylation of insulin receptor kinases. J Biol Chem 1992;31:22095–22101
89. Kohanski RA. Insulin receptor autophosphorylation. I. Autophosphorylation kinetics of the native receptor and its cytoplasmic kinase domain. Biochemistry 1993;32:5766–5772
90. King GL, Rechler MM, Kahn CR. Interactions between the receptors for insulin and the insulin-like growth factors on adipocytes. J Biol Chem 1982;257:10001–10006
91. Moxham CP, Duronio V, Jacobs S. Insulin-like growth factor I receptor beta-subunit heterogeneity: Evidence for hybrid tetramers composed of insulin-like growth factor I and insulin receptor heterodimers. J Biol Chem 1989;264:13238–13244
92. Fischer EH, Charbonneau H, Tonks NK. Protein tyrosine phosphatases: A diverse family of intracellular and transmembrane enzymes. Science 1991; 253:401–406
93. Sales GJ. Insulin receptor phosphotyrosyl protein phosphatases and the regulation of insulin receptor tyrosine kinase action. Adv Prot Phosphatases 1991; 6:159–186
94. Meyerovitch J, Backer JM, Kahn CR. Hepatic phosphotyrosine phosphatase activity and its alterations in diabetic rats. J Clin Invest 1989;84:976–983
95. Posner BI, Kahn MN, Bergeron JJ. Internalization of insulin: Structures involved and significance. Adv Exp Med Biol 1985;189:159–173
96. Duckworth WC. Insulin degradation: Mechanisms, products, and significance. Endocr Rev 1988;9:319–345
97. Marshall S. Dual pathways for the intracellular processing of insulin. Relationship between retroendocytosis of intact hormone and the recycling of insulin receptors. J Biol Chem 1985;260:13524–13531
98. Backer JM, Kahn CR, White MF. The dissociation and degradation of internalized insulin occur in the endosomes of rat hepatoma cells. J Biol Chem 1990;265:14828–14835
99. Doherty JJ, Kay DG, Lai WH, et al. Selective degradation of insulin within rat liver endosomes. J Cell Biol 1990;110:35–42
100. Khan MN, Baquiran G, Brule C, et al. Internalization and activation of the rat liver insulin receptor kinase in vivo. J Biol Chem 1989;264:12931–12940
101. Wilden PA, Kahn CR, Siddle K, White MF. Insulin receptor kinase domain autophosphorylation regulates receptor enzymatic function. J Biol Chem 1992;267:16660–16668
102. Backer JM, Shoelson SE, Haring E, White MF. Insulin receptors internalize by a rapid, saturable pathway requiring receptor autophosphorylation and an intact juxtamembrane region. J Cell Biol 1991;115:1535–1545

Diabetes Mellitus, edited by Derek LeRoith, Simeon I. Taylor, and Jerrold M. Olefsky. Lippincott–Raven Publishers, Philadelphia © 1996.

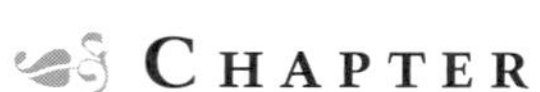

CHAPTER 16
The Role of IRS-1 During Insulin Signaling

MORRIS F. WHITE

Introduction

The identification of downstream elements controlling cellular growth and metabolism is an important question in contemporary biology. Several models for the propagation of extracellular signals through various tyrosine kinase messenger systems are rapidly coming into focus.[1] Epidermal growth factor (EGF) and platelet-derived growth factor (PDGF) receptors have led the field because they possess three intrinsic signaling elements: a specific ligand binding domain, a regulated tyrosine kinase, and autophosphorylation sites that bind *directly* to the SH2 domains in various signaling proteins (SH2 proteins) (Fig. 16-1). Several SH2 proteins bind directly to the activated PDGF or EGF receptors, including the phosphatidylinositol (PI)-3-kinase, p21^{ras}-GAP, phospholipase cγ, Grb-2, SH-PTP2, src-related kinases, and others.[2,3]

Although the recruitment of SH2 proteins directly to a receptor tyrosine kinase is the easiest coupling mechanism to characterize, most receptors employ additional subunits or cytoplasmic "docking proteins" to engage SH2 proteins.[4] Like the EGF-PDGF receptors, the receptors for insulin and insulin-like growth factor-1 (IGF-1) contain intrinsic ligand binding, catalytic domains, and multiple autophosphorylation sites; however, these tyrosine phosphorylated receptors associate poorly with SH2 signaling proteins (see Fig. 16-1). Instead, they utilize IRS signaling proteins to provide an interface between the receptor and the SH2 proteins.[5] The best characterized family member, IRS-1, contains 21 putative tyrosine phosphorylation sites at its COOH-terminus, which bind various SH2 proteins.

Although IRS-1 was originally described in insulin/IGF-1 signaling, several cytokine receptors also engage this element to mediate downstream signals. Unlike insulin/IGF-1 receptors, cytokine receptors are assembled from multiple modular components, which are frequently shared between several receptor systems.[6] Functional receptors for interleukin-4 (IL-4), IL-9, IL-13, and type I interferons (IFNα, INFβ, and IFNω, are composed of specific ligand binding subunits and shared cytoplasmic components, including tyrosine kinases in the Janus family (Jak-1, Jak-2, Jak-3, Tyk-2) (see Fig. 16-1).[6] The growth hormone receptor, a member

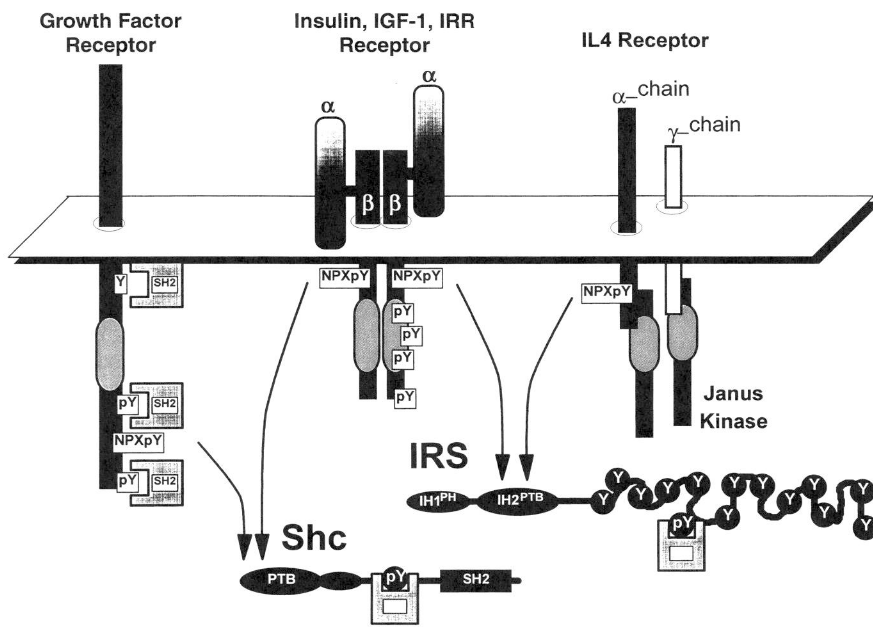

Figure 16-1. Essential elements in signal transduction by various receptors. The EGF receptor-like mechanism involves the direct association of SH2 proteins (SH2) with the COOH-terminal autophosphorylation sites. The EGF receptor also contains an NPXY motif that may interact with the phosphotyrosine binding domains (PTB) in Shc. The insulin-IGF-1 receptor model illustrates the first system found to engage IRS signaling proteins. Recent results suggest that this recognition involves two conserved modules in the NH_2-terminus of the IRS molecule, called IH-1 and IH-2. IH-1 is similar to a pleckstrin homology (PH) domain and IH-2 is similar to PTB domains. The cytokine model, illustrated with the IL-4 receptor complex, is also shown for comparison. This receptor is not a tyrosine kinase but associates with several subunits including a Janus kinase, probably Jak-3, which may mediate the phosphorylation of the NPXY motif in the receptor to mediate the association and phosphorylate IRS signaling proteins.

of the cytokine receptor superfamily, utilizes Jak-2 for signal transduction.[7,8] Additional subunits are frequently required for assembly of the functional complexes, such as the γ chain of the IL-2 receptor, which is shared by the IL-4, IL-7, IL-9, and IL-13 receptors and possibly others in this receptor superfamily.[9,10] Our interest in this subset of cytokine receptors arises from their use of IRS signaling proteins as common interfaces to engage SH2 proteins and other regulatory elements.[5]

IRS Signaling Proteins: Elements in Diabetes, Cancer, and Growth and Development

Since the discovery of insulin over 70 years ago, its effects on carbohydrate, fat, and protein metabolism have been well established.[11] The absolute lack of insulin through β-cell destruction results in insulin-dependent diabetes mellitus (IDDM), a life-threatening metabolic disease that is best treated with frequent injections of insulin. In contrast, reduced insulin sensitivity at various target tissues, together with insufficient compensation by the β-cell, causes non–insulin-dependent diabetes mellitus (NIDDM) in over 10 million Americans. Novel therapies using rationally designed drugs are essential in the future to improve the quality of these patients' lives and to reduce this burden on our health care system. A thorough knowledge of the insulin signaling system will help accomplish this goal.

A closely related polypeptide, insulin-like growth factor-1 (IGF-1) is essential for normal growth and development.[12,13] IGF-1 is essential during embryonic development, as disruption of the genes for IGF-1 or its receptor in mice causes significant developmental abnormalities.[12,13] IGF-1 also controls metabolic processes such as glucose and protein metabolism and has been tested as a replacement for insulin in patients with insulin resistance.[14] However, IGF-1 is also a potent mitogen that is implicated in the etiology of mammary carcinoma, one of the leading causes of death among women between the ages of 40 and 55. Moreover, the IGF-1 receptor is essential for SV40 transformation of murine fibroblasts.[15–17] This function may be related to antiapoptosis mediated by insulin/IGF-1 and somehow, may involve the direct interaction between IRS signaling proteins and SV40 T antigen.[18] Since IGF-1 and insulin share common signaling pathways, a full understanding of these molecular mechanisms is essential for the discovery and safe implementation of new clinical strategies to combat diabetes and cancer.

Many of the effects of growth hormone on tissues are thought to be mediated by insulin-like growth factors.[19] The overall actions of growth hormone are most clearly recognized after its administration to growth hormone–deficient children, which causes a prompt resumption of skeletal, muscular, and visceral growth. Growth hormone stimulates IGF-1 gene expression in a number of extrahepatic tissues, which can contribute locally to cell multiplication and differentiation. Moreover, many nonhepatic tissues have growth hormone receptors that mediate direct and rapid metabolic actions such as the promotion of glucose and amino acid transport in muscle and fat and the stimulation of lipolysis in fat and muscle. However, in adult liver, the effects of growth hormone are direct since hepatocytes have few type 1 IGF receptors. Recent studies in rat adipocytes or F442a adipocytes reveal that IRS-1 is phosphorylated during growth hormone stimulation.[20,21] Thus activation of IRS signaling proteins by growth hormone receptor may be an additional common element linking insulin, IGF-1, and growth hormone action.

Neurons are also sensitive to the action of insulin and IGF-1.[22] Insulin/IGF-1 may play a permissive role in the action of other neurotrophic factors in the nervous system, in particular by inhibiting apoptosis.[23] The neurotrophic actions of insulin/IGF-1 are widespread and less specific than those of other classic neurotrophic factors. Insulin and IGF-1 activate protein synthesis, stimulate neurite outgrowth, trigger the expression of the differentiated phenotypes, and generally promote survival of neurons.[24,25] During insulin stimulation of fetal chick forebrain cells, the insulin receptor is tyrosine phosphorylated and the $p70^{s6k}$ and PKCε are activated.[26,27] IRS-2 mRNA is more abundant in rat brain than IRS-1, suggesting that IRS-2 may play an important role in IGF-1 signaling.[28]

Structure and Function of the Insulin Receptor

Insulin/IGF-1 receptors are present in virtually all vertebrate tissues, although their concentrations vary. The receptors are composed of two disulfide-linked α-subunits that are each linked to a β-subunit by disulfide bonds. In each case, the α-subunits are located entirely outside the cell and contain the ligand binding site(s), whereas the intracellular portions of the β-subunits contain the regulated tyrosine protein kinase. The intracellular domains are 80% identical, reflecting some common signaling potential[29,30]; however, under certain conditions, the IFG-1 receptors transform cells, whereas the insulin receptor is weak in this regard.[18,31,32] The insulin receptor-related (IRR) receptor has a similar structure, although its ligand remains unidentified.[33,34] Interestingly, expression of the IRR receptor is closely associated with that of the NGF receptor, trk, suggesting some coordinated function.[35] IRR and trk demonstrate synchronized patterns of coexpression in neural crest–derived sensory and sympathetic neurons and in non–neural crest basal forebrain and striatal neurons.

Multiple autophosphorylation sites exist in the β-subunits of the insulin, IGF-1, and IRR receptors.[36] For the insulin receptor, autophosphorylation occurs in three regions, including the intracellular juxtamembrane region (Tyr_{960}), a regulatory region (Tyr_{1146}, Tyr_{1150}, and Tyr_{1151}), and the C-terminus (Tyr_{1316} and Tyr_{1322}).[37] Phosphorylation of the regulatory region activates the kinase. The crystal structure of the catalytic domain of the insulin receptor β-subunit suggests that Tyr_{1150} plays an important role in the activation of the receptor kinase.[38] In the unphosphorylated state this residue may inactivate the enzyme by occupying the catalytic site and inhibiting ATP binding; autophosphorylation of this tyrosine is predicted to release this inhibition. However, phosphorylation of the adjacent residues also contributes positively to the activation process, as mutations in this region have significant effects on kinase activity.[39,40]

Outside of the catalytic domain the juxtamembrane region is essential for signal transmission. This region contains a tyrosine autophosphorylation site (Tyr_{960} in the insulin receptor), which resides in an NPXY motif.[41] A similar motif exists in the IGF-1 and IRR receptors.[36] Mutations at or around Tyr_{960} inhibit insulin-stimulated tyrosine phosphorylation of IRS-1 and Shc.[37,42] The interaction between the insulin receptor cytoplasmic domains and IRS-1 in the yeast "two-hybrid" system suggests that this motif interacts with the NH_2-terminal 500 amino acids of IRS-1 and the first 200 amino acids of Shc.[43] Recently, the cloning of IRS-2 has allowed us to align the sequences of IRS-1 and IRS-2. This analysis reveals a highly conserved region in the NH_2-terminus, which is termed the IRS-homology-2 domain (IH-2) (see Fig 16-1). The IH-2 domain is similar to the PTB module in Shc and appears to be primarily responsible for binding the phosphorylated NPXY motif.[28]

Since other receptors also mediate IRS-1 phosphorylation, the question arises as to the mechanism of this interaction. Interestingly, the IL-4 receptor also contains an NPXY motif that is essential for IRS-1 phosphorylation.[44] Moreover, comparisons between the receptor for insulin, IGF-1, and IL-4 suggest that a longer amino acid sequence motif LxxxxNPXYxSxSD, may be required for IRS-1 recognition.[44] However, other receptors that phosphorylate IRS-1, for example the growth hormone receptor, do not contain an NPXY motif, suggesting that uncharacterized receptor subunits or distinct mechanisms must be involved.[21]

IRS Signaling Proteins and Other Downstream Elements

IRS-1 was initially detected in insulin-stimulated Fao hepatoma cells[45,46] and cloned from rat, human, and murine sources.[47–50] The open reading frame predicts a molecular weight of 131 kd, but IRS-1 migrates between 165 and 180 kd on SDS-PAGE owing to a high serine phosphorylation state.[47,51] Although IRS-1 is highly conserved among species, it has little extended homology to other known proteins.[47,49]

Although IRS-1 is essential for many insulin/IGF-1 and IL-4 responses, disruption of its gene is not lethal in mice.[52,53] However, IRS-1 contributes to normal development and metabolic regulation since intrauterine growth is reduced by 50% in IRS-$1^{(-/-)}$ mice, and the adults display slightly impaired glucose tolerance and decreased insulin/IGF-1-stimulated glucose uptake in vivo and in vitro.[52,53] This phenotype may be the combined result of diminished signaling through the insulin, IGF-1, and growth hormone receptors and other cytokines.

The relatively mild phenotype of the IRS-$1^{(-/-)}$ mouse suggests that other signaling proteins mediate the insulin response. One possibility is a second IRS protein (IRS-2) recently purified and cloned from a mouse cDNA library.[28] IRS-2 and IRS-1 contain regions of significant similarity at the NH_2-terminus, whereas similarity in the COOH-terminal region is weak; however, multiple tyrosine phosphorylation sites are well conserved and found in relatively similar positions, which are ideal docking sites for SH2 proteins, including the PI-3-kinase. IRS-2 is found in multiple tissues of normal and IRS-$1^{(-/-)}$ mice, mediates IRS-1-like signals, and rescues insulin-IL-4 signaling in 32D cells.[28] Thus, IRS signaling proteins are important interfaces coordinating signal transduction by insulin/IGF-1 and IL-4 receptors as well as other cytokines.

Together, IRS-1 and IRS-2 have an extensive potential to interact with downstream signaling molecules through approxi-

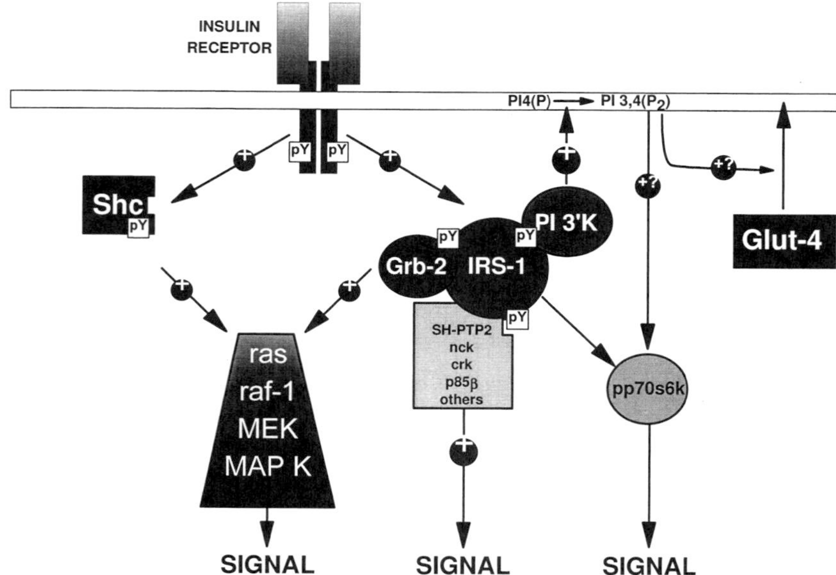

FIGURE 16-2. A model of downstream elements in insulin receptor signaling. The insulin receptor engages both IRS-1 and Shc and mediates their tyrosine phosphorylation; both molecules interact with Grb2, which regulates the MAP kinase pathway (ras, Raf-1, MEK, and MAPK). IRS-1 also interacts with other downstream signaling molecules, including the phosphatidylinositol-3 (PI-3)-kinase, which is implicated in the translocation of GLUT-4 to the plasma membrane. IRS-1 also regulates the $p70^{s6k}$ as shown. Other SH2 proteins have been shown to interact with phosphorylated IRS-1, including p85β, nck, and crk.

mately 30 unique phosphorylation motifs (see Fig. 16-2). In contrast, only a few relatively well-known SH2 proteins have been found to associate with IRS-1, including p85α/β, Grb2, SHPTP2, and nck.[5] The PI-3-kinase and SHPTP2 are activated during association with phosphorylated IRS-1.[54,55] Grb2 has also been studied extensively and is known to regulate a $p21^{ras}$ guanine nucleotide exchange factor called Sos.[56–58] The binding of the Grb2-Sos complex to phosphorylated IRS-1 plays a role in the activation of $p21^{ras}$.[59–61] Grb2-Sos also binds to phosphorylated Shc during insulin stimulation, which provides an alternate pathway and a link in common with many growth factor receptors.[61] The relative contribution of IRS-1-Grb2 and Shc-Grb2 to the regulation of ras activity may vary with the cell background; however, the significance of this distinction has not yet been revealed.[62]

In cells that lack IRS signaling protein, insulin still stimulates Shc phosphorylation and its association with GRB2, which stimulates $p21^{ras}$ GTP loading and activates the MAP kinase.[61] Thus, Shc functions independently of IRS signaling proteins during its interaction with the insulin receptor, but together with IRS-1 it converges on Grb2 (Fig. 16-2). In some cells, Shc may be the preferred pathway used by insulin to regulate ras and MAP kinase.[63] The Shc family of proteins is composed of at least three isoforms between 46 and 52 kd.[64,65] During stimulation of cells with various growth factors, including insulin/IGF-1, Shc is tyrosine phosphorylated at a YVNI motif, which binds to the SH2 domain of Grb-2.[61] Although Shc has less potential than IRS-1 to bind multiple SH2 proteins, it contains other domains that mediate protein-protein interactions (see Fig. 16-1), including an SH2 domain at its COOH-terminus, a region similar to α-1 collagen in the middle of the molecule that contains a binding motif for the SH3 domains in Grb2, and an NH_2-terminus that recognizes phosphorylated NPXY-motifs.[66,67] It is likely that the convergence of these domains in a single molecule is important for signaling.

Although Shc and IRS-1 converge at the level of $p21^{ras}$ and MAP kinase activation in certain cells, the IRS signaling proteins are an essential element in insulin/IGF-1 and IL-4 stimulated mitogenesis.[68] Overexpression of IRS-1 in Chinese hamster ovary (CHO) cells doubles the maximal response of thymidine incorporation during insulin stimulation, whereas reducing its level diminishes this response.[51,69] Moreover, microinjection of antibodies against IRS-1 into NIH-3T3 inhibits insulin-stimulated cell growth.[70] The complete absence of IRS-1 from the 32-D myeloid progenitor cells provides an ideal system for the analysis of IRS-1-IRS-2 in insulin-IL-4 signaling. 32-D cells grow in the presence of IL-3 but are insensitive to insulin, IL-4, and IGF-1; however, expression of IRS-1 or IRS-2 rescues the IGF-1 and IL-4 mitogenic response, and coexpression with the insulin receptor restores the insulin response.[28,68] Thus, IRS signaling proteins appear to be essential elements for insulin/IGF-1 and IL-4-stimulated mitogenesis and cell cycle progression in a variety of cell systems.

The Function of p85 and the PI-3-Kinase

Several experiments suggest that the PI-3-kinase is an important element in growth factor- and cytokine-regulated mitogenesis, cellular transformation, differentiation, and other biologic processes.[71] Mutant PDGF receptors that cannot engage PI-3-kinase are unable to mediate mitogenic responses.[2] Moreover, transformation defective mutants of polyoma middle T lack the ability to bind PI-3-kinase.[71] The subcellular location of the activated PI-3-kinase may be important for cellular transformation. A transformation-defective mutant of *v-abl* associates with PI-3-kinase but fails to associate with the plasma membrane or increase the cellular levels of PI-3,4-P_2 and PI-3,4,5-P_3.[72] PI-3-kinase also plays a role in NGF-stimulated differentiation of PC12 cells.[73] It is also necessary for other cellular functions, including chemotaxis, membrane ruffling, and insulin-stimulated glucose uptake.[71,74,75] PI-3-kinase is also important for growth factor and insulin-stimulated $p70^{s6k}$.[76–78] Finally wortmannin and LY294002, inhibitors of the PI-3-kinase, block insulin-stimulated glucose uptake in 3T3-L1 adipocytes.[79,80]

The PI-3-kinase is ordinarily composed of two subunits: an 85-kd regulatory subunit (p85) and a 110-kd catalytic subunit (p110).[71] Two isoforms of p85 (α and β) have been cloned, both of which are composed of 724 amino acids.[81,82] The proteins contain an NH_2-terminal Src-homology 3 (SH3) domain, a region homologous to the COOH-terminal (GAP active site) of the Bcr, and two Src-homology 2 domains (nSH2 and cSH2). The SH2 domains bind to phosphorylated YMXM motifs in various proteins, whereas the SH3 domains bind to proline-rich motifs in p85 itself or other targets.[83] The region between the SH2 domains binds to the NH_2-terminus of p110.[84,85] Thus, p85 acts as an interface between p110 and various signaling proteins, including IRS signaling proteins. Other regulatory proteins related to p85 are predicted to exist, and a third isoform of p85 (p85γ) has been discussed.[81,86]

Two isoforms of p110 have been cloned from mammalian tissues.[87,88] The p110 catalyzes phosphorylation of hydroxyl groups in the D3 position of phosphatidylinositol and its poly-phosphorylated derivatives, resulting in the production of PI-3,4-P_2 and PI-3,4,5-P_3 in cells. The p110 is homologous to the S. cerevisiae Vps34p, which also contains intrinsic PtdIns 3-kinase activity.[89] The Vps34p plays a role in targeting soluble hydrolases to the yeast vacuole and in vacuole morphogenesis during budding.[90,91] This functional similarity between Vps34p and PI-3-kinase suggests that PI-3-kinase may regulate vesicle trafficking in mammalian cells. Supporting this hypothesis, disruption of the binding of PI-3-kinase to the PDGF receptor inhibits receptor internalization.[92] Amino acid sequence similarities exist between the catalytic domains of p110 and those of protein kinases.[93] Interestingly, the PI-3-kinase displays serine-threonine kinase activity toward p85 and IRS-1.[71,94]

Several mechanisms have been proposed for the regulation of PI-3-kinase activity. During insulin/IGF-1 and IL-4 stimulation, the PI-3-kinase is activated by association with IRS signaling proteins.[54,95] In cells lacking IRS signaling proteins, insulin has no effect on PI-3-kinase activity. Although a few reports suggest that the insulin receptor can directly engage p85, it is unlikely that this is a major pathway. The binding of phosphorylated YMXM motifs in IRS-1 or other proteins to the SH2 domains of p85 causes a conformational change that stimulates the associated kinase.[96] A few studies suggest that tyrosine phosphorylation of p85 activates the PI-3-kinase, especially during PDGF and nerve growth factor stimulation, but this is difficult to show during insulin stimulation.[97] Insulin stimulates PI-3-kinase through p85α but not p85β in COS-1, CHO, and 3T3-L1 cells, suggesting that the two isoforms may not be functionally equivalent.[86] The association between the SH3 domains of c-fyn and proline-rich motifs in p85 is reported to activate the PI-3-kinase.[98] Activated ras binds to the PI-3-kinase in vitro and stimulates it.[99] In contrast, serine phosphorylation of p85 inhibits the PI-3-kinase.

The function and targets of the lipid products of the PI-3-kinase are unknown. The rapid appearance of PI-3,4-P_2 and PI-3,4,5-P_3 following growth factor stimulation and their resistance to PLC–mediated hydrolysis suggest that the lipids themselves function as second messengers. Phospholipid production probably occurs initially at the plasma membrane and later in vesicles derived from the plasma membrane that contain PI-3-kinase–tyrosine phosphorylated protein complexes. The lipid products may be involved in targeting vesicles to specific subcellular locations in which the propagation of a hormone signal takes place. In rat adipocytes, the activated PI-3-kinase is mainly found in a very-low-density internal membrane fraction.[101] Alternatively, the phospholipids may directly regulate enzyme activity: PI-3,4,5-P_3 may activate directly PKCζ and the akt-kinase which may be crucial in mitogenic signaling, possibly by regulating NFκB activity or its translocation to the nucleus.[102]

We recently identified a unique protein of 55kd that is similar to the COOH-terminal portion of p85α and p85β.[103] This protein, designated $p55^{PIK}$, associates with p110 and during insulin stimulation binds to IRS-1 and undergoes tyrosine phosphorylation.[102] It lacks several protein-binding domains found in p85, including the SH3 domain, the NH_2-terminal proline-rich motif, and the Bcr-homology region; however, $p55^{PIK}$ contains a unique NH_2-terminus and an insulin-stimulated phosphorylation site that may mediate associations with other proteins. Thus, $p55^{PIK}$ may play a unique role in growth factor signal transduction and PI-3-kinase function.

Glucose Transport, PI-3-Kinase, and pp60 in Rat Adipocytes

Blood glucose levels are maintained around 5 mM through the actions of several hormones, including insulin and IGF-1. Glucose stimulates insulin release, which promotes glucose transport in skeletal muscle, cardiac myocytes, and adipocytes. Insulin increases glucose transport by causing translocation of GLUT-4 from intracellular compartments to the plasma membrane.[104] The effect on GLUT-4 translocation reaches a maximum within minutes after insulin stimulation. Two distinct experimental approaches have converged recently, reaching the conclusion that PI-3-kinase is necessary although not necessarily sufficient for insulin-stimulated GLUT-4 (and GLUT-1) translocation. First, insulin-stimulated glucose uptake is inhibited in fat cells by wortmannin (ED_{50} = 50 nM), a poorly characterized inhibitor of the PI-3-kinase.[79] Alone, these results are questionable because it is impossible to know whether other unknown kinases are also inhibited. However, a p85 mutant (Δp85) lacking the binding site for p110 inhibits insulin-stimulated glucose uptake (translocation of GLUT-1 to the plasma membrane in this case) in CHO cells.[105] Together, these results suggest that the activation of the PI-3-kinase is necessary for insulin-stimulated glucose uptake.

Since IRS-1 is an important upstream element in the regulation of PI-3-kinase by insulin and IGF-1, IRS-1 may play an obligatory role in insulin-stimulated GLUT-4 translocation.[101] Disruption of the IRS-1 gene in mice partially supports this conclusion, since insulin-stimulated glucose uptake is reduced by 50%. In normal adipocytes, insulin-stimulated PI-3-kinase activity is found in very-low-density membrane fractions, which also contain a highly phosphorylated cohort of IRS-1. Interestingly, p85α remains largely in the cytosol during insulin stimulation, and the total amount of p85α in the subcellular fractions is unchanged.[101] The activated PI-3-kinase colocalizes with a 60-kd phosphotyrosine-containing protein that immunoprecipitates with p85 antibodies.[101,106] It is possible that pp60 contributes the regulation of the PI-3-kinase in adipocytes during insulin stimulation.

Summary

Considerable progress has been made recently in our understanding of insulin signaling. However, most of the pathways have been studied in a cell line that cannot directly address the question of interest to diabetes. This is not because of a lack of interest but rather because of the difficulty of applying molecular approaches to metabolically responsive cells. The application of homologous recombination in mouse embryonic stem cells to questions of insulin action is providing a new avenue by which to unravel the mechanisms controlling insulin's metabolic actions.

Acknowledgments

I would like to thank Jon Backer, Xiao Jian Sun, and Martin Myers for their important contributions to the evolution of these ideas. This work was supported by NIH grants DK43808 and DK38712 and generous support from the Juvenile Diabetes Foundation and the American Diabetes Association.

References

1. Pawson T, Gish GD. SH2 and SH3 domains: From structure to function. Cell 1992;71:359
2. Valius M, Kazlauskas A. Phospholipase C—gammal and phosphatidylinositol 3 kinase are the downstream mediators of the PDGF receptor's mitogenic signal. Cell 1993;73:321
3. Kazlauskas A, Feng GS, Pawson T, Valius M. The 64-kDa protein that associates with the platelet-derived growth factor receptor beta subunit via Tyr-1009 is the SH2-containing phosphotyrosine phosphatase Syp. Proc Natl Acad Sci USA 1993;90:6939
4. Pawson T. Protein modules and signalling networks. Nature 1995;373:573
5. White MF. The IRS-1 signaling system. Curr Opin Genet Devel 1994;4:47
6. Briscoe J, Guschin D, Muller M. Just another signalling pathway. Curr Biol 1994;4:1033
7. Argetsinger LS, Campbell GS, Yang X, et al. Identification of JAK2 as a growth hormone receptor-associated tyrosine kinase. Cell 1993;74:237
8. Campbell GS, Christian LJ, Carter-Su C. Evidence for involvement of the growth hormone receptor-associated tyrosine kinase in actions of growth hormone. J Biol Chem 1993;268:7427
9. Russell SM, Johnston JA, Noguchi M, et al. Interaction of IL-2Rβ and gc chains with Jak1 and Jak3: Implications for XSCID and XCID. Science 1994;266:1042
10. Kondo M, Takeshita T, Ishii N, et al. Sharing of the interleukin-2 (IL-2) receptor g chain between receptors for IL-2 and IL-4. Science 1994;262:1874
11. DeFronzo RA, Bonadonna RC, Ferrannini E. Pathogenesis of NIDDM: A balanced overview. Diabetes Care 1992;15:318
12. Baker J, Liu JP, Robertson EJ, Efstratiadis A. Role of insulin-like growth factors in embryonic and postnatal growth. Cell 1993;75:73
13. Liu JP, Baker J, Perkins JA, et al. Mice carrying null mutations of the genes encoding insulin-like growth factor I (1gf-1) and type 1 IGF receptor (1gflr). Cell 1993;75:59
14. Bach LA, Draznin B, LeRoith D, eds. Molecular Biology of Diabetes IL Insulin Action Effects on Gene Expression and Regulation, and Glucose Transport. Totowa: Humana Press;1994:393–412
15. Coppola D, Ferber A, Miura M, et al. A functional insulin-like growth factor I receptor is required for the mitogenic and transforming activities of the epidermal growth factor receptor. Mol Cell Biol 1994;14:4588
16. Sell C, Dumenil G, Deveaud C, et al. Effect of a null mutation of the insulin-like growth factor I receptor gene on growth and transformation of mouse embryo fibroblasts. Mol Cell Biol 1994;14:3604
17. Sell C, Rubini M, Rubin R, et al. Simian virus 40 large tumor antigen is unable to transform mouse embryonic fibroblasts lacking type 1 insulin-like growth factor receptor. Proc Natl Acad Sci USA 1993;90:11217
18. Baserga R. Oncogenes and the strategy of growth factors. Cell 1994;79:927
19. Daughaday WH. Growth hormone, insulin-like growth factors and acromegaly. In: DeGroot IJ, ed. Endocrinology, 3rd ed. Philadelphia: WB Saunders;1994:303–329
20. Souza SC, Frick GP, Yip R, et al. Growth hormone stimulates tyrosine phosphorylation of insulin receptor substrate-1. J Biol Chem 1994;269:30085
21. Argetsinger LS, Hsu GW, Myers MG Jr, et al. Tyrosyl phosphorylation of insulin receptor substrate-1 by growth hormone, interferon-gamma, and leukemia inhibitory factor. J Biol Chem 1995;270:14685–14692
22. Saltiel AR, Decker SJ. Cellular mechanisms of signal transduction for neurotrophins. Bio Essays 1994;16:405
23. Collins MK, Perkins GR, Rodriguez Tarduchy G, et al. Growth factors as survival factors: Regulation of apoptosis. Bio Essays 1994;16:133
24. Heidenreich KA. Insulin and IGF-I receptor signaling in cultured neurons. Ann NY Acad Sci 1993;692:72
25. Heidenreich KA, Zeppelin T, Robinson LJ. Insulin and insulin-like growth factor I induce c-fos expression in postmitotic neurons by a protein kinase C-dependent pathway. J Biol Chem 1993;268:14663
26. Heidenreich KA, Toledo SP, Kenner KA. Regulation of protein phosphorylation by insulin and insulin-like growth factors in cultured fetal neurons. Adv Exp Med Biol 1991;293:379
27. Heidenreich KA, Toledo SP, Brunton LL, et al. Insulin stimulates the activity of a novel protein kinase C, PKC-$_{1}$, in cultured fetal chick neurons. J Biol Chem 1990;265:15076
28. Sun XJ, Wang LM, Zhang Y, et al. The structure and function of IRS-2: A common element in insulin/IGF-1 and IL-4 signaling. Nature 1995;377: 173–177
29. Ullrich A, Bell JR, Chen EY, et al. Human insulin receptor and its relationship to the tyrosine kinase family of oncogenes. Nature 1985;313:756
30. Ullrich A, Gray A, Tam AW, et al. Insulin-like growth factor I receptor primary structure: Comparison with insulin receptor suggests structural determinants that define functional specificity. EMBO J 1986;5:2503
31. Baserga R, Porcu P, Rubini M, Sell C. Cell cycle control by the IGF-1 receptor and its ligands. Adv Exp Med Biol 1993;343:105
32. Baserga R, Rubin R. Cell cycle and growth control. Crit Rev Eukaryot Gene Expr 1993;3:47

33. Shier P, Watt VM. Primary structure of a putative receptor for a ligand of the insulin family. J Biol Chem 1989;264:14605
34. Jui HY, Suzuki Y, Accili D, Taylor SI. Expression of a cDNA encoding the human insulin receptor-related receptor. J Biol Chem 1994;269:22446
35. Reinhardt RR, Chin E, Zhang B, et al. Selective coexpression of insulin receptor-related receptor (IRR) and TRK in NGF-sensitive neurons. J Neurosci 1994;14:4674
36. Werner H, Beitner-Johnson D, Roberts CT, et al. Molecular comparisons of the insulin and IGF-1 receptors. In: Draznin B, LeRoith D, eds. Molecular Biology of Diabetes II. Insulin Action, Effects on Gene Expression and Regulation, and Glucose Transport. Totowa: Humana Press;1994:377–392
37. White MF, Kahn CR. The insulin signaling system. J Biol Chem 1994;269:1
38. Hubbard SR, Wei L, Ellis L, Hendrickson WA. Crystal structure of the tyrosine kinase domain of the human insulin receptor. Nature 1994;372:746
39. Wilden PA, Siddle K, Haring E, et al. The role of insulin receptor kinase domain autophosphorylation in receptor-mediated activities. J Biol Chem 1992;267:13719
40. Wilden PA, Kahn CR, Siddle K, White MF. Insulin receptor kinase domain autophosphorylation regulates receptor enzymatic function. J Biol Chem 1992;267:16660
41. Feener EP, Backer JM, King GL, et al. Insulin stimulates serine and tyrosine phosphorylation in the juxtamembrane region of the insulin receptor. J Biol Chem 1993;268:11256
42. White MF, Livingston JN, Backer JM, et al. Mutation of the insulin receptor at tyrosine 960 inhibits signal transmission but does not affect its tyrosine kinase activity. Cell 1988;54:641
43. O'Neill TJ, Craparo A, Gustafson TA. Characterization of an interaction between insulin receptor substrate-1 and the insulin receptor by using the two-hybrid system. Mol Cell Biol 1994;14:6433
44. Keegan AD, Nelms K, White M, et al. An IL-4 receptor region containing an insulin receptor motif is important for IL-4-mediated IRS-1 phosphorylation and cell growth. Cell 1994;76:811
45. White MF, Maron R, Kahn CR. Insulin rapidly stimulates tyrosine phosphorylation of a Mr 185,000 protein in intact cells. Nature 1985;318:183
46. Izumi T, White MF, Kadowaki T, et al. Insulin-like growth factor I rapidly stimulates tyrosine phosphorylation of a Mr 185,000 protein in intact cells. J Biol Chem 1987;262:1282
47. Sun XJ, Rothenberg P, Kahn CR, et al. The structure of the insulin receptor substrate IRS-1 defines a unique signal transduction protein. Nature 1991; 352:73
48. Araki E, Sun XJ, Haag BL, et al. Human skeletal muscle insulin receptor substrate-1: Characterization of the cDNA, gene and chromosomal localization. Diabetes 1993;42:1041
49. Nishiyama M, Wands JR. Cloning and increased expression of an insulin receptor substrate-1-like gene in human hepatocellular carcinoma. Biochem Biophys Res Commun 1992;183:280
50. Keller SR, Aebersold R, Garner CW, Lienhard GE. The insulin-elicited 160kDa phosphotyrosine protein in mouse adipocytes is an insulin receptor substrate 1: Identification by cloning. Bioclinica Biophysica Acta 1993; 1172:323
51. Sun XJ, Miralpeix M, Myers MG Jr, et al. The expression and function of IRS-1 in insulin signal transmission. J Biol Chem 1992;267:22662
52. Araki E, Lipes MA, Patti ME, et al. Alternative pathway of insulin signalling in mice with targeted disruption of the IRS-1 gene. Nature 1994;372:186
53. Tamemoto H, Kadowaki T, Tobe K, et al. Insulin resistance and growth retardation in mice lacking insulin receptor substrate-1. Nature 1994;372:182
54. Backer JM, Myers MG Jr, Shoelson SE, et al. The phosphatidylinositol 3′-kinase is activated by association with IRS-1 during insulin stimulation. EMBO J 1992;11:3469
55. Myers MG Jr, Backer JM, Sun XJ, et al. IRS-1 activates the phosphatidylinositol 3′-kinase by associating with the src homology 2 domains of p85. Proc Natl Acad Sci USA 1992;89:10350
56. Rozakis-Adcock M, Femley R, Wade J, et al. The SH2 and SH3 domains of mammalian Grb2 couple the EGF receptor to the Ras activator mSos1. Nature 1993;363:83
57. Li N, Batzer A, Daly R, et al. Guanine-nucleotide-releasing factor mSos1 binds to Grb2 and links receptor tyrosine kinases to Ras signalling. Nature 1993;363:85
58. Egan SE, Giddings BW, Brooks MW, et al. Association of Sos ras exchange protein with Grb2 is implicated in tyrosine kinase signal transduction and transformation. Nature 1993;363:45
59. Lowenstein EJ, Daly RJ, Batzer AG, et al. The SH2 and SH3 domain-containing proteins GRB2 links receptor tyrosine kinases to ras signaling. Cell 1992;70:431
60. Skolnik EY, Batzer A, Li N, et al. The function of GRB2 in linking the insulin receptor to ras signaling pathways. Science 1993;260:1953
61. Myers MG Jr, Wang LM, Sun XJ, et al. The role of IRS-1/GRB2 complexes in insulin signaling. Mol Cell Biol 1994;14:3577
62. Pruett W, Yuan Y, Rose E, et al. Association between GRB2/Sos and insulin receptor substrate 1 is not sufficient for activation of extracellular signal-regulated kinases by interleukin-4: Implications for ras activation by insulin. Mol Cell Biol 1995;15:1778
63. Sasaoka T, Draznin B, Leitner JW, et al. Shc is the predominant signaling molecule coupling insulin receptors to activation of guanine nucleotide releasing factor and p21ras formation. J Biol Chem 1994;269:10734
64. Pronk GJ, McGlade J, Pelicci G, et al. Insulin-induced phosphorylation of the 46- and 52-kDa Shc proteins. J Biol Chem 1993;268:5748
65. Pellici G, Lanfrancone L, Grignani F, et al. A novel transforming protein (SHC) with an SH2 domain is implicated in mitogenic signal transduction. Cell 1992;70:93
66. Kavanaugh WM, Williams LT. An alternative to SH2 domains for binding tyrosine-phosphorylated proteins. Science 1994;266:1862
67. Blaikie P, Immanuel D, Wu J, et al. A region in shc distinct from the SH2 domain can bind tyrosine-phosphorylated growth factor receptors. J Biol Chem 1994;269:32031
68. Wang LM, Myers MG Jr, Sun XJ, et al. IRS-1: Essential for insulin and IL-4-stimulated mitogenesis in hematopoietic cells. Science 1993:261:1591
69. Waters SB, Yamauchi K, Pessin JE. Functional expression of insulin receptor substrate-1 is required for insulin-stimulated mitogenic signaling. J Biol Chem 1993;238:22231
70. Rose DW, Saltiel AR, Majumdar M, et al. Insulin receptor substrate 1 is required for insulin-mediated mitogenic signal transduction. Proc Natl Acad Sci USA 1994;91:797
71. Kapeller R, Cantley LC. Phosphatidylinositol 3-kinase. Bio Essays 1994; 16:565
72. Varticovski L, Daley GQ, Jackson P, et al. Activation of phosphatidylinositol 3-kinase in cells expressing *abl* oncogene variants. Mol Cell Biol 1991; 11:1107
73. Soltoff SP, Rabin SL, Cantley LC, Kaplan DR. Nerve growth factor promotes the activation of phosphatidylinositol 3-kinase and its association with the trk tyrosine kinase. J Biol Chem 1992;267:17472
74. Kundra V, Escobedo JA, Kazlauskas A, et al. Regulation of Chemotaxis by the Platelet-Derived Growth Factor Receptor-Beta. Nature 1994;367:474
75. Ridley AJ. Membrane ruffling and signal transduction. Bio Essays 1994; 16:321
76. Cheatham B, Vlahos CJ, Cheatham L, et al. Phosphatidylinositol 3-kinase activation is required for insulin stimulation of pp70 S6 kinase. DNA synthesis and glucose transporter translocation. Mol Cell Biol 1994;14:4902
77. Chung J, Grammer TC, Lemon KP, et al. PDGF-and insulin-dependent pp70S6k activation mediated by phosphatidylinositol-3-OH kinase. Nature 1994;370:71
78. Myers MG Jr, Grammer TC, Wang LM, et al. IRS-1 mediates PI 3′-kinase and $p70^{s6k}$ signaling during insulin, IGF-1 and IL-4 stimulation. J Biol Chem 1994;269:28783
79. Okada T, Kawano Y, Sakakibara T, et al. Essential role of phosphatidylinositol 3-kinase in insulin-induced glucose transport and antilipolysis in rat adipocytes. J Biochem 1994;269:3568
80. Cheatham B, Vlahos CJ, Cheatham L, et al. Phosphatidylinositol 3-kinase activation is required for insulin stimulation of pp70 S6 kinase DNA synthesis and glucose transporter translocation. Mol Cell Biol 1994;14:4902
81. Otsu M, Hiles I, Gout I, et al. Characterization of two 85 kD proteins that associate with receptor tyrosine kinases, middle-T/$pp60^{c-src}$ complexes and PI3-kinase. Cell 1991;65:91
82. Skolnik EY. Margolis B, Mohammadi M, et al. Cloning of PI3 kinase-associated p85 utilizing a novel method for expression/cloning of target proteins for receptor tyrosine kinases. Cell 1991;65:83
83. Kapeller R, Prasad KVS, Janssen O, et al. Identification of two SH3-binding motifs in the regulatory subunit of phosphatidylinositol 3-kinase. J Biol Chem 1994;269:1927
84. Dhand R, Hara K, Hiles I, et al. PI3-kinase: Structural and functional analysis of intersubunit interactions. EMBO 1994;13:511
85. Klippel A, Escobedo JA, Hirano M, Williams LT. The interaction of small domains between the subunits of phosphatidylinositol 3-kinase determines enzyme activity. Mol Cell Biol 1994;14:2675
86. Baltensperger K, Kozma LM, Jaspers SR, et al. Regulation by insulin of phosphatidylinositol 3′-kinase bound to α- and β-isoforms of p85 regulatory subunit. [Abstract] J Biol Chem 1994;269:28937
87. Hu P, Mondino A, Skolnik EY, Schlessinger J. Cloning of a novel, ubiquitously expressed human phosphatidylinositol 3-kinase and identification of its binding site on p85. Mol Cell Biol 1993;13:7677
88. Hiles ID, Otsu M, Volinna S, et al. Phosphatidylinositol 3-kinase: Structure and expression of the 100 kd catalytic subunit. Cell 1992;70:419
89. Schu PV, Kaoru T, Fry MJ, et al. Phosphatidylinositol 3-kinase encoded by yeast *VPS*34 gene essential for protein sorting. Science 1993;260:88
90. Welters P, Takegawa K, Emr SD, Chrispeels MJ. A*t*VPS34, a phosphatidylinositol 3-kinase of *Arabidopsis thaliana,* is an essential protein with homology to a calcium-dependent lipid binding domain. Proc Natl Acad Sci USA 1994;91:11398
91. Stack JH, Herman PK, Schu PV, Emr SD. A membrane-associated complex containing the Vps15 protein kinase and the Vps34 PI3-kinase is essential for protein sorting to the yeast lysosome-like vacuole. EMBO J 1993;12:2195
92. Joly M, Kazlauskas A, Fay FS, Corvera S. Disruption of PDGF receptor trafficking by mutation of its PI-3 kinase binding sites. Science 1994;263:684
93. Hanks SK, Quinn AM, Hunter T. The protein kinase family: Conserved features and deduced phylogeny of the catalytic domain. Science 1990;241:42
94. Lam K, Carpenter CL, Ruderman NB, et al. The phosphatidylinositol 3-kinase serine kinase phosphorylases IRS-1. J Biol Chem 1994;269:20648
95. Myers MG Jr, Backer JM, Sun XJ, et al. IRS-1 activates phosphatidylinositol 3′-kinase by associating with src homology 2 domains of p85. Proc Natl Acad Sci USA 1992;89:10350
96. Shoelson SE, Sivaraja M, Williams KP, et al. Specific phosphopeptide binding regulates a conformational change in the PI3-kinase SH2 domain associated with enzyme activation. EMBO J 1993;12:795

97. Hu P, Margolis B, Skolnik EY, et al. Interactions of PI 3-kinase-associated p85 with EGF and PDGF receptors. Mol Cell Biol 1992;12:981
98. Pleiman CM, Hertz WM, Cambier JC. Activation of phosphatidylinositol 3'-kinase by Src-family kinase SH3 binding to the p85 subunit. Science 1994;263:1609
99. Rodriguez-Viciana P, Wame PH, Dhand R, et al. Phosphatidylinositol-3-OH kinase as a direct target of Ras. Nature 1994;370:527
100. Dhand R, Hiles I, Panayotou G, et al. PI-3-kinase is a dual specificity enzyme—autoregulation by an intrinsic protein-serine kinase activity. EMBO J1994; 13:522
101. Kelly KL, Ruderman NB. Insulin-stimulated phosphatidylinositol 3-kinase: Association with a 185-kDa tyrosine-phosphorylated protein (IRS-1) and localization in a low density membrane vesicle. J Biol Chem 1993;268:4391
102. Toker A, Meyer M, Reddy K, et al. Activation of protein kinase C family members by the novel polyphosphoinositides PtdIns-3,4-P_3. J Biol Chem 1994;269:32358
103. Pons S, Asano T, Glasheen E, et al. The structure and function of p55[PIK] reveals a new regulatory subunit for the phosphatidylinositol-3 kinase. Mol Cell Biol 1995;15(8):4453–4465
104. Lienhard GE, Slot JW, James DE, Mueckler MM. How cells absorb glucose. Sci Am 1992;266:86
105. Hara K, Yonezawa K, Sakaue H, et al. Phosphoinositide 3-kinase activity is required for insulin-stimulated glucose transport but not for ras activation in CHO cells. Proc Natl Acad Sci USA 1994;91(16):7415–9
106. Lavan BE, Lienhard GE. The insulin-elicited 60-kDa phosphotyrosine protein in rat adipocytes is associated with phosphatidylinositol 3-kinase. J Biol Chem 1993;268:5921
107. Haring HU, White MF, Machicao F, et al. Insulin rapidly stimulates phosphorylation of a 46-kDa membrane protein on tyrosine residues as well as phosphorylation of several soluble proteins in intact fat cells. Proc Natl Acad Sci USA 1987;84:113
108. Momomura K, Tobe K, Seyama Y, et al. Insulin-induced tyrosine phosphorylation in intact rat adipocytes. Biochem Biophys Res Commun 1988;155:1181
109. Steele-Perkins G, Roth RA. Insulin-mimetic anti-insulin receptor monoclonal antibodies stimulate receptor kinase activity in intact cells. J Biol Chem 1990;265:9458
110. Hosomi Y, Shii K, Ogawa W, et al. Characterization of a 60-kilodalton substrate of the insulin receptor kinase. J Biol Chem 1994;269:11498

Diabetes Mellitus, edited by Derek LeRoith, Simeon I. Taylor, and Jerrold M. Olefsky. Lippincott–Raven Publishers, Philadelphia © 1996.

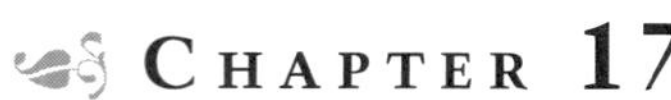

CHAPTER 17

Small GTPases and (Serine/Threonine) Protein Kinase Cascades in Insulin Signal Transduction

JOSEPH AVRUCH

Insulin is the dominant hormone regulating nutrient storage and utilization, and there has been a comprehensive understanding of the effects of insulin on fuel metabolism for some time. The discovery of cAMP in the mid 1950s and the recognition of its role as the intracellular mediator of the actions of glucagon and β-adrenergic catecholamines on glycogen and lipid metabolism refocused attention from the description of insulin's effects on nutrient and metabolite flux to the study of the regulatory mechanisms that underlie its ability to redirect cellular energy metabolism. Two general strategies were adopted. In one approach, effort was directed at characterizing the initial steps in the interaction of insulin with its target cell, examining first the binding of insulin to a putative receptor and progressing to the isolation of the receptor and its identification as a member of the receptor tyrosine kinase family. The latter finding was ultimately verified when the primary structure of the receptor was established by molecular cloning. Subsequent discoveries concerning the role of SH2 domain-containing proteins as the proximate downstream signaling element employed by tyrosine kinases, together with elucidation of the structure of the major substrates of the insulin receptor tyrosine kinase (i.e., the insulin receptor substrate [IRS] family of polypeptides) and their probable function as a platform for the assembly of multiple SH2 domain-containing polypeptides, have provided a molecular basis for understanding how the insulin-receptor interaction leads to the generation of multiple independent but coordinated intracellular signals.

Another approach to understanding insulin action developed from the study of the regulatory apparatus that controls the activity of the rate-limiting enzymes of metabolism. This approach attempted to peel back the steps composing the insulin signal transduction pathways to the earliest reactions triggered by receptor activation. Significant convergence of these two strategies has been achieved, and although the identity of all the important intracellular signals generated as a result of receptor tyrosine kinase activation is far from settled, activation of Ras and PI-3-kinase are established as crucial for a number of insulin's characteristic biologic effects. The specific biochemical steps that link these secondary intracellular signal generators together with the distal metabolic machinery of the physiologic target cells, are still incompletely understood; this area of insulin signal transduction contains most of the major outstanding questions in the reconstruction of the biochemical basis for insulin action. Nevertheless, the general nature of these linking steps has been established, and it is clear that the central elements are small GTPases and their regulatory proteins, acting in concert with a large number of protein Ser/Thr kinases, the latter arranged in parallel cascades. The evolution of information in support of this view, the current understanding of the operation of these elements at a molecular level, and their specific roles in carrying out insulin signal transduction are the primary topics of this chapter.

Insulin-Activated Protein Kinase Cascades: Early Observations

The discovery of cAMP and the concept of signal transduction emerged from the efforts of Sutherland and coworkers[1] to understand how glucagon and epinephrine induced the phosphorylation and stable activation of the enzyme glycogen phosphorylase when added to an intact liver slice but were ineffective when added to a cell-free homogenate of the same liver slice. They found that the

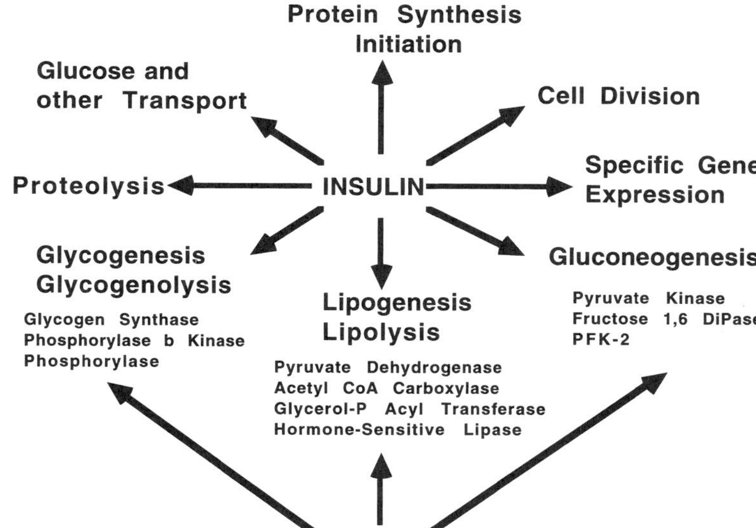

Figure 17-1. Metabolic responses to insulin and cAMP.

addition of the glycogenolytic hormones to liver membranes in the presence of Mg ATP led to the synthesis of a low-molecular-weight heat-stable substance, later identified as cAMP. When added to membrane-free liver extracts, this substance was effective in promoting the Mg ATP–dependent, stable activation of endogenous or added phosphorylase. Thus the glycogenolytic signal brought to the intact cell by the hormone had been transferred completely to an intracellular molecule (cAMP) that in turn controlled the activity of the enzymes necessary for the phosphorylation and stable activation of phosphorylase. Larner and coworkers[2] found that a similar approach could be applied to understanding the glycogenic effect of insulin; they observed that addition of insulin in vitro to intact preparations of skeletal muscle led to a rapid in situ activation of the enzyme glycogen synthase (GS). GS was stable after extraction from the tissue, much as had been found for the activation of hepatic phosphorylase by glucagon and epinephrine. Subsequent work established that hormonal regulation of GS was attributable to changes in its covalent phosphorylation on serine and/or threonine residues. Insulin activation resulted from a net dephosphorylation of the GS polypeptide, whereas cAMP-mediated GS inactivation was attributable to multisite GS phosphorylation.[3]

Building on these early findings, the biochemical basis for many of the metabolic responses to insulin and cAMP came to be understood in terms of alterations in the activity of specific enzymes and transport systems. In most of these systems (Fig. 17-1), the hormone-induced change in enzyme activity could be attributed to a change in the extent of regulatory Ser/Thr phosphorylation. In each instance, regardless of whether insulin increased or decreased enzyme activity, insulin promoted an overall dephosphorylation of the target enzyme polypeptide, an effect usually opposite to that elicited by cAMP. In many but not all instances, such antagonism could be explained by the ability of insulin to inhibit the increase in cAMP levels induced by glucagon (in liver) or β-adrenergic catecholamines (in adipose cells) as a result of insulin activation of a specific cAMP phosphodiesterase (see Chapter 20). Direct examination of the effect of insulin and cAMP on overall protein phosphorylation in intact ^{32}P-labeled rat adipocytes or hepatocytes confirmed its ability to inhibit many of the cAMP-stimulated increases in protein phosphorylation. Unexpectedly, however, when insulin was added to ^{32}P-labeled target cells as the sole hormone, the predominant response observed was the increased Ser/Thr phosphorylation of a subset of cellular proteins that was not attributable to the inhibition of (and was often partially additive with) cAMP-regulated phosphorylation.[4] Insulin-stimulated protein phosphorylation was rapid in onset and reversible on removal of hormone and occurred at physiologic insulin concentrations. Although no examples of insulin regulation of enzyme activity attributable to increased polypeptide (Ser/Thr) phosphorylation were then known, it was anticipated that these insulin-stimulated (Ser/Thr) phosphorylations reflected intermediate steps in insulin signal transduction. In effect, it was envisioned that engagement of the insulin receptor somehow led to activation of one or more protein (Ser/Thr) kinases, which phosphorylated target proteins whose activity was thereby changed. The altered activities of the insulin-stimulated phosphoproteins were presumed to underlie some subset of the more distal biochemical responses, perhaps even initiating some of the many regulatory dephosphorylations elicited by insulin.[5] Although this model is now amply confirmed, verification of the regulatory role of insulin-stimulated Ser/Thr phosphorylation was slow in forthcoming. The first several insulin-stimulated phosphoproteins identified were the lipogenic enzymes, ATP citrate lyase and acetyl CoA carboxylase, an outcome determined in part by the relatively high abundance of these enzymes in cells such as adipocytes and hepatocytes (from carbohydrate-fed rats) that carry out de novo fatty acid synthesis. The regulatory significance (if any) of the insulin-induced phosphorylation of these enzymes is still obscure.[6,7] Similar studies carried out in cultured cells consistently found the insulin-stimulated phosphorylation of a 31 kd polypeptide, identified as the 40S ribosomal protein, S6.[8,9] As with the lipogenic enzymes, the regulatory significance of insulin-stimulated ribosomal S6 phosphorylation remains poorly understood. Nevertheless, a rapid increase in S6 phosphorylation was also seen in response to numerous polypeptide growth factors and mitogens. Based on the premise that S6 phosphorylation reflected the activation in situ of protein kinase(s) that participated in insulin-mitogen signal transduction, efforts to establish assays for such insulin-activated protein kinase(s) went forward. 40S Ribosomal subunits provided a convenient, stable substrate that was phosphorylated selectively on S6 in vitro by appropriately prepared cell extracts. Moreover, insulin or mitogen treatment of cells prior to extraction greatly increased the apparent S6 kinase activity.[10] The development of reliable assays for insulin-activated S6 protein kinases enabled the ultimate purification of these enzymes and identified extraction conditions that later proved applicable to a wide array of insulin and mitogen-stimulated protein (Ser/Thr) kinases, most notably the enzymes known as the MAP kinases (Table 17-1).[11]

The first of the insulin-activated Ser/Thr kinases to be purified was an S6 kinase from *Xenopus* oocytes,[12] later named Rsk (*r*ibo-

Table 17-1. Insulin-Regulated Protein (Ser/Thr) Kinases

Stimulated	Inhibited
(Known structure)	
RSK (1, 2, ?3)	cAMP-dependent protein kinase
P70 S6 kinases (αI, αII)	5′AMP-activated protein kinase
p42 MAP kinase (erk2); p44 MAP kinase (erk1)	Glycogen synthase kinase-3
MAP kinase-kinases (1,2)	
cRaf-1/B Raf/?A Raf	
Casein kinase-2	
?PKCs (see Chapter 19)	
c-akt/PKB	
(Unknown structure)	
cAMP-Phosphodiesterase-kinase	

somal *S*6 *k*inase). A second kind of S6 kinase called the p70 S6 kinase was subsequently purified from rat liver.[13,14] Both Rsk and p70 are ubiquitously expressed in mammalian cells and are activated coordinately in response to insulin as well as a variety of growth factors and mitogens. Moreover, both kinds of S6 kinase were found to be activated through Ser/Thr phosphorylation of the enzyme polypeptide. The S6 kinases themselves thus proved to be the first "physiologic," that is, functionally regulated targets of insulin-stimulated Ser/Thr phosphorylation to be identified. Neither variety of S6 kinase is activated by autophosphorylation in situ, nor do the two kinds of S6 kinase cross-regulate each other in situ. Thus, the activation of the S6 kinases through Ser/Thr phosphorylation in situ implied the existence of at least one additional tier of protein Ser/Thr kinases interposed between the insulin receptor tyrosine kinase and the S6 kinases.

Evidence that the two S6 kinases were situated on separate limbs of the signal outflow from the activated insulin receptor was provided by the finding that the immunosuppressant drug rapamycin, added to intact cells, inhibits the activation of p70 S6 kinase (and 40S phosphorylation in situ) but not of Rsk,[15,16] indicating the existence of upstream elements required uniquely for p70 activation that are dispensable for Rsk activation. Techniques similar to those applied to the S6 kinases led to the discovery of an insulin-stimulated kinase active in vitro on the microtubule-associated protein-2 (MAP-2).[17] From this point, elucidating the signal transduction pathway interposed between the receptor and Rsk was accomplished with startling rapidity.

The MAP Kinase Pathway

Protein kinase cascades have been known for many years; the first well-characterized protein kinase, skeletal muscle phosphorylase b kinase, in addition to its regulation by Ca/calmodulin, undergoes phosphorylation and activation by the cAMP-dependent protein kinase. Subsequent work on the regulation of cholesterol metabolism led to the discovery of the enzyme known as the 5′AMP-activated protein kinase, which is activated allosterically by 5′AMP as well as by Ser/Thr phosphorylation through an upstream kinase.

Direct evidence for the operation of a protein kinase cascade downstream of the insulin receptor was first provided by the finding that the insulin-stimulated p42 MAP kinase could phosphorylate in vitro and activate the *Xenopus* S6 kinase II (Rsk-2).[18] The potential importance of the p42 MAP kinase in insulin signal transduction was further emphasized by the demonstration that activation of the enzyme in situ in response to insulin was accompanied by increased tyrosine phosphorylation of the 42 kd kinase polypeptide.[19] Moreover, tyrosine dephosphorylation in vitro, using a specific tyrosine phosphatase, resulted in deactivation of the MAP kinase.[20] The p42 MAP kinase was thus among the first enzymes shown to be regulated through tyrosine phosphorylation. Studies of growth factor–regulated protein phosphorylation had previously detected a family of low abundance 40–45 kd polypeptides that exhibited rapid increases in tyrosine phosphorylation in response to numerous growth factors; the p42 MAP kinase was shown to be one of these polypeptides.[21] These results raised the intriguing possibility that the MAP kinases were direct substrates for activated receptor tyrosine kinases. However, this idea was rapidly discarded when it was shown that the insulin-mitogen–regulated activator of the MAP kinase was not a membrane protein but another cytosolic protein kinase.[22] The MAP kinase-kinase exhibited a novel dual specificity in activating the MAP kinase, phosphorylating both a tyrosine and a threonine residue in the sequence _ _ _ TEY _ _ _ situated on a loop near the catalytic center of the MAP kinase polypeptide. Despite its unusual Tyr/Thr specificity, the MAP kinase-kinase itself proved to be regulated entirely by Ser/Thr phosphorylation.[23] Thus, in short order a cascade of three insulin-activated cytosolic protein kinases (MAPKK/MAPK/RSK) had been uncovered, with at least one additional protein (Ser/Thr) kinase situated upstream. However, the mechanism coupling this cascade to receptor activation was not yet evident.

An important insight into the overall architecture of the MAP kinase cascade was provided when the sequence of a mammalian MAP kinase, obtained by molecular cloning, was found to have a striking similarity to the sequences of a pair of protein kinases (FUS3 and KSS1) discovered in in *Saccharomyces cerevisiae* as genes required for the mating yeast response to the α/A pheromone.[24] KSS1 and FUS3, 61% identical in amino acid sequence to each other, are each approximately 52% identical to the mammalian p44 MAP kinase isoform first cloned and renamed erk1 for extracellular signal regulated kinase-1. In addition to this astonishing degree of overall identity, KSS1 and FUS3 exhibit a TEY motif corresponding to the site of activating phosphorylation in erk1. In analyzing other gene products required for the mating response in budding yeast, a variety of sterile (Ste) mutants had been selected, assigned to different complementation groups, and ordered in their sequence of action using genetic epistasis.[25] On this basis it was known that in addition to the pheromone receptor, a heterotrimeric G-protein was required for signal transduction, and the genetic evidence indicated that the βγ subunits served as the positive regulator of the mating pathway. Downstream of the G-protein, a series of genes encoding protein kinases had been uncovered whose apparent sequence of action appeared to be Ste20, Ste11, and Ste7, followed by KSS1/FUS3. A homologous set of protein kinase genes had also been identified as encoding elements critical for the mating pathway in the fusion yeast, *Schizosaccharomyces pombe*. The *S. pombe* homolog of KSS1/FUS3 is spk1, upstream of which is an Ste7 homolog known as byr1, which is activated by an Ste11 homolog known as byr2. Remarkably, spk1 has a comparable sequence identity to that of mammalian erk1 (56%) and to FUS3 (58%) and KSS1 (57%), and both the mammalian and *Xenopus* erks, when overexpressed in *S. pombe*, can partially complement spk1 deletion. Based on the amino acid sequence and functional homology between erk1 and its yeast homologs, it was anticipated the mammalian MAP kinase-kinase would be a protein kinase with structural homology to Ste7 and byr1. This expectation was borne out when peptide and subsequently cDNA sequences corresponding to mammalian MAP kinase-kinase (also called MEK, *M*AP, and *E*RK *K*inase) were analyzed.[26] In turn, given the substantial similarity in structure and regulation between the mammalian and yeast MEKs, the activator of mammalian MEK was plausibly expected to be closely related in primary sequence to the Ste11/byr2 protein kinases.

The Raf Proto-oncogenes Direct the MAP Kinase Pathway

Contrary to expectation, the mammalian MEK activator usually recruited by receptor tyrosine kinases, as well as by G-protein–linked receptors with mitogenic potential, is one of the members of the Raf family of protein (Ser/Thr) kinase proto-oncogenes, a conclusion based on considerable biochemical and genetic evidence.[27] Thus, in addition to the ability of Raf to phosphorylate and activate MEK directly in vitro,[28] independent genetic evidence gained from the study of several pathways of cellular development in *Drosophila* and *Caenorhabditis elegans* places Raf as an obligatory intermediate between receptor tyrosine kinases (RTKs) and MEK. Three Raf isoforms are known—c-Raf 1, ARaf, and BRaf—each isoform functions as an MEK activator. ARaf is found predominantly in genitourinary tissues, and BRaf is most highly expressed in the nervous system. c-Raf 1 is quite abundant in skeletal muscle but is widely expressed. Interestingly, lower eukaryotes do not have structural homologs of Raf, whose catalytic domain exhibits no sequence identity to Ste11/byr2 beyond the level (~25%) shared by the entire protein kinase superfamily. Not surprisingly, despite the ability of mammalian erk1 or erk2 to complement spk1 deficiency, mammalian MEK does not rescue byr1 deficiency unless MEK is introduced into *S. pombe* together with an active Raf.[29]

Although Raf kinases are the most ubiquitous and best established MEK activators identified thus far, other MEK activators exist. Mammalian cells express a subfamily of at least six protein kinases that bear considerable sequence similarity to Ste11/byr2. The first of these was identified by a polymerase chain reaction–based approach utilizing oligonucleotides based on amino acid sequences peculiar to and conserved between Ste11 and byr2. The kinase thus isolated was shown to be capable of activating mammalian MEK, both in situ and in vitro, and was therefore named MEK kinase (MEKK1).[30] Subsequent work, however, demonstrated that MEKK1-catalyzed activation of MEK occurs only with marked MEKK1 overexpression, and under more physiologic conditions, MEKK1 functions as an upstream element in the stress-activated protein kinase (SAPK) pathway, a parallel protein kinase cascade that is regulated independently of the MAP kinase cascade.[31,32] The SAPK pathway in most cells is activated weakly or not at all by receptor tyrosine kinases but is strongly activated in response to cellular stress and inflammatory cytokines.[33] Emerging evidence indicates that mammalian cells, like yeast, express several (at least four) independently regulated erk-based protein kinase cascades, in addition to the insulin-activated MAP kinase cascades that utilize erk1 and erk2. The members of the MEKK family identified thus far, although perhaps capable of MEK activation when greatly stimulated, probably serve primarily to regulate one or more of these functionally distinct signaling pathways.

The protein kinase product of the *c-mos* proto-oncogene can also phosphorylate and activate mammalian MEK in vitro.[34,35] Although this activation is likely to reflect a physiologic regulatory event, significant *c-mos* expression is limited to oocytes and the first several cycles of cell division after fertilization, and thus *c-mos* is unlikely to be an MEK activator of general significance.

The possibility that insulin-regulated protein kinases other than Raf serve as physiologic MEK activators remains open. Although insulin activates one or more members of the Raf family in all cells examined thus far, several reports have described insulin-activated MEK activators in adipocytes and 3T3 cells that appear to be chromatographically and immunochemically distinct from known members of the RAF family as well as from *c-mos* and MEKK.[36,37] The identity of such putative alternate insulin-responsive MEK activators is not known.

Inasmuch as MEK mutants that are constitutively active and Raf-independent are transforming when expressed in fibroblasts,[38,39] it appears quite clear that activation of MEK is sufficient explanation for RAF's transforming activity. Nevertheless, a number of instances have been observed in which introduction of activated Raf fails to induce activation of the MAP kinase pathway but nonetheless elicits a mitogenic or cell differentiation response.[40,41] The lack of measurable MEK activation implies that negative regulation of the MAP kinase cascade exists at the level of MEK, perhaps attributable to the action of protein phosphatases. The ability of Raf to direct cell fate in these circumstances indicates that Raf is capable of activating pathways other than the MAP kinase cascade. One such pathway may be mediated by cyclin-dependent kinases.

Current concepts of cell cycle regulation envision this progression to be driven by the sequential activation of cyclin-dependent kinases (cdks).[42] The cyclins are a diverse family of activating regulatory subunits for the cdks whose availability is regulated at the level of gene transcription and by control of their degradation. In addition to a requirement for cyclin binding, the kinase subunits (cdks) are further controlled by several independently regulated phosphorylation events, that is, an activating phosphorylation in catalytic subdomain VIII and an inhibitory phosphorylation within the ATP binding site in catalytic subdomain I. The final step in activation of the fully assembled cyclin-cdk complex is the removal of this inhibitory phosphorylation, a reaction catalyzed by the family of protein phosphatases known as cdc25. Recent studies[43] have shown that a stable association occurs between cRAF 1 and certain isoforms of the cdc25 protein phosphatase both in vitro and in situ. Importantly, Raf 1 phosphorylates cdc25 in vitro (primarily the A isoform, which is predominant during G_1 in mammalian cells) and activates its phosphatase activity; cdc25, in turn, dephosphorylates the inhibitory TyrP/ThrP residues in the catalytic subdomain I of the cdks, releasing the cyclin-cdk complex into an active state. This process thereby provides a second, alternate, or complementary pathway for Raf-mediated mitogenic/cell fate regulation.

The discovery that cRaf 1 (and the other Raf family members, particularly B Raf) served as the MEK activator usually recruited by receptor tyrosine kinases turned attention toward the mechanism of Raf activation by these receptors.[27] The Raf polypeptides exhibit three regions of highly conserved sequence: the catalytic domain (CR3 segment) occupies the carboxy terminal half of the polypeptides, whereas the noncatalytic amino terminal segment contains two regions (CR1 and CR2) of highly conserved sequence. A striking feature of the CR1 segment is the presence of a zinc finger structure analogous to those in the noncatalytic regulatory region of the protein kinase C polypeptides, a structure known to participate in phospholipid and/or diacylglycerol binding in that kinase family. An important clue as to the function of these Raf amino terminal domains was provided by the structure of the oncogenic forms of Raf. Spontaneously arising c-Raf 1-derived oncogenes almost always exhibit amino terminal deletion past amino acid 270 removing the CR1 and CR2 domains, with expression of Raf polypeptides either from the first inframe ATG/codon (i.e. specifying methionine) or fused inframe to viral gag sequences. Purposeful amino terminal deletion of c-Raf 1 beyond amino 270, so as to remove the CR1 and CR2 segments, results in the appearance of transforming activity; such Raf variants exhibit a constitutive kinase activity. Thus, two functions can be assigned to the Raf amino terminal noncatalytic sequences: first, this segment is necessary for suppression of the kinase activity and transforming potential of the catalytic domain. In addition, inasmuch as insulin and mitogens produce a regulated disinhibition of the Raf kinase, the amino terminal segment must also encompass the targets for the activating signals generated by receptor tyrosine kinases. Considerable genetic and mammalian transfection data indicate that an active c-Ras polypeptide was required at a step in between the receptor and Raf activation. One popular idea was that like the heterodimeric G-proteins, Ras operated by triggering some membrane-signaling element to synthesize a ligand that interacted with the Raf CR1/CR2 domains, much like diacylglycerol interacts with the regulatory domains of the PKCFs, thereby initiating Raf activation. Remarkably, the crucial signal for Raf activation is provided directly by the Ras proto-oncogene, which in its active, GTP-liganded state, binds directly to the CR1 domain of Raf and recruits the Raf kinase to the plasma membrane.

Ras Interaction with Raf and Other Downstream Effectors

v-*Ras* was discovered as the transforming agent in several rodent sarcoma viruses and subsequently as the first "spontaneous" oncogene recovered by transfection of genomic DNA from human tumors into NIH 3T3 cells.[44] The cellular Ras polypeptides are bound to the inner leaflet of the plasma membrane through the combined effects of a carboxy terminal cysteinyl-S-farnesyl moiety and a second element, slightly further amino terminal that is either a set of cysteinyl-S-palmitoyl side chains (Ha-Ras, N-Ras) or a highly basic (polylysine) segment (Ki-Ras). Localization at the inner leaflet of the plasma membrane is indispensable for the functions of both normal and oncogenic Ras proteins. Ras is a guanyl nucleotide–binding protein that is active when bound to guanosine triphosphate (GTP).[45] Cellular Ras is a GTPase that in isolation exhibits relatively slow rates of guanyl nucleotide exchange and GTP hydrolysis. Cytosolic proteins that accelerate GTP hydrolysis (GTPase activator proteins, GAPs) and the rate of guanyl nucleotide release (guanyl nucleotide exchange factors, GNEFs) are known to be important targets by which receptors regulate the relative amount of GTP-GDP bound to Ras.[46] Oncogenic versions of Ras contain mutations that impair the intrinsic and/or GAP-stimulated GTPase activity or greatly accelerate the rate of spontaneous guanyl nucleotide dissociation. The latter mutations also promote the residence of Ras in its GTP-bound, active state, because cellular levels of GTP greatly exceed those of GDP. As anticipated from its "oncogenic" origin, purposeful introduction of v-*Ras* into cultured mammalian cells leads to morphologic transformation and mitogenesis. In some cell backgrounds, however, v-*Ras* produces cell cycle arrest and terminal differentiation, as for example in the PC12 pheochromocytoma cell. An extensive analysis of the effects of mutagenesis on the transforming activity of oncogenic versions of Ras polypeptide established that transformation of NIH 3T3 cells could be abrogated by mutations near the Ras carboxy terminus that prevented polypeptide insertion in the plasma membrane as well as by mutations in a segment between Ras residues 32 and 40. The latter mutations had no demonstrable effects on Ras membrane insertion or intrinsic GTP binding and GTPase activities. Therefore the segment encompassing these inactivating mutations came to be viewed as the Ras "effector" domain, that is, a segment whose primary biochemical function was to transmit the mitogenic signal, presumably by interaction with and activation of one or more downstream cellular elements.[47] This model was strengthened when elucidation of the Ras crystal structures showed that Ras residues 32–40 were on a loop that was one of the two segments of the polypeptide whose configuration changed depending on whether the bound nucleotide was GTP or GDP. Early studies in *S. cerevisiae* indicated that adenyl cyclase served as an immediate downstream effector of yeast Ras; cyclase was rapidly eliminated as a candidate effector in mammalian cells. The discovery of the Ras GTPase activator protein (GAP) provided the first candidate mammalian Ras effector inasmuch as some effector targets of heterotrimeric Gα subunits were known to stimulate Gα GTP hydrolysis. Moreover, some inactivating mutations in the Ras effector loop interfere with the binding of GAP to Ras. Nevertheless, when examined across an array of Ras effector loop mutations, the correlation between the loss of GAP binding and the loss of v-*Ras* transforming efficiency is inconsistent. In addition, genetic evidence pointed to a negative regulatory function for Ras GAP in receptor tyrosine kinase signaling for mitogenesis. Although the specific biochemical functions of Ras remained elusive, a large body of genetic evidence in *C. elegans* and *Drosophila* indicated that the c-*Ras* proto-oncogene served as an indispensable positive regulator in the signaling pathway downstream of receptor tyrosine kinases and in the activation of Raf and the MAPKs. In mammalian systems, it was shown that inhibition of Ras function, achieved by transfection of dominant inhibitory Ras mutants or microinjection of inhibitory Ras antibodies not only prevented growth–factor induced DNA synthesis but also prevented the activation of Raf, MAP kinase, and Rsk, implying that Ras functioned upstream of these elements. Reciprocally, inactive variants of Raf (such as the c-Raf amino terminal fragment containing amino acids 1–257 or full-length Raf inactivated by mutation at the ATP binding site) blocked the ability of Ras to cause cell transformation, activation of gene transcription from specific promoters (especially serum-responsive elements), and activation of the MAP kinase pathway.

The synthesis of these findings was provided by the discovery that a segment from the amino terminal CR1 domain of cRaf-1 (encompassed within Raf amino acids 50–150) binds directly to the Ras polypeptide in vitro and in situ, and the affinity of Raf for Ras-GTP is at least 1000-fold greater than for Ras-GDP. Raf proved to have no significant GAP activity; binding of Raf to Ras has little or no effect on the rate of Ras GTPase. Nevertheless, the binding sites on Ras for Raf and GAP overlap, and because Raf has a much higher affinity for Ras-GTP than GAP, Raf binding competes with and inhibits GAP-stimulated Ras GTP hydrolysis in vitro. The designation of Raf as an authentic mitogenic effector of Ras is strongly supported by the very close correlation observed between the inhibitory effects of Ras effector domain mutations on Raf binding and on v-*Ras* transforming efficiency. This correlation, together with the ability of constitutively active mutants of Raf and MEK themselves to cause cell transformation, establishes the Raf kinases, acting in their role as MEK activators, as the crucial direct mitogenic effectors of the *Ras* proto-oncogene, at least in the specific fibroblastoid cell lines in which these transformation assays have been carried out.[48] The small GTPase Rap 1 is 50% identical in amino acid sequence to Ras and 100% identical in its effector domain sequence. Rap 1 was isolated as a cDNA capable of causing reversion of the Ras transformed phenotype and subsequently was shown to bind to Raf 1 in a manner analogous to that of Ras. The structure of a cocrystal containing the Ras binding domain of Raf 1 and a carboxy terminally truncated Rap polypeptide has been solved and demonstrates the direct contacts between the acidic and hydrophilic residues of the Rap effector loop with basic and hydrophilic amino acids in Raf's "Ras binding domain."[49] The interaction of Raf and Rap is presumably nonproductive; thus the Ras-Raf cocrystal may reveal structural elements critical for Raf activation.

In order to serve as a mitogenic effector of Ras in situ, the Raf kinase must become activated consequent to its interaction with Ras-GTP. Nevertheless, the binding of purified baculoviral recombinant Raf to Ras GTP directly in vitro does not itself activate the Raf kinase activity. Fusion of the Ras membrane localization domain, encompassing both the CAAX motif for farnesylation and the more amino terminal polylysine segment from Ki-Ras, onto the carboxy terminus of Raf (denoted Raf-CAAX) results in the direct membrane localization of the Raf polypeptide.[50,51] When expressed in situ, this modification is accompanied by a substantial increase in the specific activity of Raf-CAAX as compared with unmodified Raf. The activity of Raf-CAAX can be further augmented by activation of RTK, and this RTK-induced increase in Raf-CAAX activity is *not* suppressed if Raf-CAAX is coexpressed with dominant inhibitory (Asn 17) Ras mutants. Thus targeting of Raf to the plasma membrane by a Ras-independent mechanism activates Raf and renders it Ras-independent. These results imply that the function of Ras-GTP in Raf activation is solely to translocate Raf to the inner leaflet of the surface membrane so as to enable its stable activation in a second step through a mechanism that is as yet poorly understood in biochemical terms. Two features of the Raf amino terminal noncatalytic segment appear critical for Ras-dependent activation. The first is the integrity of the Ras binding segment, as illustrated by the loss of the Ras-Raf interaction that occurs as a result of mutation at Arg 89, a variant Raf first identified as a loss of function Raf mutation in *Drosophila*[52] and known from mutagenesis,[53] peptide competition,[54] and Raf-Rap cocrystals[49] to occur in a segment of direct interaction. In addition, the Raf zinc finger structure, immediately carboxy terminal to the Ras-binding domain, although dispensable for high-affinity binding to Ras in vitro, is required for Ras-dependent Raf-activation in situ as well as for the ability of the isolated Raf amino terminus (residues 1–257) to act as an effective inhibitor by transfection in situ of v-*Ras*–dependent MAP kinase activation.[56] It is not known whether the Raf zinc finger structure, by binding to membrane lipid, simply provides a second binding energy that is necessary for stable association of Raf at the membrane or whether it serves a more dynamic role in Raf activation. Present evidence indicates that Ras-dependent Raf activation also involves certain isoforms of the 14.3.3 polypeptides, 28–30 kd polypeptides that are tightly bound to Raf in situ as well as membrane lipids and other as yet unidentified cytosolic factors that may include phospholipases or other protein (Ser/Thr) kinases situated near the inner leaflet of the cell membrane. Ras-GTP provides the crucial template for assembly of these elements, which catalyze Raf activation in a time-limited reaction, as specified by the Ras GTPase activity.

Although the discovery of the physical association between Ras GTP and Raf established the identity of Ras' primary mitogenic effector, a number of additional candidate Ras effectors have been identified subsequently. These include a set of proteins closely related in structure to the guanyl nucleotide dissociation stimulator (GDS or GNEF) for the Ral GTPase,[55] certain isoforms or the p110 catalytic subunits of the phosphatidylinositol-3-kinase,[56] and the protein kinase MEKK1.[57] The candidate effectors all share the property of binding to Ras in vitro in a GTP-dependent manner, and this binding is abrogated by mutations in the Ras effector loop. Additional polypeptides with novel structures and unknown function have been identified by expression cloning methods; these exhibit a GTP-dependent, effector loop-mediated interaction with Ras analogous to that shown by Raf. Based on this plethora of candidate Ras partners, it appears that Ras functions as a GTP-regulated switch that makes available a surface for the assembly and activation of a variety of signal transduction molecules, in close proximity to the inner leaflet of the plasma membrane. The biochemical function carried out by each of these candidate Ras effectors, the physiologic program thereby specified, and the specific tissue and/or developmental stage wherein each Ras-regulated output is functionally relevant are all open questions, with the exception of the Raf and the MAP kinase cascade. As regards this well-established Ras effector arm, current evidence indicates that the following generalizations are defensible,

1. In fibroblastoid cell lines, inhibitors of Ras, such as anti-Ras antibodies, dominant inhibitory Ras mutants (e.g., Asn17 Ras, which binds tightly to and sequesters Ras GNEFs), or the Raf amino terminal fragment (amino acids 1–257, which binds tightly to the Ras effector domain), each shut down cell division initiated by serum, all receptor tyrosine kinase-legands, and mitogenic ligands (e.g., bombesin, lysophosphatidic acid) that act through receptors coupled to heterotrimeric G-proteins and essentially all non-nuclear oncogenes (except v-*Raf*).
2. Constitutively active Raf and MEK are each capable of transforming fibroblastic cell lines unassisted, indicating that Ras activation of the MAP kinase pathway is sufficient for Ras-induced mitogenesis, at least in fibroblasts.
3. Ras activation can be associated with proliferation or differentiation in the *same* cell, depending on the intensity of upstream stimulus. Thus overexpression of EGFR in PC12 cells converts the response to EGF from proliferation to differentiation.[58] Two mechanisms appear plausible: (1) The crucial occurrence may be the conversion of a transient activation of Ras and the MAPK pathway to a sustained activation, the latter being associated with translocation of MAPK into the nucleus.[59] (2) Alternatively, increased receptor tyrosine kinase activity and tyrosine phosphorylation may produce a stronger activation of Ras thus engaging a second lower affinity Ras directed pathway—or may engage a second receptor-initiated, Ras-independent outflow that acts in collaboration with Ras to promote differentiation.
4. Activation of Ras in some cell backgrounds can trigger mitogenesis under circumstances in which MAP kinase is not activated; thus although constitutively active forms of Raf and MEK are each capable of transforming NIH 3T3 cells, clearly Ras activates mitogenic outputs other than the Raf-MEK-MAPK pathway.

Role of Ras and the MAP Kinase Cascade in Insulin Action

The elaboration of the mechanisms by which the activated insulin receptor increases Ras-GTP charging through the IRS-1– and/or Shc–mediated recruitment of Grb2/mSOS, together with the identification of Raf as a crucial immediate downstream effector of Ras-GTP, for the first time allowed the step-by-step description of an insulin-activated signal transduction pathway that extended from the receptor, through Ras to a cascade of cytoplasmic protein kinases with identifiable physiologic targets. These protein (Ser/Thr) kinases include at least two with—broad but distinct substrate specificity, that is, the MAP kinases (erk1 and erk2) and the Rsk enzymes. Substantial preliminary evidence indicates that insulin activation of erk1, erk2 and Rsks occurs in the major insulin target tissues, examined as freshly isolated primary cells as well in vivo. Thus insulin administration in vivo activates hepatic and skeletal muscle MAP kinases in the rat, and insulin treatment of intact rat adipocytes activates MAP kinase, Rsk, and p70 S6 kinase activity.[60] Hyperinsulinemia induced in humans using the euglycemic-clamp format increases skeletal muscle 40S–S6 kinase activity (predominantly p70 but also Rsk).[61] The determination of how these signal transduction pathways contribute specifically to the physiologic programs governed by insulin requires the identification, in the relevant cell types in vivo, of the important targets for Ras-GTP and its known downstream effectors, that is, the MAP kinases and Rsk. The powerful molecular techniques that have illuminated the biologic and biochemical roles of Ras and the MAP kinase cascade face a severe limitation when applied to the study of insulin action. The transfection and transformation methodologies were developed for cultured cells, mostly fibroblasts, and such lines exhibit very few responses to insulin that are representative of those observed in insulin target tissues in vivo. Tissue culture models that faithfully recapitulate some aspects of the program of metabolic regulation activated by insulin in situ do exist, for example, 3T3-L1 adipocytes, but they are few and not always experimentally tractable. In fibroblasts, overall glucose transport increases only 30–100% within the first minutes after insulin treatment, although some later increase in GLUT-1 expression occurs at a transcriptional level. Glucose transport in fibroblasts is mediated primarily by GLUT-1, which shows virtually no translocation in response to insulin. In 3T3-L1 adipocytes, a much attenuated GLUT-4 translocation response occurs as compared to in primary rat adipocytes. Insulin regulation of cAMP metabolism is not evident in most cell lines, and in some (e.g., Swiss 3T3 cells) insulin actually increases cAMP levels. A modest activation of glycogen synthase (30–100% increase) in response to insulin is uniformly seen. However, there is little basis for anticipating that such activation occurs through biochemical mechanisms closely related to those operative in vivo in skeletal muscle, liver, or adipose tissue. Mindful of these caveats, the contribution of the Ras-MAP kinase signaling pathway to specific components of insulin's physiologic program can be assessed.

The mitogenic effects of insulin are most evident in hepatoma lines.[62] Some evidence is also available supporting a mitogenic role for insulin during hepatic regeneration in vivo.[63] Nevertheless, the mitogenic potency of the insulin receptor tyrosine kinase is very limited. Conversion of the insulin receptor to an oncogene by mutagenesis does not occur spontaneously, and the closest oncogenic receptor kinase homolog is the *Ros* oncogene, which is actually derived from another receptor subfamily.[64] The IGF-1R, although 85% identical in catalytic domain sequence to the IR, nevertheless exhibits a tenfold greater mitogenic potency in side-by-side comparisons on the same cell background.[65] Both insulin and IGF-1 lack the broad efficacy and potency of factors like platelet-derived growth factor (PDGF), fibroblast growth factor (FGF), and epidermal growth factor (EGF). Nonetheless, in the appropriate cell background mitogenicity is a real component of insulin receptor activation, and as for all other RTKs, Ras is likely to be indispensable, acting through the pathways described above.

An important but less studied physiologic function of insulin is as one of the main trophic hormones for adipose tissue. This role becomes evident in vivo only in the setting of profound insulin deficiency, when the adipose organ shrivels, reflecting not only loss of triglyceride mass as a result of unrestrained lipolysis but also loss of the ability to carry out the energy storage functions. The latter results from silencing, as a consequence of insulin deficiency, of a program of gene expression that maintains glucose transport (GLUT-4 in adipocytes) and the enzymes that provide high glycolytic capacity; the ability to synthesize fatty acids de novo from acetyl CoA; and the ability to esterify fatty acids and store them as triglyceride. The role of insulin in the development of the adipose cell and the capacity for lipogenesis and triglyceride storage is reflected by the ability of insulin to promote the differentiation in vitro of 3T3-L1 preadipocytes to the mature adipocyte phenotype. This process requires Ras.[66] Moreover, introduction of constitutively active Raf into 3T3-L1 preadipocytes promotes adipocyte differentiation, whereas mutant inactive Raf polypeptides are capable of blocking insulin-induced differentiation.[41] Interestingly, this dominant inhibitory effect of mutant Raf on adipocyte differentiation is not accompanied by an inhibition of insulin-stimulated MAP kinase or Rsk activity, suggesting that Raf-induced differentiation occurs through the engagement of an alternative Raf effector pathway. Moreover, the adipocyte phenotype evoked by Raf does not fully replicate that elicited by insulin, indicating that Raf contributes only one of several inputs required for the differentiation program. Thus present evidence indicates that insulin recruitment of Ras and Raf is important to some component of the development of the adipocyte phenotype, although the precise molecular targets cannot yet be specified.

Consideration of the role of the MAP kinases (erk1 and erk2) in insulin action is most readily approached by examining the specific substrates of these enzymes. The early delineation of the proline-directed specificity of these kinases facilitated the search for candidate substrates.[11] All high affinity-functionally regulated erk1/erk2 substrates identified thus far exhibit a proline immediately carboxy terminal to the site of Ser/Thr phosphorylation, and studies with synthetic peptides indicate that a proline at +1 is indispensable for erk1/erk2 catalyzed substrate phosphorylation. Peptide studies also indicate that a proline at −2 and basic residues adjacent to the SP/TP motif are preferred. These features overlap with the specificity determinants for the cyclin-dependent kinases, especially cdc2, which exhibits consensus site motif R/KS/T PX R/K. Interestingly, however, many proteins with SP/TP sites in a perfectly plausible context fail to be phosphorylated by erk2/erk1 at a significant rate. It appears that high-affinity substrates for erk1/erk2, such as Rsk, possess (erk1/erk2) specific binding sites that may be located adjacent to the Ser/Thr phosphorylation site or at some distance in the primary sequence. The structural elements important to the creation of an erk1/erk2 binding site are not yet known. However, the requirement of such binding sites probably explains the relatively low phosphorylation exhibited by certain erk substrates after denaturation as well as the relatively low affinity (high Km) observed for the erk-catalyzed phosphorylation of short peptides that correspond to phosphorylation sites in high-affinity protein substrates in situ (e.g., the EGFR).

A striking feature of the MAP kinase substrates identified thus far is the high prevalence of signal transduction molecules (e.g., transcription factors, kinases, phospholipase A_2, GTPase regulatory proteins). In considering these potential targets in relation to insulin, many of the transcription factors thought to be regulated by erk1/erk2, based on studies in cultured cells, are not expressed or are of unknown function in insulin target tissues and do not merit further discussion. A number of MAP kinase-catalyzed phosphorylations appear to be functionally silent (or at least quiet, e.g., as in the EGFR, Raf1) or perhaps downregulatory (e.g., as in MEK or mSOS). The MAP kinase substrates best established at this time that are relevant to insulin action are the elk1 transcription factor (p62TCF), the PHAS-1 polypeptide, and the Rsk kinases.

Prominent among the numerous transcription factors that are candidate MAP kinase substrates is the Ets family member known as the p62 ternary complex factor, p62TCF or elk1. This factor, in a complex with the serum response factor, p67SRF, binds to a DNA motif (Ets motif) located adjacent to the binding site for p67SRF, which is known as the serum response element. The insulin/serum–stimulated, Ras-dependent transcriptional activation of many genes, such as *c-Fos,* is accompanied by an increased phosphorylation of p62TCF, and substantial evidence points to the necessary participation of erk1/erk2 in the transcriptional regulatory effects of p62TCF/elk1. Both MAP kinase and Rsk also phosphorylate the serum response factor p67SRF, and thus the insulin regulation of *c-Fos* gene expression is plausibly attributable to the ability of insulin to activate this complex via recruitment of Ras/MAPK/Rsk. Numerous studies demonstrate that insulin activates *c-Fos* expression in cell culture, and this response requires Ras. It should be acknowledged, however, that insulin activation of *c-Fos* gene expression, although clearly apparent in a variety of cultured cells, does not appear to be a component of the response to insulin seen in the major target tissues in vivo. Induction of insulin-deficient diabetes with streptozocin in the rat is accompanied by an *increase* in hepatic and adipose *c-Fos* mRNA levels, which is normalized, that is *reduced,* by treatment with insulin. Reciprocally, induction of hyperinsulinemia by feeding diets high in carbohydrate to fasted rats has no effect on adipose or hepatic *c-Fos* gene expression but markedly induces the expression of several genes in adipocytes and liver encoding "anabolic" proteins, such as GLUT-4 (only in adipocytes) and a variety of glycolytic and lipogenic enzymes. Inasmuch as insulin activates Ras and the MAP kinase pathway these tissues in vivo, the failure of insulin to activate the "serum response element" in liver and adipose cells in vivo, despite a brisk response in tissue culture, is unexplained. This discrepancy indicates that the paradigms and pathways established from cell culture experiments, even in 3T3-L1 cells, each need to be examined in the relevant in vivo context.

PHAS-1 was first described by Belsham and coworkers[68] as an acidic, heat-stable 21-kd polypeptide, phosphorylated in adipocytes in situ in response to insulin. This protein was subsequently purified and cloned by Lawrence and colleagues[69] and shown to be a 12-kd polypeptide that served as an MAP kinase substrate in vitro. Sonenberg and coworkers[70] independently identified the same polypeptide as eIF 4E-BP1, a protein that bound to the protein synthesis initiation factor, eIF-4E, and inhibited its mRNA binding function. eIF-4E Binds to the 7-methylguanosine cap structure of mRNAs and acts in concert with eIF-4A and eIF 4γ (together called the eIF 4F complex) to unwind the secondary structure found in the 5′ untranslated sequences of many mRNAs so as to enable mRNA scanning by the 40S ribosomal preinitiation complex and identification of the translational start site.[71] The overall function of eIF-4F is inhibited by the overexpression of PHAS-1 in situ.

Importantly, phosphorylation of eIF-4EBP-1/PHAS-1 by MAP kinase in vitro abolishes the ability of PHAS-1 to bind to and thus inhibit eIF-4E. Activation of MAP kinase may thereby be one of the mechanisms by which eIF-4F is made available in an active form contributing to the stimulation of mRNA translation that occurs in vivo in response to insulin and all other polypeptide growth factors. The role of MAP kinase in PHAS-1 regulation is not finally established, inasmuch as the insulin-stimulated phosphorylation of PHAS-1 in situ is inhibited by rapamycin, and is unaltered by the MEK inhibitor, PO98059.[70a] Moreover, phosphorylation of PHAS-1 is not the sole mechanism by which insulin stimulates mRNA translation. Persuasive (if not compelling) evidence has also been adduced for a regulatory role for three other insulin-stimulated (Ser/Thr) phosphorylations in the regulation of translational initiation: (1)phosphorylation of ribosomal S6 (catalyzed by p70 S6 kinase—see below); (2) an insulin-growth factor-induced dephosphorylation of eIF-2B, attributable to the phosphorylation and inhibition of GSK-3[72]; and (3) an insulin-stimulated phosphorylation and activation of eIF-4E itself.[73,74]

The Rsk kinases, first purified as *Xenopus* S6 kinase II, were the first MAP kinase substrates to be identified.[18] These enzymes are now recognized as an important multifunctional protein kinase subfamily of broad range, whose substrate specificity substantially overlaps that of kinase A and the calcium calmodulin kinase-2.[11] As regards its role in insulin action, Rsk2 was independently discovered in rabbit skeletal muscle as an enzyme whose activity was stimulated two- to threefold after insulin administration in vivo and that phosphorylated in vitro the glycogen-targeting (G) subunit of the protein-phosphatase 1.[75] This phosphorylation is directed largely to a single site near the G-subunit amino terminus and results in a two and a half- to threefold increase in the activity of the glycogen-bound phosphatase-1 catalytic subunit toward glycogen synthase, without alteration in its phosphorylase or phosphatase activity. Insulin activation of phosphatase-1 coincident with G-subunit phosphorylation has also been observed in adipocytes[76] and in cultured cells. The G-subunit is also phosphorylated at site 1 by kinase A. However, kinase A efficiently phosphorylates a second site on the G-subunit, resulting in the dissociation of the phosphatase-1 catalytic subunit from the G-subunit, with a consequent five- to eightfold fall in its catalytic efficiency toward the particulate glycogen synthase. Thus, phosphorylation of the G-subunit, by Rsk (or by another insulin-sensitive kinase) and by kinase A is one of the several mechanisms through which insulin and cAMP control skeletal muscle glycogenesis in a reciprocal way. Rsk-catalyzed G-subunit phosphorylation also illustrates one of the mechanisms by which insulin, through the activation of a protein kinase (Rsk2), activates a protein phosphatase and thus causes protein dephosphorylation.

A second potential role for Rsk in the dephosphorylation and activation of GS was uncovered with the finding that GS kinase-3 (GSK-3) is inactivated in situ in response to insulin and mitogens.[77–79] GSK-3 was first purified from skeletal muscle as the most potent negative regulator of synthase activity in vitro, catalyzing the phosphorylation of four serine residues near the synthase carboxy terminus. Peptide sequence analysis of synthase purified from rabbit skeletal muscle before and after insulin administration in vivo revealed that the most extensive dephosphorylation in response to insulin occurred at the sites phosphorylated specifically by GSK-3 in vitro.[3] Thus inhibition of GSK-3 provides a plausible and attractive mechanism to account for insulin-induced dephosphorylation-activation of GS. Several studies have demonstrated that insulin and polypeptide growth factors induce a rapid transient inhibition of GSK-3 in a variety of cultured cells as well as in adipose tissue, to about 50% of initial levels.[77–79] Potent inactivation of both GSK-3 isoforms can be achieved by phosphorylation in vitro (at serine 9 in GSK-3β and at serine 21 in GSK-3α) with Rsk2, or the p70 S6 kinase.[80] Mutation of GSK-3β (ser 9 to ala) renders GSK-3β largely resistant to inhibition by insulin or mitogens or to cotransfection with Rsk1.[81] Wortmannin, a relatively selective inhibitor of PI-3-kinase, prevents GSK-3 inhibition by insulin in CHO cells S2 and L6 myoblasts,[83] concomitant with inhibition of MAP kinase, Rsk, and p70 S6 kinase. Rapamycin, a selective inhibitor of p70 S6 kinase, has no effect on the insulin inhibition of GSK-3 activity, indicating that p70 S6 kinase, although activated by insulin in situ and capable of GSK-3 phosphorylation and inactivation in vitro, does not participate in GSK-3 regulation in situ. As regards the elements upstream of GSK-3, overexpression of a dominant inhibitory MEK in NIH 3T3 cells markedly attenuates the EGF activation of Rsk and the EGF inhibition of GSK-3, indicating that GSK-3 activity is regulated by EGF through the MAP kinase cascade.[84] Taken together, these findings suggest that inhibition of Ras and/or the MAP kinase cascade mediates the epidermal growth factor–induced inhibition of GSK-3 seen in cell culture; therefore inhibition of Ras and the MAP kinase pathway should also prevent insulin activation of GS. Surprisingly, the large majority of experiments reported thus far indicate that activation of Ras does not contribute to the insulin regulation of glucose transport and GS.

The 3T3-L1 adipocyte cell line is one of the most appropriate cell culture models for the study of insulin action. In these cells, insulin activates PI-3-kinase activity, p70 S6 kinase, and the MAP kinase cascade and strongly activates GLUT-4 translocation and GS activity (about threefold). Significantly, PDGF also activates PI-3-kinase, and PDGF and EGF both activate p70 S6 kinase and the MAP kinase cascade with an intensity equal to that of insulin, but the growth factors fail to significantly alter glucose transport or GS.[85–89] Thus activation of Ras/MAP kinase and overall PI-3-kinase, individually or together, in 3T3-L1 cells is not sufficient to signal the activation of glucose transport and GS.

A variety of inhibitors have been employed to address whether input from these pathways is necessary for activation of these characteristic metabolic responses to insulin. A relatively selective inhibitor of MEK, PD98059, fails to inhibit insulin-stimulated glucose uptake, lipogenesis, and glycogen synthesis in 3T3-L1 cells or in cultured L6 myotubes,[89a] despite complete surpression of insulin-activated MAPK and Rsk activities. This provides persuasive evidence against a major role for these kinases in insulin regulation of glucose utilization, however, other Ras-regulated elements could be involved. Inhibition of Ras-GTP charging can be accomplished by overexpression of the protein tyrosine phosphatase SH-PTP-2/Syp in a mutant, catalytically inactive form[90] as well as by overexpression of a mutant, inactive version of the Ras GNEF, mSOS.[91] Expression of these inhibitors in CHO cells overexpressing the insulin receptor greatly inhibits MAP kinase activation but fails to abrogate the insulin activation of glucose transport or GS. The Asn17 mutant Ras also inhibits insulin stimulation of Ras GTP charging as well as the activation of MAP kinase and Rsk; however, it does not block insulin-IGF-1 activation of GS.[92] These studies thus provide no evidence in support of a requirement for Ras-GTP in the insulin activation of glucose transport or synthase. Several reports are somewhat at variance with these totally negative results. Lovastatin is an inhibitor of HMG CoA reductase, a reaction necessary for the synthesis of the farnesyl pyrophosphate precursor for Ras farnesylation. Lovastatin inhibits Ras GTP charging in 3T3-L1 cells and Rat1 cells overexpressing the human IR. This is accompanied by an inhibition of DNA synthesis and glucose incorporation into glycogen but no change in glucose transport or glucose-6-P levels.[93] Clonal lines of 3T3-L1 cells expressing recombinant v-*Ras* exhibit a constitutively high fraction of cellular GLUT-4 at the cell surface, and insulin does not promote further translocation of GLUT-4 to the surface membrane.[94] These lines, however, show a marked decrease in overall GLUT-4 expression, and although the distribution of GLUT-4 observed suggests that v-*Ras* promotes GLUT-4 translocation to the cell surface, the contributions of v-*Ras* per se versus clonal variation in the development of this phenotype are uncertain. Manchester and coworkers[95] used protein microinjection into isolated cardiac myocytes and a single-cell assay for glucose transport to evaluate the role of Ras. They observed that v-*Ras* polypeptide greatly increases both basal and insulin-stimulated glucose transport, whereas an inhibitory anti-Ras monclonal antibody partially inhibited both basal and insulin-activated transport by about 50%. On balance, it appears that the Ras-MAP kinase cascade, although capable of modulating GLUT-4 regulation, is neither sufficient nor necessary for insulin regulation of glucose transport. As regards the insulin regulation of GS, it is not possible at this time to provide a coherent synthesis of the conflicting evidence. Studies discounting the importance of Ras have focused mostly on fibroblastic cell lines, and more data from experiments in adipocytes and skeletal muscle are needed. If Ras can be eliminated as a component of the primary signaling pathway employed by insulin in these tissues, the role of Rsk needs further examination. The possibility exists that an enzyme with similar specificity to Rsk participates in the insulin activation of synthase and is recruited through a Ras-independent pathway perhaps involving the PI3-kinase. A Rsk3 isoform expressed in skeletal muscle has been described,[96] but its regulation is not yet characterized. Similarly, the role of GSK-3 in insulin regulation of synthase is uncertain inasmuch as it appears that the growth factor–induced inhibition of GSK-3 can be prevented by inhibitors of MAP kinase activation or Ras-GTP charging, maneuvers that do not inhibit insulin activation of synthase. This points to a Ras-independent mechanism for the insulin regulation of GSK3 (or another "site-3" kinase) or for insulin-induced phosphatase-1 activation (? via G-subunit site 1 phosphorylation). It should be noted that one report[97] finds that rapamycin substantially inhibits the insulin-stimulated incorporation of ^{14}C-glucose into glycogen in 3T3-L1 cells without inhibiting glucose transport; presumably such inhibition is independent of changes in GSK-3 activity.

Phosphatidylinositol-3-Kinase in Insulin Action

A more coherent picture emerges regarding the role of PI-3-kinase in the insulin regulation of metabolism. Although activation of the heterodimeric PI-3-kinase by PDGF/EGF in 3T3-L1 cells is not accompanied by activation of glucose transport or GS, inhibition of PI-3-kinase is consistently accompanied by inhibition of insulin action. Two classes of inhibitors have been employed to assess the requirement for PI-3-kinase in the signal transduction cascade upstream of insulin's program of metabolic regulation. Overexpression of a mutant p85 regulatory subunit of the p85/p110 PI-3-kinase that lacks the binding domain for the p110 catalytic subunit results in a marked inhibition (>80%) of insulin-stimulated PI-3-kinase activity in CHO cells overexpressing the insulin receptor.[98] This is accompanied by a comparable inhibition of insulin-activated glucose transport, but GS activation is not impaired.[90] A second class of PI-3-kinase antagonists are the low-molecular-weight inhibitors, specifically wortmannin and LY294002. These structurally unrelated compounds each give selective inhibition of PI-3-kinase; wortmannin inhibits at submicromolar concentrations, forming an irreversibly tight perhaps covalent adduct with the p110 subunit.[99] At nanomolar concentrations no effects on PI-4-kinase or receptor tyrosine kinase activity are detected, although at higher, micromolar levels, inhibition of a number of phosphotransferases becomes evident. In all reports thus far, submicromolar concentrations of wortmannin have been found to shut down nearly all aspects of insulin action (the exception being the activation of pyruvate dehydrogenase in adipocytes) concomitant with inhibition of PI-3-kinase: glucose transport and GS; antilipolysis, insulin-activation of the specific cAMP phosphodiesterase and the activation of the (Ser/Thr) kinase that mediates insulin activation of the phosphodiesterase; and insulin-activation of the p70 S6 kinase.[83,97,100–103] The ability of wortmannin to inhibit GLUT-4 translocation appears to be attributable to an inhibition of insulin signal transduction rather than to inhibition of vesicle traffic per se, inasmuch as the activation of skeletal muscle glucose transport caused by hypoxia and contraction,[104] which are also attributable in part to GLUT-4 translocation,[105] are not blocked by wortmannin. The effects of wortmannin on the Ras-MAP kinase pathway have been variable from cell to cell. In hepatoma cells, PC12 cells,[92] and 3T3-L1 cells,[97,103] wortmannin shuts down the functions enumerated above without significant inhibition of the insulin activation of MAP kinase or Rsk. In L6 myoblasts and CHO cells, wortmannin gives substantial inhibition of Raf, MAP kinase, and Rsk.[83] Interestingly, wortmannin inhibits Raf in L6 myoblasts without altering Ras GTP charging. Although not yet examined in as many systems, the effects of LY294002 on PI-3-kinase activity and insulin regulation of glucose transport, GS, and the p70 S6 kinase parallel those seen with wortmannin.[103]

1) Inhibitors of PI-3-k (wortmannin, LY294002) inhibit insulin's actions on: glucose transport
   glycogen synthase
   cAMP phosphodiesterase
   p70 S6 kinase

2) Potent activators of PI-3-k other than insulin (e.g., PDGF, EGF) strongly activate p70 S6 kinase but activate glucose transport and glycogen synthase poorly or not at all

Conclusion:
a) PI-3-k is necessary but not sufficient, or
b) PI-3-k is sufficient but functionally heterogeneous

Figure 17-2. The role phosphatidylinositide-3 kinase plays in insulin action.

On balance, it appears that PI-3-kinase provides an input necessary for the activation of glucose transport, GS, cAMP phosphodiesterase, and the p70 S6 kinase (Fig. 17-2). The inhibition of glucose transport[98] but not GS[90] by the mutant p85 polypeptide (in contrast to the ability of wortmannin to inhibit both responses) indicates that wortmannin is likely to inhibit isoforms of the PI-3-kinase in addition to those regulated by the p85 polypeptide. This implies that the receptor tyrosine kinases may also act through a variety of PI-3-kinase isoforms, and such a multiplicity of PI-3-kinases may provide the basis for understanding why the insulin receptor but not the PDGFR is able to signal to glucose transport and GS. Thus, insulin signaling to these targets may occur entirely through 3′ OH inositide phosphorylation, catalyzed by an array of independently regulated PI-3-kinases, some of which are uniquely responsive to insulin. Several isoforms of the PI-3-kinase p110 catalytic subunit have been described[106] whose activity is variously regulated by the p85 adaptor protein, which contains SH2 and SH3 domains and regions homologous to BCR as well as to rho-GAP. In addition, the activity of some p110 isoforms can be directed by Ras through direct interaction with the Ras effector domain as well as through the $\beta\gamma$ subunits of the heterotrimeric G-proteins. Alternatively, insulin may signal to GLUT-4 and synthase through PI-3-kinase and one or more additional insulin-specific signal generators with an entirely different biochemical-catalytic function, as occurs with activation of the p70 S6 kinase described below (Fig. 17-3). A comprehensive description of the PI-3-kinases is beyond the scope of this discussion. Nevertheless, better understanding of the variety within this lipid kinase family, of the mechanisms utilized by insulin in comparison to the growth factors to regulate PI-3-kinase activity, and of the biochemical steps by which lipid phosphorylation is coupled with the activation of downstream responses such as p70 S6 kinase, GLUT-4 translocation, GS, and the insulin-activated cAMP-PDE kinase is very important for the continuing advancement of knowledge concerning insulin action. At this time, understanding at a molecular level of the signaling elements downstream of PI-3-kinase is most advanced for the p70 S6 kinase.

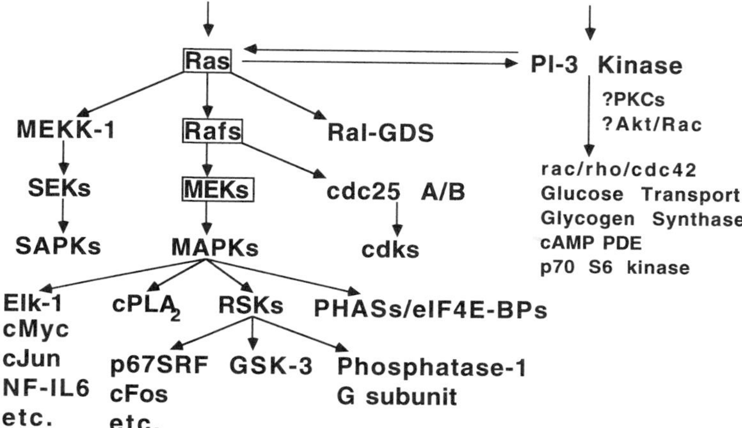

FIGURE 17-3. Signal transduction through Ras and phosphatidylinositol-3-kinase.

The p70 S6 Kinase Phosphatidylinositol-3-Kinase Pathway

In contrast to the rapid progress achieved in elucidating many of the important targets of the MAP kinases and Rsk as well as the steps interposed between the insulin receptor, Ras, and the Rsk S6 kinase, progress in understanding the biologic role and regulatory apparatus that couple the RTKs to the p70 S6 kinase has developed much more slowly. Recently, however, insight into the complex regulatory apparatus upstream of p70 has emerged, and it is now evident that p70 will provide an important model for understanding the signaling mechanisms utilized by the lipid kinases and the nature of the mitogen-regulated inputs into the cell cycle apparatus other than those flowing through Ras.

The p70 S6 kinase polypeptide is expressed from a single gene in two alternate forms denoted αI and αII, 525 and 502 amino acids in length, respectively[107–109]; this difference reflects an amino terminal extension of 23 amino acids in the αI isoform, distinctive for the presence of six consecutive Arg residues immediately after the initiator methionine. This amino terminal extension appears to localize p70αI entirely to the nucleus, whereas the shorter αII isoform is predominantly or entirely cytosolic.[110] The centrally placed p70 catalytic domain is flanked on both sides by noncatalytic sequences, each containing important regulatory elements. The catalytic domain of p70 is most closely related in structure to the amino terminal of the two catalytic domains in Rsk.[107] However, the two types of S6 kinase are largely distinct in their substrate specificity and most important, are independently regulated.[11]

The p70 S6 kinase appears to be required for progression through the G1 phase of the cell cycle, at least in some cells. Thus microinjection into REF 52 cells of anti-p70 antibodies reactive with both αI and αII arrests cell cycle progression in G1,[111] and an antibody selective for αI microinjected into the nucleus also arrests cells in G1.[112] Rapamycin, an inhibitor of p70 S6 kinase[15,16,113,114] (see below), causes cell cycle delay or arrest by prolonging or abrogating G1. Although rapamycin inhibits p70 completely in all cell backgrounds, the potency of rapamycin's inhibitory effect on G1 progression varies with the cell line. Complete blockade occurs in mature T-cells[114] but only some G1 delay occurs in NIH 3T3 cells.[15] Concomitantly, changes in cyclin E and A expression and in cdk activity are observed after addition of rapamycin, and the intensity of these changes parallels the degree of inhibition of cell cycle progression.[115] Thus the importance of p70 inhibition to the cell cycle delay induced by rapamycin is not clear; p70 inhibition may be the crucial event underlying cell cycle delay, but the importance of p70 for cell cycle progression may vary from cell to cell.

The S6 polypeptide remains the only clearly established physiologic substrate for the p70 kinase. The ability of rapamycin to inhibit 40S phosphorylation in mammalian and avian cells concomitant with the selective inhibition of p70 S6 kinase but not Rsk establishes p70 as the true insulin-regulated 40S kinase in mammalian cells. Although multisite S6 phosphorylation catalyzed in situ by p70 is a nearly universal concomitant of insulin, mitogen, and stress activation of cells, definitive evidence as to the functional role of S6 phosphorylation is not yet available. Correlative studies suggest that S6 phosphorylation parallels polysome formation[11] and may selectively facilitate translation of mRNAs containing polypyrimidine[116] tracts in their 5′ untranslated segments. Regulated S6 phosphorylation also occurs in the nucleus[117] and might be important for ribosomal biogenesis, which is known to be upregulated by insulin and other anabolic-mitogenic stimuli. Although it is likely that p70 has important physiologic substrates in addition to S6, little information on this point is available. Mitogen-regulated, rapamycin-sensitive phosphorylation of the CREM (*c*AMP-*r*esponse *e*lement *m*odulator) transcription factor in situ, at a site phosphorylated by p70 in vitro, has been reported.[118] However, the role of CREM (if any) in insulin-mitogen action is unknown. As regards substrate specificity, p70 catalyzes the phosphorylation of a cluster of five ser residues near the carboxy terminus of 40S–S6, probably in an ordered, processive reaction. The initial p70-catalyzed phosphorylation of S6 occurs at RRRLSS$_{236}$LR, and studies with synthetic peptides modeled on this sequence indicate that all three Arg residues amino terminal to Ser$_{236}$ are important in that conversion of each to Ala individually increases Km by 140×/5×/700× fold, respectively. The mechanism of the subsequent, processive phosphorylations is not yet known.[11] The ability of rapamycin to inhibit p70 selectively with no effect on MAP kinase and Rsk has enabled a rapid scan for potential p70 targets in insulin's program of metabolic regulation, which has been mostly negative thus far. Rapamycin does not alter insulin activation of glucose transport and GLUT-4 translocation[119] nor with a single exception[97] does rapamycin inhibit the insulin activation of glycogen synthase.[92] As noted above, one report finds that rapamycin inhibits insulin stimulation of glycogen deposition but not glucose transport in 3T3 L1 cells. Available information thus indicates that p70 is not upstream of elements significant to insulin regulation of glucose transport and, probably, GS. The effects of rapamycin on cAMP metabolism, protein synthesis, and specific gene expression have not yet been reported, and examination of its effects on primary cells, especially skeletal muscle, is awaited.

The major focus of effort on p70 has been to identify the upstream signals necessary for insulin activation of p70 S6 kinase activity. Both the p70 and Rsk S6 kinase subfamilies are activated maximally within 10 minutes after insulin addition, although in side-by-side comparisons p70 usually increases somewhat more slowly than Rsk. In addition to the inhibitory action of rapamycin, p70 is also inhibited selectively by treatment of cells with a variety of inhibitors of PI-3-kinase, such as wortmannin and LY294002.[103]

This implies a requirement for PI-3-kinase activity in the activation of p70, a conclusion further supported by the inability of PDGF to activate p70 when signaling through mutant PDGFRs that have selectively lost the ability to recruit PI-3-kinase by mutation of specific PDGFR intracellular Tyr residues.[120,121] Conversely, restoration of these PDGFR tyrosine residues (Tyr 740–751, located in the kinase-insert domain) alone, which restores full activation of PI-3-kinase, enables PDGF to activate endogenous p70 with a potency approaching that elicited by wild type PDGFR. These findings suggest that PI-3-kinase alone and/or some other signaling element capable of binding to these TyrP residues is sufficient to signal PDGF activation of the p70 S6 kinase. As for the biochemical mechanisms by which p70 activation is achieved, both p70[122] and Rsk S6 kinases[18,123] purified in an active form can be fully deactivated in vitro by treatment with protein phosphatase. As described above, Rsk is efficiently reactivated by phosphorylation with MAP kinase in a reaction whose pattern of multisite Rsk phosphorylation recapitulates closely the pattern seen with Rsk activation in situ by EGF or active phorbol esters (the latter acting upstream of MAP kinase rather than directly by PKC action on the Rsk).[123] In contrast, phosphatase-treated p70 is not phosphorylated by MAPK in vitro.[122] It is now evident that p70 requires at least three independent inputs for activation, directed at distinct domains of the p70 polypeptide.

Phosphorylation of a p70 S6 Kinase Autoinhibitory Domain by Proline-Directed Kinases

The carboxy terminal noncatalytic tail of the p70 contains a basic, Ser/Thr/Pro rich segment of 25 amino acids that exhibits about 30% sequence identity to the region in ribosomal S6 that encompasses the multiple sites of p70-catalyzed phosphorylation.[107] A synthetic peptide corresponding to this region of S6 is avidly phosphorylated by p70, but a peptide corresponding to the endogenous p70 segment is not phosphorylated by p70 at all.[124] Nevertheless, both peptides act as competitive inhibitors of the p70-catalyzed phosphorylation of 40S subunits. The endogenous segment in p70 thus is capable of serving as an autoinhibitory pseudosubstrate (SKAIPS, *S*6 *k*inase *a*uto*i*nhibitory *p*seudo *s*ubstrate) domain. In its unphosphorylated state, the SKAIPS domain is presumed to bind to and occlude the p70 substrate binding site. Phosphorylation of this segment by upstream insulin-activated kinases would promote its release from the catalytic domain. Amino acid sequence analysis of peptides derived from p70 activated in situ revealed that four major sites of p70 phosphorylation are clustered within the SKAIPS domain. Each of these phosphorylated Ser/Thr residues is followed by a proline residue immediately carboxy terminal.[125] The Ser/Thr phosphorylation sites in the SKAIPS domain are phosphorylated in vitro by cdc2, p54 SAP kinase, and erk2, all proline-directed kinases, but not by kinase A, kinase C, casein kinase 2, or p70 itself.[126] In addition, insulin rapidly activates in situ an array of proline-directed kinases that phosphorylate the sites in the SKAIPS domain in vitro, which include erk1 and erk2, cdc2 and some unidentified kinases reactive with erk antisera.[126] Thus although the identity of the multiple proline-directed kinases that phosphorylate this segment in situ in response to insulin-mitogen activation is not yet certain, they will clearly include erks and cdks.

Phosphorylation of the p70 Catalytic Domain by a PI-3-Kinase-Activated Protein Kinase

In spite of the strong evidence pointing to the regulatory role of SKAIPS domain phosphorylation in the insulin-mitogen activation of p70 S6 kinase, phosphorylation of the phosphatase-inactivated p70 in vitro with multiple proline-directed kinases fails to restore p70 activity despite extensive phosphorylation within the SKAIPS domain. Moreover, recombinant p70 polypeptides that lack the entire carboxy terminal tail (including the SKAIPS domain) continue to exhibit low activity in mitogen-deprived cells, a strong activation in response to insulin and mitogens, and an unaltered sensitivity to inhibition by wortmannin.[127] The last feature implies that the wortmannin-inhibitable input, presumably arising from PI-3-kinase, is directed to a region of p70 other than the carboxy terminal tail. Direct confirmation of this inference is provided by the demonstration that coexpression of such tailless p70 variants with a recombinant constitutively active PI-3-kinase results in substantial activation of p70, which is not further augmented by addition of insulin or serum, whereas Rsk activity is unaffected by overexpression of PI-3-kinase.[128] This PI-3-kinase–induced p70 activation is accompanied by a selective increase in the phosphorylation at p70 Thr252, whereas inhibition by wortmannin is associated with a selective inhibition of Thr252 phosphorylation. Thr252 is situated on a loop in subdomain VIII of the p70 catalytic domain and is homologous in location to the site at which many protein Ser/Thr and Tyr kinases undergo an activating phosphorylation, either cotranslationally (e.g., kinase A) or post-translationally (e.g., cdc2, erk1 and erk2, Rsk, Src, insulin receptor).[129] A Ser or a Thr at this site is necessary for p70 activity. The phosphorylation at p70 Thr252 appears to be catalyzed by another protein kinase rather than by p70 autophosphorylation inasmuch as Thr252 continues to be phosphorylated in situ on p70 polypeptides that contain an inactivating mutation at their ATP binding site. The p110 catalytic subunit of PI-3-kinase itself catalyzes Ser/Thr phosphorylation in vitro, both an autophosphorylation of the p110 polypeptide and a transphosphorylation of the p85 regulatory subunit. Nevertheless, the recombinant, constitutively active PI-3-kinase, although capable of a vigorous Ser/Thr autophosphorylation in vitro, is unable to directly phosphorylate p70 S6 kinase.[128] Consequently, it appears that another protein (Ser/Thr) kinase, recruited by the product of the PI-3-kinase reaction, is responsible for the phosphorylation of p70 Thr252 in situ either directly or through a protein kinase cascade. A number of potential PI-3-kinase–activated (Ser/Thr) kinases have been described. Several of the nonclassic isoforms of PKC can be activated selectively in vitro by PI lipids phosphorylated at the 3′OH, including PKC delta and epsilon, isoforms[130] that are responsive to diacylglycerol and phorbol ester but *not* to Ca^{++}; PKC zeta, a PKC isoform unresponsive to both diacylglycerol (DAG) and Ca^{++}, is also activated in vitro by PI-3 lipids as effectively as by phosphatidylserine.[131] In addition, the protein (Ser/Thr) kinase proto-oncogene known as Akt/Rac/PKB has been reported to be selectively activated by PI-3 lipids and capable of promoting activation of p70 56 kinase in situ when co-expressed as the oncogenic gag-PKB fusion protein.[132,132a] Whether one or more of these putative PI-3-kinase effector (Ser/Thr) kinases serve as upstream regulators of the p70 S6 kinase is not currently known but will certainly be ascertained in the near future.

Thus PI-3-kinase appears to engage a protein kinase cascade that includes the p70 S6 kinase. The relationship of this effector arm of PI-3-kinase to the biochemical reactions that underlie the wortmannin-sensitive insulin-activation of GLUT-4 translocation, cAMP phosphodiesterase kinase, and GS remains to be uncovered.

Rapamycin Inhibits p70 Through Inhibition of a Novel Lipid Kinase Distinct from PI-3-Kinase

Rapamycin is a macrolide of fungal origin, first identified as an antibiotic and subsequently found to have potent immunosuppressant activity. Rapamycin is structurally related to FK506, another macrolide immunosuppressant. Despite their similar structure, the two agents exhibit very different biologic effects. FK506 is a potent inhibitor of T-cell activation by the T-cell antigen receptor, whereas rapamycin does not affect T-cell activation by antigen but completely inhibits interleukin 2–mediated T-cell proliferation. In each case the active pharmacophore is not the free drug but a complex between the drug and its cellular receptor. Remarkably, despite their divergent biologic actions, FK506 and rapamycin share the same intracellular receptors, known as FK506 binding proteins (FKBPs), first identified as a family of abundant 12–13 kd basic polypeptides but now known to include polypeptides of 25 kd and 59 kd as well. The normal function of the FKBPs is not known, although each variety of FKBP exhibits a *cis-trans* prolyl isomerase activity. Both rapamycin and FK506 inhibit this catalytic function on binding to the FKBP; however, it is clear that such inhibition is not the basis for the immunosuppressant activity inasmuch as FK506 derivatives have been created that inhibit enzymatic activity but lack immunosuppressant activity.[133] The complex of FK506 bound to FKBP-12 is a potent direct inhibitor of the protein phosphatase calcineurin (protein phosphatase 2B) both in situ and in vitro, and although FKBP-12 alone can bind to calcineurin in vitro, neither FK506 nor FKBP-12 alone is inhibitory; only the FK506/FKBP complex inhibits.[134] Considerable evidence indicates that inhibition of calcineurin accounts fully for the ability of FK506 to inhibit T-cell activation.[135] Rapamycin bound to FKBP-12 has *no* effect on calcineurin in situ or in vitro. However, because rapamycin shares the same binding site on FKBP-12 as FK506, the two macrolides act as mutual antagonists in situ. Such antagonism requires micromolar concentrations of at least one drug inasmuch as the drug/FKBP complex is an active inhibitor at nanomolar concentrations, whereas the FKBPs themselves are present at micromolar levels.

Although the rapamycin/FKBP-12 complex is inert toward calcineurin, rapamycin (but not FK506) is a potent inhibitor of p70 S6 kinase in situ.[15,16,113,114] This inhibition is indirect in that the rapamycin/FKBP complex has no direct effect on p70 activity in vitro or on the rate of p70 dephosphorylation by phosphatase 2A. Inhibition of p70 by rapamycin in situ is always associated with an increase in p70 mobility on electrophoresis in polyacrylamide gels in the presence of sodium dodecylsulfate and the selective loss of the most slowly migrating band of p70 polypeptide, a response indicative of partial p70 dephosphorylation. This and other evidence[109] indicate that only this most slowly migrating (presumably fully phosphorylated) band of p70 polypeptide possesses *any* 40S kinase activity. Peptide mapping studies have not identified phosphorylation sites especially sensitive to rapamycin. Addition of rapamycin before insulin diminishes the subsequent SKAIPS domain phosphorylation, whereas addition of rapamycin after mitogen-insulin activation produces complete inhibition of p70 within minutes with little or no change in phosphorylation of the four sites in the SKAIPS domain. Thomas and coworkers described three minor ^{32}P peptides distinct from the SKAIPS sites that appear to be rapamycin-sensitive.[136] We find that Thr252 phosphorylation is susceptible to inhibition by rapamycin,[127] although it is unclear whether this is the consequence of p70 inhibition (which could lead to an increased rate of p70 dephosphorylation), inhibition of a Thr252 kinase, or activation of a p70 phosphatase.

Although the proximate biochemical mechanism for rapamycin inhibition of p70 is not known, identification of the direct target of the rapamycin-FKBP complex was first accomplished in *Saccharomyus cerevisiae*. Yeast are completely inhibited in their growth in G1 by rapamycin; deletion of the gene encoding the yeast FKBP-12 homologue rendered the organisms completely resistant to rapamycin.[137] Selection of spontaneous rapamycin-resistant variants led to the identification of a gene encoding a 280 kd polypeptide whose point mutation (Ser to Arg) confers resistance of *S. cerevisiae* to rapamycin.[138] This gene is nonessential, but additional deletion of a second gene encoding a closely related polypeptide is lethal. These polypeptides, named target(s) of rapamycin—TOR 1 and 2—contain a domain in their carboxy terminus showing homology to the catalytic domain of yeast (VSP34) and mammalian PI-3-kinases. Several groups working in mammalian systems used affinity isolation[139–141] or expression cloning[142] to identify the binding partners of the rapamycin-FKBP-12 complex, and each identified mammalian TOR homologs, variously called mTOR, c-RAFT, or FRAP. Introduction of the Ser to Arg point mutation that confers rapamycin insensitivity to yeast TOR into the mammalian TOR sequence results in a loss of the binding between FKBP 12 and mTOR.[142] Each of the TOR isoforms identified thus far exhibits the carboxy terminal lipid kinase domain. However, direct demonstration of a TOR-catalyzed lipid phosphorylation is not yet available. Consequently, the nature of the apparently indispensable input provided by TOR into p70 is obscure. Moreover, it is not known whether insulin or growth factors regulate TOR activity or if TOR provides a necessary but constitutive input. Whatever the nature of the input provided by TOR, it is entirely separate from that provided by PI-3-kinase inasmuch as deletion of a p70 amino terminal segment renders p70 highly resistant to inhibition by rapamycin without changing the susceptibility to inhibition by wortmannin or to activation by coexpressed recombinant PI-3-kinase.[127] Thus, the rapamycin-sensitive, putative lipid kinase mTOR represents a novel signaling molecule, crucial to the activation of p70 but not involved in the regulation of glucose transport.

Summary and Conclusions

Insight into the signal transduction mechanisms that operate downstream of the insulin receptor and into receptor tyrosine kinases in general accelerated dramatically in the 1990s. It is clear that regulatory protein phosphorylation is the ubiquitous chemical modification by which the signal initiated on insulin binding to its receptor is transmitted, amplified, and diversified so as to effect the complex program of cell regulation that occurs in insulin target cells. The earliest steps involve receptor catalyzed tyrosine phosphorylation, both of the insulin receptor itself and of several families of intracellular polypeptide substrates best exemplified by the IRS polypeptides. Insulin receptor autophosphorylation serves primarily to activate the receptor tyrosine kinase activity toward exogenous polypeptide substrates through the phosphorylation of a cluster of three tyrosines in subdomain VIII of the IR catalytic domain. Autophosphorylation at an NPXY motif in the IR juxtamembrane segment provides a binding site for polypeptides like IRS-1 and Shc that have so-called "phosphotyrosine binding" (PTB) domains. In turn, phosphorylation of Shc and IRS-1 creates TyrP-containing motifs that act as binding sites for the recruitment of polypeptides with SH2 domains. These polypeptides, which are themselves enzymes or are noncovalently bound to cellular enzymes, are recruited onto the insulin receptor substrates and thereby activated, either directly through the simultaneous ligation of two SH2 domains (e.g., as occurs with P85/p110 PI-3-kinase) or after tyrosine phosphorylation by the receptor or a receptor-associated tyrosine kinase (e.g., as occurs with the recruitment of PL-Cγ by the EGFR). This complex is brought into proximity with the enzymes complexed with substrate, that is, a membrane protein or lipid, or perhaps with some other newly recruited signal transduction elements, thereby enabling a new signal to be generated (e.g., active Ras GTP or 3-OH phosphorylated PI lipids), which in turn recruits a second tier of signal transducers. The major elements operating at this next level of regulation are the small GTPases and protein (Ser/Thr) kinases. Realignment of membranous components requires the participation of small GTPases of the Ras superfamily. These elements are active when bound to GTP, and their activity is specified through receptor regulation of the polypeptides that govern their relative content of GTP/GDP (i.e., GAPs and GNEFs) and perhaps their cellular location (GDIs, carboxy terminal modification). The protein kinases are organized in parallel cascades that transmit information to protein substrates in all cellular compartments. In these cascades, each protein kinase activates the next element downstream but also serves as a target for cross-regulation by parallel pathways. Most important, one or more of this sequence of kinases serve as multifunctional effectors through the phosphorylation of numerous downstream targets.

In the case of insulin it is clear that much of the program of metabolic regulation in its characteristic target cells is directly attributable to the dephosphorylation of enzymes at regulatory sites. This is accomplished by the ability of the protein kinase cascades to direct both inhibition of protein kinases such as the cAMP-dependent protein kinase and the glycogen synthase kinase 3 as well as the activation of cellular protein Ser/Thr phosphatases such as the protein phosphatase-1 bound to the glycogen particle in skeletal muscle. As described above, present information indicates that the insulin-induced dephosphorylations are governed by insulin-activated Ser/Thr kinases situated upstream.

This chapter has summarized recent information concerning the operation of the protein (Ser/Thr) kinase cascades as intermediates that couple the initial receptor-generated tyrosine phosphorylation to the immediate effectors of insulin's diverse cellular programs. At this time much more detail is available in describing the components and reactions that couple the insulin receptor to the mitogeneic and cell differentiation programs as compared with those that govern the major reactions of nutrient metabolism (e.g., activation of glucose transport, glycogen synthesis, and antilipolysis). This reflects the vastly greater number of facile systems available for the study of mitogenesis as well as the much wider interest and broader effort ongoing in the study of the signaling mechanisms underlying cell growth regulation than is currently mobilized toward understanding the regulation of nutrient metabolism. In both areas, however, present work in signal transduction is very much in the stage of identifying candidate participants and plausible mechanisms. The task remains of defining which of these candidates and which of the possible mechanisms is actually utilized to provide the dominant regulatory pathway operative in vivo that regulates the response of skeletal muscle, adipose tissue, and liver to insulin.

References

1. Robison GA, Butcher RW, Sutherland EW. Cyclic AMP. New York: Academic Press; 1971:1–23
2. Larner J. Insulin signalling mechanisms—lessons from the old testament of glycogen metabolism and from the new testament of molecular biology. Diabetes 1988;37:262
3. Cohen P. Muscle glycogen synthase. In: Boyer P, Krebs E, eds. The Enzymes. New York: Academic Press; 1986:461
4. Avruch J, Nemenoff RA, Pierce M, et al. Protein phosphorylations as a mode of insulin action. In: Czech MP, ed. Molecular Basis for Insulin Action. New York: Plenum Press; 1985:263
5. Avruch J, Witters LA, Alexander MC, et al. Insulin and the phosphorylation of intracellular proteins. Prog Clin Biol Res 1979;31:621
6. Denton RM, Brownsey RW, Belsham GJ. A partial view of the mechanism of insulin action. Diabetologia 1981;21:247
7. Avruch J, Alexander MC, Palmer JL, et al. The role of insulin-stimulated protein phosphorylation in insulin action. Fed Proc 1982;41:2629
8. Haselbacher GK, Humbel RE, Thomas G. Insulin-like growth factor: Insulin or serum increase phosphorylation of ribosomal protein S6 during transition of stationary chick embryo fibroblasts into early G1 phase of the cell cycle. FEBS Lett 1979;100:185
9. Smith CJ, Wejksnora PJ, Warner JR, et al. Insulin-stimulated protein phosphorylation in 3T3 preadipocytes. Proc Natl Acad Sci USA 1979;76:2725
10. Novak-Hofer I, Thomas G. An activated S6 kinase in extracts from serum- and epidermal growth factor-stimulated Swiss 3T3 cells. J Biol Chem 1984;259:5995
11. Kyriakis JM, Avruch J. S6 kinases and MAP kinases: Sequential intermediates in insulin/mitogen-activated protein kinase cascades. In: Woodgett JR, ed. Protein Kinases: Frontiers in Molecular Biology. Oxford: Oxford University Press; 1994:85
12. Erikson E, Maller JL. A protein kinase from *Xenopus* eggs specific for ribosomal protein S6. Proc Natl Acad Sci USA 1985;82:742
13. Price DJ, Nemenoff RA, Avruch J. Purification of a hepatic S6 kinase from cycloheximide-treated rats. J Biol Chem 1989;264:13825
14. Kozma SC, Lane HA, Ferrari S, et al. A stimulated S6 kinase from rat liver: Identify with the mitogen activated S6 kinase of 3T3 cells. EMBO J 1989;8:4125
15. Chung J, Kuo CJ, Crabtree GR, Blenis J. Rapamycin-FKBP specifically blocks growth-dependent activation of a signaling by the 70 kd S6 protein kinases. Cell 1992;69:1227
16. Price DJ, Grove JR, Calvo V, et al. Rapamycin-induced inhibition of the 70-kilodalton S6 protein kinase. Science 1992;257:973
17. Ray LB, Sturgill TW. Rapid stimulation by insulin of a serine/threonine kinase in 3T3-L1 adipocytes that phosphorylates microtubule-associated protein 2 *in vitro*. Proc Natl Acad Sci USA 1987;84:1502
18. Sturgill TW, Ray LB, Erikson E, Maller JL. Insulin-stimulated MAP-2 kinase phosphorylates and activates ribosomal protein S6 kinase II. Nature 1988;334:715
19. Ray LB, Sturgill TW. Insulin-stimulated microtubule-associated protein kinase is phosphorylated on tyrosine and threonine *in vivo*. Proc Natl Acad Sci USA 1988;85:3753
20. Anderson NG, Maller JL, Tonks NK, Sturgill TW. Requirement for integration of signals from two distinct phosphorylation pathways for activation of MAP kinase. Nature 1990;343:651
21. Rossomando AJ, Payne DM, Weber MJ, Sturgill TW. Evidence that pp42, a major tyrosine kinase target protein, is a mitogen-activated serine/threonine protein kinase. Proc Natl Acad Sci USA 1989;86:6940
22. Ahn NG, Seger R, Bratlien RL, et al. Multiple components of an epidermal growth factor-stimulated protein kinase cascade. *In vitro* activation of a myelin basic protein/microtubule-associated protein 2 kinase. J Biol Chem 1991;266:4220
23. Gomez N, Cohen P. Dissection of the protein kinase cascade by which nerve growth factor activates MAP kinases. Nature 1991;353:170
24. Boulton TG, Yancopoulos GD, Gregory JS, et al. An insulin-stimulated protein kinase homologous to yeast kinases involved in cell cycle control. Science 1990;249:64
25. Levin DE, Errede B. The proliferation of MAP kinase signaling pathways in yeast. Curr Opin Cell Biol 1995;7:197
26. Crews C, Alessandrini AA, Erikson RL. The primary structure of MEK, a protein kinase that phosphorylates the *ERK* gene product. Science 1992;258:478
27. Avruch J, Kyriakis JM, Zhang XF. Raf-1 kinase. In: Draznin B, Leroith D, eds. *Molecular Biology of Diabetes* Totowa NJ: Humana Press; 1994:179
28. Kyriakis JM, App H, Zhang X-F, et al. Raf-1 activates MAP kinase-kinase. Nature 1992;358:417
29. Hughes DA, Ashworth A, Marshall CJ. Complementation of *byr1* in fission yeast by mammalian MAP kinase kinase requires coexpression of Raf kinase. Nature 1993;364:349
30. Lange-Carter CA, Pleiman CM, Gardner AM, et al. A divergence in the MAP kinase regulatory network defined by MEK kinase and Raf. Science 1993;260:315
31. Sánchez I, Hughes RT, Mayer BJ, et al. Role of SAPK/ERK kinase-1 in the stress-activated pathway regulating transcription factor c-Jun. Nature 1994;372:794
32. Yan M, Dai T, Deak JC. Activation of stress-activated protein kinase by MEKK1 phosphorylation of its activator SEK1. Nature 1994;372:798
33. Kyriakis JM, Banerjee P, Nikolakaki E, et al. The stress-activated protein kinase subfamily of c-Jun kinases. Nature 1994;369:156
34. Posada J, Yew N, Ahn NG, et al. Mos stimulates MAP kinase in *Xeonpus* oocytes and activates a MAP kinase kinase in vitro. Mol Cell Biol 1993:13254
35. Nebreda AR, Hill C, Gomez N, et al. The protein kinase mos activates MAP kinase-kinase in vitro and stimulates the MAP kinase pathway in mammalian somatic cells in vivo. FEBS Lett 1993;333:183
36. Haystead CMM, Gregory P, Shirazi A, et al. Insulin activates a novel adipocyte mitogen-activated protein kinase kinase that shows rapid phasic kinetics and is distinct from c-Raf. J Biol Chem 1994;269:12804
37. Pang L, Zhang C-F, Guan K-L, Saltiel AR. Nerve growth factor stimulates a novel protein kinase in PC-12 cells that phosphorylates and activates mitogen-activated protein kinase kinase (MEK) Biochem J 1995;302:513
38. Mansour SJ, Matten WT, Hermann AS, et al. Transformation of mammalian cells by constitutively active MAP kinase. Science 1994;265:966
39. Cowley S, Paterson H, Kemp P, Marshall CJ. Activation of MAP kinase kinase is necessary and sufficient for PC12 differentiation and for transformation of NIH 3T3 cells. Cell 1994;77:841
40. Wood KW, Sarnecki C, Roberts TM, Blenis J. *ras* Mediates nerve growth factor receptor modulation of three signal-transducing protein kinases: MAP kinase, Raf-1 and RSK. Cell 1992;68:1041
41. Porras A, Maszynski K, Rapp UR, Santos E. Dissociation between activation of Raf-1 and the 42-kDa mitogen-activated protein kinase/90-kDa S6 kinase (MAPK/RSK) cascade in the insulin/Ras pathway of adipocytic differentiation of 3T3 L1 cells. J Biol Chem 1994;269:12741
42. Norbury C, Nurse P. Animal cell cycles and their control. Ann Rev Biochem 1992;61:441
43. Galaktino K, Jessus C, Beach D. Raf1 interaction with Cdc25 phosphatase ties mitogenic signal transduction to cell cycle activation. Genes Dev 1995;9:1046
44. Barbacid M. *ras* Genes. Ann Rev Biochem 1987;56:779
45. Kaziro Y, Itoh H, Kozasa T, et al. Structure and function of signal-transducing GTP-binding proteins. Ann Rev Biochem 1991;60:349
46. Boguski MS, McCormick F. Proteins regulating Ras and its relatives. Nature 1993;366:643
47. Marshall MS. The effector interactions of $p21^{ras}$. Trends in Biochemical Sciences 1993;18:250
48. Avruch J, Zhang X-F, Kyriakis JM. Raf meets Ras: completing the framework

of a signal transduction pathway. Trends in Biochemical Sciences 1994; 19:279

49. Nassar N, Horn G, Hermann C, et al. The 2.2.A crystal structure of the Ras-binding domain of the serine/threonine kinase c-Raf-1 in complex with Rap1A and a GTP analogue. Nature 1995;375:554
50. Leevers SJ, Paterson HF, Marshal CJ. Requirement for Ras in Raf activation is overcome by targeting Raf to the plasma membrane. Nature 1994;369:411
51. Stokoe D, Macdonald SG, Cadwallader K, et al. Activation of Raf as a result of recruitment to the plasma membrane. Science 1994;64:1463
52. Fabian JR, Vojtek AB, Cooper JA, Morrison DK. A single amino acid change in Raf-1 inhibits Ras binding and alters Raf-1 function. Proc Natl Acad Sci USA 1994;91:5982
53. Barnard D, Diaz B, Hettich L, et al. Identification of the sites of interaction between c-Raf-1 and Ras-GTP. Oncogene 1995;10:1283
54. Bruder JT, Heidecker G, Rapp U. Serum-, TPA-, and Ras-induced expression from Ap- 1/Ets-driven promoters requires Raf-1 kinase. Genes Dev 1992; 6:545
55. Kikuchi A, Demo SD, Yez N, et al. ralGDS Family members interact with the effector loop of ras p21. Mol Cell Biol 1994;14:7483
56. Rodriguez-Viciana P, Warne PH, Dhand R, et al. Phosphatidylinositol-3-3 OH kinase as a direct target of Ras. Nature 1994;370:527
57. Russell M, Lange-Carter CA, Johnson GL. Direct interaction between Ras and the kinase domain of mitogen-activated protein kinase kinase kinase (MEKK1). J Biol Chem 1995;270:11757
58. Dikic I, Schlessinger J, Lax I. PC12 cells overexpressing the insulin receptor undergo insulin-dependent neuronal differentiation. Curr Biol 1994;4:702
59. Traverse S, Seedorf K, Paterson H, et al. EGF triggers neuronal differentiation of PC12 cells that overexpress the EGF receptor. Curr Biol 1994;4:694
60. Denton RM, Tavase JM. Does mitogen-activated-protein kinase have a role in insulin action? The cases for and against. Eur J Biochem 1995;227:597
61. Sommercorn J, Fields R, Raz I, Maeda R. Abnormal regulation of ribosomal protein S6 kinase by insulin in skeletal muscle of insulin-resistant humans. J Clin Invest 1993;91:509
62. Koontz JW, Iwahashi M. Insulin as a potent specific growth factor in a rat hepatoma cell line. Science 1981;211:947
63. Bucher NLR, Patel U, Cohen S. Hormonal factors concerned with liver regeneration. CIBA Found Symp 1977;55:95
64. Wang L-H, Lin B, Jong S-MJ, et al. Activation of transforming potential of the human insulin receptor gene. Proc Natl Acad Sci USA 1987;84:5725
65. Lammers R, Gray A, Schlessinger J, Ullrich A. Differential signalling potential of insulin-and IGF-1-receptor cytoplasmic domains. EMBO J 1989; 8:1369
66. Benito M, Porras A, Nebreda AR, Santos E. Differentiation of 3T3 fibroblasts to adipocytes induced by transfection of ras oncogenes. Science 1991;253:565
67. Treisman R. Ternary complex factors: Growth factor regulated transcriptional activators. Curr Opin Gen Dev 1994;4:96
68. Belsham GJ, Brownsey RW, Hughes WA, Denton RM. Anti-insulin receptor antibodies mimic the effects of insulin on the activities of pyruvate dehydrogenase and acetylCoA carboxylase and on specific protein phosphorylation in rat epididymal fat cells. Diabetologia 1980;18:307
69. Hu C, Pang S, Kong X, et al. Molecular cloning and tissue distribution of PHAS-I, an intracellular target for insulin and growth factors. Proc Natl Acad Sci USA 1994;91:3730
70. Pause A, Belsham GJ, Donze O, et al. Insulin-dependent stimulation of protein synthesis by phosphorylation of a regulator of 5′-cap function. Nature 1994;371:762
71. Sonenberg N. Remarks on the mechanism of ribosome binding to eukaryotic mRNAs. Gene Expr 1993;3:317
72. Redpath NT, Proud CG. Molecular mechanisms in the control of translation by hormones and growth factors. Biochim Biophys Acta 1994;1220:147
73. Manzella JM, Rychlik W, Rhodes RE, et al. Insulin induction of ornithine decarboxylase. Importance of mRNA secondary structure and phosphorylation of eucaryotic initiation factors eIF-4B and eIF-4E. J Biol Chem 1991; 266:2383
74. Koromilas AE, Roy S, Barber GN, et al. Malignant transformation by a mutant of the IFN-inducible dsRNA-dependent protein kinase. Science 1992;257:1685
75. Dent P, Lavoinne A, Nakielny S, et al. The molecular mechanism by which insulin stimulates glycogen synthesis in mammalian skeletal muscle. Nature 1990;348:302
76. Begum N. Stimulation of protein phosphatase-1 activity by insulin in rat adipocytes. 1995;270:709
77. Ramakrishna S, Benjamin WB. Insulin action rapidly decreases multifunctional protein kinase activity in rat adipose tissue. J Biol Chem 1988; 263:12677
78. Hughes K, Ramakrishna SB, Benjamin WB, Woodgett JR. Identification of multifunctional ATP-citrate lyase kinase as the alpha-isoform of glycogen synthase kinase-3. Biochem J 1992;288:309
79. Welsh GI, Proud CG. Glycogen synthase kinase-3 is rapidly inactivated in response to insulin and phosphorylates eukaryotic initiation factor eIF-2B. Biochem J 1993;294:625
80. Sutherland C, Leighton I, Cohen P. Inactivation of glycogen synthase kinase-3b by MAP kinase-activated protein kinase-1 (RSK-2) and p70 S6 kinase; new kinase connections in insulin and growth factor signalling. Biochem J 1993;296:15
81. Stambolic V, Woodgett JR. Mitogen inactivation of glycogen synthase kinase-3 beta in intact cells via serine 9 phosphorylation. Biochem J 1994;303:701
82. Welsh GI, Foulstone EJ, Young SW, et al. Wortmannin inhibits the effects of insulin and serum on the activities of glycogen synthase kinase-3 and mitogen-activated protein kinase. Biochem J 1994;303:15
83. Cross DAE, Alessi DR, Vandenheede JR. The inhibition of glycogen synthase kinase-3 by insulin or insulin-like growth factor 1 in the rat skeletal muscle cell line L6 is blocked by wortmannin, but not by rapamycin: Evidence that wortmannin blocks activation of the mitogen-activated protein kinase pathway in L6 cells between Ras and Raf. Biochem J 1994;303:21
84. Eldar-Finkelman H, Seger R, Vandenheede JR, Krebs EG. Inactivation of glycogen synthase kinase-3 by epidermal growth factor is mediated by mitogen-activated protein kinase/p90 ribosomal protein S6 kinase signaling pathway in NIH/3T3 cells. J Biol Chem 1995;270:987
85. Robinson LA, Razzack ZF, Lawrence JCJ, James DE. Mitogen-activated protein kinase activation is not sufficient for stimulation of glucose transport or glycogen synthase in 3T3-L1 adipocytes. J Biol Chem 1993;268:26422
86. Fingar DC, Birnbaum MJ. Characterization of the mitogen-activated protein kinase/90-kilodalton ribosomal protein S6 kinase signaling pathway in 3T3-L1 adipocytes and its role in insulin-stimulated glucose transport. Endocrinology 1994;134:728
87. van den Berghe N, Ouwens DM, Maassen JA. Activation of the Ras/mitogen-activated protein kinase signaling pathway alone is not sufficient to induce glucose uptake in 3T3-L1 adipocytes. Mol Cell Biol 1994;14:2372
88. Lin TA, Lawrence JC. Activation of ribosomal protein S6 kinases does not increase glycogen synthesis or glucose transport in rat adipocytes. J Biol Chem 1994;269:21255
89. Wiese RJ, Mastick CC, Lazar DF, Saltiel AR. Activation of mitogen-activated protein kinase and phosphatidylinositol 3′-kinase is not sufficient for the hormonal stimulation of glucose uptake, lipogenesis, or glycogen synthesis in 3T3-L1 adipocytes. J Biol Chem 1995;270:3442

89a. Lazar DF, Wiese RJ, Brady MJ, et al. Mitogen-activated protein kinase kinase inhibition does not block the stimulation of glucose utilization by insulin. J Biol Chem 1995;270:20801

90. Sakaue H, Hara K, Noguchi T, et al. Ras-independent and wortmannin-sensitive activation of glycogen synthase by insulin in Chinese hamster ovary cells. J Biol Chem 1995;270:11304
91. Sakaue M, Bowtell D, Kasuga M. A dominant-negative mutant of mSOS1 inhibits insulin-induced Ras activation and reveals Ras-dependent and -independent insulin signaling pathways. Mol Cell Biol 1995;15:379
92. Yamamoto-Honda R, Tobe K, Kaburagi Y, et al. Upstream mechanisms of glycogen synthase activation by insulin and insulin-like growth factor-I. Glycogen synthase activation is antagonized by wortmannin or LY294002 but not by rapamycin or by inhibiting p21ras. J Biol Chem 1995;270:2729
93. Reusch JE, Bhuripanyo P, Carel K, et al. Differential requirement for p21ras activation in the metabolic signaling by insulin. J Biol Chem 1995;2700:2036
94. Kozma L, Baltensperger K, Klarlund J, et al. The ras signaling pathway mimics insulin action on glucose transporter translocation. Proc Natl Acad Sci USA 1993;90:4460
95. Manchester J, Kong X, Lowry OH, Lawrence JC. Ras signaling in the activation of glucose transport by insulin. Proc Natl Acad Sci USA 1994;91:4644
96. Moller DE, Xia C-H, Tang W, et al. Human rsk isoforms: Cloning and characterization of tissue-specific expression. Am J Physiol 1994;266:C351
97. Shepherd PR, Nave BT, Siddle K. Insulin stimulation of glycogen synthesis and glycogen synthase activity is blocked by wortmannin and rapamycin in 3T3-L1 adipocytes: Evidence for the involvement of phosphoinositide 3-kinase and p70 ribosomal protein-S6 kinase. Biochem J 1995;305:25
98. Hara K, Yonezawa K, Sakae H, et al. 1-Phosphatidylinositol 3-kinase activity is required for insulin-stimulated glucose transport but not for RAS activation in CHO cells. Proc Natl Acad Sci USA 1994;91:7415
99. Yano H, Nakanishi S, Kimura K, et al. Inhibition of histamine secretion by wortmannin through the blockade of phosphatidylinositol 3-kinase in RBL-2H3 cells. J Biol Chem 1993;268:25846
100. Kanai F, Ito K, Todaka M, et al. Insulin-stimulated GLUT4 translocation is relevant to the phosphorylation of IRS-1 and the activity of PI3-kinase. Biochem Biophys Res Comm 1993;195:762
101. Clarke JF, Young PW, Konezawn K, et al. Inhibition of the translocation of GLUT1 and GLUT4 in 3T3-L1 cells by the phosphatidylinositol 3-kinase inhibitor, wortmannin. Biochem J 1994;300:631
102. Okada T, Sakuma L, Fukui Y, et al. Blockade of chemotactic peptide-induced stimulation of neutrophils by wortmannin as a result of selective inhibition of phosphatidylinositol 3-kinase. J Biol Chem 1994;269:3563
103. Cheatham B, Vlahos CJ, Cheatham L, et al. Phosphatidylinositol 3-kinase activation is required for insulin stimulation of pp70 S6 kinase, DNA synthesis, and glucose transporter translocation. Mol Cell Biol 1994;14:4902
104. Yeh JI, Gulve EA, Rameh L, Birmbaum MJ. The effects of wortmannin on rat skeletal muscle. Dissociation of signaling pathways for insulin- and contraction-activated hexose transport. J Biol Chem 1995;270:2107
105. Barnard RJ, Youngren JF. Regulation of glucose transport in skeletal muscle. FASEB 1992;6:3238
106. Kapeller R, Cantley LC. Phosphatidylinositol 3-kinase. Bioessays 1994; 16:565
107. Banerjee P, Ahmad MF, Grove JR, et al. Molecular structure of a major insulin/mitogen-activated 70-kDa S6 protein kinase. Proc Natl Acad Sci USA 1990;87:8550

108. Kozma SC, Ferrari S, Bassand P, et al. Cloning of the mitogen-activated S6 kinase from rat liver reveals an enzyme of the second messenger subfamily. Proc Natl Acad Sci USA 1990;87:7365
109. Grove JR, Banerjee P, Balasubramanyam A, et al. Cloning and expression of two human p70 S6 kinase polypeptides differing only at their amino termini. Mol Cell Biol 1991;11:5541
110. Reinhard C, Thomas G, Kozma SC. A single gene encodes two isoforms of the p70 S6 kinase: Activation upon mitogenic stimulation. Proc Natl Acad Sci USA 1992;89:4052
111. Lane HA, Fernandez A, Lamb NJ, Thomas G. p70s6k Function is essential for G1 progression. Nature 1993;363:170
112. Reinhard C, Fernandez A, Lamb NJ, Thomas G. Nuclear localization of p85 S6k: Functional requirement for entry into S phase. EMBO J 1994;13:1557
113. Kuo CJ, Chung J, Fiorentino DF, et al. Rapamycin selectively inhibits interleukin-2 activation of p70 S6 kinase. Nature 1992;358:70
114. Calvo V, Crews CM, Vik TA, Bierer BE. Interleukin 2 stimulation of p70 S6 kinase activity is inhibited by the immunosuppressant rapamycin. Proc Natl Acad Sci USA 1992;89:7571
115. Morice WG, Brunn GJ, Wiedrirecht G, et al. Rapamycin-induced inhibition of p34cdc2 kinase activation is associated with G1/S-phase growth arrest in T lymphocytes. J Biol Chem 1993;268:3734
116. deGroot RP, Ballou LM, Sassone-Corsi P. Positive regulation of the cAMP-responsive activator CREM by the p70 S6 kinase: An alternative route to mitogen-induced gene expression. Cell 1994;79:81
117. Jefferies HBJ, Reinhard C, Kozma SC, Thomas G. Rapamycin selectively represses translation of the "polypyrimidine tract" mRNA family. Proc Natl Acad Sci USA 1994;91:4441
118. Franco R, Rosenfeld MG. Hormonally inducible phosphorylation of a nuclear pool of ribosomal protein S6. J Biol Chem 1990;265:4321
119. Fingar DC, Hausdorff SF, Blenis J, Birnbaum MJ. Dissociation of pp70 ribosomal protein S6 kinase from insulin-stimulated glucose transport in 3T3-L1 adipocytes. J Biol Chem 1993;268:3005
120. Chung J, Grammer TC, Lennon KP, et al. PDGF-and insulin-dependent pp70S6k activation mediated by phosphatidylinositol-3-OH kinase. Nature 1994;370:71
121. Ming XF, Burgering BM, Wennstrom S, et al. Activation of p70/p85 S6 kinase by a pathway independent of p21ras. Nature 1994;371:426
122. Price DJ, Gunsalus JR, Avruch J. Insulin activates a 70,000 dalton S6 kinase through serine/threonine-specific phosphorylation of the enzyme polypeptide. Proc Natl Acad Sci USA 1990;87:7944
123. Grove JR, Price DJ, Banerjee P, et al. Regulation of an epitope-tagged recombinant Rsk-1 S6 kinase by phorbol ester and erk/MAP kinase. Biochemist 1993;32:7727
124. Price DJ, Mukhopadhyay NK, Avruch J. Insulin-activated protein kinases phosphorylate a pseudosubstrate synthetic peptide inhibitor of the p70 S6 kinase. J Biol Chem 1991;266:16281
125. Ferrari S, Bannwarth W, Morley SJ, et al. Activation of $p70^{s6k}$ is associated with phosphorylation of four clustered sites displaying Ser/Thr-Pro motifs. Proc Natl Acad Sci USA 1992;89:7282
126. Mukhopadhay NK, Price DJ, Kyriakis JM, et al. An array of insulin-activated, proline-directed (Ser/Thr) protein kinases phosphorylate the p70 S6 kinase. J Biol Chem 1992;267:3325
127. Weng Q-P, Andrabi K, Kozlowski MT, et al. Multiple independent inputs are required for activation of the p70 S6 kinase. Mol Cell Biol 1995;15:2333
128. Weng Q-P, Andrabi K, Klippel A, et al. Phosphatidylinositol-3 kinase signals activation of p70 S6 kinase in situ through site-specific p70 phosphorylation. Proc Natl Acad Sci USA 1995;92:5744
129. Hanks SK, Hunter T. The eukaryotic protein kinase superfamily: Kinase (catalytic) domain structure and classification. FASEB J 1995;9:576
130. Toker A, Meyer M, Reddy K, et al. Activation of protein kinase C family members by the novel polyphosphoinositides PtdIns-3,4-P2 and PtdIns-3,4,5-P3. J Biol Chem 1994;269:32358
131. Nakanishi H, Brewer KA, Exton JH. Activation of the z isozyme of protein kinase C by phosphatidylinositol 3,4,5-triphosphate. J Biol Chem 1993;268:13
132. Franke TF, Yang SI, Chan TO, et al. The protein kinase encoded by the Akt proto-oncogene is a target of the PDGF-activated phosphatidylinositol 3-kinase. Cell 1995;81:727
132a. Burgering BM, Coffer PJ, Protein kinase B (c-akt) in phosphatidylinositol 3-kinase signal transduction. Nature 1995;376:599
133. Snyder SH, Sabatini DM. Immunophilins and the nervous system. Nature Med 1995;1:32–36
134. Liu J, Farmer JD Jr, Lane WS, et al. Calcineurin is a common target of cyclophilin-cyclosporin A and FKBP-FK506 complexes. Cell 1991;66:807
135. Liu J, Albers MW, Wandless TJ, et al. Inhibition of T cell signaling by immunophilin-ligand complexes correlates with loss of calcineurin phosphatase activity. Biochemistry 1992;31:3896
136. Ferrari S, Pearson RB, Siegmann M, et al. The immunosuppressant rapamycin induces inactivation of p70s6k through dephosphorylation of a novel set of sites. J Biol Chem 1993;268:16091
137. Heitman J, Movva NR, Hall MN. Targets for cell cycle arrest by the immunosuppressant rapamycin in yeast. Science 1991;253:905
138. Kunz J, Henriquez R, Schneider U, et al. Target of rapamycin in yeast, TOR2 is an essential phosphatidylinositol kinase homolog required for G_1 progression. Cell 1993;73:585
139. Brown EJ, Albers MW, Shin TB, et al. A mammalian protein targeted by G1-arresting rapamycin-receptor complex. Nature 1994;369:756
140. Sabatini DM, Erdjument-Bromage H, Lui M, et al. RAFT1: A mammalian protein that binds to FKBP12 in a rapamycin-dependent fashion and is homologous to yeast TORs. Cell 1994;78:35
141. Sabers CJ, Martin MM, Brunn GJ, et al. Isolation of a protein target of the FKBP12-rapamycin complex in mammalian cells. J Biol Chem 1995;270:815
142. Chiu MI, Katz H, Berlin V. RAPT1, a mammalian homolog of yeast Tor, interacts with the FKBP12/Rapamycin complex. Proc Natl Acad Sci USA 1994;91:12574

Diabetes Mellitus, edited by Derek LeRoith, Simeon I. Taylor, and Jerrold M. Olefsky. Lippincott–Raven Publishers, Philadelphia © 1996.

Chapter 18

Protein-Tyrosine Phosphatases and the Regulation of Insulin Action

Barry J. Goldstein

Although much attention has been paid over the past decade to activation of insulin signaling by tyrosyl phosphorylation of the insulin receptor and its cellular substrate proteins, interest has recently grown in the role of protein-tyrosine phosphatases (PTPases) in balancing the steady-state level of phosphorylation of proteins in the cellular insulin action pathway.[1] PTPases can impact on insulin signaling at several levels. Dephosphorylation of the active (autophosphorylated) form of the insulin receptor by PTPases attenuates the receptor kinase activity, whereas dephosphorylation of receptor substrate proteins such as insulin receptor substrate-1 (IRS-1) and Shc by cellular PTPases modulates postreceptor pathways of insulin action. Largely as a result of molecular cloning studies, PTPases have now been recognized to constitute a large superfamily of fascinating enzymes playing a variety of regulatory roles in cellular physiology. With regard to insulin action, recent work in this area has focused on mechanisms involved in the regulation of insulin signaling by dephosphorylation, the identification of specific PTPases that act on various components of the insulin action pathway, and clarifying the potential involvement of PTPases in the pathophysiology of insulin-resistant disease states. These several areas are reviewed in this chapter.

Regulation of Insulin Signaling by Dephosphorylation

The Insulin Receptor

Insulin initiates its cellular effects by binding to a specific plasma membrane receptor that encodes a tyrosyl-specific protein kinase.[2] Insulin binding elicits the rapid autophosphorylation of specific tyrosine residues in multiple domains of the cytoplasmic segment of the receptor β-subunit.[3-5] Receptor autophosphorylation occurs as a cascade involving the receptor kinase domain, the C-terminus, and the juxtamembrane domain.[3-6] Detailed studies on the activation of the insulin receptor kinase have shown that phosphorylation of two tyrosines in the kinase domain, involving Tyr^{1146} and either Tyr^{1150} or Tyr^{1151} occurs first, and that the resulting receptors with *mono-* or *bis*-phosphorylated kinase domains exhibit minimal activation of the β-subunit kinase activity. Phosphorylation of the third tyrosyl residue in the receptor "regulatory domain" follows the *bis*-phosphorylation stage rapidly and leads to full activation of the receptor kinase toward exogenous substrates.[3,5] In this way, the transition between *bis-* and *tris*-phosphorylation in the receptor regulatory domain may be considered a discrete molecular "switch" in which the steady-state level of phosphorylation in this region can determine the overall degree of receptor kinase activation[7] (Fig. 18-1).

Phosphorylation of tyrosines in the C-terminal region does not appear to influence activation of the receptor kinase; however, modification of this domain may be involved in signaling to certain distal effects of insulin.[8,9] Tyrosyl phosphorylation at the receptor juxtamembrane region[10,11] is thought to be involved in recognition

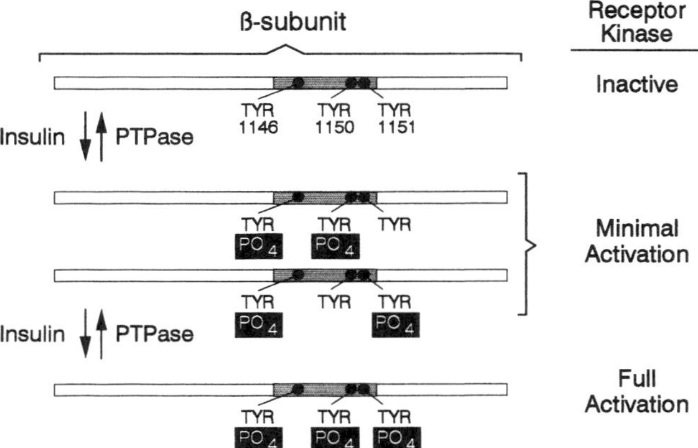

Figure 18-1. Scheme of insulin receptor activation and deactivation by a cascade of a reversible tyrosine phosphorylation events in the receptor regulatory domain. Insulin binding to the receptor α-subunit elicits the rapid autophosphorylation of two tyrosines in the receptor kinase domain involving Tyr^{1146} and Tyr^{1150} or ^{1151}. Full activation of the receptor kinase toward exogenous substrates does not occur until the third tyrosine residue in this region is phosphorylated.[3,5] PTPases may largely inactivate the receptor kinase enzyme by the discrete dephosphorylation of a single phosphotyrosine residue in the tris-phospho form of the receptor kinase and bring the receptor to the basal state by complete dephosphorylation.

and phosphorylation of substrates by the receptor kinase, in particular IRS-1.[12] The endogenous substrate Shc has also been shown to interact with the NPXpY motif in the juxtamembrane domain of several growth factor receptors.[13,14] Since the insulin receptor undergoes a complex cascade of multisite phosphorylation, the dephosphorylation by PTPases of individual receptor phosphotyrosyl residues in the kinase regulatory domain and other sites can potentially impact on signaling to various elements of the postreceptor insulin action pathway.

The physiologic role of PTPases in the reversal of insulin receptor activation has also been substantiated by the observation that purified insulin holoreceptors retain their autophosphorylation state in vitro even if insulin is removed from the ligand binding site.[15-18] Thus, the steady-state balance or the activation-deactivation of certain receptor sites by reversible tyrosyl phosphorylation appears to be an essential mechanism for the regulation of insulin action by cellular PTPases.

Insulin Receptor Substrate-1

IRS-1 is a widely expressed cellular substrate for the insulin receptor kinase that contains multiple tyrosyl residues in a sequence context that is efficiently phosphorylated by the insulin receptor kinase.[19,20] Once phosphorylated, IRS-1 is thought to act as an adapter or "docking" protein for the binding and activation of a variety of src-homology 2 (SH2) domain-containing signaling proteins, which form a tight but noncovalent association with the phosphotyrosyl domains of IRS-1. Included in the variety of proteins known to interact with IRS-1 in this way are the p85 subunit of phosphatidylinositol-3′-kinase, the adaptor proteins Grb2 and nck, and the intracellular protein-tyrosine phosphatase, SH-PTP2 (also called syp or PTP1D; see below).[21] This model of IRS-1 signaling has provided insight into the potential mechanisms by which reversible tyrosyl phosphorylation, catalyzed by the opposing effects of the insulin receptor kinase and cellular PTPases, can play a central role in the regulation of insulin action in various cell types. Furthermore, the dephosphorylation of individual sites or sets of phosphotyrosyl domains on IRS-1 may also be catalyzed by specific PTPases, adding a further element of complexity by which insulin signaling to multiple postreceptor pathways can be regulated differently in various physiologic states.

The Vanadate Connection

As PTPases are implicated in the reversal of insulin receptor activation and dephosphorylation of receptor substrate proteins, agents such as vanadate and related compounds, as potent PTPase inhibitors, can enhance insulin signaling perhaps by augmenting the phosphorylation state of the insulin receptor or receptor substrates.[22-24] The mechanism of vanadate action, however, is unclear at present. Vanadate has also been shown to enhance the activity of a cytoplasmic tyrosine kinase in adipocytes,[25] but its effects on cellular kinases and PTPases may depend on the oxidation state of the vanadium ion in the cell, which is difficult to directly assess.[26] A number of studies have shown that oral vanadate is effective in reducing hyperglycemia in diabetic animal models, and clinical trials in humans are currently under way to explore the potential effectiveness of vanadate as an antidiabetic agent.

The Protein-Tyrosine Phosphatases Superfamily of Enzymes

Molecular cloning and biochemical studies have rapidly expanded our understanding of PTPases as an extensive family of proteins that exert both positive and negative influences on a number of

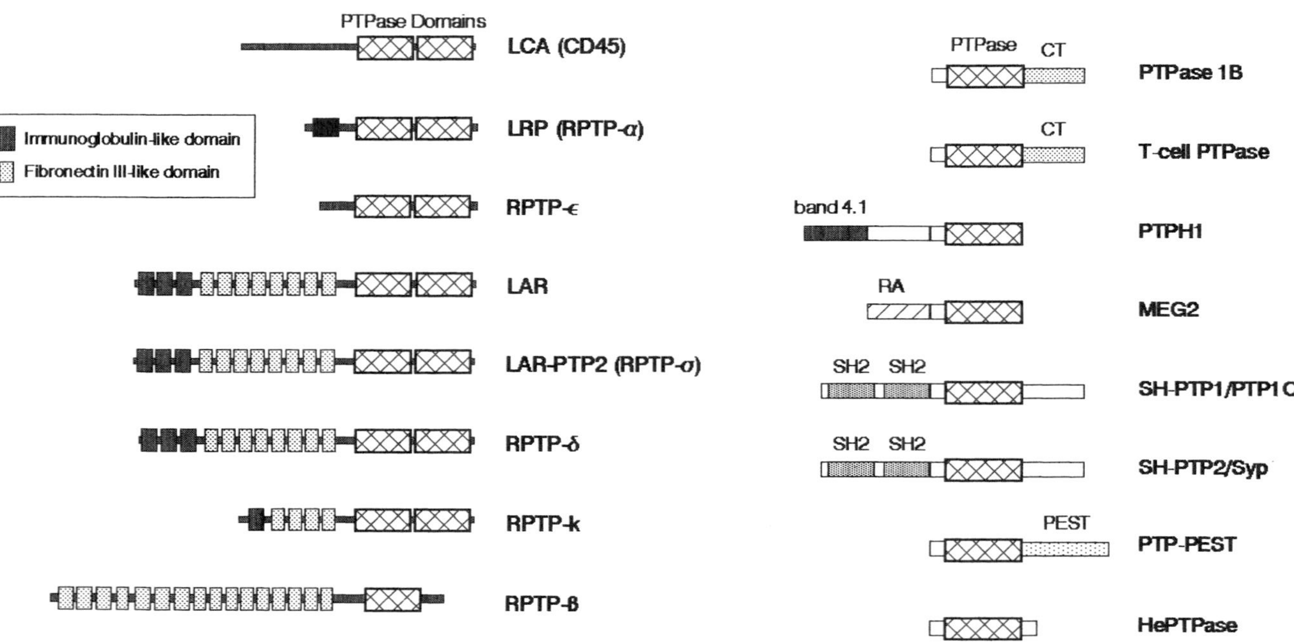

FIGURE 18-2. Representative structures of receptor-type, transmembrane PTPases (*left panel*) and nonreceptor type, intracellular PTPases (*right panel*) derived from molecular cloning studies. The receptor-type PTPases shown include: LCA, for leukocyte common antigen or CD45; LAR, for leukocyte antigen related; LAR-PTP2 or RPTP-σ; LRP, for LCA-related phosphatase or RPTP-α; RPTP-ε; RPTP-δ; RPTP-κ; and RPTP-β. The extracellular domains of several of the transmembrane enzymes shown have structural similarity to fibronectin type III repeats found in a family of cell adhesion molecules and immunoglobulin-like domains. Subfamilies of the transmembrane PTPases have exceptionally high sequence homology (e.g., LAR, LAR-PTP2/RPTP-σ, and RPTP-δ), suggesting that they may have related functional roles in the cell that can be determined by their pattern of expression in various tissues or during development. In addition to the single PTPase catalytic domain, the nonreceptor type PTPases typically have additional functional domains that are depicted and consist of the following: PTPase1B and the T-cell PTPase have C-terminal hydrophobic domains (labeled "CT") that confer an association with the endoplasmic reticulum; PTPH1 has an N-terminal domains homologous to cytoskeleton-associated proteins, such as band 4.1 and ezrin (labeled "band 4.1"); MEG2 has a domain homologous to a retinaldehyde-binding protein ("RA"); SH-PTP1/PTP1C and SH-PTP2/Syp have two N-terminal SH2 domains that promote their interaction with phosphotyrosine-containing proteins; PTP-PEST has a proline, glutamic acid, serine and threonine-rich ("PEST") domain at the C-terminus; HePTPase is unique in apparently lacking additional functional domains. See reference 1 and the text.

pathways of cellular signal transduction and metabolism.[27-29] PTPases may be divided into two broad categories (Fig. 18-2): (1) *receptor type*, which have a general structure like a membrane receptor with an extracellular domain, a single transmembrane segment, and one or two tandemly conserved PTPase catalytic domains (including LCA (CD45), LRP/RPTP-α, RPTP-ε, LAR, LAR-PTP2/RPTP-σ, RPTP-δ, RPTP-κ and RPTP-β,), and (2) *nonreceptor type*, which have a single PTPase domain and additional functional protein segments (including PTPase1B, T-cell PTPase, PTPH1, MEG2, SH-PTP1/PTP1C, SH-PTP2/Syp, PTP-PEST, and HePTPase). Although this designation helps to simplify some of the structural features of the PTPases, it fails to convey their exact subcellular localization, a key aspect to consider with regard to insulin action. Thus, transmembrane PTPases may reside in the plasma membrane or internal membranes, and "nonreceptor" PTPases are frequently found associated with internal membrane fractions either by way of complex formation with other membrane proteins or with PTPase protein segments that target the enzymes to specific intracellular sites, such as the endoplasmic reticulum.[30] Although much has been learned about the structure of cellular PTPases, it is still not known what the intracellular targets may be for many of these enzymes. In particular, the specific PTPase(s) that act on insulin and growth factor receptor pathways in intact tissues have not been conclusively identified.

Considerations for Protein-Tyrosine Phosphatases Regulating the Insulin Action Pathway

Even though insulin receptors lack intrinsic PTPase catalytic activity, significant PTPase activity can copurify with insulin receptors,[31] a factor that can complicate experiments designed to preserve the endogenous tyrosine phosphorylation state of insulin receptors. The identification of one or more of the known PTPase homologs that may coimmunoprecipitate as a high-affinity complex with insulin receptors has not been demonstrated. In order to identify candidate PTPases for the insulin action pathway, several areas of available data should be considered, including the tissue expression

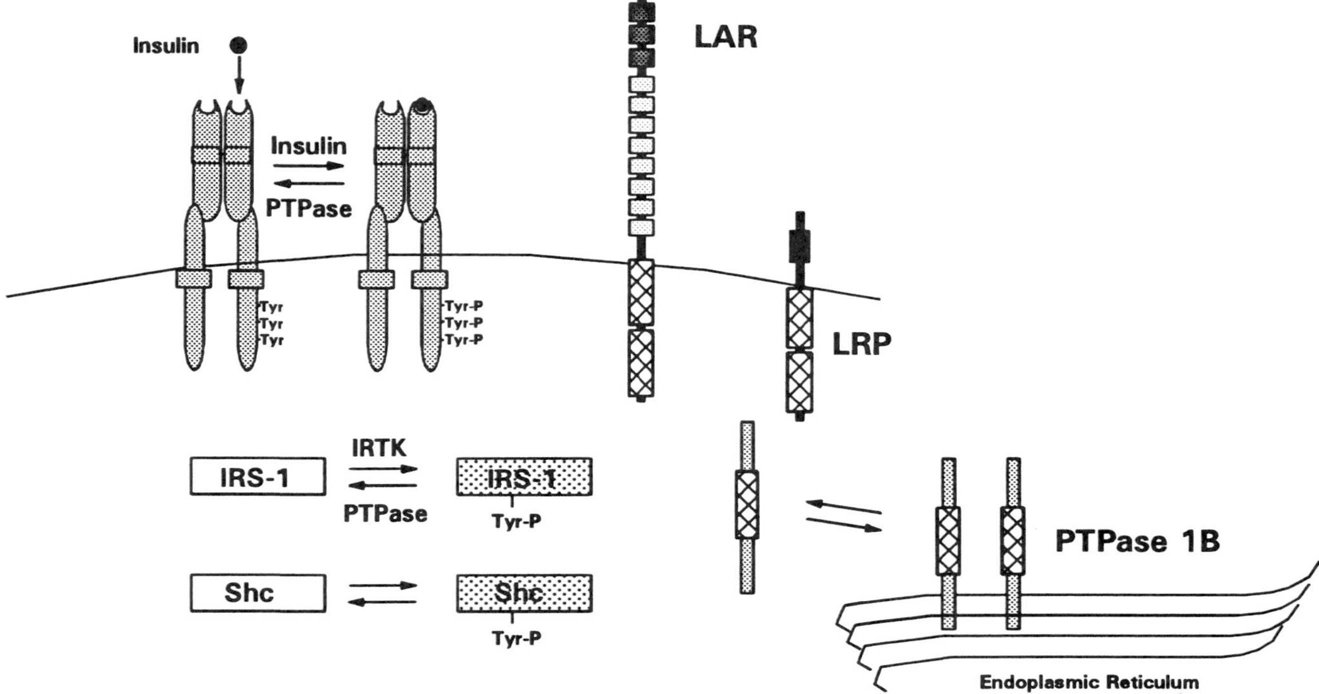

FIGURE 18-3. Access of candidate PTPases to the insulin receptor and its cellular substrate proteins in the regulation of insulin signaling. Activation of the insulin receptor tyrosine kinase by insulin leads to the phosphorylation of substrate proteins, including IRS-1 and Shc. The receptor kinase activity is reversed by PTPases that may reside in the plasma membrane compartment, such as LAR, an LAR-related PTPase such as LAR-PTP2/RPTP-σ, or another membrane-localized PTPase such as LRP/RPTP-α. Intracellular receptor substrates or the insulin receptor itself may be dephosphorylated by cytoplasmic PTPases, including SH-PTP2 (see Fig. 18-5) or PTPase1B, which is found in the free cytosol fraction as well as associated with the endoplasmic reticulum of the cell. Internalization of the insulin receptor into the cell and the association of receptor substrates with cell membrane fractions may also play a role in determining interactions that occur between candidate PTPases and tyrosine-phosphorylated proteins in the insulin action pathway.

of various PTPase homologs and their subcellular localization and catalytic specificity (Fig. 18-3). These studies have led to manipulation of the candidate enzymes in situ by molecular and cellular techniques in order to provide more direct evidence for their potential involvement in insulin receptor regulation and to explore the mechanisms of these processes in cellular physiology.

Protein-Tyrosine Phosphatases Expressed in Insulin-Sensitive Tissues

The restricted tissue distribution of some PTPases has been shown to be an important factor in determining their specialized cellular roles. For example, the lymphocyte-specific expression of CD45 (LCA) is essential for the physiologic regulation of T-cell activation.[32] When CD45 is expressed heterotopically in nonhematopoietic cells, however, it can affect receptor autophosphorylation and signaling by the platelet-derived growth factor (PDGF) and IGF-I receptor pathways.[33,34] Thus, identification of PTPases expressed in insulin-sensitive tissues, including liver, skeletal muscle, and adipose tissue, is a crucial element in designating candidate enzymes involved in the physiologic regulation of insulin signaling.

Liver tissue is a rich source of PTPase activity, and multiple enzymes have been described in particulate and soluble liver fractions that will dephosphorylate the insulin receptor.[35–37] Northern and Western blot analysis and cDNA library screening have revealed relatively high levels of expression of PTPase1B, LAR, LRP (RPTP-α) and SH-PTP2 in normal liver.[38–44] Interestingly, cDNA inserts for LAR and the insulin receptor had identical abundance in a rat liver cDNA library (seven per million), suggesting that these two proteins might have a similar level of expression in this tissue.[45] In these studies, we also identified a novel receptor-type PTPase closely related to LAR and human PTP-δ, which we termed LAR-PTP2, which is expressed in liver but is less abundant than LAR.[46] PTP-κ is also an abundant transmembrane PTPase in the liver.[47]

The identification of PTPases expressed in skeletal muscle is of particular importance, since the clinical insulin resistance associated with type II diabetes mellitus is predominantly caused by defects in insulin action in this tissue.[48] Tissue homogenates of normal rat skeletal muscle have been reported to contain approximately one-tenth of the PTPase activity found in the liver.[49] In agreement with these data, we amplified rat skeletal muscle cDNA with degenerate primers to conserved PTPase domains and found a limited set of PTPase cDNA transcripts that included LAR and LRP. Furthermore, using the LRP cDNA as a hybridization probe at reduced stringency, only a single LAR cDNA insert was identified among 10^6 plaques of a rat skeletal muscle cDNA library, indicating the rare nature of PTPase cDNAs in muscle tissue in general.[50] Direct Northern analysis of skeletal muscle RNA has confirmed the expression of PTPase1B and SH-PTP2 expression in muscle.[51–53] We have also recently purified the major peaks of PTPase activity from rat skeletal muscle particulate and cytosol fractions by column chromatographic techniques and identified some of the major PTPase enzymes by immunoblotting.[123] These included LAR

Table 18-1. Candidate Protein-Tyrosine Phosphatases Expressed in Insulin-Sensitive Tissues

PTPase	Molecular Mass	Functional Domains
Transmembrane		
LAR	212,000	A large enzyme with three immunoglobulin-like repeats and eight fibronectin type III repeats in the extracellular domain, a single transmembrane segment, and tandem cytoplasmic PTPase domains
LRP (RPTP-α)	90,000	Small extracellular domain without functional homology, single transmembrane segment, tandem cytoplasmic PTPase domains
Intracellular		
PTP1B	50,000	Single PTPase domain with hydrophobic C-terminal segment that confers association with cytoplasmic face of the endoplasmic reticulum
SH-PTP2	68,000	Single PTPase domain with two SH2 domains near N-terminus
PTP-PEST	88,000	Single PTPase domain with Pro, Glu, Ser, Thr-rich (''PEST'') domain at C-terminus

in the particulate fraction and PTPase1B and SH-PTP2, which exhibited a characteristic distribution between the cytosol and particulate fractions. Immunoblotting with an antibody that reacts with recombinant LRP (RPTP-α) failed to detect this PTPase in muscle subcellular fractions, providing further evidence that it may have a relatively low abundance in muscle.

In order to identify PTPases in adipocytes, we screened a rat cDNA library from isolated fat cells at reduced stringency with a panel of candidate PTPase probes.[54] After subcloning and sequence analysis of the positive plaques, this approach enabled us to identify the expression of LRP/RPTP-α, PTPase1B, SH-PTP2/Syp, and LAR in adipocytes at an abundance of 16, 7, 6, and 3 per million, respectively. Furthermore, an additional sequence variant of SH-PTP2/Syp was identified that may have significance in the tissue-specific activity of this enzyme (see further on).

Table 18-1 summarizes some of the available data on the expression of cloned PTPases in normal, insulin-sensitive tissues. Because of their common expression and relative abundance in insulin-sensitive tissues, the transmembrane PTPases LAR and LRP (RPTP-α) and the two ''intracellular'' PTPases—PTPase1B and SH-PTP2—have emerged to date as potential candidate PTPases for the insulin action pathway.

Subcellular Localization

In studies performed with insulin receptors in situ in permeabilized adipocytes[55,56] or Chinese hamster ovary (CHO) cells[57] essentially devoid of cytoplasmic contents, dissociation of insulin was followed by a rapid dephosphorylation of the insulin receptor, suggesting that a major tyrosine phosphatase for the insulin receptor is an integral membrane protein or one otherwise closely linked to membrane proteins or to the receptor itself. Similarly, insulin receptors are rapidly dephosphorylated in isolated liver endosomes by a process that is disrupted by solubilization of the membranes with non-ionic detergents.[58] In accordance with the notion that one or more major PTPases for the insulin receptor reside in the plasma membrane, biochemical studies in insulin-responsive tissues have shown that the bulk of PTPase activity toward insulin and IGF-I receptor dephosphorylation in fractionated liver tissue is recovered in a particulate fraction,[59] with the highest specific PTPase activity present in a glycoprotein extract of the solubilized plasma membrane fraction.[42,60] In skeletal muscle, we also confirmed that the PTPase activity toward the insulin receptor was 5.6-fold higher in the solubilized particulate fraction than in the cytosol.[123]

Following autophosphorylation of the insulin receptor in the plasma membrane, its internalization into the cell through an endosomal compartment is associated with dynamic changes in its phosphorylation state.[61] This intracellular movement of the insulin receptor influences its potential association with PTPases in various subcellular compartments. Thus, while plasma membrane PTPases may be important in the regulation of receptor phosphorylation in situ, these considerations do not exclude the possibility of additional effects of intracellular PTPases in insulin action, especially in the dephosphorylation of receptor substrates or in the deactivation of internalized insulin receptors that may associate with internal membrane pools.

The subcellular localization of known PTPases has also been characterized in a number of studies. Detailed characterization of PTPase1B protein has shown it to be associated, possibly as a high-molecular-mass complex, with the endoplasmic reticulum of the cell[62,63]; however, a significant portion of the uncleaved enzyme is also found in the cytosol of Rat 1 fibroblasts[64] and in normal rat skeletal muscle and liver tissue (Table 18-2). We have confirmed that the transmembrane PTPase LAR is localized to both plasma membranes and the microsomal fraction of liver and skeletal muscle and absent from the cell cytosol. Other enzymes, including SH-PTP2, although lacking membrane-targeting motifs, are distributed between the cytosol and particulate compartments (plasma membrane and internal membranes), perhaps associated as SH2 domain-protein-phosphotyrosyl complexes with transmembrane or membrane-bound proteins or receptors.

Table 18-2. Subcellular Distribution of PTPase1B Protein in Rat Liver and Skeletal Muscle*

Subcellular Fraction	Liver	Skeletal Muscle
Particulate fraction	35–40%	45–50%
Cytosol	60–65%	50–55%

*Protein distribution for PTPase1B was estimated by immunoblotting of the cytosol and solubilized particulate fractions from the indicated rat tissues and calculated by correcting for the total volume of each fraction derived from the crude tissue homogenate (Ahmad F, Goldstein BJ, unpublished observations, 1995).

Substrate Specificity

In vitro, PTPases dephosphorylate a number of protein and peptide substrates, although with different kinetic parameters.[65,66] Thus many PTPases have been found to be active, to a greater or lesser degree, against the autophosphorylated insulin receptor in vitro, including recombinant PTPase1B, CD45, LAR, LRP, SH-PTP2 and PTP-PEST.[42,51,67–71] The insulin receptor interaction is not specific, however, since many of these PTPases also dephosphorylate epidermal growth factor (EGF) receptors and a variety of phosphopeptide substrates.

Although a number of PTPases have been shown to catalyze the overall dephosphorylation of the insulin receptor, we investigated whether LAR, LRP, or PTPase1B, as candidate insulin receptor PTPases, differed in their relative specificity for phosphotyrosine residues in the receptor regulatory domain that is known to regulate its intrinsic tyrosine kinase activity.[72] By studying the in vitro dephosphorylation of the insulin receptor with recombinant PTPase catalytic domains from an *Escherichia coli* expression system, we found that relative to the level of overall receptor dephosphorylation, LAR deactivated the receptor kinase two to three times more rapidly than either PTPase1B or LRP. Furthermore, tryptic mapping of the insulin receptor β-subunit after dephosphorylation by PTPases showed that LAR dephosphorylated the *tris*-phosphorylated (Tyr^{1150}) receptor kinase domain three to four times more rapidly than either PTPase1B or LRP, indicating that the effect of the LAR PTPase to inactivate the receptor kinase was attributable to a preferential dephosphorylation of the receptor regulatory domain by this enzyme.[72] These studies have provided biochemical data that support a potential role for this transmembrane PTPase as a cellular regulator of the insulin receptor kinase.

Studies on Insulin Action in Intact Cells

Studies performed with PTPases in vitro can prove hazardous with regard to in vivo specificity, since subcellular localization of the enzyme or compartmentalization of substrate proteins that occurs in the intact cells is lost. Attention in recent work has thus been directed to intact cell systems in which the effects of manipulation of PTPase activities in situ can be examined. Initial work in this regard has provided some of the first evidence for direct effects of PTPases on insulin signaling in intact cells when the microinjection of purified PTPase1B (C-terminally truncated form; see below) into *Xenopus* oocytes was shown to block insulin-stimulated S6 peptide phosphorylation and to retard insulin-induced oocyte maturation.[73,74] These findings have led to recent work using expression of PTPases in various cell systems in an attempt to dissect the cellular role of the various enzymes. These studies are outlined with the individual enzymes below.

Candidate Protein-Tyrosine Phosphatases for the Insulin Receptor and Its Substrate Proteins

LAR

As discussed earlier, this large, transmembrane PTPase has emerged as a candidate enzyme for the regulation of the insulin receptor for several reasons. LAR is expressed in insulin-sensitive liver, muscle, and adipose tissue[1]; it is localized to the membrane fraction of the cell, and biochemical studies have shown that its cytoplasmic domain has catalytic preference for the regulatory phosphotyrosines in the insulin receptor kinase domain.[72] To further support the hypothesis that LAR has a role in the physiologic regulation of insulin receptor phosphorylation in intact cells, we initiated studies using transfection of LAR and other PTPase cDNAs into insulin-sensitive cells to test this hypothesis further. In CHO cells that overexpress human insulin receptors, preliminary studies have shown that transfection of the full-length LAR cDNA with overexpression of the enzyme at a transmembrane site leads to markedly reduced insulin-stimulated receptor phosphorylation (Zhang WR, Goldstein BJ, unpublished observations). Interestingly, a similar expression system generating only the soluble cytoplasmic domain of LAR does not affect receptor activation by insulin, further supporting the notion that transmembrane localization is critical for LAR action in situ. In addition, we have recently obtained compelling evidence for a physiologic role of LAR in insulin receptor regulation in studies done in collaboration with Dr. Robert Mooney[124] (Fig.18-4). Using expression of LAR antisense mRNA in hepatoma cells to reduce LAR mass by 63%, insulin receptor autophosphorylation was increased by 150% and insulin-stimulated PI-3-kinase activity was amplified to 300% over the level observed in cells transfected with the null expression vector. These studies strongly suggest that in situ LAR is a physiologic modulator of insulin signaling. Further work currently in progress will examine the specificity and mechanism of the effect of LAR overexpression as well as the reduction of LAR expression on insulin signaling.

SH-PTP2/PTP1D/Syp

This widely expressed PTPase contains two N-terminal SH2 domains, a single catalytic PTPase domain and a hydrophilic C-terminal segment with potential serine-threonine as well as tyrosine phosphorylation sites (see Fig. 18-2).[52,53,75,76] SH-PTP2 associates with autophosphorylated PDGF and EGF receptors as well as with tyrosine-phosphorylated IRS-1 by its SH2 domains.[77,78] In recombinant in vitro systems, SH-PTP2 has also been shown to associate with the insulin receptor and can be phosphorylated by the insulin receptor kinase.[79–82] However, several studies in vivo have failed to demonstrate either a direct interaction between SH-PTP2 and insulin receptors or any effects of overexpression of the native, catalytically active SH-PTP2 enzyme on the phosphorylation state of the insulin receptor or on insulin signaling in intact cells.[76,83–85]

The association of SH-PTP2 with autophospohorylated receptors for PDGF or EGF or consensus phosphopeptides derived from receptor or IRS-1 sequences can accelerate the catalytic activity of the PTPase domain up to 50-fold.[86–89] Each of the SH2 domains functions in enzyme activation, but since they have different site preferences, they may interact with alternate domains on the associated phosphoprotein to enhance the PTPase activity that is directed at a third phosphotyrosyl site. In vitro, the binding of SH-PTP2 to IRS-1 by its SH2 domains has been shown to enhance its PTPase activity, accelerate the dephosphorylation of IRS-1, and decrease the association of the p85 subunit of PI-3-kinase to IRS-1.[83] Interestingly, prior association of p85 to IRS-1 fully blocked the ability of SH-PTP2 to dephosphorylate IRS-1, suggesting that association of SH2-domain–containing proteins with IRS-1 in vivo may modulate its dephosphorylation and inactivation by cellular PTPases. A similar effect has also been demonstrated with the autophosphorylated EGF receptor where the binding of PLC-γ can block its enzymatic dephosphorylation.[90]

SH-PTP2 appears to be the mammalian homolog of the *Drosophila csw* gene product, which potentiates the action of the *Drosophila c-raf* homolog to positively transmit signals downstream of the protein receptor tyrosine kinase.[91,92] Recent evidence suggests SH-PTP2 may play a similar positive role in growth factor signaling in mammalian cells. Single-cell microinjection of SH-PTP2 antibody, a glutathione-*S*-transferase fusion construct with the SH2 domains of SH-PTP2, or IRS-1 derived phosphopeptides that bind to the SH2 domains of SH-PTP2 blocked insulin-stimulated mitogenic signaling (bromodeoxyuridine incorporation) in Rat 1 fibroblasts overexpressing the insulin receptor.[79] Responses

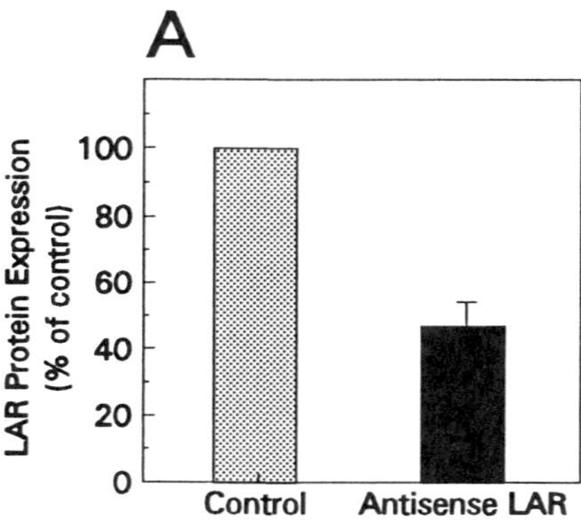

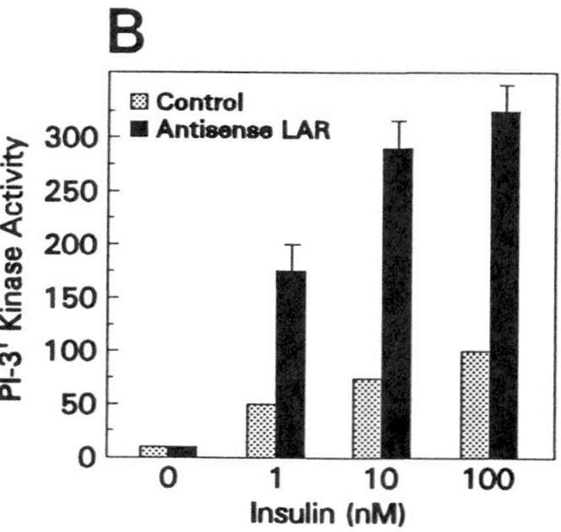

Figure 18-4. Reducing the abundance of the LAR PTPase by antisense techniques enhances insulin signaling in rat hepatoma cells. A fragment of the rat LAR cDNA flanking the translation initiation site was subcloned into the pMEP4b vector and stably expressed in antisense orientation by transfection into rat hepatoma McA-RH7777 cells. ***A,*** Western blot analysis of whole cell lysates with an antibody to the cytoplasmic domain of rat LAR demonstrates a marked reduction in the abundance of LAR protein in the cells transfected with the antisense vector. ***B,*** Antisense LAR expression augments insulin-stimulated phosphatidyl inositol (PI)-3′-kinase activity. Quiescent, transfected hepatoma cells were stimulated with insulin at the indicated concentration and PI-3′-kinase activity was measured in phosphotyrosine immunoprecipitates of cell lysates. PI-3′-kinase activity is normalized to control cells stimulated with 100 nM insulin. (From Kulas DT, Zhang WR, Goldstein BJ, Furlanetto RW, Mooney RA, J Biol Chem 1995;270:2435.)

to IGF-1 and EGF were also impaired in the microinjected cells. Related studies by Milarski and Saltiel[84] demonstrated that inducible expression of a catalytically inactive (Cys459→Ser) SH-PTP2 mutant in NIH 3T3 fibroblasts overexpressing the insulin receptor blocked insulin-stimulated mitogenesis (thymidine incorporation) as well as the phosphorylation and activation of Mitogen Activated Protein (MAP) kinase by insulin. Transfection of a catalytically inactive SH-PTP2 enzyme or of the SH2 domain segment alone has also been shown by Yamauchi[85] to block insulin-stimulated transcription of the c-Fos promoter as well as the phosphorylation of MAP kinase.[85] Interestingly, biologic responses to serum were maintained in the microinjection and transfection studies, suggesting that disruption of the SH-PTP2 signaling pathway was relatively specific for insulin and the other growth factors tested.

The site of SH-PTP2 action in the insulin signaling pathway is still uncertain (Fig. 18-5). Since overexpression of enzymatically active SH-PTP2 does not influence insulin receptor phosphorylation in intact cells,[76] SH-PTP2 most likely acts downstream of the insulin receptor. Although SH-PTP2 can dephosphorylate IRS-1 in vitro,[83] blockage of SH-PTP2 in the microinjection studies as well as by expression of the dominant-negative mutant also had no perceptible effect on the phosphorylation state of the insulin receptor, IRS-1 or Shc, or the amount of IRS-1 associated with the adaptor protein Grb2. This suggests that in intact cells, SH-PTP2 acts downstream of IRS-1 and/or Shc.[79,84,85] Milarski and Saltiel[84] have also suggested that SH-PTP2 acts upstream of MAP kinase-kinase, since the activation of this enzyme by insulin is also disrupted in the cells expressing the dominant negative mutant enzyme.

The observation that microinjection of phosphopeptides that engage and activate the PTPase activity of SH-PTP2 actually *block* insulin-stimulated mitogenesis indicates that the catalytic activity of SH-PTP2 is not sufficient to augment the signaling potential of this PTPase. Work with the dominant negative mutant enzyme and expression of its SH2 domains suggests that SH-PTP2 involvement in insulin action requires its association with docking proteins and the formation of a complex that compartmentalizes the enzyme and brings it in close proximity to appropriate substrates or downstream signaling molecules. In insulin-stimulated cells, the catalytically inactive SH-PTP2 or its isolated SH2 domains have been shown by two groups to interact with a 120 kd phosphotyrosine-containing protein.[79,84] This protein has not yet been identified, but it may provide new insights into pathways of insulin action that are regulated by SH-PTP2.

SH-PTP2 has been recently shown to undergo alternative splicing in multiple domains, which may be significant in the tissue-specific expression and signaling functions of this subfamily of PTPases (Fig. 18-6). Published sequences of SH-PTP2 have demonstrated variations in a five amino acid segment (positions 409–413) at a central location within the catalytic domain as well as significant sequence variation between SH-PTP2 and Syp at the C-terminus.[54] The insertion of four amino acids in the catalytic domain of SH-PTP2 has been shown to reduce the V_{max} of the recombinant enzyme by 8- to 20-fold, depending on the substrate.[93] In the C-terminal region, the alternatively spliced "Syp" form of the enzyme also lacks one of the potential tyrosine phosphorylation sites for the PDGF receptor kinase (Tyr^{580}). This may modulate the association of Syp with Grb2, which has been shown to result following phosphorylation of SH-PTP2 by the PDGF receptor kinase in vivo and in vitro.[94,95] Thus, sequence variations in the SH-PTP2-Syp PTPase family may have physiologic significance in the regulation of signaling pathways that involve various growth factor receptors.

PTPase1B

PTPase1B is a widely expressed enzyme that was first identified as a prominent PTPase in the cytosol fraction of placenta.[96] When its cDNA was cloned and sequenced, it was recognized that the cDNA encoded a full-length protein that has a cleavable C-terminal segment downstream from the PTPase domain that directs the association of the native protein with the endoplasmic reticulum either through a hydrophobic interaction or by attachment to a noncatalytic subunit.[38,97–100] Cleavage of the C-terminal segment of PTPase1B and activation of its PTPase activity occur in platelets in response to agonist activation and release a relatively stable 42 kd form of the enzyme.[101] During the preparation of tissue and cell homogenates, proteolytic cleavage of the susceptible C-terminus

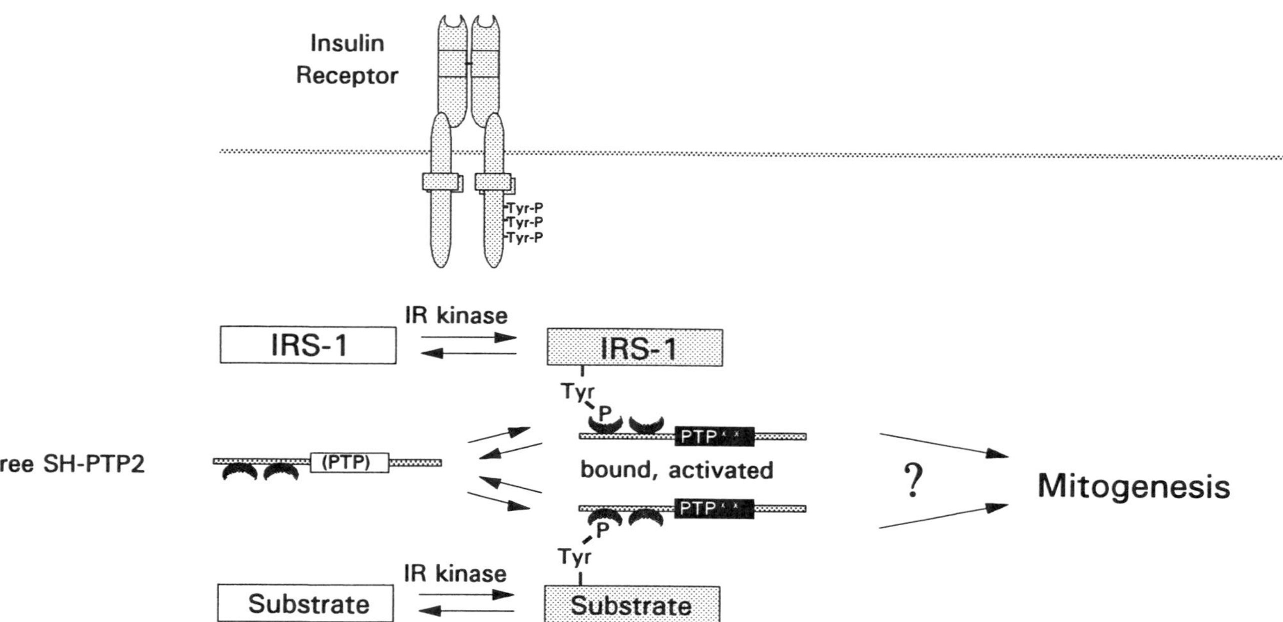

FIGURE 18-5. Modulation of insulin signaling by SH-PTP2. Recent studies have demonstrated that SH-PTP2 plays a positive role in insulin signaling to mitogenic pathways in the cell, but the mechanism of this effect is unclear. The free enzyme is relatively inactive in the cell cytosol [white box labeled "(PTP)"]. Under the influence of the insulin receptor kinase, cellular substrates become tyrosine phosphorylated and form complexes with the SH2 domains of SH-PTP2, which converts the enzyme to a highly active form (black box labeled "PTP**"). Microinjection of phosphotyrosyl peptides that activate SH-PTP2 enzyme activity block rather than activate insulin signaling, indicating that SH-PTP2 enzyme activity alone is not sufficient for enhancing insulin action. Furthermore, insulin signaling is blocked by overexpression of catalytically inactive SH-PTP2 or a protein fragment containing the SH2 domains of SH-PTP2, suggesting that for its signaling effect, SH-PTP2 must interact with appropriate phosphorylated substrate proteins by its SH2 domains. See text for references and further discussion.

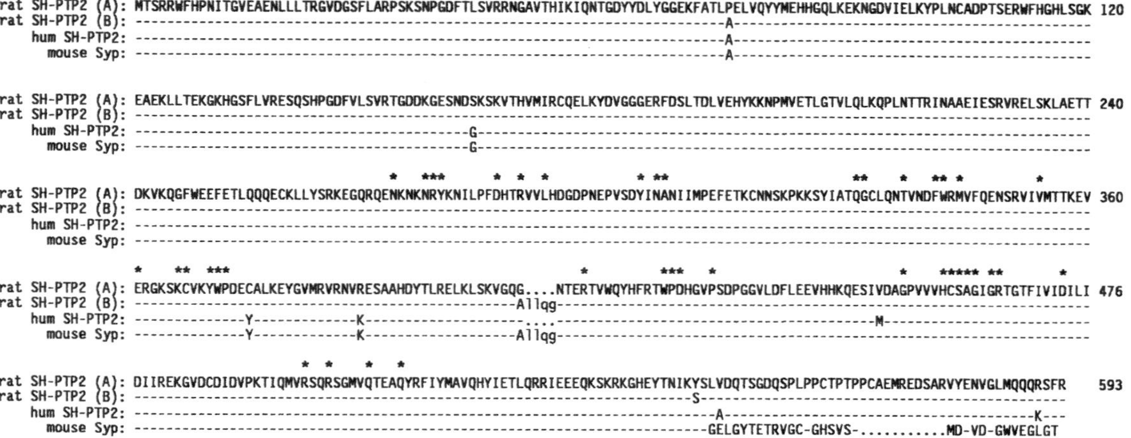

FIGURE 18-6. Sequence variation among members of the SH-PTP2/Syp PTPase subfamily. These PTPase homologs most likely result from alternative splicing of SH-PTP2 mRNA transcripts in various tissues, although this has not been rigorously proved, especially across species. Rat SH-PTP2 (A) was isolated from an adipocyte cDNA library[54] and rat SH-PTP2 (B) was cloned from a brain cDNA library.[93] Human SH-PTP2 was reported by several laboratories,[52,53,76] and the murine Syp enzyme was reported by Feng and coworkers.[75] A dash indicates residue identity with rat SH-PTP2 (A). The dotted line at position 408-411 in the rat SH-PTP2 (A) and human SH-PTP2 sequences indicates a gap where the rat SH-PTP2 (B) and mouse Syp sequences contain additional amino acids. An asterisk above a residue indicates conserved amino acids within the PTPase domain.[65] (Modified from Ding W, Zhang WR, Sullivan K, et al. Identification of protein-tyrosine phosphatases prevalent in adipocytes by molecular cloning. Biochem Biophys Res Commun 1994;202:902.)

and release of soluble truncated PTPase1B protein (~37 kd) can also occur.[62] However, as noted above, a substantial portion of the uncleaved form of PTPase1B is also present in the cytosol of rat tissues, raising the possibility that the subcellular localization of PTPase1B can be regulated in different cells and tissues and that the compartmentalization of this enzyme may be an important physiologic mechanism for its activation and interactions with specific cellular substrates.

For the insulin action pathway, PTPase1B may have access to the insulin receptor at the plasma membrane as a cytosolic enzyme or perhaps in internal membranes as the receptor is internalized into intracellular sites. In the cell cytoplasm, PTPase1B may also function in the dephosphorylation of intracellular substrates of the insulin receptor. By cotransfection of cDNAs for cell surface receptors and a panel of candidate PTPase enzymes, Lammers and coworkers[34] showed that overexpression of PTPase1B in situ resulted in almost complete dephosphorylation of insulin and IGF-1 proreceptors and β-subunits in the basal state and reduced the phosphotryosine content of the ligand-activated β-subunits to less than 50% of the control level. This effect was not specific for insulin or IGF-1 receptors, however, since PTPase1B overexpression also resulted in a significant dephosphorylation of autophosphorylated α- and β-PDGF receptors as well as EGF receptors. Although constrained by the high level of overexpression of the PTPase, these results suggest a potential role of PTPase1B in the regulation of signaling by several different types of growth factors.

LRP (RPTP-α)

This is an additional candidate PTPase for the insulin action pathway given its wide expression in insulin-sensitive tissues, its subcellular localization in the plasma membrane (which may be essential for insulin receptor regulation), and its catalytic activity toward dephosphorylating the insulin receptor.[72] LRP has been known to activate $pp60^{c\text{-}src}$ by dephosphorylation of the negative-regulatory tyrosine at position 527, which leads to transformation of rat embryo fibroblast cells[102] and may also be involved in triggering a neuronal differentiation pathway.[103] LRP itself is phosphorylated on Tyr^{789} in vivo, a site that is recognized by the SH2 domain of the adaptor protein Grb2 in intact cells.[104,105] Since Sos was not found in the LRP-Grb2 complexes, den Hertog and colleagues[104] suggested that LRP might play a role in attenuation of Grb2-mediated signaling rather than in propagating a downstream signal to the Ras pathway. Clearly, additional work is required to delineate the role of LRP in the regulation of intracellular signaling by *src* and Ras and whether it directly impacts on the insulin action cascade.

PTP1C/SH-PTP1/HCP

A recent study by Uchida and coworkers[106] demonstrated that PTP1C is phosphorylated in vitro by isolated insulin receptors as well as in vivo by insulin treatment of IM-9 lymphoblasts, CHO cells overexpressing insulin receptors, and rat H35 hepatoma cells. Tyr^{538} in the C-terminal region of PTP1C was identified as the site phosphorylated by the insulin receptor kinase, and the phosphorylation of this residue increased the enzyme activity by 1.5 to 3.5-fold. Interestingly, PTP1C was also found to bind to autophosphorylated insulin receptors not by its SH2 domains but by a 38 amino-acid region at its C-terminus, downstream from the PTP1C phosphorylation site. PTP1C lacking the C-terminal 38 amino-acid segment is not phosphorylated by the receptor kinase, suggesting that this region first associates with the activated insulin receptor, where it then undergoes tyrosyl phosphorylation and enzyme activation.

PTP1C is a prominent PTPase in hemataopoietic cells, although a low level of expression was reported in liver and lung.[107] PTP1C is also phosphorylated in a macrophage cell line in response to CSF-1 treatment,[108] and a naturally occurring mouse mutant with a disrupted PTP1C gene (the motheaten locus) has been identified and characterized.[109,110] These mice have severe combined immunodeficiency associated with impaired T-cell responses and plasma cell and macrophage hyperproliferation, suggesting that a major physiologic role of PTP1C is in the regulation of hematopoietic cell growth and function. Further studies are essential in evaluating the potential role that the tyrosyl phosphorylation, activation, and insulin receptor association of PTP1C might play in the regulation of the insulin signaling pathway in normal tissues.

Altered Protein-Tyrosine Phosphatase Activity and Expression in Diabetes and Insulin-Resistant States

Animal Models of Obesity and Diabetes

As negative regulators of the insulin action pathway, increased tissue PTPase activities have been postulated to be a pathogenetic factor in the insulin resistance associated with obesity and diabetes. In testing this hypothesis, animal and human studies have recently characterized alterations in tissue PTPase activities in insulin-resistant states. Complex profiles of PTPase activities have been observed, undoubtedly because of the variety of substrates used with different animal models that may have various types and durations of diabetes. It should be emphasized that enzymatic studies with any tissue fractions measure several PTPases simultaneously and that variation in the magnitude and direction of changes in a general PTPase assay depend on alterations in the mean abundance and activity of different PTPases toward the selected artificial substrates.

Studies in murine models of obesity with insulin resistance and diabetes have provided discrepant results with regard to changes in PTPase activities. Using a radiolabeled peptide substrate corresponding to the mono-phosphorylated insulin receptor kinase domain, PTPase activity was decreased by 50% in the cytosol and particulate liver fractions of *ob/ob* mice, and in the *db/db* mouse model, liver cytosol PTPase activity was reduced to 53% of control with no change in the particulate fraction.[22] In contrast, related studies in liver from *ob/ob* mice using a colorimetric assay based on dephosphorylation of a relatively higher concentration of a nonradioactive, tris-phosphorylated peptide from the insulin receptor kinase domain demonstrated an increase in PTPase activity up to 114% and 131% above controls in the particulate and cytosol fractions, respectively.[111] Furthermore, similar colorimetric assays with a *mono*-phosphorylated nonradioactive insulin receptor peptide demonstrated lower PTPase activities overall and no significant difference between *ob/ob* and control animals. These studies suggested that the increased PTPase activity observed in the affected animals may be specific for the tris-phosphorylated regulatory domain of the activated insulin receptor, an important result that would have been overlooked if this relevant substrate had not been employed.

In an insulin-resistant obese mouse model produced by goldthioglucose injection, PTPase activity toward the intact, autophosphorylated insulin receptor was unchanged in cytosol and particulate fractions of liver, heart, and diaphragm and in the particulate fraction of hindlimb skeletal muscle, whereas the hindlimb muscle cytosol PTPase activity was reduced to 65% of control.[112] On the other hand, elevated levels of a cytosolic PTPase activity have been demonstrated in the liver of insulin-resistant aged rats associated with defective activation of the receptor kinase in vivo.[113] These studies clearly demonstrate the heterogeneous etiology of various states of insulin resistance, some of which may not exhibit altered cellular PTPase activity.

PTPase enzyme activities in subcellular fractions of skeletal muscle in lean (+/?) and obese (*fa/fa*) Zucker and diabetic (ZDF/

Drt-*fa/fa*) Zucker rats, a well-characterized rodent model of genetically determined insulin-resistant obesity and diabetes, were recently studied in our laboratory.[44] By examining the abundance of enzyme protein for specific PTPases, we also correlated changes in overall PTPase activity with candidate enzymes that are now known to be abundant in muscle tissue. In the obese and diabetic animals, the muscle particulate fraction PTPase activity was significantly increased by 60–70% toward an artificial phosphoprotein substrate (myelin basic protein) and by 100–110% toward the autophosphorylated native insulin receptor kinase domain. These changes in PTPase activity were associated with increases ranging from 40–70% in the specific immunoreactivity of LAR, PTPase1B, and SH-PTP2 in the particulate fraction of the affected animals. Interestingly, in the diabetic muscle, increased SH-PTP2 abundance was also associated with a shift of SH-PTP2 to a plasma membrane component, which may have important consequences for the activity of this enzyme or its access to substrates or associated proteins in the insulin-resistant state.[44] These results suggest that in this genetic model that closely resembles human type II diabetes, alterations in the amount and distribution of specific enzymes may be involved in the pathogenesis of insulin resistance.

Models of Insulinopenic Diabetes

As in obesity and models of type II diabetes, the hypothesis that an alteration in tissue PTPase activities might be a pathogenetic factor in the well-characterized insulin resistance observed in insulinopenic diabetes has been examined by several laboratories. Increases in cytosol or particulate fraction PTPase activities have been demonstrated in several[35,37,114,115] but not all[116,117] studies in livers of insulin-resistant rodents with hypoinsulinemic diabetes induced by toxins. Our own studies in liver and muscle cytosol of animals made diabetic with streptozotocin showed that the PTPase activity toward the insulin receptor rose to 120–125% of control and further increased by an additional 5–10% following insulin treatment.[125] The increase in cytosolic PTPase activity is similar to the results obtained by Meyerovitch and coworkers[35] using an insulin receptor phosphopeptide substrate as well as the intact insulin receptor in liver cytosol from streptozotocin-diabetic animals. This increase in cytoplasmic PTPase activity may contribute to the insulin resistance that has been characterized in the liver and muscle in these animals. In contrast, particulate fraction PTPase activities toward the insulin receptor or artificial substrates have been shown in several studies to be significantly decreased in livers of streptozotocin[35,117] or alloxan[116] diabetic rats, with a recovery to normal levels after insulin treatment. We have also confirmed that the particulate fraction PTPase activity toward the insulin receptor in streptozotocin-treated rats was decreased to 65–70% of controls in diabetic liver and muscle and increased to 115–120% of controls following insulin treatment.

In further studies, we examined changes in the protein abundance for several candidate PTPases in the diabetic rats and found dynamic alterations in diabetes and after insulin treatment. Enzyme protein for the transmembrane PTPase LAR decreased in parallel to the changes in the PTPase activity in the solubilized particulate fraction, providing further support for this enzyme in the regulation of insulin receptor dephosphorylation in situ. Overall, SH-PTP2/Syp enzyme protein was increased in both diabetes and after insulin treatment but also demonstrated an increased ratio of particulate-cytosol enzyme abundance in diabetic liver and muscle (1.8–1.9) that was reversed after insulin treatment (0.79–0.95). Interestingly, this effect was similar to the shift of SH-PTP2/Syp to a plasma membrane component in the skeletal muscle of diabetic Zucker rats described above. PTPase1B protein was also significantly increased in both the diabetic and insulin-treated animals. Thus, the development of insulin resistance in insulinopenic diabetes is associated with changes in PTPase activity toward the insulin receptor brought about by alterations in the expression of specific major PTPases in liver and skeletal muscle. These dynamic changes in the abundance and subcellular distribution of candidate PTPases may play an essential role in the regulation of the insulin action pathway at both receptor and postreceptor sites.

Studies in Insulin-Resistant Humans

A few studies have appeared that have begun to explore the possibility that abnormal PTPase expression also plays a role in the pathogenesis of human insulin resistance. The first study used skeletal muscle biopsies from insulin-resistant Pima native American subjects and demonstrated that basal PTPase activity toward phosphorylated RCM lysozyme in the particulate fraction of muscle was 33% higher than in insulin-sensitive controls.[118] In further studies, insulin infusion in vivo produced a rapid 25% suppression of soluble PTPase activity in muscle of insulin-sensitive subjects, but this response was severely impaired in the insulin-resistant subjects. In contrast, a related study by Kusari and coworkers[119] performed with a different patient population showed that the skeletal muscle particulate fraction PTPase activity against the same RCM lysozyme substrate was actually reduced by 21–22% in obese nondiabetic and non–insulin-dependent diabetic subjects. This was associated with an average decrease of 38% in PTPase1B protein abundance in the diabetic subjects, although substantial variation was observed in both control and diabetic groups. Furthermore, the basal particulate fraction PTPase activity was positively correlated with the insulin-stimulated glucose disposal rate. These authors also went on to show that weight loss resulted in a significant increase in both the particulate fraction PTPase activity and the insulin-stimulated glucose disposal rate.[119] The conflicting data between the studies of McGuire and coworkers and Kusari and colleagues underscore the multiple factors, both genetic and environmental, in these different populations that determine the heterogeneous pathogenesis of insulin resistance in human diabetes, of which PTPase activities are likely to be one element. Further work is needed to address various PTPase activities in human tissues with additional native substrates, including the insulin receptor or IRS-1 as well as the relationship between the abundance of PTPase1B (and other candidate PTPases) and the overall tissue PTPase activity that is measured in subcellular fractions.

Regulation of PTPases by Insulin or Hyperglycemia

The regulation of cellular PTPase activities by insulin was first reported by Meyerovitch and coworkers[60] who found that treatment of Fao rat hepatoma cells with 100 nM insulin for at least 15 minutes increased the particulate fraction PTPase activity toward a phosphopeptide substrate by 40% and decreased the cytosol activity by 35%. These findings probably represent a dynamic alteration in PTPase activity that is likely to involve several distinct PTPase enzymes in both the particulate membrane and cytosolic fractions. More recently, our laboratory followed up these studies by investigating the regulation of specific PTPase mRNA transcripts by insulin in Fao cells (Fig. 18-7). The two mRNA transcripts for PTPase1B were increased by 1.6- and 3.1-fold, respectively, after treatment of cultured rat hepatoma cells with 100 nM insulin for 3 hours.[43] LAR and LRP (RPTP-α) were more constitutively expressed and not responsive to insulin treatment. In addition, treatment of the hepatoma cells with 100 ng/ml phorbol 12-myristate 13-acetate (PMA) induced expression of PTPase1B, suggesting a possible common mechanism for desensitization of the insulin action pathway by increased PTPase1B activity induced by either insulin or protein kinase C.[43] In rat L6 muscle cells, Kenner and associates[120] also demonstrated that treatment with either insulin

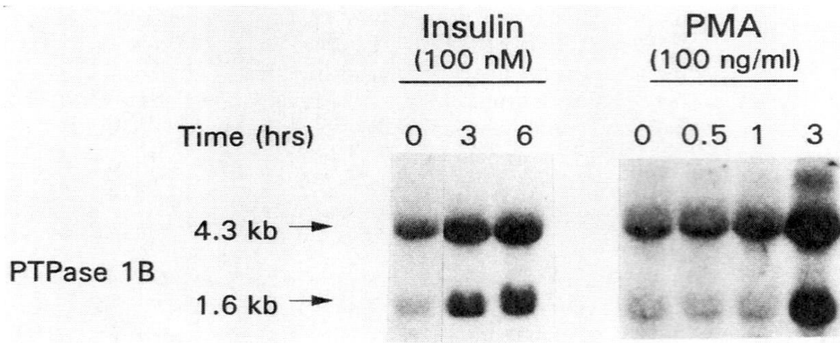

Figure 18-7. Effect of insulin and phorbol 12-myristate 13-acetate (PMA) on the expression of PTPase1B mRNA transcripts in rat Fao hepatoma cells. Total RNA was prepared from quiescent control cells and after incubation with 100 nM insulin or 100 ng/ml PMA for the indicated period of time. Twenty microgram samples of RNA were denatured and subjected to Northern blot analysis with a rat cDNA probe for PTPase1B. A representative autoradiogram is shown. (Modified from Hashimoto N, Goldstein BJ. Differential regulation of mRNAs encoding three protein-tyrosine phosphatases by insulin and activation of protein kinase C. Biochem Biophys Res Commun 1992;188:1305.)

or IGF-1 for an extended period of time, from 5–8 hours up to 32 hours, increased the PTPase activity toward a phosphopeptide substrate in the particulate fraction by 80–200%, respectively. This was associated with an induction of PTPase1B mRNA expression and increased protein abundance that roughly followed a time course similar to the increase in PTPase activity after chronic treatment with either hormone. These initial studies need to be followed up with additional data on other candidate PTPases that may be induced by insulin in these cells (e.g., PTP-PEST). The induction by insulin of PTPases that might deactivate certain components of the insulin signaling pathway might constitute a significant negative feedback control loop in these cells.

In addition to the effects of insulin, high glucose exposure can affect cellular PTPase activity. Treatment of Rat 1 fibroblasts overexpressing the insulin receptor to high glucose (27 mM) for 4 days has been shown by Ide and coworkers[64] to stimulate PTPase activity in the cell cytosol against the autophosphorylated insulin receptor as substrate by two-fold, with no significant change in the particulate fraction PTPase activity. In addition, these authors showed that the high glucose culture conditions resulted in increased abundance of PTPase1B protein in the cytosol but not the particulate fraction, suggesting that the increased insulin receptor dephosphorylating activity might be caused by increased PTPase1B enzyme expression. Since we have previously shown that activation of protein kinase C by PMA causes increased PTPase1B mRNA expression in hepatoma cells,[43] it is possible that the mechanism underlying the increase in PTPase1B in the fibroblasts treated with high levels of glucose[64] may be the activation of protein kinase C that occurs in the hyperglycemic state.[121]

PTP-PEST is an intracellular PTPase characterized by a C-terminal segment enriched in Pro, Glu, Asp, Ser, and Thr residues as a "PEST" motif that had been previously characterized in proteins with relatively short half-lives.[71] The cDNA for PTP-PEST was initially identified as a polymerase chain reaction product from amplification of human skeletal muscle cDNA, and the full cDNA was compiled from HeLa cell libraries. The mRNA for PTP-PEST is widely expressed in a variety of cultured cell lines and normal tissues, as shown by Northern blot hybridization with cDNA probe for PTP-PEST[71] as well as with an amplified fragment encoding a segment of the catalytic domain of PTP-PEST, called PTP-Ty43.[122] Chronic stimulation of human rhabdomyosarcoma A204 cells with 100 nM insulin led to a four-fold increase in PTP-PEST mRNA expression after 36 hours.[71] Further work will help define a potential physiologic role for PTP-PEST in skeletal muscle and in other tissues as well as its possible involvement in the regulation of the insulin action pathway.

Conclusions

As new information on the structure and function of PTPases has rapidly accumulated, work on these essential proteins that regulate reversible tyrosine phosphorylation in cells has appropriately included an examination of their role in the insulin action pathway. We have now identified specific candidate PTPases that are expressed in insulin-sensitive tissues, and studies are under way in several laboratories to fully characterize their potential role in the physiologic regulation of insulin signaling. An understanding of how PTPases impact on insulin signaling pathways will enable us to more fully explore their involvement in clinical insulin resistance in patients with type II diabetes as well as to develop new pharmaceuticals that might alleviate insulin resistance and enhance insulin action by modulating their enzymatic activity.

Acknowledgments

Work in the author's laboratory is supported by NIH grant DK-43396.

References

1. Goldstein BJ. Regulation of insulin receptor signalling by protein-tyrosine dephosphorylation. Receptor 1993;3:1
2. Rosen OM. After insulin binds. Science 1987;237:1452
3. White MF, Shoelson SE, Keutmann H, Kahn CR. A cascade of tyrosine autophosphorylation in the β-subunit activates the phosphotransferase of the insulin receptor. J Biol Chem 1988;263:2969
4. Tornqvist HE, Pierce MW, Frackelton AR, et al. Identification of insulin receptor tyrosine residues autophosphorylated in vitro. J Biol Chem 1987;262:10212
5. Flores-Riveros JR, Sibley E, Kastelic T, Lane MD. Substrate phosphorylation catalyzed by the insulin receptor tyrosine kinase. Kinetic correlation to autophosphorylation of specific sites in the beta subunit. J Biol Chem 1989;264:21557
6. Feener EP, Backer JM, King GL, et al. Insulin stimulates serine and tyrosine phosphorylation in the juxtamembrane region of the insulin receptor. J Biol Chem 1993;268:11256
7. King MJ, Sharma RP, Sale GJ. Site-specific dephosphorylation and deactivation of the human insulin receptor tyrosine kinase by particulate and soluble phosphotyrosyl protein phosphatases. Biochem J 1991;275:413
8. Takata Y, Webster NJG, Olefsky JM. Mutation of the two carboxyl-terminal tyrosines results in an insulin receptor with normal metabolic signaling but enhanced mitogenic signaling properties. J Biol Chem 1991;266:9135
9. Faria TN, Blakesley VA, Kato H, et al. Role of the carboxyl-terminal domains of the insulin and insulin-like growth factor I receptors in receptor function. J Biol Chem 1994;269:13922
10. Tavaré JM, Denton RM. Studies on the autophosphorylation of the insulin receptor from human placenta. Analysis of the sites phosphorylated by two-dimensional peptide mapping. Biochem J 1988;252:607
11. Kohanski RA. Insulin receptor autophosphorylation.2. Determination of autophosphorylation sites by chemical sequence analysis and identification of the juxtamembrane sites. Biochemistry 1993;32:5773
12. White MF, Livingston JN, Backer JM, et al. Mutation of the insulin receptor at tyrosine 960 inhibits signal transmission but does not affect its tyrosine kinase activity. Cell 1988;54:641
13. Prigent SA, Gullick WJ. Identification of c-erbB-3 binding sites for phosphatidylinositol 3′-kinase and SHC using an EGF receptor/c-erbB-3 chimera. EMBO J 1994;13:2831
14. Blaikie P, Immanuel D, Wu J, et al. A region in Shc distinct from the SH2 domain can bind tyrosine-phosphorylated growth factor receptors. J Biol Chem 1994;269:32031
15. Kowalski A, Gazzano H, Fehlmann M, Van Obberghen E. Dephosphorylation

of the hepatic insulin receptor: Absence of intrinsic phosphatase activity in purified receptors. Biochem Biophys Res Commun 1983;117:885

16. Rosen OM, Herrera R, Olowe Y, et al. Phosphorylation activates the insulin receptor tyrosine protein kinase. Proc Natl Acad Sci USA 1983;80:3237
17. Haring HU, Kasuga M, White MF, et al. Phosphorylation and dephosphorylation of the insulin receptor: Evidence against an intrinsic phosphatase activity. Biochemistry 1984;23:3298
18. Yu KT, Czech MP. Tyrosine phosphorylation of the insulin receptor beta subunit activates the receptor-associated tyrosine kinase activity. J Biol Chem 1984;259:5277
19. Myers MG, White MF. The new elements of insulin signaling—insulin receptor substrate-1 and proteins with SH2 domains. Diabetes 1993;42:643
20. Shoelson SE, Chatterjee S, Chaudhuri M, White MF. YMXM motifs of IRS-1 define substrate specificity of the insulin receptor kinase. Proc Natl Acad Sci USA 1992;89:2027
21. Myers MG, Sun XJ, White MF. The IRS-1 signaling system. Trends Biochem Sci 1994;19:289
22. Meyerovitch J, Rothenberg PL, Shechter Y, et al. Vanadate normalizes hyperglycemia in two mouse models of non-insulin dependent diabetes mellitus. J Clin Invest 1991;87:1286
23. Posner BI, Faure R, Burgess JW, et al. Peroxovanadium compounds—a new class of potent phosphotyrosine phosphatase inhibitors which are insulin mimetics. J Biol Chem 1994;269:4596
24. Shisheva A, Ikonomov O, Shechter Y. The protein tyrosine phosphatase inhibitor, pervanadate, is a powerful antidiabetic agent in streptozotocin-treated diabetic rats. Endocrinology 1994;134:507
25. Shisheva A, Shechter Y. Role of cytosolic tyrosine kinase in mediating insulin-like actions of vanadate in rat adipocytes. J Biol Chem 1993;268:6463
26. Elberg G, Li J, Shechter Y. Vanadium activates or inhibits receptor and non-receptor protein tyrosine kinases in cell-free experiments, depending on its oxidation state. J Biol Chem 1994;269:9521
27. Walton KM, Dixon JE. Protein tyrosine phosphatases. Annu Rev Biochem 1993;62:101
28. Brautigan DL. Great expectations—protein tyrosine phosphatases in cell regulation. Biochim Biophys Acta 1992;1114:63
29. Fischer EH, Carbonneau H, Tonks NK. Protein tyrosine phosphatases—a diverse family of intracellular and transmembrane enzymes. Science 1991; 253:401
30. Mauro LJ, Dixon JE. Zip codes direct intracellular protein tyrosine phosphatases to the correct cellular address. Trends Biochem Sci 1994;19:151
31. Formisano P, Condorelli G, Beguinot F. Antiphosphotyrosine immunoprecipitation of an insulin-stimulated receptor phosphatase activity from FRTL5 cells. Endocrinology 1991;128:2949
32. Trowbridge IS, Thomas ML. CD45: An emerging role as a protein tyrosine phosphatase required for lymphocyte activation and development. Ann Rev Immunol 1994;12:85
33. Mooney RA, Freund GG, Way BA, Bordwell KL. Expression of a transmembrane phosphotyrosine phosphatase inhibits cellular response to platelet-derived growth factor and insulin-like growth factor-1. J Biol Chem 1992; 267:23443
34. Lammers R, Bossenmaier B, Cool DE, et al. Differential activities of protein tyrosine phosphatases in intact cells. J Biol Chem 1993;268:22456
35. Meyerovitch J, Backer JM, Kahn CR. Hepatic phosphotyrosine phosphatase activity and its alteration in diabetic rats. J Clin Invest 1989;84:976
36. Gruppuso PA, Boylan JM, Smiley BL, et al. Hepatic protein tyrosine phosphatases in the rat. Biochem J 1991;274:361
37. Boylan JM, Brautigan DL, Madden J, et al. Differential regulation of multiple hepatic protein tyrosine phosphatases in alloxan diabetic rats. J Clin Invest 1992;90:174
38. Chernoff J, Schievella AR, Jost CA, et al. Cloning of a cDNA for a major human protein-tyrosine-phosphatase. Proc Natl Acad Sci USA 1990;87:2735
39. Matthews RJ, Cahir ED, Thomas ML. Identification of an additional member of the protein-tyrosine-phosphatase family: Evidence for alternative splicing in the tyrosine phosphatase domain. Proc Natl Acad Sci USA 1990;87:4444
40. Sap J, D'Eustachio P, Givol D, Schlessinger J. Cloning and expression of a widely expressed receptor tyrosine phosphatase. Proc Natl Acad Sci USA 1990;87:6112
41. Jirik FR, Janzen NM, Melhado IG, Harder KW. Cloning and chromosomal assignment of a widely expressed human receptor-like protein-tyrosine phosphatase. FEBS Lett 1990;273:239
42. Goldstein BJ, Meyerovitch J, Zhang WR, et al. Hepatic protein-tyrosine phosphatases and their regulation in diabetes. Adv Prot Phosphatases 1991;6:1
43. Hashimoto N, Goldstein BJ. Differential regulation of mRNAs encoding three protein-tyrosine phosphatases by insulin and activation of protein kinase C. Biochem Biophys Res Commun 1992;188:1305
44. Ahmad F, Goldstein BJ. Increased abundance of specific skeletal muscle protein-tyrosine phosphatases in a genetic model of obesity and insulin resistance. Metabolism 1995;44:1175
45. Goldstein BJ, Zhang WR, Hashimoto N, Kahn CR. Approaches to the molecular cloning of protein-tyrosine phosphatases in insulin-sensitive tissues. Mol Cell Biochem 1992;109:107
46. Zhang WR, Hashimoto N, Ahmad F, et al. Molecular cloning and expression of a unique receptor-like protein-tyrosine phosphatase in the leukocyte-common-antigen-related phosphatase family. Biochem J 1994;302:39
47. Jiang YP, Wang H, D'Eustachio P, et al. Cloning and characterization of R-PTP-kappa, a new member of the receptor protein tyrosine phosphatase family with a proteolytically cleaved cellular adhesion molecule-like extracellular region. Mol Cell Biol 1993;13:2942
48. DeFronzo RA, Bonadonna RC, Ferrannini E. Pathogenesis of NIDDM. A balanced overview. Diabetes Care 1992;15:318
49. Sale GJ. Insulin receptor phosphotyrosyl protein phosphatases and the regulation of insulin receptor tyrosine kinase action. Adv Prot Phosphatases 1991;6:159
50. Zhang WR, Goldstein BJ. Identification of skeletal muscle protein-tyrosine phosphatases by amplification of conserved cDNA sequences. Biochem Biophys Res Commun 1991;178:1291
51. Hashimoto N, Zhang WR, Goldstein BJ. Insulin receptor and epidermal growth factor receptor dephosphorylation by three major rat liver protein-tyrosine phosphatases expressed in a recombinant bacterial system. Biochem J 1992;284:569
52. Freeman RM, Plutzky J, Neel BG. Identification of a human src homology 2-containing protein-tyrosoine-phosphatase—a putative homolog of *Drosophila* corkscrew. Proc Natl Acad Sci USA 1992;89:11239
53. Ahmad S, Banville D, Zhao ZZ, et al. A widely expressed human protein-tyrosine phosphatase containing src homology-2 domains. Proc Natl Acad Sci USA 1993;90:2197
54. Ding W, Zhang WR, Sullivan K, et al. Identification of protein-tyrosine phosphatases prevalent in adipocytes by molecular cloning. Biochem Biophys Res Commun 1994;202:902
55. Mooney RA, Anderson DL. Phosphorylation of the insulin receptor in permeabilized adipocytes is coupled to a rapid dephosphorylation reaction. J Biol Chem 1989;264:6850
56. Mooney RA, Bordwell KL. Differential dephosphorylation of the insulin receptor and its 160 kDa substrate (pp160) in rat adipocytes. J Biol Chem 1992;267:14054
57. Bernier M, Liotta AS, Kole HK, et al. Dynamic regulation of intact and C-terminal truncated insulin receptor phosphorylation in permeabilized cells. Biochemistry 1994;33:4343
58. Faure R, Baquiran G, Bergeron JJM, Posner BI. The dephosphorylation of insulin and epidermal growth factor receptors. Role of endosome-associated phosphotyrosine phosphatase(s). J Biol Chem 1992;267:11215
59. King MJ, Sale GJ. Insulin-receptor phosphotyrosyl-protein phosphatases. Biochem J 1988;256:893
60. Meyerovitch J, Backer JM, Csermely P, et al. Insulin differentially regulates protein phosphotyrosine phosphatase activity in rat hepatoma cells. Biochemistry 1992;31:10338
61. Backer JM, Kahn CR, White MF. Tyrosine phosphorylation of the insulin receptor during insulin-stimulated internalization in rat hepatoma cells. J Biol Chem 1989;264:1694
62. Brautigan DL, Pinault FM. Activation of membrane protein-tyrosine phosphatase involving cAMP-dependent and $Ca2^{+}$ phospholipid-dependent protein kinases. Proc Natl Acad Sci USA 1991;88:6696
63. Frangioni JV, Beahm PH, Shifrin V, et al. The nontransmembrane tyrosine phosphatase PTP-1B localizes to the endoplasmic reticulum via its 35 amino acid C-terminal sequence. Cell 1992;68:545
64. Ide R, Maegawa H, Kikkawa R, et al. High glucose condition activates protein tyrosine phosphatases and deactivates insulin receptor function in insulin sensitive rat 1 fibroblasts. Biochem Biophys Res Commun 1994;201:71
65. Krueger NX, Streuli M, Saito H. Structural diversity and evolution of human receptor-like protein tyrosine phosphatases. EMBO J 1990;9:3241
66. Cho HJ, Ramer SE, Itoh M, et al. Purification and characterization of a soluble catalytic fragment of the human transmembrane leukocyte antigen related (LAR) protein tyrosine phosphatase from an *Escherichia coli* expression system. Biochemistry 1991;30:6210
67. Tonks NK, Diltz CD, Fischer EH. Characterization of the major protein-tyrosine-phosphatases of human placenta. J Biol Chem 1988;263:6731
68. Tonks NK, Diltz CD, Fischer EH. CD45, an integral membrane protein tyrosine phosphatase: Characterization of enzyme activity. J Biol Chem 1990;265:10674
69. Streuli M, Krueger NX, Thai T, et al. Distinct functional roles of the two intracellular phosphatase-like domains of the receptor-linked protein tyrosine phosphatases LCA and LAR. EMBO J 1990;9:2399
70. Tappia PS, Sharma RP, Sale GJ. Dephosphorylation of autophosphorylated insulin and epidermal-growth-factor receptors by two major subtypes of protein-tyrosine-phosphatase from human placenta. Biochem J 1991;278:69
71. Yang Q, Co D, Sommercorn J, Tonks NK. Cloning and expression of PTP-PEST—a novel, human, nontransmembrane protein tyrosine phosphatase. J Biol Chem 1993;268:6622
72. Hashimoto N, Feener EP, Zhang WR, Goldstein BJ. Insulin receptor protein-tyrosine phosphatases—leukocyte common antigen-related phosphatase rapidly deactivates the insulin receptor kinase by preferential dephosphorylation of the receptor regulatory domain. J Biol Chem 1992;267:13811
73. Cicirelli MF, Tonks NK, Diltz CD, et al. Microinjection of a protein-tyrosine-phosphatase inhibits insulin action in *Xenopus* oocytes. Proc Natl Acad Sci USA 1990;87:5514
74. Tonks NK, Cicirelli MF, Diltz CD, et al. Effect of microinjection of a low-Mr human placenta protein tyrosine phosphatase on induction of meiotic cell division in *Xenopus* oocytes. Mol Cell Biol 1990;10:458
75. Feng GS, Hui CC, Pawson T. SH2-containing phosphotyrosine phosphatase as a target of protein-tyrosine kinases. Science 1993;259:1607
76. Vogel W, Lammers R, Huang JT, Ullrich A. Activation of a phosphotyrosine phosphatase by tyrosine phosphorylation. Science 1993;259:1611

77. Kuhné MR, Pawson T, Lienhard GE, Feng GS. The insulin receptor substrate-1 associates with the SH2-containing phosphotyrosine phosphatase Syp. J Biol Chem 1993;268:11479
78. Lechleider RJ, Freeman RM, Neel BG. Tyrosyl phosphorylation and growth factor receptor association of the human corkscrew homologue, SH-PTP2. J Biol Chem 1993;268:13434
79. Xiao S, Rose DW, Sasaoka T, et al. Syp (SH-PTP2) is a positive mediator of growth factor-stimulated mitogenic signal transduction. J Biol Chem 1994;269:21244
80. Maegawa H, Ugi S, Ishibashi O, et al. Src Homology-2 domains of protein tyrosine phosphatase are phosphorylated by insulin receptor kinase and bind to the COOH-terminus of insulin receptors in vitro. Biochem Biophys Res Commun 1993;194:208
81. Maegawa H, Ugi S, Adachi M, et al. Insulin receptor kinase phosphorylates protein tyrosine phosphatase containing SRC homology 2 regions and modulates its PTPase activity in vitro. Biochem Biophys Res Commun 1994;199:780
82. Ugi S, Maegawa H, Olefsky JM, et al. Src homology 2 domains of protein tyrosine phosphatase are associated in vitro with both the insulin receptor and insulin receptor substrate-1 via different phosphotyrosine motifs. FEBS Lett 1994;340:216
83. Kuhné MR, Zhao ZZ, Rowles J, et al. Dephosphorylation of insulin receptor substrate 1 by the tyrosine phosphatase PTP2C. J Biol Chem 1994;269:15833
84. Milarski KL, Saltiel AR. Expression of catalytically inactive Syp phosphatase in 3T3 cells blocks stimulation of mitogen-activated protein kinase by insulin. J Biol Chem 1994;269:21239
85. Yamauchi K. SH-PTP2 regulates insulin-dependent transcriptional activation. Diabetes 1994;43(suppl 1):2A Abstract.
86. Lechleider RJ, Sugimoto S, Bennett AM, et al. Activation of the SH2-containing phosphotyrosine phosphatase SH-PTP2 by its binding site, phosphotyrosine-1009, on the human platelet-derived growth factor receptor b. J Biol Chem 1993;268:21478
87. Sugimoto S, Lechleider RJ, Shoelson SE, et al. Expression, purification, and characterization of SH2-containing protein tyrosine phosphatase, SH-PTP2. J Biol Chem 1993;268:22771
88. Case RD, Piccione E, Wolf G, et al. SH-PTP2/Syp SH2 Domain binding specificity is defined by direct interactions with platelet-derived growth factor beta-receptor, epidermal growth factor receptor, and insulin receptor substrate-1-derived phosphopeptides. J Biol Chem 1994;269:10467
89. Sugimoto S, Wandless TJ, Shoelson SE, et al. Activation of the SH2-containing protein tyrosine phosphatase, SH-PTP2, by phosphotyrosine-containing peptides derived from insulin receptor substrate-1. J Biol Chem 1994;269:13614
90. Rotin D, Margolis B, Mohammadi M, et al. SH2 domains prevent tyrosine dephosphorylation of the EGF receptor: Identification of Tyr992 as the high-affinity binding site for SH2 domains of phospholipase C gamma. EMBO J 1992;11:559
91. Perkins LA, Larsen I, Perrimon N. *Corkscrew* encodes a putative protein tyrosine phosphatase that functions to transduce the terminal signal from the receptor tyrosine kinase torso. Cell 1992;70:225
92. Lu X, Chou TB, Williams NG, et al. Control of cell fate determination by p21ras/Ras1, an essential component of torso signalling in *Drosophila*. Genes Dev 1993;7:621
93. Mei L, Doherty CA, Huganir RL. RNA Splicing regulates the activity of a SH2 domain-containing protein tyrosine phosphatase. J Biol Chem 1994;269:12254
94. Li W, Nishimura R, Kashishian A, et al. A new function for a phosphotyrosine phosphatase-linking Grb2-SOS to a receptor tyrosine kinase. Mol Cell Biol 1994;14:509
95. Bennett AM, Tang TL, Sugimoto S, et al. Protein-tyrosine-phosphatase SHPTP2 couples platelet-derived growth factor receptor beta to Ras. Proc Natl Acad Sci USA 1994;91:7335
96. Charbonneau H, Tonks NK, Kumar S, et al. Human placenta protein-tyrosine-phosphatase: Amino acid sequence and relationship to a family of receptor-like proteins. Proc Natl Acad Sci USA 1989;86:5252
97. Guan KL, Haun RS, Watson SJ, et al. Cloning and expression of a protein-tyrosine-phosphatase. Proc Natl Acad Sci USA 1990;87:1501
98. Woodford TA, Guan KL, Dixon JE. Expression of rat PTP1 in normal and transformed cells. Adv Prot Phosphatases 1991;6:503
99. Pallen CJ, Lai DS, Chia HP, et al. Purification and characterization of a higher-molecular-mass form of protein phosphotyrosine phosphatase (PTP 1B) from placental membranes. Biochem J 1991;276:315
100. Woodford-Thomas TA, Rhodes JD, Dixon JE. Expression of a protein tyrosine phosphatase in normal and v-src-transformed mouse 3T3 fibroblasts. J Cell Biol 1992;117:401
101. Frangioni JV, Oda A, Smith M, et al. Calpain-catalyzed cleavage and subcellular relocation of protein phosphotyrosine phosphatase-1B (PTP-1B) in human platelets. EMBO J 1993;12:4843
102. Zheng XM, Wang Y, Pallen CJ. Cell transformation and activation of pp60c-src by overexpression and activation of a protein tyrosine phosphatase. Nature 1992;359:336
103. den Hertog J, Pals CEGM, Peppelenbosch MP, et al. Receptor protein tyrosine phosphatase-a activates pp60(c-src) and is involved in neuronal differentiation. EMBO J 1993;12:3789
104. den Hertog J, Tracy S, Hunter T. Phosphorylation of receptor protein-tyrosine phosphatase a on Tyr789, a binding site for the SH3-SH2-SH3 adaptor protein GRB-2 in vivo. EMBO J 1994;13:3020
105. Su J, Batzer A, Sap J. Receptor tyrosine phosphatase R-PTP-alpha is tyrosine-phosphorylated and associated with the adaptor protein Grb2. J Biol Chem 1994;269:18731
106. Uchida T, Matozaki T, Noguchi T, et al. Insulin stimulates the phosphorylation of Tyr[538] and the catalytic activity of Ptp1C, a protein tyrosine phosphatase with Src homology-2 domains. J Biol Chem 1994;269:12220
107. Plutzky J, Neel BG, Rosenberg RD. Isolation of a src homology 2-containing tyrosine phosphatase. Proc Natl Acad Sci USA 1992;89:1123
108. Yeung YG, Berg KL, Pixley FJ, et al. Protein tyrosine phosphatase-1C is rapidly phosphorylated in tyrosine in macrophages in response to colony stimulating factor-1. J Biol Chem 1992;267:23447
109. Shultz LD, Schweitzer PA, Rajan TV, et al. Mutations at the murine motheaten locus are within the hematopoietic cell protein-tyrosine phosphatase (Hcph) gene. Cell 1993;73:1445
110. Tsui FWL, Tsui HW. Molecular basis of the motheaten phenotype. Immunol Rev 1994;138:185
111. Sredy J, Sawicki DR, Sullivan D, Flam BR. Elevation of insulin receptor phosphopeptide PTPase activity in liver of insulin-resistant ob/ob mice. Metabolism 1995;44:1074
112. Olichon-Berthe C, Hauguel deMouzon S, Peraldi P, et al. Insulin receptor dephosphorylation by phosphotyrosine phosphatases obtained from insulin-resistant obese mice. Diabetologia 1994;37:56
113. Nadiv O, Shinitzky M, Manu H, et al. Elevated protein tyrosine phosphatase activity and increased membrane viscosity are associated with impaired activation of the insulin receptor kinase in old rats. Biochem J 1994;298:443
114. Begum N, Sussman KE, Draznin B. Differential effects of diabetes on adipocyte and liver phosphotyrosine and phosphoserine phosphatase activities. Diabetes 1991;40:1620
115. Goren HJ, Boland D. The 180,000 molecular weight plasma membrane insulin receptor substrate is a protein tyrosine phosphatase and is elevated in diabetic plasma membranes. Biochem Biophys Res Commun 1991;180:463
116. Gruppuso PA, Boylan JM, Posner BI, et al. Hepatic protein phosphotyrosine phosphatase. Dephosphorylation of insulin and epidermal growth factor receptors in normal and alloxan diabetic rats. J Clin Invest 1990;85:1754
117. Hauguel deMouzon S, Peraldi P, Alengrin F, Van Obberghen E. Alteration of phosphotyrosine phosphatase activity in tissues from diabetic and pregnant rats. Endocrinology 1993;132:67
118. McGuire MC, Fields RM, Nyomba BL, et al. Abnormal regulation of protein tyrosine phosphatase activities in skeletal muscle of insulin-resistant humans. Diabetes 1991;40:939
119. Kusari J, Kenner KA, Suh KI, et al. Skeletal muscle protein tyrosine phosphatase activity and tyrosine phosphatase 1B protein content are associated with insulin action and resistance. J Clin Invest 1994;93:1156
120. Kenner KA, Hill DE, Olefsky JM, Kusari J. Regulation of protein tyrosine phosphatases by insulin and insulin-like growth factor-I. J Biol Chem 1993;268:25455
121. Considine RV, Caro JF. Protein kinase-C—mediator or inhibitor of insulin action. J Cell Biochem 1993;52:8
122. Yi TL, Cleveland JL, Ihle JN. Identification of novel protein tyrosine phosphatases of hematopoietic cells by polymerase chain reaction amplification. Blood 1991;78:2222
123. Ahmad F, Goldstein BJ. Purification, identification and subcellular distribution of three predominant protein-tyrosine phosphatase enzymes in skeletal muscle tissue. Biochim Biophys Acta 1995;1248:57
124. Kulas DT, Zhang WR, Goldstein BJ, et al. Insulin receptor signalling is augmented by antisense inhibition of the protein-tyrosine phosphatase LAR. J Biol Chem 1995;270:2435
125. Ahmad F, Goldstein BJ. Alterations in specific protein-tyrosine phosphatases accompany the insulin resistance of streptozotocin-diabetes. Am J Physiol 1995;268:E932

Diabetes Mellitus, edited by Derek LeRoith, Simeon I. Taylor, and Jerrold M. Olefsky. Lippincott–Raven Publishers, Philadelphia © 1996.

CHAPTER 19
Protein Kinase C

ROBERT V. FARESE

Insulin-Sensitive Intracellular Signaling Systems

Insulin uses multiple signaling systems to regulate metabolic processes. After initial increases in tyrosine phosphorylation of the insulin receptor and extra-receptor proteins (insulin receptor substrate 1 [IRS-1], Src homology-2–containing protein at the C-terminus [Shc], pp60, pp120), interactions occur with SH2-containing proteins (phosphatidylinositol 3-kinase, growth factor receptor–bound protein-2 [GRB2], Syp Nck, etc.) and other proteins (e.g., G_i), and various signaling systems are activated. These include (1) the GRB2/SOS*/ras/raf-1 MEK/MAP kinase cascade, (2) the phosphatidylinositol 3-kinase–dependent pathway, (3) the glycosyl-phosphatidylinositol hydrolysis system, and (4) the phosphatidylcholine hydrolysis system (Fig. 19-1). These signaling systems activate other downstream kinases and phosphatases, and thus alter the phosphorylation state and activities of many enzymes, transporters, and gene-regulating proteins. As shown, these signaling systems diverge, converge, crosstalk, and may, in some cases, be redundant. Of note, protein kinase C (PKC) can activate MAP kinase through raf-1, and PKC can directly activate many of the same factors that are activated by MAP kinase. Indeed, insulin can activate MAP kinase through, or, as is more often the case, independently of, PKC. This chapter focuses on phospholipid signaling systems, namely, phosphatidylcholine hydrolysis, glycosyl-phosphatidylinositol hydrolysis, de novo phosphatidic acid synthesis, and phosphatidylinositol 3-kinase activation, particularly as they relate to PKC signaling.

Insulin-Sensitive Phospholipid Signaling Pathways

Insulin provokes rapid changes in phospholipid metabolism in many target tissues (Table 19-1). As reviewed elsewhere,[1] the major phospholipid effects of insulin include glycosyl-phosphatidylinositol hydrolysis and phosphatidylcholine hydrolysis in the plasma membrane; de novo synthesis of phosphatidic acid in the endoplasmic reticulum; net synthesis of phosphatidylinositol and other inositol lipids, presumably in the endoplasmic reticulum; and activation of phosphatidylinositol 3-kinase in various compartments. Signaling substances that are generated from these phospholipid pathways include (1) inositol-phospho-glycan head group mediators derived from glycosyl-phosphatidylinositol hydrolysis; (2) diacylglycerol (DAG) derived from glycosyl-phosphatidylinositol hydrolysis, phosphatidylcholine hydrolysis, and de novo phosphatidic acid synthesis; and (3) D-3PO_4 derivatives of phosphatidylinositol, phosphatidylinositol-4′-PO_4 and phosphatidylinositol-4′,5′-$(PO_4)_2$. Although DAG derived from each of the three sources just named can activate PKC, PKC activation in the plasma membrane is probably different from that occurring in the endoplasmic reticulum,[2] and phosphatidylcholine hydrolysis accounts for most (80%) of the initial burst of DAG/PKC signaling that occurs in the plasma membrane in response to insulin.[3] Because of its quantitative importance and its potential relationship to the glucose transport effects of insulin, the phosphatidylcholine hydrolysis pathway is discussed in detail.

Insulin-sensitive, hydrolytic, and synthetic phospholipid pathways appear to be interrelated and integrated (Fig. 19-2). A pertussis toxin–sensitive G_i-protein apparently couples the insulin receptor to the phospholipase C that hydrolyzes glycosyl-phosphatidylinositol.[3–5] Phosphatidylcholine hydrolysis is not sensitive to pertussis toxin,[3] but may be coupled to the insulin receptor through phosphatidylinositol 3-kinase and a small G-protein, such as rho or ADP-ribosylation factor (ARF). The effect of insulin on the de novo phosphatidic acid synthesis pathway is pertussis toxin–sensitive[3,5]

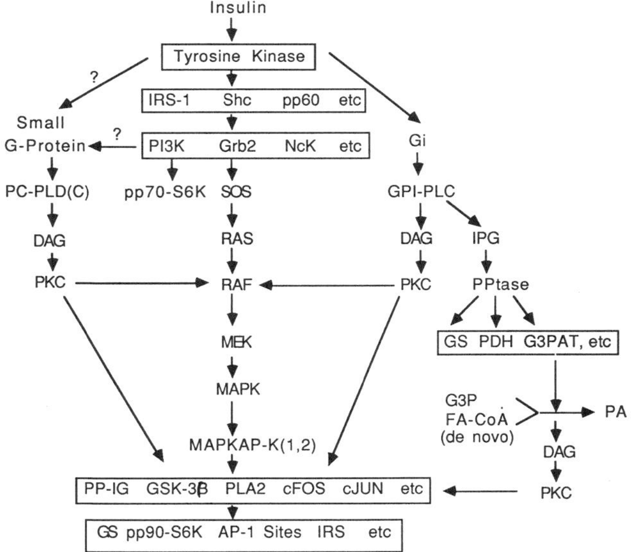

FIGURE 19-1. Phospholipid-dependent and -independent insulin signaling pathways. *IRS-1*, insulin receptor substrate-1; *Shc*, Src homology-2-containing protein at the c-terminus; *PI3K*, phosphatidylinositol 3-kinase; *Grb2*, growth factor receptor-bound protein-2; *PC-PLD(C)*, phosphatidylcholine-specific phospholipase D or phospholipase C; *GPI-PLC*, glycosyl-phosphatidylinositol-specific phospholipase C; *SOS*, son of sevenless GTP/GDP exchange factor; *DAG*, diacylglycerol; *IPG*, inositol-phospho-glycosyl head group; *PPtase*, protein phosphatase; *MAPK*, mitogen-activated protein kinase-1 and -2; *GS*, glycogen synthase; *PDH*, pyruvate dehydrogenase; *GSPAT*, glycerol-3-PO_4 acyltransferase; *FA-CoA*, fatty acyl-coenzyme A; *PA*, phosphatidic acid; *PP-IG*, glycogen-associated protein phosphatase-1; *S6K*, ribosomal S6 protein kinase.

*SOS = son-of-sevenless guanine triphosphate (GTP)/guanine diphosphate (GDP) exchange factor.

TABLE 19-1. Effects of Insulin on Phospholipid Signaling Pathways in Various Target Tissues*

	Rat Adipocytes	Rat Skeletal Muscle	Rat Liver	BC3H-1 Myocytes	CHO·IR Cells
Glycosyl-phosphatidylinositol hydrolysis	+	+	+	+	+
Phosphatidylcholine hydrolysis	+	ND	+	+	ND
De novo phosphatidic acid synthesis	+	+	+	+	+
Phosphatidylinositol synthesis	+	+	ND	+	ND
Phosphatidylinositol 3-kinase activation	+	+	+	ND	+

*See text for references.
ND = not determined.

and is the result of rapid activation of glycerol-3-PO_4 acyltransferase,[5] which transfers fatty acids to glycerol-3-PO_4. Glycerol-3-PO_4 acyltransferase is activated by inositol-phospho-glycosyl head group mediators that are released from glycosyl-phosphatidylinositol.[5,6] Accordingly, the effect of insulin on glycerol-3-PO_4 acyltransferase is blocked in intact cells by pertussis toxin,[3–5] and in cell-free systems by antibodies that inhibit G_i,[5] glycosyl-phosphatidylinositol-specific phospholipase C,[5] and inositol-phospho-glycosyl mediators.[6] Moreover, purified inositol-phospho-glycosyl mediator directly activates glycerol-3-PO_4 acyltransferase.[6] Inositol-phospho-glycosyl mediators also activate other enzymes, such as glycogen synthase and pyruvate dehydrogenase, most likely through activation of specific protein phosphatases.[6–8] Thus, insulin-induced activation of the de novo phosphatidic acid synthesis pathway is a secondary consequence of glycosyl-phosphatidylinositol hydrolysis, and inositol-phospho-glycosyl mediators serve as a biochemical link between insulin-sensitive phospholipid hydrolysis responses in the plasma membrane and phospholipid synthetic processes in the endoplasmic reticulum.

Although pertussis toxin does not inhibit phosphatidylcholine hydrolysis, it prevents the resynthesis of phosphatidylcholine through the de novo pathway during insulin action.[3,5,9] In addition, in the diabetic GK rat, insulin-stimulated glycosyl-phosphatidylinositol hydrolysis and glycerol-3-PO_4 acyltransferase activation are both impaired[6]; this lesion, like pertussis toxin, inhibits phosphatidylcholine resynthesis, but not phosphatidylcholine hydrolysis or resultant PKC activation.[6] Thus, the rapid replenishment of phosphatidylcholine during insulin action requires the concomitant activation of glycosyl-phosphatidylinositol hydrolysis and de novo phosphatidic acid synthesis. In turn, phosphatidylcholine hydrolysis and the de novo phosphatidic acid synthesis pathway provide substrate—that is, phosphatidic acid and DAG—to replenish and increase the levels of phosphatidylinositol, phosphatidylinositol-4′-PO_4, phosphatidylinositol-4′,5′-$(PO_4)_2$, and glycosyl-phosphatidylinositol,[10] and possibly, D-3PO_4 derivatives of phosphatidylinositol. To summarize, phospholipid pathways are uniquely adapted to provide for (1) rapid hydrolysis and resynthesis of both glycosyl-phosphatidylinositol and phosphatidylcholine, and (2) generation of phospholipid-derived signaling factors, namely inositol-phospho-glycosyl mediators, DAG, and D-3PO_4 derivatives of phosphatidylinositol.

Effects of Insulin on Phosphatidylcholine Hydrolysis

Hydrolysis of phosphatidylcholine by phospholipase C or phospholipase D initially yields DAG plus phosphorylcholine, or phosphatidic acid plus choline, respectively. Phosphatidic acid and DAG, in turn, are readily interconverted. The production of DAG from phosphatidylcholine hydrolysis would be expected to activate PKC, although this does not invariably occur, particularly if 1-ether diglycerides are released instead of true 1,2-*sn*-DAG. Nevertheless, in the case of insulin, PKC is activated by phosphatidylcholine-derived DAG, as PKC is activated even when other phospholipid signaling pathways (i.e., glycosyl-phosphatidylinositol hydrolysis and de novo phosphatidic acid synthesis) are completely blocked,

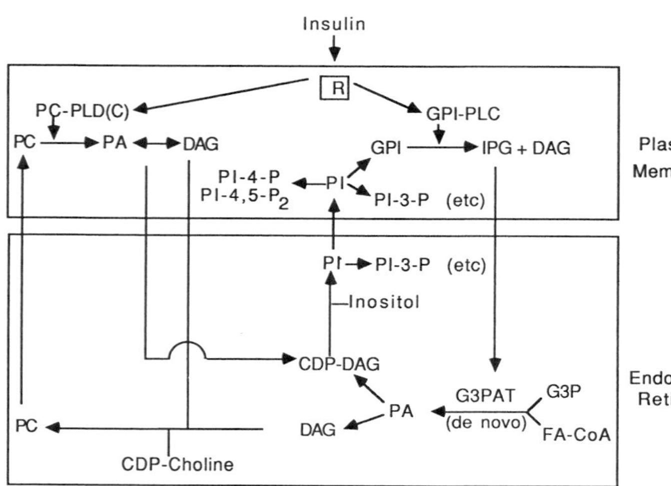

FIGURE 19-2. Insulin-sensitive phospholipid signaling pathways. *R*, receptor; *PC-PLD(C)*, phosphatidylcholine-specific phospholipase D or phospholipase C; *PC*, phosphatidylcholine; *PA*, phosphatidic acid; *GPI-PLC*, glycosyl-phosphatidylinositol-specific phospholipase C; *IPG*, inositol-phospho-glycosyl head group; *PI*, phosphatidylinositol; *DAG*, diacylglycerol; *CDP-DAG*, cytidine diphosphate-diacylglycerol; *CDP-choline*, cytidine diphosphate-choline; *G3P*, glycerol-3-PO_4; *FA-CoA*, fatty acyl-coenzyme A; and *G3PAT*, glycerol-3-PO_4 acyltransferase.

as with pertussis toxin treatment of myocytes[3,9] and in diabetic GK rat adipocytes.[6]

Insulin-induced decreases in phosphatidylcholine in rat adipocytes,[3] BC3H-1 myocytes,[3,9] and rat hepatocytes[11,12] are surprisingly large, representing 5–20% of total membrane phosphatidylcholine. Moreover, the initial decreases in phosphatidylcholine in each of these cell types are very rapid (maximal within seconds), and may be very short-lived, presumably because of the rapidity of de novo phosphatidic acid/DAG/phosphatidylcholine synthesis.[3,13,14] However, in pertussis toxin–treated myocytes,[3,9] and in diabetic GK rat adipocytes,[6] the decreases in phosphatidylcholine are exaggerated and prolonged because of defective de novo synthesis of phosphatidic acid/DAG/phosphatidylcholine.

In addition to rat adipocytes,[3] BC3H-1 myocytes,[3,9] and rat hepatocytes,[11,12] insulin stimulates phosphatidylcholine hydrolysis in C6 glioma cells,[15] Xenopus oocytes,[16] and rat skeletal muscle L6 cells[16a] (unpublished data). In C6 glioma cells, insulin increases [^{3}H]choline release from prelabeled phosphatidylcholine during a 20-minute period. In Xenopus oocytes, the effects of insulin on phosphatidylcholine hydrolysis are more delayed. In C6 glioma cells, as in BC3H-1 myocytes,[3,13,14] Swiss 3T3 cells,[17] and rat adipocytes,[3,18,18a] insulin increases phosphatidylcholine resynthesis, presumably by de novo phosphatidic acid/DAG/phosphatidylcholine synthesis.

It is not clear how the insulin receptor is coupled to a phosphatidylcholine-specific phospholipase D or phospholipase C, or both. Phosphatidylcholine hydrolysis can occur secondary to prior PKC activation or to increases in Ca^{++}, or both, but these are not the mechanisms for activation of phosphatidylcholine hydrolysis by insulin.[3,23] However, a small G-protein may be involved because, in some cells, the activation of *ras* or other small GTP-binding proteins (e.g., rho[19] and ARF[20]) leads to the activation of phosphatidylcholine hydrolysis. In rat hepatocytes,[11] C6 glioma cells,[15] BC3H-1 myocytes,[9] rat adipocytes,[18a] and L6 cells,[16a] phosphatidylcholine-phospholipase D activation (as evidenced by choline release or phosphatidylethanol formation, or both) occurs very rapidly in response to insulin. Whether or not a phosphatidylcholine-phospholipase C is also activated is less certain.

Effects of Insulin on Phosphatidylinositol 3-Kinase

Insulin increases the synthesis of phosphatidylinositol, glycosylphosphatidylinositol, and polyphosphoinositides.[10,21–23] Initially, it was assumed that the latter substances were simply 4′-PO_4 and 4′,5′-$(PO_4)_2$ derivatives of phosphatidylinositol. However, it was subsequently shown that the increases in phosphatidylinositol-PO_4 and phosphatidylinositol-$(PO_4)_2$ synthesis were partly or largely attributable to the activation of phosphatidylinositol 3-kinase,[24] leading to increases in the synthesis of phosphatidylinositol-3′-PO_4, phosphatidylinositol-3′,4′-$(PO_4)_2$, and phosphatidylinositol-3′,4′,5′-$(PO_4)_3$. These D-3PO_4 derivatives of phosphatidylinositol may function in several ways: (1) they may bind to and activate certain enzymes, such as PKC-ζ,[25] or other PKCs[26]; and (2) they may serve as docking factors to regulate the movement of organelles, such as GLUT-4 glucose transporter vesicles. Increases in phosphatidylinositol-4′-PO_4 and phosphatidylinositol-4′,5′$(PO_4)_2$ may also activate various PKCs.[27]

In addition to increasing the synthesis of D-3PO_4 derivatives of phosphatidylinositol, the activation of phosphatidylinositol 3-kinase through its SH2 domains may cause an interaction with other proteins through SH3 or other domains. Recent studies[18a] of the phosphatidylinositol 3-kinase inhibitor Wortmannin suggest that phosphatidylinositol 3-kinase may be important for the activation of phosphatidylcholine hydrolysis, as well as consequent DAG/PKC signaling, during insulin action. (By contrast, glycosyl-phosphatidylinositol hydrolysis and de novo phosphatidic acid synthesis are not inhibited by Wortmannin[18a].) The possibility that phosphatidylcholine hydrolysis may be downstream of phosphatidylinositol 3-kinase is intriguing, as it would provide a biochemical link between (1) insulin-induced activation of tyrosine kinase, IRS-1, and phosphatidylinositol 3-kinase and (2) phosphatidylcholine hydrolysis and phosphatidylcholine-dependent phosphatidylinositol synthesis. Moreover, it would provide a mechanism for the activation of PKC in specific regions of the plasma membrane or low-density microsomes, where phosphatidylinositol 3-kinase is activated.[28] Thus, the PKC activation that occurs during insulin action may be selectively targeted to regulate specific metabolic processes, in contrast to the more generalized nonspecific PKC activation that is produced by phorbol esters. This may be relevant to understanding why phorbol esters are not as effective as insulin-induced DAG in activating glucose transport (see later section).

Effects of Insulin on Diacylglycerol Production

In BC3H-1 myocytes, insulin provokes rapid increases in DAG mass and labeling of DAG by glycerol, myristate, and arachidonate.[3,13,14,22,23] Rapid increases in labeled or total DAG content, or both, have also been observed in the rat soleus,[29–31] diaphragm,[29] and gastrocnemius[31] muscles, the rat liver,[11,32] HIRC-B cells,[33] Swiss 3T3 fibroblasts,[105] CHO·IR cells,[34] and highly purified plasma membranes and microsomes of rat adipocytes[35] (Table 19-2). Insulin-induced increases in DAG production in BC3H-1 myocytes, HIRC-B cells, rat soleus muscle, and rat adipocytes do not require extracellular glucose; this is important because glucose alone can increase DAG and PKC signaling in some cell types, such as rat adipocytes, but this glucose-induced signaling is largely microsomal, and probably differs from plasma membrane DAG/PKC signaling.[2] Most of the initial burst in DAG production that occurs during the first 0.5–1 minute of insulin action is the result of phosphatidylcholine hydrolysis in the plasma membrane.[3,35] At later times of insulin action, de novo phosphatidic acid synthesis in the endoplasmic reticulum becomes increasingly important as a source of DAG.[3,35]

General Aspects of Protein Kinase C Activation

Before discussing insulin effects on PKC, it may be helpful to review some current thoughts about PKC structure and activation (Fig. 19-3). PKCs may be grouped into four types: "conventional" or "classical" cPKCs (α, β_1, β_2, γ), "novel" or nPKCs (δ, ε, η, θ), "atypical" or aPKCs (ζ, λ), and membrane-anchored PKCs (PKC-μ and PKD). Within their N-terminal regulatory domains, cPKCs have Ca^{++}-binding sites in their C_2 regions and DAG-binding and phorbol ester–binding sites (recent evidence suggests that these may be different sites) in their C_1 regions. Accordingly, the cPKCs can be activated by Ca^{++} and DAG or phorbol esters. nPKCs lack C_2/Ca^{++}-binding regions and, therefore, are not activated by Ca^{++}, but respond to DAG and phorbol esters through binding sites in their C_1 regions. aPKCs do not have C_2/Ca^{++}-binding or C_1/DAG-binding regions; however, like all PKCs, they require phospholipids (e.g., phosphatidylserine) for activation, and can be activated by unsaturated fatty acids and phospholipids, such as phosphatidylinositol-3′,4′,5′-$(PO_4)_3$ and phosphatidic acid. Membrane-anchored PKCs lack the C_2/Ca^{++}-binding regions, but have C_1/DAG-binding regions. Both cPKCs and nPKCs are activated by DAG, which is exclusively or primarily found in various cellular membranes. This explains why these PKCs are translocated from the cytosol to the membrane fraction during DAG-induced PKC activation, and why translocation is generally accepted as an

TABLE 19-2. Effects of Insulin on Diacylglycerol (DAG) and Protein Kinase C (PKC) in Various Target Tissues*

Tissue or Cell Type	DAG Increases	PKC Enzyme Activation	PKC Isoform Translocation/Activation			
			α	β	ε	θ
Rat adipocytes	+	+	+	+	+	A
Rat hepatocytes	+	+	+	+	?	A
Rat soleus muscle	+	+	+	+	+	+
Rat diaphragm	+	+	ND	ND	ND	ND
Rat gastrocnemius	+	+	+	+	+	+
Rat tensor fascia lata muscle	ND	ND	+	ND	+	ND
BC3H-1 myocytes	+	+	−	+	+	A
HIRC-B cells	+	+	−	?	+	A
3T3/L1 fibroblasts	+	+	+	+	−	A
3T3/L1 adipocytes	+	+	+	+	−	A
H4IIE hepatoma cells	ND	+	ND	?	ND	ND
CHO·IR cells	+	+	ND	ND	ND	ND
A-10 vascular smooth muscle cells	+	+	ND	+	ND	ND
Fetal chick neurons	ND	+	A	A	+	ND
Swiss 3T3/fibroblasts	+	ND	ND	ND	ND	ND
Xenopus oocytes	ND	ND	ND	+	ND	ND

*See text for references and discussion.
ND = not determined; A = absent; ? = inconclusive or mixed findings.

indicator of PKC activation. Simple increases in cellular Ca^{++} can also result in translocation of cPKCs, but not nPKCs. In the case of insulin, increases in cellular Ca^{++} are generally not present or are minimal, and insulin translocates both cPKCs and nPKCs. Therefore, it seems likely that insulin-induced PKC translocations are largely attributable to DAG or other membrane-associated lipids.

In addition to DAG, certain other lipids and phospholipids can bind to and activate certain PKCs, including oleic acid, arachidonic acid, fatty acyl-CoA, phosphatidylserine, phosphatidic acid, lysophosphatidylcholine, phosphatidylinositol-4′,5′-$(PO_4)_2$, phosphatidylinositol-3′-PO_4, phosphatidylinositol-3′,4′-$(PO_4)_2$, and phosphatidylinositol-3′,4′,5′-$(PO_4)_3$. Interestingly, insulin increases many of these PKC ligands. Several PKCs have also been found to be activated by tyrosine phosphorylation, and serine/threonine phosphorylation may be required for intrinsic PKC activity. The tyrosine phosphorylation mechanism may also be used by insulin to activate certain PKCs, such as PKC-δ and PKC-α.

Upon activation by DAG and possibly other substances, there is an unfolding of the PKC molecule at the hinge or V_3 region, and a dissociation of a V_1 inhibitory pseudosubstrate peptide sequence from the substrate binding site in catalytic domain. This allows each PKC to interact with and phosphorylate its specific substrates. Upon opening, the hinge region also becomes more vulnerable to membrane-associated proteases, (?calpains), and this may lead to cleavage and release of regulatory (30 kd) and catalytic (50 kd; "M-kinase" or PKM) fragments. Thus, prolonged activation may also lead to PKC depletion unless there is a balance between degradation and new PKC synthesis.

Effects of Insulin on Protein Kinase C Activation/Translocation

There is still considerable controversy as to whether insulin-induced increases in DAG result in PKC activation. This controversy stems partly from an initial erroneous assumption that only DAG derived from phosphatidylinositol-4′,5′-$(PO_4)_2$ hydrolysis activates PKC. However, it is now abundantly clear that DAG derived from phosphatidylcholine hydrolysis and the de novo phosphatidic acid synthesis pathway can translocate and activate PKC.[36,37] The contro-

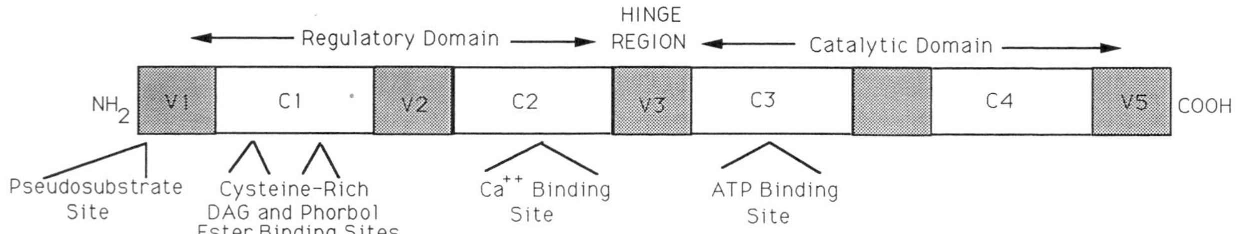

FIGURE 19-3. Structure and functional binding sites of protein kinase C (PKC) isoforms. Variable (*V*) and conserved (*C*) regions are depicted by shaded and clear areas. cPKCs (α, β_1, β_2, γ) have C_1 and C_2 regions and bind both diacylglycerol (DAG) (or phorbol esters) and Ca^{++}. nPKCs (δ, ε, η, θ) have C_1, but not C_2 regions, and only bind DAG (or phorbol esters). aPKCs lack C_2 and one of the cysteine-rich regions on C_1, and do not bind either Ca^{++} or DAG. Membrane-anchored PKCs (μ and PKD), which have recently been discovered, have extended V_1 regions that contain a transmembrane domain, a C_1/DAG-binding region, but no C_2/Ca^{++}-binding region.

versy also derives from the failure of initial studies to show that insulin stimulates the translocation of PKC from cytosol to membranes, as typically observed with phorbol esters, and originally considered to be essential as evidence for PKC activation. Moreover, even when insulin-induced increases in membrane PKC activity were observed in subsequent studies,[38,39] there were concomitant increases, rather than decreases, in PKC enzyme activity in crude or DEAE-cellulose-purified cytosolic extracts. Interestingly, it was later found that this alteration in subcellular PKC redistribution was not specific for insulin-induced PKC activation, as it was also observed with thyrotropin (TSH) in thyroid cells; concanavalin A in lymphocytes; growth hormone, vasopressin, angiotensin, and glucagon in hepatocytes; and glucose and parathyroid hormone (PTH) in islets. Nevertheless, in subsequent studies, after purifying PKC by Mono Q column chromatography to more effectively remove noncovalent PKC modulators (e.g., DAG, fatty acids, fatty acyl-CoA, phosphatidylinositol-3′,4′,5′-$(PO_4)_3$, phosphatidylinositol-4′,5′-$(PO_4)_2$, lyso-phosphatidylcholine, acidic phospholipids, and small G-proteins), we observed typical PKC translocation patterns in insulin-treated rat adipocytes,[40] BC3H-1 myocytes,[41] and various rat skeletal muscles[29–31]—that is, increases in membrane PKC enzyme activity and decreases in cytosolic PKC enzyme activity. Also, using PKC isoform-specific antisera, we observed insulin-induced translocation of PKC-α, PKC-β, PKC-ε, and/or PKC-θ from the cytosol to the membrane in each of these tissues.[9,29–31,40–42,42a,42b] Apparent PKC translocation has also been reported to occur during insulin action in CHO-IR cells,[34] A-10 vascular smooth muscle (VSM) cells,[43] H4IIE hepatoma cells,[44] 3T3/L1 cells (unpublished data, Bandyopadhyay G, Zhou X, Standaert ML, Galloway L, and Farese RV, 1995), HIRC-B cells,[33] Xenopus oocytes,[45] and L6 skeletal muscle myotubes[46] (see Table 19-2). An increase in PKC enzyme activity has also been observed in chick neurons, but this does not appear to involve translocation, and may be the result of a covalent modification of PKC.[47] More recently, we have found that insulin not only stimulates rapid increases in DAG[35,42] and PKC enzyme activity,[35] but also translocates PKC-α, PKC-β, and PKC-ε ([18a] and unpublished data, Standaert ML, Yamada K, and Farese RV, 1995) to purified plasma membranes and microsomes of rat adipocytes. Egan et al.[48] also observed similar increases in PKC enzyme activity of purified rat adipocyte plasma and microsomal membranes. These findings most likely reflect phosphatidylcholine and glycosyl-phosphatidylinositol hydrolysis in the plasma membrane, and de novo phosphatidic acid synthesis in microsomes. In keeping with this postulation, glucose primarily increases microsomal, rather than plasma membrane, DAG/PKC signaling[2]; furthermore, increases in DAG and PKC translocation to the plasma membrane occur in association with isolated phosphatidylcholine hydrolysis in these membranes in the GK rat, which is deficient in glycosyl-phosphatidylinositol hydrolysis and de novo phosphatidic acid synthesis.[6]

As in adipocytes, insulin provokes rapid biphasic increases in the translocation of (1) PKC-α, PKC-β, PKC-ε, and PKC-θ in rat soleus muscles[42a] and (2) PKC-α and PKC-β in rat hepatocyte preparations incubated in vitro (unpublished data, Standaert ML, Yamada K, Avignon A, and Farese RV, 1995). Again, these translocations of PKC are associated with increases in DAG and membrane PKC enzyme activity in both cell types.

In cultured cells, PKC translocation patterns appear to be more selective. In BC3H-1 myocytes, insulin translocates PKC-ε[42b] and PKC-β, but not PKC-α.[49] In HIRC-B cells, insulin translocates PKC-ε, but not PKC-α or PKC-δ.[33] In 3T3/L1 cells, insulin translocates PKC-α and PKC-β, but not PKC-ε (unpublished data, Bandyopadhyay G, Zhou X, Standaert ML, et al., 1995). The reason for this selectivity is not certain.

It has been noted that insulin-induced increases in membrane PKC enzyme activity have been observed in in vitro assays using a number of PKC substrates, including histone IIIs in rat adipocytes,[40] rat soleus and gastrocnemius muscles,[29–31] and CHO cells[34]; a glycogen synthase peptide in rat adipocytes[48] myristoylated alanine-rich C-kinase substrate (MARCKS) protein in rat adipocytes and rat soleus muscle[35]; and MARCKS heptapeptide in BC3H-1 myocytes.[9,50] These phosphorylations in in vitro assays clearly occur on PKC-specific sites, as they are blocked by specific PKC inhibitors, including the PKC pseudosubstrate.[9,35,50]

Effects of Insulin on Protein Kinase C Substrate Phosphorylation in Intact Cells

Another reason for doubting the importance of DAG/PKC signaling in insulin action comes from some studies of PKC substrate phosphorylation in intact BC3H-1 myocytes, HIRC-B cells, and NIH3T3/HIR3.5 cells. In these studies,[51] examination of trichloroacetic acid (TCA)–precipitable ^{32}P-labeled proteins did not reveal significant increases in the phosphorylation of an endogenous PKC substrate, namely, MARCKS. Therefore, the researchers concluded that, despite increases in DAG, PKC translocation, and membrane PKC enzyme activity as assayed in vitro, insulin did not truly activate PKC in the intact cells. However, in BC3H-1 myocytes[35] and HIRC-B cells,[33] when *equal amounts of protein* were examined for ^{32}P-labeling of immunoprecipitable MARCKS, we observed increases in the phosphorylation of immunoprecipitable MARCKS after acute insulin treatment. Equal amounts of protein were used, rather than equal amounts of ^{32}P radioactivity in TCA precipitates, because the latter, as a confounding problem, would include (1) proteins heavily labeled on tyrosine residues (e.g., the insulin receptor IRS-1, Shc, MAPK, pp60), (2) proteins labeled by GTP/GDP exchange (e.g., ras), (3) proteins labeled on ser/thr residues by non-PKC kinases (e.g., raf, MEK, MAP kinase, S6 kinases), (4) ^{32}P-labeled lipids (e.g., phosphatidic acid, phosphatidylcholine, phosphatidylinositol, phosphatidylinositol-3′,4′,5′-$(PO_4)_3$, phosphatidylinositol-4′-PO_4, phosphatidylinositol-4′,5′-PO_4), and (5) ^{32}P-labeled nucleic acids. In HIRC-B cells,[33] the effects of insulin (twofold) were less than those of phorbol esters (fourfold); however, in BC3H-1 myocytes,[35] the effects of insulin were nearly the same as those of phorbol esters (both twofold). In isolated rat adipocytes and soleus muscle preparations, insulin stimulated the phosphorylation of immunoprecipitable MARCKS nearly as well as phorbol esters.[35] Moreover, the effects of insulin and phorbol esters on adipocyte MARCKS phosphorylation were not additive, and effects were observed at physiologic insulin concentrations.[35] Thus, even by the criterion of MARCKS labeling, it appears that insulin activates DAG/PKC signaling, at least in BC3H-1 myocytes, HIRC-B cells, rat adipocytes, and rat soleus muscles.

In addition to MARCKS, insulin increases ^{32}P-labeling of other PKC substrates. In rat diaphragm, Walaas et al.[52] found that insulin and phorbol esters stimulated ^{32}P-labeling of identical tryptic peptides of a 15-kd PKC substrate. PKC also directly phosphorylated the same peptides in vitro, and insulin effects in situ were inhibited by both PKC inhibitors and phorbol ester–induced PKC downregulation. In 3T3-L1 cells, Morley and Traugh[53] found that insulin, phorbol esters, and PKC induced identical phosphorylations of phosphopeptides in tryptic digests of the protein synthesis initiation factors eukaryotic initiation factor (eIF)-4F p25 and eIF-3 p120; these effects of insulin were no longer apparent after phorbol ester–induced PKC downregulation. In rat adipocyte membranes, Graves and McDonald[54] found that insulin, phorbol esters, and PKC phosphorylated a 40-kd protein identically, as shown in phosphopeptide mapping of tryptic digests. In CHO·IR cells, Cherqui et al.[34] found that insulin and phorbol esters stimulated 40-kd protein phosphorylation, and these effects were lost after PKC downregulation. In rat adipocytes, Haystead and Hardie[55] found that insulin and phorbol esters phosphorylated acetyl-coenzyme A (CoA) carboxylase identically, as shown by phosphopeptide mapping of tryptic digests. Finally, in human mammary epithelial cells, Donaldson, Hagedorn, and Cohen[56] observed that insulin, phorbol esters, and PKC identically phosphorylated p28 and p220 subunits of eIF-4E, as shown by phosphopeptide mapping of tryptic digests. Thus, there is considerable evidence that certain insulin-stimulated protein phosphorylations in intact cells may be mediated through PKC activation. On the other hand, it is clear that other protein kinases are also activated by insulin.

On a final note concerning the use of MARCKS phosphorylation to judge PKC activation in situ, MARCKS has recently been found to contain six phosphorylation sites that are adjacent to proline and are apparently activated by MAP kinase and Cdk5 kinase.[57] These sites are distinct from three specific PKC phosphorylation sites. Because MAP kinase is usually markedly activated by phorbol esters even more intensely than by insulin, the effects of phorbol esters on MARCKS phosphorylation may provide an exaggerated estimate of PKC activation. (Note that the time-course of insulin effects on MARCKS phosphorylation[35] is decidedly different from that of MAP kinase activation[63] in rat adipocytes.)

Protein Kinase C Downregulation

Another argument that has been used to suggest that a particular biologic effect of insulin does not require DAG/PKC signaling is that the effect persists after phorbol ester–induced PKC depletion. This conclusion is correct provided that PKC enzyme activity and all relevant PKC isoforms are sufficiently depleted. However, this is not always clear-cut, as phorbol esters can change the substrate-recognizing properties of PKC[58] (e.g., histone IIIs phosphorylation may be masked), and the major phorbol ester binding site on PKC (of which there are two) appears to be distinct from the major DAG-binding site.[59] In addition, negative experiments may be difficult to interpret because only one or a few of several PKC isoforms may be retained in amounts ''sufficient'' (difficult to define) to respond to hormone-induced DAG in certain downregulated cells. For example, PKC-ε fails to diminish at all in rat adipocytes,[49,59a] or diminishes only partially in HIRC-B cells[33] after phorbol ester treatment; by contrast, PKC-α, PKC-β, and PKC-δ are markedly depleted. Thus, retention of part or all of the insulin effects on a particular biologic process in these downregulated cells could still be mediated by residual PKC-ε. Similarly, in BC3H-1 myocytes, although PKC-α,[49] PKC-β_1, and PKC-ε[42b] are fully depleted by phorbol esters, PKC-β_2 is rapidly and markedly induced by phorbol esters.[42b,60]

The failure of acute phorbol ester treatment to activate a biologic process after chronic phorbol ester treatment is frequently used to judge the completeness of functional PKC depletion. Thus, if phorbol esters are no longer effective, it is generally surmised that continued actions of a hormone are not mediated by PKC. Although this conclusion may be correct, it must be drawn cautiously for the same reasons cited earlier—namely, that phorbol esters can change substrate recognition, and that apparently there are two binding sites on purified PKC, one preferentially activated by DAG (and thus the hormone), and one preferentially activated by phorbol esters.[59] In fact, these sites seem to be independent in that phorbol ester binding is not inhibited by DAG, and the effects of DAG and phorbol esters on the enzyme activity of the same PKC molecule are additive.[59] Thus, findings with phorbol esters may not necessarily be reflective of endogenous DAG and its dependent processes.

In contrast to negative findings, many insulin-sensitive biologic processes in many different cell types are inhibited or downregulated after chronic phorbol ester treatment (Table 19-3). Although it may be argued that the downregulation of processes is attributable to nonspecific effects of phorbol esters, this does not appear to be the case in several thorough studies. For example, in rat adipocytes, insulin effects on glucose transport are inhibited by 60–90% after phorbol ester–induced PKC downregulation,[61–63] whereas receptor number[62] and insulin effects on tyrosine kinase activity,[62] MAP kinase activation,[63] and de novo phosphatidic acid synthesis[62] are not compromised. In these cells, PKC-α, PKC-β, and PKC-δ are almost completely lost, whereas PKC-ε and PKC-ζ are largely retained after phorbol ester treatment.[48a,49] It is reasonable, therefore, to postulate that, in rat adipocytes, PKC-α, PKC-β, and PKC-δ may be involved in the activation of glucose transport

TABLE 19-3. Insulin Effects that may be Protein Kinase C (PKC)–Dependent as Evidenced by Sensitivity to PKC Downregulation and Inhibition

Effect	Cell Types	PKC Downregulation	PKC Inhibitors
Glucose transport	Rat adipocytes	+[(61–63)]	+
Glucose transport	Mouse or rat soleus muscle	+[79]	+
Glucose transport	Rat heart	+[80]	ND
Glucose transport	Rat A-10 VSM Cells	+[43]	+
pp15 Phosphorylation	Rat diaphragm	+[52]	ND
Eukaryotic initiation factor (eIF) phosphorylation	3T3/L1 cells	+[53]	ND
pp40 Phosphorylation	CHO·IR cells	+[34]	ND
MAP kinase activation	L6 cells	+[46]	+
Protein phosphatase-1 activation	L6 cells	+[46]	+
Na^+/H^+ and/or Na^+/K^+ cotransport	BC3H-1 myocytes	+[102]	ND
Na^+/H^+ and/or Na^+/K^+ cotransport	Frog skin	+[103]	ND
Na^+/H^+ and/or Na^+/K^+ cotransport	Skeletal muscle	+[104]	ND
Protein synthesis	Swiss 3T3 cells	+[105]	ND
eIF Activation	Swiss 3T3 cells	+[106]	+
Pyruvate dehydrogenase activation	Rat hepatoma cells	+[107]	+
c-*Fos* gene expression	H4IIE hepatoma cells	+[44]	ND
c-*Fos* gene expression	Fetal chick neurons	+[108]	ND
p33 gene expression	H4IIE hepatoma cells	+[109]	ND
β-actin gene inhibition	H4IIE hepatoma cells	+[110]	ND
Insulin-like growth factor 1 (IGF-1) BP-1 gene inhibition	HepG2 cells	+[111]	ND
c-Ki-*ras* gene expression	Rat hepatocytes	+[112]	ND

VSM = vascular smooth muscle; ND = not determined.

by insulin. Clearly, other lines of evidence are needed to test this hypothesis.

Insulin-like Effects of Phorbol Esters

Phorbol esters, as analogues of DAG and activators of PKC, have many insulin-like effects, including:

1. Increases in glucose transport and translocation of GLUT-4 from low-density microsomes to the plasma membrane.
2. Activation of enzymes important in intracellular glucose metabolism, including phosphofructokinase, enolase, and pyruvate dehydrogenase.
3. Activation of enzymes important in fatty acid synthesis (i.e., acetyl-CoA carboxylase).
4. Increases in ion transport (e.g., the cotransport of Na^+/H^+ and activation of Na^+/K^+ATPase).
5. Increases in amino acid transport in some cell types.
6. Activation of protein synthesis initiation factors (eIFs).
7. Changes in gene expression, including increases in those encoding c-*fos,* c-*myc,* P-33, *IGF 1,* c-Ki-*ras,* lutropin, β-actin, and ornithine decarboxylase, and decreases in those encoding albumin, tyrosinase, phosphoenolpyruvate carboxykinase (PEPCK), and insulin-like growth factor 1 (IGF 1) binding protein.
8. DNA synthesis in some cell types.
9. Other metabolic processes.

Clearly, the simple demonstration that phorbol esters mimic insulin does not conclusively indicate that the insulin effects on these processes are mediated by PKC. Nevertheless, some effects of insulin appear to be PKC-dependent, as evidenced by studies with PKC inhibitors or PKC depletion (see Table 19-3). However, it should be noted that (1) only positive findings for PKC involvement are shown in Table 19-3, and (2) insulin effects on many of the same or other processes may not be PKC-dependent in other cell-types (e.g., MAP kinase).

The Potential Role of Protein Kinase C in Insulin-Stimulated Glucose Transport

Phorbol esters increase glucose transport in many cell types, including BC3H-1 myocytes, rat adipocytes, mouse soleus muscles, rat soleus muscles, rat epitrochlearis muscles, cultured L6 muscle cells, 3T3/L1 cells, Swiss 3T3 cells, BALB/c 3T3 preadipose cells, cultured glial cells, chick embryo fibroblasts, HeLa cells, brain endothelial cells, lymphocytes, polymorphonuclear leucocytes, rat heart, A-10 VSM cells, HIRC-B cells, thyroid cells, and CHO·IR cells. The effects of phorbol esters on glucose transport in some cell types, however, have been less than those of insulin. For example, in rat adipocytes, rat or mouse soleus muscle, L6 cells, and 3T3/L1 adipocytes, insulin effects on 2-deoxyglucose uptake are generally about threefold greater than those of phorbol esters. In BC3H-1 myocytes, HIRC-B cells, 3T3/L1 fibroblasts, Swiss 3T3 cells, AT-10 VSM cells, and CHO cells, phorbol ester effects on glucose transport are quantitatively comparable to those of insulin.

The failure of phorbol esters to fully mimic insulin effects on glucose transport is not understood, but the following must be considered: (1) insulin may regulate glucose transport independently of PKC, and phorbol ester effects on this process may be fortuitous; (2) insulin and phorbol esters may activate PKC differently (see earlier discussion of different binding sites for DAG and phorbol esters) and may have different substrate preferences, or different efficiencies to target specific proteins; (3) insulin, via increases in phosphatidylinositol-3′,4′,5′-$(PO_4)_3$ may activate PKC-ζ, which is not activated by phorbol esters; and (4) insulin may use both PKC-dependent and PKC-independent mechanisms (i.e., a two-step process) to activate glucose transport. In support of the last possibility, Håring's group[64–66] found that insulin effects on GLUT-4 translocation from low-density microsomes to the plasma membrane in rat adipocytes are only slightly greater than phorbol ester effects on this translocation, despite the fact that glucose transport is disproportionately greater with insulin. Our experience is similar to that of Håring's group in that we found little or no difference between insulin and phorbol ester effects on GLUT-4 translocation in rat adipocytes[67] in the presence of threefold greater increases in 2-deoxyglucose transport in response to insulin. A similar equivalence of GLUT-4 translocation in response to insulin and phorbol esters was found in GLUT-4-myc–transfected CHO cells.[68] Another research group, however, found insulin to have twofold greater effects than phorbol esters on GLUT-4 translocation in rat adipocytes, but equal effects on GLUT-1 translocation.[69,70] Whatever the case, many of these and other previously reported findings have suggested that insulin may increase the intrinsic transport activity of the GLUT-4 glucose transporter subsequent to its translocation. If so, the activation step may occur by a PKC-independent mechanism, or at least by a mechanism that is not stimulated by simple phorbol ester treatment. In keeping with this two-step translocation/activation hypothesis, cyclodextrin potentiates phorbol ester– and DAG-stimulated glucose transport (thus approaching that of insulin), both in rat adipocytes and rat soleus muscle, in the absence of a measurable change in GLUT-4 translocation.[67]

In addition to phorbol esters, DAG itself activates glucose transport in BC3H-1 myocytes[71,72] and rat adipocytes.[67,73,74] Also, phosphatidylcholine-phospholipase C, which increases DAG by hydrolyzing phosphatidylcholine, activates glucose transport in BC3H-1 myocytes,[72] rat adipocytes,[73,74] and rat skeletal muscle.[29,75] Electrically or exercise-induced DAG and resultant PKC activation also stimulates glucose transport in rat skeletal muscle.[76] A DAG kinase inhibitor—monoacylglycerol—and arachidonic acid (a PKC activator) increase DAG/PKC signaling and glucose transport in Swiss 3T3 fibroblasts.[77] Other PKC activators (mezerein and/or SC-9) increase glucose transport in BC3H-1 myocytes,[72] rat adipocytes,[73] and 3T3 fibroblasts. Although not necessarily specific for PKC, the phosphatase inhibitor okadaic acid translocates and activates PKC, and activates glucose transport in rat adipocytes[78] and rat skeletal muscle. Finally, a long list of agonists that increase DAG and activate PKC by a variety of mechanisms have been found to increase glucose transport in their target tissues. These include thyrotropin and carbachol in thyroid cells; carbachol in pancreatic acinar cells; phenylephrine in BC3H-1 myocytes; bombesin in Swiss 3T3 cells; epidermal growth factor (EGF) and IGF-1 in BC3H-1 myocytes; angiotensin II in VSM cells; and platelet-derived growth factor (PDGF), fibroblast growth factor (FGF), and serum in Swiss 3T3 cells, to name but a few.

Phorbol ester–induced PKC downregulation (see earlier discussion) concomitantly inhibits insulin-stimulated glucose transport in some cell types, including rat adipocytes,[61–63] mouse soleus,[79] rat soleus (unpublished data, Hernandez H and Farese RV, 1995), rat heart,[80] rat A-10 VSM cells,[43] and CHO·IR cells.[34] However, in other cell types, insulin effects are retained, such as in BC3H-1 myocytes,[72] HIRC-B cells,[33] 3T3/L1 cells,[81] 3T3 fibroblasts,[82] and L6 cells.[83] It is uncertain whether this reflects different regulatory mechanisms or problems with phorbol ester–induced PKC downregulation.

In addition to phorbol ester treatment, we have used antisense-DNA to deplete PKC-α and PKC-β in rat adipocytes, and this, too, has inhibited insulin-stimulated glucose transport.[84] However, a more convincing evidence in favor of a role for PKC comes from the finding that introduction (by electroporation) of pure PKC into PKC-depleted rat adipocytes restores insulin-stimulated glucose transport.[85]

All tested PKC inhibitors, including H7, staurosporine, sangivamycin, sphingosine, mellitin, polymixin B, R0 31-8220, acridine orange, bisindolemaleimide, chelerythrine, calphostin C, and the highly specific PKC pseudosubstrate[86] (see later section), inhibit insulin- and phorbol ester-stimulated glucose transport in both rat adipocytes and rat soleus muscle preparations. Some of the earlier used compounds (e.g., H7 and staurosporine) are less specific than the more recently developed PKC inhibitors, namely bisindolemaleimide, RO 31-8220, and calphostin C. We have used RO 31-8220 and calphostin C most recently,[18a] and both agents provoke similar dose-dependent inhibition of insulin- and phorbol ester–stimulated glucose transport in rat adipocytes. Moreover, using insulin-stimulated MARCKS phosphorylation to serve as a marker for inhibition of PKC activity in intact adipocytes, we have noted similar dose-related inhibitory effects of RO 31-8220 on MARCKS phosphorylation and insulin-stimulated hexose transport. (Note that, in some cases, inhibition of insulin effects on glucose transport require higher inhibitor concentrations than inhibition of phorbol ester effects. This may reflect multiple PKC isoforms separate binding sites for DAG and phorbol esters and differential inhibitor sensitivities,[58,59] or inhibition of non-PKC kinases.) From these collective findings with PKC inhibitors, it seems reasonable to suggest that PKC is required for insulin-stimulated hexose transport. A similar conclusion was also reached by Yano et al.,[87] who used electroporation to introduce low concentrations of H7 and staurosporine into rat adipocytes. Perhaps the most convincing PKC inhibitor finding comes from studies with the PKC pseudosubstrate, which is the native endogenous inhibitor of PKC in its folded inactive state. This peptide was also introduced into rat adipocytes by electroporation and was found to inhibit insulin-stimulated glucose transport in concentrations that directly inhibit PKC.[86]

Although firm conclusions on a positive role for PKC in insulin-stimulated glucose transport may not be forthcoming from PKC inhibitor and depletion studies, such studies have provided more definitive information on what effects of insulin are not PKC-dependent. For example, PKC is not required for insulin-induced activation of phosphatidylcholine hydrolysis,[3] glycosyl-phosphatidylinositol hydrolysis, or de novo phosphatidic acid synthesis,[62,84] or, in rat adipocytes, for activation of MAP kinase.[63] In addition, we have recently found that the PKC inhibitor RO 31-8220, despite fully inhibiting both insulin- and phorbol ester–stimulated glucose transport, failed to inhibit the activation of phosphatidylinositol 3-kinase by insulin.[18a] Thus, the activation of phosphatidylinositol 3-kinase, which seems to be important in insulin-stimulated glucose transport,[88,89] is not dependent upon PKC in rat adipocytes, and effects of PKC inhibitors on insulin-stimulated glucose transport must, therefore, reflect either involvement of a PKC-dependent factor that is distal to phosphatidylinositol 3-kinase, or the inhibition of a non-PKC kinase distal to phosphatidylinositol 3-kinase by PKC inhibitors. In this respect, we have also recently found[18a] that Wortmannin inhibits insulin-stimulated, but not phorbol ester–stimulated, glucose transport in rat adipocytes. This dissociation suggests that PKC effects on glucose transport are not mediated through phosphatidylinositol 3-kinase, but that PKC activation may, nevertheless, be downstream of phosphatidylinositol 3-kinase activation in the action of insulin. The latter possibility is particularly interesting, as Wortmannin inhibits insulin-stimulated phosphatidylcholine hydrolysis in rat adipocytes.[18a] Thus, both phosphatidylinositol 3-kinase and phosphatidylcholine hydrolysis-dependent PKC activation may be involved in the glucose transport effects of insulin, including those involving GLUT-4 translocation.

Although MAP kinase activation does not appear to be required for insulin-stimulated glucose transport,[90] the role of *ras* or other related small GTP-binding proteins is less certain. Some evidence favors a role for *ras* in glucose transport in 3T3/L1 adipocytes,[91] whereas in CHO cells,[89] insulin-stimulated *ras* activation can be dissociated from activation of phosphatidylinositol 3-kinase and glucose transport. One possibility is that a non-*ras*, small GTP-binding protein, such as rho, ARF, or some other factor, might serve to couple phosphatidylinositol 3-kinase activation to phosphatidylcholine hydrolysis and PKC activation (see earlier discussion). Another possibility is that phosphatidylinositol-3′,4′,5′-$(PO_4)_3$ may directly activate PKC-ζ or other PKC isoforms. However, the involvement of PKC-ζ would appear to provide only a partial answer, because insulin effects on glucose transport in phorbol ester–downregulated rat adipocytes are markedly inhibited, despite having full or large amounts of PKC-ζ remaining.[59a] These and other findings (e.g., studies using antisense-DNA, as mentioned earlier) suggest that DAG-sensitive PKC isoforms, such as PKC-α and PKC-β, are required (perhaps in addition to PKC-ζ) for insulin-stimulated glucose transport, at least in certain cell types. Clearly, more information is needed for definitive conclusions to be drawn.

Glucose-Induced Activation of Protein Kinase C

In addition to insulin, a simple increase in glucose in certain, but not all, cell types leads to an increase in de novo phosphatidic acid synthesis.[2,92] In rat adipocytes, glucose is converted to DAG in very substantial amounts within minutes,[92] and this conversion is attended by increases in DAG content, PKC enzyme activity, and translocation of PKC-α, PKC-β, PKC-ε, and PKC-δ to microsomal membranes.[2] This does not occur in all cell types, however; most importantly, we have not observed this phenomenon of significant, glucose-induced DAG/PKC signaling in rat soleus muscle.[30] In addition, in streptozotocin-induced diabetes mellitus, we have reported increases in DAG and PKC activation in rat adipose tissue, but not in rat skeletal muscles.[30] Even more recently, we have found DAG and membrane PKC levels to be increased in rat liver and heart, but not in various muscles of these diabetic rats (unpublished data, Standaert ML, Yamada K, Avignon A, and Farese RV, 1995). These increases in rat liver DAG in streptozotocin-induced diabetes may occur over a period of time, as we have not observed DAG increases in direct incubations of hepatocytes in the presence of elevated extracellular glucose concentrations (unpublished data, Standaert ML, Yamada K, Avignon A, and Farese RV, 1995); this may be similar to the pancreatic islet in which chronic, but not acute, glucose treatment leads to increases in DAG levels.[93] It is also possible that the increases in DAG and PKC activation in both liver and heart (or other tissues of streptozotocin diabetic rats) may also reflect increases in stress-type hormones and activation of phosphatidylinositol-4′,5′-$(PO_4)_2$ hydrolysis.

The glucose-induced DAG/PKC signaling that occurs in the liver, heart, and pancreatic islets may be important in producing insulin resistance in the former two tissues, or impaired glucose-stimulated insulin release in the islet. Indeed, in the islet, PKC has been found to be depleted by prolonged exposure to high glucose levels,[94] and this may impair second-phase insulin secretion, which seems to be partly dependent upon PKC.[95,96]

Increases in PKC activation have been reported in livers of rats with streptozotocin-induced diabetes,[97] and this has been postulated to cause insulin resistance. One popular idea is that persistent PKC activation in the liver (and other tissues, such as skeletal muscle) may impair insulin-induced activation of insulin receptor tyrosine kinase; this has been observed in FAO hepatoma cells,[98] but not in normal rat hepatocytes[99] or muscle. In fact, in normal rat hepatocytes, phorbol esters diminish the glycogen synthesis effects of insulin, but do not impair other metabolic effects of insulin, and do not inhibit insulin-induced activation of receptor tyrosine kinase.[99] Another possibility that should be considered is that persistent PKC activation may inhibit G_i,[97] and this may impair insulin-induced effects on glycogen synthase, pyruvate dehydrogenase, and glycerol-3-PO_4 acyltransferase that are mediated through G_i (e.g., glycosyl-phosphatidylinositol hydrolysis and inositol-phospho-glycosyl mediators; see earlier discussion). Also, in skeletal muscle, although persistent PKC activation does not appear to result from simple hyperglycemia in streptozotocin-induced diabetes, we have observed persistent PKC activation in skeletal muscles of hyperinsulinemic type II diabetic GK rats (unpublished data, Avignon A, Yamada K, Zhou X, et al., 1995). Thus, in hyperinsulinemic states, it is possible that persistent PKC activation in muscle may inhibit certain effects of insulin. Indeed, our studies of the GK rat suggest that there is an impairment of intracellular glucose metabolism[6] (i.e., conversion of glucose to glycogen and fat, and glucose oxidation), rather than impaired glucose transport.

It should be noted that, although hyperinsulinemia-induced persistent PKC activation may be a factor in insulin resistance in type II diabetes, our data[30] at this point do not support the possibility that a simple increase in blood glucose (as occurs in streptozotocin-induced or type I diabetes mellitus) is attended by increases in DAG and persistent PKC activation in rat skeletal muscle. Thus, although it may be tempting to suggest that glucose toxicity begets insulin resistance through persistent DAG/PKC signaling, decreases in insulin receptor tyrosine activity, and decreases in insulin-stimulated glucose transport in rat skeletal muscle, most available evidence disputes this hypothesis. In fact, acute phorbol ester–induced PKC activation in muscle, as in liver, fails to diminish insulin-stimulated activation of insulin receptor tyrosine kinase activity in rat skeletal muscle, and has little or no effect on insulin-stimulated glucose transport in both rat skeletal muscle and rat adipocytes. In addition, muscle DAG levels are not increased in streptozotocin-induced diabetes,[30] although presently, it is not possible to rule out an increase in a small, but important, DAG pool. Finally, it may be noted that increases in muscle DAG that occur with denervation-induced insulin resistance are attended by normal insulin receptor tyrosine kinase activation[100] and normal phosphatidylinositol 3-kinase activation.[101]

Conclusions

To summarize, there is increasing evidence that insulin increases DAG and activates PKC in many, most, or perhaps all, target tissues. This evidence has been compiled by many investigators working in diverse cell systems. It is clear that insulin increases DAG, stimulates the translocation of PKC from cytosol to membrane, and increases membrane PKC activity. Moreover, there are now considerable data to suggest that insulin increases the phosphorylation of specific PKC substrates, by PKC-dependent mechanisms, in a variety of intact cells.

Therefore, the major question that remains is the definition of the role of PKC activation in specific actions of insulin. The similarity of effects of phorbol esters and insulin on various metabolic processes suggests that PKC may play an important role. Moreover, a number of insulin effects on various metabolic processes seem to require the participation of PKC. However, the opposite may also be said of some effects, and there may be considerable redundancy in signaling, as many of the terminal pathways that are activated by PKC are also activated by the MAP kinase pathway. With respect to MAP kinase, in contrast to gene expression and cell proliferation responses, the MAP kinase pathway does not explain many of the acute metabolic effects of insulin, most notably, those related to glucose transport. Phosphatidylinositol 3-kinase does, however, seem to be involved in acute metabolic processes, and our findings suggest that phospholipase D-dependent phosphatidylcholine hydrolysis and resultant PKC activation may occur downstream of phosphatidylinositol 3-kinase activation in the action of insulin. If so, this would explain why PKC seems to be involved, perhaps along with other phospholipase/lipid factors, in the activation of glucose transport during insulin action. In addition to glucose transport, recent evidence suggests that PKC may be involved in other actions of insulin, namely, Na^+/K^+ transport processes, activation of protein synthesis, and altered expression of certain genes. However, more definitive studies will be needed to test the possibility that PKC is important in these insulin-stimulated processes.

References

1. Farese RV, Standaert ML, Arnold TP, et al. The role of protein kinase C in insulin action. Cellular Signalling 1992;4:133
2. Farese RV, Standaert ML, Arnold TP, et al. Preferential activation of microsomal diacylglycerol/protein kinase C signaling during glucose treatment (*de novo* phospholipid synthesis) of rat adipocytes. J Clin Invest 1994;93:1894
3. Hoffman JM, Standaert ML, Nair GP, et al. Differential effects of pertussis toxin on insulin-stimulated phosphatidylcholine hydrolysis and glycerolipid synthesis *de novo*. Studies in BC3H-1 myocytes and rat adipocytes. Biochemistry 1991;30:3315
4. Luttrell LM, Hewlett EL, Romero G, et al. Pertussis toxin treatment attenuates some effects of insulin in BC3H-1 murine myocytes. J Biol Chem 1988; 263:6134
5. Vila MC, Milligan G, Standaert ML, et al. Insulin activates glycerol-3-phosphate acyltransferase (*de novo* phosphatidic acid synthesis) through a phospholipid-derived mediator. Apparent involvement of Gi-α and activation of a phospholipase C. Biochemistry 1990;29:8735
6. Farese RV, Standaert ML, Yamada K, et al. Insulin-induced activation of G3PAT by a *chiro*-inositol-containing insulin is defective in adipocytes of insulin-resistant, type II diabetic, Goto-Kakizaki (GK) rats. Proc Natl Acad Sci USA 1994;91:11040
7. Larner J. Insulin-signaling mechanisms. Lessons from the Old Testament of glycogen metabolism and the New Testament of molecular biology. Diabetes 1988;37:262
8. Saltiel AR, Osterman DG, Darnell JC, et al. The role of glycoylphosphoinositides in signal transduction. Rec Prog Horm Res 1989;45:353
9. Standaert ML, Musunuru K, Yamada K, et al. Insulin-stimulated phosphatidylcholine hydrolysis, diacylglycerol/protein kinase C signalling and hexose transport in pertussis toxin-treated BC3H-1 myocytes. Cellular Signalling 1994;6:707
10. Farese RV, Cooper DR, Konda TS, et al. Insulin provokes co-ordinated increases in the synthesis of phosphatidylinositol, phosphatidylinositol phosphates and the phosphatidylinositol-glycan in BC3H-1 myocytes. Biochem J 1988;256:185
11. Baldini PM, Zannetti A, Donchenko V, et al. Insulin effect on isolated rat hepatocytes: Diacylglycerol-phosphatidic acid interrelationship. Biochim Biophys Acta 1921;1137:208
12. Petkova DH, Nikolova MN, Momchilova-Pankova AB, et al. Insulin effect on the phospholipid organization and some enzyme activities of rat liver membrane fractions. Comp Biochem Physiol 1990;95B:685
13. Farese RV, Konda TS, Davis JS, et al. Insulin rapidly increases diacylglycerol by activating *de novo* phosphatidic acid synthesis. Science 1987;236:586
14. Farese RV, Cooper DR, Konda TS, et al. Mechanisms whereby insulin increases diacylglycerol in BC3H-1 myocytes. Biochem J 1988;256:175
15. Wei JW, Yeh SR. Effects of insulin on glucose uptake in cultured cells from the central nervous system of rodent. Int J Biochem 1991;23:851
16. Garcia de Herreros A, Dominguez I, Diaz-Meco MT, et al. Requirement of phospholipase C-catalyzed hydrolysis of phosphatidylcholine for maturation of *Xenopus laevis* oocytes in response to insulin and *ras* p21. J Biol Chem 1991;266:6825

16a. Standaert ML, Bandyopadhyay G, Zhou X, et al. Insulin stimulates phospholipid D-dependent phosphatidylcholine hydrolysis, *de novo* phospholipid synthesis, and diacylglycerol/protein kinase C signalling in L6 myotubes. Endocrinology, in press, 1995.

17. Price BD, Morris JD, Hall A. Stimulation of phosphatidylcholine breakdown and diacylglycerol production of growth factors in Swiss-3T3 cells. Biochem J 1989;264:509
18. Kelly KL, Gutierrez G, Martin A. Hormonal regulation of phosphatidylcholine synthesis by reversible modulation of cytidylyltransferase. Biochem J 1988;255:693

18a. Standaert ML, Avignon A, Yamada K, et al. The phosphatidylinositol-3-kinase inhibitor, wortmannin, inhibit insulin-induced activation of phosphatidylcholine hydrolysis and associated protein kinase C translocation in rat adipocytes. Biochem J, in press, 1995.

19. Bowman EP, Uhlinger DJ, Lambeth JD. Neutrophil phospholipase D is activated by a membrane-associated rho family small molecular weight GTP-binding protein. J Biol Chem 1993;268:21509
20. Cockcroft S, Thomas GM, Fensome A, et al. Phospholipase D: A downstream effector of ARF in granulocytes. Science 1994;263:523
21. Farese RV, Larson RE, Sabir MA. Insulin acutely increases phospholipids in the phosphatidate-inositide cycle in rat adipose tissue. J Biol Chem 1982;257:4042
22. Farese RV, Barnes DE, Davis JS, et al. Effects of insulin and protein synthesis inhibitors on phospholipid metabolism, diacylglycerol levels and pyruvate dehydrogenase activity in BC3H-1 myocytes. J Biol Chem 1984;259:7094
23. Farese RV, Davis JS, Barnes DE, et al. The *de novo* phospholipid effect of insulin is associated with increases in diacylglycerol, but not inositol phosphates or cytosolic Ca^{++}. Biochem J 1985;231:269
24. Ruderman NB, Kapeller R, White MF, et al. Activation of phosphatidylinositol 3-kinase by insulin. Proc Natl Acad Sci USA 1990;87:1411
25. Nakanishi H, Brewer KA, Exton JH. Activation of the ζ isozyme of protein kinase C by phosphatidylinositol 3,4,5-trisphosphate. J Biol Chem 1993; 268:13
26. Singh SS, Chauhan A, Brockerhoff H, et al. Activation of protein kinase C

by phosphatidylinositol 3,4,5-trisphosphate. Biochem Biophys Res Commun 1993;195:104
27. Chauhan A, Chauhan VP, Brockerhoff H. Activation of protein kinase C by phosphatidylinositol 4,5-bisphosphate: Possible involvement in Na^+/H^+ antiport downregulation and cell proliferation. Biochem Biophys Res Commun 1991;175:852
28. Kelly KL, Ruderman NB. Insulin-stimulated phosphatidylinositol 3-kinase. J Biol Chem 1993;268:4391
29. Ishizuka T, Cooper DR, Hernandez H, et al. Effects of insulin on diacylglycerol-protein kinase C signaling in rat diaphragm and soleus muscles and relationship to glucose transport. Diabetes 1990;39:181
30. Hoffman JM, Ishizuka, Farese RV. Interrelated effects of insulin and glucose on diacylglycerol-protein kinase-C signalling in rat adipocytes and solei muscle *in vitro* and *in vivo* in diabetic rats. Endocrinology 1991;128:2937
31. Yu B, Standaert M, Arnold T, et al. Effects of insulin on diacylglycerol/protein kinase-C signalling and glucose transport in rat skeletal muscles *in vivo* and *in vitro*. Endocrinology 1992;130:3345
32. Cooper DR, Hernandez H, Kuo JY, et al. Insulin increases the synthesis of phospholipid and diacylglycerol and protein kinase C activity in rat hepatocytes. Arch Biochem Biophys 1990;276:486
33. Zhao L, Standaert ML, Cooper DR, et al. Effects of insulin on protein kinase C in HIRC-B cells. Specific activation of PKC-ε and its resistance to phorbol ester-induced downregulation. Endocrinology 1994;135:2504
34. Cherqui G, Reynet C, Caron M, et al. Insulin receptor tyrosine residues 1162 and 1163 control insulin stimulation of myristoyl-diacylglycerol generation and subsequent activation of glucose transport. J Biol Chem 1990;265:21254
35. Arnold TP, Standaert ML, Hernandez H, et al. Effects of insulin and phorbol esters on MARCKS (myristoylated alanine-rich C-kinase substrate) phosphorylation (and other parameters of protein kinase C activation) in rat adipocytes, rat soleus muscle and BC3H-1 myocytes. Biochem J 1993;295:155
36. Stabel S, Parker P. Protein kinase C. Pharm Ther 1991;51:71
37. Nishizuka Y. Membrane phospholipid degradation and protein kinase C for cell signalling. Neurosci Res 1992;15:3
38. Walaas SI, Horn RS, Adler A, et al. Insulin increases membrane protein kinase C activity in rat diaphragm. FEBS Lett 1987;220:311
39. Cooper DR, Konda TS, Standaert ML, et al. Insulin increases membrane and cytosolic protein kinase C activity in BC3H-1 myocytes. J Biol Chem 1987;262:3633
40. Ishizuka T, Cooper DR, Farese RV. Insulin stimulates the translocation of protein kinase C in rat adipocytes. FEBS Lett 1989;257:337
41. Cooper DR, Ishizuka T, Watson JE, et al. Protein kinase C activation patterns are determined by methodological variations. Studies of insulin action in BC3H-1 myocytes and rat adipose tissue. Biochim Biophys Acta 1990;1054:95
42. Farese RV, Standaert ML, Francois AM, et al. Effects of insulin and phorbol esters on subcellular distribution of protein kinase C isoforms in rat adipocytes. Biochem J 1992;288:319
42a. Yamada K, Avignon A, Standaert ML, et al. Effects of insulin on the translocation of protein kinase C-theta and other protein kinase C isoforms in rat skeletal muscles. Biochem J 1995;308:177
42b. Standaert ML, Avignon A, Arnold T, et al. Insulin translocates PKC-epsilon and phorbol esters induce and persistently translocate PKC-beta II in BC3H-1 myocytes. Cellular Signalling, in press, 1995.
43. Cooper DR, Khalakdina A, Watson JE. Chronic effects of glucose on insulin signaling in A-10 vascular smooth muscle cells. Arch Biochem Biophys 1993;302:490
44. Messina JL, Standaert ML, Ishizuka T, et al. Role of protein kinase C in insulin's regulation of c-*fos* transcription. J Biol Chem 1992;267:9223
45. Smith BL, Mochly-Rosen D. Inhibition of protein kinase C function by injection of intracellular receptors for the enzyme. Biochem Biophys Res Commun 1992;188:1235
46. Srinivasan M, Begum N. Stimulation of protein phosphatase-1 activity by phorbol esters. J Biol Chem 1994;269:16662
47. Heidenreich KA, Toledo SP, Brunton LL, et al. Insulin stimulates the activity of a novel protein kinase C, PKC-ε, in cultured fetal chick neurons. J Biol Chem 1990;265:15076
48. Egan JJ, Saltis J, Wek SA, et al. Insulin, oxytocin, and vasopressin stimulate protein kinase C activity in adipocyte plasma membranes. Proc Natl Acad Sci USA 1990;87:1052
49. Standaert ML, Cooper DR, Hernandez H, et al. Differential down-regulation of insulin-sensitive protein kinase-C isoforms by 12-*O*-tetradecanoylphorbol-13-acetate in rat adipocytes and BC3H-1 myocytes. Endocrinology 1993;132:689
50. Yamada K, Standaert ML, Yu B, et al. Insulin-like effects of sodium orthovanadate on diacylglycerol-protein kinase C signaling in BC3H-1 myocytes. Arch Biochem Biophys 1994;312:167
51. Blackshear PJ, Haupt DM, Stumpo DJ. Insulin activation of protein kinase C: A reassessment. J Biol Chem 1991;266:10946
52. Walaas O, Horn RS, Walaas SI. Insulin and phorbol ester stimulate phosphorylation of a 15000 dalton membrane protein in rat diaphragm in a similar manner. Biochim Biophys Acta 1991;1094:92
53. Morley SJ, Traugh JA. Differential stimulation of phosphorylation of initiation factors eIF-4F, eIF-4B, eIF-3, and ribosomal protein S6 by insulin and phorbol esters. J Biol Chem 1990;265:10611
54. Graves CB, McDonald JM. Insulin and phorbol ester stimulate phosphorylation of a 40-kDa protein in adipocyte plasma membranes. J Biol Chem 1985;260:11286
55. Haystead TAJ, Hardie DG. Insulin and phorbol ester stimulate phosphorylation of acetyl-CoA carboxylase at similar sites in isolated adipocytes. Eur J Biochem 1988;175:339
56. Donaldson RW, Hagedorn CH, Cohen S. Epidermal growth factor or okadaic acid stimulates phosphorylation of eukaryotic initiation factor 4F. J Biol Chem 1991;266:3162
57. Taniguchi H, Manenti S, Suzuki M, et al. Myristoylated alanine-rich C kinase substrate (MARCKS), a major protein kinase C substrate, is an *in vivo* substrate of proline-directed protein kinase(s). J Biol Chem 1994;269:18299
58. Robinson PJ. Differential stimulation of protein kinase C activity by phorbol ester or calcium/phosphatidylserine *in vitro* and in intact synaptosomes. J Biol Chem 1992;267:21637
59. Slater SJ, Kelly MB, Taddeo FJ, et al. Evidence for discrete diacylglycerol and phorbol ester activator sites on protein kinase C. J Biol Chem 1994;269:17160
59a. Avignon A, Standaert ML, Yamada K, et al. Insulin increases mRNA levels of protein kinase C-alpha and -beta in rat adipocytes and protein kinase C-alpha, -beta, and -theta in rat skeletal muscle. Biochem J 1995;308:181
60. Chalfant CE, McLean M, Watson JE, et al. Regulation of Alternative Splicing of Protein Kinase C by Insulin. J Biol Chem 1995;270:13326
61. Cherqui G, Caron M, Wicek D, et al. Decreased insulin responsiveness in fat cells rendered protein kinase C-deficient by a treatment with a phorbol ester. Endocrinology 1987;120:2192
62. Ishizuka T, Cooper DR, Arnold T, et al. Downregulation of protein kinase C and insulin-stimulated 2-deoxyglucose uptake in rat adipocytes by phorbol esters, glucose, and insulin. Diabetes 1991;40:1274
63. Yang Y, Farese RV. Insulin activates myelin basic protein (p42 MAP) kinase by a protein kinase C-independent pathway in rat adipocytes: Dissociation from glucose transport. FEBS Lett 1993;333:287
64. Mühlbacher C, Karnieli E, Schaff P, et al. Phorbol esters imitate in rat fat-cells the full effect of insulin on glucose-carrier translocation, but not on 3-*O*-methylglucose-transport activity. Biochem J 1988;249:865
65. Obermaier-Kusser B, Mühlbacher C, Mushack J, et al. Further evidence for a two-step model of glucose-transport regulation. Biochem J 1989;261:699
66. Vogt B, Mushack J, Seffer E, et al. The phorbol ester TPA induces a translocation of the insulin sensitive glucose carrier (GLUT4) in fat cells. Biochem Biophys Res Commun 1990;168:1089
67. Farese RV, Standaert M, Yu B, et al. 2-Hydroxypropyl-β-cyclodextrin enhances phorbol ester effects on glucose transport and/or protein kinase C-β translocation to the plasma membrane in rat adipocytes and soleus muscles. J Biol Chem 1993;268:19949
68. Kanai F, Nishioka Y, Hayashi H, et al. Direct demonstration of insulin-induced GLUT4 translocation to the surface of intact cells by insertion of a c-*myc* epitope into an exofacial GLUT4 domain. J Biol Chem 1993;268:14523
69. Holman GD, Kozka IJ, Clark AE, et al. Cell surface labeling of glucose transport isoform GLUT4 by bis-mannose photolabel. J Biol Chem 1990;265:18172
70. Saltis J, Habberfield AD, Egan JJ, et al. Role of protein kinase C in the regulation of glucose transport in the rat adipose cell. J Biol Chem 1991;266:261
71. Farese RV, Standaert ML, Barnes DE, et al. Phorbol ester provokes insulin-1like effects on glucose transport, amino acid uptake, and pyruvate dehydrogenase activity in BC3H-1 cultured myocytes. Endocrinology 1985;116:2650
72. Standaert ML, Farese RV, Cooper DR, et al. Insulin-induced glycerolipid mediators and the stimulation of glucose transport in BC3H-1 myocytes. J Biol Chem 1988;263:8696
73. Christensen RL, Shade DL, Graves B, et al. Evidence that protein kinase C is involved in regulating glucose transport in the adipocyte. Int J Biochem 1987;19:259
74. Stralfors P. Insulin stimulation of glucose uptake can be mediated by diacylglycerol in adipocytes. Nature 1988;335:554
75. Sowell MO, Boggs KP, Robinson KA, et al. Effects of insulin and phospholipase C in control and denervated rat skeletal muscle. Am J Physiol 1991;260(Endocrinol Metab 23):E247
76. Cleland PJF, Appleby GJ, Rattigan S, et al. Exercise-induced translocation of protein kinase C and production of diacylglycerol and phosphatidic acid in rat skeletal muscle *in vivo*. J Biol Chem 1989;264:17704
77. Takuwa N, Takuwa Y, Rasmussen H. Stimulation of mitogenesis and glucose transport by 1-monooleoylglycerol in Swiss 3T3 fibroblasts. J Biol Chem 1988;263:9738
78. Haystead TAJ, Sim ATR, Carling D, et al. Effects of the tumour promoter okadaic acid on intracellular protein phosphorylation and metabolism. Nature 1989;337:78
79. Tanti J-F, Rochet N, Grémeaux T, et al. Insulin-stimulated glucose transport in muscle: Evidence for a protein-kinase-C-dependent component which is unaltered in insulin-resistant mice. Biochem J 1989;258:141
80. Van De Werve G, Zaninetti D, Lang U, et al. Identification of a major defect in insulin-resistant tissues of genetically obese (*fa/fa*) rats. Impaired protein kinase C. Diabetes 1987;36:310
81. Gibbs EM, Allard WJ, Lienhard GE. The glucose transport in 3T3-L1 adipocytes is phosphorylated in response to phorbol ester but not in response to insulin. J Biol Chem 1986;261:16597
82. Kitagawa K, Nishino H, Iwashima A. Ca^{2+}-dependent stimulation of 3-0-methylglucose transport in mouse fibroblast Swiss 3T3 cells induced by phorbol-12,13-dibutyrate. Biochem Biophys Res Commun 1985;128:127

83. Klip A, Ramlal T. Protein kinase C is not required for insulin stimulation of hexose uptake in muscle cells in culture. Biochem J 1987;242:131
84. Farese RV, Standaert ML, Ishizuka T, et al. Antisense DNA downregulates protein kinase C isozymes (β and α) and insulin-stimulated 2-deoxyglucose uptake in rat adipocytes. Antisense Res Dev 1991;1:35
85. Cooper DR, Watson JE, Hernandez H, et al. Direct evidence for protein kinase C involvement in insulin-stimulated hexose uptake. Biochem Biophys Res Commun 1992;188:142
86. Standaert ML, Sasse J, Cooper DR, et al. Protein kinase C (19-31) pseudosubstrate inhibition of insulin action in rat adipocytes. FEBS Lett 1991;282:139
87. Yano Y, Sumida Y, Benzing CF, et al. Primary sites of actions of staurosporine and H-7 in the cascade of insulin action to glucose transport in rat adipocytes. Biochim Biophys Acta 1993;1176:327
88. Okada T, Kawano Y, Sakakibara T, et al. Essential role of phosphatidylinositol 3-kinase in insulin-induced glucose transport and antilipolysis in rat adipocytes. J Biol Chem 1994;269:3568
89. Hara K, Yonezawa K, Sakaue H, et al. 1-Phosphatidylinositol 3-kinase activity is required for insulin-stimulated glucose transport but not for RAS activation in CHO cells. Proc Natl Acad Sci USA 1994;91:7415
90. Robinson LJ, Razzack ZF, Lawrence JC Jr, et al. Mitogen-activated protein kinase activation is not sufficient for stimulation of glucose transport or glycogen synthase in 3T3-L1 adipocytes. J Biol Chem 1993;268:26422
91. Kozma L, Baltensperger K, Klarlund J, et al. The Ras signaling pathway mimics insulin action on glucose transporter translocation. Proc Natl Acad Sci USA 1993;90:4460
92. Ishizuka T, Hoffman J, Cooper DR, et al. Glucose-induced synthesis of diacylglycerol *de novo* is associated with translocation (activation) of protein kinase C in rat adipocytes. FEBS Lett 1989;249:234
93. Wolf BA, Easom RA, McDaniel ML, et al. Diacylglycerol synthesis *de novo* from glucose by pancreatic islets isolated from rats and humans. J Clin Invest 1990;85:482
94. Thams P. Role of protein kinase C and Ca^{2+} in glucose-induced sensitization/desensitization of insulin secretion. Experientia 1991;47:1201
95. Zawalich WS. Modulation of insulin secretion from β-cells by phosphoinositide-derived second-messenger molecules. Diabetes 1988;37:137
96. Thams P, Capito K, Hedeskov CJ, et al. Phorbol-ester-induced downregulation of protein kinase C in mouse pancreatic islets. Potentiation of phase I and inhibition of phase 2 of glucose-induced insulin secretion. Biochem J 1990;265:777
97. Tang EY, Parker PJ, Beattie J, et al. Diabetes induces selective alterations in the expression of protein kinase C isoforms in hepatocytes. FEBS Lett 1993;326:117
98. Takayama S, White MF, Kahn CR. Phorbol ester-induced serine phosphorylation of the insulin receptor decreases its tyrosine kinase activity. J Biol Chem 1988;263:3440
99. Quentmeier A, Daneschmand H, Klein H, et al. Insulin-mimetic actions of phorbol ester in cultured adult rat hepatocytes. Lack of phorbol-ester-elicited inhibition of the insulin signal. Biochem J 1993;289:549
100. Burant CF, Treutelaar MK, Buse MG. *In vitro* and *in vivo* activation of the insulin receptor in control and denervated skeletal muscle. J Biol Chem 1986;261:8985
101. Chen KS, Friel JC, Ruderman NB. Regulation of phosphatidylinositol-3-kinase by insulin in rat skeletal muscle. Am J Physiol 1993;265(Endocrinol Metab 28):E736
102. Mojsilovic LP, Rosic NK, Standaert ML, et al. The role of protein kinase C system in the mediation of insulin-stimulated (Na^+,K^+)ATPase transport activity in BC3H-1 muscle cells. Clin Res 1986;34:197A
103. Civan MM, Peterson-Yantorno K, George K, et al. Interactions of TPA and insulin on Na^+ transport across frog skin. Am J Physiol 1989;256(Cell Physiol 25):C569
104. Sampson SR, Brodie C, Alboim SV. Role of protein kinase C in insulin activation of the Na-K pump in cultured skeletal muscle. Am J Physiol 1994;266(Cell Physiol 35):C751
105. Hesketh JE, Campbell GP, Reeds PJ. Rapid response of protein synthesis to insulin in 3T3 cells: Effects of protein kinase C depletion and differences from the response to serum repletion. Biosci Rep 1986;6:797
106. Welsh GI, Proud CG. Evidence for a role for protein kinase C in the stimulation of protein synthesis by insulin in swiss 3T3 fibroblasts. FEBS Lett 1993;316:241
107. Benelli C, Caron M, de Gallé B, et al. Evidence for a role of protein kinase C in the activation of the pyruvate dehydrogenase complex by insulin in Zajdela hepatoma cells. Metabolism 1994;43:1030
108. Heidenreich KA, Zeppelin T, Robinson LJ. Insulin and insulin-like growth factor I induce *c-fos* expression in postmitotic neurons by a protein kinase C-dependent pathway. J Biol Chem 1993;268:14663
109. Weinstock RS, Messina JL. Transcriptional regulation of a rat hepatoma gene by insulin and protein kinase-C. Endocrinology 1988;123:366
110. Messina JL, Weinstock RS. Regulation of β-actin gene transcription by insulin and phorbol esters. Exp Cell Res 1992;200:532
111. Lee PDK, Abdel-Maguid LS, Snuggs MB. Role of protein kinase-C in regulation of insulin-like growth factor-binding protein-1 production by HepG2 cells. J Clin Endocrinol Metab 1992;75:459
112. Chan SO, Wong SSC, Yeung DCY. Insulin induction of *c-Ki-ras* in rat liver and in cultured normal rat hepatocytes. Comp Biochem Physiol 1993;104B:341

Diabetes Mellitus, edited by Derek LeRoith, Simeon I. Taylor, and Jerrold M. Olefsky. Lippincott–Raven Publishers, Philadelphia © 1996.

Chapter 20

A Role for Insulin-Mediated Regulation of Cyclic Guanosine Monophosphate (cGMP)–Inhibited Phosphodiesterase in the Antilipolytic Action of Insulin

Eva Degerman, Marie J. Leroy, Masato Taira, Per Belfrage, and Vincent Manganiello

Background

More than 30 years ago, Sutherland and Rall described cAMP as an intracellular messenger mediating responses of cells to a variety of hormones and neurotransmitters.[1,2] Soon thereafter, it was realized that insulin opposed the effects of several catabolic hormones that increase cAMP and regulate lipid and carbohydrate metabolism in adipose tissue and liver. A decrease in cAMP was usually associated with these actions of insulin.[3,4] Even early experiments on the biologic production of cAMP in cell homogenates indicated that, once formed, the compound was subject to rapid destruction. Butcher and Sutherland partially purified what was thought to be a ubiquitous enzyme responsible for specific hydrolysis of the 3′-5′ phosphodiester bond of cyclic nucleotides.[5] Initial attempts to demonstrate insulin activation of cAMP phosphodiesterase (PDE) were unsuccessful, mainly because the existence of multiple PDE isoforms was not recognized and the assay conditions did not detect the insulin-sensitive form.

Thompson, Appleman, and coworkers were among the first to demonstrate that several types of PDEs with different substrate specificities and affinities could be separated from various tissues.[6,7] Loten and Sneyd reported that incubation of intact rat adipocytes or fat pads with insulin resulted in activation of a "low K_m" cAMP PDE; that is, increased PDE activity was detected in homogenates assayed at low cAMP substrate concentrations.[8] Later, it was found that liver also contained insulin-sensitive cAMP PDE activity.[9] From detailed characterization of purified PDEs and molecular cloning, it has become clear that hydrolysis of intracellular cAMP and cyclic guanosine monophosphate (cGMP) is catalyzed by a diverse and complex group of structurally related PDE isoenzyme families. Seven major PDE gene families have been identified, each with distinctive properties, such as substrate specificities and affinities, physical properties, responsiveness to pharmacologic agents, and regulation by intracellular effectors (Fig. 20-1).[10–12] The adipocyte insulin-sensitive cGI-PDE belongs to the type III or cGMP-inhibited (cGI) PDE family and is predominantly found in association with adipocyte microsomal fractions.[13–19] In liver, two insulin-sensitive PDEs have been identified: a type IV or rolipram-inhibited cAMP-specific PDE associated with plasma membranes, and a type III cGI-PDE associated with the Golgi network or an incompletely characterized "dense vesicle" microsomal fraction.[20–23]

One important physiologic action of insulin—namely, its antilipolytic effect in adipocytes—has been a focus of interest for our research groups for many years.[13,24] To dissect this insulin signal transduction chain, our experimental strategy has involved starting with the final target enzyme, namely the hormone-sensitive lipase (HSL), and then analyzing each step sequentially while moving upstream toward the insulin receptor in the plasma membrane. Stimulation of adipocytes with hormones that increase cAMP results in activation of cAMP-dependent protein kinase (A-kinase) which then phosphorylates and activates HSL, the rate-controlling enzyme in lipolysis, leading to hydrolysis of stored triacylglycerols.[24,25] Although the inhibitory effects of insulin on hormone-activated lipase/lipolysis were thought to be associated with an insulin-induced reduction in cAMP,[3,4,26] initial experiments were not convincing. It is now clear that, at least under conditions of submaximal lipolysis, the antilipolytic effect of insulin can be explained by its ability to lower cAMP and A-kinase.[26–28] Furthermore, insulin-induced activation of adipocyte cGI-PDE, mediated by insulin-stimulated kinases (possibly including phosphatidylinositol-3-kinase [P13-K]),[13,29] seems to play a central role in reducing cAMP and, consequently, A-kinase.[26–28] This review concentrates on the adipocyte cGI-PDE, with emphasis on the role of this enzyme in insulin-mediated decreases in cAMP and inhibition of lipolysis.

Properties of cGMP-Inhibited Phosphodiesterases (cGI-PDEs)

Purification and Characterization of cGI-PDEs

Purification of cGI-PDEs to homogeneity has been difficult owing to their low abundance and sensitivity to proteolysis. We have used an affinity matrix composed of the *N*-(2-isothiocyanato)ethyl derivative of cilostamide, a specific inhibitor of cGI-PDEs,[10,13,30–32] to purify cGI-PDEs from several tissues, including rat and bovine adipose tissue,[19,33] bovine aortic smooth muscle,[34] human platelets,[35] and human placenta.[36] Other procedures have yielded homogenous preparations of this enzyme from rat liver, bovine heart, and human platelets.[20,21,37,38] Owing to proteolysis during purification, even in the presence of protease inhibitors, the final enzyme preparations contain, in most cases, several immunologically related polypeptides with M_r values of 60,000–135,000 (SDS-PAGE).

Immunoprecipitation or Western blotting of cGI-PDEs from different tissues has demonstrated subunit M_r values of 105,000–135,000 (SDS-PAGE); the one exception is rat liver cGI-PDE, often referred to as the "dense-vesicle" enzyme, which has an M_r of approximately 57,000.[20] It could be that rat liver contains two cGI-PDE isoforms: the "dense-vesicle" cGI-PDE and another cGI-PDE identified as a 73-kd polypeptide (with the native subunit M_r probably being higher because the enzyme was solubilized using chymotrypsin).[21] Thus, in most cases, polypeptides obtained after purification probably originate from larger native forms, which are proteolytically nicked during purification owing to the exquisite sensitivity of this enzyme to proteolysis.

cGI-PDEs can be distinguished from other PDE families by their substrate affinities for both cAMP and cGMP and their sensitivity to specific inhibitors, which are now available for most of the known PDE gene families.[10,13,30–32] cGI-PDEs have a high affinity for both cAMP and cGMP, with K_m values of 0.1–0.8 μM; the V_{max} for cAMP is higher (approximately 4–10 fold) than for cGMP. In view of the K_m values for cAMP and cGMP, it is not surprising that cGMP is a competitive inhibitor of cAMP hydrolysis (Table 20-1). A second defining characteristic of cGI-PDEs as compared

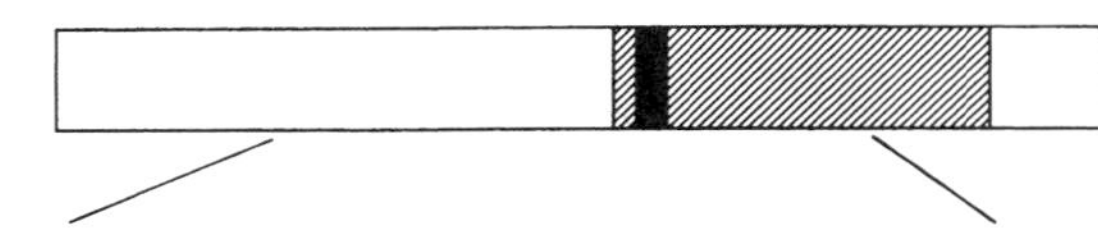

FIGURE **20-1.** Common structural pattern of PDEs. The seven PDE gene families exhibit a common domain organization. All share a conserved catalytic domain and have divergent regulatory domains.

Table 20-1. Defining Properties of cGI-PDEs

	Rat Adipose Tissue[19]	Bovine Aortic Smooth Muscle[34]	Bovine Heart[37]	Human Platelets[35]	Rat Liver		Human Placenta[36]
					Ref. 20	Ref. 21	
Catalytic Properties							
K_m (μM)							
cAMP	0.4	0.16	0.15	0.2	0.3/29	0.24	0.57
cGMP	0.3	0.09	0.10	0.3	10	0.17	15
V_{max} (μM/min/mg)							
cAMP	8.5	3.1	6.0	6.1	114/633*	6.2	0.86
cGMP	2.0	0.3	0.6	0.9	4.1*	2.1	0.47
Inhibitors (μM) IC_{50}[†]							
OPC-3911	0.04	0.054	0.005[‡]	–	–	–	0.22
Miltrinone	0.6	0.40	0.26[‡]	0.71	1	–	–
CI-930	0.4	0.40	–	0.2	–	–	–
RO 20-1724	190	30[§]	62[‡]	316	50	–	120
cGMP	0.2	0.25	0.06[‡]	0.32	2.0	0.18	0.12
Hormonal Regulation							
Insulin/cGI-PDE IK[‖]	yes[13–19,29,54]	no[¶]	–	yes[59–61]	yes[9,20–23]		–
cAMP-increasing hormones/A-kinase[#]	yes[13–19,49–53]	yes[34¶]	yes[37]	yes[47,48]	yes[20–22]		–

*nM/min/mg. †Concentration that inhibited enzyme activity by 50% at [^{3}H]cAMP < 1 μM. ‡K_I. §Inhibition with 30 μM was less than 20%. ‖Insulin-stimulated cGMP-inhibited PDE kinase. ¶Unpublished data. #cAMP-dependent protein kinase.

to other PDE families is their sensitivity to several drugs that augment myocardial contractility, inhibit platelet aggregation, and relax smooth muscle, such as cilostamide and related Otsuka Pharmaceutical (OPC) derivatives, milrinone, enoximone, CI-930 (Imazodan), LY195115 (Indolidan), Y-590, anegrelide, and IC1233188.[10,11,13,30–32] The IC_{50} values for inhibition of cGI-PDEs (at low cAMP concentrations) were less than 0.1 μM for OPC 3911 and cilostamide, and about 0.5 μM for milrinone and CI-930; by contrast, RO 20-1724 was not an effective inhibitor (IC_{50} >25 μM) (see Table 20-1).

Molecular Cloning of cGI-PDEs

The cDNAs encoding two cGI-PDE subfamilies (cGIP1 and cGIP2), products of distinct but related genes, have been cloned from rat[39] and human adipose tissue and human cardiac[40] cDNA libraries and rat and human genomic libraries (Fig. 20-2). Southern blot hybridizations of human (H) cGIP1 and HcGIP2 cDNAs with genomic digests of human-hamster somatic cell hybrids and fluorescent in situ hybridization of human metaphase chromosomes with HcGIP1 and HcGIP2 genomic clones indicate that the gene for HcGIP1 is located on human chromosome 11, whereas that for HcGIP2 is located on human chromosome 12 (unpublished data, Miki, et al., 1995; Kasuya, et al., 1995). Rat (R) cGIP1 mRNA is relatively abundant in adipocytes and increases dramatically during differentiation of cultured murine 3T3-L1 adipocytes.[39] Earlier studies had indicated that particulate 3T3-L1 adipocyte cGI-PDE activity and responsiveness to insulin also appeared or dramatically increased during differentiation of 3T3-L1 adipocytes.[41,42] RcGIP1 cDNA hybridizes weakly, if at all, with cardiac and brain mRNAs. By contrast, RcGIP2 cDNA hybridizes strongly with heart, and weakly (if at all) to rat and 3T3-L1 adipocyte mRNAs.[39] Multiple species of RcGIP2 mRNAs have been detected on Northern blots of rat heart, lung, and other tissues[39] (unpublished data, Taira, et al., 1995).

cGIP1 and cGIP2 cDNAs encode proteins with M_r values of 122,000–125,000, consistent with those of cGI-PDEs from intact rat adipocytes and human cardiac muscle microsomal preparations.[43–45] Mammalian PDE gene families, including cGI-PDEs, possess a similar domain organization, with conserved catalytic domains in C-terminal regions and N-terminal regulatory domains (see Figs. 20-1 and 20-2). Within the conserved domain of cGI-PDEs, however, there is a sequence of 44 amino acids that does not align with the sequences of other PDE families.[39,40] The regulatory domain contains hydrophobic putative membrane-association domains and several consensus substrate sequences (-RRXS-) for A-kinase. As will be discussed later, the solubilized adipocyte cGI-PDE is phosphorylated on serine 427 (based on the deduced sequence of RcGIP1[39]) in vitro by A-kinase.[46] The domain organization of cGIP1 and cGIP2 is quite similar (see Fig. 20-2). The entire deduced amino acid sequence of RcGIP1 is more closely related to that of HcGIP1 than to RcGIP2, which is similar to HcGIP2. Deduced sequences of the conserved domains of all four cGI-PDEs are very similar except for the additional region, the sequence of which is similar in HcGIP1 and RcGIP1 but different from those in HcGIP2 and RcGIP2 (which are similar). Thus, this 44–amino acid insertion, which is unique to the cGI-PDE gene family, may be important in identifying conserved members or subfamilies within the cGI-PDE gene family. The N-terminal portions of the deduced sequences of RcGIP1 and HcGIP1, including those in the hydrophobic domains and those adjacent to the consensus substrate sequences for A-kinase phosphorylation, are very similar and differ from the analogous sequences of RcGIP2 and HcGIP2, which are similar. All four cGI-PDEs have similar hydropathy plots, consistent with the notion that structural and functional domains are similar (see Fig. 20-2).

The catalytic properties of recombinant (r) cGIP1 and (r)cGIP2, as expressed in Sf9 insect cells, are similar (unpublished data, Murata, et al., 1995). Full-length and truncated (encoding a ~55-kd truncated protein, including the C-terminal portion, which contains the entire conserved catalytic domain) cDNAs have been expressed in Sf9 cells. The K_m values for cAMP (0.14–0.19 μM) are similar for full-length and truncated (r)HcGIP2 and human cardiac microsomal cGI-PDEs. K_m values (0.5 μM) are also similar for full-length (r)RcGIP1 and rat adipocyte microsomal cGI-PDE. All full-length and truncated (r)cGI-PDEs are sensitive to inhibition by cGMP and cilostamide, but not rolipram, a specific inhibitor of type IV cAMP-specific PDE. These results are entirely consistent

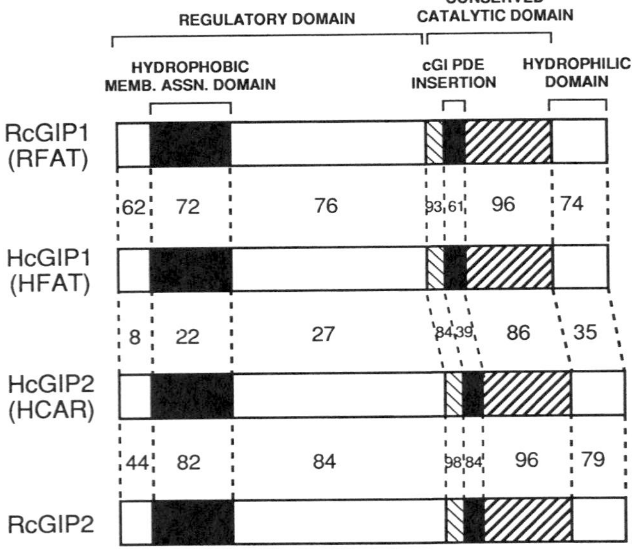

FIGURE **20-2.** Common structural pattern of cGI-PDE. cGI-PDEs representing two subfamilies have been cloned. There is a greater similarity within the same subfamily in rat and human species than between different subfamilies in the same species. All exhibit the domain organization common to PDE families. The conserved catalytic domain is followed by a hydrophilic C-terminal domain. The N-terminal region contains a hydrophobic putative membrane association domain and several consensus substrate sequences for A-kinase phosphorylation. One of those—serine 427—is phosphorylated on the solubilized cGI-PDE in vitro. Numbers refer to the percentage of amino acid identities in different domains.

with similar K_m values for cAMP and similar inhibitor sensitivities of cGI-PDEs isolated from a variety of cells and tissue.

In Sf9 cells, expressed full-length (r)RcGIP1 and full-length (r)HcGIP2 were predominantly found in particulate fractions, whereas the truncated forms were predominantly soluble (unpublished data, Murata, et al., 1995). These results suggest that determinants for cGI-PDE association with intracellular membranes may very well be located in the N-terminal portion, perhaps within the N-terminal hydrophobic domains. Based on immunoprecipitation studies, human platelet cGI-PDE, which is almost entirely cytosolic,[32,35,38,47,48] exhibits monomeric M_r values of 105,000–110,000, whereas rat adipocyte, which is predominantly microsomal, has a monomeric M_r value of 135,000.[13–19,43,44] In studies of cardiac preparations from several species, [^{32}P] cGI-PDEs immunoisolated from solubilized dog, rabbit, human, and guinea pig sarcoplasmic reticulum microsomal fractions were found to have subunit M_rs of primarily 110,000–130,000, whereas phosphorylated cytosolic forms had subunit M_rs of predominantly 80,000.[45] Although it is very likely that at least some of the lower M_r forms and cytosolic cGI-PDEs represent proteolytic fragments, it cannot be ruled out that some of them are products of other related cGI-PDE genes, or arise by alternative mRNA splicing or from alternative transcription initiation sites, especially because multiple mRNA species have been observed on Northern blots of rat tissue RNAs hybridized with RcGIP2 cDNA.[39]

All of these results are thus consistent with cGIP1 and cGIP2 being products of distinct, but related, genes. cGIP1 most likely represents the hormone-sensitive cGI-PDE found in adipocytes. Whether cGIP2 is enriched in other cells, such as cardiomyocytes or smooth muscle cells, is not certain. It is also not certain whether cGI-PDEs other than cGIP1 and cGIP2 will be found. Realizing that hormone-sensitive cGI-PDE activity is present in liver, and assuming that different cGI-PDEs may have different 44–amino acid insertions within the common conserved catalytic domain, a fragment (≈300-bp) containing the cGI-PDE insertion was cloned by reversed transcriptase-polymerase chain reaction (RT-PCR) from human hepatoma (HepG2 cells) mRNA. The sequence of this fragment was essentially identical to that of the analogous region in HcGIP1, which is consistent with the relatively strong hybridization of HepG2 poly(A)$^+$RNA with HcGIP1 cDNA and minimal hybridization with HcGIP2 cDNA (unpublished data).

Role of cGMP-Inhibited Phosphodiesterase (cGI-PDE) in Insulin Action

Activation/Phosphorylation of cGI-PDE Induced by Insulin and Agents that Increase cAMP

Incubation of rat adipocytes with insulin or agents that increase cAMP or cAMP analogues results in activation of a cGI-PDE associated with adipocyte microsomal membranes.[13–19,49–51] Virtually all results are consistent with the idea that the same cGI-PDE is activated in response to insulin and agents that increase cAMP.[13,49–51] Like adipocytes, isolated hepatocytes respond to insulin and glucagon with increases in cGI-PDE activity.[9,20–22] In liver, however, insulin alone was reported to stimulate a peripheral plasma membrane with characteristics of type IV rolipram-sensitive cAMP PDEs,[22] whereas both insulin and glucagon activated a cGI-PDE associated with the Golgi network or an incompletely characterized microsomal fraction designated as "dense vesicles."[20–23]

Activation of the cGI-PDE induced by effectors that increase cAMP results in feedback regulation of cAMP. This is not merely a response to excess cAMP because, for example, in adipocytes, activation occurs over virtually the entire range of isoproterenol-induced activation of adenylate cyclase and lipolysis, including conditions in which A-kinase is not saturated with cAMP.[28]

It may seem paradoxical that cGI-PDE is rapidly activated in response to two opposing effectors. This dual regulation of cGI-PDE has been studied in detail in rat adipocytes, where, in the presence of both insulin and lipolytic effectors, a "physiologic setting" in which insulin can reduce isoproterenol-induced increases in A-kinase and lipolysis, synergistic activation of the cGI-PDE was observed[28,44] (Fig. 20-3). The apparent paradoxical dual regulation by lipolytic effectors and the antilipolytic agent insulin may actually reflect mechanisms whereby both hormones regulate A-kinase.

Although the hormonal activation of cGI-PDEs has been well documented, the mechanism by which the enzymes are activated is only now becoming clear. With the development of specific antibodies and immunoisolation procedures, in intact [^{32}P]-labeled adipocytes, the particulate cGI-PDE was found to be phosphorylated on serine(s) in response to insulin and isoproterenol, and phosphorylation of the enzyme was found to correlate, in a time- and hormone concentration–dependent manner, with hormonal activation.[43,44] The effect of isoproterenol appeared to be more rapid than that of insulin. The exposure of adipocytes to insulin in the presence of catecholamines (i.e., the condition under which insulin exerts its antilipolytic effect) produced a synergistic activation/phosphorylation of cGI-PDE.[28,44] These results suggest that distinct phosphorylation sites on the cGI-PDE are targets for A-kinase and insulin-stimulated serine protein kinase(s) (cGI-PDE IK), respectively.[43,44]

Both A-kinase and a cGI-PDE IK have been reported to activate[52–54] and phosphorylate[29,46] the adipocyte cGI-PDE in vitro.

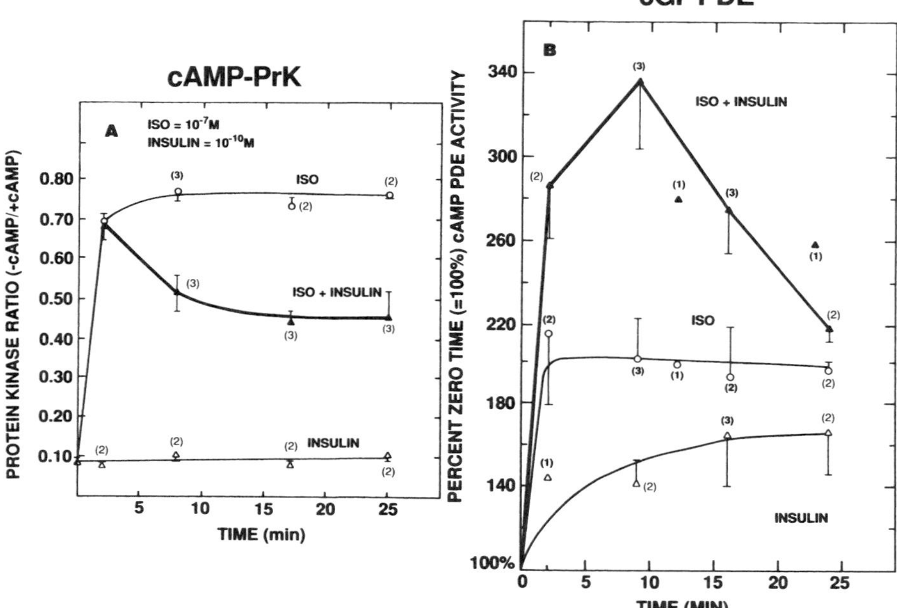

Figure 20-3. Synergistic activation of cGI-PDE in the presence of insulin and isoproterenol. Adipocytes were incubated in duplicate with 3 nM PIA plus 1 unit of ADA/mL and 100 nM isoproterenol (○), 0.1 nM insulin (△), or isoproterenol plus insulin (▲) for the times indicated. Particulate cGI-PDE activity was normalized relative to the specific activities of time-zero values. *INS*, insulin; *ISO*, isoproterenol. (Reproduced with permission from Smith CJ, Manganiello VC. The role of hormone-sensitive low K_m cAMP phosphodiesterase (PDE) in regulation of cAMP-dependent protein kinase and lipolysis in rat adipocytes. Mol Pharmacol 1988;35:381.)

Because identification by direct sequencing of proteolytic peptides from adipocyte cGI-PDE was not possible owing to insufficient amounts of purified cGI-PDE, an alternative strategy was developed to identify the peptide sequence containing the site phosphorylated by A-kinase in vitro.[46] Based on the deduced amino acid sequence of rat adipocyte cGI-PDE,[39] a peptide containing the putative A-kinase phosphorylation site was synthesized and antibodies were raised against this peptide. After phosphorylation of the synthetic peptide and the adipocyte cGI-PDE by A-kinase, the chromatographic and electrophoretic behavior of tryptic phosphopeptides from the two were compared and found to be identical. The exact location of the phosphorylated serine was then assessed by radiosequencing; from the known sequence of the synthetic phosphopeptide, serine 427 is a likely site readily phosphorylated in vitro by A-kinase.[46] The identification of the A-kinase phosphorylation site in vitro on cGI-PDE should contribute to an understanding of the mechanisms of dual hormonal regulation of this enzyme in vivo, as similar approaches can now be utilized to identify the site(s) phosphorylated in response to insulin. The availability of recombinant rat adipocyte cGI-PDE should make it possible to sequence peptides containing phosphorylation sites.

[^{32}P]cGI-PDE, isolated from unstimulated basal [^{32}P]-labeled hepatocytes, was dephosphorylated in a Mg^{++}-dependent manner.[55] In addition, activation of the hepatocyte cGI-PDE by A-kinase seemed to require prior dephosphorylation of a "basal" site.[55] Incubation of the liver "dense vesicles" with A-kinase was found to result in a time-dependent phosphorylation and activation of the cGI-PDE, provided the membranes had been previously incubated with Mg^{++}. Because phosphatase inhibitors prevented the A-kinase dependent phosphorylation and activation of the cGI-PDE, it was suggested that dephosphorylation of a specific phosphorylation site by a Mg^{++}-dependent phosphatase (with no effect on enzyme activity) was required before A-kinase could act on the cGI-PDE.[55]

Physiologic Importance of Insulin-Mediated Activation of cGI-PDE

Results of many studies are consistent with the view that insulin-mediated activation/phosphorylation of the adipocyte cGI-PDE plays a crucial role in insulin-induced reductions in cAMP and A-kinase and, therefore, inhibition of lipolysis. The concentration dependence for insulin inhibition of lipolysis is similar to that for activation of cGI-PDE, and the time course for cGI-PDE activation parallels that for reduction of A-kinase.[28] Inhibitors of cGI-PDE can block or prevent the antilipolytic effect of insulin in differentiated 3T3-L1 and rat adipocytes.[13,31,56,57] Moreover, insulin does not affect lipolysis induced by nonhydrolyzable cAMP analogues.[58] Beebe et al. reported that, of a series of cAMP analogues that activated lipolysis and glycogenolysis in intact adipocytes and hepatocytes, insulin inhibited responses to those that were substrates and competitive inhibitors of adipocyte and hepatocyte particulate cAMP PDE.[58]

Recently, stimulation of platelets with insulin, as well as effectors that increase cAMP, was found to activate platelet cGI-PDE.[47,48,59] The physiologic role for the insulin-mediated activation of the platelet cGI-PDE is not known. As is the case in adipocytes, activation of the platelet cGI-PDE by insulin correlates with serine phosphorylation of the enzyme.[59] A-kinase[47,48] and a partially purified cGI-PDE IK[60] were demonstrated to activate and phosphorylate the platelet cGI-PDE in vitro. Specific inhibition of cGI-PDE in platelets prevents platelet aggregation, suggesting an important role for this enzyme in platelet function.[10,30,32] In the diabetic state, it has been reported that platelets exhibit increased sensitivity toward aggregating agents and increased resistance to anti-aggregatory agents, perhaps indicating altered cAMP metabolism in diabetic platelets.[61] In other studies, however, insulin has been reported to reduce platelet aggregation.[62]

In Xenopus oocytes, PDE activation is associated with insulin- and insulin-like growth factor 1 (IGF1)–induced maturation; cGI-PDE inhibitors (but not inhibitors of type IV cAMP-specific PDEs) are known to block these effects.[63] These studies suggest that, in some cells, cGI-PDEs may be involved in insulin-regulated gene expression.

Insulin-Stimulated cGI-PDE Kinases

The number of insulin-stimulated serine/threonine kinases isolated from various tissues is increasing rapidly.[64,65] An insulin-stimulated kinase that phosphorylates and activates cGI-PDE was detected in cytosolic fractions of rat adipocytes and human platelets that had been incubated with insulin and in extracts of rat livers removed after administration of insulin to the animal.[29,53,54,60] The insulin-stimulated cGI-PDE kinase (cGI-PDE IK) has not yet been identified, but studies with kinase inhibitors and activators suggest that it is distinct from various other protein kinases, such as A-kinase, Ca^{++}/phospholipid protein kinase, casein kinase II, ribosomal S6 kinase, protease-activated protein kinase, Mg^{++}-specific protein kinases, and PI 3-K.[29,53,54,60] It is difficult to draw solid conclusions from such studies owing to the diversity in these kinase families, as well as to inherent limitations in the certainty of the specificity of these inhibitors. In addition, protein S-6 kinases (provided by J. Avruch), partially purified skeletal muscle insulin-stimulated protein kinase (ISPK) that phosphorylates/activates phosphatase 2A (provided by P. Cohen), immunoisolated PI3K from insulin-stimulated adipocytes (unpublished data, Rahn et al., 1994), or recombinant PKCζ (provided by P. Blumberg) did not phosphorylate cGI-PDE (unpublished data, Rahn et al., 1994). Several data indicate that the cGI-PDE IK itself is stimulated as a result of serine/threonine phosphorylation by an insulin-stimulated cGI-PDE kinase kinase (cGI-PDE IKK). For preparation and partial purification of the activated kinase, inclusion of phosphatase inhibitors in the buffers used for tissue homogenization and enzyme purification was essential.[29,53,54,60] Alkaline phosphatase treatment of cGI-PDE IK isolated from insulin-stimulated cells completely inhibits enzyme activity (unpublished data, Rahn et al., 1995) suggesting that the cGI-PDE IK is activated by phosphorylation. The kinase derived from insulin-stimulated platelets does not bind to antiphosphotyrosine agarose,[60] indicating that the cGI-PDE IK is not a direct substrate for the insulin receptor tyrosine kinase. Purification and cloning/sequencing of the cGI-PDE IK will eventually establish whether this kinase belongs to a previously described or a novel insulin-stimulated kinase family.

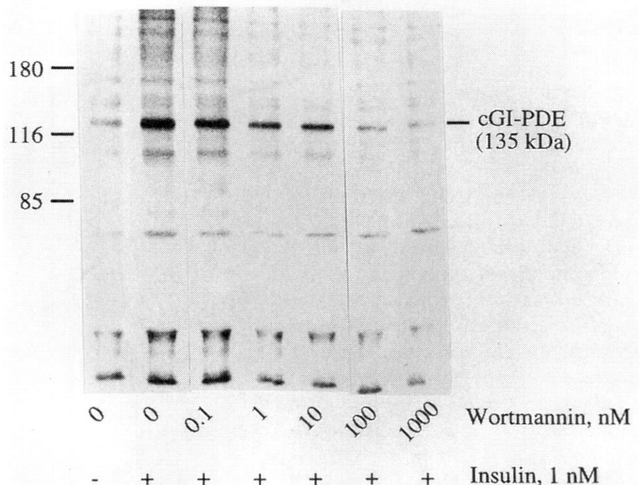

FIGURE 20-4. Effect of Wortmannin on the insulin-stimulated phosphorylation of cGI-PDE. As described in ref. 29, [^{32}P]-labeled adipocytes were incubated for 10 minutes with vehicle (dimethyl sulfoxide [DMSO]) or Wortmannin at the indicated concentrations before the addition of 1 nM of insulin. cGI-PDE was immunoprecipitated, subjected to SDS-PAGE, and then [^{32}] cGI-PDE was visualized by digital imaging. In parallel experiments using unlabeled adipocytes from the same cell preparation, 100 mM of Wortmannin was found to block, almost completely, the activation (2–3 fold) of cGI-PDE induced by 1 nM of insulin.

Phosphatidylinositol 3-Kinase and Other Upstream Regulators of cGI-PDE/cGI-PDE IK

Although no information on the regulation of the putative cGI-PDE IKK and cGI-PDE IK is available at present, the involvement and role of PI3-K in the antilipolytic signaling chain, including activation of cGI-PDE, has recently come into focus. PI3-K has been implicated in the signaling mechanisms of insulin and other mitogenic and nonmitogenic stimuli that act through tyrosine kinases.[66–70] Activation of PI3-K by insulin seems to involve primarily insulin receptor substrate-1(IRS-1).[67–69] PI3-K, a dual-specificity lipid- and protein-kinase,[70,71] consists of a 110-kd catalytic subunit and an 85-kd regulatory subunit that contain src homology-2 domains (SH2).[69–71] The activated insulin receptor tyrosine kinase phosphorylates IRS-1 on a number of tyrosines in YXXM/YMXM motifs, creating specific binding sites for SH2 domain-containing proteins.[67–71] In adipocytes, the insulin-induced association of PI3-K with tyrosine-phosphorylated IRS-1 via the p85 SH2 domains increases PI3-K activity, resulting in increased production of PI 3,4-P2 and PI 3,4,5-P3.[72]

Wortmannin, a selective PI3-K inhibitor, was reported to block the antilipolytic effect of insulin, as well as insulin-stimulated hexose uptake.[73] Thereafter, it was demonstrated that Wortmannin also blocked insulin activation of adipocyte cGI-PDE IK and activation/phosphorylation of cGI-PDE, as well as the antilipolytic effects of insulin[29] (Figs. 20-4 and 20-5). The components in the presumed signaling chain between PI3-K and cGI-PDE IK are not known. It is possible that PI3-K itself acts as a protein kinase in the antilipolytic signaling chain, as IRS-1 and the regulatory subunit of PI3-K can apparently be phosphorylated by the catalytic subunit of PI3-K.[71,74] PI 3,4,5-P3 has been reported to selectively activate PKCζ, a Ca^{++}-insensitive and phorbol ester–insensitive form of PKC,[75] and PI3-K has also been implicated in the signal chain that regulates p70S6 kinase.[76] Presently, there is no evidence that links PKCζ to regulation of cGI-PDE (unpublished data, Rahn et al., 1994). Although Wortmannin and LY294002 (another PI3-K inhibitor) block insulin activation of p70 S6 kinase and cGI-PDE IK, rapamycin, which also blocks insulin activation of p70 S6 kinase,[76] does not block activation of cGI-PDE IK (unpublished data). These

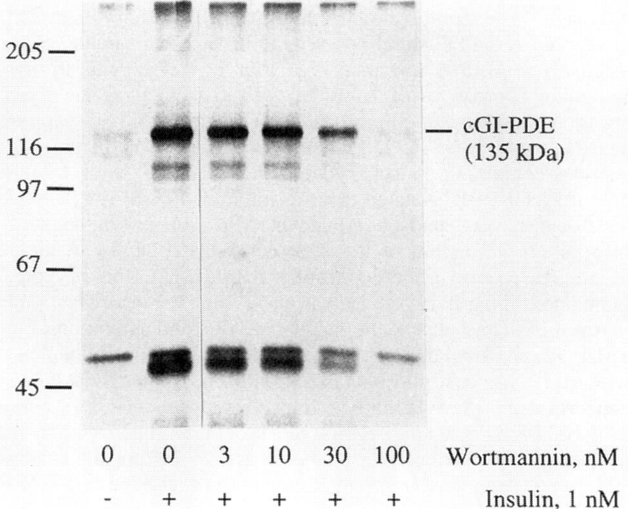

FIGURE 20-5. Effect of Wortmannin on insulin stimulation of cGI-PDE IK. As described in ref. 29, adipocytes were incubated for 10 minutes with vehicle (dimethyl sulfoxide [DMSO]) or Wortmannin at the indicated concentrations before the addition of 1 nM of insulin. Cytosolic fractions were prepared and assayed for cGI-PDE IK activity (i.e., phosphorylation of exogenous added cGI-PDE). [^{32}P]cGI-PDE was visualized by digital imaging of ^{32}P.

data suggest that activation of cGI-PDE IK and p70 S6 kinase by insulin are independent events, and that the two kinases are on different pathways, perhaps requiring different signals from PI3-K.

Hypothesis for the Antilipolytic Effect of Insulin

The mechanisms whereby insulin regulates metabolic pathways and cell proliferation are not fully understood, even though substantial progress has been made. Activation of the intrinsic tyrosine kinase of the insulin receptor is a critical event that initiates the diverse effects of the hormone.[68,77,78] The activated receptor tyrosine kinase phosphorylates specific tyrosine residues in target proteins, triggering a series of events that result in activation of serine/threonine protein kinases and phosphatases that alter the phosphorylation state/activities of key proteins involved in the regulation of cell metabolism and proliferation. Insulin opposes the effects of several catabolic hormones that increase cAMP and regulate lipid and carbohydrate metabolism in adipose tissue and liver.

Figure 20-6 represents our working hypothesis concerning mechanisms for hormonal regulation of the adipocyte cGI-PDE and its role in the antilipolytic action of insulin. IRS-1 is tyrosine phosphorylated in response to insulin activation of the intrinsic tyrosine kinase activity of the insulin receptor. This results in the association of IRS-1 with, and activation of, PI3-K, thereby initiating the antilipolytic effect of insulin. Insulin-mediated activation of PI3-K results in activation of a cGI-PDE IKK, which then phosphorylates (on serine/threonine sites) and activates cGI-PDE IK. The insulin-induced activation/phosphorylation of cGI-PDE, mediated by cGI-PDE IK, results in a reduction in cAMP/A-kinase, leading to a net dephosphorylation of HSL and inhibition of catecholamine-induced lipolysis. Activation/serine phosphorylation of cGI-PDE in response to agents that increase cAMP results in feedback downregulation of cAMP, which is important in the lipolytic signal chain; a more-than-additive activation/phosphorylation of cGI-PDE is seen in response to insulin in the presence of catecholamines (i.e., the condition under which insulin exerts its antilipolytic effect). Another important effect of insulin in the adipocyte is stimulation of glucose uptake. PI3-K activation, but not cGI-PDE activation, seems to be involved in insulin-mediated glucose uptake in adipocytes, suggesting that pathways leading to antilipolysis and glucose uptake branch at a point or points downstream of PI3-K.[56,75]

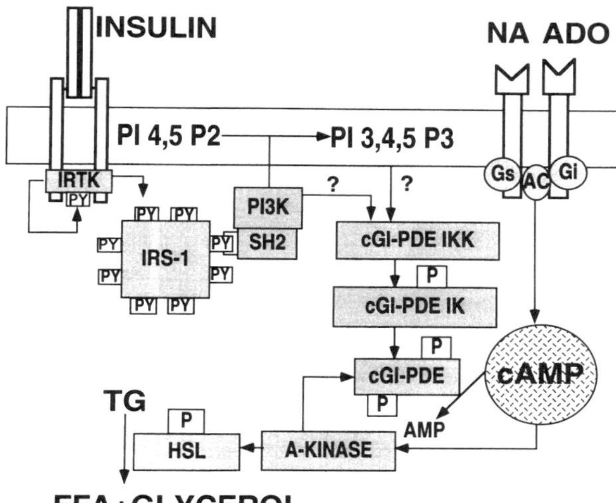

Figure 20-6. Working hypothesis concerning mechanisms for hormonal regulation of cGI-PDE and its role in the antilipolytic action of insulin. HSL, hormone sensitive lipase; A-kinase, cAMP-dependent protein kinase; cGI-PDE, cGMP-inhibited phosphodiesterase; cGI-PDE IK, insulin-stimulated cGMP inhibited phosphodiesterase kinase; cGI-PDE IKK, insulin-stimulated cGMP inhibited phosphodiesterase kinase kinase; P13K, phosphatidyl inositol 3 kinase; SH_2, Src homology 2; IRS, insulin receptor substrate 1; IRTK, insulin receptor tyrosine kinase; PI, phosphatidyl inositol; NA, noradrenaline; ADO, adenosine; TG, triacylglycerols; FFA, free fatty acids.

Acknowledgments

We thank Dr. T. Rahn and Dr. Taku Murata for allowing us to include unpublished information, and Dr. Martha Vaughan for critical reading of this manuscript. Financial support was given to some of us by the Swedish Medical Research Council (Grant 3362), the Medical Faculty, University of Lund, and the following institutions: Swedish Diabetes Association, Stockholm; Pahlssons, Malmo; Novo Nordisk, Copenhagen; Lars Hierta, Stockholm; Crafood, Lund; and the Swedish Society of Medicine, Stockholm.

References

1. Sutherland EW, Rall TW. Fractionation and characterization of a cyclic adenine ribonucleotide formed by tissue particles. J Biol Chem 1958;232:1077
2. Sutherland EW, Rall TW. The relation of adenosine-3′5′-phosphate and phosphorylase to the action of catecholamines and other hormones. Pharmacol Rev 1960;12:262
3. Jungas RL, Ball EG. Studies on the metabolism of adipose tissue. The effects of insulin and epinephrine on free fatty acid and glycerol production in the presence and absence of glucose. Biochemistry 1963;2:383
4. Butcher RW, Sneyd J, Park CR, Sutherland EW. Effect of insulin on adenosine 3′5′-monophosphate in rat epididymal fat pads. J Biol Chem 1966;241:1651
5. Butcher RW, Sutherland EW. Adenosine 3′5′-phosphate in biological material. I. Purification and properties of cyclic 3′5′-nucleotide phosphodiesterase and use of this enzyme to characterize adenosine 3′5′-phosphate in human urine. J Biol Chem 1962;237:1244
6. Thomson WJ, Appleman MM. Multiple cyclic nucleotide phosphodiesterase activities from rat brain. Biochemistry 1971;10:311
7. Thomson WJ, Appleman MM. Characterization of cyclic nucleotide phosphodiesterase of rat tissue. J Biol Chem 1971;246:3145
8. Loten EG, Sneyd JGT. An effect of insulin on adipose tissue adenosine 3′5′-cyclic monophosphate phosphodiesterase. Biochem J 1970;129:187
9. Loten EG, Assimacopoulos-Jeannet FD, Exton JH, Park CP. Stimulation of a low K_m phosphodiesterase from liver by insulin and glucagon. J Biol Chem 1978;253:746
10. Beavo JA, Reifsnyder DH. Primary sequences of cyclic nucleotide phosphodiesterase isoenzymes and design of selective inhibitors. Trends Pharmacol 1990;11:150
11. Conti M, Jin SLC, Monaco L, et al. Hormonal regulation of cyclic nucleotide phosphodiesterases. Endocrine Res 1991;12:218
12. Michaeli T, Bloom TJ, Martin T, et al. Isolation and characterization of a previously undetected human cAMP phosphodiesterase by complimentation of a cAMP deficient *Saccharomyces cerevisiae*. J Biol Chem 1993;268:12925
13. Manganiello VC, Smith CJ, Degerman E, Belfrage P. cGMP-inhibited cyclic nucleotide phosphodiesterases. In: Beavo JA, Houslay MD, eds. Cyclic Nucleotide Phosphodiesterases: Structure, Regulation, Drug Action. Chichester, UK: John Wiley and Sons;1990:87–116
14. Manganiello V, Vaughan M. An effect of insulin on cyclic adenosine 3′5′-monophosphate activity in fat cells. J Biol Chem 1973;248:7164
15. Zinman B, Hollenberg CH. Effect of insulin and lipolytic agents on fat adenosine 3′5′-monophosphate phosphodiesterase. J Biol Chem 1974;240:2182
16. Sakai T, Thompson WJ, Lavis VR, Williams RH. Cyclic nucleotide phosphodiesterase activities from isolated fat cells: Correlation of subcellular distribution with effects of nucleotides and insulin. Arch Biochem Biophys 1974;142:331
17. Kono T, Robinson FW, Sarver JA. Insulin-sensitive phosphodiesterase: Its location, hormonal stimulation, and oxidative stabilization. J Biol Chem 1975;250:7826
18. Weber HW, Appleman MM. Insulin-dependent and insulin-independent low K_m cyclic AMP phosphodiesterase from rat adipose tissue. J Biol Chem 1982;257:5339
19. Degerman E, Newman A, Rice K, et al. Purification of the putative hormone-sensitive cyclic AMP phosphodiesterase from rat adipose tissue using a derivative of cilostamide as a novel affinity ligand. J Biol Chem 1987;162:5797
20. Pyne NJ, Cooper ME, Houslay MD. The insulin- and glucagon-stimulated "dense-vesicle" high-affinity cyclic AMP phosphodiesterase from rat liver. Biochem J 1987;242:33

21. Boyes S, Loten G. Purification of an insulin-sensitive cyclic AMP phosphodiesterase from rat liver. Eur J Biochem 1988;174:303
22. Houslay MD, Kilgour E. Cyclic nucleotide phosphodiesterases in liver. A review of their characterization, regulation by insulin and glucagon and their role in controlling intracellular cyclic AMP concentrations. In: Beavo JA, Houslay MD, eds. Cyclic Nucleotide Phosphodiesterases: Structure, Regulation and Drug Action. Chichester, UK: John Wiley and Sons;1990:185–224
23. Benelli C, Desbuquois S, DeGalle B. Acute *in vivo* stimulation of low K_m cyclic AMP phosphodiesterase activity by insulin in rat liver Golgi fractions. Eur J Biochem 1986;156:211
24. Belfrage P, Donner J, Eriksson H, Stralfors P. Mechanisms for control of lipolysis by insulin and growth hormone. In: Belfrage P, Donner J, Stralfors P, eds. Mechanisms of Insulin Action. Amsterdam: Elsevier;1986:323
25. Steinberg D, Mayer SE, Khoo JC, et al. Hormonal regulation of lipase, phosphorylase and glycogen synthase in adipose tissue. Adv Cyclic Nucleotide Res 1975;5:549
26. Kono T, Barham FW. Effects of insulin on the levels of adenosine 3′5′-monophosphate and lipolysis in isolated rat epididymal fat cells. J Biol Chem 1973;248:7417
27. Londos C, Honnor RS, Dhillon GS, cAMP-dependent protein kinase and lipolysis in rat adipocytes. III. Multiple modes of insulin regulation of lipolysis and regulation of insulin responses by adenylate cyclase regulators. J Biol Chem 1985;260:15139
28. Smith CJ, Manganiello VC. The role of hormone-sensitive low K_m cAMP phosphodiesterase (PDE) in regulation of cAMP-dependent protein kinase and lipolysis in rat adipocytes. Mol Pharm 1988;35:381
29. Rahn T, Ridderstråle M, Tornqvist H, et al. Essential role of phosphatidylinositol 3-kinase in insulin-induced activation and phosphorylation of the cGMP-inhibited cAMP phosphodiesterase in rat adipocytes. FEBS Lett 1994;350:314
30. Weishaar RE, Carn MH, Bristol A. A new generation of phosphodiesterase inhibitors: Multiple molecular forms and the potential for drug selectivity. J Med Chem 1985;28:537
31. Manganiello V, Degerman E, Elks M. Selective inhibitors of specific phosphodiesterases in intact adipocytes. Methods Enzymol 1988;159:504
32. Alvarez R, Banerjee G, Bruno JJ, et al. A potent and selective inhibitor of cyclic AMP phosphodiesterase with potential cardiotonic and anti-thrombotic properties. Mol Pharmacol 1986;29:554
33. Degerman E, Manganiello VC, Newman A, et al. Purification, properties and polyclonal antibodies for the particulate cAMP phosphodiesterase from bovine adipose tissue. See Mess Phosphoprot Res 1988;12:171
34. Rascon A, Belfrage P, Lindgren S, et al. Purification and properties of the cGMP-inhibited cAMP phosphodiesterase from bovine aortic smooth muscle. Biochim Biophys Acta 1992;1134:149
35. Degerman E, Moos M Jr, Rascon A, et al. Single step purification, partial structure and properties of human platelet cGMP inhibited cAMP phosphodiesterase. Biochim Biophys Acta 1993;1205:189
36. LeBon TR, Kasuya J, Paxton RJ, et al. Purification and characterization of guanosine 3′5′-monophosphate phosphodiesterase from human placental cytosolic fractions. Endocrinology 1992;130:3265
37. Harrison SA, Reifsnyder DH, Gallis B, et al. Isolation and characterization of a bovine cardiac muscle cGMP-inhibited phosphodiesterase. Mol Pharmacol 1986;29:506
38. Grant PG, Colman RW. Purification and characterization of a human platelet cyclic nucleotide phosphodiesterase. Biochemistry 1984;23:1801
39. Taira M, Hockman SC, Calvo JC, et al. Molecular cloning of the rat adipocyte hormone-sensitive cyclic GMP-inhibited cyclic nucleotide phosphodiesterase. J Biol Chem 1993;268:18573
40. Meacci E, Taira M, Moos M Jr, et al. Molecular cloning and expression of human myocardial cGMP-inhibited cAMP phosphodiesterase. Proc Natl Acad Sci USA 1992;89:3721
41. Murray T, Russell TR. Acquisition of insulin-sensitive activity of adenosine-3′5′-monophosphate phosphodiesterase during adipose conversion of 3T3-L1 cells. Eur J Biochem 1980;107:217
42. Elks ML, Manganiello VC, Vaughan M. Hormone-sensitive particulate cAMP phosphodiesterase activity in 3T3-L1 adipocytes. J Biol Chem 1983;258:8582
43. Degerman E, Smith CJ, Tornqvist H, et al. Evidence that insulin and isoprenaline activate the cGMP inhibited low K_m cAMP-phosphodiesterase in fat cells by phosphorylation. Proc Natl Acad Sci USA 1990;87:533
44. Smith CJ, Vasta V, Degerman E, et al. Hormone-sensitive cyclic GMP-inhibited cyclic AMP phosphodiesterase in rat adipocytes. J Biol Chem 1991; 266:13385
45. Smith CJ, Krall J, Manganiello VC, Movsesian M. Cytosolic and sarcoplasmic reticulum-associated low K_m, cGMP-inhibited cAMP phosphodiesterase in mammalian myocardium. Biochem Biophys Res Commun 1993;190:516
46. Rascon A, Degerman E, Taira M, et al. Identification of the phosphorylation site *in vitro* for cAMP dependent protein kinase on the rat adipocyte cGMP-inhibited cAMP phosphodiesterase. J Biol Chem 1994;269:11962
47. Grant DG, Mannarino AF, Colman RW. cAMP-mediated phosphorylation of the low-K_m cAMP phosphodiesterase markedly stimulates its catalytic activity. Proc Natl Acad Sci USA 1988;85:9071
48. Macphee CH, Reifsnyder DH, Moore TA, et al. Phosphorylation results in activation of a cAMP phosphodiesterase in human platelets. J Biol Chem 1988;21:10353
49. Pawlson LG, Lovell-Smith CJ, Manganiello VC, Vaughan M. Effects of insulin and lipolytic agents on rat adipocyte low K_m cyclic adenosine 3′5′-monophosphate phosphodiesterase activity in fat cells. Proc Natl Acad Sci USA 1974;71:1639
50. Makino H, Kono T. Characterization of insulin-sensitive phosphodiesterase in fat cells. II. Comparison of enzyme activities stimulated by insulin and isoproterenol. J Biol Chem 1980;255:7850
51. Boyes S, Loten EG. Insulin and lipolytic hormones stimulate the same phosphodiesterase isoform in rat adipose tissue. Biochem Biophys Res Commun 1989;162:814
52. Gettys TW, Vine AJ, Simonds MF, Corbin JD. Activation of the particulate low K_m phosphodiesterase of adipose tissue by addition of cAMP-dependent protein kinase. J Biol Chem 1988;263:10359
53. Shibata H, Kono T. Cell-free stimulation of the insulin-sensitive phosphodiesterase by the joint actions of ATP and the soluble fraction from insulin-treated rat liver. Biochem Biophys Res Commun 1990;170:533
54. Shibata H, Kono T. Stimulation of the insulin-sensitive cAMP phosphodiesterase by an ATP-dependent soluble factor from insulin-treated rat adipocytes. Biochem Biophys Res Commun 1990;167:614
55. Kilgour E, Anderson NG, Houslay MD. Activation and phosphorylation of the "dense-vesicle" high-affinity cyclic AMP phosphodiesterase by cyclic AMP-dependent protein kinase. Biochem J 1989;260:27
56. Eriksson H, Ridderstråle M, Degerman E, et al. Evidence for the key role of the adipocyte cGMP-inhibited cAMP phosphodiesterase in the antilipolytic action of insulin. Biochim Biophys Acta 1995;1266:101
57. Schmitz-Peifer C, Reeves ML, Denton RM. Characterization of the cyclic nucleotide phosphodiesterase isoenzymes present in rat epididymal fat cells. Cellular Signalling 1992;4:37
58. Beebe SJ, Redmon JB, Blackmore PF, Corbin JD. Discriminative insulin antagonism of stimulatory effects of various cAMP analogs on adipocyte lipolysis and hepatocyte glycogenolysis. J Biol Chem 1985;260:15781
59. Lopez-Aparicio P, Rascon A, Manganiello V, et al. Insulin induced phosphorylation and activation of the cGMP-inhibited cAMP phosphodiesterase in human platelets. Biochem Biophys Res Commun 1992;186:517
60. Lopez-Aparicio P, Belfrage P, Manganiello V, et al. Stimulation by insulin of a serine kinase in human platelets that phosphorylates and activates the cGMP-inhibited phosphodiesterase. Biochem Biophys Res Commun 1993; 193:1137
61. Hendra T, Betteridge D. Platelet function, platelet prostanoids and vascular prostacyclin in diabetes mellitus. Prostaglandins Leukot Essent Fatty Acids 1989;35:197
62. Trovati M, Massucco P, Mattiello L, et al. Insulin increases guanosine 3′5′-cyclic monophosphate in human platelets: A mechanism involved in the insulin anti-aggregating effect. Diabetes 1994;43:1015
63. Sadler SE. Type III phosphodiesterase plays a necessary role in the growth promoting actions of insulin, insulin-like growth factor 1, and Ha21ras in *Xenopus laevis* oocytes. Mol Endocrinol 1991;5:1939
64. Denton RM, Tavare JM, Borthwick A, et al. Insulin-activated protein kinases in fat and other cells. Biochem Soc Trans 1992;20:659
65. Makino H, Manganiello VC, Kono T. Roles of ATP in insulin action. Annu Rev Physiol 1994;56:273
66. Panayotou G, Waterfield MD. The assembly of signalling complexes by receptor tyrosine kinases. BioEssays 1993;3:171
67. Keller SR, Lienhard GE. Insulin signalling: The role of insulin receptor substrate 1. Trends Cell Biol 1994;4:115
68. White MF, Kahn CR. The insulin signaling system. J Biol Chem 1994;269:1
69. Myers MG Jr, White MF. The new elements of insulin signalling: Insulin receptor substrate-1 and proteins with SH2 domains. Diabetes 1993;42: 643
70. Varticovski L, Harrison-Findik D, Keeler ML, Susa M. Role of PI-3 kinase in mitogenesis. Biochim Biophys Acta 1994;1226:1
71. Dhand R, Hiles I, Panayotou G, et al. PI 3-kinase is a dual specificity enzyme: Autoregulation by an intrinsic protein-serine kinase activity. EMBO J 1994;13:522
72. Kelly KL, Ruderman NB. Insulin-stimulated phosphatidylinositol 3-kinase. Association with a 185-kDa tyrosine-phosphorylated protein (IRS-1) and localization in a low density membrane vesicle. J Biol Chem 1993;268:4391
73. Okada T, Sakuma L, Fukui Y, et al. Essential role of phosphatidylinositol 3-kinase in insulin-induced glucose transport and antilipolysis in rat adipocytes. Studies with a selective inhibitor wortmannin. J Biol Chem 1994;269:3563
74. Lam K, Carpenter CL, Ruderman NB, et al. The phosphatidylinositol 3-kinase serine kinase phosphorylates IRS-1. Stimulation by insulin and inhibition by wortmannin. J Biol Chem 1994;269:20648
75. Nakanishi H, Brewer KA, Exton JH. Activation of the Z isozyme of protein kinase C by phosphatidylinositol 3,4,5-trisphosphate. J Biol Chem 1993; 268:13
76. Cheatham B, Vlahos CJ, Cheatham L, et al. Phosphatidylinositol 3-kinase activation is required for insulin stimulation of pp70 S6 kinase, DNA synthesis and glucose transporter translocation. Mol Cell Biol 1994;14:4902
77. Rosen O. After insulin binds. Science 1987;237:1452
78. Skolnik EY, Batzer A, Li N, et al. The function of GRB2 in linking the insulin receptor to RAS signaling pathways. Science 1993;260:1953

Diabetes Mellitus, edited by Derek LeRoith, Simeon I. Taylor, and Jerrold M. Olefsky. Lippincott–Raven Publishers, Philadelphia © 1996.

CHAPTER 21
Insulin Action on Glucose Transport

MICHAEL P. CZECH, JAMES L. ERWIN, AND MARK W. SLEEMAN

The acute stimulatory action of insulin on the uptake of glucose into muscle and fat cells is a key requirement for the maintenance of normal metabolic homeostasis in humans. This effect of insulin on glucose transport in muscle contributes, in conjunction with suppression of liver glucose output, to the amelioration of hyperglycemia in diabetes mellitus upon administration of the hormone. In both muscle and fat cells, transport of glucose across the cell surface membrane is essentially rate limiting for glucose metabolism in the basal state. Increased glucose uptake elicits increased glycolytic activity and the production of α-glycerol phosphate that is required for re-esterification of free fatty acids in adipocytes. This, in turn, helps restrain free fatty acid release that can lead to severe ketoacidosis. Thus, two of the most severely deranged metabolic parameters in uncontrolled insulin-dependent diabetes—elevated blood levels of glucose and ketone bodies—result, in part, from inappropriately low rates of sugar transport across cell surface membranes owing to deficient levels of insulin. The central importance of glucose metabolism in energy production and as provider of precursor compounds for macromolecule biosynthesis further reinforces the deleterious physiologic impact of impaired glucose transport in this disease.

The critical role of the glucose transport step in muscle and fat cells in regulating whole body metabolism explains the intense efforts by many laboratories to understand this process at the molecular level. As detailed elsewhere in this volume, much has been revealed about the insulin receptor that mediates acute stimulation of glucose uptake. Extensive information has also been obtained about the substrate proteins of the insulin receptor tyrosine kinase, and about their interactions with adaptor and signaling molecules. As will be discussed in this chapter, it is also now known that the glucose transporter protein regulated most markedly by insulin (GLUT-4) is largely localized in intracellular membranes in muscle and fat under basal conditions.[1,2] Insulin action acutely redistributes these intracellular transporter proteins to the cell surface membrane, where they can operate to catalyze uptake of extracellular sugar. Thus, one or more steps in the membrane trafficking pathway transited by these glucose transporter proteins must be regulated by insulin. However, our current understanding is least developed with regard to which specific signaling pathways initiated by the insulin receptor actually regulate membrane movements of GLUT-4, and to the underlying mechanisms that may be involved. The aim of this review is to summarize current knowledge about the life cycle and membrane dynamics of the insulin-regulated GLUT-4 glucose transporter and to provide a perspective on current attempts to define signaling elements that impact upon membrane movements of GLUT-4.

GLUT-4: The Insulin-Responsive Glucose Transporter

Several initial investigations of the response of glucose transport to insulin action have suggested that multiple glucose transporter proteins are present in insulin-sensitive fat and muscle cells. For example, Whitesell and Abumrad[3] have demonstrated that adipose cells respond to insulin with both an increased apparent affinity for glucose and an increased V_{max} of glucose uptake. These authors noted that the predominant effect of insulin was to decrease the K_m of glucose transport activity, which is consistent with the presence of two types of transporter proteins: one that contributes to basal glucose uptake and one that exhibits a lower K_m for glucose and contributes to the insulin-stimulated state. This concept has since been confirmed, and two transporter proteins—denoted GLUT-1 and GLUT-4—have been identified and shown to direct basal and insulin-stimulated transport, respectively, upon their heterologous overexpression in cultured cell systems.[4–6] Furthermore, GLUT-4 has been shown to exhibit a lower K_m (2–7 mM) than GLUT-1 (20–23 mM), although both transporters exhibit a similar turnover number (about 20,000 per minute).[4–7] Thus, at physiologic glucose concentrations, GLUT-4 exhibits higher activity than GLUT-1 per cell surface transporter protein.[6,7]

Mueckler et al.[8] first isolated a cDNA clone encoding a mammalian glucose transporter (GLUT-1), and many studies have shown that it is expressed in nearly all cell types and accounts for the high glucose uptake rate of human erythrocytes. Additional isoforms of mammalian glucose transporters (GLUT-1–5, GLUT-7) have also been cloned (for review, see refs. 9–11). The glucose transporter isoforms share 39–65% identity with each other. Although GLUT-1 is present in insulin-sensitive muscle and fat cells, initial evidence reported by Oka et al.[12] and James et al.[13] indicated that these tissues express an additional glucose transporter isoform. Oka et al.[12] raised antibodies against GLUT-1 and observed that adipocytes contained glucose transporter that did not react with these antibodies. James et al.[13] raised a monoclonal antibody against a transporter protein, expressed uniquely in adipose and muscle tissue, which was translocated from intracellular membranes to the plasma membrane fraction of adipocytes in response to insulin. This information led rapidly to the molecular cloning of the insulin-regulated glucose transporter, GLUT-4,[14–18] which reacts with the monoclonal antibody described earlier. The restriction of GLUT-4 expression to insulin-sensitive muscle and adipose cells, combined with the demonstration of its movement from intracellular membranes to the cell surface in response to insulin, provided compelling support for the idea that GLUT-4 was, indeed, the major insulin-regulated glucose transporter protein.

Zorzano et al.[19] compared levels of GLUT-1 and levels of GLUT-4 expressed in adipocytes using a combination of specific antibodies and photoaffinity labeling with [^{3}H]cytochalasin B and 3-[^{125}-I]iodo-4-azidophenethylamido-7-O-succinyldiacetyl-forskolin (IAPS-forskolin), two reagents that selectively bind to transport proteins. These investigators found that GLUT-4 represented 90% of glucose transporters within the adipocyte, based on the percentage of cytochalasin B–labeled transporters that could be immunoprecipitated from the cell. They further observed that GLUT-4 represented 75% of glucose transporters present in the plasma membrane following insulin stimulation. Marette et al.[20] reported similar results for skeletal muscle. Finally, Holman et al.[21] conducted studies using an improved transporter label—2-*N*-4-(1-azi-2,2,2-trifluoroethyl)benzoyl-1,3-bis(D-mannos-4-yloxy)-2-

propylamine (ATB-BMPA)—which is cell-impermeable and can be used to label glucose transporters present at the cell surface. These investigators reported that GLUT-4 was the predominant transporter, both in basal and in insulin-stimulated cells, and that it exhibited a higher transport activity than did GLUT-1 at low glucose concentrations.[21]

The glucose transporters display sequences similar to those of a wide range of transport proteins expressed in a diversity of organisms (for a review, see ref. 22). The amino acid sequences deduced from the cDNAs of these proteins suggest a common structural motif typified by the presence of 12 putative transmembrane α-helical domains—hence, the designation of transporter superfamily (TSF) by Henderson.[22] Evidence to support this model has best been demonstrated with the GLUT-1 transporter. Davies et al.[23,24] developed antibodies directed against epitopes predicted to reside on the intracellular and extracellular portions of GLUT-1. They were able to show that the predicted extramembranous regions of the transporter were indeed accessible to antibody binding. Moreover, they also demonstrated that the proposed orientation of the transporter with respect to the cytoplasm is also consistent with the profile of antibody binding. Holman and Rees[25] labeled GLUT-1 either with cytochalasin B or ASA-BMPA (2-*N*-[4-azidosalicoyl]-1,3-bis[D-mannos-4′-yloxy]propyl-2-amine), then caused proteolytic and chemical cleavage of the transporter protein at cysteine or tryptophan residues. ASA-BMPA cannot penetrate the intact cell membrane and is used to label the transporter at sites exposed to the extracellular space. They proposed that ASA-BMPA was bound to the transporter at the loop at amino acids between the 9th and 10th transmembrane domains, which agrees with the proposed orientation of the transporter. Cytochalasin B was bound between the 10th and 11th transmembrane domains on a site exposed to the cytoplasm. Wadzinski et al.[26] further defined cytochalasin B and IAPS-forskolin binding at tryptophan 412, which is proposed to lie near the juncture of transmembrane domain 10 and the cytoplasmic region between transmembrane domains 10 and 11. These studies are consistent with the 12 transmembrane domain model for glucose transporters.

These and other studies have also generated evidence to suggest a pore structure through which glucose is transported (see ref. 27 for review). Cytochalasin B, IAPS-forskolin, and the bismannose analogues ATB-BMPA and ASA-BMPA probably block transporter activity by occupying the pore through which glucose is transported.[25,26] Mutation of tryptophans 388 in helix 10 and 412 in helix 11 inhibits transporter activity.[28,29] Mutation of tyrosine 293 and glutamine 282 in helix seven also inhibits transporter activity.[30,31] Indeed, Hashiramoto et al.[31] proposed that helices 7 and 12 are in close proximity to one another in the membrane. Additionally, Ishihara et al.[32] reported that altering the charge of helix 11 by substituting aspartate for asparagine at residue 415 inhibited transporter function. Chin et al.[33] measured changes in intrinsic fluorescence due to pH titration (to mimic the effects of glucose binding) and proposed that trp388 and his337, trp412 and cys347, and trp412 and glu380 interact with one another to form the pore through which glucose is transported. Extrapolation of these data, described from GLUT-1 to the GLUT-4 sequence, suggests a model for the insulin-regulated glucose transporter shown in Figure 21-1.

The cloning of the glucose transporter isoforms has also provided insights into the quaternary structure of the glucose transporters. Pessino et al.[34] generated chimeras between GLUT-1 and GLUT-4 to demonstrate that GLUT-1 transporters may exist as homo-oligomers and that the region of homotypic interaction resides in the amino-terminal half of the protein. The chimeras contained varying lengths of the amino-terminal portion of GLUT-1

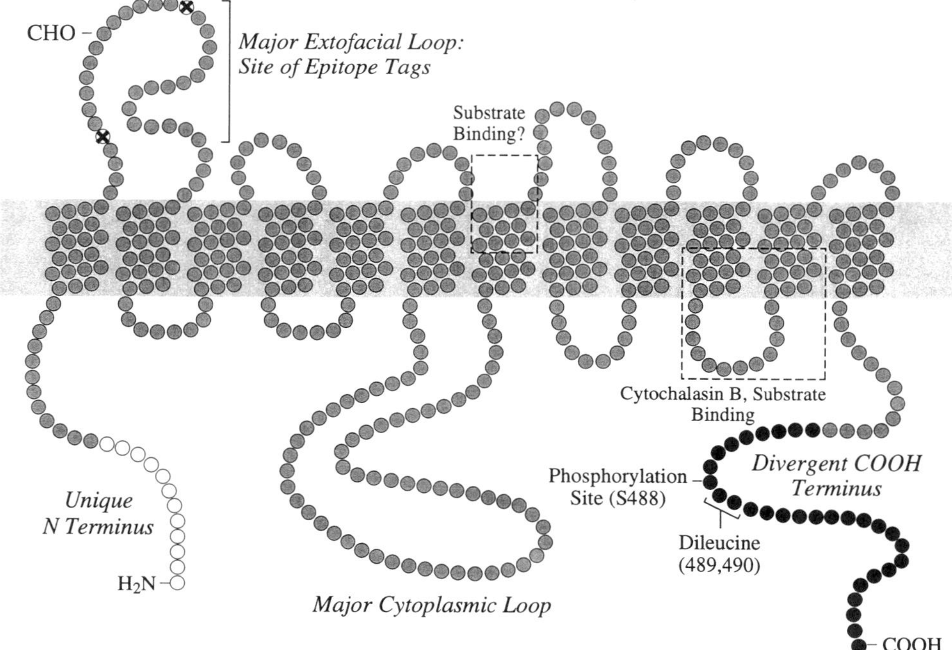

Figure 21-1. Structural domains and motifs of the human GLUT-4 glucose transporter protein. This model of GLUT-4 depicts its unique 12+ amino acid extension at the N-terminus as open circles and its divergent COOH-terminus (having only about 20% sequence identity to GLUT-1) in black circles. The latter domain contains a dileucine motif that appears to be important in the distinctive rapid endocytosis rate of GLUT-4 and its marked retention within intracellular membranes. Possible substrate-binding regions of the protein are shown, as deduced from experiments with the GLUT-1 glucose transporter. Two potential exofacial trypsin cleavage sites, identified as crossed circles, are located in the major exofacial loop, which has been the site for engineered epitope tags.

and the corresponding remainder of GLUT-4. They immunoprecipitated the expressed chimeras from CHO cells with an antibody directed against the carboxyl-terminal tail of GLUT-4 and detected endogenous GLUT-1 in the immune complexes by using an antibody directed against the carboxyl terminus of GLUT-1. Hebert and Carruthers[35] further characterized this interaction by measuring transport kinetics, cytochalasin B binding, and the reaction of GLUT-1 with a conformation-dependent antibody. This antibody recognizes GLUT-1 on intact erythrocytes and GLUT-1 purified under nonreducing conditions, but not GLUT-1 purified under reducing conditions. Based upon their experimental observations, Hebert and Carruthers[35] proposed a model whereby GLUT-1 exists as a homotetramer consisting of two homodimers, with the monomers linked in an antiparallel fashion. Thus, one monomer is outward-facing and one monomer is inward-facing. According to this hypothesis, transport of a glucose molecule into the cell switches the orientation of two monomers relative to one another. Thus, the antiparallel arrangement of the half-tetramer regenerates a glucose influx site each time a molecule of glucose is transported into the cell. Such an arrangement is energetically highly favorable (see ref. 35 for discussion). Further experimental evidence with other members of the TSF related to this issue will be important in resolving its relevance to glucose transporters in general.

Regulation of GLUT-4 Expression

High levels of GLUT-1 mRNA and protein in fetal life are repressed during the perinatal period concomitant with a triggering of GLUT-4 gene expression, such that GLUT-4 is the most abundant glucose transporter in insulin-sensitive tissues after birth.[36] Consistent with these observations, basal glucose uptake is observed to decrease during development, and the insulin-stimulated component of glucose transport dramatically increases in muscle and fat. The mouse[37] and human[38] GLUT-4 genes and their putative 5′ flanking transcriptional regulatory regions have been isolated and characterized, and there are several consensus sequences within the promoters that may contribute to tissue- and differentiation-specific expression. Studies with the rat GLUT-4 promoter have indicated that a myotube-specific activation domain lies within 517bp of the transcription start region of the promoter.[39] The helix-loop-helix myogenic factors MyoD, myogenin, Mrf 4, and myf-5 have been shown to bind to specific regulatory regions in several muscle-specific genes[40,41]; however, no specific transactivation effect has been observed by these DNA-binding proteins on the GLUT-4 gene.[39]

Studies with the mouse GLUT-4 promoter have elucidated an adipose-specific element responsive to the transcriptional factor C/EBP, which has been linked to a family of metabolic regulators of energy metabolism.[42] C/EBP can bind to and transactivate several adipocyte-specific promoters, including that for GLUT-4,[43–45] and it is only expressed following adipocyte differentiation.[46] Blocking of C/EBP expression has been reported to block terminal differentiation of 3T3-L1 cells into adipocytes.[47] No significant effect of C/EBP can be found on expression of the human GLUT-4 gene, however, reflecting either differences in gene structure or in regulation between these species.[48] Many parallels can be observed between the molecular mechanisms controlling adipogenesis and myogenesis,[49] but whether specific molecular mechanisms of GLUT-4 gene induction are common to both tissues remains elusive at present.

In addition to developmental regulation in peripheral tissues, the GLUT-4 gene is subject to long-term hormonal/metabolic regulation, and the nature of this response is cell-type–dependent. In isolated rat adipocytes from both fasting and insulin-deficient models of diabetes, the level of the GLUT-4 mRNA and protein have been found to be decreased by up to 90%.[50–53] This is attributed to a specific decrease in the transcription rate of GLUT-4,[54] and probably contributes to the impaired insulin-stimulated glucose uptake in this peripheral tissue that is associated with these altered states. Although a loss of total GLUT-4 could lead to insulin resistance, a deficiency in GLUT-4 translocation and/or sequestration mechanisms may also contribute to impaired insulin responsiveness of glucose transporters.[55] Studies in obese and non–insulin-dependent diabetic patients have correlated the decreased insulin-stimulated glucose activity in adipocytes with decreased levels of GLUT-4 mRNA and protein.[56,57] These results, combined with studies of insulinopenic states,[58] have highlighted a role for insulin, either directly or indirectly, in regulating adipocyte GLUT-4 gene transcription. In contrast to the marked alterations in GLUT-4 expression observed in adipocytes, only modest changes in GLUT-4 expression can be detected in various muscle tissues in altered metabolic states.[59,60]

Several cultured cell lines have been used to investigate both the developmental and hormonal regulation of the glucose transporter isoforms. Developmental regulation of GLUT-4, similar to endogenous expression in vivo, can be observed in the murine 3T3-L1 fibroblasts[43,46,61] and L6 myoblasts.[62] Despite the common finding of increased expression of GLUT-4 upon differentiation in these cell types, overexpression of the GLUT-4 isoform per se is insufficient to confer acute stimulation of glucose transport to fibroblasts,[63,64] Chinese hamster ovary cells,[65] or C2C12 muscle cells.[66] By contrast, overexpression of GLUT-4 in cultured L6 muscle myoblasts does result in a marked increase in the insulin-stimulated component of glucose transport,[67] suggesting that cellular components, in addition to GLUT-4, are necessary for full expression of insulin-stimulated glucose transport. Decreased expression, presumably through decreased transcription of the endogenous mouse GLUT-4 gene, has been observed in 3T3-L1 adipocytes in response to chronic elevation of cellular cAMP levels by agents such as isoproterenol, cholera toxin, and Bt_2AMP.[68,69] Another factor that has been documented to decrease the GLUT-4 mRNA and protein levels dramatically is tumor necrosis factor (TNF)-α, presumably through modulation of the transcriptional factor C/EBPα.[70] The GLUT-4 promoter also contains a thyroid hormone response element that may account for the observed T3[39] and retinoic acid[71] induction of endogenous GLUT-4 mRNA.

Membrane Trafficking of GLUT-4

The discovery by Cushman and Wardzala[1] and by Suzuki and Kono[2] of insulin-mediated glucose transporter redistribution from low-density microsomes to plasma membranes of primary adipocytes first prompted the theory that intracellular transporters were acutely translocated to the cell surface membrane. This hypothesis depended upon the assignment of transporters in the low-density microsomes to the intracellular compartment. This was confirmed by direct photoaffinity labeling of transporters in intact cells using [^{3}H]cytochalasin B and a membrane-impermeable inhibitor of the binding of cytochalasin B to glucose transporters.[72] Thus, [^{3}H]-cytochalasin B–labeling in intact cells of transporters that fractionated into the plasma membrane preparation was decreased by this inhibitor, whereas such labeling of transporters that resided in the low-density microsome fraction was not. Subsequent work by many laboratories using a variety of labeling and other biochemical detection methods have extended this paradigm to include both the GLUT-1 and GLUT-4 glucose transporter isoforms.[73–79] In the case of GLUT-4, however, almost all of the transporter protein is sequestered in intracellular membranes of fat cells and muscle in the absence of insulin. By contrast, GLUT-1 is already largely present at the cell surface (about 50%) under basal conditions. Thus, the effect of insulin to mobilize about half of the intracellular transporters to the plasma membrane leads to increases of greater than 10-fold in cell surface GLUT-4 versus increases of less than 2-fold in cell surface GLUT-1. This fact, coupled with the much larger total GLUT-4 protein content of muscle and fat cells compared to

GLUT-1, is consistent with the concept that the former contributes mostly to insulin action on cellular sugar uptake.

Important further confirmation of the marked intracellular sequestration of GLUT-4 transporters in intact cells has been achieved by immunoelectron microscopy. Slot et al.[80] and Smith et al.[81] examined rat brown adipose tissue and white adipose tissue, respectively, and found that very little GLUT-4 is at the surface in unstimulated cells, whereas about 50% of the intracellular GLUT-4 is translocated to the cell surface following insulin stimulation. Both groups also observed GLUT-4 to be associated with coated pits, suggesting that internalization of cell surface GLUT-4 occurs through clathrin-mediated endocytosis. Smith et al.[81] also noted that GLUT-4 appears to reside in invaginations near the cell surface, possibly allowing for their rapid redistribution. Evidence for localization of GLUT-4 in the tubulovesicular endosomal membrane system was also obtained.[80] Several reports have been published regarding the distribution of GLUT-4 in human skeletal muscle[82] and in rat cardiac[83] and skeletal muscle.[84–86] In both muscle types, GLUT-4 is sequestered within the sarcoplasmic reticulum and is translocated to the transverse tubule system following insulin stimulation. Because muscle fibers exist in bundles, the transverse tubules function to bring substances to the interior of the bundles. As discussed by Rodnick et al.[84] the insulin receptor in skeletal muscle is also located in the transverse tubule system. This ultrastructural arrangement may reflect an efficient utilization of muscle structure to ensure optimal distribution of glucose into the cytoplasm. Taken together, the biochemical and morphologic approaches used to define the cell biology of GLUT-4 have unequivocally validated the original recruitment hypothesis for insulin action on glucose transport, although additional effects of insulin that may regulate intrinsic activity of GLUT-4[87] cannot be ruled out at this time.

Complementing the findings of these studies, which have established the cellular distributions of GLUT-1 and GLUT-4, are important recent results defining the dynamics of movement of those proteins between cell surface and intracellular membranes. Several methods used to identify cell surface glucose transporter proteins, including trypsin cleavage,[77] affinity labeling with impermeable agents,[21,25,26,72] and antibody binding,[88] have now established that GLUT-1 and GLUT-4 recycle continuously in living cells, even in the absence of insulin. Estimates of the rates of recycling of GLUT-1 and GLUT-4 between cell surface and intracellular membranes have been based on measured rates of disappearance of cell surface transporters and of their appearance in low-density intracellular membranes. Differences in endocytosis rates between GLUT-1 and GLUT-4 appear to be small (twofold or less) compared to the difference in cellular distribution of these transporters.[88] Thus, it is thought that the major difference between the trafficking of these transporter isoforms is the extent to which they are delayed in their transit through one or more intracellular compartment during recycling.

The deduced restriction of GLUT-4 movement through internal membranes, compared to that of GLUT-1, offers a promising focal point for hypothetical regulation by insulin. Recent exciting data have defined a region of the GLUT-4 protein structure that may explain its retention in intracellular membranes. In these studies, chimera transporter proteins containing portions of GLUT-1 and GLUT-4 were used to define GLUT-4 sequences that could confer intracellular retention to the GLUT-1 protein. Czech et al.,[89] Verhey and colleagues,[90] and Marshall et al.[91] found that the carboxyl terminus of GLUT-4 (terminal 30 amino acids) is largely responsible for its intracellular sequestration under the conditions of these experiments. The former two groups expressed the chimera proteins in mammalian cells, whereas Marshall et al.[91] expressed the chimeras in Xenopus oocytes. Subsequent analysis and mutation of these chimeras by Verhey and Birnbaum[92] and Corvera et al.[88] have revealed a dileucine sequence in the GLUT-4 carboxyl-terminus functions as the signal in this domain for rapid endocytosis and retention of this transporter.

This dileucine motif has also been described as an important membrane trafficking signal for CD3-gamma chains in T lymphocytes,[93] the cation-dependent mannose 6-phosphate receptor,[94] the insulin-like growth factor 2 (IGF2) receptor,[95] and other receptors. The dileucine motifs described to date are often located near consensus sites for phosphorylation by serine/threonine kinases. Endocytosis of CD3-gamma via clathrin-coated vesicles apparently requires phosphorylation by protein kinase C.[96] The IGF2 receptor has already been shown to be phosphorylated by casein kinase II,[97,98] and phosphorylation is decreased subsequent to insulin stimulation. Phosphorylated IGF2 receptors in the plasma membrane are associated with clathrin-coated pits,[99] suggesting a possible role in directing such localization. In agreement with this observation, Meresse and Hoflack[100] have reported that phosphorylation of the IGF2 receptor coincides with its exit from the trans-Golgi network via clathrin-coated vesicles. GLUT-4 contains a consensus site for phosphorylation by protein kinase A; however, previous studies concerning the state of phosphorylation of GLUT-4 have focused

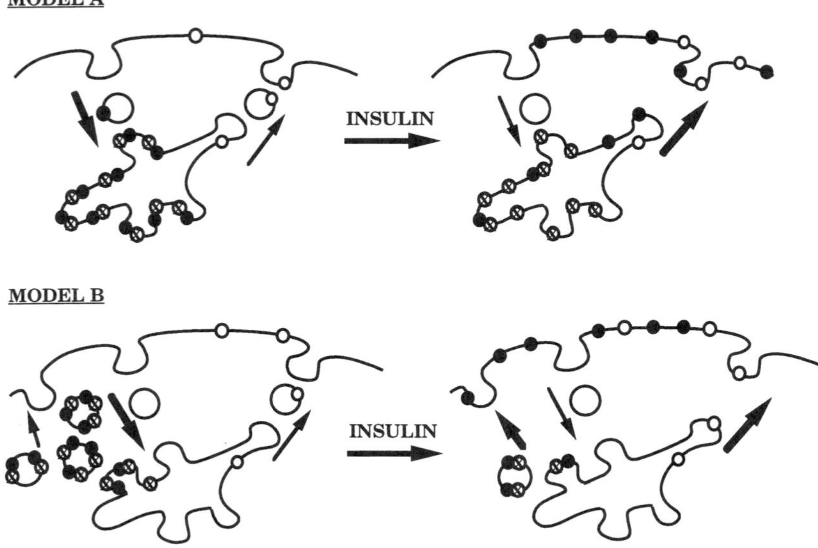

Figure 21-2. Two models by which GLUT-4 may recycle between cell surface and intracellular membrane systems of insulin-responsive cells. Model A depicts the regulated recycling mode by which GLUT-4 (*black circles*) and GLUT-1 (*open circles*) are hypothesized to transit through the normal cellular endocytosis and exocytosis pathways, involving the tubulovesicular endosomal system. In this model, insulin could translocate GLUT-4 by releasing its association with hypothetical retention receptors within the endosome, as well as by causing bulk membrane movements from intracellular endosomes to the cell surface. Model B depicts specialized vesicular structures containing GLUT-4 (*black circles*), which exclude many other recycling proteins, such as GLUT-1 (*open circles*). These vesicles are hypothesized to be mobilized to the cell surface in response to insulin, analogous to a neurotransmitter release or secretory mechanism. Thus, in this model, GLUT-4 segregates from GLUT-1 in the membrane system through which it transits.

on its transport activity,[101,102] and have not adequately addressed the state of GLUT-4 phosphorylation with respect to its distribution within the cell. It is noteworthy, however, that in insulin-stimulated cells, there is a decreased association of GLUT-4 with clathrin-coated vesicles at the plasma membrane.[103] Thus, further analysis of the phosphorylation of GLUT-4 with respect to its sorting dynamics in insulin-stimulated and unstimulated cells may be a fertile area of investigation.

Identifying the putative cellular machinery that interacts with the GLUT-4 dileucine motif is an area of intense investigation, as it may reveal the molecular mechanism of intracellular GLUT-4 retention. Other GLUT-4 domains may also be important in this mechanism. Asano et al.[65] reported that a region encompassing transmembrane domains two and three and a region including transmembrane domain seven are important for determining protein sorting of the chimeric transporter constructs. An influence of the middle region of GLUT-4 was also noted by Czech et al.[89] Piper et al.[104] have suggested that the amino terminal domain of GLUT-4 directs its sequestration. In a subsequent report, Piper et al.[105] reported that the sequence PSGFQQI, containing a critical phenylalanine and related to the NPXY motif of the transferrin receptor, was necessary for sequestration of GLUT-4. More recently, Garippa et al.[106] suggested that the N-terminus may direct internalization, but not sequestration, of GLUT-4. The differences between these results and those of the former four laboratories have not been resolved. As discussed by Verhey et al.,[90] however, the model system employed by Piper[104,105] involved lethally infected cells, which may have significant deleterious effects on the normal trafficking of GLUT-4. Further data are required to determine unequivocally which elements of GLUT-4, in addition to the dileucine, play a role in GLUT-4 trafficking.

Another critical question that has eluded resolution relates to the identity and exact cellular localization of membranes that harbor intracellular GLUT-4. As discussed in detail in previous reviews,[11,107] two distinct hypotheses have been considered. In one that we have designated Model A (Fig. 21-2, upper left panel), GLUT-4 is thought to circulate through the same endosomal tubulovesicular membrane recycling pathway traversed by many other proteins and receptors (e.g., transferrin and IGF2 receptors). This pathway, which includes endocytosis through coated pits, operates constitutively. This mode of membrane trafficking could account for intracellular GLUT-4 sequestration if retention receptors within the recycling endosome bound to dileucine and other GLUT-4 elements, retarding its movement through the pathway. Consistent with this model is the detection of GLUT-4 in apparent endosomal structures by immunoelectron microscopy and the demonstration by Corvera et al.[88] that GLUT-4 chimera protein co-localizes with transferrin in intact cells.

Alternatively, as depicted in Model B in Figure 21-2 (lower left panel), specialized vesicle structures that uniquely sequester GLUT-4 and exclude other recycling proteins, such as GLUT-1, may be operative. In this model, which is analogous to neurotransmitter or insulin release from stored granules, GLUT-4–containing vesicles are hypothesized to serve as the reservoir for intracellular GLUT-4, which can be mobilized by insulin to translocate to the cell surface. Consistent with this model are the immunoisolation of vesicles enriched in GLUT-4 from fat cell homogenates using anti–GLUT-4 antibodies and the fact that this vesicle population seems to decrease by about half in response to insulin.[108]

Insulin Regulation of GLUT-4 Trafficking

Independent of which model in Figure 21-2 best approximates the membrane cycling pathway for GLUT-4, it seems likely that a major effect of insulin is to cause intracellular membrane flow to the plasma membrane of adipocyte and muscle cells. One approach leading to this conclusion has focused on membrane proteins thought to be directly involved in the mechanism of membrane docking and fusion. One such set of proteins, which appear necessary for docking of membrane vesicles, are the SNARE receptors. These proteins appear to form docking complexes in combination with several other protein components, and are presumably a prerequisite for actual membrane fusions (see ref. 109 for review). A second set of proteins involved in this overall membrane-docking/fusion process appears to be a class of small guanosine 5′-triphosphate (GTP)–binding proteins denoted as Rab proteins (see ref. 110 for review). Rab proteins appear to be present on membranes primarily in the GTP-bound form, and are converted to the guanosine 5′-diphosphate (GDP) form upon interaction with as yet unidentified components on the target membrane. It is thought that GDP-bound Rab proteins are extracted from membranes after fusion events by cytoplasmic guanine nucleotide dissociation inhibitors, which then present the Rab proteins back to the donor membrane. Thus, at steady state in intact cells, the distribution of these proteins among donor and target membranes and cytosol remains constant. No change in this distribution would be expected if insulin action simply released retained GLUT-4 into the recycling pathway without actually altering the recycling rate of bulk membranes. Actual stimulation of bulk membrane exocytosis by insulin, however, should alter the steady-state localization of these proteins, as reflected by their cellular distributions.

Recent studies have demonstrated that both sets of proteins involved in the membrane movements just described are highly responsive to insulin in respect to their cellular distributions. Thus, for example, both the synaptobrevins (vesicle-associated membrane proteins [VAMPS]) and secretory carrier membrane proteins (SCAMPs) are markedly decreased in their association with low-density microsomes upon insulin treatment of adipocytes.[111,112] Furthermore, significant evidence indicates that both Rab 4[113] and guanine nucleotide dissociation inhibitor 2[114] are rapidly redistributed from low-density microsomes to the cytosol in response to insulin. These results are expected for a mechanism whereby insulin action causes direct promotion of membrane docking and fusion events that involve translocating GLUT-4 glucose transporters to the cell surface membrane. Although these data cannot differentiate between the two models presented in Figure 21-2, the studies also provide an explanation for the marked effect of insulin on redistribution of GLUT-1 and other recycling proteins to the surface membrane. GLUT-1 does not contain a dileucine retention motif, and it is already present largely at the cell surface membrane in the basal state. However, insulin decreases the GLUT-1 in intracellular low-density microsomes to the same extent as it does GLUT-4. Although a potential effect of insulin on GLUT-4 dileucine motif interactions with putative retention receptors remains an important possibility, the data now available strongly implicate insulin regulation of bulk membrane movements to the cell surface.

Intense efforts have been directed toward defining the signaling elements that link insulin receptor activation to regulation of glucose transport. Three recently identified signaling events triggered by the insulin receptor tyrosine kinase include activation of p21*ras* with resultant stimulation of protein kinases,[115,116] recruitment of phosphatidylinositol-3′OH-kinase (PI3-K) to tyrosine phosphorylated insulin receptor substrate 1 (IRS-1) with resultant activation of the enzyme,[117,118] and a similar modulation of the tyrosine phosphatase Syp.[119] Although some data[120,121] indicate that activated *ras* mimics the ability of insulin to stimulate glucose transport, this has not been observed in other studies,[122] and the overall results indicate that p21*ras* activation is not necessary for insulin action.[123] Definitive studies on the role of Syp in mediating insulin action on glucose transport have not yet been performed.

Recent data have strongly implicated the recruitment and activation of PI3-K activity in response to insulin as an important intermediary in the regulation of glucose transport. This enzyme, composed of a regulatory SH2 domain containing a regulatory p85

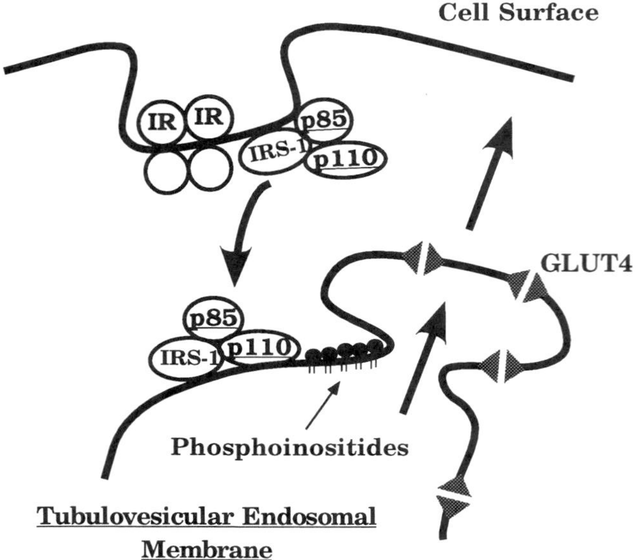

FIGURE 21-3. Hypothetical mechanism by which insulin action may stimulate movements of intracellular membranes containing GLUT-4 to the cell surface. According to this model, tyrosine-phosphorylated IRS-1, associated with PI3-K, is directed to specific sites within the tubulovesicular endosomal membrane, perhaps by its own endocytosis. Catalysis of 3′-phosphoinositide formation by IRS-1–bound PI3-K is thought to mediate budding or movements of these membranes containing GLUT-4 to the cell surface membrane. *IR,* insulin receptor.

subunit and a catalytic p110 subunit, promotes phosphorylation of the D3 position of inositol in phosphatidylinositol or its phosphorylated derivatives.[124] In yeast, a similar enzyme, denoted VPS34, has been shown to play a pivotal role in the membrane trafficking targeted to the vacuole.[125] Further indication that the formation of 3′-phosphoinositides in membranes (in response to activation of PI3-K) is involved in directing membrane movements is provided by an obligatory role of PI3-K in appropriate platelet-derived growth factor (PDGF) receptor movement to the lysosome.[126] These results linking the function of PI3-Ks with directed membrane sorting and movements, combined with the ability of insulin action to activate both PI3-Ks and movements of membranes containing GLUT-4, provide circumstantial evidence for a role of PI3-K in glucose transport regulation. This concept is greatly strengthened by recent results demonstrating blockade of insulin action on glucose transport by potent inhibitors of PI3-K.[127–129]

A useful model in further exploring the potential role of PI3-K in modulating GLUT-4–containing membrane systems is depicted in Figure 21-3. This model suggests that tyrosine phosphorylation of IRS-1 by the insulin receptor, which is known to recruit PI3-K to IRS-1, is a prerequisite for directing this signaling complex to specific sites in the intracellular endosomal system where GLUT-4 resides. Consistent with this hypothesis are recent data that have documented the localization of such IRS-1/PI3-K complexes to intracellular low-density microsomes.[130,131] Furthermore, recent data from our laboratory have led us to postulate that PI3-K–bound IRS-1 complexes, formed at the plasma membrane, are internalized and directed to specific intracellular sites as a result of their association with endosomal vesicles.[132] Taken together, the data now available provide a compelling case favoring a direct role of 3′-phosphoinositides in insulin-mediated membrane movements to the cell surface.

Glucose Transporter Expression in Transgenic Mice

Recent studies of transgenic mice carrying the human GLUT-4 (hGLUT-4) gene have demonstrated appropriate tissue-specific expression of the transporter and regulation of expression similar to that in the endogenous mouse GLUT-4 gene. In addition, all sequence information necessary for tissue-specific expression and insulin regulation of GLUT-4 appears to reside within a 2.4-kb region of DNA at the 5′ end of the hGLUT-4 gene.[133,134] Overexpression of the hGLUT-4 isoform in mice results in increased insulin-stimulated glucose transport in muscle, as well as contraction-stimulated glucose transport activity, with only mild elevation of basal uptake.[135] This is in contrast to overexpression of the GLUT-1 isoform in transgenic models,[136,137] where there is a dramatic increase in basal glucose uptake, but not insulin-stimulated uptake. These results are consistent with the view that basal glucose uptake is mediated primarily by GLUT-1 and insulin-stimulated glucose transport is primarily mediated by the GLUT-4 isoform in vivo.

Overexpression of an unregulated form of the hGLUT-4 gene, specifically in adipose tissue of mice, by use of the fat-specific aP2 promoter, results in a significantly different result.[138] These transgenic mice exhibit an enhanced net glucose disposal rate in vivo. All fat tissues sampled overexpressed GLUT-4 about five to sixfold, and basal glucose transport was elevated above non-transgenic control fat cells to a far greater extent (up to 34-fold) than the increases observed in insulin-stimulated glucose uptake (fourfold). The increased adipocity in these transgenic mice (specifically, an increase in adipose cell number) also suggests a possible role of GLUT-4 expression in the early development of obesity.

The transgenic approach to studying GLUT-4 function has also allowed examination of hormonal and metabolic influences in a physiologic context. In mice overexpressing the hGLUT-4 in muscle, normal blood plasma insulin and glucagon levels were observed; however, significantly reduced blood glucose levels were evident. Muscle hexokinase levels appear to be only moderately affected, but glycogen levels were elevated (34%), presumably owing to an increase in glycogenesis. Increased glycolysis, inferred from increased muscle lactate levels and small increases in basal glucose uptake into skeletal muscle, also suggests an increased flow of glucose into muscle in these animals. Dramatic increases are observed in basal muscle glucose uptake in transgenic mice overexpressing the GLUT-1 isoform, resulting in a marked elevation of muscle glycogen. These observations reinforce the concept that glucose transport into the muscle cell is a rate-limiting step in muscle glucose metabolism in vivo.

Studies in transgenic animals using regimens of fasting/refeeding and streptozotocin-induced insulin deficiency have shown that there are parallel changes between the overexpressed hGLUT-4 minigene and the endogenous mouse GLUT-4 mRNA. Most of the necessary elements controlling hormonal regulation, therefore, appear to reside in the 2.4-kb 5′ flanking region of the human GLUT-4 gene. Other recent studies[139] have assessed factors, such as high dietary fat intake, which are known to be associated with downregulation of the GLUT-4 gene; parallel decreases in insulin-stimulated glucose transport; and induction of insulin resistance in vivo. When fed a high-fat diet, transgenic mice overexpressing the GLUT-4 gene still exhibit the increased basal and insulin-stimulated glucose transport in adipose tissue that the non–fat-fed transgenic animals develop; however, they are unable to prevent impairment of glucose tolerance in vivo. These studies suggest that the nonregulated expression of genes critical to glucose homeostasis, in this case with a heterologous tissue promoter driving the expression of GLUT-4, may have the potential to prevent in vivo insulin resistance, if targeted to the appropriate tissue(s).

Conclusion

As highlighted in this chapter, most of the progress in understanding insulin action on glucose transport over the past several years has related to the cell biology of glucose transporter movements and the molecular biology of glucose transporter proteins, most notably, GLUT-4. Studies have identified the insulin-regulated glucose transporter GLUT-4, and have described its primary amino acid sequence. We have also learned about the roles of specific domains within the GLUT-4 transporter protein. A particularly exciting GLUT-4 motif appears to be dileucine in its COOH-terminal region, which directs its intracellular, sequestered disposition in the basal state. Also encouraging are new insights into the possible linkage of PI3-K activation by insulin and GLUT-4 translocation. The specificity of IRS-1 phosphorylation and its association with PI3-K in response to insulin and IGF1, but not other growth factors, would explain why insulin, but not epidermal growth factor (EGF), stimulates GLUT-4 translocation. Thus, IRS-1 may provide the specific targeting of PI3-K function to cellular locations that is required to promote GLUT-4 translocation.

Still, there remains much more that we do not know. Particularly elusive has been the exact membrane routing pathway transited by GLUT-4 in insulin-sensitive cells. How does it segregate itself from many other recycling proteins, and in which specific organelle does it reside under basal conditions? Most importantly, we are challenged to understand how insulin-signaling elements impact upon the membrane structures that harbor GLUT-4 and that carry it to the plasma membrane. Important answers to these questions will arise out of a greater understanding of the molecular biology of intracellular membrane composition and dynamics.

References

1. Cushman SW, Wardzala LJ. Potential mechanism of insulin action on glucose transport in the isolated rat adipocyte cell. J Biol Chem 1980;255:4758
2. Suzuki K, Kono T. Evidence that insulin causes translocation of glucose transport activity to the plasma membrane from an intracellular storage site. Proc Natl Acad Sci USA 1980;77:2542
3. Whitesell RR, Abumrad NA. Increased affinity predominates in insulin stimulation of glucose transport in the adipocyte. J Biol Chem 1985;280:2894
4. Keller K, Strube M, Mueckler M. Functional expression of the human HepG2 and rat adipocyte glucose transporters in Xenopus oocytes. J Biol Chem 1989;264:18884
5. Gould GW, Lienhard GE. Expression of a functional glucose transporter in Xenopus oocytes. Biochemistry 1989;28:9447
6. Nishimura H, Pallardo FV, Seidner GA, et al. Kinetics of GLUT1 and GLUT4 glucose transporters expressed in Xenopus oocytes. J Biol Chem 1993; 268:8514
7. Palfreyman RW, Clark AE, Denton RM, Holman GD. Kinetic resolution of the separate GLUT1 and GLUT4 glucose transport activities in 3T3-L1 cells. Biochem J 1992;284:275
8. Meuckler M, Caruso C, Baldwin SA, et al. Sequence and structure of a human glucose transporter. Science 1985;229:941
9. Gould GW, Bell GI. Facilitative glucose transporters: An expanding family. Trends Biochem Sci 1990;15:18
10. Bell GI, Burant CF, Takeda J, Gould GW. Structure and function of mammalian facilitative sugar transporters. J Biol Chem 1993;268:19161
11. Czech MP. 1995 Molecular actions of insulin on glucose transport. Ann Rev Nutr 1995;15:441
12. Oka Y, Asano T, Shibasaki Y, et al. Studies with antipeptide antibody suggest the presence of at least two types of glucose transporter in rat brain and adipocyte. J Biol Chem 1988;263:13432
13. James DE, Brown R, Navarro J, Pilch PF. Insulin-regulatable tissues express a unique insulin-sensitive glucose transport protein. Nature 1988;333:183
14. Birnbaum MJ. Identification of a novel gene encoding an insulin-responsive glucose transporter protein. Cell 1989;57:305
15. Charron MJ, Brosius FC III, Alper SL, Lodish HF. A glucose transporter protein expressed predominantly in insulin-responsive tissues. Proc Natl Acad Sci USA 1989;86:2535
16. Fukumoto H, Kayano T, Buse JB, et al. Cloning and characterization of the major insulin-responsive glucose transporter expressed in human skeletal muscle and other insulin-responsive tissues. J Biol Chem 1989;264:7776
17. James DE, Strube M, Mueckler M. Molecular cloning and characterization of an insulin-regulatable glucose transporter. Nature 1989;338:83
18. Kaestner KH, Christy RJ, McLenithan JC, et al. Sequence, tissue distribution, and differential expression of mRNA for a putative insulin-responsive glucose transporter in mouse 3T3-L1 adipocytes. Proc Natl Acad Sci USA 1989; 86:3150
19. Zorzano A, Wilkinson W, Kotliar N, et al. Insulin-regulated glucose uptake in rat adipocytes is mediated by two transporter proteins present in at least two vesicle populations. J Biol Chem 1989;264:12358
20. Marette A, Richardson JM, Ramlal T, et al. Abundance, localization and insulin-induced translocation of glucose transporters in red and white muscle. Am J Physiol 1992;263:C443
21. Holman GD, Kozka IJ, Clark AE, et al. Cell surface labeling of glucose transporter isoform GLUT4 by bis-mannose photolabel. J Biol Chem 1990; 265:18172
22. Henderson PJF. The 12-transmembrane helix transporters. Curr Op Cell Biol 1993;5:708
23. Davies A, Meeran K, Cairns MT, Baldwin SA. Peptide-specific antibodies as probes of the glucose transporter in the human erythrocyte membrane. J Biol Chem 1987;262:9347
24. Davies A, Ciardelli TL, Lienhard GE, et al. Site-specific antibodies as probes of the topology and function of the human erythrocyte glucose transporter. Biochem J 1990;266:799
25. Holman GD, Rees WD. Photolabelling of the hexose transporter at external and internal sites: Fragmentation patterns and evidence for a conformation change. Biochim Biophys Acta 1987;897:395
26. Wadzinski BE, Shanahan MF, Seamon KB, Ruoho AE. Localization of the forskolin photolabelling site within the monosaccharide transporter of human erythrocytes. Biochem J 1990;272:151
27. Mueckler M. Facilitative glucose transporters. Eur J Biochem 1994;219:713
28. Katagiri H, Asano T, Shibasaki Y, et al. Substitution of leucine for tryptophan 412 does not abolish cytochalasin B labeling but markedly decreases the intrinsic activity of GLUT1 glucose transporter. J Biol Chem 1991;266:7769
29. Garcia JC, Strube M, Leingang K, et al. Amino acid substitutions at tryptophan 388 and tryptophan 412 of the HepG2 (GLUT1) glucose transporter inhibit transport activity and targeting to the plasma membrane in Xenopus oocytes. J Biol Chem 1992;267:7770
30. Mori H, Hashiramoto M, Clark AE, et al. Substitution of tyrosine 293 of GLUT1 locks the transporter into an outward facing conformation. J Biol Chem 1994;269:11578
31. Hashiramoto M, Kadowaki T, Clark AE, et al. Site-directed mutagenesis of GLUT1 in helix 7 residue 282 results in perturbation of exofacial ligand binding. J Biol Chem 1992;267:17502
32. Ishihara H, Asano T, Katagiri H, et al. The glucose transporter activity of GLUT1 is markedly decreased by substitution of a single amino acid residue with a different charge at residue 415. Biochim Biophys Acta 1991;176:922
33. Chin JJ, Jhun BH, Jung CY. Structural basis of human erythrocyte glucose transporter function: pH effects on intrinsic fluorescence. Biochemistry 1992;31:1945
34. Pessino A, Hebert DN, Woon CW, et al. Evidence that functional erythrocyte-type glucose transporters are oligomers. J Biol Chem 1991;266:20213
35. Hebert DN, Carruthers A. Glucose transporter oligomeric structure determines transporter function. J Biol Chem 1992;267:23829
36. Santalucia T, Camps M, Castello A, et al. Developmental regulation of GLUT-1 (Erythroid/HepG2) and GLUT-4 (Muscle/Fat) glucose transporter expression in rat heart, skeletal muscle and brown adipose tissue. Endocrinology 1992;130:837
37. Kaestner KH, Christy RJ, Lane MD. Mouse insulin-responsive glucose transporter gene: Characterization of the gene and trans-activation by the CCAAT/enhancer binding protein. Proc Natl Acad Sci USA 1990;87:251
38. Buse JB, Yasuda K, Lay TP, et al. Human GLUT4/muscle-fat glucose transporter gene. Characterization and genetic variation. Diabetes 1992;41:1436
39. Richardson JM, Pessin JE. Identification of a skeletal muscle–specific regulatory domain in the rat GLUT4/muscle-fat gene. J Biol Chem 1992;268:21021
40. Weintraub H. The MyoD family and myogenesis: Redundancy, networks and thresholds. Cell 1993;75:1241
41. Rudnicki MA, Schnegelsberg PNJ, Stead RH, et al. MyoD or Myf-5 is required for the formation of skeletal muscle. Cell 1993;75:1351
42. McKnight SL, Lane MD, Gluecksohn-Waelsch S. Is CCAAT/enhancer-binding protein a central regulator of energy metabolism? Genes Dev 1989;3:2021
43. Kaestner KH, Flores-Riveros JR, McLenithan JC, et al. Transcriptional repression of the mouse insulin-responsive glucose transporter (GLUT4) gene by cAMP. Proc Natl Acad Sci USA 1991;88:1933
44. Christy RJ, Yang VW, Ntambi JM, et al. Differentiation-induced gene expression in 3T3-L1 preadipocytes: CCAAT/enhancer binding protein interacts with and activates the promoters of two adipocyte specific genes. Genes Dev 1989;3:1323
45. McKeon C, Pham T. Transactivation of the human insulin receptor gene by the CAAT/enhancer binding protein. Biochem Biophys Res Commun 1991;174:721
46. Garcia de Herreros A, Birnbaum MJ. The acquisition of increased insulin-responsive hexose transport in 3G3-L1 adipocytes correlates with expression of a novel transporter gene. J Biol Chem 1989;264:19994
47. Sammuelsson L, Stromberg K, Vikman K, et al. The CCAAT/enhancer binding protein and its role in adipocyte differentiation: Evidence for direct involvement in terminal adipocyte development. EMBO J 1991;10:3787
48. Olson AL, Liu M, Moye-Rowley WS, et al. Hormonal/metabolic regulation of the human GLUT4/muscle-fat facilitative glucose transporter gene in transgenic mice. J Biol Chem 1993;268:9839

49. Ye WC, Cao Z, Classon M, McKnight SL. Cascade regulation of terminal adipocyte differentiation by three members of the C/EBP family of leucine zipper proteins. Genes Dev 1995;9:168
50. Berger J, Biswas C, Vicario PP, et al. Decreased expression of the insulin-responsive glucose transporter in diabetes and fasting. Nature 1989;340:70
51. Garvey WT, Huecksteadt TP, Birnbaum MJ. Pretranslational suppression of an insulin-responsive glucose transporter in rats with diabetes mellitus. Science 1989;245:60
52. Kahn BB, Charron MJ, Lodish HF, et al. Differential regulation of two glucose transporters in adipose cells from diabetic and insulin-treated diabetic rats. J Clin Invest 1989;84:404
53. Sivitz WI, DeSautel SL, Kayano T, et al. Regulation of glucose transporter messenger RNA in insulin-deficient states. Nature 1989;340:72
54. Gerritis PM, Olson AL, Pessin JE. Regulation of the GLUT4/muscle-fat glucose transporter mRNA in adipose tissue of insulin-deficient diabetic rats. J Biol Chem 1993;268:640
55. Garvey WT, Maianu L, Nancock JA, et al. Gene expression of GLUT4 in skeletal muscle from insulin-resistant patients with obesity, IGT, GDM, and NIDDM. Diabetes 1992;41:465
56. Garvey WT, Maianu L, Huecksteadt TP, et al. Pretranslational suppression of a glucose transporter protein causes insulin resistance in adipocytes from patient with non–insulin-dependent diabetes mellitus and obesity. J Clin Invest 1991;87:1072
57. Sinha MK, Raineri-Maldonaldo C, Buchanan C, et al. Adipose tissue glucose transporters in NIDDM. Decreased levels of muscle/fat isoforms. Diabetes 1991;40:472
58. Kahn BB, Rossetti L, Lodish HF, Charron MJ. Decreased in vivo glucose uptake but normal expression of GLUT1 and GLUT4 in skeletal muscle of diabetic rats. J Clin Invest 1991;87:2197
59. Bourey RE, Koranyi L, James DE, et al. Effects of altered glucose homeostasis on glucose transporter expression in skeletal muscle of the rat. J Clin Invest 1990;86:542
60. Pederson O, Bak JF, Anderson PH, et al. Evidence against altered expression of GLUT-4 in skeletal muscle of patients with obesity of NIDDM. Diabetes 1990;39:865
61. Tordjman KM, Leinang KA, James DE, Mueckler MM. Differential regulation of two distinct glucose transporter species in 3T3-L1 adipocytes: Effects of chronic insulin and tolbutamide treatment. Proc Natl Acad Sci USA 1989;86:7761
62. Mitsumoto Y, Klip A. Developmental regulation of the subcellular distribution and glycosylation of GLUT1 and GLUT4 glucose transporters during myogenesis of L6 muscle cells. J Biol Chem 1992;267:4957
63. Haney PM, Slot JW, Piper RC, et cl. Intracellular targeting of the insulin-regulatable glucose transporter (GLUT4) is isoform-specific and independent of cell type. J Cell Biol 1991;114:689
64. Hudson AW, Ruiz ML, Birnbaum MJ. Isoform-specific subcellular targeting of glucose transporters in mouse fibroblasts. J Cell Biol 1992;116:785
65. Asano T, Takata K, Katagiri H, et al. Domains responsible for the differential targeting of glucose transporter isoforms. J Biol Chem 1992;267:19636
66. Kotliar N, Pilch PF. Expression of the glucose transporter isoform GLUT4 is insufficient to confer insulin-regulatable hexose uptake to cultured muscle cells. Mol Endocrinol 1992;6:337
67. Robinson R, Robinson LJ, James DE, Lawrence JC. Glucose transport in L6 myoblasts overexpressing GLUT1 and GLUT4. J Biol Chem 1993;268:22119
68. Kaestner KH, Flores-Riveros JR, McLenithan JC, et al. Transcriptional repression of the mouse insulin-responsive glucose transporter (GLUT4) gene by cAMP. Proc Natl Acad Sci USA 1991;88:1933
69. Clancy BM, Czech MP. Hexose transport stimulation and membrane redistribution of glucose transporter isoforms in response to cholera toxin, dibutyryl cyclic AMP, and insulin in 3T3-L1 adipocytes. J Biol Chem 1990;265:12434
70. Stephens JM, Pekala PH. Transcriptional repression of the C/EBP-a and GLUT4 genes in 3T3-L1 adipocytes by tumor necrosis factor-a. J Biol Chem 1992;267:13580
71. Sleeman MW, Zhou H, Rogers S, et al. Retinoic acid glucose transporter expression in L6 muscle cells. Mol Cell Endocrinol 1995;108:161
72. Oka Y, Czech MP. Photoaffinity labeling of insulin-sensitive hexose transporters in intact rat adipocytes. J Biol Chem 1984;259:8125
73. Blok J, Gibbs EM, Lienhard GE, et al. Insulin-induced translocation of glucose transporters from post-Golgi compartments to the plasma membrane of 3T3-L1 adipocytes. J Cell Biol 1988;106:69
74. Calderhead DM, Lienhard GE. Labeling of glucose transporters at the cell surface in 3T3-L1 adipocytes. J Biol Chem 1989;263:12171
75. Piper RC, Hess LJ, James DE. Differential sorting of two glucose transporters expressed in insulin-sensitive cells. Am J Physiol 1991;260:C570
76. Jhun BH, Rampal AL, Liu H, et al. Effects of insulin on steady state kinetics of GLUT4 subcellular distribution in rat adipocytes. J Biol Chem 1992;267:17710
77. Czech MP, Buxton JM. Insulin action on the internalization of the GLUT4 glucose transporter in isolated rat adipocytes. J Biol Chem 1993;268:9187
78. Kanai F, Nishioka Y, Hayashi H, et al. Direct demonstration of insulin-induced GLUT4 translocation to the surface of intact cells by insertion of a c-*myc* epitope into an exofacial GLUT4 domain. J Biol Chem 1993;268:14523
79. Quon MJ, Guerre-Millo M, Zarnowski MJ, et al. Tyrosine kinase-deficient mutant human insulin receptors (Met1153-Ile) overexpressed in transfected rat adipose cells fail to mediate translocation of epitope-tagged GLUT4. Proc Natl Acad Sci USA 1994;91:5587
80. Slot JW, Geuze HJ, Gigengack S, et al. Immunolocalization of the insulin-regulatable glucose transporter in brown adipose tissue of the rat. J Cell Biol 1991;113:123
81. Smith RM, Charron MJ, Shah N, et al. Immunoelectron microscopic demonstration of insulin-stimulated translocation of glucose transporters to the plasma membrane of isolated rat adipocytes and masking of the carboxyl-terminal epitope of intracellular GLUT4. Proc Natl Acad Sci USA 1991;88:6893
82. Friedman JE, Dudek RW, Whitehead DS, et al. Immunolocalization of glucose transporter GLUT4 within human skeletal muscle. Diabetes 1991;40:150154
83. Slot JW, Geuze HJ, Gigengack S, et al. Translocation of the glucose transporter GLUT4 in cardiac myocytes of the rat. Proc Natl Acad Sci USA 1991;88:7815
84. Rodnick KJ, Slot JW, Studelska DR, et al. Immunocytochemical and biochemical studies of GLUT4 in rat skeletal muscle. J Biol Chem 1992;267:6278
85. Bornemann A, Ploug T, Schmalbruch H. Subcellular localization of GLUT4 in nonstimulated and insulin-stimulated soleus muscle of rat. Diabetes 1992;41:215
86. Marette A, Burdett E, Douen A, et al. Insulin induces the translocation of GLUT4 from a unique intracellular organelle to transverse tubules in rat skeletal muscle. Diabetes 1992;41:1562
87. Czech MP, Clancy BM, Pessino A, et al. Complex regulation of simple sugar transport in insulin-responsive cells. Trends Biochem Sci 1992;17:197
88. Corvera S, Chawla A, Chakrabarti R, et al. A double leucine within the GLUT4 glucose transporter COOH-terminal domain functions as an endocytosis signal. J Cell Biol 1994;126:979
89. Czech MP, Chawla A, Woon CW, et al. Exofacial epitope-tagged glucose transporter chimeras reveal COOH-terminal sequences governing cellular localization. J Cell Biol 1993;123:127
90. Verhey KJ, Hausdorf SF, Birnbaum MJ. Identification of the carboxyl terminus is important for the isoform-specific subcellular targeting of glucose transporter proteins. J Cell Biol 1993;123:137
91. Marshall BA, Murata H, Hresko RC, Mueckler M. Domains that confer intracellular sequestration of the GLUT4 glucose transporter in Xenopus oocytes. J Biol Chem 1993;268:26193
92. Verhey KJ, Birnbaum MJ. A leu-leu sequence is essential for COOH-terminal targeting signal of GLUT4 glucose transporter in fibroblasts. J Biol Chem 1994;269:2353
93. Letourner F, Klausner RD. A novel di-leucine motif and a tyrosine-based motif independently mediate lysosomal targeting and endocytosis of CD3 chains. Cell 1992;69:1143
94. Johnson KF, Kornfeld S. A his-leu-leu sequence near the carboxyl terminus of the cytoplasmic domain of the cation-dependent mannose 6-phosphate receptor is necessary for the lysosomal enzyme sorting function. J Biol Chem 1992;267:17110
95. Johnson KF, Kornfeld S. The cytoplasmic tail of the mannose 6-phosphate/insulin-like growth factor-II receptor has two signals for lysosomal enzyme sorting in the Golgi. J Cell Biol 1992;119:249
96. Dietrich J, Hou X, Wegener AK, Geisler C. CD3-gamma contains a phosphoserine-dependent dileucine motif involved in down-regulation of the T cell receptor. EMBO J 1994;13:2156
97. Corvera S, Czech MP. Mechanism of insulin action on membrane protein recycling: A selective decrease in the phosphorylation state of insulin-like growth factor II receptors in the cell surface membrane. Proc Natl Acad Sci USA 1985;82:7314
98. Corvera S, Roach PJ, DePaoli-Roach AA, Czech MP. Insulin action inhibits insulin-like growth factor II (IGF-II) receptor phosphorylation in H-35 hepatoma cells. J Biol Chem 1988;263:3116
99. Corvera S, Folander K, Clairmont KB, Czech MP. A highly phosphorylated subpopulation of insulin-like growth factor II/mannose 6-phosphate receptors is concentrated in a clathrin-enriched plasma membrane fraction. Proc Natl Acad Sci USA 1988;85:7567
100. Meresse S, Hoflack B. Phosphorylation of the cation-independent mannose 6-phosphate receptor is closely associated with its exit from the trans-Golgi. J Cell Biol 1993;120:67
101. James DE, Hiken J, Lawrence JC Jr. Isoproterenol stimulates phosphorylation of the insulin-regulatable glucose transporter in rat adipocytes. Proc Natl Acad Sci USA 1989;86:8368
102. Piper RC, James DE, Slot JW, et al. GLUT4 phosphorylation and inhibition of glucose transport by dibutyryl cAMP. J Biol Chem 1993;268:16557
103. Chakrabarti R, Buxton J, Joly M, Corvera S. Insulin-sensitive association of GLUT4 with endocytic clathrin-coated vesicles revealed with the use of Brefeldin A. J Biol Chem 1994;269:7926
104. Piper RC, Tai C, Slot JW, et al. The efficient sequestration of the insulin-regulatable glucose transporter (GLUT-4) is conferred by the NH2 terminus. J Cell Biol 1992;117:729
105. Piper RC, Tai C, Kulesza P, et al. GLUT-4 NH2 terminus contains a phenylalanine-based targeting motif that regulates intracellular sequestration. J Cell Biol 1993;121:1221
106. Garippa RJ, Judge TW, James DE, McGraw TE. The amino terminus of GLUT4 functions as an internalization motif but not an intracellular retention signal when substituted for the transferrin receptor cytoplasmic domain. J Cell Biol 1994;124:705
107. James DE, Piper RC, Slot JW. Insulin stimulation of GLUT-4 translocation: A model for regulated recycling. Trends Cell Biol 1994;4:120
108. Thoidis G, Kotliar N, Pilch PF. Immunological analysis of GLUT4-enriched vesicles. J Biol Chem 1993;268:11691

109. Rothman JE. Mechanisms of intracellular protein transport. Nature 1994; 372:55
110. von Mollard GF, Stahl B, Li C, et al. Rab proteins in regulated exocytosis. Trends Biochem Sci 1994;19:164
111. Corley Cain C, Trimble WS, Lienhard GE. Members of the VAMP family of synaptic vesicle proteins are components of glucose transporter-containing vesicles from rat adipocytes. J Biol Chem 1992;267:11681
112. Laurie SM, Corley Cain C, Lienhard GE, Castle JD. The glucose transporter GLUT4 and secretory carrier membrane proteins (SCAMPs) colocalize in rat adipocytes and partially segregate during insulin stimulation. J Biol Chem 1993;268:19110
113. Cormont M, Tanti JF, Zahraoui A, et al. Insulin and okadaic acid induce Rab4 redistribution in adipocytes. J Biol Chem 1993;268:19491
114. Shisheva A, Buxton J, Czech MP. Differential intracellular localizations of GDP dissociation inhibitor isoforms. J Biol Chem 1994;269:23865
115. McCormick F. Activators and effectors of ras p21 proteins. Curr Opin Gen Dev 1994;4:71
116. Cherniack AD, Klarlund JK, Conway BR, Czech MP. Disassembly of son-of-sevenless proteins from Grb2 during $p21^{ras}$ desensitization by insulin. J Biol Chem 1995;270:1485
117. Kelly KL, Ruderman NB. Insulin-stimulated phosphatidylinositol 3-kinase. J Biol Chem 1993;268:4391
118. Backer JM, Myers Jr MG, Shoelson SE, et al. The phosphatidylinositol 3′-kinase is activated by association with IRS-1 during insulin stimulation. EMBO J 1992;11:3469
119. Sugimoto S, Wandless TJ, Shoelson SE, et al. Activation of the SH2-containing protein tyrosine phosphatase, SH-PTP2, by phosphotyrosine-containing peptides derived from insulin receptor substrate-1. J Biol Chem 1994;269:13614
120. Kozma L, Baltensperger K, Klarlund J, et al. The Ras signaling pathway mimics insulin action on glucose transporter translocation. Proc Natl Acad Sci USA 1993;90:4460
121. Manchester J, Kong X, Lowry OH, Lawrence Jr JC. Ras signaling in the activation of glucose transport by insulin. Proc Natl Acad Sci USA 1994;91:4644
122. Hausdorff SF, Frangioni JV, Birnbaum MJ. Role of $p21^{ras}$ in insulin-stimulated glucose transport in 3T3-L1 adipocytes. J Biol Chem 1994;269:21391
123. Fingar DC, Birnbaum MJ. A role for Raf-1 in the divergent signaling pathways mediating insulin-stimulated glucose transport. J Biol Chem 1994;269:10127
124. Carpenter CL, Duckworth BC, Auger KR, et al. Purification and characterization of phosphoinositide 3-kinase from rat liver. J Biol Chem 1990;265: 19704
125. Schu PV, Takegawa K, Fry MJ, et al. Phosphatidylinositol 3-kinase encoded by yeast VPS34 gene essential for protein sorting. Science 1993;260:88
126. Joly M, Kazlauskas A, Fay FS, Corvera S. Disruption of PDGF receptor trafficking by mutation of its PI-3 kinase binding sites. Science 1994;263: 684
127. Kanai F, Ito K, Todaka M, et al. Insulin-stimulated GLUT4 translocation is relevant to the phosphorylation of IRS-1 and the activity of PI3-kinase. Biochem Biophys Res Commun 1993;195:762
128. Okada T, Kawano Y, Sakakibara T, et al. Essential role of phosphatidylinositol 3-kinase in insulin-induced glucose transport and antilipolysis in rat adipocytes. J Biol Chem 1994;269:3568
129. Cheatham B, Vlahos CJ, Cheatham L, et al. Phosphatidylinositol 3-kinase activation is required for insulin stimulation of pp70 S6 kinase, DNA synthesis, and glucose transporter translocation. Mol Cell Biol 1994;14:4902
130. Kelly KL, Ruderman NB, Chen KS. Phosphatidylinositol-3-kinase in isolated rat adipocytes. Activation by insulin and subcellular distribution. J Biol Chem 1992;267:3423
131. Kublaoui B, Lee J, Pilch PF. Dynamics of signaling during insulin-stimulated endocytosis of its receptor in adipocytes. J Biol Chem 1995;270:59
132. Heller-Harrison RA, Morin M, Czech MP. Insulin regulation of membrane-associated insulin receptor substrate-1. J Biol Chem 1995;270:24442
133. Liu ML, Olson AL, Moye-Rowley WS, et al. Expression and regulation of the human GLUT4/muscle fat facilitative glucose transporter gene in transgenic mice. J Biol Chem 1993;267:11673
134. Olson AL, Liu M, Moye-Rowley WS, et al. Hormonal/metabolic regulation of the human GLUT4/muscle-fat facilitative glucose transporter gene in transgenic mice. J Biol Chem 1993;268:9839
135. Hansen PA, Gulve EA, Marshall BA, et al. Skeletal muscle glucose transport and metabolism are enhanced in transgenic mice over expressing the GLUT4 glucose transporter. J Biol Chem 1995;270:1679
136. Gulve EA, Ren JM, Marshall BA, et al. Glucose transport activity in skeletal muscles from transgenic mice overexpressing GLUT1. Increased basal transport is associated with a defective response to diverse stimuli that activate GLUT4. J Biol Chem 1994;269:18366
137. Marshall BA, Ren JM, Johnson DW, et al. Germline manipulation of glucose homeostasis via alteration of glucose transporter levels in skeletal muscle. J Biol Chem 1993;268:18442
138. Shepherd PR, Gnudi L, Tozzo E, et al. Adipose cell hyperplasia and enhanced glucose disposal in transgenic mice overexpressing GLUT4 selectively in adipose tissue. J Biol Chem 1993;268:22243
139. Gnudi L, Tozzo E, Shepherd PR, et al. High level overexpression of glucose transporter-4 driven by an adipose-specific promoter is maintained in transgenic mice on a high fat diet, but does not prevent impaired glucose tolerance. Endocrinology 1995;136:995

Diabetes Mellitus, edited by Derek LeRoith, Simeon I. Taylor, and Jerrold M. Olefsky. Lippincott–Raven Publishers, Philadelphia © 1996.

CHAPTER 22

Regulation of Glycogen Synthesis

ALEXANDER V. SKURAT AND PETER J. ROACH

Glycogen, a branched polymer of glucose, serves as a reservoir of carbohydrate in cells from bacteria, through unicellular eukaryotes, to mammals. Its accumulation and utilization are subject to intricate regulation in all species for which the process has been studied; in mammals, liver and skeletal muscle are the main sites of glycogen deposition. The biosynthesis of glycogen in liver and muscle has long been linked to the nutritional status of the organism, as represented directly by blood nutrient levels and indirectly by the concentrations of hormones, such as insulin, glucagon, catecholamines, and glucocorticoids.[1,2] An important role of insulin is to promote glycogen accumulation, and impaired glycogen metabolism is associated with diabetes.

The biosynthesis of glycogen involves at least three distinguishable stages (Fig. 22-1). The initiation step, first defined by the work of Krisman and Barrengo,[3] Whelan,[4] and Smythe and Cohen,[5] requires the formation of a glycoprotein primer, a glycosylated form of the protein glycogenin which glycogen synthase can efficiently elongate and, with the participation of the branching enzyme, can convert to a mature high-molecular-weight glycogen molecule. This review concentrates on recent molecular studies of the control of glycogen accumulation in skeletal muscle. Also discussed are recent advances in understanding the initiation process. The branching enzyme, from work on the budding yeast *Saccharomyces cerevisiae*, is essential for glycogen accumulation,[6,7] but to date, no regulatory role in mammalian cells has been identified, and so it is not included in this review. For more than three decades, considerable effort has been directed at understanding the molecular mechanisms by which insulin activates glycogen

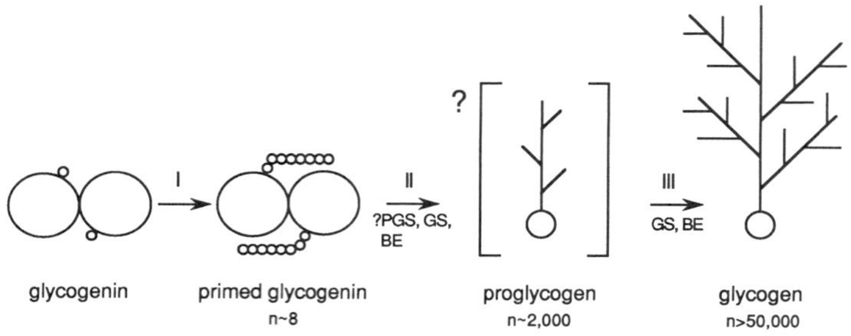

Figure 22-1. Glycogen synthesis. The small circles represent glucose residues, which are bound to a glycogenin dimer (*large circles*). The tree-like structures represent the branched polysaccharide chains of proglycogen and glycogen. *BE,* branching enzyme; *GS,* glycogen synthase; *PGS,* proglycogen synthase; *n,* number of glucose residues.

synthase; significant progress has been made, but an unequivocal mechanism has yet to be identified.

Glycogenin and the Initiation of Glycogen Synthesis

Background

The first demonstration that the initial acceptor of glucose in glycogen is a protein was made in 1975 by Krisman and Barrengo.[3] Later, in 1985, this protein was isolated from rabbit muscle glycogen and called glycogenin.[8] Glycogenin was also identified as a protein that copurified with rabbit muscle glycogen synthase.[9] The glucose chain is attached covalently to glycogenin through a tyrosine residue[2,10,11] that has been identified as Tyr-194.[12] This glucose-1-O-tyrosine linkage appears to be unique among carbohydrate-containing proteins. The protein sequence of rabbit muscle glycogenin was determined by Campbell and Cohen,[12] and a cDNA encoding this protein has since been cloned.[13] Rabbit muscle glycogenin consists of 332 amino acids and has a predicted molecular mass of 37284 Da.[12,13] The protein shows very little homology to any other UDP-sugar–utilizing enzymes.[12] Analysis of tissue distribution by Northern blot has indicated the presence of glycogenin message in most tissues, including skeletal muscle, with much weaker signals in kidney and liver.[13,14] Glycogenin purified from rabbit liver glycogen was indistinguishable from the muscle protein based on amino acid analysis, peptide mapping, or amino acid sequencing of about 20% of the protein.[15] Thus far, there is no evidence for the existence of distinct mammalian isoforms of the protein. Glycogenin comprises 0.35% muscle glycogen[8] and only 0.0025% liver glycogen.[15] This quantitative difference is consistent with the occurrence of 1 glycogenin molecule per β-particle in muscle and 1 molecule per α-particle in liver.

Glycogenin-like proteins have been sought in other species. In *S. cerevisiae,* two genes (*GLG1* and *GLG2*) that encode proteins that resemble glycogenin have recently been identified.[16] Yeast with both genes disrupted has an impaired ability to accumulate glycogen, thus providing the first evidence to date that a glycogenin-like protein is necessary for glycogen biosynthesis. A protein covalently linked to a proteoglycan fraction has been found in *Neurospora crassa* and *Escherichia coli.* However, this protein has a molecular mass of 31 kd and was found not to react with antibodies raised against chicken muscle glycogenin; moreover, the NH_2-terminal sequence of the *N. crassa* protein did not match any other protein sequences.[17]

Enzymatic Properties of Glycogenin

Besides being covalently linked to glycogen, glycogenin was found to be itself enzymatically active, catalyzing the transfer of glucose from UDP-glucose to form an oligosaccharide chain of about eight residues in length.[18,19] This self-glucosylating activity was observed in protein purified from tissue as well as recombinant glycogenin produced in *E. coli*[13] or COS cells.[20] The glucosyltransferase activities of glycogenin and glycogen synthase are quite different. Glycogen synthase activity does not require divalent cations, whereas the glucosyltransferase activity of glycogenin absolutely requires divalent cations, such as Mn^{2+} or Mg^{2+}. In addition, the apparent K_m of glycogenin for UDP-glucose (~2 μM), is 1000 times lower than that of glycogen synthase.[18]

An important question in the study of glycogenin function has been the mechanism by which the first glucose residue is attached to Tyr-194. Does glycogenin catalyze the reaction itself, or is there a separate glucosylating enzyme that mediates this reaction? This issue has been difficult to address because glycogenin purified from tissues already contains covalently attached glucose.[15,19,21] This is true even for recombinant enzyme produced in bacteria;[22,23] because *E. coli* organisms contain UDP-glucose, this finding could result from self-glucosylation or the action of some unidentified *E. coli* enzyme. The best evidence to date has come from the expression of glycogenin in an *E. coli* mutant lacking UDP-glucose pyrophosphorylase activity.[24] Hydrolysis of such glycogenin with trifluoroacetic acid did not release any detectable amount of glucose, suggesting that the protein did not contain attached carbohydrate but was able to incorporate up to 11 glucose residues (with an average of 8) in the presence of UDP-glucose.[24]

Cao et al.[22] first showed that mutation of Tyr-194 to either Phe or Thr resulted in glycogenin that was nonfunctional, as judged by its lack of activity in the self-glucosylation assay; likewise, the Phe-194 mutant expressed in COS cells did not self-glucosylate.[20] Thus, loss of Tyr-194 eliminated the one and only site of sugar attachment and Thr did not substitute. Alonso et al.[23] found similar results. It was also found that glycogenin was able to transfer sugar residues to exogenous acceptors, such as maltose,[25] *p*-nitrophenyl-α-glucoside, α-linked *p*-nitrophenyl oligosaccharides of the malto-oligosaccharide series,[26] or alkyl maltosides.[27] Replacement of Tyr-194 by Phe or Thr does not destroy the basic catalytic ability of glycogenin and does not prevent glucosylation of exogenous acceptors.[22,23,25]

The subunit structure of glycogenin is potentially quite complex and is significant with regard to the function of the protein. First, it interacts with glycogen synthase, which is also an oligomeric protein, although presumably, the glycogenin-glycogen synthase interactions would have to break up in the course of the synthesis of a glycogen molecule. Free glycogenin (i.e., that which is not covalently linked to glycogen) appears to have an oligomeric structure.[28] Some evidence has come from gel filtration experiments.[29] In other studies, x-ray diffraction of crystals of rabbit muscle glycogenin suggested the presence of dimers or possibly tetramers.[25] Kinetic experiments have indicated that the rate of self-glucosylation (or "priming"; see Fig. 22-1) is first order with respect to glycogenin,[18,22] indicative of an intramolecular reaction. If glycogenin is oligomeric, however, such an intramolecular reaction could be either intra-subunit or inter-subunit (see ref. 25). This is also consistent with the observation that glycogenin can modify exogenous acceptors. This issue is not fully settled, but an inter-subunit model, in which the catalytic site of one subunit transfers glucose to an oligosaccharide chain on an adjacent subunit, is attractive. Recently, Alonso et al.[24] reported that the first-order kinetics break down at high dilutions of glycogenin, possibly representing dissociation of the dimer (or other oligomer).

Regulation of Glycogenin

Biopolymer formation is often regulated at the initiation stage, and so glycogenin is an obvious candidate for control of glycogen accumulation. Also, whereas the other enzymes of glycogen metabolism dictate the size of glycogen molecules, glycogenin has the potential to determine their number. Our understanding of the control of glycogenin is quite limited as yet. The length of the oligosaccharide chain attached to glycogenin is an important determinant for the formation of the glycogen particle. Recently, it was shown that the electrophoretic mobility of glycogenin expressed in COS cells depends on the glucose concentration in the culture medium.[20] At high glucose levels, the glycogenin runs as a 38-kd species and is an effective substrate for elongation of glycogen synthase. At lower glucose levels, a slightly smaller 37.5-kd species is obtained, which is ineffective as a substrate for glycogen synthase. These small differences in electrophoretic mobility appear to be linked to the degree of glucosylation of the glycogenin. Indeed, the detection in cells of a lower-Mr form of glycogenin that is less than maximally glucosylated is an important observation. Unless UDP-glucose were limiting, there is no reason why the glycogenin would not be fully self-glucosylated, especially if the reaction is intramolecular. Therefore, there must be some impediment to the completion of the self-glucosylation reaction under certain conditions; one possibility is the operation of an opposing, deglucosylating activity. A candidate for such activity is glycogen phosphorylase, which has been shown in vitro to shorten the oligosaccharide chain of glycogenin by a phosphorolysis reaction.[30] In such a model, phosphorylase would not only control bulk glycogen metabolism by well-known mechanisms, but also would control the initiation phase of glycogen biosynthesis.

In resting rabbit muscle, almost all glycogenin is covalently linked to glycogen.[21,29] Acute administration of epinephrine or electrical stimulation of muscle results in degradation of glycogen, releasing glycogen-free glycogenin and glycogen synthase into the muscle cytosol.[29] These two liberated proteins reassociate very slowly, with only about 50% rebinding. Thus, it has been proposed that the process of reassociation between glycogen synthase and glycogenin may be involved in regulating the rate and extent of glycogen synthesis. This situation contrasts with isolated glycogen particles, where complete reassociation of glycogenin and glycogen synthase occurs following depletion of glycogen by phosphorolysis or digestion with α-amylase.[9,29] This discrepancy suggests the existence of some factor(s) in the cytosol controlling the reassociation of glycogenin and glycogen synthase.[29] One of the factors affecting the interaction between these two proteins could be the oligosaccharide chain of glycogenin. Expression of glycogen synthase in COS cells results in most of the enzyme being associated with insoluble cell structures.[20] Co-expression of glycogen synthase and glycogenin, however, leads to the appearance of about 40% of glycogen synthase in the soluble fraction. If the Phe-194 mutant of glycogenin, which cannot form an oligosaccharide primer, is used, however, this ''solubilization'' of glycogen synthase is eliminated.

Besides the oligosaccharide primer, glycogenin contains at least one other post-translational modification, namely, N-acetylation.[12] At present, the physiologic role of this modification is unknown, although recombinant enzyme made in bacteria, which is not NH_2-terminally blocked, is enzymatically active. It has been reported that glycogenin is phosphorylated in vitro by cAMP-dependent protein kinase[31] at a serine residue that has since been identified as Ser-43.[12] Bailey et al.[32] have reported that insulin promotes the phosphorylation of a species of similar electrophoretic mobility to glycogenin in crude extracts of cultured quail muscle cells, although the identity of the species was not demonstrated as glycogenin. Detailed studies on this issue, however, have never confirmed that native glycogenin is a substrate for cAMP-dependent protein kinase, or any of numerous other protein synthase kinases tested, when complexed to glycogen synthase.[18] When glycogenin is separated from glycogen synthase, cAMP-dependent protein kinase fails to phosphorylate Ser-43, or any other residue, at a significant rate.[12] Moreover, Ser-43 is not preceded by NH_2-terminal basic residues, as in the normal consensus motif for cAMP-dependent protein kinase.[33,34] When rabbit muscle glycogenin was expressed in COS cells labeled with [^{32}P]phosphate, no labeling of glycogenin was detected in conditions under which the ^{32}P-labeling of glycogen synthase was easily measurable.[35] Thus, the phosphorylation of glycogenin remains a controversial issue.

Intermediate Forms of Glycogen and the ''Proglycogen'' Hypothesis

When glycogenin incorporates some critical number of glucose residues as a result of self-glucosylation reaction (primed glycogenin; see Fig. 22-1), the polysaccharide chain can be elongated by glycogen synthase in the presence of branching enzyme, ultimately leading to the formation of a mature glycogen molecule. A mature muscle glycogen molecule is about 10^7 Da and is soluble in trichloroacetic acid.[36] The protein component, assumed to be glycogenin, represents 0.35% by weight. Recent studies have proposed the existence of another form of glycogen that can be precipitated by trichloroacetic acid, suggesting the presence of a larger proportion of protein relative to carbohydrate. This form, called proglycogen, has a molecular mass of about 400 kd as estimated by SDS-PAGE, and has, therefore, been named p400.[21] It has been reported that, upon storage of the muscle extract, proglycogen undergoes rapid breakdown to a p37–80-kd species, which can be labeled during incubation of the extract with UDP[^{14}C]glucose.[21,37] No additional confirmation that proglycogen or the derived species contain glycogenin has been provided. Moreover, breakdown was found to be prevented by protease inhibitors,[21] making the origin of the generated polypeptides uncertain.

Other interesting observations have come from studies in which the time courses of synthesis of proglycogen and glycogen were analyzed in astrocytes from newborn rat brain[38] or rat liver.[39] Starvation[39] or glucose deprivation[38] caused a dramatic reduction in the total glycogen level, with the appearance of a species with a molecular mass corresponding to glycogenin which could be detected by incorporation of [^{14}C]glucose from UDP[^{14}C]glucose at low concentration. Refeeding of astrocytes with glucose rapidly increased the acid-insoluble glycogen (proglycogen). Only upon completion of this process did the acid-soluble glycogen (''macroglycogen'') begin to increase. Both processes were accomplished without any significant change in glycogen synthase activity.[38] In rat liver, refeeding with glucose immediately increased the amount of the active form of glycogen synthase, with a subsequent slow increase in total glycogen level. Accumulation of the acid-insoluble glycogen (''proteoglycan,'' using the authors' terminology), however, was delayed as compared to the related process in astrocytes.[39] The authors in both studies proposed the existence of a glycogen synthase–like enzyme that can operate at a substrate concentration three orders of magnitude lower than ''classical'' glycogen synthase.[38,39] The function of this novel glycogen synthase–like enzyme would be to elongate the polysaccharide chain attached to glycogenin to some critical length before the intervention of the classical glycogen synthase activity (see Fig. 22-1). The formation of an intermediate product between glycogenin and glycogen could be an additional point of control in glycogen metabolism.[38]

The existence of an intermediate form of glycogen could have important implications for the regulation of glycogen metabolism, and so it will be interesting to monitor future developments in this area. Most lacking, however, is the isolation and chemical definition of the intermediate form of glycogen. Likewise, the postulation of the existence of two forms of glycogen synthase is an intriguing idea, but so far has not been well defined biochemically. Different mammalian isoforms are known, but thus far, these appear simply to be tissue-specific, and are not thought to coexist in cells. In *S. cerevisiae,* two different glycogen synthase genes can be expressed simultaneously, and the exact difference in functions is not yet well understood. Regulation of one gene appears to be linked to nutritional deprivation. At the same time, there is no evidence that either of these enzymes acts as a proglycogen synthase. The other possibility is that different states of a single mammalian glycogen synthase are responsible for the two putative activities. Certainly, changes in substrate kinetic parameters of several orders of magnitude owing to covalent phosphorylation have been recognized for many years.[40,41] What is needed is the purification to homogeneity of the putative proglycogen synthase so that its existence and identity can be definitively established.

Glycogen Synthase

Background

Glycogen synthase catalyzes what has usually been viewed as the rate-determining reaction in glycogen synthesis—that is, transfer of glucosyl units from UDP-glucose to the nonreducing ends of the growing glycogen molecule (reviewed in refs. 40 and 41). This enzyme has been purified from numerous sources[41] and contains a catalytic subunit of 80–90 kd.[40,41] Thus far, two distinct mammalian isoforms—from liver and muscle—have been identified. The primary structures of glycogen synthase from human[42] and rabbit[43] muscle, human[44] and rat[45] liver, and *S. cerevisiae*[46] have been determined. The enzymes exhibit significant sequence homology. The muscle and liver isoforms display about 70% sequence identity and are both 45–50% identical to the yeast enzymes. Both liver and muscle isoforms are highly conserved, with >90% identity, between mammalian species. The greatest sequence variability occurs at the NH_2- and COOH-terminals, the regions involved in control by phosphorylation. For example, a major difference in the liver isoform is that it is 34 residues shorter than the muscle enzyme[42,44,45] and also lacks the COOH-terminal phosphorylation sites 1a and 1b (Fig. 22-2). The two yeast enzymes, encoded by the *GSY1* and *GSY2* genes, lack entirely the NH_2-terminal phosphorylation domain. Glycogen synthase from rabbit skeletal muscle has been the best characterized. The native enzyme probably has a tetrameric structure, although the tetrameric species has a strong tendency to aggregate.[47] Two lysine residues—Lys-38 and Lys-300 of the rabbit muscle enzyme—have been implicated in UDP-glucose binding.[48,49]

Phosphorylation of Glycogen Synthase

In 1960, Villar-Palasi and Larner demonstrated that, after treatment of muscle with insulin, glycogen synthase in tissue extract was present in an activated state.[50] Conversion of an inactive to an active form by insulin was proposed, and this led ultimately to the currently held view that the enzyme is controlled by covalent phosphorylation; at the time, this was the third example, after phosphorylase and phosphorylase kinase, of an enzyme so regulated.[51,52] Initially, two forms of synthase were proposed, one termed D (dependent) and the other I (independent), to denote whether the allosteric activator glucose-6-P was necessary for activity.[51] The more active I form was dephosphorylated, whereas the less active D form was the phosphorylated form. Subsequent biochemical investigations over the past two decades have established that the regulation of glycogen synthase is actually more complex, involving multiple phosphorylation of the enzyme subunit and, hence, potentially more than two kinetically distinct forms (see refs. 40 and 41 for a review). This fact distinguishes synthase from its metabolic cousin phosphorylase, which is controlled by a single phosphorylation site.

Rabbit muscle glycogen synthase contains at least 9 sites that can be phosphorylated in vitro by at least 10 different protein kinases (see Fig. 22-2). Two of these sites are located in the extreme NH_2 terminus, with the remainder in the COOH-terminal 100 amino acids. cAMP-dependent protein kinase was the first enzyme reported to phosphorylate and inactivate glycogen synthase,[53,54] and it is now believed that phosphate is incorporated preferentially into three sites: sites 1a, 2, and 1b.[55–58] Site 2, which is Ser-7 and close to the NH_2 terminus, is also phosphorylated by a number of other protein kinases, including phosphorylase kinase,[59] calmodulin-dependent protein kinase II,[60,61] protein kinase C,[62] cGMP-dependent

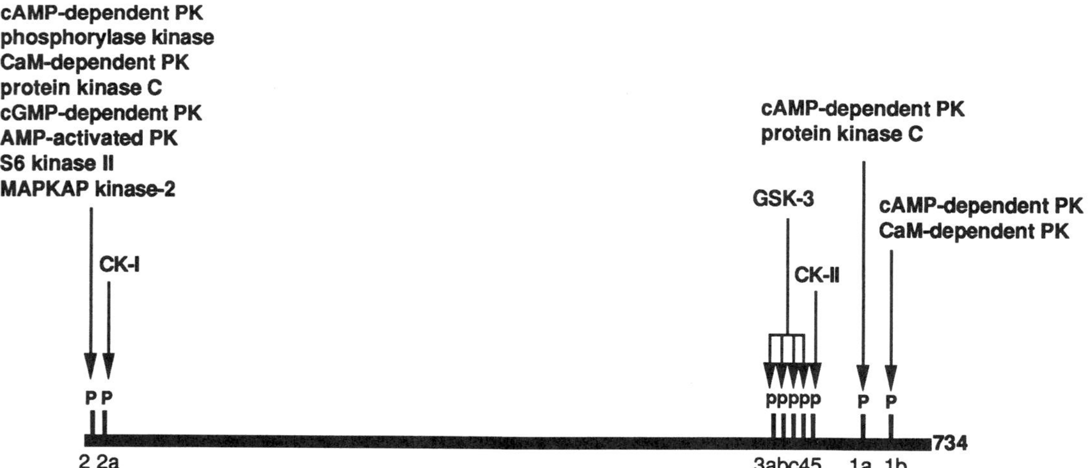

Figure 22-2. Phosphorylation of muscle glycogen synthase. The rabbit muscle glycogen synthase protein (734 amino acid residues) is depicted as a solid horizontal line with the vertical ticks corresponding to phosphorylation sites. The traditional nomenclature for these sites is indicated beneath. The protein kinases that phosphorylate these sites in vitro are also indicated. *PK,* protein kinase; *CaM,* calmodulin; *MAPKAP kinase-2,* MAP kinase–activated protein kinase-2; *CK-I,* casein kinase I; *CK-II,* casein kinase II; *GSK-3,* glycogen synthase kinase-3; *P,* covalently bound phosphate.

protein kinase,[56] glycogen synthase kinase 4,[63,64] AMP-activated protein kinase,[65] ribosomal S6 kinase 2,[66] and MAP kinase–activated protein kinase (termed MAPKAP kinase-2).[67] Some of these protein kinases also modify other sites, as indicated in Figure 22-2.

Casein kinase II phosphorylates glycogen synthase at a single residue, termed site 5.[63,68] Phosphorylation by casein kinase I is more complicated. Incubation of glycogen synthase with high concentrations of the enzyme causes the incorporation of up to 6 mol phosphates/subunit[69,70] into about 10 residues.[69] Such seemingly indiscriminate phosphorylation does not seem consistent with a specific physiologic role. Several specific residues were implicated as casein kinase I sites, including Ser-3, 7 (site 2), and 10 (site 2a) at the NH_2 terminus,[69] as well as residues 646, 651, 700, and 712 in the COOH-terminus.[71] The enzyme glycogen synthase kinase-3 (GSK-3) was also shown to modify multiple sites in glycogen synthase, including sites 3a, 3b, 3c,[63,68,72,73] and, as first suggested from studies of synthetic peptide phosphorylation, a fourth Ser termed site 4.[74]

Mechanisms of Phosphorylation of Glycogen Synthase

Phosphorylation of the multiple sites of rabbit muscle glycogen synthase does not occur completely independently; rather, modification of certain sites enhances the ability of others to be phosphorylated, in what has been called a hierarchal phosphorylation mechanism.[75] For example, GSK-3 action requires that glycogen synthase first be phosphorylated by casein kinase II.[73,76,77] Results from studies of synthetic peptides[74,78] and recombinant glycogen synthase[79] have suggested a molecular mechanism for the synergism between these two kinases. GSK-3 recognizes and phosphorylates sites in the motif -S-X-X-X-S(P)-. Phosphorylation of site 5 by casein kinase II generates the first recognition site, and then GSK-3 sequentially modifies four sites, each phosphorylation creating a new recognition site up to site 3a (Fig. 22-3). According to this hypothesis, prior phosphorylation by casein kinase II is absolutely necessary for GSK-3 to act.

A second example of hierarchal phosphorylation is derived from further investigation of the phosphorylation of glycogen synthase by casein kinase I.[71,80,81] Phosphorylation by casein kinase I was markedly stimulated by prior phosphorylation with cAMP-dependent protein kinase. Phosphates in the "primary" phosphorylation sites (sites 1a, 1b, and 2) enhanced the ability of casein kinase I to phosphorylate residues in the vicinity of these sites. For example, modification of site 2 in rabbit muscle glycogen synthase resulted in increased phosphorylation of site 2a by casein kinase I.[80] The molecular basis appears to be that casein kinase I preferentially modifies residues in the sequence motif -S(P)-X-X-S-.[71,80] This finding suggests that casein kinase 1 can modify sites

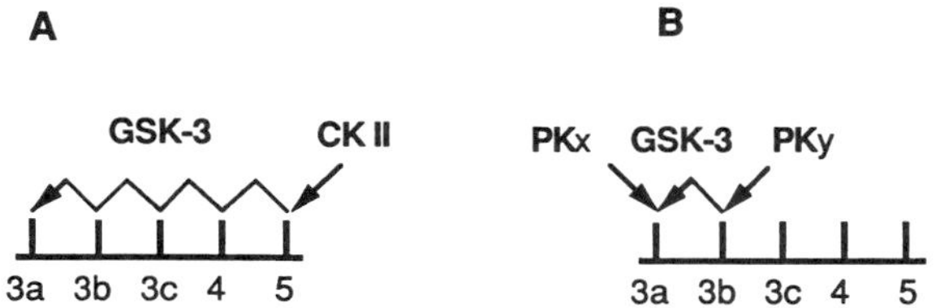

FIGURE 22-3. Mechanisms of phosphorylation of sites 3a and 3b in muscle glycogen synthase. The hierarchal mechanisms of phosphorylation of glycogen synthase by casein kinase II (CKII) and glycogen synthase kinase-3 (GSK-3) (***A***), as well as the alternative mechanisms of phosphorylation observed in the enzyme expressed in COS cells (***B***), are discussed in the text. PKx and PKy represent as yet unidentified protein kinases that independently phosphorylate site 3a and site 3b, respectively.

in glycogen synthase with considerable specificity, and that the high stoichiometries observed earlier may have been attributable to the use of relatively high levels of protein kinase. Analysis of hierarchal phosphorylation of glycogen synthase, or any other substrate, is complicated if the substrate already contains covalent phosphate in relevant sites. For this reason, synthetic peptides and recombinant protein made in bacteria have been especially useful in studies of hierarchal phosphorylation.

Effect of Phosphorylation on Glycogen Synthase Activity

In general, phosphorylation leads to a decrease in glycogen synthase activity (see refs. 40 and 41 for review). At least for the muscle isoform, however, full activity can still be elicited in the presence of the allosteric activator glucose-6-P. Alterations in the activation state can be monitored as changes in the −/+ glucose-6-P activity ratio; fully dephosphorylated enzyme has an activity ratio in the range of 0.7–0.9. Phosphorylations at different sites have different effects on the enzyme activity. Modification of sites 1a and 1b has generally been found to cause little or no inactivation.[56] Likewise, phosphorylation of site 5 does not directly affect activity[68,82] although it has the potential to influence GSK-3 action, as discussed earlier. Phosphorylation of site 2 leads to about a 50% decrease in activity ratio, with subsequent phosphorylation by casein kinase 1 at site 2a causing significant further inactivation.[77,80,81] Phosphorylation at sites 3a,b,c and 4 in the COOH-terminus by GSK-3 is also potently inactivating, decreasing the activity ratio to 0.1 or less.[63,70,73,77] Wang and Roach[79] applied site-directed mutagenesis to recombinant enzyme produced in bacteria in an effort to define which of these sites most influenced activity. Phosphorylation of site 5 by casein kinase II and sites 4 and 3c by GSK-3 did not affect activity. Additional phosphorylation of site 3b led to modest inactivation, whereas phosphorylation of all five sites (5, 4, 3c, 3b and 3a) resulted in an activity ratio of 0.1. These results implicate phosphorylation of site 3a and, to a lesser degree, site 3b in inactivation of glycogen synthase. Whether inactivation requires only 3a or all five sites to be phosphorylated was not resolved in this study (see next section). However, it is interesting that homologues of sites 3a and 3b were independently found to be important in controlling the activity of the yeast GSY2 enzyme.[83] In summary, rabbit muscle glycogen synthase can be significantly inactivated either by phosphorylation of the two NH_2-terminal sites (2 and 2a) or by COOH-terminal phosphorylation in which sites 3a and 3b have a special importance.

Analysis of Muscle Glycogen Synthase Expressed in COS Cells

An increased understanding of the phosphorylation of glycogen synthase has come from analysis of rabbit muscle enzyme transiently expressed in COS cells.[35,84] Overexpressed wild-type glycogen synthase was found to be active, but with an extremely low activity ratio (~0.01), indicating that the enzyme was in a highly phosphorylated state.[20] Under these conditions, Ser→Ala mutation at phosphorylated residues should mimic dephosphorylation of the enzyme when expressed in the COS cells. No single mutation caused significant activation of the glycogen synthase, and only by combining NH_2- and COOH-terminal mutations was significant activation achieved.[35] In fact, this is consistent with the in vitro results indicating that either NH2- or COOH-terminal phosphorylations are capable of inactivation. Also compatible with the in vitro work, the results indicate that the sites most important for regulating glycogen synthase are sites 2, 2a, 3a, and 3b. The results were also consistent with site 2 phosphorylation being a prerequisite for phosphorylation of site 2a, making casein kinase I a good candidate for phosphorylating site 2a in vivo.[35] By contrast, loss of sites 5, 4, or 3c did not affect the ability of sites 3a and 3b to be phosphorylated, and this phosphorylation was able to inactivate the enzyme.[35,84] These findings have led to the important conclusion that, in COS cells, there are alternative mechanisms for the phosphorylation of sites 3a and 3b that are independent of casein kinase II action (see Fig. 22-3). Further studies have determined that sites 3a and 3b may be phosphorylated independently of one another, although phosphorylation of 3b also influences 3a modification, leaving open the possibility that GSK-3 might also be involved in these alternative mechanisms (see ref. 85 and Fig. 22-3). More work is needed to identify the protein kinases responsible for these changes. A key question is whether this novel mechanism is unique to COS cells or is more general. Preliminary evidence suggests the presence of similar controls in Rat 1 fibroblasts (unpublished data, Skurat and Roach, 1995) and we hypothesize that multiple overlapping mechanisms may exist for the modification of sites 3a and 3b. A similar situation may apply to site 2, which has the potential to be recognized by a wide variety of protein kinases (see Fig. 22-2). The concept of redundant controls in mammalian cells is beginning to emerge from, for example, mammalian gene knockout experiments and, of course, is well known from studies of simpler organisms, such as *S. cerevisiae*.[86]

In Vivo Phosphorylation

More than 30 years ago, epinephrine and insulin were shown to modify the activity of glycogen synthase,[50,87] and this has been attributed to corresponding changes in the phosphorylation state of the enzyme. A number of studies have since attempted to quantify the changes in phosphorylation and to map, with greater or lesser precision, which phosphorylation sites are responsive to the different hormones. Parker et al.[88,89] demonstrated that treatment of normally fed rabbits with epinephrine decreased the activity ratio of glycogen synthase from 0.21 to 0.04 while increasing the total phosphate content from 2.9 to 5.1 mol/subunit. Sheorain and colleagues[90,91] reported similar results. In more recent studies, fast atom bombardment mass spectrometry[81,92] has indicated that sites 1b, 2, 2a, 3a, 3b, 3c, 4, and 5 are the only basal in vivo phosphorylation sites. Epinephrine increased the phosphate content at sites 1b, 2, 2a, and 3, but did not affect the phosphorylation state of sites 4 and 5. However, site 1a, which does not contain phosphate in the absence of epinephrine, became phosphorylated. The largest increases occurred at sites 3, 1a, and 2a. In a study conducted by Parker and co-workers,[89] insulin treatment of 24-hour-starved rabbits increased the activity ratio from 0.18 to 0.35 and decreased the total phosphate from 2.7 to 2.3 mol/subunit; it was argued that the greatest decrease was at site 3. Several other studies[93–95] have also shown that insulin promotes dephosphorylation of sites 2 and/or 2a, as well as site 1b. The islet amyloid polypeptide, or amylin, is another potential regulator of glycogen metabolism in skeletal muscle. Amylin decreased the glycogen synthase activity ratio from 0.14 to 0.08 while increasing phosphorylation by 40%.[95] Phosphorylation was increased at sites 1a, 1b, and 3(a+b+c), but not at sites 2 or 2a. This control differs from the effects of insulin or epinephrine in its being limited to the COOH-terminus of the molecule. The effects of amylin are not mediated by increased cAMP in skeletal muscle, and its mechanism of action on glycogen synthase remains unclear.

The critical question is how these hormonally induced changes in glycogen synthase phosphorylation are mediated at the molecular level. Which glycogen synthase kinases and/or phosphatases are regulated? In general, multiple sites are affected, which is not inconsistent with the idea that multiple sites affect enzyme activity. It is also noteworthy that the magnitude of the changes are relatively small; such small changes do not preclude major alterations in metabolic flux through glycogen synthase, but would seem not to represent a massive all-or-none control at the level of phosphorylation-dephosphorylation, as is seen in some signal transduction systems. For epinephrine action, activated cAMP-dependent protein kinase could account for increased phosphorylation at sites 1a and 1b, as well as site 2. However, several other protein kinases, notably phosphorylase kinase, are also candidates for mediating site 2 phosphorylation, and this role of cAMP-dependent protein kinase has been challenged.[96] Site 2a is likely to be phosphorylated by casein kinase I.[80,81] Although cAMP-dependent protein kinase can phosphorylate site 3a in vitro under what most researchers consider to be "forcing" conditions,[97] the increased phosphorylation of site 3 most likely represents indirect control by this protein kinase. No effects on GSK-3 activity by administration of epinephrine have been found so far, although one cannot exclude that as yet unidentified protein kinases (Fig. 22-4) are activated. The alternative is that the cAMP pathway suppresses phosphatase activity relevant to the dephosphorylation of site 3,[40,88,92] or, for that matter, other sites in the enzyme. For insulin action, we must invoke either the inhibition of relevant protein kinases or the activation of protein phosphatases.

Regulation by Insulin and the Role of Protein Phosphatases

Significant progress has been made in the last few years in understanding the molecular basis of insulin action, particularly as relates to events more proximal to the receptor (see Chapters 14–16). Insofar as glycogen synthase is one of the historical intracellular markers of insulin action, it is important to ask how current knowledge of glycogen synthase control fits with the recent advances in insulin signaling. As noted, what is needed are links from insulin to the control of relevant protein kinases and/or phosphatases. Insulin and other growth factors activate a protein Ser/Thr kinase cascade that results in activation of MAP kinase (or ERK). One downstream target of MAP kinase is the Rsk-2 isoform of p90 S6 kinase (also called ISPK1) which, in turn, phosphorylates (at least in vitro) two enzymes of potential relevance to glycogen synthase control. One is the enzyme GSK-3,[98] and the other is the glycogen-associated type 1 protein phosphatase.[99]

In recent studies, it has been found that GSK-3 (either the α or β isoform) is a substrate for phosphorylation by the p70 and p90 S6 kinases.[98,100] Therefore, one could postulate that insulin activation of the kinase cascade would lead to reduced GSK-3 activity with a corresponding decrease in the steady-state phosphorylation of key regulatory sites in glycogen synthase (Fig. 22-5). In support of an insulin-mediated reduction in GSK-3 activity are reports that the activity of GSK-3–like protein kinase activity is reduced in extracts from cells stimulated with insulin[101] and p90 S6 kinase, but not p70 S6 kinase,[102,103] is involved in inactivation in vivo.

Over the years, different protein Ser/Thr phosphatases (for a review, see Chapter 18) have been implicated in the dephosphorylation of glycogen synthase, but most recent evidence points to the importance of type 1 phosphatases, especially the glycogen-associated phosphatase PP1G. The enzyme is composed of a 37-kd catalytic subunit (C) complexed to a 160-kd regulatory G or R_{GI} subunit responsible for interaction with glycogen.[104,105] PP1G is much more active in dephosphorylating glycogen synthase and glycogen phosphorylase than other forms of PP1,[106] and the concentration of PP1G in muscle has been estimated to be 200 nM.[104,106] Purified PP1G binds to glycogen with high affinity (K_{app} ~6 nM) under near physiologic conditions, suggesting that, in living cells, it is likely to be bound to glycogen.[105] The primary structure of R_{GI} from rabbit[107] and human[108] muscle has been determined by

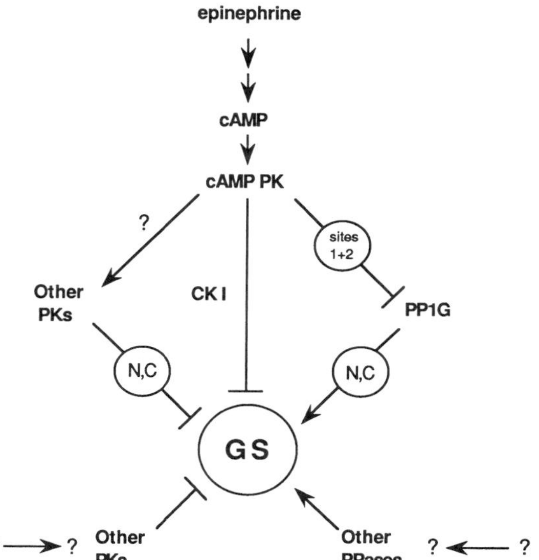

Figure 22-4. Proposed model for inactivation of glycogen synthase by epinephrine. In this model, epinephrine elevates the level of cAMP and activates cAMP-dependent protein kinase (*cAMP PK*). These events trigger (1) phosphorylation of sites 1 and 2 in PP1G that inhibits phosphatase activity of PP1G and prevents dephosphorylation and activation of glycogen synthase; (2) phosphorylation of site 2 in glycogen synthase that enhances the ability of CK I to phosphorylate site 2a and inactivate glycogen synthase; and (3) phosphorylation and activation of unidentified protein kinases which, in turn, phosphorylate and inactivate glycogen synthase. *PP1G,* glycogen-associated protein phosphatase; *PK,* protein kinase; *PPase,* protein phosphatase; *GS,* glycogen synthase; *N* and *C,* specificity for NH_2- and COOH terminal phosphorylation sites of glycogen synthase, respectively. Arrows indicate activation; bars indicate inhibition.

molecular cloning. No evidence for more than one isoform of skeletal muscle R_{GI} has been obtained. The COOH-terminus of the protein contains a putative transmembrane region that likely anchors the glycogen particle to the sarcoplasmic reticulum (for a review, see ref. 109). The NH_2-terminus of R_{GI} interacts with glycogen and the C-subunit and contains the regulatory phosphorylation sites. Co-expression of rabbit muscle glycogen synthase and R_{GI} results in activation of glycogen synthase, supporting the idea that R_{GI} specifies PP1 action on glycogen enzymes.[110] Yeast cells express a protein, GAC1,[111] which may be a functional homologue of R_{GI}, whose absence[111] or impaired interaction with the C-subunit[112] results in impaired glycogen accumulation.

R_{GI} undergoes phosphorylation at Ser-48 (site 1) and Ser-67 (site 2). Cohen and colleagues[99] have developed a model for the role of these phosphorylations in both insulin and epinephrine controls of phosphatase activity. An insulin-stimulated protein kinase, which appears to be similar to the mammalian p90 S6 kinase, phosphorylates site 1 (Ser-48) in vitro and activates PP1G.[99] Treating rabbits with insulin was found to increase phosphate in the same site in skeletal muscle PP1G, leading to the hypothesis that insulin-stimulated phosphorylation of PP1G via p90 S6 kinase is the mechanism by which insulin activates glycogen synthase (see ref. 99 and Fig. 22-5). cAMP-dependent protein kinase phosphorylates both site 1 and site 2 of R_{GI} (see Fig. 22-4). Adrenergic stimulation increases the phosphorylation of site 2 from 20% to 70%, suggesting that R_{GI} is a physiologic substrate of cAMP-dependent protein kinase.[113] Phosphorylation of site 2 reduces by a factor of 10^4 the affinity of R_{GI} for the C-subunit, causing release of the C-subunit, which is then less active toward glycogen-associated substrates.[106] In addition, cAMP-dependent protein kinase phosphorylates the phosphatase inhibitor, inhibitor-1, which then becomes a potent inhibitor of the released C-subunit.[109] By this mechanism, phosphatase activity toward the glycogen-metabolizing enzymes would be reduced, resulting in inhibition of glycogen synthesis and stimulation of glycogen breakdown.

The theory that the MAP kinase pathway links the insulin receptor to both activation of PP1G and inactivation of GSK-3 would allow for elegant control of glycogen synthase activity. However, serious questions about the operation of such a mechanism have been raised. For example, insulin and epidermal growth factor (EGF) activate MAP kinase to similar extends in 3T3-L1 adipocytes, but only insulin causes stimulation of glycogen synthesis and glucose transport.[114] Therefore, MAP kinase activation is not sufficient to stimulate synthase. Similarly, insulin stimulates glycogen synthesis in PC12 cells in the apparent absence of any stimulation of MAP kinase activity.[115] Finally, despite the fact that EGF is more effective than insulin in stimulating Rsk-2 (an isoform of p90 S6 kinase), only insulin stimulates glycogen synthase and glucose transport in rat adipocytes.[116] Likewise, activation of p70 S6 kinase, a potential regulator of GSK-3 by a separate pathway involving phosphatidylnositol 3-kinase, was found to be insufficient for activation of glycogen synthase by insulin in rat adipocytes.[116] However, this kinase was reported to be involved in the activation of glycogen synthase by insulin in 3T3-L1 adipocytes.[117] Therefore, the signal transduction pathway by which insulin exerts its metabolic effects may vary in different cell types. In conclusion, how the MAP kinases and S6 kinases fit into the activation of glycogen synthase remains somewhat obscure.

Glycogen Synthesis in Diabetes

Impaired glycogen metabolism is a well-established correlate of diabetes (see Chapter 14), and many studies have sought to identify defects in glycogen synthase, either in animal models of diabetes or in diabetics. Indeed, deficiencies in glycogen synthesis are detected in the early stages of diabetes and also occur in persons at increased risk for non–insulin-dependent diabetes mellitus (NIDDM).[118,119] In addition, it has been found that the effect of insulin on glycogen synthase from the skeletal muscle of patients with NIDDM is reduced.[120,121] In animal models of diabetes, modi-

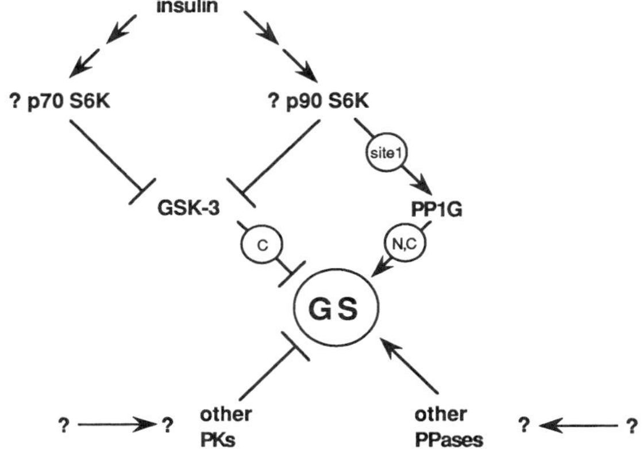

Figure 22-5. Proposed model for activation of glycogen synthase (GS) by insulin. In this model, insulin activates p70 and/or p90 S6 kinases, leading to phosphorylation and inactivation of glycogen synthase protein kinase 3 (GSK-3). Activation of p90 S6 kinase also induces phosphorylation of site 1 in glycogen-associated protein phosphatase (PP1G), which increases phosphatase activity toward glycogen synthase. Both insulin-dependent routes lead to activation of glycogen synthase.

fied glycogen synthase properties have also been observed. For example, it has been demonstrated in some studies,[122,123] but not all studies,[89] that the phosphate content of sites 3 and 2 in muscle glycogen synthase is elevated in alloxan-induced diabetic rabbits. These abnormalities are reversed by insulin treatment.[122,123] In insulin-dependent diabetic rats, the basal activity of glycogen synthase is very low in cardiac and skeletal muscle, and insulin does not increase this activity acutely, as is observed in normal animals.[124–126] These deficiencies can, at least in part, be explained by a 40–60% lower synthase phosphatase activity.[124–127] The nature of this decreased synthase phosphatase activity has not yet been investigated, but it may be attributable to a lack of functional PP1G. This view is supported by the report that the glycogen fraction from skeletal muscle of diabetic rats contains subnormal levels of immunoprecipitable R_{GI}.[128] The amount of PP1G may also be decreased, as indicated by a 40% lower trypsin-revealed phosphorylase phosphatase activity.[128,129]

Glycogen synthase has been considered to be a possible locus for genetic defects in NIDDM.[130] The human muscle glycogen synthase gene is located on chromosome 19, band q13.3,[131] and several polymorphisms in the vicinity of the gene have been identified.[131–134] To date, however, no genetic variants of glycogen synthase have been clearly implicated in NIDDM.[132–135] Mutations of other genes required for glycogen biosynthesis—notably, glycogenin and branching enzyme—may also impair glycogen accumulation, as may genetic defects that affect proteins involved in the regulation of glycogen synthase.

Several enzymes involved in the control of the phosphorylation of glycogen synthase have been studied in diabetes. Elevated casein kinase II activity[136] and cAMP-dependent protein kinase activity[137] have been reported in muscle from insulin-resistant subjects; either defect could contribute to reduced glycogen synthase activity as a result of excessive phosphorylation. Furthermore, elevated cAMP-dependent protein kinase could inhibit glycogen synthase indirectly by inactivation of PP1G. A decreased basal and insulin-stimulated activity of PP1 in skeletal muscle from insulin-resistant individuals has been reported.[138,139] Furthermore, the effect of insulin on the expression of the PP1 gene differs between insulin-sensitive and insulin-resistant skeletal muscle.[140] Analysis of the coding regions of the p90 S6 kinase gene and three isoforms of the C-subunit of PP1 genes did not reveal any structural changes in the corresponding enzymes in patients with NIDDM.[141] Analysis of the coding region of the R_{GI} subunit of PP1G has been performed in 30 insulin-resistant subjects with NIDDM.[108] Only one patient had a mutation at codon 931, which predicts a nonconservative substitution Ala→Glu in the protein molecule. It is early in the search for specific genetic defects in glycogen synthase and ancillary regulatory proteins and, although the results are negative to date, one cannot yet exclude the possibility of a causative or contributary role of such mutations in NIDDM.

References

1. Stalmans W, Bollen M, Mvumbi L. Control of glycogen synthesis in health and disease. Diabetes/Metab Rev 1987;3:127
2. Larner J. Insulin and the stimulation of glycogen synthesis. The road from glycogen structure to glycogen synthase to cyclic AMP-dependent protein kinase to insulin mediators. Adv Enzymol 1990;63:173
3. Krisman CR, Barrengo R. A precursor of glycogen biosynthesis: α-1,4-glucan-protein. Eur J Biochem 1975;52:117
4. Whelan WJ. The initiation of glycogen synthesis. BioEssays 1986;5:136
5. Smythe C, Cohen P. The discovery of glycogenin and the priming mechanism for glycogen biogenesis. Eur J Biochem 1991;200:625
6. Rowen DW, Meinke M, LaPorte DC. *GLC3* and *GHA1* of *Saccharomyces cerevisiae* are allelic and encode the glycogen branching enzyme. Mol Cell Biol 1992;12:22
7. Thon VJ, Vigneron-Lesens C, Marianne-Pepin T, et al. Coordinate regulation of glycogen metabolism in the yeast *Saccharomyces cerevisiae*. Induction of glycogen branching enzyme. J Biol Chem 1992;267:15224
8. Kennedy LD, Kirkman BR, Lomako J, et al. The biogenesis of rabbit-muscle glycogen. In: Berman MD, Gevers W, Opie LH, eds. Membranes and Muscle. Oxford: IRL Press, 1985:65
9. Pitcher J, Smythe C, Campbell DG, Cohen P. Identification of the 38-kDa subunit of rabbit skeletal muscle glycogen synthase as glycogenin. Eur J Biochem 1987;169:497
10. Rodrigues IR, Whelan WJ. A novel glycosyl-amino acid linkage: Rabbit-muscle glycogen is covalently linked to a protein via tyrosine. Biochem Biophys Res Commun 1985;132:829
11. Smythe C, Caudwell FB, Ferguson M, Cohen P. Isolation and structural analysis of a peptide containing the novel tyrosyl-glucose linkage in glycogenin. EMBO J 1988;7:2681
12. Campbell DG, Cohen P. The amino acid sequence of rabbit skeletal muscle glycogenin. Eur J Biochem 1989;185:119
13. Viskupic E, Cao Y, Zhang W, et al. Rabbit skeletal muscle glycogenin. Molecular cloning and production of fully functional protein in *Escherichia coli*. J Biol Chem 1992;267:25759
14. Rodrigues IR, Fliesler SJ. A 42,000-Da protein in rabbit tissues and in a glycogen synthase preparation cross-reacts with antibodies to glycogenin. Arch Biochem Biophys 1988;260:628
15. Smythe C, Villar-Palasi C, Cohen P. Structural and functional studies on rabbit liver glycogenin. Eur J Biochem 1989;183:205
16. Cheng C, Mu J, Farkas I, et al. Requirement of the self-glucosylating initiator proteins Glg1p and Glg2p for glycogen accumulation in Saccharomyces cerevisiae. Mol Cell Biol 1995;15:6632
17. Goldraij A, Miozzo MC, Curtino JA. Glycogen-bound protein in lower eukaryote and prokaryote. Biochem Mol Biol Int 1993;30:453
18. Pitcher J, Smythe C, Cohen P. Glycogenin is the priming glucosyltransferase required for the initiation of glycogen biogenesis in rabbit skeletal muscle. Eur J Biochem 1988;176:391
19. Lomako J, Lomako WM, Whelan WJ. The biogenesis of glycogen: Nature of the carbohydrate in the protein primer. Biochem Int 1990;21:251
20. Skurat AV, Cao Y, Roach PJ. Glucose control of rabbit skeletal muscle glycogenin expressed in COS cells. J Biol Chem 1993;268:14701
21. Lomako J, Lomako WM, Whelan WJ. The nature of the primer for glycogen synthesis in muscle. FEBS Lett 1990;269:8
22. Cao Y, Mahrenholz AM, DePaoli-Roach AA, Roach PJ. Characterization of rabbit skeletal muscle glycogenin. Tyrosine 194 is essential for function. J Biol Chem 1993;268:14687
23. Alonso MD, Lomako J, Lomako WM, Whelan WJ. Tyrosine-194 of glycogenin undergoes autocatalytic glucosylation but is not essential for catalytic function and activity. FEBS Lett 1994;342:38
24. Alonso M, Lomako J, Lomako WM, et al. Properties of carbohydrate-free recombinant glycogenin expressed in an *Escherichia coli* mutant lacking UDP-glucose pyrophosphorylase activity. FEBS Lett 1994;352:222
25. Cao Y, Steinrauf LK, Roach PJ. Mechanism of glycogenin self-glucosylation. (Manuscript submitted).
26. Lomako J, Lomako WM, Whelan WJ. Substrate specificity of the autocatalytic protein that primes glycogen synthesis. FEBS Lett 1990;264:13
27. Manzella SM, Roden L, Meezan E. A biphasic radiometric assay of glycogenin using the hydrophobic acceptor *n*-dodecyl-β-D-maltoside. Anal Biochem 1994;216:383
28. Lomako J, Lomako WM, Whelan WJ. A self-glucosylating protein is the primer for rabbit muscle glycogen biosynthesis. FASEB J 1988;2:3097
29. Smythe C, Watt P, Cohen P. Further studies on the role of glycogenin in glycogen biosynthesis. Eur J Biochem 1990;189:199
30. Cao Y, Skurat AV, DePaoli-Roach AA, Roach PJ. Initiation of glycogen synthesis: Control of glycogenin by glycogen phosphorylase. J Biol Chem 1993;268:21717
31. Lomako J, Whelan WJ. The occurrence of serine phosphate in glycogenin: A possible regulatory site. BioFactors 1988;1:261
32. Bailey JM, Lomako JP, Lomako W, Whelan WJ. The role of glycogenin in glycogen synthesis and non-insulin dependent diabetes mellitus (Abstract). Biochem Soc Trans 1993;21:124S
33. Kemp BE, Pearson RB. Protein kinase phosphorylation site sequences and consensus specificity motifs: Tabulations. Methods Enzymol 1991;200:62
34. Kennelly PJ, Krebs EG. Consensus sequences as substrate specificity determinants for protein kinases and protein phosphatases. J Biol Chem 1991; 266:15555
35. Skurat AV, Wang Y, Roach PJ. Rabbit skeletal muscle glycogen synthase expressed in COS cells. Identification of regulatory phosphorylation sites. J Biol Chem 1994;269:25534
36. Stetten D Jr, Steten MR. Glycogen metabolism. Physiol Rev 1960;40:505
37. Lomako J, Lomako WM, Whelan WJ. Proglycogen: A low-molecular-weight form of muscle glycogen. FEBS Lett 1991;279:223
38. Lomako J, Lomako WM, Whelan WJ, et al. Glycogen synthesis in the astrocyte: From glycogenin to proglycogen to glycogen. FASEB J 1993; 7:1386
39. Ercan N, Gannon MC, Nuttal FQ. Incorporation of glycogenin into hepatic proteoglycogen after oral glucose administration. J Biol Chem 1994; 269:22328
40. Cohen P. Muscle glycogen synthase. In: Boyer PD, Krebs EG, eds. The Enzymes. Orlando, FL: Academic Press, 1986;17:461
41. Roach PJ. Liver glycogen synthase. In: Boyer PD, Krebs EG, eds. The Enzymes. Orlando, FL: Academic Press, 1986;17:499
42. Browner MF, Nakano K, Bang AG, Fletterick RJ. Human muscle glycogen

synthase cDNA sequence: A negatively charged protein with an asymmetric charge distribution. Proc Natl Acad Sci USA 1989;86:1443
43. Zhang W, Browner MF, Fletterick RJ, et al. Primary structure of rabbit skeletal muscle glycogen synthase deduced from cDNA clones. FASEB J 1989;3:2532
44. Nuttall FQ, Gannon MC, Bai G, Lee EYC. Primary structure of human liver glycogen synthase deduced by cDNA cloning. Arch Biochem Biophys 1994;311:443
45. Bai G, Zhang Z, Werner R, et al. The primary structure of rat liver glycogen synthase deduced by cDNA cloning. Absence of phosphorylation sites 1a and 1b. J Biol Chem 1990;265:7843
46. Farkas I, Hardy TA, DePaoli-Roach AA, Roach PJ. Isolation of the GSY1 gene encoding yeast glycogen synthase and evidence for the existence of a second gene. J Biol Chem 1990;265:20879
47. Cohen P. The role of cyclic-AMP-dependent protein kinase in the regulation of glycogen metabolism in mammalian skeletal muscle. Curr Top Cell Regul 1978;14:117
48. Mahrenholz AM, Wang YH, Roach PJ. Catalytic site of rabbit glycogen synthase isozymes. Identification of an active site lysine close to the amino terminus of the subunit. J Biol Chem 1988;263:10561
49. Tagaya M, Nakano K, Fukui T. A new affinity labeling reagent for the active site of glycogen synthase. Uridine diphosphopyridoxal. J Biol Chem 1985; 260:6670
50. Villar-Palasi C, Larner J. Insulin-mediated effect on the activity of UDPG-glycogen transglucosylase of muscle. Biochim Biophys Acta 1960;39:171
51. Rosell-Perez M, Villar-Palasi C, Larner J. Studies on UDPG-glycogen transglucosylase. I. Preparation and differentiation of two activities of UDPG-glycogen transglucosylase from rat skeletal muscle. Biochem J 1962;1:763
52. Friedman DL, Larner J. Studies on UDPG-α-glucan transglucosylase. III. Interconversion of two forms of muscle UDPG-α-glucan transglucosylase by a phosphorylation-dephosphorylation reaction sequence. Biochemistry 1963;2:669
53. Soderling TR, Hickenbottom JP, Reimann EM, et al. Inactivation of glycogen synthase and activation of phosphorylase kinase by muscle adenosine 3′,5′-monophosphate-dependent protein kinases. J Biol Chem 1970;245:6317
54. Schlender KK, Wei SH, Villar-Palasi C. UDP-glucose: Glycogen α-4-glucosyltransferase I kinase activity of purified muscle protein kinase. Cyclic nucleotide specificity. Biochim Biophys Acta 1969;191:272
55. Proud CG, Rylatt DB, Yeaman SJ, Cohen P. Amino acid sequences at the sites on glycogen synthase phosphorylated by cyclic AMP-dependent protein kinase and their dephosphorylation by protein phosphatase-III. FEBS Lett 1977;80:435
56. Embi N, Parker PJ, Cohen P. A reinvestigation of the phosphorylation of rabbit skeletal muscle glycogen synthase by cyclic AMP-dependent protein kinase. Identification of the third site of phosphorylation at serine-7. Eur J Biochem 1981;115:405
57. Huang TS, Krebs EG. Amino acid sequence of a phosphorylation site in skeletal muscle glycogen synthase. Biochem Biophys Res Commun 1977; 75:643
58. Parker PJ, Aitken A, Bilham T, et al. Amino acid sequence of a region in rabbit skeletal muscle glycogen synthase phosphorylated by cyclic AMP-dependent protein kinase. FEBS Lett 1981;123:332
59. Roach PJ, DePaoli-Roach AA, Larner J. Ca^{++}-stimulated phosphorylation of muscle glycogen synthase by phosphorylase kinase. J Cyclic Nucleotide Res 1978;4:245
60. Payne ME, Schworer CM, Soderling TR. Purification and characterization of rabbit liver calmodulin-dependent glycogen synthase kinase. J Biol Chem 1983;258:2376
61. Ahmad Z, DePaoli-Roach AA, Roach PJ. Purification and characterization of a rabbit liver calmodulin-dependent protein kinase able to phosphorylate glycogen synthase. J Biol Chem 1982;257:8348
62. Ahmad Z, DePaoli-Roach AA, Roach PJ. Phosphorylation of glycogen synthase by the Ca^{++} and phospholipid-activated protein kinase (protein kinase C). J Biol Chem 1984;259:8743
63. Cohen P, Yellowlees D, Aitken A, et al. Separation and characterization of glycogen synthase kinase 3, glycogen synthase 4 and glycogen synthase kinase 5 from rabbit skeletal muscle. Eur J Biochem 1982;124:21
64. DePaoli-Roach AA, Roach PJ, Larner J. Multiple phosphorylation of rabbit skeletal muscle glycogen synthase. Comparison of the actions of different protein kinases capable of catalyzing phosphorylation *in vitro*. J Biol Chem 1979;254:12062
65. Carling D, Hardie DG. The substrate specificity of the AMP-activated protein kinase. Phosphorylation of glycogen synthase and phosphorylase kinase. Biochim Biophys Acta 1989;1012:81
66. Erikson E, Maller JL. Substrate specificity of ribosomal protein S6 kinase II from *Xenopus* eggs. Second Messengers Phosphoproteins 1988;12:135
67. Stokoe D, Campbell DG, Nakielny S, et al. MAPKAP kinase-2; a novel protein kinase activated by mitogen-activated protein kinase. EMBO J 1992;11:3985
68. Picton C, Aitken A, Bilham T, Cohen P. Multisite phosphorylation of glycogen synthase from rabbit skeletal muscle. Organization of the seven sites in the polypeptide chain. Eur J Biochem 1982;124:37
69. Kuret J, Woodgett JR, Cohen P. Multisite phosphorylation of glycogen synthase from rabbit skeletal muscle. Identification of the sites phosphorylated by casein kinase-I. Eur J Biochem 1985;151:39
70. Huang KP, Singh TJ, Akatsuka A, et al. Phosphorylation and inactivation of rabbit skeletal muscle glycogen synthase: Distinction between kinase Fa-, phosphorylase kinase-, and glycogen synthase (casein) kinase-1-catalyzed reactions. Arch Biochem Biophys 1984;232:111
71. Flotow H, Graves PR, Wang A, et al. Phosphate groups as substrate determinants for casein kinase I action. J Biol Chem 1990;265:14264
72. Rylatt DB, Aitken A, Bilham T, et al. Glycogen synthase from rabbit skeletal muscle. Amino acid sequence at the sites phosphorylated by glycogen synthase kinase-3, and extension of the N-terminal sequence containing the site phosphorylated by phosphorylase kinase. Eur J Biochem 1988;107:529
73. DePaoli-Roach AA, Ahmad Z, Camici M, et al. Multiple phosphorylation of rabbit skeletal muscle glycogen synthase. Evidence for interactions among phosphorylation sites and the resolution of electrophoretically distinct forms of the subunit. J Biol Chem 1983;258:10702
74. Fiol CJ, Mahrenholz AM, Wang Y, et al. Formation of protein kinase recognition sites by covalent modification of the subunit. Molecular mechanism for the synergistic action of casein kinase II and glycogen synthase kinase 3. J Biol Chem 1987;262:14042
75. Roach PJ. Control of glycogen synthase by hierarchal protein phosphorylation. FASEB J 1990;4:2961
76. Picton C, Woodgett J, Hemmings B, Cohen P. Multisite phosphorylation of glycogen synthase from rabbit skeletal muscle. Phosphorylation of site 5 by glycogen synthase kinase-5 (casein kinase-II) is a prerequisite for phosphorylation of sites 3 by glycogen synthase kinase-3. FEBS Lett 1982;150:191
77. Zhang W, DePaoli-Roach AA, Roach PJ. Mechanisms of multisite phosphorylation and inactivation of rabbit muscle glycogen synthase. Arch Biochem Biophys 1993;304:219
78. Fiol CJ, Wang A, Roeske RW, Roach PJ. Ordered multisite protein phosphorylation: Analysis of glycogen synthase kinase 3 action using model peptide substrates. J Biol Chem 1990;265:6061
79. Wang Y, Roach PJ. Inactivation of rabbit muscle glycogen synthase by glycogen synthase kinase-3. Dominant role of the phosphorylation of Ser-640 (site 3a). J Biol Chem 1993;268:23876
80. Flotow H, Roach PJ. Synergistic phosphorylation of rabbit muscle glycogen synthase by cyclic AMP-dependent protein kinase and casein kinase I: Implications for hormonal regulation of glycogen synthase. J Biol Chem 1989;264:9126
81. Nakielny S, Campbell DG, Cohen P. The molecular mechanism by which adrenalin inhibits glycogen synthesis. Eur J Biochem 1991;199:713
82. DePaoli-Roach AA, Ahmad Z, Roach PJ. Characterization of a rabbit skeletal muscle protein kinase ($PC_{0.7}$) able to phosphorylate glycogen synthase and phosvitin. J Biol Chem 1981;256:8955
83. Hardy TA, Roach PJ. Control of yeast glycogen synthase-2 by COOH-terminal phosphorylation. J Biol Chem 1993;268:23799
84. Skurat AV, Roach PJ. Phosphorylation of sites 3a and 3b (Ser-640 and Ser-644) in the control of rabbit muscle glycogen synthase. J Biol Chem 1995;270:12491
85. Skurat AV, Roach PJ. Multiple mechanisms for the phosphorylation of C-terminal regulatory sites in rabbit muscle glycogen synthase expressed in COS cells. Biochem J 1996;313:45
86. Olsen MV. Genome structure and organization in *Saccharomyces cerevisiae*. In: Broach JR, Pringle JR, Jones EW, eds. The molecular biology of the yeast *Saccharomyces cerevisiae*. CHS Press, 1991
87. Craig JW, Larner J. Influence of epinephrine and insulin on uridine diphosphate glucose-α-glucan transferase and phosphorylase in muscle. Nature 1964;202:971
88. Parker PJ, Embi N, Caudwell FB, Cohen P. Glycogen synthase from rabbit skeletal muscle. State of phosphorylation of the seven phosphoserine residues *in vivo* in the presence and absence of adrenaline. Eur J Biochem 1982;124:47
89. Parker PJ, Caudwell FB, Cohen P. Glycogen synthase from rabbit skeletal muscle. Effect of insulin on the state of phosphorylation of the seven phosphoserine residues *in vivo*. Eur J Biochem 1983;130:227
90. Sheorain VS, Khatra BS, Soderling TR. Phosphorylation of glycogen synthase in rabbit muscle. Effect of epinephrine and diabetes. FEBS Lett 1981;127: 94
91. Sheorain VS, Khatra BS, Soderling TR. Hormonal regulation of glycogen synthase phosphorylation in rabbit skeletal muscle. J Biol Chem 1982; 257:3462
92. Poulter L, Ang S, Gibson BW, et al. Analysis of the *in vivo* phosphorylation state of rabbit skeletal muscle glycogen synthase by fast atom bombardment spectrometry. Eur J Biochem 1988;175:497
93. Lawrence JC Jr, Hiken JF, DePaoli-Roach AA, Roach PJ. Hormonal control of glycogen synthase in rat hemidiaphragms. Effects of insulin and epinephrine on the distribution of phosphate between two cyanogen bromide fragments. J Biol Chem 1983;258:10710
94. Smith RL, Roach PJ, Lawrence JC Jr. Insulin resistance in denervated skeletal muscle. Inability of insulin to stimulate dephosphorylation of glycogen synthase in denervated rat epitrochlearis muscles. J Biol Chem 1988;263:658
95. Lawrence JC Jr, Zhang J. Control of glycogen synthase and phosphorylase by amylin in rat skeletal muscle. Hormonal effects on the phosphorylation of phosphorylase and on the distribution of phosphate in the synthase subunit. J Biol Chem 1994;269:11595
96. Cohen P, Hardie DG. The actions of cyclic AMP on biosynthetic processes are mediated indirectly by cyclic AMP-dependent protein kinase. Biochim Biophys Acta 1991;1094:292
97. Sheorain VS, Corbin JD, Soderling TR. Phosphorylation of sites 3 and 4 in rabbit skeletal muscle glycogen synthase by cAMP-dependent protein kinase. J Biol Chem 1985;260:1567

98. Sutherland C, Leighton IA, Cohen P. Inactivation of glycogen synthase kinase-3β by phosphorylation: New kinase connections in insulin and growth-factor signalling. Biochem J 1993;296:15
99. Dent P, Lavoinne A, Nakielny S, et al. The molecular mechanism by which insulin stimulates glycogen synthesis in mammalian skeletal muscle. Nature 1990;348:302
100. Sutherland C, Cohen P. The α-isoform of glycogen synthase kinase-3 from rabbit skeletal muscle is inactivated by p70 S6 kinase or MAP kinase-activated protein kinase-1 in vitro. FEBS Lett 1994;338:37
101. Welsh GI, Proud CG. Glycogen synthase kinase-3 is rapidly inactivated in response to insulin and phosphorylates eukaryotic initiation factor eIF-2B. Biochem J 1993;294:625
102. Welsh GI, Foulstone EJ, Young SW, et al. Wortmannin inhibits the effects of insulin and serum on the activities of glycogen synthase kinase-3 and mitogen-activated protein kinase. Biochem J 1994;303:15
103. Cross DAE, Alessi DR, Vandenheede JR, et al. The inhibition of glycogen synthase kinase-3 by insulin or insulin-like growth factor 1 in the rat skeletal muscle cell line L6 is blocked by wortmannin, but not by rapamycin: Evidence that wortmannin blocks activation of the mitogen-activated protein kinase pathway in L6 cells between Ras and Raf. Biochem J 1994;303:21
104. Stralfors P, Hiraga A, Cohen P. The protein phosphatases involved in cellular regulation. Purification and characterization of the glycogen-bound form of protein phosphatase-1 from rabbit skeletal muscle. Eur J Biochem 1985; 149:295
105. Hubbard MJ, Cohen P. The glycogen binding subunit of protein phosphatase-1_G from rabbit skeletal muscle. Further characterization of its structure and glycogen-binding properties. Eur J Biochem 1989;180:457
106. Hubbard MJ, Cohen P. Regulation of protein phosphatase-1G from rabbit skeletal muscle. 2. Catalytic subunit translocation is a mechanism for reversible inhibition of activity toward glycogen-bound substrates. Eur J Biochem 1989;186:711
107. Tang PM, Bondor JA, Swiderek KM, DePaoli-Roach AA. Molecular cloning and expression of the regulatory (R_{GI}) subunit of the glycogen-associated protein phosphatase. J Biol Chem 1991;266:15782
108. Chen YH, Hansen L, Chen MX, et al. Sequence of the human glycogen-associated regulatory subunit of type 1 protein phosphatase and analysis of its coding region and mRNA level in muscle from patients with NIDDM. Diabetes 1994;43:1234
109. DePaoli-Roach AA, Park I-K, Cerovsky V, et al. Serine/threonine protein phosphatases in the control of cell function. Adv Enzyme Regul 1994;34: 199
110. Kuntz MJ, Skurat A, Roach PJ, DePaoli-Roach AA. Activation of muscle glycogen synthase by the glycogen/SR-associated type 1 protein phosphatase transiently coexpressed in COS cells (Abstract). FASEB J 1994;8:A1437
111. François J, Thompson-Jaeger S, Skroch J, et al. *GAC1* may encode a regulatory subunit for protein phosphatase type 1 in Saccharomyces cerevisiae. EMBO J 1992;11:87
112. Skrotch SJ, Frederick DL, Varner CM, Tatchell K. The mutant type 1 protein phosphatase encoded by *glc7-1* from *Saccharomyces cerevisiae* fails to interact productively with the *GAC1*-encoded regulatory subunit. Mol Cell Biol 1994;14:896
113. Hubbard MJ, Cohen P. On target with new mechanisms for the regulation of protein phosphorylation. Trends Biochem Sci 1993;18:172
114. Robinson LJ, Razzack ZF, Lawrence JC Jr, James DE. Mitogen-activated protein kinase activation is not sufficient for stimulation of glucose transport or glycogen synthase in 3T3-L1 adipocytes. J Biol Chem 1993;268:26422
115. Ohmichi M, Pang L, Ribon V, Saltiel AR. Divergence of signaling pathways for insulin in PC-12 pheochromocytoma cells. Endocrinology 1993;133:46
116. Lin T-A, Lawrence JC Jr. Activation of ribosomal S6 kinases does not increase glycogen synthesis or glucose transport in rat adipocytes. J Biol Chem 1994;269:21255
117. Shepherd P, Nave BT, Siddle K. Insulin stimulation of glycogen synthase activity is blocked by wortmannin and rapamycin in 3T3-L1 adipocytes: Evidence for the involvement of phosphoinositide 3-kinase and p70 ribosomal protein-S6 kinase. Biochem J 1995;305:25
118. Groop LC, Bonadonna RC, DelPrato S, et al. Glucose and free fatty acid metabolism in non–insulin-dependent diabetes mellitus: Evidence for multiple sites of insulin resistance. J Clin Invest 1989;84:205
119. Eriksson J, Franssila-Kallunki A, Ekstrand A, et al. Early metabolic effects in persons at increased risk for non–insulin-dependent diabetes mellitus. N Engl J Med 1989;321:337
120. Thorburn AW, Gumbiner B, Bulacan F, et al. Multiple defects in muscle glycogen synthase activity contribute to reduced glycogen synthesis in non–insulin-dependent diabetes mellitus. J Clin Invest 1991;87:489
121. Vestergaard H, Lund S, Larsen FS, et al. Glycogen synthase and phosphofructokinase protein and mRNA levels in skeletal muscle from insulin-resistant patients with non–insulin-dependent diabetes mellitus. J Clin Invest 1993; 91:2342
122. Sheorain VS, Juhl H, Bass M, Soderling TR. Effect of epinephrine, diabetes, and insulin on rabbit skeletal muscle glycogen synthase. Phosphorylation site occupancies. J Biol Chem 1984;259:7024
123. Sheorain VS, Ramakrishna S, Benjamin WB, Soderling TR. Phosphorylation of sites 3 and 2 in rabbit skeletal muscle glycogen synthase by multiple protein kinase (ATP-citrate lyase kinase). J Biol Chem 1985;260:12287
124. Nuttall FQ, Gannon MC, Corbett VA, Wheeler MP. Insulin stimulation of heart glycogen synthase D phosphatase (protein phosphatase). J Biol Chem 1976;251:6724
125. Miller TB Jr. A dual role for insulin in the regulation of cardiac glycogen synthase. J Biol Chem 1978;253:5389
126. Miller TB Jr. Altered regulation of cardiac glycogen metabolism in spontaneously diabetic rats. Am J Physiol 1983;245:E379
127. Khatra BS. Properties of phosphoprotein phosphatase from skeletal muscle and its regulation in diabetes. Proc Soc Exp Biol Med 1984;177:33
128. Metallo A, Villa-Moruzzi E. Protein phosphatase-1 and -2A, kinase F_A, and casein kinase II in skeletal muscle of streptozotocin diabetic rats. Arch Biochem Biophys 1991;289:382
129. Villa-Moruzzi E. Effects of streptozotocin-diabetes, fasting and adrenaline on phosphorylase phosphatase activities of rat skeletal muscle. Mol Cell Endocrinol 1986;47:43
130. Beck-Nielsen H, Vaag A, Damsbo P, et al. Insulin resistance in skeletal muscles in patients with NIDDM. Diabetes Care 1992;15:418
131. Vionnet N, Bell GI. Identification of a simple tandem repeat DNA polymorphism in the human glycogen synthase gene and linkage to five markers on chromosome 19q. Diabetes 1993;42:930
132. Elbein SC, Hoffman M, Ridinger D, et al. Description of a second microsatellite marker and linkage analysis of the muscle glycogen synthase locus in familial NIDDM. Diabetes 1994;43:1061
133. Groop LC, Kankuri M, Schalin-Jantti C, et al. Association between polymorphism of the glycogen synthase gene and non–insulin-dependent diabetes mellitus. N Engl J Med 1993;328:10
134. Bjorbaek C, Echwald SM, Hubricht P, et al. Genetic variants in promoters and coding regions of the muscle glycogen synthase and the insulin-responsive GLUT4 genes in NIDDM. Diabetes 1994;43:976
135. Shimokava K, Kadowaki H, Sakura H, et al. Molecular scanning of the glycogen synthase and insulin receptor substrate-1 genes in Japanese subjects with non–insulin-dependent diabetes mellitus. Biochem Biophys Res Commun 1994;202:463
136. Maeda R, Raz I, Zurlo F, Sommercorn J. Activation of skeletal muscle casein kinase II by insulin is not diminished in subjects with insulin resistance. J Clin Invest 1991;87:1017
137. Kida Y, Nyomba BL, Bogardus C, Mott DM. Defective insulin response of cAMP-dependent protein kinase in insulin-resistant humans (Abstract). Diabetes 1990;39:254A
138. Kida Y, Esposito–Del Puente A, Bogardus C, Mott DM. Insulin resistance is associated with reduced fasting and insulin-stimulated glycogen synthase phosphatase activity in human skeletal muscle. J Clin Invest 1990;85: 476
139. Kida J, Raz I, Maeda R, et al. Defective insulin response of phosphorylase phosphatase in insulin-resistant humans. J Clin Invest 1992;89:610
140. Thompson DB, Degregorio M, Sommercorn J. Insulin resistance alters immediate early gene expression in human skeletal muscle in vivo (Abstract). Diabetes 1992;41:89A
141. Bjorbaek C, Vik TA, Echwald SM, et al. Cloning of a human insulin-stimulated protein kinase (ISPK-1) gene and analysis of coding regions and mRNA levels of the ISPK-1 and the protein phosphatase-1 genes in muscle from NIDDM patients. Diabetes 1995;44:90

Diabetes Mellitus, edited by Derek LeRoith, Simeon I. Taylor, and Jerrold M. Olefsky. Lippincott–Raven Publishers, Philadelphia © 1996.

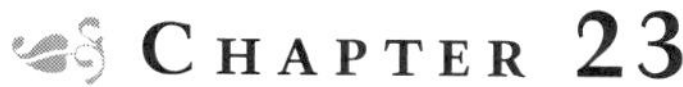

CHAPTER 23

Hormone-Sensitive Lipase and the Control of Lipolysis in Adipocytes

CONSTANTINE LONDOS

Most of the body's energy reserves are stored in adipose cells as fatty acids in triacylglycerols. Major anabolic actions of insulin include stimulating the uptake of substrates for triacylglycerol synthesis and increasing lipogenesis in the adipose cell. Another important action of insulin is inhibition of lipolysis, the process by which catabolic hormones, primarily catecholamines, stimulate hydrolysis of triacylglycerols, leading to the release of fatty acids. One complication associated with the insulin resistance of non–insulin-dependent diabetes mellitus (NIDDM) stems from unrestrained lipolysis in adipocytes, which results in elevated plasma concentrations of non-esterified fatty acids. The fatty acids are thought to both stimulate gluconeogenesis in the liver and to attenuate glucose utilization by skeletal muscle.[1] Indeed, suppression of lipolysis in adipocytes by other lipolytic inhibitors, such as agonists of the adipocyte nicotinic acid receptor, has been shown to reduce both plasma fatty acid concentrations and hyperglycemia. However, the salutary effects of nicotinic acid receptor stimulation are transitory.[2] It is anticipated that a comprehensive understanding of the lipolytic reaction may lead to improved treatment methods for NIDDM, at least with respect to suppressing fatty acid release from adipocytes.

Although many gaps remain in our understanding of the details of the lipolytic reaction, it is possible to outline the major steps in hormonal regulation of lipid hydrolysis. Lipolytic hormones increase lipolysis acutely by stimulating plasma membrane adenylyl cyclase activity, which leads to increased cAMP and activation of cAMP-dependent protein kinase (PKA). The major physiologic effectors are catecholamines, which activate the cyclase through β-adrenergic receptors coupled to the G_s subclass of heterotrimeric G-proteins. Hormone-sensitive lipase (HSL), the rate-limiting enzyme of lipolysis, is rapidly phosphorylated by PKA but, as discussed later, the mechanism by which HSL phosphorylation results in increased lipid breakdown is not fully understood. Insulin inhibits lipolysis primarily by activating a cyclic nucleotide phosphodiesterase that hydrolyzes cAMP; the hormone also increases protein phosphatases that dephosphorylate PKA substrates, including HSL. Lipolysis may also be suppressed by ligands that act at so-called inhibitory receptors—those that inhibit adenylyl cyclase by interacting with G_i, the inhibitory subclass of heterotrimeric G-proteins. Nicotinic acid uses this G_i-mediated route to suppress lipolysis, as does adenosine, by binding to adenosine A1 receptors.[3] Catecholamines, acting at α-adrenergic receptors, and prostaglandins also inhibit lipolysis via G_i. The relative importance of these various effectors under physiologic conditions is unknown. However, microdialysis studies in human subjects have shown that adenosine exerts a tonic inhibitory effect on lipolysis in situ.[4] Although other signaling systems may participate in modulating the lipolytic reaction, the pathway involving receptors, adenylyl cyclase, and protein kinase A appears to be the dominant regulator of lipid breakdown in adipocytes.

Hormone-Sensitive Lipase

Biochemical research on HSL was long hampered by lack of highly purified enzyme. In 1981, the Belfrage laboratory succeeded in isolating relatively pure and biologically active HSL from rat adipocytes.[5] The subsequent advances, which have both afforded a molecular definition of HSL and allowed cloning of the gene, have been summarized recently by others.[6–10]

Two properties set HSL apart from other lipases. First, HSL is the only known lipase whose activity is acutely regulated by reversible phosphorylation, which will be discussed in further detail later in this chapter. Second, HSL exhibits nearly equal catalytic activity against triacylglycerols and long-chain fatty acid esters of cholesterol, whereas most other triacylglycerol lipases exhibit little or no cholesteryl esterase activity. A further feature of this broad substrate specificity is the ability to hydrolyze long-chain tri-, di-, and monoacylglycerols. Because triacylglycerols are hydrolyzed considerably more slowly than diacylglycerols, the hydrolysis of triacylglycerols is thought to be rate-limiting in adipocytes.[10] The final step in triacylglycerol breakdown—hydrolysis of 2-monoacylglycerol—is catalyzed by a separate monoacylglycerol lipase in adipocytes.

Recently, cDNA clones have been isolated for both rat and human HSL, and human genomic HSL has been characterized.[6,9] Rat and human cDNAs encode proteins of 82.8 and 85.5 kd, respectively. In keeping with its unique catalytic and regulatory properties, HSL exhibits only minimal sequence similarity with enzymes of the lipase gene family.

Based on inhibition of HSL activity by diisopropyl fluorophosphate, and paralleled by covalent incorporation of this inhibitor into the molecule, HSL has been categorized as a serine esterase.[10] The Gly-X-Ser-X-Gly motif contains the catalytic serine in most lipases, and HSL contains this consensus pentapeptide (Gly-Asp-Ser-Asp-Gly). Recently, site-directed mutagenesis has confirmed that the serine of this pentapeptide is within the catalytic site of HSL.[11] The human enzyme also exhibits a region of similarity with lipase 2 of Moraxella TA144, an antarctic psychrotrophic bacterium, which catalyzes lipid hydrolysis at low temperatures. Interestingly, HSL retains far greater activity at reduced temperatures than other mammalian lipases,[9] a property most likely conferred by the lipase 2–like sequence. It is thought that the ability to hydrolyze adipocyte triacylglycerol stores at reduced temperatures has survival value in poikilotherms or hibernators.

Knowledge of the HSL amino acid sequence has not provided information on the higher order structure of the enzyme. The finding that two different functional domains—the catalytic region and the region containing sites for phosphorylation—are encoded by different exons of the human gene has led to the proposal that HSL is a mosaic protein.[9] However, the overall lack of homology with other lipases precludes assignment of specific functions to different regions of the protein. Other lipases with little primary sequence homology exhibit highly similar structural features based on crystal structure, but further information on HSL must await resolution of its crystal structure. Recent biochemical studies have provided evidence of a lipid-binding domain that is separate from the catalytic region. In addition to triacylglycerol, HSL efficiently catalyzes the hydrolysis of *p*-nitrophenyl butyrate (PNPB), a water-soluble compound. Mild proteolysis of HSL with trypsin nearly abolishes activity against trioleoylglycerol, but activity against PNPB is only minimally reduced, indicating that HSL contains a lipid-binding domain separate from its catalytic domain.[7] As trypsin treatment yields a stable 17.6-kd fragment that is relatively resistant to proteolysis, it has been speculated that HSL is composed of separately folded domains joined by short, protease-sensitive sequences. Other data providing evidence of a separate lipid-binding domain have been derived from studies on interfacial activation, a phenomenon whereby lipolytic activity is enhanced by the presence of a lipid-water interface. Intact HSL is activated by the presence of phospholipid vesicles or emulsified trioleoylglycerol, but these lipids have no effect on activity of the 17.6-kd fragment on the water-soluble substrate, suggesting that proteolysis separates the catalytic domain from the putative lipid-binding domain.[7]

Phosphorylation of HSL, both in vivo and in vitro, has been studied extensively, and two sites have been identified. The so-called regulatory site (site 1) is phosphorylated by PKA in conjunction with lipolytic activation of intact cells or by activation of the enzyme in vitro by PKA. There is little question that PKA phosphorylation at this site contributes to increased lipolytic activity, and lipolytic inhibition by insulin is most likely attributable to reduced phosphorylation of this serine. The regulatory site has been identified as ser 363 in the rat protein. The so-called basal site (site 2) is also a serine, two residues removed from site 1 (ser 365). Although site 2 may be phosphorylated by several protein kinases, the novel 5′-AMP-activated kinase is thought to phosphorylate HSL at this site in the intact cell. This site is also termed the "basal" site because phosphorylation has not been shown to affect catalytic activity. However, phosphorylation of sites 1 and 2 is apparently mutually exclusive,[12] leading to the theory that the phosphorylation of site 2 may serve to block the activation of HSL by PKA action at site 1. Recently, an analogue of 5′-AMP that activates 5′-AMP–activated kinase was shown to inhibit lipolysis in adipocytes.[13] Although these data are consistent with a role for the 5′-AMP kinase in lipolytic regulation, the physiologic relevance of phosphorylation at site 2 has yet to be determined.

Regulation of Lipolysis in the Adipocyte

Having briefly outlined our current knowledge of HSL, it is important to acknowledge that, although progress on the molecular definition of HSL represents a step forward, we are far from understanding the mechanism of cellular lipolysis. The remainder of this chapter focuses on those areas in which there are significant gaps in our understanding of the lipolytic process, as well as those areas in which current notions seem to fall short of explaining observed phenomena. New developments that may provide insights into the process of lipid metabolism are also mentioned.

Although many questions remain regarding the regulation of HSL phosphorylation, an even more pressing need is to develop an accurate description of the consequences of PKA phosphorylation at the regulatory site. Many laboratories have reported increased HSL catalysis of lipid substrates upon activation with PKA in vitro. However, in general, little more than a doubling of activity is observed, which contrasts markedly with the typical 50- to 100-fold increase in lipolysis in intact cells upon activation of PKA. An important difference between the two experimental systems is that cellular lipolysis involves activation of HSL in its natural cytoplasmic milieu, which then hydrolyzes lipids contained within native lipid storage droplets. The in vitro systems tests HSL that has been removed from its cellular environment and that usually is vastly diluted. Moreover, the in vitro system uses exogenous triacylglycerols, cholesteryl esters, or other appropriate substrates. In some cases, in vitro activity has been studied using cellular lipid droplets that have been dispersed by homogenization or sonication, and thus may no longer be considered to be native droplets. It is instructive to compare HSL activity in intact cells with activity measured against the dispersed droplets from the same cell population. Whereas unstimulated intact cells exhibit relatively low or even unmeasurable activity compared to stimulated cells, the homogenates of the *unstimulated* cells exhibit hydrolytic activity that approaches that of homogenates of stimulated cells. That is, as noted by Stralfors et al.[10] in the disrupted system with fragmented droplets, there is a great increase in lipolytic activity. Although not tested directly, it is unlikely that cellular disruption leads to phosphorylation of HSL, as the factors required for phosphorylation (ATP, magnesium, PKA) are greatly diluted by the homogenization media. What might be the basis for this large apparent activation of lipolysis upon cellular disruption? First, if HSL is restrained in its native state, cell breakage may release lipase. Second, the character of the substrate is changed; that is, the droplet is dispersed. This explanation was originally offered by Stralfors et al.,[10] who speculated that the increased lipid surface area in the mechanically dispersed (sonicated) substrate accounted for the increased lipolysis. The corollary to this argument is that lipase, whether PKA-phosphorylated or not, rapidly catalyzes lipid hydrolysis if substrate is suitably presented. Furthermore, lipids that are packaged in their native storage droplets may be protected against hydrolysis by HSL. Thus, two additional aspects of the lipolytic reaction require consideration: (1) whether the lipase is restrained from gaining access to the lipid droplet in the unphosphorylated state, and (2) whether the lipid droplet surface presents a barrier against HSL in the unstimulated cell.

Although HSL has been reported to exhibit behavior more akin to membrane-bound than to soluble proteins, the enzyme is found typically in the soluble supernatant fraction of homogenates of unstimulated adipocytes. HSL fractionates exclusively, however, with the floating lipid cake in homogenates of lipolytically stimulated primary rat adipocytes[14] or 3T3-L1 adipocytes. These data suggest that HSL translocates to the lipid droplet upon stimulation, a theory that has been confirmed by direct visualization of HSL by immunofluorescent methods (Fig. 23-1). In the unstimulated cell, the enzyme is dispersed in the cytoplasm and excluded from the droplet surface. Upon stimulation, there is a clear concentration of the enzyme at the droplet surface, indicative of translocation. An important question that remains is the basis for this redistribution of HSL. Among the factors to be considered is the disposition of cytoplasmic HSL, which does not appear to be freely soluble. Nearly all HSL remains within digitonin-treated adipocytes, in contrast to lactate dehydrogenase, which readily escapes to the medium, indicating that HSL is tethered to another cellular component. Movement to the droplet upon phosphorylation of HSL may be initiated by release from the putative component or by conformational changes in the enzyme that promote lipid binding. One must also consider the possibility that the lipid droplet actively participates in the translocation of HSL and, thus, in the lipolytic reaction, a premise based on the identification of a family of lipid droplet–associated proteins, termed perilipins.

Perilipins of Lipid Droplets

The perilipins are a family of unique proteins with properties that suggest a role in adipocyte lipid metabolism.[15,16] First, perilipins are abundant in adipocytes and are not detected in any other type of cell except those that synthesize steroid hormones, as discussed

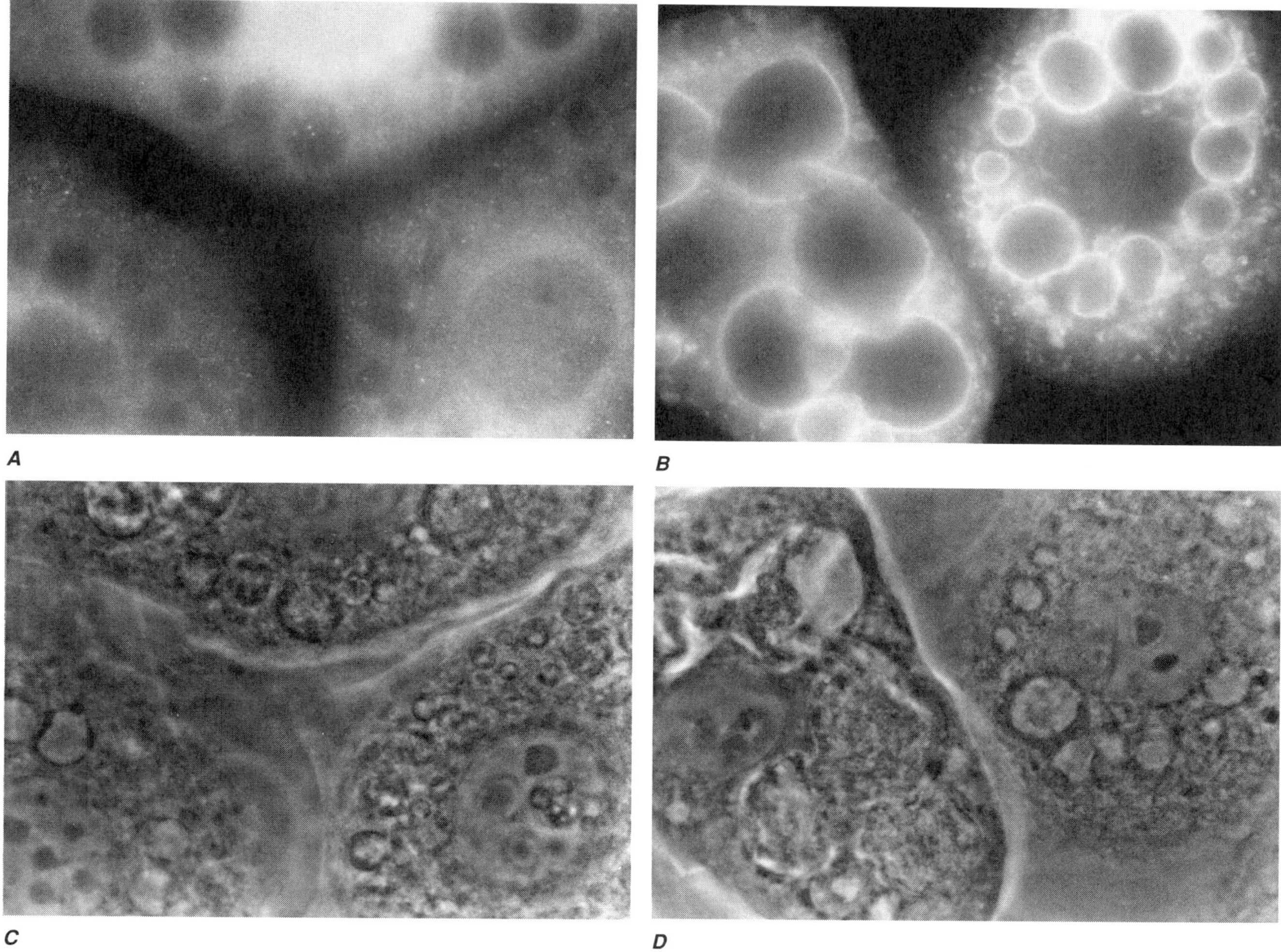

Figure 23-1. Translocation of HSL to lipid droplets in lipolytically stimulated adipocytes. ***A*** and ***B***, immunofluorescence staining of cultured 3T3-L1 adipocytes with affinity-purified anti-HSL antibodies. ***C*** and ***D***, Phase images. Panels ***A*** and ***C*** show control cells, whereas ***B*** and ***D*** are isoproterenol-stimulated. Note that HSL is diffusely distributed in the cytoplasm and excluded from the lipid droplets in the control cells (***A***). By contrast, nearly all HSL gathers at the lipid droplet surface in the stimulated cells (***B***).

later. Second, these proteins are located exclusively at the limiting surface of the lipid storage droplet (Fig. 23-2),[17] and they are the only proteins known to be intrinsic to the droplet. Third, perilipins are polyphosphorylated by PKA in concert with lipolytic activation.[18] Finally, perilipins have been shown to be expressed also in steroidogenic cells, where they also encircle lipid droplets.[19] The droplets in steroidogenic cells contain primarily cholesteryl esters which, upon hydrolysis by a cholesteryl esterase, release cholesterol, the precursor for steroid hormone synthesis. Significantly, this esterase is indistinguishable from HSL by conventional biochemical criteria, although Western and Northern analyses suggest slight differences between HSL and the cholesteryl esterase.[6,20] As in adipocytes, neutral lipid hydrolysis in steroidogenic cells is triggered by elevation of cAMP. Thus, there appears to be a strong link between the expression of perilipins and the hydrolysis of intracellular neutral lipids by the HSL-cholesteryl esterase class of hydrolases.

Perilipin cDNAs have been isolated from both rat[16] and murine adipocyte expression libraries. Perilipin is a single copy gene that, by alternative splicing, gives rise to four isoforms (A–D) in murine adipocytes and steroidogenic cells (Fig. 23-3); thus far only perilipins A and B have been identified in rat cells. Although the perilipins avidly adhere to lipid droplets from adipocytes, the primary structure contains no motifs that predict this strong lipid-binding property; this raises the possibility that perilipins associate with other, as yet unidentified, lipid droplet proteins. The largest isoform —perilipin A (~57 kd)—is by far the most heavily radiolabeled substrate for PKA found in lipolytically stimulated, $^{32}P_i$-loaded adipocytes; this species contains six consensus PKA phosphorylation sites. Although perilipin A is the most abundant isoform in both adipocytes and steroidogenic cells, the different types of cells exhibit distinct isoform specificities. For example, perilipin C (42 kd) is relatively abundant in steroid-producing cells, but this protein is not detected in adipocytes.[19] The perilipins are unique proteins bearing no extended homology to other known proteins. However, a short region of 100 amino acids in the amino terminus of perilipins A and B resembles the amino terminus of the recently discovered *a*dipocyte *d*ifferentiation *r*elated *p*rotein (ADRP). To date, ADRP has been detected only in adipocytes.[21] The significance of a common motif between the two proteins is currently unknown, but the similar and limited tissue distribution of perilipins and ADRP suggest their participation in a common process.

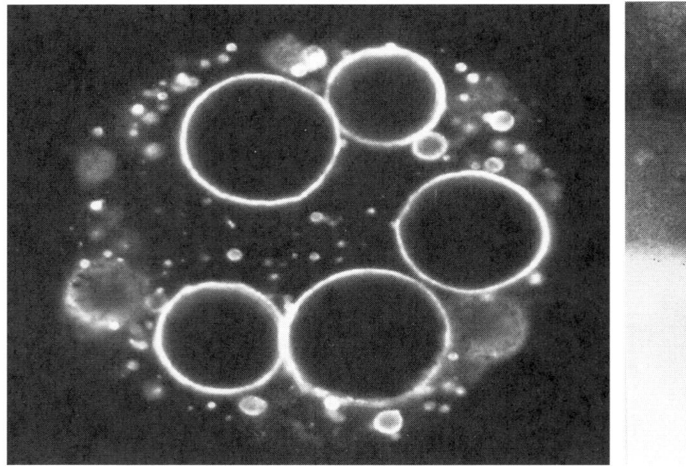

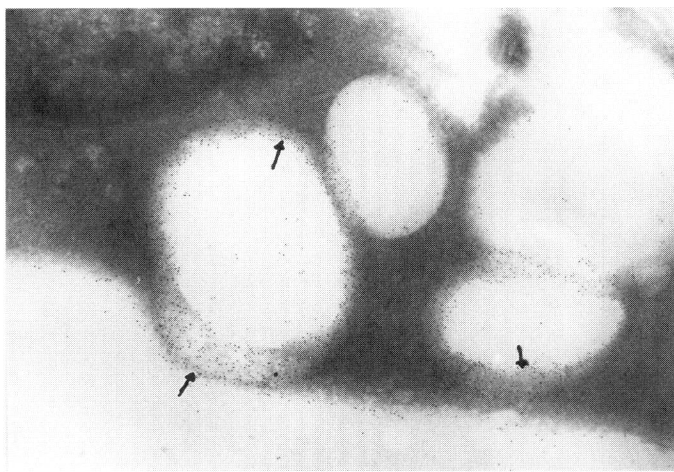

A *B*

Figure 23-2. Immunostaining of perilipins in 3T3-L1 adipocytes. Immunostaining was performed with affinity-purified anti-perilipin antibodies. ***A,*** Confocal immunofluorescence staining of lipid droplets in 3T3-L1 adipocytes. Typically, all lipid bodies detected by Nile Red staining (not shown) are surrounded by perilipin, and perilipin is only detected in association with lipid (see ref. no. 17.) ***B,*** Immunogold labeling reveals that perilipin is located on or within the limiting phospholipid monolayer (*arrows*) that surrounds the clear triacylglycerol core.

Although the function of perilipins remains unknown, their subcellular location and acute regulation by PKA point to a role in lipid metabolism. These proteins may participate in packaging of neutral lipids, their hydrolysis, or both. Certainly, the coincident expression of perilipins and HSL or HSL-like enzymes implies a catabolic action. Data gathered thus far suggest a dual role; perilipins may sequester and protect neutral lipids from hydrolysis in the absence of an appropriate signal (i.e., cAMP). Phosphorylation of perilipins by PKA ''unmasks'' the lipid and provides access for HSL.

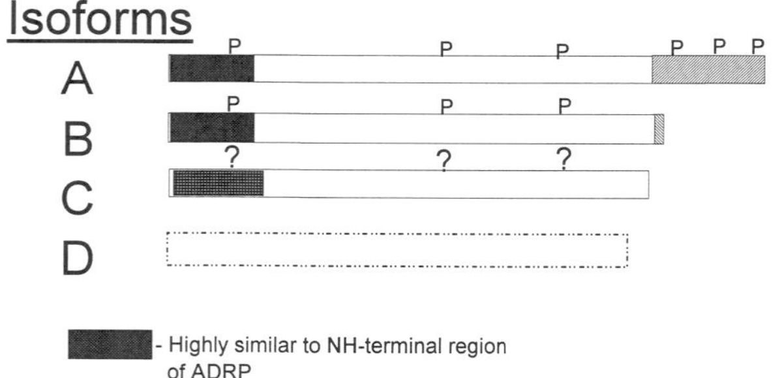

Figure 23-3. Perilipid isoforms. Perilipins A and B are found in rat adipocytes, whereas mRNAs for all four isoforms are found in murine cells. Murine adipocytes express predominantly A, B, and D perilipins, whereas steroidogenic cells express mainly A and C. Sequence data are available for only the A and B isoforms. Consensus PKA sites are labeled *"P"*; it is unknown (*?*) whether C and D isoforms contain these phosphorylation sites. A and B perilipin are identical over most of their N-terminal region, but contain unique C-termini. The composition of perilipin C has been deduced from selective probing using both Western and Northern analysis; the corresponding protein (~42 kd) is detected only in murine steroidogenic cells. The ADRP-like region of C is similar, but not identical to, the same region at the N-terminus of A and B. Perilipin D appears as a relatively prominent, 1.8-kb mRNA; no corresponding protein has been identified.

Summary and Conclusions

What emerges from this brief overview of the lipolytic process in adipocytes is that far more awaits discovery than is already known. Certainly, HSL plays a key role, as do the signaling systems that regulate cAMP concentration and, thus, PKA activity. It is likely, however, that lipolysis is governed by factors that have not yet been identified, and by those recently revealed, such as perilipins and, possibly, ADRP. Because a large percentage of food intake is cycled routinely through adipose tissue, one might expect the storage and retrieval of energy to be a highly complex process subject to elaborate control mechanisms. Carbohydrate energy stores constitute a minor percentage of energy reserves compared to lipid in adipocytes, and the glycogen granule has, at its surface, an elaborate array of enzymes and other regulatory factors that govern deposition and breakdown of glycogen. It is not unreasonable to expect, then, that the lipid droplet is subject to comparably sophisticated control processes, carried out by molecules both known and unknown.

References

1. Randle PJ, Garland PB, Hales CN, Newsholme EA. The glucose fatty acid cycle: Its role in insulin sensitivity and the metabolic disturbances of diabetes mellitus. Lancet 1963;1:785
2. Foley JE. Rationale and application of fatty acid oxidation inhibitors in treatment of diabetes mellitus. Diabetes Care 1992;15:773
3. Londos C, Cooper DM, Rodbell M. Receptor-mediated stimulation and inhibition of adenylate cyclases: The fat cell as a model system. Adv Cyclic Nucleotide Res 1981;14:163
4. Lonnroth P, Jansson P-A, Fredholm BB, Smith U. Microdialysis of intercellular adenosine concentration in subcutaneous tissue in humans. Am J Physiol 1989;256:E250
5. Fredrikson G, Stralfors P, Nilsson NO, Belfrage P. Hormone-sensitive lipase of rat adipose tissue: Purification and some properties. J Biol Chem 1981; 256:6311
6. Holm C, Kirchgessner T, Svenson K, et al. Hormone-sensitive lipase: Se-

quence, expression, and chromosomal localization to 19 cent-q13.3. Science 1988;241:1503
7. Yeaman SJ, Smith GM, Jepson CA, et al. The multifunctional role of hormone-sensitive lipase in lipid metabolism. Adv Enzyme Regul 1994;34:355
8. Holm C, Belfrage P, Osterlund T, et al. Hormone-sensitive lipase: Structure, function, evolution and overproduction in insect cells using the baculovirus expression system. Protein Eng 1994;7:537
9. Langin D, Laurell H, Holst LS, et al. Gene organization and primary structure of human hormone-sensitive lipase: possible significance of a sequence homology with a lipase of Moraxella TA144, an antarctic bacterium. Proc Natl Acad Sci USA 1993;90:4897
10. Stralfors P, Olsson H, Belfrage P. Hormone-sensitive lipase. In: Boyer PD, Krebs EG, eds. The Enzymes. 3rd ed. Vol. 18, Part B. Orlando, FL: Academic Press;1987:147–177
11. Holm C, Davis RC, Osterlund T, et al. Identification of the active site serine of hormone-sensitive lipase by site-directed mutagenesis. FEBS Lett 1994; 344:234
12. Garton AJ, Campbell DG, Carling D, et al. Phosphorylation of bovine hormone-sensitive lipase by the AMP-activated protein kinase. A possible antilipolytic mechanism. Eur J Biochem 1989;179:249
13. Corton JM, Gillespie JG, Hawley SA, Hardie DG. 5-Aminoimidazole-4-carboxamide ribonucleoside: A specific method for activating AMP-activated protein kinase in intact cells? Eur J Biochem 1995;229:558
14. Egan JJ, Greenberg AS, Chang MK, et al. Mechanism of hormone-stimulated lipolysis in adipocytes: Translocation of hormone-sensitive lipase to the lipid storage droplet. Proc Natl Acad Sci USA 1992;89:8537
15. Greenberg AS, Egan JJ, Wek SA, et al. Perilipin, a major hormonally regulated adipocyte-specific phosphoprotein associated with the periphery of lipid storage droplets. J Biol Chem 1991;266:11341
16. Greenberg AS, Egan JJ, Wek SA, et al. Isolation of cDNAs for perilipins A and B: Sequence and expression of lipid droplet-associated proteins of adipocytes. Proc Natl Acad Sci USA 1993;90:12035
17. Blanchette-Mackie EJ, Dwyer NK, Barber T, et al. Localization of perilipin in adipocytes. J Lipid Res 1995;36:1211
18. Egan JJ, Greenberg AS, Chang MK, Londos C. Control of endogenous phosphorylation of the major cAMP-dependent protein kinase substrate in adipocytes by insulin and beta-adrenergic stimulation. J Biol Chem 1990;265:18769
19. Servetnick DA, Brasaemle DL, Gruia-Gray J, et al. Perilipins are associated with cholesteryl ester droplets in steroidogenic adrenal cortical and Leydig cells. J Biol Chem 1995;270:16970
20. Holm C, Belfrage P, Fredrikson G. Immunological evidence for the presence of hormone-sensitive lipase in rat tissues other than adipose tissue. Biochem Biophys Res Commun 1987;148:99
21. Jiang H-P, Serrero G. Isolation and characterization of a full-length cDNA coding for an adipose differentiation-related protein. Proc Natl Acad Sci USA 1992;89:7856

Diabetes Mellitus, edited by Derek LeRoith, Simeon I. Taylor, and Jerrold M. Olefsky. Lippincott–Raven Publishers, Philadelphia © 1996.

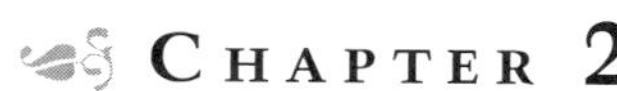

CHAPTER 24
Insulin and Intracellular Ions

BORIS DRAZNIN AND JANE E-B. REUSCH

Although insulin's main physiologic role is to maintain adequate glucose uptake and utilization by many tissues, its pleiotropic action involves regulation of protein synthesis and degradation, lipid metabolism, and ion fluxes. The latter govern the cell membrane potential and the maintenance of the intracellular milieu, which impacts greatly upon cellular function. Alterations in the concentration of intracellular ions precipitously affect signal transduction machinery and the activity of many ion-dependent and ion-sensitive intracellular enzymes. Thus, by its action upon ion pumps and channels, insulin contributes significantly to the maintenance of normal concentrations of intracellular Na^+, K^+, H^+, Ca^{++}, Mg^{++}, phosphate, and other ions.

On the other hand, concentrations of intracellular ions can be maintained and altered by numerous other mechanisms. Derangements induced by either a malfunction of ion pumps or channels themselves, or by other hormones and metabolites, can interfere with insulin action. This can occur either at the level of insulin binding (receptor defect) or at any of the numerous postbinding steps (postreceptor defects) of insulin action. Abnormalities in concentrations of intracellular ions can interrupt insulin signaling at several steps. These abnormalities may interfere with generation of the initial signal, or with transduction of this signal along the signal transduction pathways. Changes in the concentrations of the intracellular ions may affect interactions among multiple intermediates of the insulin signaling pathway, alter the magnitude of phosphorylation/dephosphorylation reactions, or influence the activity of the final substrates of insulin action. Interference at any one or at several of these steps hampers insulin action, resulting in either generalized or partial (perhaps pathway-specific) insulin resistance.

The influence of ions on insulin action can be both tissue-specific and action-specific. For example, the impact of intracellular acidification on insulin action may be more pronounced in the liver than in the muscle. Similarly, the influence of intracellular Ca^{++} on the insulin effect on glycogen metabolism in the muscle may be much stronger than its influence on the growth-promoting action of insulin in vascular smooth muscle cells.

Finally, numerous derangements in the intracellular ion concentration have been observed consistently in humans and experimental animals with diabetes.[1–15] These abnormalities include increased levels of intracellular calcium and sodium and decreased levels of intracellular magnesium and pH.[16–22] Some of these abnormalities have been also detected in patients with hypertension,[23–28] as well as those with various forms of insulin resistance.[20,29–31] Taken together, these observations have prompted several investigators to propose an intriguing "ionic hypothesis" to explain the mechanism of association of hypertension with insulin resistance and other features of the "syndrome X."[32–39]

In this chapter, three aspects of the interaction of insulin and ions are reviewed: (1) the influence of insulin upon ion fluxes and intracellular ion concentrations; (2) the influence of ions on the mechanism of insulin action; and (3) derangements in the ionic cellular milieu in diabetes.

The Influence of Insulin Upon Ion Fluxes and Intracellular Ion Concentrations

Intracellular Calcium

The resting cytosolic free calcium concentration is approximately 0.1 μM, with major pools of intracellular calcium located in the endoplasmic reticulum and mitochondria.[40] There is a wide calcium gradient across the plasma membrane, as the extracellular calcium exists in the millimolar range. Two energy-dependent processes are responsible for extruding calcium from the cells against this gradient. One is Ca^{++}/Mg^{++}-adenosine triphosphatase (ATPase) and another is Na^{++}/Ca^{++} exchanger.[41,42] The former is fairly responsive to changes in concentrations of calmodulin and calcium, whereas the latter is dependent largely upon transmembrane Na^{+} gradient.[41,43–45] The endoplasmic and sarcoplasmic reticulum membranes also contain Ca^{++}/Mg^{++}-ATPase, which pumps Ca^{++} into the intravesicular space. This enzyme is structurally and functionally distinct from the Ca^{++}/Mg^{++}-ATPase of the plasma membrane.[46,47] Calcium release from the intracellular stores is regulated by inositol triphosphate (IP_3), changes in the cytosolic calcium concentrations, and changes in membrane potential.[44,45]

Reports on the effects of insulin on calcium fluxes and intracellular concentrations have been inconsistent.[41,45,48–53] The influence of insulin on calcium fluxes and its intracellular concentration has been studied in skeletal muscle, myotubules, adipocytes, and platelets.[6–9,14,17,50,54–56] Results obtained in these studies are conflicting, with most investigators seeing either no effect of insulin or modest increases in the concentrations of cytosolic calcium.[1,41,45,48,54] The mechanism of the latter effect is not completely understood, but may be related to an inhibitory influence of insulin upon Ca^{++}/Mg^{++}-ATPase (at least in some tissues) and moderate activation of the voltage-dependent Ca^{++} channels.[31,41,57]

A calmodulin-sensitive, high-affinity plasma membrane Ca^{++}/Mg^{++}-ATPase is the primary enzyme responsible for the extrusion of calcium from the cell.[41,47,58] An enzyme that is somewhat related, but different in function and structurally distinct, is endoplasmic reticulum Ca^{++}/Mg^{++}-ATPase, which promotes movement of cytosolic calcium into the endoplasmic reticulum for storage.[47] Both phosphorylation and the activity of the adipocyte plasma membrane Ca^{++}/Mg^{++}-ATPase have been found to be inhibited by physiologic concentrations of insulin in adipocytes.[41,47,59,60] Inhibition of the major calcium extrusion machinery results in an increase in the cytosolic calcium concentration.[61] This increase, however, is also partially dependent upon calcium channels, as evidenced by experiments that have demonstrated the negation of a substantial portion of insulin effect in the presence of calcium channel blockers.[54]

In contrast to these observations, other investigators have noted a stimulatory influence of insulin on Ca^{++}/Mg^{++}-ATPase in kidney basolateral membranes and erythrocytes.[2,45,62] This stimulatory effect of insulin was seen at physiologic concentrations of insulin with clear dose-dependency.[2] Furthermore, a decrease in Ca^{++}-ATPase activity was observed in tissues of diabetic patients and animals.[2,10,63–65] Because one proposed mechanism whereby insulin stimulates Ca^{++}/Mg^{++}-ATPase involves insulin-induced alterations in the content of plasma membrane phospholipids,[64,65] some diabetic conditions that are accompanied by increases in membrane phospholipid content may be associated with increased Ca^{++}/Mg^{++}-ATPase activity.[2,9,65–67] Conceivably, tissue-specific responses to insulin may explain these seemingly contradictory findings of a stimulatory or inhibitory influence of insulin on Ca^{++}/Mg^{++}-ATPase.

Insulin has also been shown to increase the binding of calmodulin to the high-affinity site in a calcium-dependent manner.[68] Because calmodulin is a ubiquitous regulatory ligand that modulates the intracellular signaling process in all eukaryotic cells, these observations may be of fundamental significance.[41]

Another interesting aspect of insulin's effect on intracellular ions is its ability to attenuate Arginine vasopressin (AVP)-mediated calcium transients, inward calcium currents, and contractile responses in vascular smooth muscle cells (VSMCs).[69] Insulin has been shown to shift AVP dose-response curves to the right, reducing relative potency of AVP by 16-fold at 1 mU of insulin per milliliter and 220-fold at 100 mU of insulin per milliliter. Responses to AVP were significantly attenuated within 30 minutes of insulin application.[69,70] Conceivably, insulin resistance could diminish or eliminate this attenuating effect of insulin, resulting in increased levels of cytosolic calcium and an augmented contractile response of VSMCs, as typically seen in hypertension.

Intracellular pH

In the early 1970s, Manchester[71] and Moore[72] suggested that intracellular pH (pHi) might be an important intracellular signal for insulin. A kinetic analysis of the Na^{+}/K^{+} pump activation by insulin provided additional evidence in favor of an insulin effect on proton extrusion.[72] These observations also suggested that changes in pHi may be a part of the insulin signaling system. By the 1980s, the view that pHi plays a significant role in the regulation of many cell functions had gained wide acceptance and was supported by a large body of evidence.[73,74]

At the same time, the influence of insulin upon pHi has been demonstrated by several techniques in various amphibian and mammalian tissues.[74–78] The mechanism of the insulin-induced increase in pHi appears to involve insulin's ability to stimulate Na^{+}/H^{+} exchange. The effect of insulin on Na^{+}/H^{+} exchange is blocked by amiloride but not by ouabain,[74,76,78] and is largely dependent upon extracellular Na^{+} concentration.

If the physiologic role of insulin is to increase pHi by stimulating Na^{+}/H^{+} exchange, then hypoinsulinemia should be accompanied by increased intracellular Na^{+} concentrations and decreased pHi. This prediction was amply confirmed in experiments with diabetic animals. In rats with mild streptozotocin-induced diabetes with no evidence of metabolic acidosis, the soleus muscle pHi level was significantly reduced.[74]

As it is virtually impossible to change only one specific ion inside the cell, it is not surprising that alterations in pHi can elicit multiple changes in the intracellular ion profile.[74] Stimulation of Na^{+}/H^{+} exchange by insulin leads to a decrease in H^{+} concentration with an increase in Na^{+} concentration. The latter may activate the Na^{+}/K^{+} pump, which extrudes Na^{+} in exchange for K^{+}. Na^{+} can also be extruded from the cell in exchange for Ca^{++} via the Na^{+}/Ca^{++} exchange mechanism, which can become an important factor in increasing intracellular calcium concentrations.

Under pathophysiologic circumstances, such as insulin resistance, the ability of insulin to activate the Na^{+}/K^{+} pump may be lost, with a resultant activation of the Na^{+}/Ca^{++} exchange and a build-up of cytosolic calcium.

Insulin's physiologic effect upon pHi appears to be involved in the mechanism of insulin-stimulated glycolysis.[74,79] Thus, in a glucose-free Ringer's solution (30 mM HCO_3^{-}/5% CO_2), either amiloride or a 15-fold reduction in the concentration of extracellular Na^{+} blocked the effect of insulin on glycolysis and on pHi.[80] Similarly, changing the pHi by means other than insulin was found to mimic the effect of insulin on glycolysis.[77] It appears that the insulin-induced changes in pHi affect the activity of phosphofructokinase (PFK), the rate-limiting enzyme of glycolysis. Because the rates of both glycogenesis and glucogenesis are pH-sensitive (with optimal rates occurring at a pH of 6.5–7.0),[81] maintenance of a normal pH range is of great importance for insulin action. At least one other aspect of insulin action—the transport of type A amino acids—has also been linked to insulin's effect on pHi.[82]

Intracellular Na^+ and K^+

In contrast to the somewhat controversial influence of insulin on cytosolic calcium concentration, the ability of insulin to reduce serum potassium levels was one of its earliest clinically recognized effects.[83] The accumulated evidence suggests that this hypokalemic effect of insulin is secondary to enhanced uptake of K^+ into insulin-sensitive tissues. At the same time, insulin significantly alters intracellular concentrations of both Na^+ and K^+.[83]

The active transport of Na^+ and K^+ ions across the plasma membrane is mediated by Na^+/K^+-ATPase, which hydrolyzes one molecule of ATP while exchanging the influx of two K^+ ions for the efflux of three Na^+ ions.[84,85] Na^+/K^+-ATPase consists of two subunits—a larger catalytic α subunit and a smaller glycoprotein β subunit (reviewed in ref. 83)—that appear to be responsible for inserting the enzyme into the plasma membrane. There are at least three isoforms of the α subunit,[86] with αII being very sensitive to ouabain, insulin, and intracellular Na^+.[3,87,88]

Insulin stimulates Na^+/K^+ exchange in a variety of tissues, including rat skeletal muscle, adipocytes, fibroblasts, hepatocytes, and VSMCs.[83,89–91] These stimulatory effects of insulin occur in the absence of glucose or in the presence of glucose transport inhibitors,[92] indicating a direct effect of insulin. Insulin effect is inhibited by ouabain, however, suggesting that insulin stimulates Na^+/K^+-ATPase activity, which promotes Na^+/K^+ exchange.[71,90,91]

Insulin effect on the Na^+/K^+ pump (Na^+/K^+-ATPase) may involve an increase in the number of ion pumps or an activation of existing pumps. Quantitation of the number of Na^+/K^+ pumps before and after stimulation with insulin has revealed that insulin does not alter the number of active Na^+ pumps, but rather stimulates the activity of existing pumps.[93] The precise mechanism whereby insulin stimulates Na^+/K^+-ATPase activity remains unclear. It has been suggested that insulin shifts the affinity of the enzyme for Na^+ to lower values in adipocytes and muscle cells.[82,87,94]

It has been proposed that insulin-induced increases in pHi and changes in intracellular Na^+ concentrations activate Na^+/K^+-ATPase.[95] The latter facilitates Na^+ efflux and K^+ influx. The net result of insulin-induced alterations in K^+ uptake is an increase in the intracellular K^+/Na^+ ratio, with a resultant hyperpolarization of the insulin target cells. Conversely, an inadequate response of Na^+/K^+-ATPase to insulin may result in the accumulation of intracellular Na^+, activation of Na^+/Ca^{++} exchange, and an increase in intracellular Ca^{++}, which, in turn, can lead to or aggravate insulin resistance.

Influence of Intracellular Ions on Insulin Action

One consequence of the frequent permutations in intracellular ion homeostasis is that the cell's ability to respond adequately to insulin-generated signals may become impaired. In other words, alterations in the concentration of the intracellular ions may impair insulin action, leading to insulin resistance. In this regard, the influence of intracellular calcium and hydrogen ions on insulin action has been studied more extensively than the potential influence of other ions.

The mechanism whereby sustained levels of intracellular calcium cause (or potentiate) insulin resistance is only partially understood. It appears that high levels of intracellular calcium affect the postreceptor steps of insulin action, with only negligible influence on insulin binding and activation of the insulin receptor tyrosine kinase.[96] High levels of intracellular calcium alter the phosphorylation state of several enzymes and intermediates in the insulin signaling cascade, thus impairing their functional ability.[97]

Initial experiments exploring the role of calcium in the mechanism of insulin action demonstrated that chelation of intracellular calcium interfered significantly with the ability of insulin to stimulate glucose uptake.[98] Subsequently, it was determined that intracellular calcium had an optimal range for mediating insulin action,[55] and that levels higher or lower than this optimal range were associated with impaired insulin action (Fig. 24-1). A more detailed investigation of the role of intracellular calcium revealed that the duration of the elevation of intracellular calcium concentration was more important than the magnitude of this elevation. Thus, transient spikes in intracellular calcium concentration did not adversely affect insulin action, whereas sustained elevations in the level of intracellular calcium (even at the upper normal range) led to a significant diminution of the insulin effect.[96,97] Because chronic elevations in intracellular calcium levels are routinely observed in numerous tissues of patients and experimental animals affected by hypertension, obesity, and aging,[1,11,16,19,22,45,54,57] the insulin resistance associated with these conditions may be at least partially attributable to impaired homeostasis of intracellular calcium.

High levels of cytosolic calcium may be induced experimentally using several approaches. Depolarization of cell membranes with K^+ or exposure of cells to parathyroid hormone (PTH) enhances Ca^{++} influx via voltage-dependent calcium channels.[99,100] Extracellular ATP increases mobilization of intracellular calcium, whereas thapsigargin elevates cytosolic calcium by inhibiting intracellular ATPase.[101,102]

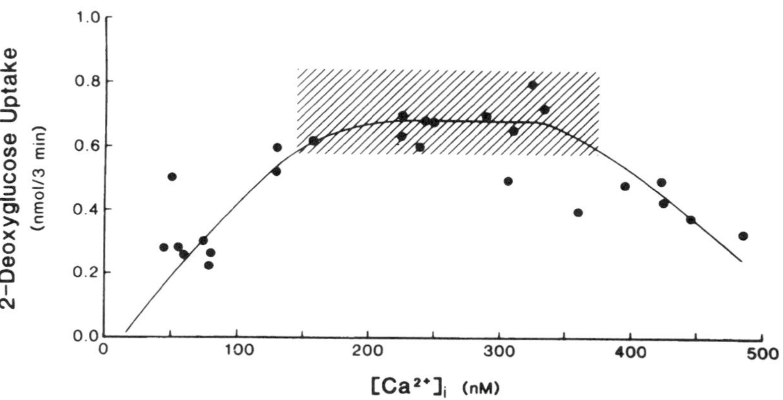

FIGURE 24-1. The rates of maximally stimulated 2-deoxyglucose uptake (at an insulin concentration of 25 ng/mL) at various levels of cytosolic free Ca^{++}. The cells, which were incubated under identical conditions (various concentrations of extracellular Ca^{++}, with or without ionomycin), were used either to study insulin-stimulated hexose uptake or to measure cytosolic free Ca^{++} concentrations. The hatched area represents the window of optimal response to insulin. Each point is a mean of duplicate determinations obtained in three separate experiments. (Reproduced with permission from Draznin B, Sussman K, Kao M, et al. The existence of an optimal range of cytosolic free calcium for insulin-stimulated glucose transport in rat adipocytes. J Biol Chem 1987;262:14385)

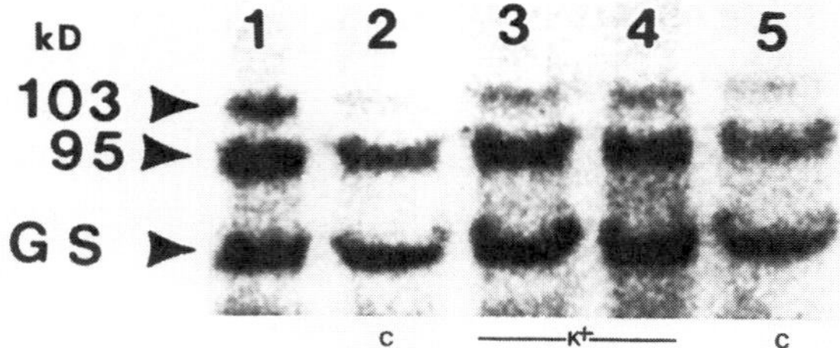

Figure 24-2. Dephosphorylation of [^{32}P]-labeled glycogen synthase (GS) by particulate fraction (PF) protein phosphatase. ***Lane 1,*** GS incubated with buffer alone; ***lanes 2 and 5,*** PF prepared from control adipocytes; ***lanes 3 and 4,*** GS incubated with two different PFs prepared from K^+-exposed cells. The 95-kd band represents a β-subunit of the insulin receptor. (Reproduced with permission from Begum N, Sussman KE, Draznin B. High levels of cytosolic free calcium inhibit dephosphorylation of insulin receptor and glycogen synthase. Cell Calcium 1991;12:423)

Using these experimental models, we recently demonstrated that high levels of cytosolic calcium inhibit insulin's ability to dephosphorylate glycogen synthase (Fig. 24-2) and insulin-regulable glucose transport (Fig. 24-3).[99,100,102,103] This results in an inhibition of glucose transport and its incorporation into glycogen. The mechanism of calcium action centers on its effect on cytosolic protein phosphatase-1 (PP-1), an enzyme activated by the insulin-initiated phosphorylation cascade.[104] PP-1 is phosphorylated by insulin in a site-specific manner in the signaling cascade involving insulin receptor substrate 1 (IRS-1), p21Ras, raf-1 kinase, mitogen-activated protein kinase kinase (MEK), mitogen-activated protein (MAP), and S6 kinases.[105–107] This site-specific phosphorylation increases PP-1 activity, resulting in dephosphorylation of glycogen synthase and GLUT-4.[108,109]

High levels of cytosolic calcium counteract insulin's effect on PP-1, presumably in a cAMP-dependent manner.[102–104,109] Thus, high levels of cytosolic calcium have been found to increase phosphorylation and the activity of inhibitor 1 (Fig. 24-4 and Table 24-1),[104] an endogenous inhibitor of PP-1.[110] At the same time, a cAMP antagonist (RpcAMP) has been found to neutralize the inhibitory effect of calcium on PP-1 activity.[110] The effect of high levels of cytosolic calcium on the phosphorylation state of GLUT-4 also appears to be mediated by cAMP,[102–104] with the cAMP antagonist restoring insulin's ability to dephosphorylate GLUT-4 (Fig. 24-5).[102]

Thus, current evidence suggests that high levels of cytosolic calcium lead to significant inhibition of PP-1 activity. This, in turn, may result in inappropriate dephosphorylation of glycogen synthase, GLUT-4, and, possibly, other insulin-sensitive substrates, thereby contributing to the development of insulin resistance.

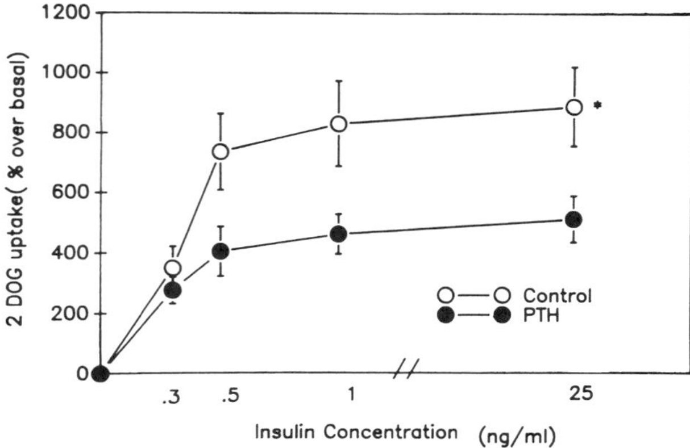

Figure 24-3. Dose-response curve of insulin-stimulated 2-deoxyglucose (2-DOG) uptake in PTH-treated adipocytes. Results represent the mean ± SEM of six experiments ($p < 0.05$). (Reproduced with permission from Reusch JE-B, Begum N, Sussman KE, Draznin B. Regulation of GLUT-4 phosphorylation by intracellular calcium in adipocytes. Endocrinology 1991;129:3269)

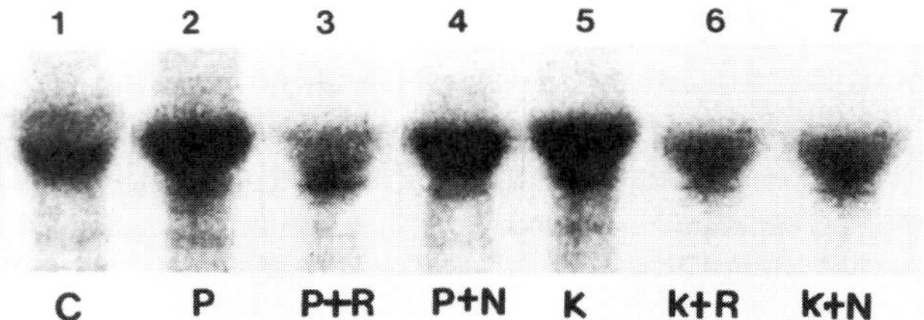

Figure 24-4. Phosphorylation of I1 by elevated intracellular Ca^{++}. Adipocytes were labeled with ^{32}P orthophosphate (0.3 mCi/mL) for 2 hours at 37°C, followed by the addition of PTH (20 ng/mL) or K^+ (40 mM, added at 0, 20, and 40 minutes) in the presence and absence of RpcAMP (10^{-4}M) or nitrendipine (30 μM), as detailed in the text. The incubation was continued for 60 minutes. Extracts of heat-stable protein were normalized for proteins or TCA-precipitable counts and immunoprecipitated with I1 Ab; the immunoprecipitates were then subjected to 12% SDS-PAGE. An autoradiogram of the gel from a representative experiment is shown. ***Lane 1,*** control; ***lane 2,*** PTH; ***lane 3,*** PTH and RpcAMP; ***lane 4,*** PTH and nitrendipine; ***lane 5,*** K^+; ***lane 6,*** K^+ and RpcAMP; ***lane 7,*** K^+ and nitrendipine. Similar results were obtained in five different experiments. (Reproduced with permission from Begum N, Sussman KE, Draznin B. Calcium-induced inhibition of phosphoserine phosphatase in insulin target cells is mediated by the phosphorylation and activation of inhibitor 1. J Biol Chem 1992;267:5959)

Table 24-1. Inhibitor 1 (I1) Activity and ^{32}P Radioactivity of Immunoprecipitated I1 from Control, K^+-, and Parathyroid Hormone (PTH)–exposed Adipocytes

I1	^{32}P Content (cpm/min)	I1 Activity (% inhibition of phosphatase 1)
Control	5014 ± 881	27.5 ± 3.57
PTH	8287 ± 993	52.5 ± 4.37[†]
PTH + RpcAMP	5590 ± 1000	27.6 ± 1.92[‡]
PTH + Nitrendipine	6362 ± 971	35.9 ± 7.98
K^+	7177 ± 208	47.9 ± 5.87[†]
K^+ + RpcAMP	5097 ± 1009	27.7 ± 0.91[‡]
K^+ + Nitrendipine	5190 ± 1000	26.9 ± 3.05[‡]
RpcAMP	5000 ± 600	27.0 ± 1.9
Nitrendipine	4995 ± 490	25.8 ± 0.22

*Method: Adipocytes were labeled with ^{32}Pi (0.3 mCi/mL) for 2 hours followed by exposure to various agents, as indicated in the text. Heat-treated extracts were prepared and equal amounts were immunoprecipitated with I1 antibody. The immunoprecipitates were subjected to sodium dodecyl sulfate/polyacrylamide gel electrophoresis (SDS-PAGE), followed by autoradiography. The corresponding bands were eluted from the gel, counted for radioactivity and tested directly for I1 activity using purified phosphatase 1 and [^{32}P]-labeled phosphorylase 'a.' The data were corrected for variations in I1 content estimated separately by Western blotting of heat-treated extracts. I1 activity is expressed as % inhibition of basal phosphatase 1 activity. Results are the mean ± SEM of three individual experiments performed in duplicate.

[†] $p < 0.05$ versus control

[‡] $p < 0.05$ versus PTH or K^+

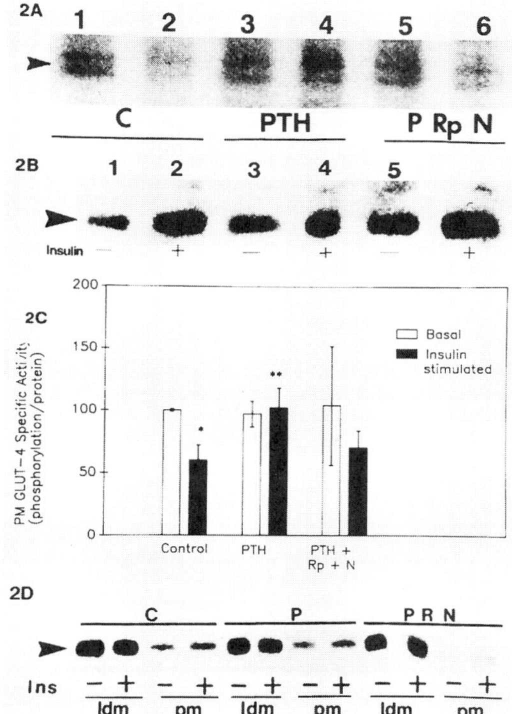

FIGURE 24-5. In vivo phosphorylation of plasma membrane GLUT-4 in control (C) and PTH-treated adipocytes. The cells were equilibrated with ^{32}P for 120 minutes and then exposed to PTH, insulin, nitrendipine (N), and RpcAMP (Rp). The cells were fractionated to isolate plasma membrane (pm) and low-density microsomal (ldm) fractions. GLUT-4 was immunoprecipitated using 1F8 antibody for measurements of phosphorylation (*A*) and for Western blotting with the R820 antibody (*B* and *D*). The arrowheads point to GLUT-4. Adipocytes exposed to insulin are designated by + (lanes 2, 4, and 6). ***Lanes 1 and 2,*** pm GLUT-4 from control cells; ***lanes 3 and 4,*** pm GLUT-4 from PTH-treated cells; ***lanes 5 and 6,*** pm GLUT-4 from the PTH (P)–treated cells preincubated with RpcAMP (Rp) and nitrendipine (N). The results of six independent experiments are summarized in part *C* (mean ± SE). GLUT-4 phosphorylation is expressed in terms of its specific activity (GLUT-4 phosphorylation/GLUT-4 content). *$p < 0.01$ versus basal controls. **$p < 0.05$ versus insulin-stimulated controls. Results of the insulin-stimulated translocation of GLUT-4 from the ldm to the pm fractions are shown in ***D.*** (Reproduced with permission from Reusch JE-B, Sussman KE, Draznin B. Inverse relationship between GLUT-4 phosphorylation and its intrinsic activity. J Biol Chem 1993;268:3348)

Although changes in extracellular pH have been shown to significantly affect both insulin binding and insulin's ability to stimulate glucose transport,[111,112] the influence of pHi on the mechanism of insulin action remains incompletely understood. An alkaline pH has been shown to promote the release of Ca^{++} from the skeletal muscle sarcoplasmic reticulum[113,114] and to stimulate glucose uptake by threefold in rat epitrochlearis muscle.[114] Interestingly, an alkaline pH has also been found to partially inhibit insulin-stimulated glucose uptake in both muscle[114] and adipocytes.[111,112] An increase in pHi may well be involved in the effect of insulin on glycolysis.[74,115] Certain changes in pHi may also be critical for DNA synthesis or protein synthesis, or both.[73,74,111] Additionally, changes in pHi are expected to affect intracellular Ca^{++} levels,[74,116] which, in turn, may alter insulin action (as described earlier).

The impact of alterations in Na^+/K^+-ATPase function on the mechanism of insulin action also remains largely undetermined. Most likely, the influence of such alterations is indirect, involving a chain of events that culminate in a rise in intracellular calcium concentration. Inhibition of Na^+/K^+-ATPase activity and an accumulation of intracellular Na^+ enhance Na^+/Ca^{++} exchange, thereby increasing the intracellular calcium concentration; this, in turn, facilitates insulin resistance.

Derangements of the Ionic Cellular Milieu in Diabetes

Although the diabetic state is known for its profound effect on intracellular ion concentrations,[1,19,22,32,45] the mechanism underlying these changes has not been elucidated completely. Levy, Gavin, and Sowers recently published an excellent review of the alterations in intracellular calcium metabolism that accompany diabetes mellitus.[1] They reported abnormal intracellular calcium regulation in the cardiac muscle, aorta, mesenteric and coronary arteries, skeletal muscle, kidney, liver, erythrocytes, lens, and osteoblasts of diabetic animals. Altered intracellular calcium metabolism has also been observed in arteries, erythrocytes, platelets, and adipocytes of patients with diabetes mellitus. The most common findings associated with both type I and type II diabetes were increases in intracellular calcium and decreases in intracellular magnesium and pH.[1,32]

Abnormalities in the regulation of the intracellular ion concentrations in diabetes have been ascribed to malfunction of the plasma membrane Ca^{++}/Mg^{++}-ATPase and Na^+/K^+-ATPase, and to the Ca^{++} channels.[1,45] At this time, it cannot be stated with certainty which of the multiple mechanisms that governs Ca^{++} homeostasis represent the primary defect in diabetes.

As mentioned earlier, insulin has been shown to attenuate AVP-mediated calcium increases and contractile responses in VSMCs.[69] Because insulin does not alter AVP binding to these cells, it appears that insulin exerts its action at a site distal to the AVP receptor. The mechanism of this attenuation remains unclear, but most likely it involves a postreceptor "cross talk" between the insulin- and AVP-dependent signaling pathways, resulting in attenuation of the AVP signaling. Diminution of this attenuation, as may occur in either diabetes or insulin resistance (either absolute or relative insulin deficiency), may lead to agonist-induced increases in intracellular calcium concentrations, independent of the insulin action of ion pumps and channels.

Chronic hyperglycemia has consistently been associated with an average increase in total body sodium of 10%.[117–119] In patients with diabetes, sodium excretion in response to a saline load or water immersion is blunted.[34,117,120] These findings indicate that hyperglycemia per se can function as an additional mechanism of chronic sodium retention, which, at the cellular level, may result in increased concentrations of intracellular calcium. Moreover, hyperglycemia, independent of insulin, has been found to elevate cytosolic calcium and suppress magnesium and pH in normal human red cells.[121] These abnormalities may then contribute to the development of insulin resistance by interfering with normal flow of insulin signaling.

Conclusions

Insulin's effect on cellular ion handling is an important factor in the overall insulin action. Insulin appears to modulate ion fluxes and, as a result, intracellular concentrations of Ca^{++}, Mg^{++}, K^+, Na^+, H^+, and phosphate (Table 24-2). These changes, in concert with the ion-independent effects of insulin, ensure proper functioning of various insulin-sensitive enzymes. Although the precise role of these ions in the mechanism of insulin action has not been established, it is clear that significant alterations in their concentrations may induce or aggravate insulin resistance. Thus, derangements in the concentrations of the intracellular ions may represent

TABLE 24-2. Effect of Insulin on Intracellular Ions

1. Increased Na^+/H^+ exchange (Na^+ in/H^+ out)
   - Decrease in pH
   - Increase in intracellular Na^+
2. Increased Na^+/K^+ exchange (Na^+ out/K^+ in)
   - Increase in intracellular K^+
3. Increased in intracellular Ca^{++}
   - Tissue-dependent* effects on Ca^{++}/Mg^{++}-ATPase
   - Voltage-dependent Ca^{++} channels
   - Activation of Na^+/Ca^{++} exchange† (Na^+ out/Ca^{++} in)
4. Maintenance of intracellular PO^-_4 and Mg^{++}‡
5. Additional effects of insulin may be mediated by its action on phospholipids or modulation of cellular responses to other hormones and metabolites (e.g., attenuation of the cellular response to vasopressin).

*Both stimulation and inhibition of Ca^{++}/Mg^{++}-ATPase have been demonstrated; the effect of insulin may be tissue-specific.
†Na^+/Ca^{++} exchange has been shown to be activated in the presence of insulin resistance or in the absence of insulin when inadequate activity of Na^+/K^+-ATPase results in an accumulation of intracellular Na^+.
‡The mechanism of low levels of intracellular phosphate and Mg^{++} in diabetes and in the presence of insulin resistance remains enigmatic.

a link between the mechanisms of hypertension and insulin resistance, an important pathophysiologic combination whose genesis continues to baffle investigators and clinicians.

Acknowledgments

This work was supported by the Research Service of the Veterans Affairs and by the Foundation for Biomedical Education and Research. Dr. Reusch is a recipient of the VA Associate Investigator Award. The authors wish to thank Ms. Gloria Smith for her excellent secretarial assistance.

References

1. Levy J, Gavin JR III, Sowers JR. Diabetes mellitus: A disease of abnormal cellular calcium metabolism? Am J Med 1994;96:260
2. Levy J, Gavin JR III, Hammerman MR, Avioli LV. Ca^{2+}-Mg^{2+}-ATPase activity in kidney basolateral membrane in non–insulin-dependent diabetic rats. Effect of insulin. Diabetes 1986;35:899
3. Nishida K, Ohara T, Johnson J, et al. Na^+/K^+-ATPase activity and its αII subunit gene expression in rat skeletal muscle: Influence of diabetes, fasting, and refeeding. Metabolism 1992;41:56
4. Allo SN, Lincoln TM, Wilson GL, et al. Non–insulin-dependent diabetes-induced defects in cardiac cellular calcium regulation. Am J Physiol 1991; 260:C1165
5. Ohara T, Sussman KE, Draznin B. Effect of diabetes on cytosolic free Ca^{2+} and Na^+-K^+-ATPase in rat aorta. Diabetes 1991;40:1560
6. Nakagawa M, Kobayashi S, Kimura I, Kimura M. Diabetic state-induced modification of Ca, Mg, Fe, and Zn content of skeletal, cardiac, and smooth muscles. Endocrinol Jpn 1989;36:795
7. Kobayashi S, Fujihara M, Hoshino N, et al. Diabetic state–induced activation of calcium-activated neutral proteinase in mouse skeletal muscle. Endocrinol Jpn 1989;36:833
8. Taira Y, Hata T, Ganguly PK, et al. Increased sarcolemmal Ca^{2+} transport activity in skeletal muscle of diabetic rats. Am J Physiol 1991;260:E626
9. Ganguly PK, Mathur S, Gupta MP, et al. Calcium pump activity of sarcoplasmic reticulum in diabetic rat skeletal muscle. Am J Physiol 1986;251:E515
10. Levy J, Grunberger G, Karl I, Gavin JR III. Effects of food restriction and insulin treatment on (Ca^{2+}-Mg^{2+})-ATPase response to insulin in kidney basolateral membranes of non–insulin-dependent diabetic rats. Metabolism 1990;39:25
11. Studer RK, Ganas L. Effect of diabetes on hormone-stimulated and basal hepatocyte calcium metabolism. Endocrinology 1989;125:2421
12. Chan KM, Junger KD. The effect of streptozotocin-induced diabetes on the plasma membrane calcium uptake activity of rat liver. Diabetes 1984;33:1072
13. Levy J, Sowers JR, Zemel MB. Abnormal Ca^{2+}-ATPase activity in erythrocytes of non–insulin-dependent diabetic rats. Horm Metab Res 1990;22:136
14. Bergh CH, Hjalmarson A, Holm G, et al. Studies on calcium exchange in platelets in human diabetes. Eur J Clin Invest 1988;18:92
15. Resnick LM. Calcium metabolism in hypertension and allied metabolic disorders. Diabetes Care 1991;14:505
16. Segal S, Lloyd S, Sherman N, et al. Postprandial changes in cytosolic free calcium and glucose uptake in adipocytes in obesity and non–insulin-dependent diabetes mellitus. Hormone Res 1990;34:39
17. Mazzanti L, Rabini RA, Faloia E, et al. Altered cellular Ca^{2+} and Na^+ transport in diabetes mellitus. Diabetes 1990;39:850
18. Ishii H, Umeda F, Hashimoto T, Nawata H. Increased intracellular calcium mobilization in platelets from patients with type 2 (non–insulin-dependent) diabetes mellitus. Diabetologia 1991;34:332
19. Resnick LM, Gupta RK, Bhargava KK, et al. Cellular ions in hypertension, diabetes, and obesity: A nuclear magnetic resonance spectroscopic study. Hypertension 1991;17:951
20. Resnick LM, Gupta RK, Gruenspan H, et al. Hypertension and peripheral insulin resistance: Mediating role of intracellular free magnesium. Am J Hypertens 1990;3:373
21. Barbagallo M, Gupta RK, Resnick LM. Cellular ionic effects of insulin in normal human erythrocytes: A nuclear magnetic resonance study. Diabetologia 1993;36:146
22. Sowers JF, Standley PR, Ram JL, et al. Insulin resistance, carbohydrate metabolism, and hypertension. Am J Hypertens 1991;4:466S
23. Erne P, Bolli P, Bürgisser E, Bühler FR. Correlation of platelet calcium with blood pressure: Effect of antihypertensive therapy. N Engl J Med 1984; 310:1084
24. Lindner A, Kenny M, Meacham AJ. Effects of a circulating factor in patients with essential hypertension on intracellular free calcium in normal platelets. N Engl J Med 1987;316:509
25. Bruschi G, Bruschi ME, Caroppo M, et al. Cytoplasmic free [Ca^{2+}] is increased in the platelets of spontaneously hypertensive rats and essential hypertensive patients. Clin Sci 1985;68:179
26. Lechi A, Lechi C, Bonadonna G, et al. Increased basal and thrombin-induced free calcium in platelets of essential hypertensive patients. Hypertension 1987;9:230
27. Haller H, Lenz T, Thiede M, et al. Platelet intracellular free calcium and hypertension. J Clin Hypertens 1987;3:12
28. Bühler FR, Resink TJ. Platelet membrane and calcium control abnormalities in essential hypertension. Am J Hypertens 1988;1:42
29. Sowers JR. At the cutting edge: Insulin resistance and hypertension. Mol Cell Endocrinol 1990;74:C87
30. Draznin B. Cytosolic calcium and insulin resistance. Am J Kidney Dis 1993;21:32
31. Reusch JE-B, Begum N, Draznin B. Cytosolic calcium as an intracellular mediator of insulin resistance. Cardiovasc Risk Factors 1994;3:1
32. Resnick LM. Ionic basis of hypertension, insulin resistance, vascular disease, and related disorders: The mechanism of "Syndrome X." Am J Hypertens 1993;6:123S
33. Resnick LM, Barbagallo M, Gupta RK, Laragh JH. Ionic basis of hypertension in diabetes mellitus: Role of hyperglycemia. Am J Hypertens 1993;6:413
34. Ferrannini E, Natali A. Insulin resistance and hypertension: Connections with sodium metabolism. Am J Kidney Dis 1993;21:37
35. Reaven GM. Insulin resistance, hyperinsulinemia, hypertriglyceridemia, and hypertension: Parallels between human disease and rodent models. Diabetes Care 1991;14:195
36. DeFronzo RA, Ferrannini E. Insulin resistance: A multifaceted syndrome responsible for NIDDM, obesity, hypertension, dyslipidemia, and atherosclerotic cardiovascular disease. Diabetes Care 1991;14:173
37. Reaven GM. Role of insulin resistance in human disease. Diabetes 1988; 37:1595
38. Aviv A, Lasker N. A common pathway for essential hypertension and non–insulin-dependent diabetes mellitus in blacks: The central role of cytosolic free calcium and the sodium-proton exchange. J Vasc Med Biol 1990;2:91
39. Ferrannini E, DeFronzo RA. The association of hypertension, diabetes, and obesity: A review. J Nephrol 1989;1:3
40. Borle AB. Control, modulation, and regulation of cell calcium. Rev Physiol Biochem Pharmacol 1981;90:113
41. McDonald JM, Pershadsingh HA. The role of calcium in the transduction of insulin action. In: Czech MP, ed. Molecular Basis of Insulin Action. New York: Plenum, 1985;6:103
42. Blaustein MP. The interrelationship between sodium and calcium ions across cell membranes. Rev Physiol Biochem Pharmacol 1974;70:33
43. Carafoli E. Intracellular calcium homeostasis. Ann Rev Biochem 1987;56:395
44. Nicholls DG. Intracellular calcium homeostasis. Br Med Bull 1986;42:353
45. Levy J, Sowers JR. Intracellular Ca^{2+} and insulin action: Possible role in the pathogenesis of Syndrome X. In: Foa PP, Walsh MF, eds. Endocrinology and Metabolism. Vol. 6. New York: Springer-Verlag; 1994:116–136
46. Pershadsingh HA, Landt M, McDonald JM. Calmodulin-sensitive ATP-dependent Ca^{2+} transport across adipocyte plasma membranes. J Biol Chem 1980;225:8983
47. McDonald JM, Chan K-M, Goewert RR, et al. The Ca^{2+}-Mg^{2+}-ATPase of adipocyte plasma membrane. Regulation of calmodulin and insulin. Ann NY Acad Sci 1982;402:381
48. Draznin B. Intracellular calcium, insulin secretion, and action. Am J Med 1988;85:44
49. Kelly KL, Deeney JT, Corkey BE. Cytosolic free calcium in adipocytes. J Biol Chem 1989;264:12754
50. Ishii H, Umeda F, Hashimoto T, Hawata H. Changes in phosphoinositide turnover, Ca^{2+} mobilization, and protein phosphorylation in platelets from NIDDM patients. Diabetes 1990;39:1561

51. Levy J, Reid I, Halstad L, et al. Abnormal cell calcium concentration in cultured bone cells obtained from femurs of obese and non–insulin-dependent diabetic rats. Calcif Tissue Int 1989;44:131
52. Kissebah AH, Clarke P, Vydelingum N, et al. The role of calcium in insulin action. Eur J Clin Invest 1975;5:339
53. Clausen T, Martin BR. The effect of insulin on the washout of [^{45}Ca] calcium from adipocytes and soleus muscle of the rat. Biochem J 1977;164:251
54. Draznin B, Sussman KE, Eckel RH, et al. Possible role of cytosolic free calcium concentrations in mediating insulin resistance of obesity and hyperinsulinemia. J Clin Invest 1988;82:1848
55. Draznin B, Sussman K, Kao M, et al. The existence of an optimal range of cytosolic free calcium for insulin-stimulated glucose transport in rat adipocytes. J Biol Chem 1987;262:14385
56. Klip A, Li G, Logan WJ. Role of calcium ions in insulin action on hexose transport in L6 muscle cells. Am J Physiol 1984;24:E297
57. Byyny RL, LoVerde M, Lloyd S, et al. Cytosolic calcium and insulin resistance in elderly patients with essential hypertension. Am J Hypertens 1992;5:459
58. Pershadsingh HA, McDonald JM. A high affinity calcium-stimulated magnesium-dependent adenosine triphosphate in rat adipocyte plasma membranes. J Biol Chem 1980;255:4087
59. Pershadsingh HA, McDonald JM. Ca^{2+}-Mg^{2+}-ATPase in adipocyte plasmalemma: Inhibition by insulin and Concanavalin A in the intact cell. Biochem Int 1981;2:243
60. Chan K-M, McDonald JM. Identification of an insulin-sensitive calcium-stimulated phosphoprotein in rat adipocyte plasma membranes. J Biol Chem 1982;257:7443
61. Pershadsingh HA, McDonald JM. Hormone receptor coupling and the molecular mechanism of insulin action in the adipocyte: A paradigm for Ca^{2+} homeostasis in the initiation of the insulin-induced metabolic cascade. Cell Calcium 1983;5:111
62. Levy J, Gavin JR III, Morimoto S, et al. Hormonal regulation of (Ca^{2+} + Mg^{2+})-ATPase activity in canine renal basolateral membrane. Endocrinology 1986;119:2405
63. Schaefer W, Priben J, Mannhold R, Gries AF. (Ca^{2+} + Mg^{2+})-ATPase activity of human red blood cells in healthy and diabetic volunteers. Klin Wochenschr 1987;65:17
64. Levy J. Insulin resistance in neonatal NIDDM: Role of abnormal cell Ca^{2+} homeostasis. In: Shafrir E, ed. Frontiers in Diabetes Research: Lessons from Animal Diabetes III. London: Smith-Gordon Press;1991:567–573
65. Levy J, Suzuki Y, Avioli LV, et al. Plasma membrane phospholipid content in non–insulin-dependent streptozotocin-diabetic rats—Effect of insulin. Diabetologia 1988;31:315
66. Borda E, Pascual J, Wald M, Sterin-Borda L. Hypersensitivity to calcium associated with an increased sarcolemmal Ca^{2+}-ATPase activity in diabetic rat heart. Can J Cardiol 1988;4:97
67. Taira Y, Hata T, Ganguly PK, et al. Increased sarcolemmal Ca^{2+} transport activity in skeletal muscle of diabetic rats. Am J Physiol 1991;260:E626
68. Goewert RR, Klaven NB, McDonald JM. Direct effect of insulin on the binding of calmodulin to rat adipocyte plasma membranes. J Biol Chem 1983;258:9995
69. Standley PR, Zhang F, Ram JL, et al. Insulin attenuates vasopressin-induced calcium transients and a voltage-dependent calcium response in rat vascular smooth muscle cells. J Clin Invest 1991;88:1230
70. Standley PR, Bakir MH, Sowers JR. Vascular insulin abnormalities, hypertension, and accelerated atherosclerosis. Am J Kidney Dis 1993;21:39
71. Manchester KL. Speculations on the mechanism of action of insulin. Hormones 1970;1:342
72. Moore RD. Effect of insulin upon the sodium pump in frog skeletal muscle. J Physiol (Lond) 1973;232:23
73. Busa WB, Nuccitelli R. Metabolic regulation via intracellular pH. Am J Physiol 1984;246:R409
74. Moore RD. The case for intracellular pH in insulin action. In: Czech MP, ed. Molecular Basis of Insulin Action. New York: Plenum Press;1985:145–170
75. Moore RD. Elevation of intracellular pH by insulin in frog skeletal muscle. Biochem Biophys Res Comm 1977;91:900
76. Moore RD. Stimulation of Na : H exchange by insulin. Biophys J 1981;33:203
77. Fidelman ML, Seeholzer SH, Walsh KB, Moore RD. Intracellular pH mediates action of insulin on glycolysis in frog skeletal muscle. Am J Physiol 1983;242:C87
78. Moolenaar WH, Tsien RY, van der Saag PT, de Laat SW. Na^+/H^+ exchange and cytoplasmic pH in the action of growth factors in human fibroblasts. Nature 1983;304:645
79. Mukherjee SP, Mukherjee C. Metabolic activation of adipocytes by insulin accompanied by an early increase in intracellular pH. Ann NY Acad Sci 1981;372:347
80. Moore RD, Fidelman ML, Seeholzer SH. Correlation between insulin action upon glycolysis and change in intracellular pH. Biochem Biophys Res Comm 1979;91:905
81. Trivedi B, Danforth WH. Effect of pH on the kinetics of frog muscle phosphofructokinase. J Biol Chem 1966;241:4110
82. Moore RD. Effect of insulin upon ion transport. Biochim Biophys Acta 1983;737:1
83. Resh MD. Insulin action on the (Na^+,K^+)ATPase. In: Czech MP, ed. Molecular Basis of Insulin Action. New York: Plenum Press;1985:451–464
84. Glynn IM, Karlish SJD. The sodium pump. Ann Rev Physiol 1975;37:13
85. Robinson JD, Flashner MS. The (Na^+ + K^+) activated ATPase: Enzymatic and transport properties. Biochim Biophys Acta 1979;549:145
86. Sweadner KJ. Isozymes of the Na^+/K^+-ATPase. Biochim Biophys Acta 1989;988:185
87. Lytton J. Insulin affects the sodium affinity of the rat adipocyte (Na^+ + K^+)-ATPase. J Biol Chem 1985;260:10075
88. Clausen T, Everts ME. Regulation of the Na,K pump in skeletal muscle. Kidney Int 1989;35:1
89. Gourley DRH, Bethea MD. Insulin effect on adipocyte tissue sodium and potassium. Proc Soc Exp Biol Med 1964;115:821
90. Resh MD. Development of insulin responsiveness of the glucose transporter and the (Na^+, K^+) adenosine triphosphatase during in vitro adipocyte differentiation. J Biol Chem 1982;257:6978
91. Fehlmann M, Freychet P. Insulin and glucagon stimulation of (Na^+-K^+)-ATPase transport activity in isolated rat hepatocytes. J Biol Chem 1981; 256:7449
92. Clausen T, Kohn PG. The effect of insulin on the transport of sodium and potassium in rat soleus muscle. J Physiol (Lond) 1977;265:19
93. Resh MD. Quantitation and characterization of the (Na^+, K^+) adenosine triphosphatase in the rat adipocyte plasma membrane. J Biol Chem 1982; 257:11946
94. Clausen T. Regulation of active Na^+/K^+ transport in skeletal muscle. Physiol Rev 1986;66:542
95. Rosic NK, Standaert ML, Pollet RJ. The mechanism of insulin stimulation of (Na^+,K^+)-ATPase transport activity in muscle. J Biol Chem 1985;260:6206
96. Draznin B, Lewis D, Houlder N, et al. Mechanism of insulin resistance induced by sustained levels of cytosolic free calcium in rat adipocytes. Endocrinology 1989;125:2341
97. Begum N, Sussman KE, Draznin B. Differential effects of diabetes on adipocyte and liver phosphotyrosine and phosphoserine phosphatase activities. Diabetes 1991;40:1620
98. Pershadsingh HA, Shade DL, Delfert DM, McDonald JM. Chelation of intracellular calcium blocks insulin action in the adipocyte. Proc Natl Acad Sci USA 1987;84:1025
99. Begum N, Sussman KE, Draznin B. High levels of cytosolic free calcium inhibit dephosphorylation of insulin receptor and glycogen synthase. Cell Calcium 1991;12:423
100. Reusch JE-B, Begum N, Sussman KE, Draznin B. Regulation of GLUT-4 phosphorylation by intracellular calcium in adipocytes. Endocrinology 1991; 129:3269
101. Lytton J, Westlin M, Hanley MR. Thapsigargin inhibits the sarcoplasmic or endoplasmic reticulum Ca-ATPase family of calcium pumps. J Biol Chem 1991;266:17067
102. Begum N, Leitner W, Reusch JE-B, et al. GLUT-4 phosphorylation and its intrinsic activity: Mechanism of Ca^{2+}-induced inhibition of insulin-stimulated glucose transport. J Biol Chem 1993;268:3352
103. Reusch JE-B, Sussman KE, Draznin B. Inverse relationship between GLUT-4 phosphorylation and its intrinsic activity. J Biol Chem 1993;268:3348
104. Begum N, Sussman KE, Draznin B. Calcium-induced inhibition of phosphoserine phosphatase in insulin target cells is mediated by the phosphorylation and activation of inhibitor 1. J Biol Chem 1992;267:5959
105. Dent P, Lavoinne A, Nakielny S, et al. The molecular mechanism by which insulin stimulates glycogen synthesis in mammalian skeletal muscle. Nature 1990;348:302
106. Moller DE, Flier JS. Insulin resistance—Mechanisms, syndromes, and implications. N Engl J Med 1991;325:938
107. Lavoinne A, Erikson E, Maller JL, et al. Purification and characterization of the insulin-stimulated protein kinase from rabbit skeletal muscle, close similarity to S6 kinase II. Eur J Biochem 1991;199:723
108. Dent P, Campbell DG, Candwell FB, Cohen P. Identification of three in vivo phosphorylation sites on the glycogen-binding subunit of protein phosphatase 1 from rabbit skeletal muscle, and their response to adrenaline. FEBS Lett 1990;259:281
109. Begum N, Olefsky JM, Draznin B. Mechanism of impaired metabolic signaling by a truncated human insulin receptor: Decreased activation of protein phosphatase 1 by insulin. J Biol Chem 1993;268:7917
110. Cohen P. Protein phosphorylation and hormone action. Proc Royal Soc (Lond) 1988;234:115
111. Sonne O, Gliemann J, Linde S. Effect of pH on binding kinetics and biological effect of insulin in rat adipocytes. J Biol Chem 1981;256:6250
112. Toyoda N, Robinson FW, Smith MM, et al. Apparent translocation of glucose transport activity in rat epididymal adipocytes by insulin-like effects of high pH or hyperosmolarity. J Biol Chem 1986;261:2117
113. Dettbarn C, Palade P. Effects of alkaline pH on sarcoplasmic reticulum Ca^{2+} release and Ca^{2+} uptake. J Biol Chem 1991;266:8993
114. Ren J-M, Youn JH, Gulve EA, et al. Effects of alkaline pH on the stimulation of glucose transport in rat skeletal muscle. Biochim Biophys Acta 1993; 1145:199
115. Bonen A, McDermott JC, Tan MH. Glycogenesis and glyconeogenesis in skeletal muscle: Effects of pH and hormones. Am J Physiol 1990;258:E693
116. Aviv A. Prospective review: The link between cytosolic Ca^{2+} and the Na^+-H^+ antiport: A unifying factor for essential hypertension. J Hypertens 1988;6:685
117. O'Hare JP, Corrall RJM. De Natrio Diabeticorum: Increase exchangeable sodium in diabetes. Diabetic Med 1988;5:22
118. Feldt-Rasmussen B, Mathiesen ER, Deckert T, et al. Central role for sodium in the pathogenesis of blood pressure changes independent of angiotensin,

aldosterone and catecholamines in Type 1 (insulin-dependent) diabetes mellitus. Diabetologia 1987;30:610

119. DeChatel R, Weidmann P, Flammer J, et al. Sodium, renin-aldosterone, catecholamines and blood pressure in diabetes mellitus. Kidney Int 1977; 12:412

120. DeFronzo RA, Cooke CR, Andres R, et al. The effect of insulin on renal sodium, potassium, calcium, and phosphate in man. J Clin Invest 1975;55:845

121. Barbagallo M, Gupta RK, Resnick LM. Independent effects of hyperinsulinemia on intracellular sodium in normal human red cells. Am J Hypertens 1990;6:264

Diabetes Mellitus, edited by Derek LeRoith, Simeon I. Taylor, and Jerrold M. Olefsky. Lippincott–Raven Publishers, Philadelphia © 1996.

CHAPTER 25
Gene Regulation

RICHARD M. O'BRIEN AND DARYL K. GRANNER

Insulin regulates metabolism by altering the concentration of critical proteins or by producing activity-altering modifications of preexisting enzyme molecules. The latter represents a well-recognized action of insulin, and it has been extensively studied for many years.[1] By contrast, it is only over the past 5 years that considerable advances have been made in understanding several aspects of insulin-regulated gene expression. This facet of insulin action is wide-ranging in that insulin affects the expression of many more genes (>100) than it does the activity of preexisting enzymes.[2,3]

Although insulin could potentially affect any of the multiple steps in the flow of information from gene to protein, to date, it appears that transcription, mRNA stability, and translation are the primary sites of insulin action. As the regulation of protein synthesis and mRNA stability by insulin have been the subjects of several recent and excellent reviews,[4–6] this chapter focuses principally on insulin-regulated gene transcription. It is clear that insulin can have positive and negative effects on the transcription of specific genes, even within the same cell.[2,3] In addition, the genes regulated by insulin encode proteins involved in a variety of biologic phenomena (Fig. 25-1). Several of these mRNAs direct the synthesis of enzymes that have a well-established metabolic connection to insulin, whereas others represent major secretory proteins/hormones, integral membrane proteins, oncogenes, transcription factors, and structural proteins (see Fig. 25-1). Not unexpectedly, this type of regulation is seen in the primary tissues associated with the metabolic actions of insulin—namely, liver, muscle, and adipose tissue—but insulin also regulates gene expression in tissues not commonly associated with these metabolic effects.[2,3]

Investigators have utilized the *cis/trans* model of transcriptional control to understand how insulin regulates gene transcription at a molecular level.[2,7] Briefly stated, the fidelity and frequency of initiation of transcription of eukaryotic genes is mediated by the interaction of *cis*-acting DNA elements with *trans*-acting factors. The specific sequence of the *cis*-acting element determines which *trans*-acting factor will bind. Several *cis*-acting elements that mediate the effect of insulin on gene transcription have recently been defined. These are referred to as insulin response sequences or elements (IRSs/IREs). To date, the general consensus is that there is no consensus IRS/IRE! In this chapter the identification of the most well-studied IRSs/IREs and the putative *trans*-acting factors with which they are associated are described in detail. When appropriate, models that describe how an insulin-regulated transcription factor might function in the particular context of a specific gene promoter are discussed. The construction and utilization of fusion genes (in which the gene promoter of interest is ligated to a reporter gene, such as that encoding the bacterial enzyme chloramphenicol acetyltransferase [CAT]), in combination with transient/stable transfection and transgenic mouse studies, for the purpose of identifying the IRSs/IREs described by various investigators, are described in detail elsewhere.[2,7]

The physiologic importance of insulin-regulated gene transcription is apparent from studies on the glycolytic and gluconeogenic pathways, which can be viewed as a series of three opposing substrate cycles.[8] As shown in Table 25-1, insulin and glucagon have antagonistic actions on the expression of the genes encoding all of the key regulatory enzymes in these three cycles.[8] The biochemical mechanisms that mediate this antagonism are of considerable interest, and it is already apparent that different mechanisms are utilized with different genes. Thus, for example, insulin inhibits the stimulation of phosphoenolpyruvate carboxykinase (*PEPCK*) gene transcription by cAMP (see the later section on PEPCK), whereas cAMP inhibits the stimulation of hepatic glucokinase gene transcription by insulin.[9] Most importantly, it now appears that defects in gene expression, although not necessarily involving insulin-regulated gene expression, may be important in the etiology of non–insulin-dependent diabetes mellitus (NIDDM). Thus, reduced expression of GLUT-2 or glucokinase may be involved in the β-cell insulin secretory defect;[10,11] increased PEPCK gene expression may lead to an increase in hepatic glucose production (HGP);[12] and reduced GLUT-4/Hexokinase II (HK II) expression and Rad overexpression may be the cause of reduced peripheral glucose utilization (PGU).[12,13] In addition, recent data have implicated altered tumor necrosis factor-α (TNF-α) and PC1 gene expression in the generation of insulin resistance.[14,15] Finally, some exciting studies on apolipoprotein CIII gene expression have revealed that a mutation in a PEPCK IRS-like element (see section on PEPCK) may be the cause of some forms of hypertriglyceridemia (HTG).[16]

One of the most important questions in the study of insulin-regulated gene transcription is how a signal passes from the insulin receptor in the plasma membrane through the cytoplasm and the nuclear membrane to a specific *trans*-acting factor binding to an IRS. The basic mechanism whereby steroid hormones activate a combined receptor/transcription factor has been understood for some time, but for peptide hormones, much less is known.[17]

The available data suggest that insulin may mediate its action on gene transcription by two basic mechanisms: (1) through plasma membrane–initiated changes in nuclear protein phosphorylation/dephosphorylation and (2) more directly, via intracellular receptors.

Intracellular Enzymes
Glucokinase (+)
Hexokinase II (+)
Malic enzyme (+)
Pyruvate kinase (+)
Fatty acid synthetase (+)
Acetyl-CoA carboxylase (+)
Tyrosine aminotransferase (−)
Phosphoenolpyruvate carboxykinase (−)
Microsomal triglyceride transfer protein (−)
Glyceraldehyde-3-phosphate dehydrogenase (+)

Integral Membrane Proteins
Thyrotropin (TSH) receptor (+)
Glucose transporter, GLUT-1 (+)
Glucose transporter, GLUT-4 (−/+)

Hormones/Secreted Proteins
Amylase (+)
Prolactin (+)
Glucagon (−)
Growth hormone (−)
Apolipoprotein CIII (−)
IGF-Binding protein-1 (−)
α_1-Acid glycoprotein (−/+)

Proto-Oncogenes/ Transcription Factors
c-*src* (+)
c-*fos* (+)
c-*jun* (+)
p21^{ras} (+)
C/EBP α, β, δ (−/+)

Reproductive Proteins
β-Casein (+)
Ovalbumin (+)

Brain Proteins
IGF II (−/+)
Neuropeptide Y (−)

Miscellaneous
Gene 33 (+)
δ1-Crystallin (+)
Thyroglobulin (+)

FIGURE 25-1. Insulin regulates the transcription of genes involved in a variety of biologic phenomena. +, insulin stimulates transcription; −, insulin inhibits transcription. (See refs. 2 and 3 for

There have been several reports indicating that internalized peptide hormones (see ref. 18 for review), including insulin,[19] directly mediate transcriptional changes in the nucleus. In addition, there have been sporadic reports of nuclear receptors for insulin (see ref. 20 and the references therein), but the mechanism by which insulin is translocated to the nucleus is unclear.

It has been known for some time that insulin stimulates the phosphorylation of certain abundant nuclear proteins, such as the lamins and nucleolin (see ref. 21 and the references therein). The identification of specific IRS-binding, low-abundance transcription factors, however, and the analysis of changes in their phosphorylation state in response to insulin, has progressed more slowly. An analysis of other peptide hormone signaling pathways suggests that insulin-stimulated changes in transcription factor phosphorylation could potentially affect transcription factor (1) nuclear translocation, (2) DNA binding activity, (3) transactivation potential, or all three.[22,23] Recent advances in the understanding of the initial events in insulin action (see Chapter 16 and refs. 6 and 24) have certainly narrowed the gap between the insulin receptor and the IRS. A link between insulin-induced changes in the activity of enzymes through the mechanism of (serine/threonine) phosphorylation/dephosphorylation and insulin-stimulated insulin receptor tyrosine kinase activity has been made through insulin receptor substrate-1 (IRS-1).[6,24] Similarly, the studies of principally Cohen and colleagues[25] have revealed how insulin can induce concomitant increases and decreases in the phosphorylation of specific proteins within the same cell. Moreover, for two IRSs—namely the c-*fos* serum response element (SRE) and the AP-1 motif (both of which are discussed in greater detail later in this chapter)—a complete pathway from the insulin receptor to an IRS is almost established. These pathways are reviewed in detail below, although it should be emphasized that neither the SRE nor the AP-1 motif mediates a signal specific for insulin, as multiple other growth factors also activate transcription through SRE/AP-1 motifs. These studies suggest, however, that the mechanism(s) involved in the action of insulin in changing enzyme activity and gene expression are not mutually exclusive; common signaling pathways may mediate both effects. Clearly, the gap between IRS-1 and the IRS is narrowing.

Identification of Positive Insulin Response Sequences

Glyceraldehyde-3-Phosphate Dehydrogenase

The glycolytic enzyme glyceraldehyde-3-phosphate dehydrogenase (GAPDH) catalyzes the conversion of glyceraldehyde-3-phosphate to 1,3-diphosphoglycerate. In their initial studies, Alexander and colleagues[26,27] demonstrated that insulin causes a threefold increase in GAPDH mRNA in the H4IIE rat hepatoma cell line and a 10-fold change in the 3T3 F442A adipocyte cell line. Using the transient transfection of GAPDH/CAT fusion genes, they then demonstrated that the stimulatory effect of insulin on human GAPDH gene expression is mediated through *cis*-acting sequences located between −488 and +21.[27] From an analysis of the effect of insulin on expression of additional GAPDH/CAT fusion gene constructs, Nasrin et al.[28] demonstrated that the GAPDH promoter contains two

TABLE 25-1. Insulin and Glucagon (cAMP) Have Opposing Actions on the Expression of Key Glycolytic/Gluconeogenic Enzyme-Encoding Genes

	Enzyme	Effect of Insulin	Effect of cAMP
↑ Glycolysis	Glucokinase	+	−
	6-Phosphofructo-1-kinase	+	−
	Pyruvate kinase	+	−
↑↓	6-Phosphofructo-2-kinase/ fructose-2,6-bisphosphatase	+	−
Gluconeogenesis ↓	Phosphoenolpyruvate carboxykinase	−	+
	Fructose-1,6-bisphosphatase	−	+
	Glucose-6-phosphatase	−	+

independent insulin response elements, designated IRE-A (located between −488 and −409) and IRE-B (located between −308 and −269). The core sequence of IRE-A is shown in Table 25-2. It has a close homology with sequences in the promoters of a number of other insulin-regulated genes.[28]

Nasrin et al.[29] used an expression screening approach to clone a protein (designated IRE-ABP) that binds to the 3′ domain of the GAPDH IRE-A. The sequence specificity of this factor overlaps that of an adipocyte nuclear protein (designated IRP-A) that binds the core IRE sequence defined in the GAPDH promoter.[28] Insulin induces the binding of IRP-A to IRE-A.[28] The present lack of knowledge about the transcription factors that bind to the IRSs/IREs in other genes prevents an assessment of whether this is a common mechanism of insulin action. IRE-ABP is a member of the HMG class of transcription factors and is 67% identical within its high mobility group (HMG) box domain to the gene encoding the testis-determining factor SRY.[29,30] GAPDH gene expression is induced 8 to 20 fold during the switch from the fasted to the refed state.[28] This same manipulation induces IRP-A binding to IRE-A[28] and IRE-ABP mRNA expression.[31] Whether insulin action on GAPDH gene expression is mediated through IRE-ABP or IRP-A, or both, however, is as yet unclear. Alexander and colleagues have suggested that insulin-stimulated phosphorylation of both IRP-A[32] and IRE-ABP[31] may be involved in the effect of insulin on GAPDH gene expression.

c-*fos*

The cellular homologue of the transforming gene of FBJ murine osteosarcoma virus is c-*fos*. Insulin stimulates c-*fos* gene transcription in H4IIE cells[33] and in their initial transient transfection experiments using c-*fos*/CAT fusion genes, Blackshear and colleagues[34] showed that the c-*fos* promoter sequence from −356 to +109 was sufficient to mediate the insulin response. Mutation of four base pairs in the c-*fos* SRE, known to abolish the response to serum, also nullified the effect of insulin on the expression of the c-*fos*/CAT construct.[34] That this region (located between −320 and −299 in the c-*fos* promoter) contains an IRS has been confirmed by demonstrating that it transfers the insulin response to a heterologous promoter.[35] The sequence of the c-*fos* SRE is compared with other IRSs in Table 25-2.

There has been considerable progress in understanding the mechanism by which insulin transmits a signal from the insulin receptor in the plasma membrane to the c-*fos* IRS (SRE) in the nucleus. A multicomponent pathway has been elucidated in which tyrosine-phosphorylated IRS-1 binds GRB2 through its SH2 domain.[6,24] GRB2 acts as an adaptor molecule and binds, through an SH3 domain, the guanine nucleotide exchange factor mSOS. In turn, mSOS promotes the formation of the active, guanosine triphosphate (GTP)–bound form of $p21^{ras}$, which leads to the activation of the serine/threonine kinase raf-1.[6,24] The dual-specificity protein kinase MAP/ERK kinase (MEK), which is phosphorylated and activated by raf-1, phosphorylates and activates members of the mitogen activated protein kinase (MAP) kinase family by phosphorylation of both tyrosine and threonine residues.[6,24] Cohen and colleagues[25] have elucidated the mechanisms whereby activation of the MAP kinase cascade may mediate the stimulation of glycogen synthesis by insulin. In addition, because MAP kinase translocates to the nucleus following stimulation of cells with serum or growth factors,[36] it may influence gene transcription directly through the phosphorylation of transcription factors. MAP kinase can phosphorylate and activate $p90^{rsk}$ MAP kinase–activated protein kinase–1 (MAPKAPK-1),[37] whereas $p90^{rsk}$ can phosphorylate and inactivate glycogen synthase kinase-3 (GSK-3).[38] Thus, the action of MAP kinase on gene transcription may be mediated indirectly via $p90^{rsk}$ or GSK-3, both of which are found in the nucleus.[36,39]

A number of studies have implicated this MAP kinase pathway in insulin-stimulated c-*fos* gene transcription.[35,40,41] For example, overexpression of wild-type ras promotes insulin-stimulated c-*fos*

TABLE 25-2. Comparison of Insulin Response Sequences*

Gene	Insulin Response Sequence	Location
Collagenase AP-1	TGAGTCA	−66
c-*fos* SRE	TTACACAGGATGTCCATATTAGGACATCTGCGTCAGC Ets SRF AP-1	−291
Pyruvate kinase	GCGCACGGGGCACTCCCGTGGTTCC E-Box E-Box	−144
Glucagon	TAGTTTTTCACGCCTGACTGAGATTGAAGGG C1A/C1B	−238
GAPDH	AAGTTCCCCAACTTTCCCGCCTCTCAGCCTTTGAAAG IRP-A IRE-ABP	−444
Prolactin	TCTTAATGACGGAAATAGATGATTGGGAGG	−77
FAS	GCCCATGTGGCGTGGCC	−52
α-Amylase	TATTTTGCGTGAGAGTTTCTAAAAGTCCATCACCTGTTCACATC IRF? PTF1 Repressor	−119
PEPCK	TCACAGCTGTGGTGTTTTGACAACCAG IRF	−399
IGFBP-1	CACTAGCAAAACAAACTTATTTTGAACAC IRF IRF	−96
TAT	GACTAGAACAAACAAGTCCTGCGTA IRF	−2420

*The identification of the various insulin response sequences shown is described in the text. The underlined regions represent either the IRS core sequence or a *trans*-acting factor binding site (see text). An Ets binding motif and AP-1 motif are located 5′ and 3′, respectively, of the core SRF binding motif in the c-*fos* SRE. The pyruvate kinase IRS is a combined insulin/glucose response element. The GAPDH IRE binds two factors: IRP-A and IRE-ABP. The PEPCK, IGFBP-1, and TAT IRSs share a common T(G/A)TTT motif that may be recognized by a common factor, IRF. This motif is also present in the amylase IRS, but 5′ of the core sequence. DNA sequences are numbered relative to the transcription start site.

gene expression,[41] whereas overexpression of dominant negative mutants of p21[ras] (and raf-1) blocks insulin-stimulated c-*fos* gene expression.[35,40] Clearly, the identification of an SRE-binding protein whose phosphorylation by a component of the MAP kinase cascade leads to a change in c-*fos* expression would complete a pathway from insulin receptor to SRE.

A number of SRE-binding proteins have been identified,[42] the most prominent of which is the 67-kd serum response factor ($p67^{SRF}$). Others include NFIL6, Phox 1, and DBF/MAPF1.[42] An Ets domain-binding motif (CAGGAT) is located just 5′ of the SRE shown in Table 25-1; this Ets motif is recognized by $p62^{TCF}$ (ternary complex factor),[42] which only binds the c-*fos* SRE as a complex with $p67^{SRF}$. In gel retardation assays, using nuclear extracts from insulin-treated cells, Blackshear and colleagues[43,44] have shown that the formation of an SRE-protein complex (designated "band 2") increases. Several lines of evidence suggest that band 2 is a ternary complex consisting of the SRE, $p67^{SRF}$, and $p62^{TCF}$,[43,44] and that insulin may stimulate its formation via phosphorylation of $p62^{TCF}$. Because MAP kinase phosphorylates Elk-1 (a protein highly homologous to $p62^{TCF}$), leading to increased binding[45] and/or transcriptional activity of the ternary complex,[46] this would appear to establish a direct connection between an insulin-stimulated protein kinase and an IRS-binding protein, thus potentially explaining the mechanism of insulin action on c-*fos* gene expression. Unfortunately, a detailed mutagenesis study by Thompson et al.[44] has demonstrated that the effect of insulin on c-*fos* gene transcription does not correlate with band 2 formation. However, Blackshear and colleagues[44] have identified a second complex (designated "band 3"), the formation of which is also increased in gel retardation assays using extracts from insulin-treated cells. The time course for formation of band 3 (and band 2) correlates with the induction of c-*fos* gene transcription by insulin.[44] The only DNA-binding protein in the band 3 complex appears to be $p67^{SRF}$, but Thompson et al.[44] have suggested that the effect of insulin is mediated indirectly via other unidentified proteins that associate with $p67^{SRF}$ through protein-protein interactions. Thus, although the MAP kinase pathway is implicated in insulin-stimulated c-*fos* gene transcription, the precise *trans*-acting factor that mediates this action of insulin (directly or indirectly) has yet to be identified conclusively.

Phorbol esters, which are known to activate certain members of the protein kinase C (PKC) family, mimic the action of insulin on several genes. For example, phorbol esters and insulin induce a similar increase in c-*fos* mRNA levels in 3T3-L1 adipocytes[47] and H4IIE hepatoma cells.[48] Similarly, phorbol esters, like insulin, inhibit both basal and glucocorticoid-stimulated PEPCK gene transcription.[49] Prolonged treatment of various tissue culture lines with phorbol esters, however, abolishes the inhibitory effect of a subsequent phorbol ester treatment on both PEPCK and c-*fos* gene expression, whereas the effect of insulin is unaltered.[47,48,50]

Even though such pretreatment with phorbol esters is now known to downregulate only some PKC family members,[51] this result would indicate that insulin and phorbol esters act through a different pathway with regard to both PEPCK and c-*fos* gene expression. These results with c-*fos* gene expression are at odds with those obtained later by Messina et al.,[52] who found that a similar phorbol ester pretreatment reduced the subsequent induction of c-*fos* gene transcription by insulin. Messina et al.[52] did not comment on the earlier c-*fos* studies, and their results have recently been challenged by Stumpo et al.[53] who were able to repeat the initial result indicating no effect of PKC downregulation on insulin-stimulated c-*fos* mRNA accumulation. Stumpo et al.[53] did acknowledge, however, that their results did not rule out the involvement of a "nonclassical," phorbol ester–insensitive form of PKC in insulin action.[51] However, insulin treatment has yet to be shown to activate such PKC isozymes in vivo and, in any case, such an activation would not explain the conflicting data with phorbol esters on c-*fos* gene expression.

Despite the considerable controversy that persists with regard to the role of PKC in insulin action (see Chapter 19), it is apparent that both insulin (Table 25-2) and phorbol esters[54] affect gene expression through multiple, distinct *cis*-acting elements. At least eight distinct phorbol ester response sequences have been identified,[54] but whether insulin can mediate transcriptional effects through these elements is largely unknown. The exceptions to date are the AP-1 motif and c-*fos* SRE, which can mediate a stimulatory effect of both phorbol esters[42,54] and insulin on gene transcription (see the later section and the earlier discussion on the AP-1 motif).

Prolactin

Insulin stimulates transcription of the prolactin gene in the GH_3 rat pituitary cell line,[55] although the increase in the rate of transcription does not entirely account for the full effect of insulin in inducing prolactin protein levels.[55] The prolactin IRS was initially mapped to a region of the promoter between −212 and +73;[56] subsequently, Stanley[57] demonstrated that deletion of the prolactin promoter sequence between −106 and −96 abolished the stimulatory effect of insulin in rat pituitary GH_4 cells. Moreover, the amount or affinity of a nuclear factor binding a region from −106 to −87 was found to be stimulated by insulin.[57] More recently, Jacob and Stanley[58] concluded, from data derived using internal deletions and a linker scanning analysis of the prolactin promoter, that the primary insulin response region is located between −97 and −87, and that the region between −76 and −67 is also required for a full insulin response. From a comparison of the DNA sequence of the two regions between −97 and −87, and between −76 and −67, Jacob and Stanley[58] suggested that the prolactin IRS is composed of the dyad repeat sequence CGGAA(A/G)(T/A)(A/G) GAT, with a 10-bp intervening sequence. The prolactin IRS (−106 to −77) functions in the context of a heterologous promoter,[58] and the sequence of the critical region from −97 to −87 is underlined in Table 25-2. Although the complement to this sequence bears some resemblance to the T(G/A)TTT IRS core sequence found in the PEPCK, TAT, and IGFBP-1 genes (see the section on negative IRSs), the induction of prolactin gene expression by insulin is, by comparison, much slower.[55] Therefore, a different mechanism of insulin action, and presumably a different *trans*-acting factor, is probably involved.

Fatty Acid Synthetase

Fatty acid synthetase (FAS) plays a central role in de novo lipogenesis in mammals. Paulauskis and Sul demonstrated that insulin increases FAS gene transcription in the livers of diabetic mice.[59] The effect is rapid (3.5 fold after 30 minutes), and reaches a maximum sevenfold increase after 2 hours of insulin treatment.[59] cAMP abolishes this stimulation, as does cycloheximide, suggesting that ongoing protein synthesis is required for this action of insulin.[59]

In their initial studies of the insulin-stimulated expression of transiently transfected FAS-CAT reporter genes in 3T3-L1 adipocytes, Sul and colleagues demonstrated that the FAS IRS is located in a region between −332 to + 67 in the FAS promoter.[60] Subsequently, Moustaid et al. precisely mapped this IRS to a region between −68 and −52.[61]

When multimerized and ligated to a heterologous promoter, the FAS IRS confers a stimulatory effect of insulin on reporter gene expression.[61] The sequence of this element is shown in Table 25-2. The FAS IRS bears some resemblance to those in the GAPDH and amylase promoters, but competition studies suggest that different proteins bind to each of these elements.[61] In addition, isolation and analysis of nuclear extracts from insulin-treated cells reveal no change in the pattern of protein binding to the FAS IRS,[61] which is also distinct from results obtained in similar experiments with the GAPDH and prolactin IRSs/IREs (see previous sections).

Amylase

Alpha-amylase catalyzes the digestion of dietary starch. Two classes of pancreas-specific amylase genes, designated Amy-2.1 and Amy-2.2, are present in the mouse genome. Expression of the Amy-2.2 gene is stimulated by insulin and carbohydrate, whereas expression of the Amy-2.1 gene is only minimally responsive to either.[62] Meisler and colleagues[63,64] have made extensive use of transgenic animals to delineate an Amy-2.2 IRS. Hybrid constructs containing sequences from the amylase promoter ligated to the insulin-unresponsive elastase promoter were coupled to the CAT reporter gene.[63,64] These heterologous constructs were introduced into the germ line of mice and the effect of diabetes on CAT expression was measured. An elastase/CAT construct containing a 30-bp fragment of the amylase promoter (from −167 to −138) was much less active in diabetic mice than in control mice.[63] Meisler and colleagues concluded, therefore, that this 30-bp fragment was an IRS.[63] More recently, three 10-bp block mutations of this 30-bp IRS were analysed in the context of the same elastase-CAT fusion gene, again in transgenic mice.[64] One of these mutants was defective in mediating the insulin response in that it gave constitutive CAT expression in diabetic animals.[64] This result suggests that the mutant sequence destroys the binding site for a repressor. Interestingly, the location of this putative repressor binding site is in the spacer region between the two half-sites required for binding of pancreatic transcription factor 1 (PTF1) (Fig. 25-2). A protein-binding activity in pancreatic nuclear extracts (distinct from PTF1) that recognizes this spacer region was detected.[64] Neither the binding activity of this factor nor PTF1 is altered when nuclear extracts from control or diabetic rats are compared.[64] Thus, Meisler and colleagues present a model in which the amylase IRS binds both a repressor and PTF1. In the absence of insulin, the repressor interferes with the transactivation potential of PTF1 (see Fig. 25-2), whereas in the presence of insulin, the repressor is disabled (see Fig. 25-2), possibly by a phosphorylation-dependent mechanism.[64]

The promoter sequence encompassing the amylase IRE is shown in Table 25-2. It contains the T(G/A)TTT motif found in the PEPCK, IGFBP-1, and TAT IRSs (see the following). However,

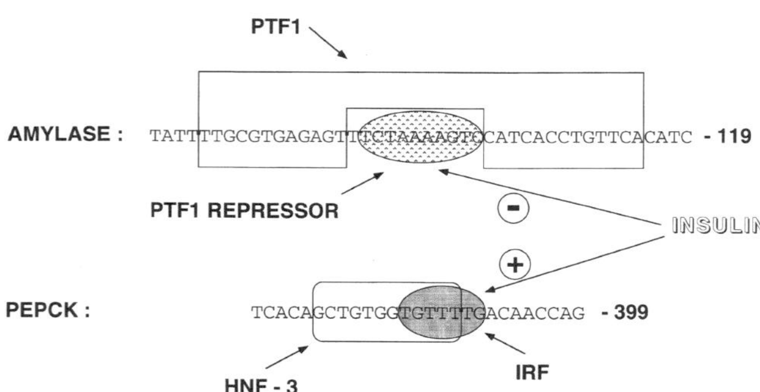

Figure 25-2. Model of insulin-regulated PEPCK and amylase gene transcription. In the PEPCK gene, insulin is hypothesized to mediate its negative effect on glucocorticoid-stimulated gene transcription via an unidentified protein IRF. Insulin is postulated to activate IRF (+), which then interferes with the binding/transactivation potential of HNF-3. In the amylase gene, insulin is hypothesized to mediate its stimulatory effect on transcription by disabling (−) a PTF1 repressor. The precise boundaries of the sequences recognized by the PTF1 repressor and IRF are unknown. Details of these models are provided in the text. DNA sequence is labeled relative to the transcription start site.

this appears to be purely coincidental, as this motif is 5′ of the IRE core sequence (Table 25-2, underlined portion).

Pyruvate Kinase

The action of insulin on both PEPCK and glucokinase is independent of the presence of glucose.[8,65] For many insulin-regulated genes, however, the action of insulin is dependent on the presence of glucose.[8,65] The regulation of gene transcription by carbohydrates has recently been the subject of intensive investigation, and the L-type pyruvate kinase gene is a paradigm for such studies (see ref. 65 for a review).

L-type pyruvate kinase catalyzes the final step in glycolysis, the conversion of phosphoenolpyruvate to pyruvate. Insulin acts in a permissive fashion, along with glucose, to increase the transcription of the L-type pyruvate kinase gene in the liver.[66,67] A combined glucose/insulin response element has been identified in the pyruvate kinase gene promoter between −168 and −144,[68,69] and the sequence of this region is shown in Table 25-2. This element consists of two imperfect E boxes (CACGGG), both of which are required for the response to glucose.[65] The pyruvate kinase E box motifs are recognized by major late transcription factor (MLTF)/upstream stimulating factor (USF), but insulin/glucose does not appear to influence the affinity of binding.[65] An adjacent hepatic nuclear factor 4 (HNF-4) binding site, located between −145 and −125, is required for the full induction of pyruvate kinase gene transcription by insulin/glucose.[65] Interestingly, the dominant negative action of cAMP on pyruvate kinase gene transcription may be mediated indirectly via the nucleoprotein complex binding both elements.[65]

The AP-1 Motif

Fos-Jun heterodimers form a major component of the transcription factor AP-1 complex.[23] The sequence recognized by AP-1 (called a TPA-responsive element or TRE) is shown in Table 25-2. Insulin can stimulate collagenase gene transcription through this element,[40] and a multimerized AP-1 motif is sufficient to confer a positive effect of insulin on the expression of a reporter gene in a heterologous context.[70]

The action of insulin through the AP-1 motif is potentially manifest at two levels. First, insulin stimulates transcription of the genes encoding both c-*fos* (see previous section) and c-*jun*.[71] Second, insulin may mediate an effect on gene transcription, via an AP-1 site, through an alteration in the phosphorylation state and transactivation potential of both c-fos and c-jun. Thus, the potential exists for insulin to have both short- and long-term effects on gene expression through the same element.

Both $p90^{rsk}$ and MAP kinase can phosphorylate c-fos in vitro,[36] but whether this occurs in vivo is unknown. Moreover, recent evidence suggests that growth factors may augment the phosphorylation and transactivation potential of c-fos via an unidentified kinase distinct from MAP kinase.[72] Although relatively little is known about the regulation of c-fos phosphorylation, the phosphorylation of c-jun by multiple kinases at multiple sites has been studied in detail (see ref. 23 for review). MAP kinase, as well as several other insulin-regulated serine kinases, including casein kinase II and GSK-3, phosphorylates c-jun in vitro; however, the precise role of these three kinases in insulin-regulated gene transcription via AP-1 sites has yet to be established (see ref. 6 for review). Moreover, several recent papers suggest that novel members of the MAP kinase family, designated JNK1 and JNK2, may mediate the phosphorylation and activation of c-jun in vivo.[23] Thus, as with the SRE, several possible mechanisms have been identified that may explain insulin-regulated gene transcription through AP-1 sites, but further experimental studies are required to provide conclusive data supporting the involvement of a specific kinase.

Identification of Negative Insulin Response Sequences

Phosphoenolpyruvate Carboxykinase

PEPCK catalyzes the conversion of oxaloacetate to phosphoenolpyruvate, which is the rate-limiting step in hepatic and renal gluconeogenesis. The mechanisms that mediate the tissue-specific and hormonally regulated expression of the hepatic cytosolic PEPCK gene have been studied in great detail (for a review, see refs. 2, 7, and 73). The rate of transcription of the hepatic cytosolic PEPCK gene is stimulated by cAMP, retinoic acid, thyroid hormone, and glucocorticoids, but is inhibited by insulin and phorbol esters.[2,7,73] In H4IIE cells, the inhibitory effects are dominant because insulin and phorbol esters prevent cAMP- and glucocorticoid-stimulated PEPCK gene transcription.[2,7] Insulin primarily inhibits the initiation of hepatic PEPCK gene transcription, but it also reduces the rate of transcript elongation.[2,7]

Detailed analysis of the PEPCK promoter by transfection of hepatoma cells with PEPCK/CAT fusion genes has shown that complex hormone response units, composed of multiple *cis*-acting elements, are required to manifest the full response to each of these hormones.[2,73] For example, in the PEPCK gene, a complex glucocorticoid response unit (GRU) mediates the stimulatory action of glucocorticoids.[74] Previous studies have shown that this GRU consists of a tandem array (5′ to 3′) of two accessory factor-binding sites (AF1, from −455 to −431; AF2, from −420 to −403) and two glucocorticoid receptor–binding sites (GR1 and GR2, from −395 to −349). AF1 and AF2 do not function as glucocorticoid response elements themselves. However, when both are mutated, the promoter is no longer responsive to glucocorticoids; thus GR1 and GR2 are inert by themselves. Similarly, Hanson and colleagues have shown that four *cis*-acting elements, designated the cAMP response element (CRE), P3[I], P3[II], and P4, are required for cAMP-stimulated PEPCK gene transcription.[73] Together, these elements form what can be termed the cAMP response unit (CRU). The CRE, located between −93 and −86 relative to the transcription start site, contains the consensus CRE sequence T(G/T) ACGTCA found in many, but not all, cAMP-regulated genes.[73] The other three elements required for the cAMP response form a complex unit located between −285 and −238 in relation to the transcription initiation site. Thus, the PEPCK promoter exemplifies an emerging paradigm: complex hormone response units, and not simple hormone response elements, are prevalent in eukaryotic promoters.[75]

At least two *cis*-acting elements are required to mediate insulin's action on PEPCK gene transcription.[2] One element is located between −437 and −402 and the other(s) between −271 and +69. The distal IRS located between −437 and −402 has been analyzed in detail in the context of a heterologous promoter.[76,77] The core sequence of the distal IRS (located between −413 and −407) is underlined in Table 25-2. This element may also mediate the negative effect of insulin on the expression of both the insulin-like growth factor binding protein-1 (IGFBP-1) and tyrosine aminotransferase (TAT) genes (see subsequent sections). In all three genes, the IRS coincides with an element required for full induction of transcription by glucocorticoids. In the case of PEPCK, this is AF2. Again, in all three genes, hepatic nuclear factor-3 (HNF-3) may be the accessory factor required for full induction of gene transcription by glucocorticoids.[77–79] However, the available data suggest that HNF-3 does not directly mediate the action of insulin.[77] We have proposed a model in which an unknown factor (designated IRF, for insulin response factor) mediates the action of insulin (see Fig. 25-2). Whether insulin induces the binding of this protein, as in the case of IRP-A and the GAPDH IRE-A element (see earlier section), or modifies the activity of a prebound factor is unclear. In vivo footprinting studies reveal no change in the footprint over the PEPCK IRS following treatment of H4IIE cells with insulin.[80] At present, no candidate IRF protein has been identified. It is envisioned that this IRF would interfere with the binding/transactivation potential of HNF-3, thus explaining the negative effect of insulin on glucocorticoid-stimulated PEPCK, IGFBP-1, and TAT gene expression (see Fig. 25-2).

As described earlier, insulin activates the p21^{ras}/MAP kinase pathway through the binding of GRB2 to tyrosine-phosphorylated IRS-1.[6,24] Because IRS-1 is phosphorylated on multiple tyrosine residues by the insulin receptor, however, it may act as a docking protein for several SH2-containing proteins. Thus, the binding of GRB2 may initiate only one of several parallel insulin-stimulated signal transduction pathways. In fact, several other IRS-1–associated proteins have already been identified, including phosphatidylinositol 3′-kinase (PI3′-K), nck, and Syp.[24]

PI3′-K is composed of two subunits: a 110-kd (p110) catalytic subunit and an 85-kd (p85) regulatory subunit. The p85 subunit interacts with tyrosine-phosphorylated IRS-1 via its two SH2 domains, leading to activation of the catalytic activity of p110.[81] This activation of PI3′-K by insulin is important for several of insulin's actions because Wortmannin, a specific inhibitor of PI3′-K, blocks many of insulin's actions in various cell types (see ref. 82 for a review).

The phosphatase inhibitor okadaic acid mimics the action of insulin on PEPCK gene transcription[83] and inhibits the action of insulin on glucokinase gene transcription,[84] suggesting that, as with most of insulin's actions, changes in protein phosphorylation are involved in these effects. Reusch et al.[85] have shown that insulin dramatically inhibits (>80%) the activity of nuclear protein phosphatase 2A (PP-2A). Thus, although the mechanism by which insulin regulates nuclear PP-2A activity is unknown, such an action might explain the observed results obtained with okadaic acid. More recently, Sutherland et al.[82] have shown that wortmannin blocks the inhibition of PEPCK gene transcription by insulin, suggesting that activation of PI3′-K is also required for this action of insulin.

Insulin-Like Growth Factor Binding Protein-1

The IGFBPs are a family of six secreted proteins, designated IGFBP-1 through IGFBP-6, which specifically bind IGF-I and IGF-II but do not bind insulin. The structure of the IGFBPs and the differential, tissue-specific, and hormonal regulation of expression of the IGFBP genes has recently been reviewed (see ref. 86).

The multihormonal regulation of the genes for PEPCK and IGFBP-1 is similar in that cAMP, thyroid hormone, and glucocorticoids stimulate the hepatic expression of both genes, whereas insulin has a dominant inhibitory effect (see ref. 86 for a review). As discussed later, the structural organization of both the PEPCK and IGFBP-1 promoters share some similarities.

A glucocorticoid response element (GRE) overlaps an IRS in both the rat and human IGFBP-1 gene promoters.[87,88] The human IGFBP-1 promoter contains a second GRE that is not present in the rat promoter; however, both promoters contain only a single IRS.[87–89] In the human promoter, the IRS is located between −120 and −96 and the two GREs are found between −110 and −84 and between −198 and −173.[87,89] In the rat promoter, the IRS is located between −109 and −85, and the single GRE is between −91 and −77.[88]

Powell and colleagues defined the human IGFBP-1 IRS by analyzing the ability of insulin to repress basal IGFBP-1 fusion gene expression.[87] A deletion that abolished the negative effect of insulin was identified. The region encompassing the deletion was then shown to confer an inhibitory effect of insulin on CAT expression directed by a heterologous promoter.[87] The sequence of the human IGFBP-1 IRS is shown in Table 25-2. The core IRS sequence—T(G/A)TTTTG—is the same as that found in the PEPCK gene, but the PEPCK promoter has a single copy of this element, whereas the IGFBP-1 promoter has two copies arranged as an inverted palindrome (see ref. 77).

The human IGFBP-1 IRS also acts as an accessory factor binding site that is required for the glucocorticoid response. Thus, mutation of the IGFBP-1 IRS abolishes the induction of human IGFBP-1 gene transcription by glucocorticoids, even though both GREs are intact.[77,89] As described in the preceding section, the accessory factor is thought to be HNF-3,[77,78] and as with the PEPCK IRS, insulin has been postulated to function by interfering with either the binding or transactivation potential of HNF-3 (see ref. 77; Fig. 25-2).

Tyrosine Aminotransferase

The TAT gene has served as a paradigm for the hormonal regulation and tissue-specific expression of hepatic genes.[90] Schutz and colleagues have defined three far-upstream enhancers that mediate this regulation.[90] An enhancer at −11 kbp mediates liver-specific TAT gene expression, whereas enhancers at −3.6 kbp and −2.5 kbp mediate the induction of TAT gene transcription by cAMP and glucocorticoids, respectively.[90] Grange and colleagues have characterized an additional glucocorticoid-dependent enhancer at −5.4 kbp.[91] As described earlier for PEPCK, all three hormone-dependent enhancers in the TAT promoter are actually hormone response units in that multiple accessory factor binding sites are required to manifest the full response to cAMP and glucocorticoids.[90,91]

Regulation of TAT gene expression by insulin has been studied in considerable detail, with several different results, depending on the cell line studied (see ref. 92 for a review). Most recently, Ganss et al.[93] has proposed that insulin mediates its negative effect on cAMP- and glucocorticoid-stimulated TAT gene transcription through the −3.6 kbp and −2.5 kbp enhancers, respectively. Ganss et al.[93] suggest that insulin acts to disable the TAT CRE in the −3.6 kbp enhancer, but this action of insulin may be mediated indirectly by its well-characterized ability to stimulate cAMP phosphodiesterase activity (see Chapter 20).

Schütz and colleagues have shown that a CCAAT box, CACCC box, and an HNF-3 binding site found in the vicinity of the −2.5-kbp TAT GRE are all required for full glucocorticoid-stimulated TAT gene transcription.[79,90] The HNF-3 binding site, and not the CCAAT box or CACCC box, is the site of insulin action in the −2.5-kbp enhancer.[93] This HNF-3 binding site contains a TGTTT motif similar to the T(G/A)TTTTG PEPCK/IGFBP-1 core IRS. We speculate that the minimum PEPCK core IRS is actually T(G/A)TTT (see Table 25-2). If this is correct, insulin may mediate its negative effect on PEPCK, IGFBP-1, and TAT gene transcription through the same *trans*-acting factor. If so, the model shown in Figure 25-2, which proposes that insulin mediates its negative effect on glucocorticoid-stimulated PEPCK gene transcription by disabling the binding/transactivation potential of HNF-3, may also be applicable to TAT.

Glucagon

Glucagon is expressed in the α-cells of the pancreatic islets where transcription of the gene is inhibited by insulin.[94] A 300-bp segment of the glucagon promoter is required for pancreas-specific expression. Within this sequence, three regions—designated G_1, G_2, and G_3—are of particular functional importance.[95] The effect of insulin on glucagon gene expression is mediated through an IRE located within G_3.[95] Ligation of this IRE (−274 to −234) onto a heterologous promoter confers a negative effect of insulin on reporter gene expression.[95] The sequence of the glucagon IRE is shown in Table 25-2. Although the prolactin IRS shares some homology with the glucagon IRE, the region of homology is outside the region known to be critical for the response of the glucagon gene to insulin (sequence underlined). By contrast, the homology between the glucagon and GAPDH IREs may be significant, as it occurs within the region considered to be critical for the effect of insulin on both genes. If so, it would be of tremendous interest to determine how the same *trans*-acting factor can mediate a positive effect of insulin on one gene (GAPDH) and a negative effect on another (glucagon). However, these elements may be distinct because whereas the binding of proteins to the GAPDH IRE is stimulated by insulin (see earlier section), this is not so with the glucagon IRE.[95] Moreover, Philippe et al.[96] have recently characterized two *trans*-acting factors—designated C1A and C1B—that bind to the glucagon IRE and have shown they are islet cell–specific. Both proteins bind the same region of the glucagon IRE between −260 and −249 (CACGCCTGACTG; see Table 25-2).[96]

Conclusions

Now that multiple IRSs/IREs have been characterized, it is apparent that a single consensus sequence does not exist (see Table 25-2). Several genes whose transcription is inhibited by insulin—namely, PEPCK, IGFBP-1, and TAT—appear to share a common IRS. An exception is the glucagon gene, in which the core IRS resembles that in the insulin-stimulated GAPDH gene (see Table 25-2). Much remains to be learned concerning the *trans*-acting factors that bind to the identified IRSs/IREs, and about the mechanism of insulin signaling to these proteins. It appears that, for a number of the IRSs/IREs identified to date, insulin may mediate its action by stimulating the binding of a *trans*-acting factor. In these cases, it will be important to establish that the time course of induced binding proceeds, or at least parallels, the induction of gene transcription by insulin. Similarly, in those instances in which insulin mediates its action through a prebound factor, it will be important to determine how an insulin-stimulated change in the phosphorylation state of such a protein alters its transactivation potential.

As the expression of so many genes (>100) is known to be regulated by insulin, the question arises as to the specificity of this action of insulin. (It should be noted, however, that not every gene is transcriptionally regulated by insulin. There are some notable exceptions; for example, insulin has little effect on the transcription of the genes encoding glycogen synthase[97] and the insulin receptor.[92]) By analogy, with the dual effects of insulin on general mRNA translation and the translation of specific mRNAs, such as that for ornithine decarboxylase,[4–6] we hypothesize that there may be a general mechanism for the regulation of gene transcription by insulin, as well as specific mechanisms utilized with a select group of genes. The general mechanism might involve an effect of insulin on the basal transcription machinery, whereas the selective effects would be manifest by specific IRSs/IREs.

In summary, the past 5 years have witnessed a tremendous leap in the understanding of insulin-regulated gene expression, although much remains to be learned. The importance of these studies is emphasized by recent evidence suggesting that defects in gene expression may be important in NIDDM and hypertriglyceridemia.[12,16]

Acknowledgments

Owing to the limitation of the number of references, we apologize to those authors whose work has not been cited. We thank Deborah Caplenor and Rachel O'Brien for preparing the manuscript. The work discussed was supported by an HHS grant (DK35107) and the Vanderbilt Diabetes Research and Training Center (DK20593).

References

1. Denton RM. Early events in insulin actions. Adv Cyclic Nucleotide Protein Phos Res 1986;20:293
2. O'Brien RM, Granner DK. Regulation of gene expression by insulin. Biochem J 1991;278:609
3. O'Brien RM, Granner DK. The regulation of gene expression by insulin. Physiol Rev. In press
4. Kimball SR, Vary TC, Jefferson LS. Regulation of protein synthesis by insulin. Annu Rev Physiol 1994;56:321
5. Redpath NT, Proud CG. Molecular mechanisms in the control of translation by hormones and growth factors. Biochim Biophys Acta 1994;1220:147
6. Denton RM, Tavare JM. Does mitogen-activated protein kinase have a role in insulin action? The cases for and against. Eur J Biochem 1995;227:597
7. O'Brien RM, Granner DK. PEPCK gene as model of inhibitory effects of insulin on gene transcription. Diabetes Care 1990;13:327
8. Granner DK, Pilkis S. The genes of hepatic glucose metabolism. J Biol Chem 1990;265:10173
9. Iynedjian PB, Jotterand D, Nouspikel T, et al. Transcriptional induction of glucokinase gene by insulin in cultured liver cells and its repression by the glucagon-cAMP system. J Biol Chem 1989;264:21824
10. Unger RH. Diabetic hyperglycemia: Link to impaired glucose transport in pancreatic β cells. Science 1991;251:1200
11. Permutt MA, Chiu KC, Tanizawa Y. Glucokinase and NIDDM. Diabetes 1992;41:1367
12. Granner DK, O'Brien RM. Molecular physiology and genetics of NIDDM. Importance of metabolic staging. Diabetes Care 1992;15:369
13. Kahn CR. Insulin action, diabetogenes, and the cause of type II diabetes. Diabetes 1994;43:1066
14. Hotamisligil GS, Spiegelman BM. Tumor necrosis factor α: A key component of the obesity-diabetes link. Diabetes 1994;43:1271
15. Maddux BA, Sbraccia P, Kumakura S, et al. Membrane glycoprotein and insulin resistance in non–insulin-dependent diabetes mellitus. Nature 1995; 373:448
16. Dammerman M, Sandkuijl LA, Halaas JL, et al. An apolipoprotein CIII haplotype protective against hypertriglyceridemia is specified by promoter and 3′ untranslated region polymorphisms. Proc Natl Acad Sci USA 1993;90:4562
17. Nigg EA. Mechanisms of signal transduction to the cell nucleus. Adv Cancer Res 1990;55:271
18. Jans DA. Nuclear signaling pathways for polypeptide ligands and their membrane receptors? FASEB J 1994;8:841
19. Miller DS. Stimulation of RNA and protein synthesis by intracellular insulin. Science 1988;240:506
20. Kim S-J, Kahn CR. Insulin induces rapid accumulation of insulin receptors and increases tyrosine kinase activity in the nucleus of cultured adipocytes. J Cell Physiol 1993;157:217
21. Csermely P, Schnaider T, Cheatham B, et al. Insulin induces the phosphorylation of nucleolin. J Biol Chem 1993;268:9747
22. Meek DW, Street AJ. Nuclear protein phosphorylation and growth control. Biochem J 1992;287:1
23. Karin M. Signal transduction from the cell surface to the nucleus through the phosphorylation of transcription factors. Curr Opinion Cell Biol 1994;6:415
24. Cheatham B, Kahn CR. Insulin action and the insulin signaling network. Endocr Rev 1995;16:117
25. Cohen P. Dissection of the protein phosphorylation cascades involved in insulin and growth factor action. Biochem Soc Trans 1993;21:555
26. Alexander M, Curtis G, Avruch J, Goodman HM. Insulin regulation of protein biosynthesis in differentiated 3T3 adipocytes. J Biol Chem 1985;260:11978
27. Alexander MC, Lomanto M, Nasrin N, Ramaika C. Insulin stimulates glyceraldehyde-3-phosphate dehydrogenase gene expression through cis-acting DNA sequences. Proc Natl Acad Sci USA 1988;85:5092
28. Nasrin N, Ercolani L, Denaro M, et al. An insulin response element in the glyceraldehyde-3-phosphate dehydrogenase gene binds a nuclear protein induced by insulin in cultured cells and by nutritional manipulations *in vivo*. Proc Natl Acad Sci USA 1990;87:5273
29. Nasrin N, Buggs C, Kong XF, et al. DNA-binding properties of the product of the testis-determining gene and a related protein. Nature 1991;354:317
30. Alexander-Bridges M, Ercolani L, Kong XF, Nasrin N. Identification of a core motif that is recognized by three members of the HMG class of transcriptional regulators: IRE-ABP, SRY, and TCF-1α. J Cell Biochem 1992;48:129
31. Alexander-Bridges M, Mukhopadhyay NK, Jhala U, et al. Growth-factor–activated kinases phosphorylate IRE-ABP. Biochem Soc Trans 1992;20:691
32. Alexander-Bridges M, Buggs C, Giere L, et al. Models of insulin action on metabolic and growth response genes. Mol Cell Biochem 1992;109:99
33. Messina JL. Insulin's regulation of c-*fos* gene transcription in hepatoma cells. J Biol Chem 1990;265:11700
34. Stumpo DJ, Stewart TN, Gilman MZ, Blackshear PJ. Identification of c-*fos* sequences involved in induction by insulin and phorbol esters. J Biol Chem 1988;263:1611
35. Yamauchi K, Holt K, Pessin JE. Phosphatidylinositol 3-kinase functions upstream of Ras and Raf in mediating insulin stimulation of c-*fos* transcription. J Biol Chem 1993;268:14597
36. Chen R-H, Sarnecki C, Blenis J. Nuclear localization and regulation of *erk*- and *rsk*-encoded protein kinases. Mol Cell Biol 1992;12:915
37. Sturgill TW, Ray LB, Erikson E, Maller JL. Insulin-stimulated MAP-2 kinase phosphorylates and activates ribosomal protein S6 kinase II. Nature 1988; 334:715
38. Sutherland C, Cohen P. The α-isoform of glycogen synthase kinase-3 from rabbit skeletal muscle is inactivated by p70 S6 kinase or MAP kinase-activated protein kinase-1 in vitro. FEBS Lett 1994;338:37
39. Plyte SE, Hughes K, Nikolakaki E, et al. Glycogen synthase kinase-3: Functions in oncogenesis and development. Biochim Biophys Acta 1992;1114:147
40. Medema RH, Wubbolts R, Bos JL. Two dominant inhibitory mutants of p21^{ras} interfere with insulin-induced gene expression. Mol Cell Biol 1991;11:5963
41. Burgering BMT, Medema RH, Maassen JA, et al. Insulin stimulation of gene expression mediated by p21ras activation. EMBO J 1991;10:1103
42. Treisman R. The serum response element. TIBS 1992;17:423
43. Malik RK, Roe MW, Blackshear PJ. Epidermal growth factor and other mitogens induce binding of a protein complex to the c-*fos* serum response element in human astrocytoma and other cells. J Biol Chem 1991;266:8576
44. Thompson MJ, Roe MW, Malik RK, Blackshear PJ. Insulin and other growth factors induce binding of the ternary complex and a novel protein complex to the c-*fos* serum response element. J Biol Chem 1994;269:21127
45. Gille H, Sharrocks AD, Shaw PE. Phosphorylation of transcription factor p62^{TCF} by MAP kinase stimulates ternary complex formation at c-*fos* promoter. Nature 1992;358:414
46. Marais R, Wynne J, Treisman R. The SRF accessory protein Elk-1 contains a growth factor–regulated transcriptional activation domain. Cell 1993;73:381
47. Stumpo DJ, Blackshear PJ. Insulin and growth factor effects on c-*fos* expression in normal and protein kinase C-deficient 3T3-L1 fibroblasts and adipocytes. Proc Natl Acad Sci USA 1986;83:9453
48. Taub R, Roy A, Dieter R, Koontz J. Insulin as a growth factor in rat hepatoma cells. J Biol Chem 1987;262:10893
49. Chu DTW, Granner DK. The effect of phorbol esters and diacylglycerol on expression of the phosphoenolpyruvate carboxykinase (GTP) gene in rat hepatoma H4IIE cells. J Biol Chem 1986;261:16848
50. Chu DTW, Stumpo DJ, Blackshear PJ, Granner DK. The inhibition of phosphoenolpyruvate carboxykinase (guanosine triphosphate) gene expression by insulin is not mediated by protein kinase C. Mol Endocrinol 1987;1:53
51. Nishizuka Y. Intracellular signaling by hydrolysis of phospholipids and activation of protein kinase C. Science 1992;258:607
52. Messina JL, Standaert ML, Ishizuka T, et al. Role of protein kinase C in insulin's regulation of c-*fos* transcription. J Biol Chem 1992;267:9223
53. Stumpo DJ, Haupt DM, Blackshear PJ. Protein kinase C isozyme distribution and downregulation in relation to insulin-stimulated c-*fos* induction. J Biol Chem 1994;269:21184
54. Rahmsdorf HJ, Herrlich P. Regulation of gene expression by tumor promoters. Pharmacol Ther 1990;48:157
55. Stanley F. Stimulation of prolactin gene expression by insulin. J Biol Chem 1988;263:13444
56. Keech CA, Gutierrez-Hartmann A. Insulin activation of rat prolactin promoter activity. Mol Cell Endocrinol 1991;78:55
57. Stanley FM. An element in the prolactin promoter mediates the stimulatory effect of insulin on transcription of the prolactin gene. J Biol Chem 1992;267:16719
58. Jacob KK, Stanley FM. The insulin and cAMP response elements of the prolactin gene are overlapping sequences. J Biol Chem 1994;269:25515
59. Paulauskis JD, Sul HS. Hormonal regulation of mouse fatty acid synthase gene transcription in liver. J Biol Chem 1989;264:574
60. Moustaid N, Sakamoto K, Clarke S, et al. Regulation of fatty acid synthase gene transcription. Biochem J 1993;292:767
61. Moustaid N, Beyer RS, Sul HS. Identification of an insulin response element in the fatty acid synthase promoter. J Biol Chem 1994;269:5629
62. Dranginis A, Morley M, Nesbitt M, et al. Independent regulation of nonallelic pancreatic amylase genes in diabetic mice. J Biol Chem 1984;259:12216
63. Keller SA, Rosenberg MP, Johnson TM, et al. Regulation of amylase gene expression in diabetic mice is mediated by a *cis*-acting upstream element close to the pancreas-specific enhancer. Genes Dev 1990;4:1316
64. Johnson TM, Rosenberg MP, Meisler MH. An insulin-responsive element in the pancreatic enhancer of the amylase gene. J Biol Chem 1993;268:464
65. Vaulont S, Kahn A. Transcriptional control of metabolic regulation genes by carbohydrates. FASEB J 1994;8:28
66. Noguchi T, Inoue H, Tanaka T. Transcriptional and post-transcriptional regulation of L-type pyruvate kinase in diabetic rat liver by insulin and dietary fructose. J Biol Chem 1985;260:14393
67. Decaux J-F, Antoine B, Kahn A. Regulation of the expression of the L-type pyruvate kinase gene in adult rat hepatocytes in primary culture. J Biol Chem 1989;264:11584
68. Thompson KS, Towle HC. Localization of the carbohydrate response element of the rat L-type pyruvate kinase gene. J Biol Chem 1991;266:8679
69. Bergot M-O, Diaz-Guerra M-JM, Puzenat N, et al. *Cis*-regulation of the L-type pyruvate kinase gene promoter by glucose, insulin and cyclic AMP. Nucleic Acids Res 1992;20:1871
70. Kim S-J, Kahn CR. Insulin stimulates phosphorylation of c-Jun, c-Fos, and Fos-related proteins in cultured adipocytes. J Biol Chem 1994;269:11887
71. Mohn KL, Laz TM, Melby AE, Taub R. Immediate-early gene expression differs between regenerating liver, insulin-stimulated H-35 cells, and mitogen-stimulated Balb/c 3T3 cells. J Biol Chem 1990;265:21914
72. Deng T, Karin M. c-Fos transcriptional activity stimulated by H-Ras-activated protein kinase distinct from JNK and ERK. Nature 1994;371:171
73. Hanson RW, Patel YM. Phosphoenolpyruvate carboxykinase (GTP): The gene and the enzyme. Adv Enzymol 1994;69:203

74. Imai E, Stromstedt PE, Quinn PG, et al. Characterization of a complex glucocorticoid response unit in the phosphoenolpyruvate carboxykinase gene. Mol Cell Biol 1990;10:4712
75. Lucas PC, Granner DK. Hormone response domains in gene transcription. Annu Rev Biochem 1992;61:1131
76. O'Brien RM, Lucas PC, Forest CD, et al. Identification of a sequence in the PEPCK gene that mediates a negative effect of insulin on transcription. Science 1990;249:533
77. O'Brien RM, Noisin EL, Suwanichkul A, et al. Hepatic nuclear factor-3 and hormone-regulated expression of the phosphoenolpyruvate carboxykinase and insulin-like growth factor-binding protein 1 genes. Mol Cell Biol 1995;15:1747
78. Unterman TG, Fareeduddin A, Harris MA, et al. Hepatocyte nuclear factor-3 (HNF-3) binds to the insulin response sequence in the IGF binding protein-1 (IGFBP-1) promoter and enhances promoter function. Biochem Biophys Res Commun 1994;203:1835
79. Nitsch D, Boshart M, Schutz G. Activation of the tyrosine aminotransferase gene is dependent on synergy between liver-specific and hormone-responsive elements. Proc Natl Acad Sci USA 1993;90:5479
80. Faber S, O'Brien RM, Imai E, et al. Dynamic aspects of DNA/protein interactions in the transcriptional initiation complex and the hormone-responsive domains of the phosphoenolpyruvate carboxykinase promoter *in vivo*. J Biol Chem 1993;268:24976
81. Backer JM, Myers MG Jr, Shoelson SE, et al. Phosphatidylinositol 3′-kinase is activated by association with IRS-1 during insulin stimulation. EMBO J 1992;11:3469
82. Sutherland C, O'Brien RM, Granner DK. Phosphatidylinositol 3-kinase, but not p70/p85 ribosomal S6 protein kinase, is required for the regulation of phosphoenolpyruvate carboxykinase (PEPCK) gene expression by insulin. J Biol Chem 1995;270:15501
83. O'Brien RM, Noisin EL, Granner DK. Comparison of the effects of insulin and okadaic acid on phosphoenolpyruvate carboxykinase gene expression. Biochem J 1994;303:737
84. Nouspikel T, Iynedjian PB. Insulin signalling and regulation of glucokinase gene expression in cultured hepatocytes. Eur J Biochem 1992;210:365
85. Reusch JE-B, Hsieh P, Klemm D, et al. Insulin inhibits dephosphorylation of adenosine 3′,5′-monophosphate response element-binding protein/activating transcription factor-1: Effect on nuclear phosphoserine phosphatase-2a. Endocrinology 1994;135:2418
86. Rechler MM. Insulin-like growth factor binding proteins. Vitam Horm 1993;47:1
87. Suwanichkul A, Morris SL, Powell DR. Identification of an insulin-responsive element in the promoter of the human gene for insulin-like growth factor binding protein-1. J Biol Chem 1993;268:17063
88. Goswami R, Lacson R, Yang E, et al. Functional analysis of glucocorticoid and insulin response sequences in the rat insulin-like growth factor-binding protein-1 promoter. Endocrinology 1994;134:736
89. Suwanichkul A, Allander SV, Morris SL, Powell DR. Glucocorticoids and insulin regulate expression of the human gene for insulin-like growth factor binding protein-1 through proximal promoter elements. J Biol Chem 1994;269:30835
90. Nitsch D, Ruppert S, Kelsey G, et al. Hormonal and liver-specific control of expression of the tyrosine aminotransferase gene. In: Cohen P, Foulkes JG, eds. The Hormonal Control Regulation of Gene Transcription. Amsterdam: Elsevier;1991:223
91. Grange T, Roux J, Rigaud G, Pictet R. Cell-type specific activity of two glucocorticoid responsive units of rat tyrosine aminotransferase gene is associated with multiple binding sites for C/EBP and a novel liver-specific nuclear factor. Nucleic Acids Res 1991;19:131
92. Granner DK, O'Brien RM. Regulation of transcription by insulin. In: Cohen P, Foulkes JG, eds. The Hormonal Control Regulation of Gene Transcription. Amsterdam: Elsevier;1991:309
93. Ganss R, Weih F, Schütz G. The cyclic adenosine 3′,5′-monophosphate- and the glucocorticoid-dependent enhancers are targets for insulin repression of tyrosine aminotransferase gene transcription. Mol Endocrinol 1994;8:895
94. Philippe J. Glucagon gene transcription is negatively regulated by insulin in a hamster islet cell line. J Clin Invest 1989;84:672
95. Philippe J. Insulin regulation of the glucagon gene is mediated by an insulin-responsive DNA element. Proc Natl Acad Sci USA 1991;88:7224
96. Philippe J, Morel C, Cordier-Bussat M. Islet-specific proteins interact with the insulin-response element of the glucagon gene. J Biol Chem 1995;270:3039
97. Vestergaard H, Andersen PH, Lund S, et al. Expression of glycogen synthase and phosphofructokinase in muscle from type 1 (insulin-dependent) diabetic patients before and after intensive insulin treatment. Diabetologia 1994;37:82

Diabetes Mellitus, edited by Derek LeRoith, Simeon I. Taylor, and Jerrold M. Olefsky. Lippincott–Raven Publishers, Philadelphia

CHAPTER 26

Insulin Degradation

ANDREW BECKER, LI DING, AND RICHARD A. ROTH

Proteases play critical roles in a wide variety of physiologic processes, including hormone processing, homeostasis, thrombosis, and signal transduction.[1,2] In recent years, there has been a dramatic increase in the study of proteolytic enzymes by both basic scientists and clinicians. The rising interest in proteases has coincided with the development of two significant classes of therapeutic agents: the angiotensin converting enzyme (ACE) inhibitors and the clot-busting tissue-plasminogen activator (TPA). This renewed focus on proteolytic enzymes on the part of biochemists, molecular biologists, and clinicians has led to new discoveries concerning the functions, physiology, and mechanisms of action of numerous proteases. These recent studies have identified new processes for protease involvement (and potential targets for therapeutic intervention), such as viral replication,[3] antigen processing,[4] and even cell death (apoptosis).[5]

In the insulin field, studies of enzymes that degrade insulin have a long and controversial history. It is well documented that every tissue and cell that responds to insulin also can degrade the insulin molecule. This process is most likely necessary for a cell to terminate its response to insulin. Evidence for the role of enzymatic degradation in terminating biologic response has been extensively documented in several other systems, including in the hydrolysis of acetylcholine by acetylcholine esterase[6] and the proteolysis of **a**-factor in *Saccharomyces cerevisiae* mating.[7] In addition, it has been suggested (but still not proven) that the processing of insulin (either as a result of the formation of fragments of the hormone or even the internalization of the whole molecule) may be required to induce various biologic responses.[8–10] The site of insulin degradation in the cell has also been contested. Early work suggested that insulin was degraded primarily in lysosomes, but subsequent studies have shown that insulin degradation begins in an earlier compartment, most likely in endosomes.[11–13] This early degradation of insulin results in a clipped insulin molecule that no longer can bind to its cell surface receptor. The enzyme(s) that degrade insulin have been studied extensively; however, it still is unclear which protease is responsible for any of the cleavages of the insulin molecule in the intact cell. Two enzymes have been most extensively studied over the years: one that interchanges the disulfide bonds in the insulin molecule (called glutathione-insulin transhydrogenase or protein disulfide isomerase) and another one that proteolytically clips the insulin molecule. The role of the former enzyme in insulin degradation has not been extensively explored recently (because of a variety of data indicating that it is not important in the degradation of insulin) and so is not discussed in this review. (The reader is referred to ref. 14 for a recent discussion of this enzyme.) The second enzyme—called insulin degrading enzyme (IDE) (also called insulinase)—was first described more than 40 years ago.[15] Recent studies have generated a variety of new information on this enzyme, but its role in the physiologic processing of insulin is still controversial. In this review, some of the new information on this enzyme is summarized and some of the questions that still remain are discussed.

Background

Most, if not all, of the varied effects of insulin appear to be initiated by the binding of insulin to its specific receptor on the plasma membrane of cells.[16,17] After insulin binds to its receptor, the receptor-insulin complex is internalized in endocytic vesicles (Fig. 26-1).[18] As the endosomes are acidified, the insulin–insulin receptor complex dissociates, with most of the receptors being recycled to the cell surface and the insulin being degraded inside the cell. Exactly where the insulin goes in the cell and the site of its degradation are still questions that warrant further study. Although early studies had indicated that insulin is mostly transported to lysosomes where it is degraded, more recent studies have indicated that insulin goes to a variety of other subcellular organelles, including the nucleus and cell cytosol.[19–21] The presence of various peptide transporters in the plasma membrane could result in the insulin molecule (or a fragment of the molecule) passing through the membrane of the endocytic vesicle and entering the cytoplasm of the cell. It could either be degraded in the cytoplasm or travel to other compartments in the cell, such as the peroxisomes or nuclei. Some studies have even argued that either the intact insulin molecule or a fragment of it could stimulate various biologic responses by interacting with other proteins in these different compartments.[8–10] More likely is the possibility that insulin degradation is a mechanism for terminating the response to insulin by removing the stimulus from the target cells. However, even this statement must be considered a working hypothesis at this time, as the data supporting a role for insulin degradation in the termination of the response to insulin are still not conclusive.

Insulin-Degrading Enzyme

History

In the 1940s, a number of studies showed that extracts of tissues that normally degrade insulin (such as the liver) had an enzymatic activity that could fairly specifically hydrolyze the peptide bonds of the insulin molecule.[15] One study at this time suggested that this activity was at least partly responsible for the normal removal of insulin, as mice with elevated levels of this activity were more resistant to elevated levels of insulin than were normal mice.[22] However, attempts at isolating this enzyme to homogeneity over the next 30 years were largely unsuccessful. Two subsequent technologic developments facilitated studies of this enzyme. The first was the demonstration that this enzyme, like the insulin receptor, could, in fact, be labeled by crosslinking radioactive insulin to it.[23] This work demonstrated for the first time that the molecular weight of the enzyme's polypeptide backbone on sodium dodecyl sulfate (SDS) gel electrophoresis was 110 kd, much higher than the previous reports indicating an Mr of 60 kd. The second development was the generation of monoclonal antibodies to the enzyme.[24] These antibodies were utilized to show that this enzyme was, indeed, responsible for most of the insulin degrading activity in total cell lysates of a variety of tissues, including liver and red blood cells. These antibodies were also utilized to provide some evidence that this enzyme might be also involved in the degradation of insulin by intact cells, as the microinjection of these antibodies into cells could partly interfere with the cellular degradation of insulin.[24] Finally, the antibodies were utilized to demonstrate that, in intact cells incubated first with labeled insulin and then with a bifunctional crosslinking agent, some labeled insulin could be crosslinked to IDE, providing further evidence that this enzyme does come in contact with insulin.[25]

Further evidence that IDE or a related enzyme degrades insulin in intact cells comes from studies showing that the degradation products of insulin from intact cells, or even in the whole organism, are nearly identical to those seen with purified IDE.[26–29] In addition, several inhibitors of IDE also inhibit insulin degradation in intact cells.[30]

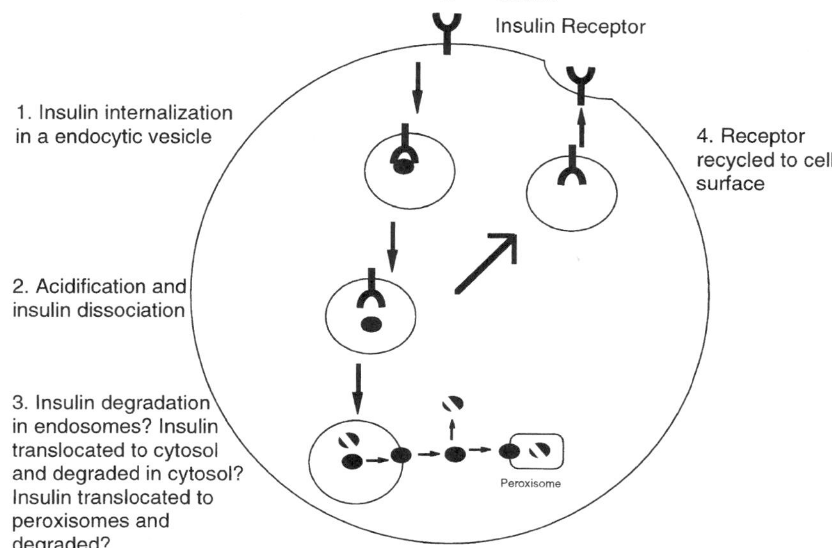

FIGURE 26-1. Potential pathways for the internalization and processing of insulin. After insulin binds to its plasma membrane receptor,[16,17] it is internalized in endocytic vesicles.[18] These vesicles then undergo acidification, which causes the insulin to dissociate from its receptor. The receptor can then recycle to the plasma membrane. In contrast, the pathway for insulin is less clear. It can, in part, be degraded in the endosomes,[11–13,29,59] or it may be transferred out of these vesicles by one of the membrane protein transporters.[60] The insulin can then be degraded in the cytoplasm of the cell or transported to other cellular compartments.

Recently, further evidence of the role of IDE in insulin degradation in the intact cell has come from the use of a cDNA encoding the human enzyme. This cDNA was used in both transient and stable transfections to increase the levels of the IDE protein in cells by approximately twofold to threefold.[31,32] Most impressive was the finding that the rate of insulin degradation by these whole cells was increased 5 to 10 fold. These authors verified that the expressed IDE was not leaking from the cells, as the media from the cells did not contain this degrading activity, but they did not test whether the uptake of the insulin in these cells was mediated by the insulin receptor, the normal process for cellular uptake and degradation of insulin.[18] The finding that the increase in insulin degradation in the intact cells matched or surpassed that measured in cell extracts is surprising, and indicates that the levels of IDE in these cells limits the rate of insulin degradation. In addition, these results further support the hypothesis that IDE is involved in the degradation of insulin by intact cells.

Structure of Insulin-Degrading Enzyme

The availability of monoclonal antibodies to IDE has allowed the purification of sufficient amounts of this protein for sequencing.[33] The amino acid sequence of various tryptic peptide fragments of the enzyme has been utilized to obtain a cDNA clone of the enzyme. This cDNA clone allows the deduction of the complete primary amino acid sequence of the human enzyme.[33] The amino acid sequence of IDE does not exhibit any of the "classical" motifs of the active sites of other known proteases, but does exhibit homology to a bacterial protease, called pi or protease III.[33] Both human and bacterial enzymes are synthesized as single polypeptide chains of similar molecular mass (approximately 100 kd), although the active mammalian enzyme appears to be a homodimer, whereas the bacterial enzyme is active as a monomer and is mainly localized in the periplasmic space of the bacteria.[34–37] There is also a related protease in Drosophila[38] and Neurospora.[39] The amino acid sequence of the bacterial protease is approximately 27% identical to the sequences of Drosophila and human enzymes, whereas the human and Drosophila proteins are 46% identical to each other.[33,38,40] Recently, the sequence of the rat enzyme was reported, and the sequences of the human and rat enzymes were found to be 95% identical, indicating the highly conserved nature of this protein.[41] The human and bacterial enzymes share three regions of high homology containing greater than 50% sequence identity, possibly indicating that these three regions are important in the function of the enzyme.[33] All of these proteases have an absolute requirement for divalent cations for activity, which characterizes them as metalloproteases.[34,37] In addition, purified protease III has been shown to contain stoichiometric amounts of zinc,[37] whereas partially purified human IDE contains high levels of zinc and significantly lower levels of manganese.[42] These findings characterize IDE as a zinc-dependent metalloprotease.

Primary sequence analyses and x-ray crystallographic data have indicated that most metalloproteases share a conserved active site.[43,44] This active site was first identified in the prototypic zinc metalloendopeptidase thermolysin and contains the sequence, HEXXH, in which the two histidines coordinate the binding of the zinc atom and the glutamate acts as a general base for catalysis.[44] However, neither the three eukaryotic IDE proteins nor bacterial protease III contain this active site motif.

Human IDE and protease III do, however, have a sequence—HXXEH—in one of the highly conserved regions which could be considered an inversion of the active site seen in other metalloendopeptidases (Fig. 26-2).[33] Mutagenesis studies of this region in protease III have demonstrated that the two histidines coordinate the binding of the zinc atom, and that glutamate is essential for catalytic activity, but not zinc binding.[45] This putative active site motif is also seen in the rat and Drosophila enzymes.[38,41] Subsequent work on human IDE has confirmed the importance of the first histidine and the glutamate in this sequence for the catalytic activity of this enzyme; however, these studies did not test the role of these residues in the binding of zinc.[46]

The identification of the HXXEH sequence as a potential active site for protease III indicates that this motif may be utilized by proteases other than those in the IDE family.[45] Recent work

ENZYME	SEQUENCE					RESIDUE NUMBERS
		*		* *		
Protease III	GLA	**H**	YL	**E H**	MSL	85-95
hIDE	GLS	**H**	FC	**E H**	MLF	64-74
dIDE	GLA	**H**	FC	**E H**	MLF	78-88
rIDE	GLS	**H**	FC	**E H**	MLF	64-74
rNRD	GLA	**H**	FL	**E H**	MVF	241-251
rMPP	GTA	**H**	FL	**E H**	MAF	98-108
		* *		*	◆	
Thermolysin	VVA	**H E**	LT	**H**	AVT	139-149
Collagenase	VAA	**H E**	LG	**H**	SLG	215-225
Serratia protease	TFT	**H E**	IG	**H**	ALG	89-99
Endopeptidase 24.11	VIG	**H E**	IT	**H**	GFD	580-590
Leukotriene A4 hydrolase	VIA	**H E**	IS	**H**	SWT	292-302

Figure 26-2. Comparison of the proposed active site residues in the IDE family, including bacterial protease III; the human (hIDE), rat (rIDE), and Drosophila (dIDE) insulin degrading enzymes; rat mitochondrial processing protease (rMPP); rat *N*-arginine dibasic convertase (rNRD); and several traditional zinc metalloendopeptidases. The three active site residues—two histidines (H) and a glutamate (E)—are marked with an asterisk (*). In the case of protease III, the two histidines were shown to be required to bind zinc and for enzymatic activity, whereas the glutamate was required only for enzymatic activity.[45] The numbering of the human and rat IDEs is based on the use of the second translation initiation codon, as mutagenesis studies have indicated that this start site is primarily utilized. The boxed residues indicate residues adjacent to the active site which are inverted in the insulin degrading enzymes and protease III relative to several other metalloendopeptidases (i.e., collagenase and Serratia protease).

has, in fact, identified this motif in at least two other proteases: the β subunit of the mitochondrial processing peptidase[47] and the *N*-arginine dibasic convertase[48] (see Fig. 26-2). It has not yet been confirmed that the residues in these two proteases are also required for activity, but this would appear to be likely, suggesting that the motif identified in the IDE class of proteases may be found in still other proteases.

Evidence Against a Role for Insulin-Degrading Enzyme in Insulin Degradation

As with many active areas of research, the role of IDE as the physiologic mediator of insulin degradation remains controversial, with opponents of this model pointing to several inconsistencies in the data obtained with this enzyme. First, IDE is known to degrade a number of substrates in addition to insulin, indicating that it is not specific for the insulin pathway. The enzyme has been shown to degrade glucagon,[49] atrial natriuretic factor,[50] transforming growth factor α,[51] and oxidatively damaged hemoglobin,[52] with affinities for some of these substrates approaching that of insulin. The finding that IDE can attack numerous substrates, however, is not inconsistent with a functional role in insulin degradation. Data derived from studies of numerous other proteases indicate that proteases often act as control points for multiple pathways simultaneously. A physiologically significant example of one such protease is ACE, which mediates the formation of angiotensin II from angiotensin I, as well as the degradation of bradykinin. Another example is neutral endopeptidase (NEP), for which more than 24 known physiologic substrates have been identified to date.[53] Finally, the finding that the interleukin–1 (IL-1) β-converting protease can also play a role in apoptosis further illustrates how a single protease can have several functions.[5]

A second argument against the role of IDE in insulin degradation comes from studies examining the levels of IDE in different tissues. Numerous tissues and cell types appear to express IDE. Indeed, Northern blot analysis and in situ hybridization have indicated that the highest levels of IDE mRNA are present in germinal epithelium in the testes (Fig. 26-3).[41,54,55] However, the IDE mRNA in this tissue appears to differ slightly from that in other tissues (being slightly larger) (see Fig. 26-3).[41,54] Thus, it is possible that the IDE protein in this tissue may be slightly different and have a different function. For example, an IDE-like enzyme has been proposed to be involved in membrane fusion.[56] These same studies have also found that levels of both IDE mRNA and its protein are high in known insulin-degrading tissues, including the liver and kidney (see Fig. 26-3).[41,54,55]

Perhaps the main argument against a role for IDE in insulin degradation in the intact cell comes from the subcellular localization of the enzyme. As mentioned earlier, insulin is thought to be degraded primarily in endosomes. Although there is some evidence that small amounts of IDE are located in endosomes,[57,58] most of the IDE in a cell is not. The deduced amino acid sequence of IDE does not contain a signal sequence that would direct it to this location. Most studies have, in fact, indicated that the major portion of IDE is found in the cytoplasm of the cell, a position consistent with its sequence.[11] The finding that the deduced IDE protein sequence contains the peroxisomal targeting sequence A/S-K-L at the carboxy terminus, however, indicates that the enzyme may be primarily located in this organelle.[41] Indeed, recent studies have indicated that a portion of IDE is present in the peroxisomes,[32,59] although it is not clear at present what fraction of IDE is actually located in this organelle. Even if a portion of IDE is present in the cytosol of cells, it remains unclear how insulin would be brought into contact with the enzyme in this part of the cell because, as noted earlier, insulin is internalized in endocytic vesicles. One hypothesis maintains that insulin would need to be pumped through the vesicle membrane by a membrane transport protein in order to come in contact with IDE. Indeed, such a process has been described. For example, in mitochondria, proteins are imported by such a mechanism.[60] These imported proteins are then cleaved via the mitochondrial processing peptidase, an enzyme which, as noted earlier, is homologous to IDE in terms of its putative active site.[61]

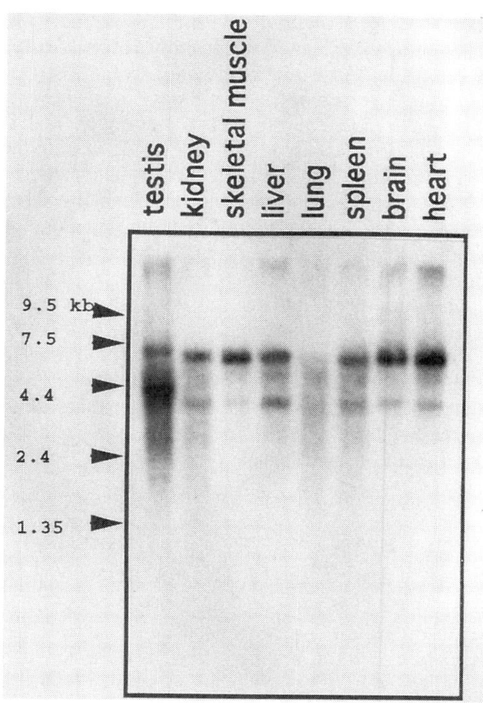

Figure 26-3. Northern blot analysis of IDE in different rat tissues. A previously described 1.2-kb cDNA encoding rat IDE (corresponding to nucleotides 400 to 1600 of human IDE cDNA)[55] was utilized to probe a Northern blot containing equivalent amounts of mRNA from the indicated tissues.

Remaining Questions Concerning Insulin-Degrading Enzyme

Although there has been some progress in our understanding of IDE, numerous questions still remain. First, Northern analyses have identified at least two mRNAs for IDE of different sizes in most tissues (a 3.7-kb form, which is most consistent with the size necessary to encode the known protein form of the enzyme and the isolated cDNAs, and a larger, 5.5-kb mRNA) (see Fig. 26-3).[41,54] It is not known whether this larger mRNA encodes a different form of the IDE protein. In addition, in testes, both of these mRNAs also appear to be slightly larger than those found in other tissues (see Fig. 26-3).[41,54] Again, it is not known whether these differences in the mRNA affect the sequence of the protein. Some differences in the 3′-terminal polyadenylation sites have been noted.[41]

Additional questions still remain as to the structure of the enzyme. For example, it is not known which regions of the enzyme are responsible for the high-affinity interaction with insulin. This could involve one of the highly conserved regions of this enzyme. A three-dimensional structure of the enzyme, as provided by x-ray crystallography, would yield important new insights into this new class of proteases, as well as possible clues as to how inhibitors could be designed to specifically inhibit this enzyme.

Two recent papers have raised new questions as to the possible roles of IDE. Kupfer et al.[62] have identified IDE as a factor capable of enhancing the binding of the androgen and glucocorticoid receptors to specific DNA sequences in vitro. Additional studies are necessary to confirm these interactions in the intact cell. If this can be done, then a role for insulin in the nucleus might be to inhibit the function of these receptors, as insulin has been shown to interfere with the interaction of the receptor complex and DNA in vitro.[62] In studies by Duckworth et al.,[63] IDE was found to be part of the multicatalytic proteinase complex (also called the 20S proteasome particle). This complex has been implicated in numerous cellular processes, including the ubiquitin-dependent pathway for intracellular degradation of proteins.[4] The presence of IDE in this complex would suggest various new roles for IDE.

Of course, the most fundamental question that still remains is whether IDE is really responsible for the degradation of insulin in intact cells. As noted earlier, evidence both for and against such a role for this enzyme has been advanced. In the future, it may be possible to obtain additional data relating to this question by decreasing the levels of this enzyme, either by a gene-knock out type of experiment or an antisense type of strategy.

Additional Enzymes Involved in Insulin Degradation and Future Directions

In part because of the questions raised as to the role of IDE in insulin degradation, some attempts have been made to identify additional enzymes that degrade insulin. Authier et al.[59] have reported an activity in rat liver endosomes that degrades insulin. This activity could be distinguished from IDE on the basis of its pH optimum (it had a more acidic pH optimum than did IDE) and the lack of crossreactivity with antibodies to IDE. This activity was similar to IDE in its partial requirement for metals for activity and its inhibition by a sulfhydryl (SH)-modifying reagent (hydroxymercuribenzoate). An attempt was made to purify this enzyme on insulin affinity columns. However, it was not clear that the two bands observed on SDS gel electrophoresis in the purified enzyme preparations were, in fact, the protease. Blache et al.[64] have progressed further in their attempts to isolate a rat liver membrane protease that cleaves both glucagon and insulin. This enzyme has a more alkaline pH optimum (more similar to IDE's optimum than to that of the endosomal protease) and a molecular weight of 100 kd on SDS gel electrophoresis. It was present at highest levels in the liver, but was also present in the kidney, pancreas, stomach, and heart. Like IDE, the enzyme was inhibited by both SH-modifying reagents and chelating agents. The amino terminal sequence of the purified protein was obtained and shown to be clearly distinct from that of IDE, although this study could not demonstrate that the amino terminal sequence obtained did in fact come from the protease as an antibody to this peptide sequence could not precipitate this proteolytic activity. Thus, it is likely that other proteases will be identified which can also degrade insulin. Depending on the subcellular location of these molecules, it may be possible that these enzymes play a greater role than IDE in the normal processing of insulin in the whole cell. However, clearly, a great deal of work remains to be done to purify these new enzymes and test their role in insulin degradation.

Acknowledgments

Work in the authors' laboratory was supported by NIH grant DK34926.

References

1. Barrett AJ. Cellular proteolysis: An overview. Ann NY Acad Sci 1992;674:1
2. Bond JS, Butler PE. Intracellular proteases. Annu Rev Biochem 1987;56:333
3. Neuzil KM. Pharmacologic therapy for human immunodeficiency virus infection: A review. Am J Med Sci 1994;307:368
4. Ciechanover A. The ubiquitin-proteasome proteolytic pathway. Cell 1994; 79:13
5. Miura M, Zhu H, Rotello R, et al. Induction of apoptosis in fibroblasts by IL-1 beta-converting enzyme, a mammalian homolog of the *C. elegans* cell death gene ced-3. Cell 1993;75:653
6. Taylor P. The cholinesterases. J Biol Chem 1991;266:4025
7. Marcus S, Xue C-B, Naider F, Becker JM. Degradation of **a**-Factor by a *Saccharomyces cerevisiae* α-mating-type-specific endopeptidase: Evidence for a role in recovery of cells from G1 arrest. Mol Cell Biol 1991;11:1030
8. Miller DS. Stimulation of RNA and protein synthesis by intracellular insulin. Science 1988;240:506
9. Purello F, Vigneri R, Clawson GA, Goldfine ID. Insulin stimulation of nucleoside triphosphatase activity in isolated nuclear envelopes. Science 1982; 216:1005
10. Lin YJ, Harada S, Loten EG, et al. Direct stimulation of immediate-early genes by intranuclear insulin in trypsin-treated H35 hepatoma cells. Proc Natl Acad Sci USA 1992;89:9691
11. Duckworth WC. Insulin degradation: Mechanisms, products, and significance. Endocr Rev 1988;9:319
12. Pease RJ, Smith GD, Peters TJ. Degradation of endocytosed insulin in rat liver is mediated by low-density vesicles. Biochem J 1985;228:137
13. Doherty J-JI, Kay DG, Lai WH, et al. Selective degradation of insulin within rat liver endosomes. J Cell Biol 1990;110:35
14. Wroblewski VJ, Masnyk M, Khambatta SS, Becker GW. Mechanisms involved in degradation of human insulin by cytosolic fractions of human, monkey, and rat liver. Diabetes 1992;41:539
15. Mirsky IA, Broh-Kahn RH. The inactivation of insulin by tissue extracts. I. The distribution and properties of insulin inactivating extracts (insulinase). Arch Biochem Biophys 1949;20:1
16. Tavare JM, Siddle K. Mutational analysis of insulin receptor function: Consensus and controversy. Biochim Biophys Acta 1993;1178:21
17. Roth RA. Insulin receptor structure. In: Cuatrecasas P, Jacobs S, eds. Handbook of Experimental Pharmacology: Insulin. Berlin/Heidelberg: Springer-Verlag;1990:169
18. Levy JR, Olefsky JM. Receptor-mediated internalization and turnover. In: Cuatrecasas P, Jacobs S, eds. Handbook of Experimental Pharmacology: Insulin. Berlin/Heidelberg: Springer-Verlag;1990:237
19. Goldfine ID, Jones AL, Hradek GT, Wong KY. Electron microscopic autoradiographic analysis of [^{125}I]iodoinsulin entry into adult rat hepatocytes in vivo: Evidence for multiple sites of hormone localization. Endocrinology 1981; 108:1821
20. Podlecki DA, Smith RM, Kao M, et al. Nuclear translocation of the insulin receptor. A possible mediator of insulin's long term effects. J Biol Chem 1987;262:3362
21. Harada S, Smith RM, Smith JA, Jarett L. Inhibition of insulin-degrading enzyme increases translocation of insulin to the nucleus in H35 rat hepatoma cells: Evidence of a cytosolic pathway. Endocrinology 1993;132:2293
22. Beyer RE. A study of insulin metabolism in an insulin tolerant strain of mouse. Acta Endocrinol 1955;19:309
23. Shii K, Baba S, Yokono K, Roth RA. Covalent linkage of ^{125}I-insulin to a cytosolic insulin-degrading enzyme. J Biol Chem 1985;260:6503
24. Shii K, Roth RA. Inhibition of insulin degradation by hepatoma cells after microinjection of monoclonal antibodies to a specific cytosolic protease. Proc Natl Acad Sci USA 1986;83:4147
25. Hari J, Shii K, Roth RA. In vivo association of ^{125}I-insulin with a cytosolic insulin-degrading enzyme: Detection by covalent cross-linking and immunoprecipitation with a monoclonal antibody. Endocrinology 1987;120:829
26. Assoian RK. Tager HS. Peptide intermediates in the cellular metabolism of insulin. J Biol Chem 1981;257:9078
27. Duckworth WC, Hamel FG, Peavy DE, et al. Degradation products of insulin generated by hepatocytes and by insulin protease. J Biol Chem 1988;263: 1826
28. Williams FG, Johnson DE, Bauer GE. [^{125}I]-insulin metabolism by the rat liver in vivo: Evidence that a neutral thiol-protease mediates rapid intracellular insulin degradation. Metabolism 1990;39:231
29. Hamel FG, Posner BI, Bergeron JJ, et al. Isolation of insulin degradation products from endosomes derived from intact rat liver. J Biol Chem 1988; 263:6703
30. Kayalar C, Wong WT. Metalloendoprotease inhibitors which block the differentiation of L6 myoblasts inhibit insulin degradation by the endogenous insulin-degrading enzyme. J Biol Chem 1989;264:8928
31. Kuo W-L, Gehm BD, Rosner MR. Regulation of insulin degradation: Expression of an evolutionarily conserved insulin-degrading enzyme increases degradation via an intracellular pathway. Mol Endocrinol 1991;5:1467
32. Kuo W-L, Gehm BD, Rosner MR, et al. Inducible expression and cellular localization of insulin-degrading enzyme in a stably transfected cell line. J Biol Chem 1994;269:22599
33. Affholter JA, Fried VA, Roth RA. Human insulin-degrading enzyme shares structural and functional homologies with *E. coli* protease III. Science 1988;242:1415
34. Cheng Y-S, Zipser D. Purification and characterization of protease III from *Escherichia coli*. J Biol Chem 1979;254:4698
35. Swamy KH, Goldberg AL. Subcellular distribution of various proteases in *Escherichia coli*. J Bacteriol 1982;149:1027
36. Dykstra CC, Kushner SR. Physical characterization of the cloned protease III gene from *Escherichia coli* K-12. J Bacteriol 1985;163:1055

37. Ding L, Becker AB, Suzuki A, Roth RA. Comparison of the enzymatic and biochemical properties of human insulin-degrading enzyme and *Escherichia coli* protease III. J Biol Chem 1992;267:2414
38. Kuo W-L, Gehm BD, Rosner MR. Cloning and expression of the cDNA for a Drosophila insulin-degrading enzyme. Mol Endocrinol 1990;4:1580
39. Kole HK, Smith DR, Lenard J. Characterization and partial purification of an insulinase from *Neurospora crassa*. Arch Biochem Biophys 1992;297:199
40. Finch PW, Wilson RE, Brown K, et al. Complete nucleotide sequence of the *Escherichia coli ptr* gene encoding protease III. Nucleic Acids Res 1986; 14:7695
41. Baumeister H, Muller D, Rehbein M, Richter D. The rat insulin-degrading enzyme: Molecular cloning and characterization of tissue-specific transcripts. FEBS Lett 1993;317:250
42. Ebrahim A, Hamel FG, Bennett RG, Duckworth WC. Identification of the metal associated with the insulin degrading enzyme. Biochem Biophys Res Commun 1991;181:1398
43. Jongeneel CV, Bouvier J, Bairoch A. A unique signature identifies a family of zinc-dependent metallopeptidases. FEBS Lett 1989;242:211
44. Matthews BW. Structural basis of the action of thermolysin and related zinc peptidases. Acc Chem Res 1988;21:333
45. Becker AB, Roth RA. An unusual active site identified in a family of zinc metalloendopeptidases. Proc Natl Acad Sci USA 1992;89:3835
46. Perlman RK, Gehm BD, Kuo W-L, Rosner MR. Functional analysis of conserved residues in the active site of insulin-degrading enzyme. J Biol Chem 1993;268:21538
47. Paces V, Rosenberg LE, Fenton WA, Kalousek F. The β subunit of the mitochondrial processing peptidase from rat liver: Cloning and sequencing of a cDNA and comparison with a proposed family of metallopeptidases. Proc Natl Acad Sci USA 1993;90:5355
48. Pierotti AR, Prat A, Chesneau V, et al. *N*-arginine dibasic convertase, a metalloendopeptidase as a prototype of a class of processing enzymes. Proc Natl Acad Sci USA 1994;91:6078
49. Kirschner RJ, Goldberg AL. A high molecular weight metalloendoprotease from the cytosol of mammalian cells. J Biol Chem 1983;258:967
50. Muller D, Baumeister H, Buck F, Richter D. Atrial natriuretic peptide (ANP) is a high-affinity substrate for rat insulin-degrading enzyme. Eur J Biochem 1991;202:285
51. Gehm BD, Rosner MR. Regulation of insulin, epidermal growth factor, and transforming growth factor-alpha levels by growth factor-degrading enzymes. Endocrinology 1991;128:1603
52. Fagan JM, Waxman L. The ATP-independent pathway in red blood cells that degrades oxidant-damaged hemoglobin. J Biol Chem 1992;267:23015
53. Erdos EG, Skidgel RA. Neural endopeptidase 24.11 (enkephalinase) and related regulators of peptide hormones. FASEB J 1989;3:145
54. Kuo W-L, Montag AG, Rosner MR. Insulin-degrading enzyme is differentially expressed and developmentally regulated in various rat tissues. Endocrinology 1993;132:604
55. Bondy CA, Zhou J, Chin E, et al. Cellular distribution of insulin-degrading enzyme gene expression. J Clin Invest 1994;93:966
56. Lennarz WJ, Strittmatter WJ. Cellular functions of metallo-endoproteinases. Biochim Biophys Acta 1991;1071:149
57. Hamel FG, Mahone MJ, Duckworth WC. Degradation of intraendosomal insulin by insulin-degrading enzyme without acidification. Diabetes 1991;40:436
58. Fawcett J, Rabkin R. Degradation of insulin by isolated rat renal cortical endosomes. Endocrinology 1993;133:1539
59. Authier F, Rachubinski RA, Posner BI, Bergeron JJM. Endosomal proteolysis of insulin by an acidic thiol metalloprotease unrelated to insulin degrading enzyme. J Biol Chem 1994;269:3010
60. Wickner WT. How ATP drives proteins across membranes. Science 1994; 266:1197
61. Rawlings ND, Barrett AJ. Homologues of insulinase, a new superfamily of metalloendopeptidases. Biochem J 1991;275:389
62. Kupfer SR, Wilson EM, French FS. Androgen and glucocorticoid receptors interact with insulin degrading enzyme. J Biol Chem 1994;269:20622
63. Duckworth WC, Bennett RG, Hamel FG. A direct inhibitory effect of insulin on a cytosolic proteolytic complex containing insulin-degrading enzyme and multicatalytic proteinase. J Biol Chem 1994;269:24575
64. Blache P, Kervran A, Le-Nguyen D, et al. Endopeptidase from rat liver membranes, which generates miniglucagon from glucagon. J Biol Chem 1993; 268:21748

PART III

Definition/ Classification

Diabetes Mellitus, edited by Derek LeRoith, Simeon I. Taylor, and Jerrold M. Olefsky. Lippincott–Raven Publishers, Philadelphia © 1996.

CHAPTER 27

Definition and Classification of Diabetes Including Maturity-Onset Diabetes of the Young

STEFAN S. FAJANS

Definition and Introduction to Classification

Diabetes mellitus is a genetic disorder in which superimposed environmental factors bring out the phenotypic expression of the disease. It is a disorder of metabolism of carbohydrate, protein, and fat associated with an absolute or relative insufficiency of insulin secretion accompanied by various degrees of insulin resistance. In its fully developed clinical expression, it is characterized by fasting hyperglycemia and, in most patients with long-standing disease, by microangiopathic and atherosclerotic macrovascular disease and neuropathy. Although major phenotypic differences in types of clinical diabetes (juvenile-onset type, maturity-onset type) have been appreciated for a century, it is only in the last 2 decades that new knowledge of the etiology and pathogenesis of diabetes, although still incomplete, has indicated that diabetes is a heterogeneous group of disorders. Differences between various forms of the disease are expressed in terms of etiology and pathogenesis (genetic, environmental, and immune factors), in natural history, and in response to treatment. Diabetes, therefore, is not a single disease but a syndrome.[1] Ideally, classification should be based on etiology and pathogenesis only. For a classification to be useful (1) for the clinician in categorizing patients for purposes of diagnosis and treatment, (2) for purposes of research, and (3) as a framework for the collection of clinical and epidemiologic data in diverse population groups, it is convenient presently to include other considerations into a classification. In 1979, an international workgroup, sponsored by the National Diabetes Data Group (NDDG) of the National Institutes of Health (NIH), published a "Classification of Diabetes Mellitus and Other Categories of Glucose Intolerance".[2] It was adopted by the World Health Organization (WHO).[3] The classification to be used in this chapter is based essentially on the work and proceedings of the NDDG workgroup with minor modifications. Indices by which other classifications could be devised have been reviewed.[4] At the present time, any classification is still arbitrary, sometimes inconsistent, not adhering ideally to what is known about the natural history of various types, and the result of a compromise to accommodate different points of view.

Classification of Diabetes Mellitus and Other Categories of Glucose Intolerance

The present classification of diabetes mellitus (Table 27-1) includes three clinical courses:

1. *Diabetes mellitus*—characterized either by fasting hyperglycemia or levels of plasma glucose that exceed defined limits during a glucose tolerance test.
2. *Impaired glucose tolerance*—characterized by plasma glucose levels, measured during a glucose tolerance test, which exceed normal but are below those defined as diabetes (Table 27-2). The levels of plasma glucose in the fasting state or during a glucose tolerance test that are defined as normal, impaired, or diabetic are also thought to be compromises and are considered not to be ideal by all investigators.
3. *Gestational diabetes*—characterized by abnormal plasma glucose levels during pregnancy.

The classification system also includes two statistical risk classes in the natural history of diabetes (for research purposes only) characterized by an absence of carbohydrate metabolism abnormalities. These classes include a previous abnormality of glucose tolerance, and a potential abnormality of glucose tolerance.[2]

The classification system was designed so that an individual could be placed in only one class at a specific point in time; the classes were to be mutually exclusive. However, an individual can change from one class to another in the natural history of the disease.

Clinical Classes

Diabetes Mellitus

Diabetes mellitus is subdivided into four different types that differ in etiology and pathogenesis. These subtypes are listed in the sections that follow.

Type I: Insulin-Dependent Diabetes Mellitus

Type I, or insulin-dependent diabetes mellitus (IDDM), occurs in approximately 10% of all diabetic patients in the Western world. Genetic factors are thought to be important in most patients with type I disease, as evidenced by the associated increased (or decreased) frequency of certain histocompatibility locus antigens (HLA) on chromosome number 6. In various Western groups of diabetic patients, the percent prevalence, particularly of DR3, DR4, and DQ, has been found to be increased as compared to control populations, whereas the frequency of DR2 and DR7 has been decreased. It is likely that, in insulin-dependent diabetes, there are one or more immune response genes in linkage disequilibrium with HLA antigens that may impart increased susceptibility to B-cell damage by permitting interaction of an environmental factor with specific cell membrane antigens. In the most common type of IDDM (type IA), it has been postulated that environmental (acquired) factors, such as certain viral infections, and possibly, nutritional or chemical agents, when superimposed on genetic factors, may lead to cell-mediated autoimmune destruction of β-cells. Thus, genetically determined abnormal immune responses (linked to HLA associations), characterized by cell-mediated and humoral autoimmunity, are thought to play a pathogenetic role after evocation by an environmental factor. Circulating cytoplasmic islet cell antibodies (ICAs) detected by immunofluorescence, insulin autoantibodies (IAAs), and antibodies to a 64K antigen (glutamic acid decarboxylase, or GAD) are present at diagnosis in approximately 80% of patients, but they disappear over the course of the next few years

TABLE 27-1. Classification of Diabetes Mellitus and Other Categories of Glucose Intolerance

Clinical Classes	Subclasses	Stages of Natural History or Evolution*	Other Information/Explanations
Diabetes Mellitus (DM)			
Type I—Insulin-dependent DM (IDDM) Types	Type IA—Classical Type IB—Primary autoimmune	1. Pre-ketosis–prone • Diabetic glucose tolerance test (GTT) • Fasting hyperglycemia 2. Ketosis-prone; insulin-dependent†	Islet-cell antibody (ICA)–positive Insulin autoantibody (IAA)–positive 64K antibody–positive
Type II—Non–insulin-dependent DM (NIDDM) Types	NIDDM in obese individuals NIDDM in nonobese individuals Maturity-onset diabetes of the young (MODY)-NIDDM in the young plus autosomal dominant inheritance	1. Non–insulin-requiring† • Diabetic GTT • Fasting hyperglycemia 2. Insulin-requiring†	MODY—chromosome 20q mutation (MODY1), chromosome 7p-glucokinase (MODY2) mutations and chromosome 12q (MODY3) mutations
Malnutrition-related diabetes mellitus (MRDM)‡	Fibrocalculous pancreatic diabetes Protein-deficient pancreatic diabetes		Insulin-dependent for health and life, not for prevention of ketosis
Other types (including DM associated with certain conditions and syndromes)	Pancreatic disease Hormonal etiology Drug- or chemical-induced Certain genetic syndromes Insulin receptor abnormalities Other miscellaneous conditions		
Impaired Glucose Tolerance (IGT)	IGT in Obese IGT in Nonobese IGT in MODY IGT associated with certain conditions and syndromes: • Pancreatic disease • Hormonal etiology • Drug- or chemical-induced • Certain genetic syndromes • Insulin receptor abnormalities • Other miscellaneous conditions		ICA-, IAA-, and 64K antibody–positive and decreased first-phase insulin response in type I DM
Gestational Diabetes (GDM)			May be precursor of type II or type I diabetes
Statistical Risk Classes			
Previous abnormality of glucose tolerance (PreAGT)			ICA-, IAA-, and 64K antibody–positive; decreased first-phase insulin response in type I DM
Potential abnormality of glucose tolerance (PotAGT)			Nondiabetic member of MODY family who has genetic marker on chromosome 7p (glucokinase) or 20q (ADA, D20S16) or 12q

*Also see IGT, GDM, and Statistical Risk Classes.
†Major clinical form of diabetes.
‡Major clinical form of diabetes in parts of Africa, Asia, and the Caribbean.
(Adapted with permission from Fajans SS. Diabetes Mellitus: Definition, Classification, Tests. In: DeGroot, LJ, ed. Endocrinology 3rd ed. Philadelphia: W.B. Saunders;1995:1412.)

in most patients. They are probably the result, rather than the cause, of an autoimmune process. (In a very small subset of patients, an overwhelming viral infection may lead to destruction of β-cells without a genetic predisposition.) Classically, this type of disease occurs most commonly in childhood and adolescence (type IA); however, it can be recognized and may become symptomatic for the first time at any age. Usually, the affected patient experiences an abrupt symptomatic onset of disease secondary to severe insulin insufficiency (polyuria, polydipsia, polyphagia, weight loss, fatigue), is prone to ketosis, and is thin. Insulin dependency implies that the administration of insulin is essential to prevent spontaneous ketosis, coma, and death. In addition to the ketosis-prone stage, this type of disease can also be recognized in an earlier symptomatic or asymptomatic stage, before the patient becomes ketotic. By prospective testing in asymptomatic siblings of insulin-dependent diabetics, one can even discover patients with diabetic glucose tolerance tests and with normal fasting plasma glucose levels.[1,5] Their diabetes progresses rapidly to the ketotic form, usually within 2 years after recognition, but occasionally after long periods of time. In nondiabetic identical twins of type I diabetic patients (with a high proportion of HLA-DR3 or HLA-DR4 positivity), circulating ICAs and IAAs and activated T lymphocytes have been found for more than 8 years with progressive β-cell dysfunction before a more profound decrease in insulin secretory activity and the appearance of fasting hyperglycemia have been noted.[6] (See later section on Potential Abnormality of Glucose Tolerance.)

A second type of insulin-dependent diabetes—type IB—occurs less commonly, affecting less than 10% of all patients with IDDM. Primary autoimmunity is thought to be involved in the pathogenesis of this form of type I diabetes. Such patients have associated autoimmune endocrine diseases, such as Hashimoto's thyroiditis, Graves' disease, Addison's disease, or primary gonadal

Table 27-2. National Diabetes Data Group (NDDG) Criteria for Interpretation of Oral Glucose Tolerance Tests Using Venous Plasma or Serum and a 75g Carbohydrate Load[*]

Fasting (F) or Hours After Glucose Load	Normal[†]	Impaired Glucose Tolerance (IGT)[‡]	Diabetes[‡§]	Gestational Diabetes[‖] (100 g glucose)	
F	<115 (6.4)	<140 (7.8)	≥140 (7.8) or	≥105	If any two or more of four values meet criteria
1/2 and/or 1 and/or 1 1/2[#]	<200 (11.1)	≥200 (11.1)	≥200 (11.1)	≥190	
2	<140 (7.8)	140–199 (7.8–11.1)	≥200 (11.1)	≥165	
3				≥145	

[*]Values are given in mg/dL; values in parentheses are in mM.
[†]Test results with glucose values above normal but below the criteria for IGT should be designated as ''nondiagnostic.''
[‡]In nonpregnant individuals.
[§]For the diagnosis of diabetes in children, the fasting value must be ≥140 mg/dL, in addition to 1- and 2-hour elevations of GTT.
[‖]Criteria of O'Sullivan and Mahan (1964).[52]
[#]WHO Study Group recommendations omit values between fasting and 2 hours.
(Adapted with permission from Fajans, SS. Diabetes Mellitus: Definition, Classification, Tests. In: DeGroot, LJ., ed. Endocrinology, 3rd ed. Philadelphia: W.B. Saunders;1995:1412)

failure, as well as associated nonendocrine autoimmune diseases, such as pernicious anemia, connective tissue diseases, celiac disease, and myasthenia gravis. These patients also have a high prevalence of a family history of endocrine and nonendocrine autoimmune disease. Primary autoimmunity is also suggested by the persistence of high titers of pancreatic ICAs during the life of the patient. Type IB diabetes occurs more frequently in female patients than in male patients and has a later onset of symptoms (usually at 30 to 50 years of age). Although diabetes may be characterized by severe insulin insufficiency, milder nonketotic forms of diabetes are also seen. Recognition of type IB diabetes is important in that it should alert the physician to the possible presence of or propensity for other autoimmune disease. Type IB diabetes is more commonly associated with histocompatibility antigen DR3, whereas classical type I diabetes is more commonly associated with DR4. Because there is an overlap in these HLA associations, however, true heterogeneity in type I diabetes mellitus in terms of HLA associations probably does not exist. Nevertheless, IDDM appears to be heterogeneous in terms of the genetic, environmental, and autoimmune factors that precipitate the disease.

Type II Non–Insulin-Dependent Diabetes Mellitus

The second type of diabetes—type II or non–insulin-dependent diabetes mellitus (NIDDM)—which affects approximately 90% of diabetics in the Western world, also has a genetic basis that is commonly expressed by a more frequent familial pattern of occurrence than is seen in IDDM. Environmental factors superimposed on genetic susceptibility are more easily identified in the evolution of NIDDM. Patients with type II diabetes may have body weights that range from normal to excessive; indeed, NIDDM has been subclassified according to its association with obesity (see Table 27-1). The intake of excessive calories leading to weight gain and obesity and resulting in or exacerbating insulin resistance is an important factor in the pathogenesis of NIDDM in most (60–80%) affected patients in Western societies. A genetic defect in the insulin secretory response to nutrients may be detected for the first time when increasing insulin resistance triggers a compensatory response that cannot be met. Fasting hyperglycemia and glucose intolerance are usually improved or corrected by weight loss. Obesity and pathologic insulin resistance are by no means essential in the evolution of NIDDM. In patients with NIDDM who are not overweight, even small increases in body weight (including normal growth in childhood and adolescence) can exacerbate glucose intolerance and precipitate fasting hyperglycemia.[1,7] Nevertheless, evidence has been presented that the absence or presence of obesity may differentiate between different forms of NIDDM. In an analysis of non–insulin-dependent diabetes, Köbberling found that the prevalence of diabetes in siblings was higher in nonobese than in obese human diabetic subjects.[8] In one Japanese study of NIDDM, Kuzuya and Matsuda[9] also found that patients with a definitive history of obesity had a lower frequency of a family history of diabetes and a lower prevalence of diabetes in their parents than did patients without obesity, supporting the concept that the presence or absence of obesity may mark heterogeneous groups of diabetics within the category of type II diabetes.

In most patients with type II diabetes, a diagnosis is made in middle age. A subclass of NIDDM includes those families in whom diabetes can be recognized in children, adolescents, and young adults, referred to as maturity-onset diabetes of the young (MODY).[1,7,10–13] Autosomal dominant inheritance of diabetes has been established in MODY; most NIDDM is not inherited in this way. Although MODY was excluded as a subclass by the NDDG classification, it is included here because MODY is the only form of diabetes in which a definite mode of inheritance has been established and a gene or genetic markers have been identified (see Table 27-1).

In contradistinction to type I diabetes, HLA associations have not been found in most populations with type II diabetes except for a weak association in three specific population groups.[5] No association has been found between specific HLA antigens and MODY.[5,7,11] Evidence of cell-mediated immunity and the presence of ICAs and IAAs characteristic of type I diabetes have not been found in type II diabetes or MODY.[7,11]

Patients with NIDDM are non–insulin-dependent for prevention of ketosis (i.e., they are ketosis-resistant or not ketosis-prone), but they may require insulin for correction of symptomatic or nonsymptomatic persistent fasting hyperglycemia if this cannot be achieved with the aid of dietary modifications, exercise or oral agents. Thus, therapeutic administration of insulin does not distinguish between IDDM and NIDDM. Occasionally, it is difficult to distinguish nonobese patients with NIDDM who are treated with insulin from truly insulin-dependent (ketosis-prone) patients (IDDM). Patients with NIDDM may even develop ketosis under circumstances of severe stress precipitated by infections or trauma. Usually, other factors, such as age of onset, family history of diabetes, clinical course, or natural history (rapidity of progression in terms of severity, fluctuations in plasma glucose, frequency of reactions, frequency of ketonuria) will aid in proper classification. In a research setting, the C-peptide response to glucose, Sustacal, or glucagon, and the presence or absence of ICA may also be helpful. In other patients with NIDDM, hyperglycemia can be corrected without the administration of insulin by diet therapy, exercise or dietary modifications plus oral agents.

In patients with type II diabetes, insulinopenia may be only relative, whereas insulin resistance may be of greater importance in the pathogenesis of hyperglycemia.[14] In such patients, the insulin response to glucose may be normal or supernormal compared to that in nonobese control subjects, particularly when they do not have hyperglycemia or have only mild fasting hyperglycemia.[14] In patients with NIDDM or MODY with similar abnormalities of glucose tolerance and fasting hyperglycemia, however, our group[1,15,16] and others[17,18] have found a wide spectrum of insulin responses to administered glucose ranging from very low insulin responses to very high insulin responses. It has become apparent that heterogeneity in pathogenesis exists even in the usual clinical forms of NIDDM.[19–23]

In the presence of moderate fasting hyperglycemia (>200 mg/dL), insulin responses to glucose are greatly diminished in NIDDM. Early in its natural history, the insulin secretory defect and insulin resistance may be reversible by treatment (e.g., weight reduction) with normalization of glucose tolerance. The typical chronic complications of diabetes—namely, macroangiopathy, microangiopathy, neuropathy, and cataracts—are seen in NIDDM as well.

Maturity-Onset Diabetes of the Young

Maturity-onset diabetes of the young (MODY) is a relatively uncommon subtype of NIDDM. Because MODY will not be discussed in the chapters on type II diabetes, a brief description of the phenotypic expression, natural history, molecular genetics, and pathogeneses of MODY is given here. MODY is defined as NIDDM characterized by an early age of onset and autosomal dominant inheritance.[7,11–13] The latter is a hallmark of MODY and distinguishes it from other types of NIDDM.

When MODY is suspected and family members are examined biochemically, a diagnosis of diabetes can be made almost invariably by the age of 25 years, and frequently by 9–13 years of age; in some families, diagnosis is possible at an even earlier age. Because of autosomal dominant inheritance and early age of onset, it is possible to collect large multigenerational pedigrees with MODY, a unique feature of this subtype of NIDDM.

An example is the RW pedigree, consisting of more than 360 family members that have been identified including 72 known subjects with diabetes distributed over five generations. This family has been studied and followed prospectively since 1958.[13] The propositus, II-5 (W branch), offspring of I-3, had diabetes diagnosed at the age of 41 years (Fig. 27-1*A*). He became blind from diabetic retinopathy at the age of 61 years and had an amputation for peripheral vascular disease. He had five brothers, four of whom had diabetes and one who did not. Macrovascular disease, including myocardial infarctions and peripheral vascular disease with gangrene and amputations, as well as microvascular disease, including retinopathy and blindness, are complications resulting from MODY in the RW pedigree (see Fig. 27-1). In addition to these, there is also evidence of neuropathy. In 1958, the 11 nonobese, apparently healthy and asymptomatic offspring of II-5 were recruited for routine blood glucose testing. Seven of the 11 were found to have abnormal glucose metabolism.[11] The older three had fasting hyperglycemia (a mean of 257 mg/dL), three others had diabetic glucose tolerance tests without diagnostic fasting hyperglycemia, and one had impaired glucose tolerance (IGT). Subsequent follow-up has revealed that fasting hyperglycemia has developed in all. Two have been treated with insulin because of eventual unresponsiveness to sulfonylurea drugs, and five have been treated successfully with sulfonylurea drugs up to the present. Subsequently, by routine blood glucose testing, diabetes has been diagnosed in 10 of the 20 members of generation IV who are offspring of diabetic subjects of generation III, as well as in four members of generation V thus far. None of them are obese. Ages at diagnosis ranged from 9 to 14 years in 12 of these patients with diabetes. Patient IV-144 has typical IDDM.

Among the offspring of II-2, three of the five diabetic members (III-3, III-4, III-8) have MODY segregating in generations III–V (see Fig. 27-1*B*). Two of the five (III-2, III-9) are obese, as well as hyperinsulinemic (although MODY subjects are generally hypo-

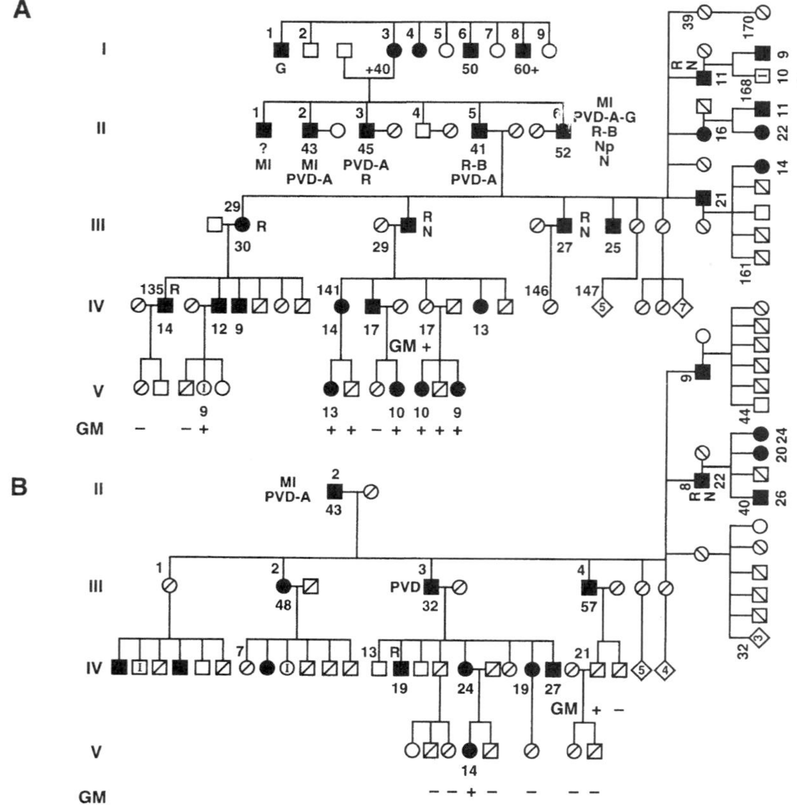

Figure 27-1. Partial pedigree of the RW family. The offspring of I-1 belong to the R branch, whereas the offspring of I-3 belong to the W branch. Only the offspring of II-5 (***A***) and II-2 (***B***) of the W branch are shown. All subjects with diabetes were or are non–insulin-dependent except IV-144, who is insulin-dependent. Diabetic or IGT offspring of II-5 of generations III–V (***A***) and diabetic offspring III-3 and III-8 (***B***) and their diabetic offspring are genetic marker (GM) (chromosome 20)–positive. In addition, nondiabetic IV-143 (***A***) and IV-21 (***B***) are GM-positive (+). In generation V, GM-positive (GM+) or -negative (−) individuals are indicated (***A, B***). The numbers above the male diabetic members (■) and female diabetic members (●) represent the number in generation, whereas those below these symbols are ages at diagnosis. *I*, impaired glucose tolerance; ○, normal glucose tolerance; □, reported normal and untested; *N*, groups of siblings untested and of unspecified sex with number of individuals given; *MI*, myocardial infarction; *PVD*, peripheral vascular disease; *A*, amputation; *G*, gangrene; *N*, neuropathy; *Ang*, angina pectoris; *R*, retinopathy; *R-B*, retinopathy and blindness; *Np*, nephropathy. All diabetic members of generations I and II, along with III-29 and III-30, are deceased. (Reprinted from Life Sciences, Volume 55, Fajans SS, Bell GI, Bowden DW, Halter JB, Polonsky KS: Maturity-onset diabetes of the young, pp. 413–422, 1994, with kind permission from Elsevier Science, Ltd, The Boulevard, Langford Lane, Kidlington 0X5 1GB, UK)

insulinemic; see later discussion); one was diagnosed with diabetes at the age of 48 years (III-2) and the other at the age of 61 years (III-9) by prospective testing. Of the 12 offspring of II-3, 6 have NIDDM. In none was the diagnosis made before the age of 43 years (although none underwent blood glucose testing at an earlier age). Moreover, none of the 44 offspring of these 6 diabetic patients who were tested have diabetes at the present time. Similarly, none of the four offspring of diabetic II-6 has diabetes, nor do any of their 15 offspring who have been tested. It appears that offspring of II-5 and some of II-2 exhibit the classic pattern of autosomal dominant inheritance characteristic of MODY, whereas the offspring of II-3 and II-6, as well as of III-2 and III-9, do not. Thus, as indicated and confirmed by molecular genetic studies (see later section), it appears that heterogeneity of inheritance and type of diabetes appears even in this large pedigree. Sibling II-4 did not have diabetes. Indeed, none of his 18 offspring of generations III–IV have NIDDM, although one granddaughter has classical IDDM. II-1 had no children.

I-1 (see Fig. 27-1*A*) had three offspring, two of whom were diagnosed as having diabetes (R branch, generation II, not shown in Figure 27-1). Among their 10 offspring in generation III, six have NIDDM or have been diagnosed as having NIDDM. Of 12 tested subjects in generation IV who are offspring of a diabetic parent, 6 have diabetes. Thus, diabetes is inherited in the autosomal pattern of MODY in the R branch as well. None of these subjects are obese.

MODY is usually asymptomatic in younger age groups, although some patients may have symptoms, particularly if stressed by an infection. Unless detected by prospective testing, either prompted by a family history of NIDDM in two or more generations, performed in a young person, or performed during a pregnancy, a clinical diagnosis of diabetes is frequently not made in many members of such families until middle or late adult life. Thus, the age of diagnosis cannot be equated to the age of onset of hyperglycemia. As demonstrated in the RW pedigree, in which MODY is linked to chromosome 20q (see discussion that follows), it can be demonstrated by repeated testing in younger members that there may be a variable rate of progression from nondiagnostic (but not normal) results on glucose tolerance tests to IGT, from IGT to diabetic glucose tolerance with normal fasting plasma glucose levels (up to 18 years), and no progression or very slow or rapid progression to fasting hyperglycemia (0.5 to 27 years). The severity of carbohydrate intolerance may fluctuate for many years, particularly in patients with mild abnormalities, before the onset of persistent fasting hyperglycemia. In contrast, other individuals with MODY from this pedigree may have fasting hyperglycemia or rapid progression from an early age. Thus, some diabetic patients with MODY may be diagnosed in their teens or early 20s by the usual symptoms of decompensated diabetes, and thus may be confused with those with type I diabetes. Among the nonobese diabetic subjects of the RW pedigree in generations III–V, approximately 80% have had fasting hyperglycemia at diagnosis or on follow-up studies. Plasma glucose levels at the time fasting hyperglycemia is first detected at ranges from 140 to 366 mg/dL. Approximately 30% have fasting hyperglycemia diagnosed between the ages of 9 and 14 years, or within a 1- to 3-year follow-up period.

Fasting hyperglycemia, even at a young age (9 to 14 years), may be responsive to either diet therapy alone, or diet plus oral agents for a few years or decades.[7,11,24] With sulfonylurea therapy, glucose-induced insulin secretion has been shown to increase an average of 68% in diabetic patients who remained responsive to chlorpropamide for up to 33 years.[24] In most patients, however, glucose-induced insulin secretion declines over time (1–4% per year). Some patients (9–13 years of age at diagnosis) become unresponsive to maximal doses of sulfonylureas after 3 to 25 years, and then demonstrate a very small or no increase in glucose-induced insulin secretion. They require treatment with insulin to normalize fasting hyperglycemia (not insulin-dependent or ketotic and ICA-negative diabetes). At that point, some of these patients have very low fasting C-peptide levels, an absence of nutrient-stimulated C-peptide levels, and an unstable type of diabetes resembling that seen in IDDM.[7,11,24] Among the known diabetic patients from generations III–V of the RW pedigree, approximately 30% have come to require insulin. Typical microangiopathic and macroangiopathic complications may occur, similar to those seen in other patients with NIDDM.[7,11] When vascular complications do occur, they frequently are not detected until middle or older age, although in some patients, they may be detected in their 30s or earlier.

In contrast to MODY that is linked to chromosome 20q (as is the case in the RW pedigree), MODY that is secondary to mutations in the glucokinase gene on chromosome 7p (see following discussion) is a relatively mild form of diabetes accompanied by mild fasting hyperglycemia and IGT that, in most affected patients, may be recognized by biochemical testing at an even younger age (mean of 7 ± 4 years; minimal age of 1 year).[25] There appears to be little progression of hyperglycemia on follow-up studies.[26,27] Severe fasting hyperglycemia and vascular complications occur infrequently. Thus, MODY that is secondary to glucokinase mutations appears to be a much milder and relatively benign form of hyperglycemia, in contrast to the more severe diabetes seen in MODY linked to chromosome 20q, which more closely resembles classical NIDDM.

MODY fulfills some of the fundamental requirements for defining the molecular genetic basis of any disorder by linkage analysis because of its established autosomal dominant inheritance and the availability of large multigenerational kindreds.[12] The RW pedigree was first used for a search of diabetes susceptibility genes by this technique. The initial linkage strategy was to search for "candidate genes"—that is, genes involved in carbohydrate and lipid metabolism. Candidate genes excluded as the cause of NIDDM in the RW pedigree include the insulin, glucagon, islet amyloid polypeptide, insulin-like growth factors 1 and 2, insulin receptor, low-density lipoprotein receptor, glucose transporters, apolipoprotein, lipoprotein lipase, and hexokinase 1 genes, as well as the major histocompatibility complex.[28] In a subsequent systematic gene mapping approach (positional cloning), DNA polymorphisms in the adenosine deaminase gene (ADA) and the anonymous locus D20S16 on the long arm of chromosome 20 were found to cosegregate with MODY[28–33] in members with diabetes of both W and R branches. There are no recombinations between these markers and MODY, and the lod score presently exceeds 17.0 at a recombination fraction of 0.00, indicating that the gene responsible for MODY in this family is tightly linked to these genes. In the W branch, the descendants of II-3 who have NIDDM do not carry the at-risk ADA and D20S16 markers, suggesting that they do not have MODY, but another form of NIDDM.[28–33] In addition, two of five diabetic offspring of II-2 (III-2 and III-9) who are obese and in whom diabetes was diagnosed at the age of 48 and 61 years, respectively, do not carry these markers.

Two subjects (IV-143 and IV-21) in the W branch of the RW pedigree who are older than 25 years of age are nondiabetic but carry the ADA and D20S16 markers. Thus, these two subjects are nonpenetrant.[28,31] IV-143 had one glucose tolerance test characteristic of IGT and one characteristic of diabetes at ages 16–17 years, but for the next 19 years, each GTT was within normal limits despite a low insulin response to orally administered glucose. She is very lean, active, and has increased sensitivity to insulin during the frequently sampled intravenous glucose tolerance test (Bergman's minimal model). During a prolonged low-dose glucose infusion, she became markedly hyperglycemic.

The identification of genetic markers for MODY in the RW pedigree has shown that linkage studies of large MODY families can uncover DNA markers for NIDDM.[12,28,30] The gene responsible for MODY in the RW pedigree is unknown, but is in the region of ADA and D20S16 on chromosome 20q. Finding genetic markers is proof at the molecular level that genetic factors play an important role in the causation of MODY. DNA typing can identify at-risk subjects; that is, genetic screening for prediabetes is possible in the RW pedigree. MODY is not fully penetrant, suggesting that environmental factors may also play a role in its development. Identification of the MODY gene on chromosome 20 may disclose previously unrecognized mechanisms controlling insulin secretion and lead us closer to an understanding of the pathogenesis of MODY in this pedigree, with possible application to NIDDM in general. Such studies may lead eventually to the prevention, improved treatment, or even cure of this and other forms of NIDDM.

NIDDM may have different causes even in a single family. Previous clinical studies have suggested heterogeneity of the diabetes in the RW pedigree, which was subsequently confirmed by molecular genetic studies. The results of these studies support the inclusion of autosomal dominant inheritance in the definition of MODY. The RW pedigree includes two patients with IDDM, one a granddaughter of II-5 and the other a granddaughter of nondiabetic II-4. Because neither of these patients carry the genetic markers for MODY, this finding provides evidence that the MODY susceptibility gene does not contribute to IDDM in this pedigree.[28] Because there was heterogeneity between MODY families in terms of hormonal and metabolic characterization,[34] it was postulated that additional NIDDM susceptibility genes or modifying determinants would be found.[28] Indeed, this occurred shortly thereafter.

Tight linkage between MODY and the glucokinase gene on chromosome 7p was found in approximately 60% of 32 French families with MODY,[25,35] in one British family,[26,36] and in two Japanese families.[37,38] Glucokinase is the first rate-limiting enzyme in the metabolism of glucose by the pancreatic β-cell. It causes the phosphorylation of glucose to glucose-6-phosphate, initiating glycolysis, which is essential for insulin secretion. This enzyme has been postulated to be the glucose-sensing mechanism for insulin secretion.[39] Subsequently, a host of different mutations (nonsense, missense, or deletions) in the glucokinase gene has been found in members of families in which MODY is linked to the glucokinase gene.[25,36–38,40–43] These mutations are believed to cause diabetes by a gene dosage mechanism with a modest decrease in glucokinase activity increasing the glucose threshold for insulin secretion. Matchinsky[39] has suggested that a 15% decrease in glucokinase activity may raise the threshold of insulin secretion from 5 to 6 mM. A correlation has been found between the degree of impairment of glucokinase activity and impairment of B-cell function.[27,43] Mutations in the glucokinase gene are the most common genetic cause of NIDDM identified to date, particularly among MODY pedigrees. In one French[35,40] and one British[36] glucokinase-linked MODY pedigree, there was also evidence for genetic heterogeneity in that some diabetic subjects had not inherited the mutant glucokinase allele. The RW pedigree is the only large pedigree in which tight linkage of MODY to chromosome 20q has been established. Evidence consistent with linkage to chromosome 20q has been found in two French[25,35] and one Canadian (D.W. Bowden and E. Colle, unpublished data) MODY pedigrees.

In addition to the glucokinase gene (MODY2) and the gene on chromosome 20 (MODY1), there must be other loci that can cause MODY, as MODY pedigrees have been described that show no evidence of linkage with glucokinase or markers on chromosome 20.[25,26,31,35,44] Recent genetic studies have identified a third locus on chromosome 12 (MODY3) that is linked to MODY in a group of French families.[45] Three MODY families from Denmark, Germany and Michigan, USA showed evidence of linkage with MODY3 and a family from Japan showed suggestive evidence of linkage.[46] The results confirm the presence of a gene contributing to the development of MODY on chromosome 12 and localizes MODY3 to a 5 cM interval between markers D12S86 and D12S807/D12S820.

In the RW pedigree, most MODY subjects who were offspring of II-2 and II-5 were found to have a delayed and subnormal insulin secretory response to orally administered glucose, strongly suggesting an impairment of B-cell function. In these individuals, impaired B-cell function, although moderate in magnitude, appears to be the major underlying pathogenetic factor for abnormal glucose levels. The low insulin secretory response to glucose may occur from childhood on, and before glucose intolerance appears. It is thought to be a manifestation of the basic genetic defect that leads to diabetes only when additional superimposed environmental factors supervene.[7,11] A number of environmental determinants superimposed on genetic factors may lead to the appearance of IGT or NIDDM in predisposed individuals. In this MODY pedigree, the important factors appear to be a decreasing physiologic insulin sensitivity, without the normally associated increase in insulin secretion, as occurs with increasing age, growth and increasing body mass, and puberty, as well as a further gain in weight without developing obesity when subjects progress from adolescence to young adult age.[7,11] In addition, as mentioned earlier, glucose-induced insulin secretion may decline further over time.[24] Pathologic insulin resistance does not appear to be an important contributing factor because of normal sensitivity to intravenously administered insulin and because of the usually low insulin requirement in insulin-treated diabetic members of the RW pedigree. In contrast, the diabetic but non-MODY offspring of II-3 and the non-MODY diabetic offspring of II-2 are hyperinsulinemic, differentiating them from the offspring of II-2 and II-5, who have MODY.

In patients with MODY that is linked to a mutation in the glucokinase gene, there is evidence of decreased insulin secretion by continuous glucose infusion,[26,27,47] although the acute insulin response to glucose remains within normal limits.[27,47] A decreased insulin secretory response to orally administered glucose has also been reported in glucokinase-linked MODY.[38] In addition, no evidence of insulin resistance has been reported[27,47] in such patients. This is in contradistinction to patients with other types of NIDDM, most of whom are obese, and in whom it has been found or postulated that insulin resistance is a more important factor than insulin deficiency in the pathogenesis of diabetes.[14,48]

Because chronic hyperglycemia has been reported to be associated with both a decrease in insulin sensitivity as well as an impairment of B-cell function, the question of which is the primary genetic defect in MODY or NIDDM is very difficult to address in diabetic patients.[14] As we now have genetic markers for MODY in the RW pedigree, we attempted to determine early abnormalities of insulin action and of insulin secretion in nondiabetic subjects of the pedigree with and without the gene markers to ascertain which of these defects might be primary. Insulin action and insulin secretion were assessed with a frequently sampled intravenous glucose tolerance test (Bergman's minimal model). Insulin secretion was further assessed during constant low-dose glucose infusion by deconvolution of plasma C-peptide and by pulse analysis. The nondiabetic marker-positive group had normal sensitivity to insulin and an unimpaired acute insulin response to intravenous glucose. However, the nondiabetic marker-positive group had decreased mean plasma C-peptide concentration and reduced absolute amplitude of insulin secretory ultradian oscillations and decreased insulin secretion rate during prolonged glucose infusion (Fig. 27-2).[49] These responses to prolonged glucose infusion were similar to those observed in the diabetic group, who, in addition, also had a decreased or absent acute insulin response to intravenous glucose.[49] Normal insulin secretion was observed in the nondiabetic marker-negative family members, as in the comparison groups. Deranged and deficient insulin secretion, and not insulin resistance, appears to be the genetic or primary abnormality that characterizes nondiabetic individuals who are predisposed to MODY in the RW pedigree. Prolonged glucose infusion studies may reveal qualitative and quantitative defects in insulin secretion that are not identified by the acute insulin response to intravenous glucose. Thus, use of the acute insulin response to glucose may not be able to exclude a primary β-cell defect in the pathogenesis of any form of NIDDM.[49]

Further qualitative and quantitative differences in insulin secretory defects between MODY subjects with glucokinase mutations and MODY subjects with chromosome 20q mutation have been confirmed by studies involving acute and prolonged intravenous infusion of glucose. MODY subjects with glucokinase muta-

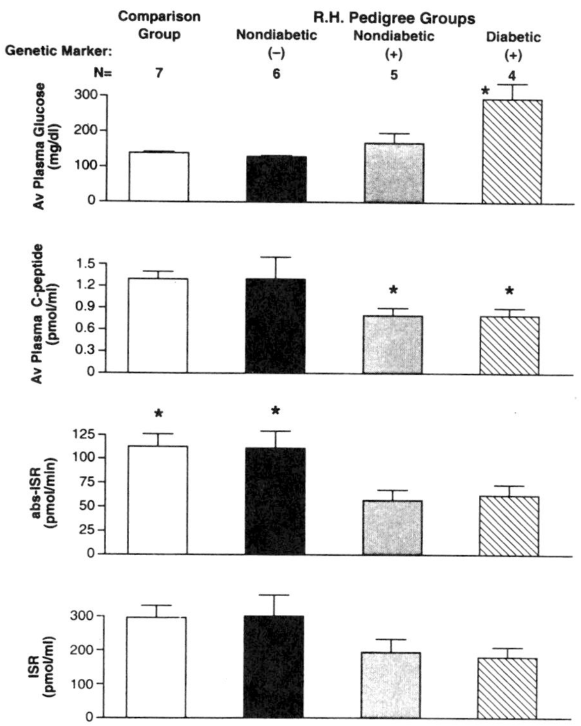

Figure 27-2. Average plasma glucose and C-peptide and ultradian oscillation of insulin secretion (abs-ISR) and insulin secretion rate (ISR) during a constant 16-hour glucose infusion.
Av. plasma glucose, $p < 0.05$ vs. other groups; Av. plasma C-peptide, $p < 0.05$ vs. comparison group; abs-ISR, $p < 0.05$ vs. nondiabetic and diabetic marker (+) groups. (Reprinted from Life Sciences, Volume 55, Fajans SS, Bell GI, Bowden DW, Halter JB, Polonsky KS: Maturity-onset diabetes of the young, pp. 413–422, 1994, with kind permission from Elsevier Science, Ltd, The Boulevard, Langford Lane, Kidlington 0X5 1GB, UK)

tions have a first-phase insulin response to glucose which is within the normal range,[27,47] whereas mildly diabetic patients with a chromosome 20, mutation have a decreased or absent acute insulin response to glucose.[49] To define the possible differences in the interaction between glucose and insulin secretion rate between MODY subjects with glucokinase mutations[47] and subjects from the RW pedigree with mutation in the diabetes susceptibility gene on chromosome 20q12 (the MODY1 locus),[50] subjects received graded IV glucose infusions during a 4-hour period on two occasions separated by a 42-hour continuous glucose infusion designed to prime the B-cell to secrete more insulin in response to glucose. In MODY1 marker-positive subjects, whether they were nondiabetic or showed mild postglucose hyperglycemia, a diminished ability of the B-cell to respond to increments in plasma glucose above 7 mM was noted, whereas these subjects had a relatively normal response to increments in glucose from basal levels to values below 7mM.[50] A downward shift in the glucose insulin secretion rate dose-response curve was noted when plasma glucose levels exceeded 7mM. By contrast, marker-negative members of the RW family demonstrated a normal steep increase in insulin secretion rate with increases in plasma glucose in the range of 5–9mM,[50] a response similar to that seen in normal control subjects.[47] After prolonged glucose infusion, the glucose priming effect on the insulin secretion rate was clearly evident in the marker-negative group, which exhibited an upward and leftward shift with a 54% increase in insulin secretion. By contrast, there was no significant increase in responsiveness in the marker-positive group. Insulin secretion failed to increase > 15% over baseline following prolonged glucose infusion in 9 of 10 marker-positive subjects.[50] Previous results in MODY subjects with glucokinase mutations, however, showed persistence of the glucose priming effect on insulin secretion rate and continued increases, albeit subnormal, in insulin secretion rate as plasma glucose concentration rose from 7 to 12 mM.[47] Although the specific genetic defect causing MODY in the RW pedigree is unknown, subjects from the RW family who have inherited the at-risk allele of the MODY1 gene appear to have a characteristic pattern of altered insulin secretory responses to glucose. These alterations are present prior to the onset of hyperglycemia, suggesting a unique mechanism of B-cell dysfunction different from the defect in MODY subjects with glucokinase mutations (Table 27-3). The data also suggest that the MODY1 gene functions in the regulation of glucose-induced insulin secretion at

Table 27-3. Differences Between Maturity-Onset Diabetes of the Young (MODY) Secondary to Mutations in the Diabetes Susceptibility Gene on Chromosome 20q and the Glucokinase Gene (Chromosome 7p)

	MODY1 Gene on Chromosome 20q	MODY2 Gene: Glucokinase Gene
Fasting hyperglycemia (>140 mg/dL)	0–++++ (~80%)	0–++
Postprandial hyperglycemia	++–++++	0–++
Progression of hyperglycemia	++–++++	0
Minimum age at diagnosis	7–9 years	1 year
Need for insulin therapy	Common (~30%)	Uncommon (2%)
Vascular complications	++	Rare
AIR_{glu}*		
Mildly diabetic subjects	↓↓–Absent	Normal–↓
Nondiabetic subjects with genetic marker	Normal	Not available
ISR† during upgraded IV glucose infusion		
Mildly diabetic subjects	↓↓↓	↓–↓↓
Nondiabetic subjects with genetic markers	↓↓↓	Not available
Reduced ISR most evident at glucose concentration	>7 mM	<7 mM
Glucose priming of ISR†		
MODY	Absent	Normal (45% increase)
Nondiabetic subjects with genetic markers	Absent	Not available
Postulated abnormality in B-cell function	Cellular level distal to glucokinase or decrease in B-cell mass	Glucose phosphorylation by glucokinase

*AIR_{glu} = acute insulin response to glucose.
†ISR = insulin secretion rate.

a cellular level distal to glucokinase or is involved in a process regulating B-cell mass.[50]

The increased severity of the insulin secretory defect in diabetic, mildly diabetic, and nondiabetic subjects with a mutation of the diabetes susceptibility gene on chromosome 20q (MODY1) correlates with the increased severity of hyperglycemia, a greater need for insulin therapy, and a greater prevalence of vascular complications in these diabetic subjects as compared to diabetic subjects with mutations in the glucokinase gene (MODY2) (Table 27-3). Diabetes associated with mutations in MODY3 resembles that due to mutation in MODY1, although hyperglycemia appears to be less severe and vascular complications may occur less frequently compared to diabetes associated with MODY1.

Malnutrition-Related Diabetes Mellitus

In certain parts of the world, malnutrition-related diabetes (MRDM) occurs far more frequently than IDDM, and may approximate the frequency of NIDDM. It is seen with particular frequency in India, certain parts of Africa, and in the West Indies. It is usually found in young people, and is characterized by severe protein malnutrition and emaciation and, in some, by evidence of pancreatic calculi on x-ray studies of the abdomen (see Table 27-1). These patients have diabetes that is characterized by severe hyperglycemia unaccompanied by ketosis. These individuals require insulin; they are dependent on insulin for preservation of health and life, although they are not dependent on insulin for prevention of ketosis. A study in southern India revealed that C-peptide concentrations were lower in patients with this type of diabetes than in patients with NIDDM, but were significantly higher than those concentrations seen in patients with classical IDDM.[51] It is quite likely that the increased insulin secretory capacity reflected by the increased C-peptide concentration is responsible for the absence of ketosis in these patients.

Other Types of Diabetes

Other types of diabetes mellitus include entities secondary to or associated with other conditions or syndromes. This subclass can be divided according to known or suspected etiologic relationships. For example, diabetes may be secondary to pancreatic disease or removal of pancreatic tissue; secondary to endocrine diseases, such as acromegaly, Cushing's syndrome, pheochromocytoma, glucagonoma, somatostatinoma, primary aldosteronism, and others; secondary to the administration of hormones causing hyperglycemia; and secondary to the administration of certain drugs (antihypertensive drugs, thiazide diuretics, preparations containing estrogen, psychoactive drugs, sympathomimetic agents, etc.).[2] Diabetes (or impaired glucose tolerance) may also be associated with a number of genetic syndromes.[2] Finally, diabetes may be associated with genetic defects of the insulin receptor, or due to antibodies to the insulin receptor, with or without associated immune disorders.

Impaired Glucose Intolerance

The NDDG workgroup recommended that a category be established for those individuals who have fasting plasma glucose levels and glucose levels during the glucose tolerance test which lie between normal and diabetic levels. It is well recognized that, in some subjects, impaired glucose tolerance (IGT) may represent a stage in the natural history of IDDM;[1,5] this is even more frequently the case in NIDDM,[1,2,7] as confirmed by prospective testing. In such patients, conversion of IGT to NIDDM, and particularly to NIDDM with fasting hyperglycemia, occurs over several years or decades. It has been found to occur in up to 50% of patients with IGT who have undergone follow-up studies for a period of 16 years. Thus, in a substantial proportion of various population groups, IGT either does not progress or it reverts to normal glucose tolerance. To avoid the psychological and socioeconomic stigma of a diagnosis of diabetes in these individuals, the category of IGT has been established. Although clinically significant renal and retinal complications of diabetes (microangiopathy) are absent or very uncommon in patients with IGT, many studies have shown in such groups an increased death rate, an increased prevalence of arterial disease and electrocardiographic abnormalities, and an increased susceptibility to atherosclerotic disease associated with other known risk factors, including hypertension, hyperlipidemia, and adiposity.[2] Thus, particularly in otherwise healthy and ambulatory individuals younger than 60 years of age (conditions appropriate for the use of the oral glucose tolerance test), IGT may have prognostic implications, and it should not be ignored or dismissed lightly. In obese individuals, IGT almost invariably reverts to normal glucose tolerance with weight reduction. IGT may also be associated with the conditions and syndromes listed under the section "Other Types of Diabetes" in Table 27-1.

Gestational Diabetes Mellitus

In patients with gestational diabetes mellitus (GDM), the detection or onset of glucose intolerance occurs during pregnancy. A known diabetic who becomes pregnant is not classified as having GDM. From a biochemical point of view (see levels of plasma glucose, Table 27-2), pregnancy-related IGT is similar but not identical to IGT. Gestational diabetes occurs in approximately 2% of all pregnant women and is associated with increased perinatal morbidity and increased frequency of loss of viable fetuses. Treatment of this mild degree of glucose intolerance can often prevent such outcomes. Patients with GDM usually return to a state of normal glucose tolerance after parturition; even so, 60% of such women develop diabetes within 15 years after parturition. Thus, after termination of pregnancy, patients with gestational diabetes should be reclassified as patients with IGT, diabetes mellitus, or a previous abnormality of glucose tolerance (see the next section).

Statistical Risk Classes

Previous Abnormality of Glucose Tolerance

The classification of previous abnormality of glucose tolerance (PreAGT) is restricted to individuals who previously had diabetic hyperglycemia or IGT, but who presently have normal glucose tolerance. Individuals who have had gestational diabetes but have returned to normal glucose tolerance after parturition are examples of this subgroup, as are individuals who were obese and whose diabetes or IGT returned to normal glucose tolerance after weight loss. Patients with IGT or mild diabetes of the NIDDM form may fluctuate between IGT, diabetes, and normal (PrevAGT) classifications, with little or no change in weight. Spontaneous remissions of type I diabetes have been described, but are usually temporary in nature. All these individuals have an increased risk of developing diabetes in the future.

Potential Abnormality of Glucose Tolerance

Individuals assigned to the classification of potential abnormality of glucose tolerance (PotAGT) have never exhibited abnormal glucose tolerance, but have a substantially increased risk for the development of diabetes. PotAGT identifies the interval of time from conception until the first demonstration of IGT in an individual predisposed to diabetes on the basis of genetic background. Factors associated with an increased risk for IDDM include being a sibling or twin of a patient with IDDM; having histocompatibility haplotypes identical to those of an IDDM first-degree relative, particularly a sibling; and having circulating ICAs and insulin antibodies and a decreased first-phase insulin response to IV glucose. Factors associated with an increased risk for NIDDM include being a first-degree relative of a type II diabetic, particularly in nondiabetic members of families with MODY carrying a genetic marker on chromosome 7, 12, or 20; being obese and having a family history of diabetes; and being a member of a racial or ethnic group with a high prevalence of diabetes (e.g., certain Native American tribes and Hispanic or African American populations). There is a particularly strong risk for developing NIDDM among monozygotic twins of an NIDDM patient or the offspring of two diabetic parents with NIDDM. Concordance of diabetes has been found in more than 90% of pairs of monozygotic twins of patients with NIDDM.

The terms "prediabetes" and "potential diabetes" have been used for individuals in this class in the past. If used at all, the term prediabetes should be reserved solely and retrospectively to refer to the period prior to the diagnosis of diabetes. It cannot be used prospectively, as it is now known that diabetes occurs primarily in those in whom a precipitating environmental factor becomes superimposed upon a genetic predisposition. The finding of ICAs in an identical twin of a type I diabetic patient cannot be taken as proof of subsequent development of diabetes at this time.

PotAGT should never be applied as a diagnosis. Rather, it is included in this classification system to identify individuals and groups of individuals for prospective research studies.

Application of the Classification

Although this classification system can be applied to most patients with diabetes mellitus, there are circumstances when it will be extremely difficult to assign an individual to one class or another with any degree of certainty. The most common example is the young adult or the young, middle-aged, nonobese individual with diabetes of recent symptomatic origin who has been treated with insulin and who has no history of ketosis. Should these individuals be classified as type I or type II diabetics? Other information may be helpful, such as a family history of type I or type II diabetes. Research procedures, such as those which establish the presence or absence of a C-peptide response to glucose or glucagon, circulating ICAs, IAAs, or GAD may be useful. It has been reported that with immunological testing approximately 10% of patients initially diagnosed as NIDDM may have a slow-onset form of IDDM that has been termed latent autoimmune diabetes in adults.[53] Fortunately, an incorrect designation is not critical in a clinical setting, as therapy will remain the same.

References

1. Fajans SS, Cloutier MC, Crowther RL. Clinical and etiological heterogeneity of idiopathic diabetes mellitus (Banting Memorial Lecture). Diabetes 1978; 27:1112
2. Harris M, Cahill G, Members of NIH Diabetes Data Group Workshop: A draft classification of diabetes mellitus and other categories of glucose tolerance. Diabetes 1979;28:1039
3. WHO Study Group: Diabetes Mellitus. World Health Organization Technical Report Series 727. Geneva: WHO, 1985
4. West KM. Standardization of definition, classification, and reporting in diabetes-related epidemiologic studies. Diabetes Care 1979;2:65
5. Fajans SS. Heterogeneity within Type II and MODY diabetes. In: Vranic M, Hollenberg CH, Steiner G, eds. Comparison of Type I and Type II Diabetes. Advances in Experimental Medicine and Biology. New York: Plenum Publishing Corp;1985:65–87
6. Srikanta S, Ganda OP, Jackson RA, et al. Type I diabetes mellitus in monozygote twins: Chronic progressive beta cell dysfunction. Ann Intern Med 1983;99:320
7. Fajans SS. Scope and heterogenous nature of maturity-onset diabetes of the young (MODY). Diabetes Care 1990;13:49. Published erratum appears in Diabetes Care 1990;13:910
8. Köbberling J. Studies on the genetic heterogeneity of diabetes mellitus. Diabetologia 1971;7:46
9. Kuzuya T, Matsuda A. Family histories of diabetes among Japanese patients with Type I (insulin-dependent) and Type II (noninsulin-dependent) diabetes. Diabetologia 1982;22:372
10. Tattersall RB, Fajans SS. A difference between the inheritance of classic juvenile-onset and maturity-onset type diabetes of young people. Diabetes 1975;24:44
11. Fajans SS. Maturity-onset diabetes of the young (MODY). In: DeFronzo RA, ed. Diabetes/Metabolism Reviews. Vol 5. New York: John Wiley & Sons; 1989:579
12. Fajans SS, Bell GI, Bowden DW. MODY: A model for the study of the molecular genetics of NIDDM. J Lab Clin Med 1992;119:206
13. Fajans SS, Bell GI, Bowden DW, et al. Maturity-onset diabetes of the young. Life Sci 1994;55:413
14. DeFronzo RA, Bonadonaa RC, Ferrannini E. Pathogenesis of NIDDM: A balanced overview. Diabetes Care 1992;15:318
15. Fajans SS, Floyd JC, Taylor CI, Pek S. Heterogeneity of insulin responses in latent diabetes. Trans Assoc Am Physicians 1974;87:83
16. Fajans SS. Heterogeneity of insulin secretion in type II diabetes. Diabetes Metab Rev 1986;2:347
17. Kosaka K, Akanuma Y. Heterogeneity of plasma IRI responses in patients with IGT (letter to the editor). Diabetologia 1980;18:347
18. Reaven GM, Olefsky JM. Relationship between heterogeneity of insulin responses and insulin resistance in normal subjects and patients with chemical diabetes. Diabetologia 1977;13:201
19. Banerji MA, Lebovitz HE. Insulin-sensitive and insulin-resistant variants in NIDDM. Diabetes 1989;38:784
20. Arner P, Pollare T, Litthell H. Different aetiologies of type 2 (non–insulin-dependent) diabetes mellitus in obese and non-obese subjects. Diabetologia 1991;34:483
21. Banerji MA, Norin AJ, Chaiken RL, Lebovitz HE. HLA-DQ associations distinguish insulin-resistant and insulin-sensitive variants of NIDDM in black Americans. Diabetes Care 1993;16:429
22. Taniguchi A, Nakai Y, Fukushima M, et al. Pathogenic factors responsible for glucose intolerance in patients with NIDDM. Diabetes 1992;41: 1540
23. Meneilly G, Dawson K, Tessier D. Alterations in glucose metabolism in the elderly patient with diabetes. Diabetes Care 1993;16:1241
24. Fajans S, Brown M. Administration of sulfonylureas can increase glucose-induced insulin secretion for decades in patients with maturity-onset diabetes of the young. Diabetes Care 1993;16:1254
25. Froguel P, Zouali H, Vionnet N, et al. Familial hyperglycemia due to mutations in glucokinase. N Engl J Med 1993;328:697
26. Hattersley AT, Turner RC, Permutt MA, et al. Linkage of Type 2 diabetes to the glucokinase gene. Lancet 1992;339:1307
27. Velho G, Froguel P, Clement K, et al. Primary pancreatic beta-cell secretory defect caused by mutations in glucokinase gene in kindreds of maturity onset diabetes of the young. Lancet 1992;340:444
28. Bell GI, Xiang K, Newman MV, et al. Gene for non–insulin-dependent diabetes mellitus (MODY subtype) is linked to DNA polymorphism on human chromosome 20q. Proc Natl Acad Sci USA 1991;88:1484
29. Cox NJ, Xiang K, Fajans SS, Bell GI. Mapping diabetes-susceptibility genes: Lessons learned from the search for a DNA marker for MODY. Diabetes 1992;41:401
30. Bowden DW, Gravius TC, Akots G, Fajans SS. Identification of genetic markers flanking the maturity-onset diabetes of the young locus on human chromosome 20. Diabetes 1992;41:88
31. Bowden DW, Akots G, Rothschild CR, et al. Linkage analysis of maturity-onset diabetes of the young (MODY): Genetic heterogeneity and non-penetrance. Am J Hum Genet 1992;50:607
32. Rothschild CB, Akots G, Fajans SS, Bowden DW. A microsatellite polymorphism associated with the PLC1 (phospholipase C) locus: Identification, mapping, and linkage to the MODY locus on chromosome 20. Genomics 1992; 13:560
33. Rothschild CR, Akots G, Hayworth R, et al. A genetic map of chromosome 20q12-q13.1: Multiply highly polymorphic microsatellite and RFLP markers linked to the maturity onset diabetes of the young (MODY) locus. Am J Hum Genet 1993;52:110
34. Fajans SS. MODY—A model for understanding the pathogenesis and natural history of Type II diabetes. Horm Metab Res 1987;19:591
35. Froguel PH, Vaxillaire M, Sun F, et al. Close linkage of glucokinase locus on chromosome 7p to early-onset non–insulin-dependent diabetes mellitus. Nature 1992;356:162
36. Stoffel M, Patel P, Lo Y-MD, et al. Missense glucokinase mutation in maturity-onset diabetes of the young and mutation screening in late-onset diabetes. Nature Genet 1992;2:153
37. Sakura H, Eto K, Kadowaki H, et al. Structure of the human glucokinase gene and identification of a missense mutation in a Japanese patient with early-onset non–insulin-dependent diabetes mellitus. J Clin Endocrinol Metab 1992;75:1571
38. Shimada F, Makino H, Hashimoto N, et al. Type 2 (non–insulin-dependent) diabetes mellitus associated with a mutation of the glucokinase gene in a Japanese family. Diabetologia 1993;36:433

39. Matchinsky FM. Glucokinase as glucose senser and metabolic signal generator in pancreatic β-cells and hepatocytes. Diabetes 1990;39:647
40. Vionnet N, Stoffel M, Takeda J, et al. Nonsense mutation in the glucokinase gene causes early-onset non–insulin-dependent diabetes mellitus. Nature 1992;356:721
41. Stoffel M, Froguel PH, Takeda J, et al. Human glucokinase gene: Isolation, characterization, and identification of two missense mutations linked to early-onset non–insulin-dependent (type 2) diabetes mellitus. Proc Natl Acad Sci USA 1992;89:7698
42. Sun F, Knebelmann B, Pueyo ME, et al. Deletion of the donor splice site of Intron 4 in the glucokinase gene causes maturity-onset diabetes of the young. J Clin Invest 1993;92:1174
43. Godh-Jain M, Takeda J, Xu LZ, et al. Glucokinase mutations associated with non–insulin-dependent (type 2) diabetes mellitus have decreased enzymatic activity: Implications for structure/function relationships. Proc Natl Acad Sci USA 1993;90:1932
44. Vaxillaire M, Vionnet N, Vigouroux C, et al. Search for a third susceptibility gene for maturity-onset diabetes of the young. Diabetes 1994;43:389
45. Vaxillaire M, Boccio V, Philippi A, et al. A gene for maturity onset diabetes of the young (MODY) maps to chromosome 12q. Nature Genet 1995;9:418–423
46. Menzel S, Yamagata K, Trabb JB, et al. Localization of MODY3 to a 5 cM region of human chromosome 12. Diabetes 1995;44:1408
47. Byrne MM, Sturis J, Clément K, et al. Insulin secretory abnormalities in subjects with hyperglycemia due to glucokinase mutations. J Clin Invest 1994;93:1120
48. Lillioja S, Mott DM, Spraul M, et al. Insulin resistance and insulin secretory dysfunction as precursors of non–insulin-dependent diabetes mellitus. N Engl J Med 1993;329:1988
49. Herman WH, Fajans SS, Ortiz FJ, et al. Insulin resistance is not the genetic or primary defect of MODY in the RW pedigree. Diabetes 1994;43:40
50. Byrne MM, Sturis J, Fajans SS, et al. Altered insulin secretory responses to glucose in subjects with a mutation in the MODY1 gene on chromosome 20. Diabetes 1995;44:699
51. Mohan V, Snehalatha C, Ramachandran A, et al. Pancreatic beta-cell function in tropical pancreatic diabetes. Metabolism 1983;32:1091
52. O'Sullivan JM, Mahan CM. Criteria for the oral glucose tolerance test in pregnancy. Diabetes 1964;13:278
53. Tuomi T, Groop LC. Zimmet PZ, et al. Antibodies to glutamic acid decarboxylase reveal latent autoimmune diabetes mellitus in adults with a non–insulin-dependent onset of disease. Diabetes 1993;42:359

Part IV

Type I Diabetes

Diabetes Mellitus, edited by Derek LeRoith, Simeon I. Taylor, and Jerrold M. Olefsky. Lippincott–Raven Publishers, Philadelphia © 1996.

CHAPTER 28

Interaction of Some Biochemical and Physiologic Effects of Insulin That May Play a Role in the Control of Blood Glucose Concentration

ERIC A. NEWSHOLME AND G. D. DIMITRIADIS

Despite an immense amount of research into the action and effects of insulin, it is still uncertain as to which is the major metabolic process that controls blood glucose concentration in response to a change in insulin concentration. Indeed it is even possible to challenge the accepted notion that changes in plasma insulin concentration normally are involved in the control of blood glucose concentration.

Because of the vast amount of information available on the effects of insulin, this chapter will focus only on those aspects that we consider to play a key role in the integration of metabolism. We use the principles of metabolic control to select more objectively those areas of metabolism that may play a major role in the control of blood glucose concentration.

First, a list of the effects of insulin on carbohydrate, fat, and protein metabolism is given.[1] These will then be used to integrate the effects of insulin into a physiologic profile of the means by which the hormone may play a role.

Summary of the Major Effects of Insulin on Metabolism

Insulin has the following effects on carbohydrate metabolism:

- It increases the rate of transport of glucose across the cell membrane in adipose tissue and muscle.
- It increases the rate of glycolysis in muscle and adipose tissue.
- It stimulates the rate of glycogen synthesis in a number of tissues, including adipose tissue, muscle, and liver. It also decreases the rate of glycogen breakdown in muscle and liver.
- It inhibits the rate of glycogenolysis and gluconeogenesis in the liver.

It must be emphasized that, although certain major tissues are largely or totally insensitive to the direct action of insulin (e.g., kidney, brain, intestine), insulin can influence the rate of glucose utilization in these tissues indirectly, that is, by affecting the mobilization of fuels from other tissues, especially adipose tissue (see below).

Insulin has the following effects on lipid metabolism:

- It inhibits the rate of lipolysis in adipose tissue and hence lowers the plasma fatty acid level.
- It stimulates fatty acid and triacylglycerol synthesis in adipose tissue and liver.
- It increases the rate of very-low-density lipoprotein formation in the liver.
- It increases lipoprotein lipase activity in adipose tissue, and this increases the uptake of triglyceride from the blood into adipose tissue.
- It decreases the rate of fatty acid oxidation in muscle and liver.
- It increases the rate of cholesterolgenesis in liver.

Insulin has the following effects on protein metabolism:

- It increases the rate of transport of some amino acids into muscle, adipose tissue, liver, and other cells.
- It increases the rate of protein synthesis in muscle, adipose tissue, liver, and other tissues.
- It decreases the rate of protein degradation in muscle (and perhaps other tissues).
- It decreases the rate of urea formation.

These insulin effects serve to encourage protein synthesis rather than amino acid oxidation especially in the young, so that the hormone produces positive nitrogen balance in the normal subject—it therefore can be considered an *anabolic hormone*.

Effect of Insulin on Glucose Utilization and Glycogen Synthesis

Glucose Transport Across the Cell Membrane

The first reaction of the glycolytic pathway in any tissue is considered to be the transport of glucose across the cell membrane. Transport involves the transient combination of a glucose molecule with the protein carrier at the outer surface of the membrane and the subsequent release of the glucose at the inner surface. In most tissues, this process of glucose transport is down a concentration gradient and is therefore a passive process. (The active transport of glucose is seen in the epithelial cells of the intestine and kidney tubule and possibly in the choroid plexus, where the cerebrospinal fluid is formed.) It has been known since 1950 that insulin increases the rate of transport of glucose across the cell membrane in both muscle and adipose tissue, and therefore this process has been a focus of attention for many years. Thus it is now known that insulin increases the number of glucose transporters (GLUT-4) in the plasma membrane, and it does this by increasing the net rate of translocation of the GLUT-4 transporter from an intracellular membrane store to the cell membrane in both skeletal muscle and adipose tissue.[2–4]

The molecular biologic approach has identified the presence of different molecular species of the transporter in different tissues, but interpretation of the function of these transporters is helped by an understanding of control-theory principles. In muscle and adipose tissue, insulin can increase the rate of glucose transport since it is a *nonequilibrium process*. If the activity of this transporter is high enough, transport of glucose will occur in both directions, the process will be *near-equilibrium*, and the net rate of transport will not be sensitive to insulin. Indeed, many of the early kinetic studies on glucose transport were carried out following the rate of outward transport of nonutilizable sugars.[5–7] In liver, by contrast, the process is always near-equilibrium, so there would be no point for this process to be stimulated by insulin. The control of the rate and direction of glucose flux in the liver therefore shifts to the enzymes glucokinase and glucose 6-phosphatase.[8]

The transport process appears also to be near-equilibrium in many cells that are undergoing proliferation; control is then transferred to the hexokinase reaction, which under these conditions is the flux-generating step for glucose utilization. This means that the rate of glycolysis in these cells can be maintained constant despite marked hypoglycemia, because the rate of glycolysis now depends on the K_m of hexokinase (<0.1 mM glucose) rather than that of the glucose transporter (>5 mM glucose). The importance of a high, yet constant, rate of glycolysis in rapidly dividing cells has been emphasized elsewhere.[9] In view of the role of glycolysis in such cells, it is not surprising that insulin has no effect on them.

Glucose Transport and Glycolysis

Insulin increases the rate of glucose transport into muscle cells as well as the rate of glycolysis (i.e., glucose conversion to lactate). How do the glycolytic enzymes respond to insulin? Is this stimulation of the glycolytic enzymes solely due to the increase in the rate of glucose transport, which then increases the concentration of intracellular glucose? In this case, this would cause an increase in the rate of all the glycolytic enzymes by internal regulation—that is, by increasing the concentration of each intermediate of glycolysis. Alternatively, in addition to its effect on transport, insulin might lead to a stimulation of one or more of other glycolytic enzymes. Such effects could not be considered to control glycolysis but would facilitate the control of those particular reactions in glycolysis. As yet, however, there is no firm evidence that insulin stimulates the activities of glycolytic enzymes.

Two candidates for such effects of insulin are hexokinase and 6-phosphofructokinase. To provide evidence that insulin affects the activity of hexokinase, it must be shown that the level of intracellular glucose decreases as the flux through hexokinase, in response to insulin, increases; this is difficult because of the problem of measuring the precise concentration of intracellular glucose in muscle. These experiments can be facilitated by the use of the compound 2-deoxyglucose, which is taken up by the same transporter for glucose and then converted to 2-deoxyglucose 6-phosphate. Thus, if radiolabeled 2-deoxyglucose is used, it may be easier to measure the muscle content of this sugar than that of glucose in order to ascertain whether its concentration in the muscle cell is influenced by insulin. Hexokinase can be bound to and released from mitochondria according to the metabolic requirements of the cell. It has been proposed that insulin promotes the binding of hexokinase to the mitochondrial membrane at a site near the generation of ATP in order to produce an increase in the efficiency of respiratory control; this would, it is claimed, facilitate the delivery of energy to all the anabolic processes.[10] However, this mechanism may be of little importance under physiologic conditions: In soleus muscle isolated from normal rats, the contents of ATP, ADP, and AMP are not affected by insulin,[11] and there is no evidence that insulin (at least at concentrations within the physiologic range) increases the activity of hexokinase other than by increasing the concentration of its substrate.[8] In soleus muscle isolated from hyperthyroid rats, however, although the rate of 2-deoxyglucose phosphorylation is increased when the concentration of insulin is increased, the content of 2-deoxyglucose remained unaltered, suggesting that insulin had increased the activity of hexokinase.[12] These findings suggest that in muscle, under conditions of increased energy requirements (e.g., the hyperthyroid state), a direct effect of insulin to increase the activity of hexokinase may supplement the effect of this hormone to increase the rate of glucose transport.

To provide evidence that insulin affects the activity of 6-phosphofructokinase, it must be shown that the level of fructose 6-phosphate decreases as the flux through this enzyme increases in response to insulin. Indeed, when insulin increases within the physiologic range, the rate of lactate formation increases but the content of glucose 6-phosphate (and presumably that of fructose 6-phosphate with which it is in equilibrium) remains unaltered; similar findings have been described for insulin-like growth factor-1 (IGF-1), which has structural and functional similarities with insulin.[11,13] These findings suggest that insulin increases the activity of 6-phosphofructokinase. Fructose 2,6-bisphosphate is a potent activator of 6-phosphofructokinase: Because it is neither a substrate nor an intermediate of glycolysis, it is an apt mediator for extracellular signals such as hormones.[14] In the soleus muscle, the changes in the content of fructose 2,6-bisphosphate in response to insulin coincide with those observed in the glycolytic rate but are opposite to those observed in the content of glucose 6-phosphate.[11] These studies suggest that, when insulin increases within the physiologic range, in addition to the increase in the rate of glucose transport, an increase in the level of fructose 2,6-bisphosphate may be part of the mechanism to increase the activity of 6-phosphofructokinase and hence aid the stimulation of the glycolytic flux. This, together with the simultaneous effect of insulin to increase the rate of glycogen synthesis, would maintain the content of glucose 6-phosphate unaltered while the rate of glucose transport is increased.[11,15]

Glucose Transport and the Flux-Generating Step for Glycolysis in Muscle

The process of glycolysis-from-glucose, in contrast to glycolysis-from-glycogen, is not a physiologic pathway according to the concept of the flux-generating step.[1] The nonequilibrium reactions in glycolysis are catalyzed by the glucose transport system, hexokinase, 6-phosphofructokinase, and pyruvate kinase; none of these reactions is saturated with substrate.[8] The flux-generating step for this process is either the absorption of glucose from the intestine or, when glucose arises endogenously, the breakdown of glycogen in the liver (Fig. 28-1). Thus, in these cases, a metabolic pathway spans more than one tissue: It includes the intestine or liver, the

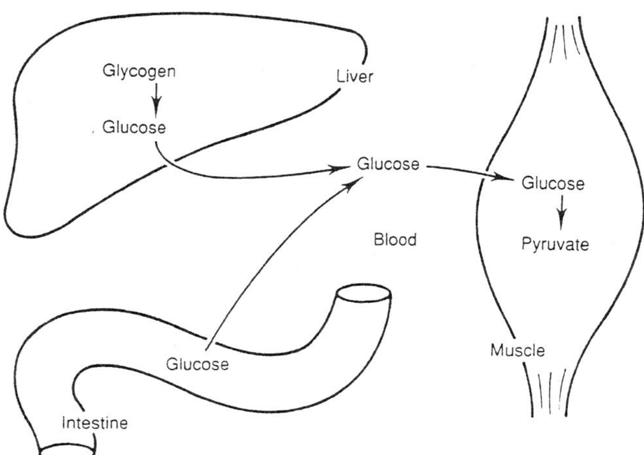

Figure 28-1. Source of glucose for glycolysis in muscle. Other glucose-utilizing tissues (e.g., brain, kidney) receive glucose from the same sources. Release of glucose from the intestine is probably important as a flux-generating step in the absorptive state, where the degradation of liver glycogen is important in the postabsorptive state. (This is taken from Biochemistry for the Medical Sciences by E. A. Newsholme and A. R. Leech, with permission of the publishers, John Wiley & Sons Ltd.)

blood, and the target tissue (e.g., muscle). The metabolic importance of this interpretation in the present context is related to the control of the rate of glucose utilization by muscle. When a meal with a high-carbohydrate content has been digested, the rate of absorption of glucose by the intestine is high, and to prevent a very large increase in the blood glucose concentration, the rate of glucose utilization by muscle is increased. (The amount of carbohydrate ingested in the average meal is approximately 20–30 times greater than that normally present in the blood, yet the normal increase in the blood glucose level is <50%.) This response cannot be due to increased demand for energy by muscle because it occurs even when muscles are resting after a meal. The response of muscle to insulin therefore can be considered physiologically abnormal: Muscle normally takes up glucose in response to a demand for energy, when the glucose will be oxidized to provide ATP. Not surprisingly, therefore, not all of the glucose taken up by muscle at the behest of insulin is oxidized to CO_2: Some, and possibly a high proportion, appears as lactate (this is best seen in isolated incubated muscle preparations[11]).

In agreement with this suggestion, studies in humans using forearm perfusion have shown that skeletal muscle is a major tissue for production and release of lactate either at basal (fasting) insulin levels (7–10 mU/L), or during hyperinsulinemia. At levels of insulin usually seen in plasma after a meal (approximately 60 mU/L), this tissue accounts for nearly 50% of systemic lactate production.[16] Measurements of the whole-body glucose metabolism in humans, however, have shown that the major pathways of glucose metabolism in skeletal muscle (estimated indirectly with the glucose-insulin clamp and indirect calorimetry) are glucose storage and oxidation rather than lactate formation.[17,18]

To understand the physiology behind this overall process, the complete metabolic pathway must be considered under the conditions of feeding. Thus, the flux-generating step is the transport of glucose across the intestine into the bloodstream. Insulin does not influence this process, but it controls the "branch" that is present in muscle, particularly the concentration of an intermediate in that pathway—an important intermediate, *blood glucose*. Insulin can be viewed as a "feed-forward" effector of the glycolytic process in muscle, which is dependent on the rate of entry of glucose into the bloodstream, and the main physiologic role of this is to prevent a massive increase in the blood glucose level. The latter would result in loss of glucose through the kidneys, and unwanted and dangerous glycosylation of proteins as a side-reaction. Therefore, secretion of insulin must be strictly related to the entry of glucose into the bloodstream from the intestine, which is known to be the case.

It follows, therefore, that a rise in the level of insulin at other times would be highly dangerous: Injection of insulin between meals can result in dangerous hypoglycemia. (Insulin is probably the only hormone that has been used as a murder weapon.)[19]

Insulin and Glycolysis in Muscle

If the insulin-stimulated increase in the rates of glucose transport and glycolysis in muscle is considered physiologically abnormal, what is the fate of the end-product of glucose metabolism? We know that an increase in the rate of glycolysis will provide more lactate, which is released from the muscle, but what happens to the end-product? There is now considerable evidence that some of the glycogen that is synthesized in the liver after a normal meal is derived not so much from glucose but from lactate, alanine, and other gluconeogenic precursors (known as the *indirect pathway*).[8,20] The conversion of glucose to lactate in muscle and the conversion of lactate to glycogen in liver may be part of an interorgan communication system designed to provide precision in regulation. The conversion in muscle controls the blood level of glucose, an excess of which could be dangerous. The increase in blood lactate concentration, together with increased hepatic blood flow, will facilitate the conversion of lactate to glycogen in the liver. Thus it is interesting to consider that the stimulation by insulin of the rate of glucose transport in muscle, via a feed-forward regulation from digestion and absorption of carbohydrate in the intestine, may lead directly, but via a long and complex intertissue metabolic pathway, to increased levels of liver glycogen (Fig. 28-2). The possible physiologic significance of this is discussed below.

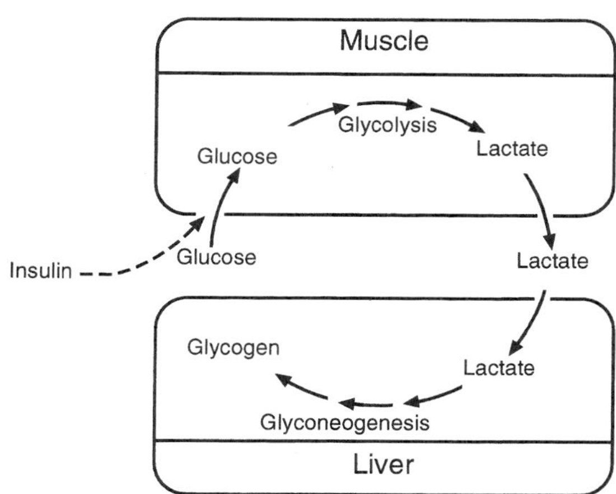

Figure 28-2. A modified Cori cycle. Insulin stimulates the conversion of glucose to lactate in muscle. The lactate is released by muscle and the blood concentration is increased (slightly). This stimulates the rate of conversion of lactate to glycogen in the liver (glyconeogenesis). In this way, insulin indirectly stimulates the rate of glycogen synthesis in the liver.

The Physiologic Pathway of Glycogen Synthesis in Muscle and the Effects of Insulin

It is known that, of the reactions involved in the process of glycogen synthesis (Fig. 28-3), hexokinase, glycogen synthase, and branching enzyme catalyze nonequilibrium reactions, whereas phospho-

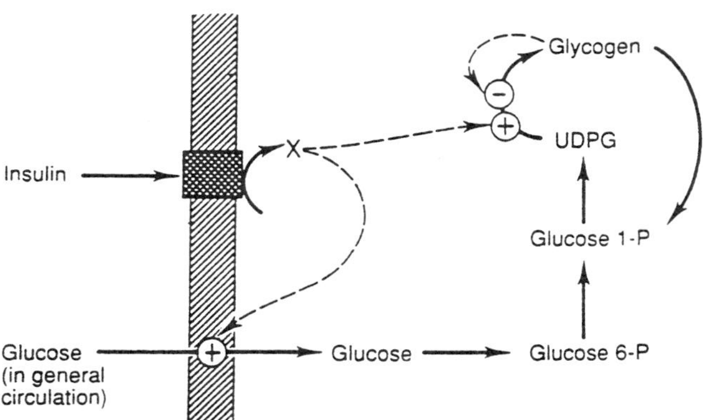

Figure 28-3. Glycogen synthesis in muscle and steps controlled by insulin. Insulin binds to its receptor, which results in the production or activation of the intracellular signaling pathway, which may be the activation of a particular protein phosphatase. This leads to activation of glucose transport and the enzyme glycogen synthase.

glucomutase and uridylyltransferase catalyze near-equilibrium reactions. Of the nonequilibrium reactions, only glycogen synthase approaches saturation with pathway substrate (uridine diphosphate [UDP]-glucose).[8] This therefore is the flux-generating reaction, so that the physiologic pathway for glycogen synthesis starts at UDP-glucose and comprises only two reactions: those catalyzed by glycogen synthase and the branching enzyme (1,6,-α-glucosyl transferase). Because the concentration of UDP-glucose is low in comparison to the rate of glycogen synthesis, however, its concentration must be maintained whenever glycogen is being synthesized. This is achieved by the reactions catalyzed by uridylyltransferase and phosphoglucomutase, both near-equilibrium reactions, utilizing glucose 6-phosphate produced via the hexokinase reaction. Of all of the reactions in the pathway, metabolic control logic predicts that glycogen synthase would be regulated by insulin; this, of course, is a well-established effect of this hormone.[8,17,21,22] It is important to appreciate that, although insulin increases the activity of glycogen synthase, this would not result in increased net glycogen synthesis unless the enzyme glycogen phosphorylase is strongly inhibited. Indeed, because the maximum catalytic capacity of phosphorylase is approximately 50-fold greater than that of glycogen synthesis in human skeletal muscle, phosphorylase must be inhibited by approximately 99% of its maximum activity when net glycogen synthesis occurs. Perhaps the complex controls of the activation of phosphorylase *a* and *b* are designed not so much for rapid and effective activation of the enzyme, but to ensure sufficient inactivity of phosphorylase to permit net glycogen synthesis. Without sufficient glycogen in muscle, physical exertion (especially sprinting, an important escape mechanism for primitive humans) would not be possible. An effective, albeit complex, mechanism for inhibition of phosphorylase activity would have survival value.

Another important principle that emerges from these considerations is that, in relation to the effects of insulin, glucose transport and glycogen synthase are independent reactions. Insulin stimulation of glucose transport does not necessarily result in a higher rate of glycogen synthesis: All of the increased glucose entering the muscle could be converted to lactate.[8,12,23] Similarly, insulin could increase markedly the rate of glycogen synthesis without affecting transport, because it would lead to more glucose residues being converted to glycogen and fewer to lactate[11,13]; this illustrates the importance of control at a branch point. (Of course, it is necessary for some glucose to enter the muscle to allow glycogen synthesis to proceed.)

In a normal, physically active animal that eats food sufficient only for maintenance, insulin may control the rate or glucose utilization primarily through its effects on glucose transport and glycogen synthesis in muscle. In this way, glycogen that had been used by the muscle during exercise would be repleted after the carbohydrate meal, and this would occur before glycogen was synthesized in the liver, because this latter process depends on control of the direction of glucose metabolism in muscle (see above). This may be an advantage of the indirect pathway for glycogen synthesis in liver and could explain why, after prolonged exercise, glycogen repletion occurs in the muscle before it occurs in the liver.[24] Indeed, glycogen is synthesized in muscle after exercise even during a period of starvation, when liver glycogen would be broken down.[25] When the amount of food ingested is above that required for repletion of muscle glycogen, however, it is suggested that insulin controls blood glucose concentration by increasing the rate of glycolysis in muscle through internal control, hence through the formation of lactate. This then, through the process of glyconeogenesis, will cause repletion of the glycogen store in the liver, and this physiologic result depends simply on the kinetic structure of the branch point at the level of glucose-6-phosphate in muscle.

In type II diabetes mellitus, insulin resistance may be the main mechanism to explain hyperglycemia.[26] In this condition, a defect in the ability of insulin to increase the rate of glycogen synthesis in muscle has been proposed as the main pathogenetic mechanism to explain insulin resistance in the liver[27] (see below). The evidence for decreased rates of glycogen synthesis in type II diabetes, is as follows. In adipocytes[28] or in the skeletal muscle of patients with type II diabetes, the stimulation of glycogen synthase by insulin is impaired; this impairment is independent of that observed in muscle glucose uptake and is compensated for by hyerglycemia or hyperinsulinemia.[29–32] In lean and obese patients with type II diabetes, impaired stimulation of nonoxidative glucose utilization by insulin (measured with indirect calorimetry) represents the major intracellular pathway responsible for the insulin resistance.[33–36] Shulman et al. used nuclear magnetic resonance spectroscopy as a direct measurement of glycogen synthesis in the gastrocnemius muscle in lean patients with type II diabetes:[37] The incorporation of [^{1}H, ^{13}C] glucose into muscle glycogen under conditions of hyperglycemia and hyperinsulinemia was markedly decreased and paralleled the decrease previously observed in total leg glucose uptake both in time and magnitude[38]; the decrease in the rate of glycogen synthesis accounted for all of the decrease in whole-body glucose disposal because the rate of glucose oxidation was normal.

Young, first-degree relatives of patients with type II diabetes, with normal oral glucose tolerance, were found to have decreased insulin-stimulated glucose metabolism in muscle (measured with glucose-insulin clamping and indirect calorimetry) due to an impairment in the rate of glycogen synthesis; in addition, the activity of glycogen synthase in extracts of muscle biopsies from these subjects was decreased.[38,40] These results suggest that impaired glycogen synthesis in response to insulin represents a major defect in patients with type II diabetes. The fact that it may be found in normal glucose tolerant first-degree relatives of patients with type II diabetes suggests that this is an early defect that may be genetically determined.

The defect in glycogen synthesis in skeletal muscle may result in an increased rate of lactate formation.[36] Indeed, in lean patients with type II diabetes, the rate of lactate formation in the forearm tissues was increased although the rate of glucose uptake was normal, supporting a redirection of glucose residues away from the pathway of glycogen synthesis towards that of glycolysis.[41] This may be facilitated by a decrease in the rate of glucose oxidation. The evidence for this is as follows. Low-dose streptozotocin-induced diabetes in rats is characterized by reduced pyruvate dehydrogenase activity and increased lactate and alanine formation in the hindlimb muscles and in the isolated adipocytes.[42] In lean patients with type II diabetes, the rate of insulin-mediated glucose oxidation measured with indirect calorimetry and the ability of insulin to stimulate pyruvate dehydrogenase activity in isolated adipocytes and muscle were impaired.[28,31,33,39,43,44] This impairment, together with the defect in glycogen synthesis directs glycolysis toward increased lactate formation.[31] Lactate thus produced may contribute to the increased rates of gluconeogenesis found in patients with overt type II diabetes.[45]

In addition to this ''role'' in overt type II diabetes, the increased rate of glycolysis (caused by a reduction in the rate of glycogen synthesis) has been proposed as the mechanism responsible for communication between skeletal muscle and liver in the early stages of this disease[27]: The increased lactate/alanine supply to the liver will increase the rate of gluconeogenesis, thus increasing the blood glucose level and hence increasing the rate of insulin secretion. At this early stage of the disease, however, mild hyperinsulinemia and hyperglycemia will manage to keep the rates of hepatic glucose production and muscle glucose uptake within normal limits.[26,27,46]

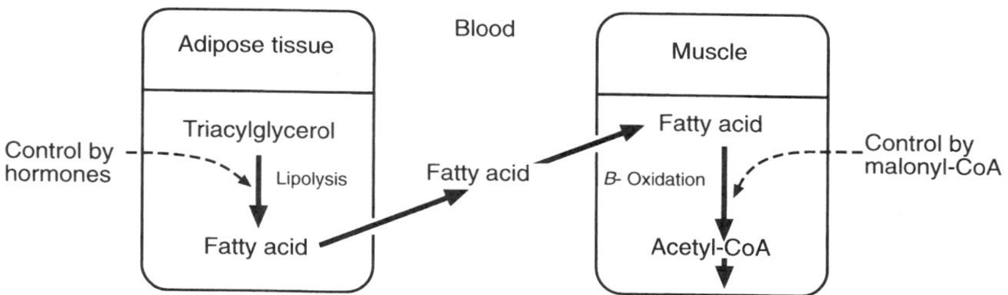

Figure 28-4. The physiologic pathway of lipid oxidation in muscle. In addition to muscle, other tissues such as kidney also oxidize fatty acids. The flux-generating step is catalyzed by triglyceride lipase within the adipose tissue, which is controlled, in part, by insulin. If the plasma fatty acid level is raised, this will facilitate fatty acid oxidation by muscle. This also can be facilitated by decreasing the level of malonyl-CoA in response to insulin. Malonyl-CoA inhibits a key enzyme of fatty acid oxidation within muscle.

Insulin and the Importance of its Antilipolytic Effect

The major store of triacylglycerol in the body is present in adipose tissue, but it is mobilized in the form of long-chain fatty acids, which are carried to other tissues via the bloodstream. Hence muscle oxidizes fatty acids derived from adipose tissue and obtains energy; however, fatty acid oxidation does more than provide energy: It specifically decreases the rate of glucose utilization and oxidation, a control mechanism known as the *glucose/fatty acid cycle* (see below).

The pathway for fatty acid oxidation in muscle involves β-oxidation and the Krebs cycle, but the flux-generating step for β-oxidation of fatty acids is lipolysis in adipose tissue because increasing the blood concentration of fatty acids increases the rate of fatty acid oxidation by muscle (and other tissues). The plasma fatty acid concentration therefore can be considered an internal regulator for the rate of β-oxidation in muscle (Fig. 28-4). The significance of this is that insulin causes inhibition of adipose tissue lipase, thus decreasing the rate of lipolysis in adipose tissue. This results in a decrease in the plasma level of fatty acid and therefore less oxidation of fatty acids by muscle. Insulin thus affects the rate of fatty acid oxidation in muscle by a direct regulatory effect on the flux-generating step in adipose tissue.

It should be noted that the increase in the amount of sustained exercise performed by muscle can increase the rate of oxidation of fatty acids without an increase in their extracellular concentration (i.e., the pathway in muscle can also be controlled by muscle itself.)[8] How is this achieved? Malonyl-coenzyme A (CoA) is an inhibitor of carnitine palmitoyltransferase-1, a key enzyme of fatty acid oxidation that catalyzes the formation of an ester of the fatty acid with carnitine; this facilitates the transport of fatty acids through the mitochondrial membrane.[8] Recently the control of this enzyme by malonyl-CoA in perfused skeletal muscle has been studied. In rats, malonyl-CoA content decreases in skeletal muscle in response to exercise, which would be expected to increase the rate of fatty acid oxidation; this decrease in malonyl-CoA content is attenuated with the infusion of glucose.[47] Further studies with the perfused rat hindlimb showed that, when glucose or insulin was not present in the perfusion medium, malonyl-CoA content was decreased; this decrease was prevented when both glucose and insulin were present.[48] These studies suggest that, in muscle, insulin could affect the rate of fatty acid oxidation by two separate means: (1) a decrease in the plasma level of fatty acids via the effect on adipose tissue lipolysis; and (2) a specific decrease in the rate of their oxidation via an increase in malonyl-Coa content within the muscle; both of these insulin effects would facilitate a decrease in the rate of fatty acid oxidation so that the rate of glucose utilization would be increased.

The Glucose/Fatty Acid Cycle

In starvation, liver glycogen is broken down to provide glucose for the tissues; measurement of the glycogen content in small samples of human liver, removed by biopsy needle, have shown that this glycogen store is largely depleted after a 24-hour starvation period.[24] Despite this, the blood glucose level remains remarkably constant, as shown by the now classic work by Cahill on starvation of Harvard divinity student volunteers.[49] One answer to the limited store of glycogen is for the tissues to use an alternative fuel—fatty acids. Mobilization of fatty acids from the adipose tissue triacylglycerol store probably begins during the overnight fast and increases particularly if breakfast is missed. It is well established, in both experimental animals and in humans, that even short periods of starvation raise the plasma fatty acid concentration.[8,50] Because both glucose and fatty acids are available in the bloodstream at the same time, the question arises: Why does muscle utilize fatty acids in preference to glucose? The answer to this question is very simple in principle. The elevated concentration of fatty acids in the bloodstream, plus a decrease in the level of malonyl-CoA in the muscle, increases the rate of fatty acid oxidation, which then decreases the rate of glucose utilization and oxidation by a specific biochemical mechanism[8] (Fig. 28-5).

The concept of the glucose/fatty acid cycle, put forward by Randle et al.,[51] provides a mechanism by which fatty acid oxidation

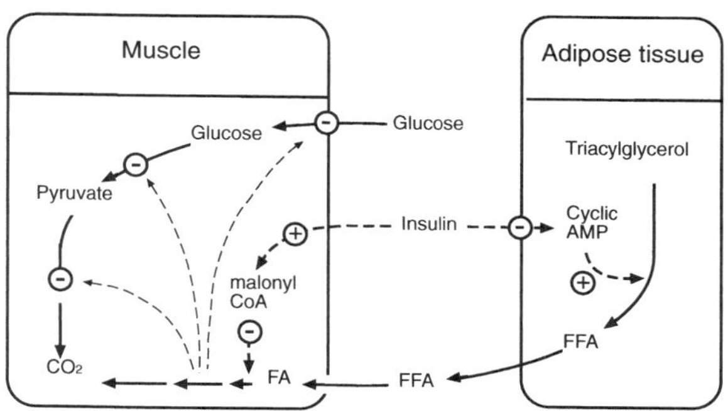

Figure 28-5. The glucose/fatty acid cycle, indicating the important role of insulin in decreasing fatty acid oxidation by muscle. Insulin decreases the AMP level in adipose tissue, which decreases the rate of lipolysis and hence lowers the plasma fatty acid level. Insulin increases the muscle content of malonyl-CoA, which inhibits the activity of carnitine palmitoyl transferase 1 and hence inhibits β-oxidation of fatty acids. This will relieve the inhibition on glucose utilization and oxidation in muscle caused by fatty acid oxidation.

decreases the rate of glucose utilization and particularly glucose oxidation by muscle. There is now considerable evidence to support the important proposal that, under conditions of "carbohydrate stress" (defined here as when the glycogen store in the liver is significantly decreased), the rate of fatty acid oxidation by muscle increases; this, in turn, decreases the rate of glucose utilization and oxidation. Conversely, when the carbohydrate stress is removed (e.g., by refeeding a starved subject) the rate of fatty acid oxidation is decreased and insulin plays an important role in changing the rate of fatty acid oxidation in muscle. In addition, increased rates of fatty acid oxidation by the liver increase the rate of hepatic glucose production,[52] the mechanism for which may be as follows: the concentration of acetyl-CoA is increased, which inhibits pyruvate dehydrogenase activity and stimulates that of pyruvate carboxylase, and the concentration ratio of oxidized:reduced nicotinamide-adenine dinucleotide (NAD^+:NADH) is decreased.[26] The regulatory effect of fatty acid on glucose utilization can be seen as a logical necessity when the small reserves of carbohydrate are taken into account, together with the fact that some tissues have an obligatory requirement for glucose (e.g., brain).

This interpretation of the role of insulin in controlling rates of glucose utilization via fatty acid oxidation is based on the application of metabolic control logic: The pathway for fatty acid oxidation in muscle starts with the flux-generating step lipolysis in adipose tissue; *this* is the key process to be controlled by insulin, but it also influences fatty acid oxidation within the muscle (Fig. 28-6).

Insulin and Gluconeogenesis

The major precursors for gluconeogenesis in the liver are lactate, glycerol, and amino acids, of which alanine is quantitatively important. The gluconeogenesis pathway can, in fact, be considered to start with the generation of alanine from muscle and the intestine, lactate from muscle (and other) tissues, and glycerol from adipose (and other) tissues. Gluconeogenesis is thus seen as a complex, branched pathway spanning more than one tissue (Fig. 28-7).

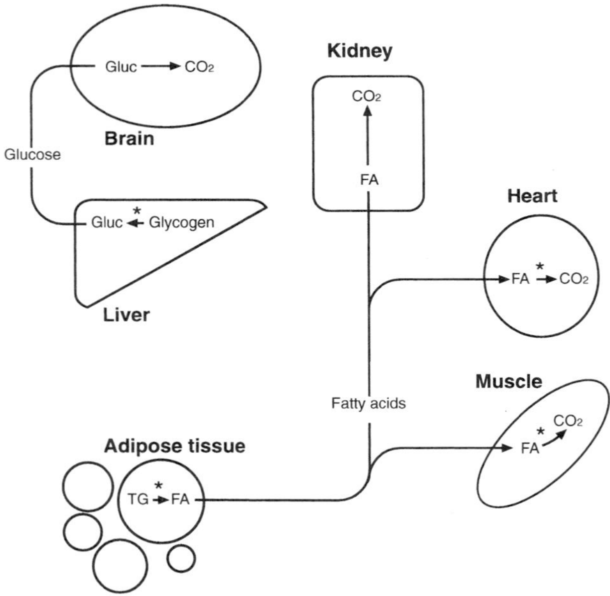

Figure 28-6. Pattern of fuel utilization during the early period of starvation, when fatty acids are beginning to be mobilized from adipose tissue. The asterisk indicates where insulin may play a direct role: The decrease in insulin concentration results in increased activity of adipose tissue lipase, increased activity of glycogenolysis and glucose release from the liver, and a stimulation of the activity of carnitine palmitoyl transferase in muscle to encourage fatty acid oxidation. FA = fatty acid; TG = triacylglycerol.

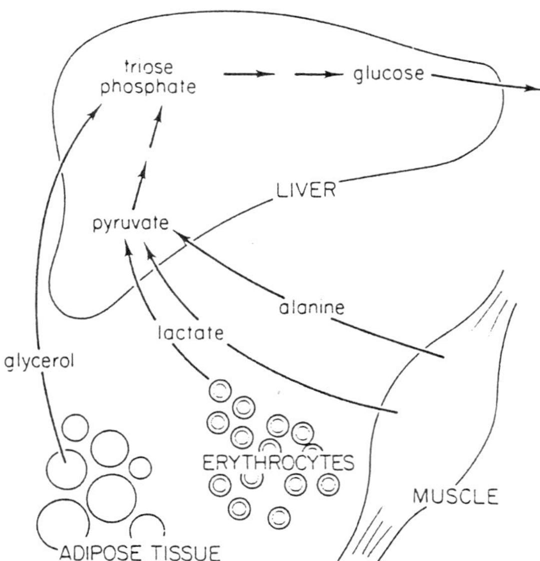

Figure 28-7. Some of the tissues involved in gluconeogenesis. The rate of gluconeogenesis is increased by increasing the concentrations of the precursors and decreased by increasing the hepatic concentration of glucose; the latter also decreases the rate of glycogenolysis. In addition to glycerol, adipose tissue may also release alanine. The process of hepatic gluconeogenesis is also used for glycogen synthesis in the liver (the indirect pathway). (Taken from Biochemistry for the Medical Sciences by E. A. Newsholme and A. R. Leech, with permission of the publishers, John Wiley & Sons Ltd.)

The normal blood lactate concentration (approximately 1 mM) represents a steady-state concentration that reflects the balance between the rates of production and utilization. Although the principal tissue for lactate utilization is liver, other tissues, such as heart and red muscles (type I and IIA fibers) can remove lactate from the bloodstream and oxidize it for energy production. Most of the lactate that is removed by the liver is converted to glucose or glycogen, via gluconeogenesis, although a small proportion may be oxidized or converted to triacylglycerol under lipogenic conditions. The conversion of lactate to glucose in the liver and the continuous formation of lactate from glucose in the other tissues of the body represents a cyclic flow of carbon that has been termed the *Cori cycle*. It may, however, have greater physiologic significance than just that of a carbon link between peripheral tissues and the liver: It may provide a basic (nonhormonal) mechanism for better control of the blood glucose concentration. By maintaining a high flux, the Cori cycle provides a dynamic buffer of key metabolic intermediates, both in the tissues and in the bloodstream, so that they can be used by tissues when required. If the rate of utilization of the intermediates is low, compared to the flux through the Cori cycle, this may provide for precision in regulation, as described and defined elsewhere.[53] This may be one reason for increased Cori cycle flux during injury, sepsis, postsurgery, burns, and hyperthyroidism—conditions where, although there is generalized resistance to insulin, muscle may have a higher rate of conversion of glucose to lactate.[12,54,55]

Glycerol is released into the bloodstream as a result of triacylglycerol hydrolysis from a number of tissues, the most important being adipose tissue. It is a very important substrate for increased rates of gluconeogenesis in patients with type II diabetes.[56]

Quantitatively, the most important amino acid precursor for gluconeogenesis is alanine; it is released from muscle, especially from branched-chain amino acid metabolism, it is released from the intestine, especially from the metabolism of glutamine and it is released from other tissues (e.g., adipose, immune cells, lung). Whether insulin can influence the rate of alanine release from adipose tissue, intestine, lung, or immune cells is not known.

Control of the gluconeogenic pathway can be achieved mainly by variations in the concentrations of the precursors (glycerol, lactate, amino acids) and of the end-product glucose: Raising the concentration of precursors will increase the rate of glucose formation, whereas raising the plasma concentration of glucose will decrease it. In addition, glucagon and glucocorticoids increase the rate of gluconeogenesis, whereas insulin counteracts the effects of these hormones and decreases it.[57,58] Insulin does not seem to affect the rate of glycogen synthesis or degradation acutely, but it suppresses glucose production mainly through its effect on glycolysis. In rats, an increase in the level of insulin (while glucose was maintained at a normal level with a clamp technique) had no effect on the activity of glycogen phosphorylase or synthetase or on the concentration of glycogen in the liver. It decreased the concentration of glucose 6-phosphate while increasing the fructose 1,6-bisphosphate, glycerol 1-phosphate, lactate, and pyruvate concentrations, suggesting that insulin had increased the activity of phosphofructokinase; indeed, the content of fructose 2,6-bisphosphate, a potent effector of this enzyme, was also increased.[59] This mechanism is the opposite of that of glucagon, which increases the rate of hepatic glucose production by decreasing the content of fructose 2,6-bisphosphate.[60]

In recent studies in humans, infusions of [U^{14}C]lactate and [U^{14}C]alanine (with plasma insulin, anti-insulin hormones, and glucose kept at normal levels) increased the rate of gluconeogenesis; however, the rate of hepatic glucose production remained unaltered, suggesting that the rate of glycogenolysis had decreased.[61] In rats, hyperglycemia (with plasma insulin kept at normal levels) was shown to suppress hepatic glucose production mainly through inhibition of glycogenolysis, with no apparent effects on the fluxes through gluconeogenesis and through glucose 6-phosphatase.[62] These studies suggest that, in the liver, changes in the plasma level of precursors for gluconeogenesis and in the plasma level of glucose may play important roles in influencing the rate of gluconeogenesis.

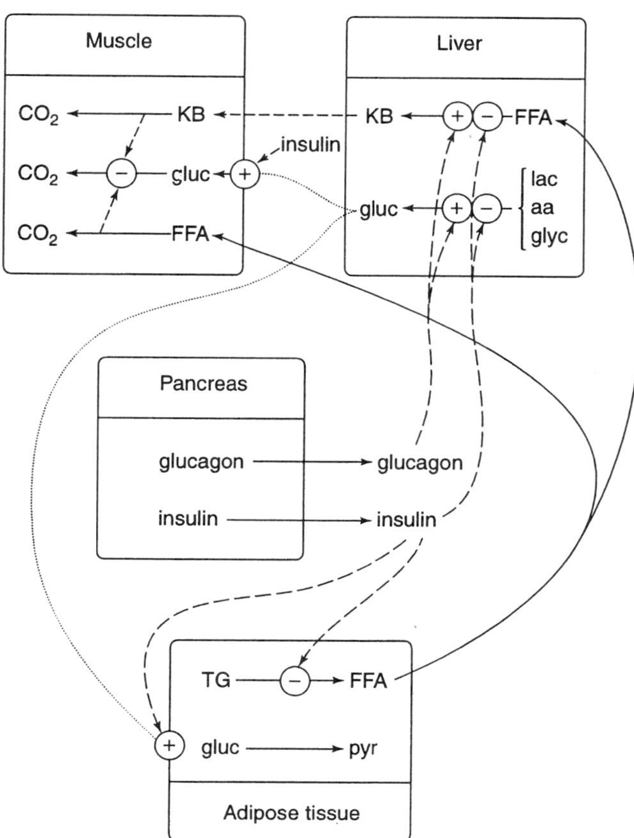

Figure 28-8. Control steps of possible importance in explaining how insulin regulates the blood glucose level. Four effects of insulin are depicted in the diagram: (1) stimulation of glucose uptake by muscle and adipose; (2) inhibition of lipolysis in adipose tissue; (3) inhibition of gluconeogenesis in the liver; (4) inhibition of ketosis in the liver. The effects on the liver are probably more chronic than acute. The acute regulation of gluconeogenesis may depend more on changes in precursor concentration and the concentrations of hexose monophosphates, and hence fructose 2-6-bisphosphate. KB = ketone bodies; gluc = glucose; lac = lactate; aa = amino acids; glyc = glycerol; pyr = pyruvate; TG = triacylglycerol. (Taken from Biochemistry for the Medical Sciences by E. A. Newsholme & A. R. Leech, with permission of the publishers, John Wiley & Sons Ltd.)

How Does Insulin Regulate the Blood Glucose Concentration?

The success of insulin in decreasing the blood glucose concentration in early work on diabetic animals stressed the important role of insulin in facilitating glucose utilization. Consequently, when it was discovered in the 1950s that insulin increased the rate of transport of glucose into the muscle cell,[63] it obviously was considered that this effect was the major means by which insulin regulated the blood glucose concentration in vivo. The advent of the concept of the glucose/fatty acid regulatory cycle in the 1960s enabled a different interpretation as to the means by which insulin regulates the blood glucose concentration. Because insulin is a potent antilipolytic hormone, an increased concentration of this hormone would decrease the rate of adipose tissue lipolysis, which would result in a decrease in the blood fatty acid concentration; this would decrease the rate of fatty acid oxidation in muscle. In addition, insulin could decrease the rate of fatty acid oxidation in muscle directly by increasing the content of malonyl-CoA (see above), and these effects would stimulate the rate of glucose utilization by muscle. This illustrates the important effect of insulin on the control of the blood glucose concentration via the glucose/fatty acid cycle. Gluconeogenesis also plays an important role in regulating blood glucose concentration. The rate of this process is regulated, in part, by the balance of glucagon and insulin, but the effect of these hormones on the concentration of precursors may be most important.

All three mechanisms described above, namely (1) stimulation of glucose transport into muscle (and adipose tissue); (2) increased rates of glucose utilization and oxidation in many tissues, depending on a decreased rate of utilization of fatty acids (decreased plasma levels of fatty acids through inhibition of adipose tissue lipase and increased content of malonyl-CoA); and (3) decreased rates of glucose production and release by the liver, could all play a role in increasing the rate, or the apparent rate, of glucose utilization when the plasma insulin concentration is increased (Fig. 28-8). The quantitative importance of each process depends on the magnitude of the response of each process in each tissue to the change in insulin concentration in vivo at that particular time. Thus it is not possible at present to provide quantitative information as to how changes in the insulin concentration, after a meal, control blood glucose concentration.

Furthermore, it is now known that the sensitivity of these processes to insulin, at least in muscle and adipose tissue, can be changed markedly by the presence of various local hormones, small molecules, and various other conditions. The above difficulties therefore are compounded by the possibility that different muscles or different adipose tissue depots, or both, may respond quantitatively differently to a change in the concentration of insulin—indeed sensitivity may change rapidly from one condition to another.

Insulin Sensivity: Its Possible Importance in Physiology

The ability of the blood glucose level to change in response to a given dose of insulin is impaired in a number of relatively common conditions (e.g., diabetes mellitus, aging, obesity, various endocrinopathies). This is described as *glucose intolerance,* a condition thought to be caused by resistance of the tissues to the effects of insulin. The frequency with which these glucose-intolerant states can occur, and the severity of the symptoms that can develop from them, has engendered massive medical interest in insulin resistance as a pathologic entity.[64] The possibility that changes in insulin sensitivity, including resistance, may also be physiologic appears to have been neglected.

If in a given condition an increase in insulin sensitivity occurred in one or more skeletal muscles, the increased entry of glucose into the body after a meal could be dealt with in the absence of a marked (or without any) change in the blood concentration of insulin; the blood glucose level would be controlled by changes in insulin sensitivity at the tissue level rather than by a change in the secretion of insulin from the pancreas and hence in the plasma insulin concentration (Fig. 28-9). In this case, it is the presence of insulin, rather than any change in its concentration, that is necessary for regulation of the blood glucose concentration.

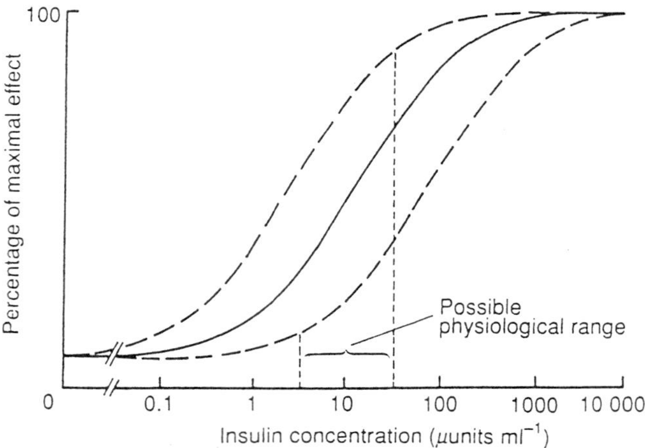

FIGURE 28-9. Effect of a change in sensitivity to insulin in relation to a physiologic change in insulin concentration. Such changes in insulin sensitivity are observed, for example, with changes in the concentration of adenosine in muscle or in the state of physical activity. It can be seen that even if the insulin concentration does not change, a marked change in the rate of glucose uptake, for example, can occur if the insulin sensitivity is changed.

Definition of Sensitivity

Sensitivity in metabolic regulation can be defined as the relationship between the change in enzyme activity and the change in the concentration of a regulator.

Let us consider a general communication, $X \rightsquigarrow Y$, where X is a stimulus (e.g., a regulator) and Y the ensuing response (e.g., a flux, concentration, reaction rate). If a given change of stimulus (ΔX) produces a response of ΔY, the strength of the communication can be expressed as the ratio of the absolute changes ($\Delta Y:\Delta X$) *or* the relative changes ($[\Delta Y/Y]:[\Delta X/X]$).

Two types of sensitivity, *absolute* and *relative,* therefore can be considered. They apply to different situations when discussing insulin sensitivity.

Absolute Sensitivity. This is used, for example, when describing the sensitivity of tissues to insulin. For the communication $X \rightsquigarrow Y$ the absolute-change sensitivity $a^Y{}_X$ is defined by the equation

(1) $$a^Y{}_X = dY/dX$$

In practice effective concentration (EC) is defined as the concentration of insulin producing 50% of the maximal response (EC_{50}). It is of importance that a change in EC_{50} alters the metabolic response produced by any given level of insulin (provided the insulin concentration chosen is not so high that it causes a maximal response) (see Fig. 28-9). The advantage of EC_{50} is that it is quantitative and can be measured in vitro or in vivo. It actually represents the insulin concentration at which a system can most readily adapt to altered (metabolic) circumstances by changing its response.

It is important to recognize what factors can alter sensitivity defined in this way. Sensitivity is affected by anything that influences the binding of insulin to a tissue or events coupling receptor binding to the insulin-sensitive process. Metabolites could, however, act allosterically on the pathway enzymes, modifying their activity and so altering the end-response to insulin; this would be described via the relative sensitivity quantitation (see below). For example, increasing the rate of substrate cycling could increase the sensitivity of the net flux to a given change in a regulator concentration: Increasing the glycogen/glucose l-phosphate cycle could increase the sensitivity of glycogen synthesis to insulin, but quantitatively this would be assessed by the mathematics applying to relative rather than absolute sensitivity. An important point is to realize that sensitivity can be modulated at different levels, even without altering the insulin-effector coupling process: There need not be a change in insulin concentration, insulin binding, or the response of the intracellular signaling pathway.

Relative Sensitivity. This is used more frequently in metabolic control discussions.[65] In the present discussion it is used to describe the role of substrate cycles. For the communication $X \rightsquigarrow Y$ the relative-change sensitivity $s^Y{}_X$ is defined by the equation:

(2) $$s^Y{}_X = (dY/Y)/(dX/X) \\ = d\ln Y/d\ln X$$

The equation for $s^Y{}_X$ can be developed further as follows:

(3) $$d\ln_Y = s^Y{}_X d\ln Y$$

so that, upon integration,

(4) $$\ln Y = s^Y{}_X \ln X + \ln k$$

where k is a constant. Therefore,

(5) $$\ln Y = \ln(kX_s)$$

or,

(6) $$Y = kX^s$$

This equation is a power equation representing the communication $X \rightsquigarrow Y$ and has been used as the basis for a quantitative algebraic analysis of control systems.[65]

If the concentration of a regular (X) changes by ΔX to produce a flux (J) change, ΔJ, the relative change is $\Delta J/J$ and the sensitivity of J to the change in concentration of (X) is given by the ratio $(\Delta J/J):(\Delta X/X)$. For example, if the concentration of a regulator increases twofold, the question arises: How large an increase in enzyme activity will this produce? The greater the response of enzyme activity to a given increase in regulator concentration, the greater the sensitivity. To understand more clearly what may be involved in providing sensitivity, it is necessary to begin with the simplest way in which a protein can interact with a small regulator, that is, via simple *equilibrium binding.*

Equilibrium Binding of a Regulator to an Enzyme. It is likely that all regulators modify the activity of an enzyme by

TABLE 28-1. Effect of Increase in Regulator Concentration on Net Flux Through a Reaction (Enzyme Activities) Controlled by a Substrate Cycle*

Concentration of Regulator	E_2	E_4	Net Flux A to B†	Relative Increase in Flux
	U/min			
Basal	10	9.8	0.2	—
Fourfold increase	90	9.8	80.2	401 times

*The activities are hypothetical.
†E_4–E_2.

binding in a reversible manner to a protein (this protein may not be the immediate ''metabolic'' or target enzyme, but may be an enzyme involved in an interconversion cycle that controls the target enzyme by covalent modification). Such binding, which is described as equilibrium binding, controls the activity of the enzyme as follows:

$$E_1R \rightleftarrows E^*R \quad (7)$$

where E is the inactive form of the enzyme, E* is the active form, and R is an activator. The asterisk indicates that the binding of the effector molecule R has changed the conformation of the catalytic site of the enzyme to produce the active form of the enzyme. The normal response of enzyme activity to the binding of the regulator is hyperbolic. The *hyperbolic response* is the simplest relationship between, for example, a protein and its regulator, a hormone and its receptor, or a neurotransmitter and its receptor. Unfortunately, this response is relatively inefficient for metabolic regulations. For example, a twofold change in regulator concentration changes the enzyme activity by less than two-fold (i.e., the maximum sensitivity is less than unity). This may be difficult to accept when simply observing the steepness of the initial part of the hyperbolic curve. It must be appreciated, however, that sensitivity is defined on the basis of relative rather than absolute changes in concentration. Not surprisingly, there are several mechanisms for improving sensitivity in control over that provided by the hyperbolic curve. One of these is the *interconversion cycle*, and this may be relevant to the mechanism by which, for example, insulin can affect glycogen synthase activity—perhaps by stimulating the activity of a protein phosphatase. Whether this would result in a control mechanism of quantitative importance depends on the kinetics of the interconnecting enzymes, phosphatase, and kinase: this theory has been provided elsewhere.[65] Another of these mechanisms that is particularly relevant to current discussions is the *substrate cycle.*

Substrate Cycles. It is possible for a reaction that is nonequilibrium in the forward direction of a pathway (i.e., A → B) to be opposed by a reaction that is nonequilibrium in the reverse direction of the pathway (i.e., B → A). Both reactions must be chemically distinct (different reactions), so they are catalyzed by separate enzymes:

$$S \xrightarrow{E_1} A \underset{E_4}{\overset{E_2}{\rightleftarrows}} B \xrightarrow{E_3} P \quad (8)$$

A substrate cycle between A and B occurs if the two enzymes (E_2 and E_4) are simultaneously catalytically active. For every molecule of A converted to B and back again to A, chemical energy must be converted to heat because these reactions are nonequilibrium, and thus heat is lost to the environment.

The advantage of this heat loss, however, is that the cycle provides an improvement in sensitivity without changing the properties or characteristics of the enzyme catalyzing the forward reaction in the pathway, and for this reason, it can be seen to differ from the other mechanisms that improve sensitivity. This has also been shown to be the case when the precise quantitative role of substrate cycles in metabolic control is considered[1,8,53,65] (Table 28-1). Figure 28-10 provides a speculative suggestion as to how the sensitivity of the translocation of GLUT-4 transporters to insulin could be increased by increasing the rate of translocation cycling between the intracellular and plasma membrane.

One advantage of the substrate-cycling mechanism in increasing sensitivity is that the sensitivity can be varied quickly, effectively, and transiently (i.e., by varying the rate of cycling) (see Table 28-1). This might, therefore, be of importance in understanding how sensitivity to insulin could rapidly change. Some factors that are known to influence insulin sensitivity are adenosine, prostaglandins, chronic elevation of catecholamines and insulin-like growth factors (IGFs).[65–67] It is not known whether these factors influence the rate of substrate cycling.

Adenosine

Adenosine is produced continuously by most tissues; when it is transported out of the tissue it can produce extracellular effects. Studies in vitro with adenosine deaminase and adenosine receptor agonists/antagonists have shown that adenosine increases the sensitivity to insulin of the rate of glucose utilization and lipolysis in adipose tissue but decreases the sensitivity of glucose utilization to insulin in skeletal muscle.[66] The adenosine receptor modulating insulin action in rat skeletal muscle has been characterized recently[67]; however, the physiologic significance of these in vitro effects will remain unclear until in vivo studies using specific adenosine receptor agonists/antagonists are carried out.

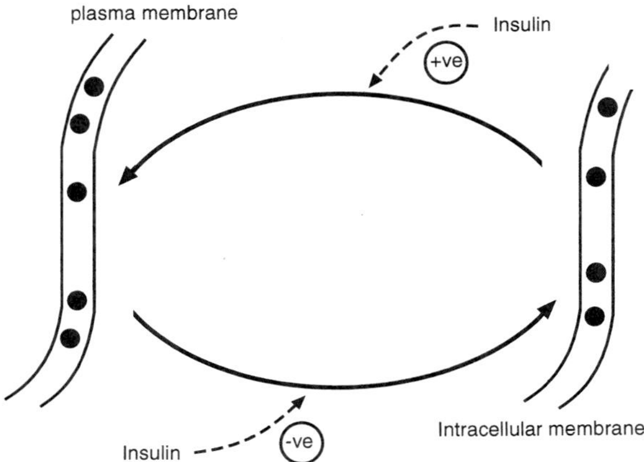

FIGURE 28-10. A suggested translocation cycle for GLUT-4 transporters and postulated effects of insulin. +ve = positive; −ve = negative.

Prostaglandins

It has been shown that prostaglandins of the E series (e.g., PGE_1, PGE_2) can improve insulin sensitivity in the isolated rat soleus muscle.[68] Because PGE_2 is produced from arachidonic acid, these findings suggest that diets that are high in polyunsaturated fatty acids could improve insulin sensitivity. Of interest is the idea that conversion of linoleic acid, a common essential fatty acid in the diet, to arachidonic acid is severely limited in humans by the activity of Δ-6-desaturase; but this limitation can be overcome by supplementation of the diet with γ-linoleic acid (GLA) which bypasses this limiting step. If this hypothesis is correct, this should allow a higher rate of synthesis of arachidonic acid, a higher level of this fatty acid in the cell membrane, and hence more substrate for PGE_2 production (provided the cyclo-oxygenase does not catalyze a flux-generating step—a process that has not been subjected to metabolic control-logic analysis). In this context, it is of possible importance that dietary supplementation with GLA improves some of the complications of type II diabetes mellitus.[69]

Catecholamines

The effect of acute injection of catecholamines is to decrease the sensitivity of glucose utilization to insulin. This probably is due to enhanced rates of glycogen breakdown and increased rates of mobilization of fatty acids. Several physiologic conditions in which catecholamines are increased, however, are associated with an increase in the sensitivity of glucose metabolism to insulin (e.g., cold-exposure, exercise-training). It has been shown that the soleus muscles removed from animals subjected to the above conditions and incubated in vitro exhibit an increased sensitivity of glucose utilization to insulin. Chronic treatment in vivo with adrenaline or β-adrenoreceptor agonists also increases the insulin sensitivity of glucose utilization by muscle incubated in vitro.[70,71]

Exercise

Endurance exercise increases the rate of utilization of all metabolic fuels. Hence, it decreases the glycogen content in muscle. The latter may result in an increase in the activity of glycogen synthase and, consequently, may decrease the requirement for insulin in the stimulation of glycogen synthesis after a carbohydrate meal. In addition, it has been shown that, in normal subjects, endurance-training markedly increases insulin sensitivity, so that very much lower concentrations of insulin are required to control blood glucose concentration after an oral glucose load.[72] It also has been shown that, in diabetic subjects who were exercised to deplete muscle glycogen stores (by 80%), the rate of glycogen synthesis in the muscles for 4-hour postexercise, after a carbohydrate-rich meal, was the same whether the subjects took their normal insulin or were deprived of it.[73]

Insulin-Like Growth Factors

Insulin-like growth factors (IGF)-1 and IGF-2 have a structural homology to proinsulin.[74] They are carried in plasma and extracellular fluids bound to specific carrier proteins. There are six types of these binding proteins (IGFBP-1–6), one with a high and several with low molecular weight. Although it is suggested that the IGFs in blood are in the bound state, there should also be a small amount of the IGFs in the free state, comprising, in part, peptides newly synthesized and released from their sites of production that have not yet been bound.[74–76] In addition, there should be a given concentration of free peptide that is in equilibrium with the complex according to the following binding constant:

$$BP - IGF \rightleftarrows BP + IGF \quad (9)$$

The high-molecular-weight binding protein (150-kd, IGFBP-3) is the predominant IGFBP in adult serum. It binds both IGF-1 and IGF-2 with a high affinity; most of the IGFs in plasma are bound to this carrier protein. It is secreted by the liver, and its rate of secretion is increased by IGF-1 and growth hormone. It does not cross the normal capillary barrier, so it is considered to act as a circulating reservoir for the IGFs in the blood. By restricting access of circulating IGFs to the tissues, IGFBP-3 prevents the intrinsic insulin-like activity of the IGFs from causing hypoglycemia.[74,77–79]

The low-molecular-weight binding proteins are synthesized by most tissues, including vascular endothelial cells; this underlines their importance as local regulators of the autocrine and paracrine effects of the IGFs in the tissues by preventing them from binding to receptors or, under some experimental conditions, by potentiating IGF activity. In addition, because they are able to cross the capillary wall, they may serve to transport the IGFs to the tissues. Their rate of secretion is not growth hormone–dependent.[74,80,81] The levels of IGFBP-1 and IGFBP-2 in plasma are mostly regulated by metabolic factors (although the evidence for IGFBP-2 is less clear than that for IGFBP-1). Experiments in humans and rats have shown that these binding proteins are suppressed during intake of oral glucose or mixed meals and are increased during fasting, insulin-induced hypoglycemia or diabetes; these changes may be controlled by changes in the plasma levels of insulin and glucose.[77,82–84] The findings suggest that these binding proteins may influence, quite markedly, the biologic effectiveness of the IGFs during physiologic or pathologic conditions. Less information exists on factors that regulate the other low-molecular-weight binding proteins; IGFBP-4 and IGFBP-5 may have a role in the regulation of the growth effects of the IGFs in neural and bone tissue. IGFBP-6 binds IGF-2 preferentially; this is in contrast to other low-molecular-weight binding proteins, which bind IGF-1 and IGF-2 with equal affinity. This suggests that IGFBP-6 may have a special role to control the effectiveness of IGF-2 on tissues.[81]

Specific receptors for IGF-1 and IGF-2 are present on membranes or cells from a large number of tissues. There is substantial cross-reactivity between these receptors and that of insulin: The IGF-1 receptor binds IGF-2 and insulin, although there is a difference in the binding affinities; similarly, the insulin receptor binds IGF-1 and IGF-2.[74,85] The metabolic effects of IGF-1 and IGF-2 on muscle, however, seem to be mediated via their own receptors.[11,86]

Effects of Insulin-Like Growth Factors on Protein and Lipid Metabolism

In general, the available information suggests that, regarding the hormonal regulation of protein anabolism, insulin acts primarily to decrease the rate of proteolysis, growth hormone to stimulate the rate of protein synthesis, and IGF-1 to influence both processes.[87] In vivo (in humans or rats) or in vitro, IGF-1 stimulates the rate of incorporation of amino acids into protein and inhibits protein degradation in muscle; on a molar basis, IGF-1 seems to be less potent than insulin.[87–89] In the studies done in vivo, these effects of IGF-1 were seen only when the plasma levels of this peptide were increased acutely, that is, the concentration of free IGF-1 was increased. On the basis of current information, it has not been possible to define whether the effects of IGF-1 on protein synthesis and degradation are mediated via IGF-1 or the insulin receptor.[87] In addition, recent studies in humans showed that infusion of IGF-1 reduced the rate of protein oxidation,[88] possibly because of a decreased rate of protein degradation.[87]

In contrast to insulin, IGF-1 does not seem to decrease the rate of lipolysis: In the rat, administration of IGF-1 for 10 days as subcutaneous injections increased the plasma level of free fatty acids, suggesting an increase in the rate of lipolysis[90]; this can be explained by the effect of IGF-1 to suppress insulin secretion.[91] In humans, infusion of IGF-1 increased the plasma levels of free fatty acids and the rate of lipid oxidation.[88]

Effects of Insulin-Like Growth Factors on Carbohydrate Metabolism

Intravenous bolus injections of IGF-1 or IGF-2 in normal or hypophysectomized rats have acute effects on glucose utilization: They lower the blood glucose concentration and increase the rate of glycogen synthesis in muscle; there is no evidence of an acute effect of IGFs on glucose release by the liver.[75,89,92,93] It appears that the IGFs cause hypoglycemia by increasing the rate of glucose utilization by peripheral tissues, probably skeletal muscle.

Skeletal muscle is considered to be quantitatively the most important tissue for disposal of glucose in response to insulin. Recently, studies have been carried out on the effects of IGF-1 on the rate of glucose utilization in this tissue. In isolated rat soleus muscle, IGF-1 increased the rates of glucose transport, glucose phosphorylation, glucose conversion to lactate (glycolysis), and glycogen synthesis[11]; however, there was no effect on the rates of glucose oxidation (measured with [^{14}C]glucose) or glycogenolysis (estimated indirectly from the differences between the rates of lactate and [^{14}C]lactate formation).[11] In these muscles, IGF-1 increased the content of fructose 2,6-bisphosphate, which is a potent activator of 6-phosphofructokinase, to a greater extent than insulin.[11,90] These results suggest that, in muscle, IGF-1 stimulates the rate of glucose utilization independent of insulin and may have a preferential effect to increase the rate of glycolysis and lactate formation. In dogs, infusion of IGF-1 increased the concentrations of lactate in plasma.[93] Because lactate is transported to the liver, where it is converted to glucose via gluconeogenesis, IGF-1 may actually increase the activity of the Cori cycle.

The fact that the increase in the rate of glucose transport by maximal concentrations of IGF-1 was similar to that produced by maximal concentrations of insulin suggests that IGF-1 increased the rate of glucose utilization by a mechanism identical to that of insulin, that is, by inducing a redistribution of all available glucose transporters from the intracellular pool to the plasma membrane.[11] Experiments with rat soleus muscle and muscle cell lines showed that IGF-1 increases the rate of glucose transport by increasing the translocation mainly of GLUT-4 but also of GLUT-1 glucose transporters to the plasma membrane.[94] In this case, insulin would not be expected to have any additive effects with IGF-1 on the rate of glucose transport. Indeed, in the presence of near-physiologic or maximal concentrations of IGF-1 insulin was less effective in increasing the rates of glucose transport and utilization in the soleus muscle.[11] This has also been shown in experiments where IGF-1 was given to rats in vivo and the soleus muscles isolated shortly after the injection: in this case, IGF-1 exceeds the capacity of the binding proteins and the level in the plasma is increased toward maximal.[90] When the concentrations of IGF-1 are lower, however, the effects of insulin to increase the rate of glucose utilization in muscle are complementary to those of IGF-1[90]; this means that, under these conditions, IGF-1 increases the apparent sensitivity of muscle to insulin. Indeed, subcutaneous administration of IGF-1 to rats in vivo for 10 days increased insulin-mediated rates of glucose utilization in the isolated soleus muscle (Fig. 28-11).[90] Therefore, IGF-1 may be a useful adjunct to insulin in treating patients with type II diabetes and insulin resistance.[95]

Somewhat in contrast to these effects of IGF-1, the IGF-2 had no effect in the absence of insulin. At low physiologic levels of insulin, however, it increased the rates of both glucose uptake and glycogen synthesis by the isolated soleus muscle, thus suggesting that it increased the sensitivity of these processes to insu-

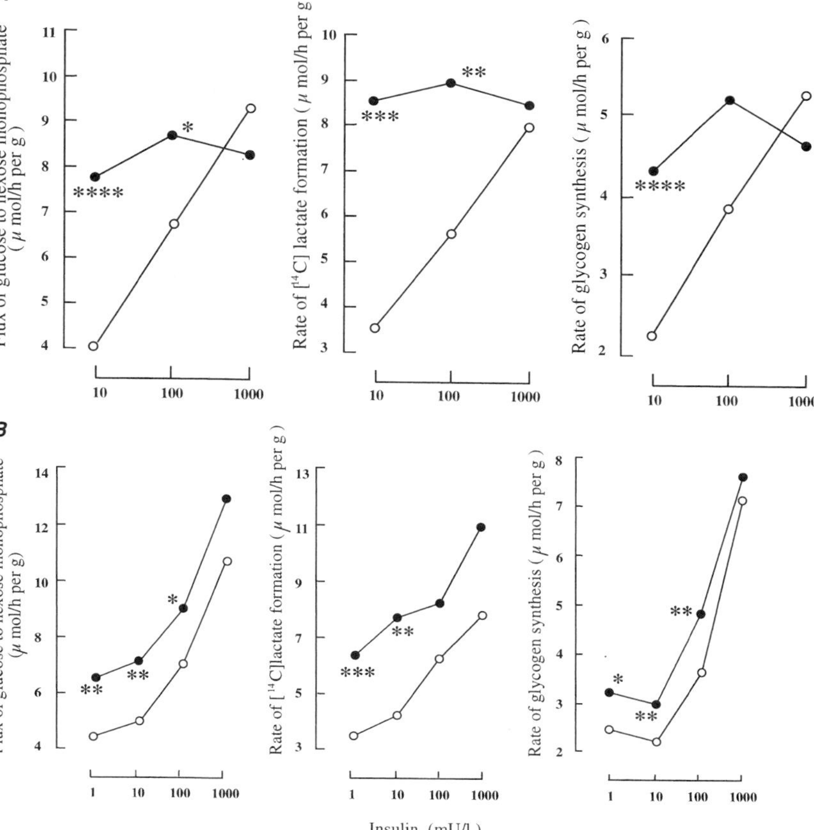

FIGURE 28-11. Effects of in vivo administration of IGF-1 on the flux of glucose to hexose monophosphate and on the rates of [^{14}C] lactate formation and glycogen synthesis in soleus muscles. Muscles were isolated from rats 1 hour after IGF-1 (●) or saline injection (○) (***A***) and 10 days after initiation of treatment with IGF-1 (●) or saline (○) injection (***B***). (Adapted with permission from Dimitriadis G, Parry-Billings M, Dunger D, et al. Effects of in vivo administration of IGF-I on the rate of glucose utilization in the soleus muscle of the rat. J Endocrinol 1992;133:37.)

lin.[96] Because these effects were observed at physiologic levels of this peptide, it is assumed to be acting on skeletal muscle via the IGF-2 receptor.

These results suggest that the IGFs may be important as regulators of glucose utilization in vivo either along with insulin or instead of insulin. Because in addition to their endocrine effects they also have paracrine and autocrine effects in the tissues,[74] they could provide local regulation for uptake of glucose by individual muscles or groups of muscles by changing their response to insulin locally. Insulin could influence the free level of the IGFs via a change in the concentration of low-molecular-weight binding proteins (see above). It is tempting to speculate that the effects of IGF-1 to increase the rate of glucose metabolism in muscle may be more important than those of insulin; the major effect of insulin overall may be its antilipolytic effect. This suggests that the list of factors presented above, under insulin sensitivity, should be increased by inclusion of IGF-1 and IGF-2. It raises the intriguing question as to whether changes in sensitivity caused by exercise, or chronic treatment with catecholamines or even adenosine, could be caused by local changes in the concentration of IGFs. Such a change could influence the rate of glucose uptake by muscle without any need for a change in the plasma level of insulin.

Finally, it is important to appreciate that, as our knowledge of biochemical physiology increases, our appreciation of how blood glucose might be controlled by insulin is expanding dramatically. Blood glucose concentration may be controlled by the action of insulin to change (1) the rate of glucose transport in muscle, (2) to change the rate of fatty acid oxidation, (3) to change the level of local hormones (4) alternatively the insulin sensitivity of glucose utilization at specific sites in the body might change under different conditions. These mechanisms suggest some new approaches to the treatment of patients with type II diabetes, such as (1) a decrease in the rate of fatty acid oxidation or fatty acid release, or (2) an increase in the effectiveness of insulin in muscle (e.g., by local changes in the concentration of factors that modify the sensitivity of muscle tissue to insulin). With this complexity of mechanisms, Renold et al. showed considerable foresight when they termed the basic cause of diabetes mellitus ''inappropriate hyperglycemia,'' as cited in Newsholme et al.[1]

References

1. Newsholme E, Bevan S, Dimitriadis G, Kelly R. In: Ashcroft F, Ashcroft S, eds. Insulin: Molecular Biology to Pathology. Oxford: IRL Press; 1992;5:155–190
2. Klip A, Paquet M. Glucose transport and glucose transporters in muscle and their metabolic regulation. Diabetes Care 1990;13:228
3. Kahn B. Facilitative glucose transporters: Regulatory mechanisms and dysregulation in diabetes. J Clin Invest 1992;89:1367
4. Gould G, Holman G. The glucose transporter family: Structure, function and tissue-specific expression. Biochem J 1993;295:329
5. Kipnis D. Regulation of glucose transport by muscle. Ann N Y Acad Sci 1959;82:354
6. Randle P, Morgan H. Regulation of glucose uptake by muscle. Vitam Horm 1962;20:199
7. Newsholme E, Start C. Regulation in Metabolism. New York, NY: John Wiley & Sons; 1973
8. Newsholme E, Leech A. Biochemistry for the Medical Sciences. New York, NY: John Wiley & Sons; 1983
9. Newsholme E, Crabtree B, Adrawi M. Glutamine metabolism in lymphocytes: Its biochemical, physiological, and clinical importance. Q J Exp Physiol 1985;70:473
10. Bessman S, Geiger P. Compartmentation of hexokinase and creatine phosphokinase: Cellular regulation and insulin action. Curr Top Cell Regul 1980;16:55
11. Dimitriadis G, Parry-Billings M, Bevan S, et al. Effects of IGF-I on the rates of glucose transport and utilization in rat skeletal muscle *in vitro*. Biochem J 1992;285:269
12. Dimitriadis GD. Studies on insulin sensitivity in muscle. Oxford: University of Oxford; 1994. Thesis
13. Rossetti L, Giaccari A. Relative contribution of glycogen synthesis and glycolysis to insulin-mediated glucose uptake. J Clin Invest 1990;85:1785
14. Hue L, Rider M. Role of fructose 2,6-bisphosphate in the control of glycolysis in mammalian tissues. Biochem J 1987;245:313
15. Wegener G, Krause U, Thuy M. Fructose 2,6-bisphosphate and glycolytic flux in skeletal muscle of swimming frog. FEBS Lett 1990;267:257
16. Consoli A, Nurjahan N, Gerich J, Mandarino L. Skeletal muscle is a major site of lactate uptake and release during hyperinsulinemia. Metabolism 1992;41:176
17. Mandarino L, Wright K, Verity L, et al. Effects of insulin infusion on human skeletal muscle pyruvate dehydrogenase, phosphofructokinase and glycogen synthase. J Clin Invest 1987;80:655
18. Kelley D, Reilly J, Veneman T, Mandarino L. Effects of insulin on skeletal muscle glucose storage, oxidation and glycolysis in humans. Am J Physiol 1990;258:E923
19. Birkinshaw V, Gurd M, Randall S, et al. Br Med J 1958;2:463
20. Shulman G, Rossetti L, Rothman D, et al. Quantitative analysis of glycogen repletion by nuclear magnetic resonance spectroscopy in the conscious rat. J Clin Invest 1987;80:387
21. Kruszynska Y, Home P, Alberti G. *In vivo* regulation of liver and skeletal muscle glycogen synthase activity by glucose and insulin. Diabetes 1986; 35:662
22. Yki-Jarvinen H, Mott D, Young A, et al. Regulation of glycogen synthase and phosphorylase activities by glucose and insulin in human skeletal muscle. J Clin Invest 1987;80:95
23. Dimitriadis G, Parry-Billings M, Leighton B, et al. Studies on the effects of growth hormone administration *in vivo* on the rates of glucose transport and utilization in rat skeletal muscle. Eur J Clin Invest 1994;24:161
24. Hultman E. Regulation of carbohydrate metabolism in the liver during rest and exercise with special reference to diet. In: Landry P, Orban W, eds. Third International Symposium on Biochemistry of Exercise. Miami, Fla: Symposia Specialist; 1978:99–126
25. Maelum S, Hermansen L. Muscle glycogen concentration during recovery after prolonged severe exercise in fasting subjects. Scand J Clin Lab Invest 1978;38:557
26. DeFronzo R, Bonnadona R, Ferrannini E. Pathogenesis of NIDDM. Diabetes Care 1992;15:318
27. Beck-Nielsen H, Hother-Nielsen O, Vaag A, Alford F. Pathogenesis of type II diabetes mellitus: The role of skeletal muscle glucose uptake and hepatic glucose production in the development of hyperglycemia. Diabetologia 1994;37:217
28. Mandarino L, Madar Z, Kolterman O, et al. Adipocyte glycogen synthase and pyruvate dehydrogenase in obese and type II diabetic subjects. Am J Physiol 1986;251:E489
29. Bogardus C, Lillioja A, Howard B, et al. Relationships between insulin secretion, insulin action and fasting plasma glucose concentrations in non-diabetic and NIDDM subjects. J Clin Invest 1984;74:1238
30. Wright K, Beck-Nielsen H, Kolterman O, Mandarino L. Decreased activation of skeletal muscle glycogen synthase by mixed meal ingestion in NIDDM. Diabetes 1988;37:436
31. Thorburn A, Gumbiner B, Bulacan F, et al. Intracellular glucose oxidation and glycogen synthetase activity are reduced in type II diabetes independent of impaired glucose uptake. J Clin Invest 1990;85:522
32. Farrace S, Rossetti L. Hyperglycemia markedly enhances skeletal muscle glycogen synthase activity in diabetic but not in normal conscious rats. Diabetes 1992;41:1453
33. Golay A, DeFronzo R, Ferrannini E, et al. Oxidative and non-oxidative glucose metabolism in non-obese Type II diabetic patients. Diabetologia 1988; 31:585
34. Golay A, Felber J, Jequier E, et al. Metabolic basis of obesity and NIDDM. Diabetes Metab Rev 1988;4:727
35. Del Prato S, Bonadonna R, Bonora E, et al. Characterization of cellular defects of insulin action in type II diabetes mellitus. J Clin Invest 1993;91:484
36. Vaag A, Alford F, Henriksen F, et al. Multiple defects of both hepatic and peripheral intracellular glucose processing contribute to the hyperglycemia of NIDDM. Diabetologia 1995;38:326
37. Shulman G, Rothman D, Jue T, et al. Quantitation of muscle glycogen synthesis in normal subjects and subjects with NIDDM by ^{13}C nulcear magnetic resonance spectroscopy. N Engl J Med 1990;322:223
38. DeFronzo R, Gunnarson R, Bjorkman O, et al. Effects of insulin on peripheral and splanchnic glucose metabolism in non-insulin dependent diabetes mellitus. J Clin Invest 1985;76:149
39. Eriksson J, Fanssila-Kallunki A, Ekstrand A, et al. Early metabolic effects in persons at increased risk for NIDDM. N Engl J Med 1989;321:337
40. Vogt B, Muhebacher C, Cassascosa J, et al. Subcellular distribution of GLUT4 in skeletal muscle of lean type II diabetic patients in the basal state. Diabetologia 1992;35:456
41. Capaldo B, Napoli R, DiBonito P, et al. Glucose and gluconeogenic substrate exchange by the forearm skeletal muscle in hyperglycemic and insulin-treated type II diabetic patients. J Clin Endocrinol Metab 1990;71:1220
42. Mondon C, Jones I, Azhar S, et al. Lactate production and pyruvate dehydrogenase activity in fat and skeletal muscle from diabetic rats. Diabetes 1992; 41:1547
43. Meyer H, Curchod B, Maeder E, et al. Modification of glucose storage and oxidation in non-obese diabetics measured by continuous indirect calorimetry. Diabetes 1980;29:752
44. Kelley D, Manarino L. Hyperglycemia normalizes insulin-stimulated skeletal muscle glucose oxidation and storage in NIDDM. J Clin Invest 1990;86:1999
45. Consoli A. Role of the liver in pathophysiology of NIDDM. Diabetes Care 1992;15:430

46. Gerich J. Is muscle the major tissue of insulin resistance in Type II diabetes? Diabetologia 1991;34:607
47. Elayan I, Winder W. Effect of glucose infusion on muscle malonyl-CoA during exercise. J Appl Physiol 1991;70:1495
48. Duan G, Winder W. Control of malonyl-CoA by glucose and insulin in perfused skeletal muscle. J Appl Physiol 1993;74:2543
49. Cahill G. Starvation in man. New Engl J Med 1970;282:668
50. Jensen M, Haymond M, Gerich J, et al. Lipolysis during fasting. Clin Invest 1987;79:207
51. Randle P, Garland P, Hales C, Newsholme E. The glucose-fatty acid cycle: Its role in insulin sensitivity and the metabolic disturbances of diabetes mellitus. Lancet 1963;1:785
52. Saloranta C, Koivisto V, Widen E, et al. Contribution of liver and muscle to glucose-fatty acid cycle in humans. Am J Physiol 1993;264:E599
53. Newsholme E, Crabtree B. Substrate cycles in metabolic regulation and in heat generation. Biochem Soc Symp 1976;41:61
54. Dimitriadis G, Baker B, Marsh H, et al. Effect of thyroid hormone excess on action, secretion and metabolism of insulin in humans. Am J Physiol 1985; 248:E593
55. Leighton B, Dimitriadis G, Parry-Billings M, et al. Effects of insulin on glucose metabolism in skeletal muscle from septic and endotoxaemic rats. Clin Sci (Colch) 1989;77:61
56. Nurjhan N, Consoli A, Gerich J. Increased lipolysis and its consequences on gluconeogenesis in non-insulin dependent diabetes mellitus. J Clin Invest 1992;89:169
57. Exton J. Gluconeogenesis. Metabolism 1972;21:945
58. Chan T. The permissive effects of glucocorticoid on hepatic gluconeogenesis. J Biol Chem 1984;259:7426
59. Terretaz J, Assimacopoulos-Jeannet F, Jeanrenaud B. Inhibition of hepatic glucose production by insulin *in vivo* in rats: Contribution of glycolysis. Am J Physiol 1986;250:E346
60. Sharp P, Johnston D. Mechanisms of hyperglycaemia and disorders of intermediary metabolism. In: Pickup J, Williams G, eds. Textbook of Diabetes, Vol. 1. Oxford: Blackwell; 1991:303–312
61. Jenssen T, Nurjhan N, Consoli A, Gerich J. Failure of substrate-induced gluconeogenesis to increase overall glucose appearance in normal humans. J Clin Invest 1990;86:489
62. Riossetti L, Giaccari A, Barzilai N, et al. Mechanism by which hyperglycemia inhibits hepatic glucose production in conscious rats. J Clin Invest 1993; 92:1126
63. Levine R, Goldstein M. On the mechanisms of action of insulin. Recent Prog Horm Res 1955;11:343
64. Moller D, Flier J. Insulin resistance: Mechanisms syndromes and implications. N Engl J Med 1991;325:938
65. Crabtree B, Newsholme E. A quantitative approach to metabolic control. Curr Top Cell Regul 1985;25:21
66. Challiss R, Leighton B, Lozeman F, Newsholme E. The hormone-modulatory effects of adenosine in skeletal muscle. In: Gerlock E, Becker B, eds. Topics and Perspectives in Adenosine Research. Berlin: Spring-Verlag; 1987:275–285
67. Challiss J, Richards S, Budohoski L. Characterization of the adenosine receptor modulating insulin action in rat skeletal muscle. Eur J Pharmacol 1992;226:121
68. Leighton B, Budohoski L, Lozeman F, et al. The effect of PGE_1, PGE_2, PGF_2 and indomethacin on the sensitivity of glycolysis and glycogen synthesis to insulin in the stripped soleus muscle of the rat. Biochem J 1985;227:337
69. Jamal G. Prevention and treatment of diabetic distal polyneuropathy by the supplementation of γ-linoleic acid. In: Horrobin D, ed. Delta-6-essential fatty acids. New York: Wiley-Liss; 1990:485–504
70. Challiss J, Budohoski L, Newsholme E, et al. Effect of a novel thermogenic β-adrenoreceptor agonist (BRL26830) on insulin resistance in soleus muscle from obese Zucker rats. Biochem Biophys Res Commun 1985;128:928
71. Budohoski L, Challiss J, Dubaniewicz A, et al. Effect of a prolonged elevation of plasma adrenaline concentration *in vivo* on insulin sensitivity in soleus muscle of the rat. Biochem J 1987;244:655
72. Bjontorp P, Fahten M, Grimb G. Carbohydrate and lipid metabolism in middle-aged physically well trained men. Metabolism 1977;21:1037
73. Maelum S, Hostmark A, Hermansen L. Synthesis of muscle glycogen during recovery after prolonged severe exercise in diabetic subjects: Effect of insulin deprivation. Scand J Clin Lab Invest 1978;38:35
74. Sara V, Hall K. IGFs and their binding proteins. Physiol Rev 1990;70:591
75. Zapf J, Hauri C, Waldvogel M, Froesch E. Acute metabolic effects and half-lives of intravenously administered IGF-I and IGF-II in normal and hypophysectomized rats. J Clin Invest 1986;77:1768
76. Guler H, Zapf J, Froesch E. Short-term metabolic effects of recombinant human IGF-I in healthy adults. N Engl J Med 1987;317:137
77. Yeoh S, Baxter R. Metabolic regulation of the growth hormone-dependent IGFBP in human plasma. Acta Endocrinol 1988;119:465
78. Zapf J, Schoenle E, Jagars G, et al. Inhibition of the action of non-suppressible insulin-like activity on isolated rat fat cells by binding to its carrier protein. J Clin Invest 1979;63:1077
79. Zapf J, Froesch E, Humbel R. The insulin-like growth factors of human serum: Chemical and biological characterization and aspects of their possible physiological role. Curr Top Cell Regul 1981;19:257
80. Ooi G, Herington A. The biological and structural characterization of specific serum binding proteins for the IGFs. J Endocrinol 1988;118:7
81. Bach L, Rechler M. Insulin-like growth factor binding proteins. Diabetes Rev 1995;3:38
82. Baxter R, Cowell C. Diurnal rhythm of growth hormone-independent binding protein for insulin-like growth factors in human plasma. J Clin Endocrinol Metab 1987;65:432
83. Holly J, Biddlecombe R, Dunger D, et al. Circadian variation of growth hormone independent IGFBP in diabetes and its relationship to insulin. Clin Endocrinol 1988;29:667
84. Suikkari A, Koivisto V, Rutanen E, et al. Insulin regulates the serum levels of low molecular weight IGFBP. J Clin Endocrinol Metab 1988;66:266
85. Werner H, LeRoith D. IGF-I receptor: Structure, signal transduction and function. Diabetes Rev 1995;3:28
86. Poggi C, LeMarchand Brustel Y, Zapf J, et al. Effects and binding of insulin-like growth factor I in the isolated soleus muscle of lean and obese mice. Endocrinology 1979;105:723
87. Fryburg D, Barrett E. Insulin, growth hormone and IGF-I regulation of protein metabolism. Diabetes Rev 1995;3:93
88. Hussain M, Schmitz O, Mengel A, et al. IGF-I stimulates lipid oxidation, reduces protein oxidation and enhances insulin sensitivity in humans. J Clin Invest 1993;92:2249
89. Jacob R, Barrett E, Plewe G, et al. Acute effects of IGF-I on glucose and amino acid metabolism in the awake fasted rat. J Clin Invest 1989;83: 1717
90. Dimitriadis G, Parry-Billings M, Dunger D, et al. Effects of *in vivo* administration of IGF-I on the rate of glucose utilization in the soleus muscle of the rat. J Endocrinol 1992;133:37
91. Rennert N, Caprio S, Sherwin R. IGF-I inhibits glucose-stimulated insulin secretion but does not impair glucose metabolism in normal humans. J Clin Endocrinol Metab 1993;76:804
92. Moxley R, Arner P, Moss A, et al. Acute effects of IGF-I and insulin on glucose metabolism *in vivo*. Am J Physiol 1990;259:E561
93. Giacca A, Gupta R, Effendic S, et al. Differential effects of IGF-I and insulin on glucoregulation and fat metabolism in de-pancreatized dogs. Diabetes 1990;39:340
94. Bilan P, Mitsumoto Y, Ramlal T, Klip A. Acute and long-term effects of IGF-I on glucose transporters in muscle cells. FEBS Lett 1992;298:285
95. Zonobi P, Jaeggi-Groisman S, Riesen W, et al. Insulin-like growth factor I improves glucose and lipid metabolism in type II diabetes mellitus. J Clin Invest 1992;90:2234
96. Bevan S, Parry-Billings M, Opara E, et al. The effect of IGF-II on glucose uptake and metabolism in rat skeletal muscle *in vitro*. Biochem J 1992; 286:561

Diabetes Mellitus, edited by Derek LeRoith, Simeon I. Taylor, and Jerrold M. Olefsky. Lippincott–Raven Publishers, Philadelphia © 1996.

CHAPTER 29

Diabetic Ketoacidosis and the Hyperglycemic Hyperosmolar Syndrome

ELIZABETH D. ENNIS AND ROBERT A. KREISBERG

Diabetic ketoacidosis (DKA) and the hyperglycemic hyperosmolar syndrome (HHS) are life-threatening forms of *decompensated diabetes*. Although DKA and HHS often are discussed as distinct entities, they appear to represent two extremes in a spectrum of diabetic decompensation (Fig. 29-1).[1] DKA and HHS differ from each other by the magnitude of hyperglycemia, the severity of acidosis/ketonemia, and the degree of dehydration. Although DKA classically occurs in young patients with insulin-dependent diabetes mellitus (IDDM), many are older and have non–insulin-dependent diabetes mellitus (NIDDM). In one epidemiologic survey, 45% of DKA patients were older than 44 years and 26% older than 65 years.[2] In another survey, 11% of patients with DKA were older than 60 years.[3] HHS typically develops in patients with NIDDM; however, some patients have features of HHS and DKA. Clearly, metabolic abnormalities can vary continuously on a continuum from one extreme to the other (see Fig. 29-1). Episodes of DKA have occurred on some occasions and HHS on other occasions in the same patient. A comprehensive review of a large number of patients with decompensated diabetes mellitus revealed that 22% had DKA, 45% had HHS, and 33% had features of both disorders (Fig. 29-2).[3]

Decompensated diabetes mellitus is an important cause of morbidity and mortality among diabetics. In 1988 in the United States there were 454,000 hospitalizations for diabetes mellitus and its complications.[4] Although 84,000 (18.5%) of these admissions were for DKA, the prevalence of DKA is actually higher because mild DKA often is managed in the ambulatory setting.[4] From 1980 to 1988, mortality due to DKA in the U.S. declined slightly from 30.6 to 27.7/100,000 patients.[4] In 1988, 2.3% of DKA admissions ended in fatalities.[4] Mortality rates were highest (~20%) in patients ≥70–75 years of age.[4,5] The highest mortality rates occurred among blacks (men > women); however, the absolute number of deaths due to DKA was greater among whites because of the higher prevalence of IDDM in the white population.[4] Unfortunately, incidence and prevalence data for HHS are not readily available, possibly because of the multiple comorbid conditions often found in these patients. In recent years, HHS mortality rates have decreased from ~58% to ~15%.[6–8] Earlier diagnosis and improved management of comorbid illnesses probably are responsible for the improved outcome.

In the past, women have been more likely than men to develop DKA, but recently increasing numbers of men have been hospitalized for DKA in the U.S. while admissions for women have declined over the last decade.[4,9] In a U.K. study spanning the years from 1971 to 1988, the female:male ratio for DKA admissions decreased from 2.79 to 1.59, reflecting a decline in episodes in female patients and an increase in episodes in male patients.[10] Female patients were slightly more likely than males to have recurrent episodes of DKA (3.3/patient vs. 2.7/patient).[10] Recurrent DKA, defined as ≥3 episodes in 4 years, was noted in 31 female and 12 male patients (199 episodes total).[10] Because female patients constitute less than one-half of IDDM patients (0.85–95:1, F:M), this suggests an excess of recurrent DKA among female patients.[10] Lack of education, hindered access to speciality care and teaching, limited personal support, and increased numbers of emergency room visits, among others, have been identified as factors that may predict a high likelihood of recurrence.[11]

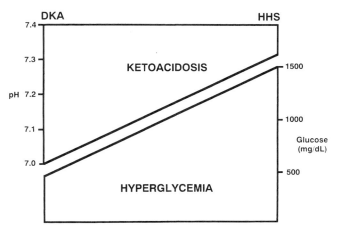

FIGURE 29-1. Severity of hyperglycemia and ketoacidosis in DKA and HHS. Classic metabolic profiles are expressed at the extreme left and right of the diagram. A continuum of combinations of hyperglycemia and ketoacidosis is possible, which is consistent with the observation that ~ 33% of patients with decompensated diabetes have features of both syndromes.

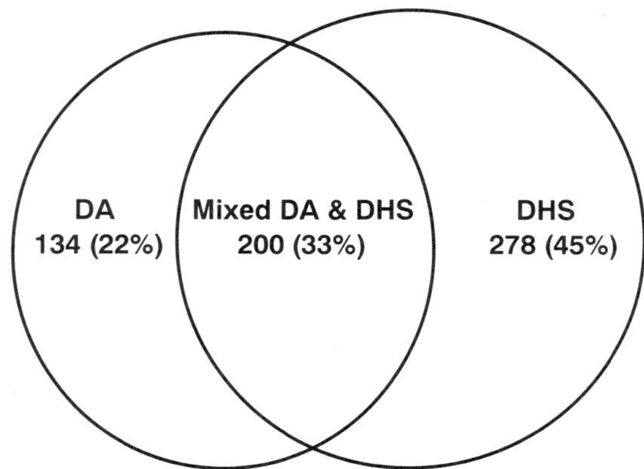

FIGURE 29-2. Overlap between diabetic acidosis (DA) and the diabetic hyperosmolar state (DHS) in patients with decompensated diabetes mellitus. (Reproduced with permission from Wachtel TJ, Tetu-Mouradjian LM, Goldman DL, et al. Hyperosmolarity and acidosis in diabetes mellitus: A three-year experience in Rhode Island. J Gen Intern Med 1991;6:495.)

Elderly persons, particularly those dependent on others for their daily care are at greatest risk for developing HHS. There appears to be no gender predilection[6]; most nursing home occupants are women, however, so a slight female predominance would be expected.[1] The relationship between being in a nursing facility and developing HHS is a reflection of the patient's level of dependence, the presence of multiple comorbid illnesses, and a predisposition to dehydration. Medical illness that limits mobility, mental function, and ability to tend to activities of daily living make the institutionalized patient dependent on others for his or her fluid requirements. Most patients who become hyperosmolar in nursing facilities have had their fluid requirements underestimated or unmet.

Pathogenesis

Diabetic ketoacidosis occurs when there is an absolute or relative deficiency of insulin and an excess of the following insulin counterregulatory hormones (ICRHs): catecholamines, glucagon, cortisol, and growth hormone.[12] When DKA occurs coincident with the initial diagnosis, of IDDM, insulin deficiency may be absolute or near absolute. Insulin levels in patients with IDDM may be within the normal range, but are inappropriate for the magnitude of hyperglycemia.[12] Insulin deficiency in NIDDM patients who develop DKA is usually relative. Measurable levels of insulin, sometimes several-fold higher than those found in IDDM patients are present, but they are clearly not high enough to prevent DKA. Stress, usually due to a coexistent medical illness, but also due to physical or mental stress, or both, provokes the release of ICRHs, which leads to the development of DKA in the presence of fixed insulin levels. When insulin levels are suboptimum, the release of and biologic responses to ICRHs are exaggerated. The degree of insulin deficiency probably determines the importance of stress as a precipitating factor. In patients with absolute or severe insulin deficiency, the release of ICRHs may be less important in causing metabolic decompensation than in patients whose insulin levels are higher but not adequate to prevent metabolic decompensation. The interaction between relative or absolute insulin deficiency and factors that increase the release of ICRHs may not be an "either/or" situation: In most situations, both insulin deficiency and ICRH release interact to precipitate decompensation. It is common, however, for a medical illness to be accompanied by omission of insulin by the patient because of a combination of reduced intake of food, fear of hypoglycemia, or a poor understanding of diabetes. In HHS, a similar sequence of events probably occurs, but insulin deficiency is less obvious since many of these patients are not previously known to have diabetes. It is unclear why decompensation in patients with HHS is expressed primarily as severe hyperglycemia and hyperosmolality with only trivial to mild ketoacidosis. This issue will be discussed in detail in the section on pathogenesis.

The role (or roles) played by cytokines and prostaglandins in the pathogenesis of DKA and HHS, particularly during medical illness, are largely unexplored at the present time but may be important because of their metabolic effects. A clearer understanding of the changes in metabolism that occur with sepsis may provide a better understanding of how medical illness causes metabolic decompensation in patients with diabetes.

Biochemistry

Insulin deficiency, alone or in combination with increased levels of ICRHs, decreases peripheral utilization of glucose by skeletal muscle and adipose tissue and increases lipolysis and proteolysis.[13] *Lipolysis* provides free fatty acids (FFAs) for ketone body production by the liver; *proteolysis* provides amino acids for increased gluconeogenesis. Insulin deficiency and increased levels of glucagon are responsible for glycogenolysis, gluconeogenesis, and ketogenesis. Although ketoacidosis is due primarily to overproduction of ketoacids, the utilization of ketone bodies by peripheral tissues also is reduced by the deficiency of insulin.

Lactate levels may be slightly increased in DKA but are seldom clinically significant.[14] The production of lactate by skeletal muscle and its utilization by the liver for gluconeogenesis are increased in diabetes and probably in DKA. Consequently lactate levels in patients with DKA may be influenced more by hemodynamic than metabolic factors. Hyperlactatemia, in patients with DKA or HHS, represents impaired tissue perfusion and oxygen delivery due to hemodynamic factors (e.g., hypovolemia, poor ventricular function, sepsis, and complicating factors such as alcoholism). Patients with normal or near-normal lactate levels before therapy may have slightly increased levels during therapy because of decreased gluconeogenesis and lactate utilization by the liver. In patients with marked volume contraction and higher initial lactate levels, therapy invariably decreases the lactate concentration by correcting volume deficits and improving tissue perfusion.

Hyperglycemia is more extreme in HHS than in DKA, but in HHS ketoacidosis appears to be milder. Whether milder ketoacidosis reflects lower levels of ICRH and decreased FFA flux to the liver for ketogenesis or higher portal levels of insulin that restrain ketogenesis is unknown. Although severe hyperosmolality inhibits peripheral glucose utilization and impairs FFA release, this is an unlikely explanation of the lower FFA levels because this would only occur during the late stages of HHS. A careful review of the average laboratory abnormalities in patients with HHS clearly indicates that β-hydroxybutyrate (βOHB) levels are elevated, but not to the extent that characterizes DKA.[15] Thus the concept that this is a nonketotic form of decompensated diabetes is incorrect.

Acid-Base Considerations

Acidosis in DKA is due to overproduction of acetoacetic acid and βOHB. The hydrogen ion (H^+) from these acids titrates bicarbonate, (HCO_3^-), leading to a decrease in the serum HCO_3^- level. Because other body buffers also are titrated, the decrease in the serum bicarbonate concentration is an underestimate of the total quantity of buffering capacity that has been lost. The ketone bodies circulate as the anionic forms (i.e., conjugate bases) of the organic acids that are the sources of the excess H^+ ions. The accumulation of these ketone bodies in the serum leads to the development of the anion-gap acidosis that typifies DKA. The *anion gap* is calculated by subtracting the sum of the chloride (Cl^-) and HCO_3^- anion concentrations from the sodium (Na^+) concentration ($Na^+ - [Cl^- + HCO_3^-]$).[16] The normal anion gap is 12 ± 2 mEq/L and represents the normal quantity of unmeasured anions. Because HCO_3^- is replaced by acetoacetic acid and βOHB in DKA, which are unmeasured anions, the sum of the HCO_3^- and Cl^- anions is reduced and the anion gap increased. A substantial quantity of the ketoacid anions is filtered and excreted in the urine. Despite substantial loss of ketoacid anions in the urine, the decrease in the serum HCO_3^- concentration and the increase in the anion gap that occurs in DKA is approximately equal. This is important because ketones are the substrate required for the regeneration of HCO_3^- after initiation of therapy: Inadequate substrate for bicarbonate regeneration due to dietourinary losses, contributes in part to the development of a hyperchloremic metabolic acidosis during recovery.[17]

The βOHB:acetoacetic acid (B:A) ratio reflects the mitochondrial redox state. Under normal circumstances, the B:A ratio is approximately 2–3:1. In uncontrolled diabetes and particularly in DKA, increased FFA oxidation leads to a more reduced mitochondrial redox state and an increase in the B:A ratio. Because the nitroprusside reagent, used for detection of ketones, detects only acetoacetate and acetone, the degree of ketosis can be underestimated if a disproportionate amount of the ketones is present as βOHB.[18] The consumption of alcohol or poor tissue oxygenation, or both, may cause a more reduced mitochondrial state, resulting in a shift of the ketoacid anions to βOHB. In rare cases, patients may develop DKA characterized by a disproportionate increase in βOHB in the absence of these factors.

Metabolic Versus Respiratory Acidosis. In metabolic acidosis, alveolar ventilation increases, initially as a result of stimulation of peripheral chemoreceptors, and later because of recruitment of the respiratory center in the brainstem. The respiratory response is predictable, and titration curves for P_{CO_2} and HCO_3^- provide an estimate of the degree of hyperventilation expected to reduce the serum HCO_3^- concentration: $P_{CO_2} = 1.5(HCO_3^-) + 8 \pm 2$.[19] It is important to remember that mixed or complex acid-base disturbances often exist in patients with DKA and HHS because of independent or associated acid-base disorders produced by medical illnesses, coexistent chronic medical problems, or various medications. This is particularly true in older patients. For example, respiratory alkalosis would be expected in patients with pneumonia and metabolic alkalosis associated with nausea and vomiting or prior use of diuretics. After successful treatment of DKA, the role played by peripheral chemoreceptors in stimulating respiration in DKA is quickly reversed, but the contribution of the respiratory center is not promptly corrected because re-equilibration of intracellular and extracellular pH occurs slowly. An important clinical consequence of this delay is continued hyperventilation, which may be sustained for 24–36 hours, and achievement of a normal pH at lower-than-normal HCO_3^- concentrations.[20] Despite having severe metabolic acidosis, most patients remain alert, emphasizing the dramatic difference in mental status between respiratory and metabolic acidosis. Because CO_2 equilibrates rapidly across cell membranes, changes in extracellular pH are communicated rapidly into the intracellular compartment in respiratory disorders. Consequently, patients with respiratory acidosis and pH values <7.2 are usually confused or obtunded, or both. In contrast, metabolic acid-base disturbances are slowly transmitted from the extracellular to the intracellular compartment; furthermore, as the P_{CO_2} decreases from hyperventilation, intracellular pH may (paradoxically) initially increase. As a result, metabolic acidosis is better tolerated than respiratory acidosis.

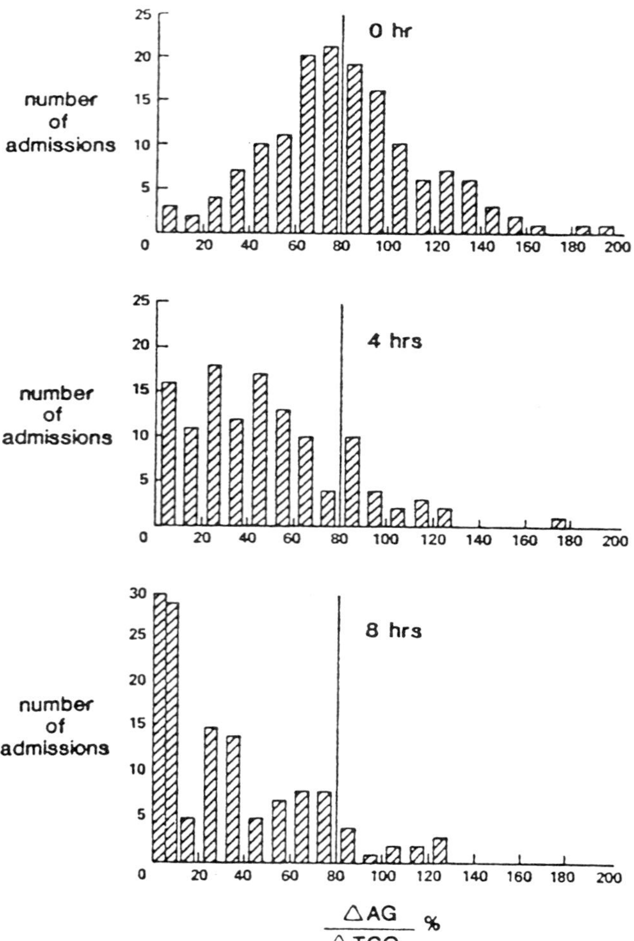

Figure 29-3. Mechanisms of metabolic acidosis in patients with DKA. The ratio of $\Delta AG/\Delta HCO_3$ (ΔTCO_2) (%) is used to reflect whether the acidosis is primarily an anion gap metabolic acidosis (>80%), a hyperchloremic metabolic acidosis (<40%), or a mixed metabolic acidosis (40–80%). On admission (0 h), 48% of patients had a ratio >80% and 41% had a ratio of 40–80%. By 4 and 8 hours of therapy 80% and 91%, respectively, had developed a component of hyperchloremic acidosis. (Reproduced with permission from Androgue HJ, Wilson H, Boyd AE, et al. Plasma acid-base patterns in diabetic ketoacidosis. N Engl J Med 1982;26:1603.)

The volume status of the patient may have a profound effect on the acid-base profile in DKA. When hydration and volume are maintained during the evolution of DKA, ketones are effectively filtered and excreted.[17] Cl^- anions are reabsorbed with Na^+ cations, and a typical anion-gap acidosis may not be present. Under these circumstances, the patient develops a hyperchloremic or a mixed metabolic acidosis partly due to an increase in the anion gap and partly due to hyperchloremia. When there is marked volume contraction, filtration and excretion of ketones in the urine are decreased and a typical anion-gap acidosis is seen. In reality, there is a spectrum of acid-base abnormalities in DKA: Some patients have a predominant hyperchloremic metabolic acidosis, some having typical anion-gap metabolic acidosis, and many have varying features of both (Fig. 29-3).[17]

During insulin and fluid therapy for DKA, there is a decrease in the level of ICRH and in FFA release from adipose tissue. Plasma ketone levels decrease due to both decreased hepatic production and increased peripheral ketone utilization. Utilization of ketones by peripheral tissues requires that they first be converted from βOHB to acetoacetic acid. This not only changes the B:A ratio, but it may initially increase the concentration of acetoacetic acid. The nitroprusside color reaction becomes more intense as acetoacetic acid increases, thus misleadingly suggesting that the severity of the ketoacidosis has worsened. Consequently, this limits the utility of the nitroprusside reaction in monitoring patients with DKA once therapy has been initiated.

Diagnosis

The diagnostic features of DKA are shown in Table 29-1.[1,21–23] It is characterized by hyperglycemia (glucose generally ≥300 mg/dL), metabolic acidosis (HCO_3^- ≤18 mEq/L, pH ≤7.30) and elevated blood ketones (βOHB and acetoacetic acid). A pH <7.35 in a patient with ketonemia and a glucose ≥300 mg/dL identifies a patient with mild DKA. HCO_3^- ≤18 mEq/L in a patient with moderate hyperglycemia should also suggest DKA. The blood glucose criterion for the diagnosis of DKA is variable: There are patients with glucose values ≥300 mg/dL who do not have ketoacidosis and patients with glucose values ≤300 mg/dL who do have ketoacidosis. Approximately 15% of DKA patients have glucose values ≤350 mg/dL at presentation; this is referred to as "euglycemic DKA."[24] This may be observed when gluconeogenesis is impaired (e.g., in liver disease, acute alcohol ingestion, prolonged fasting) or when glucose utilization is high (e.g., in pregnancy). Mild hyperglycemia can be observed in pregnant women with DKA because glucose utilization by the fetoplacental unit is insulin-independent. It is critically important to note that *these women may have severe metabolic acidosis despite relative normoglycemia.*

TABLE 29-1. Diagnostic Features of Diabetic Ketoacidosis and the Hyperglycemic Hyperosmolar Syndrome*

	DKA	HHS
Glucose (mg/dL)	≥300†	≥600
pH	≤7.3	≥7.3
HCO_3^- (mEq/L)	≤18	≥15
S_{osm} (mOsm/kg)	<320	≥320
Ketones	↑↑-↑↑↑	↑
Dehydration	↑-↑↑	↑↑↑

*Refer to refs. 1, 21, 26, and 27.
†Excluding "euglycemic DKA."
DKA = diabetic ketoacidosis; HCO_3^- = bicarbonate; HHS = hyperglycemic hyperosmolar syndrome; S_{osm} = serum osmolality; ↑ = mild; ↑↑ = moderate; ↑↑↑ = severe.

The characteristic features of HHS are shown in Table 29-1 and are as follows:

- hyperglycemia (glucose ≥600 mg/dL)
- mild acidemia (pH ≥ 7.30, HCO_3^- ≥15 mEq/L)
- profound dehydration (S_{osm} ≥320 mOsm/kg) in the absence of severe ketosis

Because urea is distributed equally in all body compartments, many only use the serum Na^+ and glucose concentrations to calculate the serum osmolality (S_{osm}) and refer to it as the *effective serum osmolality*. Published studies are variable in this regard.[1,21,25–27] At least 50% of HHS patients have mild anion-gap metabolic acidosis. When the acidosis is severe, however, other factors (e.g., lactic acidosis, acidosis due to disorders other than HHS) should be considered. Patients with HHS may have a coexistent metabolic alkalosis, caused by vomiting or the use of thiazide diuretics, that can obscure the severity of the acidosis. Alkalosis is suggested when the sum of the increment in the anion gap and the measured HCO_3^- is higher than normal.

Precipitating Factors

All patients who present with decompensated diabetes must have a rapid and thorough evaluation, and precipitating factors should be identified and treated. Coexistent medical illnesses, particularly infections, commonly precipitate DKA and HHS (Table 29-2).[1,22,23] Acute infection accounts for 30–40% of DKA and 32–60% of HHS episodes.[1,22,23] Urinary tract infection, pneumonia, and sepsis are the most common problems; Gram-negative organisms are particularly frequent.[1] Silent myocardial infarction, cerebrovascular accident, pancreatitis, and mesenteric ischemia are common precipitating factors in patients with HHS but may also be a consequence of the severe dehydration, hemoconcentration, and poor tissue perfusion that accompanies this disorder.[1] Increased catecholamine release may further compromise a previously unrecognized relative or absolute insulin deficiency (Table 29-3).[1]

A variety of medications have been associated with the development of HHS[1]; however, because patients who develop HHS are often on numerous medications (e.g., diuretics, antihypertensive agents, sedative-hypnotics), the contribution of a single medication is difficult to assess. A temporal relationship between the initiation of a diabetogenic medication and the development of HHS has been observed, but most medications probably play no specific role in the precipitating event. Nevertheless, a thorough review of medication use is essential.

Overall, DKA is the presenting illness in only 20–25% of newly diagnosed patients with IDDM.[22] Most patients in whom DKA develops are known diabetics, and the occurrence of this problem is due partly to a breakdown in the patient's education or communication, or both, concerning his or her diabetes. In patients older than 65 years, however, 30% of DKA patients and 30–40% of HHS patients have no previous history of diabetes mellitus.[6,7,28]

Insulin Omission and Eating Disorders

The patient's omission of insulin is the precipitating factor in 15–20% of DKA episodes.[22] Continuous subcutaneous insulin infusion (CSII) also increases the risk of DKA: In one series, ~30% of CSII patients developed DKA because of inadvertent insulin interruption or infection.[29] An additional 20% of recurrent ketoacidosis episodes occur in young women with psychological problems

TABLE 29-2. Predisposing or Precipitating Factors for Diabetic Ketoacidosis and the Hyperglycemic Hyperosmolar Syndrome*

HHS	DKA
Acute illness	Acute illness
Infection 32–60%	Infection 30–40%
Pneumonia	Cerebrovascular accident
Urinary tract infection	Myocardial infarction
Sepsis	Acute pancreatitis
Cerebrovascular accident	New onset diabetes 20–25%
Myocardial infarction	CSII / omission of insulin 15–20%
Acute pancreatitis	Other medical illness
Pulmonary embolus	
Intestinal obstruction	
Dialysis, peritoneal	
Mesenteric thrombosis	
Renal failure	
Heat stroke	
Hypothermia	
Subdural hematoma	
Severe burns	
Endocrine	
Acromegaly	
Thyrotoxicosis	
Cushing's disease	
Drugs/therapy	
Calcium-channel blockers	
Chlorpromazine	
Chlorthalidone	
Cimetidine	
Diazoxide	
Ethacrynic acid	
Immunosuppressive agents	
L-asparaginase	
Loxapine	
Phenytoin	
Propranolol	
Steroids	
Thiazide diuretics	
Total parenteral nutrition	
Previously undiagnosed diabetes mellitus	

*Refer to refs. 1, 21, 26, and 27.
CSII = continuous subcutaneous insulin infusion; DKA = diabetic ketoacidosis; HHS = hyperglycemic hyperosmolar syndrome.

TABLE 29-3. Average Laboratory Findings in Diabetic Ketoacidosis and the Hyperglycemic Hyperosmolar Syndrome

	DKA	HHS
Glucose (mg/dL)	475	1166
S_{osm} (mOsm/kg)	309	384
Na^+ (mEq/L)	131	143
K^+ (mEq/L)	4.8	5.0
HCO_3^- (mEq/L)	9	22
BUN (mg/dL)	21	66
Creatinine (mg/dL)	—	2.9
Anion gap (mEq/L)	29	23
Δ Gap (anion gap-12) (mEg/L)	17	11
pH	<7.3	≥7.3
Ketonuria	≥3+	≤1+
Catecholamines (ng/mL)	1.78 ± 4	6.4 ± 2.6
Cortisol (μg/dL)	49	22
Growth hormone (ng/mL)	7.9	1.1
Glucagon (pg/mL)	400–500	689
β-Hydroxybutyrate (mM)	13.7	3.6
Lactate (mM)	4.6	0.6
FFA (mM)	2.26	0.73–0.96

BUN = blood urea nitrogen; DKA = diabetic ketoacidosis; FFA = free fatty acid; HCO_3^- = bicarbonate; HHS = hyperglycemic hyperosmolar syndrome; S_{osm} = serum osmolality.
Adapted with permission from Ennis ED, Stahl EJvB, Kreisberg RA. The hyperosmolar hyperglycemic syndrome. Diabetes Rev 1994;2:115.

complicated by eating disorders and fasting.[22] Poor diabetic education places patients at risk for development of DKA/HHS. The patient may stop taking insulin because of the wrong notion that insulin should be withheld when illness interferes with eating. The importance of insulin omission as a feature of eating disorders was emphasized by a recent survey of 341 IDDM female patients, ages 13–60 years.[30] Intentional insulin omission was reported in ~31% of respondents. Frequent insulin omission was most common (16%) among females subjects 15–30 years of age.[30] Omission was also reported by older women, in whom 4.2% and 6.1% of those aged 31–45 and 46–60 years, respectively, reported frequent insulin omission.[30] Insulin omitters (13% of total subject sample; n = 44), particularly those who reported doing so to control weight, had significantly increased hemoglobin A_1C levels, more recent hospitalizations, increased emergency room visits, and a substantially higher incidence of neuropathy and retinopathy.[30] A significant number of these women reported omission of insulin and eating to the point of developing ketonuria for the purpose of controlling weight.[30] Thus, there is a strong association between insulin omission and maladaptive eating behaviors and attitudes. Factors that led to insulin omission by patients included fear of gaining weight if good control was maintained, fear of hypoglycemia, increased emotional distress, and increased diabetes-related stress.[30] Rebellion from authority by teenagers could be another important component. Although previous studies have not supported personal stress as a precipitating factor for DKA, the stress models used in these studies do not duplicate the personal nature of stress among diabetic patients.[31,32] Furthermore, the studies have been conducted in patients with well-controlled diabetes mellitus. It is important to study the effect of stress in the patient with poorly controlled diabetes mellitus. The frequent development of DKA in women at the time of menses may also reflect the importance of stress.[33] Psychologic misconceptions, body-image conflicts, and subsequent therapeutic alterations may place women at higher risk for acute diabetic decompensation. DKA and HHS may also occur in the hospital on surgical, psychiatric, and obstetrical services.

Clinical Presentation

DKA and HHS differ in presentation. At presentation, neither may be obvious. In one series, 20% of patients were not initially recognized to have DKA and were admitted for a primary diagnosis other than diabetes mellitus.[2] DKA develops within a relatively short period (hours to days). DKA patients seldom develop severe hyperglycemia or hyperosmolality because the metabolic acidosis makes them ill and prompts them to seek early medical attention; their symptoms may be due to acidosis itself or to an underlying precipitating factor.

Because many patients with HHS have no previous known history of diabetes mellitus, the diagnosis must always be considered in the elderly. In most patients with HHS, progressive dehydration and hyperglycemia develop within days to weeks. During this long prodromal period, age-related blunting of thirst, limited access to water and drinking, or receiving glucose-containing fluids may exacerbate hyperglycemia and dehydration. The absence of severe metabolic acidosis and its symptoms in HHS probably contribute to the long prodrome and the severity of dehydration. The search for and management of precipitating factors are essential for successful therapy of DKA/HHS.

Physical Examination

A thorough physical examination must be performed with particular attention to the abdomen because many patients with DKA complain of abdominal pain. The presence of abdominal pain raises the important question of whether a primary intra-abdominal problem has precipitated decompensation or whether the pain is a result of DKA. Sometimes this distinction is difficult. Isoenzyme analyses often indicate that the increased fraction of amylase seen in DKA/HHS is of salivary origin.[34,35] Therefore, unfractionated amylase levels are nonspecific for pancreatitis in the setting of DKA. Hyperamylasemia is observed in 30% of patients with acidosis other than DKA and occurs frequently in DKA without evidence of pancreatitis.[36] Formerly, lipase measurements have been used to distinguish DKA patients with pancreatitis from those with nonpancreatic amylase evaluations. Recently, three patients with lipase elevations have been described in whom neither clinical nor radiographic elevations suggested pancreatitis.[37] Close follow-up with frequent evaluation of the abdomen is required. If there is any doubt about an intra-abdominal problem, additional diagnostic studies or consultation, or both, should be promptly obtained. As a general rule, when the abdominal pain is a result of the DKA, it resolves as the DKA is corrected. Because patients with HHS are often elderly, coexistent medical problems should be suspected and a careful search should be made for precipitating factors. When abdominal pain is a presenting feature of HHS, mesenteric thrombosis due to extreme hemoconcentration, or as a precipitating factor, should be considered.

Altered sensorium in patients presenting with DKA and HHS correlates best with the magnitude of hyperosmolality rather than with the degree of acidosis or hyperglycemia. Serious alterations in sensorium, with S_{osm} <340 mOsm/kg, should suggest etiologies other than DKA or HHS (Fig. 29-4).[38] In such cases, one should have a high index of suspicion for other medical illness, including catastrophic central nervous system (CNS) events and infections.

Pathophysiology

The hyperglycemia that occurs in both DKA and HHS increases the extracellular osmolality and creates an osmotic gradient for the movement of water from the intracellular to the extracellular compartment. Hyperosmolality keeps the extracellular compart-

TABLE 29-4. Serum Electrolyte Levels at Entry and after Twelve Hours of Therapy in 28 DKA Patients (Percent Low, Normal or Elevated)

	Entry			Twelve Hours		
	% Low	% Normal	% High	% Low	% Normal	% High
Sodium	67	26	7	26	41	33
Chloride	33	45	22	11	41	48
Bicarbonate	100	0	0	46	50	4
Calcium	28	68	4	73	23	4
Potassium	18	43	39	63	33	4
Magnesium	7	25	68	55	24	21
Phosphate	11	18	71	90	10	0

Reproduced with permission from Martin HE, Smith K, Wilson ML. The fluid and electrolyte therapy of severe diabetic acidosis and ketosis. Am J Med 1958;20:376.

ment expanded relative to the intracellular compartment. The movement of water into the extracellular compartment causes the mild to modest degree of hyponatremia that exists in most patients with DKA. Consequently, hyponatremia is the expected change in the serum Na^+ concentration even when there is a deficit of body water. When hyperosmolality and dehydration are extreme and prolonged, as in HHS, the serum Na^+ concentration may normalize or reach hypernatremic levels. In DKA the expected change in the serum Na^+ level can be predicted; the serum Na^+ is decreased by 1.6–1.8 mEq/100 mg/dL increase in the glucose concentration.[39] The temporary expansion of the extracellular compartment early in DKA leads to an increase in glomerular filtration rate, which contributes to the characteristic polyuria of decompensated diabetes. Glucosuria causes an osmotic diuresis, with losses of Na^+, potassium (K^+), magnesium (Mg^{++}), and phosphate ($PO_4^{=}$) electrolytes in the urine. The urine contains 70–80 mEq of cation per liter, most of which is Na^+ and K^+.[22]

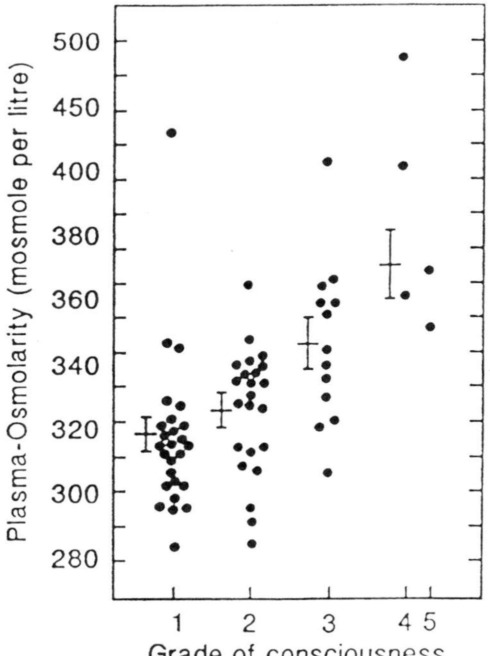

FIGURE 29-4. Individual and mean serum osmolarity values as they relate to levels of consciousness in patients with decompensated diabetes mellitus. (Reproduced with permission from Fulop M, Tannenbaum H, Dreyer N. Ketotic hyperosmolar coma. Lancet 1973;2:635.)

DKA/HHS also may be associated with hypertriglyceridemia. Insulin deficiency decreases lipoprotein lipase activity, the major enzyme responsible for triglyceride clearance from plasma. Therefore, patients with this deficiency, whether it be genetic or acquired, have difficulty clearing plasma triglycerides. The hypertriglyceridemia associated with severe lipoprotein lipase deficiency may also result in spurious levels of electrolytes and glucose because electrolytes and glucose are present only in the aqueous phase of serum and plasma, whereas their concentrations are measured and reported per total sample volume.[40] Triglyceride levels ≥1500 mg/dL are sufficient to render some methods unreliable.[40] In addition, some bedside blood glucose kits may underestimate values in lipemic samples.[41] Ultracentrifugation of lipemic samples will circumvent this problem. It is essential that the laboratory recognize and report lipemia when present.

Regardless of their measured plasma concentrations, substantial deficits of Na^+, K^+, Mg^{++}, and $PO_4^{=}$ electrolytes occur in DKA and HHS.[42] Their magnitude is related to the severity and duration of decompensation. Despite these deficits, the serum levels of K^+, Mg^{++}, and $PO_4^{=}$ are typically normal or elevated at the time of diagnosis (Table 29-4).[42] Hyperkalemia is due to insulin deficiency and perhaps a shift of K^+ from the intracellular to the extracellular compartment in exchange for H^+. Acidosis also causes $PO_4^{=}$ to move into the extracellular compartment. Hypokalemia and hypophosphatemia develop during therapy as a consequence of the continued excretion of these ions in the urine and cellular reentry. The continued loss of K^+ in the urine is due to increased aldosterone secretion and increased delivery of Na^+ to the distal tubule.

The deficits of K^+ and $PO_4^{=}$ in HHS are probably comparable to those in DKA (Table 29-5).[43] It is important to recognize that

TABLE 29-5. Deficits of Water and Electrolytes*

	DKA	HHS
Water (L)	6	9
Water (mL/kg)†	100	100–200
Na^+ (mEq/kg)	7–10	5–13‡
K^+ (mEq/kg)	3–5	5–15‡
Cl^- (mEq/kg)	3–5	3–7‡
$PO_4^{=}$ (mmol/kg)	1–1.5	1–2‡
Mg^{++} (mEq/kg)	1–2	1–2‡
Ca^{++} (mEq/kg)	1–2	1–2‡

*Refer to refs. 1, 21, 23, and 43.
†Per kilogram of body weight.
‡Approximations from balance studies done in patients with DKA.
DKA = diabetic ketoacidosis; HHS = hyperosmolar hyperglycemic syndrome; $PO_4^{=}$ = phosphate.

the deficits of water and other electrolytes may be smaller if the prodrome for the development of decompensation is short, as it is in DKA, or much greater if the prodrome is prolonged, as it is in HHS. The importance of volume in the pathogenesis of decompensated diabetes and its response to therapy should not be underestimated. Volume contraction accentuates the release of ICRHs, which precipitates and/or intensifies DKA and HHS. Failure to appreciate and correct hypovolemia may contribute to insulin resistance during treatment for DKA.[22]

Adaptation of the CNS to hyperglycemia is particularly important. Water moves from the intracellular compartment of the CNS and other tissues and enters the extracellular compartment, as extracellular osmolality increases. The CNS has adaptive mechanisms not present in other tissues, however, which allows the loss of water to be partially reversed. In experimental animals, this adaptation occurs after approximately 4 hours, and water reenters the intracellular compartment of the brain, restoring intracellular volume to near normal.[44] Exactly how this happens is unclear. The solutes in the CNS that are responsible for reversal of the osmotic gradient have not been identified clearly. Approximately one-half of the osmotically active solute probably contains K^+; the other half probably consists of amino acids, referred to as *idiogenic osmoles*. These osmoles may be responsible for the observed increase in brain water that occurs with therapy of DKA and in some way may contribute to the development of cerebral edema, particularly if the CNS is unable to adapt rapidly to the decreasing extracellular osmolality.

Treatment

Successful therapy of DKA and HHS requires the administration of insulin, fluids, and potassium (Table 29-6):

- Insulin is necessary for reversal of metabolic abnormalities.
- Fluid corrects volume deficits, improves tissue perfusion, and reduces ICRH levels.
- Potassium prevents complications associated with hypokalemia.

Deficits of K^+ must be routinely replaced, whereas deficits of $PO_4^{=}$ and Mg^{++} require replacement less often. Although there are no studies using either $PO_4^{=}$ or Mg^{++} that demonstrate benefit from routine replacement, there should be no hesitation to replace either or both if it is clinically indicated. Mg^{++} can be safely incorporated into replacement fluids[21]; there is no evidence that routine use of HCO_3^- is necessary or useful.[45–48]

It is important to address meticulously all of the medical as well as metabolic problems that exist in patients with decompensated diabetes. The only reasonable way of maintaining control of so many variables is to use a flow sheet and to assess the efficacy of the therapy frequently. ''Midstream'' corrections in the administration of fluid and electrolytes frequently are required. Most importantly, one should not become complacent or overconfident. Even in the best of hands complications occur; these must be promptly identified and addressed.

Insulin Therapy

Insulin is the cornerstone of treatment of DKA and HHS. For the majority of patients, insulin is administered as a bolus of 0.1 U/kg body weight (BW) and then at a rate of 5–10 U/h for adults. Intravenous (IV) or intramuscular (IM) routes are preferred. Smaller doses are required in children. Administration of insulin at these rates produces plasma insulin levels of 100–200 μU/mL, a range associated with its maximum biologic effect.[49,50] Insulin concentrations of 100–200 μU/mL completely suppress lipolysis and hepatic glucose production and contribute importantly toward reversal of hyperglycemia and acidosis.[22] Peripheral tissues are

Table 29-6. Therapy for Diabetic Ketoacidosis and Hyperosmolar Hyperglycemic Syndrome

Insulin

- 0.1 U/kg BW regular insulin as IV bolus followed by 0.1 U/kg/h (5–10 U/h) thereafter as a continuous infusion until glucose concentration is 250–300 mg/dL and the pH ≥7.3 or HCO_3^- ≥18 mEg/L.
  or
  10 U regular insulin IV as a loading dose followed by 5–10 U/h IM.
- Decrease administration to 2–3 U/h when the plasma glucose is 250–300 mg/dL ***and*** the HCO_3^- ≥18 mEq/L.

Fluids

- 0-1 h: 1000–2000 mL NS for prompt correction of hypotension/hypoperfusion.
- 1-4 h: 750–1000 mL/h NS or half-NS for severe volume contraction.
  or
  250–500 mL/h NS or half-NS for mild to moderate volume contraction.
- >4 h: Variable infusion rate based on intake, urinary output, and clinical assessment of volume status to replace ~50% of estimated deficit by 8 h. Composition of fluid (NS or half-NS) based on serum Na^+ and S_{osm} measurements (HHS).

Glucose

- When plasma glucose reaches 250–300 mg/dL, administer glucose at a rate of 5–10 g/h, either as a separate infusion or combined with saline.

Electrolyte replacement[§]

- Potassium (replace as the Cl^- or $PO_4^{=}$)[‡]
  Assure urinary output before K^+ supplementation.
  Maintain K^+ between 4 and 5 mEq/L.
  K^+ >5.0 mEq/L: no supplementation.
  K^+ = 4–5 mEq/L: 20 mEq/L replacement fluid.
  K^+ = 3–4 mEq/L: 30–40 mEq/L replacement fluid.
  K^+ ≤3.0 mEq/L: 40–60 mEq/L replacement fluid.
- Phosphate
  Not routinely recommended; if indicated, 30–60 mmol phosphate as potassium phosphate (K_2HPO_4) over 24 h.
- Magnesium
  If Mg^{++} <1.8 mEq/L or tetany present, give magnesium sulfate ($MgSO_4$) 5 g in 500 mL 0.45% saline over 5 h.
- Calcium
  For symptomatic hypocalcemia, give 10–20 mL of 10% calcium gluconate (100–200 mg elemental calcium as indicated).
- Bicarbonate
  Not routinely recommended in the treatment of DKA. Consider using if other indications are present.

Laboratory

- Comprehensive admission profile.
- Arterial blood gases.
- Serum/urine ketone measurements.
- q 1 h: glucose.
- q 4 h: electrolytes.[§]
- q 4 h:Ca^{++}, Mg^{++}, $PO_4^{=}$.[§]
- Cultures of blood, urine, sputum as indicated.

General care

- Electrocardiogram before administration of supplemental K^+.
- Review urine output, vital signs, neurologic status, and laboratory data q 1 h.
- Frequent assessment of clinical status and repeat physical examination.
- Protection of the airway in the unconscious patient.
- Nasogastric suction as indicated for ileus, emesis, or obtundation with vulnerable airway.
- Chest radiograph and other imaging studies as needed.
- Consider obtaining central venous pressure, Swan-Ganz catheterization in selected patients.

*Refer to refs. 1 and 23.
†Drug dosages should be modified in the patient with significant renal impairment.
‡Dosage suggested using KCl.
§Modified as necessary.
BW = body weight; CVP = central venous pressure; DKA = diabetic ketoacidosis; HCO_3^- = bicarbonate; HHS = hyperglycemic hyperosmolar syndrome; IM = intramuscular(ly); IV = intravenous(ly); $PO_4^{=}$ = phosphate; S_{osm} = serum osmolality.

markedly resistant to the action of insulin in DKA, using glucose at a rate that is approximately 10–15% of what would be expected in a normal subject with comparable insulin levels.[22] Thus increased glucose utilization by peripheral tissues does not contribute substantially to the decrease that occurs in the glucose concentration with therapy. The decrease that occurs in the blood glucose concentration in DKA is due to enhanced glucose excretion in the urine, dilution of glucose in the body by the infused fluids, and inhibition of hepatic glucose production. In HHS, where volume deficits are more extreme, dilution of glucose and glucosuria account for approximately 75% of the decrease that occurs in the glucose concentration.[51]

When insulin is used in this manner, either by the IM or the continuous IV route, the plasma glucose concentration decreases at a rate of ~75–100 mg/dL/h.[52] There may be wide interpatient variation in insulin response: Some patients may be quite resistant with a very slow glucose response to insulin, whereas in others the rate of decrease in the glucose concentration may be more rapid. The latter is more likely in patients with HHS, perhaps reflecting the importance of hypovolemia and the response to aggressive fluid replacement. The presence of infection may reduce the rate of decline in blood glucose by 50%, to approximately 50 mg/dL/h.[23] Although the rate of glucose decline may vary from patient to patient, the rate of decline, in general, will be reasonably constant within an individual.

On average, the blood glucose concentration in the typical patient with DKA will decrease from 550–650 mg/dL to the usual target of 250–300 mg/dL in approximately 4–6 hours.[52] Correction of the acidosis ($HCO_3^- \geq 18$ mEq/L; pH ≥ 7.3) occurs more slowly, taking approximately 12 hours.[52] The temporal dissociation of the correction of hyperglycemia and the correction of acidosis has important implications for management. Administration of insulin at a rate of 5–10 U/h must be *continued,* not reduced, after the glucose level reaches the target of 250–300 mg/dL. This is accomplished by adding glucose 5–10 g/h to the fluid being infused; this buffers changes in glucose that would occur with continued insulin administration. Reduction of the rate of insulin infusion prematurely will result in a deterioration of the acidosis.

The glucose and acid-base responses (decreasing glucose level and increasing HCO_3^- and pH) to insulin and fluid therapy should be detected within 2–3 hours. If the patient fails to respond, larger doses of insulin (20–100 U/h) should be used and the fluid status of the patient as well as previously unappreciated precipitating factors should be reevaluated. We recommend the use of insulin 50 U/h under these circumstances so as to not waste valuable time titrating the dose. When large doses of insulin are used, the risks of hypoglycemia and hypokalemia are increased.[52] When DKA has been corrected, the previous insulin regimen can be reimplemented or the infusion of insulin, glucose, and K^+ can be continued (2–3 U/h insulin, 10 g/h glucose, and 2.0 mEq/h K^+).

Fluid Therapy

The magnitude of the fluid deficit in DKA and HHS varies from patient to patient. Patients with DKA have milder volume depletion than patients with HHS because the prodrome is shorter and there is less time for fluid depletion. In severe DKA, water deficits of ~100 mg/kg BW can be expected, representing ~10% of BW. Deficits approaching 15% of BW are usually more common in patients with HHS, particularly those who present with hypernatremia. In patients in whom volume contraction is mild to modest, normal saline (NS) may be administered at 500 mL/h for the first 2–4 hours to produce rapid reexpansion; thereafter it should be reduced to NS 250 mL/h. Assessment of each patient's volume status and other clinical considerations should determine the rate of fluid administration. Those with marked volume contraction should receive NS 750–1000 mL/h for the first 2–4 hours to optimize hemodynamic responses; thereafter it should be NS 500 mL/h, as guided by ongoing clinical evaluation and other considerations.

There is controversy over the composition of fluids used to correct volume deficits. For the most part, there is reasonably good agreement that initial fluid therapy should be with NS so as to expand the extracellular compartment rapidly and optimally. Thereafter, whether NS or half-NS is utilized depends, to a large extent, on personal preference, the serum Na^+ concentration, and concern about a rapid decrease in osmolality. The advantage of continued use of NS is that it slows the rate at which the extracellular osmolality decreases, but it may be associated with persistent or worsening hypernatremia and the development of hyperchloremia after recovery. Use of half-NS will prevent the development of hypernatremia during resuscitation, but its use may be associated with a more rapid decrease in extracellular osmolality because both the glucose and Na^+ concentrations are decreasing. We prefer to use several liters of NS for the purposes of rapid reexpansion and then to use either NS or half-NS, depending on the rate of decrease of the glucose concentration and changes observed in the serum electrolytes. Some have recommended the routine use of a multi-electrolyte solution.

Fluid administration and urine output must be monitored carefully. Patients who are severely hypovolemic are likely to be oliguric, and an increase in urine volume can be used as an index of rehydration. If a patient has polyuria at the outset, a decrease in urine volume indicates a decrease in the plasma glucose concentration and a decrease in the severity of glucosuria. Patients who remain oliguric require careful and strict management of fluids. The role of fluid therapy in patients with anuria (acute tubular necrosis or end-stage renal disease) is limited. Insulin administration and electrolyte management form the basis of therapy in this group of patients.

Proper volume replacement is required to decrease the release of ICRH, particularly catecholamines and cortisol, and is therefore central to the management of both DKA and HHS.[22] Correction of volume deficits, without concomitant administration of insulin, decreases the glucose concentration by 15–90 mg/dL/h and may result in slight improvement in pH.[22] In one study in which patients received ~4 L fluid and no insulin over 11 hours, the glucose concentration decreased by a rate of 18 mg/dL/h and the pH improved, but patients were still hyperglycemic and acidemic.[53] Fluid replacement alone decreased the concentrations of epinephrine, norepinephrine, cortisol, glucagon, and growth hormone, emphasizing the important role of fluid administration in reversing DKA and perhaps HHS.

Electrolyte Therapy

Potassium

Replacement of K^+ deficits takes precedent over virtually all other electrolyte abnormalities. Hyperkalemia should be expected in patients with DKA or HHS. The presence of normokalemia or hypokalemia at presentation suggests that the K^+ deficit is greater than 3–5 mEq/kg and perhaps on the order of 5–10 mEq/kg. Such patients virtually always have a coexistent hypochloremic metabolic alkalosis and consequently a mixed or complex acid-base disorder. Severe hypokalemia is most frequently due to the concomitant use of diuretics, nasogastric suction, or persistent vomiting. The alkalosis may be of equal or greater magnitude than the acidosis, leading to a relatively normal pH or diabetic ketoalkalosis.

The incorporation of K^+ into replacement fluids should be delayed until urine output is known to be adequate. K^+ administration should be delayed in patients who are oliguric until there is evidence that volume has been adequately replaced and that they do not have acute tubular necrosis. Initial electrolytes, indices of renal function, and urine output will obviously influence the rate of potassium K^+ administration. Once urine output is satisfactory, K^+ should initially be administered at a rate of 20–30 mEq/h to keep the serum K^+ between 3.5 and 5.0 mEq/L. If the patient is or remains oliguric, or if $K^+ > 5$ mEq/L, K^+ should be temporarily withheld; if hypokalemia is severe, K^+ should be administered at increased rates, reaching as high as 40–60 mEq/h, but with careful monitoring. Accurate knowledge of serum K^+ at the initiation of therapy and throughout therapy, is critical. If serum K^+ is very low at the initiation of therapy, it has been suggested that K^+-containing fluids be administered for 30–60 minutes before the initiation of insulin therapy; however, we know of no data that bear on this point. Oliguric patients still require K^+ replacement because of volume expansion, correction of acidosis, and the direct effects of insulin on K^+ transport across cell membranes. Potassium replacement must be approached cautiously because 20–50% of the K^+ administered during the treatment of DKA is excreted in the urine.[43] Consequently there is a smaller margin of error in oliguric patients, and they will require substantially less K^+.

Phosphate

The phosphate deficit in DKA averages ~1.0 mmol/kg BW; there are no data for HHS.[43] This is a trivial deficiency, however, because total-body stores of phosphorus are ~6,000 moles. At presentation, most patients with DKA have hyperphosphatemia. During therapy, the serum $PO_4^{\equiv}$ concentration decreases in parallel with K^+, reaching a nadir at 4–6 hours.[42] Phosphorus deficiency is theoretically important, but there is no evidence that routine $PO_4^{\equiv}$ replacement influences morbidity or mortality in the typical patient.[54–56] However, a $PO_4^{\equiv} < 1.0$ mg/dL is associated with substantial morbidity and mortality in patients that have phosphate-depletion syndromes, and respiratory muscle function is decreased when the serum $PO_4^{\equiv}$ is below the low-normal limits.[57] Consequently, it is not unreasonable to use $PO_4^{\equiv}$ replacement therapy when concentrations reach these levels. $PO_4^{\equiv}$ is usually added to replacement fluids as potassium phosphate (K_2HPO_4) (20 mEq K^+; 16 mM $PO_4^{\equiv}$). Some investigators have recommended the routine use of potassium phosphate because they believe that it reduces the tendency to develop post-treatment hyperchloremia by limiting Cl^- anion administration. This seems irrational because the amount of $PO_4^{\equiv}$ administered is trivial and, as with K^+, a large percentage (>50%) of it is excreted in the urine. Aproximately 50% of the body deficit of $PO_4^{\equiv}$ should be replaced in the first 24 hours of therapy. Consequently only 50–75 mmol $PO_4^{\equiv}$ as the $K_2HPO_4^-$ would be infused. It is also worth noting that the use of $PO_4^{\equiv}$ may precipitate symptomatic hypocalcemia in some patients.[58] This is a situation in which Mg^{++} deficiency may be important in patients with DKA. By lowering the serum Ca^{++}, $PO_4^{\equiv}$ unmasks Mg^{++} deficiency and its consequences: impaired release of and tissue resistance to parathyroid hormone.

Bicarbonate

Despite having severe acidemia and decreased HCO_3^- concentrations, patients are usually alert and hemodynamically intact. Severe acidosis (pH <7.20) is associated with resistance to the adrenergic actions of catecholamines and impaired myocardial contractility. There is usually no need for the routine use of HCO_3^- supplements unless the clinical situation, coexistent medical problems, or the age of the patient warrants its use. The administration of HCO_3^- therapy has not been shown to be of benefit in the treatment of DKA.[45–48]

Use of HCO_3^- replacement therapy should be considered when the buffer reserve is at its limit and the respiratory response to the acidosis is maximally expressed. Under these circumstances, a further reduction in the HCO_3^- concentration or inability to maintain maximum respiratory compensation causes dramatic and serious worsening of pH.[22] Some recommend that 50–100 mEq HCO_3^- be routinely administered if the bicarbonate concentration is <8–10 mEq/L or the P_{CO_2} is 10 to 12 mmHg, with the target of raising the HCO_3^- level to 10–12 mEq/L.[22] When HCO_3^- therapy is used, it should be with the idea of "tiding the patient over" until therapy begins to reverse the acidosis. HCO_3^- is regenerated from ketone bodies; its excessive use during therapy therefore can cause rebound alkalosis and its associated adverse effects on functions such as oxygen delivery, myocardial contractility, cardiac rhythm, and ileus.

Monitoring Therapy

All patients with DKA and HHS should have a comprehensive laboratory evaluation to include a complete blood count (CBC) with a differential and a multiphasic chemistry profile including electrolytes and arterial blood gas measurements. Fluid administration and urine output should be monitored carefully and recorded hourly. An electrocardiogram should be obtained for all patients, particularly those at risk for cardiovascular disease (painless myocardial infarction). Furthermore, changes in T-wave morphology can be utilized during therapy to assess the need for K^+ fluid replacement. The blood glucose concentration should be measured at hourly intervals for the first 4–6 hours and then at 2-hour intervals thereafter until the clinical respose dictates otherwise. Frequent measurement of the blood glucose concentration is important during the course of therapy to assess the efficacy of the initial insulin dose and to change the insulin dose when the response is unsatisfactory. When the glucose concentration is 200–300 mg/dL and glucose-containing fluids are being administered, glucose measurements may be performed at less frequent intervals. The serum electrolytes should be measured at 2-hour intervals until the sixth to eighth hour of therapy. The rate of administration of K^+ depends on the rate of change of the serum K^+ concentration; the decision to use $PO_4^{\equiv}$ therapy is contingent on the absolute serum $PO_4^{\equiv}$ level. The nadir of the response in the serum K^+ and $PO_4^{\equiv}$ concentrations to therapy occurs 4–6 hours after initiation of therapy.

Complications of Therapy

During the course of therapy, the typical anion-gap metabolic acidosis of DKA resolves and the pH is restored toward, but generally not to, the normal range.[17] It is common for the HCO_3^- concentration to increase to 18 mEq/L and the pH to 7.3 with therapy, but there may be no further immediate change in either the pH or the HCO_3^- concentration thereafter. Patients frequently become hyperchloremic and develop a transient *hyperchloremic metabolic acidosis*.[17] This is a highly predictable response to therapy. It is multifactorial, due to (1) a greater loss of buffer capacity during the development of DKA than reflected by the decrease in the serum HCO_3^- concentration and the increase in anion gap; and (2) the loss of substrate in the urine (ketone bodies) from which HCO_3^- is regenerated during therapy. Not only is a substantial amount of substrate lost during the development of ketoacidosis, but optimum fluid therapy further increases urinary excretion of the ketone bodies. The HCO_3^- concentration increases during therapy, but it cannot be restored to normal because of substrate deficiency. In the presence of normal renal function, the hyperchloremic state is corrected and fluid composition adjusted within several days. Post-therapy hyperchloremia appears to be of no clinical consequence, but it is important to recognize that it occurs commonly after the treatment of DKA. When the HCO_3^- level and the pH have been corrected ($HCO_3^- \geq 18$ mEq/L; pH ≥ 7.3), the rate of insulin administration should be reduced and the patient should be switched to a transition regimen or to his or her normal insulin regimen.

Cerebral edema is a dreaded, but fortunately very rare, complication in the treatment of DKA.[59] It usually occurs during therapy of a first episode of DKA in a young child.[59] The development of headache associated with progressive drowsiness and lethargy herald this disorder and is an ominous sign. By the time papilledema, seizures, and other signs of increased intracranial pressure occur, the outlook is grim. Most patients do not survive, and those that do have permanent CNS sequelae. There are no distinguishing historical, physical, laboratory, or therapeutic features that identify patients in whom this disaster will occur, except perhaps use of hypotonic fluids.[60] Computed tomography and magnetic resonance imaging studies reveal that virtually all patients have increased cerebral water pressure associated with DKA therapy in the absence of progressive CNS signs or symptoms.[61] Cerebrospinal fluid pressure has been reported to increase during the course of DKA therapy without producing untoward side effects.[62] These observations suggest that the phenomenon of cerebral edema is perhaps more a quantitative than a qualitative abnormality. Patients with the greatest amount of cerebral edema become symptomatic; those with lesser degrees of cerebral edema do not. The aggressive use of hypotonic fluids and failure of serum Na^+ concentrations to increase with correction of hyperglycemia have been identified as potential risk factors.[60] This occurs with the excessive administration of free water and serves as the rationale against using half-NS during the DKA therapy, particularly in children.

The mechanism(s) of cerebral edema is unknown, and no theory has been completely satisfactory. There appears to be some enthusiasm for theories that propose paradoxical CNS acidosis or altered tissue oxygenation occurring as a result of a change in the extracellular pH and a shift of the oxygen-hemoglobin dissociation curve. The most popular and most frequently cited explanation is that of osmotic disequilibrium with failure of intracellular osmolality to adjust promptly to changes in extracellular osmolality, thereby creating a temporary osmotic gradient that favors the entry of water into the intracellular compartment of the CNS.[44] This theory proposes that the decrease in extracellular osmolality with treatment occurs more rapidly than the decrease in CNS intracellular osmolality, leading to an unfavorable osmotic gradient for intracellular fluid entry. CNS adaptation to extracellular hyperosmolality is associated with the creation of new or osmotically active particles that reestablish the normal distribution of water between the extracellular and the intracellular compartments of the CNS.[44] The adaptive mechanism that creates these osmoles when extracellular osmolality is increasing may be unable to respond quickly to the decrease that occurs in extracellular osmolality with therapy. As a result, unfavorable osmotic gradients are temporarily created. Insulin may also play a role in this disorder, considering that cerebral edema does not develop in rabbits when the glucose concentration is decreased by dialysis but only when insulin is used to correct the hyperglycemia.[44] This strongly suggests that insulin may have a direct effect on membrane transport of Na^+ or water, or both. It has also been suggested that the Na^+/H^+ exchanger in the cell membrane is activated in DKA.[63] High levels of H^+ within the cell activate this exchanger, leading to extrusion of H^+ from the cell and the entry of Na^+. During treatment, reduction in the extracellular concentration of H^+ allows more Na^+ to be pumped into the cell and therefore allows cerebral edema to develop. Changes in glucose levels and the fluids administered do not play a central role in this theory.[63] The decrease that occurs, however, in the serum glucose concentration during this process may further accentuate the propensity for unfavorable osmotic gradients that could interact and aggravate cerebral edema. These theories may not be mutually exclusive: Cerebral edema may be multifactorial.

During DKA therapy patients may develop progressive *hypoxemia*.[64] In most patients, oxygenation is excellent at the time of presentation, with normal or increased Po_2 values.[64] The Po_2 commonly decreases during the course of therapy, sometimes to unexpectedly low levels. This is attributed to increased lung water and decreased lung compliance. These changes may be similar to those that occur in the CNS and suggest the possibility that this may be a common biologic phenomenon among tissues. The development of increased lung water and decreased compliance may cause the adult respiratory distress syndrome. Disseminated intravascular coagulation also has been reported during DKA/HHS therapy. The incidence of these complications depends on the severity of illness and presence of comorbid illness, usually infection.

Despite aggressive therapy, patients continue to die during the course of DKA/HHS therapy. No investigations have been published to evaluate the optimum use of the laboratory in patients with these two medical emergencies. Consequently, frequent and judicious use of the laboratory is necessary with sequential measurements to monitor insulin, fluid, and electrolyte replacement therapies. The successful outcome of the DKA/HHS patient requires the clinician to take a comprehensive, compulsive approach—to anticipate, recognize, and successfully treat each complicating factor.

Conclusions

DKA and HHS are two extremes in the spectrum of decompensated diabetes mellitus. Although recent data suggest that mortality due to DKA/HHS is declining, excess mortality still occurs.[4] Improved patient and physician awareness of the precipitating conditions of DKA/HHS, as well as improved early recognition and therapy, may further decrease the incidence and improve the outcomes of DKA/HHS patients. Patient characteristics may identify those who are at increased risk for DKA, particularly recurrent DKA, thus allowing physicians and other health professionals to focus special educational efforts in these areas.

References

1. Ennis ED, Stahl EJvB, Kreisberg RA. The hyperosmolar hyperglycemic syndrome. Diabetes Rev 1994;2:115
2. Faich GA, Fishbein HA, Ellis SE. The epidemiology of diabetic acidosis: A population-based study. Am J Epidemiol 1983;117:551
3. Wachtel TJ, Tetu-Mouradjian LM, Goldman DL, et al. Hyperosmolarity and acidosis in diabetes mellitus: A three-year experience in Rhode Island. J Gen Intern Med 1991;6:495
4. Geiss LS, Herman WH, Goldschmid MG, et al. Surveillance for diabetes mellitus—United States, 1980–1989. MMWR CDC Surveill Summ 1993;42:1
5. Basu A, Close CF, Jenkins D, et al. Persisting mortality in diabetic ketoacidosis. Diabet Med 1992;10:282
6. Arieff AI, Carroll HJ. Nonketotic hyperosmolar coma with hyperglycemia: Clinical features, pathophysiology, renal function, acid-base balance, plasma-cerebrospinal fluid equilibria and the effects of therapy in 37 cases. Medicine 1972;51:73
7. Wachtel TJ, Silliman RA, Lamberton P. Predisposing factors for the diabetic hyperosmolar state. Arch Intern Med 1987;147:499
8. Khardori R, Soler NG. Hyperosmolar hyperglycemic non-ketotic syndrome. Am J Med 1984;77:899
9. Wetterhall SF, Olson DR, DeStefano F, et al. Trends in diabetes and diabetic complications, 1980–1987. Diabetes Care 1992;15:960
10. Wright AD, Hale PJ, Singh BM, et al. Changing sex ratio in diabetic ketoacidosis. Diabet Med 1990;7:628
11. Flexner CW, Weiner JP, Saudek CD, Dans PE. Repeated hospitalizations for diabetic ketoacidosis: The game of ''sartoris.'' Am J Med 1984;76:691
12. Schade DS, Eaton RP, Alberti KGMM, Johnston DG. Diabetic Coma—Ketoacidotic and Hyperosmolar. Albuquerque, NM: University of New Mexico Press;1091:59–98
13. Foster DW, McGarry JD. The metabolic derangements and treatment of diabetic ketoacidosis. N Engl J Med 1983;309:159
14. Alberti KGMM, Hockaday TDR. Blood lactic and pyruvic acids in diabetic coma [abstract]. Diabetes 1972;21:350
15. Halperin ML, Marsden PA, Singer GG, West ML. Can marked hyperglycemia occur without ketosis? Clin Invest Med 1986;8:253
16. Emmett M, Narins RG. Clinical use of the anion gap. Medicine 1977;56:38
17. Androgue HJ, Wilson H, Boyd AE, et al. Plasma acid-base patterns in diabetic ketoacidosis. N Engl J Med 1982;26:1603
18. Marliss EB, Ohman JL, Aoki TT, Kozak GP. Altered redox state obscuring ketoacidosis in diabetic patients with lactic acidosis. N Engl J Med 1970; 283:978

19. Narins RG, Emmett M. Simple and mixed acid-base disorders: A practical aproach. Medicine 1980;59:161
20. King AJ, Cooke NJ, McCuish A, et al. Acid-base changes during treatment of diabetic ketoacidosis. Lancet 1974;1:478
21. Matz R: Hyperosmolar nonacidotic diabetes (HNAD). In: Rifkin H, Porte D, eds. Ellenberg and Rifkin's Diabetes Mellitus, Theory and Practice, 4th ed. New York, NY: Elsevier; 1990:604–616
22. DeFronzo RA, Matsuda M, Barrett EJ. Diabetic ketoacidosis: A combined metabolic-nephrologic approach to therapy. Diabetes Rev 1994;2:209
23. Ennis ED, Stahl EJvB, Kreisberg RA. Diabetic ketoacidosis. In: Porte D, Sherwin R, Rifkin H, eds. Ellenberg and Rifkin's Diabetes Mellitus, Theory and Practice, 5th ed. Norwalk, Conn: Appleton & Lange; 1996. In press
24. Munro JF, Campbell IW, McCuish AC, Duncan LJP. Euglycaemic diabetic ketoacidosis. Br Med J 1973;2:578
25. Carroll P, Matz R. Uncontrolled diabetes mellitus in adults: Experience in treating diabetic ketoacidosis and hyperosmolar nonketotic coma with low-dose insulin and a uniform treatment regimen. Diabetes Care 1983;6:579
26. Lorber D. Non-ketotic hypertonicity in diabetes. Endocrinologist 1993;3:29
27. Levine SN, Sanson TH. Treatment of hyperglycemic hyperosmolar non-ketotic syndrome. Drugs 1989;38:462
28. Malone ML, Gennis V, Goodwin JS. Characteristics of diabetic ketoacidosis in older versus younger adults. J Am Geriatr Soc 1992;40:1100
29. Peden NR, Braaten JT, McKendry JBR. Diabetic ketoacidosis during long-term treatment with continuous subcutaneous insulin infusion. Diabetes Care 1984;7:1
30. Polonsky WH, Anderson BJ, Lohrer PA, et al. Insulin omission in women with IDDM. Diabetes Care 1994;17:1178
31. Kemmer FW, Bisping R, Steingrüber HJ, et al. Psychological stress and metabolic control in patients with type I diabetes mellitus. N Engl J Med 1986;314:1978
32. Carter WR, Gonder-Frederick LA, Cox DJ, et al. Effect of stress on blood glucose in IDDM. Diabetes Care 1985;8:411
33. Walsh CH, Malins JM. Menstruation and control of diabetes. Br Med J 1977;2:177
34. Warshaw AI, Feller ER, Lee KH. On the cause of raised serum-amylase in diabetic ketoacidosis. Lancet 1977;1:929
35. Vinicor F, Lehrner LM, Karn RC, Merritt AD. Hyperamylasemia in diabetic ketoacidosis: Sources and significance. Ann Intern Med 1979;91:200
36. Eckfeldt JH, Leatherman JW, Levitt MD. High prevalence of hyperamylasemia in patients with acidemia. Ann Intern Med 1986;104:362
37. Nsien EE, Steinberg WM, Borum M, Ratner R. Marked hyperlipasemia in diabetic ketoacidosis: A report of three cases. J Clin Gastroenterol 1992;15:117
38. Fulop M, Tannenbaum H, Dreyer N. Ketotic hyperosmolar coma. Lancet 1973;2:635
39. Katz MA. Hyperglycemia-induced hyponatremia—calculation of expected serum sodium depression. N Engl J Med 1973;289:843
40. Kaminska ES, Pourmotabbed G. Spurious laboratory values in diabetic ketoacidosis and hyperlipidemia. Am J Emerg Med 1993;11:77
41. Baldwin L, Price L, Henderson A, et al. Spurious euglycemia in severe diabetic ketoacidosis. Lancet 1992;340:1407
42. Martin HE, Smith K, Wilson ML. The fluid and electrolyte therapy of severe diabetic acidosis and ketosis. Am J Med 1958;20:376
43. Kreisberg RA. Diabetic ketoacidosis: New concepts and trends in pathogenesis and treatment. Ann Intern Med 1978;88:681
44. Arieff AI, Kleeman CR. Studies on mechanisms of cerebral edema in diabetic comas: Effects of hyperglycemia and rapid lowering of plasma glucose in normal rabbits. J Clin Invest 1973;52:571
45. Assal JP, Aoki TT, Manzano FM, Kozak GP. Metabolic effects of sodium bicarbonate in management of diabetic ketoacidosis. Diabetes 1974;23:405
46. Hale PJ, Crase J, Nattrass M. Metabolic effects of bicarbonate in the treatment of diabetic ketoacidosis. Br Med J 1984;289:1035
47. Lever E, Jaspan JB. Sodium bicarbonate therapy in severe diabetic ketoacidosis. Am J Med 1983;75:263
48. Morris LR, Murphy MB, Kitabchi AE. Bicarbonate therapy in severe diabetic ketoacidosis. Ann Intern Med 1986;105:836
49. Schade DS, Eaton RP. Dose response to insulin in man: Differential effects on glucose and ketone body regulation. J Clin Endocrinol Metab 1977;44:1038
50. Guerra SMO, Kitabchi AE. Comparison of the effectiveness of various routes of insulin injection: Insulin levels and glucose response in normal subjects. J Clin Endocrinol Metab 1976;42:869
51. Halperin M, Goldstein M, Richardson R, Robeson L. Quantitative aspects of hyperglycemia in the diabetic: A theoretical approach. Clin Invest Med 1980;2:127
52. Kitabchi AE, Ayyagari V, Guerra SMO. The efficacy of low-dose versus conventional therapy of insulin for treatment of diabetic ketoacidosis. Ann Intern Med 1976;84:633
53. Waldhausl W, Klemberger G, Korn A, et al. Severe hyperglycemia: Effects of rehydration on endocrine derangements and blood glucose concentration. Diabetes 1979;28:577
54. Becker DJ, Brown DR, Steranka BH, Drash AL. Phosphate replacement during treatment of diabetic ketosis: Effects on calcium and phosphorus homeostasis. Am J Dis Child 1983;137:241
55. Fisher JN, Kitabchi AE. A randomized study of phosphate therapy in the treatment of diabetic ketoacidosis. J Clin Endocrinol Metab 1983;57:177
56. Kebler R, McDonald FD, Cadnapaphornchai P. Dynamic changes in serum phosphorus levels in diabetic ketoacidosis. Am J Med 1985;79:571
57. Knochel JP. The pathophysiology and clinical characteristics of severe hypophosphatemia. Arch Intern Med 1977;137:203
58. Zipf WB, Bacon GE, Spencer ML, et al. Hypocalcemia, hypomagnesemia, and transient hypoparathyroidism during therapy with potassium phosphate in diabetic ketoacidosis. Diabetes Care 1979;2:265
59. Rosenbloom AL, Riley WJ, Weber FT, et al. Cerebral edema complicating diabetic ketoacidosis in childhood. J Pediatr 1980;96:357
60. Harris GD, Fiordalisi I, Harris WL, et al. Minimizing the risk of brain herniation during treatment of diabetic ketoacidemia: A retrospective and prospective study. J Pediatr 1990;117:22
61. Krane EJ, Rockoff MA, Wallman JK, Wolfsdorf JI. Subclinical brain swelling in children during treatment of diabetic ketoacidosis. N Engl J Med 1985;312:1147
62. Clements RS Jr, Blumenthal SA, Morrison AD, Winegrad AI. Increased cerebrospinal-fluid pressure during treatment of diabetic ketosis. Lancet 1971;2:671
63. Van der Meulen JA, Klip A, Grinstein S. Possible mechanisms for cerebral oedema in diabetic ketoacidosis. Lancet 1987;2:306
64. Fein IA, Rackow EC, Sprung CL, Grodman R. Relation of colloid osmotic pressure to arterial hypoxemia and cerebral edema during crystalloid volume loading of patients with diabetic ketoacidosis. Ann Intern Med 1982;96:570

Diabetes Mellitus, edited by Derek LeRoith, Simeon I. Taylor, and Jerrold M. Olefsky. Lippincott–Raven Publishers, Philadelphia © 1996.

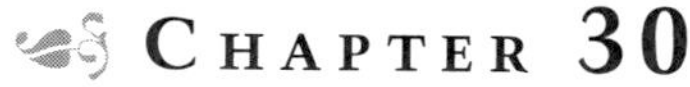

CHAPTER 30

Natural History of Autoimmunity in Type I Diabetes Mellitus

CHARLES F. VERGE AND GEORGE S. EISENBARTH

A considerable body of clinical and experimental evidence supports the conclusion that type I diabetes mellitus is a chronic autoimmune disorder.[1–4] The most telling observations relate to the appearance of a series of autoantibodies coupled with progressive loss of insulin secretion before the development of overt diabetes. Such a course is typical in a great majority of cases of what was formerly termed juvenile-onset diabetes mellitus and is now termed type I or insulin-dependent diabetes mellitus (IDDM).[5] The classification system equating IDDM with type I diabetes mellitus is likely to be altered soon on the basis of knowledge acquired during the past decade. A number of rare disorders that also lead to IDDM but are not autoimmune in etiology have been characterized (Table 30-1). In addition, a significant number of patients presenting to their physician with what appears to be non–insulin-dependent diabetes (NIDDM) actually have an early stage of type I diabetes (pseudotype II diabetes).[6] In this chapter, the term *type I diabetes mellitus* will be used to refer to autoimmune diabetes occurring at any age, irrespective of whether the diabetic individual is currently dependent on insulin for survival. This change in emphasis is now possible because of the availability of autoantibody assays for diagnosing the autoimmune form of diabetes with high sensitivity and specificity. Such accuracy cannot be approached with clinical criteria such as the age of diabetes onset, body mass index, insulin requirement, or presence of ketoacidosis.

TABLE 30-1. Genetic Approach to the Differential Diagnosis of Insulin-Dependent Diabetes Mellitus

	Locus	Insulin-Requiring
Nonautoimmune		
Wolfram's syndrome	**4p** (D4s431)[17]	Yes
Wolfram's syndrome, mitochondrial type	Mitochondrial DNA (nucleotides 6446-14134)[8,9]	Yes
Leucine tRNA mutations	Mitochondrial DNA (nucleotide 3243)[10]	Variable
MODY: Chromosome 20-linked	**20q13** (*MODY1*)[12]	Variable
MODY: *GCK*-linked	**7p15-p14** *GCK* (*MODY2*)[11]	No
MODY: Chromosome 12-linked	**12q22-qter** (*MODY3*)[170]	Yes
MODY: Other	?	?
Insulin resistance syndromes	*INSR* mutations in many **19p13.2**	Variable
Neonatal diabetes	?	Variable[174]
Transient hyperglycemia	?	No
Type II diabetes	?	Variable
Autoimmune		
APS I	**21q22.3** (D21s171)[13]	Yes
Trisomy 21	**21q** trisomy[14]	Yes
APS II	**6p21.3** (*HLA*)[15]	Yes
Type I diabetes mellitus	**6p21.3** (*HLA*)[3] **11p15.5** (*INS*)[16] **?15q26** (D15s107)[17] **?11q13** (*FGF3*)[17–19] **?2q31** (*HOXD8*)[20]	Yes

APS I and II = autoimmune polyendocrine syndromes I and II; *GCK* = glucokinase gene; *HLA* = human leukocyte antigen region; *INS* = insulin gene region; *INSR* = insulin receptor; MODY = maturity-onset diabetes of the young.

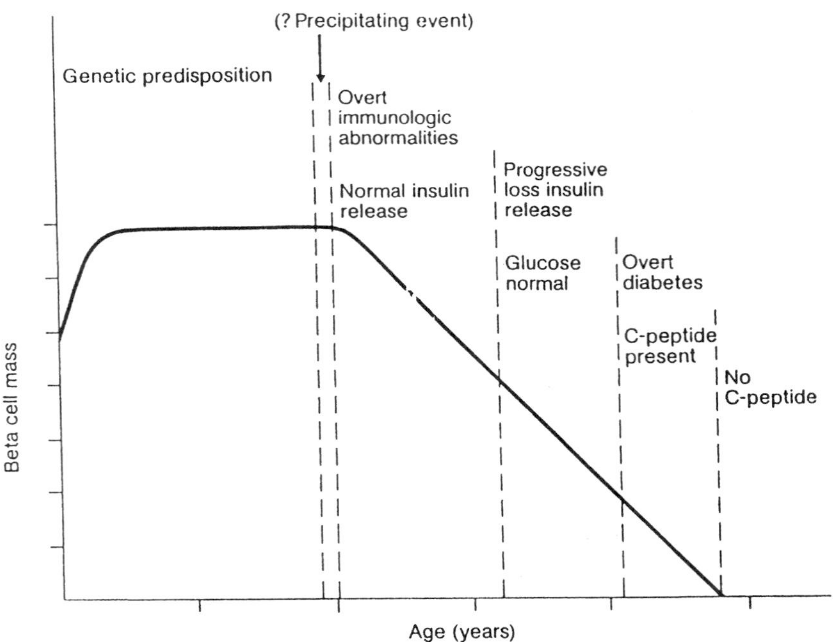

FIGURE 30-1. The natural history of type I diabetes mellitus before and after onset of overt diabetes. (Reproduced with permission from Eisenbarth GS. Type I diabetes: a chronic autoimmune disease. N Engl J Med 1986;314:1360.)

Stage I: Genetic Susceptibility

The natural history of type I diabetes mellitus begins with genetic susceptibility (Fig. 30-1). Essentially everyone who develops type I diabetes mellitus has inherited susceptibility alleles, and except for individuals with the autoimmune polyendocrine syndrome type I (APS I),[13,21] a major portion of this susceptibility maps to the human leukocyte antigen (*HLA*) region of chromosome 6.[22]

Table 30-1 includes a series of rare disorders that can be confused clinically with type I diabetes mellitus and should be considered in patients who are negative for islet autoantibodies. These disorders are now being defined on a genetic basis. Within the past 2 years, remarkable progress has been achieved in defining the genetic loci underlying these disorders by linkage analysis in multiplex pedigrees. Much of this progress has been made possible by the mapping of the human genome with microsatellite markers. These markers consist of repeated sequences that have no known genetic function; they are invaluable for linkage analysis because they are widely scattered throughout the genome and highly polymorphic. The locus defined by each marker is given a designation (e.g., D4s431), the number after the letter 'D' indicating the chromosomal location, followed by a letter indicating the complexity of the repeated sequence, and a unique identifying number for the marker. Several thousands of these markers spanning the human genome have now been identified, and most have been assigned a specific order on a given chromosome.[23]

Wolfram syndrome is a rare autosomal recessive disorder, recently linked to a locus on the short arm of chromosome 4.[7] This disease is also termed DIDMOAD syndrome, which stands for diabetes insipidus, diabetes mellitus, progressive bilateral optic atrophy and sensorineural deafness. The development of IDDM in a child is usually the first manifestation of Wolfram syndrome. Diabetes and optic atrophy are present in all cases reported, but expression of the other features is variable. In addition to the listed features, the syndrome includes a wide spectrum of neurologic and psychiatric disturbances that can lead to severe disability. Widespread atrophic changes in the brain have been detected with the use of magnetic resonance imaging.[24] Wolfram syndrome appears to be a gradually progressive neurodegenerative disorder in which there is also a nonautoimmune loss of β-cells within the pancreatic islets. The involvement of β-cells may be explained by the fact that islets share many molecules and metabolic pathways with neurons, despite their endodermal derivation. A defect in thiamine metabolism has been implicated in some cases. Borgna-Pignatti et al.[25] reported the cases of two related children with Wolfram syndrome in whom megaloblastic and sideroblastic anemia developed. These children were found to have low levels of erythrocyte thiamine pyrophosphate and thiamine pyrophosphokinase activity.[25] Thiamine treatment not only corrected the anemia, but also resulted in a marked decrease in their insulin requirement. Withdrawal of thiamine treatment was followed by relapse of the anemia, increased insulin requirement, and decreased C-peptide levels.

An even rarer form of Wolfram syndrome results from mutation of the mitochondrial DNA (see Table 30-1), with one reported case due to a 7.6 Kb deletion[8] and another due to a point mutation.[9] A syndrome of diabetes mellitus and deafness that is apparently unrelated to the Wolfram syndrome results from another mutation of the mitochondrial DNA.[10,26] This mutation affects the gene for leucine tRNA. The diabetes may be insulin-dependent or -independent.[26] Patients have sensorineural hearing loss (although their hearing abnormalities may be subtle), but the other manifestations of Wolfram syndrome are absent. Mitochondrial DNA is inherited only through the maternal germ line, and affected families are characterized by transmission of the disease from mother to offspring.

NIDDM in children and adolescents (maturity-onset diabetes of the young [MODY]) represents a heterogeneous group of genetic disorders with an autosomal dominant mode of inheritance.[27,28] Most affected individuals have mild diabetes, with no evidence of insulin resistance, and are frequently treated with diet or oral hypoglycemic agents. The best characterized form is associated with mutations of the glucokinase gene (*GCK* or *MODY2*) located on the short arm of chromosome 7.[11,29] Glucokinase, a member of the hexokinase family of enzymes, is the rate-limiting step in glucose metabolism within the β-cell. It is crucial for glucose-mediated insulin secretion and may function as the "glucose sensor" of the β-cell.[30] The mutations apparently result in an elevated set point for glucose homeostasis, and these children often present with very mild hyperglycemia. Glucokinase mutations have also been reported in a small percentage of patients with gestational[31] or apparently classic adult-onset NIDDM,[32,33] indicating that the hyperglycemia may go undetected for a long time. Froguel et al.[11] found *GCK* mutations in 18 of 32 French families with MODY.

It is likely that other genetic causes of the MODY phenotype will be defined in the future. One large North American family with MODY shows linkage to a different locus (*MODY1*) on the long arm of chromosome 20.[34] The gene responsible for this form of MODY has not yet been identified. Some families with MODY show linkage to neither GCK nor chromosome 20. Vaxillaire et al.[170] performed genome-wide linkage analysis with microsatellite markers in 12 such families and found evidence for a third MODY locus (*MODY3*) on the long arm of chromosome 12. They estimated that approximately 50% of the families studied were linked to this region, indicating that further loci remain to be discovered. Unlike other forms of MODY, *MODY3* patients have major hyperglycemia with evidence of a severe insulin secretory defect. Finally, one family with a MODY-like syndrome involving a mutant form of insulin has been described (substitution of serine for phenylalanine at position 24 of the β-chain[35]).

The autoimmune polyendocrine syndrome type I (APS I) consists of chronic mucocutaneous candidiasis, autoimmune hypoparathyroidism, and Addison's disease, usually presenting in early childhood. Approximately 5% of children with APS I develop type I (autoimmune) diabetes mellitus, and this frequency increases with follow-up into adult life.[36] Other features may include autoimmune failure of the gonads, thyroid, and gastric parietal cells; alopecia; vitiligo; chronic active hepatitis; and dystrophy of the dental enamel, nails, and cornea. The syndrome is inherited in an autosomal recessive manner associated with a locus on the tip of the long arm of chromosome 21.[13] In contrast to other forms of autoimmune diabetes, there is no association with *HLA* alleles. The presence of chronic candidiasis suggests that defective immunologic function may underlie the development of autoimmunity in this syndrome. It is noteworthy that trisomy 21 also is associated with an increased frequency of type I diabetes mellitus.[14]

APS II is a constellation of autoimmune diseases that may include: autoimmune thyroiditis, type I diabetes mellitus, celiac disease, Graves' disease, Addison's disease, myasthenia gravis, autoimmune gonadal failure, vitiligo, alopecia, hypophysitis, and pernicious anemia. Approximately 50% of affected individuals develop type I diabetes mellitus.[15,21] In contrast to APS I, the APS II is *HLA*-associated (similar to type I diabetes mellitus). Chronic mucocutaneous candidiasis is not present, and hypoparathyroidism occurs very rarely. APS II is part of a spectrum of disorders associated with type I diabetes mellitus. Among newly diagnosed diabetic children, 10% are positive for thyroid peroxidase antibodies and 2% have asymptomatic celiac disease.[37] The frequency of thyroid antibodies increases with age, and their presence in diabetic children carries a significant risk of progression to hypothyroidism over time.[38]

Table 30-2. The Lifetime Risk of Type I Diabetes Mellitus in Relatives Versus the General Population

Monozygotic twins	36%[39]
Siblings	~7%[40–45]
HLA-identical siblings	10–16%[41,46]*
Offspring of diabetic father	6%[47]*
Offspring of diabetic mother	1%[47]*
Parents	3%[40]
General population	0.7–1.5%[48,49]

*Risk to age 25 years.
HLA = human leukocyte antigen.

Several of the disorders listed in Table 30-1 have a simple Mendelian pattern of inheritance. In contrast, type I diabetes mellitus is a complex disease in which susceptibility is probably determined by the interaction of multiple genes with environmental factors. Despite familial aggregation of the disease (Table 30-2), there is no identifiable pattern of inheritance, and most cases occur in the absence of any family history. The concordance of identical twins is approximately 36%, compared with a 5–10% risk in siblings. The risk of disease is significantly higher in the offspring of diabetic fathers than in the offspring of diabetic mothers.[47] Any model of inheritance of the disease must attempt to explain these observations, as well as the association of type I diabetes mellitus with other autoimmune diseases. A major genetic determinant resides within the *HLA* region on the short arm of chromosome 6,[3] whereas the insulin gene (*INS*) region on the short arm of chromosome 11 has a weaker association.[16] Several other candidate loci have been identified recently (see Table 30-1). It is likely that other susceptibility genes will also have weak effects in comparison with *HLA*,[18] but their eventual identification will yield new information on the underlying causes of the disease.

The *HLA* region encodes class I (*A*, *B*, and *C*) and class II (*DR*, *DQ*, and *DP*) molecules (Fig. 30-2), which are involved in the presentation of antigens to T-lymphocytes (T-cells). Most *HLA* genes are highly polymorphic, resulting in wide variation in the class I and class II molecules present in different individuals. This polymorphism affects the conformation of the antigen and T-cell receptor binding site, determining how tightly certain antigens are bound. The class II alleles are most closely associated with diabetes susceptibility. Each class II molecule is a heterodimer made up of two polypeptide chains, α and β, and a number has been assigned to identify each different amino acid sequence of these polymorphic

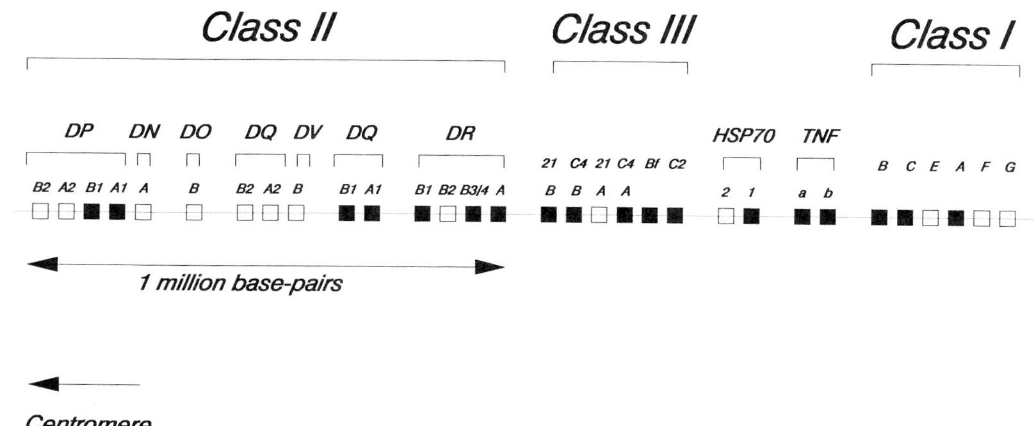

Figure 30-2. The HLA region on the short arm of chromosome 6. Expressed genes are represented by black boxes.

molecules[50] (Table 30-3). *HLA* genes also are characterized by *linkage disequilibrium* (allelic association): particular alleles at closely spaced loci do not assort independently in a population, but are present together on the same haplotype more frequently than would be expected by chance. Different haplotypes may be present in different races, however, as a result of occasional recombination events in the distant past.

Early positive associations between *HLA* and type I diabetes mellitus were found with the class I antigens *B8* and *B15;* a negative association was found with B7. Subsequently, stronger associations were found with class II genes, and it was discovered that the initial associations with class I were due to linkage disequilibrium with class II: *B8* with *DR3, B15* with *DR4,* and *B7* with *DR2.* More recent studies based in part on transracial analysis[51,52] have suggested that the strongest association within class II is with the *DQ* locus (see Fig. 30-2). For example, *DR7* is associated with susceptibility in blacks (see Table 30-3) but is neutral in Caucasians: *DR7* is associated with different *DQ* alleles in the two races. No single element within *HLA* has been found, however, that is common to all diabetes-related haplotypes. Although the presence of an amino acid other than aspartate at position 57 of the *DQ*β chain (called "non-Asp57") confers a relative risk greater than 100 in Caucasians,[53,54] this association is not present in the Japanese[55,56] (see Table 30-3). The *DQ* molecules can be encoded either in *cis* (the situation in which both α- and β-chains are encoded by alleles on the same haplotype) or in *trans* (in which they are encoded by alleles from opposite haplotypes). It is likely that the configuration of the *DQ* molecule as a whole influences susceptibility to a greater extent than the individual α- or β-chains. Ronningen et al.[57] proposed that a series of different *DQ* heterodimers, formed either in *cis* or *trans,* may confer susceptibility (see Table 30-3). The exact elements of the HLA complex responsible for susceptibility remain to be defined. It is possible that additional *HLA* susceptibility determinants other than *DQ* may be involved.

The clearest *HLA* association is the dominant protection conferred by the *DQ* molecule *DQA1*0102-DQB1*0602,* carried on *DR2* haplotypes.[58] Diabetogenic *DR2* haplotypes exist but differ from diabetes-resistant haplotypes at the *DQA1* and *DQB1* loci.[59] Approximately 20% of persons in the United States carry DQA1*0102-DQB1*0602 versus 1% of individuals with type I diabetes mellitus. There are exceptions in persons with APS I and type I diabetes. The mechanism underlying such dramatic protection is unknown, but in transgenic animal models, the introduction of a single protective class II molecule can prevent diabetes.[171] Even among islet cell antibody (ICA)-positive first-degree relatives of patients with type I diabetes mellitus, *DQA1*0102-DQB1*0602* appears to provide protection from progression to overt type I diabetes.[60] It is important to recognize that this molecule does not provide protection from all autoimmune disorders because it is a high-risk molecule for multiple sclerosis.

In Caucasians, high-risk class II molecules include *DQA1*0501-DQB1*0201* (associated with *DR3*) and *DQA1*0301-DQB1*-0302* (associated with *DR4*) (see Table 30-3). Persons carrying both *DR3* and *DR4* haplotypes (by necessity, one inherited from each parent) have the highest risk of acquiring type I diabetes mellitus. Approximately 3% of non-IDDM Caucasians are *DR3/DR4* heterozygous compared with 33% of Caucasians with type I diabetes mellitus[61] (Fig. 30-3). Assuming a 0.7% risk of type I diabetes mellitus in the general population and applying Bayes' theorem, approximately 10% of individuals in the general population with *DR3/DR4* will develop type I diabetes mellitus. Thus, programs of screening unbilical cord blood can identify persons at birth who have a risk of acquiring type I diabetes similar to the risk for first degree relatives.

The *INS* region on the short arm of chromosome 11 has been identified as a second susceptibility locus for type I diabetes mellitus.[16,62,63] The association with *INS* is much weaker than that with *HLA*. The mechanism by which the *INS* region contributes to susceptibility remains to be determined. Detailed sequencing of disease-associated haplotypes has identified many polymorphisms within the region,[64] but the *5′VNTR* appears to be most closely associated with disease.[65] It is possible that polymorphism at this locus affects the timing of insulin expression (either in the β-cell[65a] or in the thymus) during embryologic development. This in turn might affect the development of immunologic tolerance to the insulin molecule.

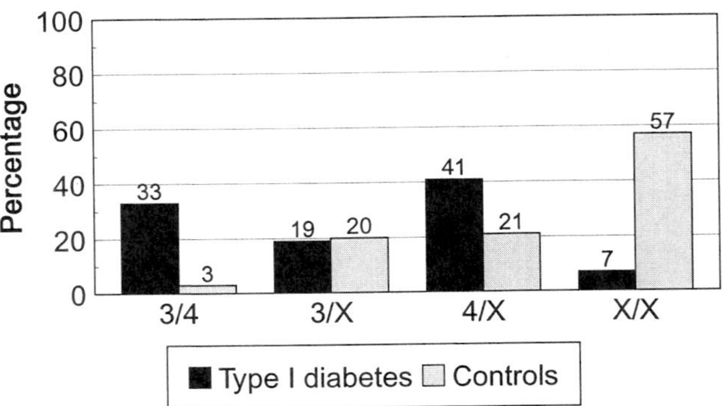

Figure 30-3. The frequency of *DR* genotypes in Caucasians with type I diabetes compared with healthy controls. *DR3/X: X* is any *DR* type except *DR4; DR4/X: X* is any *DR* type except *DR3; DRX/X: X* is neither 3 nor 4. (Data adapted from Thomson G, Robinson WP, Kuhner MK, et al. Genetic heterogeneity, modes of inheritance, and risk estimates for a joint study of Caucasians with insulin-dependent diabetes mellitus. Am Hum Genet 1988;43: 799.)

Table 30-3. The Major *HLA-DQ* Molecules (Encoded in Either *cis* or *trans*) Associated with Susceptibility to Type I Diabetes in Caucasians, Blacks and Japanese

DR	DQA1	DQB1	Position 57	Heterodimer	Race
3	0501	0201	non-Asp	*cis*	Caucasian
4	0301	0302	non-Asp	*cis*	Caucasian
3		0201	non-Asp	*trans*	Caucasian
4	0301				
7	0301	0201	non-Asp	*cis*	Black
9	0301	0201	non-Asp	*cis*	Black
4	0301	0401	Asp	*cis*	Japanese
4	0301			*trans*	Caucasian
8		0402	Asp		
9	0301	0303	Asp	*cis*	Japanese

(Reprinted with permission from Ronningen KS, Spurkland A, Iwe T, et al. Distribution of HLA-DRB1, -DQA1 and -DQB1 alleles and DQA1-DQB1 genotypes among Norwegian patients with insulin-dependent diabetes mellitus. Tissue Antigens 1991; 3:105.)

Stage II: Induction of Autoimmunity

Relatively little is known concerning the environmental determinants of type I diabetes mellitus. The strongest evidence that environmental factors may be important comes from the relatively low concordance of identical twins (~36%).[39] Such concordance estimates may be biased by a tendency for greater ascertainment of doubly affected twins in studies that are not population-based. One population-based study found a lower concordance of 23%,[66] but that study may have been biased in the opposite direction by a lack of long-term follow-up of the discordant twins. In our own studies of 30 identical twins, the follow-up period from the time of onset of type I diabetes in the index twin extends for up to 39 years. Including only 23 twin pairs who were discordant when first ascertained, survival analysis suggests that the concordance is 23% 10 years after diagnosis of the index twin and 38% 31 years after diagnosis. Our data do not support previous reports that twins who are discordant for more than 6 years are unlikely to become concordant (Fig. 30-4). Of the twins who became concordant, one-half did so more than 6 years after the diagnosis of diabetes in the index twin. In addition, two-thirds of the nondiabetic long-term discordant twins that we have studied had evidence of β-cell autoimmunity: insulin autoantibodies (IAAs), anti–glutamic acid decarboxylase (GAD) antibodies, and/or decrease in first-phase insulin release (FPIR) to below the first percentile of controls. Thus, twins discordant for diabetes often are concordant for β-cell autoimmunity.

Fewer data are available for the concordance of dizygotic twins, who are no more genetically alike than siblings but who may share environmental exposures to a greater extent. Estimates range from 5% to 16%.[66,67] This risk is not greatly different from that for siblings, suggesting that environmental factors may have a relatively weak influence on the development of type I diabetes mellitus. Nevertheless, a subset of discordant identical twins will never develop type I diabetes mellitus in their lifetime, and a smaller subset have no detectable evidence of β-cell autoimmunity. There are three possible explanations for these findings: (1) environmental factors initiating disease are lacking, (2) environmental factors that suppress disease are present, or (3) stochastic events affecting the immune system have occurred and are influencing disease activation or suppression. Such events could include somatic mutations and T-cell receptor gene rearrangement. Identical twins do not have identical T-cell repertoires because T-cell receptor genes undergo random rearrangement during T-cell differentiation. We cannot at present distinguish among the above possibilities but the identification of an avoidable environmental factor would have major implications for disease prevention. Additional evidence pointing to a role for environmental factors includes the rapidly rising incidence rates documented in several European countries[68–73] and the increased rates observed in migrant populations compared with their countries of origin.[74,75] Such changes in incidence are much too rapid to be accounted for by changes in the gene pool and indicate that factors in the environment either enhancing or suppressing diabetes are changing. It is a nearly universal observation, for example, that viral infections of NOD mouse colonies (an animal model of type I diabetes) reduce the incidence of diabetes in these inbred animals.[76,77]

The only clearly defined environmental factor associated with the development of type I diabetes mellitus in humans is congenital rubella infection.[78–80] Congenital rubella infection, although not rubella infection acquired postnatally, is responsible for a greatly increased risk of type I diabetes mellitus and an even greater risk of autoimmune thyroiditis.[81] One hypothesis relating congenital rubella infection to type I diabetes mellitus is homology between a viral protein and a 52-kd islet autoantigen.[80] An alternative hypothesis is that the congenital infection has permanently altered developing T-cells, resulting in the inability to maintain immunologic tolerance to a number of organs, including thyroid and islets.[82]

Several case-control studies[83–86] have suggested that an infant's ingestion of bovine milk or formulas manufactured from bovine milk during the first 3 months of life, as opposed to ingestion of human breast milk, increases his or her risk for acquiring type I diabetes. The increased risk found in these studies is small (~1.5 times), but it may be larger in individuals with *HLA*-susceptibility alleles. At present, there are intriguing data on two different molecules found in bovine milk that may influence the development of diabetes, namely, *bovine albumin* and *casein*. One hypothesis suggests that homology between bovine albumin[87,88] and the islet

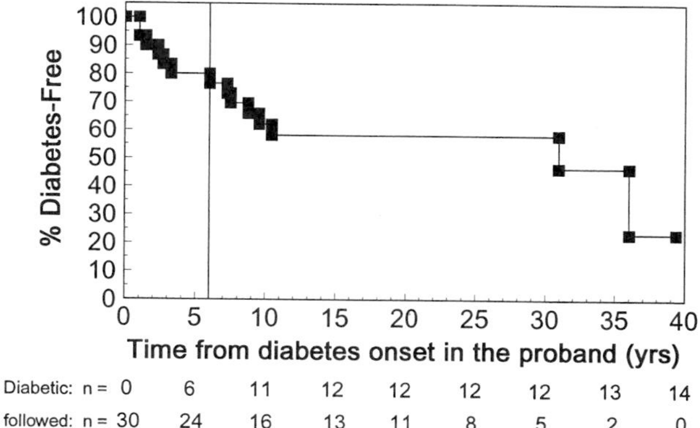

FIGURE 30-4. The concordance of 30 monozygotic twin pairs determined by survival analysis. A dashed line for the survival curve beyond 31 years indicates less than 5 twin pairs followed. One-half of the twin pairs becoming concordant did so after 6 years or more of discordance (vertical line).

molecule ICA69[89] contributes to a loss of tolerance to islets by "molecular mimicry." In this regard, type I diabetes mellitus might be analogous to celiac disease, in which ingestion of the wheat protein gliadin is pathogenic.[90] An alternative milk protein, casein, has been implicated by Elliott and coworkers.[91] This protein exists as two major variants: Casein A1 is produced by the majority of cows within the United States, western Europe, and New Zealand. In contrast, casein A2 is produced by the *Bovis indicus* strain that is common in Asia and Africa. Studies of NOD mice indicate that mice raised on an amino acid diet do not develop overt diabetes. Supplementation with casein A1 (but not A2) leads to the development of diabetes. Even in the mice raised only on amino acid diets, insulitis develops, although the frequency of progression to diabetes is reduced. Another explanation for the association in humans is that the higher caloric intake associated with formula feeding in infants may cause increased insulin secretion and increased presentation of β-cell antigens early in life. Although a causal association has not been proved, these hypotheses require further study. They have already led to proposals for a research trial to determine whether the elimination of cow's milk from the diet of infants during the first 9 months of life may prevent β-cell autoimmunity.[92]

Stage III: Expression of Autoantibodies

In many cases, the first appearance of anti-islet autoantibodies likely occurs in infancy. Studies of children less than 3 years old[93,94] presently are very limited, whereas there are several prospective long-term studies of older children and adults followed to the onset of overt type I diabetes.[4,95–98] Thus, we have an incomplete picture of the sequence, stability, and pattern of autoantibodies expressed in the first few years of life. In particular, a number of questions cannot be answered definitively, including which autoantibodies appear first, how often they appear and then disappear, and whether the genetic factors determining the presence of autoantibodies are identical to those determining the development of diabetes. In the past 2 years, the number of biochemically defined autoantigens has increased dramatically, and these questions are now much more tractable.

Table 30-4 lists three autoantigens (insulin,[99] GAD65,[100] and ICA512/IA-2[101,172,173]) for which reproducible and convenient autoantibody assays have been developed. At the Barbara Davis Center we now use recombinant protein in a radioassay format to detect the presence of autoantibodies against each of these antigens. Using this format, a single technician can assay more than 1000 samples

Table 30-4. Sensitivity and Specificity of Insulin, Glutamic Acid Decarboxylase, and ICA512bdc Autoantibodies Measured by Radioassay, and Their Use in Combination

		Sensitivity	Specificity	Specificity
Autoantibody	Age (years)	50 Relatives Subsequently Developing Diabetes	684 ICA Negative Relatives (at Low Risk for Developing Diabetes)	198 Healthy Control Subjects from the General Population
IAA	<5	100%	90%	100%
	5–15	87%	94%	100%
	>15	33%	97%	98.1%
Anti-GAD	<5	86%	86%	100%
	5–15	87%	90%	100%
	>15	100%	94%	99.0%
Anti-ICA512bdc	<5	86%	96%	100%
	5–15	68%	99.1%	100%
	>15	42%	99.0%	100%
≥1 Antibody	Overall	98.0%	88%	98.5%
≥2 Antibodies	Overall	80%	97.1%	100%
3 Antibodies	Overall	52%	99.7%	100%

GAD = glutamic acid decarboxylase; IAA = insulin autoantibodies; ICA512bdc = islet cell antigen 512 (amino acid 256-979 fragment of the IA-2 molecule); ICA = islet cell autoantibodies measured by immunohistochemistry. Percentages less than 97% are rounded to the nearest whole number.

per month. In contrast, the older cytoplasmic ICA assay is based on the reaction of antibodies in serum with undefined islet antigens present in a section of normal human pancreas, followed by incubation with fluorescently labeled anti–human IgG and detection by viewing each section with a fluorescence microscope.

The cut-off for each radioassay in Table 30-4 was determined as the 99th percentile or higher of results among 198 healthy controls with no family history of type I diabetes mellitus, thereby defining the specificity in the general population of about 99%. The figures for sensitivity among first-degree relatives are derived from data on individuals followed up to the development of type I diabetes mellitus, with a serum sample obtained 1–10 years before the onset of diabetes. For IAAs the sensitivity varies dramatically with the age at which type I diabetes mellitus develops. All persons <5 years old who progressed to diabetes mellitus were positive for IAAs. ICA512 autoantibodies also showed higher sensitivity in younger versus older relatives. GAD65 autoantibodies did not show significant variation according to the age of diagnosis, except perhaps for a slightly greater frequency among older individuals who acquired type I diabetes mellitus. As illustrated in Table 30-4, the sensitivity of the presence of any one of the three autoantibodies approaches 100%, whereas that of the combined presence of two or more autoantibodies is 80%. These figures exceed the sensitivity obtained by most laboratories with the ICA assay, especially those measuring high-titer ICA.

To assess specificity among first-degree relatives of patients with type I diabetes, we evaluated the presence of autoantibodies among cytoplasmic ICA-negative first-degree relatives. Such an analysis underestimates specificity among relatives because approximately 20% of first-degree relatives progressing to type I diabetes mellitus are ICA-negative. Nevertheless, as illustrated in Table 30-4, the specificity of the presence of any one of the three autoantibodies is lower among first-degree relatives than among the general population (88% vs. 98.5%). The higher specificity in the general population compared with first-degree relatives may offset the lower prior probability of diabetes in the general population (~0.7%, vs. 7% in first-degree relatives). If this is the case, the ability to predict type I diabetes mellitus with antibodies may be equivalent in the two groups. This is becoming an important consideration, because intervention trials to investigate the prevention of type I diabetes mellitus are now underway. More than 85% of persons who acquire type I diabetes mellitus have no affected relative. Consequently general population screening will be needed to make a major impact on the incidence of the disorder, if an effective intervention is identified by these intervention trials.

In the near future, quantitative autoantibody assays will be developed for the measurement of antibodies against other biochemically characterized autoantigens (Table 30-5). Nevertheless, the three autoantibodies discussed above already should be sufficient to replace testing for cytoplasmic ICAs. Recent studies indicate that cytoplasmic ICAs in the absence of antibodies against biochemically characterized autoantigens confer a low risk for progression to diabetes.[96,113] The cytoplasmic ICA assay has proved difficult to standardize.[114,115] In addition, different ICA subsets provide differing prognostic information. Relatives expressing "restricted" ICA[116,117] have a low risk of progression to diabetes, despite high titers of ICA.[116] The ICA reactivity of these sera can be totally absorbed by preincubation with GAD and therefore is due to the presence of autoantibodies reacting only with GAD. This form of ICA is more common among patients with APS II.

Table 30-5. β-Cell Autoantigens Associated with Type I Diabetes Mellitus

Insulin[102]
GAD65[103]
ICA512/1A-2[101,172,173]
Ganglioside GM 2-1[105]
ICA69[89]
Carboxypeptidase H[106]
37-kd antigen[107]
38-kd antigen(s)[108–110]
51-kd antigen[111]
52-kd antigen[112]

GAD = glutamic acid decarboxylase; ICA = islet cell autoantigen.

Despite the difficulties of the ICA assay, it is the standard assay on which a number of prevention trials have been and are currently based.[118,119] One can achieve a high positive predictive value for progression to diabetes by combining the ICA test with metabolic testing[120] (see below). An alternative is to accept a low predictive value for disease progression using ICA alone, requiring increased subject numbers and study duration.[121]

The ability of researchers to measure a series of autoantibodies is providing a wealth of information concerning the natural history of β-cell autoimmunity. It is already evident that expression of a single autoantibody, even if constantly present for years, is not usually associated with progression to diabetes (at least with a decade of prospective evaluation).[99,122] Some persons, such as those with the protective *HLA* haplotype *DQA1*0102-DQB1*0602*, can express high levels of GAD65 autoantibodies despite maintenance of normal FPIR.[60] These persons are unlikely ever to progress to having diabetes. In contrast, the presence of autoantibodies reacting with more than a single autoantigen usually confers a high risk for progression to diabetes.[96,113] This suggests that the immune system, especially among first-degree relatives of patients with type I diabetes mellitus, will frequently lose its tolerance to a single autoantigen but rarely will lose its tolerance to multiple islet autoantigens unless active β-cell destruction is occurring. Among relatives, we have frequently observed the occurrence of IAAs in young children, followed several years later by the appearance of additional autoantibodies (e.g., GAD65). This suggests that loss of tolerance may be progressive, especially in young children.

In older children (>8 years) and adults, the pattern of expression and even the quantitative levels of autoantibodies are often stable throughout years of prospective evaluation.[122] This suggests that after the process of autoimmunity is activated, these persons can be divided into two categories: (1) those with a single autoantibody, who have a low risk of diabetes progression, and (2) those with multiple autoantibodies, who have greater than 80% risk of acquiring type I diabetes mellitus within 10 years. The determinants of this dichotomy of immune activation are unknown. It is likely that autoreactive T-cells (not autoantibodies) destroy β-cells. This has been demonstrated clearly in animal models of type I diabetes.[123] In the NOD mouse model, CD4-positive cloned T-cells are able to destroy islets rapidly in vivo after adoptive transfer of disease. Such T-cell clones react with more than a single islet autoantigen. T-cells recognizing insulin (and other molecules yet to be characterized) are able to transfer disease. The NOD-mouse pathogenic T-cells that recognize insulin are of particular interest. These T-cells arise spontaneously within islets of NOD mice.[124] In contrast to their abundance within islets, such T-cells have been difficult to identify in peripheral lymphoid organs. This suggests that studies of T-cell autoreactivity in humans may require studies of islet infiltrating cells. Studies of peripheral T-cell responses in humans have been limited to date, and the pathogenic significance of low levels of response to known and recently characterized molecules is uncertain.[125,126] Studies of islet-infiltrating T-cells have indicated that many different T-cell receptor sequences are present, although there may be some skewing of T-cell receptor families. Such skewing has been offered as evidence that there may be a superantigen-like molecule within the islets.[127] *Superantigens* are molecules that bind to and activate whole classes of T-cells; in animal models, they can represent viruses. Evidence for T-cell receptor family skewing requires replication, and studies need to distinguish whether the skewing results from autoantigen molecules carried by islet-infiltrating cells or from the postulated viral superantigens.

Stage IV: Progressive Loss of Insulin Secretion

The first phase insulin release (FPIR) is usually calculated as the sum of the plasma insulin levels on samples drawn at one and three minutes after a standard intravenous glucose injection during an intravenous glucose tolerance test.[120] The hypothesis that type I diabetes mellitus is a chronic autoimmune disorder is based to a large extent on the observation of progressive loss of FPIR before overt diabetes.[95,120,128–132] This observation has led to the suggestion that, in the presence of islet autoantibodies, progressive loss of β-cells may occur until enough cells are destroyed to cause hyperglycemia. Despite the attractiveness of this hypothesis, there is currently little direct evidence in humans that progressive loss of β-cells occurs during the latency period of autoantibody positivity. In contrast to the availability of magnetic resonance imaging of the brain in multiple sclerosis, we do not currently have adequate tools to assess β-cell mass sequentially. Hopefully, future techniques will allow us to assess the true prediabetic course of β-cell destruction.

However, research has provided some direct information concerning the β-cell mass of diabetic and prediabetic subjects. ICA-autoantibody–negative, non-diabetic identical twins who donated a pancreatic segment to their diabetic twin mates were reported to have normal islets.[133,134] Two elderly persons with restricted ICAs (reacting only with GAD) who died without having developed diabetes were found to have normal islets with no insulitis on autopsy.[135] The lack of insulitis in these persons is consistent with the finding that first-degree relatives of patients with type I diabetes mellitus who express this form of ICA maintain normal FPIR.[116] At autopsy, persons dying at the onset of type I diabetes mellitus characteristically have markedly reduced β-cell numbers with preservation of non–β-cells.[136] In a series of Japanese patients with recent onset IDDM who underwent pancreatic biopsy,[137] about one-half lacked insulitis, probably reflecting near complete β-cell destruction. As a general rule, both in humans and in the two major animal models (BB rat and NOD mouse), islets devoid of β-cells lack insulitis.[2,134] Studies indicate that islet cells from new-onset patients express increased class I molecules[137,138] and that the most common infiltrating T-cell is *CD8*-positive. *CD8*-positive T-cells react with class I molecules, in contrast to *CD4* cells, which recognize antigen presented by class II *HLA* molecules (*DR, DP,* and *DQ*). The hypothesis that increased class II molecules[139] on β-cells are either present or important for pathogenesis generally has not been confirmed in human or animal studies,[2,140] including models of transgenic mice induced to express class II molecules on β-cells.[141]

Given the presence of anti-islet autoantibodies, the FPIR measured with an IVGTT is the best predictor of both the risk for overt diabetes and the time to onset of overt diabetes.[95] To achieve high sensitivity with the IVGTT, it must be repeated at least yearly. Approximately 80% of relatives within 1 year of diagnosis of overt diabetes will have FPIR below the 1st percentile of normal controls (48 μU/ml). Not only do severe abnormalities have a high positive predictive value, but normal FPIR has a high negative predictive value. In the absence of high levels of insulin autoantibodies,[142] individuals with an FPIR >10th percentile rarely progress to having diabetes with 3 years of follow-up.[98,99,143]

There is considerable controversy concerning the chronology of loss of FPIR during the years before the diagnosis of overt diabetes. This probably reflects the variability of the test itself, with a coefficient of variation of approximately 30%[120,132] and markedly different rates of progression in different individuals.[95] Some relatives will remain <1st percentile for up to 5 years before the onset of hyperglycemia, whereas others (usually with high IAA levels) can have a rapid decrease in FPIR <1st percentile and develop overt diabetes within 1 year. A standardized procedure for performing the IVGTT has been proposed by the Islet Cell Antibody Registry of Users (ICARUS) working group.[120] In addition, this group has served an important function by collecting and assaying sera for ICAs and IAAs as well as standardizing the insulin assays used to determine FPIR by investigators around the world. This common registry has facilitated consensus concerning the role of the IVGTT in diabetes prediction.

Stage V: Overt Diabetes

The diagnosis of type I diabetes mellitus usually is made utilizing WHO or National Diabetes Data Group (NDDG) criteria.[5] At the time diabetes is diagnosed, FPIR usually is lost, despite some preservation of responses to other secretogogues such as arginine and glucagon.[144] The FPIR was not restored even during metabolic remission in patients treated with cyclosporine.[145] Autoantibodies usually are still present at the time of diagnosis. Only 6% of newly diagnosed diabetic children are negative for ICA, IAA, and anti-GAD,[37] and this percentage is likely to decrease with the addition of new assays as other autoantigens are defined. β-Cell destruction continues after the diagnosis of type I diabetes, although a metabolic remission, termed the "honeymoon phase," may occur after the institution of insulin therapy. During this phase, very low doses of insulin may suffice to maintain normal blood glucose, and approximately 27% of patients become temporarily insulin-independent.[146]

The honeymoon phase usually ends within 1 year, but there is evidence that, compared with conventional therapy, intensive insulin therapy slows the loss of residual β-cell function.[147] Immunosuppression with cyclosporin A did not maintain long-term remission in a trial in newly diagnosed patients.[148] A number of trials utilizing agents less toxic than cyclosporin A are continuing in new-onset patients. There is general consensus that maintenance of the β-cell mass (monitored with C-peptide secretion) is a worthwhile goal if achieved with nontoxic agents. Nicotinamide, which may act as a free-radical scavenger and may protect the β-cell from the effects of autoimmune attack, preserved β-cell function in one trial[149] but failed to do so in several others.[150–152] Trials of agents such as linomide, vitamin E, the bacillus Calmette-Guerin (BCG) vaccine,[153] and interleukin-2 receptor toxins are underway.

Type I diabetes mellitus occurs at all ages, although the peak incidence is at 12 years, associated with increased insulin requirement during puberty. Data from a Danish register (with case ascertainment >99% complete) revealed that 44% of cases of type I diabetes mellitus occur after the age of 30 years.[48] The criteria for classification as type I diabetes in this study included the presence of symptoms for <6 months before diagnosis, weight loss, ketonuria or acidosis (or both), and permanent insulin treatment. With these criteria, 94% of the cases diagnosed at >30 years of age had *HLA-DR3* or DR4, or both, which is the same frequency found in the younger-onset cases.

Adult-onset type I diabetes mellitus is associated with a longer duration of symptoms before diagnosis and higher residual C-peptide secretion than childhood-onset disease, suggesting a slower rate of β-cell destruction.[154] This slow-onset presentation of type I diabetes may initially be diagnosed as type II diabetes (pseudo-type II diabetes). The diagnostic classification of adults with diabetes is likely to be improved by the measurement of islet autoantibodies. Among 102 Finnish adults diagnosed with type II diabetes, positive levels of anti-GAD antibodies were found in one-third, most of whom had low stimulated C-peptide levels.[6] Such patients are likely to progress to being insulin-dependent after diagnosis.[155] The first pilot trials of therapy with insulin versus oral agents are being carried out, and preliminary evidence suggests that early insulin therapy in such individuals may prolong their non–insulin-dependent state. Success of such therapy is associated with the maintenance of residual insulin secretion and improved metabolic control.

The failure of cyclosporin A to maintain metabolic remission in newly diagnosed patients with type I diabetes has led to intervention trials targeting at-risk individuals before the onset of diabetes. A European trial is evaluating high-dose nicotinamide, which prevents diabetes in the NOD mouse[156] but not in the BB rat model.[157] Pilot data in humans are limited. The treatment of three relatives with low FPIR did not slow their progression to becoming diabetic,[158] and follow-up data from a nonrandomized pilot trial[159] also suggests that nicotinamide is ineffective if given late in the course of progression to diabetes when the FPIR is abnormal.

Insulin prevents diabetes in both NOD mouse and BB rat animal models.[160–162] A small, nonrandomized pilot trial tested the combination of IV insulin (at 9-month intervals) and daily low-dose subcutaneous insulin. The results suggested that this may delay or prevent type I diabetes in autoantibody-positive at-risk relatives.[118] A much larger National Institutes of Health trial, the Diabetes Prevention Trial-Type I (DPT-1) is rigorously testing this intervention in a randomized fashion. This trial is now under way and will screen 60,000 first-degree relatives of patients with type I diabetes for cytoplasmic ICA over the next 5 years. Before trial entry, ICA-positive relatives are staged for diabetes risk with the parameters discussed above, including IVGTT and *HLA* typing. Those with a FPIR <10th percentile are entered into the trial, whereas those with the protective *HLA* haplotype *DQA1*0102-DQB1*0602* are excluded from entry because they have a low risk of subsequently developing diabetes.

Clinical Implications

The realization that type I diabetes mellitus is the culmination of autoimmune β-cell destruction, as well as the development of specific and sensitive assays for autoantibodies, is likely to have a significant impact on clinical practice. Below are some current recommendations and long-term possibilities for autoantibody screening and for the clinical care patients with diabetes.

Current Recommendations

Human trials are under way to evaluate nontoxic agents that have been demonstrated to prevent type I diabetes in animal models. National programs such as the DPT-1 by the National Institutes of Health provide relatives of patients with type I diabetes screening, staging, and potential trial participation without financial cost.

Patients with type I diabetes should be evaluated routinely for abnormal thyroid function because of the increased risk of autoimmune thyroid disease. Diabetic children with thyroid autoantibodies have a significant rate of acquiring hypothyroidism,[38] which may otherwise go unrecognized for some time. Patients with Addison's disease are at increased risk of acquiring type I diabetes. However, among such patients, an unusual pattern of ICA[116,117] is associated with only a minimal risk of progression to diabetes. Approximately 2% of diabetic children have asymptomatic celiac disease, which can be detected by screening for antigliadin or antiendomysial antibodies, followed by small bowel biopsy of positive individuals.[37] Children with asymptomatic celiac disease may have impaired growth and bone mineral density that improves after the institution of a gluten-free diet.[163,164] Adults found to have asymptomatic celiac disease also have evidence of osteopenia[165,166] and may have an increased risk of gastrointestinal malignancy.[167] There is no evidence, however, that the treatment of asymptomatic celiac disease improves diabetes control.

Approximately 10% of children presenting with transient hyperglycemia develop type I diabetes mellitus, and these children can be identified by the expression of autoantibodies or loss of FPIR.[168]

The majority of discordant identical twins of patients with type I diabetes (even after 6 years of discordance) are likely to become immunologically or metabolically abnormal (or both)[168a] with long-term follow-up; thus, donation of a pancreatic segment by a nondiabetic to a diabetic twin is not advisable.[133]

The measurement of islet autoantibodies will help to identify which form of diabetes is present in cases where this is uncertain on clinical grounds. In adults, the recognition that type I rather than type II diabetes is present may allow earlier institution of insulin therapy and consequent preservation of β-cell function. In children, the recognition of rare disorders such as MODY, Wolfram syndrome and mitochondrial mutations, which now are being characterized genetically, may be assisted by autoantibody testing. Approximately 5% of women with gestational diabetes[169] are actually in the early stages of type I diabetes and are likely to present within 1 year with severe hyperglycemia. Again, autoantibody detection aids in determining the prognosis and supports the early institution of insulin therapy.

Long-Term Possibilities

If current trials indicate that type I diabetes mellitus can be delayed or prevented safely, identification of at-risk individuals and preventive therapies will require implementation on an international basis.

Testing with a combination of autoantibody assays may be as predictive of diabetes risk in the general population as among first-degree relatives of patients with type I diabetes. This is despite the lower prior probability of type I diabetes in the general population. Trials for prevention of diabetes in the general population as well as among relatives of patients with diabetes should therefore be possible.

Elucidation of the genetic and environmental factors preventing or accelerating the development of type I diabetes will likely improve our understanding of autoimmunity in general and lead to safer and more effective means of prevention.

Both autoimmunity and transplant rejection appear to block successful islet transplantation and may block effective function of cells engineered to produce insulin (particularly if insulin is the primary autoantigen of this disease process[124]). To develop curative therapies, it is necessary to understand both processes.

There remain many significant questions concerning the natural history of type I diabetes. Answers to these questions will almost certainly guide efforts to prevent the disease.

References

1. Eisenbarth GS. Type I diabetes mellitus: A chronic autoimmune disease. N Engl J Med 1986;314:1360
2. Rossini AA, Greiner DL, Friedman HP, Mordes JP. Immunopathogenesis of diabetes mellitus. Diabetes Rev 1993;1:43
3. Nepom GT. Immunogenetics and IDDM. Diabetes Rev 1993;1:93
4. Palmer JP. Predicting IDDM. Diabetes Rev 1993;1:104
5. National Diabetes Data Group. Classification and diagnosis of diabetes mellitus and other categories of glucose intolerance. Diabetes 1979;28:1039
6. Tuomi T, Groop LC, Zimmet PZ, et al. Antibodies to glutamic acid decarboxylase reveal latent autoimmune diabetes in adults with a non–insulin-dependent onset of diabetes. Diabetes 1993;42:359
7. Polymeropoulos MH, Swift RG, Swift M. Linkage of the gene for Wolfram syndrome to markers on the short arm of chromosome 4. Nature Genet 1994;8:95
8. Rotig A, Cormier V, Chatelain P, et al. Deletion of mitochondrial DNA in a case of early-onset diabetes mellitus, optic atrophy, and deafness (Wolfram syndrome, MIM 222300). J Clin Invest 1993;91:1095
9. Pilz D, Quarrell OWJ, Jones EW. Mitochondrial mutation commonly associated with Leber's hereditary optic neuropathy observed in a patient with Wolfram syndrome (DIDMOAD). J Med Genet 1994;31:328
10. Kadowaki T, Kadowaki H, Mori Y, et al. A subtype of diabetes mellitus associated with a mutation of mitochondrial DNA. N Engl J Med 1994; 330:962
11. Froguel P, Zouali H, Vionnet N, et al. Familial hyperglycemia due to mutations in glucokinase: Definition of a subtype of diabetes mellitus. N Engl J Med 1993;328:697
12. Bowden DW, Gravius TC, Akots G, Fajans SS. Identification of genetic markers flanking the locus for maturity-onset diabetes of the young on human chromosome 20. Diabetes 1992;41:88
13. Aaltonen J, Bjorses P, Sandkuijl L, et al. An autosomal locus causing autoimmune disease: Autoimmune polyglandular disease type I assigned to chromosome 21. Nature Genet 1994;8:83
14. Burch PRJ, Milunsky A. Early onset diabetes mellitus in the general and Down's syndrome populations. Lancet 1969;1:554
15. Eisenbarth GS, Wilson P, Ward F, Lebovitz HE. HLA type and disease occurrence in familial polyglandular failure. N Engl J Med 1978;298:92
16. Bell GI, Horita S, Karam JH. A polymorphic locus near the human insulin gene is associated with insulin-dependent diabetes mellitus. Diabetes 1984;33:176
17. Field LL, Tobias R, Magnus T. A locus on chromosome 15q26 (IDDM3) produces susceptibility to insulin-dependent diabetes mellitus. Nature Genet 1994;8:189
18. Davies JL, Kawaguchi Y, Bennett ST, et al. A genome-wide search for human type 1 diabetes susceptibility genes. Nature 1994;371:130
19. Hashimoto L, Habita C, Beressi JP, et al. Genetic mapping of a susceptibility locus for insulin-dependent diabetes mellitus on chromosome 11q. Nature 1994;371:161
20. Owerbach D, Gabbay KH. The HOXD8 locus (2q31) is linked to type I diabetes: Interaction with chromosome 6 and 11 disease susceptibility genes. Diabetes 1995;44:132
21. Neufeld M, Maclaren NK, Blizzard BM. Two types of autoimmune Addison's disease associated with different polyglandular autoimmune (PGA) syndromes. Medicine 1981;60:355
22. Nepom GT, Erlich H. MHC class-II molecules and autoimmunity. Ann Rev Immunol 1991;9:493
23. Gyapay G, Morissette J, Vignal A, et al. The 1993-94 Genthon human genetic linkage map. Nature Genet 1994;7:246
24. Rando TA, Horton JC, Layzer RB. Wolfram syndrome: Evidence of a diffuse neurodegenerative disease by magnetic resonance imaging. Neurology 1992;42:1220
25. Borgna-Pignatti C, Marradi P, Pinelli L, et al. Thiamine-responsive anemia in DIDMOAD syndrome. J Pediatr 1989;114:405
26. Katagiri H, Asano T, Ishihara H, et al. Mitochondrial diabetes mellitus: Prevalence and clinical characterization of diabetes due to mitochondrial $tRNA^{Leu(UUR)}$ gene mutation in Japanese patients. Diabetologia 1994;37:504
27. Tattersall RB, Fajans SS. A difference between the inheritance of classical juvenile-onset and maturity-onset diabetes. Diabetes 1975;24:44
28. Bowden DW, Akots G, Rothschild CB, et al. Linkage analysis of maturity-onset diabetes of the young (MODY): Genetic heterogeneity and nonpenetrance. Am J Hum Genet 1992;50:607
29. Froguel P, Vaxillaire M, Sun F, et al. Close linkage of glucokinase locus on chromosome 7p to early-onset non-insulin-dependent diabetes mellitus. Nature 1992;356:162
30. Matschinsky FM. Glucokinase as glucose sensor and metabolic signal generator in pancreatic b-cells and hepatocytes. Diabetes 1990;39:647
31. Stoffel M, Bell KL, Blackburn CL, et al. Identification of glucokinase mutations in subjects with gestational diabetes mellitus. Diabetes 1993;42:937
32. Katagiri H, Asano T, Ishihara H, et al. Nonsense mutation of glucokinase gene in late-onset non-insulin-dependent diabetes mellitus. Lancet 1992;340:1316
33. Stoffel M, Patel P, Lo YMD, et al. Missense glucokinase mutation in maturity-onset diabetes of the young and mutation screening in late-onset diabetes. Nature Genet 1992;2:153
34. Bell GI, Xiang K, Newman MV, et al. Gene for non-insulin-dependent diabetes mellitus (maturity-onset diabetes of the young subtype) is linked to DNA polymorphism on human chromosome 20q. Proc Natl Acad Sci U S A 1991;88:1484
35. Haneda M, Chan SJ, Kwok SCM, et al. Studies on mutant human insulin genes: Identification and sequence analysis of a gene encoding (ser-B24) insulin. Proc Natl Acad Sci U S A 1983;80:6366
36. Ahonen P, Myllarniemi S, Sipila I, Perheentupa J. Clinical variation of autoimmune polyendocrinopathy–candidiasis–ectodermal dystrophy (APECED) in a series of 68 patients. N Engl J Med 1990;322:1830
37. Verge CF, Howard NJ, Rowley MJ, et al. Anti-glutamate decarboxylase and other antibodies at the onset of childhood IDDM: A population-based study. Diabetologia 1994;37:1113
38. Maclaren NK, Riley WJ. Thyroid, gastric, and adrenal autoimmunities associated with insulin-dependent diabetes mellitus. Diabetes Care 1985;8(suppl 1):34
39. Olmos P, A'Hearn R, Heaton DA, et al. The significance of concordance rate of type I (insulin dependent) diabetes mellitus in identical twins. Diabetologia 1988;31:747
40. Tillil H, Kobberling J. Age-correlated empirical genetic risk estimates for first degree relatives of IDDM patients. Diabetes 1987;36:93
41. Tarn AC, Thomas JM, Dean BM, et al. Predicting insulin-dependent diabetes. Lancet 1988;1:845
42. Chern MM, Anderson VE, Barbosa J. Empirical risk for insulin-dependent diabetes (IDD) in sibs: Further definition of genetic heterogeneity. Diabetes 1982;31:1115
43. Gavard JA, Trucco MM, Dorman JS, et al. Sex differences in secondary attack rate of IDDM to siblings of probands through older ages. Pittsburgh etiology of IDDM study. Diabetes Care 1992;15:559
44. Degnbol B, Green A. Diabetes mellitus among first and second-degree relatives of early onset diabetics. Ann Hum Genet 1978;42:25
45. Gamble DR. An epidemiological study of childhood diabetes affecting two or more siblings. Diabetologia 1980;19:341
46. Cavender DE, Wagener DK, Rabin BS, et al. The Pittsburgh insulin-dependent diabetes mellitus (IDDM) study: HLA antigens and haplotypes as risk factors for the development of IDDM in IDDM patients and their siblings. J Chron Dis 1984;37:555
47. Warram HH, Krolewski AS, Gottlieb MS, Kahn CR. Differences in risk of insulin-dependent diabetes in offspring of diabetic mothers and diabetic fathers. N Engl J Med 1984;311:149

48. Molbak AG, Christau B, Marner B, et al. Incidence of insulin-dependent diabetes mellitus in age groups over 30 years in Denmark. Diabetic Med 1994;11:650
49. Melton LJ, Palumbo PJ, Chu CP. Incidence of diabetes mellitus by clinical type. Diabetes Care 1983;6:75
50. Bodmer JG, Marsh SGE, Albert ED, et al. Nomenclature for factors of the HLA system, 1991. In: Tsuji K, Aizawa M, Sasazuki T, eds. HLA 1991: Proceedings of the 11th Histocompatibility Workshop and Conference, Vol. I. Oxford: Oxford University Press; 1992:17–31
51. Fletcher J, Mijovic C, Odugbesan O, et al. Transracial studies implicate HLA-DQ as a component of genetic susceptibility to type I (insulin-dependent) diabetes. Diabetologia 1988;31:864
52. Todd JA, Mijovic C, Fletcher J, et al. Identification of susceptibility loci for insulin-dependent diabetes mellitus by trans-racial gene mapping. Nature 1989;338:587
53. Todd JA, Bell JI, McDevitt HO. HLA-DQb gene contributes to susceptibility and resistance to insulin-dependent diabetes mellitus. Nature 1987;329:599
54. Morel PA, Dorman JS, Todd JA, et al. Aspartic acid at position 57 of the HLA-DQ beta chain protects against type I diabetes: A family study. Proc Natl Acad Sci U S A 1988;85:8111
55. Yamagata K, Nakajima H, Hanafusa T, et al. Aspartic acid at position 57 of DQ beta chain does not protect against type I (insulin-dependent) diabetes mellitus in Japanese subjects. Diabetologia 1989;32:762
56. Awata T, Iwamoto Y, Matsuda A, et al. High frequency of aspartic acid at position 57 of HLA-DQ s chain in Japanese IDDM and non-diabetic subjects. Diabetes 1989;38:90A
57. Ronningen KS, Spurkland A, Iwe T, et al. Distribution of HLA-DRB1, -DQA1 and -DQB1 alleles and DQA1-DQB1 genotypes among Norwegian patients with insulin-dependent diabetes mellitus. Tissue Antigens 1991;3:105
58. Baisch JM, Weeks T, Giles R, et al. Analysis of HLA-DQ genotypes and susceptibility in insulin-dependent diabetes mellitus. N Engl J Med 1990; 322:1836
59. Erlich HA, Griffith RL, Bugawan TL, et al. Implication of specific DQB1 alleles in genetic susceptibility and resistance by identification of IDDM siblings with novel HLA-DQB1 allele and unusual DR2 and DR1 haplotypes. Diabetes 1991;40:478
60. Pugliese A, Gianani R, Moromisato R, et al. HLA-DQB1*0602 is associated with dominant protection from diabetes even among islet cell antibody-positive first degree relatives of patients with IDDM. Diabetes 1995;44:608
61. Thomson G, Robinson WP, Kuhner MK, et al. Genetic heterogeneity, modes of inheritance, and risk estimates for a joint study of Caucasians with insulin-dependent diabetes mellitus. Am J Hum Genet 1988;43:799
62. Julier C, Hyer RN, Davies J, et al. Insulin-IGF2 region on chromosome 11p encodes a gene implicated in HLA-DR4-dependent diabetes susceptibility. Nature 1991;354:155
63. Spielman RS, McGinnis RE, Ewens WJ. Transmission test for linkage disequilibrium: The insulin gene region and insulin-dependent diabetes mellitus (IDDM). Am J Hum Genet 1993;52:506
64. Lucassen AM, Julier C, Beressi J, et al. Susceptibility to insulin dependent diabetes mellitus maps to a 4.1 kb segment of DNA spanning the insulin gene and associated VNTR. Nature Genet 1993;4:305
65. Owerbach D, Gabbay KH. Localization of a type I diabetes susceptibility locus to the variable tandem repeat region flanking the insulin gene. Diabetes 1993;42:1708
65a. Kennedy GC, German MS, Rutter WJ. The minisatellite in the diabetes susceptibility locus IDDM2 regulates insulin transcription. Nature Genet 1995;9:293
66. Kaprio J, Tuomilehto J, Koshenvuo M, et al. Concordance for type 1 (insulin-dependent) and type 2 (non-insulin-dependent) diabetes mellitus in a population-based cohort of twins in Finland. Diabetologia 1993;35:1060
67. Kumar D, Gemayel NS, Deapen D, et al. North-American twins with IDDM: Genetic, etiological, and clinical significance of disease concordance according to age, zygosity, and the interval after diagnosis in first twin. Diabetes 1993;42:1351
68. Tuomilehto J, Rewers M, Reunanen A, et al. Increasing trend in type I (insulin-dependent) diabetes mellitus in childhood in Finland: Analysis of age, calendar time, and birth cohort effects during 1965 to 1984. Diabetologia 1991;34:282
69. Drykoningen CEM, Mulder ALM, Vaandrager GJ, et al. The incidence of male childhood type 1 (insulin-dependent) diabetes mellitus is rising rapidly in the Netherlands. Diabetologia 1992;35:139
70. Green A, Andersen PK, Svendsen AJ, Mortensen K. Increasing incidence of early onset type I (insulin-dependent) diabetes mellitus: A study of Danish male birth cohorts. Diabetologia 1992;35:178
71. Joner G, Sovik O. Increasing incidence of diabetes mellitus in Norwegian children 0–14 years of age, 1973–1982. Diabetologia 1989;32:79
72. Nystrom L, Dahlquist G, Rewers M, Wall S. The Swedish childhood diabetes study: An analysis of the temporal variation in diabetes incidence, 1978–1987. Int J Epidemiol 1990;19:141
73. Rewers J, LaPorte RE, Walczak M, et al. Apparent epidemic of insulin dependent diabetes mellitus in Midwestern Poland. Diabetes 1987;36:106
74. Bodansky HJ, Staines A, Stephenson C, et al. Evidence for an environmental effect in the aetiology of insulin dependent diabetes in a transmigratory population. Br Med J 1992;304:1020
75. Elliott RB, Pilcher C, Edgar BW. Geographic IDDM in Polynesia and Macronesia: The epidemiology of insulin dependent diabetes in Polynesian children born and reared in Polynesia, compared with Polynesian children resident in Auckland, New Zealand [Abstract]. Diabetes in the Young Bulletin (Proceedings of the ISGD) 1989;20:16
76. Wilbertz S, Partke HJ, Dagnaes-Hansen F, Herberg L. Persistent MHV (mouse hepatitis virus) infection reduces the incidence of diabetes mellitus in non-obese diabetic mice. Diabetologia 1991;34:2
77. Oldstone MBA. Prevention of type I diabetes in nonobese diabetic mice by virus infection. Science 1988;239:500
78. Menser MA, Forrest JM, Bransby RD. Rubella infection and diabetes mellitus. Lancet 1978;1:57
79. Rubenstein P. The HLA system in cogenital rubella patients with and without diabetes. Diabetes 1982;31:1088
80. Karounos DG, Wolinsky JS, Thomas JW. Monoclonal antibody to rubella virus capsid protein recognizes a B-cell antigen. J Immunol 1993;150:3080
81. Clarke W, Shaver K, Bright GA, et al. Autoimmunity in congenital rubella syndrome. J Pediatr 1984;104:370
82. Rabinowe SL, George KL, Laughlin R, et al. Congenital rubella: Monoclonal antibody defined T cell abnormalities in young children. Am J Med 1986;81:779
83. Virtanen S, Rasanen L, Aro A, et al. Infant feeding in Finnish children <7 yr of age with newly diagnosed IDDM. Diabetes Care 1991;14:415
84. Verge CF, Howard NJ, Irwig L, et al. Environmental factors in childhood IDDM: A population-based, case-control study. Diabetes Care 1994;17:1381
85. Kostraba JN, Cruickshanks KJ, Lawler-Heavner J, et al. Early exposure to cow's milk and solid foods in infancy, genetic predisposition and risk of IDDM. Diabetes 1993;42:288
86. Gerstein HC. Cow's milk exposure and type I diabetes mellitus—a critical overview of the clinical literature. Diabetes Care 1994;17:13
87. Karjalainen J, Martin JM, Knip M, et al. A bovine albumin peptide as a possible trigger of insulin-dependent diabetes mellitus. N Engl J Med 1992;327:302
88. Atkinson MA, Bowman MA, Kuo-Jang K, et al. Lack of immune responsiveness to bovine serum albumin in insulin-dependent diabetes. N Engl J Med 1993;329:1853
89. Pietropaolo M, Castano L, Babu S, et al. Islet cell autoantigen 69 kDa (ICA69): Molecular cloning and characterization of a novel diabetes associated autoantigen. J Clin Invest 1993;92:359
90. Marsh MN. Gluten, major histocompatibility complex, and the small intestine: A molecular and immunobiologic approach to the spectrum of gluten sensitivity ('celiac sprue'). Gastroenterology 1992;102:330
91. Elliott RB, Reddy SN, Bibby NJ, Kida K. Dietary prevention of diabetes in the non-obese diabetic mouse. Diabetologia 1988;31:62
92. Akerblom HK, Paganus A, Teramo K, et al. Primary prevention of type I diabetes by nutritional intervention: Description of a pilot study [Abstract]. Autoimmunity 1993;15(suppl):58
93. Lesile DG, Elliott RB. Early environmental events as a cause of IDDM: Evidence and implications. Diabetes 1994;43:843
94. Pilcher CC, Elliott RB. Ontogeny of islet cell and insulin autoantibodies in first degree relatives of IDDM [Abstract]. Autoimmunity 1993;15:78
95. Vardi P, Crisa L, Jackson RA, et al. Predictive value of intravenous glucose tolerance test insulin secretion less than or greater than the first percentile in islet cell antibody positive relatives of type I (insulin-dependent) diabetic patients. Diabetologia 1991;34:93
96. Bingley PJ, Christie MR, Bonifacio E, et al. Combined analysis of autoantibodies improves prediction of IDDM in islet cell antibody-positive relatives. Diabetes 1994;43:1304
97. Schatz D, Krischer J, Horne G, et al. Islet cell antibodies predict insulin-dependent diabetes in United States school age children as powerfully as in unaffected relatives. J Clin Invest 1994;93:2403
98. Thai A, Eisenbarth GS. Natural history of IDDM. Diabetes Rev 1993;1:1
99. Ziegler AG, Ziegler R, Vardi P, et al. Life table analysis of progression to diabetes of anti-insulin autoantibody-positive relatives of individuals with type I diabetes. Diabetes 1989;38:1320
100. Grubin CE, Daniels T, Toivola B, et al. A novel radioligand binding assay to determine diagnostic accuracy of isoform-specific glutamic acid decarboxylase antibodies in childhood IDDM. Diabetologia 1994;37:344
101. Rabin DU, Pleasic SM, Shapiro JA, et al. Islet cell antigen 512 is a diabetes-specific islet autoantigen related to protein tyrosine phosphatases. J Immunol 1994;152:3183
102. Palmer JP, Asplin CM, Clemons P, et al. Insulin antibodies in insulin-dependent diabetics before insulin treatment. Science 1983;222:1337
103. Baekkeskov S, Aanstoot H, Christgau S, et al. Identification of the 64K autoantigen in insulin-dependent diabetes as the GABA-synthesizing enzyme glutamic acid decarboxylase. Nature 1990;347:151
104. Heaton DA, Millward BA, Gray IP, et al. Increased proinsulin levels as an early indicator of beta-cell dysfunction in non-diabetic twins of type I (insulin-dependent) diabetic patients. Diabetologia 1988;31:182
105. Dotta F, Previti M, Tiberti C, et al. Identification of the GM2-1 islet ganglioside: Similarities with a major neuronal autoantigen. Diabetes 1992;41:365A
106. Castano L, Russo E, Zhou L, et al. Identification and cloning of a granule autoantigen (carboxypeptidase H) associated with type I diabetes. J Clin Endocrinol Metab 1991;73:1197
107. Christie MR, Richard YM, Tun RYM, et al. Antibodies to GAD and tryptic fragments of islet 64K antigen as distinct markers for development of IDDM: Studies with identical twins. Diabetes 1992;41:782
108. Roep BO, Arden SD, deVries RP, Hutton JC. T-cell clones from a type-1 diabetes patient respond to insulin secretory granule proteins. Nature 1990;345:632

109. Pak CY, Cha CY, Rajotte RV, et al. Human pancreatic islet cell specific 38 kilodalton autoantigen identified by cytomegalovirus-induced monoclonal islet cell autoantibody. Diabetologia 1990;33:569
110. Honeyman MC, Cram DS, Harrison LC. Transcription factor jun-B is target of autoreactive T-cells in IDDM. Diabetes 1993;42:626
111. Velloso LA, Winqvist O, Gustafsson J, et al. Autoantibodies against a novel 51 kDa islet antigen and glutamate decarboxylase isoforms in autoimmune polyendocrine syndrome type I. Diabetologia 1994;37:61
112. Karounos DG, Thomas JW. Recognition of common islet antigen by autoantibodies from NOD mice and humans with IDDM. Diabetes 1990;39:1085
113. Eisenbarth GS. Combinatorial autoantibody screening for prediction of type I diabetes. Clin Res 1993;41:154A
114. Bonifacio E, Dawkins RL, Lernmark A. Immunology and diabetes workshops: Report of the second international workshop on the standardization of cytoplasmic islet cell antibodies. Diabetologia 1987;30:273
115. Landin-Olsson M. Precision of the islet-cell antibody assay depends on the pancreas. J Clin Lab Anal 1990;4:289
116. Gianani R, Pugliese A, Bonner-Weir S, et al. Prognostically significant heterogeneity of cytoplasmic islet cell antibodies in relatives of patients with type I diabetes. Diabetes 1992;41:347
117. Genovese S, Bonifacio E, McNally JM, et al. Distinct cytoplasmic islet cell antibodies with different risks for type I (insulin-dependent) diabetes mellitus. Diabetologia 1992;35:385
118. Keller RJ, Eisenbarth GS, Jackson RA. Insulin prophylaxis in individuals at high risk of type I diabetes. Lancet 1993;341:927
119. Gale EAM, Bingley PJ. Can we prevent IDDM? Diabetes Care 1994;17:339
120. Bingley PJ, Colman P, Eisenbarth GS, et al. Standardization of IVGTT to predict IDDM. Diabetes Care 1992;15:1313
121. Eisenbarth GS, Verge CF, Allen H, Rewers MJ. The design of trials for prevention of IDDM. Diabetes 1993;42:941
122. Yu L, Gianani R, Eisenbarth GS. Quantitation of glutamic acid decarboxylase autoantibody levels in prospectively evaluated relatives of patients with type I diabetes. Diabetes 1994;43:1229
123. Bradley BJ, Haskins K, La Rosa FG, Lafferty KJ. CD8 T cells are not required for islet destruction induced by a CD4+ islet-specific T-cell clone. Diabetes 1992;41:1603
124. Wegmann D, Norbury-Glaser M, Daniel D. Insulin-specific T cells are a predominant component of islet infiltrates in pre-diabetic NOD mice. Eur J Immunol 1994;24:1853
125. Atkinson MA, Bowman MA, Campbell L, et al. Cellular immunity to a determinant common to glutamate decarboxylase and Coxsackie virus in insulin-dependent diabetes. J Clin Invest 1994;94:2125
126. Harrison LC, Honeyman MC, De Aizpurua HJ, et al. Inverse relationship between humoral and cellular immunity to glutamic acid decarboxylase in subjects at risk of insulin-dependent diabetes. Lancet 1993;341:1365
127. Conrad B, Weidmann E, Trucco G, et al. Evidence for superantigen involvement in insulin-dependent diabetes mellitus aetiology. Nature 1994;371:351
128. Srikanta S, Ganda OP, Jackson RA, et al. Type I diabetes mellitus in monozygotic twins: Chronic progressive beta cell dysfunction. Ann Intern Med 1983;99:320
129. Srikanta S, Ganda OP, Gleason RE, et al. Pre-type I diabetes: Linear loss of beta cell response to intravenous glucose. Diabetes 1984;33:717
130. McCulloch DK, Bingley PJ, Colman PG, et al. Comparison of bolus and infusion protocols for determining acute insulin response to intravenous glucose in normal humans. Diabetes Care 1993;16:911
131. McNair PD, Colman PG, Alford FP, Harrison LC. Reproducibility of the first phase insulin response (FPIR) in the intravenous glucose tolerance test (IVGTT) is not improved by retrograde cannulation and arterialisation or by the use of a lower glucose dose [Abstract]. Autoimmunity 1993;15(suppl):62
132. Smith CP, Tarn AC, Thomas JM, et al. Between and within subject variation of the first phase insulin response to intravenous glucose. Diabetologia 1988;31:123
133. Kendall DM, Sutherland DER, Najarian JS, et al. Effects of hemipancreatectomy on insulin secretion and glucose tolerance in healthy humans. N Engl J Med 1990;322:898
134. Sutherland DE, Sibley R, Xu X, et al. Twin to twin pancreas transplantation: Reversal and reenactment of the pathogenesis of type I diabetes. Trans Assoc Am Phys 1984;97:80
135. Wagner R, McNally JM, Bonifacio E, et al. Lack of immunohistological changes in the islets of nondiabetic, autoimmune, polyendocrine patients with B-Selective GAD-specific islet cell antibodies. Diabetes 1994;43:851
136. Foulis AK, Clark A. Pathology of the pancreas in diabetes mellitus. In: Kahn CR, Weir GC, eds. Joslin's Diabetes Mellitus. 13th ed. Philadelphia: Lea & Febiger; 1994:281
137. Hanafusa T, Miyazaki A, Miyagawa J, et al. Examination of islets in the pancreas biopsy specimens from newly diagnosed type I (insulin-dependent) diabetic patients. Diabetologia 1990;33:105
138. Bottazzo GF, Dean BM, McNally JM, et al. In situ characterization of autoimmune phenomena and expression of HLA molecules in the pancreas in diabetic insulitis. N Engl J Med 1985;313:353
139. Bottazzo GF, Pujol-Borrell R, Hanafusa T, Feldmann M. Role of aberrant HLA-DR expression and antigen presentation in induction of endocrine autoimmunity. Lancet 1983;2:1115
140. Trucco M, Ricordi C, Weidman E, et al. Involvement of superantigens in the etiology of IDDM. Diabetes 1993;42(suppl 1):4A
141. Campbell IL, Harrison LC. Molecular pathology of type I diabetes. Mol Biol Med 1989;6:1
142. Eisenbarth GS, Jackson RA. Insulin autoimmunity: The rate limiting factor in pre-type I diabetes. J Autoimmun 1992;5(suppl A):241
143. Jackson RA, Vardi P, Herskowitz RD, et al. Dual parameter linear model for prediction of onset of type I diabetes in islet cell antibody positive relatives. Clin Res 1988;36:585A
144. Ganda OP, Srikanta S, Brink WJ, et al. Differential sensitivity to beta cell secretagogues in "early" type I diabetes mellitus. Diabetes 1984;33:516
145. Hramiak IM, Dupre J, Finegood DT. Determinants of clinical remission in recent-onset IDDM. Diabetes Care 1993;16:125
146. Martin S, Pawlowski B, Greulich B, et al. Natural course of remission in IDDM during 1st year after diagnosis. Diabetes Care 1992;15:66
147. Shah SC, Malone JI, Simpson NE. A randomized trial of intensive insulin therapy in newly diagnosed insulin-dependent diabetes mellitus. N Engl J Med 1989;320:550
148. Martin S, Schernthaner G, Nerup J, et al. Follow-up of cyclosporin A treatment in type I (insulin-dependent) diabetes mellitus: Lack of long-term effects. Diabetologia 1991;34:429
149. Vague P, Picq R, Bernal M, et al. Effect of nicotinamide treatment on the residual insulin secretion in type I (insulin-dependent) diabetic patients. Diabetologia 1989;32:316
150. Chase HP, Butler-Simon N, Garg S, et al. A trial of nicotinamide in newly diagnosed patients with type 1 (insulin-dependent) diabetes mellitus. Diabetologia 1990;33:444
151. Lewis CM, Canafax DM, Sprafka JM, Barbosa JJ. Double-blind randomized trial of nicotinamide on early-onset diabetes. Diabetes Care 1992;15:121
152. Mendola G, Casamitjana R, Gomis R. Effect of nicotinamide therapy on β-cell function in newly diagnosed type 1 (insulin-dependent) diabetic patients. Diabetologia 1989;32:160
153. Shehadeh N, Calcinaro F, Bradley BJ, et al. Effect of adjuvant therapy on development of diabetes in mouse and man. Lancet 1994;343:706
154. Karjalainen J, Salmela P, Ilonen J, et al. A comparison of childhood and adult type I diabetes mellitus. N Engl J Med 1989;320:881
155. Hagopian WA, Karlsen AE, Gottsater A, et al. Quantitative assay using recombinant human islet glutamic acid decarboxylase (GAD65) shows that 64K autoantibody positivity at onset predicts diabetes type. J Clin Invest 1993;91:368
156. Yamada K, Nonaka K, Hanafusa T, et al. Preventive and therapeutic aspects of large dose nicotinamide injections on diabetes associated with insulitis: An observation in non-obese diabetic (NOD) mice. Diabetes 1982;31:749
157. Hermitte L, Viallettes B, Atlef N. High dose nicotinamide fails to prevent diabetes in BB rats. Autoimmunity 1989;5:79
158. Herskowitz RD, Jackson RA, Soeldner JS, Eisenbarth GS. Pilot trial to prevent type I diabetes: Progression to overt IDDM despite oral nicotinamide. J Autoimmun 1989;2:733
159. Elliott RB, Chase HP. Prevention or delay of type I (insulin-dependent) diabetes mellitus in children using nicotinamide. Diabetologia 1991;34:362
160. Gotfredsen CF, Buschard K, Frandsen EK. Reduction of diabetes incidence of BB Wistar rats by early prophylactic insulin treatment of diabetes prone animals. Diabetologia 1985;28:933
161. Atkinson M, Maclaren N, Luchetta R, Burr I. Insulitis and diabetes in NOD mice reduced by prophylactic insulin therapy. Diabetes 1990;39:933
162. Zhang JZ, Davidson L, Eisenbarth GS, Weiner HL. Suppression of diabetes in nonobese diabetic mice by oral administration of porcine insulin. Proc Natl Acad Sci U S A 1991;88:10252
163. Mora S, Weber G, Barera G, et al. Effect of gluten-free diet on bone mineral content in growing patients with celiac disease. Am J Clin Nutr 1993;57:224
164. Barera G, Bianchi C, Calisti L, et al. Screening of diabetic children for coeliac disease with antigliadin antibodies and HLA typing. Arch Dis Child 1991; 66:491
165. Lindh E, Ljunghall S, Larsson K, Lavo B. Screening for antibodies against gliadin in patients with osteoporosis. J Intern Med 1992;231:403
166. Mazure R, Vazquez H, Gonzalez D, et al. Bone mineral affection in asymptomatic adult patients with celiac disease. Am J Gastroenterol 1994;89:2130
167. Holmes GKT, Prior P, Lane MR, et al. Malignancy in coeliac disease—effect of a gluten free diet. Gut 1989;30:333
168. Herskowitz RD, Wolfsdorf JI, Ricker AT, et al. Transient hyperglycemia in childhood: Identification of a subgroup with imminent diabetes mellitus. Diabetes Res 1988;9:161
168a. Verge CF, Gianni R, Yu L, et al. Late progression to diabetes and evidence for chronic β-cell autoimmunity in identical twins of patients with type I diabetes. Diabetes 1995;44:1176
169. Ratner RE. Gestational diabetes mellitus: After three international workshops do we know how to diagnose and manage it yet? J Clin Endocrinol Metab 1993;77:1
170. Vaxillaire M, Boccio V, Philiip A, et al. A gene for maturity onset diabetes of the young (MODY) maps to chromosome 12q. Nature Genet 1995;9:418
171. Lund T, O'Reilly L, Hutchings P, et al. Prevention of insulin-dependent diabetes mellitus in non-obese diabetic mice by transgenes encoding modified I-A beta chain or normal I-E alpha chain. Nature 1990;345:727
172. Gianani R, Rabin DU, Verge CF, et al. ICA512 autoantibody radioassay. Diabetes 1995;44:1340
173. Payton MA, Hawkes CJ, Christie MR. Relationship of the 37,000- and 40,000-MR tryptic fragments of islet antigens in insulin-dependent diabetes to the protein tyrosine phosphatase-like molecule 1A-2 (ICA512). J Clin Invest 1995;96:1506
174. von Muhlendahl KE, Herkenhoff M. Long-term course of neonatal diabetes. N Engl J Med 1995;333:704

Diabetes Mellitus, edited by Derek LeRoith, Simeon I. Taylor, and Jerrold M. Olefsky. Lippincott–Raven Publishers, Philadelphia © 1996.

Chapter 31
Humoral Autoimmunity

Alberto Falorni and Åke Lernmark

Insulin-dependent (type 1) diabetes mellitus (IDDM) is associated with a number of immune abnormalities. Insulitis is present in many but not in all patients at the time of clinical diagnosis.[1–3] The specific loss of β-cells is substantial and reflects a disease process that is impressive in its ability to eradicate one cell type in the complex endocrine pancreas. The hypothesis that IDDM is an autoimmune disorder was further supported by a high frequency of organ-specific autoimmune disorders in addition to autoantibodies—in particular thyroid antibodies.[4,5] Additional indirect support has been provided by the observations that human lymphocyte antigen (HLA)-B15[6] and -B8[7] increased the risk for IDDM. Later, this association was found to be secondary to DR4 and DR3, respectively,[8] followed by the demonstration that the risk for IDDM is higher for DQ8 than for DR4.[9–14] It has still not been possible to distinguish DR3 from DQ2.[15,16] The autoimmune hypothesis also has been supported by the demonstration of a genetic link to IDDM.[17–19] After failing to demonstrate the presence of antibodies against the islets in IDDM, researchers since have gained technical advances in tissue preparation and epifluorescence microscopy; these have resulted in the identification of *islet cell antibodies* (ICAs) by indirect immunofluorescence.[20,21] This finding was a critical piece of evidence to support the hypothesis that IDDM is an organ-specific autoimmune disorder belonging to the family of autoimmune endocrinopathies that includes Hashimoto's thyroiditis, Graves' disease, atrophic gastritis, and Addison's disease.

The mere demonstration of ICAs, however, did not prove that there was an immune-cell attack on the β-cells in IDDM. First, the presence of ICAs in relation to insulitis was not understood. Do ICAs play a role in cellular infiltrations? Second, although in these studies,[20,21] ICAs reacted with all endocrine cell types, only the β-cells seemed to be lost. Third, the ICA reaction was intracellular, and ICAs therefore sometimes are referred to as islet cell cytoplasmic antibodies. How could an antibody be of pathogenic significance if it is binding to an intracellular antigen (or antigens)? The notion was that in vivo endocrine islet cell plasma membrane is not permeable to immunoglobin G (IgG), the common immunoglobulin form of ICA. Therefore, if islet cell antibodies were of pathogenic importance they would react with the cell surface either to affect β-cell function or to produce *complement-dependent antibody-mediated cytotoxicity* (C′AMC). It was also possible that β-cell membrane antibodies would be secondary to β-cell destruction. In this case, the antibodies would be formed as a result of a primary β-cell destruction, resulting in processing of numerous β-cell autoantigens, antigen peptide presentation and T-cell reactivity, B-lymphocyte activation, and the formation of islet cell autoantibodies to quite a number of autoantigens. In this model, the ICAs would represent a bystander phenomenon to mark injury, but they would be of little or no pathogenetic importance.

Because cellular and humoral mechanisms are dependent on and interact with each other, it is difficult to accept the argument that a condition such as IDDM is solely a T-cell–mediated disease, whereas another disorder such as myasthenia gravis is antibody mediated. Not surprisingly, recent investigations of myasthenia gravis have documented a pathogenetic role for T-lymphocytes in this disorder as well, which has been viewed dogmatically as an antibody-mediated disease.[22,23] Most likely, although it has not been proved, chronic autoantibody production would not take place unless T-cells were also involved and perhaps continuously recruited in an autoreactivity cycle involving B-lymphocyte–driven antigen presentation and T-cell activation. In this chapter, we discuss the effect of ICAs on β-cell function, mediating complement, and cell-dependent cellular toxicity, as well as the autoantigen(s) detected by serum from subjects studied before and after the onset of IDDM. Different antibody assays and their use to predict IDDM is discussed in Chapter 32.

Effects on β-Cell Function

There are at least three methods that can be used to determine possible effects of antibodies on the function of β-cells (Table 31-1). Results obtained in each one of the methods will be reviewed below. Each method has its own advantages and disadvantages in terms of interpretation of results and possible relevance to the pathogenesis of IDDM. A major problem is to prove that ICAs bind to an antigen on the β-cells. The antigen would be accessible immediately if it were expressed on the cell surface. For instance, there are several well-documented examples of receptor antibodies such as those acting against the receptors for insulin, acetyl choline, and thyroid-stimulating hormone in which the antibodies are shown to interfere directly with ligand binding. In vivo as well as in vitro, these receptors may be directly reached by circulating antibodies. In the islets of Langerhans, however, the antibodies have to pass the following:

1. The fenestrated endothelial cells in the pancreatic islets
2. The basal membrane of the endothelial cells
3. An interstitial matrix of unknown composition
4. The basal membrane of the β-cells before the β-cell plasma membrane is reached.

The mechanisms of transport of antibodies across these four membranous barriers are not known. This is also true for antibody-mediated immunologic reactions such as C′AMC. The several complement proteins necessary to induce the complement cascade also must cross these membranes. Little is known about mechanisms of permeation of these barriers not only for humoral factors but also for immunocytes—that is, whether they are monocytes, T- or B-lymphocytes. In the following discussion, we will review results obtained in three different systems: islet cell suspensions, isolated islets, and the in vitro perfused pancreas.

Islet Cell Suspensions

Methods to prepare islet cell suspensions have been in use since 1974.[24] First, single cell suspensions were prepared by mechanical disruption of collagenase-isolated islets.[24] Subsequently, mechani-

TABLE 31-1. In Vitro Effects of Islet Cell (Surface) Antibodies on β-Cell Function

Method	Islet Preparation	Serum Tested	Effects
Islet Cell Suspensions			
Insulin release	Mouse (ob/ob) rat	IDDM and controls	Inhibition of glucose-stimulated insulin release
Glucose transport	Rat	IDDM and controls	Inhibition of initial glucose uptake by the GLUT2 transporter
Ca^{++} transport	Mouse (ob/ob)	IDDM and controls	Activation of L-type Ca^{++} channels
Isolated Islets			
Insulin release and Rb^{+} uptake	Mouse (ob/ob) rat	Homologous or autologous	Activation of the alternative pathway is cytotoxic
Insulin release	Mouse rat	IDDM and controls	Inhibition of insulin release
In Vitro Perfused Pancreas			
Insulin release	Mouse	IDDM and controls	Inhibition of glucose-stimulated insulin release
Insulin release	BB rat	Non-diabetics and diabetics	Stimulation of insulin release

IDDM = insulin-dependent diabetes mellitus.

cal disruptions were followed by fractionation efforts, first by flow sorting[25] and later by gradient centrifugations, as well as fluorescence-activated cell sorting.[26] The most advanced techniques, which have been developed by Pipeleers,[26] permit studies on purified islet cell subpopulations. In these cell preparations, it is possible to study antibody binding directly to the β-cell plasma membrane without interfering barriers (Table 31-2). Islet cells were prepared initially from ob/ob mouse islets,[24] which are easy to isolate in large quantities, and later (with the development of improved islet isolation techniques) from rat, monkey, and human islets. Islet cell surface antibodies (ICSAs) were first detected in about 70% of new-onset IDDM patients.[27] The frequency among controls was 2–5%. Initially, the surface-bound antibodies were detected by indirect immunofluorescence, but later other more quantitative and objective techniques (e.g., ^{125}I-protein-A) have been used.[28]

The demonstration of ICSAs made it possible to test whether antibody binding to the cell surface affects β-cell function. The methods used involved perfusion of islet cells.[29] Using immunoglobulin fractions of sera, it was found that glucose-stimulated insulin release was inhibited by IDDM immunoglobulin compared to controls.[29] It was concluded from these data that ICSAs interfere with the mechanism of glucose-stimulated insulin release. In subsequent experiments it was found that amino acid– or sulphonylurea–induced insulin release was not affected by ICSA-positive IDDM.[22] This suggests that ICSA might specifically and selectively interfere with glucose-stimulated insulin release. It therefore became of particular importance to test whether a membrane-associated autoantigen was specifically immunoprecipitated by IDDM sera (see below). A clue to a possible target antigen (or antigens) came, however, from additional in vitro experiments with islet cell suspensions and cell lines.

The single cell suspension proved an excellent system to study initial glucose transport.[30] It was not until 1990 however, that this system was used to test whether IDDM serum affected initial glucose transport.[31] In 26 of 27 (96%) IDDM serum IgG preparations, the initial 3-*O*-methyl glucose uptake was inhibited compared to normal or NIDDM serum IgG. The rat β-cells were shown to express the GLUT2 transporter,[32] and absorption of the IDDM IgG with liver membranes containing this transporter abolished the inhibitory effect. Furthermore, in subsequent experiments, IDDM IgG also was found to inhibit initial glucose transport into AtT-20ins cells transfected with the GLUT2 but not in cells transfected with the GLUT1 transporter.[33] Taken together, these results suggest that IDDM IgG may recognize and interfere with the GLUT2 transporter and therefore may be of pathogenetic importance. This assay system has yet to be applied to larger population-based studies to determine disease sensitivity and specificity. Using in vitro transcribed and translated ^{35}S-methionine–labeled glucose transporters GLUT1–5 in immunoprecipitation experiments, we found no evidence that 10 IDDM-standard sera immunoprecipitated any of the five glucose transporters (H Bärmeier, S Seino, G Bell, and Å Lernmark, unpublished observations, 1991). This does not exclude the possibility that IDDM sera may contain antibodies that interfere with the function but are unable to precipitate the entire transport molecule. Other membrane molecules that have been implicated are Ca^{++} transport and a non-IgG fraction of IDDM serum has been reported to interfere with L-type Ca^{++} channels.[34]

To study effects of IDDM sera on living islet cell preparations, serum samples from early-onset IDDM patients may not be useful because a higher frequency of autoantigen-specific antibodies was detected in patients in whom diabetes developed at an older age.[35] Late-onset latent autoimmune diabetes in the adult (LADA),[36] or slow-onset autoimmune diabetes,[37] may represent a chronic state of β-cell autoimmunity. A long duration of β-cell autoreactivity may be associated with not only increased levels of glutamic acid decarboxylase (GAD65) antibodies but also spreading to other autoantigens such as transporters and receptors.

TABLE 31-2. Tests for Islet Cell Surface Antibodies

Method	Cells
Complement-dependent antibody-mediated cytotoxicity	Mouse islet
	Rat islet
	Cell lines
$125_{\text{I-protein-A}}$	Rat islet
	Cell lines
$125_{\text{I-IgG}}$	Cell lines
Indirect immunofluorescence	Rat islet
	Human islet
	Cell lines
CELISA	Cell lines
ELISA	Islet cell membranes

CELISA = cell-enzyme-linked immunoabsorbent assay; ELISA = enzyme-linked immunoassay.

The isolated purified β-cells therefore offer a means to detect antibody binding directly to cells without complicating diffusion barriers. The cell surface is directly accessible. ICSAs may directly affect glucose-stimulated insulin release. Perhaps this effect is mediated by antibodies affecting the β-cell GLUT2 transporter without directly precipitating the transporter itself. The mechanisms of ICSA interaction with β-cell function are unclear, and it remains to be determined whether antibody binding takes place to one or several autoantigens. Epitope-specific antibodies will be needed to probe the β-cell surface in order to establish the possible role of antibody interference in autoimmune diabetes.

Isolated Islets

Islets of Langerhans have also been used to explore effects of IDDM and normal sera on β-cell function. The first study involved the ability of heterologous and homologous sera to induce the complement cascade, either the classical or the alternative pathway.[38] The alternative pathway was activated by islets incubated with either homologous or heterologous sera. Serum effects on isolated islets also were identified, demonstrating profound effects of IL-1 and other cytokines alone or in combination on β-cell survival, growth, and function.[39,40] The use of intact, isolated islets to demonstrate antibody effects[41] is, however, questionable because of the diffusion problems for the antibodies to reach the individual endocrine cells. Most of the antibody reactivity would occur on the islet surface, rather than on the surface of individual cells. The column-perifusion system, initially developed for single-cell suspensions,[29] but also used later for islets, is ideally suited for studying the kinetics of insulin release from islets. The ability of isolated human islets to respond to ICAs has not yet been explored. Batch-type incubation of islets suffers from being less sensitive: Factors accumulating in the medium during incubation or prolonged islet culture is a problem. Experiments with IDDM and control sera in batch-type experiments also have been difficult to reproduce.

Isolated islets therefore have been less useful in studying effects of IDDM sera or ICSAs on β-cell function. This is most likely due to the poor permeability of macromolecules in the disrupted capillary system of the islets and diffusion (if any) of macromolecules in the interstitial spaces.

In Vitro Perfused Pancreas

The in vitro perfused pancreas is advantageous for the analysis of the dynamics of insulin release in a denervated organ with an intact capillary system. The pancreas may be perifused both from the arterial to the venous side (forward) and from the venous to the arterial side. There are no data on the effects of direct perfusion of human IDDM serum in the perfused pancreas of the mouse or the rat. BB rat serum perfused in the isolated pancreas of normal Wistar rats had a stimulating effect on insulin release.[42] It is unclear whether this effect is mediated by antibodies or by other factors that may be present in the serum of diabetes-prone BB rats.

Passive transfer of serum, immunoglobulin fractions, or purified IgG is another approach to test a possible effect of ICAs on β-cell function. The problem in such experiments is to distinguish acute effects from long-term effects experienced by the recipient animal in response to the heterologous serum. In one series, immunoglobulin fractions of IDDM sera were injected into cyclophosphamide-immunosuppressed mice.[43] The pancreata of the recipient mice were perfused in the presence of low or high glucose. In four of five IDDM sera, glucose-stimulated insulin release was decreased in comparison to the response noted in mice injected with immunoglobulin from healthy controls. Although there was an effect produced by the injected IDDM immunoglobulin, it could not be determined whether this was an acute effect of the last injection preceding perfusion or a chronic effect of multiple injections. Further experiments are needed to understand the possible effect of human IDDM and control immunoglobulins on insulin release in the perfused pancreas.

Complement-Dependent Antibody-Mediated Cytotoxicity

A specific way to kill cells is by complement-dependent antibody-mediated cytotoxicity. Antibodies to cell-surface antigens bind, and the resulting immune complex initiates the complement pathway. The complement will render the cell permeable by punching holes in the plasma membrane. C′AMC is easily demonstrated in vitro, but the possible in vivo correlate is difficult to demonstrate. So-called complement-fixing ICAs (CF-ICAs) are used in the indirect immunofluorescence test to demonstrate antibodies bound to islet antigens, including cytoplasmic antigens, by their ability to bind or "fix" complement. An animal antiserum against human complement component C3b then is used to visualize bound antibody. Hence, it is unclear how CF-ICAs, which seem to represent high-titer ICAs, relate to ICAs or ICSAs other than by the fact that they are an alternative ICA assay with less diagnostic sensitivity.

The CF-ICAs in an in vitro test for C′AMC are detected in a variety of assays. Typically, a preparation of living cells, sometimes islets, are incubated with serum from IDDM patients and controls. The cells are washed to remove an excess of serum and then are incubated with fresh serum carefully collected to preserve complement; often animal sera (e.g., rabbit, guinea pig) are used as a source of complement. The complement will induce a leaky cell, and intracellular markers, typically ^{51}Cr-labeled cells, are measured in the supernatant fluid. The assay is both sensitive and quantitative.

Using rat islet cells or insulin-producing rat islet tumor (RIN) cells as targets, C′AMC was first demonstrated in new-onset IDDM patients.[44,45] There was also a high frequency of C′AMC-positive sera among first-degree relatives. C′AMC tended to decrease with increasing duration during follow-up but was not related to ICA.[46] The C′AMC reaction is complicated, however, by an altered reactivity, depending on whether the target islet cells were kept at low or high glucose in vitro.[47] High glucose and C′AMC produced the highest β-cell deterioration. Plasmapheresis decreased C′AMC, but the activity returned between repeated plasma exchanges.[46] The cellular specificity of the islet cell C′AMC reaction is still unclear. In sorted subpopulations of islet cells, β-cell specificity was suggested.[48] The specificity of the C′AMC reaction is complicated, however, by the observation that bound ICSA may activate both the classical and the alternative pathways for complement.[49]

In the spontaneously diabetic BB rat, ICSAs (*not* ICAs) are demonstrated.[42,50] Using neonatal rat islet cells, rat serum, and rabbit complement, investigators reported that approximately 50% of new-onset IDDM BB rats had C′AMC. Although insulin treatment had no effect, cyclosporin A maintained both C′AMC and relative β-cell volume density.[51] Some C′AMC inhibitory activity was present in the serum from diabetic BB rats, which might have been due to interference with the alternative complement pathway.[52] The BB rat C′AMC activity was detected, however, as early as day 10, with all diabetes-prone animals being affected by day 30.[53] C′AMC therefore seems to be a reliable marker for IDDM in the BB rat, although the concomitant cytotoxic antibodies against lymphocytes are not understood. The generation of ICSAs by immunizing rabbits[54] or mice,[55] in addition to preparing monoclonal antibodies from immunized rodents or from spontaneously diabetic BB rats, has resulted in ICSAs with C′AMC activity in vitro.[54–57] Further studies are needed to determine whether C′AMC in spontaneous human or BB rat IDDM is of pathogenetic importance. Taken together, C′AMC seems to represent a reproducible marker for β-cell autoimmunity, although a standardized cell preparation is needed for studies on diagnostic sensitivity and specificity.

Antibody-Dependent Cellular Cytotoxicity

Antibody-dependent cellular cytotoxicity in IDDM was first tested in xenogenic systems.[41,58] The test system is complicated by the fact that human islet cells are not readily available and that human effector cells may show high spontaneous reactivity against rodent islet cells, which often are used as the target cells in an ADCC reaction. In early experiments with cells from a human islet tumor, an increased rosetting between the target cells and IDDM lymphocytes was also reported.[59] Such studies are badly needed; however, the lack of suitable normal human β-cells has hampered our understanding of T-cells directly reactive with islet β-cells or of cells in the peripheral blood that mediate ADCC. In the spontaneously diabetic BB rat, however, ADCC was not a toxic factor additional to C′AMC or antibody-independent cellular cytotoxicity.[60]

Islet Cell Surface Antibodies

The lack of human insulin–producing cell lines has hampered the development of precise and reproducible ICSA assays. Mostly rodent islet cells[27,28,48] and tumor islet cell lines[45,61] have been used to detect cell-surface–bound antibodies by immunofluorescence,[27] ^{125}I-protein-A,[28] or rabbit antihuman IgG.[62] The ICSA assays have not been subjected to standardization, as is the case with ICA,[63] insulin autoantibody (IAA),[64] and GAD65-Ab[65] assays.

In attempts to use human islet cell preparations, in a limited number of sera ICSAs either were not found to be specific to β-cells[66,67] or were barely detected.[68] Exposing human islet cells[66] or rat islet cells to different glucose-concentrations did not seem to affect ICSAs, but it did influence the cell-surface binding of monoclonal antibodies specific to cell-surface gangliosides.[69,70] A study of sorted rat islet cells and splenocytes showed an increase in IgM binding and concentration, suggesting that IDDM onset may be associated with polyclonal activation of natural autoantibodies.[71]

The possible role of ICSA and their antigen (or antigens) has not been clarified despite the fact that they were described approximately 20 years ago. Several methods have been developed to detect ICSAs in human serum[72–74]; attempts have been made to prepare monoclonal antibodies against ICSAs.[75–78] The focus of research, however, has moved away from the phenomenon itself to the identification of (auto)antigens. The same is true for ICAs (discussed below).

Islet Cell Antibodies

Islet cell antibodies were described in 1974 by indirect immunofluorescence of frozen sections of human pancreas.[20] During the first decade, numerous studies were published using a nonstandardized assay. The first Immunology of Diabetes serum exchange workshop was carried out in 1985,[79] and subsequent standardization efforts identified a world standard allowing ICAs to be expressed in common units.[80] Although interlaboratory precision is still poor, the possibility of comparing results between laboratories has improved dramatically.[81] As discussed in Chapter 32, ICAs are being used to screen first-degree relatives for immune intervention trials.

In the remainder of this chapter, we will therefore only briefly review (1) the association between ICAs and the onset of IDDM; (2) the association between ICAs and loss of endogenous insulin production; (3) ICAs and altered β-cell function in nondiabetic subjects; and (4) the autoantigens that may explain the ICA reaction.

The diagnostic sensitivity of ICA for IDDM is approximately 80% and the specificity 2–4%.[82] The predictive value of ICA for IDDM in the general population is therefore low because the prevalence of IDDM is only 0.2–0.3%. The 2–3% ICA frequency among the healthy consists of persons with transient ICAs[83] and persons who stay healthy despite having ICAs.[84] Several large investigations have been completed among first-degree relatives of IDDM patients.[63,85] These studies indicate that approximately 30% of ICA-positive relatives go on to develop IDDM. ICAs are detected among 4% of healthy school children[83,86]; at a higher cut-off level, it is detected among 0.6%.[87] The estimated risk among ICA-positive school children for the development of IDDM was found to be 45%, which is comparable to the risk among first-degree relatives. The ICA test is, however, sensitive to numerous factors that affect assay reliability.[88] In addition, it is cumbersome to use in large screening efforts.

After the clinical onset of IDDM, it is well known that ICAs are evanescent. In attempts to test whether ICAs are associated with the continuous loss of endogenous insulin production, several prospective studies have been carried out without[89] or with[90] immunosuppression with cyclosporin A. High-titer ICAs seemed to predict a more rapid loss of C-peptide. In addition, the duration of residual β-cell function over time was affected by age, gender, and C-peptide level at diagnosis.[91] If the presence of ICAs after diagnosis predicted an increased rate of loss of residual β-cell function, the next question was whether ICAs affected β-cell function in healthy relatives. In the Seattle family study the presence of ICAs did not always indicate loss in β-cell function.[84,92] Among first-degree relatives with ICAs, however, increased levels of proinsulin were found, possibly reflecting β-cell dysfunction perhaps related to the islet cell autoimmunity.[93] In school children screened for ICA and HLA, β-cell dysfunction was detected in ICA-positive children who had the high-risk HLA alleles DQB1*0302 or DQB1*0201.[94] In ICA-positive individuals, altered T-cell CD4:CD8 ratios have been reported before the clinical onset of IDDM. This supports the hypothesis that an abnormality in T-cells is associated with progression to clinical onset of IDDM.[95,96] Further studies are needed to fully understand the mechanisms that control ICA formation and why these antibodies in only some persons are associated with clinical onset of IDDM. The isolation of autoantigens such as insulin and GAD65 has made it possible to develop reliable and reproducible assays; therefore, it is important to isolate the major autoantigen for ICA. Currently, part of the ICA reaction is explained by antibodies against GAD65. In fact, some IDDM patients have ICAs that are GAD65 specific, and they exhibit so-called restricted ICA in the immunofluorescence test. In most ICA-positive sera, the GAD65 reactivity is only a minor part. The ICA antigen does not seem to depend on proteolysis. Biotechnical analyses suggest that the ICA autoantigen has the properties of a monoasialo-ganglioside migrating between GM2 and GM1 standards.[97] It will be necessary, however, to isolate and characterize the ICA antigen. A number of approaches primarily using immunoprecipitation and immunoblotting have been used to identify islet cell autoantigens (see below).

Islet Cell Autoantigen-Specific Antibodies

The first autoantigen to be described was the 64K protein, which was detected by immunoprecipitation with IDDM sera of ^{35}S-methionine–labeled human islet proteins solubilized in detergent.[98–101] Before the discovery that the 64K protein was GAD and recombinant GAD became available,[102] insulin was used as a candidate autoantigen; it was demonstrated in a radioligand binding assay that approximately 50% of newly diagnosed but untreated IDDM patients have insulin autoantibodies (IAAs).[103] These IAAs have been standardized, and the measurements carried out in fluid-phase radioimmunoassay was found to be closer to IDDM than solid-phase enzyme-linked immunosorbent assay (ELISA) analyses.[104] It has been proposed that IAAs predict IDDM better in children than in adults[105] and that IAAs are related to a linear loss of β-cell function, leading to IDDM.[106] The disease sensitivity and specificity as well as predictive value are discussed in Chapter 32. It is unclear why IAAs are found earlier in childhood and are less frequently found in adults.[83,105] IAAs were positively associated with DR4,[107] perhaps because they are in linkage disequilibrium with DQ8. In families[108] and in a population-based study, IAAs also were associated with the DQ8 (DQB1*0302-DQA1*0301) but not with the DQ2 (DQB1*0201-DQA1*0501) haplotype.[109,110] Because more patients with the DQ2/8 genotype develop diabetes before the age of 15 than after,[111–113] the increased frequency of IAA among children may not be explained simply by the HLA association, but by other factors. The rate of β-cell destruction could be accelerated in the DQ2/8 genotype, which may favor the formation of IAAs rather than ICAs and GAD65-Ab. A first analysis of the IAA epitope indicates that the amino acids B1-B3 and A8-A13 are included[114]; however, further site-directed mutagenesis and use of insulin analogs will be necessary to map IAAs in relation to diagnostic sensitivity and specificity. The only data so far indicate that first-degree relatives of IDDM patients, in whom IAAs are found, share common epitopes with their IDDM relatives.[114] There is a strong association between the methimazole-induced insulin autoimmune syndrome, and the presence of the DR4 subtype DRB1*0406 (more than 14 different subtypes of DR4 are now known), which may exhibit preferential binding of a linear fragment of the α-chain of insulin and may be associated with the activation of self-insulin T-helper lymphocytes.[115] Prospective, population-based studies of school children therefore are required to determine the possible association between HLA, including the DR4 subtypes, and the production of IAAs. In addition, prospective studies would be useful to clarify the predictive value for IDDM in the general population, considering that many more healthy children will have the IAA marker than will develop IDDM.

The availability of a pure antigen such as insulin was critical for the successful development of a standardized assay and reference standards.[64,104] This also was true for the molecular cloning of human islet GAD65[116] and the rapid development of a standardized radioligand binding assay.[65,117–120] GAD65 as well as its isoform GAD67 are enzymes that convert glutamate to the neuroinhibitor gamma-amino butyric acid (GABA). GABA is present in the brain but also at extraneuronal sites.[121,122] The role of GABA in the islets of Langerhans remains to be clarified.[123–125] It cannot be excluded that GABA may be more important as a source of ATP[124] than as a neurotransmitter. An agent that is able to release GABA from the islet β-cells has yet to be identified.[123] A major unanswered question is why GAD65 is autoantigenic and what triggers the autoimmune reaction to this antigen. It is assumed, but not yet proved, that GAD65 linear peptides are presented by HLA class II molecules. This antigen presentation leads to the activation of T-helper lymphocytes whose T-cell receptors are specific for the trimolecular complex of the class II molecule α- and β-chains, with the peptide loaded between the two chains. The activation of T-helper cells would stimulate B-lymphocytes with anti-GAD65 membrane-bound IgM molecules. Such B-lymphocytes would then produce IgG GAD65 antibodies. The series of events that leads to the formation of GAD65-antibody IgG, which may be stable for many years before the clinical onset of IDDM, requires further investigation. A first step is to determine the IDDM serum specificity for GAD65; a second step is to determine the IDDM serum specificity for GAD65; a second step is to determine the possible existence of a unique IDDM epitope.

Several recent studies have addressed the specificity of IDDM antibodies for GAD65 (Table 31-3). Analyses of GAD expression in human islets resulted in the cloning of a novel GAD transcript, GAD65[116] that was different from previously known GAD transcripts cloned in the brain.[126,127] The two GAD transcripts were encoded by two different genes: *GAD1*, transcribed to the GAD67 3.7-Kb transcript, is encoded on human chromosome 2; the *GAD2* 5.6-Kb transcript is encoded on chromosome 10.[116,128] A sequence comparison revealed that 65% of the amino acids are identical. The major structural differences between the two molecules are found at the N-terminal, where the sequence homology is only 40%. Approximately 80% of the amino acids are identical at the C-terminal. The different structures are reflected in different subcellular distribution,[129,130] reflecting membrane association for GAD65 and cytoplasmic location for GAD67.[131,132] The structural homology also includes sequences that seem to control the formation of dimers.[133,134] Such dimers may be of pathogenetic importance. In the human pancreatic β-cells, however, GAD65 (not GAD67) is primarily expressed.[135,136] The unique β-cell expression of GAD65 underlines the possible role of this molecule in β-cell–specific destruction in IDDM. Using the novel specific radioligand binding assays for GAD65 and GAD67, it is also demonstrated that IDDM antibodies are directed against GAD65.[117,137–141] In large population-based studies, the average GAD65 reactivity in new-onset IDDM patients amounted to 80%, compared to 10–20% for GAD67.[35,117,118] Most GAD67-reactive sera in IDDM had high-titer GAD65 antibodies, and the GAD67 binding also was displaced by an excess of human recombinant GAD65.[118] The conclusion is that GAD65 antibodies are the best autoantibody markers for IDDM particularly in older persons.[35,119,142] How this response is generated and whether it is specific for IDDM has been studied by epitope mapping and by comparison of the GAD65 antibody response with that observed in Stiff Man syndrome (SMS)—another autoimmune neurologic disorder that shares GAD65 as the autoantigen.

It is not clear to what extent the GAD65 antibody response is monoclonal, oligoclonal, or polyclonal. This question was first analyzed in elegant experiments by Richter and coworkers,[143,144] who developed several human GAD-reactive monoclonal antibodies from IDDM patients. The epitopes of some of these monoclonal antibodies were located toward the C-terminal and central part of the GAD65 molecule,[143] but they did not seem to react with the portion of the molecule with sequence homologies to candidate environmental factors such as a Coxsackie virus antigen or heat-shock protein sequence.[145] This location of an IDDM-specific epitope has been confirmed in experiments involving deletion mutants and chimeric molecules between GAD65 and GAD67.[143,146–148] Some of these results of deletion mutants are difficult to interpret because the IDDM GAD65 antibodies require a conformational epitope.[100,101] However, studies of the intact molecules in fluid phase assay seem to support the notion that the C-terminal end of the molecule has a major epitope and that there is possibly one more in the central portion.[146] These results are important because these regions do not seem to be detected in sera from SMS patients. First, these patients have antibodies that are able to detect a linear GAD65 epitope.[147,149,150] Second, the autoantibody levels are much higher in SMS patients.[119,147] Third, on immunoblotting SMS sera detect only GAD65, whereas both GAD65 and GAD67 are detected in the fluid-phase assay.[149,151] Finally, the SMS[152] (not IDDM[100,153]) autoantibodies tend to inhibit the GAD65 enzymatic activity—an effect also observed in patients with autoimmune polyendocrine syndrome I.[152] Other neurologic diseases, however, may also show GAD65 autoreactivity.[154] Taken together, these data indicate that the GAD65 molecule may be the target for three different disease entities. Patients with both IDDM and SMS may have autoantibodies against two different epitopes, but in the unique IDDM patient, the frequency of autoantibodies against the part of the molecule reactive with SMS antibodies will be rare. It will be important to determine whether epitope-specific GAD65-antibody immunoassays increase the predictive value for the different GAD65-antibody–associated diseases, including IDDM. The reader is referred to Chapter 32 for a discussion of the sensitivity and specificity of GAD65 antibodies and their relative merits compared to other islet cell autoantibody assays to predict IDDM.

Future studies will include detailed investigations on the control of GAD65 antibody formation. Initial studies on thymidine incorporation into human peripheral blood cells in response to GAD and GAD peptides are controversial.[155–159] The major problem in these thymidine incorporation studies is the absence of (1) T-cell purification, (2) an independent demonstration of cytokine production, and (3) NK-cell incorporation of the label. The association between GAD65 antibodies and HLA is found primarily with DQ2 in Swedish children,[109] with DQ8 in non-DQ2 patients[109] or in other populations.[160] Further experiments therefore are needed to determine the ability of GAD65 peptides to bind to different HLA class II molecules associated (or not) with IDDM as well as to elute peptides from class II antigen–presenting cells that have been allowed to internalize and process GAD65.

The demonstration of insulin and GAD65 as the major antigens in IDDM has resulted in experiments aimed at identifying additional autoantigens (Table 31-4). These autoantigens can be divided into those that are available as recombinant proteins (e.g., insulin, GAD, ICA69, carboxypeptidase-H) and those that are seen as band on a sodium dodecyl sulphate (SDS) gel after immunoprecipitation or Western blotting (37K, 38K, 155K).

The ICA512 antigen was detected by screening an islet expression library with human IDDM sera.[161] The antigen was found to react with approximately 50% of IDDM sera.[162] This transmembrane molecule[161] belongs to the protein phosphatase family and is confirmed to be expressed in islets and the brain.[163,164] Currently, experiments are aimed at determining to what extent the ICA512 autoantibodies will be useful predicting IDDM.

The ICA69 or p69 autoantigen was isolated after screening a rat islet lambda-expression library with sera from ICA-positive first-degree relatives.[165] Although the ICA69 molecule has a deduced molecular mass of Mr 54,600, this molecule apparently migrates on an SDS-polyacrylamide gel at Mr 69,000 which suggests the presence of significant post-translational modification. The cellular localization of ICA69 indicates both islet and exocrine localization. It was reported that approximately 80% of IDDM patients and 50% of first-degree relatives in whom IDDM later developed were ICA69-antibody positive.[165] ICA69 does not share any significant homology with other proteins, but a weak 4-5 amino acid homology to bovine serum albumin (BSA) was proposed because BSA antibodies often are found to be increased in IDDM.[166,167] The initial interest in IDDM-associated molecular mimicry to BSA has been dampened, however, by the inability of investigators to reproduce these results.[168]

The Mr 64,000 (64K) protein tryptic digests has been found to generate three fragments that are immunoprecipitated by IDDM sera.[169,170] The Mr 37,000 (37K) and Mr 40,000 (40K) fragments seem to be generated from a non-64K source, whereas the 50K fragment seems to be derived from 64K or GAD65. The precursors of the 37K and 40K component therefore should be identified. One possibility is that the 37K component is derived from the ICA512 antigen. Further analyses of these fragments will be necessary to define their role in the pathogenesis of IDDM. Analysis of both new-onset patients and persons at risk for IDDM suggest that the 37K component primarily appears close to the clinical onset of IDDM in approximately 50% of patients.[169,171]

The Mr 38,000 (38K) antigen was first described by Baekkeskov et al.[172] The identity of this molecule remains to be determined. It may be reactive with T-cells in IDDM,[173] but proof is lacking the 38K antigen is the same as the Mr 38,000 component which stimulate T cells. Jun-B also was proposed to represent the 38K molecule. Another 38K component was identified by immunoblotting with a monoclonal antibody produced after the immunization of mice with cytomegalovirus.[174] Sequence homology was noted between a cytomegalovirus antigen and Jun-B.[174] This observation may be comparable to the finding that retrovirus may react with IAA[175] and that antirubella antibodies cross-react with a 52K protein detected by IDDM antibodies in some patients.[176,177]

TABLE 31-3. Glutamic Acid Decarboxylase Isoforms and Insulin-Dependent Diabetes Mellitus

	GAD65	*GAD67*
Gene (human)	*GAD2*	*GAD1*
Chromosome	10	2
mRNA (Kb)	5.6	3.7
Protein (molecular weight × 10^3)	65	67
Brain	+	+
Testes	+	–
Islets	+	–
Human β-cells	+	–
Human non-β-cells	±	–
Liquid phase assay		
IDDM serum (%)	+ (70)	+ (10–20)
SMS serum (%)	+++	+++
Western Blot assay		
IDDM serum	–	–
SMS serum	++	–

GAD = glutamic acid decarboxylase; IDDM = insulin-dependent diabetes mellitus; SMS = Stiff Man syndrome.

The 155K RIN cell membrane protein was identified by the reactivity with monoclonal antibody 1A2.[178] This assay is an indirect competing assay in which IDDM and control sera are allowed to compete with the binding of 1A2 to RIN cell lines. The 155K protein has yet to be sequenced and tested for IDDM sensitivity and specificity.

Thus, the number of islet cell autoantigens has increased, but several of these autoantigens have not withstood the test of disease sensitivity and specificity. The humoral immune response in human IDDM to several autoantigens underscores the utility of these antibodies as markers for a disease process that often, but not always, results in clinical IDDM associated with significant β-cell destruction. The molecular mimicry between autoantigens and virus antigens is an attractive hypothesis. For example, there is a significant homology between GAD65 and a Coxsackie virus antigen.[156,179,180] Whether this sequence, which is not part of the molecule recognized by IDDM autoantibodies,[147] initiates the IDDM autoimmune process[156] needs to be the subject of further intense research.

Summary

Insulin-dependent diabetes mellitus is strongly associated with the presence of specific autoantibodies (Table 31-4). The pathogenesis is a marked destruction of pancreatic β-cells. It is not yet resolved, however, whether ICAs cause diabetes, or whether they mark an ongoing autoimmune reaction against insulin-producing cells. The autoreactivity against the GAD65 isoform is pronounced both before and at the clinical onset of IDDM. GAD65 autoantibodies showed highest predictive value, especially among older persons. Although the GAD65 autoantibodies may represent an initiating autoantigen, the features of the humoral immune response would rather indicate a second effect due to β-cell destruction. This speculation is underscored by the presence of autoantibodies to numerous other β-cell autoantigens. The reactivity to other antigens may represent either the autoreactive genetic background of the IDDM patient or the spreading out of antigens during a sustained autoimmune attack on β-cells. The role of T-cells in the human IDDM autoantibody–β-cell reaction is yet to be defined. GAD65 and other islet autoantibodies have a low positive predictive value for IDDM in the general population. Therefore, it will be necessary to further determine ways by which IDDM can be predicted and prevented in the general population.

Table 31-4. Autoantigens in Insulin-Dependent Diabetes Mellitus*

	Newly Diagnosed Diabetes (%)	Relatives† (%)	General Population (%)
IAAs	40–60	1–3	1
GAD65	60–90	8	1.2
GAD67	10–20	2	2–3
155K/160K RIN cell membrane antigen	92	25	5
ICA69	21	45	1–6
ICA512	50	TBD	2
52K RIN cell secretory granule antigen	58	TBD	5
Carboxypeptidase-H	TBD	25	0
38K	17	TBD	0
37/40K	78		0
GM2-1 antibodies	TBD	67	4
Antisulphatide antibodies	88	TBD	0

*More than 500 subjects studied in each category. For details see reference 82.
†ICA-positive relatives.
GAD = glutamic acid decarboxylase; IAAs = autoantibodies; ICA = islet cell antibody; TBD = to be determined.

Acknowledgments

We thank Sue Blaylock for assistance and our many colleagues for stimulating and fruitful discussions. Research was supported by National Institutes of Health grants DK42654, DK46620, DK41801, and DK17047; the Swedish Medical Research Council (19X-10408); the Swedish Diabetes Association; the Nordisk Insulin Fund; and the Petrus and Augusta Hedlunds Fund; and fellowships from the Karolinska Institute and the Juvenile Diabetes Foundation International (A. F.).

References

1. Gepts W. Pathologic anatomy of the pancreas in juvenile diabetes mellitus. Diabetes 1965;14:619
2. Pipeleers D, Ling Z. Pancreatic beta cells in insulin-dependent diabetes. Diabetes Metab Rev 1992;8:209
3. Lernmark Å, Klöppel G, Stenger D, et al. Heterogeneity of human islet pathology in newly diagnosed childhood insulin-dependent diabetes mellitus: Macrophage infiltrations and expression of HLA-DQ and glutamic acid decarboxylase. Virchows Archiv 1995;425:631
4. MacCuish AC, Irvine WJ. Autoimmunological aspects of diabetes mellitus. Clin Endocrinol Metab 1975;4:435
5. Drell DW, Notkins AL. Multiple immunological abnormalities in patients with type 1 (insulin-dependent) diabetes mellitus. Diabetologia 1987;30:132
6. Singal DP, Blajchman MA. Histocompatibility (HL-A) antigens, lymphocytotoxic antibodies and tissue antibodies in patients with diabetes mellitus. Diabetes 1973;22:429
7. Nerup J, Platz P, Anderssen OO. HL-A antigens and diabetes mellitus. Lancet 1974;2:864
8. Platz P, Jakobsen BK, Morling M, et al. HLA-D and DR-antigens in genetic analysis of insulin-dependent diabetes mellitus. Diabetologia 1981;21:108
9. Nepom BS, Palmer J, Kim SJ, et al. Specific genomic markers for the HLA-DQ subregion discriminate between DR4+ insulin-dependent diabetes mellitus and DR4+ seropositive juvenile rheumatoid arthritis. J Exp Med 1986;164:345
10. Owerbach D, Lernmark Å, Platz P, et al. HLA-D region β-chain DNA endonuclease fragments differ between HLA-DR identical healthy and insulin-dependent diabetic individuals. Nature 1983;303:815
11. Todd JA, Bell JI, McDevitt HO. HLA DQ β gene contributes to susceptibility and resistance to insulin-dependent diabetes mellitus. Nature 1987;329:599
12. Baisch JM, Weeks T, Giles R, et al. Analysis of HLA-DQ genotypes and susceptibility in insulin-dependent diabetes mellitus. New Engl J Med 1990;322:1836
13. Khalil I, d'Auriol L, Gobet M, et al. A combination of HLA-DQβ Asp57–negative and HLA-DQ alpha Arg52 confers susceptibility to insulin-dependent diabetes mellitus. J Clin Invest 1990;85:1315
14. Sanjeevi CB, Lybrand TP, DeWeese C, et al. Polymorphic amino acid variations in HLA-DQ are associated with systematic physical property changes and occurrence of insulin-dependent diabetes mellitus. Diabetes 1995;44:125
15. Kockum I, Wassmuth R, Holmberg E, et al. HLA-DQ primarily confers protection and HLA-DR susceptibility in type 1 (insulin-dependent) diabetes studied in population-based affected families and controls. Am J Hum Genet 1993;53:150
16. Kockum I, Sanjeevi CB, Eastman S, et al. HLA-DR and DQ gene susceptibility in a population-based study of newly diagnosed Swedish insulin-dependent diabetes children and controls. Eur J Immunogenetics 1995; in press
17. Risch N. Genetics of IDDM: Evidence for complex inheritance with HLA. Genet Epidemiol 1989;6:143
18. Rich SS, Green A, Morton NE, Barbosa J. Combined segregation and linkage analysis of insulin-dependent diabetes mellitus. J Hum Genet 1987;40:237
19. Davies JL, Kawaguchi Y, Bennett ST, et al. A genome-wide search for human type 1 diabetes susceptibility genes. Nature 1994;371:130
20. Bottazzo GF, Florin-Christensen A, Doniach D. Islet cell antibodies in diabetes mellitus with autoimmune polyendocrine deficiencies. Lancet 1974; 2:1279
21. MacCuish AC, Barnes EW, Irvine WJ, Duncan LJP. Antibodies to pancreatic islet-cells in insulin-dependent diabetics with coexistent autoimmune disease. Lancet 1974;2:1529
22. Yi Q, Ahlberg R, Pirskanen R, Lefvert AK. Acetylcholine receptor-reactive T cells in myasthenia gravis: Evidence for the involvement of different subpopulations of T helper cells. J Neuroimmunol 1994;50:177
23. Yi Q, Lefvert AK. Idiotype- and anti-idiotype-reactive T lymphocytes in myasthenia gravis: Evidence for the involvement of different subpopulations of T helper lymphocytes. J Immunol 1994;153:3353
24. Lernmark Å. The preparation of, and studies on, free cell suspensions from mouse pancreatic islets. Diabetologia 1974;10:431
25. Nielsen DA, Lernmark Å, Berelowitz M, et al. Sorting of pancreatic islet cell subpopulations by light scattering using a fluorescence-activated cell sorter. Diabetes 1982;31:299
26. Pipeleers D. The biosociology of pancreatic B cells. Diabetologia 1987; 30:277
27. Lernmark Å, Freedman ZR, Hofmann C, et al. Islet-cell-surface antibodies in juvenile diabetes mellitus. N Engl J Med 1978;299:375
28. Huen AH-J, Haneda M, Freedman Z, et al. Quantitative determination of islet cell surface antibodies using ^{125}I-protein A. Diabetes 1983;32:460
29. Kanatsuna T, Baekkeskov S, Lernmark Å, Ludvigsson J. Immunoglobulin from insulin-dependent diabetic children inhibits glucose-induced insulin release. Diabetes 1983;32:520
30. Lernmark Å, Sehlin J, Täljedal I-B. The use of dispersed pancreatic islet cells in measurements of transmembrane transport. Anal Biochem 1975;63:73
31. Johnson JH, Crider BP, McCorkle K, et al. Inhibition of glucose transport into rat islet cells by immunoglobulins from patients with new-onset insulin-dependent diabetes mellitus. N Engl J Med 1990;322:653
32. Johnson JH, Newgard CB, Milburn JL, et al. The high km glucose transporter of islets of Langerhans is structurally and functionally similar to the high km glucose transporter of the liver. J Biol Chem 1990;265:6548
33. Inman LR, MaAllister CT, Chen L, et al. Autoantibodies to the GLUT-2 glucose transporter of beta cells in insulin-dependent diabetes mellitus of recent onset. Proc Natl Acad Sci 1993;90:1281
34. Juntti-Berggren L, Larsson O, Rorsman P, et al. Increased activity of L-type Ca^{2+}-channels exposed to serum from patients with type 1 diabetes. Science 1993;261:86
35. Vandewalle CL, Falorni A, Svanholm S, et al. High diagnostic sensitivity of glutamate decarboxylase autoantibodies in IDDM with clinical onset between age 20 and 40 years. J Clin Endocrinol Metab 1995;80:846

36. Zimmet PZ, Tuomi T, Mackay IR, et al. Latent autoimmune diabetes mellitus in adults (LADA): The role of antibodies to glutamic acid decarboxylase in diagnosis and prediction of insulin dependency. Diabet Med 1994;22:53
37. Kobayashi T, Tamemoto K, Nakanishi K, et al. Immunogenetic and clinical characterization of slowly progressive IDDM. Diabetes Care 1993;16:780
38. Idahl LA, Sehlin J, Taljedal IB, Thornell LE. Cytotoxic activation of complement by mouse pancreatic islet cells. Diabetes 1980;29:636
39. Mandrup-Poulsen T, Bendtzen K, Nerup J, et al. Affinity-purified interleukin-1 is cytotoxic to isolated islets of Langerhans. Diabetologia 1986;29:63
40. Eizirik DL, Sandler S, Palmer JP. Repair of pancreatic β-cells: A relevant phenomenon in early IDDM? Diabetes 1993;42:1383
41. Boitard C, Sai P, Debray-Sachs M, et al. Antipancreatic immunity: *In vitro* studies of cellular and humoral immune reactions directed toward pancreatic islet. Clin Exp Immunol 1984;55:571
42. Crisá L, Mordes JP, Rossini AA. Autoimmune diabetes mellitus in the BB rat. Diabetes Metab Rev 1992;8:9
43. Svenningsen A, Dyrberg T, Gerling I, et al. Inhibition of insulin release after passive transfer of immunoglobulin from insulin-dependent diabetic children to mice. J Clin Endocrinol Metab 1983;57:1301
44. Dobersen MJ, Scharff JE, Ginsberg-Fellner F, Notkins AL. Cytotoxic autoantibodies to beta-cells in the serum of patients with insulin-dependent diabetes mellitus. N Engl J Med 1980;303:1493
45. Eisenbarth GS, Morris MA, Scearce RM. Cytotoxic antibodies to cloned rat islet cells in serum of patients with diabetes mellitus. J Clin Invest 1981; 67:403
46. Rabinovitch A, MacKay P, Ludvigsson J, Lernmark Å. A prospective analysis of islet cell cytotoxic antibodies in insulin-dependent diabetic children: Transient effects of plasmapheresis. Diabetes 1984;33:224
47. Schroeder D, Kohnert KD, Hehmke B, et al. Modulation of the effect of humoral-mediated cytotoxicity on isolated rat pancreatic islets by glucose. APMIS 1993;101:387
48. van de Winkel M, Smets G, Gepts W, Pipeleers DG. Islet cell surface antibodies from insulin-dependent diabetics bind specifically to pancreatic β-cells. J Clin Invest 1982;70:41
49. Okada S, Ichiki K, Sato K, et al. Complement activation pathways associated with islet cell surface antibody (ICSA) derived from child patients with insulin-dependent diabetes mellitus (IDDM). Acta Med Okayama 1991; 45:185
50. Dyrberg T, Poussier P, Nakhooda F, et al. Islet cell surface and lymphocyte antibodies often precede the spontaneous diabetes in the BB rat. Diabetologia 1984;26:159
51. Hehmke B, Lucke S, Schroder D, et al. Complement-dependent antibody-mediated cytotoxicity in the spontaneously diabetic BB/OK rat: Association with beta cell volume density. Eur J Immunol 1990;20:1091
52. Hehmke B, Shroder D, Kloting I, Kohnert KD. Complement-dependent antibody-mediated cytotoxicity (C′AMC) to pancreatic islet cells in the spontaneously diabetic BB/OK rat: Interference from cell-bound and soluble inhibitors. J Clin Lab Immunol 1991;35:71
53. Hehmke B, Schroder D, Kloting I. Early appearance of complement-dependent antibody mediated cytotoxicity (C′AMC) to islet cells in serum of diabetes-prone BB/OK rats. Diabetes Res 1990;13:183
54. Lernmark Å, Kanatsuna T, Patzelt C, et al. Antibodies directed against the pancreatic islet cell plasma membrane: Detection and specificity. Diabetologia 1980;19:445
55. Ziegler B, Lucke S, Kohler E, et al. Monoclonal antibody-mediated cytotoxicity against rat beta cells detected *in vitro* does not cause beta-cell destruction *in vivo*. Diabetologia 1992;35:608
56. Augstein P, Kohnert KD, Ziegler B, et al. Induction of islet cell surface and insulin antibodies in Balb/c mice by application of porcine insulin and Freund's adjuvant is not associated with insulitis. Horm Metab Res 1993; 25:344
57. Tanguay KE, Amano K, Hart DA, Yoon JW. A cytotoxic monoclonal autoantibody from the BB rat which binds an islet cell surface protein. Diabetes Res Clin Pract 1990;8:23
58. Charles MA, Suzuki M, Waldeck N. Immune islet killing mechanisms associated with insulin-dependent diabetes: In vitro expression of cellular and antibody-mediated islet cell cytotoxicity in humans. J Immunol 1983; 130:1189
59. Huang S-W, MacLaren NK. Insulin-dependent diabetes: A disease of autoaggression. Science 1976;192:64
60. Koevary SB. *In vitro* lysis of islet cells by lymphocytes from diabetic BB/Wor rats is not antibody mediated. Diabetes Res 1990;13:133
61. Matsuba I, Lernmark Å. A novel microwell indirect immunofluorescence assay to detect antibodies against islet cell surface antigens in insulin-dependent diabetes mellitus. Reg Immunol 1990;3:23
62. Hellerström S, Ludvigsson J. Islet cell surface antibodies in diabetic children determined with ^{125}I-labelled anti-IgG as tracer. Diabetes Res 1992;20:1
63. Bonifacio E, Bingley PJ, Shattock M, et al. Quantification of islet cell antibodies and prediction of insulin dependent diabetes. Lancet 1990;335:147
64. Greenbaum CJ, Palmer JP, Kuglin B, Kolb H. Insulin autoantibodies measured by radioimmunoassay methodology are more related to insulin-dependent diabetes mellitus than those measured by enzyme-linked immunosorbent assay: Results of the Fourth International Workshop on the Standardization of Insulin Autoantibody measurement. J Clin Endocrinol Metab 1992;74:1040
65. Schmidli RS, Colman PG, Bonifacio E, et al. High level of concordance between assays for glutamic acid decarboxylase antibodies: The First International Glutamic Acid Decarboxylase Antibody Workshop. Diabetes 1994; 43:1005
66. Björk E, Kämpe O, Grawe J, et al. Modulation of beta-cell activity and its influence on islet cell antibody (ICA) and islet cell surface antibody (ICSA) reactivity. Autoimmunity 1993;16:181
67. Peterson C, Campbell IL, Harrison LC. Lack of specificity of islet cell surface antibodies (ICSA) in IDDM. Diabetes Res Clin Pract 1992;17:33
68. Vives M, Somoza N, Soldevila G, et al. Reevaluation of autoantibodies to islet cell membrane in IDDM: Failure to detect islet cell surface antibodies using human islet cells as substrate. Diabetes 1992;41:1624
69. Kjaer TW, Rygaard J, Bendtzen K, et al. Interleukins increase surface ganglioside expression of pancreatic islet cells *in vitro*. APMIS 1992;100:509
70. Aaen K, Rygaard J, Josefsen K, et al. Dependence of antigen expression on functional state of beta-cells. Diabetes 1990;39:697
71. Decraene T, Vandewalle C, Pipeleers D, Gorus FK. Increased concentrations of total IgM at clinical onset of type 1 (insulin-dependent) diabetes: Correlation with IgM binding to cells: The Belgian Diabetes Registry. Clin Chem 1992;38:1762
72. Peakman M, Vergani D. A new ELISA measuring antibodies to islet cell membranes: Levels are increased in type I diabetes. Horm Metab Res Suppl 1992;26:117
73. Betterle C, Presotto F, Magrin L, et al. Islet cell surface antibodies by an ELISA method in diabetic and nondiabetic patients. J Endocrinol Invest 1991;14:293
74. Bizzarro A, DeBellis A, Florio A, et al. A new ELISA assay for islet cell surface antibodies: Determination in type 1 diabetes mellitus of recent onset. Horm Metab Res Suppl 1992;26:119
75. Ziegler AG, Strandl E, Lander T, et al. Cell-mediated autoimmunity at the onset of insulin-dependent diabetes mellitus (IDDM). Klin Wochenschr 1987;65:546
76. Ziegler R, Alper CA, Awdeh ZL, et al. Specific association of HLA-DR4 with increased prevalence and level of insulin autoantibodies in first-degree relatives of patients with type 1 diabetes. Diabetes 1991;40:709
77. Ziegler B, Schlosser M, Furll B, et al. CELISA for rapid screening of monoclonal islet cell surface antibodies using living rat insulinoma cells as target. Diabetes Res 1991;16:41
78. Ziegler B, Witt S, Kohnert KD, et al. Characterization of monoclonal islet cell reactive autoantibodies from the diabetic biobreeding (BB/OK) rat. Acta Diabetol 1993;30:201
79. Bottazzo GF, Gleichmann H. Workshop report: Immunology and diabetes workshops: Report of the first international workshop on the standardisation of cytoplasmic islet cell antibodies. Diabetologia 1986;29:125
80. Bonifacio E, Lernmark Å, Dawkins RL. Serum exchange and use of dilutions have improved precision of measurement of islet cell antibodies. J Immunol Methods 1988;106:83
81. Greenbaum CJ, Palmer JP, Nagataki S, et al. Improved specificity of ICA assays in Fourth International Immunology of Diabetes Serum Exchange Workshop. Diabetes 1992;41:1570
82. Greenbaum CJ, Brooks-Worrell BM, Palmer JP, Lernmark Å. Autoimmunity and prediction of insulin dependent diabetes mellitus. Diabetes Annual 1994;8:21
83. Landin-Olsson M, Palmer JP, Lernmark Å, et al. Predictive value of islet cell and insulin autoantibodies for type 1 (insulin-dependent) diabetes mellitus in a population-based study of newly-diagnosed diabetic and matched control children. Diabetologia 1992;35:1068
84. McCulloch DK, Klaff LJ, Kahn SE, et al. Nonprogression of subclinical β-cell dysfunction among first degree relatives of IDDM patients: 5-yr follow-up of the Seattle family study. Diabetes 1990;39:549
85. Riley WJ, Maclaren NK, Krischer J, et al. A prospective study of the development of diabetes in relatives of patients with insulin-dependent diabetes. N Engl J Med 1990;323:1167
86. Levy-Marchal C, Tichet J, Fajardy I, et al. Islet cell antibodies in normal French school-children. Diabetologia 1992;35:577
87. Schatz D, Krischer J, Horne G, et al. Islet cell antibodies predict insulin-dependent diabetes in United States school age children as powerfully as in unaffected relatives. J Clin Invest 1994;93:2403
88. Landin-Olsson M. Precision of the islet cell antibody assay depends on the pancreas. J Clin Lab Anal 1990;4:289
89. Marner B, Agner T, Binder C, et al. Increased reduction in fasting C-peptide is associated with islet cell antibodies in type I (insulin-dependent) diabetic patients. Diabetologia 1985;28:875
90. Mandrup-Poulsen T, Stiller CR, Bille G, et al. Disappearance and reappearance of islet cell cytoplasmic antibodies in cyclosporin-treated insulin-dependent diabetics. Lancet 1985;2:599
91. Schiffrin A, Ciampi A, Hendricks L, et al. Evidence for different clinical subtypes of type 1 diabetes mellitus: A prospective study. Diabetes Res Clin Pract 1994;23:95
92. Bärmeier H, McCulloch DK, Neifing JL, et al. Risk for developing type 1 (insulin-dependent) diabetes mellitus and the presence of islet 64K antibodies. Diabetologia 1991;34:727
93. Spinas GA, Snorgaard O, Hartling SG, et al. Elevated proinsulin levels related to islet cell antibodies in first-degree relatives of IDDM patients. Diabetes Care 1992;15:632
94. Rowe RE, Leech NJ, Nepom GT, McCulloch DK. High genetic risk for IDDM in the Pacific Northwest: First report from the Washington State Diabetes Prediction Study. Diabetes 1994;43:87

95. Schatz DA, Riley WJ, Maclaren NK, Barrett DJ. Defective inducer T-cell function before the onset of insulin-dependent diabetes mellitus. J Autoimmun 1991;4:125
96. Al-Sakkar L, Pozzilli P, Bingley PJ, et al. Early T-cell defects in pre-type 1 diabetes. Acta Diabetol 1992;28:189
97. Dotta F, Tiberti C, Previti M, et al. Rat pancreatic ganglioside expression: Differences between a model of autoimmune islet B cell destruction and a normal strain. Clin Immunol Immunopathol 1993;66:143
98. Lernmark Å, Baekkeskov S. Islet cell antibodies—theoretical and practical implications. Diabetologia 1981;212:431
99. Lernmark Å, Hägglöf B, Freedman Z, et al. A prospective analysis of antibodies reacting with pancreatic islet cells in insulin-dependent diabetic children. Diabetologia 1981;20:471
100. Baekkeskov S, Aanstoot HJ, Christgau S, et al. Identification of the 64K autoantigen in insulin-dependent diabetes as the GABA-synthesizing enzyme glutamic acid decarboxylase. Nature 1990;347:151
101. Baekkeskov S, Warnock G, Christie M, et al. Revelation of specificity of 64K autoantibodies in IDDM serums by high-resolution 2-D gel electrophoresis. Diabetes 1990;38:1133
102. Karlsen AE, Michaelsen BK, Pedersen JK, et al. Glutamic acid decarboxylase: An autoantigen in insulin-dependent diabetes mellitus. Diabetes Nutr Metab 1992;5:97
103. Palmer JP, Asplin CM, Clemons P, et al. Insulin antibodies in insulin-dependent diabetics before insulin treatment. Science 1983;222:1337
104. Kuglin B, Kolb H, Greenbaum C, et al. The fourth international workshop on the standardisation of insulin autoantibody measurement. Diabetologia 1990;33:638
105. Eisenbarth GS, Jackson GS. Insulin autoimmunity: The rate limiting factor of pre-type 1 diabetes. J Autoimmun 1992;5:214
106. Vardi P, Ziegler AG, Matthews JH, et al. Concentration of insulin autoantibodies at onset of type 1 diabetes: Inverse log-linear correlation with age. Diabetes Care 1988;9:736
107. Pugliese A, Bugawan R, Moromisato R, et al. Two subsets of HLA-DQA1 alleles mark phenotypic variation in levels of insulin autoantibodies in first degree relatives at risk for insulin-dependent diabetes. J Clin Invest 1994;93:2447
108. Gorus FK, Vandewalle CL, Dorchy H, et al. Influence of age on the associations among insulin autoantibodies, islet cell antibodies, and HLA DQA1*0301-DQB1*0302 and siblings of patients with type 1 (insulin-dependent) diabetes mellitus. J Clin Endocrinol Metab 1994;78:1172
109. Hagopian WA, Sanjeevi CB, Kockum I, et al. Glutamate decarboxylase-, insulin- and islet cell-antibodies and HLA typing to detect diabetes in a general population-based study of Swedish children. J Clin Invest 1995;95:1505
110. Vandewalle CL, Decraene T, Schuit FC, et al. Insulin autoantibodies and high titre islet cell antibodies are preferentially associated with the HLA DQA1*0301-DQB1*0302 haplotype at clinical type 1 (insulin-dependent) diabetes mellitus before age 10 years, but not at onset between age 10 and 40 years: The Belgian Diabetes Registry. Diabetologia 1993;36:1155
111. Knip M, Ilonen J, Mustonen A, Åkerblom HK. Evidence of an accelerated B-cell destruction in HLA-Dw3/Dw4 heterozygous children with type 1 (insulin-dependent) diabetes. Diabetologia 1986;29:347
112. Caillat-Zucman A, Garchon H-J, Timsit J, et al. Age-dependent HLA genetic heterogeneity of type 1 insulin-dependent diabetes mellitus. J Clin Invest 1992;90:2242
113. Karjalainen J, Salmela P, Ilonen J, et al. A comparison of childhood and adult type 1 diabetes mellitus. N Engl J Med 1989;320:881
114. Castano L, Ziegler A, Ziegler R, Shoelson S, Eisenbarth GS. Characterization of insulin autoantibodies in relatives of patients with insulin-dependent diabetes mellitus. Diabetes 1993;42:1202
115. Matsushita S, Takahashi K, Motoki M, et al. Allele specificity of structural requirement for peptides bound to HLA-DRB1*0405 and -DRB1*0406 complexes: Implication for the HLA-associated susceptibility to methimazole-induced insulin autoimmune syndrome. J Exp Med 1994;180:873
116. Karlsen AE, Hagopian WA, Grubin CE, et al. Cloning and primary structure of a human islet isoform of glutamic acid decarboxylase from chromosome 10. Proc Natl Acad Sci U S A 1991;88:8337
117. Grubin CE, Daniels T, Toivola B, et al. A novel radioligand binding assay to determine diagnostic accuracy of isoform-specific glutamic acid decarboxylase antibodies in childhood IDDM. Diabetologia 1994;37:344
118. Falorni A, Grubin CE, Takei I, et al. Radioimmunoassay detects the frequent occurrence of autoantibodies to the Mr 65,000 isoform of glutamic acid decarboxylase in Japanese insulin-dependent diabetes. Autoimmunity 1994; 113
119. Falorni A, Örtqvist E, Persson B, Lernmark Å. Radioimmunoassays for glutamic acid decarboxylase (GAD65) and GAD65 autoantibodies using ^{35}S or ^{3}H recombinant human ligands. J Immunol Meth 1995; in press
120. Petersen JS, Hejnaes KR, Moody A, et al. Detection of GAD65 antibodies in diabetes and other autoimmune diseases using a simple radioligand assay. Diabetes 1994;43:459
121. Erdö SL, Joo F, Wolff JR. Immunohistochemical localization of glutamate decarboxylase in the rat oviduct and ovary: Further evidence for non-neural GABA system. Cell Tissue Res 1989;255:431
122. Erdö SL, Wolff JR. Gamma-aminobutyric acid outside the mammalian brain. J Neurochem 1990;54:363
123. Michalik M, Nelson J, Erecinska M. GABA production in rat islets of Langerhans. Diabetes 1993;42:1506
124. Vincent ST, Hökfelt T, Wu J-Y, et al. Immunohistochemical studies of the GABA system in the pancreas. Neuroendocrinology 1983;36:197
125. Gilon P, Bertrand G, Loubatieres-Mariani MM, et al. The influence of γ-aminobutyric acid on hormone release by the mouse and rat endocrine pancreas. Endocrinology 1991;129:2521
126. Kobayashi Y, Kaufman DL, Tobin AJ. Glutamic acid decarboxylase cDNA: Nucleotide sequence encoding as enzymatically active fusion protein. J Neurosci 1987;7:2768
127. Julien J-F, Legay F, Dumas S, et al. Molecular cloning, expression and *in situ* hybridization of rat brain glutamic acid decarboxylase messenger RNA. Neurosci Lett 1987;73:173
128. Bu D-F, Erlander MG, Hitz BC, et al. Two human glutamate decarboxylases, 65-kDa GAD and 67-kDa GAD, are each encoded by a single gene. Proc Natl Acad Sci U S A 1992;89:2115
129. Christgau S, Aanstoot HJ, Schierbeck H, et al. Membrane anchoring of the autoantigen GAD65 to microvesicles in pancreatic β-cells by palmitoylation in the NH_2-terminal domain. J Cell Biol 1992;118:309
130. Shi Y, Veit B, Baekkeskov S. Amino acid residues 24-31 but not palmitoylation of cysteines 30 and 45 are required for membrane anchoring of glutamic acid decarboxylase, GAD65. J Cell Biol 1994;124:927
131. Solimena M, Dirkx R, Jr., Radzynski M, et al. A signal located within amino acids 1-27 of GAD65 is required for its targeting to the Golgi complex region. J Cell Biol 1994;126:331
132. Solimena M, Aggujaro D, Muntzel C, et al. Association of GAD-65, but not of GAD-67, with the Golgi complex of transfected Chinese hamster ovary cells mediated by the N-terminal region. Proc Natl Acad Sci U S A 1993; 90:3073
133. Dirkx R, Jr., Thomas A, Linsong L, et al. Targeting of the 67-kDa isoform of glutamic acid decarboxylase to intracellular organelles is mediated by its interaction with the NH2-terminal region of the 65-kDa isoform of glutamic acid decarboxylase. J Biol Chem 1995;270:2241
134. Christgau S, Schierbeck H, Aanstoot H-J, et al. Pancreatic β cells express two autoantigenic forms of glutamic acid decarboxylase, a 65-kDa hydrophilic form and a 64-kDa amphiphilic form which can be both membrane-bound and soluble. J Biol Chem 1991;286:21257
135. Karlsen AE, Hagopian WA, Petersen JS, et al. Recombinant glutamic acid decarboxylase representing a single isoform expressed in human islets detects IDDM associated 64K autoantibodies. Diabetes 1992;41:1355
136. Petersen JB, Russel S, Marshall MO, et al. Differential expression of glutamic acid decarboxylase in rat and human islets. Diabetes 1993;42:484
137. Hagopian WA, Michelsen B, Karlsen AE, et al. Autoantibodies in IDDM primarily recognize the 65,000-Mr rather than the 67,000-Mr isoform of glutamic acid decarboxylase. Diabetes 1993;42:631
138. Mauch L, Abney CC, Berg H, et al. Characterization of a linear epitope within the human pancreatic 64-kDa glutamic acid decarboxylase and its autoimmune recognition by sera from insulin-dependent diabetes mellitus patients. Eur J Biochem 1993;212:597
139. Seissler J, Amann J, Mauch L, et al. Prevalence of autoantibodies to the 65- and 67-kD isoforms of glutamate decarboxylase in insulin-dependent diabetes mellitus. J Clin Invest 1993;92:1394
140. Velloso LA, Kämpe O, Hallberg A, et al. Demonstration of GAD-65 as the main immunogenic isoform of glutamate decarboxylase in type 1 diabetes and determination of autoantibodies using a radioligand produced by eukaryotic expression. J Clin Invest 1993;91:2084
141. Lühder F, Woltanski K-P, Mauch L, et al. Detection of autoantibodies to the 65KDa isoform of glutamate decarboxylase by radioimmunoassay. Eur J Endocrinol 1994;130:575
142. Yu L, Gianani R, Eisenbarth GS. Quantitation of glutamic acid decarboxylase autoantibody levels in prospectively evaluated relatives of patients with type 1 diabetes. Diabetes 1994;43:1229
143. Richter W, Shi Y, Baekkeskov S. Autoreactive epitopes defined by diabetes-associated human monoclonal antibodies are localized in the middle and C-terminal domains of the smaller form of glutamate decarboxylase. Proc Natl Acad Sci U S A 1993;90:2832
144. Richter W, Scißler J, Wolfahrt S, Scherbaum WA. Human monoclonal islet specific autoantibodies share features of islet cell and 64 kDa antibodies. Diabetologia 1993;36:785
145. Richter W, Mertens T, Schoel B, et al. Sequence homology of the disease-associated autoantigen glutamate decarboxylase with Coxsackie B4-2C protein and heat shock protein 60 mediates no molecular mimicry of autoantibodies. J Exp Med 1994;180:721
146. Ujihara N, Daw K, Gianani R, et al. Identification of glutamic acid decarboxylase autoantibody heterogeneity and epitope regions in type I diabetes. Diabetes 1994;43:968
147. Kim J, Namchuck M, Bugawan T, et al. Higher autoantibody levels and recognition of a linear NH_2-terminal epitope in the autoantigen GAD65, distinguish stiff-man syndrome from insulin-dependent diabetes mellitus. J Exp Med 1994;180:595
148. Daw K, Powers AC. Two distinct glutamic acid decarboxylase auto-antibody specificities in IDDM target difference epitopes. Diabetes 1995;44:216
149. Li L, Hagopian WA, Brashear HR, et al. Identification of autoantibody epitopes of glutamic acid decarboxylase in Stiff-Man syndrome patients. J Immunol 1994;152:930
150. Solimena M, De Camilli P. Autoimmunity to glutamic acid decarboxylase (GAD) in Stiff Man syndrome and insulin-dependent diabetes mellitus. Trends Neurosci 1991;14:452

151. Butler MH, Solimena M, Dirkx R Jr, et al. Identification of a dominant epitope of glutamic acid decarboxylase (GAD-65) recognized by autoantibodies in Stiff-Man syndrome. J Exp Med 1993;178:2097
152. Velloso LA, Winqvist O, Gustafsson J, et al. Autoantibodies against a novel 51 kDa islet antigen and glutamate decarboxylase isoforms in autoimmune polyendocrine syndrome type I. Diabetologia 1994;37:61
153. Martino G, Tappaz M, Braghi S, et al. Autoantibodies to glutamic acid decarboxylase (GAD) detected by an immunotrapping enzyme activity assay: Relation to insulin-dependent diabetes mellitus and islet cell antibodies. J Autoimmun 1991;4:915
154. Nemni R, Braghi S, Natali-Sore MG, et al. Autoantibodies of glutamic acid decarboxylase in palatal myoclonus and epilepsy. Ann Neurol 1994;36:665
155. Atkinson MA, Kaufman DL, Campbell L, et al. Response of peripheral-blood mononuclear cells to glutamate decarboxylase in insulin-dependent diabetes. Lancet 1992;339:458
156. Atkinson M, Bowman M, Campbell L, et al. Cellular immunity to determinant common to glutamate decarboxylase and Coxsackie virus in insulin dependent diabetes. J Clin Invest 1994;94:2125
157. Armstrong NW, Jones DB. Epitopes of GAD 65 in insulin-dependent diabetes mellitus. Lancet 1994;343:1607
158. Lohmann T, Leslie RDG, Hawa M, et al. Immunodominant epitopes of glutamic acid decarboxylase 65 and 67 in insulin-dependent diabetes mellitus. Lancet 1994;343:1607
159. Harrison LC, Honeyman MC, Deaizpurua HJ, et al. Inverse regulation between humoral and cellular immunity to glutamic acid decarboxylase in subjects at risk of insulin-dependent diabetes. Lancet 1993;341:1365
160. Serjeantson SW, Kohonen-Corish MRJ, Rowley MJ, et al. Antibodies to glutamic acid decarboxylase are associated with HLA-DR genotypes in both Australians and Asians with type 1 (insulin-dependent) diabetes mellitus. Diabetologia 1992;35:996
161. Rabin DU, Pleasic SM, Palmer-Crocker R, Shapiro JA. Cloning and expression of IDDM-specific human autoantigens. Diabetes 1992;41:183
162. Rabin DU, Pleasic SM, Shapiro JA, et al. Islet cell antigen 512 is a diabetes-specific islet autoantigen related to protein tyrosine phosphatases. J Immunol 1994;152:3183
163. Lu J, Notkins AL, Lan MS. Isolation, sequence and expression of a novel mouse brain cDNA, mIA-2, and its relatedness to members of the protein tyrosine phosphatase family. Biochem Biophys Res Commun 1994;204:930
164. Lan MS, Lu J, Goto Y, Notkins AL. Molecular cloning and identification of a receptor-type protein tyrosine phosphatase, IA-2, from human insulinoma. DNA Cell Biol 1994;13:505
165. Pietropaolo M, Castano L, Babu S, et al. Islet cell autoantigen 69KDa (ICA69): Molecular cloning and characterization of a novel diabetes-associated autoantigen. J Clin Invest 1993;92:359
166. Krokowski M, Caillat-Zucman S, Timsit J, et al. Anti-bovine serum albumin antibodies: Genetic heterogeneity and clinical relevance in adult-onset IDDM. Diabetes Care 1995;18:170
167. Karjalainen J, Martin JM, Knip M, et al. A bovine albumin peptide as a possible trigger of insulin-dependent diabetes mellitus. N Engl J Med 1992;327:302
168. Atkinson MA, Bowman MA, Kao K-J, et al. Lack of immune responsiveness to bovine serum albumin in insulin-dependent diabetes. N Engl J Med 1993;329:1853
169. Christie MR, Tun RYM, Lo SSS, et al. Antibodies to GAD and tryptic fragments of islet 64K antigen as distinct markers for development of IDDM. Diabetes 1992;41:782
170. Christie MR, Hollands JA, Brown TJ, et al. Detection of pancreatic islet 64,000 Mr autoantigens in insulin-dependent diabetes distinct from glutamate decarboxylase. J Clin Invest 1993;92:240
171. Christie MR, Genovese S, Cassidy D, et al. Antibodies to islet 37K antigen, but not to glutamate decarboxylase, discriminate rapid progression to IDDM in endocrine autoimmunity. Diabetes 1994;43:1254
172. Baekkeskov S, Nielsen JH, Marner B, et al. Autoantibodies in newly diagnosed diabetic children immunoprecipitate human pancreatic islet cell proteins. Nature 1982;298:167
173. Roep BO, Kallan AA, Hazenbos WLW, et al. T-cell reactivity to 38 kD insulin-secretory-granule protein in patients with recent-onset type 1 diabetes. Lancet 1991;337:1439
174. Pak CY, Cha CY, Rajotte RV, et al. Human pancreatic islet cell specific 38 kilodalton autoantigen identified by cytomegalovirus-induced monoclonal islet cell autoantibody. Diabetologia 1990;33:569
175. Serreze DV, Leiter EH, Kuff EL, et al. Molecular mimicry between insulin and retroviral antigen p73: Development of cross-reactive autoantibodies in sera of NOD and C57BL/KsJ db/db mice. Diabetes 1988;37:351
176. Karounos DG, Wolinsky JS, Thomas JW. Monoclonal antibody to rubella virus capsid protein recognizes a β-cell antigen. J Immunol 1993;150:3080
177. Karounos DG, Nell LJ, Thomas JW. Autoantibodies present at onset of type 1 diabetes recognize multiple islet cell antigens. Autoimmunity 1990; 6:79
178. Thomas NM, Ginsberg-Fellner F, McEvoy RC. Strong association between diabetes and displacement of mouse anti-rat insulinoma cell monoclonal antibody by human serum *in vitro*. Diabetes 1990;39:1203
179. Kaufman DJ, Erlander MG, Clare-Salzler M, et al. Autoimmunity to two forms of glutamate decarboxylase in insulin-dependent diabetes mellitus. J Clin Invest 1992;89:283
180. Hou J, Said C, Franchi D, et al. Antibodies to glutamic acid decarboxylase and P2-C peptides in sera from Coxsackie virus B4-infected mice and IDDM patients. Diabetes 1994;43:1260

Diabetes Mellitus, edited by Derek LeRoith, Simeon I. Taylor, and Jerrold M. Olefsky. Lippincott–Raven Publishers, Philadelphia © 1996.

CHAPTER 32

Autoantibodies and the Disease Process of Insulin-Dependent Diabetes Mellitus

CARLA J. GREENBAUM AND JERRY P. PALMER

Within the past two decades investigators have established that type I (insulin-dependent) diabetes mellitus (IDDM) occurs as a result of autoimmune destruction of pancreatic β-cells. This destructive process may occur over a long period of time before the development of clinical symptoms from hyperglycemia. During the period of time in which the individual is clinically healthy, antibodies to pancreatic antigens and abnormalities in pancreatic β-cell function often are detected. Investigators have capitalized on this information, using antibodies and β-cell function assessments to predict who will develop clinical IDDM, with the goal of preventing the disease in these high-risk subjects. In this chapter, we review the use of antibodies for prediction of IDDM, including discussion of measurement techniques and usefulness of the tests among various population groups.

Islet Cell Antibodies

In 1974, it was reported that when serum from patients with polyendocrine disease and IDDM was applied to a section of pancreas and tagged with a fluorescent second antibody to human immunoglobulin G (IgG), fluorescence could be seen throughout the pancreatic islet.[1] Termed islet cell antibodies (ICAs), since it was not clear what the antigen was, ICAs were subsequently measured in patients with IDDM and later in relatives of IDDM patients.[2–4] From current studies of IDDM patients, it has been shown that ICAs are present in approximately 80% of these subjects. The natural history of ICAs after diagnosis is such that in many patients, ICAs diminish over time in association with diminishing islet function. In patients clinically diagnosed with non–insulin-dependent diabetes (NIDDM) or gestational diabetes, the presence of ICAs appears to predict the subsequent need for insulin treatment, suggesting that ICAs are associated with acute destruction of the pancreatic β-cell. Nevertheless, ICAs are not β-cell specific, and despite two decades of study, the antigen (or antigens) for ICA are still unknown.

Though all ICA antibodies are of the IgG class, it is likely that reaction to more than one islet antigen causes certain sera to be ICA-positive. There are reports that two distinct ICA staining patterns can be seen:

1. The fluorescence appears predominantly on β-cells (β-cell–selective, or *restricted ICAs*).
2. The entire islet fluoresces (*whole-islet ICAs*).

It has been suggested that a major antigen for restricted ICAs is glutamic acid decarboxylase (GAD) (see below), as preabsorption with GAD can block some ICA reactions.[5] Nonetheless, in newly diagnosed IDDM subjects, those with antibodies to GAD are not exclusively a subset of those who are ICA-positive. Another antigen is probably a ganglioside, considering that preabsorption with GM2-1 blocks some ICA binding,[6] and the antiganglioside antibody GM2-1 has been measured in two-thirds of a small number of ICA-positive relatives of patients with IDDM.[7] In nonobese diabetic (NOD) mice, both diabetes onset and β-cell destruction are associated with a significant decrease in GM2-1,[8] and both diabetes-prone and resistant Bio Breeding (BB) rats express GM2-1, a finding that parallels the presence of ICAs in these strains.[9]

Islet Cell Antibody Assay

The assay requires a supply of snap frozen pancreas processed into cryostat sections of 4–5 mm thickness. Although human type O pancreas from organ donors is used most often, some laboratories use pancreas from other species. It is important that the pancreas have a sufficient number of easily identified islets per field. Serum can be preabsorbed with rat liver powder to remove the nonspecific binding and then applied to the section and incubated; laboratories report incubation times ranging from 20 minutes to overnight. After the specimens are washed, fluorescein isothiocyanate-labeled antihuman IgG is added. The slides are then read and evaluated on the basis of the fluorescence of the islet. Because of the difficulties in determining immunofluorescence, it is imperative that the slides be read masked and that both positive and negative control sera be used with each assay. Reproducibility difficulties often occur at low levels of fluorescence. False-positives can occur in the presence of other antibodies in the subjects' serum (e.g., antinuclear antibodies), and false-negatives when the background exocrine tissue has a high degree of fluorescence.

Possibly because of the mixture of antigens involved in the ICA reaction or because of the variability among pancreases, the ICA assay has been difficult to standardize. Under the auspices of the Juvenile Diabetes Foundation International and the Immunology of Diabetes Workshops, a series of workshops to work toward standardization of ICA assays worldwide was begun about a decade ago. A reference serum was set as 80 JDF (Juvenile Diabetes Foundation) units and made available to participating laboratories. Laboratories now performing the ICA assay serially dilute the JDF standard serum, determine the end-point titer at each point, and construct a standard curve. The dilution at which test serum remain fluorescent can then be compared to the standard curve and expressed in JDF units. This quantification of ICA measurements using JDF units has improved the precision and concordance of laboratories worldwide; however, some technical difficulties persist. The University of Florida at Gainesville, under the auspices of the International Diabetes Workshop, has established a yearly proficiency test, available to any ICA laboratory, to evaluate the sensitivity, specificity, and validity of its individual assay.

Insulin Autoantibodies

Defined as antibodies that bind to insulin in subjects that are insulin-naive, insulin autoantibodies (IAAs) were initially described in 1963 by Pav et al.,[10] who found IAAs in 34% of a mixed group of type I and type II untreated patients and in 4% of controls. These data and other scattered reports were largely ignored until 1983, when Palmer et al.[11] reported that at least 18% of newly diagnosed, untreated subjects with IDDM had IAAs. More recent studies of larger groups have indicated that approximately 60% of newly diagnosed IDDM patients are IAA-positive. Unlike that for ICAs, the IAA antigen is known (insulin), and it is β-cell–specific. Nonetheless, it is not known why IAAs develop.

Insulin Autoantibody Assay

During the 1980s, there appeared conflicting reports on the prevalence of IAAs in various subject groups, the association of IAAs with the clinical course of IDDM, and the predictive value of IAAs for the development of clinical disease. It subsequently became apparent that many of the differences in these studies were due to the different methods used to measure IAAs.[12] IAAs were measured by either a fluid-phase radioimmunoassay (RIA) or a solid-phase enzyme-linked immunoabsorbent assay (ELISA). As with ICA assays, International Diabetes Workshops were held to compare IAA assays from numerous laboratories. The Fourth International Workshop on the Standardization of Insulin Autoantibody Measurement compared results from RIA and ELISA laboratories on sera from newly diagnosed patients, nondiabetic subjects who subsequently developed IDDM, first-degree relatives of IDDM patients, and normal controls. Although both techniques had a very low frequency of IAA in control sera, laboratories using RIA methods found a much higher percentage of sera from newly diagnosed patients and nondiabetic individuals who later developed diabetes to be IAA-positive than did laboratories that used ELISA methods[13] (Fig. 32-1).

It is not surprising that these methods appear to measure different antibodies. In a solid-phase assay, a conformational epitope required for IAA recognition may be lost by insulin coating of ELISA plates. Additionally, RIA assays could be expected to measure antibodies of higher affinity than ELISA assays.

These workshop data strongly suggest that IAAs measured by RIA methods are more disease-related than those measured by ELISA and therefore should be used to predict subsequent IDDM or to assign individual risk.[13] It is important to note, however, that the ELISA laboratories were very specific in their measurements (i.e., very few controls were positive), and that they also measure antibodies in relatives of IDDM subjects, although these are distinct from those seen by RIA laboratories. The significance of the

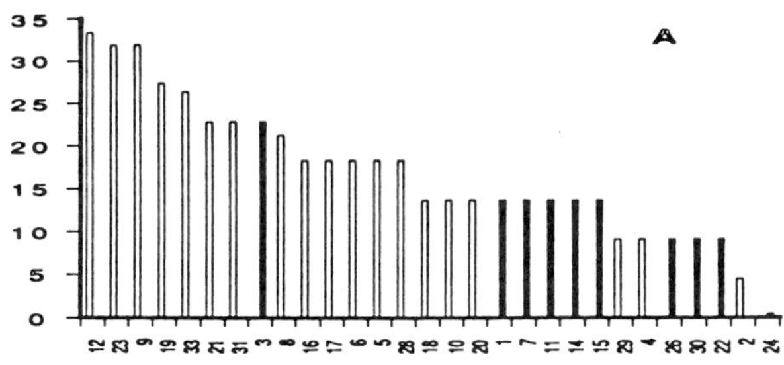

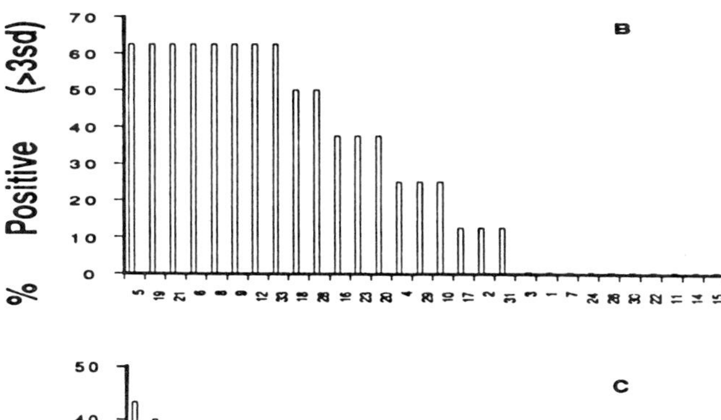

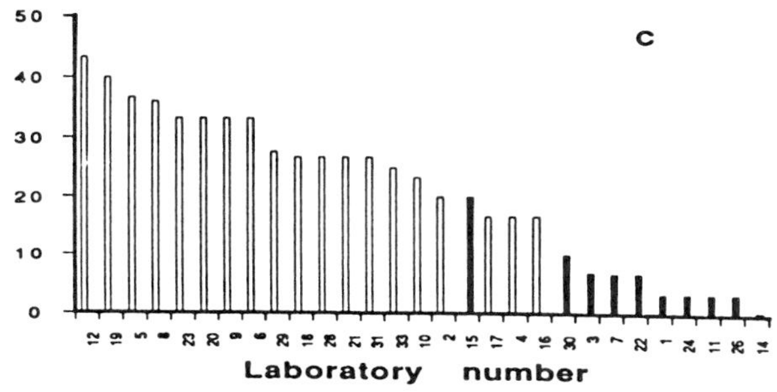

FIGURE 32-1. Percentage of IAA-positive (> 3 SD from mean of controls) sera from first-degree relatives of IDDM patient probands (*A*, n = 22), healthy subjects who later developed IDDM (*B*, n = 8) and newly diagnosed IDDM patients (*C*, n = 30) in 19 RIA (□) and 10 ELISA (■) laboratories. ELISA = enzyme-linked immunosorbent assay; RIA = radioimmunoassay. (Reproduced with permission from Greenbaum CJ, Palmer JP, Kuglin B, et al. Insulin autoantibodies measured by radioimmunoassay methodology are more related to insulin-dependent diabetes mellitus than those measured by enzyme-linked immunoabsorbent assay: Results of the Fourth International Workshop on the Standardization of Insulin Autoantibody Measurement. J Clin Endocrinol Metab 1992;74: 1040.)

ELISA-measured IAAs is currently unknown; however, it is possible that these antibodies form preferentially in patients who are able to arrest the immune destructive process.

There are at least two different methods used to measure IAAs by RIA. Despite the methodologic differences between these two RIA assays (Table 32-1), when one compares results expressed as standard deviations from a control population, there is good correlation between these two methods. A major reason for this correlation is that both use a displacement step in which much of the nonspecific binding is removed. The importance of a displacement step in an RIA assay is also illustrated by IAA measurements in subjects with thyroid disease. It has been reported that a large number of persons with thyroid disease are IAA-positive; however, when a cold displacement step is added to IAA determination, removing much of the nonspecific binding, many apparently IAA-positive thyroid patients become IAA-negative.[14]

TABLE 32-1. Comparison Between Two RIA Methods for Insulin Autoantibody Assays

	Method A	Method B
Amount of test sera	160 λ	600 λ
Acid charcoal extraction	Yes	No
Amount of labeled insulin	20,000 cpm	10,000 cpm
Incubation time	Overnight	7 days
γ-counter time	3 min	9 min

Glutamic Acid Decarboxylase

In 1982, antibodies to a 64-kd islet protein in IDDM patients were identified by immunoprecipitation of radiolabeled human islet proteins with IDDM sera.[15] At the time of diagnosis approximately 80% of IDDM patients had antibodies to the 64-kd antigen, but these antibodies were not present in patients with other autoimmune disorders or in healthy controls.[16] These antibodies were subsequently found in subjects at risk for clinical IDDM[17] as well as in animal strains that develop diabetes.[18,19]

In 1990, the 64kd antigen was shown to have glutamic acid decarboxylase (GAD) activity.[20] Antibodies to GAD were initially described in stiff man syndrome (SMS), a rare neurologic disorder characterized by progressive rigidity due to impaired gamma–amino butyric acid (GABA) neurotransmission. GAD is the enzyme required for GABA synthesis and is expressed in neurons of the central nervous system, in pancreatic islets, and in the testes and ovaries. All SMS patients with GAD antibodies are ICA-positive, and about one-third of these also have IDDM. A study by Baekkeskov et al.[15] equating GAD with the 64-kd antigen demonstrated (1) that antibodies to GAD from IDDM and SMS patients immunoprecipitated islet proteins that migrated with islet 64-kd antigen, and (2) that IDDM patient sera precipitated GAD enzyme activity from islet and brain extracts.

Important data from animal studies have pointed to GAD as possibly the key antigen relevant to the IDDM disease process. Simultaneous reports by two groups[21,22] indicate that antibody and T-cell proliferative responses to GAD precede proliferation to other antigens and occur as early as 4 weeks of age in the NOD mouse, just when insulitis is first apparent. Early injection of GAD produced tolerance in these animals and prevented both IDDM development and subsequent T-cell responses to other antigens.

Two genes for GAD have been identified (*GAD1* and *GAD2*), with about 65% amino acid sequence identity.[23,24] Part of the amino acid sequence shared by both forms of GAD is similar to the P2-C protein of the Cocksackie virus. The possibility of molecular mimicry between GAD and the Cocksackie virus has led to speculation that the virus could be responsible for initiation of autoimmunity in IDDM. Others have evidence, however, that this linear sequence homology is less relevant than similarity in conformational epitopes.[25]

In humans, *GAD1* is on chromosome 2 and it is transcribed into a 3.7-Kb mRNA with a long untranslated sequence at the 3′ end. *GAD2*, on chromosome 10, has a 5.6-Kb mRNA with a long untranslated region at the 5′ end. *GAD2* mRNA is present in human brain and islet tissues.[26] It is translated into GAD65 (the 64-kd protein) and is predominantly found in the human β-cell, where it is associated with synaptic-like membrane vesicles. *GAD1* mRNA has been reported only in human brain tissue. It is translated into GAD67, which generally is not detected in human islets.[26] There are marked species differences, however. In the rat and mouse both *GAD1* and *GAD2* mRNA are found in the islet as well as the brain, and mouse islets have a predominance of GAD67[27,28] (Fig. 32-2).

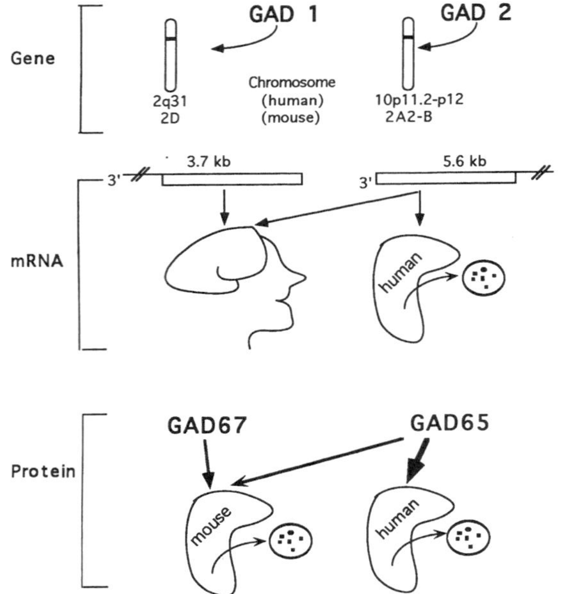

Figure 32-2. The *GAD1* gene is found on human chromosome 2. It has an untranslated 3′ end. *GAD1* mRNA is found in the human brain. *GAD1* is translated to GAD67 protein, which is present in mouse islets. The *GAD2* gene is found on human chromosome 10. It has an untranslated 5′ end. *GAD2* mRNA is present in human brain and islets. It is translated into GAD65 protein, which is present in human and (to a lesser extent) mouse islets.

Glutamic Acid Decarboxylase Assay

Although initial studies have pointed to the association between IDDM and GAD by measuring enzyme activity, this sort of assay has not been sensitive enough to detect the presence of GAD antibodies in every case. Assays that measure GAD antibodies by other techniques were therefore developed. In the recently released report of the First International Glutamic Acid Decarboxylase Antibody Workshop, the majority of assays that immunoprecipitated radiolabeled GAD had a high degree of sensitivity and specificity. In the immunoprecipitated radiolabeled GAD assay, the antigen-antibody complex is precipitated by protein A-Sepharose and quantified by scintillation counting or by sodium dodecyl sulfate-polyacrilamide gel electrophoresis (SDS-PAGE) and fluorography. In contrast, enzyme-linked immunosorbent assays and assays using immunofluorescence were generally less sensitive.[29] Recombinant technology promises to produce a large amount of specific antigen for continued development of assays. Studies using recombinant proteins have shown that IDDM sera preferentially recognize GAD65 over GAD67.

Although the number of subjects studied remains much smaller than the number screened for ICAs or IAAs, when measured by immunoprecipitant assays with recombinant protein, GAD antibodies appear to be present in up to 80% of newly diagnosed white IDDM subjects.[30–33] In Asian IDDM patients, the prevalence of GAD antibodies appear to be much lower, although the number of subjects studied is small.[34] Importantly, GAD antibodies appear to be stable after diagnosis, such that patients with IDDM of >10 years' duration continue to have GAD antibodies present in their sera,[30,35] indicating that GAD antibodies remain despite the absence of functional β-cells. Similarly, analysis of sera samples from up to 10 years before the onset of IDDM indicates that once GAD antibodies are produced, their levels do not fluctuate.[31] One report indicates that higher GAD antibodytiters are present in subjects with thyroid disease in association with IDDM[36]; another indicates that GAD titers are higher and more prevalent in women.[30] GAD-antibody–positive sera also have been reported in patients whose clinical presentation was of NIDDM,[37] and although GAD antibodies were found to be absent in black NIDDM subjects with diabetic ketoacidosis,[38] it has been suggested that GAD positivity may identify NIDDM subjects who will subsequently require insulin treatment.[37]

Other Antibodies

ICA, IAA, and GAD antibodies can be distinguished from a second group of antibodies that have been reported to be associated with the IDDM disease process in that these three antibodies have been studied extensively and reported on by a large number of investigators (Table 32-2). In contrast, the second group of antibodies (discussed below) have been less well characterized; some have been investigated by only one or a few research groups.

The identification of GAD as the major 64-kd antigen involved in IDDM temporarily obscured research on the presence of other proteins of similar molecular weight, which subsequently have been identified as autoantigens in IDDM. Heat-shock proteins (HSPs) of

Table 32-2. Antibody Comparisons*

	ICAs	IAAs	64-kd
Year of first report	1974	1983	1982
Antigen	Still unknown, likely multiple antigens including, GAD and GM2-1	Insulin	GAD (reported 1990), possibly others
Assay methods	Immunofluorescence of sera on islets	RIA	Immunoprecipitation
% of newly diagnosed cases of IDDM in whites with this one antibody	~80%	~60%	~80%
Risk of relative acquiring IDDM if relative is positive for only this one antibody	Moderately high	Very low	Unknown
Persistence in IDDM patients after diagnosis	Unusual	N/A[†]	Yes

*Comparisons of ICAs, IAAs, and GAD antibodies.
[†]Assay cannot distinguish from antibodies that develop from insulin treatment.
GAD = glutamic acid decarboxylase; IAAs = insulin autoantibodies; ICAs = islet cell antibodies; IDDM = insulin-dependent diabetes mellitus; RIA = radioimmunoassay; GM2-1 = monosialoganglioside 2-1.

this molecular weight are thought to be involved in arthritis, systemic lupus erythematosus, and the immune response in general. In NOD mice, HSP65 has been identified as a potential antigen, and when injected into prediabetic animals, it can prevent disease.[39] Antibodies to HSP65 have not been demonstrated, however, in IDDM patient sera, and therefore their relevance to human disease is unclear.

Antibodies to bovine serum albumin (BSA) have been reported to be associated with IDDM,[40] and a portion of BSA, termed the *ABBOS peptide,* has sequence homology with another protein of similar molecular weight, ICA69. ICA69 was initially identified by screening cDNA libraries with IDDM patient sera.[41] Its expression in islet cells increases after exposure to interferon gamma. It has been proposed that early exposure to cow's milk could sensitize a person to BSA. A subsequent pancreatic viral infection would then increase the interferon gamma production and ICA69 expression with its peptide, with homology to the ABBOS peptide. This peptide then elicits a response by the T-cells, already primed by their exposure to BSA, which leads to β-cell destruction. Although this hypothesis is interesting, another group failed to find an association between IDDM and anti-BSA or -ABBOS antibodies.[42]

Another protein of similar molecular weight, but distinct from GAD and BSA, has been reported that can be immunoprecipitated by antibodies from IDDM patient sera.[43] Christie et al.[44] reported that partial tryptic proteolysis of a 64-kd antigen generated fragments of 50, 40, and 37 kd. Although antibodies to the 50-kd fragment precipitate GAD enzyme activity and are blocked with recombinant GAD65, the 40- and 37-kd fragments do not precipitate this activity, indicating that these fragments are from a distinct, unidentified protein (37-kd antigen). This same group reported in a previous study that antibodies to the 37-kd fragment are more closely associated with IDDM than those to the 64-kd antigen.[45]

Other antibodies reported to be associated with IDDM include those that bind a human islet protein of approximately 30 kd, which appears to be chymotrypsinogen. These antibodies were found in 4 of 16 subjects with newly diagnosed IDDM.[46] Carboxypeptidase-H, which is responsible for processing proinsulin to insulin, has been identified as a 38-kd protein precipitated by IDDM patient sera.[47] A 38-kd protein that may be distinct from carboxypeptidase-H has been identified by antibody and T-cell responses in some newly diagnosed patients, but has not been further characterized.[48,49] An antigen of approximately 52 kd and probably located in secretory granules has been reported to have bound antibodies in the sera of 58% of newly diagnosed IDDM patients.[50] Interestingly, this antigen is also recognized by a monoclonal antibody to the rubella virus, suggesting molecular mimicry.[51] Another antigen approximately 118 kd in human islet cells (~ 155 kd in the rat) is thought to be a glycoprotein. Antibodies to this antigen have been reported in approximately 90% of a sample of 300 IDDM patients and in only 4% of 1600 controls.[52] These antibodies, however, are widely present in first-degree relatives of IDDM patients, implying that these antibodies are not specific enough to be used in a screening program (R. McEvoy, M.D., personal communication, 1993).

Predictive Value of Antibodies for the Development of Clinical Insulin-Dependent Diabetes Mellitus

Because clinical IDDM has a prevalence of only approximately 0.3% in the general population of whites, in practical terms our ability to prevent the disease in this group will depend on our ability to define subjects at high risk for IDDM. Investigators therefore have concentrated on studying family members of IDDM patients because the prevalence rate of diabetes among this group is at least 10 times greater than in the general population. Nonetheless, without a completely safe, inexpensive, and effective intervention, prevention efforts administered to all family members will remain an impracticality. Additional screening tests also are needed to identify high risk subjects.

To date, the most effective screening test for family members to determine their risk of acquiring IDDM is the cumbersome ICA assay. Cross-sectional analysis indicates that approximately 5% of family members are ICA-positive. Relatives who share human lymphocyte antigen type with their affected family member are more likely to be ICA-positive. Long-term prospective studies of family members confirm that many of the ICA-positive relatives will develop IDDM. Data from several independent studies and pooled data have shown that ICA titer is an important determinant of risk: Subjects with ICA titers >80 JDF units have a 40–50% risk of developing IDDM within 5 years as determined by life table analysis (Fig. 32-3). In contrast, family members who remain ICA-negative on prospective testing have a markedly diminished risk of developing the disease (estimated as the same as that of the general population). The ICA test is therefore useful as an initial screen in family members because the use of this test alone will identify persons with about a 50/50 chance of developing IDDM within 5 years. The importance of ICA as a screening test is underscored by its use to select relatives for intervention for both the European Nicotinamide Diabetes Intervention Trial (ENDIT) and the United States Diabetes Prevention Trial (DPT-1).

It is not known whether the 50% of ICA-positive relatives who do not develop IDDM within 5 years will remain free of disease throughout their lifetime, or whether the ICA positivity marks them as being at high risk forever. A small number of ICA-positive family members have been followed prospectively for ten years and still remain free of clinical disease, although some have abnormal pancreatic function.[53] It is possible that this abnormal pancreatic function will become clinically relevant only in later years, when insulin resistance increases insulin demand and these subjects appear to manifest NIDDM.

Those ICA-positive relatives who are also IAA-positive have an increased risk of developing IDDM compared to those who are only ICA-positive.[54] The utility of the IAA test, however, in screening relatives for risk for IDDM has been questioned. In the Diabetes Prevention Trial under way in the United States, although IAAs are being measured, this measurement is not being used as a screening test to identify subjects in the highest risk group. The IAA measurement is being used instead to identify subjects at intermediate risk: that is, ICA-positive subjects whose β-cell function is not severely impaired are classified in this group if they are IAA-positive.

Importantly, however, relatives who are IAA-positive alone have only a slightly increased risk of developing IDDM[54] and do not appear to have any abnormalities in pancreatic function compared to relatives who are both ICA- and IAA-negative.[55] This group of relatives may represent persons in whom the autoimmune process has stopped, and thus study of this group may be of great utility in the understanding of the pathophysiology of the disease. IAA measurements also may be used as a measure of effect of therapy in subjects participating in intervention trials. In a pilot study of insulin treatment to prevent IDDM in high-risk first-degree relatives, IAA values rose in some subjects who did not acquire IDDM and fell in those in whom intervention failed (R. Jackson, M.D., personal communication, 1994). These observations will be (i.e., the ongoing Diabetes Prevention Trial Type I) tested in investigations in larger intervention studies.

Because most studies of the natural history of IDDM were done before the availability of an assay for GAD antibodies, few data are available to discern how useful GAD testing alone will be as a screening test for risk in relatives of IDDM patients. Interestingly, the very high levels of GAD antibody seen in patients with polyglandular autoimmune syndrome or SMS is not associated with a high incidence of IDDM.[56] It is possible that when the immune system's response to GAD creates high levels of antibodies, as it does in SMS, it does not create the cellular immune response necessary for IDDM. With the availability of recombinant

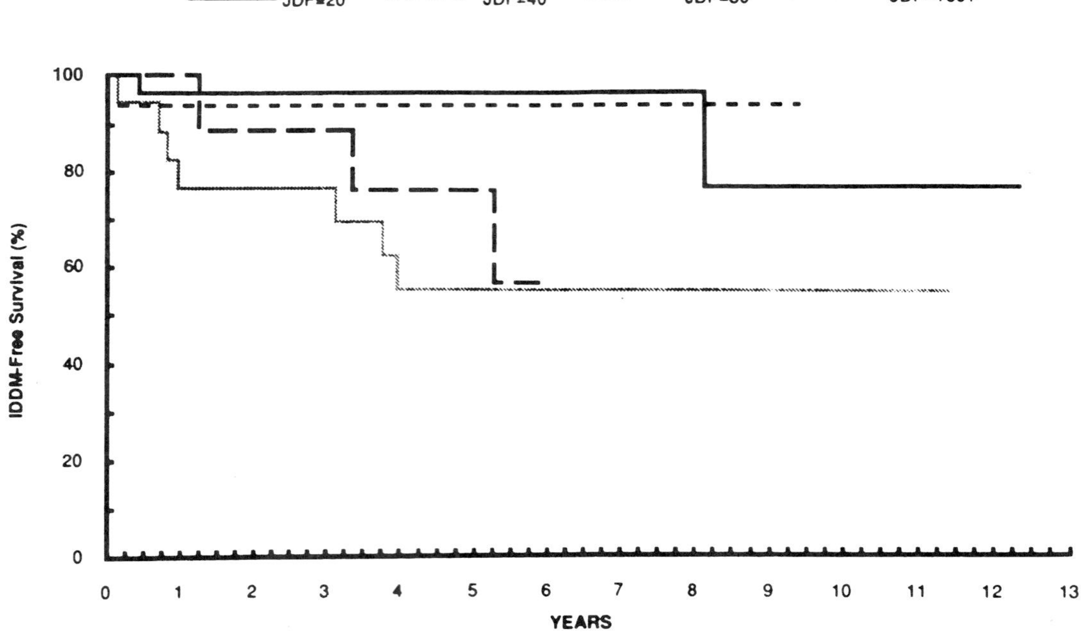

Figure 32-3. Probability of remaining IDDM-free stratified by JDF titers for relatives who are IAA-negative. (Reproduced with permission from Krischer JP, Schatz D, Riley WJ, et al. Insulin and islet cell autoantibodies as time-dependent covariates in the development of insulin-dependent diabetes: A prospective study in relatives. J Clin Endocrinol Metab 1993;77:743.)

GAD, it is possible that assays with good reproducibility, sensitivity, and specificity will become widely available, and when sufficient data are accumulated, the GAD assay could replace the ICA assay as an initial screening test. For now, however, the primary utility of GAD in determining risk of IDDM will be in association with testing for other antibodies. For example, ICA relatives that also are GAD-positive have a higher risk of developing IDDM than those that are ICA-positive alone.[45,57] It may be, however, that there is nothing particular about GAD in terms of the increased risk over ICA positivity alone. Rather, it is likely that relatives positive for more than one β-cell or islet antibody of any specificity are in a higher risk group. In a recently published prospective study of ICA-positive relatives,[57] 36 had ICA alone, of which 3% acquired IDDM. In contrast, 16% of ICA- and GAD-positive relatives and 67% of ICA and 37-kd–positive relatives developed IDDM. IDDM developed in 42% of ICA-, GAD-, and IAA-positive subjects and in 100% of ICA, GAD, and 37-kd–positive individuals. The concept that combinations of antibodies are better predictors of IDDM than any one or two individual tests needs further evaluation.

As stated above, for practical reasons investigators have focused on predicting who will get IDDM among the population of relatives of IDDM patients. It is important to keep in mind, however, that most people who develop IDDM have no family history of the disease (Fig. 32-4). The assumption has been made that the disease in these two groups does not differ, and that choosing family members is essentially a "free" genetic screening test. According to this hypothesis, antibody positivity in persons from the general population should confer the same risk as it does in antibody-positive relatives. This hypothesis assumes that islet-relevant antibodies occur only in subjects who carry the genetic background for development of IDDM. Rowe et al.[58] reported that 69 (1.7%) of approximately 4000 high school students in Washington State without a family history of IDDM were ICA-positive. In several students with multiple antibodies, IDDM developed, suggesting that antibody-positive subjects from the general population are at the same risk of developing IDDM as relatives. Also in support of equivalent risk was a study of ICA-positive Florida school children.[59] The risk of IDDM development in ICA-positive children without a family history of diabetes was found to be 28% at 5 years, compared to a 38% 5-year risk in ICA-positive relatives. Several studies, however, indicate that ICA positivity in the general population has a higher rate than the prevalence of IDDM, thus arguing that many ICA-positive persons with no family history of the disease will never develop IDDM. Whether the ICA-positive tests in subjects who do not develop IDDM represent a group of

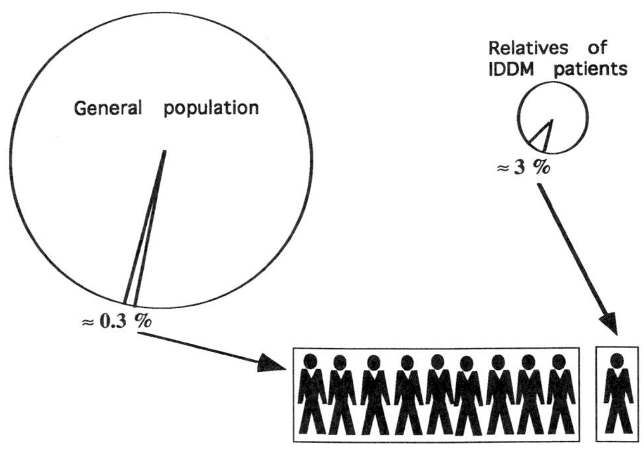

Figure 32-4. Although approximately 3% of relatives will develop IDDM, because the pool of relatives is much smaller than the pool of the remainder of the population, only 1 of every 10 newly diagnosed persons with IDDM will have had a relative with the disease. The remaining nine IDDM patients will have no family history of the disease, for although the risk in this group is low (0.3%), it is multiplied by the large size of the general population pool.

persons with an arrested autoimmune process, or whether these tests are true false-positives, needs further investigation. It is likely that many healthy individuals have low levels of circulating autoantibodies; by increasing the threshold of positivity in the ICA test, these persons might no longer be identified as being at risk for IDDM. Further investigation on the predictive value of antibody screening in the general population is needed.

Summary

Antibodies to ICAs can be identified in the sera of subjects throughout the natural history of the diabetes disease process. Although these antibodies are not the effectors of β-cell destruction (a role ascribed to the cellular arm of the immune system), they have proven utility in identifying individuals at risk of developing clinical IDDM. The ICA assay is currently used as a first screening test in relatives of IDDM patients for initial identification of those subjects at highest risk. Because the GAD antibody assay may prove to be easier to perform, it may replace the ICA assay as an initial screening test in the near future. At this time, both GAD and IAA measurements are generally used only in conjunction with the ICA test. It is likely that assays for other antibodies that have reported associations with IDDM will be further developed when their measurements are proved to be cheaper and more easily performed than ICA. At that time, it is probable that a combination of antibody tests will be used to identify relatives in whom there is a high risk of IDDM development. The utility of antibody screening in the general population awaits the development of such tests and the demonstration that effective preventive therapy is available to treat subjects who have a high risk of acquiring the disease.

Acknowledgments

This work was supported in part by the Medical Research Service of the Department of Veterans Affairs and by National Institutes of Health grants DK17047 and DK02456.

References

1. Bottazzo G, Lorin-Christensen A, Doniach D. Islet cell antibodies in diabetes mellitus with autoimmune polyendocrine deficiencies. Lancet 1974;2:1279
2. Bruining GJ, Molenaar JL, Grobbee DE, et al. Ten-year follow-up study of islet-cell antibodies and childhood diabetes mellitus. Lancet 1989;1:1100
3. Tarn AC, Thomas JM, Dean BM, et al. Predicting insulin-dependent diabetes. Lancet 1988;1:845
4. Karjalainen JK. Islet cell antibodies as predictive markers for IDDM in children with high background incidence of disease. Diabetes 1990;39:1144
5. Atkinson MA, Kaufman DL, Newman D, et al. Islet cell cytoplasmic autoantibody reactivity to glutamate decarboxylase in insulin-dependent diabetes. J Clin Invest 1993;91:350
6. Colman PG, Nayak RC, Campbell IL, Eisenbarth GS. Binding of cytoplasmic islet cell antibodies is blocked by human pancreatic glycolipid extracts. Diabetes 1988;37:645
7. Dotta F, Gianani R, Dionisi S, et al. Expression of anti-GM2-1 islet ganglioside antibodies in ICA+ relatives of type 1 diabetics [Abstract]. Autoimmunity 1993;15:70
8. Dotta F, Peterson LB, Previti M, et al. Pancreatic islet ganglioside expression in nonobese diabetic mice: Comparison with C57BL/10 mice and changes after autoimmune beta-cell destruction. Endocrinology 1992;130:37
9. Dotta F, Tiberti C, Previti M, et al. Rat pancreatic ganglioside expression: Differences between a model of autoimmune islet B cell destruction and a normal strain. Clin Immunol Immunopathol 1993;66:143
10. Pav J, Prague MD, Jexokova Z, Skrha F. Insulin antibodies. Lancet 1963;2:221
11. Palmer J, Asplin C, Clemons P. Insulin autoantibodies in insulin-dependent diabetes before insulin treatment. Science 1983;222:1337
12. Wilkin T, Palmer J, Kurta A, et al. The second international workshop on the standardization of insulin autoantibody (IAA) measurement. Diabetologia 1988;31:449
13. Greenbaum CJ, Palmer JP, Kuglin B, et al. Insulin autoantibodies measured by radioimmunoassay methodology are more related to insulin-dependent diabetes mellitus than those measured by enzyme-linked immunosorbent assay: Results of the Fourth International Workshop on the Standardization of Insulin Antibody Measurement. J Clin Endocrinol Metab 1992;74:1040
14. Hegewald MJ, Schoenfeld SL, McCulloch DR, et al. Increased specificity and sensitivity of insulin autoantibody measurements in autoimmune thyroid disease and type I diabetes. J Immunol Methods 1992;154:61
15. Baekkeskov S, Nielsen J, Marner B, et al. Autoantibodies in newly diagnosed diabetic children immunoprecipitate human pancreatic islet cell proteins. Nature 1982;298:167
16. Christie M, Landin-Olsson M, Sundkvist G, et al. Antibodies to a Mr-64,000 islet cell protein in Swedish children with newly diagnosed type 1 (insulin-dependent) diabetes. Diabetologia 1988;31:597
17. Atkinson MA, Maclaren NK, Scharp DW, et al. 64,000 Mr autoantibodies as predictors of insulin-dependent diabetes. Lancet 1990;9:1357
18. Atkinson MA, Maclaren NK. Autoantibodies in nonobese diabetic mice immunoprecipitate 64,000-Mr islet antigen. Diabetes 1988;37:1587
19. Baekkeskov S, Dyrberg T, Lernmark Å. Autoantibodies to a 64-kilodalton islet cell protein precede the onset of spontaneous diabetes in the BB rat. Science 1984;224:1348
20. Baekkeskov S, Aanstoot HJ, Christgau S, et al. Identification of the 64kD autoantigen in insulin-dependent diabetes as the GABA-synthesizing enzyme glutamic acid decarboxylase. Nature 1990;347:151
21. Kaufmann DL, Clare-Salzer M, Tian J, et al. Spontaneous loss of T-cell tolerance to glutamic acid decarboxylase in murine insulin-dependent diabetes. Nature 1993;366:69
22. Tisch R, Yang X-D, Singer SM, et al. Immune response to glutamic acid decarboxylase correlates with insulitis in non-obese diabetic mice. Nature 1993;366:72
23. Erlander M, Tillakaratne N, Feldblum S, et al. Two genes encode distinct glutamate decarboxylases with different responses to pyridoxal phosphate. Neuron 1991;7:91
24. Edelhoff S, Grubin CE, Karlsen AE, et al. Mapping of glutamic acid decarboxylase (GAD) genes. Genomics 1993;17:93
25. Richter W, Mertens T, Schoel B, et al. Sequence homology of the diabetes-associated autoantigen glutamate decarboxylase with Coxsackie B4-2C protein and heat shock protein 60 mediates no molecular mimicry of autoantibodies. J Exp Med 1994;180:721
26. Karlsen AE, Hagopian WA, Grubin CE, et al. Cloning and primary structure of a human islet isoform of glutamic acid decarboxylase from chromosome 10. Proc Natl Acad Sci U S A 1991;88:8337
27. Petersen JS, Dryberg T, Markholst H, et al. Analysis of GAD 65 autoantibodies in NOD mice and GAD expression in the pancreas: Evidence of low antibody frequency and low expression [Abstract]. Autoimmunity 1993;15:77
28. Velloso LA, Eizirik DL, Karlsson FA, Kampe O. Absence of autoantibodies against glutamate decarboxylase (GAD) in the non-obese diabetic (NOD) mouse and low expression of the enzyme in mouse islets. Clin Exp Immunol 1994;96:129
29. Schmidli RS, Colman PG, Bonifacio E, et al. High level of concordance between assays for glutamic acid decarboxylase antibodies: The First International Glutamic Acid Decarboxylase Antibody Workshop. Diabetes 1994; 43:1005
30. Schmidli RS, DeAizpurua HJ, Harrison LC, Colman PG. Antibodies to glutamic acid decarboxylase in at-risk and clinical insulin-dependent diabetic subjects: Relationship to age, sex and islet cell antibody status, and temporal profile. J Autoimmun 1994;7:55
31. Tuomilehto J, Zimmet P, Mackay IR, et al. Antibodies to glutamic acid decarboxylase as predictors of insulin-dependent diabetes mellitus before clinical onset of disease. Lancet 1994;343:1383
32. Chen QY, Rowley MJ, Byrne GC, et al. Antibodies to glutamic acid decarboxylase in Australian children with insulin-dependent diabetes mellitus and their first-degree relatives. Pediatr Res 1993;34:785
33. Petersen JS, Hejnaes KR, Moody A, et al. Detection of GAD65 antibodies in diabetes and other autoimmune diseases using a simple radioligand assay. Diabetes 1994;43:459
34. Zimmet PZ, Rowley MJ, Mackay IR, et al. The ethnic distribution of antibodies to glutamic acid decarboxylase: Presence and levels of insulin-dependent diabetes mellitus in Europid and Asian subjects. J Diabetes Complications 1993;7:1
35. Christie MR, Daneman D, Champagne P, Delovitch TL. Persistence of serum antibodies to 64,000-Mr islet cell protein after onset of type I diabetes. Diabetes 1990;39:653
36. Kawasaki E, Takino H, Yano M, et al. Autoantibodies to glutamic acid decarboxylase in patients with IDDM and autoimmune thyroid disease. Diabetes 1994;43:80
37. Tuomi T, Groop LC, Zimmet PZ, et al. Antibodies to glutamic acid decarboxylase reveal latent autoimmune diabetes mellitus in adults with a non-insulin-dependent onset of disease. Diabetes 1993;42:359
38. Banerji MA, Chaiken RL, Huey H, et al. GAD antibody negative NIDDM in adult black subjects with diabetic ketoacidosis and increased frequency of human leukocyte antigen DR3 and DR4: Flatbush diabetes. Diabetes 1994; 43:741
39. Elias D, Reshef T, Birk O, et al. Vaccination against autoimmune mouse diabetes with a T-cell epitope of human 65kDa heat shock protein. Proc Nat Acad Sci U S A 1991;88:3088
40. Karjalainen J, Martin JM, Knip M, et al. A bovine albumin peptide as a possible trigger of insulin-dependent diabetes mellitus. N Engl J Med 1992;327:302
41. Pietropaolo M, Castano L, Babu S, et al. Islet cell autoantigen 69kD (ICA69). J Clin Invest 1993;92:359
42. Atkinson MA, Bowman MA, Kao K-J, et al. Lack of immune responsiveness

to bovine serum albumin in insulin dependent diabetes. N Engl J Med 1993; 329:1853
43. Christie MR, Vohra G, Champagne P, et al. Distinct antibody specificities to a 64-kD islet cell antigen in type 1 diabetes as revealed by trypsin treatment. J Exp Med 1990;172:789
44. Christie MR, Hollands JA, Brown TJ, et al. Detection of pancreatic islet 64,000 M autoantigens in insulin-dependent diabetes distinct from glutamate decarboxylase. J Clin Invest 1993;92:240
45. Christie MR, Tun RY, Lo SS, et al. Antibodies to GAD and tryptic fragments of islet 64K antigen as distinct markers for development of IDDM: Studies with identical twins. Diabetes 1992;41:782
46. Kim YJ, Zhou Z, Hurtado J, et al. IDDM patients' sera recognize a novel 30 kD pancreatic autoantigen related to chymotrypsinogen. Immunol Invest 1993;22:219
47. Castano L, Russo E, Zhou L, et al. Identification and cloning of a granule autoantigen (carboxypeptidase-H) associated with type I diabetes. J Clin Endocrinol Metab 1991;73:1197
48. DeAizpurua HJ, Honeyman MC, Harrison LC. A 64 kDa antigen/glutamic acid decarboxylase (GAD) in fetal pig pro-islets: Co-precipitation with a 38 kDa protein and recognition by T cells in humans at risk for insulin dependent diabetes. J Autoimmun 1992;5:759
49. Roep BO, Kallan AA, Hazenbos WL, et al. T-cell reactivity to 38 kD insulin-secretory-granule protein in patients with recent-onset type 1 diabetes. Lancet 1991;337:1439
50. Karounos DG, Simmerman L, Hickman SL, Jacob RJ. Identification of the p52-rubella related autoantigen as an insulin secretory granule protein [Abstract]. Autoimmunity 1993;15:73
51. Karounos D, Wolinsky J, Thomas J. Monoclonal antibody to rubella virus capsid protein recognizes a beta cell antigen. J Immunol 1993;150:3080
52. Thomas NM, Ginsberg-Fellner F, McEvoy RC. Strong association between diabetes and displacement of mouse anti-rat insulinoma cell monoclonal antibody by human serum in vitro. Diabetes 1990;39:1203
53. McCulloch DK, Klaff LJ, Kahn SE, et al. Nonprogression of subclinical beta-cell dysfunction among first-degree relatives of IDDM patients. 5-yr follow-up of the Seattle Family Study. Diabetes 1990;39:549
54. Krischer JP, Schatz D, Riley WJ, et al. Insulin and islet cell autoantibodies as time-dependent covariates in the development of insulin-dependent diabetes: A prospective study in relatives. J Clin Endocrinol Metab 1993;77:743
55. Neifing JL, Greenbaum CJ, Kahn SE, et al. Prospective evaluation of B-cell function in insulin-autoantibody-positive relatives of insulin-dependent diabetic patients. Metabolism 1993;42:482
56. Velloso LA, Wingvist O, Gustafsson J, et al. Autoantibodies against a novel 51 kDa islet antigen and glutamate decarboxylase isoforms in autoimmune polyendocrine syndrome type 1. Diabetologia 1994;37:61
57. Bingley PJ, Christie MR, Bonfanti R, et al. Combined analysis of autoantibodies improves prediction of IDDM in islet cell antibody positive relatives. Diabetes 1994;43:1304
58. Rowe RE, Leech NJ, Nepom GT, McCulloch DK. High genetic risk for IDDM in the Pacific Northwest: First report from the Washington State Diabetes Prediction Study. Diabetes 1994;43:87
59. Riley WJ, Maclaren WK, Krischer J, et al. A prospective study of the development of diabetes in relatives of patients with insulin-dependent diabetes. N Engl J Med 1990;323:1167

Diabetes Mellitus, edited by Derek LeRoith, Simeon I. Taylor, and Jerrold M. Olefsky. Lippincott–Raven Publishers, Philadelphia © 1996.

CHAPTER 33

Roles of Cell-Mediated Immunity and Cytokines in the Pathogenesis of Insulin-Dependent Diabetes Mellitus

ALEX RABINOVITCH

Insulin-dependent diabetes mellitus (IDDM) is a disease characterized by specific destruction of the insulin-producing β-cells in the pancreatic islets of Langerhans. It is not clear, however, what causes β-cell destruction. Current evidence favors the concept that β-cells are destroyed by an *autoimmune response* directed against certain β-cell constituents (*autoantigens*). This autoimmune response is thought to occur in genetically predisposed persons who possess certain "susceptibility" alleles and who lack other "protective" alleles of the major histocompatibility (MHC) gene complex, which regulates immune responses. In addition, non-MHC genes may contribute to the autoimmune response. The traditional concept is that environmental factors (e.g., microbial, chemical, dietary) may trigger an autoimmune response against β-cells in a genetically diabetes-prone phenotype. Recent studies in animal models with spontaneous autoimmune diabetes, however, have revealed that environmental factors (particularly microbial agents) may either *promote or protect against* diabetes development. Therefore, the current concept being explored is that both environmental and genetic inputs may be either pathogenic (i.e., IDDM-promoting) or protective against IDDM, and that disease appearance is influenced by the net effects of genetic and environmental factors on immunoregulatory responses. According to this concept, IDDM, like other organ-specific autoimmune diseases, results from a disorder of immunoregulation. This posits that T-lymphocytes (T-cells) specific for islet β-cell molecules (i.e., autoantigens) exist normally, but are restrained by immunoregulatory mechanisms (*the self-tolerant state*); and that IDDM develops when one or another immunoregulatory mechanism fails, allowing β-cell autoreactive T-cells to become activated, to expand clonally, and to entrain a cascade of immune/inflammatory processes in the islet (*insulitis*), culminating in β-cell destruction (Fig. 33-1). In this chapter, current information regarding mechanisms by which T-cells lead to islet β-cell injury and IDDM is integrated in accordance with the paradigm that autoimmune disease is a disorder of immunoregulation. Because cytokines are essential regulators of the immune response, their roles in IDDM pathogenesis are reviewed. Present information on the roles of T-cells and cytokines in human IDDM pathogenesis is limited, so most of the evidence reviewed here is drawn from studies of animals, the nonobese diabetic (NOD) mouse and the Bio Breeding (BB) rat, that develop forms of spontaneous autoimmune diabetes that resemble the disease in humans.

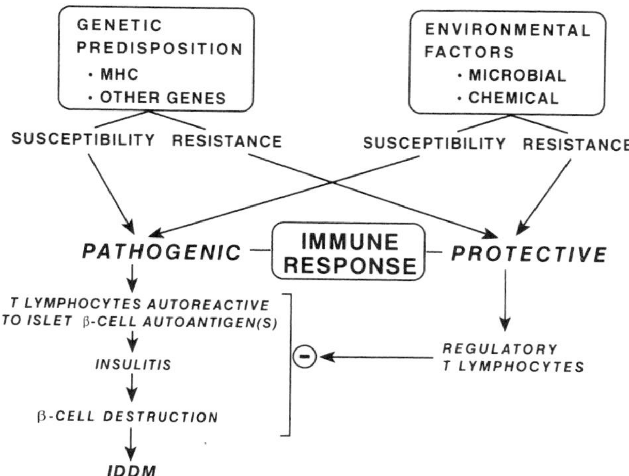

FIGURE 33-1. A current formulation of the pathogenesis of IDDM. Both genetic and environmental factors influence IDDM development, and these inputs may confer either susceptibility or resistance to disease. Genetic and environmental factors that confer *susceptibility* to IDDM may elicit a pathogenic immune response, which involves activation of T-cells that are reactive to islet β-cell self-antigen(s), infiltration of pancreatic islets by immune or inflammatory cells (insulitis), followed by β-cell destruction and IDDM. Genetic and environmental factors that confer *resistance* to IDDM, however, may elicit a protective immune response, which involves activation of T-cells that regulate (suppress) the pathogenic immune response at some point, thereby preventing IDDM.

Insulin-Dependent Diabetes Mellitus as a T-Cell–Mediated Autoimmune Disease

Autoimmune diseases are caused by the pathogenic effects of autoantibodies or autoreactive T-cells that provoke functional or structural alterations (usually destruction) of organs or cells. Four criteria usually have to be met for a disease to be defined as autoimmune[1]

1. The disease can be transferred by the patient's antibodies or T-cells.
2. The disease can be slowed or prevented by immunosuppressive therapy.
3. The disease is associated with manifestations of humoral or cell-mediated autoimmunity directed against a target organ.
4. The disease can be experimentally induced by sensitization against an autoantigen present in the target organ, which presupposes knowledge of the target autoantigen.

Human IDDM fulfills the first three of these criteria, and indirect evidence for the fourth has been seen in animal models. The evidence that IDDM is a T-cell–mediated autoimmune disease is summarized in Figure 33-2 and discussed below.

Diabetes Transfer and Disease Recurrence

There are case reports of IDDM developing in subjects who have received allogeneic bone marrow transplantation from donors with IDDM. In one report, a patient with severe aplastic anemia received a bone marrow transplant from his human lymphocyte antigen (HLA)-identical diabetic sibling and acquired IDDM with islet cell antibodies (ICAs) 5 years after transplantation.[2] In another report, a patient received a bone marrow transplant for acute lymphocytic leukemia from a histocompatible brother with IDDM and developed hypothyroidism and ICA-positive IDDM 3 years after the operation.[3] DNA restriction fragment length polymorphism analysis showed full hematologic chimerism of the recipient after bone marrow transplantation. Thus, it is likely that the production of anti-ICA and antithyroid antibodies and the destruction of the target cells in both pancreas and thyroid were due to bone marrow cells from the donor, presumably lymphoid cells; however, this was not proved. A worldwide survey utilizing the International Bone Marrow Transplant Registry disclosed three other similar cases; in one case, IDDM developed in the recipient only 3 years post-transplant, whereas the donor became ICA-positive 5 years post-transplant.[4] These clinical case reports directly demonstrate that IDDM can be transferred in human subjects by bone marrow cells; however, the responsible cells have not been identified. Peripheral blood mononuclear cells (PBMCs)—lymphocytes and monocytes—have been transferred from humans with IDDM to immunoincompetent mice in attempts to identify human lymphoid cells that can destroy islet β-cells. In one study,[5] athymic CD-1 nu/nu mice injected with PBMCs from newly diagnosed IDDM patients showed evidence of a mononuclear cell infiltrate around islets (peri-insulitis) as well as some islet disruption, but the mice did not develop glucose intolerance or diabetes. In another study,[6] mice with severe combined immunodeficiency disease were reconstituted with PBMCs from an IDDM patient positive for ICAs and glutamic acid decarboxylase (GAD). The reconstituted mice produced human ICAs (made by the transferred human B-lymphocytes [B-cells]) but did not develop islet cell damage, glucose intolerance, or diabetes. This demonstrates that IDDM-associated autoantibodies alone do not appear to be sufficient to induce islet β-cell destruction, which is in agreement with abundant evidence in animals with spontaneous autoimmune diabetes (NOD mice and BB rats), whose β-cell destruction is mediated by T-cells rather than B-cells.[7]

The mirror image of adoptive transfer of IDDM by bone marrow or T-cells from a diabetic donor is the recurrence of IDDM after transplantation of normal islets into a diabetic patient. Islets in pancreatic grafts from a nondiabetic twin or HLA-identical sibling were infiltrated with mononuclear cells, islet β-cells were destroyed, and IDDM recurred in the pancreatic graft recipients.[8] This study provides strong evidence that normal islet β-cells can be the targets of an autoimmune response, at least one that is presumably reactivated by reexposure to a β-cell autoantigen (or autoantigens). This does not exclude the possibility that some β-cell abnormality (intrinsic or acquired) may have participated in *initiating* an autoimmune response. Once established, however, it is clear that the immune response is the cause of β-cell destruction.

- *bone marrow cells from IDDM subjects transfer IDDM in HLA-compatible siblings*
- *IDDM recurs after pancreas transplantation from a non-diabetic twin or HLA-identical sibling*
- *immunosuppressive therapy acting mainly at the T cell level (e.g. CsA) arrests decreasing β-cell function (insulin secretion) in recent-onset IDDM subjects*
- *serum antibodies to islet cells, insulin, and other β-cell proteins (? antigens) precede clinical disease*
- *the "insulitis" lesion consists of lymphocytic and monocytic cells infiltrating the pancreatic islets*

FIGURE 33-2. Evidence that human IDDM is a T-cell–mediated autoimmune disease. CsA = Cyclosporin A.

Effects of Immunosuppression

Immunosuppressive agents have been demonstrated to slow the progression of islet β-cell damage in patients with recent-onset IDDM. These agents act mainly at the T-cell level and include cyclosporin[9–11] and azathioprine plus steroids.[12] Also, a large variety of immunosuppressive and immunomodulatory agents, acting mostly on T-cells, have been reported to prevent or arrest IDDM in autoimmune diabetes-prone NOD mice and BB rats.

Manifestations of Anti–β-Cell Autoreactivity

Both islet-reactive autoantibodies and T-cells have been detected in patients with IDDM. The autoantibodies do not appear to be damaging to β-cells. Rather, they serve as markers of autoimmune responses to the β-cells. As discussed above, diabetes can be transferred in humans by bone marrow cells but not by plasma from patients with IDDM.[2–4] Although T-cells appear to play the central roles in IDDM pathogenesis, there are few data on T-cell reactivity to islet antigens in humans. Of note are pioneering studies using the leukocyte migration assay with islet extracts[13] and, more recently, proliferation assays using human islets, fetal pig islets,[14,15] and GAD.[16,17] The anti-islet T-cell response has been documented best in the NOD mouse and BB rat models, in which transfer of diabetes can be obtained with purified T-cell populations[18–20] and islet-specific T-cell clones.[21,22] Successful transfer requires the simultaneous presence of CD4+ and CD8+ T-cells when using irradiated recipients that are the most immunoincompetent.[20,23,24]

Immunization and Tolerance

The fourth criterion of autoimmune diseases (i.e., reproduction of the disease by sensitization against an autoantigen) cannot be met in human diabetes and has been met only partially in animal models, probably because of insufficient knowledge about the target autoantigen. Interestingly, rather than sensitizing to disease, putative β-cell autoantigens (e.g., GAD, insulin) have been reported to prevent insulitis and diabetes in animal models, possibly by inducing immune tolerance to the autoantigen (see section on Immunostimulatory Procedures to Prevent Insulin-Dependent Diabetes Mellitus).

Indirect Evidence for IDDM as an Autoimmune Disease

Additional evidence exists to support the concept that human IDDM is an autoimmune disease:

- Insulitis: infiltration of the islets of Langerhans by mononuclear cells of the immune system, mainly lymphocytes and macrophages or monocytes[8,25–29]
- Common association of IDDM with other classic autoimmune diseases, notably thyroiditis[30]
- Association of IDDM with HLA genes,[31,32] which are known to be associated with most autoimmune diseases.

Immunoregulatory Defects May Underlie Development of Insulin-Dependent Diabetes Mellitus

The above lines of evidence support the concept of IDDM as an autoimmune disease caused by the pathogenic effects of autoreactive T-cells on islet β-cells. This implies that IDDM is a disease in which the immune system inappropriately attacks healthy β-cells. It has not been excluded, however, that a primary β-cell lesion (possibly viral or chemical) might be involved in initiating an autoimmune response.[33] At present there is no evidence in IDDM, as in other organ-specific autoimmune diseases, that the target autoantigen is abnormal. On the contrary, diabetes transfer studies discussed above[2–7,18–24] demonstrate that bone marrow–derived cells can transfer β-cell–destructive insulitis to non–diabetes-prone human, mouse, or rat pancreas, thereby indicating that the abnormality resides in the immune system.

Autoimmunity is generally viewed as a failure of the immune system to develop tolerance or nonreactivity to self molecules (potential antigens). Self-tolerance may be established by a variety of mechanisms. T-cell self-tolerance is controlled mainly in the thymus, where self-reactive T-cell clones that expand after contact with self MHC molecules present on the thymic epithelium and stroma (*positive selection*) are eliminated by autoantigen-driven apoptosis (*negative selection*).[34,35] This phenomenon does not, however, eliminate all autoreactive clones, particularly those reacting to subdominant or cryptic epitopes[36] and autoantigens not present in sufficient concentrations in the thymus. These autoreactive clones are controlled either by a phenomenon known as *T-cell anergy* (the autoreactive cells are present but are not activated after binding the antigen) or by suppressor mechanisms.[34–36] Thus, the breakdown of self-tolerance that characterizes autoimmune diseases can occur through three major mechanisms:

- Insufficient intrathymic negative selection
- Bypass of peripheral anergy
- Defective suppression

These mechanisms have all been considered to play roles in the immunopathogenesis of IDDM.[37]

T-cells play a central role in IDDM pathogenesis. Thus, disease is prevented in NOD mice and BB rats by neonatal thymectomy, backcross to athymic animals, and administration of various anti–T-cell antibodies.[37] Conversely, diabetes can be transferred to nondiabetic syngeneic animals by purified T-cells from diabetic NOD mice[19,20] or BB rats[18] or by T-cell clones[21,22] derived from diabetic NOD mice. The question then arises as to whether the abnormality is located at the T-cell precursor level (in the bone marrow) or in the thymus. Bone marrow precursor cells contain the "germ" of diabetogenicity: Transplantation of NOD mouse or BB rat bone marrow to nondiabetic strains (after irradiation) leads to diabetes,[38,39] and bone marrow transplantation from human diabetics may lead to rapid diabetes onset in the recipient.[2–4] Conversely, transplantation of normal allogeneic bone marrow prevents diabetes in BB rats[39] and NOD mice.[40] This does not rule out an intrinsic thymus defect, several of which have been identified in the NOD mouse.[37] There is little evidence, however, of a failure of negative selection of islet β-cell–reactive T-cells.[37] In fact, islet-reactive T-cells having escaped negative selection are present in normal individuals, as demonstrated by the onset of diabetes in non–autoimmune-prone rats after adult thymectomy and sublethal irradiation[41,42] or in athymic rats by transfer of normal spleen cells.[43]

Therefore, most evidence regarding autoimmune diabetes emergence in rodents points to failures of immune regulatory mechanisms to restrain islet-autoreactive T-cells from activation and clonal expansion. Autoreactive T-cells may become activated by a bypass (or breakdown) of T-cell anergy due to molecular mimicry. In this mechanism, an environmental agent may serve as a carrier for the "tolerated" cross-reactive T-cell epitopes of the autoantigen, leading to a bypass of self-tolerance. For example, Coxsackie B viral protein possesses antigen cross-reactivity with the islet β-cell autoantigen, GAD[44]; bovine serum albumin (in cow's milk) may exhibit cross-reactivity with the islet β-cell autoantigen, p69 peptide.[45] It remains to be proved, however, whether these or any other environmental agents can trigger islet β-cell–directed autoimmune responses by molecular mimicry or other mechanisms.

Whatever may trigger loss of self-tolerance to islet antigens in IDDM, defective immunoregulatory (suppressor) mechanisms appear to be necessary for the autoimmune state to progress to a pathologic level and cause β-cell destruction. There is now abundant evidence that suppressor cell defects may contribute to diabetes development in rodent models of IDDM. In the NOD mouse, diabetes onset is accelerated by thymectomy performed at 3 weeks of age[46] and by administration of cyclophosphamide,[47,48] a drug known for its selective effects on suppressor T-cells. Diabetes transfer is obtained only in immunodeficient recipients, that is, neonates[20] and adults that have been sublethally irradiated[21] or thymectomized and treated with a monoclonal antibody to CD4+ T-cells.[49] One can prevent diabetes transfer by spleen cells from diabetic mice by preinfusion of CD4+ spleen cells from nondiabetic syngeneic mice.[50] CD4+ and CD8+ suppressor clones have been reported,[51–53] as has the production of a suppressor factor.[53] Treatment of young NOD mice with an anti-MHC class II monoclonal antibody protects them from diabetes, and this protection is transferable to non–antibody-treated mice by infusion of CD4+ T-cells from protected mice.[54] In the BB rat, diabetes is accelerated by the administration of a monoclonal antibody to RT 6.1+ T-cells[55] and prevented by transfusion of lymphoid cells from diabetes-resistant BB rats.[56] Finally, the mechanisms by which islet-autoreactive T-cells may be suppressed are unknown; however, recent studies have pointed to cytokines as important immunoregulatory molecules.

Immune Responses: Roles of Cytokines

The Immune Response to an Antigen

The initial event in an immune response is the uptake and processing of antigen by macrophages, dendritic cells, or B-cells, which are termed collectively as *antigen-presenting cells* (APCs) because they present processed antigens to T-cells in association with MHC class I or II molecules at the surface of the APC. T-cell antigen receptors (i.e., T-cells with specific receptors that recognize the antigen) bind to the antigen-MHC complex. T-cells that respond to antigens complexed with MHC class I molecules are of the CD8+ phenotype (the CD8 molecule on the T-cell binds to the MHC class I molecule on the APC); T-cells that respond to antigens complexed to MHC class II molecules are of the CD4+ phenotype (the CD4 molecule on the T-cell binds to the MHC class II molecule on the APC). T-cells also bind, by other ligands, to accessory (adhesion or costimulatory) molecules on APCs. T-cell binding to the antigen-MHC complex and to accessory molecules on APCs leads to activation of the T-cells. An important functional property of activated T-cells is cytokine production.

Characteristics of Cytokines

Cytokines are peptide molecules synthesized and secreted by activated lymphocytes (*lymphokines*), macrophages or monocytes (*monokines*), and cells outside the immune system (e.g., endothelial cells, bone marrow stromal cells, fibroblasts). Cytokines are used mainly by immune system cells to communicate with each other and to control local and systemic events of immune and inflammatory responses. More than 30 immunologically active cytokines exist and are generally grouped as interleukins (ILs), interferons (IFNs), tumor necrosis factors (TNFs), and colony-stimulating factors (CSFs).[57] Both the production of cytokines by cells and the actions of cytokines on cells are complex: A single cell can produce several different cytokines, a given cytokine can be produced by several different cell types, and a given cytokine can act on one or more cell types. Also, cytokine actions are usually local: It can act (1) between two cells that are conjugated to one another, (2) on neighboring cells (paracrine), and (3) on the cell that secretes the cytokine (autocrine). In some cases (notably the macrophage-derived inflammatory cytokines, such as IL-1, IL-6 TNFα) cytokines exert actions on distant organs (endocrine).

Interpretation of the actions of cytokines in general is complicated by the very nature of cytokine biology. First, large amounts of a cytokine often are produced when a cell is stimulated by an antigen, mitogen, or other cytokines (e.g., up to 2% of cell protein synthesis can be devoted to a single cytokine). Second, cytokine receptors have high affinities for their specific cytokine ligands, so most cytokines have very high specific activity. The consequences of these properties of cytokines and cytokine receptors is that one activated cell can produce enough cytokine to activate 1000–10,000 other cells (i.e., a very small number of antigen-reactive cells can have widespread effects).[58] Cytokine synthesis is regulated by the differentiation of cells into the various cytokine-secreting phenotypes and by the selective activation of different cell types to produce some or all of their characteristic set of cytokines.

T-Cell Subsets, Cytokine Profiles, and Immune Response Regulation

Antigen-activated T-cells are termed T-helper (Th) cells because they help to mediate both cellular and humoral (antibody) immune responses. Th cells are generally identified as CD4+, but CD8+ Th cells also exist.[59] At least two distinct Th cell types, Th1 and Th2, have been described in both mice[58,60–62] and humans.[59] Th1 and Th2 cells are distinguished by their distinct cytokine secretion patterns (Table 33-1). Th1 cells produce IL-2 IFNγ, and TNFβ (lymphotoxin), whereas Th2 cells produce IL-4, IL-5, and IL-10. Other cytokines are produced by both Th1- and Th2-cell populations. Also, Th-cell phenotypes other than Th1 and Th2 exist and have other patterns of cytokine secretion.[58–62]

The functional significance of Th1- and Th2-cell subsets is that their distinct patterns of cytokine secretion lead to strikingly different T-cell actions.[58–62] Th1 cells and their cytokine products (IL-2, IFNγ, TNFα, and TNFβ) are the mediators in *cell-mediated immunity* (formerly termed delayed-type hypersensitivity). Th1-cell–derived IFNγ, TNFα, and TNFβ activate vascular endothelial cells to recruit circulating leukocytes into the tissues at the local site of antigen challenge, and they activate macrophages to eliminate the

TABLE 33-1. Cytokines Produced by Th1- and Th2-Cell Subsets of T-Cells*

Cytokine Produced	Th1-Cell Subset		Th2-Cell Subset	
	Mouse	Human	Mouse	Human
IL-2	+	++	—	—
IFNγ	++	++	—	—
TNFβ	++	++	—	—
TNFα	++	++	+	+
GM-CSF	++	+	+	++
IL-3	++	+	++	++
IL-4	—	—	++	++
IL-5	—	—	++	++
IL-10	—	+	++	++

*Values for mouse Th1- and Th2-cell subsets are proportions of mouse CD4+ T-cell clones producing a given cytokine.[61] Values for human Th1- and Th2-cell subsets are proportions of human T-cell clones producing a given cytokine.[59]
CSF = colony-stimulating factor; GM = granulocyte-macrophage; IL = interleukin; TNF = tumor necrosis factor; ++ = large proportion; + = small proportion; — = none.

antigen-bearing cell. In addition, Th1-cell–derived IL-2 and IFNγ activate (1) cytotoxic T-cells to destroy target cells expressing the appropriate MHC-associated antigen, and (2) natural killer cells to destroy target cells in an MHC-independent fashion. Thus, Th1 cytokines activate cellular immune responses. In contrast, Th2 cytokines are much more effective stimulators of humoral immune responses: that is, immunoglobulin (antibody) production, especially immunoglobulin E, by B-cells. Furthermore, responses of Th1 and Th2 cells are mutually inhibitory. Thus, the Th1 cytokine IFNγ inhibits the production of the Th2 cytokines IL-4 and IL-10; these, in turn, inhibit Th1 cytokine production.

Among signals that may orient the immune response in the direction of either a Th1- or Th2-cell response, the macrophage-derived cytokines IL-10[63] and IL-12[64] have been discovered to play important roles. IL-12 is a potent stimulant of Th1 cells and cytokines, notably IFNγ. Thus, IL-12 can initiate cell-mediated immunity. In contrast, IL-10 (derived from macrophages or Th2 cells) exerts anti-inflammatory effects by inhibiting production of IL-12 and other proinflammatory macrophage cytokines (e.g., IL-1, IL-6, IL-8, TNFα), by increasing macrophage production of IL-1 receptor antagonist, and by inhibiting the generation of oxygen and nitrogen free radicals by macrophages. In addition, IL-10 may favor Th2- over Th1-cell differentiation and function by inhibiting expression of MHC class II molecules and the B7 accessory molecule on macrophages, a major costimulator of T-cells.[65] The combination of IL-4 and IL-10 is particularly effective in inhibiting Th1-effector function (i.e., cell-mediated immunity) in vivo.[66]

It is evident, then, that the activation of Th1 or Th2 cells will result in cellular or humoral immune responses, respectively. Protective responses to pathogens depend on activation of the appropriate Th subset accompanied by its characteristic set of immune effector functions. For example, human Th1 cells are produced in response to intracellular bacteria and viruses, whereas Th2 cells are generated in response to allergens and helminth components.[59] Th1 and Th2 cells play different roles not only in protection against exogenous offending agents, but also in immunopathology. Th1 cells are involved in contact dermatitis, organ-specific autoimmunity, and allograft rejection, whereas Th2 cells are responsible for initiation of the allergic cascade.[59]

Evidence is accumulating that the islet β-cell–directed autoimmune response in IDDM may be mediated via a Th1-cell response, and that prevention of IDDM by immunostimulatory procedures may result from activation of an opposing Th2-cell response. Because cytokines are essential mediators of Th1 and Th2 immune responses, current information on cytokines implicated in IDDM pathogenesis will be reviewed first.

Cytokines: Friends or Foes?

Studies published during the past decade have examined the possible involvement of cytokines in the autoimmune pathogenesis of IDDM through several different approaches (Table 33-2).

Cytokine Studies in Isolated Islets

It is now well documented that cytokines can be cytotoxic to pancreatic islets in vitro.[67,68] IL-1, TNFα, TNFβ, and IFNγ (in piconanomolar concentrations) are *cytostatic* to β-cells: that is, the individual cytokines inhibit insulin synthesis and secretion, but these largely recover after the cytokine is removed. In addition, the cytokines may be *cytocidal:* that is, IL-1, TNFα, TNFβ, and IFNγ, usually when added in combination, destroy the β-cells in both rodent and human islets. Because the cytodestructive effects of cytokines on islet β-cells in vitro are not specific to β-cells (e.g., α-cells in the islets are also damaged),[68] cytokines may not qualify as mediators of β-cell destruction in IDDM, which is β-cell specific. Even agents with known β-cell specificity in vivo (e.g., alloxan, streptozocin), however, can damage other islet endocrine cells in vitro,[69] possibly because of nonspecific damage to the non–β-cells adjacent to damaged β-cells in vitro. For example, β-cells separated from non–β-cells in islets are destroyed by streptozocin and alloxan, but non–β-cells are not.[70] Similarly, IL-1 is cytotoxic to both β- and α-cells in isolated rat islets, but it selectively inhibits β-cell secretion of insulin and not α-cell secretion of glucagon in separated purified preparations of these islet endocrine cells.[71]

Moreover, cytokine applications to islets in vitro may not mimic the molecular pathology of the pancreatic insulitis lesion in vivo. Polar release of cytokines by Th cells conjugated B-cells has been reported,[72] and membrane forms of IL-1[73] and TNFα[74] may contribute to macrophage-mediated cytotoxicity. Similarly, cytokine products of islet-infiltrating macrophages and T-cells could be delivered in a targeted fashion into the microenvironment of the β-cell or even directly into the β-cell by contiguous cytotoxic T-cells. Highly localized and directed delivery of cytokines from T-cells and macrophages to β-cells might explain why rejection of islet allografts in rats was found not to destroy syngeneic islets mixed in with the allogeneic islets (whole islets, not single cell preparations, were admixed).[75] Also, syngeneic islets were not destroyed after cotransplantation with allogeneic or xenogeneic islets in mice; however, insulin secretory responses from the syngeneic islets cotransplanted with xenogeneic islets were severely

TABLE 33-2. Cytokines Implicated in the Pathogenesis of Insulin-Dependent Diabetes Mellitus

Cytokine Action or Production (NOD mice/BB rats)	IL-1	IL-2	IL-4	IL-6	IL-10	TNFα/β	IFNα	IFNγ
Inhibits insulin secretion and may destroy β-cells in vitro	Yes	No	No	No	No	Yes	Yes	Yes
Present in insulitis lesion	Yes	Yes	Yes	Yes	Yes	Yes	Yes	Yes
Transgenic β-cell expression leads to diabetes in normal mice	?	Yes*	?	?	Yes†	Yes‡	Yes	Yes
Cytokine production in diabetes-prone rodents	↓	↓	↓	?	?	↓	?	↑
Effect of cytokine administration on diabetes incidence	↓ or 0	↓ ↑	↓	?	↓	↓ ↑§	↑	?
Effect of blocking cytokine action on diabetes incidence	?	↓	?	↓	?	↑‖	↓#	↓

*Insulitis; IDDM if mice express both copies of the IL-2 transgene.
†Insulitis; IDDM if IL-10 transgenic mice are backcrossed to NOD mice.
‡Insulitis; IDDM if additional molecules to TNFα are expressed on β-cells (e.g., B7).
§TNFα decreases IDDM in NOD mice after age 3 weeks, but increases IDDM before age 3 weeks.
‖Anti-TNFα antibody increases insulitis in NOD mice.
#Anti-IFNα antibody prevents IDDM in IFNα transgenic mice.
IFN = interferon; IL = interleukin; TNF = tumor necrosis factor; ↓ = decreased; ↑ = increased; 0 = no change; ? = not determined.

impaired, suggesting inhibitory effects of xenogeneic macrophage-derived products (e.g., IL-1, TNFα, nitric oxide) on islet β-cell function.[76]

Cytokine Studies in Vivo

A variety of cytokines implicated in the pathogenesis of IDDM have been found to be expressed at the gene or protein level, or both, in the insulitis lesion of NOD mice and BB rats, and in the pancreata of IDDM patients (Table 33-2).[77] The simple presence of a cytokine in the insulitis lesion, however, does not identify the role of that cytokine in IDDM pathogenesis. Thus, a cytokine might be either proinflammatory or, alternatively, it may be responding to regulate (i.e., suppress) the inflammatory process. In recent studies of cytokine gene expression in pancreatic islet-infiltrating mononuclear cells of NOD mice, IFNγ mRNA expression was found to correlate with β-cell destructive insulitis.[78,79] Further evidence for a β-cell cytotoxic role for IFNγ comes from the findings that transgenic expression of IFNγ by β-cells in normal mice leads to an autoimmune, lymphocyte-dependent infiltration of the islets by mononuclear cells (insulitis), β-cell destruction, and IDDM.[80,81] Also, monoclonal antibodies to IFNγ protect against diabetes development in NOD mice[82,83] and BB rats.[84] In addition, IFNγ has been detected in lymphocytes infiltrating islets of human subjects with recent-onset IDDM.[85] Interestingly, another proinflammatory cytokine, IFNα, has been detected in β-cells of human subjects with recent-onset IDDM,[86] and IFNα mRNA expression is significantly increased in the pancreata of IDDM patients as compared to control pancreata.[87] Also, islet expression of IFNα precedes insulitis and diabetes in BB rats.[88] Furthermore, islet β-cell transgenic expression of IFNα in normal mice elicits an immune-mediated destruction of the β-cells, and anti-IFNα antibody prevents this β-cell damage and IDDM.[89] Because IFNα is a product of many cells that are virally infected or otherwise stressed, these findings suggest that an initial β-cell stress (possibly viral) may induce IFNα production, which would recruit immune system cells and these, in turn, could damage the IFNα-producing islet β-cells. Other studies in transgenic mice that ectopically express immunoregulatory cytokines in islet β-cells suggest proinflammatory roles for IL-2,[90] IL-10,[91] TNFα,[92,93] and TNFβ[94] produced locally in the islet, in addition to IFNα[89] and IFNγ.[80,81]

In contrast to the actions of cytokines as mediators of β-cell injury, suggested from the in vitro and transgenic studies described above, studies involving systemic administration of cytokines to diabetes-prone NOD mice and BB rats in vivo have revealed that several cytokines can *prevent* diabetes development: these include IL-1,[95,96] IL-2,[97,98] IL-4,[99] IL-10,[100] TNFα,[96,101,102] and TNFβ.[103,104] Because deficiencies in the endogenous production of IL-1,[105] IL-2,[99,105] IL-4,[99] TNFα[96,101,106] and TNFβ[104] have been reported in diabetes-prone NOD mice and/or BB rats, the diabetes-preventive effects of chronic administrations of these cytokines may result from corrections of specific deficits in cytokine production in the diabetes-prone animals. Systemically administered cytokines, however, may act on targets outside the immune system. For example, IL-1 and TNF can stimulate the hypothalamic-pituitary axis, leading to secretion of adrenocorticotropic hormone and consequently adrenal corticosteroids, which suppress inflammatory cells and cytokines.[107] Also, although IL-1 may decrease IDDM incidence in BB rats,[95] this effect might not be observed if controlled for the effects of IL-1 on decreased food intake.[108] These findings highlight the pleiotropic effects of cytokines that complicate interpretations of their actions. Cytokines are highly interdependent; therefore, a given cytokine may affect the production and action of other cytokines, resulting in physiologic or pathologic changes different from those induced by the original cytokine. For example, IL-1, TNFα, TNFβ, and IL-2 appear to be cytotoxic to islet β-cells in the islet microenvironment (in studies in vitro and in transgenic studies), whereas systemic administration of these cytokines may *prevent* an islet β-cell–directed autoimmune response by acting on immunologic circuits outside the islet or possibly on neuroendocrine cells (in studies in vivo). Finally, studies using NOD mice and BB rats to examine the effects on diabetes incidence of administering antibodies to cytokines or cytokine receptors to block cytokine actions in vivo (see Table 33-2) have supported diabetes-promoting roles for IL-2,[109,110] IL-6,[82] and IFNγ.[82,83]

It is important to recognize that most of our current information on cytokines implicated in IDDM pathogenesis comes from studies using NOD mouse and BB rat models. There is evidence, however, for cytotoxic actions of IL-1, TNFα, and IFNγ on human islets in vitro, and IFNα and IFNγ have been detected in islets of patients with recent-onset IDDM (see Table 33-2). Reports on plasma levels of IL-1, TNFα and IFNγ, as well as secretion of these cytokines by peripheral blood mononuclear cells from patients with IDDM, have not provided consistent results, and it is not clear whether changes in cytokine levels preceded or resulted from IDDM.[111,112] Also, peripheral blood cells probably do not adequately represent the cell infiltrate within the islet. Because the pancreas may not be accessible for immunologic investigation in humans, and considering that immunoregulatory actions of cytokines are exerted at short distances (paracrine and autocrine), it may be difficult to study the intraislet roles of cytokines in the evolution of β-cell destructive insulitis in human IDDM.

Autoimmune Diabetes: A Th1-Cell–Mediated Immune Process?

Abundant evidence now suggests that autoreactive T-cells are present in the normal immune system but are prevented from expressing their autoreactive potential by other regulatory (suppressor) T-cells.[113] The opposing actions of autoreactive and regulatory T-cells are regulated by their respective cytokine products[58–61]; one study has provided direct evidence for the operation of such a cytokine immunoregulatory balance in the avoidance of autoimmune diabetes.[41] Diabetes was induced in a nonautoimmune rat strain by rendering the animals relatively T-cell deficient using a protocol of adult thymectomy and sublethal γ-irradiation. Importantly, these researchers were able to prevent insulitis and diabetes in these rats by injecting them with a particular CD4+ T-cell subset that is isolated from healthy syngeneic donors and produces IL-4 and IL-2, but not IFNγ. In another study, CD4+ T-cell lines that react to rat insulinoma cells and secrete either IFNγ or IL-4 were developed from spleens of diabetic NOD mice.[114] The IFNγ-secreting CD4+ T-cells (Th1-like phenotype) adoptively transferred β-cell destructive insulitis and diabetes in neonatal NOD mice, whereas the IL-4-secreting CD4+ T-cells (Th2-like phenotype) induced a nondestructive peri-islet insulitis.[114] Similarly, Th1 cells expressing a diabetogenic T-cell receptor adoptively transferred β-cell destructive insulitis and diabetes in neonatal NOD mice, whereas Th2 cells expressing the same T-cell receptor did not; however, the Th2 cells could not prevent the Th1 cells from transferring diabetes.[115] Nevertheless, the protective effects against insulitis and diabetes of IL-4,[99] IL-4–producing CD4+ T-cells,[41] and IL-10[100] suggest that Th2 cells producing IL-4 and IL-10 may be responsible for preventing β-cell–destructive insulitis, possibly by suppressing IFNγ-producing Th1 cells. Thus, suppression of IFNγ production is a recognized action of both IL-4 and IL-10,[60–63] and IFNγ is a mediator of islet β-cell destruction in vitro as well as β-cell-destructive insulitis and IDDM (see Table 33-2). These findings have formed the concept that the autoimmune response in IDDM involves some disturbance (or disturbances) in immunoregulatory circuits that leads to a dominance of Th1 cells and their cytokine products over Th2 cells and their cytokines (Fig. 33-3).

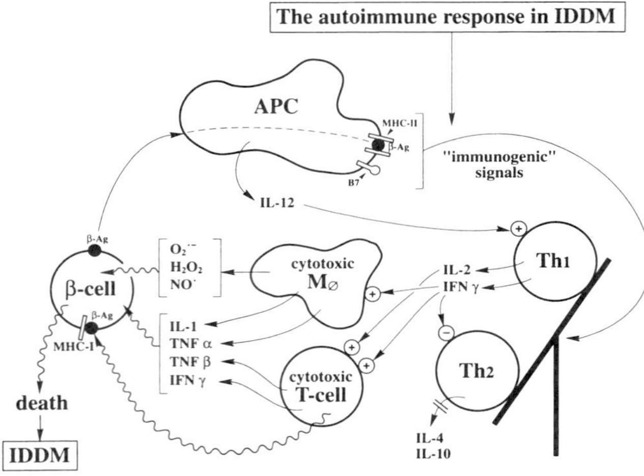

FIGURE 33-3. A scheme of the proposed circuitry of immune system cells and cytokines that may be involved in the autoimmune response leading to destruction of pancreatic islet β-cells and IDDM. The concept illustrated posits that certain β-cell proteins act as autoantigens (β-Ag) after being processed by antigen-presenting cells (APC), such as macrophages and dendritic cells, and presented in a complex with MHC class II molecules on the surface of the APC. Collectively, the β-Ag-MHC II complex, accessory molecules on the APC (e.g., the B7 molecule), APC-derived IL-12, and perhaps other signals would constitute immunogenic signals that activate T-cells, predominantly of the Th1 subset. Antigen-activated Th1 cells produce IL-2 and IFNγ, which inhibit Th2-cell production of IL-4 and IL-10. Also, IL-2 and IFNγ activate macrophages (Mϕ) and cytotoxic T-cells, and these effector cells may kill islet β-cells by a variety of mechanisms, including (1) antigen-specific cytotoxic T-cells that interact with a β-cell autoantigen-MHC class I complex on the β-cell and (2) nonspecific inflammatory mediators such as oxygen free radicals ($O_2^{\cdot -}$ and H_2O_2), nitric oxide ($NO^{\cdot}$), and cytokines (IL-1, TNFα, TNFβ, IFNγ) acting as direct β-cell toxins. (Reproduced from Rabinovitch A. Immunoregulatory and cytokine imbalances in the pathogenesis of IDDM: Therapeutic intervention by immunostimulation? Diabetes 1994;43:613, with permission of the American Diabetes Association.)

According to the scheme, depicted in Figure 33-3, certain β-cell proteins act as autoantigens after being processed by macrophages or other APCs (e.g., dendritic cells, possibly endothelial cells) and presented in a complex with MHC class II molecules on the surface of the APC. The immunogenicity of a β-cell protein may depend on the peptide fragment derived from processing by the APCs,[116] the amino acid sequences of the MHC class II molecules that bind and present the β-cell peptide (antigen), and the precursor frequency of autoreactive T-cells with T-cell receptors to match the MHC-antigen complex.[117]

In addition to the MHC-antigen complex interaction with T-cell receptors, costimulation of T-cells by interaction with APC accessory molecules is necessary for full T-cell activation.[118] For example, expression of the costimulator molecule B7-1 in pancreatic β-cells, by the transgenic approach, has been shown to accelerate the course of diabetes in NOD mice.[119] Also, pancreatic islet grafts have been shown to survive xenogeneic transplantation (from rats to streptozocin-induced diabetic mice) when the mice were treated with an immunoligand that binds the B7 molecule on APCs.[120] Importantly, the direction taken by the T-cell response, in terms of Th phenotype, is largely regulated by cytokines. Thus, naive T-cells are not precommitted to any particular Th phenotype: The Th phenotype varies with the cytokines in the microenvironment. The presence of IL-12, a macrophage and B-cell product, favors Th1 cell differentiation, and anti–IL-12 antiserum blocks expression of the Th1 phenotype.[121,122] Indeed, administration of IL-12 to prediabetic NOD female mice was found to accelerate diabetes onset, and this was associated with (1) enhanced IFNγ and decreased IL-4 production by islet-infiltrating lymphocytes and (2) selective β-cell destruction.[123] IL-4, a Th2 and possibly a mast cell product,[122] favors Th2 cell differentiation, and anti–IL-4 monoclonal antibody promotes expression of a Th1 phenotype.[124,125] The results of Th1 cell activation are induction of IL-2 and IFNγ production, inhibition of Th2 cytokine production, and activation of macrophages, cytotoxic T-cells, and natural killer cells. These activated "effector" cells may be cytotoxic to islet β-cells through a variety of antigen-specific and nonspecific mechanisms (described below).

In addition to their actions as cytotoxic effector molecules, IL-1, TNFα, TNFβ, and IFNγ can provide a positive feedback loop to the autoimmune response shown in Figure 33-3 by increasing the expression of (1) MHC class II proteins and adhesion molecules (e.g., B7, intercellular adhesion molecule [ICAM-1]) on APCs and (2) MHC class I proteins on islet β-cells. Indeed, immunohistochemical studies of the pancreas in subjects with recent-onset IDDM,[28] as well as in patients with disease recurrence after pancreas transplantation,[27] have revealed increased expression of MHC class I molecules on β-cells, other islet endocrine cells, and vascular endothelium of islets and small vessels near the islets. MHC class II and ICAM-1 molecules were expressed on vascular endothelium; MHC class II molecules also were expressed on islet-infiltrating macrophages and T-cells (mostly CD8+). Islet β-cells did *not* express MHC class II or ICAM-1 molecules in these studies.[27,28] Therefore, the evidence for aberrant presentation of an islet β-cell putative autoantigen (or autoantigens) directly to Th cells by the β-cells themselves remains incomplete.[26]

Antigen-Specific and Nonspecific Mechanisms of Islet β-Cell Destruction

Both antigen-specific and nonspecific immune or inflammatory responses appear to be involved in mediating islet β-cell destruction in IDDM.[126] Antigen-specific β-cell destruction would involve binding of CD8+ cytotoxic T-cells, through T-cell receptors specific for β-cell antigens, to the β-cell antigen-MHC class I complex on β-cells (see Fig. 33-3). Antigen-specific CD8+ T-cell–mediated cytotoxicity as a mechanism for islet β-cell destruction is supported by several lines of evidence[37]:

1. CD8+ T-cells are predominant in human IDDM-associated insulitis.[26,28]
2. CD8+ T-cells are necessary to transfer diabetes to fully immunoincompetent irradiated or neonatal NOD mice[20,22,23,127,128] and BB rats.[24]
3. NOD mice backcrossed with CD8+ T-cell–deprived mice whose MHC class I genes have been inactivated by homologous recombination do not develop diabetes.[129]

There is some evidence that CD8+ T-cells from diabetic patients and animals lyse β-cells,[22,130] but these results have been difficult to reproduce. CD8+ T-cells expressing the cytolytic mediator perforin are found in NOD mouse insulitis,[131] but this mediator is found in most cytotoxic cells, not exclusively in antigen-specific cytolytic T-cells. CD8+ T-cells also have been shown to inhibit insulin release by islet cells cultured in vitro,[132] but the interpretation is complicated by the absence of MHC restriction in this model.

In addition to antigen-specific CD8+ T-cell–mediated cytotoxicity, antigen-nonspecific β-cell destruction could result from free radicals ($O_2^{\cdot -}$, H_2O_2, $NO^{\cdot}$), cytokines (IL-1, TNFα, TNFβ, IFNγ), and other inflammatory products of activated macrophages and T-cells, both CD4+ Th1 cells and CD8+ cytotoxic T-cells (see Fig. 33-3). Antigen-nonspecific mechanisms for islet β-cell destruction are supported by several lines of evidence.[37] Diabetes can be transferred to young NOD mice by CD4+ T-cell clones alone,[21,22] even after administration of an anti-CD8 monoclonal antibody to rule out any involvement of host CD8+ T-cells.[128,133] This observation is at variance with previously mentioned evidence that CD8+ T-cells are necessary for diabetes transfer. Perhaps young NOD mice (3–4 weeks) used for T-cell clone transfer have some CD8+ T-cells (even after anti-CD8 antibody treatment) that cooperate with the CD4+ T-cell clones. CD8+ T-cell clones have not proved capable of transferring the disease,[22] but the addition of polyclonal CD8+ T-cells from diabetic mice accelerates diabetes transfer by CD4+ T-cell clones in irradiated recipients.[22] Also favoring a role for non–MHC-restricted β-cell destruction is the recurrence of diabetes after transplantation of MHC-incompatible islet grafts in NOD mice[134] or BB rats[135] under conditions excluding allogeneic rejection (e.g., prior islet culture in vitro). Also, anti-CD4 monoclonal antibodies prevent recurrence of diabetes in islets grafted in NOD mice, whereas anti-CD8 monoclonals do not.[134]

CD4+ T-cells could mediate antigen-nonspecific β-cell destruction by secreting various cytokines (IFNγ, TNFα, TNFβ) that can be directly toxic to β-cells, or can attract into the islets and activate other cell types such as monocytes and macrophages, or both. These cells could, in turn, produce β-cell–toxic mediators such as IL-1, TNFα, oxygen free radicals ($O_2^{\cdot -}$, H_2O_2) and nitric oxide (NO˙). Selective destruction of β-cells in islets might occur if these inflammatory mediators are more toxic to β-cells than to other islet cell types; however, data on this question are inconclusive.[68,71] Prevention of diabetes in rodent models by treatment with antioxidants and nicotinamide[136,137] fits with the hypothesis that oxygen free radicals and possibly nitric oxide may contribute to immune or inflammatory cell-mediated destruction of islet β-cells in IDDM.[67,68]

In conclusion, both CD4+ and CD8+ T-cell subsets are needed for diabetes because elimination of either subset can prevent diabetes in NOD mice and BB rats. It is still not clear, however, which cell(s) are the final effector(s) of islet β-cell destruction, and exactly how each cell type regulates the other. Nor is it known whether the CD4+ and CD8+ T-cells recognize the same, or different, autoantigens. Nevertheless, it appears that both islet antigen-specific CD8+ T-cells and antigen-nonspecific cytotoxic mechanisms induced by islet antigen-specific CD4+ T-cells may contribute to β-cell injury in IDDM.

In addition to T-cells and macrophages, other cellular elements in and around the islet (not shown in Fig. 33-3) are likely participants in the insulitis lesion. For example, vascular endothelial cells may contribute cytokines (IL-1 and IL-6) and may respond to inflammatory cytokines (IL-1, TNF, and IFNγ) by expressing adhesion molecules to circulating leukocytes.[138] This response would permit migration of macrophages and lymphocytes from the circulation into the islet. Also, endothelial cells may respond to inflammatory cytokines (IL-1, TNF, and IFNγ) by expressing MHC class II molecules,[139] which could allow endothelial cells to act as APCs and possibly present β-cell autoantigen (or antigens) to T-cells. Thus, intra- and peri-islet vascular endothelial cells could participate actively in amplifying the β-cell–directed autoimmune process.[140]

Immunostimulatory Procedures to Prevent Insulin-Dependent Diabetes Mellitus

The concept has been presented above that the autoimmune response in IDDM involves disturbances in immunoregulatory circuits that may be manifested as dominance of Th1 over Th2 T-cell subset function and cytokine production (see Fig. 33-3). A corollary of this proposition is that measures leading to reversal of this Th subset balance, with Th2 cells/cytokines dominating over Th1 cells/cytokines, should block the autoimmune response and prevent IDDM (Fig. 33-4). Evidence is building to support

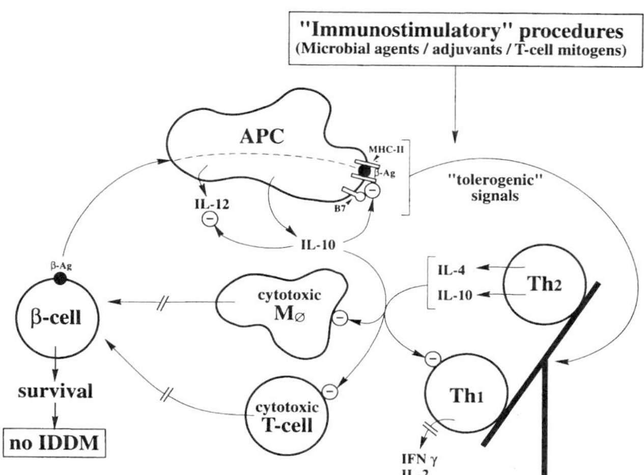

Figure 33-4. A scheme of the proposed mechanisms by which different immunostimulatory procedures (e.g., microbial agents, adjuvants, T-cell mitogens) may prevent or block the autoimmune response in IDDM. These immunostimulatory procedures may act at some point in the APC-T-cell interaction to convert immunogenic signals (see Fig. 33-2) to tolerogenic signals, which activate a Th2 subset of T-cells producing IL-4 and IL-10, and downregulate Th1 cells producing IFNγ and IL-2. In addition to IL-10 from the Th2 cells, IL-10 production by APCs may be upregulated by these immunostimulatory procedures. IL-10 inhibits expression of MHC class II molecules and the B7 costimulatory molecule on APCs, leading to altered β-Ag presentation and reinforcement of a tolerogenic signal for recognition of β-Ag as self by the immune system. In addition, IL-10 inhibits production of IL-12, a Th1-cell activator. The combination of upregulated IL-4 and IL-10 production and downregulated IFNγ and IL-2 production would inhibit cytotoxic Mϕ and T-cell activities and thereby prevent β-cell damage and IDDM. (Reproduced from Rabinovitch A. Immunoregulatory and cytokine imbalances in the pathogenesis of IDDM: Therapeutic intervention by immunostimulation? Diabetes 1994;43:613, with permission of the American Diabetes Association.)

this possibility. Thus, a number of immunostimulatory procedures have been discovered to prevent the development of insulitis, β-cell destruction, and IDDM in genetically diabetes-prone animals, including administration of certain microbial agents and extracts, immune adjuvants, and T-cell mitogens.[141–162] Importantly, these immunostimulatory procedures prevent diabetes development in genetically diabetes-prone NOD mice and BB rats without structural changes or complete remodeling of the immune system—unlike procedures that involve bone marrow, thymic, or lymphoid-cell replacement or deletion (e.g., antilymphocyte serum, cyclosporine, monoclonal antibodies to T-cells, silica, antimacrophage antibodies.)[7] Rather, the diabetes-preventive effects of immune adjuvants have been attributed to stimulation of T-regulatory (suppressor) cells and cytokines whose effects were to suppress[157,158] or render dormant[156] autoreactive T-cells. Taken together, these studies suggest that certain immunostimulatory procedures may provide tolerogenic signals that substitute for the immunogenic signals operant in autoimmune diabetes, thereby resetting the Th subset balance so that Th2 cells/cytokines now dominate over Th1 cells/cytokines (see Fig. 33-4).

The hypothesis that immunostimulatory procedures may prevent IDDM in autoimmune diabetes-prone rodents by upregulating Th2 cells/cytokines is supported by several lines of evidence. Protection against β-cell–destructive insulitis and diabetes in NOD mice, provided by injecting the mice with the immune adjuvant complete Freund's adjuvant (CFA), was reported to be associated with a relative increase in IL-4–producing T-cells and a decrease in IFNγ-producing T-cells recovered from sentinel syngeneic islet grafts placed under the renal capsule in NOD mice.[163] In another study, treatment of already diabetic NOD mice with CFA at the time of syngeneic islet transplantation also prevented destruction of β-cells in the islet graft, and diabetes did not recur.[155] Lymphocytes and monocytes/macrophages still accumulated around the transplanted islets (peri-islet insulitis) in the CFA-treated NOD mice, but these mononuclear cells did not invade the islets and β-cells remained intact. In yet another study, IL-10 mRNA expression was significantly increased, and expressions of IL-2 and IFNγ mRNA significantly decreased, in syngeneic islet grafts of CFA-injected NOD mice compared with saline-injected NOD mice.[164] This suggested that CFA treatment upregulated IL-10 production (possibly from Th2 cells, macrophages, or other cells in the islet graft), and this may have downregulated Th1 cytokines (IL-2 and IFNγ) and converted a β-cell–destructive islet infiltrate into a nondestructive peri-insulitis lesion. This interpretation was supported in a subsequent study, in which the combined administration of IL-10 plus IL-4 (Th2 cytokines) was found to produce significantly prolonged survival of syngeneic islet grafts in diabetic NOD mice.[165] These effects of IL-4 and IL-10 are in accord with the known actions of these cytokines to downregulate inflammatory responses mediated by monocytes/macrophages and their cytokine products, as well as to downregulate cell-mediated immune responses triggered by Th1 cells and their cytokine products.[63,66]

Interestingly, transgenic expression of IL-10 by islet β-cells in nonautoimmune diabetes–prone mice leads to pronounced vascular endothelial cell changes and leukocyte extravasation into the pancreas, and NOD mice backcrossed to these IL-10 transgenic mice were found to produce NOD progeny with accelerated onset and increased prevalence of diabetes.[91] Whereas these transgenic studies suggest a proinflammatory role for IL-10 in the pathogenesis of IDDM, this is not borne out by (1) the protective effect of IL-10 against diabetes development in NOD mice[100]; (2) the protective effects of IL-10 plus IL-4 against disease recurrence after syngeneic islet transplantation in NOD mice[165]; and (3) the correlation of IL-10 mRNA expression with syngeneic islet graft survival in NOD mice.[164]

Collectively, these studies suggest that immunostimulatory procedures, such as certain microbial agents and immune adjuvants, may stimulate the production of regulatory cytokines, such as IL-4 (by Th2 or mast cells, or both) and IL-10 (by Th2 or macrophages, or both). These cytokines could contribute to tolerogenic signals (i.e., signals for the immune system to recognize islet β-cell potential autoantigens as self), thereby avoiding an autoimmune response. Thus, IL-4 and IL-10 would favor T-cell differentiation along a Th2 pathway, downregulate Th1 cells and cytokines (IFNγ, IL-2, TNFβ), inhibit cytotoxic macrophages and T-cells, and consequently preserve islet β-cells and avoid the onset of IDDM (see Fig. 33-4).

Future Prospects: Clinical Considerations

The clinical hope from the observations that certain immunostimulatory procedures prevent autoimmune diabetes development in genetically diabetes-prone animals is that clinically safe means of immune stimulation may be similarly effective in preventing IDDM in human subjects at risk for this disease. *Immunostimulatory agents* that have a broad spectrum of immune stimulation affecting macrophages and T-cells (e.g., the immune adjuvant bacille Calmette-Guérin [BCG] vaccine) and *polyclonal T-cell activators* (e.g., microbial superantigens, lectins) may not be optimal for clinical trials because of possible undesirable side effects from generalized immunostimulation.

Recent findings, however, demonstrate that more selective immunostimulation may be at hand. Thus, administration of the peptide GAD65, an islet β-cell autoantigen, can prevent autoimmune diabetes development in NOD mice, and this prevention is associated with the induction of specific tolerance to this peptide.[166–168] Moreover, GAD-responsive T-cells from diabetes-prone NOD mice were characterized in one study as Th1, IFNγ-producing,[167] whereas IFNγ production in antigen-stimulated spleen cell cultures from GAD65-tolerant (and diabetes-protected) NOD mice was reduced significantly in another study, indicating that tolerance may result from suppression of GAD65-responsive Th1 cells.[168] Because this effect was not accompanied by a corresponding reduction of the humoral (antibody) response to GAD and to other IDDM autoantigens, a GAD65 induction of Th2 cells with suppression of Th1 cells has been suggested.[168] These findings are directly relevant to the observation that in humans there is an inverse relation between humoral (Th2-cell–mediated) and cellular (Th1-cell–mediated) autoimmunity to GAD in subjects at risk for IDDM[169]; also, a strong humoral response to GAD correlates with a slow progression to IDDM.[169,170] Administration of β-cell candidate autoantigens other than GAD may also induce self-tolerance and prevent IDDM. For example, insulin (and insulin B-chain) can prevent diabetes development in NOD mice and BB rats, and possibly in human subjects at high risk for IDDM.[171] The protective effects of insulin in NOD mice have been attributed to regulatory cells that have been found to inhibit intraislet expression of IFNγ-producing T cells.[79] In another study, diabetes-inducing, IFNγ-secreting CD4+ T-cell lines and clones from NOD mice were reported to recognize a 38-kd protein in a rat insulinoma membrane fraction,[114] possibly the 38-kd protein islet antigen against which T-cell reactivity has been described in human subjects with IDDM.[172] Collectively, these recent studies of cytokine production by T-cells reactive to islet candidate autoantigens (GAD, insulin, 38-kd protein) suggest that cytokine production profiles of peripheral blood T-cells specifically reactive to islet autoantigens may serve as predictors of IDDM development.

In summary, the paradigm of autoimmune diabetes as a Th1-cell–mediated immune response is based on recent evidence in autoimmune diabetes-prone animal models. Evidence in human IDDM remains to be obtained. There is some evidence for involvement of Th1 cells and cytokines in the pathogenesis of other organ-specific autoimmune disorders, including Hashimoto's thyroiditis[173] and progressive multiple sclerosis.[174] In the final analysis, the concept that imbalances of T-cell subsets and their respective cytokine products are involved in the autoimmune response of IDDM will be judged by its ability to predict and guide various forms of clinical intervention. First, however, there must be further identification of immunologic cells and cytokines that may mediate or suppress the autoimmune response in animal models with IDDM and, most importantly, in human subjects at risk for the disease. Whereas this review has focused on the presently best characterized Th1 and Th2 subsets of T-cells and their respective cytokine products, it is likely that other subsets of immune system cells and their cytokine products will be added to the list of cells and cytokines involved in IDDM pathogenesis. For example, recent studies suggest roles for TGFβ[51,175] and other as yet unidentified T-cell–derived immunosuppressive factors[53] in abrogating diabetogenic autoimmunity. The hope is that as our knowledge of the biology of immunoregulatory cytokines continues to grow, it may be possible to use this information to divert the immune response in IDDM from autoimmunity to self-tolerance by intervening in the cytokine network. This may be achieved through cytokine-based therapies involving cytokines, antibodies to cytokines or to cytokine receptors, soluble cytokine receptors, and receptor antagonists. Alternatively, balances of endogenous cytokine levels may be altered by the manipulation of the expression of costimulatory molecules (e.g., B7) on APCs, thereby influencing T-cell signaling pathways.

References

1. Rose NR, Bona C. Defining criteria for autoimmune diseases (Witebsky's postulates revisited). Immunol Today 1993;14:426
2. Lampeter EF, Homberg M, Quabeck K, et al. Transfer of insulin-dependent diabetes between HLA-identical siblings by bone marrow transplantation. Lancet 1993;341:1243
3. Vialettes B, Maraninchi D, San Marco MP, et al. Autoimmune polyendocrine failure—type 1 (insulin-dependent) diabetes mellitus and hypothyroidism—after allogeneic bone marrow transplantation in a patient with lymphoblastic leukaemia. Diabetologia 1993;36:541
4. Lampeter EB. Discussion remark to Session 24: BMT in autoimmune diseases. Exp Hematol 1993;21:1155
5. Calcinaro F, Hao L, Chase HP, et al. Detection of cell-mediated immunity in type I diabetes mellitus. J Autoimmun 1992;5:137
6. Petersen JS, Marshall MO, Bækkeskov S, et al. Transfer of type 1 (insulin-dependent) diabetes mellitus associated autoimmunity to mice with severe combined immunodeficiency (SCID). Diabetologia 1993;36:510
7. Rossini AA, Greiner DL, Friedman HP, Mordes JP. Immunopathogenesis of diabetes mellitus. Diabetes Rev 1993;1:43
8. Sibley RK, Sutherland DER, Goetz F, Michael AF. Recurrent diabetes mellitus in the pancreas iso- and allograft. Lab Invest 1985;53:132
9. Feutren G, Papoz L, Assan R, et al. Cyclosporin increases the rate and length of remissions in insulin-dependent diabetes of recent onset: Results of a multicentre double-blind trial. Lancet 1986;328:119
10. The Canadian-European Randomized Control Trial Group. Cyclosporin-induced remission of IDDM after early intervention: Association of 1 yr of cyclosporin treatment with enhanced insulin secretion. Diabetes 1988;37:1574
11. Bougneres PF, Carel JC, Castano L, et al. Factors associated with early remission of type I diabetes in children treated with cyclosporine. N Engl J Med 1988;318:663
12. Silverstein J, MacLaren N, Riley W, et al. Immunosuppression with azathioprine and prednisone in recent-onset insulin-dependent diabetes mellitus. N Engl J Med 1988;319:599
13. Nerup J, Andersen OO, Bendixen G, et al. Antipancreatic cellular hypersensitivity in diabetes mellitus. Diabetes 1971;20:424
14. Harrison LC, de Aizpurua H, Loudovaris T, et al. Reactivity to human islets and fetal pig proislets by peripheral blood mononuclear cells from subjects with preclinical and clinical insulin-dependent diabetes. Diabetes 1991;40:1128
15. Harrison LC, Chu SX, de Aizpurua HJ, et al. Islet-reactive T cells are a marker of preclinical insulin-dependent diabetes. J Clin Invest 1992;89:1161
16. Atkinson MA, Kaufman DL, Campbell L, et al. Response of peripheral-blood mononuclear cells to glutamate decarboxylase in insulin-dependent diabetes. Lancet 1992;339:458.
17. Honeyman MC, Cram DS, Harrison LC. Glutamic acid decarboxylase 67-reactive T cells: A marker of insulin-dependent diabetes. J Exp Med 1993;177:535
18. Koevary S, Rossini A, Stoller W, et al. Passive transfer of diabetes in the BB/W rat. Science 1983;220:727
19. Wicker LS, Miller BJ, Mullen Y. Transfer of autoimmune diabetes mellitus with splenocytes from nonobese diabetic (NOD) mice. Diabetes 1986;35:855
20. Bendelac A, Carnaud C, Boitard C, Bach JF. Syngeneic transfer of autoimmune diabetes from diabetic NOD mice to healthy neonates: Requirement for both L3T4+ and Lyt−2+ T cells. J Exp Med 1987;166:823
21. Haskins K, McDuffie M. Acceleration of diabetes in young NOD mice with a CD4+ islet-specific T cell clone. Science 1990;249:1433
22. Shimizu J, Kanagawa O, Unanue ER. Presentation of beta-cell antigens to CD4+ and CD8+ T cells of non-obese diabetic mice. J Immunol 1993;151:1723
23. Miller BJ, Appel MC, O'Neil JJ, Wicker LS. Both the Lyt-2+ and L3T4+ T cell subsets are required for the transfer of diabetes in nonobese diabetic mice. J Immunol 1988;140:52
24. Edouard P, Hiserodt JC, Plamondon C, Poussier P. CD8+ T-cells are required for adoptive transfer of the BB rat diabetic syndrome. Diabetes 1993;42:390
25. Gepts W, Lecompte PM. The pancreatic islets in diabetes. Am J Med 1981;70:105
26. Bottazo GF, Dean BM, McNally JM, et al. *In situ* characterization of autoimmune phenomena and expression of HLA molecules in the pancreas in diabetic insulitis. N Engl J Med 1985;313:353
27. Santamaria P, Nakhleh RE, Sutherland DE, Barbosa JJ. Characterization of T lymphocytes infiltrating human pancreas allograft affected by isletitis and recurrent diabetes. Diabetes 1992;41:53
28. Hänninen A, Jalkanen S, Salmi M, et al. Macrophages, T-cell receptor usage, and endothelial cell activation in the pancreas at the onset of insulin-dependent diabetes mellitus. J Clin Invest 1992;90:1901
29. Itoh N, Hanafusa T, Miyazaki A, et al. Mononuclear cell infiltration and its relation to the expression of major histocompatibility complex antigens and adhesion molecules in pancreas biopsy specimens from newly diagnosed insulin-dependent diabetes mellitus patients. J Clin Invest 1993;92:2313
30. Rotter JI, Vadheim CM, Rimoin DL. Genetics of diabetes mellitus. In Rifkin H, Porte D (eds). Diabetes Mellitus: Theory and Practice, 4th ed. Amsterdam: Elsevier; 1990:378–413
31. Nepom GT. Immunogenetics and IDDM. Diabetes Rev 1993;1:93
32. Thorsby E, Ronningen KS. Particular HLA-DQ molecules play a dominant role in determining susceptibility or resistance to type 1 (insulin-dependent) diabetes mellitus. Diabetologia 1993;36:371
33. Wilkin TJ. The primary lesion theory of autoimmunity: A speculative hypothesis. Autoimmunity 1990;7:225
34. Nossal GJ, Herold KC, Goodnow CC. Autoimmune tolerance and type 1 (insulin-dependent) diabetes mellitus. Diabetologia 1992;35(suppl 2):S49
35. Shehadeh NN, Gill RG, Lafferty KJ. Mechanism of self-tolerance to endocrine tissue. Springer Semin Immunopathol 1993;14:203
36. Ametani A, Sercarz EE. The nature of B- and T-cell determinants. In: Bach JF, ed. Monoclonal Antibodies and Peptide Therapy in Autoimmune Diseases. New York: Marcel Dekker; 1993:13–28
37. Bach JF. Insulin-dependent diabetes mellitus as an autoimmune disease. Endocr Rev 1994;15:516
38. Stein PH, Rees MA, Singer A. Reconstitution of (BALB/c × B6)F1 normal mice with stem cells and thymus from nonobese diabetic mice results in autoimmune insulitis of the normal hosts' pancreases. Transplantation 1992;53:1347
39. Nakano K, Mordes JP, Handler ES, et al. Role of host immune system in BB/Wor rat: Predisposition to diabetes resides in bone marrow. Diabetes 1988;37:520
40. Leiter EH, Serreze DV. Autoimmune diabetes in the nonobese diabetic mouse: Suppression of immune defects by bone marrow transplantation and implications for therapy. Clin Immunol Immunopathol 1991;59:323
41. Fowell D, Mason D. Evidence that the T cell repertoire of normal rats contains cells with the potential to cause diabetes: Characterization of the CD4+ T cell subset that inhibits this autoimmune potential. J Exp Med 1993;177:627
42. Stumbles PA, Penhale WJ. IDDM in rats induced by thymectomy and irradiation. Diabetes 1993;42:571
43. McKeever U, Mordes JP, Grenier DL, et al. Adoptive transfer of autoimmune diabetes and thyroiditis to athymic rats. Proc Natl Acad Sci U S A 1990;87:7618
44. Kaufman DL, Erlander MG, Clare-Salzler M, et al. Autoimmunity to two forms of glutamate decarboxylase in insulin-dependent diabetes mellitus. J Clin Invest 1992;89:283
45. Karjalainen J, Martin JM, Knip M, et al. A bovine albumin peptide as a possible trigger of insulin-dependent diabetes mellitus. N Engl J Med 1992;327:302
46. Dardenne M, Lepault F, Bendelac A, Bach JF. Acceleration of the onset of diabetes in NOD mice by thymectomy at weaning. Eur J Immunol 1989;19:889
47. Harada M, Makino S. Promotion of spontaneous diabetes in non-obese diabetes-prone mice by cyclophosphamide. Diabetologia 1984;27:604
48. Yasunami R, Bach JF. Anti-suppressor effect of cyclophosphamide on the development of spontaneous diabetes in NOD mice. Eur J Immunol 1988;18:481
49. Sempé P, Richard MF, Bach JF, Boitard C. Evidence of CD4+ regulatory T cells in the nonobese diabetic male mouse. Diabetologia 1994;37:337
50. Boitard C, Yasunami R, Dardenne M, Bach JF. T cell-mediated inhibition of the transfer of autoimmune diabetes in NOD mice. J Exp Med 1989;169:1669
51. Pankewycz OG, Guan JX, Benedict JF. A protective NOD islet-infiltrating CD8+ T cell clone, I.W. 2.15, has *in vitro* immunosuppressive properties. Eur J Immunol 1992;22:2017
52. Pankewycz O, Strom TB, Rubin-Kelley VE. Islet-infiltrating T cell clones from non-obese diabetic mice that promote or prevent accelerated onset diabetes. Eur J Immunol 1991;21:873
53. Diaz-Gallo C, Moscovitch-Lopatin M, Strom TB, Rubin-Kelley V. An anergic, islet-infiltrating T-cell clone that suppresses murine diabetes secretes a factor that blocks interleukin 2/interleukin 4–dependent proliferation. Proc Natl Acad Sci U S A 1992;89:8656
54. Boitard C, Bendelac A, Richard MF, et al. Prevention of diabetes in nonobese diabetic mice by anti-I-A monoclonal antibodies: Transfer of protection by splenic T cells. Proc Natl Acad Sci U S A 1988;85:9719
55. Greiner DL, Mordes JP, Handler ES, et al. Depletion of RT6.1+ T lymphocytes induces diabetes in resistant biobreeding/Worcester (BB/W) rats. J Exp Med 1987;166:461
56. Rossini AA, Faustman D, Woda BA, et al. Lymphocyte transfusions prevent diabetes in the bio-breeding/Worcester rat. J Clin Invest 1984;74:39
57. Thorpe R, Wadhwa M, Bird CR, Mire-Sluis AR. Detection and measurement of cytokines. Blood Rev 1992;6:133
58. Mosmann TR, Coffman RL. TH1 and TH2 cells: Different patterns of lymphokine secretion lead to different functional properties. Annu Rev Immunol 1989;7:145
59. Romagnani S. Lymphokine production by human T cells in disease states. Annu Rev Immunol 1994;12:227
60. Fitch FW, McKisic MD, Lancki DW, Gajewski TF. Differential regulation of murine T lymphocyte subsets. Annu Rev Immunol 1993;11:29
61. Powrie F, Coffman RL. Cytokine regulation of T-cell function: Potential for therapeutic intervention. Immunol Today 1993;14:270
62. Seder RA, Paul WE. Acquisition of lymphokine-producing phenotype by CD4+ T-cells. Annu Rev Immunol 1994;12:635
63. Moore KV, O'Garra A, de Waal Malefyt R, et al. Interleukin 10. Annu Rev Immunol 1993;11:165
64. Trinchieri G. Interleukin-12: A proinflammatory cytokine with immunoregulatory functions that bridge innate resistance and antigen-specific adaptive immunity. Annu Rev Immunol 1995;13:251

65. Ding L, Linsley PS, Huang L-Y, et al. IL-10 inhibits macrophage costimulatory activity by selectively inhibiting the upregulation of B7 expression. J Immunol 1993;151:1224
66. Powrie F, Menon S, Coffman RL. Interleukin-4 and interleukin-10 synergize to inhibit cell-mediated immunity in vivo. Eur J Immunol 1993;23:2223
67. Mandrup-Poulsen T, Helqvist S, Wogensen LD, et al. Cytokines and free radicals as effector molecules in the destruction of pancreatic β-cells. Curr Top Microbiol Immunol 1990;164:169
68. Rabinovitch A. Roles of cytokines in IDDM pathogenesis and islet β-cell destruction. Diabetes Rev 1993;1:215
69. Bolaffi JL, Nowlain RE, Cruz L, Grodsky GM. Progressive damage of cultured pancreatic islets after single early exposure to streptozotocin. Diabetes 1986;35:1027
70. Pipeleers D, Van de Winkel M. Pancreatic β cells possess defense mechanisms against cell-specific toxicity. Proc Natl Acad Sci U S A 1986;83:5267
71. Ling Z, Veld PA, Pipeleers DG. Interaction of interleukin-1 with islet β-cells. Distinction between indirect, aspecific cytotoxicity and direct, specific functional suppression. Diabetes 1993;42:56
72. Poo W-J, Conrad L, Janeway CA. Receptor-directed focusing of lymphokine release by helper T cells. Nature 1988;332:378
73. Kurt-Jones EA, Beller DI, Mizel SB, Unanue ER. Identification of a membrane associated interleukin-1 in macrophages. Proc Natl Acad Sci U S A 1985;82:1204
74. Kriegler M, Perez C, DeFay K, et al. A novel form of TNF/cachetin is a cell surface cytotoxic transmembrane protein: Ramifications for the complex physiology of TNF. Cell 1988;53:45
75. Sutton R, Gray DWR, McShane P, et al. The specificity of rejection and the absence of susceptibility of pancreatic islet β-cells to nonspecific immune destruction in mixed strain islets grafted beneath the renal capsule in the rat. J Exp Med 1989;170:751
76. Korsgren O, Jansson L. Characterization of mixed syngeneic-allogeneic and syngeneic-xenogeneic islet-graft rejections in mice: Evidence of functional impairment of the remaining syngeneic islets in xenograft rejections. J Clin Invest 1994;93:1113
77. Rabinovitch A. Immunoregulatory and cytokine imbalances in the pathogenesis of IDDM: Therapeutic intervention by immunostimulation? Diabetes 1994;43:613
78. Rabinovitch A, Suarez-Pinzon WL, Sorensen O, et al. IFN-γ gene expression in pancreatic islet-infiltrating mononuclear cells correlates with autoimmune diabetes in nonobese diabetic mice. J Immunol 1995;154:4874
79. Muir A, Peck A, Clare-Salzler M, et al. Insulin immunization of nonobese diabetic mice induces a protective insulitis characterized by diminished intraislet interferon-γ transcription. J Clin Invest 1995;95:628
80. Sarvetnick N, Liggit D, Pitts SL, et al. Insulin-dependent diabetes mellitus induced in transgenic mice by ectopic expression of class II MHC and interferon-gamma. Cell 1988;52:773
81. Sarvetnick N, Shizuru J, Liggitt D, et al. Loss of pancreatic islet tolerance induced by β-cell expression of interferon-γ. Nature 1990;346:844
82. Campbell IL, Kay TWH, Oxbrow L, Harrison LC. Essential role for interferon-γ and interleukin-6 in autoimmune insulin-dependent diabetes in NOD/Wehi mice. J Clin Invest 1991;87:739
83. Debray-Sachs M, Carnaud C, Boitard C, et al. Prevention of diabetes in NOD mice treated with antibody to murine IFN-γ. J Autoimmun 1991;4:237
84. Nicoletti F, Meroni PL, Landolfo S, et al. Prevention of diabetes in BB/Wor rats treated with monoclonal antibodies to interferon-γ [Abstract]. Lancet 1990;336:319
85. Foulis AK, McGill M, Farquharson MA. Insulitis in type 1 (insulin-dependent) diabetes mellitus in man: Macrophages, lymphocytes, and interferon-γ containing cells. J Pathol 1991;165:97
86. Foulis AK, Farquharson MA, Meager A. Immunoreactive α-interferon in insulin-secreting β cells in type I diabetes mellitus. Lancet 1987;330:1423
87. Huang X, Yuan J, Goddard A, et al. Interferon expression in the pancreases of patients with type 1 diabetes. Diabetes 1995;44:658
88. Huang X, Hultgren B, Dybdal N, Stewart TA. Islet expression of interferon-α precedes diabetes in both the BB rat and streptozotocin-treated mice. Immunity 1994;1:469
89. Stewart TA, Hultgren B, Huang X, et al. Induction of type I diabetes by interferon-α in transgenic mice. Science 1993;260:1942
90. Allison J, Oxbrow L, Miller JFAP. Consequences of in situ production of IL-2 for islet cell death. Int Immunol 1994;6:541
91. Wogensen L, Lee M-S, Sarvetnick N. Production of interleukin 10 by islet cells accelerates immune-mediated destruction of β cells in nonobese diabetic mice. J Exp Med 1994;179:1379
92. Ohashi PS, Oehen S, Aichele P, et al. Induction of diabetes is influenced by the infectious virus and local expression of MHC class 1 and tumor necrosis factor-α. J Immunol 1993;150:5185
93. Guerder S, Picarella DE, Linsley PS, Flavell RA. Costimulator B7-1 confers antigen-presenting-cell function to parenchymal tissue and in conjunction with tumor necrosis factor α leads to autoimmunity in transgenic mice. Proc Natl Acad Sci U S A 1994;91:5138
94. Picarella DE, Kratz A, Li C-B, et al. Insulitis in transgenic mice expressing tumor necrosis factor β (lymphotoxin) in the pancreas. Proc Natl Acad Sci U S A 1992;89:10036
95. Wilson CA, Jacobs C, Baker P, et al. IL-1β modulation of spontaneous autoimmune diabetes and thyroiditis in the BB rat. J Immunol 1990;144:3784
96. Jacob CO, Asiso S, Michie SA, et al. Prevention of diabetes in nonobese diabetic mice by tumor necrosis factor (TNF): Similarities between TNF-α and interleukin-1. Proc Natl Acad Sci U S A 1990;87:968
97. Serreze DV, Hamaguchi K, Leiter EH. Immunostimulation circumvents diabetes in NOD/Lt mice. J Autoimmun 1989;2:759
98. Zielasek J, Burkart V, Naylor P, et al. Interleukin-2–dependent control of disease development in spontaneously diabetic BB rats. Immunology 1990;69:209
99. Rapoport MJ, Jaramillo A, Zipris D, et al. IL-4 reverses T-cell proliferative unresponsiveness and prevents the onset of diabetes in NOD mice. J Exp Med 1993;178:87
100. Pennline KJ, Roque-Gaffney E, Monahan M. Recombinant human IL-10 (rHU IL-10) prevents the onset of diabetes in the nonobese diabetic (NOD) mouse. Clin Immunol Immunopathol 1994;71:169
101. Satoh J, Seino H, Abo T, et al. Recombinant human tumor necrosis factor-α suppresses autoimmune diabetes in nonobese diabetic mice. J Clin Invest 1989;84:1345
102. Satoh J, Seino H, Shintani S, et al. Inhibition of type I diabetes in BB rats with recombinant human tumor necrosis factor-α. J Immunol 1990;145:1395
103. Seino H, Takahashi K, Satoh J, et al. Prevention of autoimmune diabetes with lymphotoxin in NOD mice. Diabetes 1993;42:398
104. Takahashi K, Satoh J, Seino H, et al. Prevention of type I diabetes with lymphotoxin in BB rats. Clin Immunol Immunopathol 1993;69:318
105. Serreze DV, Leiter EH. Defective activation of T suppressor cell function in nonobese diabetic mice: Potential relation to cytokine deficiencies. J Immunol 1988;140:3801
106. Lapchak PH, Guilbert LJ, Rabinovitch A. Tumor necrosis factor production is deficient in diabetes-prone BB rats and can be corrected by complete Freund's adjuvant: A possible immunoregulatory role of tumor necrosis factor in the prevention of diabetes. Clin Immunol Immunopathol 1992;65:129
107. Reichlin S. Neuroendocrine-immune interactions. N Engl J Med 1993;329:1246
108. Reimers JI, Mørch L, Markholst H, et al. Interleukin-1β (IL-1) does not reduce the diabetes incidence in diabetes-prone BB rats. Autoimmunity 1994;17:105
109. Kelley VE, Gaulton GN, Hattori M, et al. Anti-interleukin 2 receptor antibody suppresses murine diabetic insulitis and lupus nephritis. J Immunol 1988;140:59
110. Pacheco-Silva A, Bastos MG, Muggia RA, et al. Interleukin-2 receptor targeted fusion toxin (DAB480-IL-2) treatment blocks diabetogenic autoimmunity in non-obese diabetic mice. Eur J Immunol 1992;22:697
111. Cavallo MG, Pozzilli P, Bird C, et al. Cytokines in sera from insulin-dependent diabetic patients at diagnosis. Clin Exp Immunol 1991;86:256
112. Ciampolillo A, Guastamacchia E, Caragiulo L, et al. In vitro secretion of interleukin-1β and interferon-γ by peripheral blood lymphomononuclear cells in diabetic patients. Diabetes Res Clin Pract 1993;21:87
113. Fowell D, McKnight AJ, Powrie F, et al. Subsets of CD4+ T-cells and their roles in the induction and prevention of autoimmunity. Immunol Rev 1991;123:37
114. Healey D, Ozegbe P, Arden S, et al. *In vivo* activity and *in vitro* specificity of CD4+ Th1 and Th2 T cells derived from the spleens of diabetic NOD mice. J Clin Invest 1995;95:2979
115. Katz JD, Benoist C, Mathis D. T helper cell subsets in insulin-dependent diabetes. Science 1995;268:1185
116. Shimizu J, Kanagawa O, Unanue ER. Presentation of β-cell antigens to CD4+ and CD8+ T-cells of nonobese diabetic mice. J Immunol 1993;151:1723
117. Nepom GT, Erlich H, MHC class-II molecules and autoimmunity. Annu Rev Immunol 1991;9:493
118. van Seventer GA, Shimizu Y, Shaw S. Roles of multiple accessory molecules in T-cell activation. Curr Opin Immunol 1991;3:294
119. Wong S, Guerder S, Visintin I, et al. Expression of the co-stimulator molecule B7-1 in pancreatic β-cells accelerates diabetes in the NOD mouse. Diabetes 1995;44:326
120. Lenschow DJ, Zeng Y, Thistlethwaite JR, et al. Long-term survival of xenogeneic pancreatic islet grafts induced by CTLA4 Ig. Science 1992;257:789
121. Hsieh C-S, Macatonia SE, Tripp CS, et al. Development of TH1 CD4+ T-cells through IL-12 produced by *Listeria*-induced macrophages. Science 1993;260:547
122. Scott P. IL-12: Initiation cytokine for cell-mediated immunity. Science 1993;260:496
123. Trembleau S, Penna G, Bosi E, et al. Interleukin 12 administration induces T helper type 1 cells and accelerates autoimmune diabetes in NOD mice. J Exp Med 1995;181:817
124. Hsieh C-S, Heimberger AB, Gold JS, et al. Differential regulation of T helper phenotype development by interleukins 4 and 10 in an αβ T-cell-receptor transgenic system. Proc Natl Acad Sci U S A 1992;89:6065
125. Seder RA, Paul WE, Davis MM, Fazekas de St. Groth B. The presence of interleukin 4 during in vitro priming determines the lymphokine-producing potential of CD4+ T-cells from T-cell receptor transgenic mice. J Exp Med 1992;176:1091
126. Kolb H, Kolb-Bachofen V, Roep BO. Autoimmune *versus* inflammatory type I diabetes: A controversy? Immunol Today 1995;16:170
127. Matsumoto M, Yagi H, Kunimoto K, et al. Transfer of autoimmune diabetes from diabetic NOD mice to NOD athymic nude mice: The roles of T cell subsets in the pathogenesis: Cell Immunol 1993;148:189

128. Christianson SW, Shultz LD, Leiter EH. Adoptive transfer of diabetes into immunodeficient NOD-scid/scid mice. Relative contributions of CD4+ and CD8+ T cells from diabetic *versus* prediabetic NOD.NON-Thy-la donors. Diabetes 1993;42:44
129. Katz J, Benoist C, Mathis D. Major histocompatibility complex class I molecules are required for the development of insulitis in non-obese diabetic mice. Eur J Immunol 1993;23:3358
130. Nagata M, Yokono K, Hayakawa M, et al. Destruction of pancreatic islet cells by cytotoxic T lymphocytes in nonobese diabetic mice. J Immunol 1989;143:1155
131. Young LH, Peterson LB, Wicker LS, et al. *In vivo* expression of perforin by CD8+ lymphocytes in autoimmune disease: Studies on spontaneous and adoptively transferred diabetes in nonobese diabetic mice. J Immunol 1989;143:3994
132. Boitard C, Chatenoud L, Debray-Sachs M. *In vitro* inhibition of pancreatic B cell function by lymphocytes from diabetics with associated autoimmune diseases: A T cell phenomenon. J Immunol 1982;129:2529
133. Bradley BJ, Haskins K, La Rosa FG, Lafferty KJ. CD8 T cells are not required for islet destruction induced by a CD4+ islet-specific T-cell clone. Diabetes 1992;41:1603
134. Wang Y, Pontesilli O, Gill RG, et al. The role of CD4+ and CD8+ T cells in the destruction of islet grafts by spontaneously diabetic mice. Proc Natl Acad Sci U S A 1991;88:527
135. Weringer EJ, Like AA. Immune attack on pancreatic islet transplants in the spontaneously diabetic biobreeding/Worcester (BB/W) rat is not MHC restricted. J Immunol 1985;134:2383
136. Rabinovitch A, Suarez WL, Power RF. Lazaroid antioxidant reduces incidence of diabetes and insulitis in nonobese diabetic mice. J Lab Clin Med 1993;121:603
137. Mandrup-Poulsen T, Reimers JI, Andersen HU, et al. Nicotinamide treatment in the prevention of insulin-dependent diabetes mellitus. Diabetes Metab Rev 1993;9:295
138. Bevilacqua MP. Endothelial-leukocyte adhesion molecules. Annu Rev Immunol 1993;11:767
139. Pober JS, Cotran RS. Immunologic interactions of T lymphocytes with vascular endothelium. Adv Immunol 1991;50:261
140. Doukas J, Mordes JP. T lymphocytes capable of activating endothelial cells in vitro are present in rats with autoimmune diabetes. J Immunol 1993;150:1036
141. Oldstone MB. Prevention of type I diabetes in nonobese diabetic mice by virus infection. Science 1988;239:500
142. Dyrberg T, Schwimmbeck PL, Oldstone MBA. Inhibition of diabetes in BB rats by virus infection. J Clin Invest 1988;81:928
143. Wilberz S, Partke HJ, Dagnaes-Hansen F, Herberg L. Persistent MHV (mouse hepatitis virus) infection reduces the incidence of diabetes mellitus in non-obese diabetic mice. Diabetologia 1991;34:2
144. Hermitte L, Vialettes B, Naquet P, et al. Paradoxical lessening of autoimmune processes in nonobese diabetic mice after infection with the diabetogenic variant of encephalomyocarditis virus. Eur J Immunol 1990;20:1297
145. Takei I, Asaba Y, Kasatani T, et al. Suppression of development of diabetes in NOD mice by lactate dehydrogenase virus infection. J Autoimmun 1992;5:665
146. Toyota T, Satoh J, Oya K, et al. Streptococcal preparation (OK-432) inhibits development of type I diabetes in NOD mice. Diabetes 1986;35:496
147. Satoh J, Shintani S, Oya K, et al. Treatment with streptococcal preparation (OK-432) suppresses anti-islet autoimmunity and prevents diabetes in BB rats. Diabetes 1988;37:1188
148. Kawamura T, Nagata M, Utsugi T, Yoon J-W. Prevention of autoimmune type I diabetes by CD4+ suppressor T-cells in superantigen-treated nonobese diabetic mice. J Immunol 1993;151:4362
149. Kino K, Mizumoto K, Sone T, et al. An immunomodulating protein Ling Zhi-8 (LZ-8) prevents insulitis in nonobese diabetic mice. Diabetologia 1990;33:713
150. Elias D, Markovits D, Reshef T, et al. Induction and therapy of autoimmune diabetes in the nonobese diabetic (NOD/Lt) mouse by a 65-kDa heat shock protein. Proc Natl Acad Sci U S A 1990;87:1576
151. Sadelain MWJ, Qin H-Y, Lauzon J, Singh B. Prevention of type I diabetes in NOD mice by adjuvant immunotherapy. Diabetes 1990;39:583
152. Sadelain MWJ, Qin H-Y, Sumoski W, et al. Prevention of diabetes in the BB rat by early immunotherapy using Freund's adjuvant. J Autoimmun 1990;3:671
153. McInerney MF, Pek SB, Thomas DW. Prevention of insulitis and diabetes onset by treatment with complete Freund's adjuvant in NOD mice. Diabetes 1991;40:715
154. Pearce RB, Peterson CM. Studies of concanavalin A in nonobese diabetic mice: I. Prevention of insulin-dependent diabetes. J Pharmacol Exp Ther 1991;258:710
155. Wang T, Singh B, Warnock GL, Rajotte RV. Prevention of recurrence of IDDM in islet-transplanted diabetic NOD mice by adjuvant immunotherapy. Diabetes 1992;41:114
156. Ulaeto D, Lacy PE, Kipnis DM, et al. A T-cell dormant state in the autoimmune process of nonobese diabetic mice treated with complete Freund's adjuvant. Proc Natl Acad Sci U S A 1992;89:3927
157. Qin H-Y, Suarez WL, Parfrey N, et al. Mechanisms of complete Freund's adjuvant protection against diabetes in BB rats: Induction of non-specific suppressor cells. Autoimmunity 1992;12:193
158. Qin H-Y, Sadelain MWY, Hitchon C, et al. Complete Freund's adjuvant-induced T-cells prevent the development and adoptive transfer of diabetes in nonobese diabetic mice. J Immunol 1993;150:2072
159. Harada M, Kishimoto Y, Makino S. Prevention of overt diabetes and insulitis in NOD mice by a single BCG vaccination. Diabetes Res Clin Pract 1990;8:85
160. Yagi H, Matsumoto M, Suzuki S, et al. Possible mechanism of the preventive effect of BCG against diabetes mellitus in NOD mice: I. Generation of suppressor macrophages in spleen cells of BCG-vaccinated mice. Cell Immunol 1991;138:130
161. Yagi H, Matsumoto M, Kishimoto Y, et al. Possible mechanism of the preventive effect of BCG against diabetes mellitus in NOD mice: II. Suppression of pathogenesis by macrophage transfer from BCG-vaccinated mice. Cell Immunol 1991;138:142
162. Lakey JRT, Warnock GL, Singh B, Rajotte RV. BCG adjuvant therapy prevents recurrence of diabetes in islet grafts transplanted into NOD mice. Transplantation 1994;57:1213
163. Shehadeh N, LaRosa F, Lafferty KJ. Altered cytokine activity in adjuvant inhibition of autoimmune diabetes. J Autoimmun 1993;6:291
164. Rabinovitch A, Sorensen O, Suarez-Pinzon WL, et al. Analysis of cytokine mRNA expression in syngeneic islet grafts of NOD mice: Interleukin 2 and interferon gamma mRNA expression correlate with graft rejection and interleukin 10 with graft survival. Diabetologia 1994;37:833
165. Rabinovitch A, Suarez-Pinzon WL, Sorensen O, et al. Combined therapy with interleukin-4 and interleukin-10 inhibits autoimmune diabetes recurrence in syngeneic islet-transplanted nonobese diabetic mice: Analysis of cytokine mRNA expression in the graft. Transplantation 1995;60:368
166. Solimena M, De Camilli P. Spotlight on a neuronal enzyme. Nature 1993;366:15
167. Kaufman DL, Clare-Salzler M, Tian J, et al. Spontaneous loss of T-cell tolerance to glutamic acid decarboxylase in murine insulin-dependent diabetes. Nature 1993;366:69
168. Tisch R, Yang X-D, Singer SM, et al. Immune response to glutamic acid decarboxylase correlates with insulitis in nonobese diabetic mice. Nature 1993;366:72
169. Harrison, LC, Honeyman MC, DeAizpurua HJ, et al. Inverse relation between humoral and cellular immunity to glutamic acid decarboxylase in subjects at risk of insulin-dependent diabetes. Lancet 1993;341:1365
170. Yu L, Gianani R, Eisenbarth GS. Quantitation of glutamic acid decarboxylase autoantibody levels in prospectively evaluated relatives of patients with type I diabetes. Diabetes 1994;43:1229
171. Ramiya V, Muir A, Maclaren N. Insulin prophylaxis in insulin-dependent diabetes mellitus: Immunological rationale and therapeutic use. Clin Immunother 1995;3:177
172. Roep BO, Kallan AA, Hazenbos WLW, et al. T-cell reactivity to 38kd insulin-secretory-granule protein in patients with recent-onset type 1 diabetes. Lancet 1991;337:1439
173. Del Prete GF, Tiri A, De Carli M, et al. High potential to tumor necrosis factor-α (TNF-α) production of thyroid-infiltrating T lymphocytes in Hashimoto's thyroiditis: A peculiar feature of destructive thyroid autoimmunity. Autoimmunity 1989;4:267
174. Brod SA, Benjamin D, Hafler DA. Restricted T-cell expression of IL-2/IFNγ mRNA in human inflammatory disease. J Immunol 1991;147:810
175. Zhang ZJ, Davidson LE, Eisenbarth G, Weiner HL. Suppression of diabetes in NOD mice by oral administration of porcine insulin. Proc Natl Acad Sci U S A 1991;88:10252

Diabetes Mellitus, edited by Derek LeRoith, Simeon I. Taylor, and Jerrold M. Olefsky. Lippincott–Raven Publishers, Philadelphia © 1996.

CHAPTER 34

Major Histocompatibility Locus and other Genes that Determine the Risk of Development of Insulin-Dependent Diabetes Mellitus

SUSAN FAAS AND MASSIMO TRUCCO

Human Leukocyte Antigen Genes

Studies aimed at identifying susceptibility genes for insulin-dependent (type I) diabetes mellitus (IDDM) as well as for many other autoimmune diseases initially have focused on those encoding the highly polymorphic human leukocyte antigen (HLA) molecules. In humans, the major histocompatibility complex (MHC) comprises a cluster of genes[1] that encode MHC class I (HLA-A, -B, -C) and class II (HLA-DR, -DQ, -DP) molecules; genes in the class III region of the MHC encode such unrelated products as tumor necrosis factor, complement, and 21 hydroxylase (Fig. 34-1).[1] Both MHC class I and class II protein products consist of separately encoded α- and β-chains. The class I α-chain is noncovalently associated with its monomorphic β-chain, β_2-microglobulin.[2] In contrast, class II molecules contain highly variable α- and β-chains, each encoded by polymorphic genes within the HLA complex. Class I proteins are expressed on virtually all nucleated cells, whereas class II molecules are found on selected cell types such as B-lymphocytes, macrophages, dendritic cells, and activated T-cells. Both class I and class II proteins function similarly to "present" antigen to T-cells; cytotoxic T-cells primarily recognize antigen in the context of class I,[3] whereas helper/inducer cells usually recognize antigen associated with class II molecules.

Early studies suggested that persons with IDDM were significantly more likely to express HLA-B8 and -B15 alleles than nondiabetic controls.[4,5] More significant associations between HLA-DR and IDDM became apparent once these HLA class II molecules were identified with HLA-DR3 and -DR4 alleles found to be strongly linked with IDDM susceptibility.[6,7] (The original association with the HLA-B locus is now thought to be a function of linkage disequilibrium between DR3/4 and B8/15 locus antigens, respectively.) Subsequent studies revealed that approximately 95% of patients with IDDM were heterozygous for DR3/4 or expressed at least one of these alleles.[7,8] Persons with heterozygosity at these loci appeared to be most susceptible to IDDM development. Expression of the HLA-DR2 allele, by contrast, was highly associated with resistance to IDDM development.

The application of newly developed molecular techniques to studies of the genetic basis of disease has permitted a more detailed analysis of the association between HLA genes and IDDM susceptibility. Restriction fragment length polymorphism (RFLP) analysis was the first such method to be used.[9] During RFLP analysis, a set of restriction enzymes cleave the genomic DNA of interest. The resulting fragments are separated by size with gel electrophoresis and are immobilized on a nitrocellulose filter. Particular sequences contained within the fragments are recognized by specific DNA probes, which reveal a "fingerprint" characteristic of each person's DNA. RFLP analysis of DNA from IDDM patients and nondiabetic controls revealed an even stronger association between the HLA-DQ locus and disease susceptibility than had been described previously for DR.[10,11] The importance of DQ in IDDM susceptibility was underscored by DNA sequencing analysis of the MHC (H-2) genes of the nonobese diabetic (NOD) mouse strain.[12] In addition to their susceptibility to diabetes development, these mice also have an unusual MHC expression pattern that permits an experimental dissection of the potential role of different class II gene products in IDDM development. Due to a mutation within the class II I-E locus (the murine homologue of DR), mice of this strain express only class II I-A molecules (equivalent to the human HLA-DQ). The nucleotide sequences of the I-A α- and β-chain genes from NOD mice were compared with those from nonobese normal (NON) control mice. Nucleotide differences between the two strains were found only at codons 56 and 57 of the I-Aβ gene; these changes permitted a serine residue at position 57 in NOD mice, whereas aspartic acid was found at the same position in NON mice.[12] Subsequent analysis of the DNA sequences of specific human DQα- and β-chains confirmed that position 57 of the DQβ-chain was strongly associated with IDDM incidence[13,14]; a negatively charged aspartic acid at position 57 (Asp-57) correlated with "resistance" to IDDM, whereas alleles in which a neutral amino acid such as alanine, valine, or serine was present (non–Asp-57) correlated with increased susceptibility to the disease.

DNA sequencing, although precise, is a costly and laborious technique unsuited for studies of large numbers of persons. The development of the polymerase chain reaction[15] (PCR) enabled researchers to perform the first large-scale characterization of the DQ alleles of persons whose families have multiple members with IDDM. Twenty-seven multiplex families were examined with the use of PCR and allele-specific oligonucleotide probes able to distinguish a single base difference.[16] Among the families examined, approximately 96% of the diabetic haplotypes contained non–Asp-

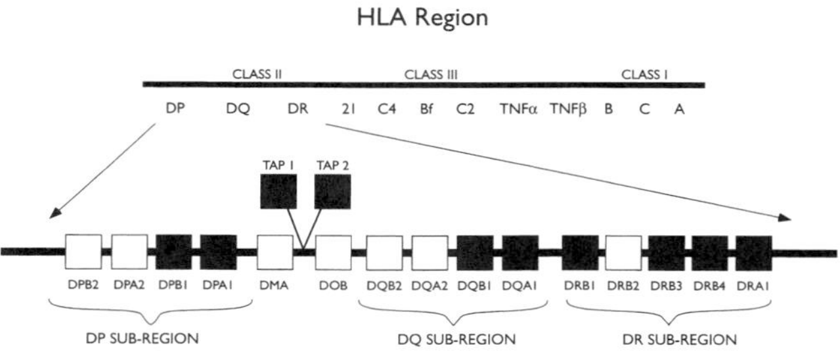

FIGURE 34-1. Schematic representation of the human leukocyte antigen (HLA) complex on chromosome 6. The genes that encode a protein product are indicated in black; the genes encoding nonfunctional products, or products that have not been characterized, are indicated in white.

57 sequences, compared with 19% of nondiabetic haplotypes ($P<0.0001$). In probands homozygous for non–Asp-57, the relative risk of developing diabetes was calculated as 107, an order of magnitude higher than the risk predicted by the best serologic markers, DR3 and DR4.[16]

The importance of Asp-57 in conferring resistance to disease was underscored as additional studies were performed on diabetic and nondiabetic individuals in populations with differing incidences of IDDM.[17,18] Molecular typing revealed the genotypic frequency of non–Asp-57 alleles among these groups; this calculation was then compared with data collected through epidemiologic IDDM registries. The non–Asp-57 marker was highly associated with IDDM incidence in all populations studied (as measured by relative risk). These studies also demonstrated a positive correlation between the frequency of the disease and the frequency of the marker in almost every population examined.[17–22] The Japanese were the only group to exhibit a higher than expected frequency of Asp-57 in IDDM patients relative to nondiabetic controls.[23,24] These and other studies[25,26] suggested that susceptibility or resistance to IDDM is a polygenic phenomenon, with HLA-DQ being the most sensitive genetic marker available for determining risk.

The contribution of the DQα chain to IDDM susceptibility or resistance was also examined in a study by Khalil et al.,[27] who used PCR and specific oligonucleotide probes to molecularly type 50 unrelated IDDM patients and 75 randomly selected healthy controls. These results implicated a role for the Arg-52 residue of the DQα chain in disease susceptibility and confirmed the importance of DQβ Asp-57. Further, this study as well as others[28–30] suggested that susceptibility to disease was increased in patients bearing DQ alleles that could form multiple ''diabetogenic'' dimers through the association of DQ chains encoded on the same chromosome (in *cis*) or on separate chromosomes (in *trans*). The pairing of *cis*-encoded and *trans*-encoded α- and β-chains permits highly polymorphic class II molecules to achieve even greater diversity[31,32] (shown schematically in Fig. 34-2). In the Khalil study, subjects were grouped on the basis of their genetic potential to form four possible heterodimeric DQ molecules through either *cis* or *trans* pairing. Susceptible dimers (αS-βS) were defined as DQβ non–Asp-57-DQα Arg-52, and protective dimers (αP-βP) were defined as DQβ Asp–57-DQα non–Arg-52. The frequency of subjects with IDDM correlated closely with the expected frequency of the formation of the αS-βS heterodimer. Thus, subjects who could form only αS-βS heterodimers were all affected with IDDM, whereas the disease was not observed in any subjects who could generate only S-P or P-P DQ molecules.[27] The formation of hybrid DQ molecules

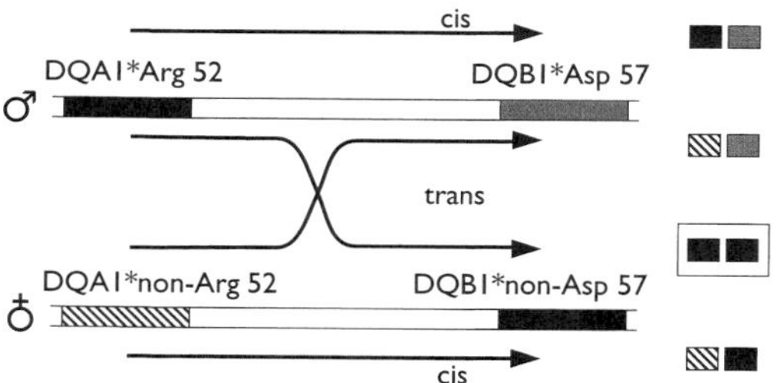

Figure 34-2. Associations of DQα- and DQβ-chains encoded either in *cis* or in *trans* can result in the formation of different DQ heterodimers, some of which may be "diabetogenic" (e.g., Arg-52α, non–Asp-57β). In this example, only one diabetogenic heterodimer (indicated by the double black boxes) can be formed by the association in *trans* of the α-chain encoded by the paternal (♂) haplotype (Arg-52) with the β-chain encoded by the maternal (♀) haplotype (non–Asp-57). (Adapted from Trucco M. To be or not to be Asp 57, that is the question. Diabetes Care 1992;15:705.)

through the association of α- and β-chains encoded in *trans* was also implicated in the development of disease in an analysis of a multiplex family.[28] The incidence of IDDM (which occurred in three of six offspring of the nondiabetic parents) could be traced only to the diabetogenic DQ heterodimer formed in these children through the pairing of the father's α-chain (Arg-52) with the mother's β-chain (non–Asp-57).

The ability to form hybrid diabetogenic class II molecules may also help explain the apparent discrepancies observed between HLA haplotype, the presence of islet cell antibodies (ICAs) in the patients' sera (a classic ''prediabetes'' marker used to follow relatives of IDDM probands[33]) and IDDM incidence. In a study of 151 first-degree relatives of probands from the Pittsburgh IDDM registry,[29] 74 were ICA-positive (irrespective of their HLA haplotype), but only 23% of these ICA-positive individuals went on to develop IDDM within the 4.9-year duration of the study. A comparison of ICA positivity, the potential to generate diabetogenic HLA dimers, and the incidence of disease in these subjects indicated that the greater the possible number of diabetogenic heterodimers, the higher the incidence of disease. Relatives who were ICA-positive αS-βS homozygotes were estimated to be 229.3 times more likely to develop IDDM than those who were antibody-negative and could not form diabetogenic heterodimers.[29] Similarly, a study in Spain examined the annual incidence of IDDM relative to the expression of non–Asp-57 and Arg-52 alleles[30] (Table 34-1). Subjects who could not generate any diabetogenic heterodimers experienced an incidence of disease roughly similar to that among subjects who could generate only one (1.94 versus 0.8/100,000/year). The annual incidence increased among those who could generate two (12.8/100,000/year) or four diabetogenic heterodimers (101.7/100,000/year). This is an extraordinarily high value when compared with the incidence calculated in the same area by conventional epidemiologic methods (11.8/100,000/year)[34] that do not fractionate the population based on HLA phenotypes. These studies, taken together, suggest that the genetic predisposition to IDDM increases, in a dose-dependent fashion, as the number of susceptible alleles in a given person increases. Thus, persons whose haplotypes comprise two non–Asp-57 alleles and two Arg-52 alleles would appear to have the greatest probability of generating diabetogenic molecules and developing the disease.

In 1987, Bjorkman et al.[35] succeeded in deciphering the precise structure of the crystallized HLA-A2 molecule, a triumph that shed considerable light on the molecular implications of amino acid changes at various positions in these class I molecules. Their analysis revealed that the antigenic peptide, processed by the antigen-presenting cell from which the A2 molecules were purified, was still intact within the molecular pocket (the so-called *Bjorkman's groove*) that functions as the antigen-binding site (Fig. 34-3). It appeared that changes in the amino acids deep within the groove might alter the structural pockets that accommodate particular peptide side chains. Such changes would thus inhibit or enhance peptide binding, and in turn, recognition by a given T-cell. Conversely, changes in amino acids on the exposed surface of the alpha helices that actually form the groove might interfere with the molecular interactions between the HLA molecule/peptide complex and the T-cell receptor. The recent characterization of the crystal structure of various forms of the DR1 class II molecule[36–38] permitted closer scrutiny of the potential implications of amino acid changes at certain positions. A schematic representation of the antigen-binding groove is shown in Fig. 34-4. Residue 57 of the DR1β-chain faces the inside of the groove at one end of the peptide binding site; an amino acid change at this position could easily translate into a critical conformational modification of the antigen-binding site. Asp-57 is involved in hydrogen and salt bonding with both the peptide main chain and the DRα Arg-76 side chain[36,37]; thus, changes in the DRα Arg-76 residue would also be expected to alter the antigen-binding site. DQ molecules have yet to be crystallized and their structure analyzed, but it is likely that these critical residues will be positioned similarly in these class II molecules.

Table 34-1. The Influence of HLA-DQα and HLA-DQβ Genotypes and the Possible Formation of Diabetogenic Heterodimers or the Risk of Development of Insulin-Dependent Diabetes Mellitus*

Genotype			Diabetic Patients (N = 102)		Nondiabetic Subjects (N = 87)		Risk	
DQβ57	+	DQα52	n	Freq.	n	Freq.	Relative	Absolute
■ ■	+	■ ■	66	0.65	6	0.07	30.7	101.3
■ ■	+	■ ▨	16	0.15	9	0.10	5.2	17.2
■ ■	+	▨ ▨	2	0.02	10	0.11	0.7	2.3
■ ▒	+	■ ■	11	0.11	12	0.14	2.8	9.2
■ ▒	+	■ ▨	1	0.01	17	0.20	0.3	1.0
■ ▒	+	▨ ▨	0	0.00	16	0.18	0.1	0.3
▒ ▒	+	■ ■	3	0.03	6	0.07	1.6	5.3
▒ ▒	+	■ ▨	3	0.03	10	0.12	1.0	3.3
▒ ▒	+	▨ ▨	0	0.00	1	0.01	1.0	3.3
Possible Diabetogenic Heterodimers								
4			66	0.65	6	0.07	52.4	101.7
2			27	0.26	21	0.24	6.6	12.8
1			1	0.01	17	0.20	0.4	0.8
0			8	0.08	43	0.49	1.0	1.94

*The genotype of subjects at positions DQβ57 and DQα52 are indicated (see Fig. 34-2) as follows: susceptibility loci DQβ non–Asp-57 (black boxes), or DQα Arg-52 (black boxes); protective loci DQβ Asp-57 (grey boxes) and DQα non–Arg-52 (striped boxes).
Absolute = absolute risk × 100,000 per year; Freq. = frequency of the genotype among the population studied; n = number of persons (subgroup).
Adapted from Gutierrez-Lopez MD, Bertera S, Chantres MT, et al. Susceptibility to type I diabetes in Spanish patients correlates quantitatively with expression of HLA-DQα Arg 52 and HLA-DQβ non–Asp 57 alleles. Diabetologia 1992;35:583.

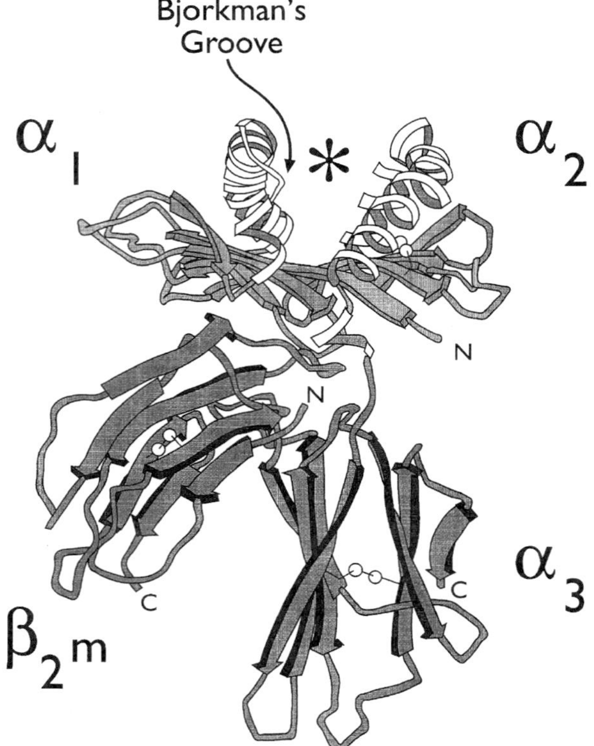

Figure 34-3. Schematic representation of the crystallized HLA-A2 class I molecule. The peptide antigen present within the antigen-binding site (Bjorkman's groove) is indicated with an asterisk. (Adapted with permission from Bjorkman P, Saper M, Samraoni W, et al. Structure of the human class I histocompatibility antigen, HLA-A2. Nature 1987;329:512.)

Small structural changes, then, may result in large functional changes in the antigen-presenting capabilities of the class II molecules. One might imagine that the cells from a person who is heterozygous for both DQα and DQβ would contain all four chain combinations on their surface. Competition for binding the processed antigen could take place, with effective antigen binding dictated by the conformation of the antigen-binding site on the DQ dimer. Changes at either amino acid DQα Arg-52 or DQβ Asp-57, located at opposite ends of the alpha helices that form the antigen-binding groove, could alter the configuration of the groove. Changes at both positions, however, would likely inflict a much

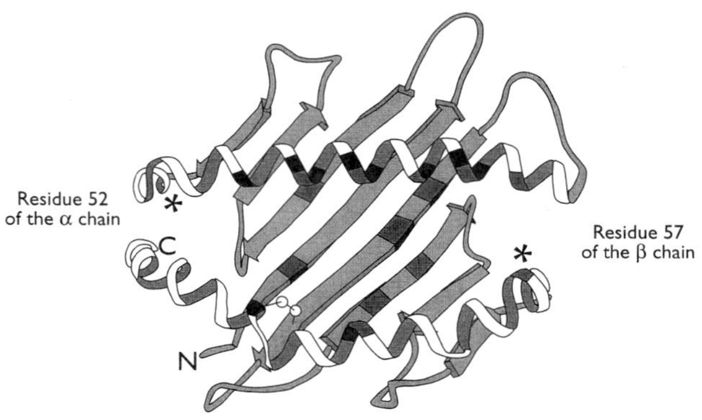

Figure 34-4. The antigen binding site of an HLA class II DR1 molecule, shown from the top. (Adapted with permission from Stern LJ, Brown JH, Jardetzky TS, et al. Crystal structure of the human class II MHC protein HLA-DR1 complexed with an influenza peptide. Nature 1994;368:215.)

greater conformational effect on the molecule's antigen-presentation capability. Such conformational differences may be partially responsible for the observed hierarchy in the degree of susceptibility within the group of non–Asp-57 alleles, and for the differences in the degree of protection afforded by each allele within the group of Asp-57 alleles. For example, the protective effect of the Asp-57 allele DQB1*0502 prevails over that of certain susceptible alleles, such as non–Asp-57 DQB1*0501. Conversely, the susceptible allele non-Asp-57 DQB1*0302 dominates over the protective effect of Asp-57 DQB1*0301.[39]

Competition for antigen binding would also be influenced by the relative abundance of each form of heterodimer on the cell surface, which in turn is likely influenced by several factors:

1. Certain DQα and DQβ molecules appear to be under structural constraints that limit the formation of dimers between them. For example, the β-chain of the DQB1*0501 allele does not couple efficiently with α-chains of the DQA1*0301 or DQA1*0501 alleles.[40] Thus, persons who are heterozygous for these alleles would not be expected to readily form significant numbers of hybrid molecules from the *trans*-encoded genes.
2. Studies of the promoter regions of these genes suggest that the levels of transcription of the DQα- and β-chain genes may differ among allelic variants.[41,42] These studies imply that a chain encoded by one gene may be synthesized in larger amounts than a chain encoded by the other allele, thereby increasing the probability of its participating in dimerization.

Although the actual ratio of *cis*-encoded versus *trans*-encoded DQ heterodimers at the cell surface remains to be determined experimentally, it is possible that moderate differences in chain production translate into large functional differences with respect to antigen presentation and T-cell activation. Relatively few class II molecules appear to be required on the surface of an antigen-presenting cell to cross-link the T-cell antigen receptor (TCR) efficiently and initiate a T-cell response.[43] Thus the dose-response relationship observed between HLA and IDDM susceptibility[17–19] may be the consequence of a complex interplay between a number of elements affecting DQ expression and function.

To date, the influence of HLA on IDDM susceptibility remains unquestioned, although it still does not appear to account for all cases of IDDM. A number of other candidate genes also have been examined for their potential role in influencing disease susceptibility. A genome-wide search for other genes affecting IDDM susceptibility has been undertaken recently by several groups, who are using microsatellite markers to construct high-resolution human genetic linkage maps[44,45] and fluorescence-based DNA fragment analysis.[44] As expected, the results of these studies suggest a strong link between IDDM and HLA. These studies also have revealed a positive link between IDDM and the *INS* region (discussed below), and they have identified at least 18 other chromosomal regions that may contain susceptibility loci. The majority of these remain uncharacterized at present, but several others map in close proximity to previously identified gene candidates, such as *MDU1* and *ZFM1* (genes encoding cell-surface and nuclear proteins expressed in the pancreas),[45] *GAD1* and *GAD2* (genes that encode the enzyme glutamic acid decarboxylase, a pancreatic β-cell autoantigen in IDDM),[44] *SOD* (the gene encoding superoxide dismutase),[44] and a gene (or genes) near or within the Kidd blood group locus.[44] The exact identity of these susceptibility loci is currently under investigation.

Transporters for Antigen Processing, 5′ Human Insulin, and Immunoglobulin Gm Genes

TAP1 (previously *PSF1* or *RING4*) and *TAP2* (previously *PSF2* or *RING11*) are genes that encode subunits of the transporter proteins required for the delivery of antigenic peptides to class I molecules in the endoplasmic reticulum.[46] The *TAP* genes are located within the HLA class II region 5′ to DQ (see Fig. 34-1). Polymorphisms within the *TAP2* gene in rats result in an altered repertoire of peptides bound by cell-surface class I molecules, which in turn affects their recognition by allogeneic T-cells.[47] Their critical role in antigen processing, their allelic polymorphism, and their physical location in the MHC have made these loci attractive targets for studies aimed at defining IDDM susceptibility genes. Thus far, however, studies investigating IDDM incidence and *TAP1* allelic distribution have not revealed a strong positive or negative association.[48] Conflicting results also have been reported by several groups investigating the potential association between *TAP2* alleles and IDDM,[48–50] with the suggestion that strong linkage disequilibrium between *TAP2* alleles and certain IDDM-associated HLA haplotypes might account for observations of disease association.[50,51] A more extensive allelic dissection of this genetic locus in IDDM multiplex families among different ethnic groups will likely shed more light on the potential involvement of the *TAP2* gene in the development of diabetes.

The tyrosine hydroxylase–*INS*–insulin-like growth factor II gene cluster on the short arm of chromosome 11 (*5′INS* region) also has received considerable attention as a possible susceptibility locus for both type I and type II diabetes. Initial studies suggested an association between this region and NIDDM but did not reveal a significant association between these genes and IDDM.[52–55] This conclusion was disputed by the results of other studies that indicated a significant association between the *5′INS* region and IDDM.[56–58] Differences in analysis may account for the contradictory conclusions of these studies: Population-association studies detect *5′INS* as a susceptibility locus; linkage-analysis studies do not.[59,60] The allelic forms within this region that may confer susceptibility or resistance to IDDM have not been precisely identified. The relevant DNA sequences or genes appear to be in strong linkage disequilibrium with the variable number of tandem repeats (VNTR) of *5′INS*. This polymorphic region, detected by virtue of its varying number of repetitive genetic elements, may or may not contain the actual gene.

The genes encoding the immunoglobulin (Ig) heavy chains are located on the long arm of chromosome 14. Serologically defined allotypes of the IgGγ heavy chains (called Gm allotypes) have been described and examined for their association with a number of diseases, including IDDM.[60] Although these Gm antigens are strictly defined as IgG heavy-chain epitopes, the genetic region that is the object of disease association studies (by linkage analysis) also includes loci that encode the other Ig heavy chains (IgA, IgD, IgE, and IgM). Thus far, numerous association studies have offered little evidence that Gm-region genes directly influence IDDM susceptibility.[61] However, a number of studies suggest that these genes, or unrelated loci in strong linkage disequilibrium with them, may indirectly affect susceptibility to IDDM. For example, diabetics heterozygous for DR3 and DR4 have a significantly higher frequency of non-G2m(23) allotypes than do diabetics with other HLA genotypes.[61] The absence of the G2m(23) allotype also appears to be associated with certain TCRβ alleles in patients with IDDM compared with their unaffected siblings.[60] The precise interactions, however, between the Gm region and these associated alleles must be further characterized, and their overall effect on IDDM susceptibility remains to be determined.

T-Cell Antigen Receptor (TCR) Genes

The study of any autoimmune disease must acknowledge the role of the T-cell, specifically the role of particular TCRs in mediating disease. The TCR on a given peripheral T-cell is composed of separately encoded α- and β-chains that are disulfide linked; these dimers must form a molecular complex with the multichain CD3 molecule to be functionally expressed at the cell surface. T-cells undergo a maturation process that occurs primarily in the thymus during fetal life. During this process, precursor stem cells from the fetal liver enter the thymic *anlage,* where they are induced to rearrange their germline TCRα and TCRβ genes.[62] (The sequential steps involved in TCR gene rearrangement are outlined in Figure 34-5, and result in the junction of a variable [V], diversity [D], joining [J], and constant [C] region gene segment. TCR gene rearrangements are essentially random, and most are nonproductive as a result of out-of-frame joints; however, these rearrangements are requisite for the expression of a functional TCR at the cell surface, and their essentially random nature ensures an extremely large ($\sim 10^{10}$–10^{15}) repertoire of distinct antigen specificities present in the unselected thymocyte pool.

Once a T-cell expresses its TCR at the cell surface, it is subject to either positive or negative selection events in the thymus.[63,64] Both positive selection and negative selection depend on interactions between the TCR, MHC, and peptide. *Positive selection* occurs as thymic stromal cells bearing MHC molecules (containing self-peptide fragments) engage TCR molecules on the developing thymocytes and direct their continued maturation into functionally mature T-cells. T-cells with "useless" receptors (i.e., those that cannot bind antigen in the context of MHC) are not driven to mature and expand, and these cells eventually die. *Negative selection* refers to the poorly understood set of events that specifically eliminates or alternatively "anergizes" potentially autoreactive cells, thereby inducing "tolerance" to self (i.e., self-tolerance). During negative selection, factors such as affinity for antigen and antigen load likely influence the final outcome of cell death or clonal anergy. Thus the peripheral T-cell repertoire of each person (including identical twins) is unique[65] and is a consequence of both the random generation of TCRs in the initial unselected thymocyte pool as well as of positive and negative selection events.

Autoimmune diseases such as IDDM result from a breakdown in self-tolerance, but the precipitating antigen that leads to the onset of disease remains unknown. Tolerance may be "broken" in affected individuals simply because of a cross-reactivity between an initial benign foreign antigen and an islet β-cell epitope. Destruction of the islets would rapidly occur through a process of *molecular mimicry*[66]: The memory T-cell clones, primed by the initial antigen, would recognize a structurally similar (but unrelated) antigenic molecule on the islet β-cells and initiate a secondary immune response that would destroy them. In a recently described autoimmunity model,[67] specific nonresponsiveness to a self-antigen (U1 small nuclear ribonucleoprotein particle, snRNP) after repeated immunizations was clearly demonstrated in mice. Both the T-cell and B-cell tolerance to this self-antigen was overcome, however, by immunization with a mixture of human and murine snRNP. Thus according to results of this model, a foreign, cross-reacting antigen could elicit an autoimmune T-cell response in a previously tolerant person.

IDDM also may develop as a consequence of "virgin" T-cells reacting against a newly exposed antigen on the islet β-cells to which the T-cells have never been tolerized. "Self-ignorance" rather than self-tolerance may be the operative mechanism under conditions where antigens are developmentally restricted or site-restricted.[64] For example, self-antigens in tissues with limited accessibility to the thymus, or intracellular proteins that do not reach the circulation in significant levels, may become the target of an immune response should they encounter T-cells with specific autoreactivity as a result of trauma or inflammation.

The two functionally opposite processes, *tolerance induction* and *immune responsiveness,* each depend on the presence of class I and class II molecules with appropriate structures (dictated by the genes encoding them) that are able to present the critical peptide antigens. In genetically susceptible individuals, certain class I or class II molecules may ineffectively present these self-peptides or exogenous antigens, thereby leading to inadequate negative selection of T-cell populations that could later become activated to manifest an autoimmune response. Similarly, T-cells with appropriate antigen receptors that can recognize the critical MHC-antigen complex must also be present; their availability in the periphery is dictated by both genetic (the TCR variable region genes themselves) and somatic (gene rearrangements and thymic selection) events.

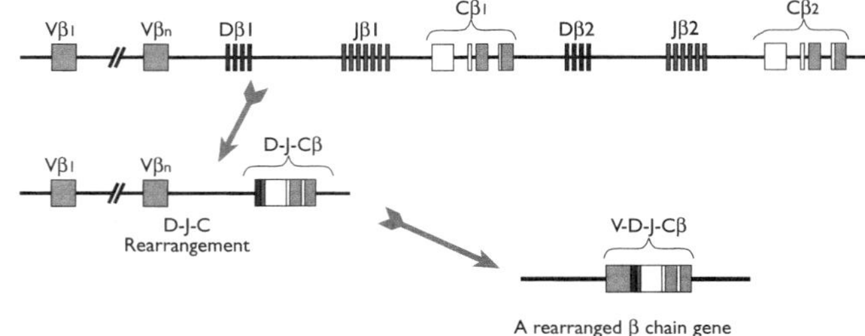

FIGURE 34-5. The rearrangement of TCRβ chain genes is accomplished in two steps. The first rearrangement event results in the random joining of a D (diversity), J (joining), and C (constant region) segment to result in D-J-C joining. The second rearrangement event allows a V (variable) region segment to align with the previously rearranged D-J-C gene segments.

Data from our laboratory suggest that a special class of antigens, called *superantigens,* may be involved in the pathogenesis of IDDM.[68] Superantigens are proteins derived from both bacterial and viral sources, the latter including endogenous retroviruses as well as exogenous agents.[69] These superantigens can activate a broad spectrum of T-cells based on their use of particular TCR Vβ genes and regardless of their precise antigen specificity. Approximately 1–30% of the entire peripheral pool of T-cells can become activated by an initial encounter with certain described superantigens,[70] in contrast to approximately 1 in 10^5 T-cells typically activated by conventional antigens.[71] Superantigens bind as unprocessed, intact proteins to MHC class II molecules outside of the peptide-binding groove,[38,72] and they appear to interact primarily with the TCR Vβ-chain and the HLA class II α-chain, rather than with the antigen-binding sites of the TCR or HLA molecules. A schematic view of this molecular association between an HLA molecule, superantigen, and TCR is depicted in Figure 34-6. Because superantigens do not activate T-cells in a classic MHC-restricted fashion, the positive and negative selection events that normally occur in the thymus may not effectively constrain a population of T-cells with potential reactivity to these antigens. Thus T-cells that can respond normally to a given foreign antigen with no ill-effects (e.g., no self-reactivity) may also be activated via their TCR Vβ-chain by a superantigen. Similarly, potentially autoreactive T-cells that remain in the periphery in an anergized state may become superantigen-reactivated, via their Vβ-chain, to carry out their effector functions.

Our data suggest that superantigen-activated Vβ7+ T-cells are present in large numbers in the pancreatic islets of several patients with early-onset IDDM.[68] In addition, the membrane proteins from the islets of these patients preferentially expand Vβ7+ T-cells from the peripheral blood of nondiabetic individuals, suggesting that either the islets themselves or the infiltrating lymphocytes are infected and express the superantigen. Destruction of the β-cells might occur in an antigen-specific manner, that is, if rare T-cells bearing Vβ7+ antigen receptors specific for self-antigens in the pancreas were among the pool of superantigen-activated cells. In studies of rheumatoid arthritis,[73] a superantigen appeared to be responsible for the broad infiltration of T-cells into the synovium, of which a small subset was clonally selected in response to the synovial autoantigen. Thus the presence of but a few T-cell clones in the snovial fluid were sufficient to mediate disease.[73] Alternatively, the β-cells may be bystanders rather than targets of the immune response, possibly destroyed as a consequence of their exquisite sensitivity to cytokines[74,75] produced during superantigen-induced T-cell activation.

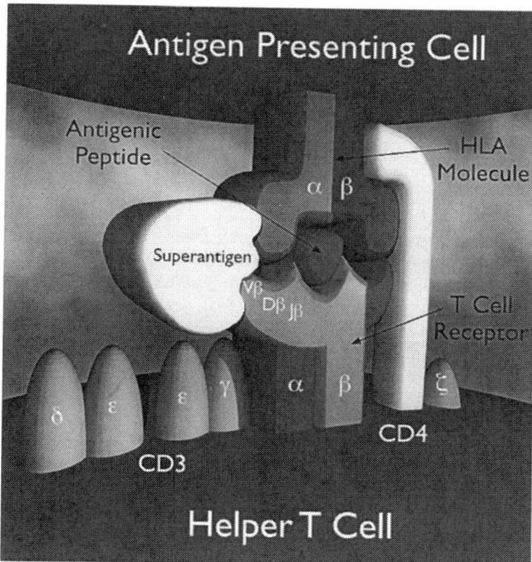

Figure 34-6. A schematic representation of the interactions among the T-cell receptor (TCRαβ), CD3 components (δ, ε, γ, and ζ), HLA class II molecule, peptide, accessory molecule (CD4) and superantigen during T-cell activation by an antigen-presenting cell. (Adapted with permission from Trucco M, LaPorte R. Exposure to superantigens as an immunogenetic explanation of type I diabetes mini-epidemics. J Pediatr Endocrinol & Metabol 1995; 8:3–10.)

Viruses have been implicated previously in MHC-associated susceptibility to IDDM[76,77] and are likely candidates for the source of the superantigen in these IDDM patients. The first and most complete characterization of a retroviral superantigen was reported in a study on the milk-borne infectious murine mammary tumor virus (MMTV).[78] This superantigen, normally transferred in the milk from C3H/Hej mothers to the pups during nursing, is responsible for clonal deletion of $V\beta^{14}$-expressing T-cells in the offspring.[79] Interestingly, the superantigen MIs-1, encoded by the Mtv-7 *sag* gene of MMTV, is presented with varying degrees of efficiency by HLA class II molecules bearing β-chains encoded by different alleles.[80] The most efficient among the alleles of the tested HLA genes were DR1 and 4, whereas DR2 and DQ1 presented the superantigen very poorly. (Note that DR1, DR3, and DR4 are the alleles most associated with IDDM susceptibility, whereas DR2 and DR2-linked DQ1 alleles confer resistance to the disease[81]). Such a hierarchy of antigen presentation of superantigen-derived peptides by different HLA alleles may directly explain the well-characterized but loose association between HLA class II alleles and IDDM susceptibility or resistance.

Although an analogous retroviral superantigen has not been described in human breast milk, the MMTV model offers an illustrative example of clonal deletion and functional immune tolerance to a viral superantigen encountered early in life. It is tempting to speculate that immune tolerance to a superantigen involved in development of IDDM might protect against onset of disease. Specific T-cell clones able to participate in the pathogenic process leading to IDDM could be deleted or inactivated through negative selection. The absence or silencing of such "dangerous" T-cell clones would therefore protect against the development of the disease. Although the complete absence of an entire *V*β family has not been described consistently in nondiabetics,[82–84] it is possible that only critical clones among those from the same TCR Vβ family are eliminated, whereas other clones belonging to the same family are spared. Alternatively, the relevant T-cell clones could still be present, but anergic, in such persons. Tolerance to the superantigen might be broken by a subsequent infection with a similar virus, or by reactivation of a dormant virus or endogenous retroviral gene. A breakdown in peripheral tolerance was responsible for β-islet cell destruction in a transgenic mouse model, in which the lymphocytic choriomeningitis viral (LCMV) glycoprotein was expressed on the surface of the β-islet cells of the pancreas. LCMV-reactive T-cells remained immunologically nonresponsive in these animals unless they were challenged with an acute LCMV infection.[85]

If, instead, the first exposure to the relevant superantigen were years after birth, specific tolerance to the superantigen would not occur and a potentially large pool of different T-cell clones expressing the same relevant TCR Vβ would be available to become activated in the periphery. Perhaps several viral infections would be required to inflict substantial pancreatic tissue damage. Any breakdown in the integrity of the pancreatic tissue would reveal new self-determinants (e.g., GAD65) which would, in turn, become simultaneous or subsequent targets for immune attack.[86,87] This anti-self attack, mediated by "conventional" HLA-restricted clones, would eventually bring a person to the point of disease onset by further reducing the number of available β-cells below a critical threshold, after which the body's need for insulin could no longer be met.

Thus, at the population level, a person's encounter with a potentially diabetogenic superantigen would have different outcomes (with respect to diabetes), based on his or her genetic predisposition and whether or not the person had been immunologically tolerized against the critical superantigen determinants. In tolerant individuals who are genetically susceptible to IDDM, exposure to the superantigen during the course of an infection would have no harmful outcome. Similarly, in genetically nonsusceptible individuals, constraints mediated by the HLA or TCR molecules themselves would protect against the pathologic consequences of superantigen exposure, and specific immune tolerance would not be obligatory for disease prevention.

This hypothesis may explain apparently conflicting or inconsistent observations in the epidemiology of IDDM on subjects such as genetic predisposition, the importance of the environment, the time of disease onset, the variety of agents considered to be involved with the disease, and the absence of an agent consistently found to be chronologically linked to the disease. The involvement of a virus may also explain the rapid "spikes" in the incidence of IDDM demonstrated in population studies worldwide.[88] It is conceivable that in at least some cases IDDM epidemics are caused by exposure to a single virus at the population level. The identification of the source of the superantigen that precipitated disease in our patients[68] would constitute an essential step forward in our understanding of IDDM etiology. Characterization of the superantigen itself may enable us to design strategies to inactivate or delete potentially dangerous T-cell clones in genetically predisposed individuals through tolerization programs, using peptide vaccines to circumvent the development of IDDM.

References

1. Campbell RD, Trowsdale J. Map of the human MHC. Immunol Today 1993;14:349
2. Grey HM, Kubo RT, Colon SM, et al. The small subunit of HLA antigens is beta-2 microglobulin. J Exp Med 1973;138:1608
3. Zinkernagel R, Doherty P. Immunological surveillance against altered self-components by sensitized T-lymphocytic choriomeningitis. Nature 1974; 248:701
4. Nerup J, Platz P, Anderson O, et al. HLA antigens and diabetes mellitus. Lancet 1974;2:864
5. Cudworth AG, Woodrow JC. Genetic susceptibility in diabetes mellitus: Analysis of the HLA association. Br Med J 1976;2:846
6. Wolf E, Spencer KM, Cudworth AG. The genetic susceptibility to type I (insulin-dependent) diabetes: Analyses of the HLA-DR associations. Diabetologia 1983;23:224
7. Bertram J, Baur M. Insulin-dependent diabetes mellitus. In: Albert ED, Baur MP, Mayr WR, eds. Histocompatibility Testing. Heidelberg: Springer-Verlag; 1984:348–358

8. Thomson G. HLA DR antigens and susceptibility to insulin-dependent diabetes mellitus. Am J Hum Genet 1984;36:1309
9. Trucco M, Ball E. RFLP analysis of DQ beta chain gene: Workshop report. In: Histocompatabitility Testing. Heidelberg: Springer-Verlag;1989:860–867
10. Schreuder G, Tilanus M, Bontrop R, et al. HLA-DQ polymorphism associated with resistance to type I diabetes detected with monoclonal antibodies, isoelectric point differences and restriction fragment length polymorphism. J Exp Med 1986;164:938
11. Owerbach D, Gunn S, Ty G, et al. Oligonucleotide probes for HLA-DQA and DQB genes define susceptibility to type 1 (insulin-dependent) diabetes mellitus. Diabetologia 1988;31:751
12. Acha-Orbea H, McDevitt HO. The first external domain of the non-obese diabetic mouse class II, 1-A beta chain is unique. Proc Natl Acad Sci U S A 1987;84:2435
13. Todd JA, Bell JI, McDevitt HO. HLA-DQ-beta gene contributes to susceptibility and resistance to insulin-dependent diabetes mellitus. Nature 1987;329:559
14. Horn GT, Bugawan TL, Long C, Erlich HA. Allelic sequence variation of the HLA-DQ loci: Relationship to serology and insulin-dependent diabetes susceptibility. Proc Natl Acad Sci U S A 1988;85:6012
15. Mullis KB, Faloona FA. Specific synthesis of DNA *in vitro* via a polymerase-catalyzed chain reaction. In: Diego RW, ed. Methods in Enzymology. San Diego, Calif: Academic Press;1987:335–350
16. Morel PJ, Dorman JS, Todd JA, et al. Aspartic acid at position 57 of the DQB chain protects against type I diabetes: A family study. Proc Natl Acad Sci U S A 1988;85:8111
17. Trucco G, Fritsch R, Giorda R, Trucco M. Rapid detection of IDDM susceptibility using amino acid 57 of the HLA-DQ beta chain as a marker. Diabetes 1989;38:1617
18. Dorman J, LaPorte R, Stone R, Trucco M. World-wide differences in the incidence of type I diabetes are associated with amino acid variation at position 57 of the HLA-DQ beta chain. Proc Natl Acad Sci U S A 1990;87:7370
19. Bao MZ, Wang JX, Dorman JS, Trucco M. HLA-DQ beta non-ASP-57 allele and incidence of diabetes in China and the USA. Lancet 1989;2:497
20. Carcassi C, Trucco G, Trucco M, Contu L. A new HLA-DR2 extended haplotype is involved in IDDM susceptibility. Hum Immunol 1991;31:159
21. Contu L, Carcassi C, Trucco M. Diabetes susceptibility in Sardinia. Lancet 1991;338:65
22. Ronningen LS, Iwe T, Halstensen TS, et al. The amino acid at position 57 of the HLA-DQ beta chain and susceptibility to develop insulin-dependent diabetes mellitus. Hum Immunol 1991;26:215
23. Yamagata K, Nakajima H, Hanfusa T, et al. Aspartic acid at position 57 of DQ beta chain does not protect against type I (insulin-dependent) diabetes mellitus in Japanese subjects. Diabetologia 1989;32:763
24. Awata T, Kuzuya T, Matusda A, et al. High frequency of aspartic acid at position 57 of HLA-DQ beta-chain in Japanese IDDM patients and non-diabetic subjects. Diabetes 1990;39:266
25. Erlich HA, Bugawan TL, Scharf S, et al. HLA-DQβ sequence polymorphism and genetic susceptibility to insulin-dependent diabetes. Diabetes 1990;39:96
26. Balsch JM, Weeks T, Giles R, et al. Analysis of HLA-DQ genotypes and susceptibility in insulin-dependent diabetes mellitus. N Engl J Med 1990; 322:1836
27. Khalil I, d'Auriol L, Gobet M, et al. A combination of HLA-DQ beta Asp 57-negative and HLA-DQ alpha Arg 52 confers susceptibility to insulin-dependent diabetes mellitus. J Clin Invest 1990;85:1315
28. Erlich HA, Griffith RL, Bugawan TL, et al. Implication of specific DQB1 alleles in genetic susceptibility and resistance by identification of IDDM siblings with novel HLA-DQB1 allele and unusual DR2 and DR1 haplotypes. Diabetes 1991;40:478
29. Lipton RB, Kocova M, LaPorte RE, et al. Autoimmunity and genetics contribute to the risk of insulin-dependent diabetes mellitus in families: Islet cell antibodies and HLA DQ heterodimers. Am J Epidemiol 1992;136:503
30. Gutierrez-Lopez MD, Bertera S, Chantres MT, et al. Susceptibility to type I diabetes in Spanish patients correlates quantitatively with expression of HLA-DQαArg 52 and HLA-DQβ non-Asp 57 alleles. Diabetologia 1992;35:583
31. Charron PJ, Lotteau V, Turmel P. Hybrid HLA-DC antigens provide molecular evidence for gene *trans*-complementation. Nature 1984;312:157
32. Nepom BS, Schwarz D, Palmer JP, Nepom GT. *Trans*-complementation of HLA genes in IDDM. HLA-DQα and β chains produce hybrid molecules in DR3/DR4 heterozygotes. Diabetes 1987;36:114
33. Bottazzo GF, Florin-Christensen A, Doniach D. Islet cell antibodies in diabetes mellitus with autoimmune polyendocrine deficiency. Lancet 1974;2:1279
34. Serrano-Rios M, Moy CS, Martin-Serrano R, et al. Incidence of type I diabetes mellitus in subject 0–14 years of age in the Comunidad of Madrid, Spain. Diabetologia 1990;33:422
35. Bjorkman P, Saper M, Samraoni W, et al. Structure of the human class I histocompatibility antigen, HLA-A2. Nature 1987;329:512
36. Brown JH, Jardetzky TS, Gorga JC, et al. Three-dimensional structure of the human class II histocompatibility antigen HLA-DR1. Nature 1993;364:33
37. Stern LJ, Brown JH, Jardetzky TS, et al. Crystal structure of the human class II MHC protein HLA-DR1 complexed with an influenza peptide. Nature 1994;368:215
38. Jardetzky TS, Brown JH, Gorga JC, et al. Three-dimensional structure of a human class II histocompatibility molecule complexed with superantigen. Nature 1994;368:711
39. Rudert WA, Trucco M. New insights in autoimmune mechanisms and the pathogenesis of IDDM. In: Scherbaum WA, Bogner V, Weinheimer B, Bottazzo GF, eds. Autoimmune Thyroiditis: Approaches Towards Its Etiological Differentiation. Heidelberg: Springer-Verlag;1991:3–11
40. Kwok WW, Nepom GT. Structural and functional constraints on HLA class II dimers implicated in susceptibility to insulin-dependent diabetes mellitus. In: Harrison LC, Tart BD, eds. Bailliere's Clinical Endocrinology and Metabolism. Philadelphia: Balliere Tindall;1991;5:375–393
41. Turco E, Manfras BJ, Ge L, et al. The x boxes from promoters of HLA class II B genes at different loci do not compete for nuclear protein-specific binding. Immunogenetics 1990;32:117
42. Anderson LC, Beaty JS, Nettles JW, et al. Allelic polymorphisms in transcriptional regulatory regions of HLA-DQB genes. J Exp Med 1991;173:181
43. Demotz S, Grey HM, Sette A. The minimal number of class II MHC-antigen complexes needed for T cell activation. Science 1990;249:1028
44. Davies JL, Kawaguchi Y, Bennett ST, et al. A genome-wide search for human type 1 diabetes susceptibility genes. Nature 1994;371:130
45. Hashimoto L, Habita C, Beressi JP, et al. Genetic mapping of a susceptibility locus for insulin-dependent diabetes mellitus on chromosome 11q. Nature 1994;371:161
46. Spies T, Bresnahan M, Bahram S, et al. A gene in the human major histocompatibility complex class II region controlling the class I antigen presentation pathway. Nature 1990;348:744
47. Powis SH, Mockridge I, Kelly A, et al. Polymorphism in a second ABC transporter gene located within the class II region of the human major histocompatibility complex. Proc Natl Acad Sci U S A 1992;89:1463
48. Caillat-Zucman S, Bertin E, Timsit J, et al. Protection from insulin-dependent diabetes mellitus is linked to a peptide transporter gene. Eur J Immunol 1993;23:1784
49. Colonna M, Bresnahan M, Bahran S, et al. Allelic variants of the human putative peptide transporter involved in antigen processing. Proc Natl Acad Sci U S A 1992;89:3932
50. Ronningen KS, Undlien DE, Ploski R, et al. Linkage disequilibrium between TAP^2 variants and HLA class II alleles; no primary association between TAP^2 variants and insulin-dependent diabetes mellitus. Eur J Immunol 1993;23:1050
51. van Endert P, Lopez M, Patel S, et al. Genomic polymorphism, recombination, and linkage disequilibrium in human major histocompatibility complex-encoded antigen-processing genes. Proc Natl Acad Sci U S A 1992;89:11594
52. Bell GI, Karam JH, Rutter WJ. Polymorphic DNA region adjacent to the 5′ end of the human insulin gene. Proc Natl Acad Sci U S A 1981;78:5759
53. Rotwein P, Chyn R, Chirgwin J, et al. Polymorphism in the 5′ flanking region of the human insulin gene and its possible relation to type 2 diabetes. Science 1981;213:1117
54. Owerbach D, Nerup J. Restriction fragment length polymorphism of the insulin gene in diabetes mellitus. Diabetes 1982;31:275
55. Rotwein PS, Chirgwin J, Province M, et al. Polymorphism of the 5′ flanking region of the human insulin gene: A genetic marker for non-insulin-dependent diabetes. N Engl J Med 1983;308:65
56. Bell GI, Horita Sand Karam JH. A polymorphic locus near the human insulin gene is associated with insulin-dependent diabetes mellitus. Diabetes 1984; 33:176
57. Hitman GA, Tarn AC, Winter RM, et al. Type I (insulin-dependent) diabetes and a highly variable locus close to the insulin gene on chromosome 11. Diabetologia 1985;28:218
58. Julier C, Hyer RN, Davies J, et al. Insulin-IgF_2 region on chromosome 11p encodes a gene implicated in HLA-DR4-dependent diabetes susceptibility. Nature 1991;354:155
59. Cox NJ, Baker L, Spielman RS. Insulin gene sharing in sub-pairs with insulin-dependent diabetes mellitus: No evidence for linkage. Am J Hum Genet 1988;42:167
60. Field LL. Non-HLA region genes in insulin-dependent diabetes mellitus. In: Harrison LC, Tait BD, eds. Bailliere's Clinical Endocrinology and Metabolism. Philadelphia: Balliere Tindall;1991;5:413–438
61. Field LL, Stephure DK, McArthur RG. Association between HLA-DR and G2m (23) in insulin-dependent diabetes. Am J Hum Genet 1989;45:A239
62. Haars R, Kronenberg M, Gallaten WM, et al. Rearrangement and expression of T cell antigen receptor and γ-genes during thymic development. J Exp Med 1986;164:1
63. von Boehmer H. Positive selection of lymphocytes. Cell 1994;76:219
64. Nossal GJV. Negative selection of lymphocytes. Cell 1994;76:229
65. Davey MP, Meyer MM, Bakke AC. T cell receptor Vb gene expression in monozygotic twins: Discordance in CD8 subset and in disease states. J Immunol 1994;152:315
66. Oldstone MB. Molecular mimicry and autoimmune disease. Cell 1987;50:819
67. Mamula MJ. The inability to process a self-peptide allows autoreactive T cells to escape tolerance. J Exp Med 1993;177:567
68. Conrad B, Weidmann E, Trucco G, et al. Evidence for superantigen involvement in insulin-dependent diabetes mellitus etiology. Nature 1994;371:351
69. Marrack P, Kappler J. The streptococcal endotoxins and their relatives. Science 1990;248:705
70. Herman A, Kappler JW, Marrak P, Pullen AM. Superantigens: Mechanism of T-cell stimulation and role in immune responses. Annu Rev Immunol 1991;9:745
71. Davis NM, Bjorkman PJ. T-cell antigen receptor genes and T-cell recognition. Nature 1988;334:395
72. Choi YW, Herman A, DiGiusto D, et al. Residues of the variable region of the T-cell receptor β chain that interact with *S. aureas* toxin superantigens. Nature 1990;324:163

73. Paliard X, West SG, Lafferty JA, et al. Evidence for the effects of a superantigen in rheumatoid arthritis. Science 1991;253:325
74. Mandrup-Paulsen T, Bendtzen K, Dinarello CA, Nerup J. Human tumor necrosis factor potentiates human interleukin 1-mediated rat pancreatic β-cell cytotoxicity. J Immunol 1987;12:4077
75. Mandrup-Paulsen T, Helqvist S, Molvig J, et al. Cytokines as immune effector molecules in autoimmune disease with special reference to insulin-dependent diabetes mellitus. Autoimmunity 1989;4:191
76. Notkins AL, Yoon JW. Virus-induced diabetes mellitus. In: Notkins AL, Oldstone MBA, eds. Concepts in Viral Pathogenesis. New York: Springer Verlag;1984:241–247
77. Oldstone MBA, Nerenberg M, Southern P, et al. Virus infection triggers insulin-dependent diabetes mellitus in a transgenic model: Role of anti-self (virus) immune response. Cell 1987;3:819
78. Marrack P, Kasonir E, Kappler J. A naturally inherited superantigen encoded by a mammary tumor virus. Nature 1991;350:203
79. Acha-Orbea H, Shakhov AN, Scapellino L, et al. Clonal deletion of Vβ14-bearing T cells in mice transgenic for mammary tumor virus. Nature 1991;350:207
80. Subramanyam M, McLellan B, Labrecque N, et al. Presentation of the Mls-1 superantigen by human HLA class II molecules to murine T cells. J Immunology 1993;151:2538
81. Trucco M. To be or not to be Asp 57, that is the question. Diabetes Care 1992;15:705
82. Robinson MA. Usage of human T-cell receptor Vβ, Jβ, Cβ and Vα gene segments is not proportional to gene number. Hum Immunol 1992;35:60
83. Weidmann E, Whiteside TL, Giorda R, et al. The T cell receptor Vβ usage in tumor-infiltrating lymphocytes and blood of patients with hepatocellular carcinoma. Cancer Res 1992;52:5913
84. Hall BL, Finn OJ. PCR-based analysis of the T-cell receptor Vβ multigene family: Experimental parameters affecting its validity. Biotechniques 1992; 2:248
85. Ohashi PS, Oehen S, Buerki K, et al. Ablation of "tolerance" and induction of diabetes by virus infection in viral antigen transgenic mice. Cell 1991;65:305
86. Tisch R, Yan X-D, Singer SM, et al. Immune response to glutamic acid decarboxylase correlates with insulitis in non-obese diabetic mice. Nature 1993;366:72
87. Kaufman DL, Clare-Salzler M, Tian J, et al. Spontaneous loss of T-cell tolerance to glutamic acid decarboxylase in murine insulin-dependent diabetes. Nature 1993;366:69
88. Trucco M, LaPorte R. Exposure to superantigens as immunogenetic explanation of type I diabetes mini-epidemics. J Pediatr Endocrinol & Metabol 1995;8:3–10

Diabetes Mellitus, edited by Derek LeRoith, Simeon I. Taylor, and Jerrold M. Olefsky. Lippincott–Raven Publishers, Philadelphia © 1996.

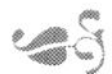

CHAPTER 35

Association Between Insulin-Dependent Diabetes Mellitus and Other Autoimmune Diseases

PINA L. BALDUCCI-SILANO, ELLEN CONNOR, AND NOEL K. MACLAREN

Historical Background

During the past two decades, researchers have been accumulating a large body of evidence indicating that insulin-dependent diabetes mellitus (IDDM), as well as other endocrine diseases associated with it, has an autoimmune pathogenesis[1–3] (Fig. 35-1).

Since the inception of modern immunology, immune responses directed against self-structures have been considered potentially harmful. It was believed initially that autoimmune responses are restricted to disease states and do not occur under normal conditions. This idea soon needed modification because autoimmune phenomena were subsequently found to greatly exceed disease-associated states in their occurrences. In normal individuals, the destruction of autoreactive T-cells occurs in the thymus for all self-antigens (autoantigens) that are able to be expressed in this gland as restricted by human leukocyte antigen (HLA) molecules *(central tolerance)*. Many self-antigens, however, are expressed only in peripheral tissues. At this level, an individual's T-lymphocytes will only recognize foreign antigens in conjunction with autologous HLA molecules presented on the surfaces of antigen-presenting cells, but in the absence of coexpression of accessory molecules, anergy is usually induced *(peripheral tolerance)*. A new model of autoimmune diseases therefore proposes that the disease state represents a breakdown of normal self-tolerance, a complex balance maintained by several mechanisms within the immune system, both central and peripheral.

Immunologic recognition of self-structures is not by itself a pathologic event, but one that is essential for the normal function of the immune system. However, excessive anti-self reaction and production of high amounts of autoantibodies of autoreactive T-lymphocytes with high affinity for self-molecules may ultimately lead to an autoimmune or self-attack.

The fact that IDDM has an autoimmune pathogenesis is supported by considerable direct as well as indirect evidence. Direct evidence includes: autoantibodies specific for islet cells, cell-mediated immune abnormalities detected in the peripheral blood, lymphocytic infiltrations of the pancreatic islets (insulitis lesions), and an immunogenetic susceptibility reflected mainly by HLA-class II gene associations.[4,5] Some of the earliest and most compelling indirect evidence for abnormal immune mechanisms in IDDM has been provided by the clinical observations of associations between IDDM and other disorders of putative or established autoimmune etiology (Table 35-1).

In 1849, Addison[6] first described the clinical and pathologic features of adrenocortical failure in patients, some of whom also appeared to have pernicious anemia. Ogle[7] reported the first instance of coexisting IDDM and adrenal insufficiency in 1866. In 1908, Claude and Gourgerot[8] suggested a common pathogenesis for the simultaneous expression of polyglandular insufficiencies involving pancreatic islet, thyroid, gonadal, adrenal, and anterior hypophysis, a fascinating and correct assertion. Parkinson,[9] in 1910 was the first to note an association between pernicious anemia and IDDM. Mononuclear leukocyte infiltrates of goitrous thyroid glands were first noted by Hashimoto[10] in 1912; a similar lesion of pancreatic islets, termed *insulitis,* was described by von Meyenburg[11] in 1940. The association between adrenocortical failure and thyroiditis was documented by Schmidt[12] in 1926, and the syndrome complex was extended by Carpenter et al.[13] in 1964 to include IDDM. It wasn't

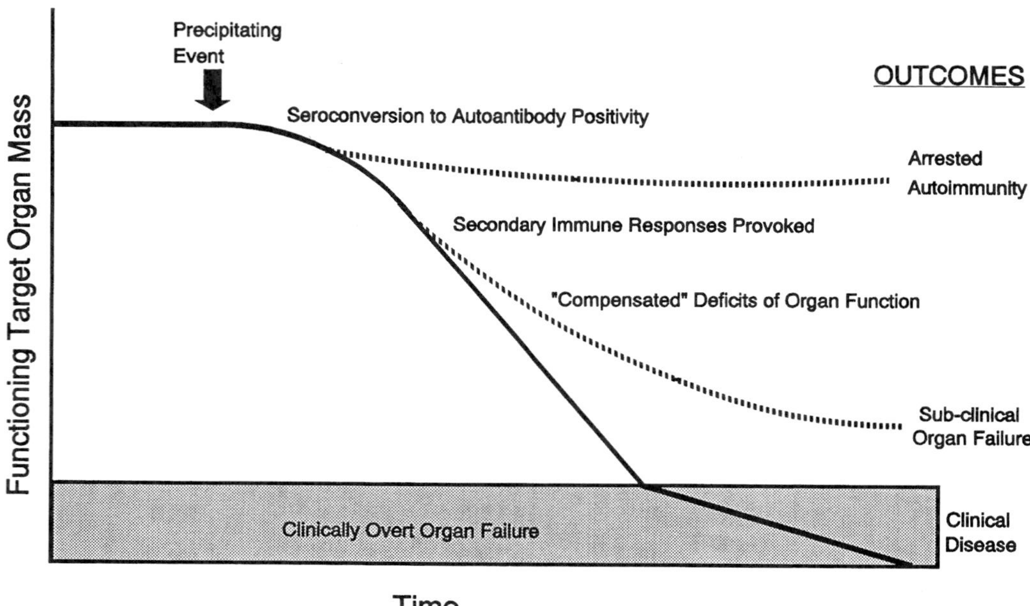

FIGURE 35-1. The proposed natural history of endocrine autoimmunity. Autoimmune attack of target organs often begins after an unknown precipitating event in persons who have a genetic predisposition (*arrow*). The early process manifests itself by provoking autoantibody production, and it may arrest at that stage (*top broken line*). Progressive disease, associated with secondary responses against antigens released by damaged tissue, is initially detectable by minimal biochemical abnormalities, such as elevations of trophic hormones. Organ function loss may plateau before the threshold of critical organ mass is reached (*lower broken line*), or it may progress to clinically overt disease (*solid line*). Hormone replacement therapy may decelerate the destruction of surviving tissue, but at this late stage, complete organ atrophy is inevitable. (Reproduced with permission from Muir A, Schatz DA, Maclaren NK. Polyglandular failure syndromes. In: DeGroot LJ, Leslie J, eds. Endocrinology. 3rd ed. Philadelphia, Pa: WB Saunders; 1995:3013.)

until 1956 that the *autoimmune pathogenesis* of these disorders began to become documented, beginning with the discovery of circulating precipitating autoantibodies to thyroglobulin in patients with Hashimoto's thyroiditis by Roitt et al.[14]

The ability to detect organ-specific humoral antibodies with methods developed by Anderson et al.[15] (1957) and Blizzard and Kyle[16] (1963) confirmed the clinical association between diabetes and idiopathic (autoimmune) adrenalitis. Solomon et al.[17] (1965) demonstrated the coexistence of adrenal atrophy in diabetics with thyroid and adrenal dysfunction. A body of literature clearly supports an increased incidence of autoimmune thyroid disease, either Graves' disease or Hashimoto's thyroiditis, in diabetics as well as an increased incidence of IDDM in autoimmune thyroid disease. An increased incidence of overt thyroid autoimmune disease as well as thyroid autoantibodies occurs in IDDM patients and their family members. Irvine et al.[18] (1970) reported that both pernicious anemia and thyroid disorders occur with significant frequency in first-degree relatives of diabetic patients. Autoantibodies to specific thyroid and gastric antigens,[19–23] as well as to adrenal and islet cell antigens,[24–29] in diabetic patients have been studied extensively. Cellular autoimmunity to thyroid antigens in IDDM has also been reported.[30] Neufeld et al.,[31,32] from our own group, distinguished the two major autoimmune polyglandular syndromes (APS I and II) summarized in Table 35-2. APS I and APS II are at present well-circumscribed entities, whereas APS III represents a group that may be a subset of APS II.

APS I is diagnosed when a patient presents with at least two of its three key features:

- Hypoparathyroidism
- Hypoadrenocorticism
- Recurrent mucocutaneous candidiasis.

The more common APS II is characterized by adrenocortical insufficiency occurring in conjunction with thyroiditis or IDDM, or both. APS III does not include adrenal insufficiency but does include the association between IDDM, lymphocytic thyroiditis, and pernicious anemia, sometimes with vitiligo. Finally, an association among IDDM, myasthenia gravis,[33] and vitiligo[34] also has been documented. The clinical associations between IDDM and autoimmune diseases are impressive, as are findings of strikingly high prevalences of certain organ-specific autoantibodies in diabetic sera (Table 35-3). The presence of these additional autoantibodies suggest that IDDM patients have a generalized tendency toward autoimmunity involving multiple endocrine glands and specific organs. It remains unclear at present, however, whether these apparently unrelated humoral specificities play any direct role in the pathogenesis of the disease. Most evidence suggests that T-lymphocyte–mediated processes play a more important role. In 1974, two independent studies have confirmed the existence of an antibody directed against the islet cells (islet cell antibodies [ICAs]) of endocrine pancreas in the sera of diabetic patients who had other coexistent autoimmune endocrine disorders.[35,36] Insulin autoantibodies (IAAs) also have been described, first in untreated newly diagnosed diabetic patients[37] and subsequently in first-degree relatives of diabetics, with the use of either radioimmunoassay (RIA)[38] or enzyme-linked immunosorbent assay (ELISA).[39]

In 1982, Baekkeskov et al.[40] first described a pancreatic islet cell protein considered an islet cell autoantigen recognized by disease-specific antibodies and autoreactive T-cells. This protein of 64 kd could be precipitated from human and rodent islets with the use of sera containing autoantibodies from IDDM patients and prediabetic subjects.[41] In 1990, this protein was identified to be a lower molecular weight isoform of the glutamic acid decarboxylase (GAD) enzyme.[42]

Table 35-1. Insulin-Dependent Diabetes Mellitus and other Organ-Specific Autoimmune Diseases: Historical Background

Year	Author(s)	Event
1849	Addison	Adrenocortical atrophy and pernicious anemia
1866	Ogle	Coexistence of IDDM and adrenal insufficiency
1908	Claude and Gourgerot	Polyglandular insufficiencies
1910	Parkinson	Pernicious anemia and IDDM
1912	Hashimoto	Lymphocytic infiltrates of goitrous thyroid glands
1926	Schmidt	Association between adrenocortical failure and thyroiditis
1940	von Meyenburg	Lymphocyte infiltrates of pancreatic islets
1956	Roitt et al.	Thyroid autoantibodies
1964	Carpenter et al.	Schmidt's syndrome with IDDM
1965	Solomon et al.	Adrenal atrophy pattern in IDDM combined with thyroid and adrenal dysfunction
1969	Osserman	Myasthenia gravis and IDDM
1970	Irvine et al.	Pernicious anemia and autoimmune thyroid disease in first-degree relatives of IDDM patients
1970	Goldstein et al.	Prevalence of thyroid and gastric antibodies in IDDM patients
1974	Bottazzo et al. MacCuish et al.	ICAs in IDDM combined with other autoimmune disorders
1974	Moulias et al.	Cellular thyroid autoimmunity and IDDM
1980, 1981	Neufeld et al.	Clinical classification of APS
1982	Baekkeskov et al.	Spontaneous autoantibodies to human pancreatic islet cell protein
1983	Palmer et al.	Spontaneous IAAs in untreated IDDM patients
1987, 1990	Baekkeskov et al.	Identification of 64-kd antigen in human pancreatic islets as GAD enzyme
1992	Kauffman et al.	Autoimmunity to two isoforms of GAD in IDDM
1992	Atkinson et al.	Cellular autoimmunity to GAD in IDDM

APS = autoimmune polyglandular syndrome; GAD = glutamic acid decarboxylase; IAAs = insulin autoantibodies; ICAs = islet cell antibodies; IDDM = insulin-dependent diabetes mellitus.

Table 35-2. The Autoimmune Polyglandular Syndromes

Features	APS I	APS II	APS III
Diagnostic features			
	Addison's disease	Addison's disease	
	Hypoparathyroidism	Hashimoto's thyroiditis	Hashimoto's thyroiditis
	Candidiasis	IDDM	IDDM
		Graves' disease	Pernicious anemia (late)
Associated diseases			
	Pernicious anemia (early)	Pernicious anemia (late)	
	Hypogonadism	Hypogonadism	
	Vitiligo	Vitiligo	Vitiligo
	Alopecia	Alopecia	
	Malabsorption	Myasthenia gravis	
	Chronic active hepatitis	Celiac disease	
	Myopathy		
	Sjögren's syndrome		
Mendelian inheritance	Recessive or sporadic	Dominant Female bias	Dominant Female bias

APS = autoimmune polyglandular syndrome; IDDM = insulin-dependent diabetes mellitus.

Table 35-3. Autoantigens in Autoimmune Polyglandular Syndrome

Disease	Autoantigen(s)
Insulin-dependent diabetes mellitus	ICA, IAA, GAD65, 38-kd
Hashimoto's thyroiditis	Thyroid peroxidase, thyroglobulin
Graves' disease	Thyroid peroxidase, thyroglobulin, TSH receptor
Pernicious anemia	H^+, K^+-ATPase, intrinsic factor
Addison's disease	21-hydroxylase, 17-hydroxylase, side-chain cleavage enzyme (?)
Vitiligo	Tyrosinase

GAD = glutamic acid decarboxylase; H^+, K^+-ATPase = the parietal cell proton pump; IAA = insulin autoantibody; ICA = islet cell antigen; TSH = thyroid-stimulating hormone.

Kaufman et al.[43] recently demonstrated that two specific isoforms of GAD, GAD65 and GAD67 (65 kd and 67 kd, respectively), could be immunoprecipitated by using the sera of IDDM patients. Human islets have been found to express GAD65, but lower levels of GAD67.[44]

In summary, the study of the etiopathogenesis of Type I diabetes and human autoimmunity in general has attracted a great deal of interest among immunologists. The common association of multiple endocrine disorders in the same patient family, or both, as well as the association of multiple endocrine disorders with genes in the immune response region, specifically the HLA-DR and HLA-DQ genes, have been used as evidence of a common autoimmune origin for these multiple disorders.

The Genetics of Insulin-Dependent Diabetes Mellitus

How and why IDDM develops remains an area of fervent research effort. Clearly, however, IDDM development depends greatly on multiple genetic predispositions, coupled with some inductive event from the environment. Inherited susceptibility to IDDM is associated with genes in the major histocompatibility complex (MHC), especially those located on the HLA-D or HLA-class II region on the short arm of chromosome 6.[45–49] In 1973, an association between IDDM and HLA-class I antigens B8 and B15 (B62) was observed.[50,51] Later, this association was explained by the existence of these alleles in linkage disequilibrium with HLA-class II DR3 and DR4.[52,53] Of IDDM patients in the United States, 95% carry either DR3 or DR4 (versus 45% in the normal population). The following DRB1 alleles also confer susceptibility: DRB1*01, DRB1*16, DRB1*08, and DRB1*1302.[45,54] In contrast, the alleles DRB1*1301, DRB1*15, and DRB1*11 are protective against IDDM.[45,55]

Class II HLA genes are clearly more closely linked with IDDM than class I HLA genes.[56] In recent years, the strongest class II association described has been between the DQB genes that contain a neutral amino acid (serine, valine, or alanine) at position 57 and the DQA genes that contain arginine at position 52.[57–61] Because both *cis*- and *trans*-complementation forms of DQα/β dimers are encoded, persons with DQ in whom all possible dimers conform to the above, are those most susceptible to acquiring IDDM.

In whites, susceptibility to IDDM is strongly associated with particular HLA-DQA1-DQB1 combinations, mainly those in linkage disequilibrium with DR3 and DR4 antigens, rather than single DQA1 or DQB1 alleles.[60,62] In white populations, the highest risk is found in DQA1*0501-DQB1*0201/DQA1*0301-DQB1*0302 heterozygotes, which might be due to their capacity to encode four different susceptibility HLA-DQ heterodimers, in both *cis*- and *trans*-complementation.[58,63] HLA-DQ heterodimers encoded by DQA1 with Arg position 52 (Arg-52+) and DQB1 with non-Asp at position 57 (Asp-57−) alleles confer susceptibility of various strengths.[63,64]

The importance of these DQ residues could be in the maintenance of islet cell relevant antigen-binding site conformation.[46] HLA-DR and -DQ genes seem to have similar impact on IDDM susceptibility or resistance, although their relative importance varies considerably depending on the ethnic group studied.[65,66,67] Associations between HLA-DP antigens and several autoimmune diseases[68,69,70] including IDDM[71,72,73] have been described. However, the role of HLA-DP antigens in the pathogenesis of IDDM remains to be solved. HLA class II molecules are usually involved in the presentation of foreign peptides to the immune system. Thus, the HLA-D associations with IDDM could result from a unique immunoresponse to a foreign antigen, such as from an enteric virus, with an antigen found on β-cells that has molecular mimicry with the environmental immunogen.

Mode of Inheritance

Computer modeling of IDDM genetics suggests that many non-HLA genes are involved in IDDM pathogenesis. Specifically, it has been suggested that DRB1*03 is linked with a recessive diabetes susceptibility gene and that DRB1*04 is linked to a dominant gene.[74] Further evidence that there is gene interplay is given by the preferential paternal transmission of IDDM to offspring of either sex.[75]

The nonobese diabetic (NOD) mouse model of IDDM indicates that there are as many as 10 distinct genes involved in its susceptibility; in studies of men, at least 5 genes will soon be identified.[76]

Genetic Associations Between Insulin-Dependent Diabetes Mellitus and Other Autoimmune Endocrinopathies

Whereas the HLA class II associations with IDDM are well described, less is known about the genetics leading to the development of other autoimmune diseases found, in turn, to be associated with IDDM. IDDM is most frequently seen as a component of APS III, in which autoimmune insulitis and thyroiditis frequently coexist. Fully one-third of female IDDM patients have or will develop autoimmune thyroiditis in their lifetime. We recommend routine screening for this disorder among such patients.

Genetic susceptibility to APS III is not well understood. Hashimoto's thyroiditis has been ambiguously associated with HLA DRB1*03, DRB1*04, and DRB1*05 in various studies,[77,78] whereas DRB1*03/DQA1*0501/DQB1*0201 has been linked more strongly to Grave's disease.[79] Because none of these associations adequately explain the multiplex families affected by thyroiditis, as is commonly seen by the clinician, evidence of genetic loci outside the HLA locus is currently being studied.

The genetics of Addison's disease occurring with IDDM also are not well understood. Previous reports have associated Addison's disease with HLA DRB1*03 and DRB1*04 in populations of patients with thyroiditis or IDDM, or both.[80,81] Our own studies indicate that the degree to which HLA-DR and HLA-DQ are associated in APS II is similar to that found in IDDM (Table 35-4). For example, APS II is also strongly associated with the same HLA-DR genes, DR3 and DR4. In fact, there are more patients with APS II HLA-DR3 and HLA-DR4 heterozygotes than patients who are affected only by IDDM; however, patients with APS I do not have elevated frequencies of these alleles (7% DR3/DR4 heterozygosity, compared to 3% in normal controls and nearly 40% in APS II of IDDM). Most of the DR3/DR4 heterozygotic patients with APS II are also ICA-positive. Thus, the strength of DRB1*03 and

Table 35-4. HLA-DRB1 Association in Autoimmune Polyglandular Syndrome*

Disease	DRB1*03/DRB1*04
Isolated Addison's	No association
APS I and APS II	Significant association[†]
APS I	No association
APS II	Significant association[†]
APS II and ICA +	Significant association[†]
APS II and ICA −	No association

*E.L. Connor, P.L. Balducci-Silano, Y.-H. Song, and N.K. Maclaren, unpublished data, 1994.
[†]$P \geq 0.05$.
APS = Autoimmune polyglandular syndrome.

DRB1*04 associations with IDDM precludes knowing whether the association with Addison's disease is real or merely a reflection of these patients' underlying β-cell autoimmunity. Clearly, further genetic studies of patients with IDDM in combination with thyroiditis or Addison's disease, or both, are indicated.

Clinical Relevance

Given the interrelationship between IDDM and other endocrinopathies in the polyglandular syndromes, how should the clinician monitor the IDDM patient? Clearly, accurate and early diagnosis of other endocrinopathies, particularly Addison's disease, can significantly reduce morbidity and mortality. All patients with IDDM should be screened for the presence of adrenal, steroidal, gastric parietal, thyroid microsomal, and thyroglobulin antibodies at the time of their diagnosis, which itself should be confirmed with ICA and IAA testing when clinical presentations are not classic. Family members of a proband with IDDM should also undergo ICA and IAA studies, and those who are positive or who have family members with other endocrinopathies should have full autoantibody profiles performed. The necessity of further workup of IDDM patients or their family members depends on their panel results. ICA screening should be repeated annually in children younger than 10 years and every 2 years in relatives younger than 20 years because these age groups are at higher risk for developing pancreatic β-cell autoimmunity; the risk of conversion from negative to positive markedly falls with increasing age.

Thyroiditis. All patients with thyroid autoantibodies should have thyroid panel determinations performed annually. Thyroid-stimulating hormone (TSH) levels are the most diagnostically helpful. Those with hypothyroidism should be chemically treated with thyroid hormone replacement therapy. Any IDDM patient developing a goiter should have thyroid studies and antibodies determined. If a patient is found to have thyroiditis, family members should be screened for thyroid autoantibodies and goiter also.

Addison's Disease. Patients with adrenal or steroidal antibodies should be carefully evaluated for clinical signs and symptoms of adrenal insufficiency; they should have annual basal plasma adrenocorticotrophic hormone (ACTH) and renin levels studied because these will become elevated before the onset of electrolyte abnormalities and most clinical symptoms. A history of weight loss, hyperpigmentation (often described as "dirty" pigmentation of the neck or elbows), easy fatigability, muscular weakness, dehydration, emesis, or malaise should be sought at each clinical visit. Patients should be educated to recognize and report these symptoms immediately. Addison's disease may be present in as many as every 250 patients with IDDM. It should be recognized and treated as it occurs; left unrecognized, this disease poses an absolute risk to patients.

Atrophic Gastritis. Patients found to have gastric parietal antibodies should have annual B12 and ferritin levels determined. If abnormalities are found, monthly B12 injections should be administered. Most patients reach mid life before this becomes necessary. Any IDDM patient with new onset of paresthesia should notify his or her endocrinologist promptly.

Steroidal Antibodies. Patients with steroidal antibodies may develop both Addison's disease and hypogonadism. Thus, antibody-positive patients should be admonished to recognize the symptoms of adrenal insufficiency described above; they also should be monitored for secondary amenorrhea, pregnancy loss, and signs of infertility. Annual determinations of follicle-stimulating hormone (FSH) and luteinizing hormone (LH) may permit prediction of gonadal failure. Patients also should be examined for evidence of mucocutaneous candidiasis or for hypoparathyroidism, if these autoantibodies are detected.

Recommendations for Screening

Appreciating that IDDM often occurs with other autoimmune endocrinopathies, we recommend screening for those diseases both in patients with IDDM and in their relatives. Such screening is not an esoteric exercise: The consequences of undiagnosed endocrinopathies can involve significant morbidity or mortality. One could argue that the clinician certainly would recognize the onset of a new endocrinopathy in an IDDM patient or the symptoms of endocrine insufficiency in a relative of a patient; however, disease onset may be insidious and easily missed unless specifically and routinely thought of and tested for.

Thyroid Screening. Fully one-third of IDDM patients develop autoimmune thyroiditis (e.g., Hashimoto's thyroiditis, Grave's disease), most commonly recognized after the diagnosis of IDDM. The consequences of untreated hypothyroidism include congestive heart failure, dyslipidemia, infertility, growth retardation, and rarely, slipped capital femoral epiphysis. Grave's disease can cause significant weight loss, weakness, and congestive heart failure. We would suggest screening for thyroid microsomal antibodies when IDDM is diagnosed and whenever a goiter is noted. Patients with thyroid autoantibodies or goiter should have TSH screening annually and careful monitoring of vital signs at each examination.

Adrenal Screening. Any IDDM patient showing family pedigree including Addison's disease should be screened for adrenocortical and steroidal cell antibodies. Adrenocortical autoantibodies of relevance to Addison's disease recently have been shown to include those to the p450 enzyme 21-hydroxylase with antibody reactivity, preferentially directed to the conserved humoral binding site of the enzyme.[27,28] Steroidal cell autoantibodies have been suggested to include those directed at the side chain cleavage enzyme.[28] Similar screening should be sought in patients with unexplained weight loss, refractory hypoglycemia, hyperpigmentation, or unexplained hypovolemia. Patients with adrenocortical antibodies should have determinations of ACTH, 8:00 AM serum cortisol, and supine renin levels annually. Electrolyte abnormalities are a late finding, and normal electrolytes do not exclude disease.

Gastric Parietal Antibodies. IDDM patients with (1) strong family histories of thyroiditis or pernicious anemia, (2) megaloblastic anemia, or (3) unexplained fatigue should be screened for gastric parietal cell antibodies. Any patient with these antibodies should have yearly determinations of ferritin and B12 levels.

Ovarian, Testicular, and Placental Autoantibodies. Impaired fertility may result from inadequate glycemic control in IDDM. Gonadal autoimmunity, however, particularly in patients with steroidal cell antibodies, has been well documented in patients with IDDM. A history of amenorrhea (usually secondary), oligomenorrhea, or infertility should alert the clinician to the possibility of autoimmune ovarian or testicular failure. Determination of serum steroidal cell antibodies, LH, FSH, estrogen, and testosterone levels will facilitate diagnosis.

Summary and Conclusions

IDDM often occurs in the context of other autoimmune endocrinopathies. Its most common presentation with other autoimmunity is as part of APS III, which is the constellation of IDDM and autoimmune thyroiditis, sometimes with pernicious anemia, vitiligo, and/or hypogonadism. The association of IDDM with Addison's disease in the context of APS II carries the greatest risk of mortality and requires rapid recognition and specific replacement therapies to prevent fatalities. The possible genetic explanations for the association between other endocrinopathies and IDDM remain unclear. Until the issue of genetics has been resolved, the clinician must rely entirely on the recognition of subtle symptoms and a knowledge of serum autoantibody profiles to swiftly diagnose and treat polyglandular autoimmunity.

At present, there appear to be no common antigens shared uniquely among organs targeted by the autoimmune processes underlying APS. Indeed, the putative antigens of pathogenic importance appear to be distinctively different (see Table 35-3). We recently were able to add the enzyme tyrosinase, as targeted by autoimmune vitiligo, to this list.[34] Further, there are no known common genes to explain the concomitant development of the autoimmune endocrinopathies seen in APS. HLA associations did not offer such an explanation. APS I, which is associated with autoantibodies to denatured peptides of GAD65 but rarely diabetes, appears to be due to a single recessive, albeit unknown, gene that has yet to be identified. The genetic predispositions evident in APS II and III, however, affect each successive generation as would multiple dominant and interactive genes, which have yet to be identified.

References

1. Maclaren N, Riley W. Thyroid, gastric and adrenal autoimmunities and insulin dependent diabetes. Diabetes Care 1985;8:34
2. Maclaren N, Riley W. Polyglandular autoimmunity: Autoimmune diseases of the parathyroid and adrenal glands. In: Samter M, Claman H, eds. Immunological Diseases. Boston: Little Brown and Company; 1988:1737–1746
3. Muir A, Schatz DA, Maclaren NK. Polyglandular failure syndromes. In: DeGroot, Leslie J, ed. Endocrinology 3rd ed. Philadelphia Pa: WB Saunders; 1995;3013–3024
4. Schatz D, Winter W, Maclaren N. Immunology of insulin dependent diabetes. In: Volpè R, ed. Autoimmune Diseases of the Endocrine System. Boca Raton, Fla: CRC Press; 1990:241–296
5. Bottazzo GF, Todd J, Mirakian R, et al. Organ-specific autoimmunity: A 1986 overview. Immunol Rev 1986;94:137
6. Addison T. Anaemia—Disease of the suprarenal capsules. Lond Med Gaz 1849;8:517
7. Ogle JW. On disease of the brain as a result of diabetes mellitus. St George's Hosp Rep 1866;1:157
8. Claude H, Gourgerot H. Insuffisance pluriglandulaire endocrinienne. J Physiol Pathol Gen 1908;10:469
9. Parkinson J. A case of pernicious anaemia terminating in acute diabetes. Lancet 1910;2:543
10. Hashimoto H. Zur Kenntnis der lymphomatosen veranderung der schilddruse (struma lymphomatosa). Acta Klim Chir 1912;97:219
11. von Meyenburg H. Uber "Insulitis" bei diabetes. Schweitz Med Wochenschr 1940;21:554
12. Schmidt MB. Eine biglandulare Erkrankung (Nebennieren und Schilddrusse) bei Morbus Addisonii. Verh Dtsch Ges Pathol 1926;21:212
13. Carpenter CCJ, Solomon N, Silverberg SG, et al. Schmidt's syndrome (thyroid and adrenal insufficiency): A review of the literature and a report of fifteen new cases including ten instances of coexistent diabetes mellitus. Medicine (Baltimore) 1964;43:153
14. Roitt IM, Doniach D, Campbell PN, et al. Autoantibodies in Hashimoto's disease (lymphadenoid goitre). Lancet 1956;2:820
15. Anderson JR, Goudie RB, Gray K, Timbury GC. Auto-antibodies in Addison's disease. Lancet 1957;1:1123
16. Blizzard RM, Kyle M. Studies of the adrenal antigens and antibodies in Addison's disease. J Clin Invest 1963;42:1653
17. Solomon N, Carpenter CJC, Bennett IL, Harvey AM. Schmidt's syndrome (thyroid and adrenal insufficiency) and coexistent diabetes mellitus. Diabetes 1965;14:300
18. Irvine WJ, Clarke BF, Scarth L, et al. Thyroid and gastric autoimmunity in patients with diabetes mellitus. Lancet 1970;2:163
19. Goldstein RE, Drash A, Gibbs J, Blizzard RM. Diabetes mellitus: The incidence of circulating antibodies against thyroid, gastric and adrenal tissue. J Pediatr 1970;77:304
20. Pinchera A, Mariotti S, Vitti P, et al. Thyroid autoantigens and their relevance in the pathogenesis of thyroid autoimmunity. Biochimie 1989;71:237
21. Jeffries GH, Hosking DW, Sleisenger MH. Antibody to intrinsic factor in serum from patients with pernicious anaemia. J Clin Invest 1962;41:1106
22. De Aizpurua HJ, Toh BH, Ungar B. Parietal cell surface reactive autoantibody in pernicious anaemia demonstrated by indirect membrane immunofluorescence. Clin Exp Immunol 1983;52:341
23. Karlsson FA, Burman P, Lööf L, Mårdh S. Major parietal cell antigen in autoimmune gastritis with pernicious anaemia is the acid producing H, K-adenosin triphosphatase of the stomach. J Clin Invest 1988;81:475
24. Krohn K, Perheentupa J, Heinonen E. Precipitating anti-adrenal antibodies in Addison's disease. Clin Immunol Immunopathol 1974;3:59
25. Krohn K, Uibo R, Aarik E, et al. Identification by molecular cloning of an autoantigen associated with Addison's disease as 17 hydroxylase. Lancet 1992;339:770
26. Winquist O, Karlsson AF, Kämpe O. 21 Hydroxylase, a major autoantigen in idiopathic Addison's disease. Lancet 1992;339:1559
27. Song Y-H, Connor E, Muir A, et al. Autoantibody epitope mapping of the 21-hydroxylase antigen in autoimmune Addison disease. J Clin Endocrinol Metab 1993;78:1108
28. Uibo R, Aavik E, Peterson P, et al. Autoantibodies to cytochrome P450 enzymes P450scc, P450c17, and P450c21 in autoimmune polyglandular disease types I and II and in isolated Addison's disease. J Clin Endocrinol Metab 1994;78:323
29. Atkinson MA, Maclaren NK. Islet cell autoantigens in insulin-dependent diabetes. J Clin Invest 1993;92:1608
30. Moulias R, Goust JM, Bernard S, et al. Humoral and cellular thyroid autoimmunity and diabetes mellitus. In: Bastenie PA, Gepts W, eds. Immunity and Auto-immunity in Diabetes Mellitus. Amsterdam: Excerpta Medica; 1974:140
31. Neufeld M, Maclaren N, Blizzard R. Autoimmune polyglandular syndromes. Pediatr Ann 1980;9:154
32. Neufeld M, Maclaren NK, Blizzard RM. Two types of autoimmune Addison's disease associated with different polyglandular autoimmune (PGA) syndromes. Medicine (Baltimore) 1981;60:355
33. Osserman KE. Muscles (myasthenia gravis). In: Mieschar PA, Muller-Eberhard M, eds. Textbook of Immunopathology. 2nd ed. New York: Grune and Stratton; 1969:607
34. Song Y-H, Connor EL, Li Y, et al. Tyrosinase is an autoantigen in autoimmune vitiligo. Lancet 1994;344:1049
35. Bottazzo GF, Florin-Christensen AF, Doniach D. Islet-cell antibodies in diabetes mellitus with autoimmune polyendocrine deficiencies. Lancet 1974;2:1279
36. MacCuish AC, Barnes EW, Irvine WJ, Duncan LJP. Antibodies to pancreatic islet-cells in insulin-dependent diabetes with coexistent autoimmune disease. Lancet 1974;2:1529
37. Palmer JP, Asplin CM, Clemons P, et al. Insulin antibodies in insulin-dependent diabetics before insulin treatment. Science 1983;222:1337
38. Srikanta S, Ricker AT, McCulloch DK, et al. Autoimmunity to insulin, beta cell dysfunction, and development of insulin dependent diabetes mellitus. Diabetes 1986;35:139
39. Dean BM, Becker F, McNally JM, et al. Insulin autoantibodies in the prediabetic period: Correlation with islet cell antibodies and development of diabetes. Diabetologia 1986;29:339
40. Baekkeskov S, Neilsen JH, Marner B, et al. Autoantibodies in newly diagnosed diabetic children with immunoprecipitate human pancreatic islet cell proteins. Nature 1982;298:167
41. Baekkeskov S, Landin S, Kristensen JK, et al. Antibodies to a 64,000 M_r human islet cell antigen precede the clinical onset of insulin-dependent diabetes. J Clin Invest 1987;79:926
42. Baekkeskov S, Aanstoot JH, Christgau S, et al. The 64kD autoantigen in insulin-dependent diabetes is the GABA synthesizing enzyme glutamic acid decarboxylase. Nature 1990;347:151
43. Kaufman D, Erlander M, Clare-Salzler M, et al. Autoimmunity to two forms of glutamate decarboxylase in insulin-dependent diabetes mellitus. J Clin Invest 1992;89:283
44. Atkinson M, Kaufman D, Campbell L, et al. Response of peripheral blood mononuclear cells to glutamate decarboxylase in insulin dependent diabetes. Lancet 1992;339:458
45. Todd JA. Genetic control of autoimmunity type I diabetes. Immunol Today 1990;11:122
46. Nepom GT, Erlich H. MHC class-II molecules and autoimmunity. Ann Rev Immunol 1991;9:493
47. Bach FH, Rich SS, Barbosa RS, Segall M. Insulin-dependent diabetes associated HLA-D region encoded determinants. Hum Immunol 1985;12:59
48. Todd JA, Acha-Orbea H, Bell JI, et al. A molecular basis for MHC class II autoimmunity. Science 1988;240:1003
49. Todd JA, Bain SC. A practical approach to identification of susceptibility genes for IDDM. Diabetes 1992;41:1029
50. Singal DP, Blajchman MA. Histocompatibility (HLA) antigens, lymphocytotoxic antibodies and tissue antibodies with diabetes mellitus. Diabetes 1973;22:429
51. Nerup J, Platz P, Ortred-Anderson M, et al. HLA antigens and diabetes mellitus. Lancet 1974;2:864
52. Wolf E, Spencer KM, Cudworth AG. The genetic susceptibility to type I (insulin-dependent) diabetes: Analysis of the HLA-DR association. Diabetologia 1983;24:224
53. Rotter J, Vadheim C, Raffel L, et al. Genetic etiologies of diabetes. In: Laron Z, Tikva P, eds. Pediatric and Adolescent Endocrinology. New York: S. Karger; 1986:1–11
54. Maclaren N, Riley W, Skordis N, et al. Inherited susceptibility to insulin dependent diabetes is associated with HLA-DR1, while DR5 is protective. Autoimmunity 1988;1:197

55. Sheehy MJ. HLA and insulin-dependent diabetes: A protective perspective. Diabetes 1992;41:123
56. Todd JA, Aitman TJ, Cornall RJ, et al. Genetic analysis of a complex, multifactorial disease, autoimmune type 1 (insulin-dependent) diabetes. Res Immunol 1991;142:483
57. Ronningen KS, Iwe T, Halstensen TS, et al. The amino acid at position 57 of the HLA-DQ beta chain and susceptibility to develop insulin dependent diabetes mellitus. Hum Immunol 1989;26:215
58. Nepom BS, Schwarz D, Palmer JP, Nepom GT. Transcomplementation of HLA genes in IDDM: HLA-DQ alpha- and beta-chains produce hybrid molecules in DR3/4 heterozygotes. Diabetes 1987;36:114
59. Nepom GT. A unified hypothesis for the complex genetics of HLA associations with IDDM. Diabetes 1990;39:1153
60. Khalil I, D'Auriol L, Gobet M, et al. A combination of HLA-DQβ Asp57-negative and HLA DQα Arg 52 confers susceptibility to insulin-dependent diabetes mellitus. J Clin Invest 1990;85:1315
61. Todd JA, Bell JI, McDevitt HO. HLA-DQ beta gene contributes to susceptibility and resistance to insulin-dependent diabetes mellitus. Nature 1987; 329:599
62. Todd JA, Mijovic C, Fletcher J, et al. Identification of susceptibility loci for insulin-dependent diabetes mellitus by trans-racial gene mapping. Nature 1989;338:587
63. Khalil I, Deschamps I, Lepage V, et al. Dose effect of cis- and trans-encoded HLA-DQαβ heterodimers in IDDM susceptibility. Diabetes 1992;41:378
64. Ronningen KS, Spurkland A, Iwe T, et al. Distribution of HLA-DRB1, DQA1 and DQB1 alleles and DQA1-DQB1 genotypes among Norwegian patients with insulin-dependent diabetes-mellitus. Tissue Antigens 1991;37:105
65. Easteal S, Vigwanathan M, Serjeantson SW. HLA-DP, -DQ and -DR RFLP types in South Indian insulin dependent diabetes mellitus patients. Tissue Antigens 1990;35:71
66. Sanjeevi CB, Zeidler A, Shaw S, et al. Analysis of HLA-DQA1 and DQB1 genes in Mexican Americans with insulin dependent diabetes mellitus. Tissue Antigens 1993;42:72
67. Balducci-Silano PL, Layrisse Z, Domínguez E, et al. HLA-DQA1 and DQB1 allele and genotype contribution to IDDM susceptibility in an ethnically mixed population. Eur J Immunogen 1994;21:405
68. Begovich AB, Bugawan TL, Nepom BS, et al. A specific HLA-DP beta allele is associated with pauciarticular juvenile rheumatoid arthritis but not adult rheumatoid arthritis. Proc Natl Acad Sci 1989;86:9489
69. Bugawan TL, Angelimi G, Larrick J, et al. A combination of a particular HLA-DPβ allele and an HLA-DQ heterodimer confers susceptibility to coeliac disease. Nature (London) 1989;339:470
70. Caffrey C, Hitman A, Niven MJ, et al. HLA-DP and coeliac disease: Family and population studies. Gut 1990;31:663
71. Easteal S, Kohenen-Corish RJM, Zimmet P, Serjeantson SW. HLA-DP variation as additional risk factor in IDDM. Diabetes 1990;39:855
72. Baish JM, Capra JD. Analysis of HLA genotypes and susceptibility to insulin dependent diabetes mellitus. Association maps telomeric to HLA-DP. Scand J Immunol 1992;36:331
73. Balducci-Silano PL, Layrisse ZE. HLA-DP and susceptibility to insulin-dependent diabetes mellitus in an ethnically mixed population. Associations with other HLA-alleles. J Autoimmunity 1995;8:425
74. Louis EJ, Thomson G. Three-allele synergistic mixed model for insulin dependent diabetes. Diabetes 1986;35:958
75. Warram JH, Krolewski AS, Gottlieb MS, Kahn CR. Differences in risk of insulin-dependent diabetes in offspring of diabetic mothers and diabetic fathers. N Engl J Med 1984;311:149
76. Davies JL, Kawaguchi Y, Bennett ST, et al. A genome-wide search for human type 1 diabetes susceptibility genes. Nature 1994;371:130
77. Tachi J, Amino N, Tamaki H, et al. Longterm follow-up and HLA association in patients with post-partum hypothyroidism. J Clin Exp Med 1988;66:480
78. Thompson C, Farid NR. Post partum thyroiditis and goitrous (Hashimoto's) thyroiditis are associated with HLA-DR4. Immunol Lett 1985;11:301
79. Yanagawa T, Manglclabruks A, Chang Y-B, et al. Human histocompatibility leukocyte antigen-DQA1*0501 allele associated with genetic susceptibility to Grave's disease in a Caucasian population. J Clin Exp Med 1993;76:1569
80. Latinne D, Vandeput Y, DeBruyere M, et al. Addison's disease: Immunological aspects. Tissue Antigens 1987;30:23
81. Maclaren N, Riley W. Inherited susceptibility to autoimmune Addison's disease is linked to human leukocyte antigens-DR3 and/or DR4, except when associated with type 1 autoimmune polyglandular syndrome. J Clin Endocrinol Metab 1986;62:455

Diabetes Mellitus, edited by Derek LeRoith, Simeon I. Taylor, and Jerrold M. Olefsky. Lippincott–Raven Publishers, Philadelphia © 1996.

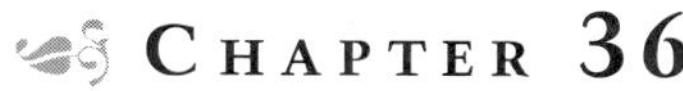

CHAPTER 36

Role of Viruses in the Pathogenesis of Insulin-Dependent Diabetes Mellitus

JI-WON YOON

It is believed that genetic predisposition is necessary for the development of insulin-dependent diabetes mellitus (IDDM)[1]; however, because the concordance rate for IDDM between genetically identical, monozygotic twins approaches only 40%,[2] researchers have turned their attention to elucidating the environmental factors affecting the penetrance of susceptibility genes. In this chapter, I will briefly review viruses as one environmental factor, as well as the various pathogenic mechanisms by which viruses may act either to induce or to prevent diabetes.

Viruses have been considered for many years to be associated with the development of some cases of IDDM.[3] There appears to be a seasonal variation in the onset of acute IDDM, with a peak in the autumn,[4,5] and diseases with seasonal incidences often are caused by viral infections. There also have been numerous anecdotal reports of a temporal association between viral infections and the development of diabetes by some individuals.[3] It is thought that, in some cases, viruses directly destroy insulin-producing pancreatic β-cells by cytolytic infection; in other cases, viruses are thought to trigger or somehow contribute to β-cell-specific autoimmunity, leading to the development of IDDM[3] (Fig. 36-1). In addition, there is evidence that viruses can also protect against the development of diabetes by the spontaneously diabetic BioBreeding (BB) rat and nonobese diabetic (NOD) mouse.[6,7]

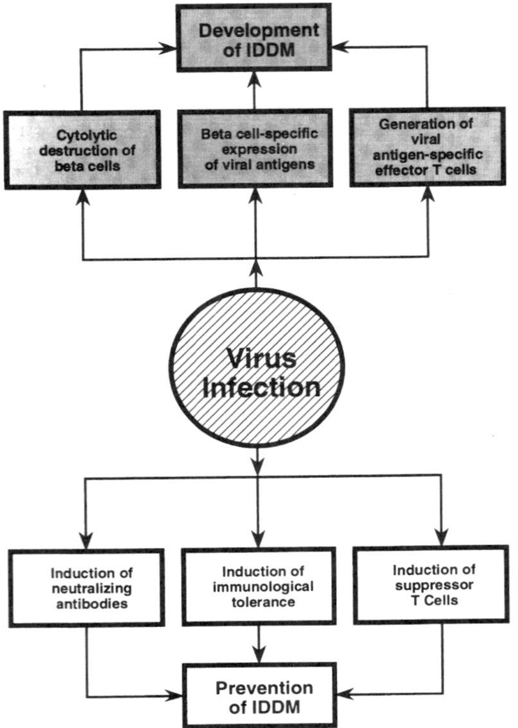

Figure 36-1. The role of viruses in the pathogenesis of IDDM. Genetic susceptibility appears to be a prerequisite for the development of IDDM. However, environmental factors such as viruses may act as inducing or preventive agents. Some viruses, including EMC-D virus and Coxsackie B4 virus, can induce diabetes by infecting and destroying β-cells in a genetically susceptible host (cytolytic destruction of β-cells). Other viruses (e.g., retrovirus in NOD mice, rubella virus in hamsters and humans) may alter a normally existing β-cell antigen into an immunogenic form or might induce a new antigen that may trigger β-cell–specific autoimmune IDDM (β-cell–specific expression of viral antigens). Furthermore, other viruses (e.g., KRV in DRBB rats) may generate antigen-specific effector T-cells that may cross-react with β-cell–specific autoantigens, leading to autoimmune IDDM (generation of antigen-specific T-cells cross-reacting with β-cell antigens). As preventive agents, viruses may act in several ways. Vaccination with nondiabetogenic EMC-B virus can prevent diabetogenic EMC-D virus–induced diabetes in mice (neutralization of infectious virus). Other viruses may induce suppressor T-cells, which can prevent T-cell–mediated autoimmune IDDM (induction of suppressor T-cells). Some other viruses, such as LCMV, may prevent IDDM in NOD mice by selectively depleting the CD4+ T-cell subset (disordering of lymphocyte subsets). In these ways, as environmental factors, viruses may affect the penetrance of susceptibility genes.

Virus-Induced Diabetes in Animals

Studies using experimental animal models of IDDM have provided valuable information indicating that viruses can cause IDDM. Several viruses have been clearly demonstrated to cause diabetes in animals, including encephalomyocarditis (EMC) virus,[8] Coxsackie B4 virus,[9,10] and Kilham's rat virus.[11] Other viruses, such as rubella virus,[12,13] retrovirus,[14,15] and bovine viral diarrhea-mucosal disease virus,[16] are suspected of causing diabetes in hamsters and rabbits, NOD mice, and cattle, respectively.

Encephalomyocarditis Virus-Induced Diabetes in Mice

Encephalomyocarditis virus-induced diabetes[8,17] is the best experimental animal model for diabetes brought on by viral infection. Genetically susceptible strains of mice infected with the M variant of EMC virus (EMC-M) develop a diabetes-like syndrome, characterized by hypoinsulinemia, hyperglycemia, glycosuria, polydipsia, and polyphagia[8]; however, EMC-M virus does not consistently induce diabetes.[18,19] The incidence of diabetes induced by this virus varies greatly, ranging from 10–30% of infected mice developing diabetes in some experiments to 40–60% in others.

Plaque purification of EMC-M virus has resulted in the isolation of two antigenically indistinguishable variants, which cannot be differentiated by either a sensitive plaque neutralization assay or a competitive radioimmunoassay. One variant, designated EMC-D, is highly diabetogenic, producing diabetes in more than 90% of the animals it infects by destroying β-cells (Fig. 36-2). The other variant, EMC-B, is completely nondiabetogenic.[17] Genomes of mutant viruses generated from the two variants were sequenced, and comparison of the sequences revealed that only the 776th amino acid on the polyprotein alanine is critical for the diabetogenicity of the EMC virus.[20] All diabetogenic variants of EMC have a ''G'' base at nucleotide position 3155 (Ala [GCC]-776 on the polyprotein), whereas an ''A'' base at the same position (Thr[ACC]-776 on the polyprotein) is identical in all nondiabetogenic variants. Changing the amino acid at nucleotide position 3155 by point mutation from alanine to threonine or vice versa changes the diabetogenicity of the virus.[20] It appears that changing the amino acid at this position influences the rate of attachment of the two variants to β-cells, possibly through changes in the hydrophilicity of the variants.

The genetic background of the host also contributes to the development of EMC-D virus–induced diabetes: Only certain inbred strains of mice are susceptible to this form of the disease.[17] Studies suggest that susceptibility to EMC-D virus–induced diabetes is determined by a single autosomal recessive gene inherited in a mendelian mode,[20] which may operate by modulating the expression of viral receptors on β-cells.[21]

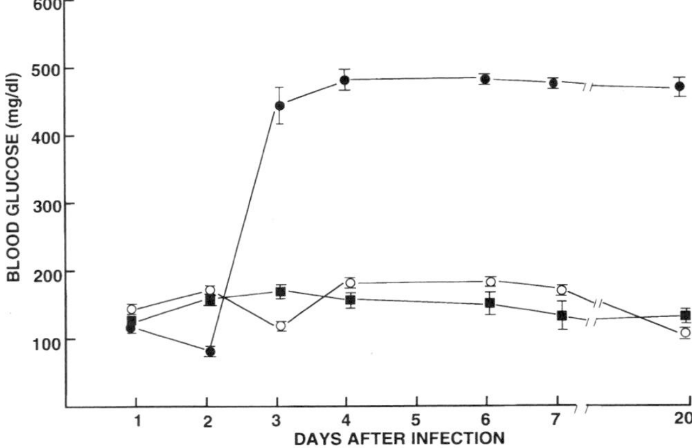

Figure 36-2. Blood glucose levels of mice infected with EMC-D or EMC-B virus: Mice infected with 10^6 PFU of diabetogenic EMC-D virus (●) or nondiabetogenic EMC-B virus (○), or phosphate buffered saline-injected, uninfected control mice (■). At the times indicated, mice were bled and their nonfasting blood glucose levels determined. Each point represents a mean of 10 animals. The vertical bars represent the standard error of the mean.

Coxsackie B Virus–Induced Diabetes in Mice

In mice, Coxsackie B4 virus can also induce diabetes by infecting and destroying β-cells (Fig. 36-3), after it has been repeatedly passaged in murine-enriched pancreatic β-cell cultures.[22] As with EMC-D virus, however, only certain inbred strains of mice are susceptible to this form of disease induction. In the majority of animals, hyperglycemia, is transient and a sufficient number of β-cells may remain intact to result in metabolic compensation. This was seen when Coleman et al.[23] infected CD1 mice with a passaged Coxsackie B4 isolate and only 20–30% of the animals developed hyperglycemia. It may be that varying degrees of viral β-cell damage are responsible for the observed differences in the metabolic response of individual animals. All six B serotypes of Coxsackie virus, once repeatedly passaged in β-cells, were subsequently shown to be capable of inducing diabetes in SJL/J mice.[9]

Mechanisms other than cytolytic infection have been suggested for the induction of diabetes by Coxsackie B viruses. The expression of the 64-kd autoantigen, glutamic acid decarboxylase (GAD), in Coxsackie B4 virus-infected SJL/J and CD1 mice was found to increase twofold to threefold before the onset of hyperglycemia, and 90% of Coxsackie B4 virus-infected mice developed antibodies to GAD by 4-6 weeks after infection,[24,25] indicating that Coxsackie B4 viral infection may possibly initiate or enhance an autoimmune reaction. Homology is known to exist between GAD and the Coxsackie B4 noncapsid protein P2-C.[26] It was initially proposed by Kaufman and coworkers[26] that molecular mimicry between the P2-C protein and GAD could be involved in the viral induction of IDDM, whereby antibodies directed against the viral protein could cross-react with GAD on the β-cells. Further murine studies have shown, however, through peptide mapping of GAD for the fine specificity of T-cell responses, that the region of sequence similarity between GAD and Coxsackie B4 virus is a region that reacts with T-cells in a later stage of the autoimmune process.[27] This study and another[28] do suggest, however, that GAD may play a critical role in the initial development of IDDM in NOD mice.

Recently Hou et al.[29] raised peptide antibodies against the P2-C protein and against human GAD65 and GAD67. Using enzyme-linked immunosorbent assays (ELISA) and immunoblotting techniques they examined the immunoreactivity of these antibodies to each other and to GAD extracted from the brains and pancreata of SJL and CD1 mice. In addition, Hou et al. also assessed the presence of antibodies to these peptide antigens in sera from humans with IDDM, nondiabetic subjects, and Coxsackie B4 virus–infected mice. Using ELISA, they found strong cross-reactivity of the Coxsackie B4 P2-C protein with GAD65, but not GAD67, even though GAD65 and GAD67 are themselves quite cross-reactive. All three peptides were also recognized by antibodies present in sera from diabetic patients and Coxsackie B4 virus–infected mice.[29] More recently, Richter et al.[30] isolated six diabetes-associated GAD-specific monoclonal antibodies from a newly diagnosed IDDM patient. Of these six monoclonal antibodies, four required the P2-C homology region to be present in GAD65 to bind to the GAD65 molecule; however, these monoclonal antibodies cross-reacted neither with Coxsackie B4 viral antigens, nor with the P2-C protein, suggesting no evidence for molecular mimicry between GAD and the P2-C protein. Any possible role that the homology between GAD and the Coxsackie B4 P2-C protein plays in the viral induction of diabetes remains to be determined.

Coxsackie B4–Induced Diabetes in Nonhuman Primates

We determined glucose and insulin levels in cynomoglus, rhesus, cebus and patas monkeys infected with Coxsackie B4 virus passaged in monkey β-cell cultures[10] (Fig. 36-4). The glucose and insulin levels after viral infection in cynomoglus, rhesus, and cebus monkeys were normal. The Coxsackie B4 virus–infected patas monkeys, however, had glucose tolerance curves that were clearly elevated and insulin secretion curves that were markedly depressed.[10] These results clearly show that genetic factors play a critical role in the development of diabetes in Coxsackie B4 virus–infected monkeys.

Retrovirus and Autoimmune Diabetes in Nonobese Diabetic Mice

β-Cell–specific expression of endogenous retroviruses appears to be associated with the development of insulitis and autoimmune diabetes in NOD mice. Electron microscopic examination of thin sections of islets from cyclophosphamide-treated NOD mice, which had received silica for the inhibition of insulitis, frequently revealed clusters of endogenous retrovirus particles in β-cells, but not in α-, δ-, pancreatic polypeptide–producing, or exocrine acinar cells.[14] Retrovirus particles also were not found in other organs of either the treated or the control mice. We recently found, however, that

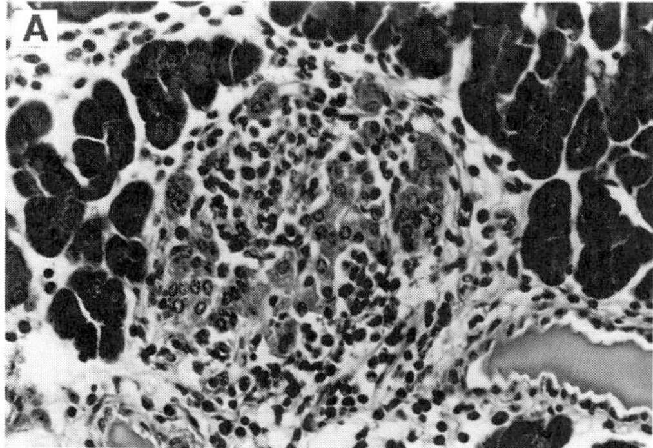

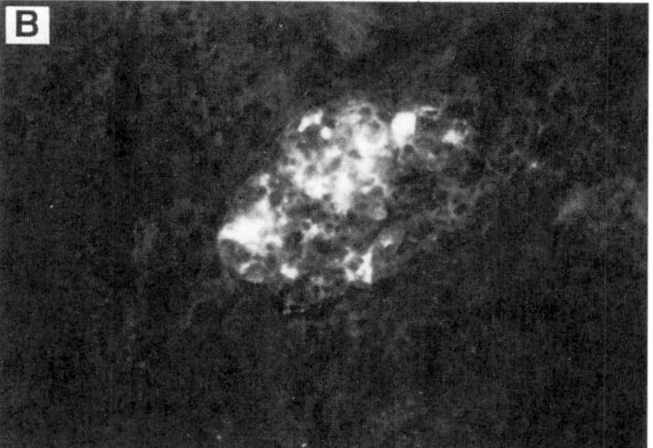

Figure 36-3. Histopathologic changes of islets after infection with Coxsackie B4 and viral-specific antigens in the islets. *A,* Section of pancreas from SJL/J mouse 5 days after infection with pancreatic β-cell–passaged Coxsackie B4 virus, showing extensive infiltration of the islet by mononuclear and occasional polymorphonuclear leukocytes (H&E × 550). *B,* Coxsackie B4 viral antigens in islets of Langerhans from Coxsackie B4 virus-infected SJL/J mice. Frozen sections of pancreas taken 4 days after infection with Coxsackie B4 virus and staining with fluorescein-labeled anti-Coxsackie B4 antibody.

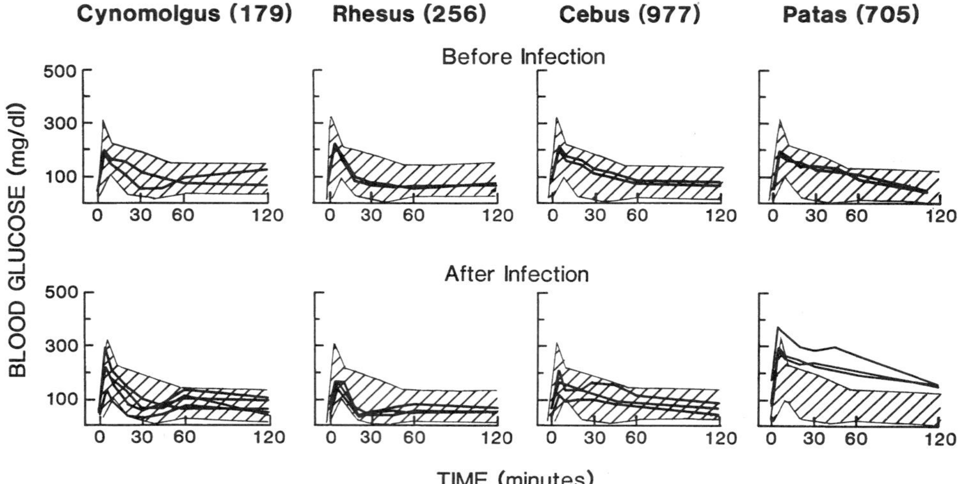

Figure 36-4. Blood glucose levels after intravenous tolerance tests in monkeys before infection (*top*) and after infection (*bottom*) with Coxsackie B4 virus. Hatched areas represent mean ± SD of 11 monkeys before infection. Samples were obtained two times (−7 and −14 days) before infection and three to five times (+7, +14, +21, +31, and +38 days) after infection.

retroviral genomes are present in all tested tissues and organs from both NOD mice and their nondiabetic parental strain, ICR mice, but that retroviral mRNAs for *gag, pol,* and *env* genes are expressed in only NOD pancreatic islet cells. Group-specific antigen p73 of A-type retrovirus (*gag* gene product) was found to be expressed in only NOD β-cells.[31] Serreze et al.[32] had previously found that the peak titer of autoantibodies against p73 in NOD mice developed only shortly before, or concomitant with, the development of hyperglycemia. Further investigation revealed that the autoantibodies against p73 recognized a common epitope on insulin and immunoglobulin E (IgE)-binding factor, possibly suggesting a role for molecular mimicry between insulin and retroviral antigen p73. Other groups have found the presence of both A-type and C-type retrovirus particles in pancreatic β-cells of NOD mice[15,33,34] and have considered the presence of retrovirus particles to be associated with the development of autoimmune IDDM in these animals.

It is not certain if or how retroviruses are involved in the pathogenesis of autoimmune IDDM in NOD mice. The presentation of a retroviral antigen on the β-cells by antigen-presenting cells, such as macrophages, to CD4+ T-cells may be the initial step in the autoimmune destruction of β-cells. Our previous experimental results support this possibility: Elimination of macrophages resulted in the prevention of β-cell–specific autoimmune processes in NOD mice.[35] Another possible mechanism whereby retroviruses could be involved in the initiation of autoimmune IDDM in NOD mice, is the alteration of cellular gene expression by retroviral genomes in the β-cells, possibly resulting in a β-cell–specific altered antigen (or antigens). An altered antigen might be recognized as foreign by immunocytes, leading to β-cell–specific autoimmunity.

Kilham's Rat Virus–Induced Diabetes in Diabetes-Resistant BB Rats

Another virus that has been implicated recently in animal diabetes is Kilham's rat virus (KRV), which has been shown to cause autoimmune diabetes in diabetes-resistant BB (DRBB) rats derived from diabetes-prone progenitors.[11] Unlike DPBB rats, which are lymphopenic, DRBB rats have normal lymphocyte numbers and phenotypes and do not normally develop diabetes. When 3-week-old DRBB rats were infected with KRV, approximately 30% of the animals developed autoimmune diabetes within 2–4 weeks, without distinct infection of β-cells, and an additional 48% showed evidence of lymphocytic insulitis without diabetes.[11] It is speculated that KRV infection may generate viral antigen-specific effector T-cells, which may recognize β-cells by cross-reaction with β-cell–specific autoantigens, leading to β-cell–specific autoimmunity. Alternatively, a recent study has suggested that widespread infection of peripancreatic and other lymphoid tissue, but not pancreatic β-cells, by KRV may trigger autoimmune diabetes by perturbing the immune system of the animals.[36]

Bovine Viral Diarrhea Mucosal Disease Virus and Diabetes in Cattle

In a 1992 study,[16] IDDM was reported to have developed in eight bovine viral diarrhea mucosal disease (BVD-MD) virus–infected cattle. The viral infection was diagnosed by isolation of the virus from serum samples. When pancreata from these animals were examined, lymphocytic infiltration of the islets was observed. Because there was no genetic relationship among the cattle, and the cattle had been bred in eight different places, the investigators concluded that the development of IDDM in these animals may have been caused by the BVD-MD viral infection. A further study[37] of pancreata from four BVD-MD-infected diabetic cattle has revealed that in all of the pancreata there were lesions, a reduction in the number of beta cells, and the residual beta cells were severely degranulated. No definitive mechanism for the induction of IDDM by BVD-MD virus has been postulated, but since BVD-MD viral infection is known to affect immunoregulation, the disease most likely has an autoimmune basis.[16]

Rubella Virus and Diabetes in Rabbits and Hamsters

Rubella virus–induced diabetes has been studied in both rabbits and hamsters. Offspring of rubella virus–infected rabbits were found to have lower serum insulin and blood glucose levels than those of uninfected dams.[13] Histopathologic examination of the pancreata from the experimental group showed β-cell degranulation and other β-cell changes.[13] When neonatal golden Syrian hamsters are infected with β-cell–passaged rubella virus, they develop hyperglycemia and hypoinsulinemia at 7–10 days of age.[12] Islets from these animals reveal mononuclear cell infiltration, and their β-cells show positive immunofluorescence for rubella virus antigen. In 40% of infected animals, cytoplasmic islet cell antibodies have been detected and insulitis has been observed in 34.5% of the hamster islets examined.[12] It is therefore speculated that the rubella virus may cause autoimmune diabetes in golden Syrian hamsters under certain circumstances.

Studies on the Pathogenesis of Autoimmune Diabetes Using Mice Transgenic for Viral Antigens

Because the target antigen involved in the immunopathogenesis of autoimmune IDDM has not yet been identified,[38] studies using transgenic mice that express novel surface antigens, including viral proteins, have been undertaken. This strategy has primarily employed mice transgenic for Simian virus 40 (*SV40*) antigens,[39] influenza viral proteins,[40] and lymphocytic choriomeningitis viral (LCMV) proteins,[41–44] and the Epstein-Barr viral (EBV) receptor.[45]

Adams et al.[39] showed that delayed expression of an *SV40* transgene in β-cells resulted in failure to establish self-tolerance and consequently produced autoimmune lesions in the pancreatic islets of several lines of mice. In contrast, mice that expressed this transgene early in life were tolerant. Several lines of transgenic mice expressing the influenza viral protein hemagglutinin on their β-cells exhibited hyperglycemia, lymphocytic infiltration of the pancreatic islets, and a humoral response against β-cell antigens, including hemagglutinin.[40] Oldstone et al.[41] developed LCMV-transgenic mice (expressing LCMV glycoprotein [LCMV-gp] in β-cells) to investigate the potential association between viruses and IDDM. They found that LCMV-gp expression in β-cells at an early age does not produce tolerance when the host is exposed to the same virus later in life. The viral antigen–specific cytotoxic T-lymphocyte (CTL) response led to the selective and progressive destruction of β-cells in these transgenic mice.[41]

Similar studies were carried out by Ohashi et al.[42] in mice transgenic for a LCMV-gp. In this model, self-reactive T-cells remained functionally silent, apparently due to the inability of the β-cells to activate an immune response properly. As a result of data from their further studies[43] in which double transgenic mice (i.e., transgenic for both LCMV-gp and α-tumor necrosis factor (αTNF) or LCMV-gp and an LCMV-specific T-cell receptor) were used, they suggest that the induction of diabetes in these transgenic animals is influenced by the major histocompatibility complex (MHC) haplotype, the infectious agent (LCMV vs. vaccinia virus), the expression of αTNF, the level of MHC class I expression, and induction of a threshold number of self-reactive CTLs.[43] CD8+ T-cells in LCMV-transgenic mice also could be tolerized in vivo with a synthetic peptide corresponding to the immunodominant epitope of LCMV, thus preventing the autoimmune destruction of β-cells in this model.[46]

Virus-Induced Diabetes in Humans

Coxsackie B Viruses and Human Diabetes

A great number of epidemiologic studies have found statistically significantly higher levels of anti-Coxsackie B virus-specific antibodies in recent-onset IDDM patients than in nondiabetic healthy control subjects, although a few studies have found a negative or reverse correlation.[47] The contrasting results from these studies do not necessarily negate a relationship between Coxsackie B viral infection and IDDM. Diabetogenic and nondiabetogenic variants of Coxsackie B viruses are cross-reactive, therefore, if a person is exposed to a more common nondiabetogenic variant of Coxsackie B4 virus before being exposed to a rarer diabetogenic variant of the same serotype, the person already will have developed antibodies that will neutralize the diabetogenic variant during the subsequent infection and the person will not become diabetic, even if genetically predisposed to the disease. If this person is a subject in an epidemiologic study, the results will not be meaningful because the lack of diabetes seen will not be a result of lack of exposure to a diabetogenic Coxsackie B4 virus, and no correlation between Coxsackie B4 viral infection and the incidence of diabetes would be found. In contrast, in certain geographic areas, outbreaks of diabetogenic virus before outbreaks of nondiabetogenic viruses would result in a high correlation between Coxsackie B viral infection and the development of diabetes. Thus the correlation found between Coxsackie B viral infection and IDDM development in some studies, in contrast to the lack of correlation found in other studies, is a reflection of variations in genetic makeup of the virus, as well as the genetic backgrounds of the subjects.[47]

In addition to epidemiologic studies, there also have been many anecdotal reports describing the development of IDDM in patients with a recent or concurrent Coxsackie B viral infection.[47] β-Cell damage and destruction have been observed in the pancreata of children who have died of severe Coxsackie B viral infections.[48,49] The isolation of viruses from the pancreata of children with acute-onset IDDM, or the presence of viral antigens in their pancreata, provides further evidence of an etiologic role for the virus. In 1976, Gladisch et al.[50] reported the case of a 5-year-old girl in whom myocarditis and diabetes developed 2 weeks after open heart surgery. At necropsy, her islets showed a lymphocytic infiltrate and β-cell necrosis. Coxsackie B4 antigens were detected in the islets by immunofluorescence, and high levels of antibody against Coxsackie B4 virus were present in the child's serum. Three years later, we obtained pancreatic tissue from a previously healthy 10-year-old boy who died 7 days after being hospitalized for diabetic ketoacidosis; the boy was admitted less than 3 days after the onset of an influenza-like illness.[49] At autopsy, lymphocytic infiltration of the islets of Langerhans and β-cell necrosis were observed (Fig. 36-5). The condition of the child's islets was very similar to that seen in murine islets after EMC or Coxsackie B4 viral infection. When several inbred strains of mice were inoculated with the Coxsackie B4 variant isolated from the diabetic child, SJL/J male mice became diabetic, whereas CBA/J, C57BL/6J, and BALB/c mice did not.[49] Champsaur et al.[51] reported the case of a 16-month-old girl with a Coxsackie B5 viral infection in whom IDDM developed. In this case, the virus isolated from the girl's feces caused glucose intolerance in infected DBA/2, SJL/J, and Swiss mice, but not in BalbC/c or C3H mice. Islet cell antibodies were found in the child 1 week before the onset of diabetes, and immunogenetic analysis revealed that the child had markers indicating a high risk for IDDM development.[51] Clements et al.[52] recently found by polymerase chain reaction (PCR) that 9 of 14 (64%) serum samples taken from children at the onset of IDDM contained enteroviral RNA, whereas serum samples from only 2 of 45 control subjects were positive for enteroviral RNA. Sequence analysis showed that the RNA from 6 of 9 of the positive patients had a high degree of homology with Coxsackie B3 and Coxsackie B4 viruses, providing additional evidence for a role for Coxsackie B viruses in human IDDM.

A recently published prospective study[53] examining IDDM development by children after intrauterine exposure to Coxsackie B viruses and by initially nondiabetic siblings of IDDM patients, reported that anti-enteroviral (including anti-Coxsackie B) antibodies were statistically significantly elevated in pregnant mothers whose children subsequently developed IDDM and that serologically verified enteroviral infections were almost twice as frequent in siblings in whom IDDM developed than in those who remained nondiabetic.

Although the Coxsackie B viruses normally are considered to be lytic viruses, there is some evidence that, in certain cases, they may establish a persistent infection.[47] Foulis et al.,[54] using an antiserum raised to the VP1 capsid protein of recombinant Coxsackie B3 virus, tested autopsy specimens of heart and pancreas tissue from patients who had died of acute Coxsackie B myocarditis. In 7 of 12 cases where the heart was available for study, the pancreata displayed insulitis, and in all seven of these pancreata, islet endocrine cells contained Coxsackie B VP1 proteins. When pancreata from 88 patients who had died of acute-onset diabetes were examined, none were found to contain Coxsackie B VP1 protein. Foulis et al. believed that these results suggested the possibility that a persistent infection of β-cells by a defective enterovirus might have resulted in their destruction by an autoimmune mechanism. This hypothesis is not incompatible with findings of continuing Coxsackie B viral infection in other diseases. Earlier, Foulis et al.[55] found that in three of four cases of infantile viral pancreatitis known to be caused by Coxsackie B viral infection, only the pancreata showed α-interferon (αIFN) related to hyperexpression of MHC class I antigens. Coxsackie B viral infection of the β-cells might therefore result in the synthesis and release of αIFN, which in turn could induce MHC class I hyperexpression on adjacent endocrine cells. See and Tilles[56] recently reported that prolonged persistence of Coxsackie B4 viral RNA in the pancreata of Coxsackie B4-infected CD-1 mice was associated with development of diabetes in the animals.

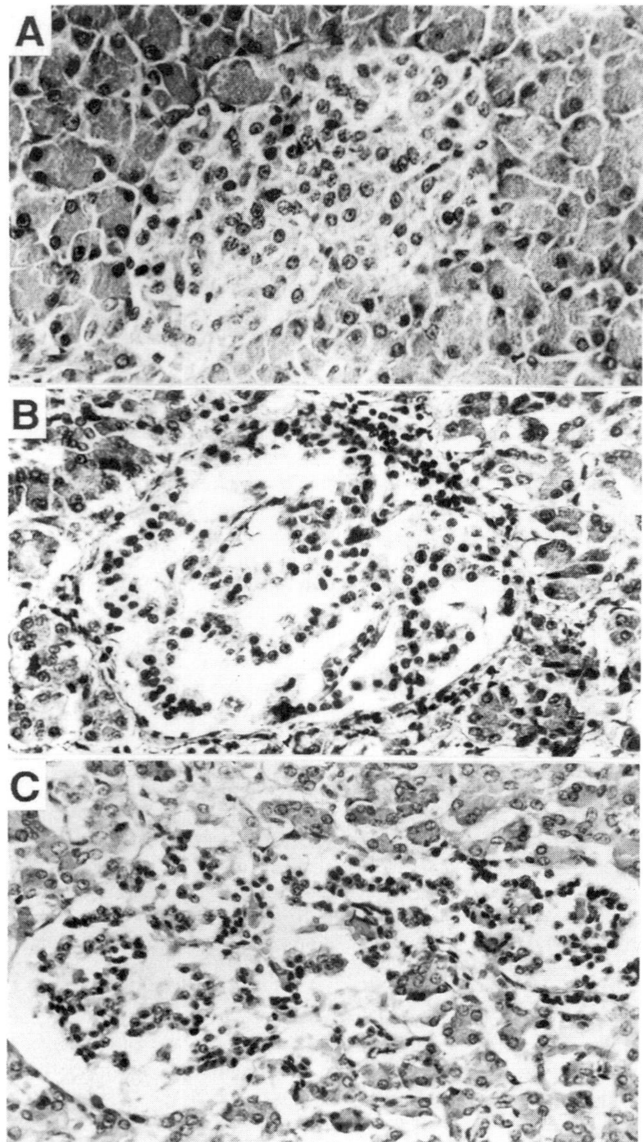

Figure 36-5. Pancreatic sections from a non-diabetic subject and a diabetic, Coxsackie B4 virus–infected patient. ***A,*** Section of a pancreas from a nondiabetic subject, showing a single intact islet of Langerhans surrounded by acinar cells (× 160). ***B,*** Section of pancreas from a Coxsackie B4 virus–infected 10-year-old boy who died after acute onset of IDDM. The section shows moderate accumulation of inflammatory cells at the periphery of the islets (× 230). ***C,*** Additional section from the same diabetic patient showing extensive inflammatory infiltrate, loss of islet architecture, and severe islet cell degeneration, with little inflammation in surrounding acinar tissue (× 160).

Peripheral blood mononuclear cells (PBMC) from people with, or at risk for, IDDM, show an elevated reactivity to GAD. Atkinson et al.[57] identified the T-cell-reactive determinants of GAD and found that the major determinant of GAD in persons at risk for developing IDDM had significant sequence homology with the Coxsackie B4 viral protein P2-C. PMBC from individuals responding to GAD also responded to the P2-C protein, supporting molecular mimicry as an etiologic mechanism for human IDDM, as had been previously postulated for Coxsackie B virus-infected mice.

Coxsackie B viral infection also may be involved in the pathogenesis of IDDM by acting as the final insult in an ongoing β-cell-specific autoimmune process.[3] In this situation, Coxsackie B4 viral infection may destroy residual β-cells in persons who have already undergone some β-cell loss through an autoimmune process. The destruction of residual β-cells by Coxsackie B viral infection would result in the clinical onset of IDDM.

Rubella Virus and Human Insulin-Dependent Diabetes Mellitus

In persons diagnosed with congenital rubella syndrome (CRS), diabetes develops in approximately 12–20% within 5-20 years.[58,59] Because islet cell antibodies (ICAs) and insulin autoantibodies (IAAs) have been found in at least 20% of nondiabetic patients with CRS and in 50-80% of diabetic patients with CRS, the endocrine abnormalities in CRS might have an autoimmune basis. The majority of CRS patients also have an abnormal carbohydrate metabolism.[58,60] As a togavirus, rubella virus might insert, expose, or alter antigens in the plasma membrane of the host cell during infection as it buds through the host cell membrane. Rubella viral antigens on β-cells or rubella virus–altered antigens on the surface of β-cells may act as foreign to the host's immune system, leading to β-cell–specific autoimmunity. Alternatively, rubella virus might be involved in the induction of autoimmune IDDM by generating viral antigen–specific cytotoxic T-cells that recognize β-cell–specific antigens by molecular mimicry. This second mechanism is plausible: Karounos et al.[61] examined a panel of monoclonal antibodies that recognize rubella virus capsid and envelope glycoproteins for reactivity with islet cell antigens and found that one monoclonal antibody that recognizes a domain within the rubella virus capsid protein reacts with extracts from rat and human islets, as well as extracts from a rat insulinoma line. The shared epitope was shown to be on a 52-kd protein. Rubella virus exposure therefore may lead to a β-cell antigen response in susceptible persons. There has been a case report of Still's disease and IDDM developing simultaneously in an adult after a recent rubella infection.[62] The patient showed an isolated persistent increase of serum antibodies against rubella virus, and the simultaneous onset of the two diseases does suggest that they were triggered by the same cause, possibly the rubella infection.

Cytomegalovirus and Human Insulin-Dependent Diabetes Mellitus

Like rubella, human cytomegalovirus (CMV) can also be transmitted before birth, either transplacentally or through the sperm or ovum from an infected parent. CMV infections also can be transmitted perinatally or postnatally through close maternal contact or breast milk. Although the initial infection usually takes place very early in life, disease may not appear until later. CMV also has been implicated in IDDM, as evidenced by a case report of a 13-month-old child with a congenital CMV infection in whom IDDM developed.[63] An additional case report has described a 27-year-old woman infected with CMV, in whom rhabdomyolysis and renal failure developed, as well as pancreatitis leading to diabetes.[64] It has been suggested that in certain situations, pan-pancreatitis in which whole islets and acini are destroyed can initiate IDDM.[65] In other reports, characteristic inclusion bodies have been found in the β-cells of infants and children who died with disseminated CMV infections.[48]

Using both dot and in situ hybridization techniques, Pak et al.[66] showed that 20% of IDDM patients appear to have CMV genomic material in their pancreatic islets. Of the patients who had both anti-CMV antibodies and CMV genome, 80% also had islet cell autoantibodies.[67] The monoclonal islet cell antibody induced by CMV has been shown to react with a 38-kd autoantigen isolated from other human pancreatic islets.[67] This reaction probably results from the sharing of similar epitopes by islet cell-specific proteins and antigenic determinants of CMV. Nicoletti et al.[68] found that there was a statistically significant correlation between high titers of anti-CMV IgG antibodies and ICAs in nondiabetic siblings of IDDM patients, but no correlation between CMV IgG and HLA-DR antigens. They suggested that a chronic CMV infection may be associated with ICA production, but that other factors may be needed for the development of clinical IDDM. A Swedish study following 73 infants with congenital CMV infection found that IDDM subsequently developed in only one infected child, compared to 38 of 19,483 noninfected control subjects.[69] While not statistically significant, these data suggest that CMV infection and the subsequent development of IDDM may be associated in occasional cases.

The association between persistent CMV infection and autoimmune IDDM may be explained in several ways. Autoimmune disease can result from an immune response to viral antigens in host cells, or from an immune response to host cell–specific antigens that are exposed as a result of infection. If CMV infection persists in the β-cells, under certain circumstances, such as a particular genetic background or the presence of environmental factors (e.g., drugs, diet), viral antigens may be expressed or β-cell–specific autoantigens induced, triggering β-cell–specific autoimmunity. Alternatively, CMV may generate viral antigen-specific T-cells that recognize β-cell–specific autoantigens by molecular mimicry, leading to β-cell–specific autoimmune IDDM.

Mumps Virus and Human Insulin-Dependent Diabetes Mellitus

Mumps virus was one of the first viruses implicated in the development of IDDM,[70] and there continue to be cases in which mumps infection appears to precede the onset of IDDM.[71,72] It has been hypothesized that an infection by mumps virus may induce autoimmunity because some children appear to develop ICAs during parotiditis.[72] In an investigation into whether vaccination against mumps has had any impact on antimumps antibody activity in children with IDDM or on the incidence of IDDM, Hyöty et al.[73] concluded that the elimination of natural mumps viral infection by vaccination may have been responsible for the decreased risk of IDDM development observed. Furthermore, Cavallo et al.[74] found that mumps infection of a human insulinoma cell line induced the release of IL1 and IL6 and also upregulated the expression of HLA class I and II antigens; Parkkonen et al.[75] found that pancreatic β-cells infected in vitro with mumps virus had increased expression of only HLA class I molecules. These observations suggest that cytokine release by mumps virus–infected cells and increased expression of HLA molecules by β-cells may somehow lead to an immune response against the β-cells or may increase preexisting autoimmune processes directed against β-cells.

Epstein–Barr Virus and Human Insulin-Dependent Diabetes Mellitus

A temporal link between EBV infection and the onset of IDDM has been reported in a rare number of cases, including one in which the child also had concurrent adenovirus and Coxsackie B viral infections.[76] In children with new-onset IDDM, EBV capsid antigen IgG antibody levels were significantly lower than in age-matched nondiabetic controls, suggesting that the diabetic children had abnormalities in their EBV-specific immune responses.[77] In 1991, the EBV BOLF1 molecule (residues 497-513-AVTPL RIFIVP-PAAEY) was found to have an 11-amino-acid sequence with homology to the HLA-DQw8 β-chain peptide (residues 49-60-AVTPL GPPAAEY [including the Asp-57 site]), although sera from diabetic patients did not bind to DQw8 β (residues 44-63) or BOLF1 (residues 496-515) peptides.[78] Recently, it was found that a 5-amino-acid sequence GPPAA, in the same region of the HLA-DQ β-chain (near Asp-57) is successively repeated six times in the EBV BERF4-encoded epitope.[79,80] Two patients who produced antibodies against this epitope during acute EBV infections soon developed IDDM, whereas five individuals who were also acutely infected, but who did not produce antibodies against this epitope, did not exhibit IDDM development.[81] This recent consideration of EBV as a candidate virus possibly capable of triggering autoimmune IDDM by molecular mimicry is interesting and worthy of further investigation.

Retrovirus and Human Insulin-Dependent Diabetes Mellitus

Retroviruses may be associated with the development of human IDDM. A recent report showed that IAAs from human IDDM patients and nondiabetic first-degree relatives cross-reacted with retroviral antigen p73.[81] Two-thirds of sera from newly diagnosed patients that bound insulin in ELISA, also bound retroviral protein p73. Sera from 75% of IAA-positive, nondiabetic first-degree relatives also bound p73. In contrast, only 2.7% of sera from nondiabetic healthy controls bound p73. These results indicate that IAA-positive sera contain antibodies that recognize both insulin and p73 and suggest that endogenous retroviruses may be involved in the pathogenesis of autoimmune IDDM in humans. Circumstantial evidence for retroviral involvement in the pathogenesis of human IDDM comes from a 1994 report by Conrad et al.,[82] who found that islet-infiltrating T cells from two diabetic patients showed a selective expansion in TCR Vβ7 gene expression, indicating that a superantigen, quite possibly retroviral in origin, and not a conventional antigen, is involved in the etiology of IDDM.

Our recent data from electron microscopic studies the presence of retroviruses in the cytoplasm of pancreatic β-cells of four IDDM patients who died shortly after the onset of the disease (Fig. 36-6B, C, D). In contrast, we did not find retrovirus particles in the β-cells in pancreata from any of 10 deceased nondiabetic control subjects (Fig. 36-6A). Histologic examination of the pancreata from the four IDDM patients revealed islet destruction and lymphocytic infiltration. Staining with monoclonal antibodies against macrophages (Leu M1, CD15), CD8+ T-cells (Leu 2), NK cells (Leu

7, CD57), and CD4+ T-cells (Leu 3) revealed that the majority of infiltrating immunocytes were macrophages, CD8+ T-cells, and NK cells, whereas only a minor number of CD4+ T-cells were found. In contrast, histologic examination of the pancreata from the deceased nondiabetic subjects showed no lymphocytic infiltration of the islets.

Very recently, through sequence analysis, we identified a 48-nucleotide region of the *pol* gene (which encodes a 16-amino-acid peptide) expressed only in pancreatic islets from the above four IDDM patients, but neither in the islets from the above nondiabetic control subjects nor in any other tissues from either group. We synthesized this 16-amino-acid peptide and found that sera from nearly 70% of 260 new-onset IDDM patients reacted with this peptide, whereas none of the sera from 46 nondiabetic control subjects reacted. On the basis of the above observations, we speculate that humoral immune responses in IDDM patients may be induced by β-cell–specific expression of this retroviral gene and may result from the presence, in the sera of IDDM patients, of antibodies directed against a β-cell–specific autoantigen cross-reacting with the retroviral peptide if there is homology between the two proteins. Alternatively, sera from 70% of recent-onset IDDM patients may contain antibodies against the retroviral peptide itself.

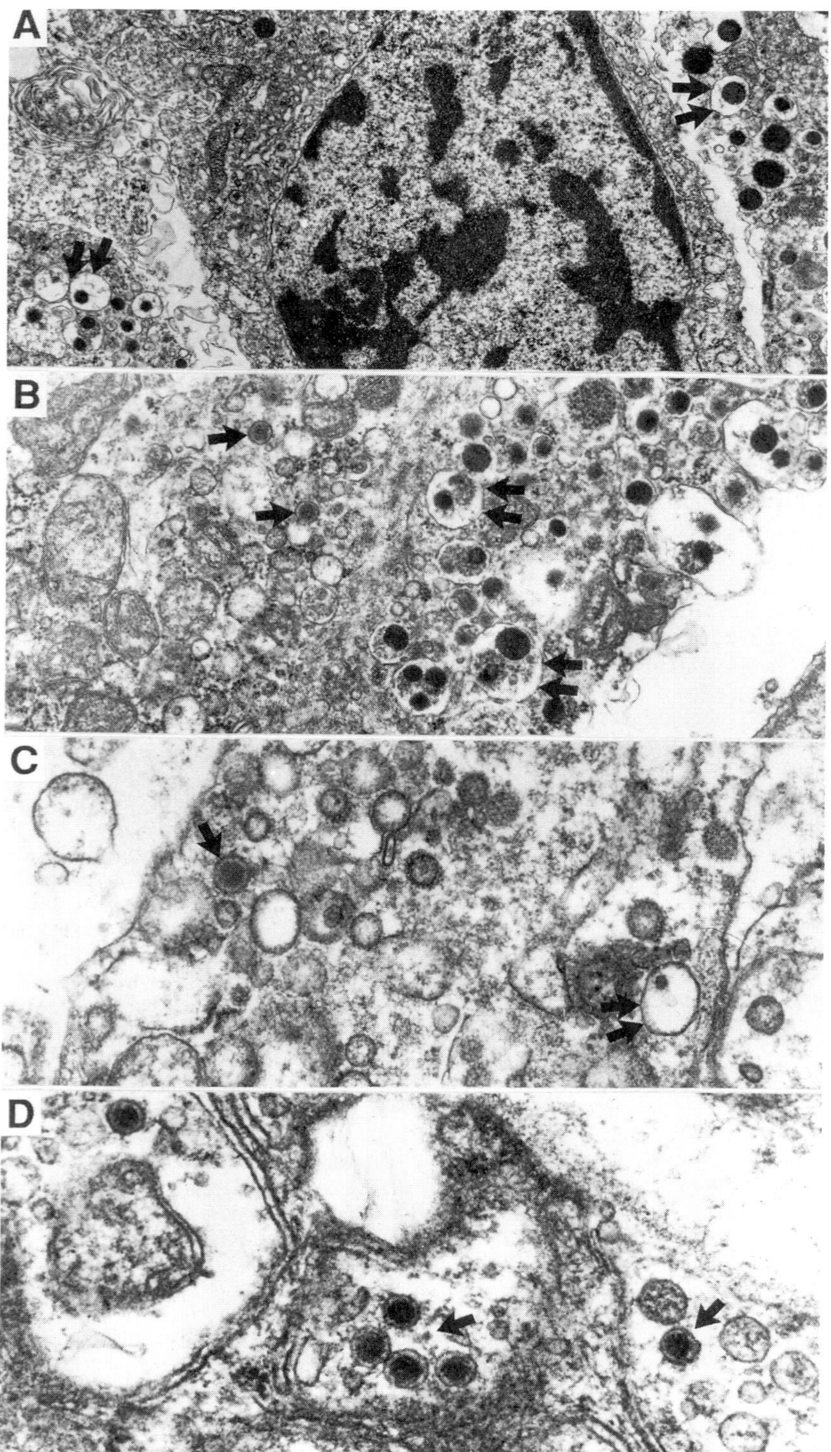

Figure 36-6. Electron micrographs of pancreatic β-cells from a nondiabetic subject and from IDDM patients. ***A,*** Human pancreatic β-cells from a nondiabetic control subject. Retrovirus particles are not found in these β-cells, and insulin secretory granules (*double arrows*) are distinct. ***B,*** Pancreatic β-cells from an IDDM patient, showing partial degranulation and degeneration. Retrovirus particles are visible in these β-cells (*single arrows*), and insulin secretory granules appear (*double arrows*). ***C,*** Pancreatic β-cells from an IDDM patient, showing severe degranulation and degeneration. Retrovirus particles are visible in these β-cells (*single arrow*), and the β-cells contain some residual insulin secretory granules (*double arrows*). ***D,*** Islet from an IDDM patient, showing almost complete degranulation and degeneration of β-cells; only vesicles and some degenerated cellular components remain. Retrovirus particles are visible (*single arrows*).

Other Viruses and Human Insulin-Dependent Diabetes Mellitus

There is indirect, circumstantial evidence that several other viruses may be associated with the onset of IDDM in humans. These viruses include Coxsackie A and echoviruses,[83,84] hepatitis A virus,[85] varicella zoster,[86] measles,[87] polio,[87] and influenza.[87]

Prevention of Insulin-Dependent Diabetes Mellitus by Viruses

Viral antibody–free BB rats show an increased frequency and accelerated onset of diabetes, suggesting that infection may have a protective effect against the development of diabetes by these animals.[88] In addition, diabetogenic EMC-D virus–induced diabetes can be prevented by vaccination with the nondiabetogenic EMC-B virus.[89] In the spontaneously diabetic NOD mouse, viral infection sometimes paradoxically prevents the development of IDDM, as is the case with NOD mice infected with EMC-D virus,[90] mouse hepatitis virus,[91] lactate dehydrogenase virus (LDV),[92] or LCMV.[93]

Regarding the prevention of diabetes by LCMV, it is thought that the virus may infect and deplete a subpopulation of CD4+ T-cells given that selective suppression of some CD4+ T-cells has been observed during LCMV infection.[94] Oldstone et al.[95] have further shown that various strains of LCMV, including Armstrong 53b, Traub, WE, and Pasteur, prevent diabetes in NOD mice, whereas other strains of LCMV do not. A strain of LCMV that established a persistent infection lasting for the life span of the animals was not able to prevent IDDM. Further investigation using recombinant strains of LCMV to infect NOD mice showed that the portion of the viral genome responsible for the prevention of IDDM mapped to the small RNA segment of LCMV Pasteur.[95] Inoculation of BB rats with LCMV (Armstrong strain clone) also reduced their incidence of diabetes and prevented mononuclear cell infiltration into the islets by somehow disordering particular lymphocyte subsets.[7]

Thus, we speculate that viral infection or other immune stimulation in humans may also reduce the penetrance of susceptibility genes (see Fig. 36-1), which could account for the low concordance rate between identical twins for the development of IDDM.[2]

Conclusions

Although a genetic predisposition appears to be necessary for the development of IDDM, nongenetic environmental factors play a critical role in the expression of the disease. Viruses, as one environmental factor, may directly infect and destroy pancreatic β-cells or trigger β-cell–specific autoimmunity. Certain viruses, such as retrovirus and rubella virus, may alter normally existing β-cell antigens into immunogenic forms or may induce new antigens leading to β-cell–specific autoimmunity. In this situation, viral antigens or virus-induced autoantigens may be released from β-cells, and then processed and presented by macrophages, in conjunction with MHC class II molecules, to CD4+ helper T-cells, which then secrete IL2. During this process, viral antigen–specific CD8+ effector T-cells would be generated, which would then recognize the cross-reactive autoantigen expressed on unaffected β-cells, and then act to destroy the cells as final effectors, working synergistically with cytokines released from macrophages and other lymphocytes.

Other viruses, such as KRV, may generate viral antigen–specific effector T-cells. The viral antigen, which generates the effector T-cells, may have homology with the β-cell–specific autoantigen, and in this way the effector T-cells may mistakenly recognize the β-cell–specific autoantigen. Still other viruses, such as EMC-D and some variants of Coxsackie B viruses, can induce IDDM by infecting and destroying β-cells in genetically susceptible hosts.

In contrast to viral induction of diabetes, several viruses, including EMC, MHV, LDV, and LCMV, can prevent the development of autoimmune IDDM in NOD mice and BB rats, most likely by immunomodulation (via induction of suppressor T-cells, depletion of certain T-cell subpopulations, or both). Thus, as an environmental factor, viruses can influence the penetrance of susceptibility genes.

Acknowledgments

Research was supported by grant MA9584 from the Medical Research Council of Canada to Ji-Won Yoon. Ji-Won Yoon is a Heritage Medical Scientist Awardee of the Alberta Heritage Foundation for Medical Research. The editorial assistance of Helen Kominek is greatly appreciated.

References

1. Todd JA, Bain SC. A practical approach to identification of susceptibility genes for IDDM. Diabetes 1992;41:1029
2. Barnett A, Eff C, Leslie R, Pyke D. Diabetes in identical twins: A study of 200 pairs. Diabetologia 1981;20:87
3. Yoon JW. Viruses as triggering agents of insulin-dependent diabetes mellitus. In: Leslie RDG, ed. The Causes of Diabetes. London: John Wiley and Sons;1993:83–103
4. Adams SF. The seasonal variation in the onset of acute diabetes. Arch Intern Med 1926;37:861
5. Gamble DR, Taylor KW. Seasonal incidence of diabetes mellitus. Br Med J 1969;3:631
6. Oldstone MBA. Prevention of type 1 diabetes in nonobese diabetic mice by virus infection. Science 1988;239:500
7. Dyrberg T, Schwimmbeck PL, Oldstone MBA. Inhibition of diabetes in BB rats by viral infection. J Clin Invest 1988;81:928
8. Craighead JE, McLane MF. Diabetes mellitus: Induction in mice by encephalomyocarditis virus. Science 1968;162:913
9. Toniolo A, Onodera T, Jordan G, et al. Virus induced diabetes mellitus: Glucose abnormalities produced in mice by all six members of the Coxsackie B virus group. Diabetes 1982;31:496
10. Yoon JW, London WT, Curfman BL, et al. Coxsackie virus B_4 produces transient diabetes in nonhuman primates. Diabetes 1986;35:712
11. Guberski DL, Thomas VA, Shek WR, et al. Induction of type 1 diabetes by Kilham's rat virus in diabetes-resistant BB/Wor rats. Science 1991;254:1010
12. Rayfield E, Kelly K, Yoon JW. Rubella virus-induced diabetes in hamsters. Diabetes 1986;35:1276
13. Menser MA, Forrest JM, Bransby RD. Rubella infection and diabetes mellitus. Lancet 1978;1:211
14. Suenaga K, Yoon JW. Association of beta cell-specific expression of endogenous retrovirus with the development of insulitis and diabetes in NOD mice. Diabetes 1988;37:1722
15. Gaskins H, Prochazka M, Hamaguchi K, et al. Beta cell expression of endogenous xenotropic retrovirus distinguishes diabetes-susceptible NOD/Lt from resistant NON/Lt mice. J Clin Invest 1992;90:2220
16. Tajima M, Yazawa T, Hagiwara K, et al. Diabetes mellitus in cattle infected with bovine viral diarrhea mucosal disease virus. J Vet Med Assoc 1992;39:616
17. Yoon JW, McClintock PR, Onodera T, Notkins AL. Virus-induced diabetes mellitus: Inhibition by a non-diabetogenic variant of encephalomyocarditis virus. J Exp Med 1980;152:878
18. Ross ME, Onodera T, Brown KS, Notkins AL. Virus-induced diabetes mellitus IV: Genetic and environmental factors influencing the development of diabetes after infection with the M variant of encephalomyocarditis virus. Diabetes 1976;25:190
19. Yoon JW, Onodera T, Notkins AL. Virus-induced diabetes mellitus: IX. Studies on virus passage and dose in susceptible and resistant strains of mice. J Gen Virol 1977;27:225
20. Yoon JW, Bae YS. Development of insulin-dependent diabetes in animals: Control by a single gene of the host and a single amino acid of the virus. In: Shafrir E, ed. Frontiers in Diabetes Research: Lessons from Animal Diabetes III. London: Smith-Gordon;1993:51–60
21. Kang Y, Yoon JW. A genetically determined host factor controlling susceptibility to encephalomyocarditis virus-induced diabetes in mice. J Gen Virol 1993;74:1203
22. Yoon JW, Onodera T, Notkins AL. Virus-induced mellitus: XV. Beta cell damage and insulin-dependent hyperglycemia in mice infected with Coxsackie virus B4. J Exp Med 1978;148:1068
23. Coleman TJ, Taylor KW, Gamble DR. The development of diabetes following Coxsackie B virus infection in mice. Diabetologia 1974;10:755

24. Gerling I, Nejman C, Chatterjee NK. Effect of coxsackievirus B4 infection in mice on expression of 64,000 Mr autoantigen and glucose sensitivity of islets before development of hyperglycemia. Diabetes 1988;37:1419
25. Gerling I, Chatterjee NK, Nejman C. Coxsackievirus B4-induced development of antibodies to 64,000 Mr islet autoantigen and hyperglycemia in mice. Autoimmunity 1991;10:49
26. Kaufman DL, Erlander MG, Clare-Salzler MJ, et al. Autoimmunity to two forms of glutamate decarboxylase in insulin-dependent diabetes mellitus. J Clin Invest 1992;89:283
27. Kaufman DL, Clare-Salzler MG, Tian J, et al. Spontaneous loss of T-cell tolerance to glutamic acid decarboxylase in murine insulin-dependent diabetes. Nature 1993;366:69
28. Tisch R, Yang X, Singer S, et al. Immune response to glutamic acid decarboxylase correlates with insulitis in non-obese diabetic mice. Nature 1993;366:72
29. Hou J, Said C, Franchi D, et al. Antibodies to glutamic acid decarboxylase and P2-C peptides in sera from coxsackie virus B4-infected mice and IDDM patients. Diabetes 1994;43:1260
30. Richter W, Mertens T, Schoel B, et al. Sequence homology of the diabetes-associated autoantigen glutamate decarboxylase with Coxsackie B4-2C protein and heat shock protein 60 mediated no molecular mimicry of autoantibodies. J Exp Med 1994;180:721
31. Pak CY, Jun HS, Lee M, Yoon JW. Beta cell-specific expression retroviral mRNAs and group-specific antigen and the development of beta cell-specific autoimmunity in non-obese diabetic mice. Autoimmunity 1995;20:19
32. Serreze DV, Leiter EH, Kuff EL, et al. Molecular mimicry between insulin and retroviral antigen p73: Development of cross-reactive autoantibodies in sera of NOD and C57BL/KsJ db/db mice. Diabetes 1988;37:351
33. Fukino-Kurihara H, Fujita H, Hakura A, et al. Morphological aspects on pancreatic islets of non-obese diabetic (NOD) mice. Virchows Arch 1985; 49:107
34. Nakagawa C, Hanafusa T, Miyagawa J, et al. Retrovirus gag protein p30 in the islets of nonobese diabetic mice: relevance for pathogenesis of diabetes mellitus. Diabetologia 1992;35:614
35. Lee KU, Amano K, Yoon JW. Evidence for initial involvement of macrophages in development of insulitis in NOD mice. Diabetes 1988;37:1989
36. Brown DW, Welsh RM, Like AA. Infection of peripancreatic lymph nodes but not islets precedes Kilham's rat virus-induced diabetes in BB/Wor rats. J Virol 1993;67:5873
37. Taniyama H, Ushiki T, Tajima M, et al. Spontaneous diabetes mellitus associated with persistent bovine diarrhea (BVD) virus infection in young cattle. Vet Pathol 1995;32:221
38. Rossini AA, Greiner DL, Friedman HP, Mordes JP. Immunopathogenesis of diabetes mellitus. Diabetes Rev 1993;1:43
39. Adams TE, Alpert S, Hanahan D. Non-tolerance and autoantibodies to a transgenic self antigen expressed in pancreatic beta cells. Nature 1987;325:223
40. Roman L, Simons L, Hammer R, et al. The expression of influenza virus hemagglutinin in the pancreatic beta cells of transgenic mice results in autoimmune diabetes. Cell 1990;61:383
41. Oldstone MBA, Nerenberg M, Southern P, et al. Virus infection triggers insulin-dependent diabetes mellitus in a transgenic model: Role of anti-self (virus) immune response. Cell 1991;65:319
42. Ohashi P, Oehen S, Buerki K, et al. Ablation of tolerance and induction of diabetes by virus infection in viral antigen transgenic mice. Cell 1991;65:305
43. Ohashi PS, Oehen S, Aichele P, et al. Induction of diabetes is influenced by the infectious virus and local expression of MHC class I and tumor necrosis factor-α. J Immunol 1993;150:5185
44. Laufer TM, von Herrath MG, Grusby MJ, et al. Autoimmune diabetes can be induced in transgenic major histocompatibility complex class II-deficient mice. J Exp Med 1993;178:589
45. Holers VM, Hollis GF, Schwartz BD, et al. Induction of peri-insulitis but not diabetes in islet transplants expressing a single foreign antigen: A multi-stage model of disease. J Immunol 1993;151:5041
46. Aichele P, Kyburz D, Ohashi PS, et al. Peptide-induced T-cell tolerance to prevent autoimmune diabetes in a transgenic mouse model. Proc Natl Acad Sci U S A 1994;91:444
47. Yoon JW, Kominek HI. Role of Coxsackie B viruses in the pathogenesis of diabetes mellitus. In: Rose NR, Friedman H, eds. Microbial Infections and Pathogenesis. New York: Plenum Press;1995:In press
48. Jenson A, Rosenberg H, Notkins AL. Pancreatic islet cell damage in children with fatal viral infections. Lancet 1980;2:354
49. Yoon JW, Austin M, Onodera T, Notkins AL. Virus-induced diabetes mellitus: Isolation of a virus from the pancreas of a child with diabetic ketoacidosis. N Engl J Med 1979;300:1173
50. Gladisch R, Hoffmann W, Waldherr R. Myocarditis and insulitis in Coxsackie virus infection. Z Kardiol 1976;65:873
51. Champsaur H, Bottazzo G, Bertrams J, et al. Virologic, immunologic and genetic factors in insulin-dependent diabetes mellitus. J Pediatr 1982;100:15
52. Clements GB, Galbraith DN, Taylor KW. Coxsackie B virus infection and onset of childhood diabetes. Lancet 1995;346:221
53. Hyöty H, Hiltunen M, Knip M, et al. A prospective study of the role of Coxsackie B and other enterovirus infections in the pathogenesis of IDDM: Childhood Diabetes in Finland Study Group. Diabetes 1995;44:652
54. Foulis AK, Farquharson MA, Cameron SO, et al. A search for the presence of the enteroviral capsid protein VP1 in pancreases of patients with type 1 (insulin-dependent) diabetes and pancreases and hearts of infants who died of coxsackieviral myocarditis. Diabetologia 1990;33:290
55. Foulis AK, Farquharson MA, Meager A. Immunoreactive α-interferon in insulin-producing β cells in type I diabetes mellitus. Lancet 1987;2:1423
56. See DM, Tilles JG. Pathogenesis of virus-induced diabetes in mice. J Infect Dis 1995;171:1131
57. Atkinson MA, Bowman MA, Campbell L. Cellular immunity to a determinant common to glutamate decarboxylase and coxsackie virus in insulin-dependent diabetes. J Clin Invest 1994;94:2125
58. Ginsberg-Fellner F, Witt ME, Fedun B. Diabetes mellitus and autoimmunity in patients with congenital rubella syndrome. Rev Infect Dis 1985;7(suppl 1):S170
59. Ginsberg-Fellner F, Fedun B, Cooper Z, et al. Interrelationships of congenital rubella and type 1 insulin-dependent diabetes mellitus. In: Jaworski MA, Molnar GD, Rajotte RV, Singh B, eds. The Immunology of Diabetes Mellitus. Amsterdam: Elsevier Science Publishers;1986:279–286
60. Ginsberg-Fellner F, Witt ME, Yagihaski S. Congenital rubella-syndrome as a model for type 1 (insulin-dependent) diabetes mellitus: Increased prevalence of islet cell surface antibodies. Diabetologia 1984;27:87
61. Karounos DG, Wolinsky JS, Thomas JW. Monoclonal antibody to rubella virus capsid protein recognizes a beta-cell antigen. J Immunol 1993;150:3080
62. Sibley JT. Concurrent onset of adult onset Still's disease and insulin dependent diabetes mellitus. Ann Rheum Dis 1990;49:547
63. Ward KP, Galloway WH, Auchterlonie IA. Congenital cytomegalovirus infection and diabetes. Lancet 1979;1:497
64. Yasumoto N, Hara M, Kitamoto YU, et al. Cytomegalovirus infection associated with acute pancreatitis, rhabdomyolysis and renal failure. Intern Med 1992;31:426
65. Kimura N, Fujiya H, Yamaguchi K, et al. Vanished islets with pancreatitis in acute-onset insulin-dependent diabetes mellitus in an adult. Arch Pathol Lab Med 1994;118:84
66. Pak CY, Eun HM, McArthur RG, Yoon JW. Association of cytomegalovirus infection with autoimmune type I diabetes. Lancet 1988;2:1
67. Pak CY, Cha CY, Rajotte RV, et al. Human pancreatic islet cell-specific 38 kD autoantigen identified by cytomegalovirus-induced monoclonal islet cell autoantibody. Diabetologia 1990;33:569
68. Nicoletti F, Scalia G, Lunetta M, et al. Correlation between islet cell antibodies and anti-cytomegalovirus IgM and IgG antibodies in healthy first-degree relatives of type 1 (insulin-dependent) diabetic patient. Clin Immunol Immunopathol 1990;55:139
69. Ivarsson SA, Lindberg B, Nilsson KO, et al. The prevalence of type 1 diabetes mellitus at follow-up of Swedish infants congenitally infected with cytomegalovirus. Diabet Med 1993;10:521
70. Harris HF. A case of diabetes mellitus quickly following mumps on the pathological alterations of salivary glands, closely resembling those found in pancreas, in a case of diabetes mellitus. Boston Med Sur J 1899;140:465
71. Gamble DR. Relation of antecedent illness to development of diabetes in children. Br Med J 1980;2:99
72. Helmke K, Otten A, Willems W. Islet cell antibodies in children with mumps infection. Lancet 1980;2:211
73. Hyöty H, Hiltunen M, Reunanen A, et al. Decline of mumps antibodies in type 1 (insulin-dependent) diabetic children and a plateau in the rising incidence of type 1 diabetes after introduction of the mumps-measles-rubella vaccine in Finland: Childhood Diabetes in Finland Study Group. Diabetologia 1993; 36:1303
74. Cavallo MG, Baroni MG, Toto A, et al. Viral infection induces cytokine release by beta islet cells. Immunology 1992;75:664
75. Parkkonen P, Hyöty H, Koskinen L, Leinikki P. Mumps virus infects beta cells in human fetal islet cell cultures upregulating the expression of HLA class I molecules. Diabetologia 1992;35:63
76. Surcel HM, Ilonen J, Kaar ML, et al. Infection by multiple viruses and lymphocyte abnormalities at the diagnosis of diabetes. Acta Paediatr Scand 1988; 77:471
77. Hyöty H, Rasanen L, Hiltunen M, et al. Decreased antibody reactivity to Epstein-Barr virus capsid antigen in type 1 (insulin dependent) diabetes mellitus. APMIS 1991;99:359
78. Sairenji T, Daibata M, Sorli CH, et al. Relating homology between the Epstein-Barr virus BOLF1 molecule and HLA-DQw8 beta chain to recent onset type 1 (insulin-dependent) diabetes mellitus. Diabetologia 1991;34:33
79. Horn G, Bugawan T, Long C, Erlich H. Allelic sequence of the HLA-DQ loci: relationship to serology and to insulin-dependent diabetes susceptibility. Proc Natl Acad Sci U S A 1988;85:6012
80. Parkkonen P, Hyöty H, Ilonen J, et al. Antibody reactivity to an Epstein-Barr virus BERF4-encoded epitope occurring also in Asp-57 region of HLA-DQ8 β chain. Clin Exp Immunol 1994;95:287
81. Hao W, Serreze DV, McCulloch DK, et al. Insulin (auto) antibodies from human IDDM cross-react with retroviral antigen p73. J Autoimmun 1993;6:787
82. Conrad B, Weldmann E, Trucco G, et al. Evidence for superantigen involvement in insulin-dependent diabetes mellitus aetiology. Nature 1994;371:351
83. Frisk G, Nilsson E, Tuvemo T, et al. The possible role of Coxsackie A and echo viruses in the pathogenesis of type I diabetes mellitus studied by IgM analysis. J Infect 1992;24:13
84. Uriarte A, Cabrera E, Venture R, Vargas J. Islet cell antibodies and ECHO-4 virus infection [Abstract]. Diabetologia 1987;30:590A
85. Makeen AM. The association of infective hepatitis type A (HAV) and diabetes mellitus. Trop Geogr Med 1992;44:362
86. Jali MV, Shankar PS. Transient diabetes following chickenpox. J Assoc Physicians India 1990;38:663

87. Notkins AL. Virus-induced diabetes mellitus: Brief review. Arch Virol 1977; 54:1
88. Guberski DL, Butler L, Like AA. Environmental agents influence spontaneous and RT6 depletion induced diabetes (DB) in the BB/Wor rat. Diabetes 1990;39:97A
89. Notkins AL, Yoon JW. Virus-induced diabetes in mice prevented by a live attenuated vaccine. N Engl J Med 1983;306:486
90. Hermitte L, Vialettes B, Naquet P, et al. Paradoxical lessening of autoimmune processes in non-obese diabetic mice after infection with the diabetogenic variant of encephalomyocarditis virus. Eur J Immunol 1990;20:1297
91. Wilberz S, Partke HJ, Dagnaes-Hansen F, Herberg L. Persistent MHV (mouse hepatitis virus) infection reduces the incidence of diabetes mellitus in non-obese diabetic mice. Diabetologia 1991;34:2
92. Takei I, Asaba Y, Kasatani T, et al. Suppression of development of diabetes in NOD mice by lactate dehydrogenase virus infection. J Autoimmun 1992;5: 665
93. Oldstone MBA. Prevention of type 1 diabetes in nonobese diabetic mice by virus infection. Science 1988;239:500
94. Oldstone MBA. Viruses as therapeutic agents: I. treatment of nonobese insulin-dependent diabetes mice with virus prevents insulin-dependent diabetes mellitus while maintaining general immune competence. J Exp Med 1990;101: 2077
95. Oldstone MB, Ahmed R, Salvato M. Viruses as therapeutic agents: II. Viral reassortments map prevention of insulin-dependent diabetes mellitus to the small RNA of lymphocytic choriomeningitis virus. J Exp Med 1990;171: 2091

Diabetes Mellitus, edited by Derek LeRoith, Simeon I. Taylor, and Jerrold M. Olefsky. Lippincott–Raven Publishers, Philadelphia © 1996.

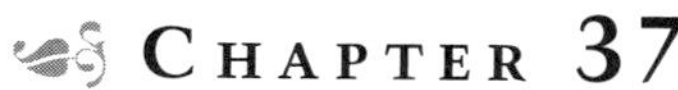

Animal Models of Autoimmune Diabetes Mellitus

John P. Mordes, Dale L. Greiner, and Aldo A. Rossini

Rationale for Studying Insulin-Dependent Diabetes Mellitus in Animals

Insulin-dependent diabetes mellitus (IDDM) results from destruction of pancreatic β-cells in the context of inflammatory infiltration of the islets of Langerhans (insulitis).[1] Strongly associated with the major histocompatibility complex (MHC) and ameliorated by immunosuppression, IDDM is believed to be a T-lymphocyte–dependent autoimmune disorder that reflects islet-specific loss of self-tolerance. Our understanding of its natural history, genetics, and pathophysiology has expanded steadily, but the disease remains refractory to cure or prevention.[2,3] This intractability reflects the difficulty of studying IDDM in humans, particularly in children. The diseased organ is inaccessible; identification of those at risk is costly and imprecise; the genetics of susceptible populations cannot be manipulated; and new therapies, particularly those targeted at prevention in otherwise healthy individuals, must be implemented cautiously.

To circumvent these limitations, investigators have sought animal models of IDDM.[4] The strategy substantially leverages our ability to acquire information. Diabetic animals can be tested, biopsied, and autopsied. They can be bred to study and manipulate inheritance; their genome can be altered. Provocation of IDDM constitutes a fruitful line of animal research, and innovative therapies to prevent or reverse the disease can be tested at greatly reduced cost and risk.

Principal Animal Models of IDDM

Animals with Spontaneous Onset of Insulitis and Hyperglycemia

The scientific database derived from studies of diabetic animals is remarkably extensive. Two animals in particular have yielded useful data relevant to human IDDM: the BioBreeding (BB) rat[5–8] and the nonobese diabetic (NOD) mouse.[8–10] The clinical presentation and underlying microscopic pathology in both animals are similar to that observed in humans. Spontaneous *insulitis* is followed by *selective β-cell destruction with ensuing insulin deficiency* and *hyperglycemia*, all of which can be prevented by immunosuppression and immunomodulation (Tables 37-1 and 37-3). Figure 37-1 illustrates the archetypal pathology of IDDM in an example taken from the BB rat. The figure typifies the underlying inflammatory pathologic lesion found in the animal models of IDDM, but it is important to stress that the presence of insulitis alone does not equate with the presence of autoimmune diabetes mellitus. Selective β-cell destruction, hyperglycemia, and ketoacidosis due to absolute insulin deficiency are also required to establish this diagnosis.

The striking pathology and pathophysiology observed in BB rats and NOD mice have engendered exhaustive programs of investigation, and few facets of the immune systems of these rodents have escaped scrutiny. The information gathered has led directly to experimental human therapeutics. Studies of cyclosporine in children with new-onset IDDM[12] were engendered in this way, as have other studies of tolerance induction and disease prevention.[3]

Another inbred rat strain that develops spontaneous insulitis and diabetes was reported from Japan in 1991.[13,14] This animal has been designated LETL, for Long Evans Tokushima lean. A cross of the BB and Zucker fatty rats, designated BBZ/Wor, has yielded an animal with both obesity and insulitis.[15] As yet, neither of these strains has been analyzed in detail.

Animals with Induced Diabetic Syndromes

IDDM in animals can also be induced rather than spontaneous, and many strategies have been used to generate insulitis and hyperglycemia. One class of induced IDDM models has been produced by manipulation of environmental factors, including toxins and infectious agents.[16] An inducible model of this type is the mouse treated with multiple subdiabetogenic doses of the β-cell toxin

TABLE 37-1. Clinical and Genetic Features of Autoimmune Diabetes

	Human	NOD Mouse[8–10]	DP-BB Rat[5–8]	Induced Diabetes in DR-BB Rats[5,7]	Low-Dose STZ Induced[11]
Onset:	Spontaneous	Spontaneous	Spontaneous	Inducible	Inducible
Latency:	Years	Up to 6 months	1–2 months	2–4 weeks	10–14 days
Ketosis:	Severe	Mild	Severe	Severe	None
Insulin Deficiency:	Absolute	Mild to severe	Severe	Severe	Mild
Associated Autoimmune Diseases:	Thyroiditis; adrenalitis; vitiligo; PA; polyendocrine syndromes	Sialoadenitis, thyroiditis	Thyroiditis	Thyroiditis	None
Autoantibodies:	Insulin, GAD, ICA, ICSA, BSA, CPH, EC	Insulin, GAD, ICA, ICSA	GAD, ICSA, insulin, smooth muscle, gastric parietal cells, EC	EC	Unknown
MHC Genes:	HLA-DQα and β	Unique I-A; absent I-E	$RT1^u$	$RT1^u$	None
Non-MHC Genes:	At least 2 loci	>12 loci	At least 2 loci; *lyp* causes lymphopenia	Not known	Strain-specific
Gender Effect:	♀=♂	♀>♂	♀=♂	♀=♂	♂>♀
Response to General Immunosuppression:	Cyclosporine prolongs endogenous insulin production if given at onset	Cyclosporine, FK506 prevent diabetes	Cyclosporine, FK506, thymectomy, ALS, radiation prevent diabetes and thyroiditis	Cyclosporine prevents diabetes and thyroiditis	Attenuated by ALS; cyclosporine ineffective; FK506 ameliorates

Low-dose STZ = rodent treated with multiple subdiabetogenic doses of streptozocin; MHC = major histocompatibility complex; HLA = human leukocyte antigen; PA = pernicious anemia; ALS = antilymphocyte serum; GAD = glutamic acid decarboxylase; EC = endothelial cell; CPH = carboxypeptidase H; ICA = islet cell cytoplasmic antibody; ICSA = islet cell surface antibody; BSA = bovine serum albumin. Additional incompletely characterized autoantibodies are present in humans, NOD mice, and BB rats.[7,50,141]

streptozocin (STZ).[11] Another is the encephalomyocarditis virus–infected mouse.[17] A second class of induced IDDM models has been generated by manipulations of the immune system. IDDM has been produced in normal PVG strain rats by combining thymectomy and sublethal irradiation[18,19] and in the diabetes-resistant subline of BB rats by depletion of regulatory T-cell subsets.[7] Insulitis and occasionally hyperglycemia have also been induced by immunizing various species with homologous or heterologous insulin plus adjuvant.[20] A third class of induced models is the product of contemporary biotechnology, transgenic mice.[21,22] These provide tools for dissecting and studying in isolation various components of the immune system hypothesized to be relevant to IDDM.

General Considerations: Autoreactivity, Immunoregulation, and the Issue of Extrapolation

Selective β-cell destruction in human IDDM and its animal models appears to require the interplay of multiple contributory factors. The first factor is the generation of autoreactive cells, a process that involves both genetic predisposition and environmental influences that activate or amplify that predisposition. A second factor is the capability of an individual to regulate peripheral autoreactive cell populations.

The cellular and molecular biology of the processes underlying the generation and regulation of autoreactivity is not completely understood in either human or animal IDDM. The available animal data do, however, suggest that autoimmune diseases such as IDDM can be understood in terms of the equilibrium between these two processes. As diagrammed in Figure 37-2, IDDM may occur as the result of forces that unmask or amplify autoreactivity or of forces that impair regulatory function, or as the result of a combination of both. Much of the animal data reviewed here can usefully be analyzed in the context of this "balance hypothesis."

A final consideration in this review is an analysis of the limitations of the animal models of IDDM. The extent to which it is appropriate to extrapolate from rodents to children is always an open question. Albert Renold and Eleazar Shafrir, early proponents of the study of animal models of complex metabolic disorders, emphasized that there are limits to the identity between animals and humans, which in turn limit the extent to which animal disease can "model" human disease.[4] To emphasize this point, Tables 37-1 and 37-2 both summarize and contrast various cardinal features of IDDM as they appear in humans and in some of the principal animal models.

Diabetes-Prone and Diabetes-Resistant BB Rats

Natural History and Pathology

Routine surveillance at the BioBreeding Laboratories in Ottawa, Canada, revealed the presence of spontaneous hyperglycemia and ketoacidosis in a colony of outbred Wistar rats in the 1970s.[5–8]

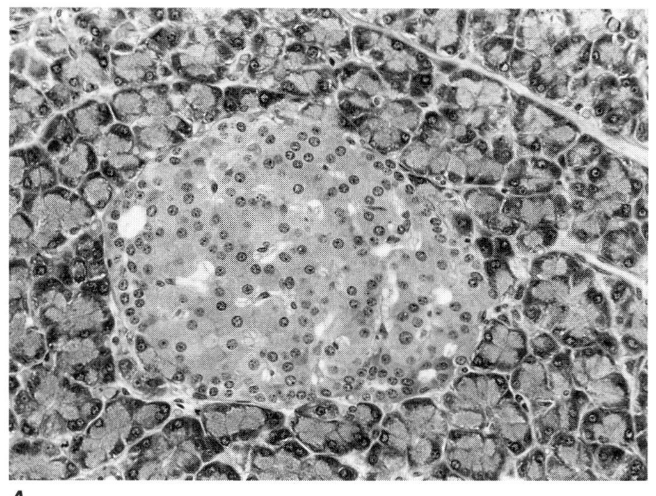

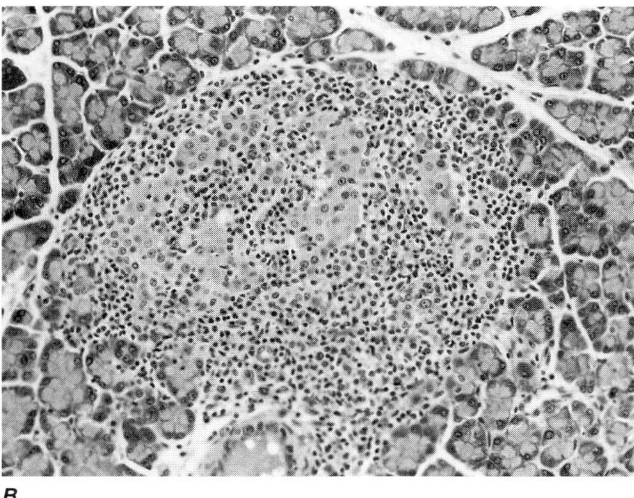

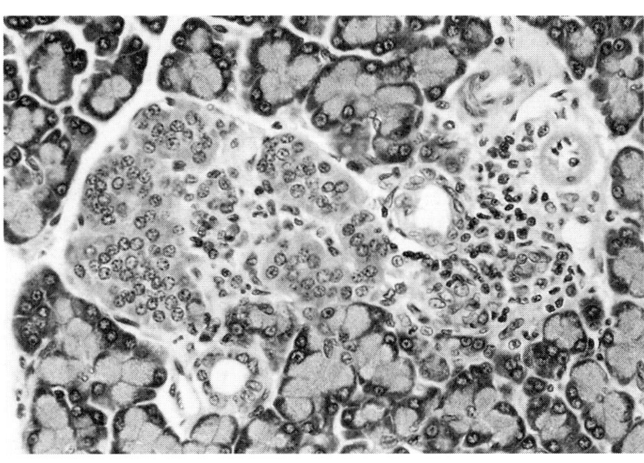

Figure 37-1. Hematoxylin and eosin stained sections of DP-BB rat pancreatic islets of Langerhans. ***A*** shows a normal islet from a young adult animal before the onset of disease (× 310). ***B*** shows the insulitis lesion; the islet has been extensively infiltrated by mononuclear cells (× 305). ***C*** shows an end-stage islet from an animal with longstanding diabetes that had been treated with a daily injection of exogenous insulin to prevent ketoacidosis (× 390). The islet is shrunken and its architecture has been distorted; immunohistochemical staining would demonstrate the selective absence of β-cells from the islet with preservation of α-, δ-, and pancreatic polypeptide cells.[174] Phenotyping of the cells that compose the infiltrate in ***B*** would reveal the presence of CD4$^+$ and CD8$^+$ T-lymphocytes, natural killer (NK) cells, B-lymphocytes, and macrophages.[175] There is evidence for the expression of multiple genes encoding cytokines in the inflammatory lesion but no evidence of any intrinsic abnormality of the β-cells themselves. Comparable pathology is observed in the islets of humans[176,177] and in NOD mice.[178,179] (Photomicrographs courtesy of Dr. Arthur Like.)

Affected animals became the founders of the inbred diabetes-prone (DP) BB rat strain. In the international resource colony sponsored by the National Institutes of Health, >90% of DP-BB rats of both sexes develop pancreatic insulitis (see Fig. 37-1) that is rapidly followed by selective destruction of β-cells and frank diabetes between 50 and 90 days of age.[23] After the onset of hyperglycemia, the residual "end-stage" islets are small, distorted, and composed predominantly of non–β-cells. Unless treated with exogenous insulin, the disease of hyperglycemic BB rats quickly progresses to diabetic ketoacidosis, dehydration, and death. DP-BB rats also develop spontaneous lymphocytic thyroiditis but not clinical hypothyroidism.[24]

At the sixth generation of inbreeding, a subpopulation of nondiabetic BB rats was selected to start a control subline. Now

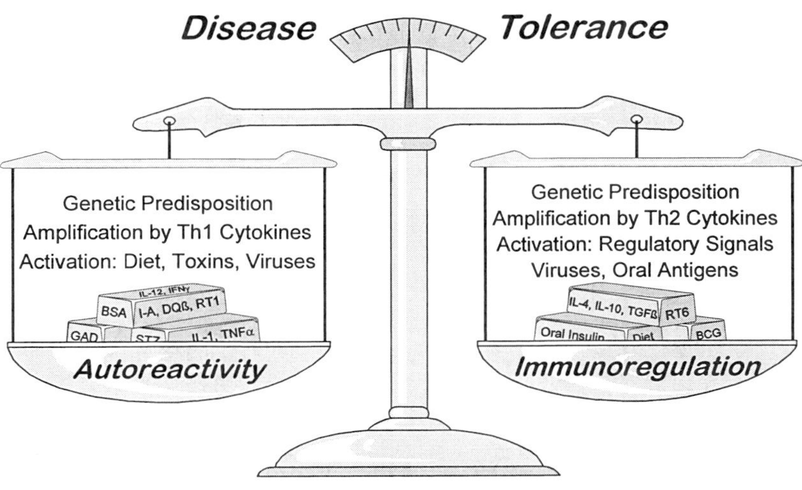

Figure 37-2. Schematic representation of the balance hypothesis of autoimmunity. The factors listed on each side of the scale have been implicated in the expression of human or animal IDDM. Details are given in the text. GAD = glutamic acid decarboxylase; STZ = streptozocin; IFN-γ = interferon gamma; BSA = bovine serum albumin; BCG = bacillus Calmette-Guérin; IL = interleukin; TNF-α = tumor necrosis factor alpha; TGF-β = transforming growth factor β; RT6 = a rat T-cell alloantigen. I-A, DQβ, and RT1 refer to IDDM-associated major histocompatibility loci in mouse, humans, and rat, respectively.

TABLE 37-2. Environment and Autoimmune Diabetes

	Human	NOD Mouse[8-10]	DP-BB Rat[5-8]	Induced Diabetes in the DR-BB Rat[5,7]	Low-Dose STZ[11]
Diet:	Unknown; suspected association with BSA	Preventable by removal of protein or calorie restriction	Prevented by removal of casein or by restriction of essential fatty acids	Prevented by restriction of essential fatty acids	Prevented by restriction of essential fatty acids
Habitat:	No known effects	Prevented by high temperature; gnotobiosis increases incidence	Gnotobiosis does not prevent IDDM; incidence higher and onset earlier in VAF colonies	Induction by depletion of RT6$^+$ T-cells does not occur in VAF animals	No known effects
Virus Prevention:	Unknown	Sendai; LCMV; LDHV Pichinde; MHV; vaccinia	LCMV	Unknown	Unknown
Virus Induction/ Association:	Mumps; rubella; coxsackie virus B4	Unknown; retroviruses present	Unknown	KRV	Unknown; retroviruses induced

ALS = anti-lymphocyte serum; LCMV = lymphocytic choriomeningitis virus; LDHV = lactate dehydrogenase virus; MHV = murine hepatitis virus; BSA = bovine serum albumin; VAF = viral antibody free; KRV = Kilham rat virus.

designated as diabetes-resistant (DR) BB rats, these coisogenic descendants of DP-BB forebears have a cumulative incidence of spontaneous diabetes that is now 0%,[23] but they retain susceptibility to IDDM induction.[7]

Immunopathogenesis

IDDM in both DP and DR-BB rats involves at least one gene, designated *iddm2*, associated with the rat major histocompatibility complex (MHC). Expression of diabetes is independent of class I haplotype but requires the presence of at least one class II RT1^u allele.[25-28] Intercross studies indicate that the *u* allele of the BB rat is not a unique diabetogenic variant, since *u* alleles derived from normal rat strains also confer susceptibility.[25,29,30]

The region around position 57 of the class II β chains of normal LEW and BUF rats is identical to that found in both DP and DR-BB rats.[31] The enrichment for DQβ alleles with uncharged amino acids at position 57 observed in diabetic white humans[32] and in NOD mice[33] does not appear to apply to the BB rat.

In the DP-BB rat a second locus designated *iddm1* has been identified. This gene is believed to be responsible for lymphopenia in these animals. DP-BB rats are severely T-cell–deficient, particularly with respect to the CD8$^+$ and RT6$^+$ phenotypes. RT6 is a rat maturational T-cell alloantigen that appears to identify cells with immunoregulatory properties.[7] DP-BB rats are susceptible to infections, prone to B-cell lymphomas, and able to reject allografts only poorly. The gene responsible for lymphopenia, *lyp*, has been mapped to chromosome 4 (RNO_4).[34] The mechanism underlying T-cell lymphopenia in the DP-BB rat is unknown. The expression of peripheral T-cell lymphopenia favors the expression of spontaneous hyperglycemia.[35]

The presence of a resistance gene designated *iddm3* has been inferred from crosses between diabetic DP-BB and resistant, nonlymphopenic non-BB rats.[34,36] Recently, a heritable defect in thymic epithelium has been identified in BB rats and may point to a new unmapped susceptibility locus.[37]

In addition to islet and thymic histopathology and lymphopenia, many other observations suggest a role for the immune system in the pathogenesis of spontaneous DP-BB rat diabetes.[5,7] Neonatal thymectomy and injections of antilymphocyte serum prevent the disease, as do many standard immunosuppressive drugs and immunomodulatory modalities (Tables 37-1 and 37-3). Mitogen-activated spleen cells from acutely diabetic donors accelerate disease in young DP rats and transfer it to MHC-compatible naive recipients. Anti-islet cell, antiglutamic acid decarboxylase, and other autoantibodies occur in these animals (see Table 37-1), but the identity of the primary autoantigen or autoantigens is not certain.

The Balance Hypothesis of IDDM in the BB Rat

As is the case with human IDDM, the inciting event that leads to β-cell autoreactivity in the BB rat is not known. The BB rat has, however, provided insight into the processes that determine whether autoreactivity progresses to overt disease or remains dormant. As shown schematically in Figure 37-3, we hypothesize that the expression of IDDM in the BB rat is a function of the relative balance between RT6$^-$ autoreactive (T_A) cells and RT6$^+$ regulatory (T_R) cells that should normally prevent β-cell destruction.[38] Supportive observations include the fact that lymphocyte transfusions prevent disease in lymphopenic, RT6-deficient DP rats if RT6$^+$ donor T-cells become engrafted.[39] IDDM can also be prevented by islet-derived DP-BB CD4$^+$ autoreactive T-cell lines.[40] In addition, mitogen-activated spleen cells from diabetic DP rats adoptively transfer the disease to naive recipients, but cells from transfused nondiabetic animals do not.[41,42] DR-BB rats have normal numbers of RT6$^+$ T-cells. They normally do not become diabetic, but in vivo depletion of these cells induces diabetes in >90% of treated animals.[43] In addition, spleen cells from RT6-depleted DR rats can transfer diabetes to naive recipients even before the onset of IDDM.[44,45] Diabetes in DR rats can also be induced using low-dose irradiation or cyclophosphamide, agents thought to deplete regulatory cell populations.[7]

An important extension of this hypothesis was provided by the discovery of autoreactive T-cells in normal rat strains with no known predisposition to autoimmunity.[45] Such cells were detectable in an adoptive transfer paradigm provided that donors were depleted of RT6$^+$ T-cells. The data suggest that cell populations with autoreactive potential may be present in small numbers or in a functionally inactive state and that some degree of risk for development of autoimmune IDDM may be relatively common.

There is no known human equivalent of the RT6$^+$ T-cell. The primate equivalent of the RT6 gene appears to be a pseudogene.[46]

Table 37-3. Experimental Immunotherapies for IDDM

	NOD Mouse[8–10]	DP-BB Rat[5–8]	Induced DR-BB Rat Diabetes[5,7]	Low-Dose STZ Diabetes[11]
Selective Immunosuppression with Monoclonal Antibodies	Prevention by antibodies against CD3, the TCR, Vβ8, CD4, CD8, MHC class I, MHC class II, CD45, IFN-γ, IL-6, the IL-2 receptor, L-selectin	Prevention by antibodies against CD8, ASGM1, CD3	Prevention by anti-CD8	Prevention by antibodies against *Thy-1*, CD3, CD4, CD8, IL-2r, I-A, I-E, ICAM-1, LFA-1, VCAM-1
Cytokine Therapy	IL-1, IL-4, TNFα, IFN-γ, IL-10 prevent	Unknown	Unknown	IL-1, IFN-γ enhance
Immunostimulation				
Poly I:C	Prevents diabetes	Accelerates onset	Induces diabetes	Polyribocytidylic acid delays
CFA	Prevents diabetes	Prevents diabetes	Unknown	Potentiates
HSP65	Prevents diabetes	Unknown	Unknown	Potentiates
BCG	Prevents diabetes	Prevents diabetes	Unknown	Unknown
Ciamexone	Prevents diabetes	Controversial	Unknown	Ameliorates
Peptide Immunization	HSP, insulin-α and -β chains, glucagon, GAD, viral peptides prevent diabetes	Unknown	Unknown	Unknown
Miscellaneous				
Nicotinamide	Prevents diabetes	Does not prevent diabetes	Unknown	Prevents
Parenteral insulin	Prevents diabetes even at doses that do not produce hypoglycemia	Prevents IDDM at doses that cause hypoglycemia	Same as DP	Unknown
Oral insulin	Prevents diabetes	Unknown	Unknown	Unknown
Vitamins	D, E prevent diabetes	Unknown	Unknown	Unknown
Caramel food coloring	Prevents diabetes	Unknown	Unknown	Unknown
Androgen	Prevents diabetes in ♀	Does not prevent diabetes	Unknown	Potentiates disease in ♀
NO inhibitors	Unknown	Delays onset	Unknown	Prevents diabetes

IL = interleukin; TNF = tumor necrosis factor; Poly I:C = polyinosinic polycytidylic acid; CFA = complete Freund's adjuvant; HSP = heat shock protein; BCG = bacillus Calmette-Guérin; TcR = T-cell receptor; IFN = interferon; ASGM1 = asialoGM1; ALS = antilymphocyte serum; IL-2r = interleukin 2 receptor; NO = nitric oxide. ICAM-1, LFA-1, and VCAM-1 are intercellular adhesion molecules.

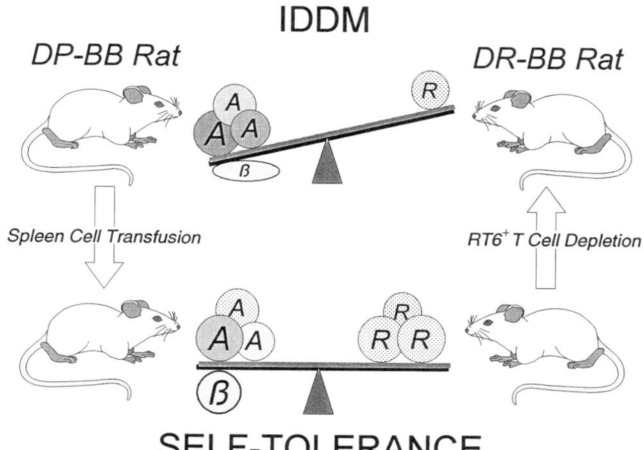

Figure 37-3. The balance hypothesis of autoimmunity as applied to IDDM in the DP and DR-BB rat disease models. A = Autoreactive cell; R = regulatory cell; β = pancreatic β-cell; DP-BB = spontaneously hyperglycemic diabetes-prone BB rat; DR = diabetes-resistant BB rat.

Which cell populations may subserve the equivalent function in humans is unknown. There is as yet no evidence for a mouse RT6$^+$ regulatory T-cell, but other data have nonetheless suggested the applicability of the balance model for disease expression in the NOD mouse.[47]

NOD Mice

Natural History and Pathology

Makino and colleagues discovered this mouse model of spontaneous autoimmune diabetes in the late 1970s.[48–50] These nonobese diabetic animals develop pancreatic insulitis when 4 or 5 weeks old. By 7 months of age, ≈80% of female and ≈20% of male mice typically become diabetic. These animals are widely available, but the cumulative frequency of diabetes can vary substantially in different colonies.[51] Ketoacidosis in affected animals is mild. Diabetic mice can survive for up to a month without exogenous insulin, although eventually it becomes required for survival. Morphologically, "nests" of lymphocytes are observed juxtaposed to pancreatic islets at ≈5 weeks of age. As NOD mice mature, these mononuclear cells appear to migrate toward the islets, and by the time hyperglycemia occurs, frank insulitis is present. NOD mice also develop sialoadenitis and thyroiditis. As summarized in Tables 37-1 and 37-3, IDDM in NOD mice is preventable by an extensive repertoire of immunosuppressive and immunomodulatory interventions.[49]

Immunopathogenesis

In addition to insulitis and the response to immunosuppression, many additional lines of evidence suggest that NOD mouse diabetes is an autoimmune disorder. Splenocytes from adult NOD mice can adoptively transfer disease to MHC-compatible, immunodeficient recipients; both $CD4^+$ and $CD8^+$ lymphocytes appear to be required.[52] Recently, islet specific T-cell clones have been obtained from affected NOD mice; these can induce diabetes in appropriate recipients.[53] Extensive investigations of the T-cell receptor have failed to reveal evidence of TcR Vβ clonality or allelic polymorphism of Vβ coding regions in the islet-infiltrating T-cells of NOD mice.[54]

Efforts to understand the origin of autoreactive cell populations in the NOD mouse have led to extensive genetic investigations. Both MHC and non-MHC genes have been linked to IDDM in these animals. Analyses indicate at least 15 loci on five different chromosomes that associate with diabetes or insulitis.[55,56] These loci are found on chromosomes 1, 3, 9, 11, and 17. The chromosome 17 locus is MHC-associated. Another report, using an interspecific cross of NOD mice with *Mus spretus,* implicated markers on at least four chromosomes: 3, 6, 15, and 17 (MHC-associated).[57] Analogous to the human *IDDM1* locus, *idd-1* in the mouse has been assigned to an MHC class II–associated region located between the class I K and class III *bat5* genes.[58] Additional MHC-associated candidate genes include those encoding tumor necrosis factor alpha (TNF-α), lymphotoxin-α, and heat shock proteins.[59] As in humans, diabetes susceptibility in NOD mice is associated with MHC class II alleles with uncharged amino acids at position 57.[33] Non-MHC IDDM loci have been associated with candidate genes such as *Nramp* (possibly important in nitric oxide metabolism),[56] *Fcgr1* (high-affinity receptor for IgG Fc-γ-R1),[60] *IL-2* (interleukin 2, T-cell growth factor), *glut-2* (a glucose transporter), *Ins-1* (insulin gene),[55] and *Bcl-2*.[61] NOD mice lack expression of I-E. Restoration of I-E expression in transgenic NOD has yielded conflicting reports of prevention[62,63] and failure to prevent[64] IDDM. NOD mice express a unique I-A haplotype on chromosome 17.

All of these genes represent candidate susceptibility loci, but they are not the only genetic associations in NOD diabetes. Of particular interest in the context of the balance hypothesis (Fig. 37-2) is the discovery of non-MHC linked loci that appear to confer resistance to diabetes.[65] Designated *Idd3* and *Idd10,* homozygosity for either resistance allele confers partial protection, and the expression of resistance alleles at both loci confers nearly complete protection from IDDM.

As in the human and BB rat, anti-islet cell and anti-GAD autoantibodies are found in the NOD mouse. The relationships among these many genetic and humoral immune factors remain to be determined, but some possible connections are beginning to be discerned. A recent study has demonstrated, for example, the existence of T-cell cross-reactivity between a coxsackievirus protein and glutamate decarboxylase associated with the unique NOD I-A diabetes susceptibility allele.[66]

The preponderance of diabetes in female as compared with male NOD mice has prompted speculation that androgens exert a protective effect. Male castration does increase the frequency of NOD diabetes, but sex-specific differences in antioxidant enzyme activities have also been described and could contribute to differential susceptibility.[67] In human IDDM both sexes are affected about equally.[68,69] In the BB rat neither neonatal gonadectomy nor hypophysectomy changes the frequency of diabetes.[5]

The Balance Hypothesis and the NOD Mouse

The identification of both susceptibility and resistance genes in the NOD mouse has been noted above. Parallel findings at the cellular level have also been reported. In addition to T-cells capable of adoptively transferring IDDM, the islets of diabetic NOD mice contain islet populations capable of preventing IDDM.[70] Cell lines with this capability, similar to lines obtained from DP-BB rats,[40] were autoreactive. These results suggest that, as in the DP-BB rat (Fig. 37-3), a failure of peripheral immunoregulation may play an important role in disease expression.

This concept has recently gained additional support from studies of transgenic NOD mice. Singer and coworkers produced animals that expressed both the unique $I\text{-}A^{NOD}$ and a transgenic $I\text{-}A^{d}$.[71] These animals developed insulitis, but the frequency of IDDM was reduced, and T-cells from these animals interfered with the adoptive transfer of IDDM by nontransgenic NOD T-cells.

An attractive concept derived from studies in the NOD mouse, BB rat, and humans holds that the balance between autoreactive and regulatory cell populations may in part represent a balance between the Th1 and Th2 subsets of the $CD4^+$ T-cell population.[72] The former function principally to mediate proinflammatory reactions and secrete interferon gamma (IFN-γ) and interleukin-2 (IL-2); the latter subserve a suppressor function, secrete IL-4 and IL-10, and can downregulate a Th1 cell–mediated immune response. These subsets function in an agonist-antagonist fashion, and it is possible that the outcome of an autoreactive process reflects the balance between these two Th subtypes (see Fig. 37-2). Biasing the system in favor of immunoregulation is the underlying goal of several interventions designed to prevent IDDM. One strategy being tested is the oral administration of islet-specific antigen. In the NOD mouse, for example, orally administered insulin prevents disease,[73] possibly as the result of generating populations of islet T-cells that secrete immunosuppressive cytokines such as transforming growth factor β.[74]

Toxin-Induced IDDM: The Low-Dose STZ Model

DP-BB rats and NOD mice provide models of spontaneous IDDM. The RT6-depleted DR-BB rat provides a model of induced IDDM based on alteration of peripheral T-cell phenotypes. Additional models have emerged from the discovery that β-cells are susceptible to environmental toxins. Alloxan,[75] streptozocin (STZ),[75] and the rodenticide Vacor[76] at high doses are all selective β-cell cytotoxins. STZ is used as chemotherapy for insulinomas; Vacor has been ingested with suicidal intent, leaving some survivors with IDDM. There is no epidemiologic evidence to suggest that these or other environmental agents commonly cause IDDM by killing β-cells directly. It remains possible, however, that occult chemical alteration of β-cells might render them immunogenic.[16] In the context of the balance hypothesis (see Fig. 37-2), environmental toxins would initiate, activate, or amplify autoreactivity against β-cells. This process has been modeled in studies of low-dose STZ diabetes.

When mice receive multiple small subdiabetogenic doses of STZ, pancreatic insulitis, selective β-cell destruction, and diabetes ensue after a delay of several days.[77] Insulitis in mice treated with low doses of STZ is composed of T-cells and macrophages.[11,77,78] Various MHC associations have been identified, including one in the I-A subregion,[79] but no one haplotype uniformly confers resistance or susceptibility to all strains. Exogenous IL-1 can overcome the inherent resistance of some strains.[80]

Islet autoantibodies appear after STZ treatment, but there is no evidence for an etiologic role for humoral immunity. Treatment with low-dose STZ is also associated with the induction of pancreatic retroviruses, but there is no evidence that they play an active role in pathogenesis.[81] Athymic mice are resistant to low-dose STZ diabetes,[82] but this resistance can be reversed by T-cell reconstitution from normal donors.

Many immunosuppressive interventions ameliorate low-dose STZ diabetes (see Tables 37-1 and 37-3). These include radiation, antilymphocyte serum, anti-inflammatory compounds, silica, IL-1 receptor antagonist, and various antibodies that recognize *Thy-1*, CD3, CD4, CD8, the IL-2 receptor, I-A, I-E, ICAM-1, LFA-1, and VCAM-1.[9,11,83–87] Cyclosporine does not prevent diabetes after administration of low-dose STZ, but this apparent failure of immunosuppression may be caused by the direct toxicity of this agent on mouse β-cells.[88] The immunosuppressive drug FK506 does inhibit β-cell damage caused by low-dose STZ.[89]

Investigations of the primary pathogenesis of low-dose STZ diabetes suggest strongly that the immunologic process described above is dependent on chemical alteration of the β-cell. Adoptive transfer of low-dose STZ diabetes requires pretreatment of recipients with low "priming" doses of STZ.[90,91] Treatment with 5-thio-D-glucose prevents high-dose STZ-induced cytotoxicity but does not prevent the inflammatory events associated with low-dose STZ.[92] Finally, *scid/scid* mice that lack both T- and B-cells are susceptible to low-dose STZ diabetes induction,[93] emphasizing that on at least some genetic backgrounds the combination of reagent and protocol that was employed is inherently β-cell cytotoxic.

The data indicate that the low-dose STZ model has two distinct components. One is a direct β-cytotoxic effect. The other is the generation of immunologic recognition of residual, altered β-cells—irrespective of whether or not those β-cells have been lethally injured by STZ. The latter event has been characterized as the stimulation of "natural cytotoxicity" by non-MHC–restricted macrophages and natural killer cells.[94,95]

Islet transplantation data have also provided insights into the induction of IDDM by low-dose STZ treatment.[96] Syngeneic islet transplants in low-dose STZ diabetic mice develop insulitis if transplanted 10–14 days before the injection of the drug. In contrast, there is no graft insulitis if the transplants are done 3 days after injection of STZ, indicating that some exposure to STZ is needed to facilitate immunologic recognition of islet grafts. These and other data suggest that pre-exposure of transplant recipients to STZ is essential to the development of insulitis and are consistent with the concept that low-dose STZ induces autoimmunity in susceptible hosts by altering β-cells and inducing autoantigenicity. What determines an individual host's susceptibility and what precisely is the β-cell alteration induced by STZ remain important unanswered questions.

Viruses and IDDM in Animals

In humans the temporal relationship of viral infection to diabetes is well documented, but the exact role of this environmental agent in pathogenesis is unknown.[17] Both direct β-cell cytotoxicity and processes of molecular mimicry have been implicated as pathogenic mechanisms.[97] These hypotheses have been modeled extensively in animals, particularly the mouse infected with the M variant of encephalomyocarditis virus.[17] Diabetes induced by encephalomyocarditis and other viruses in animals is discussed extensively in Chapter 35. Here we briefly review the diverse influence of certain viruses on the expression of IDDM in NOD mice and BB rats.

Compared with mice raised in conventional animal facilities, cesarian-derived NOD mice reared in a gnotobiotic environment become diabetic more often and at a younger age.[98] Vaccinia, lactate dehydrogenase virus, lymphocytic choriomeningitis virus, mouse hepatitis virus, and sendai and Pichinde viruses all decrease the incidence of IDDM in NOD mice.[50] Complicating these observations is the issue of vertically transmitted genomic retroviral infection and activation (see Chapter 35), which remains a controversial area in studies of the NOD mouse.[99–101]

In the DP-BB rat, diabetes occurs in gnotobiotic (germ-free) animals,[102] but viral pathogens do modulate the frequency and age at onset of spontaneous disease.[103] Rederivation of the National Institutes of Health resource colony of DP-BB rats into a viral antibody-free environment has increased the frequency of diabetes and lowered the age at onset.[103] As in the NOD mouse, lymphocytic choriomeningitis viral infection decreases the frequency of IDDM in DP-BB rats.[104] This virus is hypothesized to function by directly infecting and downregulating a subset of peripheral helper T-cells.[104,105]

DR-BB rats housed in viral antibody-free facilities remain free of spontaneous diabetes, but DR-BB rats infected with Kilham's rat virus become diabetic.[103,106] Naturally occurring infection, transmitted by close contact, induces diabetes in ≈1–2% of animals; direct injection of Kilham's rat virus induces ≈30% of animals to become diabetic.[106] Disease induction does not involve infection of the pancreatic β-cells.[107] Kilham's rat virus may trigger diabetes in DR rats by altering the balance between autoreactive T-cells and $RT6^+$ regulatory T-cells (see Fig. 37-2). Interestingly, diabetes in DR rats can also be induced by administration of polyinosinic:polycytidylic acid (poly I:C), a synthetic double-stranded polyribonucleotide that elicits immune responses analogous to those observed during viral infection.[108]

These findings in NOD mice and BB rats provide an instructive example of the interaction of genetics and environment. They also re-emphasize the need for rigorous definition of animal environmental status in evaluating results that address any area of pathogenesis.

Transgenic Mouse Models of IDDM

Transgene technology has been applied to the study of IDDM by expressing genes of interest in the pancreatic β-cells of normal and NOD mice, by engineering T-cell transgenic mice, and by testing the effects of gene knockouts in both normal and NOD mice. Table 37-4 summarizes the varied outcomes of these genetic manipulations.

The most obvious lesson from studies of transgenic mice has been that the mere presence of a neoantigen or hyperexpression of a self-antigen on β-cells is by itself insufficient to trigger IDDM. Whereas some antigens are completely quiescent, others are associated with islet pathology. Transgenic animals have been used successfully to test the hypothesis that aberrant expression of MHC molecules on β-cells predisposes to IDDM.[109] Mice engineered to hyperexpress class I antigen on β-cells[110] become diabetic, but in the absence of an inflammatory lesion. Mice that express class II molecules on the β-cell surface develop islet atrophy without an inflammatory component.[111–113] Rather than induce autoreactivity, transgenic class II expressing islets may, in fact, induce antigen-specific unresponsiveness in T-cells, altering the balance of forces in the immune system (Fig. 37-2) and playing a role in the maintenance of self-tolerance.[114]

The transgenic approach has also enabled investigators to dissect elements of the immune system and to test specific hypotheses concerning relevance of those elements. Transgenic animals expressing high concentrations of cytokines in pancreatic islets have been created (Table 37-4). Transgenics expressing the proinflammatory Th1 cytokines IFN-γ[115] or IL-2[116] develop IDDM, and the latter accelerates IDDM in NOD mice.[117] In contrast, those expressing either TNF-α[118] or TNF-β[119] develop insulitis without diabetes. Transgenics expressing the Th2 cytokine IL-10 on a normal background develop pancreatitis without insulitis or diabetes,[120] but NOD mice transgenic for islet expression of IL-10 experience accelerated disease.[121] In their aggregate these data demonstrate the capabilities of supraphysiologic concentrations of cytokines in the islets without implicating any one cytokine as the determinant of the balance between autoreactivity and immunoregulation.

TABLE 37-4. Transgenic and Knockout Mice Used to Study Autoimmune Diabetes

Category	Transgene	Insulitis + Hyperglycemia	Other Outcomes
Foreign Antigen	SV40 T antigen[142–144]	No	Neoplasia; insulitis; autoantibodies; tolerance
	LCMV GP + viral infection[124–126]	Yes	No disease from transgene without viral infection
	Influenza virus hemagglutinin[145]	Yes	Diabetes in only 13–27% of animals
	H-ras[146,147]	No	Hyperglycemia with islet degeneration
	Yeast hexokinase[148]	No	Enhances insulin secretion
	Human E-B virus receptor[149]	No	Peri-insulitis
Native Antigen	Class I[110,150]	No	Hyperglycemia without insulitis
	I-A[112,113]	No	Hyperglycemia with islet atrophy and no insulitis
	I-E[111,151]	No	Hyperglycemia with islet atrophy and no insulitis
	β_2-Microglobulin[152]	No	Defective insulin secretion
	Insulin[153]	No	Compensated gene hyperexpression
	Amylin[154,155]	No	Increased insulin storage/secretion
	Superoxide dismutase[156]	No	Reduced oxidative stress diabetes
	Calmodulin[157]	No	Nonimmune β-cell destruction at birth
	GLUT-2 antisense RNA expression[158]	?	Reduced insulin; hyperglycemia; no histology reported
Cytokine	IL-2[159]	No	Inflammation of exocrine and endocrine pancreas
	IFN-γ[113,115]	Yes	Hyperglycemia with insulitis
	IFN-α[160]	Yes	Hyperglycemia with insulitis
	TNF-α[118]	No	Insulitis without diabetes
	TNF-β[119]	No	Insulitis without diabetes
	IL-10[120]	No	Exocrine pancreatic inflammation without insulitis
Multiple	Influenza virus HA + HA-specific TCR[161]	Yes	IDDM depended on non-MHC background genes
	LCMV + TNF-α[162]	Yes	TNF-α enhanced diabetes induction
	LCMV + viral TCR + viral infection[125]	Yes	No IDDM in the absence of infection
	B7 + TNF-α[122]	Yes	Neither transgene alone sufficient for IDDM
	B7, islet viral GP, + GP-specific TCR[123]	Yes	No IDDM in the absence of B7
	IL-2 + MHC class I + MHC-specific TCR[116]	Yes	No IDDM without IL-2
Transgenic NOD Mice	$I\text{-}A^{d}$ [71]	No	Prevents IDDM
	$I\text{-}A^{k}$ [163–165]	No	Prevents IDDM
	Modified I-Aβ[63]	No	Prevents IDDM
	$I\text{-}E^{C57BL/6}$ [62]	No	Prevents IDDM
	$I\text{-}E\alpha^{d}$ [63]	No	Prevents IDDM
	$I\text{-}E\alpha^{k}$ [166]	No	Prevents IDDM
	L^{d} [167]	No	Prevents IDDM
	IL-10 in NOD[121]	Yes	Accelerates IDDM
	Non-NOD TCR in NOD[168]	Yes	Did not prevent IDDM
	Diabetogenic NOD TCR[169]	Yes	Accelerates IDDM; TCR from diabetogenic T-cell clone
Knockouts	Class I in NOD[170]	No	No insulitis
	Class II in LCMV transgenic[171]	Yes	$CD4^+$ T-cells absent in insulitis
	β2 Microglobulin in NOD[172,173]	No	Prevents IDDM

Transgenes other than T-cell receptor genes were generally coupled to a rat or human insulin promoter for targeting to pancreatic β-cells. The summary column labeled insulitis plus hyperglycemia indicates that at minimum both islet inflammation and diabetes were observed, suggesting an autoimmune diathesis; selective β-cell destruction, absolute insulin deficiency, and sparing of non–β-islet cells were not reported in some cases. Diabetes without insulitis and *vice versa* are reported as other outcomes. Many other transgenes have been investigated, not all of which have been formally reported.[22] TCR = T-cell receptor; LCMV = lymphocytic choriomeningitis virus; GP = glycoprotein; E-B virus = Epstein-Barr virus; HA = hemagglutinin; GLUT-2 = glucose transporter GLUT-2.

Another interesting avenue for animal IDDM research exploits the development of multiply transgenic animals. For example, islet transgenic mice that express both TNF-α and the B7 costimulatory molecule develop insulitis and diabetes, whereas neither transgene alone is effective.[122] Similarly, mice transgenic for islet B7 and a viral glycoprotein become diabetic in the presence of a glycoprotein-specific transgenic T-cell receptor.[123] In the absence of B7, there is no disease. These studies provide promising models for the dissection of candidate diabetogenic processes. It must be remembered, however, that tactics that require the expression of a costimulatory molecule like B7 on a β-cell are inherently artificial and should engender cautious interpretation.

A final use of transgenic models has been to explore the concept of virus-induced molecular mimicry. The expression of lymphocytic choriomeningitis virus glycoprotein on the surface of β-cells does not by itself induce insulitis or diabetes,[124–126] even if T-cells expressing a T-cell receptor specific for the glycoprotein are present.[125] Actual infection with lymphocytic choriomeningitis virus in both model systems does, however, induce diabetes,[124–126] but again a cautionary note should be sounded. These results in genetically engineered rodents contrast starkly with the protection from IDDM that is induced by naturally occurring lymphocytic choriomeningitis virus infection in both NOD mice[105] and BB rats.[104]

Lessons, Limits, and Cautions

Variation in Phenotype

Many differences between human and rodent IDDM are obvious. DP-BB rats, for example, are severely lymphopenic; humans and NOD mice are not. The risk of IDDM in NOD mice is far greater in females; this is not true of humans or BB rats. Ketoacidosis in humans and BB rats is more severe than in NOD mice. In the case of diabetic transgenic animals, important caveats are also obvious. Transgenes can alter intracellular metabolism, affecting insulin secretion, and induce the expression of molecules that do not naturally occur in β-cells. Reports of transgenic models of IDDM often lack convincing proof that β-cells are selectively destroyed, rather than degranulated, and that non–β-islet cell populations are preserved and functional. Differences in phenotype between human and animal IDDM limit the interspecific analogy that can be ascribed to the disease states. Several other issues should be considered when assessing analogies among models.

Genetic Variation

Heterogeneity among various rodent colonies around the world affects the interpretation of animal model data. Sublines can vary substantially with respect to their frequency, severity, and immunobiologic characteristics.[51,127,128] At least 24 inbred and 2 outbred lines of the BB rat exist.[129] In some substrains of NOD mice, the frequency of diabetes can be >90% in females and 50% in males, whereas in other substrains the frequency in both sexes can be less than 5%.[51] The possibility also exists that variations among mouse colonies may affect the expression of low-dose STZ diabetes. These idiosyncracies need to be considered before generalizing observations that may apply only to unique combinations of locale, substrain, and environment.

Environmental Idiosyncracy

In addition to genetic variation, the geographic distribution of animal models introduces other variables.[59] These include idiosyncratic exposure to diet, viruses, and other environmental factors (see Table 37-2). For example, increasing the room temperature in one colony of NOD mice has been reported to lower the frequency of IDDM.[130] This observation suggests that difficult to control local variables may indirectly affect NOD mouse experimentation. In the study just cited, higher ambient temperature was associated with lower food intake.

The importance of diet, particularly protein that is derived from cow's milk, is currently under intensive study.[131,132] In part, this line of research has been driven by the finding that the type of protein in food influences the onset of diabetes in the NOD mice.[133] Pregestimil, a cow milk–free diet, prevents diabetes in female NOD mice; extracts of commercial mouse chow added to Pregestimil increase the incidence of diabetes.[134] These observations argue that some ingredients of "chow" are diabetogenic and can be eliminated from semipurified diets, but other dietary findings are more perplexing. Feeding NOD mice a conventional diet but giving them access to it only every other day decreases the incidence of IDDM.[135]

Dietary protein also affects the expression of BB rat IDDM.[133] Wheat gluten flour and soybean meal–containing diets maximize the frequency of diabetes,[136] whereas semisynthetic diets and diets based on hydrolyzed casein reduce the incidence of IDDM and delay its onset.[136,137] The mechanisms are unknown. Diets deficient in essential fatty acids also prevent IDDM in both DP and RT6-depleted DR rats[138] and in the low-dose STZ model.[139]

The effects of dietary protein are being explored to define disease mechanisms that may be common to IDDM in humans and rodents.[133] It must be borne in mind, however, that variation in diet from colony to colony and from season to season (according to the availability of raw materials) can affect the expression of animal IDDM.

Conclusion

Useful analogies exist between human IDDM and similar disorders in rodents. These analogies have engendered creative experimentation and powerful insights into the processes that generate autoreactivity and those that regulate it. IDDM is not the same across species, however. From a clinical perspective, mice and rats sometimes seem to be teaching different lessons about human IDDM. Particularly with respect to the generation of human therapeutics,[140] animal data need to be interpreted with caution and prudence.

References

1. Gepts W. Pathology and anatomy of the pancreas in juvenile diabetes mellitus. Diabetes 1965;14:619
2. Bach J-F. Insulin-dependent diabetes mellitus as an autoimmune disease. Endocr Rev 1994;15:516
3. Atkinson MA, Maclaren NK. Mechanisms of disease: The pathogenesis of insulin-dependent diabetes mellitus. N Engl J Med 1994;331:1428
4. Renold AE, Porte D Jr, Shafrir E. Definitions for diabetes types: Use and abuse of the concept 'animal models of diabetes mellitus'. In: Shafrir E, Renold AE, eds. Frontiers in Diabetes Research. Lessons from Animal Diabetes II. London: John Libbey;1988:3–7
5. Mordes JP, Desemone J, Rossini AA. The BB rat. Diabetes/Metab Rev 1987;3:725
6. Parfrey NA, Prud'homme GJ, Colle E, et al. Immunologic and genetic studies of diabetes in the BB rat. CRC Crit Rev Immunol 1989;9:45
7. Crisá L, Mordes JP, Rossini AA. Autoimmune diabetes mellitus in the BB rat. Diabetes/Metab Rev 1992;8:9
8. Serreze DV, Leiter EH. Insulin dependent diabetes mellitus (IDDM) in NOD mice and BB rats: Origins in hematopoietic stem cell defects and implications for therapy. In: Shafrir E, ed. Lessons from Animal Diabetes V. London: Smith Gordon;1994:59–73
9. Kolb H. Mouse models of insulin dependent diabetes: Low-dose streptozotocin induced-diabetes and nonobese diabetic (NOD) mice. Diabetes/Metab Rev 1987;3:751
10. Kikutani H, Makino S. The murine autoimmune diabetes model: NOD and related strains. Adv Immunol 1992;51:285
11. Kolb H, Kröncke K-D. IDDM: Lesson from the low-dose streptozocin model in mice. Diab Rev 1993;1:116
12. Mahon JL, Dupre J, Stiller CR. Lessons learned from use of cyclosporine for insulin-dependent diabetes mellitus: The case for immunotherapy for insulin-dependent diabetics having residual insulin secretion. Ann NY Acad Sci 1993;696:351
13. Kawano K, Hirashima T, Mori S, et al. New inbred strain of Long-Evans Tokushima lean rats with IDDM without lymphopenia. Diabetes 1991; 40:1375
14. Shi K, Mizuno A, Sano T, et al. Sexual difference in the incidence of diabetes mellitus in Otsuka-Long-Evans-Tokushima-fatty rats: Effects of castration and sex hormone replacement on its incidence. Metabolism 1994;43:1214
15. Guberski DL, Butler L, Manzi SM, et al. The BBZ/Wor rat: Clinical characteristics of the diabetic syndrome. Diabetologia 1993;36:912
16. Leslie RDG, Elliott RB. Early environmental events as a cause of IDDM: Evidence and implications. Diabetes 1994;43:843
17. Yoon J-W. Role of viruses in the pathogenesis of IDDM. Ann Med 1991; 23:437
18. Penhale WJ, Stumbles PA, Huxtable CR, et al. Induction of diabetes in PVG/c strain rats by manipulation of the immune system. Autoimmunity 1990;7:169
19. Stumbles PA, Penhale WJ. IDDM in rats induced by thymectomy and irradiation. Diabetes 1993;42:571
20. Klöppel G. "Insulin" induced insulitis. In: Ortved Andersen O, Deckert T, Nerup J, eds. Immunological Aspects of Diabetes Mellitus. International Symposium. Steno Memorial Hospital, Denmark, Copenhagen: Acta Endocrinologica;1976:107–121

21. Goodnow CC. Transgenic mice and analysis of B-cell tolerance. Annu Rev Immunol 1992;10:489
22. Shizuru JA, Sarvetnick N. Transgenic mice for the study of diabetes mellitus. Trends Endocrinol Metab 1991;2:97
23. Guberski DL. Diabetes-prone and diabetes-resistant BB rats: Animal models of spontaneous and virally induced diabetes mellitus, lymphocytic thyroiditis, and collagen-induced arthritis. ILAR News 1994;35:29–37
24. Rajatanavin R, Appel MC, Reinhardt W, et al. Variable prevalence of lymphocytic thyroiditis among diabetes-prone sublines of BB/Wor rats. Endocrinology 1991;128:153
25. Colle E, Guttmann RD, Fuks A. Insulin-dependent diabetes mellitus is associated with genes that map to the right of the class 1 RT1.A locus of the major histocompatibility complex of the rat. Diabetes 1986;35:454
26. Colle E, Guttmann RD, Fuks A, et al. Genetics of the spontaneous diabetic syndrome. Interaction of MHC and non-MHC-associated factors. Mol Biol Med 1986;3:13
27. Colle E. Genetic susceptibility to the development of spontaneous insulin-independent diabetes mellitus in the rat. Clin Immunol Immunopathol 1990; 57:1
28. Fuks A, Ono SJ, Colle E, Guttmann RD. A single dose of the MHC-linked susceptibility determinant associated with the $RT1^u$ haplotype is permissive of insulin-dependent diabetes mellitus in the BB rat. Exp Clin Immunogenet 1990;7:162
29. Ono SJ, Colle E, Guttmann RD, Fuks A. MHC association of IDDM maps to permissive immune response genes. In: Jaworski MA, Molnar GD, Rajotte RV, Singh B, eds. The Immunology of Autoimmune Diabetes Mellitus. Amsterdam: Elsevier; 1986:51–57
30. Colle E, Guttmann RD, Seemayer TA, Michel F. Spontaneous diabetes mellitus syndrome in the rat. IV. Immunogenetic interactions of MHC and non-MHC components of the syndrome. Metabolism 1983;32(Suppl 1):54
31. Chao NJ, Timmerman L, McDevitt HO, Jacob CO. Molecular characterization of MHC class II antigens (beta 1 domain) in the BB diabetes-prone and -resistant rat. Immunogenetics 1989;29:231
32. Todd JA, Bell JI, McDevitt HO. HLA-DQ_β gene contributes to susceptibility and resistance to insulin-dependent diabetes mellitus. Nature 1987; 329:599
33. Acha-Orbea H, McDevitt HO. The first external domain of the nonobese diabetic mouse class II I-A beta chain is unique. Proc Natl Acad Sci USA 1987;84:2435
34. Jacob HJ, Pettersson A, Wilson D, et al. Genetic dissection of autoimmune type I diabetes in the BB rat. Nature Genet 1992;2:56
35. Markholst H, Eastman S, Wilson D, et al. Diabetes segregates as a single locus in crosses between inbred BB rats prone or resistant to diabetes. J Exp Med 1991;174:297
36. Colle E, Fuks A, Poussier P, et al. Polygenic nature of spontaneous diabetes in the rat: Permissive MHC haplotype and presence of the lymphopenic trait of the BB rat are not sufficient to produce susceptibility. Diabetes 1992;41:1617
37. Doukas J, Mordes JP, Swymer C, et al. Thymic epithelial defects and predisposition to autoimmune disease in BB rats. Am J Pathol 1994;145:1517
38. Rossini AA, Greiner DL, Friedman HP, Mordes JP. Immunopathogenesis of diabetes mellitus. Diab Rev 1993;1:43
39. Burstein D, Mordes JP, Greiner DL, et al. Prevention of diabetes in the BB/ Wor rat by a single transfusion of spleen cells: Parameters that affect the degree of protection. Diabetes 1989;38:24
40. Nagata M, Yoon J-W. Prevention of autoimmune type I diabetes in BioBreeding (BB) rats by a newly established, autoreactive T cell line from acutely diabetic BB rats. J Immunol 1994;153:3775
41. Koevary S, Rossini AA, Stoller W, et al. Passive transfer of diabetes in the BB/W rat. Science 1983;220:727
42. Koevary SB, Williams DE, Williams RM, Chick WL. Passive transfer of diabetes from BB/W to Wistar-Furth rats. J Clin Invest 1985;75:1904
43. Thomas VA, Woda BA, Handler ES, et al. Exposure to viral pathogens alters the expression of diabetes in BB/Wor rats. Diabetes 1991;40:255
44. Greiner DL, Mordes JP, Handler ES, et al. Depletion of $RT6.1^+$ T lymphocytes induces diabetes in resistant BioBreeding/Worcester (BB/W) rats. J Exp Med 1987;166:461
45. McKeever U, Mordes JP, Greiner DL, et al. Adoptive transfer of autoimmune diabetes and thyroiditis to athymic rats. Proc Natl Acad Sci USA 1990; 87:7718
46. Haag F, Koch-Nolte F, Kühl M, et al. Premature stop codons inactivate the RT6 genes of the human and chimpanzee species. J Mol Biol 1994;243:537
47. Rashba EJ, Reich E-P, Janeway CA, Sherwin RS. Type 1 diabetes mellitus: An imbalance between effector and regulatory T cells? Acta Diabetol 1993;30:61
48. Makino S, Kunimoto K, Munaoko Y, et al. Breeding of a non-obese diabetic strain of mice. Exp Anim 1980;29:1
49. Bowman MA, Leiter EH, Atkinson MA. Prevention of diabetes in the NOD mouse: Implications for therapeutic intervention in human disease. Immunol Today 1994;15:115
50. Karasik A, Hattori M. Use of animal models in the study of diabetes. In: Kahn CR, Weir GC, eds. Joslin's Diabetes Mellitus. Malvern, Pa: Lea & Febiger; 1994:317–350
51. Pozzilli P, Signore A, Williams AJK, Beales PE. NOD mouse colonies around the world—recent facts and figures. Immunol Today 1993;14:193
52. Christianson SW, Shultz LD, Leiter EH. Adoptive transfer of diabetes into immunodeficient NOD-*scid/scid* mice: Relative contributions of $CD4^+$ and $CD8^+$ T-cells from diabetic versus prediabetic NOD.NON-*Thy-1*^{a} donors. Diabetes 1993;42:44
53. Peterson JD, Pike B, McDuffie M, Haskins K. Islet-specific T cell clones transfer diabetes to nonobese diabetic (NOD) F_1 mice. J Immunol 1994; 153:2800
54. Sarukhan A, Gombert J-M, Olivi M, et al. Anchored polymerase chain reaction based analysis of the Vβ repertoire in the non-obese diabetic (NOD) mouse. Eur J Immunol 1994;24:1750
55. Ghosh S, Palmer SM, Rodrigues NR, et al. Polygenic control of autoimmune diabetes in nonobese diabetic mice. Nature Genet 1993;4:404
56. Garchon H-J. Non-MHC-linked genes in autoimmune diseases. Curr Opin Immunol 1993;5:894
57. De Gouyon B, Melanitou E, Richard MF, et al. Genetic analysis of diabetes and insulitis in an interspecific cross of the nonobese diabetic mouse with *Mus spretus*. Proc Natl Acad Sci USA 1993;90:1877
58. Ikegami H, Kawaguchi Y, Ueda H, et al. MHC-linked diabetogenic gene of the NOD mouse: Molecular mapping of the 3′ boundary of the diabetogenic region. Biochem Biophys Res Commun 1993;192:677
59. Todd JA, Steinman L. Autoimmunity. The environment strikes back. Curr Opin Immunol 1993;5:863
60. Prins J-B, Todd JA, Rodrigues NR, et al. Linkage on chromosome 3 of autoimmune diabetes and defective Fc receptor for IgG in NOD mice. Science 1993;260:695
61. Garchon H-J, Luan J-J, Eloy L, et al. Genetic analysis of immune dysfunction in non-obese diabetic (NOD) mice: Mapping of a susceptibility locus close to the *Bcl-2* gene correlates with increased resistance of NOD T cells to apoptosis induction. Eur J Immunol 1994;24:380
62. Nishimoto H, Kikutani H, Yamamura K, Kishimoto T. Prevention of autoimmune insulitis by expression of I-E molecules in NOD mice. Nature 1987;328:432
63. Lund T, O'Reilly L, Hutchings P, et al. Prevention of insulin-dependent diabetes mellitus in non-obese diabetic mice by transgenes encoding modified I-A β-chain or normal I-E α-chain. Nature 1990;345:727
64. Podolin PL, Pressey A, DeLarato NH, et al. $I\text{-}E^+$ nonobese diabetic mice develop insulitis and diabetes. J Exp Med 1993;178:793
65. Wicker LS, Todd JA, Prins J-B, et al. Resistance alleles at two non-major histocompatibility complex-linked insulin-dependent diabetes loci on chromosome 3, *Idd3* and *Idd10*, protect nonobese diabetic mice from diabetes. J Exp Med 1994;180:1705
66. Tian J, Lehmann PV, Kaufman DL. T cell cross-reactivity between coxsackievirus and glutamate decarboxylase is associated with a murine diabetes susceptibility allele. J Exp Med 1994;180:1979
67. Cornelius JG, Luttge BG, Peck AB. Antioxidant enzyme activities in IDD-prone and IDD-resistant mice: A comparative study. Free Radic Biol Med 1993;14:409
68. Karvonen M, Tuomilehto J, Libman I, LaPorte R. A review of the recent epidemiological data on the worldwide incidence of type 1 (insulin-dependent) diabetes mellitus. Diabetologia 1993;36:883
69. Green A, Gale EAM, Patterson CC. Incidence of childhood-onset insulin-dependent diabetes mellitus: The EURODIAB ACE study. Lancet 1992; 339:905
70. Reich E-P, Scaringe D, Yagi J, et al. Prevention of diabetes in NOD mice by injection of autoreactive T-lymphocytes. Diabetes 1989;38:1647
71. Singer SM, Tisch R, Yang X-D, McDevitt HO. An *Ab*^{d} transgene prevents diabetes in nonobese diabetic mice by inducing regulatory T cells. Proc Natl Acad Sci USA 1993;90:9566
72. Rabinovitch A. Immunoregulatory and cytokine imbalances in the pathogenesis of IDDM: Therapeutic intervention by immunostimulation. Diabetes 1994;43:613
73. Zhang ZJ, Davidson L, Eisenbarth G, Weiner HL. Suppression of diabetes in nonobese diabetic mice by oral administration of porcine insulin. Proc Natl Acad Sci USA 1991;88:10252
74. Weiner HL, Friedman A, Miller A, et al. Oral tolerance: Immunologic mechanisms and treatment of animal and human organ specific autoimmune diseases by oral administration of autoantigens. Ann Rev Immunol 1994; 12:809
75. Dulin WE, Soret MG. Chemically and hormonally induced diabetes. In: Volk BW, Wellmann KF, eds. The Diabetic Pancreas. New York: Plenum; 1977:425–465
76. Karam JH, Lewitt PA, Young CW, et al. Insulinopenic diabetes after rodenticide (Vacor) ingestion: A unique model of acquired diabetes in man. Diabetes 1980;29:971
77. Like AA, Rossini AA. Streptozotocin-induced pancreatic insulitis: New model of diabetes mellitus. Science 1976;193:415
78. Kolb-Bachofen V, Epstein S, Kiesel U, Kolb H. Low-dose streptozocin-induced diabetes in mice. Electron microscopy reveals single-cell insulitis before diabetes onset. Diabetes 1988;37:21
79. Tanaka S-I, Nakajima S, Inoue S, et al. Genetic control by *I-A* subregion in *H-2* complex of incidence of streptozocin-induced autoimmune diabetes in mice. Diabetes 1990;39:1298
80. Zunino SJ, Simons LF, Sambrook JF, Gething MJH. Interleukin-1 promotes hyperglycemia and insulitis in mice normally resistant to streptozotocin-induced diabetes. Am J Pathol 1994;145:661
81. Appel MC, Rossini AA, Williams RM, Like AA. Viral studies in streptozotocin-induced pancreatic insulitis. Diabetologia 1978;15:327

82. Paik SG, Fleischer N, Shin S. Insulin-dependent diabetes mellitus induced by subdiabetogenic doses of streptozotocin: Obligatory role of cell-mediated autoimmune processes. Proc Natl Acad Sci USA 1980;77:6129
83. Rossini AA, Like AA, Chick WL, et al. Studies of streptozotocin-induced insulitis and diabetes. Proc Natl Acad Sci USA 1977;74:2485
84. Wilson GL, Leiter EH. Streptozotocin interactions with pancreatic β cells and the induction of insulin-dependent diabetes. In: Dyrberg T, ed. The Role of Viruses and the Immune System in Diabetes Mellitus-Experimental Models. Berlin: Springer Verlag;1989:1
85. Hatamori N, Yokono K, Hayakawa M, et al. Anti-interleukin 2 receptor antibody attenuates low-dose streptozotocin-induced diabetes in mice. Diabetologia 1990;33:266
86. Herold KC, Bluestone JA, Montag AG, et al. Prevention of autoimmune diabetes with nonactivating anti-CD3 monoclonal antibody. Diabetes 1992;41:385
87. Herold KC, Vezys V, Gage A, Montag AG. Prevention of autoimmune diabetes by treatment with anti-LFA-1 and anti-ICAM-1 monoclonal antibodies. Cell Immunol 1994;157:489
88. Kolb H, Oschilewski M, Schwab E, et al. Effect of cyclosporin A on low-dose streptozotocin diabetes in mice. Diabetes Res 1985;2:191
89. Papaccio G, Latronico M, Baccari GC. The immunosuppressant FK506 inhibits the damage to mouse pancreatic islets induced by low dose streptozocin. Cell Tissue Res 1994;277:573
90. Kim YT, Steinberg C. Immunologic studies on the induction of diabetes in experimental animals: Cellular basis for the induction of diabetes by streptozotocin. Diabetes 1984;33:771
91. Buschard K, Rygaard J. Passive transfer of streptozotocin induced diabetes mellitus with spleen cells. Acta Pathol Microbiol Scand 1977;85:469
92. Wang Z, Dohle C, Friemann J, et al. Prevention of high- and low-dose STZ-induced diabetes with D-glucose and 5-thio-D-glucose. Diabetes 1993; 42:420
93. Gerling IC, Friedman H, Greiner DL, et al. Multiple low-dose streptozocin-induced diabetes in NOD-*scid/scid* mice in the absence of functional lymphocytes. Diabetes 1994;43:433
94. Kantwerk-Funke G, Burkart V, Kolb H. Low dose streptozotocin causes stimulation of the immune system and of anti-islet cytotoxicity in mice. Clin Exp Immunol 1991;86:266
95. Andrade J, Conde M, Sobrino F, Bedoya FJ. Activation of peritoneal macrophages during the prediabetic phase in low-dose streptozotocin-treated mice. FEBS Lett 1993;327:32
96. Weide LG, Lacy PE. Low-dose streptozocin-induced autoimmune diabetes in islet transplantation model. Diabetes 1991;40:1157
97. Yoon J-W. The role of viruses and environmental factors in the induction of diabetes. Curr Top Microbiol Immunol 1990;164:95
98. Suzuki T, Yamada T, Takao T, et al. Diabetogenic effects of lymphocyte transfusion on the NOD or NOD nude mouse. In: Rygaard MBJ, Graem N, Sprang-Thomsen M, eds. Immune-Deficient Animals in Biomedical Research. Basel: Karger;1987:112–116
99. Fujino Kurihara H, Fujita H, Hakura A, et al. Morphological aspects of pancreatic islets of non-obese diabetic (NOD) mice. Virchows Arch B Cell Pathol 1985;49:107
100. Suenaga K, Yoon J-W. Association of beta-cell-specific expression of endogenous retrovirus with development of insulitis and diabetes in NOD mouse. Diabetes 1988;37:1722
101. Tsumura H, Wang J-Z, Ogawa S, et al. The character of endogenous retrovirus in pancreatic β-cells of NOD mice. Lab Anim Sci 1994;44:47
102. Rossini AA, Williams RM, Mordes JP, et al. Spontaneous diabetes in the gnotobiotic BB/W rat. Diabetes 1979;28:1031
103. Like AA, Guberski DL, Butler L. Influence of environmental viral agents on frequency and tempo of diabetes mellitus in BB/Wor rats. Diabetes 1991; 40:259
104. Dyrberg T, Schwimmbeck PL, Oldstone MBA. Inhibition of diabetes in BB rats by virus infection. J Clin Invest 1988;81:928
105. Oldstone MBA. Viruses as therapeutic agents. I. Treatment of nonobese insulin-dependent diabetes mice with virus prevents insulin-dependent diabetes mellitus while maintaining general immune competence. J Exp Med 1990;171:2077
106. Guberski DL, Thomas VA, Shek WR, et al. Induction of type 1 diabetes by Kilham's rat virus in diabetes resistant BB/Wor rats. Science 1991;254: 1010
107. Brown DW, Welsh RM, Like AA. Infection of peripancreatic lymph nodes but not islets precedes Kilham rat virus-induced diabetes in BB/Wor rats. J Virol 1993;67:5873
108. Doukas J, Cutler AH, Mordes JP. Polyinosinic:polycytidylic acid is a potent activator of endothelial cells. Am J Pathol 1994;145:137
109. Bottazzo GF, Foulis AK, Bosi E, et al. Pancreatic β-cell damage. In search of novel pathogenetic factors. Diab Care 1988;11(Suppl 1):24
110. Allison J, Campbell IL, Morahan G, et al. Diabetes in transgenic mice resulting from over-expression of class I histocompatibility molecules in pancreatic beta cells. Nature 1988;333:529
111. Lo D, Burkly LC, Widera G, et al. Diabetes and tolerance in transgenic mice expressing class II MHC molecules in pancreatic beta cells. Cell 1988; 53:159
112. Böhme J, Haskins K, Stecha P, et al. Transgenic mice with I-A on islet cells are normoglycemic but immunologically tolerant. Science 1989;244:1179
113. Sarvetnick N, Liggitt D, Pitts SL, et al. Insulin-dependent diabetes mellitus induced in transgenic mice by ectopic expression of class II MHC and interferon-gamma. Cell 1988;52:773
114. Markmann J, Lo D, Naji A, et al. Antigen presenting function of class II MHC expressing pancreatic beta cells. Nature 1988;336:476
115. Sarvetnick N, Shizuru J, Liggitt D, et al. Loss of pancreatic islet tolerance induced by β-cell expression of interferon-gamma. Nature 1990;346:844
116. Heath WR, Allison J, Hoffmann MW, et al. Autoimmune diabetes as a consequence of locally produced interleukin-2. Nature 1992;359:547
117. Allison J, McClive P, Oxbrow L, et al. Genetic requirements for acceleration of diabetes in non-obese diabetic mice expressing interleukin-2 in islet β-cells. Eur J Immunol 1994;24:2535
118. Higuchi Y, Herrera P, Muniesa P, et al. Expression of a tumor necrosis factor α transgene in murine pancreatic β cells results in severe and permanent insulitis without evolution towards diabetes. J Exp Med 1992;176:1719
119. Picarella DE, Kratz A, Li C, et al. Insulitis in transgenic mice expressing tumor necrosis factor β (lymphotoxin) in the pancreas. Proc Natl Acad Sci USA 1992;89:10036
120. Wogensen L, Huang X, Sarvetnick N. Leukocyte extravasation into the pancreatic tissue in transgenic mice expressing interleukin 10 in the islets of Langerhans. J Exp Med 1993;178:175
121. Wogensen L, Lee M-S, Sarvetnick N. Production of interleukin 10 by islet cells accelerates immune-mediated destruction of β cells in nonobese diabetic mice. J Exp Med 1994;179:1379
122. Guerder S, Picarella DE, Linsley PS, Flavell RA. Costimulator B7-1 confers antigen-presenting-cell function to parenchymal tissue and in conjunction with tumor necrosis factor α leads to autoimmunity in transgenic mice. Proc Natl Acad Sci USA 1994;91:5138
123. Harlan DM, Hengartner H, Huang ML, et al. Mice expressing both B7-1 and viral glycoprotein on pancreatic beta cells along with glycoprotein-specific transgenic T cells develop diabetes due to a breakdown of T-lymphocyte unresponsiveness. Proc Natl Acad Sci USA 1994;91:3137
124. Oldstone MBA, Nerenberg M, Southern P, et al. Virus infection triggers insulin-dependent diabetes mellitus in a transgenic model: Role of anti-self (virus) immune response. Cell 1991;65:319
125. Ohashi PS, Oehen S, Buerki K, et al. Ablation of "tolerance" and induction of diabetes by virus infection in viral antigen transgenic mice. Cell 1991; 65:305
126. Aichele P, Kyburz D, Ohashi PS, et al. Peptide-induced T-cell tolerance to prevent autoimmune diabetes in a transgenic mouse model. Proc Natl Acad Sci USA 1994;91:444
127. Butler L, Guberski DL, Like AA. Genetics of diabetes production in the Worcester colony of the BB rat. In: Shafrir E, Renold AE, eds. Frontiers in Diabetes Research: Lessons from Animal Diabetes II. London: John Libbey;1988:74–78
128. Klöting I, Vogt L, Stark O, Fisher U. Genetic heterogeneity in different BB rat subpopulations. Diabetes Res 1987;6:145
129. Prins J-B, Herberg L, Den Bieman M, Van Zutphen BFM. Genetic characterization and interrelationship of inbred lines of diabetes-prone and not diabetes-prone BB rats. In: Shafrir E, ed. Frontiers in Diabetes Research. Lessons from Animal Diabetes III. London: Smith-Gordon;1991:19–24
130. Williams AJK, Krug J, Lampeter EF, et al. Raised temperature reduces the incidence of diabetes in the NOD mouse. Diabetologia 1990;33:635
131. Karjalainen J, Martin JM, Knip M, et al. A bovine albumin peptide as a possible trigger of insulin-dependent diabetes mellitus. N Engl J Med 1992;327:302
132. Atkinson MA, Bowman MA, Kao K-J, et al. Lack of immune responsiveness to bovine serum albumin in insulin-dependent diabetes. N Engl J Med 1993;329:1853
133. Scott FW, Marliss EB. Conference summary: Diet as an environmental factor in development of insulin-dependent diabetes mellitus. Can J Physiol Pharmacol 1991;69:311
134. Coleman DL, Kuzava JE, Leiter EH. Effect of diet on incidence of diabetes in nonobese diabetic mice. Diabetes 1990;39:432
135. Yoon J-W, Elliott RB. Discussion: Environmental factors: Viruses and diet. In: Shafrir E, ed. Frontiers in Diabetes Research. Lessons from Animal Diabetes III. London: Smith-Gordon;1991:198–203
136. Scott FW, Hoorfar J, Cloutier HE. Lymphocytes and macrophages in BB rats fed diabetes-retardant or promoting diets. In: Shafrir E, ed. Frontiers in Diabetes Research. Lessons from Animal Diabetes III. London: Smith-Gordon;1991:192–194
137. Scott FW, Mongeau R, Kardish M, et al. Diet can prevent diabetes in the BB rat. Diabetes 1985;34:1059
138. Lefkowith J, Schreiner G, Cormier J, et al. Prevention of diabetes in the BB rat by essential fatty acid deficiency. Relationship between physiological and biochemical changes. J Exp Med 1990;171:729
139. Wright JR Jr, Lefkowith JB, Schreiner G, Lacy PE. Essential fatty acid deficiency prevents multiple low-dose streptozotocin-induced diabetes in CD-1 mice. Proc Natl Acad Sci USA 1988;85:6137
140. Rossini AA, Mordes JP, Handler ES, Greiner DL. Human autoimmune diabetes mellitus: Lessons from BB rats and NOD mice—*Caveat emptor*. Clin Immunol Immunopathol 1995;74:2
141. Harrison LC. Islet cell antigens in insulin-dependent diabetes: Pandora's box revisited. Immunol Today 1992;13:348
142. Adams TE, Alpert S, Hanahan D. Non-tolerance and autoantibodies to

a transgenic self antigen expressed in pancreatic β cells. Nature 1987;325:223

143. Skowronski J, Jolicoeur C, Alpert S, Hanahan D. Determinants of the B-cell response against a transgenic autoantigen. Proc Natl Acad Sci USA 1990;87:7487
144. Jolicoeur C, Hanahan D, Smith KM. T-cell tolerance toward a transgenic β-cell antigen and transcription of endogenous pancreatic genes in thymus. Proc Natl Acad Sci USA 1994;91:6707
145. Roman LM, Simons LF, Hammer RE, et al. The expression of influenza virus hemagglutinin in the pancreatic β cells of transgenic mice results in autoimmune diabetes. Cell 1990;61:383
146. Efrat S, Fleischer N, Hanahan D. Diabetes induced in male transgenic mice by expression of human H-*ras* oncoprotein in pancreatic β cells. Mol Cell Biol 1990;10:1779
147. Efrat S. Sexual dimorphism of pancreatic β-cell degeneration in transgenic mice expressing an insulin-*ras* hybrid gene. Endocrinology 1991;128:897
148. Epstein PN, Boschero AC, Atwater I, et al. Expression of yeast hexokinase in pancreatic β cells of transgenic mice reduces blood glucose, enhances insulin secretion, and decreases diabetes. Proc Natl Acad Sci USA 1992; 89:12038
149. Holers VM, Hollis GF, Schwartz BD, et al. Induction of peri-insulitis but not diabetes in islet transplants expressing a single foreign antigen: A multistage model of disease. J Immunol 1993;151:5041
150. Morahan G, Allison J, Miller JF. Tolerance of class I histocompatibility antigens expressed extrathymically. Nature 1989;339:622
151. Götz J, Eibel H, Köhler G. Non-tolerance and differential susceptibility to diabetes in transgenic mice expressing major histocompatibility class II genes on pancreatic β cells. Eur J Immunol 1990;20:1677
152. Allison J, Malcolm L, Culvenor J, et al. Overexpression of β_2-microglobulin in transgenic mouse islet β cells results in defective insulin secretion. Proc Natl Acad Sci USA 1991;88:2070
153. Schnetzler B, Murakawa G, Abalos D, et al. Adaptation to supraphysiologic levels of insulin gene expression in transgenic mice: Evidence for the importance of posttranscriptional regulation. J Clin Invest 1993;92:272
154. Verchere CB, D'Alessio DA, Palmiter RD, Kahn SE. Transgenic mice overproducing islet amyloid polypeptide have increased insulin storage and secretion in vitro. Diabetologia 1994;37:725
155. De Koning EJP, Höppener JWM, Verbeek JS, et al. Human islet amyloid polypeptide accumulates at similar sites in islets of transgenic mice and humans. Diabetes 1994;43:640
156. Kubisch HM, Wang J, Luche R, et al. Transgenic copper/zinc superoxide dismutase modulates susceptibility to type I diabetes. Proc Natl Acad Sci USA 1994;91:9956
157. Epstein PN, Overbeek PA, Means AR. Calmodulin-induced early-onset diabetes in transgenic mice. Cell 1989;58:1067
158. Valera A, Solanes G, Fernández-Alvarez J, et al. Expression of GLUT-2 antisense RNA in β cells of transgenic mice leads to diabetes. J Biol Chem 1994;269:28543
159. Allison J, Malcolm L, Chosich N, Miller JFAP. Inflammation but not autoimmunity occurs in transgenic mice expressing constitutive levels of interleukin-2 in islet β cells. Eur J Immunol 1992;22:1115
160. Stewart TA, Hultgren B, Huang X, et al. Induction of type I diabetes by interferon-α in transgenic mice. Science 1993;260:1942
161. Scott B, Liblau R, Degermann S, et al. A role for non-MHC genetic polymorphism in susceptibility to spontaneous autoimmunity. Immunity 1994;1:73
162. Ohashi PS, Oehen S, Aichele P, et al. Induction of diabetes is influenced by the infectious virus and local expression of MHC class I and tumor necrosis factor-α. J Immunol 1993;150:5185
163. Slattery RM, Kjer-Nielsen L, Allison J, et al. Prevention of diabetes in non-obese diabetic I-A^k transgenic mice. Nature 1990;345:724
164. Miyazaki T, Uno M, Uehira M, et al. Direct evidence for the contribution of the unique I-A^{NOD} to the development of insulitis in non-obese diabetic mice. Nature 1990;345:722
165. Slattery RM, Miller JFAP, Heath WR, Charlton B. Failure of a protective major histocompatibility complex class II molecule to delete autoreactive T cells in autoimmune diabetes. Proc Natl Acad Sci USA 1993;90:10808
166. Böhme J, Schuhbaur B, Kanagawa O, et al. MHC-linked protection from diabetes dissociated from clonal deletion of T cells. Science 1990;249:293
167. Miyazaki T, Matsuda Y, Toyonaga T, et al. Prevention of autoimmune insulitis in nonobese diabetic mice by expression of major histocompatibility complex class I L^d molecules. Proc Natl Acad Sci USA 1992;89:9519
168. Lipes MA, Rosenzweig A, Tan K-N, et al. Progression to diabetes in nonobese diabetic (NOD) mice with transgenic T cell receptors. Science 1993;259:1165
169. Katz JD, Wang B, Haskins K, et al. Following a diabetogenic T cell from genesis through pathogenesis. Cell 1993;74:1089
170. Katz J, Benoist C, Mathis D. Major histocompatibility complex class I molecules are required for the development of insulitis in non-obese diabetic mice. Eur J Immunol 1993;23:3358
171. Laufer TM, Von Herrath MG, Grusby MJ, et al. Autoimmune diabetes can be induced in transgenic major histocompatibility complex class II-deficient mice. J Exp Med 1993;178:589
172. Wicker LS, Leiter EH, Todd JA, et al. β2-microglobulin-deficient NOD mice do not develop insulitis or diabetes. Diabetes 1994;43:500
173. Serreze DV, Leiter EH, Christianson GJ, et al. Major histocompatibility complex class I-deficient NOD-$B2m^{null}$ mice are diabetes and insulitis resistant. Diabetes 1994;43:505
174. Nakhooda AF, Like AA, Chappel CI, et al. The spontaneously diabetic Wistar rat. Metabolic and morphologic studies. Diabetes 1977;26:100
175. Hosszufalusi N, Chan E, Teruya M, et al. Quantitative phenotypic and functional analyses of islet immune cells before and after diabetes onset in the BB rat. Diabetologia 1993;36:1146
176. LeCompte PM, Gepts W. The pathology of juvenile diabetes. In: Volk BW, Wellmann KF, eds. The Diabetic Pancreas. New York: Plenum Press; 1977:325–363
177. Itoh N, Hanafusa T, Miyazaki A, et al. Mononuclear cell infiltration and its relation to the expression of major histocompatibility complex antigens and adhesion molecules in pancreas biopsy specimens from newly diagnosed insulin-dependent diabetes mellitus patients. J Clin Invest 1993; 92:2313
178. Fujita T, Yui R, Kusumoto Y, et al. Lymphocyte insulitis in a 'non-obese diabetic (NOD)' strain of mice: An immunohistochemical and electron microscope investigation. Biochem Res 1982;3:429
179. Kay TWH, Campbell IL, Harrison LC. Characterization of pancreatic T lymphocytes associated with beta cell destruction in the non-obese diabetic (NOD) mouse. J Autoimmun 1991;4:263

Diabetes Mellitus, edited by Derek LeRoith, Simeon I. Taylor, and Jerrold M. Olefsky. Lippincott–Raven Publishers, Philadelphia © 1996.

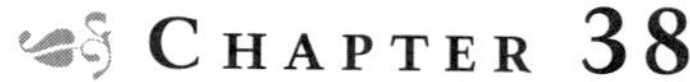

Chapter 38

Transgenic and Gene Targeting Strategies in Insulin-Dependent Diabetes

Leonard C. Harrison and Thomas W. H. Kay

Introduction

Insulin-dependent diabetes mellitus (IDDM) results from the selective destruction of the insulin-producing β-cells in the islets of the pancreas. There is considerable evidence in the rodent models of spontaneous IDDM, in the nonobese diabetic (NOD) mouse and the BioBreeding (BB) rat, that β-cell destruction is an autoimmune process mediated primarily by autoreactive T cells.[1] The islet pathology of human IDDM, revealed by examination of pancreas tissue obtained at post mortem[2,3] or by needle biopsy,[4] is similar to although less florid than that of the "insulitis" lesion in the rodent models, being characterized in the end stage by a mixed mononuclear cell infiltrate containing predominantly CD8+ T cells. Indirect evidence of the autoimmune nature of IDDM in humans includes the presence of circulating IgG antibodies and T cells reactive with islet antigens and the effect of immunosuppressive agents to induce and/or prolong remission from insulin dependence in newly diagnosed patients.[1]

Genetic susceptibility to IDDM maps to the major histocompatibility complex (MHC) in the rodent models and in humans. The significant association between IDDM and class II MHC alleles implies a direct role for class II MHC proteins in presenting peptide antigens to diabetogenic autoreactive T cells. However, the molecular pathology of IDDM remains poorly defined. What triggers the breakdown of immune tolerance to the β-cell? What β-cell antigen or antigens are the target of the initial autoimmune response? What types of T cells are pathogenic or regulatory in the immune response to β-cells? What sustains the autoimmune response?

Within the last decade, the ability to manipulate the expression of individual genes and define the role of specific gene products in vivo in mice and other animals has been strengthened enormously by the advent of transgenic and gene targeting techniques. These have rapidly been applied to many areas of biology, particularly in immunology to address the central issue of self-tolerance. In this regard, β-cell autoimmunity has served as the major model system.

The Transgenic Strategy

Transgenic expression involves introducing functional genes into the germ line, in most cases to obtain expression of a specific gene in a target tissue of interest. The experimental method is only summarized here; for further details the reader is referred to several excellent reviews.[5–7]

Microinjection of cloned DNA directly into the male pronuclei of recently fertilized one-cell stage oocytes is the most common method used for generating transgenic mice (Fig. 38-1). The DNA transgene may contain both the coding sequence and the promoter-enhancer sequence that normally directs tissue-specific expression of the gene. Alternatively, the coding sequence can be ligated to another gene's promoter-enhancer sequence specific for the tissue of interest to which the coding sequence is to be targeted. Expression of these latter artificial gene constructs is enhanced if they include some noncoding intron and 3′ polyadenylation sequences to mimic normal genomic DNA. After microinjection of several hundred copies of DNA, eggs are implanted into the oviducts of gonadotropin-primed pseudopregnant foster mothers. This germ line injection results in random chromosomal integration of the DNA into all cells of the offspring, but gene expression to RNA and protein should normally occur only in the tissue for which the promoter-enhancer sequence is active. Integration of multiple DNA copies is thought to be organized in a tandem head-to-tail manner by the process of homologous recombination. Postnatally, the presence of the transgene in the offspring is detected by analysis of DNA extracted from a segment of the mouse tail or from blood cells, by the Southern blot test, or the polymerase chain reaction technique, respectively. Transgene-positive "founder" mice can then be mated with nontransgenic mice to establish separate transgenic lineages. To ensure that the phenotype of the transgenic offspring is consistent and due to expression of the transgene (not an artifact of random integration), it is important to establish several founder lines. The transgene is normally inherited as a simple mendelian trait, but the developmental timing and level of its expression may vary greatly from one founder to another; this is thought to depend primarily on the chromosomal integration site rather than gene copy number. Expression within each transgenic lineage is uniform.

The transgenic approach has many applications to the study of autoimmunity (Table 38-1). As an example, two transgenic lines can be made, one expressing a T-cell receptor of known specificity and the other the target antigen of the T-cell receptor in a selected tissue (e.g., the β-cell). The lines can then be crossed and several questions asked about the effect of the antigen on T cells expressing the transgene-encoded T-cell receptor: Are the T cells stimulated? Is tolerance induced in the T cells and, if so, by what mechanism? Alternatively, do the T cells ignore the antigen and, if so, can this be overcome by modifying the presentation of the antigen or priming the immune system to the antigen?

Transgenes and the β-Cell

Like most breakthroughs in the biologic sciences, the ability to complement a mammalian genotype transgenically depended on technologic advances, first in oocyte harvesting, manipulation, and reimplantation as pioneered by veterinary scientists seeking to accelerate cattle breeding programs through in vitro fertilization, and second in the general ability to isolate and clone DNA and identify promoter-enhancer sequences of tissue-specific genes. The history of transgenes and the β-cell began with the isolation of the rat insulin II promoter (RIP) sequence by Douglas Hanahan at Cold Spring Harbor in the mid-1980s. He demonstrated that the RIP

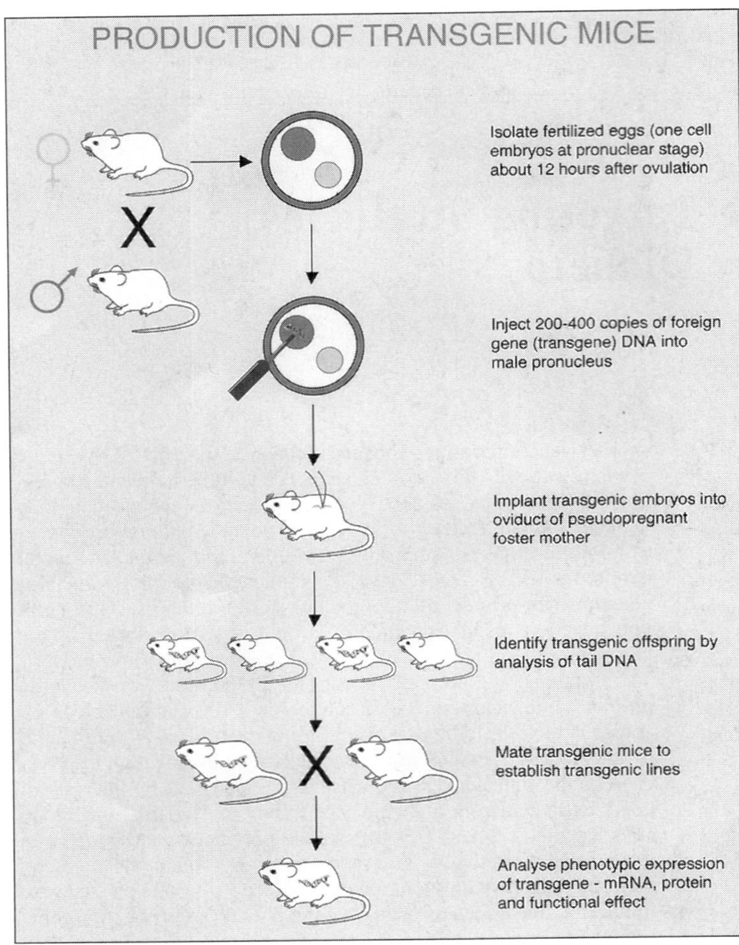

Figure 38-1.

could be used to selectively direct the expression of the large T (transforming) antigen (Tag) of simian virus (SV) 40 in the β-cells.[8] Several lineages of RIP-Tag mice were generated in C57BL/6J × DBA/2J mice. Some lineages expressed Tag at high levels early in fetal life and others not until after birth. Early expression was associated with immunologic tolerance to Tag and the later development of β-cell tumors, whereas later expression was associated with antibodies to Tag and lymphocytic infiltration of the islets, although without the development of diabetes.[9] Apart from establishing the model, these experiments immediately told us about a window of tolerance induction and yielded a unique (explanted) transformed β-cell line, βTC, which has been used to study β-cell growth and function. Later, the hybrid RIP-SV40 Tag construct was used by Hamaguchi and coworkers[10] to generate β-cell tumors in NOD mice from which the very useful NOD β-cell line, NIT-1, was established.

Hanahan generously provided the RIP to many investigators and spawned a plethora of studies, not primarily by mainstream diabetes researchers (many of whom had never heard of a transgene) but by immunologists and cell biologists who saw the power of the transgenic approach and lost no time becoming acquainted with the β-cell as a convenient target for transgene expression.

Table 38-1. Potential Applications of Transgenic Models for Studying Autoimmunity

1. Express gene for an immune protein, e.g., MHC molecule, cytokine, adhesion molecule, in a tissue-specific, even, regulatable manner to investigate the function of the protein in the normal site of endogenous gene expression or in an ectopic site.
2. Express gene for a foreign antigen at a particular stage of development to investigate the ontogeny of tolerance development.
3. Express gene for a foreign antigen in a tissue-specific manner extrathymically to ask if peripheral tolerance occurs when the antigen is not present in the thymus during development.
4. Express gene for an antigen in the thymus to ask if tolerance occurs when developing T cells are exposed to the antigen.
5. Express a tissue-specific autoantigen in an ectopic site to demonstrate the pathogenicity of the autoantigen by its ability to direct the autoimmune response to the ectopic site.
6. Express a rearranged T-cell receptor gene or immunoglobulin gene that codes for an anti–self-antigen to investigate mechanisms of tolerance to self-antigen.

Transgenic Mouse Models of Insulin-Dependent Diabetes Mellitus

More than 20 transgenic mouse models of IDDM based on the RIP have been described[11,12] (Table 38-2).[13-39] The first RIP transgenics were made to establish a simple mouse model of IDDM by expressing either class I MHC (K^b) or class II MHC (A^d, A^k, $E\alpha^d/E\beta^d$) alloantigens in the β-cells (Table 38-2). There were surprises in store. The foreign antigens, apparently expressed outside of the tolerizing influence of the thymus, did not evoke the expected immune response in the islets. Instead, in some cases a novel nonimmune form of β-cell destruction was observed. This phenomenon was subsequently also observed in thyrocytes when the transgenic expression of K^b was directed in them by the promoter for thyroglobulin.[40] Although disruption of insulin biosynthesis in

TABLE 38-2. Transgenic Mouse Models of Insulin-Dependent Diabetes Mellitus Based on the Insulin Promoter

Transgene	Strain	Insulitis	Diabetes	Reference
SV40 TAg	(B6×DBA/2)FI	No/yes	No	9
SV40 TAg	NOD	No	No	10
K^b	B10.BR	No	Yes	13
A^d	BALB/c	No	Yes	14
A^d	C57BL/6	No	No	15
A^k	C57BL/6	No	No	16
$E\alpha^d\beta^b$	(B6×SJL)F2	No	Yes	17
$E\alpha^k\beta^d$	(B6×SJL)F1	No	Yes	18
$E\alpha^d\beta^b$ + B7-1	C57BL/6	Yes	Yes	19
K^b - IL-2 + T-cell receptor	B10.BR	Yes	Yes	20
β2 microglobulin	CBA	No	Yes	21
Calmodulin	FVB/N	No	Yes	22
Harvey-ras	(C57BL/6×DBA/$_2$)F2	No	Yes	23
IFN-γ	(CD1×BALB/c)F1	Yes	Yes	14
IFN-α	CD1	Yes	Yes	24
TNF-α	NMRI, NMRI-SCID	Yes	No	25
TNF-α	C57BL/6	Yes	No	26
IL-2	CBA,C57BL/6^{bm1}	Yes (pancreatitis)	No	27
IL-10	BALB/c	No (pancreatitis)	No	28
IL-10	NOD	Yes	Yes	29
LCMVgp + LCMV infection	C57BL/6, H-2^{bxd}	Yes	Yes	30
LCMVgp × TNFα + vacc-gp	C57BL/6, B10.BR	Yes	Yes	31
Influenza hemagglutinin	B10.D2	Yes	Yes	32
Hemagglutinin + flu infection	B10.D2	No	No	33
Influenza hemagglutinin + T-cell receptor	BALB/c	Variable	No	34
Influenza hemagglutinin + T-cell receptor	B10.D2	Yes	Yes	34
Influenza hemagglutinin + T-cell receptor + flu infection	B10.D2	Yes	Yes	35
LCMVgp × TCR + virus infection	C57BL/6	Yes	Yes	36
IL-10 × LCMVgp + virus infection		Yes	Yes	37
LCMVgp × B7-1 × T-cell receptor	H-$2^{b\times q}$	Yes	Yes	38
B7-1; B7-1 × TNF-α	(C57BL/6×CBA/CA)F2	No; yes	No; yes	39

the β-cell is regarded by many as an artifact of transgene expression and not necessarily MHC-specific, it is conceivable that the detrimental intracellular effect of overexpressing particular MHC proteins may have a parallel in the pathophysiology of IDDM.[11,41] For example, overexpression of class I MHC proteins is a characteristic direct response to many viral infections as well as to certain immunoinflammatory cytokines, for example, tumor necrosis factor (TNF)-α and interferon (IFN)-γ,[41,42] and is the earliest observed abnormality of islet cells in IDDM.[43,44] Viral infection might therefore induce β-cell damage via overexpression of class I MHC; furthermore, this preimmune response might even directly trigger β-cell autoimmunity. Transgenic models do not always behave as predicted and sometimes raise more questions than answers.

The inferences from these first RIP allo-MHC transgenics were that foreign antigen simply expressed on an epithelial (β) cell without costimulator or accessory molecules required for a normal immune response was either not recognized in this context (later referred to as ignorance) or induced T-cell anergy. A detailed account of the immunology of this controversial area is not appropriate here, but the types of transgenic experiments subsequently undertaken to further investigate the nature of immune unresponsiveness is described. Significantly, it was later shown that in some cases the RIP was leaky, resulting in cryptic expression outside the β-cell, notably in the thymus. Thymus transplant experiments into nontransgenic mice then demonstrated that high-affinity K^b-reactive T cells were actually being deleted in the thymus in the RIP-K^b mice.[20,45] Nevertheless, experiments by different investigators in which transgenic mice were crossed to generate double or triple transgenic lines indicated that autoreactive T cells do ignore antigens in the β-cell but may be triggered to cause IDDM when provided with help from cytokines or costimulator proteins. This was shown with foreign antigen and either the cytokine interleukin (IL)-2 or the costimulator protein B7-1 in the β-cell or with foreign antigen and IL-2 in the β-cell and T-cell receptor to the antigen (see Table 38-2).

The concept of a multistage process of β-cell autoimmunity has evolved from a different type of transgenic experiment in which a viral protein from lymphocytic choriomeningitis virus (LCMV) was expressed on the RIP. In this experiment, there was a lack of response in vivo to the LCMV protein without demonstrable thymic leakiness of the transgene or unresponsiveness of LCMV-specific T cells. These mice were crossed with T-cell receptor transgenic mice in which the T-cell receptor was specific for the LCMV protein in the context of the class I MHC of the LCMV transgenic mice.[31,36] As mentioned, transgenic mice expressing the mature, rearranged T-cell receptor for a specific antigen are a powerful means to analyze the role of antigen-specific T cells, which normally are present at a frequency of only 1 in 10^4 to 10^5 T cells. Because of the almost complete allelic exclusion of the endogenous T-cell receptor β-gene loci and the partial exclusion of the T-cell receptor α-loci, mice bearing a transgenic T-cell receptor have a T-cell repertoire that is highly skewed for the transgene-encoded specificity. In the double transgenic mice expressing LCMV protein in the β-cell and the T-cell receptor specific for this protein, islet infiltration and diabetes did not occur until the mice were infected with native LCMV. Thus, the CD8 T cells bearing the transgenic T-cell receptor required activation by natural LCMV infection before they were capable of attacking "self" LCMV protein expressed in the non–antigen-presenting context of β-cells. In a similar double transgenic experiment, mice expressing influenza hemagglutinin in β-cells were crossed with mice expressing a transgenic T-cell receptor that reacts with hemagglutinin.[34,35] Clonal ignorance was also observed but in this case could not be reversed by infection with influenza virus.[35] Part of the reason for this difference may be that the balance between ignorance and autoimmunity is affected by different background genes in the respective mouse strains.[46]

It has also been shown that the transgenic coexpression of TNF-α with the LCMV protein in the β-cell enhances β-cell destruction by anti-LCMV CD8 T cells.[31] On the other hand, IL-10, a cytokine that might be expected to be immunosuppressive for cell-mediated immunity, when transgenically coexpressed with LCMV in the β-cell, did not retard β-cell destruction by anti-LCMV CD8 T cells triggered by LCMV infection.[37] Transgenic expression of TNF-α alone caused only patchy insulitis,[25,26] but when coexpressed with B7-1 in β-cells it resulted in islet infiltration and diabetes.[39] In the double LCMV, anti-LCMV T-cell receptor transgenic, coexpression of B7-1 or B7-2 on β-cells in the absence of LCMV infection was sufficient to induce CD8 T-cell responsiveness, leading to β-cell destruction and diabetes.[38]

The idea that epithelial cells are normally unable to provide costimulation signals with antigen to active T cells is not new. Lafferty and coworkers[47] showed that thyroid tissue or islets depleted of lymphoid cells, including antigen-presenting cells, could be transplanted across MHC barriers. Nevertheless, the series of experiments culminating in triple transgenic models elegantly support the second signal/costimulator concept. The implication is that β-cell antigen-reactive T cells, which can be detected in normal individuals,[48–50] can be activated to destroy β-cells either indirectly via their response to a cross-reactive antigen presented in an immunogenic context or possibly even directly if the β-cell can acquire the costimulator properties of an antigen-presenting cell. The latter idea was originally proposed by Bottazzo and coworkers[51] and found some support in the demonstration that IFN-γ, particularly in combination with TNF-α, could induce expression of both class I and class II MHC proteins[42] and intercellular adhesion molecule 1 (ICAM-1)[52] in islet cells. However, there is no evidence[53] that islet cells in the insulitis lesion or islet cells exposed to these cytokines express the critical costimulator protein, B7.

It can be argued that the transgenic models in which only class I or class II proteins are (over)expressed in the β-cell cannot adequately test the proposition that β-cells could present antigen. Expression of a foreign protein in the β-cell before the development of immune tolerance is not analogous to its upregulation or induction de novo in an animal with a mature T-cell repertoire. There are other problems as well. Studies have now revealed a crucial role for the invariant chain (Ii) to facilitate peptide binding to class II proteins within intracellular vesicles. The class II transgenics did not incorporate Ii. Importantly, it is now apparent that class II MHC expression alone does not confer all the properties of an antigen-presenting cell; coexpression of costimulator proteins such as B7, other adhesion proteins such as ICAM-1, and cytokines are necessary for effective T-cell activation. In following up the effects of cytokines on islets in vitro and in an attempt to mimic host responses to local islet infection, for example with virus, Sarvetnick and colleagues[14] generated transgenic mice expression IFN-γ on the human insulin promoter. In contrast to mice expressing transgenic MHC molecules, these mice developed diabetes preceded by insulitis consisting predominantly of T cells. Syngeneic islets transplanted into the transgenic mice were also infiltrated by T cells and their β-cells were (selectively) destroyed. Thus, local overproduction of IFN-γ resulted in loss of T-cell tolerance to islets. This result is consistent with a role for IFN-γ in the induction of expression of a variety of molecules required for antigen presentation and T-cell activation as well as for the transmigration of T cells through endothelium. It also demonstrates an essential role for IFN-γ in β-cell destruction in the NOD mouse.[54] Whether the apparently selective destruction of β-cells is attributable to their specific targeting by T cells or to their differential sensitivity to inflammatory mediators remains enigmatic. Nevertheless, the result is consistent with although not proof of the ability of the β-cell to act as an antigen-presenting cell. If the β-cells could acquire the functionality of an antigen-presenting cell, it must be asked, from where does the stimulus come? What is the primary event that directly or indirectly (via cytokines) initiates the autoimmune attack?

Transgenic Models in the NOD Mouse

The NOD mouse is the most widely used model of spontaneous IDDM. Like the human disease, diabetes in the NOD mouse is strongly associated with class II MHC. In fact, the NOD mouse has only one expressed class II MHC, the unique I-A^{g7}, the haplotype that is essential for insulitis.[55,56] NOD mice do not express I-E because of a deletion in the promoter region of the I-Eα gene,[55] with the result that the unpaired I-E β-chain does not get to the cell surface. Following the first wave of transgenic experiments in which the insulin promoter was used in attempts to generate new models of IDDM in normal mice, beginning in 1990 investigators turned their attention to the natural NOD model and in a series of experiments demonstrated that the lack of I-E and the unique I-A^{g7} each contribute to diabetes susceptibility in the NOD mouse.

A relative impediment with NOD mice was the low yield of transgenic founders, which has caused some investigators to avoid direct NOD oocyte injections and take the more predictable but slower path of back-crossing from transgenic mice made in other strains. However, it is possible to achieve conditions of ovulation induction, oocyte harvesting, and transfer that result in reasonably efficient yields after direct injection of NOD oocytes[57] (M. French, J. Allison, and L.C. Harrison, unpublished data, 1994).

NOD mice that transgenically express self-, modified self-, or foreign class II MHC proteins were generated by different investigators (Table 38-3) to examine the significance of I-E deficiency and/or I-A^{g7} in the development of insulitis and diabetes. These studies used complete genomic sequences of the class II genes containing their own promoter-enhancer regions. Direct introduction of the $E\alpha^d$ gene into NOD mice[59,61,63] prevented insulitis. Clearly, a lack of I-E is not the only cause of insulitis because NOD mice are not unique in lacking I-E. They are distinguished, however, by their I-A^{g7} which, analogous to the human IDDM susceptibility allele HLA-DQβ*0302,[70] is non-Asp at position β57.[71] In what could be called transgene therapy, two groups simultaneously reported[57,60] that complementing NOD mice with the Asp57-containing class II protein I-A^k dramatically reduced insulitis and diabetes. The diabetes susceptibility conferred by I-A^{g7} is therefore recessive and can somehow be overridden by the presence of either I-E^d or I-A^k. Subsequently, Singer and coworkers[66] reported that an I-$A\beta^d$ transgene, although not altering the histologic appearance of insulitis, significantly decreased the incidence of diabetes in NOD mice. Prevention of insulitis was complete in the I-E^d transgenic mice but not in the I-A^k or I-$A\beta^d$ mice, which suggests that these transgenes may operate by different mechanisms.

Miyazaki and coworkers[60] produced NOD transgenic mice carrying either $A\alpha^k$ or $A\beta^k$ and then mated these lines to obtain $A\alpha^k$-$A\beta^k$ double transgenics. They found that the β-chain of I-A^k prevented insulitis in diabetes only when it associated with the α-chain of I-A^k and not with the α-chain of the NOD (which is identical to that of I-A^d). This demonstrates that the α-chain of

Table 38-3. Transgenic Models in the NOD Mouse

Transgene	Strain	Insulitis	Diabetes	Reference
$E\alpha^d$	NOD	No	No	58
$A\alpha^k\beta^k$	NOD	Reduced	No	57
$A\beta^k$	NOD	Yes	Yes	59
$A\alpha^k\beta^k$; β^k (Ser57)	NOD	Reduced	No	60
$A\beta^{g7}$ Pro56; $E\alpha^d$	NOD	Reduced	No	61
$E\alpha^k$	NOD	Reduced	No	62
L^d	NOD	Reduced	No	64
$A\beta^d$	NOD	Yes	Reduced	66
T-cell receptor (anti-conalbumin)	NOD	Yes	Yes	67
T-cell receptor BDC2.5 (anti-islet)	NOD	Increased	Yes	69

I-A also contributes to disease susceptibility, again in an analogous fashion to DQα in human IDDM.[70] Peptide presentation by the αβ dimer of I-A^{g7} could be involved either in driving pathogenic β-cell autoreactive T cells or in failing to drive protective regulatory T cells. Which if either alternative is operating and just what is happening at the molecular-atomic level remains unclear, but presumably it has to do with which peptides are or are not presented by I-A^{g7}.

The polymorphic residues in I-$A\beta^{g7}$ contribute to the peptide-binding groove, and site-directed mutagenesis is the logical way to define their contribution to disease susceptibility. Miyazaki and coworkers[60] found that transgenic I-A^k with Asp replaced by Ser at position β57 was in fact more protective than I-A^k, indicating that the single non-Asp substitution at β57 is not sufficient for causing disease. In a somewhat complementary approach, Lund and colleagues[61] generated transgenic NOD mice that expressed a mutated I-A^{g7} with Pro for His at the polymorphic β56 position (β57 was still the unique non-Asp, Ser). This single substitution converted I-A^{g7} to a class II protein that conferred dominant protection against disease. This was therefore also a demonstration that Asp57 is not essential for protection against insulitis.

Not surprisingly, the first explanations offered for the protective effects of class II transgenes in NOD mice were that islet autoreactive T cells were deleted in the thymus and/or rendered anergic as a result of their affinity for I-A^k. However, in their transgenic I-A^k model, Slattery and associates[65] ruled out these explanations by demonstrating that T cells from transgenic I-A^k NOD mice could transfer protection. The nature of these T cells was not further explored. Another hypothesis for the protective effect of I-A^k was that coexpression of I-A^k and I-A^{g7} on peripheral antigen-presenting cells allowed I-A^k to capture a relevant peptide otherwise presented by I-A^{g7} to autoreactive T cells.[72] Experimental evidence in support of this determinant capture as a mechanism of protection afforded by I-$E\alpha^d$ has been reported.[73] However, in the case of I-A^k at least, Slattery and coworkers[65] showed that NOD mice were protected from diabetes by neonatal injection of bone marrow cells from transgenic I-A^k NOD mice which, although expressing both I-A^k and I-A^{g7}, constitute less than 10% of the recipient's total lymphoid pool. Thus, the majority of antigen-presenting cells expressed I-A^{g7} only and would be capable of processing and presenting peptides without competition from coexpressed I-A^k. Despite this, activation of islet-reactive T cells was absent. Böhme and colleagues[62] found that transgenic expression of different I-$E\alpha^d$ mutants in NOD mice mediated thymic deletion of T cells bearing antigen receptors with variable regions that recognized I-E. However, in contrast to wild type I-E, no mutant protected against diabetes. This implies that transgenic I-$E\alpha^d$ does not protect NOD mice from diabetes by inducing deletion of autoreactive T cells. In the transgenic I-$A\alpha^d$ NOD mice,[66] splenic T cells still reacted in vitro to islet antigens and at the same time inhibited the transfer of diabetes by spleen cells from diabetic female mice to young, irradiated NOD males. The conclusion, which fits also with the I-A^k results of Slattery,[65] is that these class II MHC transgenes induce regulatory T cells that suppress pathogenic autoreactive T cells. Conceptually, we can say that the nature of a T-cell response, whether it is pathogenic or protective, is a function of the class II MHC. Whether the peptides seen by T cells in the context of I-A^{g7} versus other class II MHC transgene products are identical or, as seems more likely, are not identical but are derived from the same islet antigens is unknown at present. In either case, protective T cells might colocalize with pathogenic T cells in the islet and exert a bystander suppressor effect, for example by the secretion of cytokines such as IL-4 or transforming growth factor-β.[74]

Toward Better Transgenic Models of Insulin-Dependent Diabetes Mellitus

In the earlier transgenic models, the antigen expressed in the β-cell, for example allo-MHC or viral protein, was not an authentic β-cell autoantigen. Further progress in the application of transgenic technology to IDDM came, therefore, when Katz and coworkers[69] generated transgenic mice carrying the rearranged T-cell receptor genes from a diabetogenic T-cell clone (BDC 2.5) derived from a NOD mouse. Transgenic expression of a rearranged T-cell receptor normally results in a T-cell repertoire that is highly skewed for the transgene-coded specificity, thereby enabling study of antigen-specific T cells that would normally be present at such low frequency as to preclude their analysis.

The BDC 2.5 CD4 clone derived by Haskins and colleagues[75] from an NOD mouse proliferates and releases IL-2 when challenged with islet cells from any mouse strain and antigen-presenting cells from NOD mice but not with cells from other tissues or other strains. When transferred into young, asymptomatic NOD mice, the clone rapidly provoked insulitis and diabetes.[76] Although the target islet antigen is unknown, BDC 2.5 is clearly islet antigen-specific, I-A^{g7}-restricted, and diabetogenic. It was therefore an ideal candidate from which to select T-cell receptor genes and express them transgenically. The transgenic T-cell receptor was shown to be expressed on the majority of CD4+ CD8− T cells in the thymus and periphery. These T cells were neither tolerized to islet antigens nor ignorant of them. They reacted to islets in vitro; in vivo, they infiltrated both the islets and submandibular salivary glands earlier and more rapidly than the natural infiltration seen in nontransgenic NOD mice. Interestingly, the phenotype of these BDC 2.5 TCR transgenic mice was unchanged by crossing them with the I-$E\alpha^d$ NOD transgenics, a maneuver that completely prevented diabetes in T-cell receptor transgene-negative control mice. Perhaps this is not surprising; transgenic I-$E\alpha^d$ may not be able to induce regulatory T cells when the T-cell repertoire is restricted to one clone.

The study of Katz and coworkers[69] demonstrates, perhaps not unexpectedly, the pathogenicity of a T-cell receptor from a known pathogenic T-cell clone. That CD4 T cells bearing the T-cell receptor were not deleted implies that the islet antigen recognized by BDC 2.5 is not "expressed" in the thymus. The spontaneous aggression of this TCR contrasts with the anti-LCMV transgenic TCR,[30,31,36] but there are key differences between the two models. The BDC 2.5 clone was selected as being not only self-reactive but also pathogenic, and therefore it would be surprising if the result of the transgenic experiment had not been self-fulfilling. It was also expressed in NOD mice and not in C57BL6 mice, which may be intrinsically less prone to develop β-cell autoimmunity. The BDC 2.5 T-cell receptor is class II MHC-restricted and the islet antigen that it recognizes may be expressed outside the islets, for example, on endothelium or by antigen-presenting cells after being shed from the islets. CD4 cells, once activated, would then be more likely to enter the islet. How the barriers to T-cell activation by islet antigen are overcome in both the BDC 2.5 model and in the NOD mouse remains unanswered. The anti-LCMV T-cell receptor is expressed in a CD8 cell that, in the absence of LCMV infection, would require endogenous processing and presentation of antigen peptide on β-cell class I MHC protein expressed with costimulator molecules. This is likely to be a stronger requirement for activation. Finally, transfer experiments indicate that CD4 cells alone can infiltrate islets, whereas CD8 cells generally require cotransfer with CD4 cells.[76] Thus, "the failure of T cells in the LCMV model to infiltrate the islets and initiate disease may be more because they are helpless rather than ignorant."[69]

Caveats on Transgenic Models

Transgenic models must be designed carefully if the intention is to draw inferences about natural mechanisms. Analyzing the outcome after injecting multiple copies of a DNA molecule that integrate randomly may not simply be analogous to analyzing a mass spectrum after a compound has been bombarded with fast atoms. Unlike physics, the complexity of biology in space and time does not always allow either simple or reproducible conclusions.

A retrospective of the short history of transgenes and immunology reveals a subtle shift in long cherished immunologic paradigms. The effects of transgenically expressing alloantigen ectopically (in the β-cell) or anti-self T-cell receptor or immunoglobulin were interpreted from the outset as evidence for either peripheral or central thymic (clonal deletion) mechanisms of tolerance, respectively. They had to fit the all or none premise of self versus nonself rooted in Burnet's seminal clonal selection theory. The fact that self and nonself in practice overlap and are likely to represent a quantitative continuum was then acknowledged as results from some of the earlier transgenic studies failed to conform to immunologic dogma. Lymphocytes that recognize self are present in normal individuals who do not have autoimmune disease. In retrospect, transgenic models have told us that ignorance reigns in the face of autoreactive T-cell receptors. Transgenically expressing an antigen in the thymus that normally is not present there or is present only at low levels may demonstrate deletion of developing T cells reactive with that antigen, but this is not necessarily physiologic. Likewise, transgenes that encode antigen receptors derived from highly selected mature lymphocyte clones and then are deliberately expressed in developing lymphocytes that do not normally display these receptors cannot be said to mimic physiology. Analysis of not only the spatial but also the temporal expression of a transgene is essential. Apart from the specific encounter of transgene product with T-cell receptors envisaged to account for clonal deletion, the outcome of transgene expression in the thymus during ontogeny might also reflect an effect of the transgene to nonspecifically arrest T-cell development. Some transgenic models of tolerance can now be interpreted in a more realistic post-Burnetian perspective in light of recent evidence that positive and negative selection in the thymus operate on a continuum of affinity of T-cell receptors for antigen,[77] with only high-affinity and anti–self-peptide interactions resulting in negative selection (clonal deletion). This leaves room for overlap between self and nonself and the escape into the periphery of the potentially self-reactive mature T cells that must normally either be ignorant of self-antigen in the physiologic context or under the control of other regulatory cells.

Apart from these conceptual issues, a very practical problem with transgenic models has been leakiness of the transgene, that is, expression at unexpected sites of minute or even immunochemically undetectable amounts of transgene-encoded protein. When transgenic expression of alloantigen on the RIP failed to elicit immunoreactivity against pancreatic β-cells, this was interpreted as evidence for a peripheral mechanism of tolerance.[78] However, this interpretation required revision when it became evident that the RIP was leaky and could be active in other tissues, including the thymus. Although expression in the thymus of alloantigen protein under the control of the RIP was too low to be detected immunochemically, the presence of sufficient antigen to delete alloreactive T cells was demonstrated by thymus transplantation from transgenic to nontransgenic littermates.[20] Thus, ironically, the transgenic model of peripheral tolerance turned out to be one of central thymic deletion.

Sometimes, transgenic experiments come up with different answers from traditional breeding experiments. For example, although both Miyazaki's group[58] and Lund and colleagues[61] showed that expression of I-E after introduction of an I-Eα^d transgene protected against insulitis and diabetes in the NOD mouse, Podolin and coworkers[68] failed to show this by breeding mice of various I-E$^+$ and I-E$^-$ MHC haplotypes onto the NOD background. They crossed the resulting NOD-MHC congenic mice with the NOD strain to produce the F1 generation in which both I-E$^+$ and I-E$^-$ mice developed insulitis and diabetes. This appears to demonstrate that I-E expression is not in itself sufficient to prevent disease. Is this a case in which the transgenic experiment is cleaner because I-E manipulation is not influenced by other undefined MHC-linked genes?

A seemingly trivial but important variable in all NOD experiments that can account for different results between laboratories is environment. Frequent early handling, crowded housing conditions, higher temperatures, endogenous viral infection, and dietary manipulation have all been shown to significantly decrease the expression of disease. Podolin and coworkers[68] remind us that the effect of transgenic I-E in mice in different laboratories ranges from complete protection from insulitis and diabetes[59,61] to mild insulitis in a low percentage of mice[62] to insulitis and diabetes,[68] which could reflect differences in environment.

The Gene-Targeting Strategy

There are limitations of transgenic technology. These include the potential for nonspecificity and unpredictable effects owing to random integration of foreign DNA, the inability of limited promoter sequences to mimic complex natural regulatory sequences that may be much longer or dispersed, and in some cases pathologic effects of overexpression of the transgene that may not reflect the usual functions of the gene product in health or disease. These considerations, plus the realization that foreign DNA injected into normal cells is processed and integrated into the host DNA by the machinery of homologous recombination, stimulated the development of technology variously called gene targeting, gene knockout, or gene replacement.[79,80] In this technology, a normal sequence of interest is replaced by sequences engineered in the laboratory to ablate the gene or to potentially alter it in a defined way. When the engineered DNA contains stretches of DNA homologous to normal cellular DNA, it manages to find its complementary endogenous sequence at a low but detectable frequency resulting in homologous recombination.

Engineered DNA molecules (called targeting vectors) designed to carry such altered genes into cells contain sequences encoding selectable markers that allow cells containing the foreign DNA to be distinguished from cells that do not. A typical example of a selectable marker is the gene-encoding resistance to the neomycin analogue G418, an antibiotic active in mammalian cells. A second selectable marker, typically the herpes simplex virus thymidine kinase (HSV-TK) gene that makes cells susceptible to ganciclovir, is used to determine whether recombination has been random or homologous. In homologous recombination the HSV-TK gene, positioned at the extreme of one end of the targeting vector, is not integrated (being outside the regions of homology) and is degraded, leaving cells resistant to ganciclovir. In contrast, nonhomologous recombination typically includes the ends of the vector allowing the TK gene to be integrated and expressed so that the cells are susceptible to ganciclovir. The neomycin resistance gene is usually expressed from the locus where the target gene was previously present. Instead of the neomycin-resistance gene, however, a mutated copy of the gene can be introduced with retained flanking base pairs to aid homologous recombination. This then constitutes gene replacement rather than gene knockout.

The targeting vector is inserted into embryonic stem cell lines, usually by electroporation (Fig. 38-2). Embryonic stem cell lines were originally derived from day 4.5 mouse blastocysts[81,82] and are kept in an undifferentiated state by culture with leukemia inhibitory factor or with cells that produce it. Following electroporation, embryonic stem cells are grown in a medium containing G418, and resistant clones are then tested for the presence of the electroporated DNA by the polymerase chain reaction (PCR). Embryonic stem cells with homologous integration of the foreign DNA are reintroduced into blastocysts. Crucially, the embryonic stem cells containing the targeted locus are from a mouse strain of different coat color than the strain from which the recipient blastocysts are obtained. Embryonic stem cells from the 129/SV strain with its dominantly inherited Agouti coat color are usually used. The reconstituted blastocysts are placed in the uterus of a pseudopregnant foster mother, and the ensuing chimeric progeny are identifiable by their chimeric coat color. With luck, not only the coat color but also the mouse germ cells are chimeric. Chimeric mice are then bred with normal mice, and heterozygote knockout animals result and are then mated to produce homozygote knockout mice.

Gene Targeting in Immunology

There has been rapid utilization of this technology to dissect the function of individual genes or to create models of human genetic disorders where the mutation in the model is exactly analogous to that in the human disease. Its application has been so widespread that one cannot help feeling that all newly cloned cDNAs of biologic interest will be knocked out as a ''routine.'' Cytokines and their receptors, components of the T- and B-cell receptors for antigen, MHC molecules, costimulatory molecules, transcription factors, and effector molecules are included in the long list of immunologically relevant genes that have been targeted. In elucidating the function of a cloned gene, homologous recombination has certain advantages compared with transgenic overexpression, as indicated above. In particular, because recombination is homologous, there are no effects caused by insertion of the transgene close to a power-

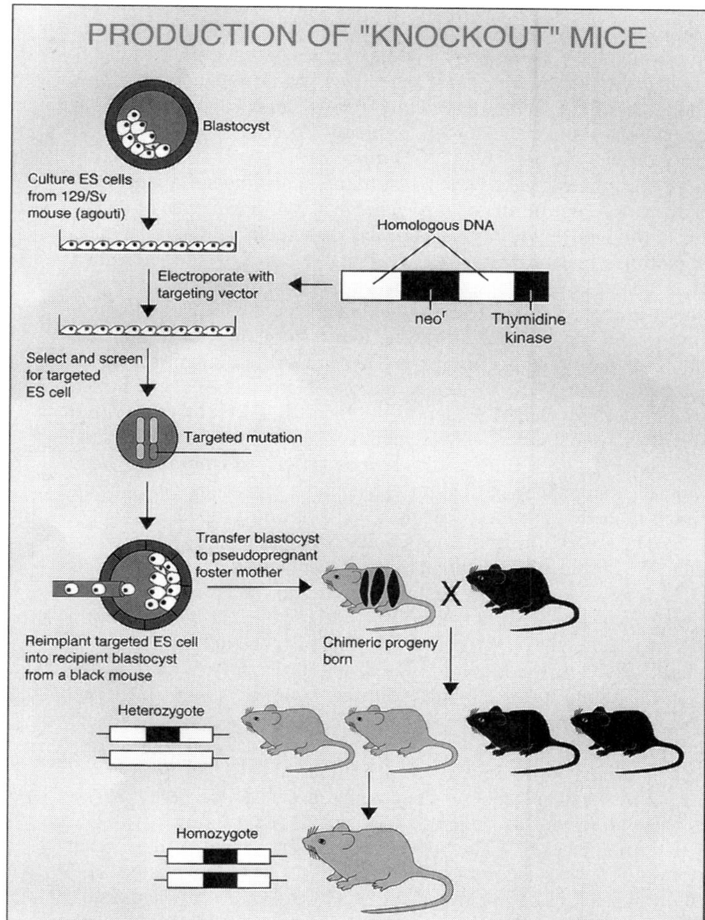

Figure 38-2.

ful heterologous promoter or in a site where an endogenous gene might be disrupted.

On the other hand, homologous recombination may create its own distortions of physiology. The absence of function of a molecule from early in development can stimulate the compensatory expression of a related molecule. For example, mice made deficient in CD8+ cytotoxic T cells owing to β2-microglobulin knockout (described below) have been shown to resist lymphocytic choriomeningitis virus infection with CD4+ CTL, cells which are of minor importance in wild-type mice.[83] Thus the phenotypes seen after gene knockout may not faithfully reflect the normal function of the gene product. Examples of no phenotype after gene knockout have also revealed the existence of previously unsuspected related family members. The existence of the costimulatory molecule B7-2 and the IL-2-like cytokine IL-15 was deduced from the lack of phenotype of B7-1 and IL-2 knockout mice, respectively. Not surprisingly, prior insight into the biology of a protein is frequently critical in demonstrating the characteristic phenotype of its gene knockout. Certain molecules may be necessary to resist particular infections but not for healthy survival in a germ-free facility or for resistance to other infections. Conversely, IL-2 and IL-10 knockout mice, both of which develop colitis with conventional housing, have highlighted the critical role played by the immune system in providing a barrier to ubiquitous but normally nonpathogenic organisms.[84]

Gene Knockout Models in the NOD Mouse

There is enormous potential for applying defined mutant strains created by gene targeting to the study of autoimmune diabetes, for example by back-crossing onto the NOD genotype. Several knockouts have also been applied to transgenic models of diabetes such as the LCMV transgenic model to indicate dependence of this model on CD8+ rather than CD4+ T cells[85] and the requirement for interferon-γ and its receptor. Typically, between four and eight back-crosses are done with NOD mice before brother-sister mating to produce homozygous knockout animals carrying sufficient NOD diabetes susceptibility genes to achieve a high prevalence of diabetes in the wild-type littermates of the knockouts. A theoretical and sometimes real problem occurs when the targeted gene is linked to a diabetes susceptibility locus. The allele from the nondiabetic strain is passed on with the knockout locus, and it is difficult or impossible to split the knockout locus from the nonsusceptible allele of the diabetogenic gene. This is a particular problem, for example, with MHC or tumor necrosis factor genes (both linked to the strongest IDDM susceptibility locus, IDDM1, located within the MHC) and the IL-2 gene, which is linked to another susceptibility locus, IDDM3. Embryonic stem cells derived from NOD mice would enhance the application of knockout technology to autoimmune diabetes, but these have not yet been developed.

The study of mice made deficient in a particular gene product can provide surprising insights into the function of that protein, as shown by inherited disorders in humans and mice that are experiments of nature. This is amply illustrated by the β2 microglobulin (β2-m)–deficient NOD mouse. β2-m is the constant light chain of class I MHC that is required in addition to the polymorphic heavy chain for stability of the heterodimeric complex. β2-m–Deficient mice were generated independently by two groups[86,87] and were among the first gene knockout experiments in mice. The targeting vector used had 10 kilobases of homology to β2-m but exon 2 of β2-m was replaced by the neomycin-resistance gene. β2-m-Knockout results in deficient cell surface expression of class I MHC molecules.[88,89] The resulting homozygous mice developed normally but were completely deficient in CD8+ T cells because of the absence of cell surface class I MHC expression in the thymus. These mice have been used to dissect the role of CD8+ T cells in many models of infection and transplantation as well as of autoimmune disease. Interestingly, although there is some leakiness of the phenotype of these knockouts with a few CD8+ T cells being detectable, the combination of the absent T cell subset and its class I MHC recognition complex leads to solid functional CD8+ T-cell deficiency, which is perhaps more profound than occurs with direct knockout of the CD8 molecule itself.

Back-crossing of these knockout mice onto the NOD background, reported by four groups,[90-93] showed that NOD mice homozygous for the β2-m knockout were completely free of insulitis and protected from diabetes. This was a truly dramatic result that has contributed to a paradigm shift in the understanding of the pathogenesis of diabetes in the NOD mouse. Prior to these experiments and to some other experiments involving transfer of cell populations into the NOD scid mouse, CD4 T cells were believed by some investigators to have a preeminent role in diabetes pathogenesis in this model and CD8 T cells were thought to have a supporting role, possibly as effectors of β-cell destruction. It had been known that both CD4 and CD8 cells were required for efficient transfer of diabetes to nondiabetic recipient mice, but the knockout mice showed that CD8+ T cells are absolutely required for initiation of autoimmunity in this model. Additionally, these animals, when used as recipients for T cells from diabetic NOD mice, develop diabetes very slowly several months after transfer compared with rapid transfer achieved in wild-type NOD mice. This implies that there is likely to be a role for CD8+ T cells in the efferent as well as the afferent phase of diabetes. When β2-m is replaced in β-cells of the knockout mice using a RIP-β2-m transgene, insulitis is reconstituted, showing that class I MHC protein expression on the β-cell is absolutely required for initiation of diabetes and implying direct recognition of the β-cell by CD8+ T cells (T.W.H. Kay and J. Allison, unpublished observations, 1995). Of great interest will be the outcome in NOD mice with knockout of the perforin gene, which encodes an essential component of the cytotoxicity mechanism of CD8+ T cells.[94] These mice will reveal whether the role of CD8+ T cells in initiation of diabetes is dependent on cytotoxic function or whether another function such as cytokine secretion is important.

Reports of other knockout models relevant to diabetes have been slow to appear in print, although there are likely to be a large number in the next few years. NOD mice in which the IFN-γ gene has been knocked out have delayed and reduced the prevalence of diabetes, although they are not absolutely protected (T.A. Stewart, personal communication, 1995). Many other knockout back-crossing experiments are known to be in progress, including knockouts of the IFN-γ receptor; the interferon-regulated transcription factor IRF-1; the tumor necrosis factor receptors; the cytokines IL-10, IL-12, and GM-CSF; cell surface molecules on T cells including CD4 and CD28; and the cytotoxic T lymphocyte effector molecule perforin. No doubt many others are in progress or are planned.

Transgenes, Knockouts, and Insulin-Dependent Diabetes Mellitus—The Future

This chapter will probably be dated in the near future. Transgenic and gene targeting approaches to understanding the pathogenesis of IDDM continue to be applied by an increasing number of investigators, limited only by funds and good animal facilities. The next transgenics off the production line will include mice carrying T-cell receptor genes to defined islet antigens such as proinsulin and glutamic acid decarboxylase; mice expressing islet antigens in the thymus to demonstrate that autoreactive T cells can be deleted or in other peripheral sites to demonstrate that these antigens can redirect autoimmune responses; and mice expressing a variety of immune proteins in the β-cell to determine if these proteins increase or decrease β-cell autoimmunity. It can be envisioned that transgenic expression will be refined by the use of regulatable promoters to allow transgene expression to be switched on or off, for example at different stages of development. A recent development with great potential to regulate transgene expression utilizes the tetracycline (tet) resistance genes from the tet resistance operon of *Escherichia coli* that are normally inhibited by the tet repressor protein (tetR). In the presence of tetracycline, tetR is inactivated and the tet resistance genes are transcribed. TetR has been linked to the powerful transcriptional activator VP16 from herpes simplex virus. This converts tetR into a strong activator, inhibited by tetracycline, of promoters with tet operator sequences. The tetR-VP16 fusion protein was expressed in β-cells under the control of RIP and in a separate transgenic line SV40 Tag was expressed under the control of tet operator sequences and a weak promoter.[95] When the two transgenic lines were mated, the progeny had expression of Tag in β-cells that could be switched off by tetracycline in vitro and in vivo. Many transgene experiments will have implications for the prevention and cure of IDDM. For instance, potential growth factor or immunosuppressive proteins could be tested by their targeted expression in the β-cell. Plans are under way to generate pigs that transgenically express immunosuppressive proteins in their β-cells as a source of islets for transplantation into people with established IDDM.

Transgenic and homologous recombination technology will be used to perform in vivo gene targeting in specific cell types. Using sequence-specific recombinases (including the CRE recombinase from bacteriophage P1 or the FLP recombinase from yeast) expressed in a tissue-specific manner (e.g., in the β-cell using RIP), it is possible to ''edit'' DNA that contains the appropriate target sequences.[96] The recombinase target sequences (called lox sequences in the case of CRE) are inserted on either side of the DNA to be excised using the homologous recombination technology described previously. The recognition sites are in targeting vectors similar to those used to target genes for conventional knockouts, and mice carrying the DNA flanked by recognition sequences are made exactly the same way. These mice are then mated with mice carrying the recombinase transgene. Recombination resulting in deletion of the sequences bracketed by recognition sequences then occurs in cells expressing the recombinase transgene. Again, in the case of application to the NOD model this would require backcrossing of mice carrying the targeted DNA, but the RIP-CRE transgene could be injected directly into NOD eggs. These and many other applications of transgene technology to IDDM will come to fruition over the next decade.

Acknowledgments

We thank Drs. George Rudy, Margo Honeyman, and Michelle French for reviewing this work and Margaret Thompson for secretarial assistance. The authors' work is supported by the National Health and Medical Research Council of Australia.

References

1. Honeyman MC, Harrison LC. The immunologic insult in type 1 diabetes. Springer Semin Immunopathol 1993;14:253
2. Bottazzo GF, Dean BM, McNally JM, et al. In situ characterization of autoimmune phenomena and expression of HLA molecules in the pancreas in diabetic insulitis. N Engl J Med 1985;313:353
3. Foulis AK, McGill M, Farquharson MA. Insulitis in type 1 (insulin-dependent) diabetes mellitus in man—macrophages, lymphocytes, and interferon-gamma containing cells. J Pathol 1991;165:97
4. Itoh N, Hanafusa T, Miyazaki A, et al. Mononuclear cell infiltration and its relation to the expression of major histocompatibility complex antigens and adhesion molecules in pancreas biopsy specimens from newly diagnosed insulin-dependent diabetes mellitus patients. J Clin Invest 1993;92:2313
5. Palmiter RD, Brinster RL. Germ line transformation of mice. Annu Rev Genet 1986;20:465
6. Jaenisch R. Transgenic animals. Science 1988;240:1468
7. Hanahan D. Transgenic mice as probes into complex systems. Science 1989; 246:1265
8. Hanahan D. Heritable formation of pancreatic β-cell tumours in transgenic mice expressing recombinant insulin/simian virus 40 oncogenes. Nature 1985;315:115
9. Adams TE, Alpert S, Hanahan D. Non-tolerance and autoantibodies to a transgenic self antigen expressed in pancreatic β cells. Nature 1987;325:223
10. Hamaguchi K, Gaskins HR, Leiter EH. NIT-1, a pancreatic beta-cell line established from a transgenic NOD/Lt mouse. Diabetes 1991;40:842
11. Harrison LC, Campbell IL, Allison J, Miller JFAP. MHC molecules and β-cell destruction: Immune and nonimmune mechanisms. Diabetes 1989;38:815
12. Allison J, Harrison LC, Campbell IL, Miller JFAP. Major histocompatibility complex molecules and the beta cell: Inferences from transgenic models. Curr Top Microbiol Immunol 1990;156:121
13. Allison J, Campbell IL, Morahan G, et al. Diabetes in transgenic mice resulting from over-expression of class 1 histocompatibility molecules in pancreatic β cells. Nature 1988;333:529
14. Sarvetnick N, Liggitt D, Pitts SL, et al. Insulin-dependent diabetes mellitus induced in transgenic mice by ectopic expression of class II MHC and interferon-gamma. Cell 1988;52:773
15. Miller J, Daitch L, Rath S, Selsing E. Tissue-specific expression of allogeneic class II MHC molecules induces neither rejection nor clonal inactivation of alloreactive T cells. J Immunol 1990;144:344
16. Böhme J, Haskins K, Stecha P, et al. Transgenic mice with I-A islet cells are normoglycemic but immunologically intolerant. Science 1989;244:1179
17. Lo D, Burkly LC, Widera G, et al. Diabetes and tolerance in transgenic mice expressing class II MHC molecules in pancreatic beta cells. Cell 1988;53:159
18. Gotz J, Eibel H, Kohler G. Non-tolerance and differential susceptibility to diabetes in transgenic mice expressing major histocompatibility class II genes on pancreatic β cells. Eur J Immunol 1990;20:1677
19. Guerder S, Meyerhoff J, Flavell R. The role of the T cell costimulator B7-1 in autoimmunity and the induction and maintenance of tolerance to peripheral antigen. Immunity 1994;1:155
20. Heath WR, Allison J, Hoffmann MW, et al. Autoimmune diabetes as a consequence of locally produced interleukin-2. Nature 1992;359:547
21. Allison J, Malcolm L, Culvenor J, et al. Overexpression of B2-microglobulin in transgenic mouse islet beta cells results in defective insulin secretion. Proc Natl Acad Sci USA 1991;88:2070
22. Epstein PN, Overbeek PA, Means AR. Calmodulin-induced early-onset diabetes in transgenic mice. Cell 1989;58:1067
23. Efrat S, Fleischer N, Hanahan D. Diabetes induced in male transgenic mice by expression of human H-ras oncoprotein in pancreatic beta cells. Mol Cell Biol 1990;10:1779
24. Stewart TA, Hultgren B, Huang X, et al. Induction of type 1 diabetes by interferon-alpha in transgenic mice. Science 1993;260:1942
25. Higuchi Y, Herrara P, Muniesa P, et al. Expression of a tumor necrosis factor alpha transgene in murine pancreatic beta cells results in severe and permanent insulitis without evolution towards diabetes. J Exp Med 1993;176:1719
26. Picarella DE, Kratz A, Li CB, et al. Transgenic tumor necrosis factor (TNF)-alpha production in pancreatic islets leads to insulitis, not diabetes. J Immunol 1993;150:4136
27. Allison J, Malcolm L, Chosich N, Miller JFAP. Inflammation but not autoimmunity occurs in transgenic mice expressing constitutive levels of interleukin-2 in islet beta cells. Eur J Immunol 1992;22:1115
28. Wogensen L, Huang X, Sarvetnick N. Leukocyte extravasation into the pancreatic tissue in transgenic mice expression interleukin 10 in the islets of Langerhans. J Exp Med 1993;178:175
29. Wogensen L, Lee MS, Sarvetnick N. Production of interleukin 10 by islet cells accelerates immune-mediated destruction of beta cells in nonobese diabetic mice. J Exp Med 1994;179:1379
30. Oldstone MBA, Nerenberg M, Southern P, et al. Virus infection triggers insulin-dependent diabetes mellitus in a transgenic model: Role of anti-self (virus) immune response. Cell 1991;65:319
31. Ohashi PS, Oehen S, Aichele P, et al. Induction of diabetes is influenced by the infection virus and local expression of MHC class I and tumor necrosis factor alpha. J Immunol 1993;150:5185
32. Roman LM, Simons LF, Hammer RE, et al. The expression of influenza virus hemagglutinin in the pancreatic beta cells of transgenic mice results in autoimmune diabetes. Cell 1990;61:383
33. Freedman J, Hesse S, Palmiter RD, et al. Peripheral tolerance to an islet cell-specific hemagglutinin transgene affects both CD4+ and CD8+ T cells. Eur J Immunol 1992;22:1013
34. Scott B, Liblau R, Degermann S, et al. A role for non-MHC genetic polymorphism in susceptibility to spontaneous autoimmunity. Immunity 1994;1:73
35. Degermann S, Reilly C, Scott B, et al. Eur J Immunol: 1994;24:3155
36. Ohashi PS, Oehen S, Buerki K, et al. Ablation of ''tolerance'' and induction of diabetes by virus infection in viral antigen transgenic mice. Cell 1991;65:305
37. Lee MS, Wogensen L, Shizuru J, et al. Pancreatic islet production of murine interleukin-10 does not inhibit immune-mediated tissue destruction. J Clin Invest 1994;93:1332
38. Harlan DM, Hengartner H, Huang ML, et al. Mice expressing both B7-1 and viral glycoprotein on pancreatic beta cells along with glycoprotein-specific transgenic T cells develop diabetes due to a breakdown of T-lymphocyte unresponsiveness. Proc Natl Acad Sci USA 1994;91:3137
39. Guerder S, Picarella DE, Linsley PS, Flavell RA. Costimulator B7-1 confers

antigen-presenting-cell function to parenchynal tissue and in conjunction with tumor necrosis factor alpha leads to autoimmunity in transgenic mice. Proc Natl Acad Sci USA 1994;91:5138
40. Frauman AG, Chu P, Harrison LC. Nonimmune thyroid destruction results from transgenic overexpression of an allogeneic major histocompatibility complex class I protein. Mol Cell Biol 1993;13:1554
41. Campbell IL, Harrison LC. Molecular pathology of type 1 diabetes. Mol Biol Med 1990;7:299
42. Campbell IL, Oxbrow L, West J, Harrison LC. Regulation of MHC protein expression in pancreatic beta-cells by interferon-gamma and tumor necrosis factor-alpha. Mol Endocrinol 1988;2:101
43. Foulis AK, Farquharson MA, Hardman R. Aberrant expression of class II major histocompatibility complex molecules by B cells and hyperexpression of class I major histocompatibility complex molecules by insulin-containing islets in type 1 (insulin-dependent) diabetes mellitus. Diabetologia 1987;30:333
44. Foulis AK, Farquharson MA, Meagher A. Immunoreactive alpha-interferon in insulin-secreting beta cells in type 1 diàbetes mellitus. Lancet 1987;2:1423
45. Miller JFAP, Heath W. Self-ignorance in the peripheral T-cell pool. Immunol Rev 1993;133:131
46. Benoist C, Mathis D. Transgenes and knock-outs in autoimmunity. Curr Opin Immunol 1993;5:900
47. Lafferty KJ, Prowse SJ, Simeonovic CJ. Immunology of tissue transplantation: A return to the passenger leukocyte concept. Annu Rev Immunol 1983;1:143
48. Harrison LC, De Aizpurua H, Loudovaris T, et al. Reactivity to human islets and fetal pig proislets by peripheral blood mononuclear cells from subjects with preclinical and clinical insulin-dependent diabetes. Diabetes 1991;40:1128
49. Harrison LC, Chu SX, DeAizpurua HJ, et al. Islet-reactive T cells are a marker of preclinical insulin-dependent diabetes. J Clin Invest 1992;89:1161
50. Honeyman MC, Cram DS, Harrison LC. Glutamic acid decarboxylase 67-reactive T cells: A marker of insulin-dependent diabetes. J Exp Med 1993;177:535
51. Bottazzo GF, Pujol-Borrell R, Hanafusa T. Role of aberrant HLA-DR expression and antigen presentation in induction of endocrine autoimmunity. Lancet 1983;2:1115
52. Campbell IL, Cutri A, Wilkinson D, et al. Intercellular adhesion molecule 1 is induced on isolated endocrine islet cells by cytokines but not by reovirus infection. Proc Natl Acad Sci USA 1989;86:4282
53. Stephens LA, Kay TWH. Pancreatic expression of B7 costimulatory molecules in the non-obese diabetic (NOD) mouse. Int Immunol 1995:in press
54. Campbell IL, Kay TW, Oxbrow L, Harrison LC. Essential role for interferon-gamma and interleukin-6 in autoimmune insulin-dependent diabetes in NOD/Wehi mice. J Clin Invest 1991;87:739
55. Hattori M, Buse JB, Jackson RA, et al. The NOD mouse: Recessive diabetogenic gene in the major histocompatibility complex. Science 1986;231:733
56. Prochazka M, Serreze DV, Worthen SM, Leiter EH. Genetic control of diabetogenesis in NOD/Lt mice. Diabetes 1989;38:1446
57. Slattery RM, Kjer-Nielsen L, Allison J, et al. Prevention of diabetes in non-obese diabetic I-Ak transgenic mice. Nature 1990;345:724
58. Nishimoto H, Kikutani H, Yamamura K, Kishimoto T. Prevention of autoimmune insulitis by expression of I-E molecules in NOD mice. Nature 1987;328:432
59. Uehira M, Uno M, Kurner T, et al. Development of autoimmune insulitis is prevented in E-alpha-d but not in A-beta-k NOD transgenic mice. Int Immunol 1989;1:209
60. Miyazaki T, Uno M, Uehira M, et al. Direct evidence for the contribution of the unique I-Anod to the development of insulitis in non-obese diabetic mice. Nature 1990;345:722
61. Lund T, O'Reilly L, Hutchings P, et al. Prevention of insulin-dependent diabetes mellitus in non-obese diabetic mice by transgenes encoding modified I-A beta chain or normal I-E alpha chain. Nature 1990;345:727
62. Böhme J, Schubaur B, Kanagawa O, et al. MHC-linked protection from diabetes dissociated from clonal deletion in T cells. Science 1990;249:293
63. Uno M, Miyazaki T, Uehira M, et al. Complete prevention of diabetes in transgenic NOD mice expressing I-E molecules. Immunol Lett 1991;31:47
64. Miyazaki T, Matsuda Y, Toyonaga T, et al. Prevention of autoimmune insulitis in nonobese diabetic mice by expression of major histocompatibility complex class I L^d molecules. Proc Natl Acad Sci USA 1992;89:9519
65. Slattery RM, Miller JF, Heath WR, Charlton B. Failure of a protective major histocompatibility complex class II molecule to delete autoreactive T cells in autoimmune diabetes. Proc Natl Acad Sci USA 1993;90:10808
66. Singer SM, Tisch R, Yang XD, McDevitt HO. An Ab^d transgene prevents diabetes in nonobese diabetic mice by inducing regulatory T cells. Proc Natl Acad Sci USA 1993;90:9566
67. Lipes MA, Rosenzweig A, Tan K-N, et al. Progression to diabetes in nonobese diabetic (NOD) mice with transgenic T cell receptors. Science 1993;259:1165
68. Podolin PL, Pressey A, DeLarato NH, et al. I-E+ nonobese diabetic mice develop insulitis and diabetes. J Exp Med 1993;178:793
69. Katz JD, Wang B, Haskins K, et al. Following a diabetogenic T cell from genesis through pathogenesis. Cell 1993;74:1089
70. Todd JA. The role of MHC class II genes in susceptibility to insulin-dependent diabetes mellitus. Curr Top Microbiol Immunol 1990;164:17
71. Acha-Orbea H, McDevitt HO. The first external domain of the nonobese diabetic mouse class II I-A beta chain is unique. Proc Natl Acad Sci USA 1987;84:2435
72. Nepom GT. A unified hypothesis for the complex genetics of HLA associations with IDDM. Diabetes 1990;39:1153
73. Deng H, Apple R, Clare-Salzler M, et al. Determinant capture as a possible mechanism of protection afforded by major histocompatibility complex class II molecules in autoimmune disease. J Exp Med 1993;178:1675
74. Weiner HL, Friedman A, Miller A. Oral tolerance: Immunologic mechanism and treatment of animal and human organ-specific autoimmune disease by oral administration of autoantigens. Annu Rev Immunol 1994;12:809
75. Haskins K, Portas M, Bergman B, et al. Pancreatic islet-specific T-cell clones from non-obese diabetic mice. Proc Natl Acad Sci USA 1989;86:8000
76. Haskins K, McDuffie M. Acceleration of diabetes in young NOD mice with a CD4+ islet-specific T cell clone. Science 1990;249:1433
77. Ashton-Rickardt PG, Bandeira A, Delaney JR, et al. Evidence for a differential avidity model of T cell selection in the thymus. Cell 1994;76:651
78. Miller JFAP, Morahan G, Slattery R, Allison J. Transgenic models of T-cell self tolerance and autoimmunity. Immunol Rev 1990;118:21
79. Capecchi MR. The new mouse genetics: Altering the genome by gene targeting. Trends Genet 1989;5:70
80. Capecchi MR. Targeted gene replacement. Sci Am 1994;270:52
81. Evans MJ, Kaufman MH. Establishment in culture of pluripotential cells from mouse embryos. Nature 1981;292:154
82. Martin GR. Isolation of a pluripotent cell line from early mouse embryos cultured in medium conditioned by teratocarcinoma stem cells. Proc Natl Acad Sci USA 1981;78:7634
83. Muller D, Koller BH, Whitton JL, et al. LCMV-specific, class II-restricted cytotoxic T cells in beta 2-microglobulin-deficient mice. Science 1992;255:1576
84. Strober W, Ehrhardt RO. Chronic intestinal inflammation: An unexpected outcome in cytokine or T-cell receptor mutant mice. Cell 1993;75:203
85. Laufer TM, VonHerrath MG, Grusby MJ, et al. Autoimmune diabetes can be induced in transgenic major histocompatibility complex class II-deficient mice. J Exp Med 1993;178:589
86. Zijlstra M, Li E, Sajjadi F, et al. Germ-line transmission of a disrupted beta 2-microglobulin gene produced by homologous recombination in embryonic stem cells. Nature 1989;342:435
87. Koller BH, Smithies O. Inactivating the beta 2-microglobulin locus in mouse embryonic stem cells by homologous recombination. Proc Natl Acad Sci USA 1989;86:8932
88. Zijlstra M, Bix M, Simister NE, et al. Beta 2-microglobulin deficient mice lack CD4-8+ cytolytic T cells. Nature 1990;344:742
89. Koller BH, Marrack P, Kappler JW, Smithies O. Normal development of mice deficient in beta 2-M, MHC class I proteins, and CD8+ T cells. Science 1990;248:1227
90. Wicker LS, Leiter EH, Todd JA, et al. Beta 2-microglobulin-deficient NOD mice do not develop insulitis or diabetes. Diabetes 1994;43:500
91. Serreze DV, Leiter EH, Christianson GJ, et al. Major histocompatibility complex class I-deficient NOD-B_2mnull mice are diabetes and insulitis resistant. Diabetes 1994;43:505
92. Sumida T, Furukawa M, Sakamoto A, et al. Prevention of insulitis and diabetes in beta 2-microglobulin-deficient non-obese diabetic mice. Int Immunol 1994;6:1445
93. Katz J, Benoist C, Mathis D. Major histocompatibility complex class I molecules are required for the development of insulitis in non-obese diabetic mice. Eur J Immunol 1993;23:3358
94. Kagi D, Ledermann B, Burki K, et al. Cytotoxicity mediated by T cells and natural killer cells is greatly impaired in perforin-deficient mice. Nature 1994;369:31
95. Efrat S, Fusco-DeMane D, Lemberg H, et al. Conditional transformation of a pancreatic β-cell line derived from transgenic mice expressing a tetracycline-regulated oncogene. Proc Natl Acad Sci USA 92:3576
96. Zou YR, Muller W, Gu H, Rajewsky K. Cre-loxP-mediated gene replacement: A mouse strain producing humanized antibodies. Curr Biol 1994;4:1099

Part V

Type I Diabetes: Therapeutics

Diabetes Mellitus, edited by Derek LeRoith, Simeon I. Taylor, and Jerrold M. Olefsky. Lippincott–Raven Publishers, Philadelphia © 1996.

Chapter 39

The Treatment of Diabetes to Prevent and Delay Long-Term Complications: The Diabetes Control and Complications Trial

David M. Nathan

Background

After more than 60 years of active debate and 10 years of study, the Diabetes Control and Complications Trial (DCCT) determined the salutary effects of intensive diabetes management on the development and progression of the microvascular and neurologic complications of insulin-dependent diabetes mellitus (IDDM).[1] The debate regarding the relationship between metabolic control and the genesis of long-term complications in diabetes mellitus began soon after the introduction of insulin therapy.[2–4] During the first decades of insulin use, clinicians began to observe previously unrecognized microvascular and neurologic complications.[5,6] These long-term complications, including retinopathy, neuropathy, and nephropathy, were previously unknown because the rapid fatal course of IDDM in the pre-insulin era precluded the development of the complications, which only occur after more than 5 to 10 years of diabetes duration.

Numerous explanations for the occurrence of the complications were advanced; however, the most popular hypothesis was that imperfect glucose control was the cause. The "glucose hypothesis," as it was called, gained support from studies in animal models of diabetes. Classic studies by Engerman and colleagues demonstrated a decrease in the development of retinopathy in diabetic dogs whose glucose levels were maintained at a level that prevented glycosuria compared with the occurrence of retinopathy in less intensively treated diabetic dogs.[7] Other studies in animal models demonstrated decreased development of nephropathy and neuropathy in the setting of intensive therapy.[8,9] Although these studies almost uniformly supported the glucose hypothesis, they suffered from the limitation of being performed in animal models. Whether the benefits documented in animal models would apply in human diabetes remained an open question; however, epidemiologic studies lent further support to the glucose hypothesis. A durable and consistent positive association between chronic glycemia (assessed either with indices of glycemic control or with glycosylated hemoglobin measurements) and long-term complications was demonstrated in IDDM and non–insulin dependent diabetes mellitus (NIDDM).[10–12]

Although committed proponents of the glucose hypothesis espoused "tight" metabolic control, no definitive clinical data supported the efficacy of any mode of therapy in preventing the development or slowing the progress of complications. Moreover, there was no consensus regarding the specific therapy necessary to establish and maintain normal or near-normal levels of glycemia over time. Finally, the absence of clinical trial data prevented an examination of the balance between putative benefits and adverse consequences and costs of intensive therapy, that is, the cost : benefit ratio.

The tools to achieve long-term, near-normal glucose control, such as blood glucose self-monitoring and intensive insulin therapy regimens, became available in the late 1970s.[13] Objective methods to measure long-term glycemia and complications were developed at the same time.[14] These developments made possible the design and conduct of clinical experiments to settle the debate. The first such studies were of generally brief duration and underpowered, with too few patients to avoid a type two error.[15–18] Despite meta-analyses that suggested a beneficial effect of intensive therapy,[19,20] no conclusive studies demonstrated a benefit that outweighed the risks and costs that accompanied such therapy. Another study of similar duration to the DCCT but considerably smaller in size was conducted in Sweden during the same period as the DCCT.[21] Although the Swedish study altered conventional therapy to be more intensive at the third year, the investigators continued to follow the patients for as long as 8 years.

Design of the DCCT

The DCCT, initiated in 1983, was designed to answer definitively whether intensive diabetes management would affect the development and/or progression of long-term complications in IDDM, and at what cost.[22] The DCCT asked and provided remarkably clear answers to the following questions: (1) Will intensive therapy aimed at achieving glycemic levels as close to the nondiabetic range as possible prevent the development or slow the progression of complications in IDDM patients with no complications at baseline (primary prevention)? (2) Will intensive therapy prevent the progression of complications in IDDM patients who already have some evidence of complications at baseline (secondary intervention)? (3) What are the adverse events associated with intensive compared with conventional therapy?

In order to answer these questions, the DCCT selected two separate cohorts of patients. The Primary Prevention cohort was 13–39 years of age with 1 to 5 years of diabetes duration and no evidence of retinopathy or nephropathy. The Secondary Intervention cohort was similarly aged but could have had IDDM for as long as 15 years. They had to have at least one microaneurysm but no more than moderate nonproliferative retinopathy, and they could have as much as 200 mg of albumin excretion per 24 hours. The baseline characteristics of the two study cohorts are shown in Table 39-1. Study patients were selected not only on the basis of demographic, clinical, and biochemical criteria but also based on an assessment that they would accept random assignment of therapy and that they were likely to continue to participate in a long-term study. On average, these patients were probably more motivated than the usual patient with IDDM.

DCCT Intensive Treatment and Metabolic Goals

The Primary Prevention and Secondary Intervention cohorts were randomly assigned either to conventional therapy (designed to mimic the usual diabetes therapy with one or two daily injections

TABLE 39-1. Baseline Characteristics of the Study Population

	Primary Prevention (n=726)	Secondary Intervention (n=715)
Age (years)	27 ± 7	27 ± 7
Gender (% male)	52	53
Duration of IDDM (years)	2.6 ± 1.4	8.7 ± 3.7
Retinopathy		
None	100%	0%
Very minimal NPDR*	0	63%
Minimal NPDR	0	20%
Moderate NPDR	0	17%
Nephropathy albumin excretion (mg/24 h)	12 ± 8	20 ± 24
HbAlc (%)	8.8 ± 1.6	8.9 ± 1.5

*NPDR = nonproliferative diabetic retinopathy.

of insulin and daily glucose monitoring) or to intensive therapy (designed to normalize blood glucose control). Conventional therapy had the clinical goals of avoiding any symptoms of hyper- or hypoglycemia, but no specific numeric blood glucose targets. Intensive therapy had the goal of achieving blood glucose control as close to the nondiabetic range as possible, including premeal blood glucose levels between 70 and 120 mg/dL (3.9 to 6.7 mMol/L), peak postprandial levels less than 180 mg/dL (10 mMol/L), and hemoglobin (Hb)A1c levels in the nondiabetic range (<6.05%). In order to reach these goals, patients assigned to intensive therapy used three or more insulin injections per day or insulin pump therapy, guided by frequent self-monitoring of blood glucose levels

TABLE 39-2. Intensive Therapy

Insulin	Multiple daily injection (MDI)—≥3 injections per day (once or twice per day long- or intermediate-acting insulin plus premeal rapid-acting insulin) or Continuous subcutaneous insulin infusion (CSII) with external pumps All doses adjusted by algorithms based on glucose results, diet, and exercise
Monitoring	
Blood glucose	≥4 tests per day—premeal and prebed
Urine ketones	During illness or if blood glucose level- >16.7 mM
HbAlc	Monthly
Diet	Extensive instruction and frequent reinforcement stressing understanding of carbohydrate content and effect of specific meals on glucose control (i.e., insulin requirements for meals)
Exercise	Exercise encouraged. Patients taught to adjust insulin based on anticipated exercise and during exercise
Supervision	Monthly clinic visits with nurse-educator and physician Weekly phone contact to review results and help adjust regimen

(Table 39-2). Insulin therapy was adjusted frequently in response to ambient blood glucose levels, diet, and exercise.

DCCT Results

The results of intensive compared with conventional therapy in the DCCT have been reported in a series of reports.[1, 23–33] The initial report[1] summarized the major results whereas subsequent reports presented more detailed, expanded analyses of the effects of intensive therapy on long-term complications, including retinopathy,[23,24] nephropathy,[25] neuropathy,[26] and macrovascular disease and its risk factors.[27] It also examined the effect of intensive therapy on quality of life[28] and neurobehavioral outcome[29]; the implementation[30] and adverse effects of intensive therapy[31]; and the cost : benefit analysis of intensive therapy compared with conventional therapy.[32]

Adherence and Metabolic Results

Over the 6.5-year mean follow-up time of the study (range 3–9 years), compliance was excellent with 99% of the cohort completing the trial. In addition, there was virtually no cross-over between assigned treatments. Subjects adhered to their assigned treatment more than 97% of study time. Intensive therapy decreased HbA1c to a nadir of approximately 6.9% by 6 months and maintained mean HbA1c levels during the remainder of the trial that were approximately 2% lower than with conventional treatment (9% versus 7%) (Fig. 39-1). Of note, intensive therapy did not lower mean HbA1c to the nondiabetic range.

Retinopathy

Retinopathy was evaluated every 6 months by 7-field stereoscopic fundus photography. The photographs were graded in a central facility, with the graders masked to patient identity. Although many analytic levels of retinopathy were assessed, the principal outcome

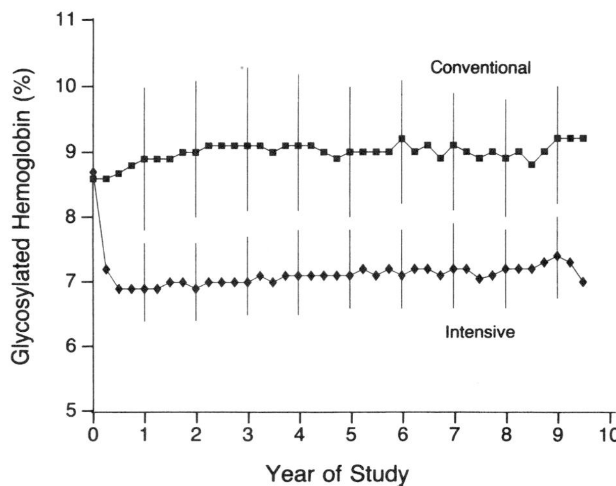

FIGURE 39-1. Median hemoglobin A1c levels for conventional (squares) and intensive (diamonds) treatment groups during the study. The vertical lines represent the middle quartiles (25th to 75th percentile) for each group. The differences between treatment groups were highly significant (p<.0001) from 3 months onward. (Reprinted with permission from DCCT Research Group. The effect of intensive treatment of diabetes on the development and progression of long-term complications in insulin-dependent diabetes mellitus. N Engl J Med 1993;329:977.)

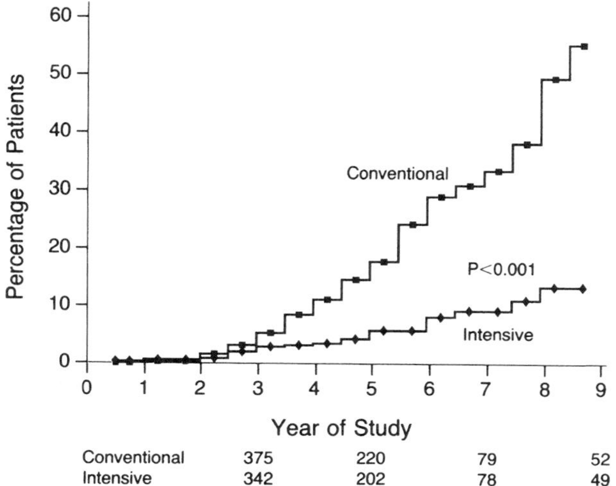

Figure 39-2. Cumulative incidence of sustained three-step progression of retinopathy for conventional and intensive treatment groups of primary prevention cohort (symbols same as in Fig. 39-1). (Reprinted with permission from DCCT Research Group. The effect of intensive treatment of diabetes on the development and progression of long-term complications in insulin-dependent diabetes mellitus. N Engl J Med 1993;329:977.)

in the primary prevention study was the development of a sustained (seen on two consecutive exams) three-step or greater progression on a retinopathy severity scale adopted from the Early Treatment of Diabetic Retinopathy Study (ETDRS).[33] Similarly, the principal outcome in the secondary intervention study was a sustained progression of three or more steps from the baseline level. Intensive therapy reduced the development of these end points by 76% in the Primary Prevention study and by 54% in the Secondary Intervention study compared with conventional therapy (Figs. 39-2 and 39-3). Other retinopathy outcomes and the effects of intensive therapy are shown in Table 39-3.

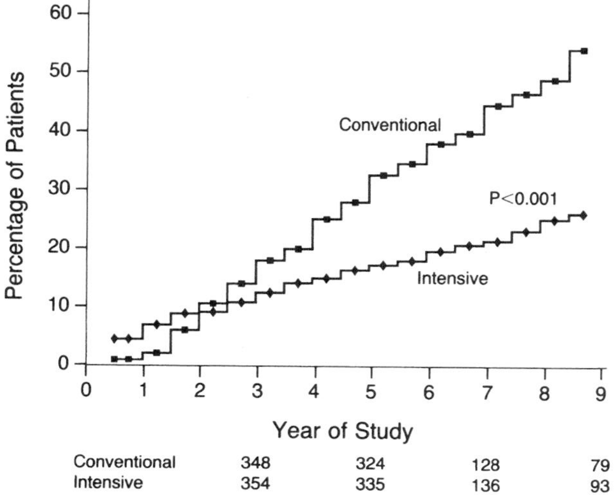

Figure 39-3. Cumulative incidence of sustained three-step progression of retinopathy for conventional and intensive treatment groups of Secondary Intervention cohort (symbols same as in Figs. 39-1 and 39-2). (Reprinted with permission from DCCT Research Group. The effect of intensive treatment of diabetes on the development and progression of long-term complications in insulin-dependent diabetes mellitus. N Engl J Med 1993;329:977.)

Table 39-3. Effect of Intensive Therapy for Diabetes on Long-Term Complications

Complication	Percent Reduction in Risk (Intensive vs. Conventional) Primary Prevention	Secondary Intervention
Retinopathy		
3-step progression	76*	54*
Preproliferative or proliferative†		47*
Laser treatment†		56*
Nephropathy		
Microalbuminuria (≥28 μg/min=40 mg/24 h)	34*	43*
Albuminuria (≥208 μg/min=300 mg/24 h)	44	56*
Neuropathy	69*	57*

*p<0.05, intensive versus conventional therapy.
†Too few events to analyze in Primary Prevention cohort.

The overall effect of intensive therapy was to decrease all stages of retinopathy included in the DCCT. However, intensive therapy was relatively more effective when initiated early in the course of diabetes (shorter versus longer duration) and when retinopathy was less severe at baseline.[23,24] Although intensive therapy reduced the risk somewhat less for more advanced stages of retinopathy than for earlier stages, patients with more advanced retinopathy still benefited from intensive therapy. Their retinal status was much more likely to stabilize or even to improve with intensive compared with conventional therapy. The beneficial effects of intensive therapy were not seen for the first 3 years of therapy, presumably because of the natural ''momentum'' of diabetic complications. In addition, intensive therapy was associated with a transient worsening of retinopathy during the first year of therapy. Both of these factors conspired to delay the beneficial effects of intensive therapy, which were similar in almost all subgroups of patients defined by age, gender, and other baseline characteristics.

Nephropathy

Nephropathy was assessed by measurements of albumin excretion and standard creatinine clearance, based on an annual standardized 4-hour collection and by periodically measured iothalamate clearance. The primary analytic end points for nephropathy are shown in Table 39-3 and Figures 39-4 and 39-5. As with retinopathy, the risk for progression of nephropathy was reduced by intensive therapy. This included reduction in the development of microalbuminuria (≥40 mg/24 h) and clinical grade albuminuria (≥300 mg/24 h). The small number of patients developing clinical nephropathy, defined as a creatinine clearance <70 mL/min/1.73 m^2 with albumin excretion ≥300 mg/24 hours, precluded a statistically valid analysis of any difference between treatment groups. However, the number of conventional treatment patients who developed this level of renal dysfunction (n=5) was more than twice the number of intensive treatment patients (n=2).

The relatively small number of secondary intervention patients who had microalbuminuria at baseline (n=70) made it difficult to demonstrate a benefit of intensive therapy with regard to slowing progression to clinical grade albuminuria once microalbuminuria had occurred.[25] However, the Steno study had previously demonstrated such a benefit with only 36 patients. Their success may have been rooted in the very frequent measurement of repeated 24-hour albumin excretion rates, which decreased the variance of

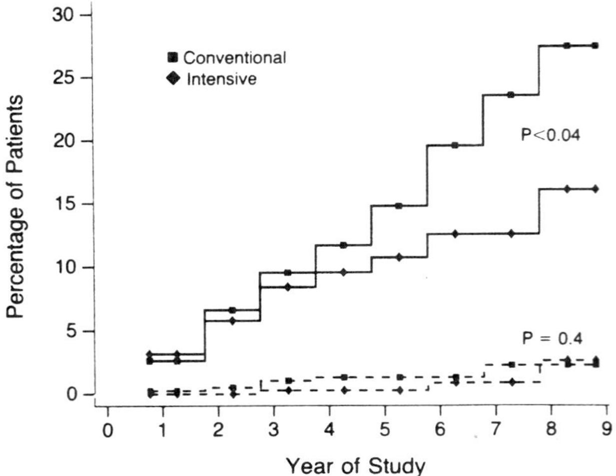

FIGURE 39-4. Cumulative incidences of development of microalbuminuria (≥40 mg/24 h), shown by solid lines, and clinical grade albuminuria (≥300 mg/24 h), shown by dashed lines, for conventional and intensive treatment groups in Primary Prevention cohort. Symbols same as in previous figures. (Reprinted with permission from DCCT Research Group. The effect of intensive treatment of diabetes on the development and progression of long-term complications in insulin-dependent diabetes mellitus. N Engl J Med 1993;329:977.)

the measurements.[34] In any case, the results of the DCCT, which showed a decrease in virtually all levels of renal dysfunction,[25] in conjunction with the Steno study results, conclusively support the role of intensive therapy in delaying and perhaps preventing diabetic nephropathy.

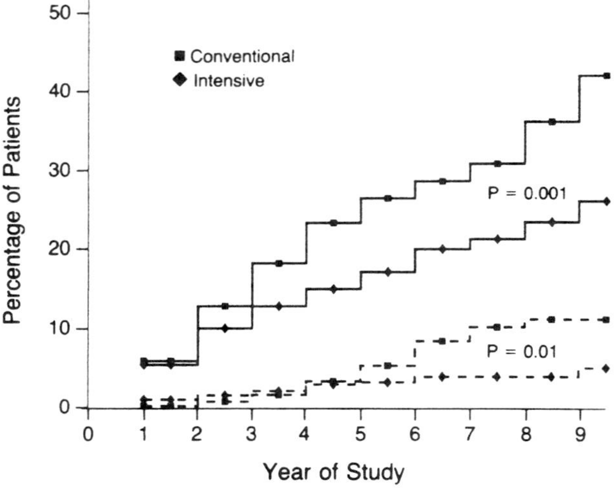

FIGURE 39-5. Cumulative incidences of development of microalbuminuria and clinical grade albuminuria for conventional and intensive treatment groups in Secondary Intervention cohort. Symbols same as in Fig. 39-4. (Reprinted with permission from DCCT Research Group. The effect of intensive treatment of diabetes on the development and progression of long-term complications in insulin-dependent diabetes mellitus. N Engl J Med 1993; 329:977.)

Neuropathy

Confirmed clinical neuropathy was defined as the presence of signs or symptoms of peripheral neuropathy plus either abnormal nerve conduction in at least two peripheral nerves or unequivocally abnormal autonomic nerve testing. Intensive therapy reduced the risk of developing clinical neuropathy 60% in the combined cohorts.[1,26] In addition to the decreased development of confirmed clinical neuropathy, the most stringent of the neurologic outcomes, intensive therapy reduced the risk of deterioration of nerve function, as measured with electrophysiologic methods, that occurred with conventional therapy.[26] The decline in autonomic nerve function that occurred with conventional therapy was significantly reduced with intensive therapy in the Primary Prevention but not in the Secondary Intervention cohort.

Macrovascular

The DCCT did not demonstrate a significant difference in major macrovascular outcomes (death from cardiovascular disease, myocardial infarction, and major peripheral vascular events) between treatment groups.[27] Although the risk for these combined events was reduced by 41% with intensive therapy, the difference between groups failed to achieve conventional levels of statistical significance (p=0.06). However, several risk factors for cardiovascular disease were improved with intensive therapy, including a 34% reduction in low-density lipoprotein cholesterol (p=0.02). Further study is required to ascertain whether intensive therapy improves the risk of macrovascular disease that accompanies IDDM. It was reassuring to note that intensive therapy, which included modestly higher insulin doses (.01 to .05 U/kg/day more insulin with intensive than with conventional therapy),[30] did not increase cardiovascular disease.

Other Outcomes and Adverse Events

Accompanying the salutary effects of intensive therapy on long-term complications was an approximately three-fold increase in severe hypoglycemia, defined as an episode that required assistance to treat.[1,31] Although the majority of these episodes were clinically benign, the incidence of hypoglycemia resulting in coma and seizures or requiring Emergency Room treatment was also increased by approximately two- to three-fold. The more severe hypoglycemic reactions, such as those resulting in seizure or coma, were relatively rare (16 versus 5 episodes per 100 patient-years in the intensive and conventional treatment groups, respectively). Other adverse events that accompanied intensive therapy included an increased risk for weight gain, secondary in part to the decrease in caloric wasting with decreased glycosuria, and catheter-related infections in patients using insulin pumps. Taken together, none of these adverse events caused significant morbidity or mortality. There were no patient deaths or macrovascular events ascribed to hypoglycemia. Moreover, the increased frequency of hypoglycemia had no adverse effects on neurocognitive function as judged by frequent testing in both treatment groups.[29] Finally, despite the demands of intensive therapy, quality of life, measured yearly by self-report,[28] did not differ between the two treatment groups.

Treatment Recommendations

The DCCT Research Group, the American Diabetes Association, and other groups have concluded that the significant and consistent effects of intensive therapy in reducing the risk of development and progression of long-term complications of diabetes outweigh its costs, the considerable effort to implement it, and the increased

Table 39-4. Treatment Regimens for IDDM

Level of Therapy	Self-Monitoring of Blood Glucose (Times per Day)	Insulin Regimen (Injections/Day)	Diet	Exercise	Complications of Therapy	Expected Hemoglobin A1C Level (%)*
Minimal	0–1	1 or 2 (I without R)	45–50% carbohydrate <30% fat <300 mg cholesterol Protein, 0.8 g/kg Limited sucrose Regular meals	Patient preference; snack to prevent hypoglycemia	Hypoglycemia	≥9.5
Average	1–3 (Fasting and before supper or bed)	2 (I plus R)	Same diet as used in minimal level of therapy Patients may also use carbohydrate exchange list	Same precautions as used in minimal level	Hypoglycemia	7.5–9.5
Intensive	4–7 (Before meals and bed; at 3:00 AM once a week; postprandial as needed)	≥3 (I or UL plus R or continuous subcutaneous insulin infusion)	Use glycemic indices when appropriate for more accurate carbohydrate exchange	Adjust insulin, meals, or both to prevent hypoglycemia	Threefold increase in hypoglycemia; catheter inflammation and infections; weight gain	>7.5†

*Nondiabetic range, 3.8–6.4%.
†In the Diabetes Control and Complications Trial, the goal was to achieve a nondiabetic range of HbAlc. Intensive therapy accomplished a mean hemoglobin A1c level of 7.1%.
I=Intermediate-acting (neutral protamine Hagedorn [NPH] or Lente) insulin; UL=Ultralente insulin; R=rapid-acting (CZI) insulin.

patient risk for hypoglycemia.[1,33] Intensive therapy has been endorsed as the treatment of choice for most patients with IDDM. This conclusion is further supported on the basis of the projected economic impact of intensive therapy.[32] Although the annual cost of intensive therapy exceeds the cost of conventional therapy and must be incurred for at least 3 years before a benefit is seen, the long-term benefits of intensive therapy, in the form of reducing loss of vision and the need for laser therapy, reducing the incidence of end-stage renal disease and the need for dialysis and transplantation, and reducing the number of amputations, and the costs associated with all these problems make intensive therapy an economically viable therapy.

Realistically, not all IDDM patients are able to implement intensive therapy; however, the goal for all patients should be to lower glycemia as close to the normal range as safety and lifestyle allow. For patients who cannot implement intensive treatment, therapies of variable intensity are available (Table 39-4). All patients should be evaluated and advised to increase the intensity of their therapy as needed. Any reduction in HbA1c level is likely to provide a benefit with regard to long-term complications. Intensive therapy has been mandatory for more than a decade in women with IDDM who are trying to conceive and during pregnancy based on the demonstrated improvement in neonatal outcome.[34–36]

Future Considerations

Many questions and challenges remain in the wake of the DCCT. First, although intensive therapy was highly effective in the DCCT, the research volunteers were selected, in part, for their anticipated high level of compliance. Whether and to what extent nonresearch IDDM patients can implement intensive therapy remains to be seen. The added motivation provided by the DCCT results, which were not available to DCCT participants during the trial, should help motivate patients with IDDM and their health care providers to implement intensive therapy. Second, remarkable resources were made available to implement intensive therapy in the DCCT. Whether satisfactory resources are or can be made available in the nonresearch setting is unknown. Expert treatment teams must be established and financial barriers must be abrogated as early steps in making intensive therapy as widely available as possible. Third, intensive therapy in the strictest sense and not normoglycemia was proved to be effective in preventing the development and slowing the progression of diabetic complications. Whether all methods of treatment designed to achieve normoglycemia will similarly improve complications is not clear. It is likely that attainment of normoglycemia is the major reason why intensive therapy was effective. Similar treatment methods, such as artificial pancreases (implantable pumps with built-in glucose sensors), are likely to provide similar benefits. However, methods that introduce different treatment principles may need to be considered carefully. For example, pancreas transplantation, which can normalize blood glucose levels very effectively,[37] introduces variables such as immunosuppression that might have independent effects on outcome. Such therapy may need to be evaluated to determine its cost-to-benefit ratio. Finally, no patients with NIDDM, the most common form of diabetes, were included in the DCCT; therefore the applicability of DCCT results to NIDDM is speculative. Although the similarity between complications in IDDM and NIDDM[38] and the similar relationship between progression of retinopathy and levels of chronic glycemia in IDDM and NIDDM[10–12] suggest that intensive therapy should be effective in preventing and/or delaying progression of complications in NIDDM, there are no direct data available. Moreover, there are no long-term studies that establish the relative risks of different therapies to achieve normoglylcemia in NIDDM. The concern that the high insulin doses that are ultimately required to treat many patients with NIDDM may be atherogenic tempers enthusiasm for the widespread implementation of intensive therapy in NIDDM.[39]

References

1. DCCT Research Group. The effect of intensive treatment of diabetes on the development and progression of long-term complications in insulin-dependent diabetes mellitus. N Engl J Med 1993;329:977

2. Cahill GF Jr, Etzwiler DD, Freinkel N. "Control" and diabetes [Editorial]. N Engl J Med 1976;294:1004
3. Siperstein MD, Foster DW, Knowles HC Jr, et al. Control of blood glucose and diabetic vascular disease [Editorial]. N Engl J Med 1977;296:1060
4. Ingelfinger FJ. Debates on diabetes. N Engl J Med 1977;296:1288
5. Ballantyne AJ, Loewenstein A. The pathology of diabetic retinopathy. Trans Ophthalmol UK 1943;63:95
6. Kimmelstiel P, Wilson C. Intercapillary lesions in the glomeruli of the kidney. Am J Pathol 1936;12:83
7. Engerman R, Bloodworth JMB Jr, Nelson, S. Relationship of microvascular disease in diabetes to metabolic control. Diabetes 1977;26:760
8. Gray BN, Watkins E. Prevention of vascular complications of diabetes by pancreatic islet transplantation. Arch Surg 1976;111:254
9. Steffes MW, Brown DM, Basgen JM, Mauer M. Amelioration of mesangial volume and surface alterations following islet transplantation in diabetic rats. Diabetes 1980;29:509
10. Pirart J. Diabetes mellitus and its degenerative complications: A prospective study of 4400 patients observed between 1947 and 1973. Diabetes Care 1978;1:168
11. Klein R, Klein BEK, Moss SE, et al. JAMA 1988;260:2864
12. Nathan DM, Singer DE, Godine JE, et al. Retinopathy in older type II diabetics: Association with glucose control. Diabetes 1986;35:797
13. Nathan DM. Modern management of insulin-dependent diabetes mellitus. Med Clin North Am 1988;72:1365
14. Nathan DM, Singer DE, Hurxthal K, Goodson JD. The clinical information value of the glycosylated hemoglobin assay. N Engl J Med 1984;310:341
15. Kroc Collaborative Study Group. Blood glucose control and the evolution of diabetic retinopathy and albuminuria. N Engl J Med 1984;311:365
16. Feldt-Rasmussen B, Mathiesen ER, Deckert T. Effect of two years of strict metabolic control on progression of incipient nephropathy in insulin dependent diabetes. Lancet 1986;2:1300
17. Dahl-Jorgensen K, Brinchmann-Hansen O, Hanssen KF, et al. Effect of near normoglycemia for two years on progression of early diabetic retinopathy, nephropathy, and neuropathy: The Oslo study. Br Med J 1986;293:1195
18. Brinchman-Hansen O, Dahl-Jorgensen K, Hanssen KF, Sandvik L. The response of diabetic retinopathy to 41 months of multiple daily injections, insulin pumps and conventional insulin therapy. Arch Ophthalmol 1988;106:1242
19. Hansssen KF, Dahl-Jorgensen K, Lauritzen T, et al. Diabetic control and microvascular complications: The near-normoglycaemic experience. Diabetologia 1986;29:677
20. Wang PH, Lau J, Chalmers TC. Meta-analysis of effects of intensive blood-glucose control on late complications of type I diabetes. Lancet 1993;341:1306
21. Reichard P, Nilsson B-Y, Rosenqvist U. The effect of long-term intensified insulin treatment on the development of microvascular complications of diabetes mellitus. N Engl J Med 1993;329:304
22. DCCT Research Group. The Diabetes Control and Complications Trial: Design and methodologic considerations for the feasibility phase. Diabetes 1986; 35:530
23. DCCT Research Group. The effect of intensive diabetes treatment on the progression of diabetic retinopathy in insulin-dependent diabetes mellitus: The Diabetes Control and Complications Trial. Arch Ophthalmol 1995;113:36
24. DCCT Research Group. Progression of retinopathy with intensive vs conventional therapy in the Diabetes Control and Complications Trial. Ophthalmology 1995;102:647
25. DCCT Research Group. The effect of intensive therapy on the development and progression of diabetic nephropathy in the Diabetes Control and Complications Trial. Kidney Int 1995;47:1703
26. DCCT Research Group. The effect of intensive diabetes therapy on the development and progression of neuropathy. Ann Int Med 1995;122:561
27. DCCT Research Group. The effect of intensive diabetes therapy on macrovascular disease and its risk factors in the Diabetes Control and Complications Trial. Am J Cardiol 1995;75:894
28. DCCT Research Group. The effect of intensive therapy on quality of life outcome in the Diabetes Control and Complications Trial. Diabetes Care 1995;in press
29. DCCT Research Group. The effect of intensive therapy on neurobehavioral outcomes in the DCCT. Ann Int Med 1995;in press
30. DCCT Research Group. Implementation of treatment protocols in the Diabetes Control and Complications Trial. Diabetes Care 1995;18:361
31. DCCT Research Group. Treatment related adverse events in the Diabetes Control and Complications Trial. Diabetes Care 1995;18:1415
32. DCCT Research Group. Lifetime benefits of intensive therapy as practiced in the Diabetes Control and Complications Trial: An economic evaluation. In preparation
33. American Diabetes Association. Position statement: Implications of the Diabetes Control and Complications Trial. Diabetes Care 1993;16:1517
34. American College of Obstetrics and Gynecology. Management of diabetes mellitus in pregnancy. ACOG Technical Bull 1986;92:1
35. Jovanovic L, Druzin M, Peterson CM. Effect of euglycemia on the outcome of pregnancy in insulin-dependent diabetic women as compared with normal control subjects. Am J Med 1981;71:921
36. Fuhrmann K, Reiher H, Semmler K, et al. Prevention of congenital malformations in infants of insulin-dependent diabetic mothers. Diabetes Care 1983;6:219
37. Nathan DM, Fogel H, Norman D, et al. Long-term metabolic and quality of life results with pancreatic/renal transplantation in IDDM. Transplantation 1991;52:85
38. Nathan DM. Long-term complications of diabetes mellitus. N Engl J Med 1993;328:1676
39. Nathan DM. Inferences and implications: Do the DCCT results apply in NIDDM? Diabetes Care 1995;18:25

Diabetes Mellitus, edited by Derek LeRoith, Simeon I. Taylor, and Jerrold M. Olefsky. Lippincott–Raven Publishers, Philadelphia © 1996.

CHAPTER 40

Translation of the Diabetes Control and Complications Trial

SAUL GENUTH

Introduction

The Diabetes Control and Complications Trial (DCCT) has ended any further debate as to whether the level of metabolic control of diabetes influences the development of long-term complications.[1] The DCCT was a prospective randomized trial that compared the effects of intensive treatment with those of conventional treatment on retinopathy, nephropathy and neuropathy in insulin-dependent diabetes mellitus (IDDM) subjects. Intensive treatment was aimed at producing normoglycemia and consisted of 3–4 daily injections or continuous subcutaneous infusion of insulin, frequent blood glucose monitoring, and close contact with the treatment team. Conventional treatment was aimed at producing day-to-day clinical well-being and consisted of no more than 2 insulin injections per day, urine or blood glucose monitoring, and routine quarterly contact with the clinic.

The results of the DCCT were presented in detail in the preceding chapter. In summary, they showed that intensive treatment of IDDM aimed at producing near-normal blood glucose levels reduces the risk of retinopathy, nephropathy, and neuropathy by

50–75% when compared with conventional treatment aimed at producing day-to-day clinical well-being. These risk reductions were evident in both a Primary Prevention cohort of patients with 2.5 years average IDDM duration and no detectable retinopathy at entry and in a Secondary Intervention cohort of patients with 8.5 years average duration of IDDM and minimal to moderate background retinopathy at baseline. The benefits of intensive treatment relative to conventional treatment did not become evident until approximately 3 years had elapsed, but they became progressively greater as patients were followed to 9 years. The lower rates of complications in intensively treated patients were associated with a median hemoglobin (Hb)A1c of 7.2% compared with 8.9% in the conventionally treated patients (nondiabetic range 4.0–6.0%). The difference of 1.7% in HbA1c corresponded to a difference in mean daytime blood glucose levels of 4.2 mM (8.6–12.8 mM). These lower (but still above normal) levels of glycemia were achieved with intensive treatment at the expense of a threefold greater risk of hypoglycemia and an increased risk of weight gain.

The purpose of this chapter is to discuss issues raised relative to the translation of these results into the general management of IDDM and non–insulin-dependent diabetes mellitus (NIDDM) in the community. The DCCT was, all after, a research study. The subjects were not a random sample of the IDDM population.[2] No NIDDM patients were studied. Treatment teams in each DCCT clinic were ample, professionally diverse, and included physicians, nurses, dietitians, mental health professionals, and social workers. All diabetes care and supplies were free to the patients with the generous support of the National Institute of Diabetes, Digestive and Kidney Diseases and supplementary assistance from industry. A common and constantly emphasized research goal, frequent telephone and clinic contact, and a variety of adherence activities all created strong bonding between the DCCT personnel and the patient volunteers. This was clearly evidenced by a high degree of compliance with assigned treatment and by a 99% participation in final follow-up measurements. All of the above considerations make it fair to ask whether the DCCT results are widely applicable and capable of being generally implemented.

Translation to Insulin-Dependent Diabetes Mellitus in General

To what extent can the IDDM subjects of the DCCT be considered atypical and to what extent representative of the general IDDM population? Of note is that the sample size was rather large, composing 0.2–0.3% of the estimated available IDDM population. Although the subjects' mean age of onset of their IDDM was 18 years, beyond the usual peak, 18% of the Primary Prevention cohort and 10% of the Secondary Intervention cohort were adolescents aged 13–18 at entry. Therefore, typical onset patients were certainly represented. Moreover, the adolescent subjects showed the same reduction in the risk of retinopathy, nephropathy, and neuropathy as did the adult subjects.[3] On the other hand, the patients were above average IQ, there was over-representation of better educated individuals, and there was a low percentage of economically disadvantaged and minority persons.[4] Although these factors might have influenced the success with which intensive therapy was carried out, there is no reason to believe they should have affected the biologic responses to treatment. Subjects with pre-existing hypertension, nondiabetic hyperlipemia, and in the Primary Prevention cohort with significant microalbuminuria were screened out.[2] To the extent that such factors might independently increase the risk of developing retinopathy or nephropathy, the DCCT subjects could be considered less vulnerable than the general IDDM population. However, it is not likely that the excluded individuals would have shown no response to intensive therapy, since other smaller clinical trials, which have included some such subjects, did show trends toward benefit from intensive treatment.[5,6] Moreover, the rate of progression of retinopathy in the conventional treatment group was very similar to that of a matched subset of IDDM subjects from the population-based Wisconsin Epidemiology Study of Diabetic Retinopathy (WESDR).[7] Most important, the benefits of intensive treatment with respect to retinopathy and nephropathy were evident in all subgroups of DCCT subjects stratified according to the following baseline characteristics: age, gender, duration of IDDM, HbA1c level, degree of retinopathy, blood pressure, or albumin excretion rate.[1] In addition, risk reductions for retinopathy with intensive treatment were observed across the spectrum of 29 participating clinics throughout the United States and Canada. These facts all give assurance that the conclusions of the DCCT have both external and internal validity and that the benefits of near normal glycemia should be observable generally.

A related issue is whether the implementation of intensive therapy in the DCCT was successful because of special characteristics of the cohort. This does not seem likely for two principal reasons. First, the DCCT subjects were not unusual in their prior history of metabolic control, which is itself an important factor in predicting both the subsequent HbA1c and the development of complications.[8] Their entry level of HbA1c ranged from 6.6–15.4%, with a mean of 9.0%. This level was similar to that of a contemporaneous reference group of non-DCCT IDDM subjects.[2] Second, all prospects had to agree to accept either intensive or conventional treatment on a random basis. Those individuals indicating a desire for intensive treatment assignment were eliminated from further consideration. The subjects who were randomly assigned to conventional treatment stayed with it through 97% of the follow-up time and most of the deviations to intensive treatment in this group were mandated by pregnancy.[4] These facts support the conclusion that the DCCT cohort was not unusually amenable to achieving glycemic goals with intensive treatment. Therefore, given adequate resources and motivation, the diabetes care delivery system should be able to achieve glycemic levels at least approaching those achieved by the DCCT.

Another particular concern is whether the DCCT results should be applied to children, since the eligibility criteria excluded subjects under age 13. It has been suggested that the complications clock does not usually start ticking until puberty[9] so that intensive treatment might not be needed before then. Furthermore, the vulnerability of young children to central nervous system damage from hypoglycemia is thought to be considerable.[10,11] Therefore, the benefit-to-risk ratio of intensive treatment in childhood may not warrant advising it in that age group. On the other hand, it has also been pointed out that in well-trained, motivated, and functional families, frequent insulin injections and blood glucose monitoring may be the best form of diabetes treatment for young children, both to minimize hypoglycemia and maximize consistency.[12] Therefore, a blanket injunction against employing the elements of intensive treatment under age 13 also does not seem wise. Given the lag time between starting intensive treatment and observing its benefits[1] and given the putative initiating-accelerating effect of puberty on the microvascular complications, a prudent position would be to encourage patients to begin seeking near-normal glycemia around age 10 or 11, at least pending further information. This would also offer the advantage of inculcating the intensive treatment approach before the beginning of the stormy years of adolescence when instituting any form of regimentation is known to be more difficult.

Translation to Non–Insulin-Dependent Diabetes Mellitus

Because up to 90% of all diabetic patients have NIDDM, a major public health issue is whether the DCCT conclusions and treatment recommendations that were derived from studying IDDM can be extrapolated to NIDDM. There is no totally supportable simple answer to this question at the present time. Most commentators have taken the position that with certain reservations and cautions, the DCCT results do apply to NIDDM, at least in some respects.[13–16] Considerable evidence buttresses this point of view, at least with regard to the DCCT outcomes in retinopathy, nephropathy, and neuropathy.

To begin with, there are no significant qualitative differences between the clinical or pathologic characteristics of the microvascular complications in IDDM and NIDDM. Although proliferative retinopathy is somewhat less prevalent in NIDDM, these patients show the progression from microaneurysm to diabetic retinopathy study high-risk characteristics—as well as the occurrence of macular edema—typical of IDDM.[17] Neuropathy is likewise clinically and pathologically indistinguishable between the two forms of diabetes. The classic pathologic picture of IDDM (e.g., glomerulosclerosis) is seen, although hypertension, nephrosclerosis, and pyelonephritis also contribute significantly to the development of full-blown renal failure in NIDDM.[18] In animal models of diabetes, hyperglycemia per se has been associated with all three complications, and plausible pathogenetic mechanisms by which the glucose molecule may cause damage to the retina, kidney, and peripheral nerves have been discovered.[19–24] There is no reason why these mechanisms should not be relevant to both NIDDM and IDDM. More direct evidence can be adduced. In NIDDM, a significant correlation between the HbA1c level and the prevalence of retinopathy, independent of age or treatment modality, has been shown in cross-sectional studies.[25] In subjects found on screening to have NIDDM or impaired glucose tolerance, the subsequent appearance of retinopathy has been related to the degree of baseline hyperglycemia.[26] In the WESDR study, the rate of appearance of any retinopathy and the progression of already existing nonproliferative retinopathy were similar in patients with established IDDM or NIDDM, suggesting a common pathogenesis.[17] Furthermore, in this population-based sample, the 4-year incidence and 10-year incidence and progression of retinopathy in both insulin-treated and non–insulin-treated NIDDM patients was predicted by the baseline HbA1c in a manner similar to that for IDDM subjects.[27,28] HbA1c is also a powerful predictor of the incidence of retinopathy in Pima Indians.[29]

With regard to nephropathy, studies in Pima Indians,[26] Oklahoma Indians,[30] and Rochester, Minnesota, Caucasians[31] with NIDDM have suggested that the long-term prevalence of proteinuria is positively correlated with the fasting glucose level at diagnosis, and in WESDR subjects[32] with the entry level HbA1c. The initial fasting blood glucose level may even be a weak risk factor for end-stage renal disease many years later.[33,34] In addition, reduction of blood glucose levels with diet or oral drug treatment[35] or insulin treatment[36] decreases albumin excretion rate in NIDDM as it does in IDDM patients.[1,5] In the case of neuropathy, nerve conduction velocities are inversely related to fasting plasma glucose and glycohemoglobin levels in NIDDM subjects.[37] Moreover, motor nerve conduction velocity improves when blood glucose is lowered either by sulfonylurea drugs or insulin treatment.[38] Thus a strong case can be made that treatment that normalizes blood glucose levels should reduce the risks of retinopathy, nephropathy, and neuropathy in NIDDM.

Nevertheless, as a counterpoint to the above, the following observations must also be considered. Whereas retinopathy and nephropathy are not seen at the time of clinical diagnosis in IDDM, they are found then in as many as 20% of NIDDM patients,[39–42] and microalbuminuria may even precede glucose intolerance.[42] A reasonable and widely accepted explanation for this is that NIDDM probably began 5–10 years prior to clinical presentation in these individuals, and their lack of awareness of glycosuric symptoms permitted hyperglycemic damage to the retina to occur before they saw a physician.[39] But this observation is at least theoretically open to other interpretations. In contrast to the case in IDDM, insulin resistance with accompanying hyperinsulinemia plays a major role in the pathogenesis of NIDDM, although insulin deficiency assumes increasing importance as fasting hyperglycemia develops.[43] It is not inconceivable that endogenous hyperinsulinism or even elevated plasma proinsulin levels might augment the damaging effect of hyperglycemia on certain target cells, for example, by activating insulin-like growth factor receptors.[44]

Of great importance is the fact that macrovascular disease in the form of myocardial infarction, stroke, and ischemic ulcer or amputation is the dominant cause of morbidity and mortality in NIDDM. These may already be present at the time of NIDDM diagnosis.[39] There is thus much less certainty that hyperglycemia is as important pathogenetically in causing these macrovascular complications.[45,46] Of recent concern is the specter that hyperinsulinemia or hyperproinsulinemia might actually foster atherosclerosis in NIDDM, and this has led to the greatest expressions of caution in recommending intensive insulin treatment for NIDDM subjects.[13,16] In longitudinal studies of nondiabetic and diabetic subjects, insulin levels, c-peptide levels, and insulin dose have been identified as risk factors for future cardiovascular disease and mortality.[43] Potential pathogenetic connections exist between accelerated cardiovascular disease and a variety of insulin effects on endothelial cells, lipid metabolism, and thrombogenic or fibrinolytic processes.[43] The notion that hyperinsulinemia is intrinsically related to the high prevalence of hypertension, hyperlipidemia, and cardiovascular disease in NIDDM has been given great currency and termed syndrome X, or the insulin resistance syndrome.[47] This concern that intensive insulin treatment might be more harmful than beneficial in NIDDM has been sharpened by other recent observations: an unexplained excess of myocardial infarcts and deaths during therapeutic clinical trials of proinsulin in NIDDM[48] and an increased incidence of cardiovascular events (though of borderline statistical significance) in a group of overweight NIDDM patients being treated intensively with insulin and glipizide as compared with a control group on standard insulin treatment.[49] In contrast to the latter observation, the DCCT noted a reduction in cardiovascular events and lipid risk factors with intensive as compared to conventional treatment.[1] However, the total daily dose of insulin was not significantly greater with intensive treatment than conventional treatment[4]; therefore it is not certain that the DCCT intensive treatment group was preferentially exposed to hyperinsulinemia.

This issue can only be completely resolved by a prospective, randomized, long-term clinical trial in typical NIDDM patients comparing intensive insulin treatment to diet therapy and sulfonylurea drugs, ideally aimed at similar glycemic levels in all treatment groups. The only such completed trial, the University Group Diabetes Program, showed neither increased nor decreased cardiovascular disease in a somewhat more vigorously insulin-treated group than in a standard insulin-treated group or in a diet only group.[50] However, the insulin doses used were relatively low, and many of the NIDDM subjects were only minimally hyperglycemic at the outset. No benefits from intensive treatment were seen with regard to retinopathy or nephropathy.

A recent small prospective randomized study from Japan demonstrated that intensive insulin treatment reduced the risks of development and progression of retinopathy, nephropathy, and neuropathy in NIDDM patients when compared to conventional treatment.[51] No effect on cardiovascular disease was reported. However, the subjects were not obese and their daily insulin secretion, as assessed by urinary C-peptide excretion, was only 30% of average nondiabetic levels. Thus, while this study is probably applicable to a minority of the NIDDM population, it leaves the major question unanswered for the majority of NIDDM subjects who are obese.

Our current best hope for a definitive answer lies in the ongoing United Kingdom Prospective Diabetes Study.[52] This multifactorial prospective randomized study has accrued approximately 5000 newly diagnosed NIDDM subjects with median fasting plasma glucose of 203 mg/dl. They have been randomly assigned to diet only, sulfonylurea, metformin, or insulin treatment groups. Some of the subjects already had some evidence of cardiovascular disease at entry. Yet, after a median follow-up of over 9 years, neither significant benefit with regard to microvascular complications nor significantly increased risk of cardiovascular events has been observed from insulin treatment that has kept mean blood glucose and HbA1c levels below those of the intensive treatment group in the DCCT.[52] This at least suggests that regardless of whether exogenous insulin treatment proves to be beneficial or harmful in NIDDM, the quantitative effect may be small and difficult to establish within a practical time span of study.

Given all of the above, for the present the most prudent course is to treat NIDDM patients by aiming for similar blood glucose and HbA1c targets that the DCCT now mandates for IDDM patients.[1] There is, however, one very important proviso. Diet and exercise should be used to their utmost to lower blood glucose levels in NIDDM patients. To some extent, such advice still begs the question because many patients do not maintain their initial response to these modalities.[53] When diet and exercise fail, a choice must be made between sulfonylurea drugs or exogenous insulin if the hyperglycemic contribution to the microvascular (and possibly macrovascular) complications of NIDDM is to be abolished. Sulfonylurea drugs may seem less worrisome than insulin because they may lower glucose without markedly raising peripheral plasma insulin levels.[54] But portal vein insulin levels still may be elevated and exert atherogenic effects via hepatic mechanisms. Sulfonylurea drugs may also never completely escape the shadow of the University Group Diabetes Program report incriminating them in cardiovascular death,[50] even though experience since 1970 does not seem to have substantiated such a markedly adverse effect. Metformin has now been approved for use in the United States and adds another oral drug alternative that increases responsivity to insulin but does not have notable β-cell stimulatory action.[55] Eventually, however, many NIDDM patients lose responsiveness to oral drugs.[56] This often forces an unpalatable choice: (1) either to employ intensive insulin treatment that may require very high doses in obese patients to achieve near-normal glycemia and that carries the putative risk of accelerating atherosclerosis, or (2) to accept persistent hyperglycemia.[56] Enthusiasts for combination therapy with sulfonylurea drugs and insulin offer that approach as at least a partial escape from the dilemma,[57] but there is insufficient evidence of long-term effective control of glycemia when compared with intensive insulin treatment alone.[58,59] At this juncture, physicians can only follow their own judgment, assess the evidence, and determine the appropriateness of intensive insulin treatment in each of their NIDDM patients.

Translation into Glycemic Targets and Treatment Method

Can the DCCT results with intensive treatment be translated into a specific operational target for controlling glycemic levels short of strict normality? Is there a HbA1c level in the diabetic range below which no further beneficial effect on complications is seen? It is important to remember that the DCCT was an intervention trial, designed to test the comparative efficacy and safety of two treatment regimens in IDDM. It was not designed to determine the mechanism through which one regimen might prove superior to the other or to determine whether differences in blood glucose levels were specifically instrumental in affecting rates of complications. Even if glycemia is the culprit, the study was not designed to define the optimum level of glucose to maintain. In a sense, the blood glucose profiles and the HbA1c levels that were measured regularly can be considered simply parallel treatment outcomes to the measured complications. However, because the HbA1c levels were being actively driven down in the intensive treatment group, in another sense they can be considered to reflect the ''dose of intensive treatment'' received by those subjects. But in any case the DCCT did not prospectively, in a randomized design, study the quantitative relationship between the incidence of microvascular complications and various intentionally produced and prespecified levels of glycemia such as 7.0, 8.0, or 9.0%. Therefore, the DCCT results cannot *rigorously* define an optimal blood glucose or HbA1c target for all clinicians and patients to aim for.

Nonetheless, this is such a practical translation question that it must be addressed. Therefore, the DCCT carried out a retrospective analysis of the data to determine the relationship between the incidence of retinopathy events and the mean HbA1c up to the time of each event. Within the *intensive treatment group*, a positive *curvilinear* relationship was observed (Fig. 40-1A,B). Thus, the lower the HbA1c

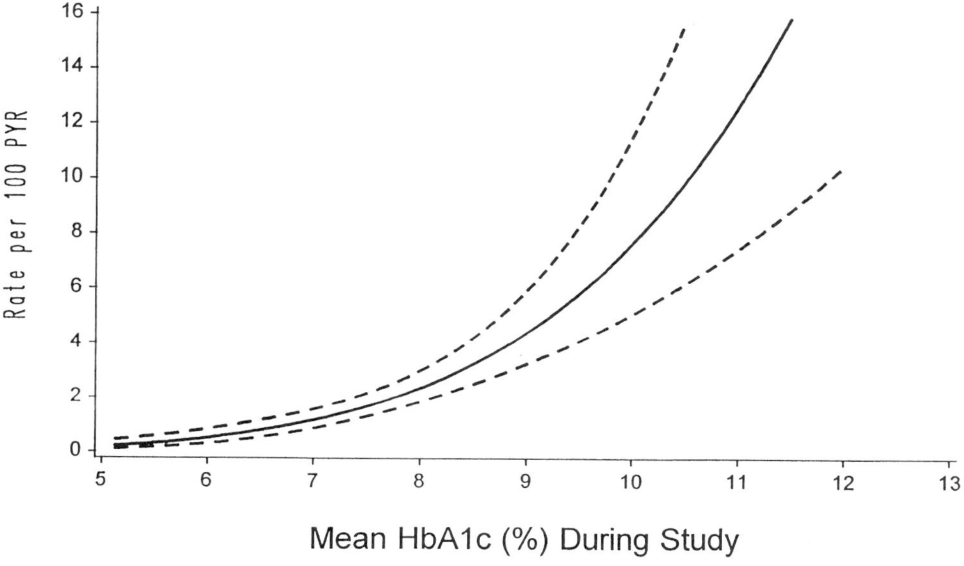

FIGURE **40-1A.** The absolute risk of a sustained progression in retinopathy is plotted against the mean HbA1c during the DCCT up to the time of the retinopathy event. A Poisson regression model was used to calculate the curve. Data are from the intensive treatment group combining the primary prevention and secondary intervention cohorts. The risk gradient is a 43% reduction in retinopathy progression for each 10% decrement in mean HbA1c (e.g., 8.0% to 7.2%). PYR = person years.

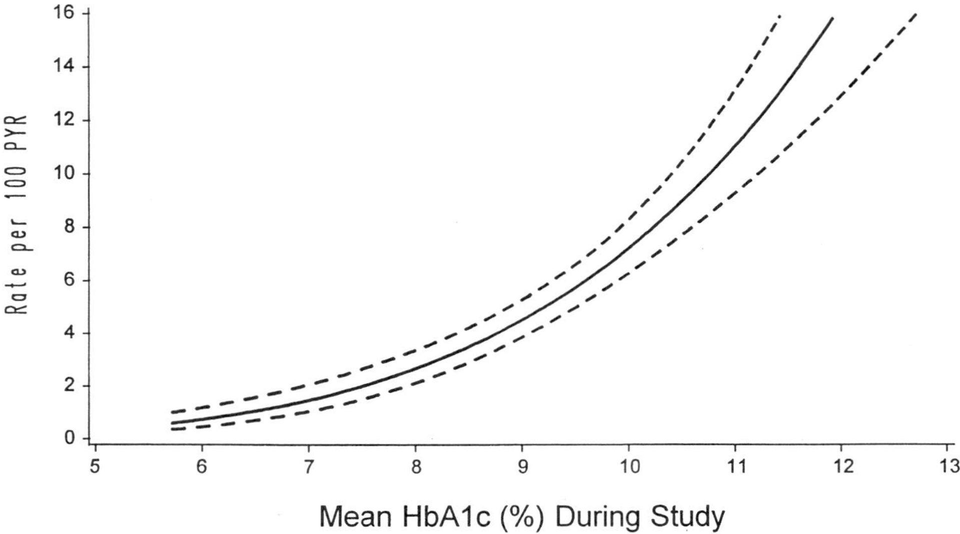

FIGURE 40-1B. The absolute risk of a sustained progression in retinopathy is plotted against the mean HbA1c during the DCCT up to the time of the retinopathy event. A Poisson regression model was used to calculate the curve. Data are from the conventional treatment group combining the primary prevention and secondary intervention cohorts. The risk gradient is a 37% reduction in retinopathy progression for each 10% decrement in mean HbA1c (e.g., 8.0% to 7.2%). PYR = person years. Figure reproduced with permission of the American Diabetes Association from the DCCT Research Group. Relationship of glycemic exposure (HbA1c) to the development and progression of retinopathy in the Diabetes Control and Complications Trial. Diabetes, 1995;44:968.

achieved with intensive treatment, the lower the corresponding risk of retinopathy. If HbA1c is looked at as an indicator of the dose of intensive treatment delivered, then the reduction in risk of retinopathy is proportional to the intensity of such treatment. This remains the most important operational conclusion of the DCCT.

The DCCT data were also modeled in a number of ways so as to explore other potential influences on the risk of retinopathy. These included the entry-level HbA1c prior to intensive treatment, the duration of IDDM, the baseline degree of retinopathy, and interactions between these and other baseline factors.[8] A higher baseline or entry level of HbA1c and a longer duration of IDDM independently increased the risk of progression of retinopathy during the trial in both groups. In addition, the entry level HbA1c predicted the mean HbA1c value during the trial. Thus, the patient's prior history of metabolic control influences events for at least some time after intensive treatment is begun. Nonetheless, once intensive treatment was established, the patient's subsequent mean HbA1c became the most important identifiable quantitative factor that determines future progression of microvascular complications.

The DCCT analyses do not show a statistically significant break point or inflection in the curve of Figure 40-1A that could be interpreted as a hyperglycemic threshold below which there is no risk of retinopathy. That is, there appears to be a continuous decrease in risk of retinopathy down to the nondiabetic range of HbA1c, implying that only complete normal glycemia with intensive treatment would yield a zero rate of retinopathy (and presumably of other complications). However, it is very difficult to maintain this utopian goal in most patients with current techniques of insulin administration (only 4% of DCCT subjects did so throughout the trial in a research setting). Furthermore, the incidence of severe hypoglycemia increases as the HbA1c is lowered (Fig. 40-2). Given these considerations, is there a practical HbA1c target that would provide most of the benefit of intensive treatment without too much of the accompanying risk of hypoglycemia? One candidate target would be the median HbA1c of the DCCT intensively treated group, that is, 7.2% (nondiabetic range 4.0–6.0%). In a population sense, this level would reduce the risk of complications 50–75% from that associated with the conventional treatment median HbA1c of 9.0%. But it must be remembered that to achieve a median HbA1c value of 7.2% and the associated average benefit, half of the patients in the DCCT intensive treatment group had to maintain HbA1c levels lower than 7.2%. Furthermore, this HbA1c was attained by a treatment program relentlessly directed toward a goal of less than 6.0%, not a goal of 7.2%. If the latter value had been the target, the final median HbA1c with intensive treat-

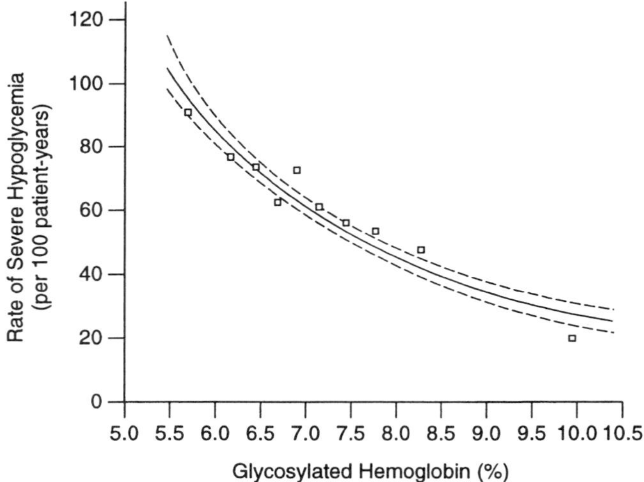

FIGURE 40-2. The rate of severe hypoglycemia is plotted against the mean HbA1c during the DCCT. Data are from the intensive treatment group combining the primary and secondary intervention cohorts. Reprinted by permission of the *New England Journal of Medicine* and Massachusetts Medical Society from the DCCT Research Group. The effect of intensive treatment of diabetes on the development and progression of long-term complications in insulin-dependent diabetes mellitus. N Engl J Med 1993;329:984.

ment may well have been higher than 7.2% and the benefit less. Finally, our knowledge of the quantitative pathogenetic association between hyperglycemia and microvascular disease does not permit us to assume that it is identical in each individual; more likely the relationship is affected by genetic[60] and environmental factors which, if we could identify them, would create a family of curves in Figure 40-1A.

For the above reasons, it is preferable with intensive treatment to strive for an HbA1c below 7.0% and as close to 6.0% as safety considerations, patient commitment, and resources permit. In terms of home-monitored blood glucose, conservative targets are 4.4–6.7 mM premeal, less than 10.0 mM postprandially, and 5.6–7.8 mM at bedtime. Such goals have been suggested in the recent American Diabetes Association Standards of Care for patients with insulin dependent and non-insulin dependent diabetes mellitus.[61] They are similar to those recently recommended by a European consensus group.[62]

A more broadly biologic interpretation of the curve in Figure 40-1A is that the risk of retinopathy increases continuously with the degree of hyperglycemia. This has been further substantiated by demonstrating a similar positive relationship in the *conventional treatment group* of the DCCT (see, Fig. 40-1B). Furthermore, in the conventionally treated group, the risk of sustained progression in retinopathy increased 37% compared with 43% in the intensively treated group for each 10% increase in the mean HbA1c (e.g., 8.0–8.8%; 9.0–9.9%). The close similarity of the quantitative relationships between the risk of retinopathy and glycemia in two separate groups of patients managed differently supports the inference that intensive treatment exerted its beneficial effects in major part by lowering blood glucose levels. Similar relationships between HbA1c and the risks of developing microalbuminuria, albuminuria, and clinical neuropathy during the trial were also demonstrated.[8] Thus, to put it succinctly, lower is better. *However, similar risk gradients do not mean that conventional treatment, as practiced in the DCCT, is as good as intensive treatment,* particularly when striving for the important lower range of HbA1c. Whereas 50% of intensively treated patients maintained a mean HbA1c of less than 7.2% throughout the study, only 5% of conventionally treated patients did so. By this criterion, the DCCT intensive treatment regimen was ten times as effective as the DCCT conventional treatment regimen in diminishing the risk of complications. Hence, these secondary analyses do not blunt the major conclusion of the DCCT Study Group, that is, intensive treatment is the superior and preferred method of managing IDDM. The analysis in the conventional group does, however, emphasize that if intensive treatment is unavailable or the goal unattainable, any significant lowering of HbA1c in an IDDM patient should be of considerable benefit in reducing the risk of complications. Conversely, if a particular patient is fortunate enough to maintain a desirable HbA1c level on a conventional regimen of two insulin injections per day, there is little reason to switch to more daily injections or to continuous subcutaneous insulin infusion (CSII).

Also of relevance to the glycemic target and treatment issue is an important time factor. The reduction in risk with intensive treatment compared to conventional treatment did not clearly become evident for either retinopathy or nephropathy until about 3 years of follow-up.[1] For retinopathy, this was accounted for in part by a transient "early worsening" phenomenon with intensive treatment[1] seen in 10% of DCCT patients during the first year. But as time went on, the cumulative incidence curves of the two treatment groups separated dramatically,[1] and the absolute risk increased far more in the conventional than in the intensive group.[8] Even when compared at similar mean HbA1c levels, the absolute risk of retinopathy increased with follow-up time in the conventional treatment group but remained stable with intensive treatment. Finally, the reduction in risk of retinopathy with intensive treatment was inversely related to IDDM duration at baseline, and it was significantly greater in the Primary Prevention cohort than in the Secondary Intervention cohort. These observations all emphasize that early intervention with intensive treatment is also important in order to halt the momentum with which retinopathy develops in the presence of hyperglycemia.

In summary, the DCCT data suggest that the nature of the relationship between glycemic exposure and the risks of complications is not determined by which form of insulin treatment is used. However, the absolute risks of developing complications is markedly lowered by employing intensive insulin treatment. Hence, all efforts should be made to engage IDDM patients in intensive treatment regimens and as early in their course of disease as possible. Near normoglycemia should also be the goal of treatment in NIDDM. Public health policy should be directed at providing the resources necessary to accomplish this.

Translation to Individual Patients

Although the DCCT results should be broadly translated, a number of therapeutic caveats are in order. The benefit-to-risk ratio for intensive treatment regimens that aim for near-normal glycemia may not be as favorable in a number of individual circumstances. (1) The most important exception is the IDDM patient with defective glucose counter-regulatory mechanisms, hypoglycemia unawareness, and/or a history of repeated severe hypoglycemic reactions. Patients who absolutely require treatment with beta-blockers and those who habitually drink large quantities of alcohol also fall into this category. Although all efforts should be made to lessen the threefold increased risk of severe hypoglycemia by preventive education and meticulous frequent adjustment of insulin regimens, diet, and exercise, it is best to raise the glycemic targets to a safer zone in these especially vulnerable individuals. (2) There is no evidence that patients who already have renal insufficiency and vision-threatening proliferative retinopathy are likely to benefit from intensive insulin treatment. However, if an IDDM patient has far advanced retinopathy but only microalbuminuria, intensive insulin treatment may still be justified to reduce the risk of future renal insufficiency. (3) A patient with 20–25 years' duration of IDDM who has developed only a few microaneurysms and no microalbuminuria with conventional treatment may not be very susceptible to hyperglycemic damage, for example, because of his or her genotype.[60] Such unusual patients could be monitored regularly and intensive treatment instituted only if complications begin to progress. (4) With advanced patient age, especially if accompanied by debilitating conditions such as Alzheimer's disease, intensive treatment would not be warranted for NIDDM or IDDM. (5) In a similar vein, individuals with malignancies or other life-shortening diseases such as acquired immunodeficiency syndrome are not good candidates for intensive treatment if they are unlikely to survive long enough to be harmed by microvascular complications. (6) Patients with active coronary artery or cerebrovascular disease on rare occasions may suffer a myocardial infarction or stroke because of hypoglycemia. This, along with their already reduced life expectancy, argues against intensive insulin treatment. (7) Individuals who live alone and/or have poor family or social support systems as well as those who have irremediably erratic behavior patterns or lifestyles may be poor candidates for intensive treatment, both on grounds of safety and a low likelihood of success.

Principles of Implementing Intensive Insulin Treatment

The case for translation of the DCCT results depends on its feasibility in real life. Although detailed discussion of all aspects of implementing intensive treatment of IDDM is beyond the scope of this chapter, the fundamental principles and key components employed by the DCCT are summarized below:

1. Self monitoring of blood glucose at least 3–4 times per day.
2. Basal delivery of insulin day and night.
3. Premeal delivery of short-acting regular insulin adjusted each time for blood glucose levels and often for anticipated carbohydrate intake as well.
4. Close attention to diet and quantitative knowledge of carbohydrate-containing foods in particular.
5. As much regularity of meal times and exercise as possible.
6. Real patient motivation to seek normal glycemia and to adjust behavior toward that end.
7. Patient acceptance of some increase in the frequency of symptomatic and asymptomatic hypoglycemia and of some weight gain.
8. A treatment team of physician, nurse, dietitian, and (as needed) a mental health professional willing to train patients in self-management, constantly remind them of glucose targets, and actively support them through interfering life situations. Although after achieving glycemic goals some patients can maintain them with less guidance from the treatment team, most require frequent contact.

Routine blood glucose self-measurements should be supplemented with extra ones to monitor unplanned exercise periods or to distinguish hypoglycemia from other causes of the symptoms. Postprandial blood glucose levels must be measured when preprandial levels are in target but HbA1c is not. Patients should also observe postprandial blood glucose responses to specific carbohydrates. Occasional 3.00 AM determinations help monitor the safety of nocturnal basal insulin doses. Reports of blood glucose levels must be reviewed regularly for adjustment of the regimen by the treatment team.

A wide variety of multiple daily injections (MDI) regimens may be used. In these, basal delivery can be provided as Ultralente, NPH (neutral protamine Hagedorn), or Lente preparations of human insulin, which is rapidly replacing animal insulin. Each of these can be given at bedtime alone or twice daily to provide the basal underpinning to premeal doses of insulin. Algorithms for premeal regular insulin boluses may have to begin at blood glucose levels as low as 60 or 70 mg/dl. Both patients and treatment teams must be willing to practice such pre-emptive administration of insulin in order to avoid undue postprandial hyperglycemia. Three injections may be enough if morning NPH or Lente, plus the regular insulin dose, covers the after lunch period adequately or if human Ultralente, given with the regular insulin dose at supper, maintains a fasting blood glucose level in the target range. When intensive regimens replace conventional ones, the total daily dose of insulin usually changes little,[4] emphasizing the importance of the flexibility of insulin doses and their coordination with blood glucose and carbohydrate intake. The same principles apply to continuous subcutaneous infusion of insulin (CSII) by external pump in which the basal insulin delivery is with regular insulin. In either MDI or CSII regimens, no more than 40–50% of the day's total insulin should usually be in the basal form. CSII offers the advantage that basal insulin delivery can be precisely tailored to different times of the day. For example, the rate can be increased at 4:00 or 5:00 AM to counter the dawn phenomenon. In a retrospective analysis of the DCCT experience with MDI and CSII as chosen and implemented treatment regimens for at least 5 years, CSII resulted in an average 0.2–0.4% lower HbA1c levels than MDI.[4] These small differences are rather similar to comparisons found in the literature.[63–65] In general, the choice of CSII versus MDI should be made based on patient desire for more lifestyle flexibility and both patient and treatment team comfort with pump use.

Implications for Delivery of Diabetes Care in the Community

Perhaps the most difficult translation issue of all is how to create a diabetes care delivery system that makes intensive treatment available to all who could benefit from it. Replication of enough DCCT-like treatment teams and resources to accomplish this, even for all IDDM patients, is currently impracticable because of cost and limitations in trained personnel. For all NIDDM patients this would essentially be out of the question. Yet, if a number of initiatives were adopted, many patients could practice intensive treatment and others could improve their regimens, the average level of glycemia in the United States could be significantly reduced, and complications could be decreased.

First, endocrinologist/diabetologist-led intensive treatment teams must learn to amplify their effectiveness by comanagement or shared arrangements with internists, pediatricians, general practitioners, and family practitioners. Managed care systems as they grow in dominance must make such cooperation economically viable, understanding that long-term savings will accrue from the preventive practices of excellent glycemic control. Second, primary care physicians who probably will continue to care for many NIDDM patients and at least some IDDM patients must be provided with reinforced education and enhanced motivation. The system should make it possible for them to commit the greatly increased time and effort required. Third, patient training in self-management provided by diabetes educators must be accepted as an integral part of any private or governmental health care reimbursement system. Time spent on the telephone or in review of blood glucose levels between visits, with corresponding adjustment of treatment regimens, must also be reimbursed in some manner. If these operational changes in the delivery of diabetes care are not brought about in a widespread fashion, the outstanding scientific achievements of the DCCT may lose their potentially huge humanitarian value.

References

1. DCCT Research Group. The effect of intensive treatment of diabetes on the development and progression of long-term complications in insulin-dependent diabetes mellitus. N Engl J Med 1993;329:977
2. DCCT Research Group. The Diabetes Control and Complications Trial (DCCT). Design and methodological considerations for the feasibility phase. Diabetes 1986;35:530
3. DCCT Research Group. The effect of intensive diabetes treatment on the development and progression of long-term complications in adolescents with insulin-dependent diabetes mellitus: The Diabetes Control and Complications Trial. Jour Pediatrics 1994;125:177
4. DCCT Research Group. Implementation of treatment protocols in The Diabetes Control and Complications Trial. Diabetes Care 1995;18:361
5. Feldt-Rasmussen B, Mathiesen ER, Deckert T. Effect of two years of strict metabolic control on progression of incipient nephropathy in insulin-dependent diabetes. Lancet 1986;2:1300
6. Reichard P, Berglund B, Britz A, et al. Intensified conventional insulin treatment retards the microvascular complications of insulin-dependent diabetes mellitus (IDDM): The Stockholm Diabetes Intervention Study (SDIS) after 5 years. J Int Med 1991;230:101
7. Klein, R and The DCCT Research Group. A comparison of the study populations in the Diabetes Control and Complications Trial and the Wisconsin Epidemiologic Study of Diabetic Retinopathy. Arch Int Med 1995;155:745
8. The DCCT Research Group. Relationship of glycemic exposure (HbA1c) to the risk of progression of complications in the Diabetes Control and Complications Trial. Diabetes 1995;44:968
9. Kostraba JN, Dorman JS, Orchard TJ, et al. Contribution of diabetes duration before puberty to development of microvascular complications in IDDM subjects. Diabetes Care 1989;12:686
10. Ryan CM, Atchison J, Puczynski S, et al. Mild hypoglycemia associated with deterioration of mental efficiency in children with insulin dependent diabetes mellitus. J Pediatrics 1990;117:32
11. Ryan C, Vega A, Drash A. Cognitive deficits in adolescents who developed diabetes early in life. Pediatrics 1985;75:921
12. Tamborlane WV, Gatecomb P, Held N, Ahern J. Implications of the DCCT results in treating children and adolescents with diabetes. Clin Diabetes 1994;12:115
13. Lasker R. The Diabetes Control and Complications Trial: Implications for policy and practice. N Engl J Med 1993;329:1035
14. Eastman RC, Seibert CW, Harris M, Gorden P. Clinical review 51: Implications for the Diabetes Control and Complications Trial. J Clin Endocrinol Metab 1993;77:1105
15. American Diabetes Association. Implications of the Diabetes Control and Complications Trial. Diabetes Care 1993;16:1517

16. Lebovitz HE. The DCCT and its implications for NIDDM. Clin Diabetes 1994;12:3
17. Davis MD. Diabetic retinopathy. Diabetes Care Review Issue 1992;15:1844
18. Parving HH, Gall MA, Skott P, et al. Prevalence and causes of albuminuria in non-insulin dependent diabetic patients. Kidney Int 1992;41:758
19. Engerman R, Bloodworth JMB Jr, Nelson S. Relationship of microvascular disease in diabetes to metabolic control. Diabetes 1977;26:760
20. Kern TS, Engerman RL. Kidney morphology in experimental hyperglycemia. Diabetes 1987;36:244
21. Engerman RL, Kern TS. Experimental Galactosemia produces diabetic-like retinopathy. Diabetes 1984;33:97
22. Kinoshita JH, Nishimura C. The involvement of abuse reductase in diabetic complications. Diabetes Metab Rev 1988;4:323
23. Brownlee M. Glycation products and the pathogenesis of diabetic complications. Diabetes Care 1992;15:1835
24. Mandarino LJ. Current hypothesis for the biochemical basis of diabetic retinopathy. Diabetes Care 1992;15:1892
25. Nathan D, Singer DE, Godine JE, et al. Retinopathy in older type II diabetics. Association with glucose control. Diabetes 1986;35:797
26. Pettitt DJ, Knowler WV, Lisse JR, Bennett PH. Development of retinopathy and proteinuria in relation to plasma-glucose concentrations in Pima Indians. Lancet 1980;2:1050
27. Klein R, Klein BEK, Moss SE, et al. Glycosylated hemoglobin and progression of diabetic retinopathy. JAMA 1988;260:2864
28. Klein R, Klein B, Moss S, et al. Relationship of hyperglycemia to the long-term incidence and progression of diabetic retinopathy. Arch Intern Med 1994;154:2169
29. Liu QZ, Pettitt DJ, Hanson RL, et al. Glycated haemoglobin, plasma glucose and diabetic retinopathy: Cross-sectional and prospective analyses. Diabetologia 1993;36:428
30. West KM, Erdreich LJ, Stober JA. A detailed study of risk factors for retinopathy and nephropathy in diabetes. Diabetes 1980;29:501
31. Ballard DJ, Humphrey LL, Melton LJ, et al. Epidemiology of persistent proteinuria in type II diabetes mellitus: Population-based study in Rochester, Minnesota. Diabetes 1988;37:405
32. Klein R, Klein BEK, Moss S. Incidence of gross proteinuria in older-onset diabetes: A population based perspective. Diabetes 1993;42:381
33. Humphrey LL, Ballard DJ, Frohnert PP, et al. Chronic renal failure in non-insulin-dependent diabetes mellitus: A population-based study in Rochester, Minnesota. Ann Int Med 1989;111:788
34. Lee ET, Lee VS, Min L, et al. Incidence of renal failure in NIDDM: The Oklahoma Indian Diabetes Study. Diabetes 1994;43:572
35. Vora JP, Dolben J, Williams JD, et al. Impact of initial treatment on renal function in newly-diagnosed type 2 (non–insulin-dependent) diabetes mellitus. Diabetologia 1993;36:734
36. Jungmann E, Carlberg C, Schumm-Draeger PM. Impact of glycaemic control on urinary albumin excretion in patients with type 2 (non–insulin-dependent) diabetes mellitus. Diabetologia 1994;37:441
37. Graf RJ, Halter JB, Halar E, Porte D. Nerve conduction abnormalities in untreated maturity-onset diabetes; relation to levels of fasting plasma glucose and glycosylated hemoglobin. Ann Int Med 1979;90:298
38. Graf RJ, Halter JB, Pfeifer MA, et al. Glycemic control and nerve function abnormalities in non-insulin dependent diabetic subjects. Ann Int Med 1981; 94:307
39. Harris MI. Undiagnosed NIDDM: Clinical and public health issues. Diabetes Care 1993;16:642
40. Morgensen CE, Damsgaard EM, Froland A, et al. Microalbuminuria in non-insulin-dependent diabetes. Clin Nephrol 1992;38:5
41. Olivarius N de F, Andreasen AH, Keiding N, Mogensen CE. Epidemiology of renal involvement in newly-diagnosed middle-aged and elderly diabetic patients: Cross-sectional data from the population-based study, ''Diabetes Care In General Practice: Denmark.'' Diabetologia 1993;36:1007
42. Mykkänen L, Haffner SM, Kuusisto J, et al. Microalbuminuria precedes the development of NIDDM. Diabetes 1994;42:552
43. Genuth S. Insulin use in NIDDM. Diabetes Care 1990;13:1240
44. Merimee TJ. Mechanisms of disease: Diabetic retinopathy—a synthesis of perspectives. New Engl J Med 1990;322:978
45. Donahue RP, Orchard TJ. Diabetes mellitus and macrovascular complications: An epidemiological perspective. Diabetes Care 1992;15:1141
46. Singer DE, Nathan DM, Anderson KM, et al. Association of HbA2c with prevalent cardiovascular disease in the original cohort of the Framingham heart study. Diabetes 1992;41:202
47. Reaven GM. Syndrome X. Clinical diabetes 1994;12:32
48. Galloway JA, Hooper SA, Spradlin CT, et al: Biosynthetic proinsulin: Review of chemistry, in vitro and in vivo receptor binding, animal and human pharmacology studies, and clinical trial experience. Diabetes Care 1992;15: 666
49. Abraira C, Johnson N, Colwell J, et al. VA cooperative study on glycemic control and complications in type II diabetes (VA CSOM): Results of the completed feasibility trial. Diabetes 1994;43:59A
50. University Group Diabetes Program. A study of the effects of hypoglycemic agents on vascular complications in patients with adult-onset diabetes. I. Design, methods, and baseline results. II. Mortality results. Diabetes 1970;19: 747
51. Ohkubo Y, Kishakawa H, Araki E, et al. Intensive insulin therapy prevents the progression of diabetic microvascular complications in Japanese patients with non–insulin-dependent diabetes mellitus: A randomized prospective 6-year study. Diabetes Research and Clinical Practice 1995;28:103
52. UK Prospective Diabetes Study Group. UK Prospective Diabetes Study (UKPDS): VIII. Study design, progress and performance. Diabetologia 1991; 34:877
53. Sonksen PH, Lowy C, Perkins JR, Slim HS. Non–insulin-dependent diabetes: 10-year outcome in relation to initial response to diet and subsequent sulfonylurea therapy. Diabetes Care 1984;7:59
54. Chu PC, Conway MJ, Krous HA, Goodner CJ. The pattern of response of plasma insulin and glucose to meals and fasting during chlorpropamide therapy. Ann Int Med 1968;68:757
55. Vigneri R, Goldfine ID. The role of metformin in treatment of diabetes mellitus. Diabetes Care 1987;10:118
56. Genuth SM. Management of the adult onset diabetic with sulfonylurea drug failure. Endocrinol Metab Clin North Am 1992;21:351
57. Riddle MC. Combined insulin and sylfonylurea therapy: A practical way to start insulin therapy for people with NIDDM. Clin Diabetes 1994;12: 57
58. Gutniak M, Karlander SG, Efendic S. Glyburide decreased insulin requirement, increases β-cell response to mixed meal, and does not affect insulin sensitivity: Effects of short- and long-term combined treatment in secondary failure to sylfonylurea. Diabetes Care 1987;10:545
59. Peters AL, Davidson MB. Insulin plus sulfonylurea agent for treating type II diabetes. Ann Int Med 1991;45:115
60. Doria A, Warram JH, Krolewski AS. Genetic predisposition to diabetic nephropathy: Evidence for a role of the angiotensin T-converting enzyme gene. Diabetes 1994;43:690
61. American Diabetes Association. Standards of medical care for patients with diabetes mellitus. Diabetes Care 1994;17:616
62. European IDDM Policy Group. Consensus guidelines for the management of insulin-dependent (type 1) diabetes. Diabetic Med 1993;10:990
63. Schiffrin AD, Desrosiers M, Aleyassine H, Belmonte MM. Intensified insulin therapy in type I diabetic adolescent: A controlled trial. Diabetes Care 1984;7:107
64. Haakens K, Hanssen KF, Dahl-Jorgensen K, et al. Continuous subcutaneous insulin infusion (CSII), multiple injection (MI) and conventional insulin therapy (CT) in self-selecting insulin-dependent diabetic patients. A comparison of metabolic control, acute complications and patient preferences. J Int Med 1990;228:457
65. Dusseldorf Study Group. Comparison of continuous subcutaneous insulin infusion and intensified conventional therapy in the treatment of type I diabetes: A two year randomized study. Diab Nutr Metab 1990;3:203

Diabetes Mellitus, edited by Derek LeRoith, Simeon I. Taylor, and Jerrold M. Olefsky. Lippincott–Raven Publishers, Philadelphia © 1996.

CHAPTER 41
Diet Therapy in Type I Diabetes

CHRISTINE BEEBE

Results of the Diabetes Control and Complications Trial (DCCT) reinforce the importance of nutrition therapy in the intensive management of type I diabetes.[1] Self-reported adherence to a prescribed diet plan was inversely related to glycosylated hemoglobin levels.[2] Specific nutrition-related behaviors associated with improved control were adhering to the prescribed snack regimen, that is, no extra snacks, and appropriate treatment of hypoglycemia. Individuals who reported adjusting insulin dose to food intake the majority of the time also had better control, although this relationship lacked statistical significance. Adherence to the nutrition regimen has repeatedly been identified as the single behavior most positively correlated with good blood glucose control in children.[3,4]

Advances in nutrition research and experience obtained from clinical trials such as the DCCT have enhanced our ability to design and implement an effective nutrition plan in diabetes. Just as diabetes is recognized as a heterogeneous disease, the nutritional management of the disease is emerging as equally heterogeneous. Individuals with type I diabetes respond to nutrient modifications differently from those with type II diabetes. Genetics, age, duration of diabetes, and the presence of complications are only a few of the factors that contribute to individual blood glucose responses to nutrient modification.

Much of the challenge associated with translating nutrition research into clinical practice involves making modifications and recommendations sufficiently reasonable so that they fit into the lifestyle of an average person. Food and eating are deeply rooted in our cultural, emotional, and physiologic well-being. Although daily self–blood glucose testing and insulin injections are imposing and unpleasant tasks, they represent new behaviors about which there are no preconceived notions or attitudes that require changing. Eating, on the other hand, is a behavior that is established early in life and is not easily changed. Indeed, clinicians and patients alike identify adhering to the diet plan as the most difficult self-management behavior necessary in treatment and control of diabetes.[5]

Altering food intake to successfully improve metabolic control is an ongoing process that requires patience, practice, skills, and knowledge before it can become a permanent behavior. Several psychosocial factors such as chronic lifestyle stress, health locus of control, attitude, support systems, and self-efficacy have been identified as influencing adherence to diet in both adults[6] and children[4] with type I diabetes. Effective implementation of any meal plan must consider such factors. Techniques for helping persons develop the necessary coping and self-efficacy skills have been described.[7]

The Nutrition Plan

Implementing the nutrition plan (Table 41-1) begins with an accurate assessment of usual food intake, including the quantity and pattern of consumption (i.e., number of meals and snacks eaten daily). Dramatic alterations in usual eating patterns produce large lifestyle changes that almost certainly result in failure to adhere to the meal plan. Fortunately, insulin regimens can be modified to adjust to almost any desired eating pattern. Calories, particularly from fat, protein, and alcohol, need to be examined and then modified only if found to be problematic. Frequency of hypoglycemic reactions and the manner in which they are treated should be assessed to aid in establishing a cause of weight gain or fluctuating blood glucose values.

Individuals with type I diabetes seek counseling at various ages and at various stages of the duration of their diabetes. Consequently, each individual has specific goals of nutrition therapy. In addition to achieving near-normal blood glucose values, these goals generally include establishing normal weight in adults and normal growth and development in children. Preventing or delaying development of complications such as cardiovascular disease and nephropathy is also a desired medical outcome that has a nutritional component. Establishing and discussing individualized goals with patients helps them understand why specific dietary modifications are necessary.

Following the nutrition assessment and goal setting process, usual food intake is modified to produce the desired medical outcomes. This process needs to be individualized to enhance learning and adherence. One of the most valuable outcomes of the DCCT was reaffirmation that a variety of teaching tools can be used to modify a person's diet successfully. The choice of which tool to use should be based on the cognitive abilities and lifestyle of the individual. Carbohydrate counting provides flexibility in quantity and types of food choices, although some individuals may need and desire the kind of structure provided by an exchange system. Several approaches may have to be implemented, recognizing that needs and priorities change throughout the lifespan.

TABLE 41-1. Implementing the Nutrition Plan

Assess usual food intake:
- Calories
- Carbohydrate, protein, fat
- Alcohol
- Supplements
- Pattern of intake

Develop nutrition goals:
- Optimal blood glucose levels
- Normal growth
- Weight gain, maintenance
- Normal serum lipids
- Reduced proteinuria
- Normal blood pressure

Implement nutrition strategies:
- General guidelines—Food Pyramid
- Exchange system
- Carbohydrate exchanges
- Carbohydrate counting

Evaluate outcome:
- Blood glucose testing
- Glycated hemoglobin
- Serum lipids
- Proteinuria
- Body weight
- Frequency of reactions

Table 41-2. 1994 American Diabetes Association Nutrition Goals, Principles, and Recommendations

Calories	* Sufficient to maintain reasonable body weight in adults * Normal growth/development in children * Adequate nutrition for pregnancy/lactation
Protein	10–20% of daily calories No less than adult RDA (0.8 g/kg/day)
Fat	Total amount varies with treatment goals Saturated fat <10% of calories, <7% with high low-density lipoprotein Polyunsaturated fat up to 10% of calories Monounsaturated fats preferred
Cholesterol	<300 mg/day
Carbohydrate	Difference after protein and fat Total amount varies with treatment goals/preferences
Sweeteners	Sucrose—not restricted in context of healthy diet, substitute as carbohydrate Nutritive sweeteners—no advantage over sucrose, substitute as carbohydrate Nonnutritive sweeteners—can be useful
Fiber	20–35 g/day, same as general population
Sodium	<3000 mg/day for overall health <2400 mg/day if hypertensive
Alcohol	No more than two alcoholic beverages/day
Vitamins/Minerals	Same as general population. Individualize if at high risk

Periodic evaluation of the efficacy of any nutrient modification is necessary to direct changes and reinforce behaviors. The DCCT experience, spanning several years, illustrated how achieving intensive metabolic control (including dietary adherence) is an ongoing process. Changes in lifestyle, cognitive and physical abilities (as with children), and in attitude toward the management regimen necessitate regular assessments and fine-tuning sessions. Glycated hemoglobin and daily blood glucose values, along with other measures of metabolic control such as lipid and urine protein levels, provide the feedback that drives adjustments in the nutrition regimen.

Clearly, the diet in type I diabetes is a dynamic component of the intensive management regimen. The DCCT reinforced the well-known concept that there is no single diet plan for managing diabetes. A nutrition plan that is well balanced and healthy, produces desired medical outcomes, and is acceptable to the person it is designed for is the best diet for that time. The American Diabetes Association's Nutrition Recommendations for individuals with diabetes published in 1994 (Table 41-2) emphasize the importance of individualizing the nutrition plan based on desired medical outcomes.[8]

Calories and Body Weight

One of the primary goals of nutrition therapy in type I diabetes is to promote normal growth in children and a reasonable body weight in adults. Since most individuals with type I diabetes are thin adults or children, there is less of a need to focus on calories as there is in type II diabetes. If weight loss has occurred prior to diagnosis, most individuals (provided they have not had a previous weight problem) consume enough calories to reach a steady state if enough insulin is available to cover food intake.

Daily caloric requirements are a composite of calories used for basal energy expenditure (nearly 70% of daily energy needs) plus the amount needed for physical activity. Age, body weight, and body composition influence basal energy expenditure and therefore daily calorie needs. Basal calorie requirements are greatest in infants and children in whom growth and development are occurring and then gradually decrease with age.

Despite the fact that body weight does not accurately reflect body composition, it is generally used when determining daily calorie needs. Several formulas exist for calculating basal energy requirements for both adults and children. The Harris-Benedict equation is considered one of the most precise methods for determining basal calorie needs, since it factors in gender, weight, height, and age. Weight is measured in kilograms, height in centimeters, and age in years:[9]

$$\text{Males: REE} = 66.47 + (13.75 \times \text{wt}) + (5.03 \times \text{ht}) - (6.75 \times \text{age})$$

$$\text{Females: REE} = 655.1 + (9.56 \times \text{wt}) + (1.85 \times \text{ht}) - (4.68 \times \text{age})$$

Actual and not ideal body weight should be used in these calculations, since the majority of individuals with type I diabetes are at or near a reasonable body weight. Confusion over whether to use ideal body weight or actual weight occurs when working with the obese patient, for whom this formula overestimates by 12% when actual weight is used and underestimates by as much as 38% when ideal body weight is used.[10] This formula can also be used in children, although the equation for males is recommended for both sexes in children under 10 years of age.[11]

Daily physical activity greatly influences total calorie needs. Despite the fact that basal energy expenditure decreases with age, a very physically active older adult may have the same daily caloric needs as a younger, less active person. The amount of calories burned in daily physical activity must be added to basal energy expenditure when calculating total calorie requirements. Simple factors can be used but all are merely estimates.[12] Children and infants expend large amounts of energy in relationship to their body weight; therefore, the physical activity factor decreases with age.

The majority of clinicians agree that the best way to estimate daily caloric needs is by asking the person what he or she eats. A food dairy or 24-hour food recall, when compiled by an experienced professional, can provide a good estimate of daily calorie needs.

Most of the time calorie intake does not need to be calculated or changed if the nutrition assessment indicates a reasonable body weight and food intake. The United States Department of Agriculture food pyramid serves as a useful guide to making daily food choices in individuals with type I diabetes.[13] Even if body weight is less than desired, individuals can be guided to increase usual intake by a few hundred calories each day with the addition of one or two food items. If glycosuria is reduced through improved blood glucose control, calorie retention will increase. Eventually, body weight will stabilize as food intake stabilizes.

As the DCCT illustrated, good diabetes control often leads to weight gain.[14] Weight gain can occur with decreased glycosuria and/or when frequent bouts of hypoglycemia occur. Treating hypoglycemia with 15–30 g of a carbohydrate food minimally contributes 60–120 kcal or more to the day's intake. Many individuals have a tendency to overtreat a hypoglycemic reaction[14] and as a result consume two or more times this amount of calories. Frequent overconsumption can eventually lead to weight gain when you consider that as few as 100 additional calories/day can result in nearly 1 lb of body fat/month. Daily food and blood glucose records assist in identifying problems with food intake. Whenever intensive management is being initiated and promoted, food intake should be assessed through routine visits to the dietitian.

Providing enough calories for growth has always been a concern when developing the nutrition plan for children with diabetes. Historically, children with diabetes are in the lowest percentiles on the growth curves.[15] This can be attributed to a combination of less than optimal diabetes control and withholding of food by parents concerned about elevated blood glucose values. Logic would imply that a child who exhibits increasing hunger may be involved in more physical activity than usual or is experiencing a growth spurt. In either case, more calories are needed if energy balance is to be maintained. Parents of children with type I diabetes need to be guided in adjusting the insulin dose to the child's increasing energy needs and be warned against withholding food or substituting noncaloric foods in an effort to keep blood glucose levels under control.

Recent concern over the increasing incidence of obesity in American children and teens[16] should be of concern when counseling children with type I diabetes. Promoting physical activity, sports, and healthy but not restrictive eating should assist in this battle. Teens, in particular, are more likely to consume large amounts of high fat-high calorie snack foods and to participate in sedentary activities. Dietary adherence and exercise correspond to lower glycated hemoglobin levels and better metabolic control in youths aged 13–18.[3] Adherence to a dietary regimen appears to decrease with the age of the youth and increasing parental nagging.[4] Health care professionals have a special obligation to work with youth to develop knowledge and self-efficacy regarding their diets and to educate parents in the appropriate management of dietary issues.

Protein

There is no scientific evidence that individuals with type I diabetes require more or less protein than the general population.[8] The nutrition plan should be individualized based on food preferences and desired medical outcomes. The recommendation for protein in the diet of persons with diabetes is thus broad at 10–20% of total daily caloric intake.

Amino acids derived from dietary protein provide substrates for cellular synthesis and new tissue formation. Such anabolic processes are greatest during periods of rapid growth such as occurs in infancy and childhood. Protein requirements are greatest at birth (2.2 g/kg) and gradually diminish until age 4 (1.2 g/kg), after which they remain stable at the adult RDA of 0.8 g/kg body weight/day.[17] This represents approximately 10% of total daily caloric intake for most individuals. Daily or periodic physical training as seen in athletes, in whom muscle tissue is continuously broken down and rebuilt, increases protein and energy needs slightly.[18] These needs are generally met by the more than adequate appetites of athletes in training.

Most individuals in the United States find it extremely easy to obtain the RDA for protein. Food consumption surveys suggest that the average protein intake varies from 14–20% of total daily calories. This represents 70–100 g daily for an individual consuming 2000 kcal. The RDA for this reference man of 76 kg would be 61 g. About 65% of dietary protein is derived from animal sources such as meat, fish, poultry, eggs, and cheese, each of which provide 7 g/oz. Remaining protein in the diet is derived from vegetables and grains, which contain an average of 3 g/serving. Thus the United States Department of Agriculture food pyramid guide of around 6 oz of meat protein daily would provide 42 g of protein; the addition of only six servings of grains and vegetables would be needed to meet the RDA of 61 g.

Since animal fat is a major source of saturated fatty acids, there is concern that reliance on meat protein contributes to increased risk of atherosclerosis and heart disease. Animal protein is considered to be of the highest biologic value to humans because it contains all the essential amino acids not made by the human body. Although this is true, the majority of world populations maintain positive nitrogen balance without consuming animal proteins. Vegetable proteins are missing one or more essential amino acids. However, if consumed from a variety of sources, these incomplete proteins can provide all the essential amino acids. Such amino acids need not be consumed simultaneously to be utilized. A vegetarian diet plan is acceptable in persons with type I diabetes.

Excessive protein consumption has been implicated in the pathogenesis of diabetic nephropathy.[19] High protein intakes increase glomerular filtration rates and renal plasma flow. Restricting protein intake in type I individuals with established proteinuria appears to retard the progression of renal disease by proteinuria and to improve hemodynamic factors.[20,21] However, responses show this effect of protein restriction to be marginal. The Modification of Diet in Renal Disease (MDRD) study[22] compared two protein levels in 585 nondiabetic patients with glomerular filtration rates (GFRs) of 25–55 mL/minute and serum creatinine levels of 1.5–3 mg/dL (equivalent to 25–50% of kidney function). Patients consumed either 1.3 g protein/kg/day or 0.58 g/kg/day. The GFR declined faster in the group consuming the lower protein diet and having the lowest blood pressures. Rate of decline was fastest in the first 4 months of the diet. Overall, this study did not show a significant difference in the rate of progression of renal disease.

These and other studies[23] imply that protein restriction may be advantageous for the person with type I diabetes. Yet confounding issues such as blood pressure control, brevity of the study periods, and inability to adhere to restricted diet regimens make it difficult to suggest protein restriction as a preventive measure or to suggest a restriction less than the RDA. Furthermore, protein undernutrition, as measured by decreased muscle strength, increased adiposity, and negative nitrogen balance, has been observed in type I patients consuming 0.6 g/kg/day for 12 weeks.[24] More research is needed on the long-term effects of protein restriction as well as how early in the course of diabetes a benefit may be derived.

Amino acids from various sources (meat, eggs, vegetables, and proteins) may differ in their effect on renal function. Meat, fish, and poultry appear to have a greater hemodynamic effect than do egg, vegetable, or soy protein.[25,26] If this is true, restricting only animal protein may be the primary protein modification necessary in persons with type I diabetes and mild albuminuria. Since severe protein restriction is difficult for patients to adhere to, this may enhance compliance. Although more research is required to differentiate the effect of different amino acids on kidney function, emphasis on moderate consumption of animal and fish proteins may be judicious for those adults who have had diabetes for over 10 years. The United States Department of Agriculture food pyramid serves as a valuable guide for nutrition prescriptions in type I diabetes.

Protein is often used in the evening snack of diabetes patients to prevent night-time hypoglycemia. During digestion, protein is broken down into amino acids that are transported via the hepatic portal vein to the liver, where they are used either in metabolic processes or converted to glucose or fat. During the fasted state specific amino acids stored in tissues are released to provide the substrate for gluconeogenesis. It is generally accepted that about 50% of protein ingested is converted to glucose via gluconeogenesis. However, this theory is based on data from 1936[27] that has never been substantiated. More recently, adding three times a standard amount of protein to a meal was found to increase the late postprandial glucose response (150–300 minutes) in persons with type I diabetes.[28] This effect is not seen with similar amounts of fat. Although prolonged hyperglycemia following a high-protein snack may be clinically advantageous in treating and preventing hypoglycemia, it is not clear how much protein is required or what ratio of protein to carbohydrate is necessary to achieve the desired outcome. Moreover, this suggests that consuming larger than usual amounts of protein at a meal or in a snack may increase insulin needs and require a patient either to decrease the carbohydrate content of the meal or to increase the premeal insulin dose.

Fat

Since protein contributes 10–20% of total calories for the day, the remaining calories are derived from a combination of fat and carbohydrates. The heterogeneity of the diabetic diet is particularly evident in the prescription for calories provided by fat and carbohydrates. The actual percentage of calories that either nutrient contributes should be based on desired level of glucose control, serum lipid levels, and food preferences of the person with diabetes.

Dietary fat does not elevate blood glucose levels. Fat slows digestion of foods and shifts the glucose response curve to the right.[28] Thus a high-fat meal or snack may appear to raise blood glucose levels when in truth the peak response is most likely delayed because of slowed absorption of carbohydrate. The purpose of fat restriction in the nutrition plan of a person with diabetes is to improve serum lipid levels in the hope of reducing the risk of cardiovascular disease.

The amount and type of fat in the diet influence serum lipid levels in the general population and in those with diabetes. The average American derives 36–37% of his or her diet from fat.[8] Restricting total fat intake to less than 30% is part of a nationwide goal to reduce both serum lipid levels and incidence of obesity.[17,29,30] Saturated fat should be restricted to under 10% of calories and dietary cholesterol to less than 300 mg/day. The atherogenic properties of saturated fat and cholesterol are well documented.[29] More recently, trans-fatty acids formed from the hydrogenation of vegetable oils have been shown to elevate serum cholesterol levels to the same extent as does saturated fat.[31]

Although it would appear that the two- to fourfold increased risk for cardiovascular disease in diabetic patients would warrant adherence to the same guidelines for fat restriction as the general population, the recommended level of total fat intake for persons with diabetes remains controversial. The controversy originates in research suggesting that substituting carbohydrate for total and saturated fat may worsen blood glucose control and serum triglyceride levels in insulin-resistant individuals with type II diabetes.[8] However, given the obscure lines of definition among the classifications of diabetes and the heterogeneity of populations, individual nutrition prescriptions for fat intake are best based on existing lipid abnormalities.

Poorly controlled type I diabetes is associated with elevated plasma lipid levels that are characterized by hypertriglyceridemia, hypercholesterolemia, and low high-density lipoprotein cholesterol levels. Adequate insulin therapy and optimal blood glucose control usually restore lipid levels to normal. Therefore, people with type I diabetes who are of relatively normal weight and have good blood glucose control have the same lipid levels as the general population of the same age and sex. Indeed, their high-density lipoprotein cholesterol levels are often higher than those of the general population.[32] However, the composition and size of the lipoprotein particles may be abnormal.[33] Such abnormalities may play a role in the increased risk for coronary atherosclerosis seen in populations with normal cholesterol levels.

The NCEP focuses on the low-fat diet as the means to reduce hypercholesterolemia and risk of coronary heart disease. The nutrition plan is driven by serum lipid levels and may contain as little as 10% of total calories from fat or as many as 35% of calories from fat. Persons with type I diabetes who have an elevated low-density lipoprotein cholesterol level despite good blood glucose control should be guided to reduce total fat intake to less than 30% of calories. Considerable evidence links saturated fat intake with coronary heart disease.[34,35] Saturated fat should be restricted to fewer than 8–10% of calories. Those with known coronary heart disease should follow the NCEP Step 2 Diet that restricts saturated fat to less than 7% of calories. Since the major source of saturated fat in the American diet is animal products, such reduction can be accomplished by decreasing intake of red meat, cheese, butter, and cream (Table 41-3).

Table 41-3. Composition of Common Dietary Fats (%)

Type	Monounsaturated Fatty Acids	Polyunsaturated Fatty Acids	Saturated Fatty Acids
Avocado	73	12	15
Canola	58	36	6
Safflower	13	78	9
Sunflower	20	69	11
Corn	25	62	13
Olive	77	9	14
Soybean	24	61	15
Sesame	41	44	15
Peanut	48	34	18
Cottonseed	19	54	27
Lard	47	12	41
Palm	39	10	41
Beef	44	4	52
Butterfat	30	4	66
Coconut	6	2	92
Chicken	45	25	30

Replacing saturated fat with 7–10% polyunsaturated fat is considered acceptable. Vegetable oils such as corn, safflower, and soy are the major sources of polyunsaturated fat in the American diet. They are considered good substitutes for saturated fat because of their serum cholesterol lowering properties.[36] Two major limitations to their use, however, have been observed. First, substituting polyunsaturated oils for saturated fat reduces not only total and low-density lipoprotein cholesterol but also high-density lipoprotein cholesterol. Second, there is concern that diets high in polyunsaturated fatty acid compromise the immune system and may contribute to cancer, although this has not been proved.

Another source of polyunsaturated fat is marine lipids or fish oils. These omega-3 fatty acids are found primarily in cold-water fish such as salmon, mackerel, halibut, albacore tuna, and herring. Epidemiologic data suggest that consumption of fish oils is negatively associated with heart disease risk.[37] Approximately 8–10 oz of fish per week has been identified as the minimum consumption needed to reduce risk. The mechanism involves lowering triglycerides (decreasing very low-density lipoprotein production), decreasing blood pressure, increasing high-density lipoprotein, and decreasing platelet aggregation.[38] Studies examining the use of fish oil supplements in reducing the hypertriglyceridemia of type II diabetes find an increase in low-density lipoprotein cholesterol and a worsening of glycemic control.[39] This effect is not seen with fish itself. Since fish is low in saturated fat and calories and contains omega-3 fatty acids, it may be prudent to recommend at least 8 oz/week. Even shellfish, which was previously restricted because of its cholesterol content, is being encouraged as a low-fat alternative to chicken and turkey because it contains similar amounts of cholesterol (75 mg/3.5 oz).

The remaining 10–16% of calories derived from fat should come from monounsaturated fat. Monounsaturated fats predominate in olive oil, peanut oil, canola oil, and avocadoes (see Table 41-3). They are the primary source of fat in the "Mediterranean diet" that has achieved popularity because of epidemiologic data linking monounsaturated fat to reduced risk of cardiovascular disease.[40] The majority of the research examining the impact of a high monounsaturated fat diet in diabetes is performed in persons with type II diabetes in whom hypertriglyceridemia is reduced when monounsaturated fats are substituted for carbohydrate in the meal plan.[41,42] Polyunsaturated fat does not appear to have the same lowering effect on very low-density lipoprotein and triglyceride as monounsaturated fat.

Probably the greatest obstacle to increasing monounsaturated fat in the American diet is the fact that foods most commonly contributing fat to the American diet do not readily lend themselves to easy incorporation of olive oil—the most concentrated source of monounsaturated fatty acids. Use of olive oil and herb mixtures for breads and olive oil and olives in pastas and salads should be encouraged. However, this type of plan may not be practical for the American culture. Canola oil can be used in baked products prepared at home, and nuts can be added to recipes. Since individuals with type I diabetes are often children or adults of normal weight, nuts (almonds, peanuts, and cashews) can be incorporated into the nutrition plan as snacks without concern for the excessive consumption that could occur with obese individuals.

Recommended dietary cholesterol intake for the general population is currently 300 mg/day. There is no evidence at the present time that persons with diabetes need to be more restrictive.[8] Control of serum lipid levels, that is, low-density lipoprotein cholesterol, should be the primary medical outcome measure driving the dietary restriction of cholesterol. Since many persons with type I diabetes have normal serum lipid values, severe restriction of dietary cholesterol may not be necessary. More scientific data are emerging that suggest heterogeneity in individual responses to cholesterol intake, that is, some persons can consume more than 300 mg cholesterol/day without detrimental effects to their serum cholesterol levels.[43] Saturated fats play a greater role in elevating serum cholesterol levels than does dietary cholesterol intake. Since eggs are considered an excellent source of protein in the diet, are low in saturated fat, and are easy to prepare and eat, their use can be beneficial in the diets of small children and older adults with diabetes.

Implementing a fat-restricted meal plan for patients with type I diabetes may not require either the structure or the strict limitations that are needed for patients with type II diabetes. Consistency in daily fat intake is not required for good blood glucose level control. Therefore, general guidelines to reduce total and saturated fat can be discussed with the patient. It is not necessary to distribute the fat grams or fat exchanges between meals and snacks. Frequently parents of children with diabetes become overwhelmed and confused by low-fat guidelines often intended for individuals with type II diabetes. Maintaining the same healthy goals for dietary fat intake as the general population should be the initial dietary goal for the person with type I diabetes. Further restrictions are warranted only if serum lipid levels are found to be abnormal.

Carbohydrates

Carbohydrates constitute the remainder of the diet after dietary protein and fat preferences have been met. Carbohydrate makes up the bulk of most nutrition plans and is the nutrient primarily responsible for the rise in blood glucose levels following ingestion of food. Carbohydrates occur as simple sugars—monosaccharides and disaccharides—and starch and fiber—polysaccharides. The digestion of carbohydrates into individual monosaccharides occurs rapidly in the mouth and small intestine; these are then absorbed into the bloodstream and transported to the hepatic portal vein. Traditionally, it has been thought that simple sugars, particularly the disaccharide sucrose, are more rapidly digested and absorbed than starches. Hence simple sugars were assumed to yield a higher glycemic response. However, scientific research has not shown this to be true.

Simple carbohydrates do not appear to raise blood glucose levels more dramatically than an equal amount of carbohydrate in the form of starch. If sucrose is fed as a single nutrient, it produces a glycemic response similar to that of bread, rice, or potatoes.[44] Furthermore, simple carbohydrates consumed as fruit, milk, or candy have lower glycemic responses than many starches. Studies substituting sugar for starch in the diet of persons with either type I[46] or type II[46] diabetes do not demonstrate a detrimental effect of sucrose.

Thus the 1994 nutrition recommendations for persons with diabetes do not advocate sugar restriction for the purposes of blood glucose control.[8] Clearly, sugar and many sugar-rich foods may need to be restricted because of their high calorie content and lack of nutritional value; however, a modest amount can be considered allowable in the context of nearly any healthy diet. If a person with type I diabetes wishes to use sucrose-containing foods, they can be substituted for another carbohydrate food in the meal plan. The total amount of carbohydrate consumed at a meal determines insulin requirements for that meal. Alterations in the carbohydrate content of a given meal require alterations in insulin dose if blood glucose levels are expected to remain constant. For example, a child consuming 30 g of carbohydrate from 2 cups of unsweetened breakfast cereal each morning may wish to substitute a sweetened breakfast cereal. Since approximately 1 cup of an average sweetened cereal provides 30 g of carbohydrate, only one cup of such cereal could be consumed. If more than 30 g of carbohydrate from either cereal were desired, the breakfast insulin dose could be increased based on a predetermined insulin-to-carbohydrate ratio.

If the type of carbohydrate does not seem to affect blood glucose response, what is responsible for differing glucose responses seen in response to foods consumed by diabetics? The glycemic index of foods (a stratification of foods based on their effect on postprandial blood glucose levels) has not proved clinically useful, but the research itself has expanded our knowledge in this area.[44] Factors such as how a food is prepared, the extent of processing, the amount and type of fiber it contains, and how it is consumed (e.g., as a liquid or solid, with or without fat) all contribute to the glycemic response. Furthermore, individual variability makes it difficult to predict a glycemic response based on the glycemic index. Recommending a food based solely on the glycemic response could compromise the nutritional value of the diet. Potato chips, for example, yield a flatter glycemic response than a baked potato because they are coated with fat. Any nutrition guideline that restricts food choices increases the risk of not providing nutrients known to be part of a healthy diet.

Since carbohydrate-rich foods have the greatest impact on postprandial blood glucose response, the primary nutrition strategy for controlling blood glucose in type I diabetes is balancing carbohydrate intake and insulin dose. Accomplishing this requires determining the amount of insulin necessary to produce a desired blood glucose response. Most individuals with type I diabetes benefit from intensive insulin therapy whereby regular insulin is taken with each meal either through separate injections or via an insulin pump. This approach allows for a more flexible food consumption pattern than previously possible with conventional therapy. Insulin dose can be adjusted to correspond to the total amount of carbohydrate consumed at the meal. Increases or decreases in carbohydrate can be accommodated with alterations in the insulin dose.

If conventional two-shot therapy is used, as in some smaller children, carbohydrate intake must be more consistent from meal to meal with little deviation. Many persons learn to adjust the Regular Insulin dose at both breakfast and dinner, but the technique is less precise than with multiple injections. Adjusting NPH insulin is difficult because it is affected by unforeseen variables in food and physical activity.

Implementing such a carbohydrate-monitored nutrition plan is usually accomplished either by carbohydrate counting[47] or by an exchange system that focuses on carbohydrate-containing foods only (Table 41-4). Once usual or desired food intake is determined for each meal and snack, insulin dose is estimated using body weight. Insulin doses are adjusted from blood glucose testing results until desired blood glucose levels are achieved. Once this evaluation is performed, an insulin-to-carbohydrate ratio can be established and used for future adjustments in insulin. Using exchanges is less precise than actually counting grams of carbohydrate because each carbohydrate exchange must be equivalent to a specific amount of

Table 41-4. Implementing Carbohydrate Counting

1. Determine goal for grams of carbohydrate to be eaten at each meal and snack (negotiate with patient)
   Example: Breakfast 45 g
   Lunch 75 g
   Snack 30 g
   Dinner 75 g
   Snack 15 g
2. Discuss how to approximate goal using:
   Food labels
   Exchange lists for carbohydrate foods
3. Estimate insulin-to-carbohydrate ratio
   Approximately 10–15 g carbohydrate/1 unit R
   Less in children under 100 lb (20–30 g/1 R)
4. Collect SMBG records for 2-hour postprandial testing
5. Adjust insulin ratio to optimize glucose response
   Decrease grams/R if blood glucose level higher than goal
   Increase gram/R if blood glucose level lower than goal
6. Teach patient how to increase or decrease insulin in relation to changes in carbohydrate intake

insulin, that is, one unit of R equals one exchange or 1/2 unit R equals 1 exchange.

Carbohydrate counting provides a level of flexibility in meal composition that has previously been absent in the diet of young individuals with type I diabetes. Focusing on carbohydrate alone also simplifies a nutrition plan for both parent and child that may enhance compliance and lead to better glycemic control. Carbohydrate counting is also useful during times of illness when carbohydrate-containing liquids need to be substituted for solid forms of carbohydrate.

Fiber

Dietary fiber, a nondigestible form of carbohydrate, appears to have an insignificant effect on glycemic control in persons with diabetes.[8] Insoluble fibers such as cellulose, lignin, and hemicellulose make up the majority of total daily fiber intake since they are found in fruits, vegetables, breads, and cereals. Insoluble fibers increase stool volume and decrease intestinal transit times, properties that make them beneficial in the treatment of constipation, hemorrhoids, and diverticulitis. Colon cancer may in fact be prevented by a high-fiber diet.[48] However, there are no data suggesting that insoluble fibers reduce either serum cholesterol levels or blood glucose levels.

Selected soluble fibers such as guar and oat gums have been reported to reduce fasting hyperglycemia and postprandial blood glucose response in type II diabetes.[49] The most widely accepted mechanism of action proposed is that soluble fibers inhibit absorption of glucose from the small intestine. Soluble fibers tend to slow the rate of gastric emptying and intestinal transit. Chronic consumption would be required to be beneficial to glycemic control. This is difficult in the American diet, since beans, lentils, and oat bran are not readily consumed at each meal.

Clinical trials indicate that chronic consumption of soluble fibers (20 g/day) modestly reduces total and low-density lipoprotein blood cholesterol levels in nondiabetic[50,51] and type II populations.[52] Problems seen in studies of persons with either type I or type II diabetes are confounding variables such as changes in body weight and insulin doses, which may contribute to improvements in blood lipid levels and glycemic control.

The lack of a strong glycemic benefit and the difficulty in routinely obtaining significant amounts of soluble fibers in the American diet have prompted the recommendation that persons with diabetes should aim for the same fiber intake as the goal set for the general population. Persons should be advised to consume fiber-rich foods with a goal of consuming approximately 20–35 g/day from a variety of sources. The United States Department of Agriculture Food Pyramid serves as a good guide. Daily consumption of five to nine servings of fruits and vegetables could provide 15–30 g, with whole grains and legumes making up the difference. Whole fruits are encouraged over juices because of their fiber content.

Sugar and Sweeteners

The average per capita consumption of sugar from all sources is approximately 95 g/day or 17–21% of total calorie intake.[53] Sucrose itself represents 9% of total calorie intake or about 41 g per person. Other commonly used sweeteners include fructose, corn sweeteners, fruit juice, fruit juice concentrate, honey, molasses, dextrose, maltose, sorbitol, mannitol, xylitol, and starch hydrolysates. They are classified as nutritive sweeteners because they provide 4 calories/g just as sucrose does. Therefore, from the standpoint of calories, these sweeteners offer no advantage over sucrose and must be accounted for in meal planning. The three polyols (sorbitol, mannitol, and xylitol) and hydrogenated starch hydrolysates are thought to be incompletely digested and absorbed and therefore may provide fewer calories than other sugars. Studies are conflicting, as the caloric values of these sugar alcohols have been defined as between 2.4 kcal/g and 3.5 kcal/g.[54,55]

Sugar alcohols produce a lower glycemic response than sucrose and other carbohydrates. However, they are often not the sole source of carbohydrate in a food, and their slightly smaller effect on postprandial blood glucose levels may be negated by the presence of these other carbohydrates. Excessive consumption of the polyols (over 50 mg/day) may have a laxative effect and produce abdominal bloating.[54] This is of particular concern with children who may consume large quantities in relation to their body weight. For the most part, products made with these sweeteners offer little advantage to persons with type I diabetes.

Fructose, a monosaccharide commonly found in fruits and vegetables, contains 4 kcal/g and produces a slightly lower blood glucose response than an equal amount of sucrose or glucose. Studies conducted in individuals with type I diabetes who substituted fructose for other forms of carbohydrate resulted in lower postprandial blood glucose responses and better blood glucose control.[56,57] The practicality of achieving improved blood glucose control from chronic substitution of fructose for sugar and concern over the hyperlipidemic effect of large fructose intakes may temper the widespread use or recommendation for this sugar at present. Increased low-density lipoprotein cholesterol levels have been demonstrated in studies of persons with diabetes.[57]

Non-nutritive sweeteners such as saccharin, aspartame, and acesulfame K do not contribute calories to the food products in which they are contained. Thus these products can be useful in sugar-free drinks, frozen treats, and gelatin products, which can be consumed freely. The Food and Drug Administration has established an acceptable daily intake for these sweeteners which is defined as the amount that can be safely consumed daily throughout one's lifetime without adverse effects.[58] It includes a 100-fold safety factor; thus, actual intake is only a small portion of the acceptable daily intake. People with diabetes consume approximately 2 to 4 mg/kg/day of these sweeteners, which is well below the US acceptable daily intake of 50 mg/kg.[59]

Micronutrients

Vitamins and minerals are utilized in small quantities by the human body, yet they play a highly specific role in facilitating energy transfer and tissue synthesis. The relationship between diabetes and micronutrients is unclear and surrounded by controversy. More studies are required that investigate the role of individual micronutrients in persons with diabetes. Many studies that exist are inconclusive because of the differences in patient populations and methodological problems with accurately measuring micronutrient status. Plasma levels do not always reflect tissue pools of micronutrients, making it difficult to identify deficiencies, particularly marginal ones.

The reciprocal nature of the micronutrient issue in diabetes is that many of these substances can directly affect blood glucose homeostasis and, in turn, poor blood glucose control can significantly alter the status of the micronutrients.[60] Poorly controlled diabetes can result in excessive loss of water-soluble vitamins and minerals. Serum magnesium levels, for example, may be low during and following diabetic ketoacidosis because of excessive urinary losses of magnesium.[61] This hypomagnesemia can potentially cause insulin resistance.[62] A study of children with diabetes found that magnesium levels decrease with increasing duration of diabetes.[63] Increased urinary excretion of the B vitamins also occurs in poorly controlled diabetes.[60] Each of these B vitamins plays a role in homeostasis and can affect glucose tolerance.

Acute and chronic complications of diabetes may be influenced by micronutrient status. Thiamine (vitamin B_1) and pyridoxine (vitamin B_6) have been implicated as both improving[64] and worsening[65] diabetic neuropathy. The antioxidant vitamins (vitamins C, E, and beta carotene) have been studied in nondiabetic populations with favorable although controversial results. Epidemiologic data and clinical studies associate a higher level of antioxidant consumption with reduced cardiovascular risk.[66] Vitamin E, the antioxidant linked most strongly to reduced risk of cardiovascular disease, is thought to function by reducing low-density lipoprotein oxidation and lipid deposits in the arteries. Plasma vitamin E levels are found to be elevated in persons with diabetes,[67] and supplementation has been found to normalize platelet aggregation[68] and reduce glycosylated hemoglobin.[69]

Deficiencies in the antioxidant vitamins do not generally exist in the United States population, but their role in reducing free radical formation is considered valuable in potentially preventing heart disease, cataracts, and cancer. Evidence suggesting that diabetes is a state of increased free radical formation indicates that these vitamins may be therapeutic.[60] More studies involving individuals with diabetes are necessary to draw conclusions regarding the efficacy of supplemental antioxidant therapy in diabetes. Increased turnover of vitamin C in type II diabetes and the high incidence of cardiovascular disease in diabetics has some clinicians wondering if the supplemental requirements for persons with diabetes may be elevated. Supplementation with the antioxidant vitamins is considered safe and to have few side effects, although long-term studies have not examined this issue directly.

People who are at greatest risk for antioxidant vitamin deficiency include people on weight-reducing diets who consume fewer than 1200–1500 kcal/day, strict vegetarians, the elderly, pregnant or lactating women, people taking medications that affect vitamin and mineral status, people in critical care environments, and people with poor metabolic control. A nutrition assessment that includes a food frequency evaluation can assist in evaluating intake.

In general, individuals who consume a healthy, well-balanced diet that mimics the United States Department of Agriculture Food Pyramid should ingest the Recommended Dietary Allowances (RDAs) for vitamins and minerals without taking supplements. The recommendation for five to nine servings of fruit and vegetables each day is targeted at providing the antioxidant vitamins C and beta carotene. Whole-grain breads and cereals as well as nuts and legumes are good sources of many of the vitamins and minerals (Table 41-5). Food preparation can have an impact on retention of water-soluble vitamins; overcooking or cooking in excess water should be discouraged in order to reduce vitamin loss.

Nutritional supplements are not necessary except in cases in which deficiencies are identified or a therapeutic trial is considered potentially beneficial. Elemental zinc has been reported to aid in wound healing in patients with leg ulcers.[70] Calcium and iron supplementation may be necessary in many women. It has been suggested that persons with type I diabetes may be at risk for significant changes in vitamin D and calcium metabolism associated with reduced bone mass.[71] Yet, epidemiologic studies do not show a higher incidence of fractures in individuals with diabetes.

Table 41-5. Selected Micronutrient Sources and Recommendations

	Food Sources	Adult RDA	Potential Role in Diabetes	Supplementation
Chromium	Brewer's yeast, liver, wheat germ	50–200 mg	Part of glucose tolerance factor	No effect unless deficient; 20 μg
Zinc	Meat, whole grains	15 mg men 12 mg women	Insulin secretion Insulin action	No effect 250 mg for wound healing
Copper	Organ meats, seafood, nuts, seeds	1.5 mg	None in humans	
Magnesium	Nuts, legumes, grains	350 mg men 280 mg women	Glucose oxidation and transport	Poor control, diabetic ketoacidosis Dose unclear
Selenium	Seafood, organ meats, grains	70 μg men 55 μg women	Antioxidant	18 mg
Iron	Meat, eggs, cereals	10 mg men 15 mg women	Minor	Toxic
Beta carotene	Carrots, sweet potatoes, cantaloupe	None 5–6 mg recommended	Antioxidant	6–15 mg
Vitamin C	Citrus fruits, strawberries, tomatoes, potatoes	60 mg	Antioxidant	250–500 mg
Vitamin E	Vegetable oils, nuts, wheat germ	15 IU men 12 IU women	Antioxidant	200–800 IU
Thiamine (vitamin B_1)	Grains, beans, meats, nuts	1.5 mg men 1.0 mg women	Carbohydrate metabolism	Not recommended 50 mg in neuropathy
Pyridoxine (vitamin B_6)	Meat, rice, eggs	2.0 men 1.6 women	Carbohydrate metabolism	Not recommended 50 mg in neuropathy

Sodium

Average sodium consumption in the general population is around 4000 to 6000 mg/day. The American Diabetes Association recommends no more than 3000 mg/day in normotensive individuals and 2400 mg/day in hypertensive persons. Although sodium has been identified as playing a role in the maintenance of blood pressure, it is apparent that the magnitude of that role differs across the spectrum of individuals with and without hypertension. Sensitivity to sodium seems greater in the Afro-American population[72] and in persons with diabetes.[73] Diabetics may have reduced sodium excretion as a result of enhanced tubular reabsorption of sodium. Since sensitivity to sodium is not easily measured, a modest approach to sodium intake is warranted.

Given the clear importance of modifying fat and carbohydrates in the diets of persons with diabetes, sodium restriction should be put into perspective. Many persons become so overwhelmed by the dietary restrictions in diabetes that long-term adherence is compromised. Dietary recommendations must be driven by desired medical outcomes. If hypertension is not a problem, as in an adolescent for example, sodium intake may need to be accorded a lower priority, at least temporarily, than other dietary modifications.

A teaspoon of salt contains about 2300 mg of sodium. Most individuals do not obtain the majority of their sodium from table salt. In fact, restricting table salt is easier for many individuals than restricting food sources of salt. Cheese, snack items, and prepared foods such as luncheon meats, soups, and convenience meals provide a great deal of salt in the diet. A good rule of thumb is that a main entree should supply less than 800 mg of sodium/day. An average snack should contain fewer than 400 mg of sodium if the day's total is to be close to 3000 mg.

Alcohol

Moderate use of alcoholic beverages is considered safe and without effect on blood glucose levels in persons with well-controlled diabetes. Nutritional guidelines published by the United States Department of Agriculture and the United States Department of Health and Human Services define moderate as a daily consumption of no more than one drink for women and two for men.[13] One drink is defined as a 12-oz beer, 5 oz of wine, or 1.5 oz of 80-proof spirits.

Alcohol increases the risk of hypoglycemia if consumed in the fasting state. This hypoglycemia is caused by impaired gluconeogenesis and is not ameliorated by glucagon. Ingestion of alcohol and alcoholic beverages should occur only with a meal or snack to reduce the likelihood of a hypoglycemic reaction. Since most individuals with type I diabetes are of normal weight, the extra calories from moderate alcohol consumption are not of major concern. Persons following a calorie-controlled meal plan can figure the calories from alcohol directly into their meal plan. Chronic alcohol ingestion may aggravate glycemic control and hypertriglyceridemia and worsen neuropathies. Individuals with a history of alcohol abuse or pregnant women should be discouraged from drinking. The effect of alcohol on blood glucose control should be discussed during nutrition counseling of everyone, but particularly in adolescents and young adults, who may be more prone to experimenting. Serious hypoglycemia can be avoided by common sense and warning discussions.

Team Approach

Diabetes is a chronic disease that requires major modifications in lifestyle, particularly in situations and conditions that include eating. The role of the team in managing diabetes should not be underestimated. Certified diabetes dietitians and nurse educators can assist the patient and the physician in implementing the necessary skills and behaviors to achieve desired medical outcomes. This needs to be an ongoing process performed throughout the life span of the individual. Type I diabetes, which can cover the entire life span from the infant to the octogenarian, is particularly challenging as patient needs are different and continuously evolving.

References

1. The Diabetes Control and Complications Trial Research Group. The effect of intensive treatment of diabetes on the development and progression of long-term complications in insulin-treated diabetes mellitus. N Engl J Med 1993; 329:977
2. Delahanty L, Halford B. The role of diet behaviors in achieving improved glycemic control in intensively treated patients in the Diabetes Control and Complications Trial. Diabetes Care 1993;16:1453
3. Burroughs TE, Pontious SL, Santiago JV. The relationship among six psychosocial domains, age, health care adherence, and metabolic control in adolescents with IDDM. Diabetes Educator 1993;19:396
4. Charron-Prochownik D, Becher MH, Brown MB, et al. Understanding young children's health beliefs and diabetes regimen adherence. Diabetes Educator 1993;19:409
5. Lockwood D, Frey ML, Hladish NA, Hiss R. The biggest problem in diabetes. Diabetes Educator 1986;12:30
6. Peyrot M, McMurry JF. Psychosocial factors in diabetes control: Adjustment of insulin-treated adults. Psychosom Med 1985;47:542
7. Rubin RR, Peyrot M. Saudek CD. The effect of a diabetes education program incorporating coping skills training on emotional well-being and diabetes self efficacy. Diabetes Educator 1993;19:210
8. Franz MJ, Horton ES, Bantle JP, et al. Nutrition principles for the management of diabetes and related complications. Diabetes Care 1994;17:490
9. Harris JA, Benedict FG. Biometric studies of basal metabolism in man. Washington DC: Carnegie Institute of Washington;1919:publication number 297
10. Feurer ID, Crosby LO, Buzby GP, et al. Resting energy expenditure in morbid obesity. Ann Surg 1983;197:17
11. Pellett PL. Food energy requirements in humans. Am J Clin Nutr 1990;51:711
12. Powers MA, ed. Nutrition Guide for Professionals. American Diabetes Association and American Dietetic Association;1988:30
13. U.S. Department of Agriculture. The Food Guide Pyramid. Hyattsville MD: USDA's Human Nutrition Information Service;1992
14. Wing RR, Klein R, Moss SE. Weight gain associated with improved glycemic control in population-based sample of subjects with type I diabetes. Diabetes Care 1990;13:1106
15. Jackson RL, Holland E, Chatman ID, et al. Growth and maturation of children with insulin-dependent diabetes mellitus. Diabetes Care 1978;1:96
16. Gortmaker SL, Dietz WH, Sobol AM, Wehler CA. Increasing pediatric obesity in the United States. Am J Disab Child 1987;141:535
17. U.S. Department of Agriculture, U.S. Department of Health and Human Services. Nutrition and Your Health: Dietary Guidelines for Americans, 3rd ed. Hyattsville, MD: USDA's Human Nutrition Information Service;1990
18. Lenon PWR. Effect of exercise on protein requirements. J Sports Sci 1991;9:53
19. Brenner BM, Meyer TW, Hostetter TH. Dietary protein intake and the progressive nature of kidney disease: The role of hemodynamically mediated glomerular injury in the pathogenesis of progressive glomerular sclerosis in aging, renal ablation and intrinsic renal disease. N Engl J Med 1982;308:652
20. Zeller K, Whittaker E, Sullivan L, et al. Effect of restricting dietary protein on the insulin-dependent diabetes mellitus. N Engl J Med 1991;324:78
21. Walker JD, Dodds RA, Murrells TJ, et al. Restriction of dietary protein and progression of renal failure in diabetic nephropathy. Lancet 1989;ii:1411
22. Klahr S, Levey AS, Beck GJ, et al. The effects of dietary protein restriction and blood pressure control on the progression of chronic renal disease. N Engl J Med 1994;330:877
23. Henry RR. Protein content of the diabetic diet. Diabetes Care 1994;17:1502
24. Brodsky IG, Robbins DC, Hiser E, et al. Effects of low protein diets on protein metabolism in insulin-dependent diabetes mellitus patients with early nephropathy. J Clin Endocrinol Metab 1992;75:351
25. Dheene M, Sabot JP, Philippart Y, et al. Effects of acute protein loads of different sources on glomerular filtration rate. Kidney Int 1987;32:S25
26. Kontessis P, Jones S, Dodds R, et al. Renal, metabolic and hormonal responses to ingestion of animal and vegetable proteins. Kidney Int 1990;38:136
27. Conn JW, Newburgh LH. The glycemic response to isoglucogenic quantities of protein and carbohydrate. J Clin Invest 1936;15:665
28. Peters AL, Davidson MG. Protein and fat effects on glucose responses and insulin requirements in subjects with insulin-dependent diabetes mellitus. Am J Clin Nutr 1993;58:555
29. Expert Panel on Detection, Evaluation and Treatment of High Blood Cholesterol in Adults: Summary of the second report of the National Cholesterol Education Program (NCEP) expert panel on detection, evaluation and treatment of high blood cholesterol in adults. JAMA 1993;269:3015
30. The Expert Panel on Blood Cholesterol Levels in Children and Adolescents. Report of the expert panel on blood cholesterol levels in children and adolescents. Pediatrics 1992;89:525

31. Mensink RP, Katan MB. Effect of dietary trans fatty acids on high-density and low-density lipoprotein cholesterol levels in healthy subjects. N Engl J Med 1990;323:439
32. Nikkila EA, Hormila P. Serum lipids and lipoprotein in insulin-treated diabetes: Demonstration of increased high density lipoprotein concentrations. Diabetes 1978;27:1078
33. Dunn FL. Plasma lipid and lipoprotein disorders in IDDM. Diabetes 1992; 41:102
34. Barr SL, Ramakrisknan R, Johnson C, et al. Reducing total dietary fat without reducing saturated fatty acids does not significantly lower total plasma cholesterol concentration in normal values. Am J Clin Nutr 1992;55:675
35. Stone NJ. Diet, blood cholesterol levels and coronary heart disease. Coronary Artery Dis 1993;4:871
36. Jacobs DR, Anderson JT, Hannan P, et al. Variability in individual serum cholesterol response to change in diet. Arteriosclerosis 1983;3:349
37. Kromhout D, Bosschieter EB, DeLezzane Coulander C. The inverse relation between fish consumption and twenty year mortality from coronary heart disease. N Engl J Med 1985;312:1205
38. Levine P, Fisher M, Schenlider P, et al. Dietary supplementation with omega 3 fatty acids prolongs platelet survival in hyperlipidemic patients with atherosclerosis. Arch Intern Med 1989;149:1115
39. Malasanos T, Stocpoole P. Biological effects ω-3 fatty acids in diabetes mellitus. Diabetes Care 1991;41:1160
40. Ginsberg H, Barr S, Gilbert A, et al. Reduction of plasma cholesterol levels in normal men on an American Heart Association step 1 diet or a step 1 diet with added monounsaturated fat. N Engl J Med 1990;322:574
41. Garg A, Bonanome A, Grundy S, et al. Comparison of a high-carbohydrate diet with high monounsaturated fat diet in patients with non-insulin dependent diabetes mellitus. N Engl J Med 1988;391:829
42. Coulston A, Hollenbeck C, Swislock A, Reaven G. Persistence of hypertriglyceridemic effect of low fat, high carbohydrate diets in NIDDM patients. Diabetes Care 1989;12:94
43. Hegsted DM, Nicolosi RJ. Individual variation in serum cholesterol levels. Proc Natl Acad Sci USA 1987;84:6259
44. Jenkins D, Wolener T, Jenkins A, et al. The glycemic response to carbohydrate foods. Lancet 1984;2:388
45. Loghmani E, Rickard K, Washburne L, et al. Glycemic response to sucrose-contaminating mixed meals in diets of children with insulin dependent diabetes mellitus. J Pediatr 1991;119:531
46. Abraira C, Derler J. Large variations of sucrose in constant carbohydrate diets in type II diabetes. Am J Med 1988;84:193
47. Gregory R, Davis D. Use of carbohydrate counting for meal planning in type I diabetes. Diabetes Educator 1994;20:406
48. National Research Council, Committee on Diet and Health, Food and Nutrition Board. Diet and health: Implications for reducing chronic disease risk. Washington DC: National Academy;1989:291
49. Blackburn NA, Redfern J, Jarjis H, et al. The mechanism of action of guar gum in improving glucose tolerance in man. Clin Sci 1984;66:329
50. Kay RM. Dietary fiber. J Food Res 1992;23:221
51. Ripsin CM, Keenan JM, Jacobs DR, Elmer PJ. Oat products and lipid lowering: A meta-analysis. JAMA 1992;267:3317
52. Aro A, Usitupa M, Voutilainen E, et al. Improved diabetic control and hypocholesterolemia effect induced by long term dietary supplementation with guar gum in type II diabetes. Diabetologia 1981;21:29
53. Glinsmann W, Irausquin H, Park Y. Evaluation of health aspects of sugars contained in carbohydrate sweeteners: Report of sugars task force, 1986. J Nutr 1986;116:21
54. Beaugerie L, Flourie B, Marteau P, et al. Digestion and absorption in the human intestine of three sugar alcohols. Gastroenterology 1990;99:717
55. Nguyen N, Dumoulin G, Henriet M, et al. Carbohydrate metabolism and urinary excretion of calcium and oxalate after ingestion of polyol sweeteners. J Clin Endocrinol Metab 1993;77:338
56. Bantle J, Laine C, Thomas J. Metabolic effects of dietary fructose and sucrose in types I and II diabetic subjects. JAMA 1986;256:3241
57. Crapo P, Kolterman O, Henry R. Metabolic consequence to two-week fructose feeding in diabetic subjects. Diabetes Care 1986;9:111
58. Morgan R, Wong O. A review of epidemiological studies on artificial sweeteners and bladder cancer. Food Chem Toxicol 1985;23:529
59. Butchko H, Kotsonis F. Acceptable intake vs actual intake: The aspartame example. J Am Coll Nutr 1991;10:258
60. Mooradian A, Failla M, Hoogwerf B, et al. Selected vitamins and minerals in diabetes. Diabetes Care 1994;17:464
61. McNair P, Christensen M, Christensen C, et al. Renal hypomagnesemia in human diabetes mellitus: Its relation to glucose homeostasis. Eur J Clin Invest 1982;12:81
62. Jain A, Gupta N, Kumar A. Some metabolic effects of magnesium in diabetes mellitus. J Assoc Physicians India 1976;24:827
63. Ewald U, Gebre-Medhin M, Luvemo T. Hypomagnesemia in diabetic children. Acta Paediatr Scand 1983;72:367
64. Kaplan W, Abourigk N. Diabetic peripheral neuropathies affecting the lower extremity. J Am Podiatr Med Assoc 1981;71:356
65. Schamberg H, Kaplan J, Windebank A, et al. Sensory neuropathy from pyridoxine abuse: A new mega vitamin syndrome. N Engl J Med 1983;309:445
66. Rim E, Stampfer M, Ascherio A, et al. Vitamin E consumption and the risk of coronary heart disease in men. N Engl J Med 1993;328:1450
67. Vatassery G, Morley H, Kuskowski M. Vitamin E in plasma and platelets of human diabetic patients and control subjects. Am J Clin Nutr 1983;37: 641
68. Kunisaki M, Umeda F, Inoguchi T, et al. Effects of vitamin E administration on platelet function in diabetes mellitus. Diabetes Res 1990;14:37
69. Ceriello A, Giugliano D, Quatraro H, et al. Vitamin E reduction of protein glycosylation in diabetes: New prospect for prevention of diabetic complications? Diabetes Care 1991;14:68
70. Hallbook T, Lanner E. Serum-zinc and healing of venous leg ulcers. Lancet 1972;2:780
71. Hui S, Epstein S, Johnston C. A prospective study of bone mass in patients with type I diabetes. J Clin Endocrinol Metab 1985;60:74
72. American Diabetes Association. Treatment of hypertension in diabetes. Diabetes Care 1993;16:1394
73. Trevisan R, Loiretto P, Semplicini A, et al. Role of insulin and a trial natriuretic peptide in sodium retention in insulin treated IDDM patients during isotonic volume expansion. Diabetes 1990;39:289

Diabetes Mellitus, edited by Derek LeRoith, Simeon I. Taylor, and Jerrold M. Olefsky. Lippincott–Raven Publishers, Philadelphia © 1996.

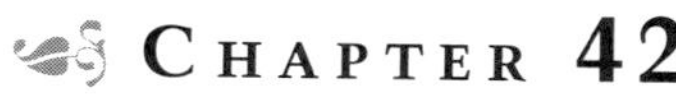

Chapter 42

Exercise for the Patient with Insulin-Dependent Diabetes Mellitus

Edward S. Horton

Introduction

Before the discovery of insulin, diet and exercise were the principal therapies used in the treatment of diabetes mellitus. In patients with insulin-dependent diabetes mellitus (IDDM), however, the ability to exercise was often severely limited because of the associated metabolic abnormalities, including muscle wasting, dehydration, and ketosis. With the advent of insulin therapy, vigorous exercise became possible for patients with IDDM, although difficult to manage. It was soon recognized that exercise potentiates the hypoglycemic effect of injected insulin,[1] and that the combination of insulin and exercise may lead to acute or delayed symptomatic hypoglycemia and decreased insulin requirements. More recently, it has also been recognized that exercise may result in a further rise in blood glucose and the rapid development of ketosis in insulin-deficient diabetics with poor metabolic control,[2] and that even in patients with well-controlled blood glucose, high-intensity exercise may result in sustained hyperglycemia.[3] Even today, standard medical teaching is that optimum blood glucose control in patients with IDDM depends on a carefully managed interaction among food intake, physical exercise, and insulin administration. Before the availability of self–blood glucose monitoring, many people with IDDM found it difficult to participate in sports or other recreational activities in which physical exercise was intermittent, and of varied intensity and duration, because of problems with the regulation of blood glucose during or after exercise. Not uncommonly, in the past, physically active and otherwise healthy persons with IDDM were not allowed to participate in organized athletics and were discouraged from participating in potentially dangerous recreational sports because of these risks.

As knowledge has increased about the multiple endocrine and neural factors that regulate blood glucose and other metabolic fuels during and after exercise, it has become both possible and safe for persons with IDDM to participate in sports or other forms of vigorous physical activity. Today, many diabetics are achieving the same level of athletic training and success in competition as their nondiabetic peers. In cross-sectional studies, however, children and young adults with IDDM tend to be less physically fit and have lower aerobic capacity than their peers without diabetes. It is not clear whether this is due to a lower average level of physical training in those with diabetes (because of inherent problems in blood glucose regulation with exercise) or to subclinical autonomic neuropathy with an impaired cardiovascular response to exercise. Most persons with IDDM show normal cardiovascular and peripheral adaptations to physical training, with the possible exception of deficient proliferation of capillaries in skeletal muscle,[4] and many have become world-class athletes. Nevertheless, the appropriate role of physical exercise in the treatment of IDDM is still somewhat controversial: Should all persons with IDDM be instructed to exercise regularly as an integral part of their treatment plan or should the role of health care professionals be to develop strategies and instruct patients to make it possible for them to participate in exercise and sports only if they wish? In recent years, the latter approach has gained favor, with the realization that there are both benefits and significant risks of exercise for patients with IDDM and that appropriate advice depends on careful evaluation of each patient with regard to personal desires, the types of exercise to be performed, and the relative benefits and risks involved. Most diabetologists now believe that the goal should be to develop educational programs for those with diabetes who want to participate in sports or other forms of physical exercise but not to recommend exercise for everyone. Educational programs should be designed to enable those with IDDM to maintain good metabolic control before, during, and after exercise and to avoid or minimize the various complications of exercise.

Benefits of Exercise

Regular physical exercise is recognized to have several benefits to health, not only for those with diabetes but for everyone. Potential benefits of exercise for patients with IDDM are listed in Table 42-1.

In addition to lowering blood glucose acutely[2,5] and increasing insulin sensitivity,[6–8] regular exercise improves several of the recognized risk factors for cardiovascular disease. Serum cholesterol and triglyceride concentrations decline with physical training due to decreases in low density and very low density lipoproteins,[9,10] and high density lipoprotein cholesterol increases.[11–13] Also, mild to moderate hypertension is reduced,[14] resting pulse rate and cardiac work are decreased, and physical working capacity, usually measured as maximal aerobic capacity (VO_2max), is increased with physical training. Since persons with diabetes are at increased risk of developing long-term complications, including premature cardiovascular disease, retinopathy, nephropathy, and neuropathy,

Table 42-1. Benefits of Exercise for Patients with Insulin-Dependent Diabetes Mellitus

1. Lower blood glucose concentration during and after exercise
2. Improved insulin sensitivity and decreased insulin requirement
3. Improved lipid profile
   a. Decreased triglycerides
   b. Slightly decreased low density lipoprotein cholesterol
   c. Increased high density lipoprotein 2 cholesterol
4. Improvement in mild to moderate hypertension
5. Increased energy expenditure
   a. Adjunct to diet for weight reduction
   b. Increased fat loss
   c. Preservation of lean body mass
6. Cardiovascular conditioning
7. Increased strength and flexibility
8. Improved sense of well-being and enhanced quality of life

all these effects of regular physical exercise may have long-term benefits for health and provide the rationale for encouraging exercise as part of daily life. Psychological benefits of exercise such as an increased sense of well-being, improved self-esteem, and an enhanced quality of life are also important for persons with diabetes, who have to cope with the anxieties and limitations of living with a chronic disease.

Despite the acute blood glucose–lowering effects of exercise and increased insulin sensitivity, some studies have failed to demonstrate a beneficial effect of regular exercise on long-term glycemic control in patients with IDDM,[15,16] although others have shown that a program of regular exercise *does* result in improved glucose control.[17,18] This may be due to the observation that persons with IDDM increase their food intake to compensate for the increased energy expenditure of exercise and that average blood glucose concentrations during a 24-hour period may not be altered.[16] Thus, an exercise program should not be prescribed for persons with IDDM for the sole purpose and expectation of improving long-term glycemic control. Individual preferences and the desire to participate in recreational exercise or sports, as well as the more general health benefits of exercise, should be the primary considerations in initiating an exercise program for a person with IDDM.

Risks of Exercise

Exercise also presents several risks for diabetics (Table 42-2), and these risks must be weighed against the potential benefits when advising persons with IDDM about participation in vigorous physical activity. As noted above, hypoglycemia may occur during or after exercise. Further, when exercise is superimposed on the insulin-deficient state, a rapid increase in blood glucose concentration and the development of ketosis may occur. Even in persons with well-controlled IDDM, brief periods of high-intensity exercise may cause hyperglycemia.

In adults, exercise may precipitate angina pectoris, myocardial infarction, cardiac arrhythmias, or sudden death if there is underlying coronary artery disease. In addition, several of the long-term complications of diabetes may be worsened by exercise. Individuals who have proliferative retinopathy are at increased risk of developing retinal or vitreous hemorrhages during vigorous exercise, and retinal detachment may occur. Vigorous exercise also increases proteinuria,[19,20] although this is probably a transient hemodynamic response, and it has not been shown that exercise leads to the progression of renal disease.

In patients with peripheral neuropathy, soft tissue and joint injuries are more likely to occur. In those with autonomic neuropathy, physical working capacity may be significantly decreased.[21] This is associated with an increased resting pulse rate and a decreased cardiovascular response to exercise,[22–24] lower maximal aerobic capacity (VO_2max),[25] and an impaired response to dehydration. Gastroparesis with an altered rate of gastric emptying may affect the absorption of food, fluid, and electrolytes.

In adults, careful screening for long-term complications of diabetes is essential before starting an exercise program of moderate to vigorous intensity. In addition to a complete history and physical examination, a dilated retinal examination to identify proliferative retinopathy, renal function tests including a screen for microalbuminuria, and a neurologic examination for peripheral and autonomic neuropathy should be completed. For persons aged 35 or more, an exercise stress test is recommended to screen for ischemic cardiac disease that may not have been previously diagnosed.

One further note: Epidemiologic data from long-term follow-up of children with type I diabetes suggest that regular physical activity early in life is not associated with an adverse effect on health. In fact, it maybe beneficial.[26]

Table 42-2. Risks of Exercise for Patients with Insulin-Dependent Diabetes Mellitus

1. Hypoglycemia
   a. Exercise-induced hypoglycemia
   b. Late-onset postexercise hypoglycemia
2. Hyperglycemia after very strenuous exercise
3. Hyperglycemia and ketosis in insulin-deficient patients
4. Precipitation or exacerbation of cardiovascular disease
   a. Angina pectoris
   b. Myocardial infarction
   c. Arrhythmias
   d. Sudden death
5. Worsening of long-term complications of diabetes
   a. Proliferative retinopathy
      - Vitreous hemorrhage
      - Retinal detachment
   b. Nephropathy
      - Increased proteinuria
   c. Peripheral neuropathy
      - Soft tissue and joint injuries
   d. Autonomic neuropathy
      - Decreased cardiovascular response to exercise
      - Decreased maximum aerobic capacity
      - Impaired response to dehydration
      - Postural hypotension
      - Altered gastrointestinal function

Regulation of Metabolic Fuels During Exercise

During the past 15 years, much has been learned about the hormonal and metabolic adaptations that occur during physical exercise, and several excellent reviews have been written on exercise and diabetes.[27–29] As more is learned about the physiology of exercise in normal subjects and the alterations that occur in diabetes mellitus, it is becoming clear that much can be done to make it possible for persons with IDDM who wish to exercise to do so with minimum risks. In this section, the regulation of metabolic fuels during exercise will be summarized and comparisons made between normal responses and the abnormalities observed in IDDM. This information can be used to develop strategies for the management of exercise in persons with diabetes who wish to participate in sports or other vigorous recreational activities.

During exercise, numerous cardiovascular, hormonal, and neural responses occur in a highly integrated fashion to ensure the delivery of oxygen and metabolic fuels to working muscle groups and to remove metabolic end products. Increased oxygen delivery and carbon dioxide removal from tissues are accomplished by increased respiration, increased cardiac output, redistribution of blood flow, and increased capillary perfusion of working muscles. Metabolic fuels are made available by a more complex system that involves breakdown of glycogen and triglyceride stores within muscle and increased delivery of substrates via the blood. Glucose and fatty acids, the major metabolic fuels for muscle, are released into the circulation from the liver and adipose tissue, respectively, and amino acids are made available by increased release from muscle.

In the resting, postabsorptive state, the blood glucose concentration is maintained at a constant level by a balance between glucose utilization and hepatic glucose production. Approximately 50% of glucose turnover is accounted for by uptake in the brain; 30–35% is taken up by other tissues, including blood cells, the kidney, and the splanchnic bed; and only 15–20% is used by the muscles. Hepatic glucose production results from a breakdown of hepatic glycogen stores through glycogenolysis and the formation of new glucose by gluconeogenesis. In normal subjects in the postprandial state, hepatic glucose production occurs predominantly by glycogenolysis; by contrast, in persons with diabetes, gluconeogenesis may account for as much as 40% of hepatic glucose production. The major gluconeogenic precursors (lactate, pyruvate, alanine, and glycerol) are derived from glycolysis and oxidation of amino acids in muscle and other peripheral tissues and from lipolysis in adipose tissue. Free fatty acids (FFA) are also released by lipolysis and provide a major substrate for energy production.

At rest, approximately 10% of the energy generated in skeletal muscle comes from glucose oxidation, 85–90% is from the oxidation of fatty acids, and only 1–2% is from amino acids.[30] With the onset of exercise, carbohydrate utilization in muscle increases abruptly and is associated with the rapid breakdown of muscle glycogen stores. The marked increase in glycolysis results in the formation of lactate, which accumulates in muscle and is released into the circulation. Within the first few minutes of exercise, blood flow to the muscles is increased, glucose uptake from the circulation occurs, and lactate release declines as aerobic metabolism is established. The increase in glucose uptake by exercising muscles is closely matched by increased hepatic glucose production, and blood glucose concentrations stay relatively constant for up to several hours during sustained, moderate-intensity exercise.

Exercise is also associated with the activation of lipolysis in adipose tissue and the release of FFA and glycerol into the circulation. FFA concentrations rise, and FFA are taken up and utilized by exercising muscle in proportion to their concentration in plasma. Lactate, pyruvate, alanine, and other gluconeogenic amino acids released from both exercising and nonexercising muscles, and glycerol released from adipose tissue, are extracted by the liver and utilized for gluconeogenesis.

Several factors influence the relative amounts of carbohydrate and FFA utilized during exercise. These include the intensity and duration of exercise, the level of physical training, the antecedent diet, and the effects of meals taken shortly before or during exercise.

As the *intensity* of exercise is increased, carbohydrate becomes a progressively more important substrate for energy production. During exercise of moderate intensity, that is, at 50% of VO_2max, muscle derives approximately 50% of its energy from carbohydrate oxidation. At intensities of 70–75% of VO_2max, carbohydrate becomes the predominant metabolic fuel. When exercise is at or near 100% of VO_2max, nearly all of the energy is derived from carbohydrate oxidation. Amino acids contribute only 1–2% of the energy required for muscular contraction at all intensities of exercise, and oxidation of lipids makes up the difference.[31] Thus, during very high intensity exercise, the carbohydrate oxidation rate is markedly increased, muscle glycogen stores are depleted rapidly, and glucose uptake from the circulation is high. If hepatic glycogen stores are adequate, hepatic glucose production is able to match or exceed peripheral utilization, and the blood glucose concentration remains constant or may actually increase.

With increasing *duration* of low- to moderate-intensity exercise, muscle and hepatic glycogen stores decline and the plasma FFA concentration increases in conjunction with increased lipolysis in adipose tissue. Fatty acid oxidation by exercising muscles increases gradually and carbohydrate oxidation decreases, so that after 2 or 3 hours of continuous exercise, FFA become the major substrate for energy production. With increasing duration of exercise, hepatic glucose production decreases and becomes progressively more dependent on gluconeogenesis, but it is usually sufficient to maintain normal blood glucose concentrations. Hypoglycemia rarely develops, but it may occur during prolonged, exhaustive exercise such as long-distance running or cycling. This hypoglycemia is usually associated with depletion of muscle and hepatic glycogen stores and with the inability of hepatic glucose production to keep up with the high rate of peripheral glucose utilization.

Physical training has a major effect on the pattern of metabolic fuel utilization during exercise. Compared to untrained persons, trained subjects perform the same amount of work at a lower percentage of VO_2max and thus utilize less carbohydrate and more FFA. Even when exercising at the same relative intensity, that is, the same percentage of VO_2max, trained subjects utilized less carbohydrate and more FFA than untrained subjects. This results in a slower rate of decline of muscle and liver glycogen stores and is associated with greater endurance.

The *antecedent diet* is also an important factor in determining substrate utilization during exercise and endurance. A carbohydrate-rich diet is associated with an increased rate of carbohydrate oxidation during exercise, and endurance is greater after a high-carbohydrate diet compared to a high-fat diet. The dietary effects on endurance during prolonged exercise are correlated with the pre-exercise muscle glycogen content, an observation that has led to the practice of "carbohydrate loading" by some participants in endurance sports.

Following exercise, glucose uptake by muscle continues to be increased, and this glucose is utilized to rebuild muscle glycogen stores. Without feeding, muscle glycogen stores are replenished rather slowly, depending on continued hepatic glucose production and maintenance of normal plasma glucose concentrations. With feeding, particularly during the first 2 hours after exercise, muscle glycogen stores are replenished more rapidly, reaching normal levels within 12–14 hours. Ingested glucose is taken up preferentially by previously exercised muscle groups, whereas hepatic glycogen stores recover at a slower rate.

The hormonal response to exercise is a complex, highly integrated system that involves activation of the sympathetic nervous system and the hypothalamic pituitary axis, as well as the suppression or release of a large number of hormones that regulate the mobilization and/or metabolism of glucose, FFA, and amino acids or alter fluid and electrolyte balance. The magnitude and pattern of the hormonal adaptation to physical activity depend on multiple factors, including the intensity and duration of the exercise; the level of physical training; and the physiologic state in which the exercise is performed, including body and environmental temperature, hydration, the supply of oxygen, and the availability of glucose and other metabolic substrates to working muscles. These responses have been reviewed extensively by Galbo[32] and Sutton and Farrell.[33]

The major physiologic effects of sympathetic nervous system activation during exercise are an increased heart rate and the development of vasoconstriction in the vascular beds supplying the splanchnic circulation, kidneys, and nonexercising muscles. These effects result in a redistribution of blood flow away from these areas and an increase in flow to exercising muscle groups. Norepinephrine and epinephrine also play major roles in the regulation of metabolic fuel mobilization and utilization, both by direct and indirect mechanisms.[34] Insulin secretion is suppressed by alpha-adrenergic stimulation, lipolysis is stimulated by beta-adrenergic stimulation, and catecholamines stimulate glycogenolysis in both liver and muscle tissue, making glucose available to provide energy for muscular contraction.

Insulin plays a key role in the regulation of metabolic fuel delivery and utilization during exercise. Its secretion is suppressed during physical activity in response to alpha-adrenergic inhibitory effects on the pancreatic β-cells. In addition, increased blood flow to working muscles results in increased insulin delivery to these tissues. The falling insulin concentration in plasma has major effects on glucose, lipid, and amino acid metabolism, making these fuels more readily available for energy production. Insulin is the major inhibitor of hepatic glucose production, and the fall in plasma insulin concentration during exercise, coupled with no change or a rise in plasma glucagon concentration, results in increased hepatic glucose output. This is closely correlated with peripheral glucose utilization and maintenance of blood glucose concentration within a normal range. In addition, the falling insulin concentration decreases the inhibitory effects on lipolysis in adipose tissue and the release of amino acids from muscle. Since little or no insulin is needed for glucose uptake in exercising muscle,[35] the fall in plasma insulin concentration does not impair glucose utilization during exercise.

Glucagon secretion increases during exercise, primarily in response to the falling glucose concentration. Glucagon responses are minimal during mild to moderate-intensity exercise. However, with very high intensity or prolonged exercise, glucagon concentration increases and plays a role in maintaining glucose homeostasis. Glucagon responses are greater in untrained than in trained individuals. The major role of glucagon is to increase the uptake of amino acids in the liver and, along with epinephrine, is the major glucose counter-regulatory hormone during exercise.[36]

During physical activity, *growth hormone* and *cortisol* concentrations also increase and are important in maintaining glucose concentrations during prolonged exercise. Cortisol and growth hormone antagonize insulin action in peripheral tissues and may limit glucose utilization in nonexercising, insulin-sensitive tissues, making more glucose available to working muscles. Several other hormones also increase during physical activity, although much less is known about their physiologic roles or their relevance to metabolic homeostasis during exercise in diabetes mellitus.

Exercise Effects on Glucose Regulation in Insulin-Dependent Diabetes Mellitus

Exercise-Induced Hypoglycemia

Whereas changes in blood glucose are very small in normal subjects during exercise, several factors may complicate glucose regulation during and after exercise in patients with IDDM. Exercise potentiates the hypoglycemic effect of injected insulin, and regular physical activity leads to a decreased insulin requirement and an increased risk of hypoglycemic reactions in insulin-treated patients. Several studies have confirmed that physical training increases sensitivity to insulin. Athletes have normal or increased tolerance to oral glucose in conjunction with low basal and glucose-stimulated insulin responses,[37] and physical inactivity results in rapidly decreased glucose tolerance.[38] Both normal control subjects and patients with diabetes have been shown to have a 30–35% increase in insulin-stimulated glucose disposal after physical training when studied by the hyperinsulinemic-euglycemic clamp technique.[39] This increase in insulin sensitivity correlates well with the training-induced increase in VO_2max and is due primarily to increased glucose uptake by muscle, associated with an increase in skeletal muscle GLUT-4 content.[40]

Acute exercise in untrained subjects is also associated with increased insulin sensitivity and glucose metabolism that persist for several hours after exercise.[41] These effects are related both to the need for replenishment of decreased muscle and liver glycogen stores and to increased glucose metabolism in muscle.

One major problem for persons with IDDM is that the plasma insulin concentration does not respond to exercise in a normal manner, thus upsetting the balance between peripheral glucose utilization and hepatic glucose production. In normal persons, the plasma insulin concentration decreases to a low level during exercise. This decrease, in conjunction with the constant or increasing plasma concentration of glucagon, promotes increased hepatic glucose production to match the increased rate of peripheral glucose utilization. The low insulin concentration during exercise also increases the lipolytic response to catecholamines, making FFA available for oxidation by exercising muscle and making glycerol available to the liver for gluconeogenesis. In IDDM, plasma insulin concentrations do not decrease during exercise and may even increase substantially if exercise is undertaken shortly after an insulin injection due to increased absorption of insulin from the subcutaneous tissue. This effect of exercise on insulin absorption is most marked if regular insulin is used and if the injection site is in a part of the body being exercised.[42] At rest, soluble human insulin is absorbed more rapidly than porcine insulin, but during exercise this difference disappears, both being absorbed more rapidly than in the resting condition. The increased absorption rate during exercise is not associated with increased cutaneous blood flow but may be due to mechanical stimulation of the injection site.[43]

Enhanced insulin absorption during exercise is most likely to occur when the insulin injection is given shortly before exercise begins. The longer the interval between injection and exercise, the less significant this effect will be and the less important it is to choose the site of injection to avoid an exercising area. Since there is considerable variation in the insulin absorption rate from different injection sites, such as the thigh, abdomen, or arm, the site may have a greater effect on the rate of insulin absorption than the exercise itself. To avoid this problem, vigorous exercise should be postponed for at least 60–90 minutes after an insulin injection. However, even with this precaution, the plasma insulin concentration does not fall normally during exercise in insulin-treated patients, and glucose homeostasis may be impaired.

The sustained insulin concentration during exercise may enhance peripheral glucose uptake and stimulate glucose oxidation by exercising muscle. However, the major effect is an inhibition of hepatic glucose production.[16] Both glycogenolysis and gluconeogenesis are inhibited by the high insulin concentration, and even though counter-regulatory hormone responses may be normal or even enhanced, the hepatic glucose production rate cannot match the rate of peripheral glucose utilization and the blood glucose concentration decreases. During mild to moderate exercise of short duration, this may be considered a beneficial effect of exercise, but during more prolonged exercise, hypoglycemia may result. This is particularly true in some diabetics in whom glucagon deficiency coexists, since the combination of high insulin and low glucagon concentrations may result in decreased gluconeogenesis and impaired hepatic glucose production.

Several factors may affect the epinephrine response to hypoglycemia in IDDM. It is now well recognized that one of the trade-offs in intensive metabolic control is an increased incidence of severe hypoglycemic reactions, many of which are associated with exercise. One possible mechanism of the increased incidence of exercise-induced hypoglycemia in patients on intensive insulin therapy is a subnormal response of epinephrine, growth hormone, and cortisol when blood glucose is lowered to 50 mg/dL.[44] This observation, coupled with the finding that epinephrine secretion is stimulated in diabetics but not in normal persons when blood glucose is decreased rapidly from 200 to 100 mg/dL, is consistent with the hypothesis that the preceding plasma glucose concentration has a major effect on the magnitude of the counter-regulatory hormone response to a falling blood glucose concentration. Furthermore, it has been clearly demonstrated that strict control of blood glucose by insulin pump therapy results in a significant decrease in the threshold glucose concentration of epinephrine and growth hormone release, as well as an increase in the sensitivity of the liver to insulin for inhibition of glucose production.[45] Thus, intensively treated patients achieve much lower blood glucose concentrations before counter-regulatory mechanisms become activated and hepatic glucose production increases.

Another factor that may contribute to exercise-induced hypoglycemia is autonomic neuropathy. Defective autonomic nervous system function has been associated with decreased catecholamine responses to and inadequate glucose counter-regulation of insulin-induced hypoglycemia in a group of patients who experienced frequent hypoglycemic reactions during intensive insulin therapy.[46] In addition, patients with autonomic neuropathy often do not show the classic warning signs of hypoglycemia before developing severe neuroglucopenia, which further compounds the problem of exercise-induced hypoglycemia.

Strategies to avoid hypoglycemia during prolonged, vigorous exercise include decreasing the insulin dose prior to exercise and taking supplemental carbohydrate feedings before and during exercise. For example, insulin should be injected at least 60 minutes before exercise and the dose decreased by 25–50%. If blood glucose is less than 100 mg/dL, supplemental feedings should be taken before and during exercise. In exhaustive, competitive events such as marathon running, insulin-dependent diabetics may omit their usual insulin dose altogether and start with an elevated blood glucose concentration that gradually falls to the normal range during the first 60 to 90 minutes of the run. As long as insulin deficiency is not severe enough to result in ketosis before exercise, metabolic fuel regulation during exercise is fairly normal, although lactate and pyruvate concentrations are greater and several of the glucose counter-regulatory hormones, including glucagon, catecholamines, growth hormone, and cortisol, increase more in diabetics than in normal persons.[47] This counter-regulatory response is probably a key factor in preventing hypoglycemia.

Because the vast majority of persons with IDDM do not participate in marathon running or similar exhausting events, it is important to develop strategies for managing more moderate forms of exercise. In persons with IDDM treated with a closed-loop "artificial endocrine pancreas," blood glucose responses following breakfast and exercise are similar to those in normal control subjects, and there is an appropriate 30% decrease in the insulin requirement during exercise. When insulin is infused at a constant rate, that is, not decreased during exercise, symptomatic hypoglycemia occurs, further demonstrating the interaction between insulin and exercise in lowering the blood glucose concentration in insulin-treated persons.[48]

The metabolic responses to moderate intensity exercise performed 30 minutes after breakfast have been studied in persons with IDDM and compared to those in normal persons.[49] In normal subjects, the expected postprandial rise in blood glucose and insulin concentrations is rapidly reversed by exercise, returning to fasting levels within 45 minutes. When exercise is stopped, there is a moderate rebound increase in glucose and insulin concentrations, which do not exceed those occurring after breakfast alone. Thus, 45 minutes of cycle exercise started 30 minutes after a meal produces a significant but transient lowering of blood glucose concentration.

In diabetic patients treated with subcutaneous insulin, responses to exercise started 30 minutes after breakfast are variable, with the majority having an improved blood glucose concentration that persists through lunch. Some patients, however, show an improved glucose concentration during lunch only, and a few show no significant improvement at all.[49] Thus, the effect of exercise after meals on blood glucose concentration and the appropriate adjustments in insulin dosage may vary considerably. Therefore, individual responses should be determined to achieve improved glucose control and avoid symptomatic hypoglycemia.

Postexercise Hypoglycemia

Another major problem for persons with IDDM is the occurrence of postexercise hypoglycemia. Many diabetics experience increased insulin sensitivity and have hypoglycemic reactions several hours after exercise, in some cases even the following day. In one study,[50] 16% of 300 young patients with IDDM who were followed prospectively for 2 years experienced postexercise, late-onset hypoglycemia, usually occurring at night 6 to 15 hours after the completion of unusually strenuous exercise or play. Although the mechanism of postexercise hypoglycemia is not well understood, it is most likely due to increased glucose uptake and glycogen synthesis in the previously exercised muscle groups, associated with increased insulin sensitivity and activation of glycogen synthase in skeletal muscle.[41] Hepatic glycogen stores also recover following exercise, but at a slower rate than occurs in muscle, so that increased requirements for dietary carbohydrate may persist for up to 24 hours after prolonged glycogen-depleting exercise. Various strategies have been used to prevent postexercise hypoglycemia, including decreasing pre-exercise doses of intermediate- or short-acting insulin and taking supplemental feedings after exercise, but no universal guidelines are totally effective and treatment regimens must be individualized.

Exercise-Induced Hyperglycemia

In contrast to moderate-intensity, sustained exercise during which the blood glucose concentration remains constant or decreases slightly, short-term, high-intensity exercise at 80% of VO_2-max or greater is normally associated with a transient increase in blood glucose concentration.[3] The rise in blood glucose during exercise reaches a peak 5 to 15 minutes after exercise is stopped and then gradually returns to the pre-exercise level within 40 to 60 minutes. This glycemic response to intense exercise is due to marked stimulation of hepatic glucose production that exceeds the rate of glucose uptake in muscle and is associated with activation of the sympathetic nervous system; a sharp rise in the concentration of glucose counter-regulatory hormones, particularly epinephrine; and suppression of insulin secretion. The energy for muscular contraction is provided predominantly by glycolysis and oxidation of glucose derived from breakdown of muscle glycogen stores, and glucose uptake from the circulation increases only gradually. Hepatic glucose production, by contrast, is stimulated rapidly by the decrease in portal vein insulin concentration, the increase in the glucagon:insulin ratio, and the rapid rise in plasma epinephrine. When exercise is stopped, there is a rapid two- to threefold increase in plasma insulin concentration, which inhibits hepatic glucose production and increases postexercise glucose uptake in muscle. As a result, the transiently elevated blood glucose concentration returns rapidly to normal.[51]

In IDDM, this highly integrated response to brief, high-intensity exercise is abnormal and sustained hyperglycemia may occur. Mitchell et al.[3] have studied the effects of exercise to exhaustion at 80% of VO_2max on glucose and hormone responses in diabetics treated with insulin pumps and in normal control subjects. In contrast to the normal subjects, blood glucose rose to much higher concentrations during postexercise recovery in the diabetic subjects and remained elevated for the entire 2-hour postexercise observation period. The pattern of postexercise hyperglycemia was influenced by the initial, pre-exercise glucose concentration, being considerably greater when the pre-exercise level was elevated. The most likely mechanism of the sustained hyperglycemic response to the high-intensity, exhausting exercise is intense autonomic nervous system stimulation of hepatic glucose production and the absence of any increase in plasma insulin during postexercise recovery in the diabetic subjects.

Since many sports and recreational activities require relatively short periods of very high intensity exercise, the sustained hyperglycemic response to this type of exercise may present a problem for persons with diabetes. At present, there are no clear guidelines for prevention or management of this response, although the administration of small doses of insulin following exercise may shorten the period of hyperglycemia. Careful self-monitoring of blood glucose levels before, during, and after exercise of different intensities and durations may provide useful information that will allow the individual patient to develop strategies to minimize the risks of either hyper- or hypoglycemia.

Exercise-Induced Ketosis

Another problem in insulin-treated diabetics occurs when exercise occurs in the presence of severe insulin deficiency. In this situation, plasma insulin concentrations are very low or absent, and hyperglycemia and ketosis are present. With the onset of exercise, peripheral glucose utilization is impaired, lipolysis is enhanced, and hepatic glucose production and ketogenesis are stimulated. In this situation the already poor metabolic control rapidly worsens, and instead of lowering blood glucose, the exercise results in a rise in blood glucose and the development of ketosis.[2] The mechanism for the rapid development of ketosis is not altogether clear, but recent studies suggest that there is a defect in peripheral clearance of ketones rather than a marked increase in ketogenesis during exercise in insulin-deprived persons.[52] To avoid this, the person with IDDM should check the blood glucose concentration and urine ketones before beginning vigorous physical activity. If blood glucose is greater than 250 md/dL and ketones are present in urine or blood, the exercise should be postponed and supplemental insulin taken to re-establish good metabolic control.

Strategies for Management of Exercise in Insulin-Dependent Diabetes Mellitus

A list of factors to consider before beginning exercise is provided in Table 42-3. Obviously, it is impossible to predict all situations because physical exercise is often spontaneous, intermittent, and varying greatly in intensity and duration from one time to the next. A number of strategies that may be useful to avoid either hypo- or hyperglycemia are outlined in Table 42-4. If exercise can be anticipated, ideally it should occur 1–3 hours after a meal when the starting blood glucose concentration is above 100 mg/dL. If exercise is prolonged and vigorous, frequent carbohydrate feedings should be taken during the activity, as well as extra food afterward to avoid postexercise hypoglycemia. If exercise is intermittent, of high intensity, and of short duration, hyperglycemia may be a problem, and small supplemental doses of insulin may be needed during postexercise recovery.

Table 42-3. Checklist Before Starting Exercise

1. *The Exercise Plan*
   a. Will the exercise be habitual or unusual?
   b. What is the anticipated intensity of exercise?
   c. How does it relate to the level of physical training?
   d. How long will it last?
   e. Will it be continuous or intermittent?
   f. How many calories will be expended?
2. *The Plan for Meals and Supplemental Feedings*
   a. When was the last meal eaten?
   b. Should a high-carbohydrate snack be eaten before starting?
   c. Should supplemental carbohydrate feedings be taken during exercise? If so, how much and how often?
   d. Will extra food be required after exercise to avoid postexercise hypoglycemia?
3. *The Insulin Regimen*
   a. What is the usual insulin mixture and dosage? Should it be decreased before or after exercise?
   b. When was the last insulin injection?
   c. Should the injection site be changed to avoid exercising areas?
4. *The Pre-Exercise Blood Glucose Concentration*
   a. Is the blood glucose concentration in a safe range to exercise (100–250 mg/dL)?
   b. If the blood glucose concentration is less than 100 mg/dL, a pre-exercise carbohydrate snack should be taken to decrease the risk of exercise-induced hypoglycemia.
   c. If the blood glucose concentration is greater than 250 mg/dL, urine ketones should be checked. If they are negative and the high glucose is due to recent food intake, it is generally safe to exercise. If they are positive, supplemental insulin should be taken and exercise delayed until ketones are negative and blood glucose is less than 250 mg/dL.

Table 42-4. Suggested Strategies to Avoid Hypo- or Hyperglycemia During and After Physical Exercise

1. *Adjustments to the Insulin Regimen*
   a. Take insulin at least 1 hour before exercise. If less than 1 hour before exercise, inject in a nonexercising area of the body.
   b. Decrease the dose of both short- and intermediate-acting insulin before exercise.
   c. Alter the daily insulin schedule.
2. *Meals and Supplemental Feedings*
   a. Eat a meal 1 to 3 hours before exercise and check to see that blood glucose is in a safe range (100–250 mg/dL) before starting exercise.
   b. Take supplemental carbohydrate feedings during exercise (at least every 30 minutes if exercise is vigorous and of long duration). Monitor blood glucose during exercise if necessary to determine the size and frequency of feedings needed to maintain a safe glucose concentration.
   c. Increase food intake for up to 24 hours after exercise, depending on the intensity and duration of exercise, to avoid late-onset postexercise hypoglycemia.
3. *Self-Monitoring of Blood Glucose and Urine Ketones*
   a. Monitor blood glucose before, during, and after exercise to determine the need for and effect of changes in insulin dosage and feeding schedule.
   b. Delay exercise if blood glucose is less than 100 mg/dL or greater than 250 mg/dL and ketones are present. Use supplemental feedings or insulin to correct glucose concentration and metabolic control before starting exercise.
   c. Learn individual glucose responses to different types, intensities, and conditions of exercise. Determine effects of exercise at different times of the day (e.g., morning, afternoon, or evening) and effects of training versus competition on blood glucose responses.

There are no precise guidelines regarding how much carbohydrate should be eaten during prolonged exercise to avoid hypoglycemia. Still, one can make some estimate of energy requirements based on the intensity and duration of the physical exercise to be performed. For example, if one is planning to go jogging, cycling, backpacking, or swimming, it might be estimated that the activity will require 600 kcal/h or 10 kcal/min. This might represent 50% of the patient's maximum aerobic capacity, an exercise intensity at which about 50% of the energy would be derived from carbohydrate oxidation. Thus, the energy requirement from carbohydrate would be approximately 5 kcal/min, equivalent to 1.25 g/min of glucose. A 30-minute period of exercise at this intensity would utilize 37.5 g of carbohydrate, partly from glycogen breakdown in muscle and partly from circulating glucose. Since glucose uptake by muscle can range from 0.2 to 0.8 g/min in a 70-kg person during cycling for up to 40 minutes[53] and up to 1.1 g after 3 hours of cycling at 70% VO_2max,[52] the precise amount of exogenous carbohydrate needed to maintain a normal blood glucose concentration is difficult to determine. Children, because of their smaller muscle mass, generally require less exogenous carbohydrate during exercise than adults. Based on an estimated glucose uptake of 0.5 to 0.8 g/min in the example given, the patient might be instructed to eat a carbohydrate snack containing 15 to 25 g carbohydrate every 30 minutes to maintain a normal blood glucose concentration during exercise.

Obviously, this kind of calculation is only approximate. Actual carbohydrate requirements depend on multiple factors, such as the intensity and duration of exercise, the level of physical conditioning, the antecedent diet, the circulating insulin concentration, and the relative need for exogenous carbohydrate to maintain blood glucose concentration in a normal range. For example, lower-intensity exercise would decrease the requirement initially, but if exercise is continued for several hours, muscle and liver glycogen levels will become depleted and more exogenous carbohydrate will be required to prevent hypoglycemia. The most practical approach is to monitor blood glucose at frequent intervals during exercise of different types and durations to determine individual responses and learn from experience.

If exercise is planned in advance, the insulin dosage and schedule may be altered to decrease the likelihood of hypoglycemia during or after exercise. Persons who take a single dose of intermediate-acting insulin may decrease the dose by 30–35% on the morning before exercise or may change to a split-dose regimen, taking two-thirds of the usual dose in the morning and one-third before the evening meal if supplemental insulin is needed after the exercise. Those who are taking a combination of intermediate- and short-acting insulin may decrease the short-acting insulin by 50% or omit it altogether before exercise. They may also decrease the intermediate-acting insulin before exercise and take supplemental doses of short-acting insulin if needed.

For those on multiple daily injections (MDI) of short-acting insulin, the dose before exercise may be decreased by 30–50% and postexercise doses adjusted based on glucose monitoring and experience with postexercise hypoglycemia. If an insulin pump is used, the basal infusion rate may be decreased during exercise and the premeal boluses decreased or omitted. If this is not done, hypoglycemia may occur during exercise,[53] although this has not been a universal finding in studies of the effects of moderate-intensity exercise on glucose homeostasis in patients treated with insulin pumps. In practice, both the intra- and postexercise basal infusion rates and premeal boluses can be adjusted based on glucose monitoring and personal experience. In advising a patient regarding these strategies, it is important to stress the individual nature of the problem and the need for careful glucose monitoring and experience. If exercise patterns are relatively consistent with respect to time of day and the intensity and duration of exercise, a routine program can often be developed to avoid either hypo- or hyperglycemia during or after exercise. If exercise is unusual, then frequent glucose monitoring will be helpful to make adjustments in insulin dosage and in the frequency and size of supplemental feedings.

Summary

Although exercise has long been recommended as an important part of the treatment of diabetes, it has often been difficult to manage by patients with IDDM because of problems with metabolic regulation and/or the presence of diabetic complications. In recent years, much has been learned about the regulation of metabolic fuel homeostasis during and after exercise. This information, combined with self–blood glucose monitoring (SBGM) and the use of MDI or insulin pump therapy, has made it possible for persons with IDDM to participate successfully and safely in a wide variety of recreational and competitive sports. Increasing numbers of diabetic athletes have found success and enjoyment in sports performance, and many have achieved world-class status or became professional athletes.

Recommendations about exercise for persons with IDDM should be made on an individual basis, taking into consideration the patient's personal attitudes and desires about exercise, his or her knowledge and skills in blood glucose management, and the presence or absence of diabetic complications that might pose risks or limitations to exercise. Based on individual assessment, education regarding the risks and benefits of exercise and the development of strategies to manage exercise safely and successfully should be provided by the health care team.

References

1. Lawrence RH. The effects of exercise on insulin action in diabetes. Br Med J 1926;1:648
2. Berger M, Berchtold P, Cuppers HJ, et al. Metabolic and hormonal effects of muscular exercise in juvenile type diabetics. Diabetologia 1977;13:355
3. Mitchell TH, Abraham G, Shiffrin A, et al. Hyperglycemia after intense exercise in IDDM subjects during continuous subcutaneous insulin infusion. Diabetes Care 1988;11:311
4. Mandroukas K, Krotkiewski M, Holm G, et al. Muscle adaptations and glucose control after physical training in insulin-dependent diabetes mellitus. Clin Physiol 1986;6:39
5. Kemmer FW, Berchtold P, Berger M, et al. Exercise-induced fall of blood glucose in insulin-treated diabetics unrelated to alteration of insulin mobilization. Diabetes 1979;28:1131
6. Bjorntorp P, de Jounge K, Sjostrom L, Sullivan L. The effect of physical training on insulin production in obesity. Metabolism 1970;19:631
7. Sato Y, Iguchi A, Sakamoto N. Biochemical determination of training effects using insulin clamp technique. Horm Metab Res 1984;16:483
8. Soman VJ, Koivisto VA, Deibert D, et al. Increased insulin sensitivity and insulin binding to monocytes after physical training. N Engl J Med 1979; 301:1200
9. Huttunen JK, Lanisimies E, Voutilainen E, et al. Effect of moderate physical exercise on serum lipoprotein. Circulation 1979;60:1220
10. Lipson LC, Bonow RW, Schaefer EJ, et al. Effect of exercise condition on plasma high-density lipoprotein and other lipoproteins. Atherosclerosis 1980; 37:529
11. Ruderman NB, Ganda OP, Johansen K. The effect of physical training on glucose tolerance and plasma lipids in maturity-onset diabetes mellitus. Diabetes 1979;28(suppl 1):89
12. Wood PD, Haskell W, Klein H, et al. Distribution of plasma lipoproteins in middle-aged male runners. Metabolism 1976;25:1249
13. Wood PD, Haskell WL. Effect of exercise on plasma high density lipoproteins. Lipids 1979;14:417
14. Horton ES. The role of exercise in the treatment of hypertension in obesity. Int J Obes 5(suppl 1);1979:89
15. Wallberg-Henriksson H, Gunnarsson R, Rossner S, Wahren J. Long-term physical training in female type I (insulin-dependent) diabetic patients: Absence of significant effect on glycemic control and lipoprotein levels. Diabetologia 1986;29:53
16. Zinman B, Murray FT, Vranic M, et al. Glucoregulation during moderate exercise in insulin treated diabetics. J Clin Endocrinol Metab 1977;45:641
17. Marrero DG, Fremion AS, Golden MP. Improving compliance with exercise in adolescents with insulin-dependent diabetes mellitus: Results of a self-motivated home exercise program. Pediatrics 1988;81:519
18. Stratton R, Wilson DP, Endres RK, Goldstein DE. Improved glycemic control after supervised 8-wk exercise program in insulin-dependent diabetic adolescents. Diabetes Care 1987;10:589
19. Mogensen CE, Vittinghus E. Urinary albumin excretion during exercise in juvenile diabetes. Scand J Clin Lab Invest 1975;35:295
20. Viberti GC, Jarrett RJ, McCartney M, Keen H. Increased glomerular permeability to albumin induced by exercise in diabetic subjects. Diabetologia 1978;14:293
21. Storstein L, Jervell J. Response to bicycle exercise testing of long-standing juvenile diabetes. Acta Med Scand 1979;205:227
22. Hilsted J, Galbo H, Christensen NJ. Impaired cardiovascular responses to graded exercise in diabetic autonomic neuropathy. Diabetes 1979;28:313
23. Kahn JK, Zola B, Juni JE, Vinik AI. Decreased exercise heart rate and blood pressure response in diabetic subjects with cardiac autonomic neuropathy. Diabetes Care 1986;9:389
24. Margonato AP, Gerundini G, Vicedomini MC, et al. Abnormal cardiovascular response to exercise in young asymptomatic diabetic patients with retinopathy. Am Heart J 1986;112:554
25. Rubler S. Asymptomatic diabetic females—exercise testing. NYS J Med 1981;81:1185
26. LaPorte RE, Dorman JS, Tajima N, et al. Pittsburgh insulin-dependent diabetes mellitus morbidity and mortality study: Physical activity and diabetic complications. Pediatrics 1986;78:1027
27. Horton ES. Role and management of exercise in diabetes mellitus. Diabetes Care 1988;11:201
28. Zinman B, Vranic M. Diabetes and exercise. Med Clin North Am 1985;69:145
29. Wallberg-Henriksson H. Exercise and diabetes mellitus. Exerc Sports Sci Rev 1992;20:339
30. Ahlborg G, Felig P, Hagenfeldt L, et al. Substrate turnover during prolonged exercise. J Clin Invest 1974;53:1080
31. Felig P, Wahren J. Fuel homeostasis in exercise. N Engl J Med 1975;293: 1078
32. Galbo H. Hormonal and Metabolic Adaptation to Exercise. New York, Thieme Stratton, 1983
33. Sutton JR, Farrell PA. Endocrine responses to prolonged exercise. In: Lamb DR, Murray R, eds. Perspectives in Exercise Science and Sports Medicine, Vol. 1: Prolonged Exercise. Indianapolis: Benchmark Press;1988:153–212
34. Clutter WE, Rizza RA, Gerich JE, Cryer PE. Regulation of glucose metabolism by sympathochromaffin catecholamines. Diabetes Metab Rev 1988;4:1

35. Richter EA, Ploug T, Galbo H. Increased muscle glucose uptake following exercise: No need for insulin during exercise. Diabetes 1985;34:1041
36. Wasserman DH, Lickley HLA, Vranic M. Interactions between glucagon and other counterregulatory hormones during normoglycemic and hypoglycemic exercise in dogs. J Clin Invest 1984;74:1401
37. Lohmann D, Liebold F, Heilmann W, et al. Diminished insulin response in highly trained athletes. Metabolism 1978;27:521
38. Lipman RL, Raskin P, Love T, et al. Glucose intolerance during decreased physical activity in man. Diabetes 1972;21:101
39. DeFronzo RA, Ferrannini E, Koivisto V. New concepts in the pathogenesis and treatment of non-insulin dependent diabetes mellitus. Am J Med 1983; 74:52
40. Goodyear LJ, Hirshman MF, Valyou PM, Horton ES. Glucose transporter number, function and subcellular distribution in rat skeletal muscle after exercise training. Diabetes 1992;41:1091
41. Bogardus C, Thuillez P, Ravussin E, et al. Effect of muscle glycogen depletion in vivo in insulin action in man. J Clin Invest 1983;72:1605
42. Kovisto V, Felig P. Effects of leg exercise on insulin absorption in diabetic patients. N Engl J Med 1978;298:77
43. Fernqvist E, Linde B, Ostman J, Gunnarsson R. Effects of physical exercise on insulin absorption in insulin-dependent diabetics. A comparison between human and porcine insulin. Clin Physiol 1986;6:489
44. Simonson DC, Tamborlane WV, DeFronzo RA, Sherwin RS. Intensive insulin therapy reduces the counterregulatory hormone responses to hypoglycemia in patients with type 1 diabetes. Ann Intern Med 1985;103:184
45. Amiel SA, Tamborlane WV, Simonson DC, Sherwin RS. Defective glucose counterregulation after strict control of insulin-dependent diabetes mellitus. N Engl J Med 1987;316:1376
46. White NH, Skor D, Cryer PE, et al. Identification of type I diabetic patients at increased risk for hyperglycemia during intensive therapy. N Engl J Med 1983;308:485
47. Meinders AE, Willekens FLA, Heere LP. Metabolic and hormonal changes in IDDM during long-distance run. Diabetes Care 1988;11:1
48. Nelson JD, Poussier P, Marliss EB, et al. Metabolic response of normal man and insulin-infused diabetics to postprandial exercise. Am J Physiol 1982; 242:E309
49. Caron D, Poussier P, Marliss EB, Zinman B. The effect of postprandial exercise on meal-related glucose intolerance in insulin-dependent diabetic individuals. Diabetes Care 1982;5:364
50. MacDonald MJ. Postexercise late-onset hypoglycemia in insulin-dependent diabetic patients. Diabetes Care 1987;10:584
51. Calles J, Cunningham JJ, Nelson L, et al. Glucose turnover during recovery from intensive exercise. Diabetes 1983;32:734
52. Fery F, deMaertalaer V, Balasse EO. Mechanism of the hyperketonaemic effect of prolonged exercise in insulin-deprived type I (insulin-dependent) diabetic patients. Diabetologia 1987;30:298
53. Schiffrin A, Parikh S, Marliss EB, Desrosier MM. Metabolic response to fasting exercise in adolescent insulin-dependent diabetic subjects treated with continuous subcutaneous insulin infusion and intensive conventional therapy. Diabetes Care 1984;7:255

Diabetes Mellitus, edited by Derek LeRoith, Simeon I. Taylor, and Jerrold M. Olefsky. Lippincott–Raven Publishers, Philadelphia © 1996.

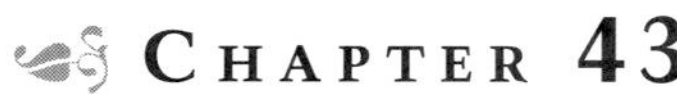

CHAPTER 43
Immune Intervention

JAY S. SKYLER AND JENNIFER B. MARKS

Type I diabetes mellitus arises as a consequence of immunologically mediated pancreatic islet β-cell destruction in genetically susceptible individuals.[1,2] The disease process evolves over a period of years, during which there appear a number of immune markers that indicate the presence of ongoing β-cell damage, accompanied by a progressive decline in β-cell function. The clinical syndrome of type I diabetes becomes evident when a majority of β-cells have been destroyed and hyperglycemia supervenes. Yet, even at disease onset, 10–20% of β-cells remain. Improvement in their function accounts for the ''honeymoon'' period often seen during the first year after the onset of type I diabetes. Moreover, the potential ''rescue'' of those residual β-cells from immune destruction was the basis for the first studies of immune intervention in human type I diabetes. The goal of intervention at disease onset is to halt the destruction of β-cells, perhaps allowing residual β-cells to recover their function, thus modifying the severity of clinical manifestations. More recently, intervention trials have been initiated during the period of evolution of the disease before the development of clinical hyperglycemia. The goals of intervention before disease onset are to arrest the immune destruction and thus delay or prevent clinical disease.

A review of immune intervention studies in human type I diabetes can be divided into three categories—pilot studies, clinical trials in new-onset diabetes, and clinical trials aimed at prevention of overt diabetes. It should be mentioned, too, that the scientific basis for all of the intervention strategies tested in human beings has been well established in animal models. In particular, there have been extensive studies in the NOD (nonobese diabetic) mouse and the BB (Biobreeding) rat, two models of spontaneous type I diabetes.

Most of the animal studies have been aimed at disease prevention.[2] In contrast, all of the early human studies were initiated at the time of clinical diagnosis.[3–5] This was done to ensure that the subjects participating in the clinical investigations clearly had the disease. Yet, the trade-off is that by the time of disease onset, most β-cell function has been lost, making the demonstration of successful intervention more difficult. In fact, it is quite possible that interventions that might be successful if applied early would fail to be effective when tested so late in the course of the disease. Appreciation of this dilemma, coupled with better predictors of disease development, has led to the newer approach of controlled trials designed to test interventions that might delay or prevent the development of clinical hyperglycemia. However, interventions used in these otherwise healthy persons must be confined to ones with a very favorable safety profile.

During the stage of disease evolution, predicting which persons are destined to develop the disease is crucial in testing any intervention strategy. For ease of implementation, attention has focused on first-degree relatives of patients with type I diabetes, because such relatives have a 10–20-fold increased empiric risk of developing type I diabetes (about 3–6% among first-degree relatives) compared to the general population (prevalence of about 0.25–0.3%). Nevertheless, perhaps as many as 80–90% of persons with new-onset type I diabetes do not have a first-degree relative previously known to have the disease. Consequently, all of these persons would be missed by an approach confined to relatives. In the long run, there are two options for these nonrelatives: either to identify combinations of genetic and immune markers suitable for screening of the general population to identify those at risk of developing the disease or to develop a simple prevention strategy (e.g., a vaccine) that could be used in the entire population.

This chapter will review the pivotal immune intervention studies that have been conducted and are currently in progress or planned.

Pilot Studies

Pilot studies have been conducted in persons with established diabetes, usually of recent onset. Most of these studies involved insufficient numbers of subjects to draw any firm conclusions, at least with the endpoints used. Thus, although many assume that these were apparently ineffective in altering the clinical course of type I diabetes, no firm conclusions can be reached about their potential effectiveness.

Combination Therapy

In what was probably the first use of immune intervention in type I diabetes, Leslie, Pyke, and Denman,[6,7] working with five subjects (aged 19 to 33 years), used a vigorous combination immunotherapy approach that included prednisone, antilymphocyte globulin, and plasmapheresis (in three of the subjects). No effect was seen in the two subjects not undergoing plasmapheresis. The other three subjects maintained insulin-free remissions for 3–26 months but subsequently resumed insulin therapy. Thus, in the first attempt at immune intervention, some benefit was seen and was maintained even after the cessation of therapy.

Glucocorticoids

Several groups began experimenting with glucocorticoid therapy in the late 1970s and early 1980s. Elliott and coworkers[8,9] compared the administration of prednisone in a group of 17 children aged 2–13 years to a comparison group of 8 children who declined steroids plus 15 recent historical controls. They found increased urinary C-peptide excretion at 12, 18, and 24 months after diagnosis, and decreased insulin dosage at 24 months, in the treated group versus the comparison group. This was the first report of immune intervention that included a comparison group. It gave impetus to the study of immune intervention in type I diabetes. A subsequent report included a total of 32 children treated with steroids (including the 17 initial patients previously reported, 7 others, and 8 randomly allocated to the steroid therapy group) and 32 control subjects (24 patients "best matched" for age, gender, and concurrent time of onset to the treated subjects, plus an additional group of 8 randomly allocated to the control group).[10] The data suggested that there was a better response in children over the age of 11, with increased urinary C-peptide and decreased insulin dosage in the treated group.

A number of other small studies were performed with glucocorticoids, with minor effects when used for short periods. Longer-term usage of steroids showed some benefit in terms of C-peptide response and insulin dosage. Because of potential side effects, particularly the risk of growth limitation in children, steroid therapy has not been pursued.

More recently, Yilmaz[11] has reported prolongation of the honeymoon period by initiating glucocorticoid during that remission period.

Plasmapheresis

Plasmapheresis was performed by Ludvigsson and colleagues[12] in 10 subjects, and the outcome was contrasted to that of an age-matched comparison group. The treatment group had increased C-peptide and improved metabolic control up to 36 months after treatment, suggesting a small but perceptible, sustained benefit from plasmapheresis.

Photophoresis

Phototherapy entails extracorporeal irradiation with ultraviolet-A light of lymphocytes treated with 8-methoxypsoralen. The treated cells are reinfused into the subject. This approach is being studied in Australia and Sweden, principally in new-onset type I diabetes.[13,14] No clear outcome data have yet emerged.

Interferon

Two studies examined the effects of human leukocyte α-interferon.[15,16] In neither of these studies could a beneficial effect of interferon be ascertained.

Methisoprinol

Four studies have examined the effects of methisoprinol (inosine pranobex, inosiplex), an immune modulator that enhances production of interleukin-2 (IL-2).[17–19] The results were insufficient to produce a beneficial effect.

Ciamexone

Ciamexone, an immune modulator, was used in a randomized pilot study in 20 subjects.[20] At the end of 1 year, three of the treated subjects and none of the control subjects were in remission. A full-scale trial was planned but never completed.

Antithymocyte Globulin

Antithymocyte globulin was used in 10 subjects in two studies.[21,22] There was no sustained clinical benefit, and there was a high risk of thrombocytopenia. Therefore, further trials were abandoned.

Monoclonal Antibodies and Related Anti–T-Cell Therapies

Several monoclonal antibodies have been evaluated for potential effectiveness in pilot studies of new-onset type I diabetes. Preliminary experience with these agents generally suggests that β-cell function is preserved. For example, an anti-CD5 immunoconjugate coupled to the A chain of ricin toxin was given as a short course (5 days of intravenous infusion) to 15 subjects with relatively recent-onset type I diabetes.[23] Over 12 months of follow-up, β-cell function was preserved in this group. Also, an anti–IL-2 receptor (IL-2R) monoclonal antibody has been used (for 14 days) in combination with cyclosporine (for 9 months) to induce better preservation of C-peptide production in the treated group ($n = 18$) versus the control group ($n = 20$) given cyclosporine alone, demonstrating a synergistic effect of the two intervention strategies.[24] An IL-2R-targeted fusion protein, consisting of a diphtheria toxin–related protein linked to IL-2, DAB_{486}–IL-2, was used in 18 subjects with recent-onset type I diabetes for 7 days as induction immunotherapy, followed by a tapering dose of cyclosporine.[25] There was preservation of β-cell function. Other antibodies used have included an antiblast antibody (CBL1), an anti-CD3 antibody (OKT3), an anti-CD4 antibody, and a humanized chimeric anti-CD4 antibody. Unfortunately, full-scale, controlled trials of these or similar therapies have not yet been reported.

Miscellaneous Immune Therapies

A number of immune therapies have been used in very small pilot trials, generally without much success, although that may be an unfair interpretation because large numbers of subjects may be needed to demonstrate a substantial effect. The approaches studied have included levamisole, gamma globulin, theophylline, ketotifen, leukocyte or lymphocyte transfusions; tacrolimus (previously called FK506); the thymic hormones thymostimulin and thymopoietin; localized pancreatic irradiation by a linear accelerator; and transfusion. An ongoing study is examining a combination of antioxidants (which act as free radical scavengers), including nicotinamide, vitamin C, vitamin E, β-carotene, and selenium, in new-onset type I diabetes.[14] Under consideration for study are sirolimus (rapamycin) and mycophenolate mofetil.

Clinical Trials in New-Onset Diabetes

Several controlled clinical trials have been conducted in new-onset type I diabetes. These are summarized below.

Azathioprine

Azathioprine is a purine antagonist that prevents the generation of cytotoxic T cells and NK cells. It is widely used as an immunosuppressive drug in transplantation and other immune conditions, such as rheumatoid arthritis. It has been studied in four randomized, placebo-controlled clinical trials in new-onset diabetes.

One trial involved 24 subjects (aged 15–50) treated either with (n = 13) or without (n = 11) azathioprine.[26] Subjects treated with azathioprine had more insulin-free "remissions," a lower insulin requirement, and higher glucagon-stimulated C-peptide concentrations.

The second study involved 49 children (aged 2–20) treated with either azathioprine or placebo.[27] None of the subjects achieved remission, and there were no significant differences in insulin dosage, glycemic control, or stimulated C-peptide response between the groups.

The third study evaluated 46 subjects (aged 4–32), half treated with azathioprine plus steroids and half with placebo.[28] Twenty subjects in each group completed the 1-year study. Insulin was able to be discontinued in 50% of the treated subjects versus 10% of the control subjects. Treated subjects showed higher meal-stimulated peak C-peptide:glucose ratios and required lower insulin dosages than control subjects at 1 year.

The fourth study compared azathioprine alone to the combination of azathioprine and glucocorticoids.[29,30] Four treatment regimens were evaluated in 57 subjects with new-onset type I diabetes: steroids and azathioprine, steroids and placebo, azathioprine alone, and placebo alone. Subjects treated with azathioprine alone had better metabolic status than did the other three groups.

Although the data available to date on juvenile rheumatoid arthritis subjects show that azathioprine is generally well tolerated and is associated with few side effects, it may result in severe leukopenia (which can be avoided with careful monitoring and dose titration), and there is an unquantitated concern about oncogenic potential. As a consequence of fears about potential toxicity, azathioprine is no longer currently being studied as therapy in type I diabetes.

Cyclosporine

Cyclosporine (cyclosporin A) is a potent immunosuppressive drug that selectively acts on T cells, both helper and cytotoxic, to inhibit the secretion of IL-2 and thus suppress cell-mediated immunity. Cyclosporine has been evaluated in two large and two small double-masked, placebo-controlled studies in new-onset diabetes, and subsequently in additional open studies.

The French Study[31,32] involved 122 subjects (aged 15–40) randomly assigned to receive cyclosporine (n = 63) or placebo (n = 59) for 1 year. At 9 and 12 months the cyclosporine group had a greater frequency of complete remissions. Yet, the response was not sustained on discontinuation of the drug. Moreover, 81% of the cyclosporine-treated subjects showed acute nephrotoxicity.

The Canadian/European Study[33,34] included 188 subjects (aged 9–35) randomized to receive either cyclosporine or placebo for 1 year. Responses included complete remission and/or preservation of islet cell function, defined as a stimulated C-peptide level ≥0.6 ng/mL with near-normal glycemic control. The rate of response was significantly greater at both 6 months and 12 months in the cyclosporine-treated group compared to the control group. Subjects with a shorter duration of symptoms before entry had a better chance of response. Loss of cyclosporine effect was observed over 2 years of follow-up whether the drug was continued or not.

In a small study from Denver, 43 subjects (aged 8–36) were randomized to receive either cyclosporine or placebo for 4 months and were followed for 3 years.[35] No significant differences were found between the two groups.

A small study from Miami randomized 23 subjects (aged 9–38) to either cyclosporine or placebo.[36] In spite of the small study size, the cyclosporine group had greater preservation of β-cell function (meal-stimulated C-peptide response) over the duration of the study.

The French group subsequently initiated several additional open studies. In one, cyclosporine was given to 79 children (aged 7–15).[37,38] Insulin-free remissions were attained in 67.5% after 4 months and in 50% at 12 months. Yet, by 24 months, there were no sustained remissions despite continuation of cyclosporine therapy. Subjects who had experienced a previous remission had better glycemic control, similar insulin dosages, and higher C-peptide levels than nonremission subjects.

A small study from London, Ontario, involved 14 very young children (aged 22–95 months).[39] Four patients (29%) became insulin independent for some period. This study showed that immune mechanisms contribute to the pathogenesis of type I diabetes even in very young children.

Thus, in patients with new-onset diabetes, it has been shown that cyclosporine preserves β-cell function and reduces the insulin requirement. Yet, the responses have been transient, ending after withdrawal of cyclosporine or despite continued immunosuppression with cyclosporine.

Potential nephrotoxicity is the major concern with cyclosporine usage.[40,41] Although some nephrotoxicity is reversible, an irreversible, dose-dependent, chronic interstitial nephritis may develop. Whether this can be minimized by titration of the dosage or by combination with another induction immunotherapy remains uncertain. The toxicity of cyclosporine is such that it cannot safely be considered in usual dosages in new-onset type I diabetes.

Nicotinamide

Nicotinamide (niacinamide, nicotinic acid amide) is a water-soluble vitamin (B_6) derived from nicotinic acid. In animal models of spontaneous and induced diabetes, it has been shown to improve β-cell regeneration; to cause an increase in insulin synthesis; and, if administered before onset, to prevent the development of clinical diabetes in animal models.[42,43] There are a number of potential mechanisms by which nicotinamide may be beneficial in preventing β-cell destruction: by returning the β-cell content of nicotinamide adenine dinucleotide (NAD) toward normal by inhibiting poly-ADP-ribose polymerase (a major route of NAD metabolism); by serving as a free radical scavenger, thereby limiting DNA and β-cell damage; and/or by inhibiting cytokine-induced islet nitric oxide production.

Nicotinamide has been used in several studies in new-onset diabetes. The results have been mixed, with some studies showing marginal beneficial effects of nicotinamide and others being without effect.[44–51] The studies that have demonstrated some apparent improvement in β-cell function suggest that nicotinamide might be effective in earlier attempts at disease prevention, perhaps if utilized in the prodromal stage of the disease process.

Insulin

Several studies have suggested that early and more aggressive insulin treatment may result in preservation of β-cell function, better metabolic control, and/or a prolonged honeymoon period. However, the results have been inconsistent.

A study from Tampa randomized 26 newly diagnosed adolescent subjects with diabetes to either conventional insulin therapy or a 2-week course of intravenous insulin delivered via an artificial pancreas to maintain blood glucose concentrations in the low normal range.[52] There was preservation of β-cell function (meal-stimulated C-peptide concentrations) for at least 1 year.

Adjuvant Therapy

Vaccination with complete Freund's adjuvant or the bacillus Calmette-Guerin (BCG) strain of *Mycobacterium bovis* prevents diabetes in animals,[53] presumably by activating protective components of the immune system, thus decreasing the immune attack on β-cells. A pilot study in new-onset diabetes suggested better preservation of β-cell function, warranting a full-scale clinical trial.[54] This has led to the initiation of several full-scale clinical trials of BCG in new-onset diabetes in Edmonton, Denver, Ann Arbor, Rome, and Israel.

Linomide

Linomide, quinoline-3-carboxamide, is a synthetic immunomodulator.[55] Linomide administration to young nonobese diabetic (NOD) mice results in complete protection from insulitis and diabetes for over 40 weeks.[56,57] Linomide also suppresses autoreactivity in NODs with established insulitis. Therefore, linomide is now being tested in new-onset type I diabetes.

Clinical Trials Aimed at Prevention of Overt Diabetes

Pilot studies have been performed in an attempt to prevent type I diabetes.

In a single subject predicted to be within months of developing clinical diabetes, azathioprine has been used for over 5 years without the appearance of diabetes.[58] Cyclosporine has been used in at least two subjects before the clinical onset of diabetes, one with impaired glucose tolerance; both showed some improvement in β-cell function.[59,60]

Nicotinamide

Nicotinamide has been used in prediabetes. No effect was seen in one tiny pilot study.[61] In two others, subjects given nicotinamide appeared to fare better than untreated historical control subjects.[62]

The largest nicotinamide study to date was done in Auckland, New Zealand.[63] In this study, during the period 1988–1991, school children aged 5–8 (with no immediate family history of diabetes) were randomized by school to receive islet cell antibody (ICA) testing. A total of 33,658 children were offered testing; 20,195 accepted and 13,463 declined. Of those tested, 150 were treated with nicotinamide (maximum dose 1.5 g/day) on the basis of either ICA concentrations of ≥10 JDF units and first-phase insulin release <25th percentile of normal or those with ICA concentrations of >20 JDF units. Another 48,335 children were neither screened nor treated and served as controls. The rate of development of diabetes was $8.1/10^5$ per year in the nicotinamide-treated group versus $20.1/10^5$ per year in the comparison group ($p = 0.03$). The rate in those who refused testing was $15.1/10^5$ per year. No adverse effects were seen in treated subjects.

Given that nicotinamide is both inexpensive and has a benevolent side effect profile, coupled with the Auckland observations and the array of animal studies with nicotinamide, it seems reasonable for nicotinamide to be tested in human beings for the prevention of type I diabetes. Therefore, two large multicenter randomized, double-masked, controlled clinical trials are evaluating the effects of nicotinamide in high-risk relatives of persons with type I diabetes: the European Nicotinamide Diabetes Intervention Trial (ENDIT) and the German (Deutsch) Nicotinamide Diabetes Intervention Study (DENIS).

Neonatal and Early Infant Nutrition

In epidemiologic and case-control studies, a reciprocal relationship has been found between infant breast-feeding and subsequent development of type I diabetes.[64,65] In Finland, a small prospective study suggests that exclusive breast-feeding reduces the risk of diabetes development.[66] It has been proposed that breast-feeding may be a surrogate for the absence of consumption of cow milk proteins (CMP). An array of evidence has been cited in support of the CMP hypothesis—epidemiologic data, disease rates in animal models, humoral and cellular immune markers directed against CMP in patients with new-onset type I diabetes, and identification of a peptide sequence on bovine serum albumin with homology to a sequence on the islet cell protein ICA-69 (or p69) (''molecular mimicry''). The notion is that consumption of CMP, particularly during a critical period of vulnerability early in life, may lead to initiation of the immunologic attack on pancreatic islet β-cells and increase susceptibility to type I diabetes.[67] To test this hypothesis, a multinational experiment is being planned to determine whether the frequency of type I diabetes can be reduced by preventing exposure to CMP during early life. This randomized, prospective trial will involve over 5000 infants, who will be newborns with first-degree relatives with type I diabetes. They will receive either a conventional CMP formula or a formula in which CMP has been replaced with casein hydrolysate. The intervention will be for 6 months, with follow-up for 10 years. If successful, this would be a true primary prevention strategy.

Insulin

Insulin injections (subcutaneously or intraperitoneally) have been shown to delay the development of diabetes and to inhibit the appearance and progression of insulitis in animal models (Biobreeding [BB] rats or nonobese diabetic [NOD] mice) of type I diabetes.[68–74]

One hypothesis is that insulin may be acting metabolically, by resting β-cell function, and thereby reducing antigen expression associated with endogenous insulin secretion, thus making β-cells less susceptible to immune attack.[75–77] Indeed, in vitro, actively secreting β-cells are more susceptible to cytotoxic actions of cytokines than are resting β-cells.

A more likely explanation, however, is that insulin acts immunologically—by immunization, tolerization, or immune modulation. Many lines of evidence support this conclusion: (1) insulin injections prevent adoptive transfer of diabetes in NOD mice and BB rats.[78,79] (2) Insulin-specific T lymphocytes predominate in islet infiltrates in NOD mice,[80] and insulin-specific T-cell clones propagated from islet infiltrates mediate β-cell destruction on adoptive transfer.[81] (3) Insulin or insulin B-chain immunization, by periodic vaccination in incomplete Freund's adjuvant, prevents the development of insulitis and diabetes in NOD mice.[82,83] (4) Oral administration of insulin to young NOD mice decreases insulitis and delays the onset of diabetes.[82,84–86] Also, spleen cells from animals treated with oral insulin prevent adoptive transfer of diabetes. (5) A 15-residue peptide of the insulin B chain (B9–23) given nasally to young NOD mice prevents the development of insulitis and diabetes.[87]

In human beings, there have been four pilot studies of insulin use in high-risk relatives of persons with type I diabetes. (1) In the first pilot study, from Boston, insulin therapy was offered to 12 subjects, 5 of whom accepted; 7 declined and served as a comparison group.[88] In this study, insulin therapy consisted of 5 days of continuous intravenous insulin use every 9 months coupled with twice daily subcutaneous insulin. Life table analysis suggested that this treatment may delay the appearance of diabetes. (2) A combined Boston-Denver pilot study continued the combined intravenous-subcutaneous approach while enrolling subjects in a randomized fashion, with similar results. (3) A pilot study from Munich randomized 10 subjects to 7 days of intravenous insulin every 12 months, combined with subcutaneous insulin for the first 6 months.[89] Preliminary results suggest that diabetes may be delayed. (4) Another pilot study, from Gainesville, Florida, has treated relatives of patients with diabetes with daily subcutaneous insulin injections and report the approach to be safe, with encouraging preliminary results.[82]

The preliminary results from these pilot studies suggest that in high-risk relatives, insulin has the potential to delay or prevent the development of overt diabetes. In contrast to other interventions, insulin (1) is β-cell specific; (2) does not have generalized effects on the immune system; (3) has well-understood effects on persons; and (4) has known side effects that are controllable. This has led to the Diabetes Prevention Trial of Type I Diabetes (DPT-1), a randomized, controlled, multicenter clinical trial conducted throughout the United States. DPT-1 is designed to test whether intervention with insulin during the prodromal period of the disease can delay the appearance of overt clinical diabetes.[90] In high-risk relatives (i.e., ≥50% risk over 5 years), the protocol will test whether parenteral insulin therapy, combining yearly 4-day courses of continuous intravenous insulin with daily subcutaneous, long-acting human ultralente insulin, will decrease the expected rate of development of type I diabetes over 5 years. Meanwhile, simultaneously identified relatives with intermediate risk (i.e., 26–50% risk over 5 years) will be offered enrollment in a randomized, placebo-controlled, double-masked, clinical trial to test whether oral recombinant human insulin (7.5 mg/day) can modify immune tolerance and thus decrease the rate of development of type I diabetes.[91]

Ironically, the idea of using insulin to prevent diabetes is not new. In 1940, Haist, Campbell, and Best,[92] writing in the *New England Journal of Medicine,* stated: "The prophylactic administration of insulin to potential diabetic patients may become an accepted clinical procedure in the future. We suggest that the incidence of diabetes should be investigated in two large and comparable groups of children with a family history of this disease. . . . [One] group might receive insulin in the limited amounts which may be safely given under these conditions. We appreciate the difficulties inherent in this type of clinical investigation, but believe that the goal justifies the endeavor." Fifty-five years later, such a protocol is underway.

Conclusions

The last one and a half decades have witnessed dramatic progress in immune intervention in type I diabetes mellitus. The first experiments, demonstrating preservation of β-cell function in new-onset diabetes with a variety of immune strategies, served to confirm that type I diabetes is indeed an immunologically mediated disease. Yet, the use of immune interventions did not greatly alter the clinical course of the disease. Moreover, many of the earlier interventions were associated with unwanted side effects. As a consequence, the focus of investigation has shifted in two critical ways. First, the strategies being tested are ones with less severe side effects. Second, the emphasis is being placed on studies designed to delay or prevent diabetes, with the hope that intervention earlier in the course of the disease will offer a better chance of preventing β-cell destruction because of increased β-cell mass and potentially less aggressive immune destructive responses. Nevertheless, experiments at the time of disease onset continue, both because such individuals are readily identified and with the hope that prolonging the remission period will result in a milder course of diabetes in terms of both glycemic control and development of chronic complications. Yet, in the long run, efforts to prevent diabetes are likely to be the predominant effort. Our prediction is that there soon will be wide-scale investigation of vaccination programs to prevent type I diabetes mellitus. Eventually, this will prove to be a preventable disease.

References

1. Atkinson MA, Maclaren NK. The pathogenesis of insulin dependent diabetes mellitus. N Engl J Med 1994;331:1428
2. Bach JF. Insulin-dependent diabetes mellitus as an autoimmune disease. Endocrine Rev 15:516
3. Skyler JS. Immune intervention studies in insulin-dependent diabetes mellitus. Diabetes Metab Rev 1987;3:1017
4. Skyler JS, Marks JB. Immune intervention in type I diabetes mellitus. Diabetes Rev 1993;1:15
5. Pozzilli P, Kolb H, Ilkova HM. New trends for prevention and immunotherapy of insulin dependent diabetes mellitus. Diabetes Metab Rev 1993;9:237
6. Leslie RDG, Pyke DA. Immunosuppression of acute insulin-dependent diabetics. In: Irvine WJ, ed. Immunology of Diabetes. Edinburgh, Teviot Scientific Publications; 1980:345–347
7. Leslie RDG, Pyke DA, Denman AM. Immunosuppressive therapy in diabetes. Lancet 1985;i:516
8. Elliott RB, Crossley JR, Berryman CC, James AG. Partial preservation of pancreatic beta-cell function in children with diabetes. Lancet 1981;2:1
9. Elliott RB, Crossley JR, Berryman CC, James AG. Partial preservation of pancreatic beta-cell function in children with diabetes (letter). Lancet 1981;2:631
10. Elliott RB, Pilcher CC, Edgar BW. Long-term outcome of children with insulin dependent diabetes mellitus treated with prednisone. Pediatr Adolescent Endocrinol 1986;15:345
11. Yilmaz MT. The remission concept in type I diabetes and its significance in immune intervention. Diabetes Metab Rev 1993;9:337

12. Ludvigsson J, Heding L, Lieden G, et al. Plasmapheresis in the initial treatment of insulin-dependent diabetes mellitus in children. Br Med J 1983;286: 176
13. Harrison LC, Honeyman M, Steele C, Graham M. Photophoresis trial in IDDM: An interim report. Proc Aust Diabetes Soc 1992:91
14. Ludvigsson J. Intervention at diagnosis of type I diabetes using either antioxidants or photophoresis. Diabetes Metab Rev 1993;9:329
15. Rand KH, Rosenbloom AL, Maclaren NK, et al. Human leukocyte interferon treatment of two children with insulin dependent diabetes. Diabetologia 1981; 21:116
16. Koivisto VA, Aro A, Cantell K, et al. Remissions in newly diagnosed type I (insulin dependent) diabetes mellitus: Influence of interferon as an adjunct to insulin therapy. Diabetologia 1984;27:193
17. Greulich B, Lander T, Standl E, et al. Immune intervention trial in early diabetes mellitus type I: Effects of inosiplex on metabolic and immunological parameters. Pediatr Adolescent Endocrinol 1986;15:350
18. Mirouze J, Rodier M, Richard JL, et al. Effect of inosiplex on remission obtained in recent acute onset diabetes (abstract). Immunology in Diabetes 84—International Symposium Abstracts, Rome; March 15–17, 1984:82
19. Galluzzo A, Giordano C, Caruso C, et al. Methisoprinol therapy in the early phases of type I (insulin-dependent) diabetes mellitus (abstract). Immunology in Diabetes 84—International Symposium Abstracts, Rome; March 15–17, 1984:42
20. Usadel KH, Teuber J, Schmeidl R, et al. Management of type I diabetes with ciamexone. Lancet 1986;2:567
21. Eisenbarth GS, Srikanta S, Jackson R, et al. Anti-thymocyte globulin and prednisone immunotherapy of recent onset type I diabetes mellitus. Diabetes Res 1985;2:271
22. Silverstein J, Riley W, Barrett D, et al. Immunosuppressive therapy for newly diagnosed insulin dependent diabetes mellitus with anti-thymocyte globulin and prednisone. Pediatr Res 1983;71:295A
23. Skyler JS, Lorenz TJ, Schwartz S, et al. Effects of an anti-CD5 immunoconjugate (CD5-plus) in recent onset type I diabetes mellitus—a preliminary investigation. J Diabetes Complications 1993;7:224
24. Vialettes B, Vague P. Treatment of diabetes by monoclonal antibodies. Lessons from a pilot study using anti-IL-2 receptor MoAb in recently diagnosed diabetic patients. Diabetes Prev Ther 1991;5:21
25. Boitard C, Timsit J, Assan R, et al. Treatment of type I diabetes mellitus with DAB_{486}–IL-2, a toxin conjugate which targets activated T-lymphocytes. Diabetologia 1992;35(suppl 1):A218
26. Harrison LC, Colman PG, Dean B, et al. Increase in remission rate in newly diagnosed type I diabetic subjects treated with azathioprine. Diabetes 1985;34:1306
27. Cook JJ, Hudson I, Harrison LC, et al. A double-blind controlled trial of azathioprine in children with newly-diagnosed type I diabetes. Diabetes 1989; 38:779
28. Silverstein J, Maclaren N, Riley W, et al. Immunosuppression with azathioprine and prednisone in recent onset insulin-dependent diabetes mellitus. N Engl J Med 1988;319:599
29. Silverstein J, Maclaren N, Riley W, et al. Double blind trial with azathioprine and steroids in newly-diagnosed IDD. Diabetes 1990;39(suppl 1):294A
30. Silverstein J, Maclaren N, Riley W, et al. Lymphopenia dictates metabolic response to azathioprine in new onset IDD. Diabetes Res Clin Practice 1991; 14(suppl 1):S52
31. Feutren G, Papoz L, Assan R, et al. Cyclosporin increases the rate and length of remissions in insulin dependent diabetes of recent onset: Results of a multicentre double-blind trial. Lancet 1986;2:119
32. Bach JF, Feutren G, Boitard C. Immunoprevention of insulin-dependent diabetes by cyclosporin. In: Adreani D, Kolb H, Pozzilli P, eds. Immunotherapy of Type I Diabetes. Chichester: Wiley;1989:125–136
33. The Canadian-European Randomized Control Trial Group. Cyclosporin-induced remission of IDDM after early intervention: Association of 1 year of cyclosporin treatment with enhanced insulin secretion. Diabetes 1988;37: 1574
34. Martin S, Schernthaner G, Nerup J, et al. Follow-up of cyclosporin A treatment in type I (insulin dependent) diabetes mellitus: Lack of long-term effects. Diabetologia 1991;34:429
35. Chase HP, Butler-Simon N, Garg SK, et al. Cyclosporin A for the treatment of new-onset insulin-dependent diabetes mellitus. Pediatrics 1990;85:241
36. Skyler JS, Rabinovitch A, Miami Cyclosporine Diabetes Study Group. Cyclosporine in recent onset type I diabetes mellitus: Effects on islet beta cell function. J Diabetes Complications 1992;6:77
37. Bougneres PF, Carel JC, Castano L, et al. Factors associated with early remission of type I diabetes in children treated with cyclosporine. N Engl J Med 1988;318:663
38. Bougneres PF, Landais P, Boisson C, et al. Limited duration of remission of insulin dependency in children with recent overt type I diabetes treated with low-dose cyclosporine. Diabetes 1990;39:1264
39. Jenner M, Bradish G, Stiller C, Atkison P, for the London Diabetes Study Group. Cyclosporine A treatment of young children with newly-diagnosed type I (insulin dependent) diabetes mellitus. Diabetologia 1992;35:884
40. Myers BD, Ross J, Newton L, et al. Cyclosporin associated chronic nephropathy. N Engl J Med 1984;311:699
41. Feutren G, Mihatsch MJ. Risk factors for cyclosporine-induced nephropathy in patients with autoimmune diseases. N Engl J Med 1992;326:1654
42. Pozzilli P, Andreani D. The potential role of nicotinamide in the secondary prevention of IDDM. Diabetes Metab Rev 1993;9:219
43. Mandrup-Poulsen T, Riemers JI, Andersen HU, et al. Nicotinamide treatment in the prevention of insulin-dependent diabetes mellitus. Diabetes Metab Rev 1993;9:295
44. Vague P, Viallettes B, Lassman-Vague V, Vallo JJ. Nicotinamide may extend remission phase in insulin dependent diabetes. Lancet 1987;i:619
45. Vague P, Picq R, Bernal M, et al. Effect of nicotinamide on the residual insulin secretion of type I (insulin-dependent) diabetic patients. Diabetologia 1989;32:316
46. Mendola G, Casamitgana R, Gomis R. Effects of nicotinamide therapy upon B-cell function in newly diagnosed type I (insulin-dependent) diabetes mellitus patients. Diabetologia 1989;32:160
47. Pozilli P, Visalli N, Ghirlanda G, et al. Nicotinamide increases C-peptide secretion in patients with recent onset type I diabetes. Diabetic Med 1989; 6:568
48. Chase HP, Butler-Simon N, Garg S, et al. A trial of nicotinamide in newly diagnosed patients with type I (insulin-dependent) diabetes mellitus. Diabetologia 1990;33:444
49. Lewis MC, Canafx DM, Sprafka JM, Barbosa JJ. Double-blind randomized trial of nicotinamide on early onset diabetes. Diabetes Care 1992;15:121
50. Viallettes B, Picq R, du Rostu M, et al. A preliminary multicentre study of the treatment of recently diagnosed type I diabetes by combination nicotinamide-cyclosporin therapy. Diabetic Med 1990;7:731
51. Pozilli P, Marozzi G, Pisano L, et al. A multicenter randomised control trial of nicotinamide vs. nicotinamide and cyclosporin in IDDM at diagnosis. Diabetes Res Clinical Practice 1991;14(suppl 1):S61
52. Shah SC, Malone JI, Simpson NE. A randomized trial of intensive insulin therapy in newly diagnosed type I insulin-dependent diabetes mellitus. N Engl J Med 1989;320:550
53. Vardi P. Adjuvant administration modulates the process of beta cell autoimmunity and prevents IDDM: Introduction to human trials. Diabetes Metab Rev 1993;9:317
54. Shehadeh N, Calcinaro F, Bradley BJ, et al. Effects of adjuvant therapy on development of diabetes in mouse and man. Lancet 1994;343:706
55. Kalland T, Alm G, Stalhandske T. Augmentation of mouse natural killer cell activity by LS 2616. A new immunomodulator. J Immunol 1985;134: 3956
56. Slavin S, Sidi H, Weiss L, et al. Linomide, a new treatment for autoimmune diseases: The potential in type I diabetes. Diabetes Metab Rev 1993;9:329
57. Gross D, Sidi H, Weiss L, et al. Prevention of diabetes mellitus in non-obese diabetic mice by linomide, a novel immunomodulating drug. Diabetologia 1994;37:1195
58. Riley WJ, Maclaren NK, Spillar R. Reversal of deteriorating glucose tolerance with azathioprine in prediabetes. Transplant Proc 1986;18:819
59. Levy-Marchal C, Czernichow P, Quiniou MC, et al. Cyclosporin administration reversed abnormalities in a prediabetic child. Diabetes 1984;33(suppl 1): 183A
60. Assan R, Feutren G, Bougneres PH, Carel JC. Treatment of a glucose intolerant pre–type I diabetic twin with cyclosporin. Diabetes Res Clinical Practice 1991;14(suppl 1):S51
61. Dumont-Herskowitz R, Jackson RA, Soeldner JS, Eisenbarth GS. Pilot trial to prevent type I diabetes: Progression to overt IDDM despite oral nicotinamide. J Autoimmunity 1989;2:733
62. Elliott RB, Chase HP. Prevention or delay of type I (insulin-dependent) diabetes mellitus in children using nicotinamide. Diabetologia 1991;34:362
63. Elliott RB, Pilcher CC, Stewart A, et al. The use of nicotinamide treatment in the prevention of type I diabetes. Ann NY Acad Sci 1993;696:333
64. Borch-Johnsen K, Joner G, Mandrup-Paulsen T, et al. Relationship between breastfeeding and incidence rates of insulin dependent diabetes mellitus. Lancet 1984;2:1083
65. Gerstein H. Cow's milk exposure and type I diabetes mellitus. Diabetes Care 1994;17:13
66. Virtanen SM, Rasanen L, Aro A, et al. Infant feeding in Finnish children <7 yr of age with newly diagnosed IDDM. Diabetes Care 1991;14:415
67. Akerblom HK, Savilahti E, Saukkonen TT, et al. The case for elimination of cow's milk in early infancy in prevention of type I diabetes: The Finnish experience. Diabetes Metab Rev 1993;9:269
68. Gotfredsen GF, Buschard K, Frandsen EK. Reduction of diabetes incidence of BB Wistar rats by early prophylactic insulin treatment of diabetes-prone animals. Diabetologia 1985;28:933
69. Like AA. Morphology and mechanisms of autoimmune diabetes as revealed by studies of the BB/Wor rat. In: Hanahan D, McDevitt HO, Cahill GJ, eds. Perspectives on the Molecular Biology and Immunology of the Pancreatic Beta Cell. Cold Spring Harbor, N.Y.;1989:81–91
70. Like AA. Insulin injections prevent diabetes in Bio-breeding/Worcester (BB/Wor) rats. Diabetes 1986;35(suppl 1):74A
71. Vlahos WD, Seemayer TA, Yale JF. Diabetes prevention in BB rats by inhibition of endogenous insulin secretion. Metabolism 1991;40:825
72. Gottlieb PA, Handler ES, Appel MC, et al. Insulin treatment prevent diabetes mellitus but not thyroiditis in RT6-depleted diabetes resistant BB/Wor rats. Diabetologia 1991;34:296
73. Atkinson MA, Maclaren NK, Luchetta R. Insulitis and insulin dependent diabetes in NOD mice reduced by prophylactic insulin therapy. Diabetes 1990;39:933

74. Stubbs M, Like A. Insulin-releasing implants protect against KRV-induced diabetes in BB/Wor rats. Diabetes 1995;44(suppl 1):164A
75. Aaen K, Rygard J, Josefson K, et al. Dependence of antigen expression on functional state of cells. Diabetes 1990;39:697
76. Bjork E, Kampe O, Andersson A, Karlsson FA. Expression of the 64K/glutamic acid decarboxylase rat islet autoantigen is influenced by the rate of insulin secretion. Diabetologia 1992;35:490
77. Bjork E, Kampe O, Karlsson FA, et al. Glucose regulation of the autoantigen GAD65 in human pancreatic islets. J Clin Endocrinol Metab 1992;75:1574
78. Thiovet CH, Goillot E, Bedossa P, et al. Insulin prevents adoptive cell transfer of diabetes in the autoimmune non-obese diabetic mouse. Diabetologia 1991;34:314
79. Bertrand S, de Paepe M, Vigant C, Yale JF. Prevention of adoptive transfer in BB rats by prophylactic insulin treatment. Diabetes 1992;41:1273
80. Wegmann DR, Norbury-Glaser M, Daniel D. Insulin-specific T cells are a predominant component of islet infiltrates in pre-diabetic NOD mice. Eur J Immunol 1994;24:1853
81. Daniel D, Gill RG, Schloot N, Wegmann DR. Epitope specificity, cytokine production profile and diabetogenic activity of insulin-specific T cell clones isolated from NOD mice. Eur J Immunol 1995;25:1056
82. Muir A, Schatz D, Maclaren M. Antigen-specific immunotherapy: Oral tolerance and subcutaneous immunization in the treatment of insulin-dependent diabetes. Diabetes Metab Rev 1993;9:279
83. Muir A, Peck A, Clare-Salzler M, et al. Insulin immunization of nonobese diabetic mice induces a protective insulitis characterized by diminished intraislet interferon-γ transcription. J Clin Invest 1995;95:628
84. Zhong ZJ, Davidson L, Eisenbarth GS, Weiner HL. Suppression of diabetes in non-obese diabetic mice by oral administration of porcine insulin. Proc Natl Acad Sci 1991;88:10252
85. Dong J, Muir A, Schatz D, et al. Oral administration of insulin prevents diabetes in NOD mice. Diabetes Res Clin Practice 1991;14(suppl 1):S55
86. Bergerot I, Fabien N, Maguer V, Thivolet C. Oral administration of human insulin to NOD mice generates CD4+ T cells that suppress adoptive transfer of diabetes. J Autoimmunity 1994;7:655
87. Daniel D, Wegmann DR. Intranasal administration of insulin peptide B:9-23 protects NOD mice from diabetes. Submitted for publication.
88. Keller RJ, Eisenbarth GS, Jackson RA. Insulin prophylaxis in individuals at high risk of type I diabetes. Lancet 1993;341:927
89. Ziegler A, Bachmann W, Rabl W. Prophylactic insulin treatment in relatives at high risk for type I diabetes. Diabetes Metab Rev 1993;9:289
90. DPT-1 Study Group. The Diabetes Prevention Trial of Type 1 Diabetes (DPT-1): Implementation of screening and staging of relatives. Diabetes 1995; 44(suppl 1):129A
91. Schatz D for the DPT-1 Study Group. The Diabetes Prevention Trial of Type 1 Diabetes (DPT-1): Design and implementation of the oral antigen (insulin) protocol. Diabetes 1995;44(suppl 1):230A
92. Haist RE, Campbell J, Best CH. The prevention of diabetes. N Engl J Med 1940;223:607

Diabetes Mellitus, edited by Derek LeRoith, Simeon I. Taylor, and Jerrold M. Olefsky. Lippincott–Raven Publishers, Philadelphia © 1996.

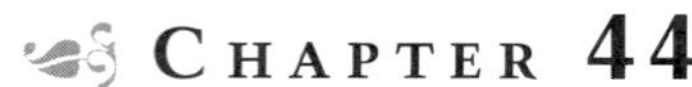

Chapter 44
Islet Cell Transplantation

Norma S. Kenyon, Camillo Ricordi, and Daniel H. Mintz

Introduction

In the last decade, significant advances have been made in the recovery of islets harvested from human cadaveric pancreata.[1,2] The availability of large numbers of relatively purified human islets has encouraged several centers to resume clinical trials of islet cell transplantation in patients with insulin-dependent diabetes mellitus.[3–7]

Insulin independence has been achieved in several patients and has persisted in some cases for over 4 years posttransplant.[8] The majority of recipients of islet allografts, however, either never became insulin independent or, having been so, eventually required a return to insulin therapy. The causes of graft failure have been attributed mainly to rejection, insufficient β-cell mass, and/or problems related to islet engraftment at the ectopic transplant site.

Although the limited functional capacity of many islet allografts resulted in a requirement for supplemental treatment with greatly reduced doses of exogenous insulin, glycemic control was distinctly improved compared to the pretransplant conditions. An analysis of islet allograft recipients with partial graft function clearly indicates that the degree of long-term metabolic control obtained is substantially better than that observed in patients undergoing intensive insulin therapy, as exemplified by the insulin regimens used in the DCCT[9] (Fig. 44-1). As reported from several centers, including our own, patients with long-term partial graft function have had normal or near-normal glycosylated hemoglobin levels for over 4 years. Moreover, in contrast to an intensive insulin treatment, the superior metabolic control achieved in some islet transplant recipients has also been associated with absence of the severe hypoglycemic episodes reported to occur in patients treated under intensive insulin regimens. Also, the hyperinsulinemia that accompanies systemic venous drainage in whole organ pancreas transplantation is eliminated. We have previously shown in dogs that hyperinsulinemia following pancreas transplantation is accompanied by changes in aortic lipid metabolism that could be precursors of atherogenic lesions in the aortas of recipient dogs.[10] By contrast, lipid metabolic indices in canine recipients of islet autografts are unchanged.[11]

Even though progress in clinical islet transplantation during the last 5 years has been clearly superior to that reported in the two preceding decades, there are still critical issues that need to be resolved to allow wide clinical application of this procedure to the treatment of diabetes mellitus. In this chapter, we will address the problems that are limiting and examine recent advances that continue to fuel enthusiasm for this approach.

Islet Isolation

Since islets comprise only 1–2% of the total mass of the pancreas, the challenge has been to define methods that result in the isolation of viable, functionally intact islets that have been liberated from the surrounding acinar tissue. The technical advances have, in fact, been few since Moskalewski[12] first introduced the use of collagenase to disrupt guinea pig pancreas enzymatically and liberate cellular fractions. Lacy and Kostianovsky[13] improved the procedure by utiliz-

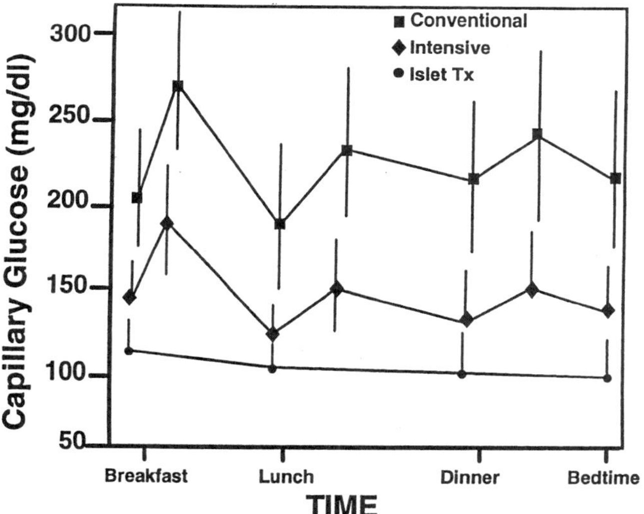

Figure 44-1. The upper two lines (■———■) and (♦———♦) represent preprandial (breakfast, lunch, and dinner) and prebedtime mean of seven capillary blood glucose measurements in a 24-hour period in each patient in the DCCT trial, with the 25th and 75th percentiles indicated by the vertical lines. The lower line (●———●) represents the mean of seven capillary blood glucose measurements in a 24-hour period over the previous 6 months in patient 4 (see Table 44-1). Patient 4 received an islet after kidney transplant. The patient takes 2–3 units of regular insulin before meals and 9 units of NPH at bedtime. (Modified with permission from The Diabetes Control and Complications Trial Research Group. The effect of intensive treatment of diabetes on the development and progression of long-term complications in insulin-dependent diabetes mellitus. N Engl J Med 1993;329:977.)

ing intraductal distention to percolate Hanks solution through the pancreatic ducts. This resulted in distention and disruption of the exocrine component of the pancreas, thus enhancing collagenase digestion of the pancreas to a cell slurp. However, the techniques developed for islet separation from the pancreata of rodents were found to be inadequate for scaled-up isolation of islets from the glands of larger mammals, including humans. The gradual evolution of technologies that allowed the digested components to be separated led to a parallel improvement in islet yield from the pancreata of dogs,[14] pigs,[15] and human donors.[16] All of these procedures, however, still involved a significant mechanical component during the digestion process (i.e., tissue maceration or forced passage of the digesting tissue through needles of decreasing size). For this reason, it was generally not possible to obtain enough islets from large animal pancreata to reverse diabetes following islet allotransplantation from a single donor. A further development of islet isolation technology was the introduction of the automated method,[1] in which the whole pancreas was loaded into a digestion chamber and the islets were progressively released during a continuous digestion process that did not involve any significant mechanical component. This method is now widely used for islet separation from the pancreata of multiple species, including humans. With the introduction of the automated method, there was still a problem related to the subsequent purification step that was manually performed by centrifugation on discontinuous density gradients using tubes or specially made high-volume syringes. This problem was solved by Lake and colleagues[17] and by Alejandro and colleagues,[18] who adapted existing technology for the separation of hematopoietic cells to the requirement of islet purification from nonendocrine tissue. The purification procedure utilized low-temperature centrifugation for large-volume ficoll gradients and a computerized cell separator, thus leading to reduced processing time, minimal handling, and a decreased risk of contamination. These improvements in islet separation and purification techniques allowed for the retrieval of a greater number of viable, functionally competent islets.[18–20]

Despite recent progress, however, the number of islets obtained from a human pancreas is still considerably less than the total islet content of the native human pancreas. The latter number varies considerably but has been considered to approximate 1,000,000.[21,22] Several donor variables can affect the outcome of islet isolation, including age, gender, previous medical history, the presence of obesity, and premorbid conditions. In addition, conditions surrounding the harvesting and preservation of cadaveric pancreata can play a key role in determining the outcome of islet isolation.[23] Nevertheless a key variable remains the availability of enzyme blends that allow reproducible digestion of the pancreatic tissue. Although some progress has been made in identifying critical components of the collagenase enzyme complex that are responsible for optimal digestion and liberation of islets, the most important qualities have not yet been thoroughly established. The enormous variability in the yield of islets from a cadaveric human pancreas is primarily attributable to the absence of knowledge that would allow for standardization of enzyme preparations.[24,25] Collagenase is usually produced from extracts of *Clostridium histolytica;* strain-to-strain variation in the content of the enzyme complex, as well as potentially toxic properties of the extract, have been major concerns. Some progress in defining species-specific enzymatic mixtures to optimize islet yield has been made by an increasing number of commercial enterprises interested in solving this problem. Alternatives under investigation include recombinant DNA technology that may provide an answer to this dilemma by enabling the production of highly purified, recombinant components that can be mixed together to define the optimal composition of enzymes for effective digestion.

The earliest reports on islet isolation procedures involved hand picking to obtain an enriched islet preparation; these approaches were impractical for the retrieval of islets from large mammal pancreas digests. A difference in density between endocrine and nonendocrine tissues allowed for the development of density gradient centrifugation techniques that led to substantial enrichment of islets.[18] If the density of the nonendocrine tissues is not decreased by degranulation (e.g., related to prolonged warm and/or cold ischemia), islet preparations can be enriched by these techniques to a purity of 90% or greater. Highly enriched preparations are contained in packed cell volumes of less than 1.5 mL.

The volume of the transplant should be as small as possible to minimize occlusion of the portal venous radicles and ischemic infarction of the liver that might be associated with it; minimize inflammatory responses that are provoked initially by cells and cellular products at the transplantation site; prevent intravascular coagulation that has been reported with relatively large-volume cellular implants delivered intraportally[26]; and, theoretically, minimize the antigenicity of the transplant by limiting the amount of nonislet tissue that is cotransplanted with the islets.

The absolute requirement for a pure islet inoculum remains controversial.[27] With the rationale that the manipulation required to obtain a highly enriched preparation of islets actually results in the loss of functional endocrine tissue, Sutherland and his colleagues have utilized impure preparations, infused into the portal vein or into the portal vein and peritoneal cavity, in their recent clinical trials.[27] Although no apparent complications from this approach have been reported, the concern remains that high cell volumes could lead to portal vein thrombosis, as suggested earlier. Alternatively, ultrapurification of islets may result in decreased islet yield and fragmentation, thus resulting in preparations for use in transplantation that comprise an inadequate mass of functionally competent islets. Infusion of intact islets that are juxtaposed by a layer of non-insulin-producing cells, thus forming a mantle around the islet, may provide a middle ground between these extremes. Moreover, the so-called mantle islets may confer an advantage to islet survival. Our longest-surviving islet allograft, which maintained insulin independence for almost 5 years, was transplanted with a preparation comprised of these mantle islets.[28]

Since the procedures for islet isolation are directed to separation and subsequent infusion of large quantities of islets, another area of concern is the loss of islets that occurs with maintenance, in either short- or long-term cultures or with cryopreservation. Although limited progress has been made in these areas, many islet transplant centers, still concerned with islet losses associated with maintenance techniques, have chosen to transplant fresh islets to obviate the need for ex-vivo maintenance of islets. However, it is not known whether islets that have been exposed to trauma and noxious conditions associated with both mechanical and enzymatic forces can survive another fresh insult associated with infusions into a new heterotopic site.

Islet Transplantation

The liver has been the major site for islet transplantation in patients. Several reasons have dictated this choice. For one, islets within the portal triad were thought, on theoretical grounds, to be upstream from the hepatic veins. If this were so, it would have limited systemic insulinization. Hyperinsulinemia is a consistent finding with systemic drainage sites, such as occurs after subcutaneous insulin injections or pancreatic whole organ transplants. Also, the site, considered to be immunologically privileged,[29] is easily accessible by percutaneous transhepatic catheterization, as we first showed.[30] Percutaneous transhepatic catheterization, which obviated the need for an operating room procedure, proved to be simple, relatively inexpensive, and without significant morbidity. Moreover, in contrast to an open surgical transplant procedure, islet transplantation might be conducted entirely on an outpatient basis.

We showed that islet autografts engrafted within the livers of dogs would eventually all fail to produce insulin, and hyperglycemia induced initially by pancreatectomy would recur.[31] These observations seemed to dim enthusiasm for islet cell transplantation in humans or, at the least, raised questions about the longevity of survival of islets sited heterotopically within the liver. The liver site was further questioned by the observations of Warnock and his colleagues,[32] who demonstrated that islet autografts placed in the spleens of pancreactomized dogs did not suffer the same fate.

In contrast to the limited survival of intrahepatic islet autografts in dogs, the experience in the human liver with islet allografts demonstrated that they survive for long periods, during which functional competence is sustained and islet structural integrity is maintained. We have, in fact, observed intact islets (that contain well-granulated β-cells) in the liver of a patient who had a combined liver-islet transplant almost 5 years before the specimen was obtained. This patient had the longest-surviving islet allograft reported, up to the time of her demise from recurrent malignancy. In addition, the patient remained insulin independent throughout life, although a total pancreatectomy had been performed at the time of her initial islet transplant.

One unique histologic feature of canine islet autografts that fail over time is the observation that the α-cells, but not the β-cells, are present,[31] similar to the lesions observed histologically in patients with type I diabetes mellitus and islet-directed autoimmunity.

An interpretation of these findings was that intrahepatic islets were exposed to waves of portal hyperglycemia each time the animals were fed, unlike the situation that exists when islets are in the native pancreas, where they are exposed to the much lower glycemic levels contained in the systemic arterial blood. Thus, there was concern that transplantation into the liver would enhance the possibility that islets exposed to high portal glucose concentrations would experience glucose-mediated β-cell damage.[31]

Although this consideration cannot be excluded, we were perplexed by the peculiar β-cell specificity observed in the failed canine intrahepatic islet autograft. As the story unfolded concerning the vulnerability of β-cells to damage by cytokine-induced generation of nitric oxide, a more plausible explanation for our findings in the dogs seemed to be on hand. It was observed that the pancreatectomized dogs experienced bacterial translocation to portal lymph nodes.[33] Seemingly, this could result in seeding of the liver and activation of hepatic macrophages to release interleukin-1 and tumor necrosis factor.[33] Because of the failure of α-cells to express nitric oxide synthase, a downstream intracellular target for these cytokines, activated macrophages that are present in abundance in the liver could induce β- but not α-cell death.

All of these considerations combined lead us to conclude that reservations concerning intrahepatic islet transplantation in patients is mostly based on findings unique to the dog model used in these original studies.[31] Because we know that functionally competent human islets can survive for prolonged periods of time in the liver, we are not reluctant to accept the advantages of this site in ongoing clinical trials of islet cell transplantation in patients. Of the islets that are embolized to the liver, only some survive. Some are lost through attrition before the islets are vacularized, and others are lost through what has been termed *primary nonfunction*. Primary nonfunction implies that the implanted islets are viable, at least temporarily, but that their function is restrained by a reversible process. Primary nonfunction appears to respond to immunosuppression.[34]

We and others have proposed that the inflammatory response that encircles a freshly implanted islet is comprised of cells that release cytokines. At first, cytokines limit insulin secretion before ultimately inducing cell death. Although there are still conflicting reports about whether human islets are vulnerable to nitric oxide damage, results obtained in collaboration with the Nerup group[35] and by Corbett and colleagues[36] suggest that this is the case. Thus, an interesting possibility is that inhibition of nitric oxide generation in the microenvironment at the transplantation site should reduce primary nonfunction and result in more efficient engraftment. This notion will undoubtedly be thoroughly evaluated in the near future.

Tolerance Induction

One primary obstacle to the broad-based application of islet cell transplantation as a cure for type I diabetes mellitus is the requirement for chronic administration of potent immunosuppressive agents to the recipient. The side effects of generalized immunosuppression, including an increased incidence of both infection and malignancy, plus decreased kidney and islet function, are considered to be more harmful to the patient than administration of exogenous insulin. Islet cell transplantation has therefore been available only to individuals who are already receiving immunosuppressive agents for a previous or concurrent solid organ transplant. One focus of the entire transplant community has been to delineate antirejection strategies that, alone or via multifaceted approaches, result in the development of donor-specific tolerance, thus obviating the need for chronic, generalized immunosuppression of the recipient. Single approaches to the induction and maintenance of donor-specific tolerance have often proved uniformly successful in rodent models of solid organ or cellular transplantation. Although such approaches have not transferred well to large animal models, the rodent studies have led to the development of clinical protocols that include immunointerventions first defined in small animal studies. As detailed below for islet transplantation, therapeutic manipulation of the recipient, as well as immunomodulation of the graft itself, have been explored as means to achieve graft acceptance.

Islet Immunomodulation

Although multiple cell types have been implicated in the pathogenesis of rejection, the effector mechanisms that mediate graft rejection all require the recognition of donor major histocompatibility complex antigens, known as *alloantigens,* by recipient T cells. The donor MHC antigens must be displayed to recipient T lymphocytes by specialized antigen presenting cells (APC) that possess costimulatory molecules critical to the process of T-cell activation. APC take up antigen and, through a series of intracellular processing steps, degrade it into a series of peptides. These antigenic peptides are then expressed, in association with MHC antigens, on the APC cell surface. It is this complex of histocompatibility antigen and peptide that is recognized by the T-cell receptor. Only APC that express the appropriate costimulatory molecules can then actually activate T cells; in the absence of these molecules, T cells can be rendered nonresponsive (anergy) or eliminated (clonal deletion). In the case of histocompatibility antigens, which are highly expressed on the surface of both donor and recipient APC, recipient T cells can either directly recognize MHC antigens on the surface of mature donor APC (without processing) or, after liberation of donor alloantigen (via shedding or cell death and disintegration), can recognize donor allopeptides complexed with MHC on the surface of recipient APC. Historically, the direct pathway has been considered to be the primary avenue to recipient anti-donor specific T-cell responses, especially in the early post-transplant period. These activated T cells then release soluble factors that recruit and activate a variety of cell types, which can then act in concert to destroy grafted tissue.[37,38]

One area of active investigation in the past has therefore been to remove, or functionally inactivate, the directly immunogenic donor APC from islets prior to transplantation.[39] All nucleated cells in the body express class I MHC molecules; however, only mature APC and a few other specialized cell types express class II histocompatibility antigens. Freshly isolated rat, dog, pig, and human islets contain 0–15 APC per islet,[40,41] and monoclonal antibodies specific for donor class II antigens have been utilized, in combination with complement, to lyse and deplete donor APC from islets. Other immunomodulatory protocols, which are thought to result in the functional inactivation of APC, are irradiation with ultraviolet light and culture in low-oxygen conditions or at room temperature.[39,42] In particular strain combinations, all of these procedures have resulted in the indefinite prolongation of rodent islet allograft survival, but translation to large animal models has been less successful. In our model of canine islet allotransplantation, we can consistently prolong allograft survival with a short course of high-dose cyclosporin A (CSA) treatment. Inclusion of immunomodulation, with either ultraviolet irradiation[42] or anti–class II plus complement treatment,[43] allowed us to transplant in the presence of significantly lower levels of CSA. Unlike the rodent studies, however, the prolongation achieved was neither indefinite nor uniform, thus highlighting the probable need for multifaceted approaches in large animals and humans.

In addition to actual manipulation of islets to alter immunogenicity, many groups continue to explore the area of immunoisolation.[44–46] Islets have been encapsulated in various materials that allow for the entry of glucose and the efflux of insulin. Large molecular weight molecules, such as antibodies, and cells cannot gain access to the islet. Although much progress has been made, obstacles remain that limit this approach, such as fibrotic responses to capsule material, the size of the device required for full islet replacement, the need for recharging with fresh islets, and small molecular weight molecules that can still traverse the encoating capsule to injure the islets.

Recipient Immunotherapy

With the advent of monoclonal antibody (moab) technology in the early 1980s and the subsequent development of moab that recognize various cells and key functional molecules in the immune system came the idea of using these reagents to deplete, or functionally inactivate, the recipient cells and molecules that participated in the afferent or efferent arms of the rejection response. Moab specific for T cells and T-cell subsets, adhesion molecules, growth factor receptors, and so on have all been utilized, with varying degrees of success, to manipulate the recipient's immune system.[38,47] Similar to what was found with immunomodulation techniques, application of such approaches in large mammals, including dogs, primates, and humans, has led to more limited successes in the prolongation of graft survival. Clinically, the best example of successful exploitation of moab therapy is OKT3, a moab specific for the human CD3 complex, associated with the T-cell receptor. In vivo administration of OKT3 is routinely used, either as induction therapy during the peritransplant period (e.g., as in our clinical trials of islet cell transplantation) or as antirejection therapy. Initially, the antibody causes depletion of circulating mature T cells, followed by a phase in which the T-cell receptor is modulated off the surface of T cells that could potentially mediate rejection. These lymphocytes are therefore unable to recognize and respond to antigen. The end result, however, is still generalized immunosuppression. Our experiences with a pan-T-cell–specific moab, in the canine model of islet cell transplantation, have revealed that moab therapy alone will not prevent rejection, but similar to our results with immunomodulation, moab treatment can result in graft prolongation in the presence of subimmunosuppressive doses of CSA.

Another reagent that has been used extensively in both clinical and experimental studies is antithymocyte or antilymphocyte globulin (ATG or ALG). These powerful agents can effectively deplete mature, circulating T cells in rodents and mammals.[38,48] ATG alone will not suffice to prolong graft acceptance in large animals and humans; however, by eliminating the mature T cells that would recognize and respond to donor alloantigen, the drug provides an opportunity in time for the recruitment of putative tolerogenic mechanisms. Depleting agents will, therefore, probably continue to play key roles in future approaches to tolerance induction.

Intrathymic Administration of Donor Cells or Antigen

T cells learn to discriminate between self and nonself primarily through a process known as *thymic education,* in which T cells reactive with self antigens undergo programmed cell death.[49] Depleting agents result in the elimination of mature T cells from the periphery, thus stimulating emigration of immature T lymphocytes from the bone marrow to the thymus. One area of active investigation has therefore been the possible induction of donor-specific tolerance via intrathymic administration of donor cells or antigen to a recipient preconditioned with, for example, ATG.[38] We and others have demonstrated indefinite prolongation of rodent islet allograft survival with this strategy.[50,51] Thymic atrophy occurs with age, and the potential application of this approach to the clinic remains a topic of debate, because it would be technically difficult to place donor cells or antigen accurately and consistently into the intact thymic tissue. Should these technological issues be resolved, however, intrathymic administration of donor antigen could prove to be a powerful tool for exploitation of naturally occurring mechanisms of tolerance induction.

Chimerism

Hematopoietic reconstitution of cytoablated mice, via transplantation of bone marrow from an allogeneic donor, results in the production of a chimeric animal that, depending on the transplant protocol, possesses varying degrees of both host- and donor-derived hematopoietic cells. It has long been known that such animals develop donor-specific tolerance and accept subsequent tissue or organ grafts from mice of the same strain as the original bone marrow donor.[38] Translation of this approach to clinical solid organ or cellular transplantation, however, has been hampered by the perceived requirement for cytoablation of the recipient, through chemotherapy or irradiation, to make space for donor hematopoietic cells. This paradigm has recently been challenged by the demonstration that chimerism can be achieved in the absence of cytoablation via multiple infusions of donor bone marrow to recipient mice.[52]

Studies of long-term human transplant recipients who have discontinued their immunosuppressive medications have yielded evidence of microchimerism, thus leading Starzl, Ricordi, and their colleagues[53,54] to propose that the establishment of chimerism may be a prerequisite for the induction and maintenance of donor-specific tolerance. Analysis of recipient tissues has revealed the presence of donor-derived dendritic cells (DC). Since DC are the most potent antigen-presenting cells in the body, and have long been thought to be responsible for direct stimulation of the rejection response, it was postulated that non-antigen-presenting, progenitor DC may somehow be critical to the tolerogenic process.[53,54]

Historically, it has been easier to achieve graft acceptance for the liver than for other organs, and it is well known that the liver has a large hematopoietic component; the concept was therefore born that the liver serves as a mini–bone marrow transplant. With the idea that infusion of donor bone marrow may increase the chances for the development of chimerism, clinical trials have been initiated to test this hypothesis.[55–57] Although the concept that chimerism is a prerequisite for the establishment and/or maintenance of donor-specific tolerance remains to be proved, clinical data from the University of Miami clearly show that donor bone marrow infusion significantly decreases acute rejection episodes in the first 6 months post-transplant and results in improvement in liver allograft survival.[56] Chimerism has been documented in all recipients of donor bone marrow, but it is too early to determine if the presence and/or level of chimerism is correlated with the frequency of rejection and/or the long-term survival of the organ.[56] For those patients who demonstrate donor-specific nonreactivity, we await an assessment of whether tapering of immunosuppressive medications will be possible.

Should it prove possible to establish chimerism, induce a state of donor-specific tolerance, and ultimately either discontinue or markedly reduce the dosages of long-term immunosuppressive therapy, the implications for transplantation will be far-reaching. One could envision that islet cell transplantation as a cure for type I diabetes would become a clinical reality; furthermore, patients with new-onset diabetes who do not yet have diabetic complications would be eligible for the procedure. Theoretically, an added benefit would be tolerization to islet antigens, thus preventing the recurrence of autoimmunity in the transplanted islets.

Clinical Trials of Human Islet Allotransplantation

Islet-Kidney Combined Allografts

Since January 1990, we have transplanted 29 patients in trials performed in collaboration with the University of Pittsburgh.[8,28] In upper abdominal exenteration and combined liver-islet allotransplantation, six of nine patients who survived the extensive surgery became insulin independent until they eventually died of recurrent metastatic disease. The first patient, who remained insulin independent for over 5 years after a liver islet allograft, died recently. Insulin-containing islets were readily detected in specimens of the liver. The documentation of islet allografts 5 years after transplantation has never before been observed.

In the absence of proper inductive immunosuppression, all type I diabetic recipients of combined kidney-islet allografts experienced at least one rejection episode.[58] In a trial in collaboration with the University of Milan, it was possible, however, to achieve prolonged insulin independence in patients treated with an inductive course of antilymphocyte globulin (ALG),[59] similar to our experience with OKT3. Despite the encouraging results demonstrating that it is possible to reverse diabetes with an islet cell transplant, prolonged insulin independence after human islet allotransplantation has been rare.

Since September 1990, at the University of Miami, we have transplanted seven patients with long-term (17–29 years duration) type I diabetes mellitus. None were able to attain normal HgbAlc levels despite intensive insulin regimens, and all experienced recurrent, moderate to severe hypoglycemia before islet cell transplantation. Six of the patients had stable kidney allografts placed 1–11 years before islet cell transplantation, except patient 5 (Table 44-1), who received a simultaneous kidney-islet allograft, with one of the three islet donors also serving as the kidney donor. To ensure an adequate β-cell mass, two to five islet donors were used per recipient. The donor pancreata experienced a mean cold ischemia time of 8 hours (range, 3–14 hours), and the islets were isolated via automated methods and administered through a catheter into a mesenteric vein.[7,30] All patients received a 14–16-day course of OKT3 (5 mg daily), starting 3–5 days before islet transplantation. Each patient received 500–1000 mg methylprednisolone daily for the first 3 days of OKT3 therapy in an attempt to ameliorate the symptoms of cytokine storm. The first four patients subsequently received their usual established maintenance dose of methylprednisolone. The following patients were treated by maintaining the higher doses of the drug, followed by gradual tapering, as would normally be done for a primary kidney transplant in this center. All patients received azathioprine and cyclosporin A (CSA); the azathioprine dose was adjusted according to the white blood cell count, and the CSA dose was adjusted to achieve blood trough concentrations of 250–300 ng/mL. Blood glucose concentrations were maintained at 80–140 mg/dL by continuous insulin infusion, followed by conversion to subcutaneous insulin. Sufficient insulin was administered to maintain euglycemia and avoid hypoglycemia for 30–60 days after transplantation. The clinical outcomes are depicted in Table 44-1.

Two patients (1 and 3) were euglycemic and insulin independent for 36 and 38 days, respectively, with normalization of HgbAlc levels. Graft failure occurred 125 and 154 days after transplantation, respectively. Patients 4 and 6 take 2 or 3 units of regular insulin before meals and 3 to 12 units NPH, respectively, at bedtime. Evidence of C-peptide secretion from these islet allografts has been documented for over 48 and 42 months, respectively, by serial oral Sustacal challenges. HgbAlc levels are normal and near normal (5.5% and 6.1%, respectively), and the glycemic concentrations (pre- and postprandial) are within normal limits (see Fig. 44-1). To this date, neither patient has experienced hypoglycemia for over 4 years. In our experience, these are remarkable results that strongly support the notion that islet replacement, even if incomplete, is associated with very beneficial effects (e.g., normalization of HgbAlc levels for over 4 years) and with the absence of hypoglycemia requiring assistance. Patient 5 lost graft function approximately 16 months post-transplant; the HgbAlc levels remained normal until that time. Patient 7, who received the lowest number of islets, showed a transient improvement in glucose control, but C-peptide levels are no longer detectable. The development of cytotoxic antibodies against donor lymphocytes was observed in the four patients who were so tested and who rejected the islets. Documentation of the presence of these antibodies was correlated temporally with graft failure.[7]

Although complete insulin independence was not achieved in all patients, the normalization of HgbAlc levels, even in recipients with partial graft function, encourages us, and investigators at

TABLE 44-1. Quantification of Islet Mass* and Clinical Outcome

Case	Number of Donors	Islets* per Kilogram	Graft Survival (Days)	Insulin Independence (Days)	Insulin Pre-Tx (Units)	Insulin Current (Units)	HgbAlc§ Pre-Tx (%)	Current HgbAlc (%)
1	3	18,699	125	36	51	37	7.5	8.3
2	4	21,185	23	0	30	30	8.2	8.6
3	3	18,858	154	38	52	54	11.2	10.8
4	3	18,044	>1255†	‡	44	19	7.3	5.5
5	3	12,664	756	‡	34	28	11.6	11.0
6	2	10,559	>1129†	‡	57	12	8.5	6.1
7	2	8,318	356	‡	40	26	10.5	9.4

*Islet equivalents.
†As of April 30, 1994.
‡No attempt to discontinue insulin.
§Normal range, 3.5–6.2%.

many other centers (Table 44-2), to continue to improve islet cell engraftment, so that one donor can provide sufficient numbers of islets, and to evaluate intervention strategies that might permit either low-dose maintenance immunosuppression or discontinuation of immunosuppressive drugs entirely.

TABLE 44-2. Number of Transplants at Various Centers Involved in Islet Cell Transplantation from 1990 to 1994

Location	1990	1991	1992	1993	1994	Total
Brussels					1	1
Charlestown		2				2
Edmonton	2		1		1	4
Giessen			1	5	5	11
Giessen/Wurzburg				1		1
Hamburg				1		1
Leicester		2	1			3
London, Ontario					1	1
Los Angeles I			3	1		4
Los Angeles II				1	1	2
Madrid			2	1	1	4
Miami	4	2	1	1	2	10
Milan	4	3	3	4	4	18
Minneapolis	1	4	5	5	2	17
Omaha					1	1
Oxford		1	1	1	1	4
Paris	3	1				4
Perugia	1	1			1	3
Pittsburgh	17	6	4	3	4	34
St. Louis	3	3	2	4	2	14
St. Louis/London	2	1	1			4
Verona				1		1
					Total:	144

Islets Before Kidney

With the knowledge that bone marrow infusion combined with solid organ transplants can result in fewer rejection episodes (supra vitae), and might even facilitate donor-specific tolerance, several centers are organizing clinical trials in carefully selected patients with islet cell transplants before kidney transplants. The rationale for these clinical investigative initiatives rests on two fundamental notions. One is that although islet cell transplants can clearly result in insulin independence, the grafts are quite vulnerable to allo- and (even recapitulated) autoreactivity, thus leading to early graft failure. Thus, interventions that offer the hope of reducing alloreactivity and recurrent autoimmunity should be viewed favorably because, if the hypothetical considerations are correct, the procedure should be associated with a higher degree of long-term success of islet cell transplants. It was stated earlier that although insulin independence is the ultimate goal for this type of serious intervention, sustained graft function is accompanied by a level of metabolic improvement not yet achievable and/or demonstrable in patients with type I diabetes mellitus who accept intensive treatment with insulin therapy. The second notion is that there are patients whose lives are devastated by unmanageable disease and who suffer side effects (e.g., hypoglycemia, autonomic neuropathy) that are themselves life-threatening.

Islets Before Kidney: Patient Selection

Patients with insulin-dependent diabetes mellitus for more than 10 years who are 21–50 years of age will be selected for these clinical trials. The inclusion criteria for entrance into such a clinical trial should be similar to those recommended by the American Diabetes Association for pancreas-only transplants.[60,61] These patients have very poorly controlled diabetes, not resulting from psychogenic factors, in which the day-to-day metabolic problems of diabetes are severe enough to be incapacitating. Therapeutic approaches have consistently failed to ameliorate the situation. These patients tend to have (1) recurrent episodes of ketoacidosis or severe hyperglycemia, often requiring hospitalization and/or (2) multiple episodes of severe hypoglycemia. Severe hypoglycemia is defined as hypoglycemia requiring the assistance of another person, with a frequency in our protocol of four such episodes in 1 year, documented by patient history and self-monitored blood glucose records. The majority of these patients have the clinical syndrome of hypoglycemia unawareness in the setting of defective glucose counterregulation. After 5–10 years of insulin-dependent diabetes mellitus, most patients have no glucagon responses to hypoglycemia and reduced epinephrine responses to a given degree of hypoglycemia.[62] They no longer have the warning symptoms that previously allowed them to recognize developing hypoglycemia and act (eat) to prevent its progression to severe hypoglycemia.[62] Others suffer from intractable postural hypotension due to autonomic neuropathy. Patients suffering from these diabetic complications have a higher risk of death[63,64] than those not afflicted with these complications. Patients should be excluded if they have proteinuria, since there is a risk of drug-induced nephrotoxicity that could accelerate renal failure.

Exclusion criteria are planned as follows: positive pregnancy test, proteinuria, creatinine clearance <60 mL/min, significant coronary artery disease, mentally unfit, active peptic ulcer disease, malignancy, previous malignancy, hypertension or a family history of hypertension or end-stage renal disease, hypersensitivity to rabbit proteins, active infections, hepatitis B or C, duration of diabetes mellitus of less than 10 years, portal hypertension, and acute peptic ulcer disease.

Islet Transplant Registry

Through December 1994, 242 adult islet transplant procedures have been performed, starting with the first attempt to implant pancreatic fragments from a sheep into a 15-year-old diabetic boy in 1893.[65] Following this first attempt, which also represented the first xenogeneic islet graft, all other adult islet transplants were allografts. A few hundred fetal islet allografts and xenografts have been reported, but without detailed information. The results of clinical islet allotransplantation have improved significantly since 1990. The number of cases reported to the registry is presented in Table 44-2. In fact, compared to the previous era (1985–1989), both the percentage of grafts resulting in prolonged insulin production (63% vs. 21% in 1985–1989) and the percentage of patients achieving insulin independence (29% vs. 7% in 1985–1989) have improved. Detailed data are available from the international registry[65] on 55 patients, with documented absence of C-peptide plasma concentrations, who received an islet allograft between 1990 and 1992. One-year patient survival, graft survival, and insulin independence percentages were 93%, 33%, and 11%, respectively. Long-term graft survival associated with insulin independence reported to the registry is depicted in Table 44-3. Graft survival did not appear to correlate with recipient age, sex, or duration of diabetes. Also, the number of donor pancreata and islet purity did not appear to affect 1-year graft survival. A few factors, however, appeared to be associated with the cases in which insulin independence was obtained. These variables included intraportal infusion as the route of islet administration and a relatively short cold preservation time of the pancreas before processing of the gland to harvest the insulin-producing tissue. In fact, only transplantation of islets obtained from pancreata that were stored for less than 8 hours ultimately resulted in insulin independence in the recipients. The minimal number of islets per kilogram was 6000 islet equivalents (number of islets if all had a diameter of 150 μm), and an inductive phase of immunosuppression with an anti–T-cell agent was associated with the best results. Islet allografts in type I diabetic recipients in whom all of the above-mentioned criteria were met resulted in 53% graft function; 60% had HbAlc levels <7%, and 47% were insulin independent at 1 year of follow-up. It is not yet possible to determine what factors prevent successful long-term function after adult islet allotransplantation in almost half of the transplanted patients. Variables that have not been well quantitated include islet viability and function at the time of infusion and the determination of the percentage of islets that can successfully engraft at the ectopic transplant site, as discussed earlier.

Table 44-3. Longest Period of Insulin Independence After Islet Transplantation (as of January 1995)

	Type of Graft	Center	No. of Years
Islet	Autograft	Minneapolis	>10.0
Liver-islet	Allograft	Pittsburgh	4.8
Islet after kidney	Allograft	Milan	3.2
Islet and kidney	Allograft	Edmonton	2.3

Summary

Islet cell transplantation has held the promise of a cure for insulinopenic diabetes mellitus for over three decades. The failure to reach this goal has been an enormous disappointment to clinicians and patients alike. But those investigators who have continued to work in this field have recently witnessed increasing success. The long-term results in patients with even partial graft function are still far better than those achievable with any of the intensive insulin regimens in use today. Inducing insulin independence, the gold standard of success, has also been achieved in several of the more recent clinical trials. But the excitement that fuels great enthusiasm now is the possibility that recipients can be made to accept islet allografts even in the absence of immunosuppressive therapy. This hypothesis is being actively pursued at a number of centers. If these trials can confirm that islets can completely restore metabolism, in the absence of a persistent requirement for immunosuppression, a new era in islet transplantation will be upon us, with the renewed promise that this approach can provide a permanent biologic replacement for the destroyed endocrine pancreas.

Acknowledgments

This work has been supported by the National Institutes of Health Grants DK25802 and 5R32 DK07346.

References

1. Ricordi C, Lacy PE, Finke EH, et al. Automated method for isolation of human pancreatic islets. Diabetes 1988;37:413
2. Ricordi C, Digon BJ III, Mintz DH, Alejandro R. Human islet separation. In: Lanza RP, and Chick UW, eds. Procurement of Pancreatic Islets, vol. 1. Austin, Tex.: R.G. Landes;1994:97
3. Scharp DW, Lacy PE, Santiago JV, et al. Results of our first nine intraportal islet allografts in type I, insulin-dependent diabetic patients. Transplantation 1991;51:76
4. Warnock GL, Kneteman NM, Ryan E, et al. Normoglycemia after transplantation of freshly isolated and cryopreserved pancreatic islets in type I (insulin-dependent) diabetes mellitus. Diabetologia 1991;34:55
5. Socci C, Falqui L, Davalli AM, et al. Fresh human islet transplantation to replace pancreatic endocrine function in type I diabetic patients. Acta Diabetologia 1991;28:151
6. Warnock G, Kneteman NM, Ryan EA, et al. Long-term follow-up after transplantation of insulin-producing pancreatic islets into patients with type I (insulin-dependent) diabetes mellitus. Diabetologia 1992;35:89
7. Alejandro R, Burke G, Shapiro ET, et al. Long-term survival of intraportal islet allografts in type I diabetes mellitus. In Ricordi C, ed. Pancreatic Islet Cell Transplantation. Austin, Tex.: R.G. Landes;1992:410
8. Ricordi C, Tzakis A, Carroll P, et al. Human islet transplantation in 22 consecutive cases. Transplantation 1992;53:407
9. DCCT Research Group. The effect of intensive treatment of diabetes on the development and progression of long-term complications in insulin-dependent diabetes mellitus. N Engl J Med 1993;329:977
10. Falholt K, Cutfield R, Alejandro R, et al. The effects of hyperinsulinemia on arterial wall and peripheral muscle metabolism in dogs. Metabolism 1985; 34:1146
11. Falholt K, Cutfield R, Alejandro R, et al. Influence of portal delivery of insulin on intracellular glucose and lipid metabolism. Metabolism 1991;40:122
12. Moskalewski S. Isolation and culture of the islets of Langerhans of the guinea pig. Gen Comp Endocrinol 1965;5:342

13. Lacy PE, Kostianovsky M. Method for the isolation of intact islets of Langerhans from the rat pancreas. Diabetes 1967;16:35
14. Noel J, Rabinovitch A, Olson L, et al. A method for large-scale, high-yield isolation of canine pancreatic islets of Langerhans. Metabolism 1982;31:184
15. Ricordi C, Finke EH, Lacy PE. A method for the mass isolation of islets from the adult pig pancreas. Diabetes 1986;35:649
16. Gray DWR, McShane P, Grant A, Morris PJ. A method for isolation of islets of Langerhans from the human pancreas. Diabetes 1984;33:1055
17. Lake SP, Bassett D, Larkins A, et al. Large-scale purification of human islets utilizing discontinuous albumin gradient on IBM 2991 cell separator. Diabetes 1989;38:143
18. Alejandro R, Strasser S, Zucker P, Mintz DH. Isolation of pancreatic islets from dogs: Semi-automated purification on albumin gradients. Transplantation 1990;50:207
19. Robertson GSM, Chadwick DR, Contractor H, et al. The optimization of large scale density gradient human islet isolation. Acta Diabetol 1993;30(2):93–98
20. London NJM, Robertson GSM, Chadwick DR. Purification of human pancreatic islets by large scale continuous density gradient centrifugation (abstract). Horm Metab Res 1993;25:61
21. Hellman B. The frequency of distribution and the number and volume of islets of Langerhans in man. Acta Soc Med Upsalien 1959;64:432
22. Saito K, Iwama N, Takahashi T. Morphometrical analysis of topographical differences in size distribution, number and volume of islets in the human pancreas. Tohoku J Exp Med 1978;124:177
23. Ricordi C. Qualitative and quantitative assessment of islet isolation in man and large mammals. Pancreas 1991;6:242
24. Ricordi C, Gray DWR, Hering BJ. Islet isolation assessment in man and large animals. Acta Diabetol Lat 1990;27:185
25. Benhamou PY, Watt PC, Mullen Y, et al. Human islet isolation in 104 consecutive cases. Transplantation 1994;57:1804
26. Mehigan DG, Bell WR, Zuidema GD, et al. Disseminated intravascular coagulation and portal hypertension following pancreatic islet autotransplantation. Ann Surg 1980;191:287
27. Gores PF, Sutherland DER. Pancreatic islet transplantation: Is purification necessary? Am J Surg 1993;166:538–542
28. Tzakis AG, Ricordi C, Alejandro R, et al. Pancreatic islet transplantation after upper abdominal exenteration and liver replacements. Lancet 1990;336:402
29. Qian J-H, Hashimoto T, Fujiwara H, Hamaoka T. Studies on the induction of tolerance to alloantigens. I. The abrogation of potentials for delayed-type-hypersensitivity responses to alloantigens by portal venous inoculation with allogeneic cells. J Immunol 1985;134:3656
30. Alejandro R, Mintz DH, Noel J, et al. Islet cell transplantation in type I diabetes mellitus. Transplant Proc 1987;19:2359
31. Alejandro R, Cutfield RG, Shienvold FL, et al. Natural history of intrahepatic canine islet cell autografts. J Clin Invest 1986;78:1339
32. Warnock GL, DeGroot T, Untch D, et al. The natural history of pure canine islet autografts in hepatic or splenic sites. Transplant Proc 1989;21:2617
33. Strasser S, Martinez O, Alejandro R. Bacterial translocation in pancreatectomized beagles. Transplantation 1993;56:247
34. Kaufman DB, Rabe F, Platt JL, et al. On the variability of outcome after islet allotransplantation. Transplantation 1988;45:1151
35. Zumsteg U, Reimers J, Pociot F, et al. Differential interleukin-1 receptor antagonism on pancreatic beta and alpha cells. Studies in rodent and human islets and in normal rats. Diabetologia 1993;36:759
36. Corbett JA, Wang JL, McDaniel ML. Nitric oxide mediates cytokine-induced inhibition of insulin secretion by human islets of Langerhans. Proc Natl Acad Sci USA 1993;90:1731
37. VanBuskirk AM, Brown DJ, Adams PW, Orosz CG. The MHC and allograft rejection. In: Mohanakumar T, ed. The Role of MHC and Non-MHC Antigens in Allograft Immunity. Georgetown, Tex.: R.G. Landes;1994:27
38. Charlton B, Auchincloss H Jr, Fathman CG. Mechanisms of transplantation tolerance. Annu Rev Immunol 1994;12:707
39. Lafferty KJ, Prowse SJ, Simeonovic CJ, Warren HS. Immunobiology of tissue transplantation: A return to the passenger leukocyte concept. Annu Rev Immunol 1983;1:143
40. Shienvold FL, Alejandro R, Mintz DH. Identification of Ia-bearing cells in rat, dog, pig and human islets of Langerhans. Transplantation 1986;41:364
41. Alejandro R, Shienvold FL, Hayek SV, et al. Immunocytochemical localization of HLA-DR in human islets of Langerhans. Diabetes 1982;31:17
42. Kenyon NS, Strasser S, Alejandro R. Ultraviolet light immunomodulation of canine islets for prolongation of allograft survival. Diabetes 1990;39:305
43. Alejandro R, Latif Z, Noel J, et al. Effect of anti-Ia antibodies, culture and cyclosporin on prolongation of canine islet allograft survival. Diabetes 1987;36:269
44. Soon-Shiong P, Heintz RE, Merideth N, et al. Insulin independence in a type 1 diabetic patient after encapsulated islet transplantation. Lancet 1994;343:950
45. Lanza RP, Sullivan SJ, Chick WL. Perspectives in diabetes. Islet transplantation with immunoisolation. Diabetes 1992;41:1503
46. Sullivan SJ, Maki T, Borland KM, et al. Biohybrid artificial pancreas: Long-term implantation studies in diabetic, pancreatectomized dogs. Science 1991;252:718
47. Waldmann TA. Immune receptors: Targets for therapy of leukemia/lymphoma, autoimmune diseases and for the prevention of allograft rejection. Annu Rev Immunol 1992;10:675
48. Rebellato LM, Gross U, Verbanac KM, Thomas JM. A comprehensive definition of the major antibody specificities in polyclonal rabbit antithymocyte globulin. Transplantation 1994;57:685
49. Robey E, Fowlkes BJ. Selective events in T cell development. Annu Rev Immunol 1994;12:675
50. Qian T, Schachner R, Brendel M, et al. Induction of donor specific tolerance to rat islet allografts by intrathymic inoculation of solubilized spleen cell membrane antigens. Diabetes 1993;42:1544
51. Posselt AM, Barker CF, Tomaszewski JE, et al. Induction of donor-specific unresponsiveness by intrathymic islet transplantation. Science 1990;249:1293
52. Stewart FM, Crittenden RB, Lowry PA, et al. Long-term engraftment of normal and post-5-fluorouracil murine marrow into normal nonmyeloablated mice. Blood 1993;81:2566
53. Starzl TE, Demetris AJ, Murase N, et al. Donor cell chimerism permitted by immunosuppressive drugs: A new view of organ transplantation. Immunol Today 1993;14:241
54. Starzl TE, Demetris AJ, Trucco M, et al. Cell migration and chimerism after whole-organ transplantation: The basis of graft acceptance. Hepatology 1993;17:1127
55. Fontes P, Rao A, Demetris AJ, et al. Augmentation with bone marrow of donor leukocyte migration for kidney, liver, heart, and pancreas islet transplantation. Lancet 1994;344:151
56. Ricordi C, Karatzas T, Selvaggi G, et al. Effect of two infusions of donor bone marrow on the incidence of liver allograft rejection. Ann NY Acad Sci in press
57. McDaniel DO, Naftilan J, Hulvey K, et al. Peripheral blood chimerism in renal allograft recipients transfused with donor bone marrow. Transplantation 1994;57:852
58. Rilo HR, Carroll PB, Shapiro R, et al. Effect of intraportal human islet transplantation on kidney graft survival in simultaneous kidney-islet allografts. Transplant Proc 1993;25:955
59. Socci C, Falqui L, Davalli AM, et al. Fresh human islet transplantation to replace pancreatic endocrine function in type I diabetic patients. Acta Diabetol 1991;28:151
60. Milde FK, Hart LK, Zehr PS. Pancreatic transplantation: Impact on the quality of life of diabetic renal transplant recipients. Position statement. Diabetes Care 1995;18:93
61. Pancreas transplantation for patients with diabetes mellitus. Technical review, ADA. Diabetes Care 1992;15:1673
62. Cryier PE, Fisher JN, Shamoon H. Hypoglycemia. Diabetes Care 1994;17:734
63. Kent LA, Gill GV, Williams G. Mortality and outcome of patients with brittle diabetes and recurrent ketoacidosis. Lancet 1994;344:778
64. Rathmann W, Ziegler D, Jahnke M, et al. Mortality in diabetic patients with cardiovascular autonomic neuropathy. Diabetic Med 1993;10:820
65. Hering BJ, Geier C, Schultz AO, et al. International Islet Transplant Registry Newsletter. Summary. 1995;5:1

Diabetes Mellitus, edited by Derek LeRoith, Simeon I. Taylor, and Jerrold M. Olefsky. Lippincott–Raven Publishers, Philadelphia © 1996.

Chapter 45
Pancreas Transplantation

David E. R. Sutherland, Rainer W. G. Gruessner, Kenneth Brayman, and Angelika Gruessner

History and Purpose of Pancreas Transplantation

In 1966, the first human pancreas transplant was performed at the University of Minnesota.[1,2] During the following decade, only a few surgeons performed pancreas transplants.[3–7] In recent years, however, the number of institutions offering transplants and the number of recipients have increased rapidly.[8] More than 6500 pancreas transplants, performed in more than 200 institutions, had been reported to the International Pancreas Transplant Registry (IPTR) by mid-1994.[9] Of these, about two-thirds were simultaneous pancreas-kidney (SPK) transplants, slightly more than one-sixth were pancreas after kidney (PAK) transplants, and a little less than one-sixth were pancreas transplants alone (PTA). Thus far, most pancreas transplants (nearly two-thirds) have been performed in the United States, and about one-fourth have been performed in Europe. The number of U.S. and non-U.S. cases tabulated by year as of May 1995 are shown in Figure 45-1.[10]

The establishment of an insulin-independent, euglycemic state with amelioration of secondary diabetic complications, as well as improvement in the quality of life of patients with type I diabetes mellitus, has been the main purpose of pancreas transplantation.[11] In addition, pancreas transplantation has also been used occasionally to correct exocrine, as well as endocrine, deficiency in a few patients after total pancreatectomy for benign disease.[12] For most transplant recipients, however, the objective is simply to transplant the insulin-producing β-cells within the islets of Langerhans.

Islets may also be transplanted as a free graft,[13] and clinical attempts date back to the 1970s.[7] The clinical success rate with islets, however, has been low[14] compared to that achieved with immediately vascularized, intact organ grafts.[15] Enthusiasm for the free graft approach has been sustained by the appeal of performing less surgery, as well as the hope that it will bestow an immunologic advantage, although thus far it has had just the opposite effect.[16] The results to date with clinical islet transplantation are summarized in Chapter 44.

The only treatment of type I diabetes that has been able to induce insulin independence consistently is pancreas transplantation.[16] Normalization of glycosylated hemoglobin levels is observed in patients undergoing pancreas transplantation during the period of graft function.[17] This correction of diabetes, however, necessitates immunosuppression of these transplant patients.[18] Thus, pancreas transplants are performed in nonuremic patients only when the problems of diabetes are perceived to be more serious than the potential side effects of antirejection drugs.[19]

For uremic diabetic patients who are candidates for kidney transplantation, the addition of a pancreas has become routine.[20] Because renal allograft recipients require immunosuppression (usually a combination of cyclosporine, azathioprine, and corticosteroids for maintenance, with anti–T-cell agents for induction therapy or treatment of rejection episodes), there is usually no reason not to make them insulin-independent as well as dialysis-free.

The etiology of type I diabetes mellitus in most patients is an autoimmune process directed specifically against the β-cells within the islets of Langerhans.[21–23] Thus, following pancreas transplantation, rejection, as well as recurrence of autoimmune isletitis, must be thwarted. Adequate immunosuppression will accomplish both in most patients.[24] The propensity for the disease to recur within the graft, independent of rejection, in non-immunosuppressed or minimally immunosuppressed recipients is an interesting story in

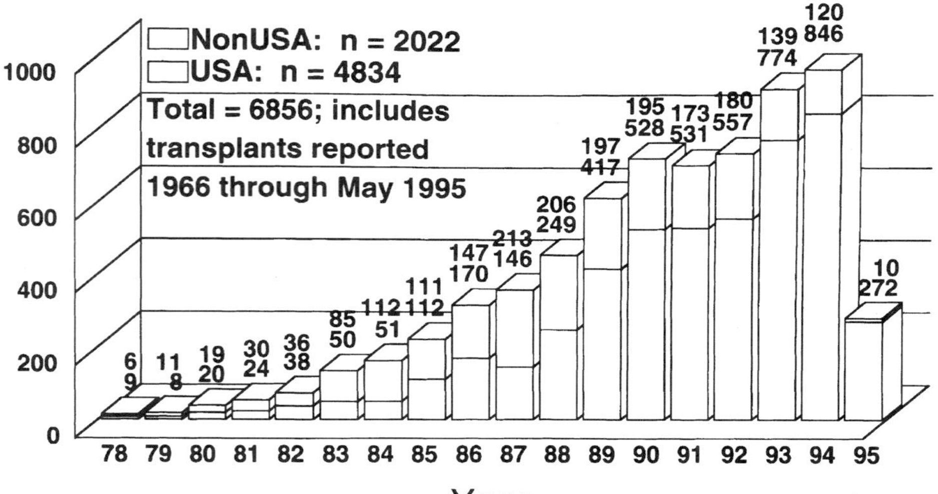

Figure 45-1. Number of pancreas transplants reported annually for the International Pancreas Transplant Registry, through May 31, 1995, with comparison of USA and non-USA categories. Reproduced with permission from the International Pancreas Transplant Registry Newsletter. 1995;8(1):1–16.

the history of pancreas transplantation,[25–27] and so is reiterated here. First, however, the indications for and current results of pancreas transplantation are summarized.

Patient Selection and Recipient Categories

After decades of debate,[28] the Diabetes Control and Complications Trial (DCCT) has now shown unequivocally that the incidence and severity of diabetic complications are related to the degree that glycemia is controlled by exogenous insulin from the onset of the disease.[29] Ideally, pancreas transplants should be performed early in the course of diabetes, as perfect control of diabetes in all patients cannot be obtained by any method of insulin administration. Even with imperfect control, however, not all diabetic patients get secondary complications, and it is difficult to predict who is at risk. Thus, most recipients to date have had diabetes for several years before transplantation, and have already shown a propensity for developing complications. At some stage, the lesions are too advanced to help or are self-perpetuating. In such patients, the main benefit of a pancreas transplant may simply be the improvement in quality of life that accompanies insulin independence.

It is generally accepted that quality of life is better for people who are immunosuppressed and dialysis-free than for those who are not immunosuppressed but are dialysis-dependent.[30] Thus, uremia in patients with diabetes is best treated by a kidney transplant. In such patients, correction of diabetes can be achieved, and only the surgical risks of adding a pancreas graft need to be considered.[20,31] If the patient does not have a living donor for the kidney, a pancreas can be transplanted simultaneously with a kidney from a cadaver donor.[20] If the patient has a living donor for a kidney,[32] a kidney alone can be transplanted first (which is less likely to be rejected than a cadaver kidney) and then a cadaver (or living donor) pancreas can be transplanted subsequently. This approach maximizes the probability of remaining dialysis-free for a prolonged period (even more important, in terms of quality of life, than insulin independence). Even if the nonrenal secondary complications of diabetes are too advanced to be treated successfully, achieving insulin independence in a diabetic renal allograft recipient will improve the quality of life over and above that achieved by simple correction of uremia.[33]

The situation is different for nonuremic patients, as posttransplant immunosuppression is given only for the purpose of correcting diabetes. There are two main questions for candidate recipients:

1. How do the risks of complications from the immunosuppression required to prevent rejection of a pancreas graft compare to the risks of developing or having secondary complications of diabetes progress in the absence of a transplant?
2. Will the improvement in quality of life achieved by being nondiabetic offset the penalties of being immunosuppressed?

Although the DCCT results indicate that complete correction of the diabetic state will prevent the development of complications,[29] the effects of reversal of diabetes on the course of established secondary complications is less predictable.[34] Thus, early application of pancreas transplants to the general diabetic population awaits either the development of a benign antirejection strategy (tolerance) or the organization of a randomized trial of insulin versus pancreas transplantation using the immunosuppression modalities currently available. It is an open question as to whether the incidence and severity of problems associated with long-term immunosuppression would be less, the same, or more than the morbidity associated with long-standing diabetes. The impetus to perform a randomized trial of early transplantation versus continued exogenous insulin will increase as new and less toxic antirejection drugs[35] are introduced into the field of transplantation.

Currently, pancreas transplantation is routinely performed in diabetic renal allograft recipients at many centers.[20,36] Some centers restrict its application to young uremic patients without cardiovascular disease,[37] whereas others are more liberal.[38,39] Multivariate analysis at the University of Minnesota,[40] an institution with liberal criteria, shows that the outcome is better in recipients younger than 45 years of age who do not have cardiovascular disease than in older patients with disease, but the presence of blindness or peripheral vascular disease is not a risk factor.

Nonuremic patients undergo transplantation less often than uremic patients, but those with severe metabolic problems are appropriate candidates for a pancreas transplant.[19] A successful pancreas transplant completely obviates diabetic control problems, such as hypoglycemic unawareness.[41] The new pancreas compensates for the impaired counterregulatory mechanisms that exist in some patients with long-standing diabetes.[42,43]

For any patient in whom the management of diabetes is so difficult as to seriously interfere with day-to-day living, pancreas transplants are a therapeutic option. It is a judgment call as to whether the problems encountered in managing their diabetes are more than those usually associated with being immunosuppressed. Retrospective studies in recipients of solitary pancreas transplants, however, have revealed a nearly unanimous opinion that being immunosuppressed and insulin-independent afforded a better quality of life than before the transplant.[44]

Clinical Management of Pancreas Transplant Recipients

Surgical Approaches

Many aspects of the surgical approach to pancreas transplantation are similar to those involved in kidney transplantation.[45,46] Usually, the graft vessels are anastomosed to the recipient iliac vessels, resulting in systemic drainage of the graft venous effluent. Techniques to direct the venous drainage to the portal system have been devised,[47–53] but they are technically difficult, and a metabolic advantage for the patient is not apparent.[54] Systemic insulin levels are higher with systemic versus portal venous drainage, but euglycemia can be achieved with either approach.

Most pancreas transplants have been from cadaver donors, but more than 80 have been segmental grafts from living related donors.[55] As with kidney transplants from living related donors,[56] rejection is less likely to occur with the latter.[57] The only reason to use living related donors for segmental pancreas transplants is the immunologic advantage, as currently the number of pancreas transplants being performed is less than the number of cadaver donors theoretically available.[58] For highly sensitized patients, this may well be their only practical option. Overall, long-term functional survival rates are higher for grafts from related donors than from cadaver donors.[2,59] Hemi-pancreatectomized donors experience changes in the results of metabolic tests of their endocrine function[60,61] that are similar in magnitude to the changes seen in renal function test results in uni-nephrectomized living kidney donors.[62] Follow-up studies to determine the long-term sequelae of hemi-pancreatectomy in donors are ongoing.[63]

Several surgical techniques have been used to manage the graft exocrine secretions in pancreas transplant recipients, including enteric drainage, polymer injection, or urinary drainage.[45] Urinary drainage is currently the most popular,[15] but enteric drainage[64] and duct injection[5] still predominate at some European centers. Enteric drainage is the most physiologic method,[65] and duct injection is very safe,[66] but both suffer from not allowing exocrine function to be monitored, making early diagnosis of pancreas graft rejection difficult. Urinary drainage was introduced early in the history of pancreas transplants. Originally, this was accomplished using segmental grafts with duct anastomosis of the pancreas duct to the recipient ureter.[67] Sollinger et al.[68] modified the technique of urinary drainage in the early 1980s by direct anastomosis of the pancreas to the bladder. In the mid-1980s, Nghiem and Corry[69] further modified the technique by using whole pancreaticoduodenal grafts with side-to-side anastomosis of an intact segment of graft duodenum to the recipient bladder (Fig. 45-2). This can be accomplished by either hand-sewing or stapling.[70]

Currently, in the United States, the technique of exocrine drainage established via the bladder is used in more than 90% of the pancreas transplants.[15] The technique is associated with a relatively low complication rate, but a small percentage of patients develop problems, such as dysuria or metabolic acidosis, from bicarbonate secreted by the graft and not reabsorbed as it would be in the intestine.[71] If symptoms develop, the problem can be corrected by conversion from bladder to enteric drainage[72–75] or duct injection.[76]

With SPK transplants from the same donor, the kidney can be used as a surrogate marker for rejection involving the pancreas as well,[77] so monitoring of exocrine function by bladder drainage is less critical than with solitary pancreas transplants. For example, the Stockholm group has reported an 83% 1-year pancreas graft survival rate in SPK recipients (n=36) of whole pancreaticoduodenal grafts anastomosed directly to the bowel.[65]

Application of proper organ procurement and preservation techniques is critical to pancreas transplant success. Surgical techniques to reconstruct the pancreatic vasculature are standard.[46] The most common method is to connect the superior mesenteric and splenic arteries of the pancreas with a Y-graft of donor iliac vessels, and then to anastomose the latter to the recipient's iliac artery.[78–81]

The pancreas of most cadaver donors is suitable for transplantation.[82] With the stress of brain trauma, many donors are at least mildly hyperglycemic, but in the absence of a history of diabetes mellitus, this finding does not appear to influence early outcome in the recipient.[83] It is uncertain, however, whether late results are affected by donor hyperglycemia.[82,84] A higher functional survival rate has been observed for pancreas grafts from younger donors than from older donors,[84] but there is no definitive test for identifying those that are unsuitable when no gross pathology is present. Probably a good conservative approach would be not to use donors older than 50 years of age who exhibit hyperglycemia with the stress of brain death.[32]

Either plasma-based solutions[85,86] or the University of Wisconsin (UW) solution[86,87] can be used for preservation of pancreas grafts for up to 30 hours. This duration of preservation allows nearly all pancreases to be retrieved and used for recipients locally or at hospitals distant to the site of procurement.

Diagnosis and Treatment of Rejection Episodes

The use of urinary drainage for pancreas grafts is advantageous for detecting pancreas rejection episodes early (before hyperglycemia) as it allows monitoring of amylase that is excreted directly into the urine by the graft.[88] Antirejection treatment, begun as soon as urine amylase activity decreases, can usually reverse the process, allowing endocrine function to be maintained.[89] Urine amylase activity is essential for monitoring episodes of rejection in solitary pancreas transplants (PTA and PAK transplants) (i.e., those performed without a concomitant kidney transplant).[90,91]

In SPK transplants, both grafts come from the same donor, and a rise in serum creatinine as a manifestation of rejection usually occurs before pancreatic function changes from concomitant rejection.[20,91,92] Thus, for SPK transplant recipients, the method of pancreas graft duct management is not so critical from a long-term standpoint, as the kidney can be used as a surrogate indicator of rejection affecting both organs.[77] Reversal of rejection in the kidney is nearly always associated with maintenance of pancreas graft function.

In animal models, the physiologic manifestations of rejection have been observed to appear earlier in the kidney than in the pancreas graft.[93,94] Histologic manifestations of rejection are usually demonstrated in both when concomitant biopsy studies are performed[93,95] but the severity is often discordant.[94] This is usually the case in human SPK transplants as well,[96] but occasionally, rejection occurs in the kidney without appearing in the pancreas, or vice versa.[97] Thus, markers of function or dysfunction of both organs should be monitored, but if nonbladder drainage techniques are used for management of the exocrine secretions, or if a bladder-drained graft has to be converted to enteric drainage for whatever reason,[72–74] monitoring of the kidney without monitoring pancreatic graft exocrine function can continue, with little, if any, change in the probability of remaining insulin-independent over time.[75] (Endocrine function can, of course, still be monitored.)

For bladder-drained solitary pancreas transplants, urine amylase is an organ-specific marker of pancreas function that can be measured by any laboratory and is, therefore, a practical test. A decrease will occur during rejection episodes (Fig. 45-3). An increase in serum levels of pancreatic enzymes may also occur early

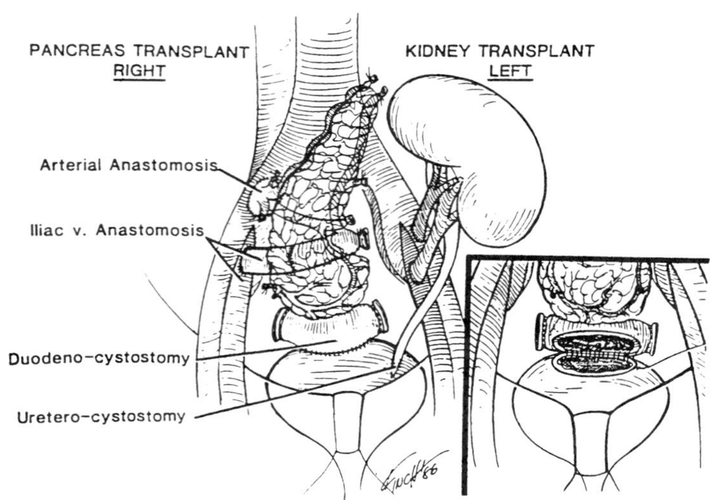

Figure 45-2. Technique of whole pancreas-duodenal transplantation with bladder drainage. The donor duodenum is simply used as a conduit for delivery of pancreas exocrine secretions to the bladder via a duodenocystostomy. A kidney transplant is also illustrated, as performed in patients who also have diabetic nephropathy. (Reproduced with permission from Prieto M, Sutherland DER, Goetz FC, et al. Pancreas transplant results according to the technique of duct management: Bladder versus enteric drainage. Surgery 1987;102:680.)

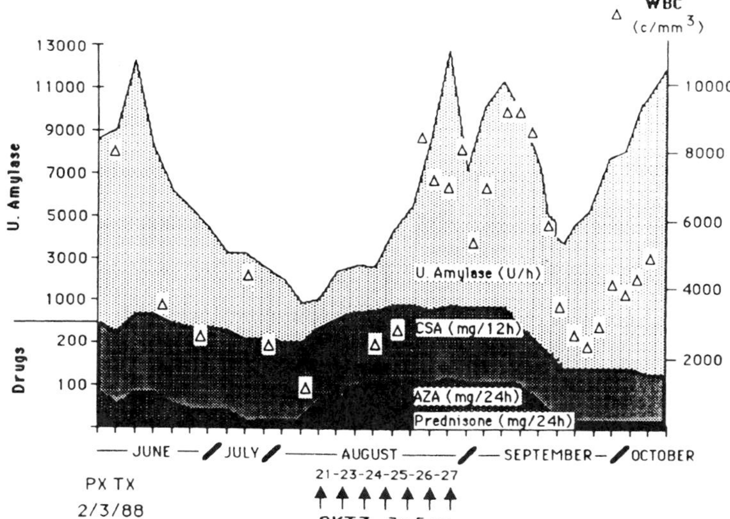

Figure 45-3. Urinary amylase levels in relation to antirejection treatment in a nonuremic recipient of a bladder-drained pancreas transplant. The urine amylase level declined without a rise in plasma glucose. A pancreas graft biopsy showed rejection. Treatment with anti-OKT3 was followed by an increase in urine amylase levels, and the patient has remained normoglycemic. *AZA,* azathioprine; *CSA,* cyclosporine A; (Reproduced with permission from Sutherland DER, Dunn DL, Goetz FC, et al. A 10-year experience with 290 pancreas transplants at a single institution. 1989; Ann Surg 210:274.)

during pancreas rejection episodes,[98,99] but as with hypoamylasuria, has to be differentiated from other causes, such as graft pancreatitis.[100] An initial rise in serum enzyme levels, followed by a decrease in urinary levels (directly reflecting decreased secretion), however, is characteristic of rejection.[89] By monitoring both serum and urine enzymes levels, rejection episodes are most likely to be detected early; when in doubt, pancreas graft biopsies can also be performed.[95,101–105]

Various serum and radiologic parameters have been proposed as markers for pancreas rejection), but these are not specific and have not been shown to correlate precisely with the results of a biopsy. Thus, serum and urinary or radiologic aberrations consistent with rejection may justify treatment, but to avoid overtreating the patient based on false-positive test results, a biopsy is necessary, just as it is for other organ transplants.[77]

In the early post-transplant period, rejection episodes are frequent, but if treatment is initiated promptly, normal pancreas graft endocrine function can be preserved.[106] Biopsy of the organ can be undertaken using open[101] or percutaneous[102,105] techniques, wherever located and no matter what method of duct management was used, or transcystoscopically if the graft was bladder-drained[103,104] and if doubt exists as to whether rejection is the cause of pancreas graft dysfunction. Various causes of graft dysfunction can be diagnosed by pathologic examination.[105,107–111] Biopsy of the graft duodenum can also be performed, and if there is evidence of rejection, treatment can be initiated promptly.[112–114] The absence of rejection in the duodenum, however, does not rule out rejection in the pancreas.[115] If clinical suspicion is high, either pancreatic tissue must be obtained or treatment must be initiated in the absence of a diagnostic biopsy.[77]

In SPK transplants, the concordance rate for simultaneous rejection in both organs is high, but not 100%.[94,95] The presence of rejection in either organ demands treatment. A decrease in urine amylase levels with no change in serum creatinine levels may signify isolated rejection of the pancreas, but a biopsy must be performed to confirm this. Discordant total rejection of one organ with maintenance of function in the other has also been described.[116] The pancreas is more likely to be retained in the presence of kidney failure than vice versa, but both patterns may be seen.

It should also be noted that chronic rejection of pancreas grafts (solitary or with a kidney) has been described in patients in whom endocrine function has been maintained.[107,117] In bladder-drained grafts, if good endocrine function (allowing insulin independence) has persisted for 1 month after loss of urine amylase, the probability of being insulin-independent 1 year later is 50%.[117]

Immunosuppression

The approach to immunosuppression for pancreas transplants is also very similar to that for other solid organs.[18] Since the mid-1980s, nearly every program has used cyclosporine in combination with azathioprine and prednisone for maintenance immunosuppression, and most also use anti–T-cell agents for induction immunosuppression.[118]

According to an analysis of data from the IPTR,[118] the results are best when an anti–T-cell agent and cyclosporine are both used for induction. Indeed, when anti–T-cell agents are not used for induction, and cyclosporine is used only for maintenance, the graft survival rates are not as high. The new drug FK506 is just beginning to be used in pancreas transplant recipients.[119]

Rejection episodes are treated as for the kidney, with either an increase in steroids, in anti–T-cell antibody administration, or a combination of the two. With other solid organs, anti–T-cell treatment is usually reserved for "steroid-resistant" rejection, but in pancreas transplantation, the incidence of steroid resistance rejection episodes has been high, so many groups use anti–T-cell agents at the onset of antirejection therapy.[18,120] Several groups have also reported a higher incidence of rejection episodes in recipients of combined kidney/pancreas transplants than in recipients of kidney transplants alone.[31,121] The incidence of rejection episodes in recipients of pancreas transplants alone has also been higher than for recipients of kidney transplants alone treated with cyclosporine.[90] Preliminary observations suggest that the incidence of rejection episodes is lower in pancreas transplant recipients treated with FK506 than in those treated with cyclosporine.[119]

The pancreas may be more immunogenic and have a greater potential for surgical complications than some of the other organs commonly transplanted. Nevertheless, the results of pancreas transplantation have steadily improved to the point that they now approximate those achieved with other solid organ transplants when combined with a kidney, or when a good human leukocyte antigen (HLA) match is obtained for a solitary graft.

Clinical Results

Patient and Graft Survival Rates

Registry Data

The results of pancreas transplantation progressively improved following the introduction of cyclosporine and the refinement of surgical techniques, as has been documented by several reports from the IPTR.[15] The most recent analyses of IPTR data were done on more than 6800 cadaver donor cases reported worldwide between October 1987 and May 1995.[9,10] The overall 1-year patient survival rate was 91%, and the overall 1-year insulin-independent (graft functional survival) rate was 74%.[9]

Separate analyses were conducted to determine the influence of several variables on outcome, including recipient category, duct management technique, organ preservation time prior to implantation, HLA matching, and year of transplantation. The influence of a pancreas transplant on kidney graft survival in SPK recipients was also assessed.

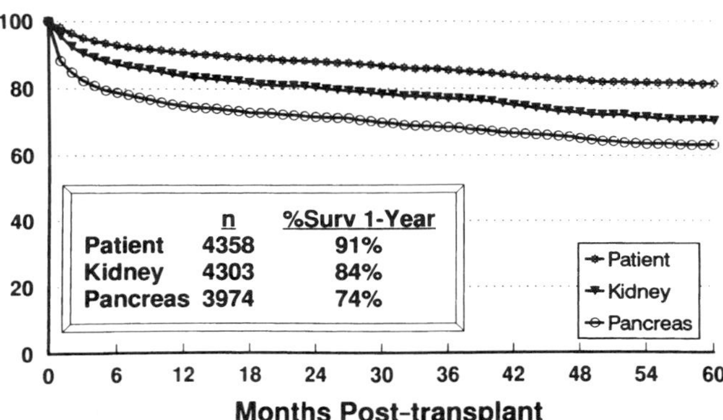

Figure 45-4. Patient, kidney, and pancreas graft survival (*Surv*) rates worldwide in recipients of bladder drained SPK transplants from cadaver donors reported to the IPTR from October 1, 1987 to May 31, 1995. (Reproduced with permission from International Pancreas Transplant Registry Newsletter. 1995;8(1):1.)

Category

The simultaneous pancreas-kidney category of recipients was the largest (N=4358). Worldwide,[9] the 1-year pancreas graft functional survival rate was 74%, and the 1-year kidney graft functional survival rate was 84%, with a 3–5% per year loss rate after the first year (Fig. 45-4). The patient survival rate for SPK recipients was 91% at 1 year.

A comparison of outcome by category (Fig. 45-5) was restricted to U.S. cases[10] because so few PAK and PTA transplants have been done elsewhere (86% of PAK and 77% of PTA cases in the IPTR are from the United States). Patient survival rates are identical between the three groups (Fig. 45-5*A*). Pancreas graft functional survival rates, however, were significantly higher for SPK recipients, with 75% being insulin-independent at 1 year, compared to only 50% of the recipients of solitary (PAK and PTA) grafts (Fig. 45-5*B*).

The ability to detect pancreas graft rejection episodes by surrogate monitoring of kidney graft function in SPK recipients (in whom both organs are from the same donor) may be the reason why functional survival rates are higher in this category. An increase in serum creatinine levels during rejection episodes almost always occurs before a detectable change in pancreas graft function, either exocrine or endocrine, allowing early treatment and reversal.[77] In the PAK and PTA groups, renal function bears no relation to rejection episodes involving the pancreas. If only endocrine function is monitored, rejection episodes may not be detected until it is too late to effect a reversal.[77]

Individual centers have achieved better results with solitary pancreas transplants[122,123] than those reflected in the analysis of IPTR data. These centers have used the bladder drainage technique and have measured urine amylase levels to detect a decrease in exocrine function and the need for treatment or biopsy. By monitoring urinary amylase levels, a decrease in exocrine function can be detected before endocrine dysfunction as a consequence of rejection, and treatment can be initiated early enough to reverse the process in solitary pancreas transplant recipients, as is usually true when serum creatinine levels are monitored in SPK recipients.[77]

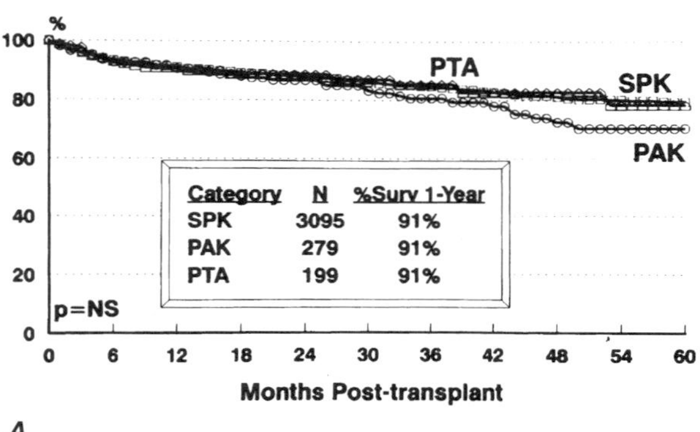

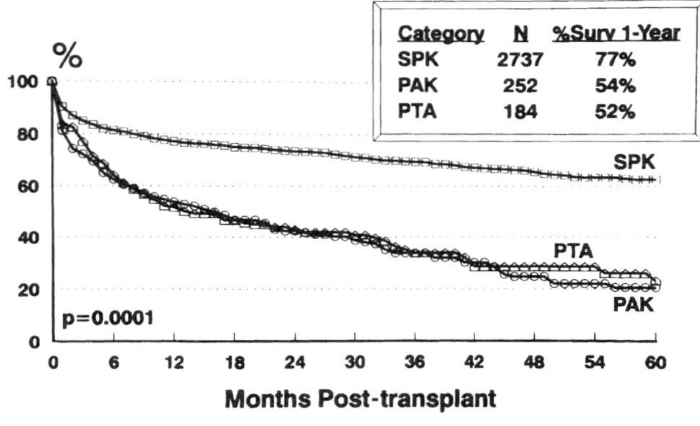

Figure 45-5. Patient (*A*) and pancreas graft (*B*) survival rates according to recipient category for U.S. bladder-drained cadaveric transplants reported to IPTR/UNOS from October 1, 1987 to May 31, 1995. (Reproduced with permission from the International Pancreas Transplant Registry Newsletter. 1995;8(1):1.)

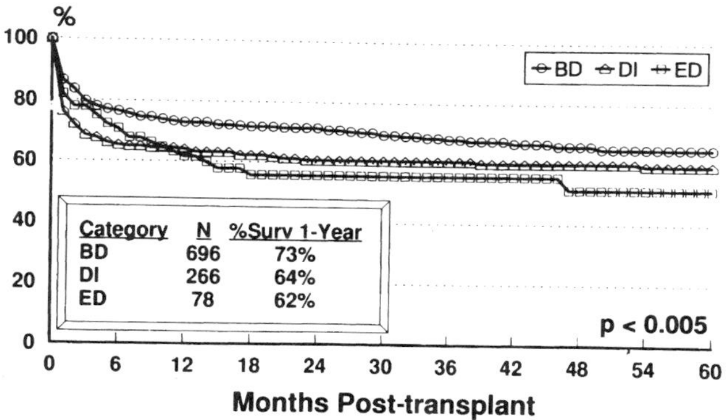

Figure 45-6. Pancreas graft functional survival (*Surv*) rates in Europe according to method of duct management in recipients of SPK transplants reported to the IPTR from October 1, 1987 to May 31, 1995. *BD*, bladder-drained; *DI*, duct injection; *ED*, enteric drained. (Reproduced with permission from International Pancreas Transplant Registry Newsletter 1995;8(1):1.)

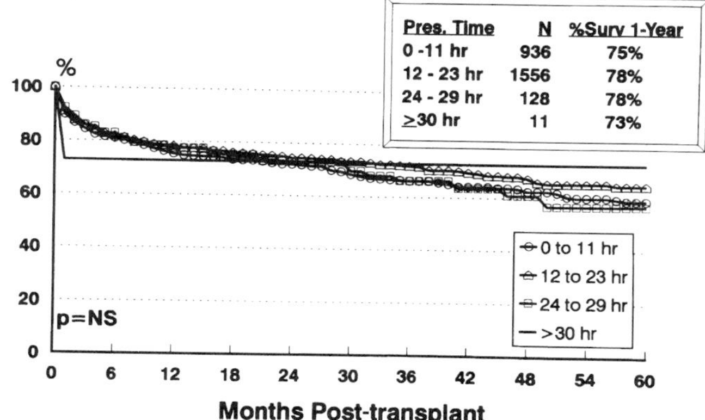

Figure 45-7. Pancreas graft functional survival (*Surv*) rates worldwide according to preservation time for bladder-drained (BD) cadaveric SPK transplants reported to IPTR/UNOS from October 1, 1987 to May 31, 1995. (Reproduced with permission from International Pancreas Transplant Registry Newsletter. 1995; 8(1):1.)

Duct Management

Assessment of differences in pancreas transplant outcome according to duct management was done for European cases only,[9] as 95% of the transplants performed in the United States were managed by bladder drainage. In Europe, from 1987 to 1995, nearly one-third of the cases were managed using the alternative techniques of either enteric drainage (in about 10% of the cases) or duct injection (about 25% of the cases).

Nearly all pancreas transplants in Europe are in the SPK category. Thus, analysis of outcome by duct management was done in this set of patients (Fig. 45-6). In SPK European cases, bladder drainage was associated with a 73% graft functional survival at 1 year, compared to 64% and 62% for enteric drainage and duct injection cases, respectively.

Again, however, there are institutions in which the enteric drainage[65] or duct injection[124–126] techniques was associated with results as good, or nearly as good, as those reported by others using bladder drainage,[38,123,127,128] and at least equal to or superior to those in the overall IPTR analysis of SPK results. Most likely, good results can be obtained with all techniques in the SPK category as long as the group is an expert in that technique. Monitoring urine amylase levels was less important for SPK than for PAK or PTA cases, and the fact that individual institutions achieved SPK pancreas graft functional survival rates similar to the overall IPTR results indicates that monitoring of kidney function is generally adequate for detecting rejection that may be going on in a simultaneously transplanted pancreas.[77]

Preservation

With regard to pancreas graft preservation, univariate analyses of IPTR world data[9] show no significant differences in graft survival rates for storage times of 30 hours or less (Fig. 45-7). However, a previous multivariate analysis showed a slight, but statistically significant, detrimental effect on outcome when preservation time was increased.[129] In general, then, the graft should be transplanted as soon as possible after procurement.

Human Leukocyte Antigen Matching

The impact of HLA matching was analyzed separately for each recipient category in the latest IPTR analysis,[10] and thus could be assessed only for U.S. cases (Fig. 45-8). In each category, two analyses were done. In the first (Fig. 45-8*A, B, C*), graft survival rates were calculated with all causes of failure included (i.e., surgical losses [technical] and death with function as well as rejection). In the other analysis (Fig. 45-8*D, E, F*), only technically successful cases were included, and if the graft was functioning at the time the patient died, it was censored (i.e., not counted as a failure). The second analysis was done in order to assess the immunologic effect of matching on the probability of rejection.

In the overall analysis, recipients who were not mismatched for any HLA-A, HLA-B, or HLA-DR antigens had superior results (Fig. 45-8*A, B, C*). Indeed, no grafts from donors without a mismatch were rejected during the first year posttransplant (Fig. 45-8*D, E, F*). In the PAK (Fig. 45-8*B*) and PTA (Fig. 45-8*C*) categories, recipients of grafts from donors mismatched for one HLA antigen had graft survival rates that were intermediate between those mismatched for no antigens and those mismatched for two to six antigens in the SPK category. In the SPK category, recipients of pancreases from donors mismatched for two to six antigens had functional survival rates as good as those mismatched for one antigen (Fig. 45-8*A*).

In the SPK category, very few pancreases were lost from rejection, no matter what the degree of mismatching (see Fig. 45-8*D*), whereas in the PAK (Fig. 45-8*E*) and PTA (Fig. 45-8*F*) categories, nearly one-third of the grafts were rejected in those mismatched for two to six antigens.

Thus, HLA matching has its greatest impact in the solitary pancreas transplant categories. With a mismatch of no antigens or one antigen, the results approach those in the SPK category. In the SPK category, graft survival rates were high no matter what the degree of mismatch; indeed, only a perfect match was found to have a graft survival advantage over a less good match. Whether the introduction of FK506 will obviate the need for a good match in solitary pancreas transplant recipients remains to be determined.[119] Meanwhile, in the PAK and PTA categories, every effort should be made to obtain a good match.

Influence of a Pancreas Transplant on Kidney Graft Survival Rates in SPK Recipients

Previous IPTR analyses compared patient and renal allograft function survival rates in diabetic recipients of a kidney transplant alone with those in patients receiving SPK transplants.[130,131] One analysis was done in collaboration with the United States Renal

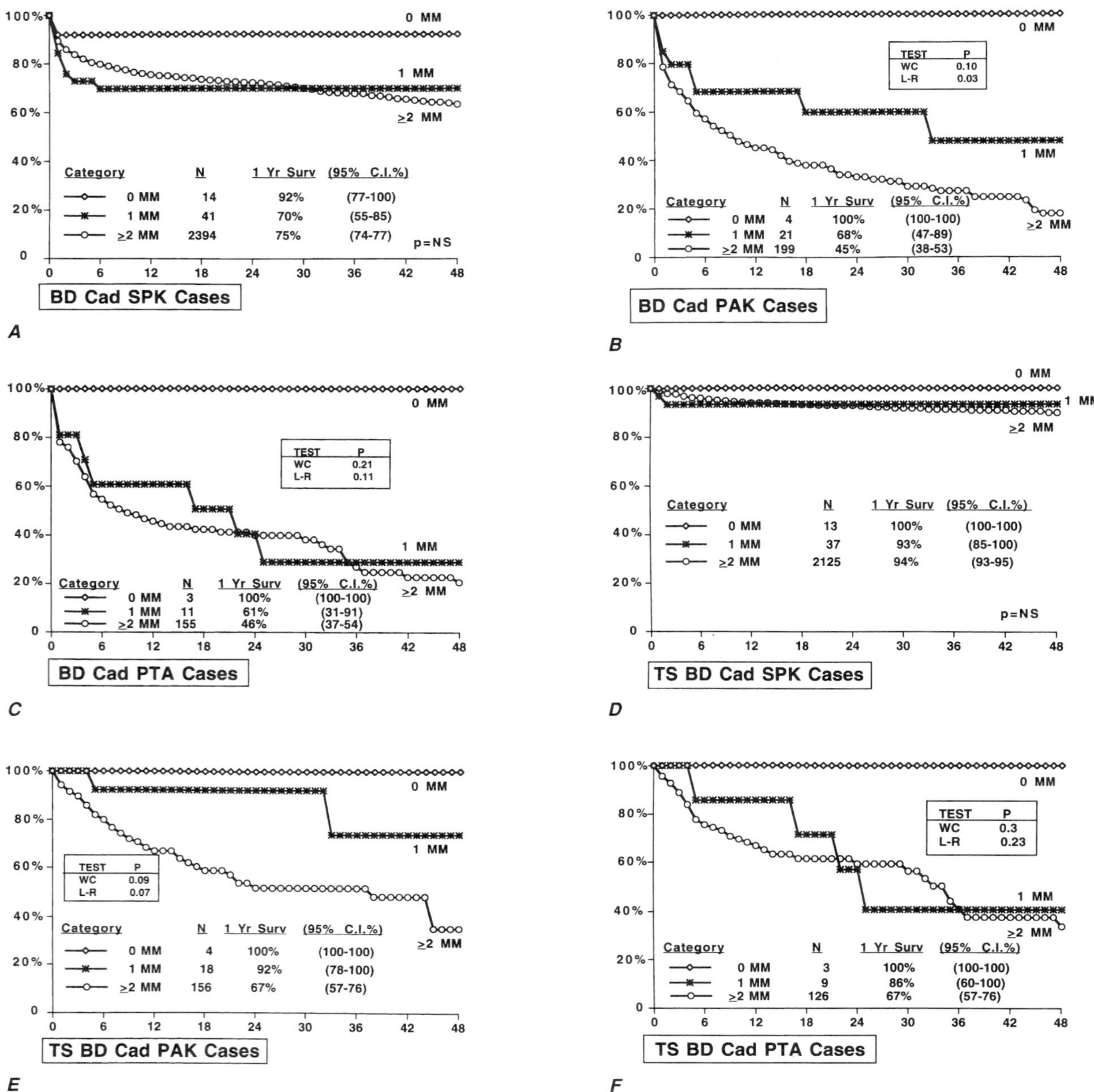

FIGURE **45-8.** Graft functional survival (*Surv*) rates according to number of HLA-A, HLA-B, and HLA-DR mismatches for bladder-drained (BD) cadaveric (cad) pancreas tranplants in recipients of SPK transplants, ***A,*** PAK transplants, ***B,*** and PTAs, ***C,*** reported to IPTR/UNOS from October 1, 1987 to April 30, 1994, with all causes of graft loss counted. In panels ***D*** (SPK), ***E*** (PAK), and ***F*** (PTA), only technically successful (TS) cases were analyzed, and deaths with functioning grafts were censored at the time of death, leaving only rejection as a cause of failure. (Reproduced with permission from Gruessner AC, Sutherland DER. Pancreas Transplant Registry, United Network for Organ Sharing and International Data Report. In: Terasaki PI, Ceka JM, eds. Clinical Transplants—1994. Los Angeles: UCLA Tissue Typing Laboratory;1995:47–68.)

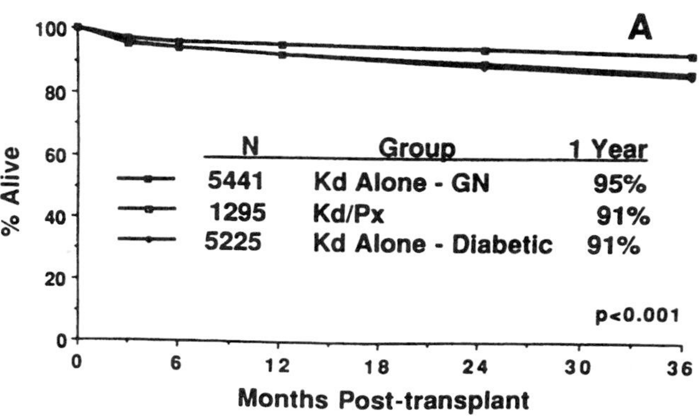

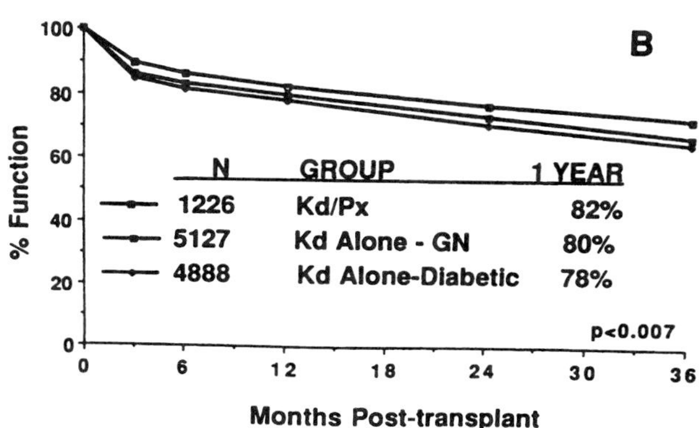

FIGURE 45-9. Patient (*A*) and kidney graft (*B*) survival rates for diabetic and nondiabetic glomerulonephretic recipients of cadaveric kidney transplants alone (*Kd Alone*) or simultaneous pancreas/kidney (*Kd/Px*) transplants in the United States as reported to UCLA/UNOS. (Reproduced with permission from Sutherland DER, Gruessner AC, Moudry-Munns KC, Cecka M. Tabulation of cases from the International Pancreas Transplant Registry and analysis of United Network for Organ Sharing U.S. Pancreas Transplant Registry data according to multiple variables. Transplant Proc 1993;25:1707.)

Disease System.[131] The other, done in conjunction with the University of California at Los Angeles (UCLA)/UNOS Kidney Transplant Registry on U.S. cases of renal allotransplantation from cadaver donors in recipients with type I diabetes reported to the IPTR from October 1987 to November 1992[130] is resummarized here.

The recipients were divided into two groups: those who underwent a kidney transplant alone (KTA-D; n=5853) versus those who, as identified by the IPTR, received an SKP transplant (n=1772). The results in both groups were compared to a nondiabetic cohort who underwent cadaver kidney transplants alone to treat renal failure from glomerulonephritis (KTA-GN; n=6615). The patient survival rate curves for the two diabetic groups were superimposed (Fig. 45-9*A*), with 92% of SKP and 91% of KTA-D recipients alive at 1 year, whereas renal allograft survival rates were slightly, but significantly ($p<0.001$), higher (Fig. 45-9*B*) in the SKP than in the KTA group (83% versus 78%, respectively, at 1 year). Patient survival rates were slightly higher for the KTA-GN group than for either the SKP or KTA-D group, but interestingly, the KTA-GN renal allograft survival rates were lower than in the SKP group.

Thus, there was no apparent difference in mortality risks for uremic diabetic patients undergoing an SPK transplant and those receiving KTA. If anything, those selected for an SKP transplant had a lower risk of renal allograft loss. This was true in all categories, with 1-year kidney graft survival rates for SPK and KTA recipients being 84% (n=425) and 80% (n=670), respectively, in those 21–30 years old; 83% (n=831) and 79% (n=1714), respectively, in those 31–40 years old, and 82% (n=437) and 78% (n=3176), respectively, in those older than 40 years of age.

Effect of Era

The latest analyses[9] show a trend for an improvement in pancreas transplants results over time worldwide (Fig. 45-10). The incidence of technical failure and rejection losses have both decreased, contributing to the higher graft survival rates in recent years.[10]

In summary, the IPTR data show that the graft function survival rates for pancreases transplanted in combination with the kidney are in a range similar to those for solid organ transplants.[132] Patient and kidney graft functional survival rates are actually higher in SPK than in diabetic KTA recipients. To achieve equivalent results with solitary pancreas transplants requires that the donors and recipients be well matched for HLA antigens.

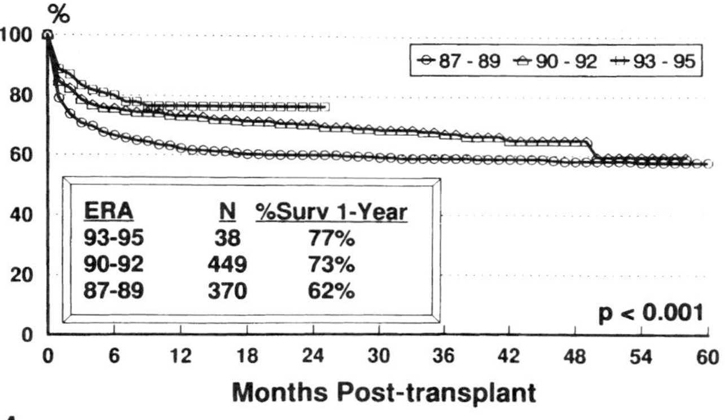

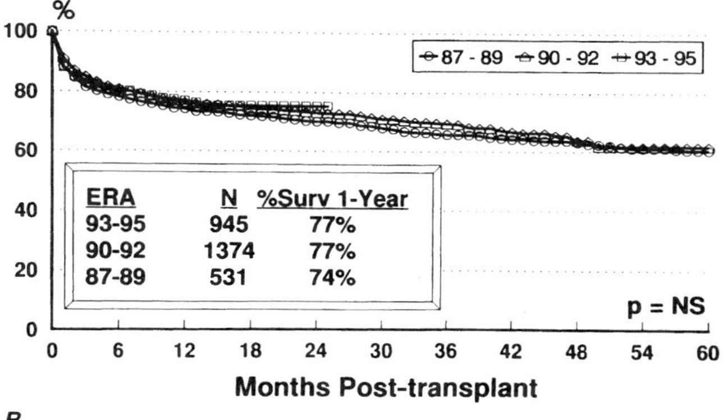

FIGURE 45-10. Pancreas graft functional survival (Surv) rates *A,* in Europe and *B,* in the U.S.A. according to year of transplant for bladder-drained (BD) SPK transplants reported to the IPTR from October 1, 1987 to May 31, 1995. (Reproduced with permission from International Pancreas Transplant Registry Newsletter. 1995;8(1):1.)

Individual Institutional Data

Simultaneous pancreas/kidney transplant in uremic diabetic patients are routinely performed at many transplant centers, several of which have published the results of their experience.[37–39,52,92,121,124–126,128,133–140] The results at these centers are similar to or better than those summarized in the IPTR statistics.

The experience with solitary pancreas transplantation (PAK and PTA) is much less widespread, and is routine at only a few centers.[123,141] However, at these centers, the results are better than those reported in the IPTR analysis of all cases. For example, the University of Nebraska Transplant Center in Omaha reported a 1-year graft survival rate of 75% for solitary pancreas transplants (n=20).[123]

The center with the longest history and largest series of solitary pancreas transplants is the University of Minnesota.[2,90,120] Of the more than 500 pancreas transplants reported at this institution through 1992,[2] two-thirds were solitary, being nearly equally divided between PAK (n=142) and PTA (n=188) recipients. In recipients of solitary pancreas transplants, HLA matching (or mismatching) has had a significant impact on the results.[122,142] Of 133 solitary bladder-drained cadaver donor pancreas transplants performed between November 1984 and August 1991 at the University of Minnesota,[120] the actuarial 1-year graft functional survival rate was 80% for those mismatched for zero or one HLA-A, HLA-B, or HLA-DR antigen (n=15), versus only 56% for those mismatched for two to three antigens (n=44) and 44% for those mismatched for four to six antigens (n=74). In an analysis of all bladder-drained solitary pancreas transplants performed between 1984 and 1991 in recipients mismatched for zero or only one HLA-A, HLA-B, or HLA-DR antigens, the 1-year insulin-independent rates were 91% in the SPK (n=11), 88% in the PAK (n=8), and 71% in the PTA (n=7) categories. In a later analysis of cases done between July 1986 and the end of 1992,[143] the 1-year PTA graft survival rate was 70% in recipients mismatched for zero or one antigen (n=13) versus 47% in those mismatched for two to six antigens (n=71; p=0.07).

In an effort to improve results achieved with solitary pancreas transplants, the protocols at Minnesota were changed in 1987.[18] The changes included the acceptance of only well-matched pancreases (< 3 HLA mismatches), induction immunosuppression consisting of 2 weeks of treatment with antilymphocyte globulin, the use of a decrease in urine amylase activity of 25% as an indication for antirejection therapy, and the performance of graft needle biopsies for confirmation of rejection if doubt existed. In December of 1991, 170 consecutive transplant recipients, representing all categories of primary grafts transplanted since October 1987 using this new protocol, were analyzed.[32] The 1-year graft functional survival rate (actuarial) for nonuremic or preuremic recipients of primary PTA was 61% (n=42); for posturemic recipients of primary PAK transplants, the rate was 70% (n=31).

The results with all PTA cases (n=102) from 1986 to 1993 were recently reanalyzed.[59] Although the 1-year functional survival rate was only 54% overall (65% for living donors and 52% for cadaveric grafts), it was 80% for cadaver grafts mismatched for zero or one HLA antigen (n=11).

Thus, it appears that, by minimizing HLA mismatches and treating rejection episodes early, the results in nonuremic, preuremic, or posturemic diabetic recipients of solitary pancreas grafts are similar to those obtained in uremic recipients of SPK transplants treated with cyclosporine. FK506 is just beginning to be used for solitary pancreas transplants, and whether it will obviate the need for good HLA matches remains to be seen.[119]

Because HLA matching reduces the incidence of solitary pancreas graft loss from rejection and enhances graft functional survival rates, there is an impetus to share well-matched organs between centers and regions.[81] Sharing is logistically feasible, as pancreas grafts can be preserved for up to 30 hours with minimal impact on functional outcome.[15,86]

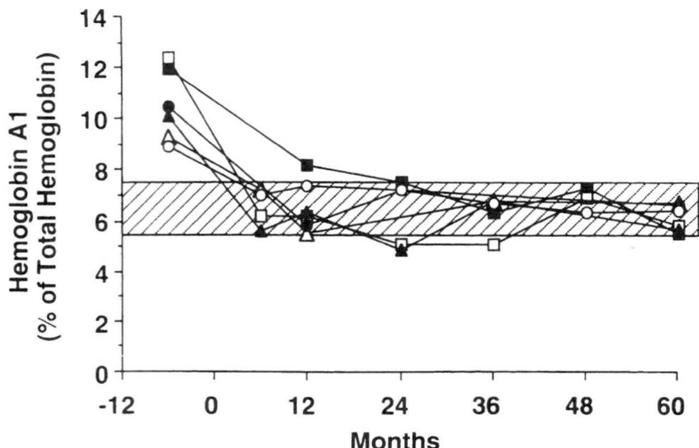

Figure 45-11. Serial glycosylated hemoglobin A1 levels in six selected recipients of successful (functioning for 5 years) pancreas transplants. The 0 value on the *x* axis indicates the time of pancreas transplant. The target range (*striped area*) is between 5.4% and 7.4%. (Reproduced with permission of Morel P, Goetz FC, Moudry-Munns KC, et al. Long-term glucose control in patients with pancreatic transplants. Annals of Internal Medicine 1991; 115:694.)

Metabolic Effect of Pancreas Transplantation

It has been well documented that successful pancreatic transplantation results in normalization of blood glucose and glycosylated hemoglobin levels[11,134,144,145] (Fig. 45-11). Normal endocrine function can be sustained following successful treatment of rejection episodes.[106] Some patients who have undergone follow-up studies for more than a decade have shown no diminution in graft β-cell function.[43] Although pancreas transplantation is the only treatment of diabetes that consistently achieves this objective, there are many metabolic details that are of interest.

Diem et al.,[54] from Minnesota, evaluated β-cell function in recipients of pancreas transplants with systemic venous drainage by measuring insulin and C-peptide responses to the intravenous administration of glucose and arginine. Basal insulin levels were elevated in pancreas transplant recipients compared to the levels in age- and sex-matched controls and compared to nondiabetic kidney transplant recipients receiving similar immunosuppressive drugs. Acute insulin responses to intravenous glucose were approximately twofold to threefold greater than those observed in control subjects and approximately 50% than those observed in nondiabetic kidney recipients. However, integrated acute C-peptide responses to glucose were not statistically different when comparing pancreas recipients with kidney recipients and control subjects. Similar insulin and C-peptide results were obtained with both intravenous glucose and intravenous arginine. It was concluded that recipients of pancreas allografts managed with systemic venous drainage had elevated basal and stimulated insulin levels, and that these alterations were primarily attributable to alterations of first-pass hepatic insulin clearance, although insulin resistance secondary to immunosuppressive therapy (including prednisone) probably played a role. The hyperinsulinemia was not considered equivalent to that which is seen in some individuals in the absence of a transplant. Other groups have reported similar results.[146–149] There are no data showing that transplantation of pancreas allografts into sites with portal rather than systemic venous drainage has a practical advantage for the patient, and even the theoretical advantages have been challenged.[150]

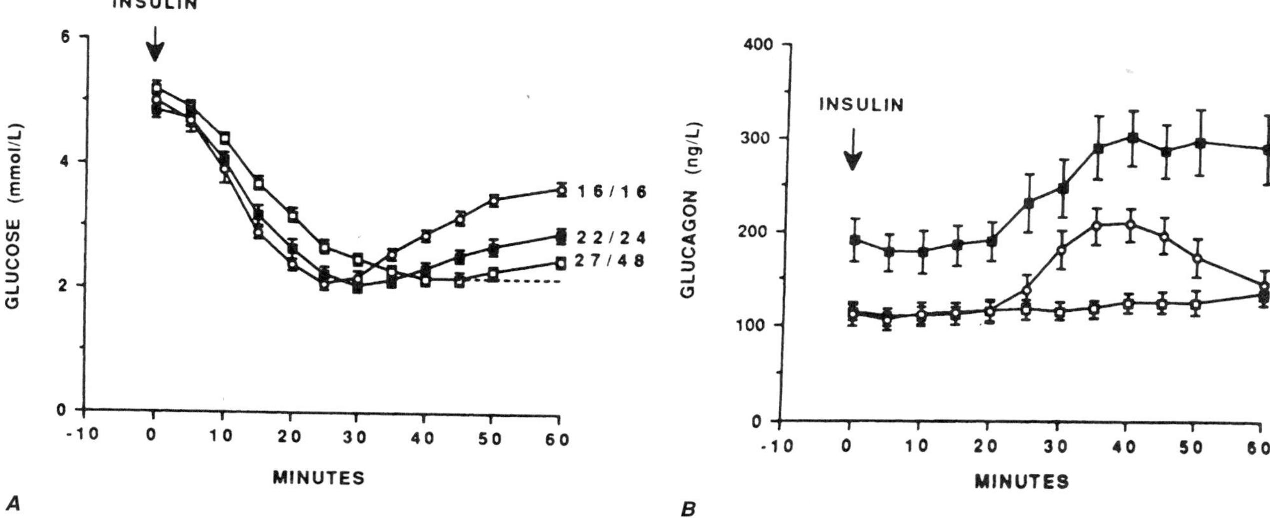

Figure 45-12. Circulating glucose and glucagon levels before and during insulin-induced hypoglycemia in 24 type I diabetic recipients of pancreas allografts (*closed squares*), 48 type I diabetic nonrecipients (*open squares*), and 16 nondiabetic normal control subjects (*open circles*). The test was completed in 22 of 24 type I diabetic recipients, 27 of 48 type I diabetic nonrecipients, and 16 of 16 normal controls. The dashed line represents an estimation of the theoretical 60-minute glucose level that would have been achieved had the 21 of 48 nonrecipients completed their test. This estimation was made based upon the last three plasma glucose levels before premature discontinuation of this test by injection of intravenous glucose owing to severe patient discomfort. Plasma glucose recovery in recipients of pancreas allografts was significantly improved compared with that in type I diabetic nonrecipients ($P<0.0001$), but was still significantly lower than that observed in normal control subjects ($P<0.00001$). Basal levels of glucagon were significantly elevated in pancreas recipients compared with those in nonrecipients ($P<0.001$) and controls ($P<0.01$). The maximal incremental glucagon responses in recipients were significantly different than those controls. (Reproduced with permission from Diem P, Redmon JB, Abid M, et al. Glucagon, catecholamine, and pancreatic polypeptide secretion in type I diabetic recipients of pancreas allografts. J Clin Invest 1990;86:2008.)

In a separate set of studies, Diem et al.[42] also examined glucagon, catecholamine, and pancreatic polypeptide secretion in pancreas transplant recipients. They observed that successful pancreas transplantation resulted in an improvement in glucose recovery after insulin-induced hypoglycemia (Fig. 45-12*A*). It was further noted that basal glucagon levels were significantly higher in transplant recipients when compared with those in type I diabetic patients not receiving pancreas transplantation and in normal subjects. Glucagon responses to insulin-induced hypoglycemia were significantly greater in the pancreas transplant recipients than in the control subjects (Fig. 45-12*B*). No differences were observed, however, in epinephrine and pancreatic polypeptide responses to hypoglycemia. The authors concluded that type I diabetic recipients of pancreas transplantation had significant improvement in glucose recovery after hypoglycemia, associated with improved glucagon secretion. The lack of improvement in pancreatic polypeptide secretion was interpreted as evidence that the allograft remained denervated post-transplantation.

Further studies by the Minnesota group have shown normalization of hepatic glucose production following pancreas transplantation, even with systemic venous drainage.[43] A comparison to diabetic recipients of KTA demonstrated that the improved counterregulation was the result of the transplant and not of immunosuppression.[43]

Immunosuppressive drugs can increase the need for insulin secretion (corticosteroids) while at the same time diminishing secretory reserves (cyclosporine).[151] In SPK transplant recipients of segmental pancreas grafts, basal C-peptide levels were elevated compared to those in normal individuals, while at the same time, maximal insulin secretion and glucose disposal were reduced compared to nondiabetic immunosuppressed recipients of kidney transplants alone.[152] Nevertheless, even half a pancreas (segmental transplant) is sufficient to establish insulin independence and euglycemia in a diabetic transplant recipient.[151,152] (The redundant islet mass of a pancreas may be one reason this method of transplantation has worked so much better than free grafts of allogenic islets. The number of islets engrafted, if not transplanted, may be much less than that contained in even half of a pancreas, and too little to overcome the diabetogenic effects of the antirejection drugs.[153])

The improved counterregulation has led the Minnesota group to conclude that pancreas transplants should be considered as a therapeutic option in type I diabetic patients who have repeated episodes of insulin-induced hypoglycemia and who demonstrate refractoriness to conventional medical management with diet and alteration of insulin dosage.[42,154] Patients with frequent insulin reactions who have high glycohemoglobin levels are usually not being overtreated with insulin, and indeed, may be undertreating themselves. Even a small dose of insulin may cause hypoglycemia if gastroenteropathy is present with erratic and unpredictable absorption of food. In such patients, a successful pancreas transplant abolishes the need for exogenous insulin, preventing the insulin reactions even if gastrointestinal problems persist.[19]

Lipid[150,155] and protein[156] metabolism have also been studied in pancreas transplant recipients. Lipid profiles have been found to be more favorable after SPK transplants than after kidney transplants alone,[155] and are improved compared to pretransplant profiles.[150] Indeed, one group has postulated that systemic hyperinsulinemia is responsible for the increased lipoprotein lipase activity, increasing triglyceride clearance and promoting high levels of HDL cholesterol.[150] According to this hypothesis, the peculiar form of hyperinsulinemia induced by systemically drained pancreas transplants may attenuate the risk of cardiovascular disease that these patients might otherwise have. SPK transplant recipients also have normalization of insulin-mediated protein kinetics, whereas protein metabolism is not normalized in diabetic patients with uremia who undergo kidney transplantation alone.[156]

Overall, a pancreas transplant has a profoundly beneficial effect on metabolic parameters in diabetic recipients. Metabolic disturbances can be detected by some tests, but are trivial compared to those that exist in type I diabetics who are treated with exogenous insulin.

Effect of Pancreas Transplantation on Secondary Complications of Diabetes

In general, for either patients with end-stage nephropathy undergoing PAK transplantation, or for nonuremic patients who are selected for PTA, any benefits derived from establishment of constant normoglycemia (in terms of secondary complications of diabetes) are an incidental bonus.[34]

In nonuremic patients, a successful pancreas transplant can induce regression of early,[157] but not advanced,[158] microscopic lesions of diabetic nephropathy.[159] Renal function usually stabilizes,[160,161] but progressive deterioration can occur because of the nephrotoxic effect of the cyclosporine necessary to prevent rejection.[162] In renal allograft recipients, a successful pancreas transplant, performed either simultaneously with[163,164] or within a few years after kidney transplantation,[165] will prevent recurrence of diabetic nephropathy in the new graft. In this situation, immunosuppression is necessary in order to have renal function at all; by keeping diabetic lesions from being superimposed on those caused by cyclosporine or graft rejection, long-term renal graft function is likely to be improved.

With regard to retinopathy, one study in patients with advanced disease did not show a difference in the probability of progression during the first 3 years after successful pancreas transplantation versus after failed pancreas transplantation.[166] However, in patients with long-term functioning grafts, retinopathy tended to stabilize, whereas in those with failed grafts, it continued to progress.[90,166] Another study that compared the course of retinopathy in diabetic recipients of SPK transplants and in those undergoing KTA revealed that progression rates were lower in those who had a successful pancreas transplant.[167] Because disease was already advanced in these patients, it was hard to show a benefit, and no data exist with regard to the effect of pancreas transplants on patients with early retinopathy.

Neuropathy improves or stabilizes in most pancreas transplant recipients.[41,90,168–172] Nerve conduction velocities and evoked muscle action potentials have been found to increase,[169,170] and even advanced polyneuropathy may improve in some patients after successful transplantation.[172] Autonomic parameters also improve.[171] Indeed, in patients with severe autonomic neuropathy or severe conduction abnormalities, those who undergo a successful pancreas transplant have a significantly higher probability of survival than those who are not transplant recipients or who have unsuccessful transplants.[173]

Vasculopathy may also improve after pancreas transplantation, as evidenced by increased transcutaneous oxygen levels[174] and decreased capillary leakage.[175] The clinical benefit of these findings is uncertain, but there are no data to suggest that pancreas transplantation has a detrimental effect on the vascular system, even in cases of systemic hyperinsulinemia. It should also be remembered that exogenous insulin (absorbed systemically) causes hyperinsulinemia without euglycemia, whereas pancreas transplantation results in both, both of which can be beneficial, according to Königsrainer, et al.[150]

Effect of Pancreas Transplantation on Quality of Life

Although the potential for pancreas transplantation to have a favorable effect on the secondary complications of diabetes is important, it is its overall impact on quality of life—including that associated with insulin independence per se—that should be emphasized. The studies conducted thus far are nearly unanimous in finding that patients undergoing successful transplantation rate their quality of life as improved in comparison to that before their transplant.[33,44,59,143,176–186]

In the largest study to date on PTA recipients,[44,182] 131 patients were analyzed 1 to 10 years post-transplantation, 50% of whom had functioning grafts (n=65) and 50% of whom had grafts that ultimately failed (n=66). Overall, 92% stated that managing immunosuppression was easier than managing diabetes.[44] When asked which was more demanding on their family's time and energy—the transplant or their diabetes—63% responded that their diabetes was more demanding, 29% responded that the two were equally demanding, and 9% responded that the transplant was more demanding. Of the 65 patients with functioning grafts, 89% stated that they were healthier after the transplant than before. Indices of well-being were quantified by standard tests, and were significantly higher in patients with functioning grafts than in those without.[182] Moreover, 100% of the patients with continuous graft function and 85% of those whose grafts ultimately failed stated that they would encourage others with similar complications of diabetes to consider pancreas transplantation.[44] In addition, most of the patients with failed grafts desired retransplantation, and those with functioning grafts said that they would undergo a retransplant if their current graft failed.

If the original indications for pancreas transplant are present after graft failure, retransplantation should be considered.[187] The University of Minnesota experience has shown the results with retransplants of a pancreas alone are similar to those for primary transplantation.[59] Careful donor selection and good HLA matching yield a high probability of success with pancreas retransplantation.[82]

Pancreas transplants in patients with hyperlabile diabetes and extreme difficulty with metabolic control can improve quality of life simply by inducing insulin independence.[41,44] Kidney transplants also improve quality of life in uremic patients by obviating the need for dialysis.[30] For diabetic patients with both problems, the effect of a double transplant can be dramatic.[33,176,181] SPK recipients rate their quality of life higher than do diabetic KTA recipients on almost all scales.[183] With one surgical procedure, two difficult clinical problems are corrected for as long as rejection is prevented by immunosuppression. For diabetic patients without nephropathy, however, the price (i.e., immunosuppression) is the same simply to be rid of their diabetes. Whether the benefit is worth the "price" has been debated,[188,189] but pancreas transplant recipients have emphatically stated that it is.[190,191]

β-Cell Autoimmunity and Recurrence of Diabetes in Pancreas Transplant Recipients

Autoimmunity is sometimes the cause of disease leading to the need for total replacement therapy of organs other than the endocrine pancreas,[192] but the proportion of pancreas transplant recipients whose original disease—type I diabetes mellitus—has an autoimmune etiology is uniquely high (nearly all).[193] A few pancreas transplants have been successfully performed in patients who are diabetic as a result of total pancreatectomy for benign disease[12] (usually chronic pancreatitis),[194] in whom the etiology of diabetes is surgical ablation of the islets. However, the demographics of the entire pancreas transplant population, as reported to the Pancreas Transplant Registry,[193] is nearly identical to that of diabetic patients documented to have immunoreactivity directed against islet cells.[195] Nearly 90% of recipients of pancreas transplants type positive for HLA-DR3 or -DR4, the alleles strongly associated with type I diabetes mellitus.[195]

The immunosuppressive regimens currently used to prevent rejection of pancreas allografts are similar to those used for other solid organ transplants.[18] The new organs may be as susceptible to the autoimmune process as the one being replaced (whether it be pancreas, liver, heart, lung, or kidney), but in practical terms, the amount of immunosuppression required to prevent allograft rejection is nearly always sufficient to prevent autoimmune damage of the graft as well.[196] If an identical twin is the organ donor (as was the case with the very first successful kidney transplant[197]), immunosuppression is not necessary to prevent rejection. Moreover, if the original disease has a nonautoimmune etiology, as is the case in many renal disorders, immunosuppression is not necessary to prevent recurrence of disease either.[198] However, if the disease that destroyed the native kidneys has an autoimmune etiology, the same disease can recur in the new (transplanted) kidney (including isografts) unless adequate immunosuppression is given.[198,199]

Immunosuppression has been used to treat a variety of autoimmune diseases,[192] including type I diabetes mellitus.[200] However, if immunosuppression is used to treat an autoimmune disease, the benefits, or the degree to which the disease is ameliorated, must exceed the detriments associated with immunosuppression.[201] Because most of the β-cell mass has been destroyed by the time type I diabetes mellitus becomes clinically apparent, immunosuppression has only a minimal impact on the course of the disease in most patients receiving such therapeutic attempts.[202] Thus, if immunosuppression is to be given, it is best to do so in conjunction with a pancreas or islet transplant, so the β-cell mass is restored to normal. Because immunotherapy can prevent recurrence (in isografts or allografts), as well as rejection (in allografts), a clinical "cure" is possible with transplantation.

As for kidney transplants, nondiseased (nondiabetic) identical twins have been donors of segmental pancreas isografts to their diabetic twin counterparts.[55] Of nine cases at the University of Minnesota Hospital, seven were technically successful.[58] The early courses of the first four twin recipients have been reported in detail.[25,27] All of the twin pairs in the Minnesota series had been discordant for diabetes for more than 15 years at the time of transplantation; thus, the donors themselves were at very low risk to develop the disease.[203] The twin donors were normal metabolically before organ donation, and all have remained disease-free since donation.[63]

It was initially assumed that the risk of recurrence of disease in the pancreas isografts, even in the absence of recipient immunosuppression, would be low because of the long interval between the onset of the original disease and the transplant.[25] This assumption has not been supported by experience, however.[26] Indeed, the need for immunosuppression to prevent isletitis (not rejection), even in diabetic recipients of segmental pancreas transplants from nondiabetic identical twin donors, has been underscored by the Minnesota experience.[27]

The first three twin recipients of technically successful isografts from identical twin donors in the Minnesota series were not given prophylactic immunosuppression.[25] Diabetes recurred within 6 to 12 weeks, and pathologic examination showed isletitis with specific β-cell destruction.[26] In the third patient, immunosuppression with azathioprine was instituted at the time that graft dysfunction first occurred and isletitis (recurrence of disease) was confirmed by graft biopsy. This patient has retained β-cell function for a long period (10 years), with persistence of the ability to increase serum C-peptide levels upon stimulation, as well as demonstration of β-cells on follow-up pancreas graft biopsies (the latest biopsy being performed 7 years posttransplantation).[26,109] However, as is usually the case when patients with new-onset diabetes are given immunosuppression, normal metabolism was not restored, and the patient has required exogenous insulin since 1 year after recurrence of disease was diagnosed.

The next four recipients of technically successful segmental pancreas isografts from identical twin donors in the Minnesota series were treated with prophylactic immunosuppression. The first of these (fourth in the entire series) was treated with azathioprine only; the last three (fifth, sixth, and seventh in the series) were treated with a combination of cyclosporine and azathioprine. The patient treated with azathioprine alone was normoglycemic for 4 years; she then was found to have recurrence of disease, with selective loss of islet β-cells confirmed by biopsy, and had to resume insulin therapy.[27]

Of the three twin recipients treated with cyclosporine and azathioprine, all were insulin-independent as of 1994, and all have been insulin-independent for at least 4 years, the longest period now being 7 years. The grafts of all three have been subjected to biopsy one or more times between 6 months and 5 years posttransplant. All biopsy results except one have shown absolutely normal histologic findings with no isletitis and with a normal proportion of β-cells within the islets. The one graft in this trial that showed mild isletitis on biopsy (at 6 months) did not have isletitis at a 3½-year follow-up biopsy, but β-cell mass was reduced. The other two had normal β-cell mass at the time of biopsies performed 2 and 5 years posttransplant, respectively.[58]

It is apparent that isletitis and recurrence of disease in pancreas grafts can be prevented by adequate prophylactic immunosuppression. The need for prophylaxis, however, also means that, to be a candidate for a pancreas isograft, the problems associated with diabetes have to be severe enough so that immunosuppression is an acceptable trade-off for their correction.

Recurrence of disease (isletitis with selective β-cell destruction in the absence of vasculitis or other histologic features of rejection) has not been seen in cadaveric pancreas grafts.[26,107] Most likely, the degree of immunosuppression necessary to prevent rejection of HLA-mismatched grafts is always able to overcome autoimmunity. The identical twin recipients at Minnesota received much less immunosuppression than recipients of cadaveric pancreas grafts, based on the assumption that the autoimmune process is easier to suppress than allograft rejection. Recurrence of disease in the absence of rejection has been seen in allografts from HLA-identical sibling allografts transplanted to recipients treated with minimal immunosuppression, as not much is required to prevent rejection.[24,26,204,205]

T-cells, present in biopsies from pancreas grafts showing either rejection[206] or isletitis,[205] have been cloned. The characteristics of the cells derived from an HLA-identical sibling allograft with isletitis and selective β-cell destruction[205] differ from those of the cells derived from biopsies in patients who simply showed allograft rejection.[206] There were no features of rejection in the pancreas allograft of the one patient with isletitis and selective β-cell destruction in whom the T-cells were cloned.[205] The fact that a renal allograft in the same sibling donor was normal, both functionally and histologically, was further evidence that the process observed was not secondary to an alloimmune response, but a reenactment of the original anti-immune process in a patient receiving only low-dose azathioprine and prednisone. Rejection episodes in recipients of dual transplants (kidney and pancreas), or outright rejection of one organ without rejection of the other when both are derived from the same donor, have been described,[91,97,116] but such occurrences are the exception rather than the rule.[193] For the case in question, rejection was shown to be absent in both organs.[205]

Recurrence of disease has only been observed in segmental pancreas grafts from donors that are HLA-identical with the recipient, but this does not mean that the process is major histocompatibility complex (MHC)–restricted.[107] The recipients of HLA-mismatched grafts receive relatively more immunosuppression, and the lack of recurrence in such grafts may be attributable to this reason.[26] Furthermore, studies using transplants in animal models of autoimmune diabetes indicate that the process is not MHC-restricted.[207,208]

The main lessons to be derived from the clinical experience with segmental pancreas transplants from HLA-identical siblings or discordant identical twin (syngenic) donors to their diabetic counterparts are that (1) immunologic memory for autoreactivity against β-cells in type I diabetes mellitus is life-long, (2) adequate immunotherapy can prevent recurrence of disease in the graft, and (3) the immune response to autoantigens can be stronger than to the minor histocompatibility antigens (e.g., some recipients of HLA-identical sibling allografts who were receiving minimal immunosuppression developed recurrence of disease in the absence of rejection). The fact that adequate immunosuppression could prevent recurrence of disease in pancreas isografts means that the same treatment, initiated before extensive β-cell destruction in the native pancreas of patients with preclinical type I diabetes mellitus, would almost certainly allow normal metabolism to be preserved.

Summary

Currently, pancreas transplantation is most widely applied as an adjunct to kidney transplantation in preuremic, uremic, or post-uremic diabetic patients,[36] but its application to nonuremic patients, particularly those with hyperlabile diabetes, has increased in recent years.[59] Because current immunosuppressive regimens have many side effects,[18] however, the recipients must be carefully selected.[209]

HLA matching improves the probability of long-term success, but does not eliminate the need for immunosuppression.[193] At least some immunosuppression is required, even for recipients of a segmental graft from a nondiabetic identical twin donor; if immunosuppression is not afforded, the original autoimmune process will recur in the graft.[24] Immunosuppression that is sufficient to prevent rejection is nearly always able to prevent recurrence of disease.[107] Again, the recipient's problems with diabetes should be of a sufficient magnitude so that the potential side effects of immunosuppression are an acceptable trade-off.[44]

Whether islet transplantation will eventually supersede pancreas transplantation as a method of endocrine replacement therapy for the treatment of type I diabetes remains to be determined.[210] Prevention of rejection of islet allografts appears to be even more difficult than prevention of pancreas rejection.[211] The fact that the main problem to solve with islet transplants is immunologic is readily apparent. Insulin independence has been preserved with intraportal islet autotransplantation following total pancreatectomy for benign disease.[212] In this situation (in which there is no possibility of rejection), normoglycemia can be maintained with a relatively small number of intrahepatic islets.[213,214]

For diabetic patients who wish to undergo a procedure with the highest probability of inducing an insulin-independent, euglycemic state, pancreas transplantation is the preferred choice at this time.[154] Nearly all uremic diabetic candidates for a kidney transplant are also candidates for a pancreas or islet transplant. The best treatment option is to receive a living related donor kidney transplant first, followed later by a pancreas transplant from either a living related (segmental graft) or cadaver (whole organ or segmental) donor.[56,58] In uremic patients who do not have a living related donor for a kidney, a pancreas transplant can be performed simultaneously with a kidney transplant from a cadaver donor.[20,215]

Living related donor kidneys have the highest long-term renal allograft functional survival rates.[30] When coupled with a subsequent pancreas transplant from either a cadaver or related donor, this approach promotes the best overall outcome for the patient.[216] The incentive to perform a living related donor kidney transplant first is more compelling than ever, as the insulin independence rates achieved with a PAK transplant can be as good as those derived from an SPK transplant as long as the donor is a good HLA match.[120] The approach taken must be tailored, however, to the individual patient.

The arguments for performing pancreas transplants differ[188,217] according to whether the prospective recipient does or does not need a kidney transplant.[218–221] The rationale for performing pancreas transplants in diabetic kidney transplant recipients is clear.[154,209,218,220,222] For nonuremic diabetic patients, the selection criteria are less certain.[41,90,154,209,219,221,222] In general, such patients must have problems correctable by transplantation that exceed those that are associated with chronic immunosuppression.[19] Patients with labile diabetes and hypoglycemia unawareness are currently the best candidates, as the problem is correctable by a pancreas transplant and the qualify of life is improved in spite of the need for immunosuppression.[59] This situation is analogous to the conclusion that, for a patient with renal failure, immunosuppression to eliminate uremia is preferred to dialysis.[30]

When antirejection strategies become available that have fewer consequences than the present regimens, there will be an incentive to use pancreas transplants as a treatment for nonlabile diabetes, before any predisposition to secondary complications is evident. For now, pancreas transplantation constitutes routine therapy for renal allograft recipients with type I diabetes. It is also used to treat selected nonuremic patients with labile diabetes or other diabetic problems that are not well-served by alternative therapeutic methods. Further expansion of this role will depend upon advances in specific immunosuppression and upon donor availability. Currently, approximately 4500 cadaver donors are available annually in the United States (equivalent to about 25% of the annual incidence of type I diabetes in the United States), and this may closely approximate the number for whom exogenous insulin is unsatisfactory as a treatment. If all cadaver donors were used for pancreas transplants, the impact on type I diabetes would be considerable.

References

1. Kelly WD, Lillehei RC, Merkel FK, et al. Allotransplantation of the pancreas and duodenum along with the kidney in diabetic nephropathy. Surgery 1967;61:827
2. Sutherland DER, Gores PF, Farney AC, et al. Evolution of kidney, pancreas, and islet transplantation for patients with diabetes at the University of Minnesota. Am J Surg 1993;166:456
3. Lillehei RC, Simmons RL, Najarian JS. Pancreatico-duodenal allotransplantation: Experimental and clinical experience. Diabetes Care 1970;172:405
4. Gliedman ML, Tellis VA, Soberman R. Long-term effects of pancreatic transplant function in patients with advanced juvenile onset diabetes. Diabetes Care 1978;1:1
5. Dubernard JM, Treaeger J, Neyra P, et al. A new method of preparation of segmental pancreatic grafts for transplantation: Trials in dogs and in man. Surgery 1978;84:633
6. Groth CG, Lundgren G, Arner P, et al. Rejection of isolated pancreatic allografts in patients with diabetes. Surg Gynecol Obstet 1976;143: 933
7. Sutherland DER. International human pancreas and islet transplant registry. Transplant Proc 1980;12:229
8. Sutherland DER, Moudry-Munns KC, Gillingham KJ. Report from the International Pancreas Transplant Registry. Diabetologia 1991;34:S28
9. International Pancreas Transplant Registry Newsletter. 1995;8(1):1
10. Gruessner AC, Sutherland DERC. Pancreas Transplant Registry, United Network for Organ Sharing and International Data Report. In: Terasaki PI, Cecka JM, eds. Clinical Transplants—1994. Los Angeles: UCLA Tissue Typing Laboratory;1995:47–68
11. Morel P, Goetz FC, Moudry-Munns KC, et al. Long-term glucose control in patients with pancreatic transplants. Ann Intern Med 1991;115:694
12. Gruessner RWG, Manivel DC, Dunn DL, Sutherland DER. Pancreaticoduodenal transplantation with enteric drainage following native total pancreatectomy for chronic pancreatitis: A case report. Pancreas 1991;6:479

13. Hering BJ, Browatzki CC, Schultz A, et al. Clinical islet transplantation—Registry report, accomplishments in the past and future research needs. Cell Transplant 1993;2:269
14. Federlin KF, Bretzel RG, Hering BJ, et al. International Islet Transplant Registry Newsletter. 1994;5(1):1–28
15. Sutherland DER, Moudry-Munns KC, Gruessner AC. Pancreas Transplant Registry, United Network for Organ Sharing and International Data Report. In: Terasaki PI, ed. Clinical Transplants—1993. Los Angeles: UCLA Tissue Typing Laboratory;1994:47
16. Lacy PE. Status of islet cell transplantation. Diabetes Care 1993;1:76
17. Morel P, Goetz FC, Moudry-Munns KC, et al. Serial glycosylated hemoglobin levels in diabetic recipients of pancreatic transplants. Transplant Proc 1990;22:649
18. Sutherland DER. Immunosuppression for clinical pancreas transplantation. Clin Transplant 1991;5:549
19. Sutherland DER. Present status of pancreas transplantation alone in nonuremic diabetic patients. Transplant Proc 1994;26:379
20. Sollinger HW. Current status of simultaneous pancreas-kidney transplantation. Transplant Proc 1994;26:375
21. Eisenbarth GS. Type I diabetes mellitus: A chronic autoimmune disease. N Engl J Med 1986;314:1360
22. Bottazzo GF. Banting Lecture. On the honey disease: A dialogue with Socrates. Diabetes 1993;42:778
23. Atkinson MA, Maclaren NK. The pathogenesis of insulin-dependent diabetes mellitus. N Engl J Med 1994;331:1428
24. Sutherland DER, Sibley RK. Recurrence of Disease in Pancreas Transplants. Amsterdam: Elsevier Science Publishers B V;1988:60
25. Sutherland DER, Sibley RK, Xu XZ, et al. Twin-to-twin pancreas transplantation: Reversal and reenactment of the pathogenesis of type I diabetes. Trans Assoc Am Physicians 1984;97:80
26. Sibley RK, Sutherland DER, Goetz FC, Michael AF. Recurrent diabetes mellitus in the pancreas iso- and allograft: A light and electron microscopic and immunohistochemical analysis of four cases. Lab Invest 1985;53:132
27. Sutherland DER, Goetz FC, Sibley RK. Recurrence of disease in pancreas transplants. Diabetes 1989;38:85
28. Hanssen KF, Dahl-Jorgenson K, Lauritzen J. Diabetic control and microvascular complications: The near normoglycemic experience. Diabetologia 1986; 10:677
29. DCCT Research Group. Diabetes control and complications trial (DCCT): The effect of intensive diabetes treatment on long-term complications in IDDM. N Engl J Med 1993;329:977
30. Jacobson SH, Fryd DS, Sutherland DER, Kjellstrand CM. Treatment of the diabetic patient with end-stage renal failure. Diabetes Metab Rev 1988;4:191
31. Cheung AHS, Sutherland DER, Gillingham KJ, et al. Simultaneous pancreas-kidney (SPK) transplant versus kidney transplant alone (KTA) in diabetic patients. Kidney Int 1992;41:924
32. Gruessner AC, Gruessner RWG, Moudry-Munns KC, et al. Influence of multiple factors (age, transplant number, recipient category, donor source) on outcome of pancreas transplantation at one institution. Transplant Proc 1993;25:1303
33. Gross CR, Zehrer CL. Impact of the addition of a pancreas to quality of life in uremic diabetic recipients of kidney transplants. Transplant Proc 1993;25: 1293
34. Sutherland DER. Effect of pancreas transplants on secondary complications of diabetes: Review of observations of a single institution. Transplant Proc 1992;24:859
35. Morris RP. Rapamycins: Antifungal, antitumor, antiproliferative, and immunosuppressive macrolides. Transplant Rev 1992;6(1):39
36. Sutherland DER. Pancreatic transplantation: State of the art. Transplant Proc 1992;24:762
37. Perkins JD, Frohner PP, Service FJ, et al. Pancreas transplantation at Mayo. III. Multidisciplinary. Mayo Clin Proc 1990;65:496
38. Sutherland DER, Dunn DL, Goetz FC, et al. A 10-year experience with 290 pancreas transplants at a single institution. Ann Surg 1989;210:274
39. Stratta RJ, Taylor RJ, Ozaki CF, et al. A comparative analysis of results and morbidity in type I diabetics under-going preemptive versus post-dialysis combined pancreas-kidney transplantation. Transplantation 1993;55(5):1097
40. Gruessner RWG, Dunn DL, Gruessner AC, et al. Recipient risk factors have an impact on technical failure and patient and graft survival rates in bladder-drained pancreas transplants. Transplantation 1994;57:1598
41. Bolinder J, Wahrenberg H, Linde B, et al. Improved glucose counterregulation after pancreas transplantation in diabetic patients with unawareness of hypoglycemia. Transplant Proc 1991;23:1667
42. Diem P, Redmon JB, Abid M, et al. Glucagon, catecholamine and pancreatic polypeptide secretion in type I diabetic recipients of pancreas allografts. J Clin Invest 1990;86:2008
43. Barrou Z, Seaquist ER, Robertson RP. Pancreas transplantation in diabetic human normalizes hepatic glucose production during hypoglycemia. Diabetes 1994;43:661
44. Zehrer CL, Gross CR. Quality of life of pancreas transplant recipients. Diabetologia 1991;34:S145
45. Dubernard JM, Martin X, Sanseverino R, Gelet A. Surgical techniques and complications. In: Dubernard JM, Sutherland DER, eds. International Handbook of Pancreas Transplantation. Dordrecht: Kluwer Academic Publishers;1988:71
46. Brayman KL, Najarian JS, Sutherland DER. Current Surgical Therapy. Toronto: BC Decker;1994:458
47. Calne RY. Paratopic segmental pancreas grafting: A technique with portal venous drainage. Lancet 1984;1:595
48. Gilbert-Vernet JM, Fernandez-Cruz L, Andreu J, et al. A clinical experience with pancreaticopyelostomy for exocrine pancreatic drainage and portal venous drainage in pancreas transplantation. Transplant Proc 1985;17:342
49. Tydén G, Wilczek H, Lundgren G. Experience with 21 intraperitoneal segmental pancreatic transplants with enteric or gastric exocrine diversion in humans. Transplant Proc 1985;17:331
50. Sutherland DER, Goetz FC, Moudry KC, et al. Use of recipient mesenteric vessels for revascularization of segmental pancreas grafts: Technical and metabolic considerations. Transplant Proc 1987;19:2300
51. Müehlbacher F, Gnant MF, Auinger M. Pancreatic venous drainage to the portal vein: A new method in human pancreas transplantation. Transplant Proc 1990;22:636
52. Rosenlof LK, Earnhardt RC, Pruett TL, et al. Pancreas transplantation: An initial experience with systemic and portal drainage of pancreatic allografts. Ann Surg 1992;215:586
53. Gaber AO, Shokouh-Amiri MH, Grewal HP, Britt LG. A technique for portal pancreas transplantation with enteric drainage. Surg Gynecol Obstet 1993; 177(4):417
54. Diem P, Manuir A, Redmon JB. Systemic drainage of pancreas allografts as independent cause of hyperinsulinemia in type I diabetic recipients. Diabetes 1990;39:534
55. Sutherland DER, Goetz FC, Gillingham KJ, et al. Medical Risks and Benefit of Pancreas Transplants from Living Related Donors. In: Land W, Dossetor JB, eds. Organ Replacement Therapy: Ethics, Justice, and Commerce. Berlin: Springer-Verlag;1991:93–101
56. Cheung AHS, Matas AJ, Gruessner RWG, et al. Should uremic diabetic patients who want a pancreas transplant receive a simultaneous cadaver kidney-pancreas transplant or a living related donor kidney first, followed by cadaver pancreas transplant? Transplant Proc 1993;25:1184
57. Sutherland DER, Goetz FC, Najarian JS. Pancreas transplants from related donors. Transplantation 1984;38:625
58. Sutherland DER, Gruessner RWG, Dunn DL, et al. Pancreas transplants from living related donors. Transplant Proc 1994;26(6):443
59. Sutherland DER, Gruessner RWG, Moudry-Munns KC, et al. Pancreas transplants alone in nonuremic patients with labile diabetes. Transplant Proc 1994;26:446
60. Kendall DM, Sutherland DER, Goetz FC, Najarian JS. Metabolic effects of hemipancreatectomy in donors. Preoperative prediction of postoperative oral glucose tolerance. Diabetes 1989;38(suppl):101
61. Kendall DM, Sutherland DER, Najarian JS, et al. Effects of hemipancreatectomy on insulin secretion and glucose tolerance in healthy humans. N Engl J Med 1990;322:898
62. Williams SL, Oler J, Jorkasky DK. Long-term renal function in kidney donors: A comparison of donors and their siblings. Ann Intern Med 1986;106:1
63. Seaquist ER, Robertson RP. Effects of hemipancreatectomy on pancreatic alpha and beta cell function in healthy human donors. J Clin Invest 1992;89:1761
64. Tydén G, Tibell A, Bolinder J, et al. Pancreatic transplantation with enteric exocrine diversion: Experience with 120 cases. Transplant Proc 1992;24:771
65. Tibell A, Brattström C, Wadström J, et al. Improved results using whole organ pancreatico-duodenal transplants with enteric exocrine drainage. Transplant Proc 1994;26:412
66. Martin X, Lefrancois N, Dawahra M, et al. Pancreas transplantation in the uremic patient: A random trial of total pancreas with bladder drainage versus duct obstruction of segmental grafts. Transplant Proc 1993;25:1182
67. Gliedman ML, Gold M, Whittaker J, et al. Clinical segmental pancreatic transplantation with ureter-pancreatic duct anastomosis for exocrine drainage. Surgery 1973;74:171
68. Sollinger HW, Cook K, Kamps D. Clinical and experimental experience with pancreaticocystostomy for exocrine pancreatic drainage in pancreas transplantation. Transplant Proc 1984;16:749
69. Nghiem DD, Corry RJ. Technique of simultaneous pancreaticoduodenal transplantation with urinary drainage of pancreatic secretion. Am J Surg 1987;153:405
70. Pescovitz MD, Dunn DL, Sutherland DER. Use of the circular stapler in construction of the duodenoneocystostomy for drainage into the bladder in transplants involving the whole pancreas. Surg Gynecol Obstet 1989;169: 169
71. Sollinger HW, Messing EM, Eckhoff DE, et al. Urological complications in 210 consecutive simultaneous pancreas-kidney transplants with bladder drainage. Ann Surg 1993;218:561
72. Burke GW, Gruessner RWG, Dunn DL, Sutherland DER. Conversion of whole pancreaticoduodenal transplants from bladder to enteric drainage for metabolic acidosis or dysuria. Transplant Proc 1990;22:651
73. Sollinger HW, Sasaki TM, D'Alessandro AM, et al. Indications for enteric conversion after pancreas transplantation with bladder drainage. Surgery 1992;112:842
74. Stephanian E, Gruessner RWG, Brayman KL, et al. Conversion of exocrine secretions from bladder to enteric drainage in recipients of whole pancreaticoduodenal transplants. Ann Surg 1993;216(6):663
75. Gruessner RWG, Stephanian E, Dunn DL, et al. Cystoenteric conversion

after whole pancreaticoduodenal transplantation: Indications, risk factors, and outcome. Transplant Proc 1993;25:1179
76. Martin X, Jemni N, Lefrancois N, et al. Conversion of total bladder-drained pancreas into total injected grafts. Transplant Proc 1994;26:460
77. Gruessner RWG, Sutherland DER. Clinical diagnosis of pancreas allograft rejection. In: Solez K, Racusen LC, Billingham M, eds. Pathology and Rejection Diagnosis in Solid Organ Transplantation. New York: Marcel Dekker, 1995. In press
78. Sutherland DER, Moudry KC, Najarian JS. Pancreas transplantation. In: Cerilli J, ed. Organ Transplantation and Replacement. Philadelphia: JB Lippincott; 1987:535
79. Marsh CL, Perkins JD, Sutherland DER, et al. Combined hepatic and pancreaticoduodenal procurement for transplantation. Surg Gynecol Obstet 1989; 168:254
80. Delmonico FL, Jenkins RL, Auchincloss H Jr, et al. Procurement of a whole pancreas and liver from the same cadaveric donor [see comments]. Surgery 1989;105:718
81. Dunn DL, Schlumpf RB, Gruessner RWG, et al. Maximal use of liver and pancreas from cadaveric organ donors. Transplant Proc 1990;22:423
82. Gores PF, Gillingham KJ, Dunn DL, et al. Donor hyperglycemia as a minor risk factor and immunologic variables as major risk factors for pancreas allograft loss in a multivariate analysis of a single institution's experience. Ann Surg 1992;215:217
83. Shaffer D, Madras PN, Sahyoun AI, et al. Cadaver donor hyperglycemia does not impair long-term pancreas allograft survival or function. Transplant Proc 1994;26(2):439
84. Gruessner RWG, Troppmann C, Barrow B, et al. Assessment of donor and recipient risk factors on pancreas transplant outcome. Transplant Proc 1994;26(2):437
85. Florack G, Sutherland DER, Heise JW, Najarian JS. Successful preservation of human pancreas grafts for 28 hours. Transplant Proc 1987;19:3882
86. Morel P, Moudry-Munns KC, Najarian JS, et al. Influence of preservation time on outcome and metabolic function of bladder-drained pancreas transplants. Transplantation 1990;49:294
87. Belzer FO. Clinical organ preservation with UW solution. Transplantation 1989;47:1097
88. Prieto M, Sutherland DER, Fernandez-Cruz L, et al. Experimental and clinical experience with urine amylase monitoring for early diagnosis of rejection in pancreas transplantation. Transplantation 1987;43:71
89. Prieto M, Sutherland DER, Goetz FC, et al. Pancreas transplant results according to the technique of duct management: Bladder versus enteric drainage. Surgery 1987;102:680
90. Sutherland DER, Kendall DM, Moudry KC, et al. Pancreas transplantation in nonuremic, type I diabetic recipients. Surgery 1988;104:453
91. Gruessner RWG, Dunn DL, Tzardis PJ, et al. Simultaneous pancreas and kidney transplants versus single kidney transplants and previous kidney transplants in uremic patients and single pancreas transplants in nonuremic diabetic patients: Comparison of rejection, morbidity, and long-term outcome. Transplant Proc 1990;22:622
92. Sollinger HW, Stratta RJ, D'Alessandro AM, et al. Experience with simultaneous pancreas-kidney transplantation. Ann Surg 1988;208:478
93. Nakai I, Kaufman DB, Field MJ, et al. Differential effects of preexisting uremia and a synchronous kidney graft on pancreas allograft functional survival in rats. Transplantation 1992;54:17
94. Gruessner RWG, Nakhleh RE, Tzardis PJ, et al. Rejection in single versus combined pancreas and kidney transplantation in pigs. Transplantation 1993;56:1053
95. Barr D, Bronner MP, Marsh CL, et al. Concordance of histologic rejection in human kidney and pancreas transplantation. Transplantation 1995. In press
96. Davis CL, Alpers CE, Bacchi CE, Marsh CL. Protocol biopsies of kidney-pancreas transplant recipients. J Am Soc Nephrol 1992;3:855
97. Reinholt FP, Tydén G, Bohman SO, et al. Pancreatic juice cytology in the diagnosis of pancreatic graft rejection. Clin Transplant 1988;2:127
98. Fernstad R, Skoldefors H, Pousette A, et al. A novel assay for pancreatic cellular damage. III. Use of a pancreas-specific protein as a marker of pancreatic graft dysfunction in humans. Pancreas 1989;4:44
99. Marks WH, Borgstrom A, Sollinger HW, Marks C. Serum immunoreactive anodal trypsinogen and urinary amylase as biochemical markers for rejection of clinical whole-organ pancreas allografts having exocrine drainage into the urinary bladder. Transplantation 1990;49:112
100. Munn SR, Engen DE, Barr D, et al. Differential diagnosis of hypoamylasuria in pancreas allograft recipients with urinary exocrine drainage. Transplantation 1990;49:359
101. Sutherland DER, Casanova D, Sibley RK. Role of pancreas graft biopsies in the diagnosis and treatment of rejection after pancreas transplantation. Transplant Proc 1987;19:2329
102. Allen RD, Wilson TG, Grierson JM, et al. Percutaneous biopsy of bladder-drained pancreas transplants. Transplantation 1991;51:1213
103. Perkins JD, Munn SR, Marsh CL, et al. Safety and efficacy of cystoscopically directed biopsy in pancreas transplantation. Transplant Proc 1990;22:665
104. Brayman KL, Moss AA, Morel P, et al. Exocrine dysfunction evaluation of bladder-drained pancreaticoduodenal transplants using a transcystoscopic biopsy technique. Transplant Proc 1992;24:901
105. Gaber AO, Gaber LW, Shokouh-Amiri MH, Hathaway DK. Percutaneous biopsy of pancreas transplants. Transplantation 1992;54:548
106. Morel P, Brayman KL, Goetz FC, et al. Long-term metabolic function of pancreas transplants and influence of rejection episodes. Transplantation 1991;51:990
107. Sibley RK, Sutherland DER. Pancreas transplantation: An immunohistologic and histopathologic examination of 100 grafts. Am J Pathol 1987;128:151
108. Carpenter HA, Engen DE, Munn SR, et al. Histologic diagnosis of rejection by using cystoscopically directed needle biopsy specimens from dysfunctional pancreatoduodenal allografts with exocrine drainage into the bladder. Am J Surg Pathol 1990;14:837
109. Nakhleh RE, Gruessner RWG, Swanson PE, et al. Pancreas transplant pathology: A morphologic, immunohistochemical, and electron microscopic comparison of allogeneic grafts with rejection, syngeneic grafts, and chronic pancreatitis. Am J Surg Pathol 1991;15:246
110. Nakhleh RE, Sutherland DER. Pancreas rejection: The significance of histopathologic findings with implications for the classification of rejection. Am J Surg Pathol 1992;16:1098
111. Casanova D, Gruessner RWG, Brayman KL, et al. Retrospective analysis of the role of pancreatic biopsy (open and transcystoscopic technique) in the management of solitary pancreas transplants. Transplant Proc 1993;25:1192
112. Nakhleh RE, Gruessner RWG, Tzardis PJ, et al. Pathology of transplanted human duodenal tissue: A histological study, with comparison to pancreatic pathology in resected pancreaticoduodenal transplants. Clin Transplant 1991; 5:241
113. Nakhleh RE, Sutherland DER, Benedetti E, et al. Diagnostic utility and correlation of duodenal and pancreas biopsy tissue in pancreaticoduodenal transplants with emphasis on therapeutic use. Transplant Proc 1995;27:1327
114. Benedetti E, Nakhleh RE, Sutherland DER, et al. Correlation between transcystoscopic biopsy results and hypoamylasuria in bladder-drained pancreas transplants. Surgery 1995;118:864
115. Nakhleh RE, Sutherland DER, Tzardis PJ, et al. Correlation of rejection of the duodenum with rejection of the pancreas in a pig model of pancreaticoduodenal transplantation. Transplantation 1993;56:1353
116. Sutherland DER, Gruessner RWG, Moudry-Munns KC, Gruessner AC. Discordant graft loss from rejection of organs from the same donor in simultaneous pancreas-kidney recipients. Transplant Proc 1995;27:907
117. Barrou B, Barrou Z, Gruessner AC, et al. Probability of retaining endocrine function (insulin-independence) after definitive loss of exocrine function in bladder-drained pancreas transplants. Transplant Proc 1994;26(2):473
118. Sutherland DER, Moudry-Munns KC, Gruessner AC. Pancreas transplant outcome with or without biological anti-T-cell therapy for induction immunosuppression with use of cyclosporine. Transplant Proc 1994;26(5):2752
119. Gruessner RWG, Sutherland DER, Drangstveit MB, et al. Use of FK506 in pancreas transplantation. Transplant Int 1995. In press
120. Sutherland DER, Gruessner RWG, Gillingham KJ, et al. A single institution's experience with solitary pancreas transplantation. In: Terasaki PI, ed. Clinical Transplants—1991. Los Angeles: UCLA Tissue Typing Laboratory; 1992:141
121. Tesi RJ, Henry ML, Elkhammas EA, et al. The frequency of rejection episodes after combined kidney-pancreas transplant—the impact on graft survival. Transplantation 1994;58:424
122. Sutherland DER. Pancreas transplants in non-uremic and post-uremic diabetic patients. Transplant Proc 1992;24:780
123. Stratta RJ, Taylor RJ, Bynon JS, et al. Surgical treatment of diabetes mellitus with pancreas transplantation. Ann Surg 1994;220(6):809
124. Dawahra M, Cloix P, Martin X, et al. Simultaneous transplantation of kidney and pancreas in diabetes patients. Transplant Proc 1993;25:2227
125. Drexel H, Palos G, Konigsrainer A, et al. Long-term follow-up of glycaemic control and parameters of lipid transport after pancreas transplantation. Diabetologia 1991;34:S47
126. Illner WD, Schleibner H, Schneeberger R, et al. Pancreatic transplantation—A single center experience over a period of one decade. Transplant Proc 1994;26:420
127. Sollinger HW, Ploeg RJ, Eckhoff DE, et al. Two hundred consecutive simultaneous pancreas-kidney transplants with bladder drainage. Surgery 1993; 114:736
128. Henry ML, Elkhammas EA, Tesi RJ, Ferguson RM. Evolution of combined kidney/pancreas transplantation in a single center. Transplant Proc 1994; 26:419
129. Sutherland DER, Moudry-Munns KC, Gruessner AC. Pancreas preservation. In: Collins G, Dubernard JM, Land W, Persijn G, eds. Procurement and Preservation of Vascularized Organs. Amsterdam: Kluwer-Academic Publishers; 1995. In press
130. Sutherland DER, Gruessner AC, Moudry-Munns KC, Cecka M. Tabulation of cases from the International Pancreas Transplant Registry and analysis of United Network for Organ Sharing United States Pancreas Transplant Registry data according to multiple variables. Transplant Proc 1993;25:1707
131. United States Renal Disease System. Simultaneous kidney-pancreas transplantation versus kidney transplantation alone: Patient survival, kidney graft survival, and posttransplant hospitalization. Am J Kidney Dis 1992;20(5):61
132. Cecka M, Belle SH, Sutherland DER, Kay MP. Registries in Clinical Transplants—1991. Los Angeles: UCLA Tissue Typing Laboratory; 1992:1(1)
133. Garvin PJ, Castaneda M, Carney K. Simultaneous cadaver renal and pancreas transplantation in type I diabetes. Arch Surg 1987;122:274
134. Cosimi AB, Auchincloss H Jr, Delmonico FL. Combined kidney and pancreas transplantation in diabetics. Arch Surg 1988;123:621

135. Wright FH, Smith JL, Ames SA. Function of pancreas allografts more than one year following transplantation. Arch Surg 1989;124:796
136. Henry ML, Ketel BL, Elkhammas EA, et al. The role of transplantation in diabetics with end-stage renal disease. Los Angeles: UCLA Tissue Typing Laboratory;1991:31
137. Hathaway DK, Abel T, Cardoso S, et al. Improvement in autonomic function following pancreas-kidney versus kidney alone transplantation. Transplant Proc 1993;25:1306
138. Castoldi R, Ferrari G, Staudacher C, et al. Segmental duct-injected versus whole bladder drained pancreas transplantation: The San Raffaele Hospital experience. Transplant Proc 1994;26:450
139. Hughes CB, Crewal HP, Shokouh-Amiri MH, Gaber AO. Solid organ pancreas transplantation: A review of the current status and report of one institution's experience. Am Surg 1994;60:669
140. Schulak JA, Mayes JT, Hricik DE. Kidney transplantation in diabetic patients undergoing combined kidney-pancreas or kidney-only transplantation. Transplantation 1992;53:685
141. Sutherland DER, Moudry-Munns KC, Gillingham KJ, et al. Solitary pancreas transplantation: Alone in nonuremic and after a kidney in uremic diabetic patients. Transplant Proc 1991;23:1637
142. So SKS, Moudry-Munns KC, Gillingham KJ, et al. Short-term and long-term effects of HLA matching in cadaveric pancreas transplantation. Transplant Proc 1991;23:1634
143. Hathaway DK, Hartwig M, Milstead D, et al. Improvement in quality of life reported by diabetic recipients of kidney-only and pancreas-kidney allografts. Transplant Proc 1994;26:512
144. Sutherland DER, Najarian JS, Greenberg BZ, et al. Hormonal and metabolic effects of a pancreatic endocrine graft: Vascularized segmental transplantation in insulin-dependent diabetic patients. Ann Intern Med 1981;95:537
145. Robertson RP, Abid M, Sutherland DER, Diem P. Glucose homeostasis and insulin secretion in human recipients of pancreas transplantation. Diabetes 1989;38:97
146. Secchi AV, Pontiroli AE, Bosi E. Effects of arginine and arginine plus somatostatin infusion on insulin release in diabetic patients submitted to pancreas allotransplantation. Diabetes Metab Rev 1987;13:422
147. Ostman J, Bolinder J, Gunnarsson R. Metabolic effects of pancreas transplantation: Effects of pancreas transplantation on metabolic and hormonal profiles in IDDM patients. Diabetes 1989;38(suppl 1):88
148. Osei K, Henry ML, O'Dorisio TM. Physiological and pharmacological stimulation of pancreatic islet hormone secretion in type I diabetic pancreas allograft recipients. Diabetes 1990;39:1235
149. Bosi E, Piatti PM, Secchi AV. Response of glucagon and insulin secretion to insulin-induced hypoglycemia in type I diabetic recipients after pancreatic transplantation. Diabetes Nutr Metab 1988;1:21
150. Königsrainer A, Föger BH, Miesenbock G, et al. Pancreas transplantation with systemic endocrine drainage leads to improvement in lipid metabolism. Transplant Proc 1994;26:501
151. Teuscher AU, Seaquist ER, Robertson RP. Diminished insulin secretory reserve in diabetic pancreas transplant and nondiabetic kidney transplant recipients. Diabetes 1994;43:593
152. Christiansen E, Andersen HB, Rasmussen K, et al. Pancreatic B-cell function and glucose metabolism in human segmental pancreas and kidney transplantation. Am J Physiol 1993;264:E441
153. Gores PF, Sutherland DER. Pancreatic islet transplantation: Is purification necessary? Am J Surg 1993;166(5):32767
154. Robertson RP. Pancreas and islet transplantation for diabetes: Cures or curiosities? N Engl J Med 1993;327:1861
155. Hughes TA, Gaber AO, Amiri HS, et al. Lipoprotein composition in insulin-dependent diabetes mellitus with chronic renal failure: Effect of kidney and pancreas transplantation. Metabolism 1994;43:333
156. Luzi L, Battezzati A, Perseghin G, et al. Combined pancreas and kidney transplantation normalizes protein metabolism in insulin-dependent diabetic-uremic patients. J Clin Invest 1994;93:1948
157. Bilous RW, Mauer SM, Sutherland DER, Steffes MW. Glomerular structure and function following successful pancreas transplantation for insulin-dependent diabetes mellitus. Diabetes 1987;36:43A
158. Fioretto P, Mauer SM, Sutherland DER, Steffes MW. Effect of solitary pancreas transplantation on the progression of diabetic nephropathy. Diabetologia 1992;35:A74
159. Fioretto P, Mauer SM, Bilous RW, et al. Effects of pancreas transplantation on glomerular structure in insulin-dependent diabetic patients with their own kidneys. Lancet 1993;342:1193
160. DeFrancisco AM, Mauer SM, Steffes MW, et al. The effects of cyclosporine on native renal function in non-uremic diabetic recipients of pancreatic transplants. J Diabetic Complic 1987;1:128
161. Morel P, Sutherland DER, Almond PS, et al. Assessment of renal function in type I diabetic patients after kidney, pancreas or combined kidney-pancreas transplantation. Transplantation 1991;51:1184
162. Wang TL, Stevens RB, Fioretto P, et al. Correlation of preoperative renal function and identification of risk factors for eventual native renal failure in cyclosporine-treated nonuremic diabetic recipient of pancreas transplants alone. Transplant Proc 1993;25:1291
163. Bohman SO, Tydén G, Wilczek H. Prevention of kidney graft diabetic nephropathy by pancreas transplantation in man. Diabetes 1987;34:306
164. Wilczek H, Jaremko G, Tydén G, Groth CG. Evolution of diabetic nephropathy in kidney grafts. Evidence that a simultaneously transplanted pancreas exerts a protective effect. Transplantation 1995;59:51
165. Bilous RW, Mauer SM, Sutherland DER, et al. The effects of pancreas transplantation on the glomerular structure of renal allografts in patients with insulin-dependent diabetes. N Engl J Med 1989;321:80
166. Ramsay RC, Goetz FC, Sutherland DER, et al. Progression of diabetic retinopathy after pancreas transplantation for insulin-dependent diabetes mellitus. N Engl J Med 1988;312:208
167. Wang Q, Klein R, Moss SE, et al. The influence of combined pancreas-kidney transplantation on the progression of diabetic retinopathy. A case series. Ophthalmology 1994;101:1071
168. van der Vliet JA, Navarro X, Kennedy WR, et al. The effect of pancreas transplantation on diabetic polyneuropathy. Transplantation 1988;45:368
169. Kennedy WR, Navarro X, Goetz FC, et al. Effects of pancreatic transplantation on diabetic neuropathy. N Engl J Med 1990;322:1031
170. Solders G, Tydén G, Persson A, Groth CG. Improvement of nerve conduction in diabetic neuropathy: A follow-up study 4 years after combined pancreatic and renal transplantation. Diabetes 1992;41:946
171. Gaber AO, Cardoso S, Pearson S. Improvement in autonomic function following combined pancreas-kidney transplantation. Transplant Proc 1991;23:1660
172. Muller-Felber W, Landgraf R, Sheuer R, et al. Diabetic neuropathy three years after successful pancreas and kidney transplantation. Diabetes 1993;42:1482
173. Navarro X, Kennedy WR, Loewensen RB, Sutherland DER. Influence of pancreas transplantation on cardiorespiratory reflexes, nerve conduction, and mortality in diabetes mellitus. Diabetes 1990;39:802
174. Abendroth D, Illhmer VD, Landgraf R, Land W. Are late diabetic complications reversible after pancreatic transplantation? A new method of follow-up of microcirculatory changes. Transplant Proc 1987;19:2325
175. Cheung ATW, Perez RV, Cox KL, et al. Microangiopathy reversal in successful simultaneous pancreas-kidney transplantation. Transplant Proc 1994;26:493
176. Nakache R, Tydén G, Groth CG. Quality of life in diabetic patients after combined pancreas-kidney or kidney transplantation. Diabetes 1991;39:802
177. Voruganti LNP, Sells RA. Quality of life of diabetic patients after combined pancreatic renal transplantation. Clin Transplant 1989;3:78
178. Zehr PS, Milde FK, Hart LK, Corry RJ. Pancreas transplantation: Assessing secondary complications and life quality. Diabetologia 1991;34:S138
179. Nathan DM, Fogel H, Norman D, et al. Long-term metabolic and quality of life results with pancreatic/renal transplantation in insulin-dependent diabetes mellitus. Transplantation 1991;52:85
180. Secchi AV, Di Carlo S, Martinenghi S, et al. Effect of pancreas transplantation on life expectancy, kidney function and quality of life in uremic type I (insulin-dependent) diabetic patients. Diabetologia 1991;34:S141
181. Wheeler SJ, Sollinger HW, Pirsch JD. Quality of life in diabetics following simultaneous pancreas/kidney and kidney transplants (abstract). Presented at the American Society of Transplant Surgeons, Chicago, and the International Congress of the Transplantation Society, Paris, 1992
182. Gross CR, Zehrer CL. Health-related quality of life outcomes of pancreas transplant recipients. Clin Transplant 1992;6:165
183. Zehrer CL, Gross CR. Comparison of quality of life between pancreas/kidney transplant recipients and kidney transplant recipients: One year follow-up. Transplant Proc 1993;26(2):508
184. Schareck WD, Hopt UT, Geisler F, et al. Quality of life after combined pancreas/kidney transplantation. Transplant Proc 1994;26:518
185. Nakache R, Tydén G, Groth CG. Long-term quality of life in diabetic patients after combined pancreas-kidney transplantation or kidney transplantation. Transplant Proc 1994;26:510
186. Kiebert GM, von Oosterhour ECAA, Lemkes HPJ, et al. Quality of life after combined renal-pancreatic transplantation. Transplant Proc 1994;26(2):517
187. Morel P, Schlumpf RB, Dunn DL, et al. Pancreas retransplants compared with primary transplants. Transplantation 1991;51:825
188. Pyke DA. A critique of pancreas transplantation. Clin Transplant 1990;4:235
189. Ramirez LC, Rios JM, Rosenstock J, Raskin P. Is pancreas transplantation in nonuremic patients a viable option? (Letter). Diabetes Care 1989;12:511
190. Harmer N. Nonuremic pancreas transplantation (Letter). Diabetes Care 1990;13:452
191. Loseke C. Quality of life after transplantation (Letter). Diabetes Care 1990;13:541
192. Keown PA. Emerging indications for the use of cyclosporine in organ transplantation and autoimmunity. Drugs 1990;40:315
193. Sutherland DER. Pancreas transplantation. Curr Opin Immunol 1989;1:1195
194. Farney AC, Sutherland DER. Pancreas and islet transplantation. In: Go VLW, ed. The Pancreas: Biology, Pathobiology, and Disease. 2nd ed. New York: Raven Press;1993:815
195. Nerup J, Mandrup-Poulsen T, Molvig J. The HLA-IDDM association: Implications of etiology and pathogenesis of IDDM. Diabetes Metab Rev 1987;3:779
196. Sanchez-Urdazpal L, Czaja AJ, van Hoek G, et al. Prognostic features and role of liver transplantation in severe corticosteroid-treated autoimmune chronic active hepatitis. Hepatology 1992;15:215
197. Merrill JP, Murray JE, Harrison JH, Guild WR. Successful transplantation of a human kidney between identical twins. JAMA 1956;160:277
198. Tilney NL. Renal transplantation between identical twins: A review. World J Surg 1986;10:381

199. Glassock RJ, Feldman D, Reynolds EG, et al. Human renal isografts: A clinical and pathological analysis. Medicine 1968;47:411
200. Canadian-European Randomized Control Trial Group. Cyclosporin-induced remission of IDDM after early intervention. Diabetes 1988;37:1574
201. Skyler JS, Marks JB. Immune intervention in type I diabetes mellitus. Diabetes Rev 1993;1(1):15
202. Bougners PF, Carel JC, Castano L, et al. Factors determining very early remission of type I diabetes in children treated with cyclosporin A. N Engl J Med 1988;318:663
203. Olmos P, A'Hern R, Heaton DA, et al. The significance of the concordance rate for type I (insulin-dependent) diabetes in identical twins. Diabetologia 1988;31:747
204. Sutherland DER, Goetz FC, Elick BA, Najarian JS. Experience with 49 segmental pancreas transplants in 45 diabetic patients. Transplantation 1982;34:330
205. Santamaria P, Nakhleh RE, Sutherland DER, Barbosa JJ. Characterization of T lymphocytes infiltrating a human pancreas allograft affected by isletitis and recurrent diabetes. Diabetes 1992;41:53
206. Binimelis J, Sibley RK, Sutherland DER, et al. Characterization and cloning of alloreactive T lymphocytes from pancreas allografts transplanted into diabetics. Transplantation 1987;44:453
207. Roza A, Markmann JF, Brayman K, et al. Isolated islet cells are more vulnerable to recurrent diabetes than vascularized pancreas grafts. Surg Forum 1987;38:373
208. Nakai I, Oka T, Field MJ, et al. Occurrence and prevention of graft-vs-host disease after pancreaticoduodenal transplantation in the BB rat. Transplant Proc 1993;25:965
209. Lebebvre PH. Pancreatic transplantation: Why, when, and who? Diabetologia 1992;35:494
210. Warnock GL, Rajotte RV. Human pancreatic islet transplantation. Transplant Rev 1992;6:195
211. Ricordi C, Tzakis AG, Carroll PB, et al. Human islet isolation and allotransplantation in 22 consecutive cases. Transplantation 1992;53:407
212. Farney AC, Najarian JS, Nakhleh RE, et al. Autotransplantation of dispersed pancreatic islet tissue combined with total or near-total pancreatectomy for treatment of chronic pancreatitis. Surgery 1991;110:427
213. Pyzdrowski KL, Kendall DM, Halter JB, et al. Preserved insulin secretion and insulin independence in recipients of islet autografts. N Engl J Med 1992;327:220
214. Farney AC, Najarian JS, Nakhleh RE, et al. Long-term function of islet autotransplants. Transplant Proc 1992;24:969
215. London NJM, Robertson GSM, Chadwick DR, et al. Human pancreatic islet isolation and transplantation. Clin Transplant 1994;8(5):421
216. Najarian JS, Kaufman DB, Fryd DS, et al. Long-term survival following kidney transplantation in 100 type I diabetic patients. Transplantation 1989;47:106
217. Sutherland DER. Indications for pancreas transplantation: A commentary. Clin Transplant 1990;4:242
218. Pyke DA. Pancreas transplantation. Diabetes Metab Rev 1991;7:3
219. Sutherland DER. Commentary on pancreas transplantation. Diabetes Metab Rev 1991;7:129
220. Nerup J. Is there a need for pancreas transplantation? Transplant Proc 1993;25:52
221. Sutherland DER. Is there a need for pancreas transplantation? Transplant Proc 1993;25:47
222. Robertson RP. Pancreas transplantation in humans with diabetes. Diabetes 1991;40:1085

Diabetes Mellitus, edited by Derek LeRoith, Simeon I. Taylor, and Jerrold M. Olefsky. Lippincott–Raven Publishers, Philadelphia © 1996.

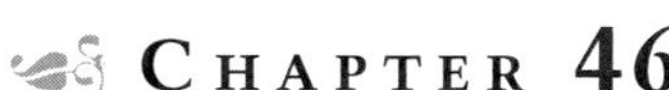

Chapter 46
Gene Therapy for Metabolic Disease

Daniel J. Rader, Steven Raper, and James M. Wilson

Somatic gene therapy refers to the introduction of genetic material into a specific organ or tissue in order to treat an inherited or acquired disease. Many metabolic diseases, such as diabetes mellitus, are potential candidates for treatment with somatic gene therapy. This chapter presents an overview of the current status of somatic gene therapy for metabolic disease. It focuses on liver-directed gene transfer for the purpose of illustration and uses homozygous familial hypercholesterolemia as a model. A final section of this chapter discusses some of the issues related to somatic gene therapy for type I diabetes mellitus.

An important concept in somatic gene therapy is that of ex vivo vs. in vivo gene delivery. An ex vivo approach involves removing a portion of the targeted tissue from the patient, transferring the genetic material into cells in culture, and then reintroducing the genetically modified cells into the patient. This approach has the advantage of gene transfer directly into the targeted cells under controlled conditions, but has the disadvantage of the need to obtain tissue, which, for the liver, requires partial surgical resection. In contrast, an in vivo approach involves the administration of a vector systemically or locally without removal of the targeted tissue. It has the advantage of circumventing the need for surgical resection, but has the attendant technical problem of targeting to the appropriate tissue. Both ex vivo and in vivo approaches are currently being investigated for application to liver-directed gene transfer.

Potential Vectors for Liver-Directed Gene Transfer

Because the liver is a key target for gene therapy of many diseases, much effort has been expended in the development of vectors for liver-directed gene transfer. A list of some potential vectors is shown in Table 46-1, and the vectors are discussed in more detail in the following sections.

Retroviral Vectors

Retroviral vectors have a broad host spectrum, can accommodate up to 7 kb of foreign DNA, and can integrate into the host genome, resulting in persistent transgene expression (reviewed in ref. 1). For these reasons, they have been developed for use in therapeutic

Table 46-1. Potential Vectors for Liver-Directed Gene Therapy

Vector	Application		Stability
	Ex vivo	In vivo	
Viral			
Retrovirus	+	−	+
Adenovirus	−	+	−
Adeno-associated virus	+	+	+
Nonviral			
DNA/protein complexes	−	+	−
Liposomes	−	+	−

+, strong possibility for application or reasonable stability of expression with current vectors;
−, unlikely application or poor stability of expression with current vectors.

gene transfer. However, active host cell replication is required in order for the DNA to integrate. In vivo, hepatocytes are generally relatively quiescent cells, and therefore are not a good target for in vivo liver-directed gene transfer using retroviral vectors. By contrast, primary hepatocytes in culture undergo cell division and, if infected with a recombinant retrovirus, can support stable integration of viral genetic material. Methods for ex vivo liver-directed gene transfer, therefore, have been developed using recombinant retroviruses. In this approach, part of the liver is resected, primary hepatocytes are infected with a recombinant retrovirus, and the engineered cells are reintroduced into the host liver (reviewed in ref. 2). The first application of this approach was in a rabbit model of low density lipoprotein (LDL) receptor deficiency.[3] Alternatively, hepatocyte replication can be induced by partial hepatectomy or hepatotoxic drugs, followed by in vivo delivery of the retroviral vector.[1] However, this approach is unlikely to be utilized for human clinical trials. For liver-directed gene therapy, the major disadvantage of retroviral vectors is the need to induce hepatocyte replication.

Adenoviral Vectors

Recombinant adenoviral vectors have been used for gene transfer to multiple tissue types in animals (reviewed in refs. 4 and 5). A major advantage of these vectors over retroviral vectors is their ability to transfer genetic material into nonreplicating cells. Adenoviruses are double-stranded DNA viruses that are normally tropic for respiratory epithelium in humans, but have the capability of infecting many types of cells. Replication-defective recombinant adenoviruses have a deletion of most of the E1 region required for replication,[4] and thus can result in transgene expression without active viral replication. When injected intravenously, recombinant adenoviruses efficiently infect the liver, resulting in a high level of hepatic transgene expression.[6] Recombinant adenoviruses have been used successfully for in vivo liver-directed gene transfer and the expression of several different genes in mice,[7-13] rats,[14,15] and rabbits.[16]

One disadvantage of recombinant adenoviral vectors for in vivo gene transfer is that, with current adenoviral vectors, gene expression does not persist beyond several weeks. In most species, recombinant adenoviruses stimulate a cellular immune response as a result of some degree of adenoviral protein expression, leading to hepatic inflammation and destruction of the genetically modified hepatocytes.[17] A second-generation virus, which has had another essential adenoviral gene (E2a) inactivated, results in less inflammation and substantially longer transgene expression in mouse liver.[18] Second administration of a recombinant adenovirus in rabbits failed to result in further transgene expression, probably because of neutralizing antibodies to the first dose.[16] Therefore, the humoral immune response may limit the ability to administer adenoviral vectors more than once. Many laboratories are currently working to engineer recombinant adenoviruses in order to achieve greater persistence of transgene expression after in vivo liver-directed gene transfer.

Adeno-Associated Virus Vectors

Adeno-associated virus (AAV) is a human parvovirus that has not been associated with human disease. Wild-type AAV has the ability to infect a broad range of cell types and to integrate with high frequency into a defined region of human chromosome 19,[19] even in nondividing cells.[20] Because of these properties, AAV has been proposed to be a potentially useful vector for somatic gene therapy (reviewed in ref. 21). Recombinant AAV vectors have been utilized to express transgenes in vitro in human hematopoietic cells; for example, phenotypic correction of the Fanconi anemia defect in primary human hematopoietic progenitor cells[22] and expression of the human ∂-globin gene in human primary erythroid cells[23] were demonstrated using recombinant AAV vectors. Recombinant AAV has also been demonstrated to result in gene transfer and expression in rabbit lung airway epithelium,[24] and in rat brain neurons and glial cells.[25] Recombinant AAV gene transfer to liver has not yet been reported.

Although AAV is a promising vector, several issues must be resolved before AAV can be utilized for human somatic gene therapy (reviewed in ref. 21). First, replication of AAV requires the presence of "helper" adenovirus, which must then be fully removed from the recombinant AAV stocks. The methods for complete purification of recombinant AAV, at high titer free of adenovirus, have yet to be fully developed. Second, recombinant AAV may not integrate as frequently or as site-specifically as wild-type AAV, and the implications for persistence of expression are unclear. Third, the success of recombinant AAV in establishing stable gene expression in vivo in animals has not been fully established. Efforts are ongoing in many laboratories to address these and other issues related to the use of recombinant AAV for somatic gene therapy.

DNA/Protein Complexes

DNA could theoretically be targeted to the liver in vivo by coupling the DNA with a specific protein ligand to form DNA/protein complexes. Certain liver-specific cell surface receptors, such as the asialoglycoprotein receptor and the transferrin receptor, have been proposed as targets for liver-directed gene transfer (reviewed in ref. 26). This approach has been used successfully in rats using asialorosomucoid to target genes to the liver.[27,28] It has also been used to target the delivery of the LDL receptor gene to the livers of rabbits deficient in the LDL receptor following partial hepatectomy,[29] which resulted in greater stability of gene expression. After gene transfer using DNA/protein complexes, the transgene DNA remains episomal and is not integrated into the host genome.[30]

DNA/protein complexes generally result in transient, low-level expression of transgenes in the liver. One major reason is that the complexes are targeted to the lysosome after receptor-mediated endocytosis and are degraded.[26] One approach to overcome this problem has been the use of replication incompetent adenovirus for endosomal lysis. When adenovirus is cointernalized with the DNA/protein complexes, either separately[31] or directly coupled to the complexes,[32,33] gene expression is considerably enhanced. It has also been reported that condensation of the DNA/protein complexes to form small unimolecular complexes results in more prolonged, higher level transgene expression.[34] Investigation is ongoing in several laboratories to modify DNA/protein complexes further in order to achieve increased levels of persistent expression in liver and other tissues.

Liposomes

Liposomes are macromolecular structures composed primarily of phospholipids, which orient themselves so that the polar head groups interact with the aqueous environment and the fatty acyl chains point inward, toward a hydrophobic core. DNA can be placed within the liposome core and protected from degradation in the plasma. Liposomes are nontoxic, nonimmunogenic, and stable in plasma, making them attractive potential vehicles for delivery of DNA to cells (reviewed in ref. 35). When cationic cholesterol derivatives are complexed with the phospholipids, the liposomes can mediate escape of associated DNA from the endosome and entry into the cytosol.[36] Cationic liposomes are effective in promoting gene expression in hepatocytes in vitro.[35] Liposomes have been used for in vivo gene transfer and expression in the liver in rats[37,38] and after tail vein injection in mice.[39] However, targeting to hepatocytes in vivo is difficult because liposomes are avidly taken up by Kupffer cells. The lack of tissue specificity and the low levels of gene expression have thus far limited the applicability of liposomes to in vivo liver-directed gene transfer. Nevertheless, the surface of cationic liposomes may be able to be modified with proteins that will enhance both targeting and endosomal escape, making liposomes potential vectors for liver-directed gene therapy.

Liver-Directed Gene Transfer for Familial Hypercholesterolemia: A Paradigm for the Development of Gene Therapy for Metabolic Disease

Familial Hypercholesterolemia

Plasma concentrations of LDL cholesterol are strongly influenced by heritable factors. Based on multiple epidemiologic studies, the genetic heritability of LDL cholesterol levels has been estimated to be approximately 50%. Genetic defects in the LDL receptor are among the most common familial cause of elevated LDL and result in a condition known as familial hypercholesterolemia (FH).[40] FH is an autosomal codominant condition; the heterozygous form is associated with LDL cholesterol levels in the 250–500 mg/dL range, whereas the homozygous form of the disease causes LDL cholesterol levels in the 500–1000 mg/dL range. Heterozygous FH has a population frequency of approximately 1 in 500 and results in tendon xanthomas and premature coronary heart disease in the fourth to sixth decades. Homozygous FH, which occurs in about 1 in a million individuals, is a clinical syndrome characterized by generalized tendon and cutaneous xanthomas, aortic and supravalvular aortic stenosis, and markedly premature atherosclerotic cardiovascular disease, often occurring in childhood or adolescence.

Patients with heterozygous FH can often be treated with medication to lower the LDL cholesterol to acceptable levels. By contrast, therapeutic options for those with homozygous FH are limited. Liver transplantation has been shown to be effective in nearly normalizing LDL cholesterol levels, but is associated with significant morbidity and mortality related to the need for immunosuppression. The current standard of care for patients with homozygous FH is plasma exchange or LDL apheresis, in which the LDL is physically removed from the blood on a regular basis.[41] However, in young children, this procedure usually requires permanent intravenous access, which has been associated with frequent line sepsis, and places patients at risk for aortic valve endocarditis. Furthermore, even if treated with LDL apheresis, patients with homozygous FH remain at high risk for premature atherosclerotic vascular disease. Therefore, there remains a significant need for more effective therapy for this disease. Because of the need for improved therapy and because the molecular etiology and pathophysiology of this disease are so well understood, homozygous FH serves as a valuable paradigm for the development of somatic gene therapy for metabolic disease.

Liver-Directed LDL Receptor Gene Transfer in Animals

Another reason that FH has been a valuable paradigm for the investigation of liver-directed gene transfer is the existence of a natural animal model of homozygous FH, the Watanabe heritable hyperlipidemic (WHHL) rabbit. These rabbits are homozygous for a mutation in the LDL receptor that results in impaired receptor activity, severe hypercholesterolemia, and accelerated atherosclerosis. Ex vivo gene transfer of the LDL receptor gene using recombinant retroviruses was successfully achieved in WHHL rabbits, resulting in temporary[3] and, ultimately, long-term[42] improvement in hypercholesterolemia. A similar ex vivo protocol was used to express the human LDL receptor gene in dog[43] and baboon[44] hepatocytes. These studies eventually led to the development and implementation of a clinical protocol for ex vivo gene therapy for homozygous FH in humans.

Liver-directed LDL receptor gene transfer and expression in vivo has been accomplished using recombinant adenoviral vectors. Injection of normal mice with a recombinant adenovirus containing the human LDL receptor cDNA resulted in transient human LDL receptor expression in the liver and accelerated LDL catabolism.[7] Injection of a recombinant adenovirus containing the LDL receptor gene into LDL receptor gene knockout mice successfully reduced cholesterol levels.[8] The human LDL receptor gene was expressed in WHHL rabbit livers using recombinant adenovirus, and this resulted in substantial decreases in cholesterol level.[16] Livers harvested 3 days after adenovirus infusion were found to have 50% of hepatocytes positive for the recombinant-derived human LDL receptor transgene. The treated rabbits were shown to have an increased rate of LDL catabolism compared with that in controls.

Liver-Directed LDL Receptor Gene Transfer in Humans

A pilot study of ex vivo liver-directed gene therapy for homozygous FH was initiated by Wilson and colleagues in 1992[45] (Fig. 46-1). The protocol was initially approved by the FDA for three patients, and this was later extended to five. Eligibility for the clinical protocol required documented coronary artery disease confirmed by coronary angiography. After serial baseline lipid tests, the patients underwent surgical resection of the left lateral segment of the liver with placement of a Hickman catheter in the inferior mesenteric vein at the time of surgery. Primary hepatocytes were isolated, and after 2 days in culture, were infected with a recombinant murine retrovirus containing the human LDL receptor cDNA. Hepatocytes were harvested the following day and immediately reinfused into the patient via the Hickman catheter in three separate infusions,

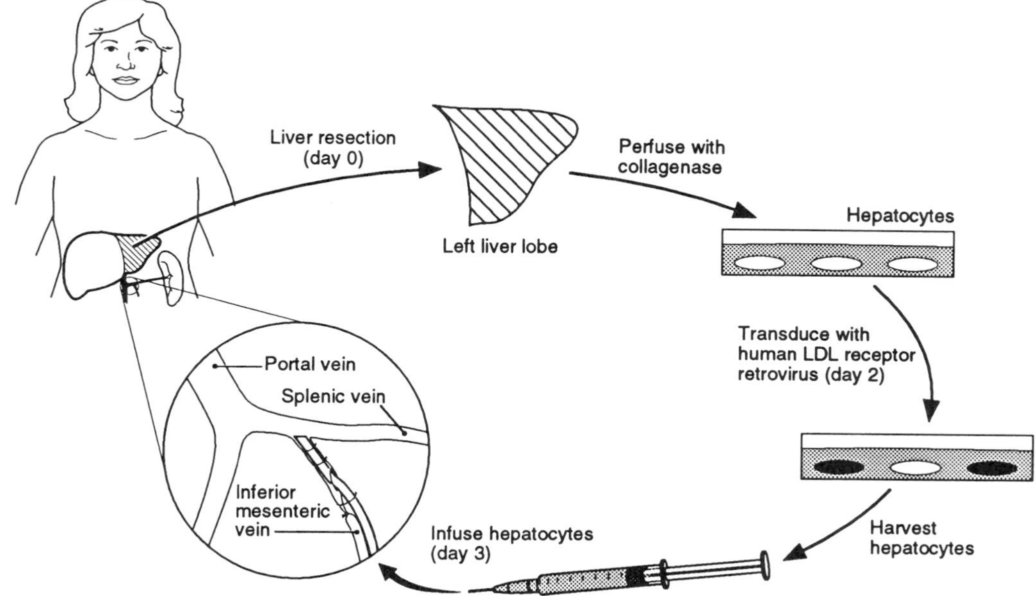

Figure 46-1. Schematic diagram of the strategy for ex vivo liver-directed gene therapy for homozygous familial hypercholesterolemia.

each lasting approximately 30 minutes. Blood was drawn serially after therapy and assayed for cholesterol and other lipids in a blinded fashion by an outside reference laboratory. Patients returned after 3 to 4 months for a percutaneous liver biopsy to evaluate transgene expression by in situ hybridization.

A total of five patients with homozygous FH underwent this ex vivo gene therapy procedure in an initial pilot study. The first patient to be treated using this protocol, a 29-year old French Canadian woman, was reported in the scientific literature in early 1994,[46] and the results in all 5 patients were subsequently reported.[46a] All five patients tolerated the reinfusion of autologous hepatocytes well, without significant complications. Liver tissue harvested 4 months later by percutaneous liver biopsy showed definite evidence of LDL receptor transgene expression by in situ hybridization in a limited number of hepatocytes in all five patients. Significant reductions in LDL cholesterol were demonstrated in three patients. One receptor negative patient had a reduction of LDL cholesterol of 150 mg/dl accompanied by a 50% increase in the rate of in vivo LDL catabolism.

The experience with ex vivo liver-directed gene therapy for homozygous FH has provided some important information for the further development of somatic gene therapy. First, it has demonstrated that infusion of up to 3×10^9 autologous hepatocytes into the portal system during a 12-hour period is safe and well tolerated, and is not accompanied by the development of acute or subacute portal hypertension. Second, it has demonstrated that ex vivo liver-directed gene transfer is feasible and can result in persistent gene expression for at least four months. Third, it has demonstrated that this approach can result in stable modification of a biologic and therapeutic endpoint in humans. This experience has provided the groundwork for further developments in somatic gene transfer.

Efforts to develop in vivo methods for targeting the LDL receptor to human liver are ongoing. As noted earlier, recombinant adenoviruses have been used to target the LDL receptor gene to the livers of LDL receptor–deficient mice[8] and WHHL rabbits.[16] A recombinant adenovirus was also utilized successfully to transfer the LDL receptor cDNA into human FH hepatocytes ex vivo.[47] New and more effective protocols for liver-directed gene therapy for homozygous FH will be developed over the next several years.[48]

Some Future Directions for Liver-Directed Gene Therapy for Metabolic Diseases

Once the technology for effective targeting and persistent gene expression is developed, liver-directed gene therapy will be applied to a variety of human diseases. In Table 46-2 are listed some of the disorders that may be candidates for treatment with liver-directed gene therapy. Two of these are discussed below as examples of the different approaches that may be used.

Gene Therapy for an Acute Complication of an Inherited Metabolic Disorder

Stable long-term correction of a monogenic disorder like homozygous FH by genetic reconstitution using ex vivo or in vivo gene transfer is one approach to gene therapy for metabolic disease. A different concept is that of short-term gene therapy for an acute complication of an inherited metabolic disorder. An example of such an approach is gene therapy for the hyperammonemic crises seen in children with ornithine transcarbamylase deficiency (OTCD). OTCD is the most common inborn error of urea cycle synthesis and is inherited as an X-linked disorder. Most affected patients experience life-threatening hyperammonemic crises starting in infancy; these crises are associated with a 50% mortality rate.[49] The five-year survival rate of male patients with OTCD is less than 25%, and most of those who survive have significant developmental disabilities that correlate with the number and duration of hyperammonemic crises.[49] If hyperammonemic coma persists longer than 3 days, mental retardation is almost inevitable. Therefore, acute therapy to shorten the duration of hyperammonemic coma could lead to decreased morbidity and mortality of this disease.

There exist two animal models of OTCD; the sparse fur (spf) mouse and the abnormal skin and hair (ash) mouse. Both have mutations in the OTC gene and share many of the biochemical and phenotypic features of the human disease. Gene transfer of the human OTC gene into primary hepatocytes from spf mice

Table 46-2. Some Examples of Diseases for which Liver-Directed Gene Therapy May Be Indicated

Disease	Potential Therapeutic Gene
Monogenic Disorders	
Homozygous familial hypercholesterolemia	LDL receptor
Ornithine transcarbamylase (OTC) deficiency	OTC
Phenylketonuria	Phenylalanine hydroxlase
Hereditary tyrosinemia	Fumarylacetoacetate hydrolase
$Alpha_1$-antitrypsin deficiency	$Alpha_1$-antitrypsin
Hemophilia A and B	Factors VIII and IX
Some lysosomal storage diseases	Various
Polygenic or Multifactorial Disorders	
Premature atherosclerosis	Apolipoprotein A-I
Severe hyperlipidemia	Apolipoprotein E
Diabetes mellitus	Insulin; others
Anemia	Erythropoietin
Infectious Diseases	
Viral hepatitis	Uncertain
Malignant Diseases	
Hepatic metastases	Various

can increase hepatic OTC activity and improve the biochemical alterations.[50] Clinical trials are planned involving the use of recombinant adenovirus vectors for in vivo liver-directed gene transfer of the OTC gene as acute treatment for hyperammonemic coma.

Modulation of Metabolic Pathways to Influence Multifactorial Chronic Diseases

Another potential application of liver-directed gene therapy is for the modulation of metabolic pathways in order to influence favorably the course of a multifactorial chronic disease. An example of this approach is gene transfer to raise circulating levels of high-density lipoprotein (HDL) cholesterol in order to prevent progression or cause regression of coronary atherosclerosis. Epidemiologic studies have consistently demonstrated a strong inverse correlation between plasma concentrations of HDL cholesterol and the incidence of coronary heart disease.[51] Apolipoprotein A-I (apoA-I) is the major protein component of HDL. Plasma concentrations of apoA-I are highly correlated with HDL levels and are also inversely associated with the risk of coronary heart disease.[52] The epidemiologic and clinical data suggest that HDL and apoA-I may be ''antiatherogenic,'' or directly protective against the development of coronary heart disease. Further supporting the concept that HDL and apoA-I may protect against atherosclerosis is the observation that genetic syndromes of high HDL and apoA-I—termed familial hyperalphalipoproteinemia—are associated, in some cases, with increased apoA-I production and decreased incidence of coronary heart disease.[53] This suggests that therapy to increase endogenous apoA-I production could raise HDL levels and may protect against the development or progression of CHD. However, no such therapy currently exists.

Animal studies have provided some support for the concept that raising levels of HDL and apoA-I is directly protective against atherosclerosis. Intravenous infusion of HDL in cholesterol-fed rabbits, for instance, resulted in decreased atherosclerosis.[54] Overexpression of human apoA-I in transgenic C57BL/6 mice fed an atherogenic diet has been found to raise HDL levels and decrease the degree of atherosclerosis.[55] Mice that are deficient in apolipoprotein E (apoE), in which atherosclerosis normally develops when the mice are fed a chow diet, developed much less atherosclerosis when made transgenic for overexpression of apoA-I.[56,57] However, more animal data are required regarding the issue of whether intervention to raise HDL or apoA-I levels will cause regression or halt progression of atherosclerosis.

It was recently demonstrated that the injection of mice with a recombinant adenovirus containing the gene for human apoA-I resulted in expression of human apoA-I and increased levels of HDL cholesterol.[13] In the absence of specific HDL-raising drugs, the first clinical trial of the specific effect of raising HDL on the development or progression of atherosclerosis in humans may require the use of apoA-I gene transfer, rather than a pharmacologic agent. However, data must first be generated in animal models to demonstrate that apoA-I gene transfer can have a favorable impact on the progression of atherosclerosis.

Approaches to Gene Therapy for Diabetes Mellitus

The demonstration that liver-directed gene transfer in humans can lead to stable genetic reconstitution is critical to the potential application of somatic gene therapy to diabetes mellitus. One potential target for gene therapy for diabetes is the pancreatic β-cell. Rat islets transplanted as isografts into diabetic rats have been shown to result in reversal of the diabetic state to normal and to prevent or reverse early diabetic complications.[58] Pancreas transplantation has been shown to be a viable clinical approach to rendering type I diabetic patients euglycemic.[59] As in liver transplantation for homozygous FH, the success of pancreatic islet transplantation in correcting the underlying metabolic defect in type I diabetes suggests that selective somatic gene transfer and stable, regulated expression of the insulin gene should be sufficient for metabolic correction of type I diabetes mellitus.

Recombinant adenoviruses have been shown to efficiently accomplish gene transfer and expression in pancreatic islets ex vivo. Adenoviral transfer of a marker gene (β-galactosidase) into freshly isolated rat islet cells resulted in transgene expression in up to 70% of the cells, and gene expression persisted for up to 21 days.[60] Normal functions of the islets were not altered by infection with recombinant adenovirus or expression of the transgene. Utilizing a recombinant adenovirus, hexokinase I was expressed in pancreatic islets ex vivo, resulting in increased basal levels of insulin release and glucose usage.[61] These studies demonstrate that recombinant adenoviruses can infect islet cells with high efficiency, resulting in transgene expression with the expected physiologic and biochemical effects.

Although pancreatic islet cells are the natural site of insulin synthesis and secretion, regulated expression of the insulin gene in an extrapancreatic tissue could theoretically be effective therapy for insulin-deficient diabetes mellitus. For example, transgenic mice expressing human insulin in the liver are relatively resistant to streptozotocin-induced diabetes.[62] Both insulin-producing pituitary cells[63] and fibroblasts[64] have been demonstrated to attenuate hyperglycemia in streptozotocin-diabetic mice. Therefore, gene transfer of a regulated insulin gene to extrapancreatic cells, such as hepatocytes, could be utilized as therapy for type I diabetes mellitus (reviewed in ref. 65).

Most of the issues relating to the successful development of gene therapy for diabetes mellitus are technical issues similar to those encountered in other diseases: targeting of the transgene to the appropriate tissue and achieving stable, regulated expression of the transgene. Another important issue for diabetes mellitus is the choice of gene for gene transfer. For most patients with type I diabetes, the insulin gene would appear to be the appropriate therapeutic gene for transfer. Another approach would be to transduce immunomodulatory cytokines into the pancreatic islets to prevent the autoimmune destruction that causes type I diabetes. Finally, those forms of diabetes caused by defects in the glucose-sensing pathway might be treatable through reconstitution of gene expression of the specific defective gene. For example, glucokinase deficiency has been demonstrated to be a cause of type II diabetes mellitus as a result of a defective sensing mechanism.[66] Gene transfer of the glucokinase gene into β-cells could be expected to correct the metabolic defect in these individuals. This hypothesis remains to be tested in animal models.

In summary, effective gene therapy for complex metabolic diseases such as diabetes mellitus, will take longer to develop than for monogenic disorders of metabolism, such as familial hypercholesterolemia or OTCD. However, development of effective gene therapy for diabetes will benefit from the technologic advances made in the development of vectors for gene transfer into other tissues, such as the liver.

Summary

Somatic gene therapy carries great promise for the treatment of a variety of metabolic diseases, including not only rare monogenic disorders, but also more common polygenic and multifactorial diseases. However, improved technology for safe and effective in vivo gene transfer in humans is required. Ultimately, the efficacy of somatic gene therapy in treating many types of metabolic diseases will be determined in human clinical trials utilizing a variety of vectors to target genes to different tissues.

References

1. Salmons B, Günzburg WH. Targeting of retroviral vectors for gene therapy. Human Gene Ther 1993;4:129
2. Raper SE, Wilson JM. Cell transplantation in liver-directed gene therapy. Cell Transplant 1993;2:381
3. Wilson JM, Chowdhury NR, Grossman M, et al. Temporary amelioration of hyperlipidemia in low-density lipoprotein receptor-deficient rabbits transplanted with genetically modified hepatocytes. Proc Natl Acad Sci USA 1987;87:8437
4. Kozarsky K, Wilson JM. Gene therapy: Adenovirus vectors. Curr Opin Genet Devel 1993;3:499
5. Brody S, Crystal R. Adenovirus-mediated in vivo gene transfer. Ann NY Acad Sci 1994;716:90
6. Stratford-Perricaudet L, Levero M, Chasse JF, et al. Evaluation of the transfer and expression in mice of an enzyme-encoding gene using a human adenovirus vector. Hum Gene Ther 1990;1:241
7. Herz J, Gerard R. Adenovirus-mediated transfer of the low-density lipoprotein receptor gene acutely accelerates clearance in normal mice. Proc Natl Acad Sci USA 1993;90:2812
8. Ishibashi S, Brown M, Goldstein J, et al. Hypercholesterolemia in low-density lipoprotein receptor knockout mice and its reversal by adenovirus-mediated gene delivery. J Clin Invest 1993;92:883
9. Smith T, Mehaffey M, Kayda D, et al. Adenovirus-mediated expression of therapeutic plasma levels of human factor IX in mice. Nat Genet 1993;5:397
10. Fang B, Eisensmith RC, Li X, et al. Gene therapy for phenylketonuria: Phenotypic correction in a genetically deficient mouse model by adenovirus-mediated hepatic gene transfer. Gene Ther 1994;1:247
11. Descamps V, Blumenfeld N, Villeval J, et al. Erythropoetin gene transfer and expression in adult normal mice: Use of an adenovirus vector. Human Gene Ther 1994;5:979
12. Willnow T, Sheng Z, Ishibashi S, Herz J. Inhibition of hepatic chylomicron remnant uptake by gene transfer of a receptor antagonist. Science 1994;264:1471
13. Kopfler W, Willard M, Betz T, et al. Adenovirus-mediated transfer of a gene encoding human apolipoprotein A-I into normal mice increases circulating high-density lipoprotein cholesterol. Circulation 1994;90:1319
14. Jaffe H, Danel C, Longenecker G, et al. Adenovirus-mediated in vivo gene transfer and expression in normal rat liver. Nat Genet 1992;1:372
15. Drazen K, Shen X, Csete M, et al. In vivo adenoviral-mediated human p53 tumor suppressor gene transfer and expression in rat liver after resection. Surgery 1994;166:197
16. Kozarsky KF, McKinley DR, Austin LL, et al. In vivo correction of LDL receptor deficiency in the Watanabe heritable hyperlipidemic rabbit with recombinant adenoviruses. J Biol Chem 1994;269:13695
17. Yang Y, Nunes F, Berencs K, et al. Cellular immunity to viral antigens limits E1-deleted adenoviruses for gene therapy. Proc Natl Acad Sci USA 1994;91:4407
18. Engelhardt JF, Ye X, Doranz B, Wilson JM. Ablation of E2a in recombinant adenoviruses improves transgene persistence and decreases inflammatory response in mouse liver. Proc Natl Acad Sci USA 1994;91:6196
19. Samulski R, Zhu X, Xiao X, et al. Targeted integration of adeno-associated virus (AAV) into human chromosome 19. EMBO J 1991;10:3941
20. Podsakoff G, Wong K, Chatterjee S. Efficient gene transfer into nondividing cells by adeno-associated virus-based vectors. J Virol 1994;68:5656
21. Kotin R. Prospects for the use of adeno-associated virus as a vector for human gene therapy. Human Gene Ther 1994;5:793
22. Walsh C, Nienhuis A, Samulski RJ, et al. Phenotypic correction of Fanconi anemia in human hematopoietic cells with a recombinant adeno-associated virus vector. J Clin Invest 1994;94:1440
23. Miller J, Donahue R, Sellers S, et al. Recombinant adeno-associated virus (rAAV)-mediated expression of a human ∂-globin gene in human progenitor-derived erythroid cells. Proc Natl Acad Sci USA 1994;91:10183
24. Flotte T, Afione S, Conrad C, et al. Stable in vivo expression of the cystic fibrosis transmembrane regulator with an adeno-associated virus vector. Proc Natl Acad Sci USA 1993;90:10613
25. Kaplitt M, Leone P, Samulski RJ, et al. Long-term gene expression and phenotypic correction using adeno-associated virus vectors in the mammalian brain. Nat Genet 1994;8:148
26. Michael S, Curiel D. Strategies to achieve targeted gene delivery via the receptor-mediated endocytosis pathway. Gene Ther 1994;1:223
27. Wu CH, Wilson JM, Wu GY. Targeting gene delivery and persistent expression of a foreign gene driven by mammalian regulatory elements in vivo. J Biol Chem 1989;264:16985
28. Wu GY, Wilson JM, Shalaby F, et al. Receptor-mediated gene delivery in vivo. J Biol Chem 1991;266:14338
29. Wilson JM, Grossman M, Wu CH, et al. Hepatocyte-directed gene transfer in vivo leads to transient improvement of hypercholesterolemia in low-density lipoprotein receptor-deficient rabbits. J Biol Chem 1992;267:963
30. Wilson JM, Grossman M, Wu CH, et al. A novel mechanism for achieving transgene persistence in vivo after somatic gene transfer into hepatocytes. J Biol Chem 1992;267:11483
31. Cristiano RJ, Smith LC, Woo S. Hepatic gene therapy: Adenovirus enhancement of receptor-mediated gene delivery and expression in primary hepatocytes. Proc Natl Acad Sci USA 1993;90:2122
32. Michael S, Huang C, Romer M, et al. Binding-incompetent adenovirus facilitates molecular conjugate-mediated gene transfer by the receptor-mediated endocytosis pathway. J Biol Chem 1993;268:6866
33. Cristiano RJ, Smith LC, Kay MA, et al. Hepatic gene therapy: Efficient gene delivery and expression in primary hepatocytes utilizing a conjugated adenovirus-DNA complex. Proc Natl Acad Sci USA 1993;90:11548
34. Perales JC, Ferkol T, Beegen H, et al. Gene transfer in vivo: Sustained expression and regulation of genes introduced into the liver by receptor-targeted uptake. Proc Natl Acad Sci USA 1994;91:4086
35. Hug P, Sleight R. Liposomes for the transformation of eukaryotic cells. Biochim Biophys Acta 1991;1097:1
36. Farhood H, Gao X, Son K, et al. Cationic liposomes for direct gene transfer in therapy of cancer and other diseases. Ann NY Acad Sci 1994;716:23

37. Kaneda Y, Iwai K, Uchida T. Increased expression of DNA cointroduced with nuclear protein in adult rat liver. Science 1989;243:375
38. Leibiger I, Leibiger B, Sarrach D, et al. Genetic manipulation of rat hepatocytes in vivo: Complications for a therapy model of type-1 diabetes. Biomed Biochem Acta 1990;49:1193
39. Zhu N, Liggitt D, Liu Y, Debs R. Systemic gene expression after intravenous DNA delivery into adult mice. Science 1993;216:209
40. Brown MS, Goldstein JL. A receptor-mediated pathway for cholesterol homeostasis. Science 1986;232:34
41. Gordon BR, Kelsey SF, Bilheimer DW, et al. Treatment of refractory familial hypercholesterolemia by low-density lipoprotein apheresis using an automated dextran sulfate cellulose adsorption system. Am J Cardiol 1992;70:1010
42. Chowdhury JR, Grossman M, Gupta S, et al. Long-term improvement of hypercholesterolemia after ex vivo gene therapy in LDLR-deficient rabbits. Science 1991;254:1802
43. Grossman M, Wilson JM, Raper S. A novel approach for introducing hepatocytes into the portal circulation. J Lab Clin Med 1993;121:472
44. Grossman M, Raper S, Wilson JM. Transplantation of genetically modified autologous hepatocytes in nonhuman primates: Feasibility and short-term toxicity. Human Gene Ther 1992;3:501
45. Wilson JM, Grossman M, Raper SE, et al. Clinical protocol: Ex vivo gene therapy of familial hypercholesterolemia. Human Gene Ther 1992;3:179
46. Grossman M, Raper S, Kozarsky K, et al. Successful ex vivo gene therapy directed to the liver in a patient with familial hypercholesterolemia. Nat Genet 1994;6:335
46a. Grossman M, Rader DJ, Muller D, et al. A pilot study of ex vivo gene therapy for homozygous familial hypercholesterolemia. Nature Medicine 1995;1:1148
47. Kozarsky K, Grossman M, Wilson JM. Adenovirus-mediated correction of the genetic defect in hepatocytes from patients with familial hypercholesterolemia. Somatic Cell Molec Genet 1993;19:449
48. Wilson JM, Grossman M. Therapeutic strategies for familial hypercholesterolemia based on somatic gene transfer. Am J Cardiol 1993;72:59D
49. Batshaw ML. Inborn errors of urea synthesis. Ann Neurol 1994;35:133
50. Grompe M, Jones S, Louseged H, Caskey T. Retroviral-mediated gene transfer of human ornithine transcarbamylase into primary hepatocytes of spf and spf-ash mice. Hum Gene Ther 1992;3:35
51. Gordon DJ, Rifkind BM. High-density lipoprotein—The clinical implications of recent studies. N Engl J Med 1989;321:1311
52. Rader DJ, Hoeg JM, Brewer HB Jr. Quantitation of plasma apoliproproteins in the primary and secondary prevention of coronary artery disease. Am Intern Med 1994;120:1012
53. Rader DJ, Schaefer JR, Lohse P, et al. Increased production of apolipoprotein A-I associated with elevated levels of high-density lipoproteins and apolipoprotein A-I in a patient with familial hyperalphalipoproteinemia. Metabolism 1993;42:1429
54. Badimon JJ, Badimon L, Fuster V. Regression of atherosclerotic lesions by high-density lipoprotein plasma fraction in the cholesterol-fed rabbit. J Clin Invest 1990;85:1234
55. Rubin EM, Krauss RM, Spangler EA, et al. Inhibition of early atherogenesis in transgenic mice by human apolipoprotein AI. Nature 1991;353:265
56. Paszty C, Maeda N, Verstuyft J, Rubin E. Apolipoprotein AI transgene corrects apolipoprotein E deficiency-induced atherosclerosis in mice. J Clin Invest 1994;94:899
57. Plump A, Scott C, Breslow J. Human apolipoprotein A-I gene expression increases high-density lipoprotein and suppresses atherosclerosis in the apolipoprotein E-deficient mouse. Proc Natl Acad Sci USA 1994;91:9607
58. Mauer S, Sutherland DER, Steffes MW, et al. Pancreatic islet transplantation. Effects on the glomerular lesions of experimental diabetes in the rat. Diabetes 1974;23:748
59. Lacy PW. Status of islet transplantation. Diabetes Rev 1993;1:76
60. Csete ME, Afra R, Mullen Y, et al. Adenoviral-mediated gene transfer to pancreatic islets does not alter function. Transplant Proc 1994;26:756
61. Becker TC, BeltrandelRio H, Noel RJ, et al. Overexpression of hexokinase I in isolated islets of Langerhans via recombinant adenovirus: Enhancement of glucose metabolism and insulin secretion at basal but not stimulatory glucose levels. J Biol Chem 1994;269:21234
62. Valera A, Fillat C, Costa C, et al. Regulated expression of human insulin in the liver of transgenic mice corrects diabetic alterations. FASEB J 1994;8: 440
63. Stewart C, Taylor N, Green I, et al. Insulin-releasing pituitary cells as a model for somatic cell gene therapy in diabetes mellitus. J Endocrinol 1994;142:339
64. Kawakami Y, Yamaoka T, Hirochika R, et al. Somatic gene therapy for diabetes with an immunological safety system for complete removal of transplanted cells. Diabetes 1992;41:956
65. Newgard C. Cellular engineering and gene therapy strategies for insulin replacement in diabetes. Diabetes 1994;43:341
66. Matschinsky F, Liang Y, Kesavan P, et al. Glucokinase as pancreatic β-cell glucose sensor and diabetes gene. J Clin Invest 1993;92:2092

Diabetes Mellitus, edited by Derek LeRoith, Simeon I. Taylor, and Jerrold M. Olefsky. Lippincott–Raven Publishers, Philadelphia

CHAPTER 47
Engineering the Pancreatic β-Cell

SHIMON EFRAT AND NORMAN FLEISCHER

The success of segmental pancreatic transplantation in humans and progress in experimental studies of islet transplantation highlight the potential of utilizing pancreatic β-cells for the treatment of type I and insulin-requiring type II diabetes. This approach is limited by a variety of obstacles, not the least of which is the limited supply of donor material and the difficulty in isolating large numbers of islets from the pancreas. Insulin-producing cell lines could provide a readily available and virtually unlimited source of donor cells with well-defined and reproducible properties. To be considered as donor cells for transplantation therapy of diabetes, such cell lines would have to fulfill minimal requirements, including the following:

1. Efficient growth in culture, to allow propagation of large numbers of cells
2. Production of insulin in amounts similar to those of normal β-cells
3. Regulated synthesis and secretion of insulin in response to physiologic secretagogues in a manner similar to normal islets
4. Phenotypic stability in culture and in vivo
5. The ability to control cell proliferation when transplanted in vivo. This is essential to prevent overproliferation, which may lead to hypoglycemia. Withdrawal from the cell cycle may also enable the cells to better focus on their differentiated functions.
6. Finally, the cells need to be nonimmunogenic to escape rejection, as well as the autoimmune attack characteristic of type I diabetes.

Recent and future advances in cell encapsulation techniques may alleviate the need for the last two requirements by providing a physical barrier to unlimited proliferation as well as to immunologic attack. The use of human cell lines may not be essential, depending on the effectiveness of genetic engineering or encapsulation, or both, to allow xenograft tolerance. Even if nonhuman cell lines were to be used, it might be beneficial to engineer them to produce human insulin to limit generation of anti-insulin antibodies in the host.

In this chapter, we describe the work in our laboratories, as well as in other laboratories, directed toward the development and evaluation of pancreatic β-cell lines with these desired properties.

β-Cell Immortalization

Adult β-cells do not proliferate in vivo or in culture, although they include a small percentage of cells that maintain a proliferative capacity.[1] Embryonic islets contain a larger proportion of proliferating cells; however, these are not fully differentiated and may coexpress other islet hormones. Because of the difficulties in obtaining sufficient numbers of islet cells, many investigators have relied on immortalized or transformed β-cell lines for β-cell studies. To produce continuous β-cell lines, several groups have introduced oncogenes into rodent β-cells. Unfortunately, human β-cells have thus far been resistant to transformation by these approaches.

Two β-cell lines—RIN, a line derived from an x-ray-induced rat insulinoma,[2] and HIT, a line derived by infecting hamster islets with the SV40 virus[3]—have been widely used in β-cell research. However, upon prolonged culture, these cells deviate considerably from normal β-cells in terms of insulin production and secretion. In addition, the transformation events that give rise to these lines are difficult to reproduce, making it difficult to replace cells that dedifferentiate following prolonged propagation in culture.

In principle, oncogenes can be introduced into β-cells by transfection, by the use of viral vectors, or by transgenic approaches. However, the first two techniques are difficult to apply for stable gene integration into nonproliferating cells. The transgenic approach has proven to be more productive in generating a renewable source of transformed β-cells. The gene encoding the active oncoprotein of SV40—large T antigen (Tag)—has been found to be efficient in transforming mouse β-cells when stably introduced into the mouse genome by transgenic techniques.[4-6] Placing the Tag gene under control of the rat insulin II gene regulatory elements (RIP) targets the expression of the oncoprotein in these mice specifically to β-cells. RIP-Tag transgenic mice, first generated by Hanahan,[4] exhibit heritable insulinomas.[4] These tumors can be cultured to derive continuous cell lines, denoted β tumor cells (βTC).[7] Other groups have subsequently developed similar lines from transgenic tumors[5,6] and from pre–tumor-stage hyperplastic islets[8] of RIP-Tag mice.

βTC cells contain, on average, 30% of the insulin concentration found in normal islets.[7] Histologically, they resemble normal β-cells (Fig. 47-1). In both static incubations and perifusion assays, they secrete low basal levels of insulin and are induced by all of the major insulin secretagogues—most notably glucose—to increase their insulin output. The insulin secretory characteristics of βTC cells are similar to those of normal pancreatic β-cells. Glucose-induced insulin secretion is potentiated by a number of β-cell incretins that are known either to elevate cellular levels of cAMP or to promote phosphatidylinositol (PI) turnover, but they are not active in the absence of glucose (Fig. 47-2). Under maximal stimulating conditions, insulin secretion rises to a level many times greater than basal levels.[9] βTC lines manifest two different patterns of glucose sensitivity. In some lines, the glucose concentration dependency for insulin secretion is in the physiologic range that stimulates insulin secretion from the normal islet (e.g., 4–20 mM). In other lines, maximal insulin release is attained at subphysiologic glucose concentrations. Understanding the underlying cause for the difference in glucose sensitivity between various βTC cell lines has been important in our attempts to generate correctly regulated cell lines and has provided an opportunity to study the mechanism of glucose sensing by the β-cell.

Glucose-Induced Insulin Secretion in βTC Cells

Glucose must be metabolized in β-cells to induce insulin secretion, and the rate of insulin secretion is proportional to the rate of glucose metabolism.[10] Glucose metabolism—possibly by increased production or flux of ATP, or increased ATP/ADP ratios—inhibits ATP-sensitive K^+ channels in the β-cell. The resulting plasma membrane depolarization opens voltage-gated Ca^{++} channels and induces an influx of Ca^{++}, which triggers the fusion of prestored insulin vesicles with the plasma membrane. Other intracellular second messengers also play a role in coupling glucose metabolism to insulin secretion.[11] Proteins that control the metabolic flux of glucose in β-cells function as "glucose sensors" that couple changes in the extracellular glucose concentrations to insulin secretion.

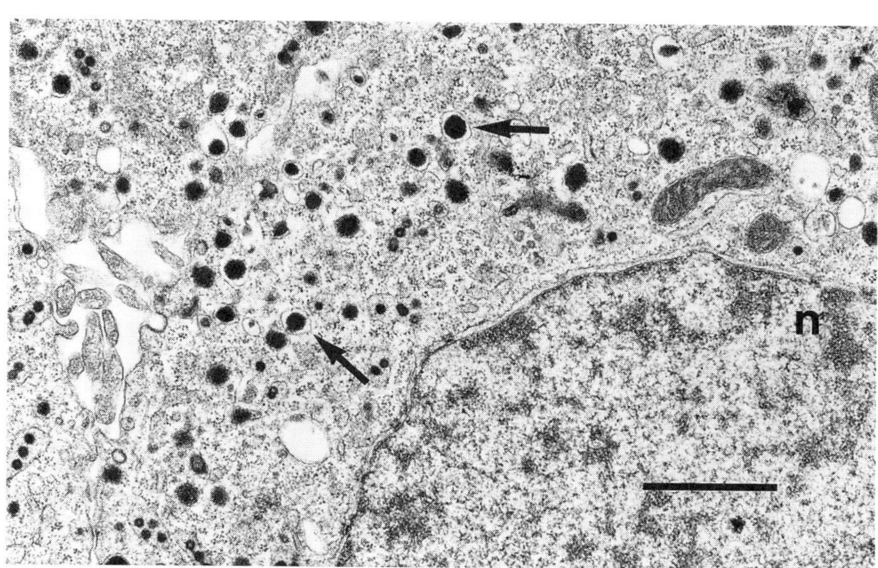

Figure 47-1. Electron micrograph of βTC6-F7 cells. The arrows point to mature insulin secretory granules. *n*, cell nucleus. Bar scale represents 1 μm. (Reproduced with permission from Knaack D, Fiore DM, Surana M, et al. Clonal insulinoma cell line which stably maintains correct glucose responsiveness. Diabetes 1994;43:1413.)

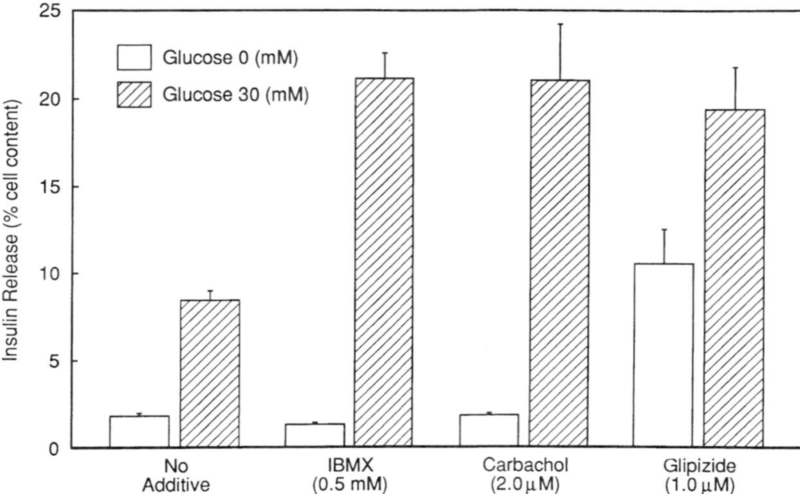

Figure 47-2. The effect of various incretins on insulin release from βTC6-F7 cells in the absence (*open bars*) or presence (*hatched bars*) of 30 mM of glucose. Glucose alone stimulates insulin release. Isobutylmethylxanthine (IBMX), which elevates cellular levels of cAMP, and the cholinergic agonist carbachol are ineffective secretagogues in the absence of glucose, but they do potentiate the effect of glucose. The sulfonylurea glipizide is active as a secretagogue in the absence of glucose. These secretory dynamics are similar to those reported for normal islets. (Modified with permission from Knaack D, Fiore DM, Surana M, et al. Clonal insulinoma cell line which stably maintains correct glucose responsiveness. Diabetes 1994;43:1413.)

β-Cells express two specialized proteins that have been considered as candidates for the glucose sensor: the glucose transporter isotype GLUT-2[12,13] and the glucose phosphorylating enzyme glucokinase.[14] The K_m of GLUT-2 for glucose is approximately 17 mM, which is considerably higher than that of the ubiquitously expressed GLUT-1 or of the fat/muscle-specific isoform GLUT-4. This high K_m results in a rate of glucose influx into β-cells that is proportional to the extracellular glucose concentration, up to 10 mM. Similarly, glucokinase (also termed hexokinase IV) has a K_m for glucose in the 8-mM range, which is significantly higher than the 10- to 50-μM range that is characteristic of hexokinases I, II, and III.[10] The K_m values of both GLUT-2 and glucokinase are in the range of physiologic changes in blood glucose concentrations. Although either could function as the "physiologic glucose sensor," abundant experimental evidence, some of which has been provided by studies of βTC and related cell lines, suggests that the production of glucose-6-phosphate, catalyzed by glucokinase, the rate-limiting step in β-cell glycolysis,[10] is the predominant reaction that couples increases in extracellular glucose levels to insulin secretion. Glucose transport into β-cells is not rate-limiting for glycolysis and does not appear to play an important regulatory role in insulin secretion under normal circumstances (see ref. 15 for review).

Transformed β-cells often manifest decreased GLUT-2 and increased GLUT-1 expression.[16] Several β-cell lines, however, have been developed that maintain the normal expression of GLUT-2 and express little, if any, GLUT-1.[5,8,17-19] Two examples of such are the βTC6 and βTC7 lines, which respond to glucose concentrations in the physiologic range.[17,19] This phenotype is associated with activities of glucokinase and hexokinase similar to those of normal islets. Following prolonged propagation in culture (about 20 passages), these cells acquire responsiveness to subphysiologic concentrations of glucose (Fig. 47-3). This shift occurs without major changes in the expression of glucose transporters or in the rates of glucose uptake.[17] Glucokinase activity remains stably expressed. However, hexokinase activity is markedly increased.[17]

Increased hexokinase activity is the only consistent change we have noted in a variety of βTC lines that have acquired secretory responsiveness to subphysiologic glucose levels. The elevation in activity of the low-K_m hexokinase accelerates the rate of glucose metabolism at low glucose concentrations, thus enabling low levels of glucose to induce insulin secretion. Partial inhibition of hexokinase activity with 2-deoxyglucose, a glucose analogue that can be phosphorylated but not further metabolized, shifts the maximal insulin secretory response to glucose to a higher glucose concentration (Leiser M, Surana M, Efrat S, and Fleischer N, unpublished data, 1994; Fig. 47-4). Hexokinase, unlike glucokinase, is inhibited by the accumulating 2-deoxyglucose-6-phosphate. These results demonstrate that the elevated hexokinase activity is the major cause for the response of βTC cells to subphysiologic glucose levels. The hexokinase isotype which is upregulated, appears to be hexoki-

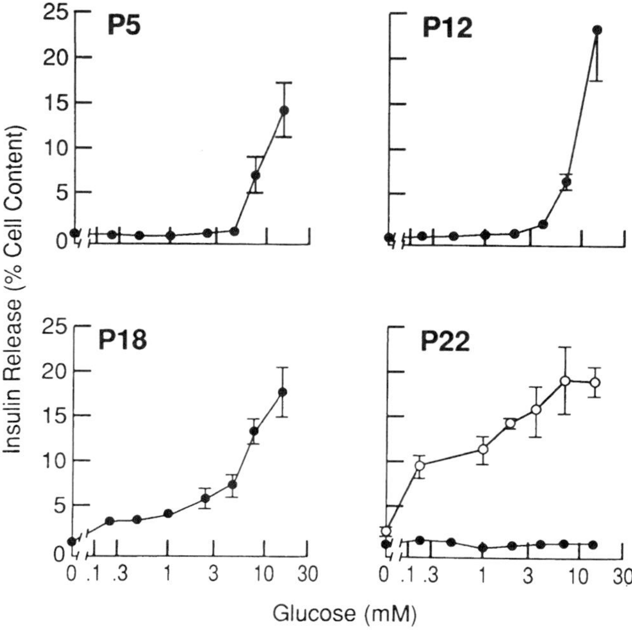

Figure 47-3. Effect of passage number on glucose-induced insulin release in βTC6 cells. At low passages, insulin release is not stimulated by glucose concentrations of less than 5 mM. At passage 18, a small response is noted at low glucose concentrations. At passage 22 or higher, two types of response are noted. Either no response to glucose (*closed symbols*) or a robust secretory response at low glucose concentrations (*open symbols*). Although the closed symbol response was seen several times during serial passage of these cells, the response shown by the open symbols was also seen on several occasions, and with multiple other cell types. (Modified with permission from Knaack D, Fiore DM, Surana M, et al. Clonal insulinoma cell line which stably maintains correct glucose responsiveness. Diabetes 1994;43:1413.)

nase-I, as judged by fractionation of βTC extracts on DEAE-Cibacron Blue F3GA agarose columns (Leiser M, Efrat S, and Fleischer N, unpublished data, 1994). There is a correlation between increased hexokinase-I activity and increased hexokinase-I mRNA levels, suggesting that the induction represents increased transcription or mRNA stability (Lemberg H, Efrat S, Leiser M, Fleischer N, unpublished data, 1994).

In some RIP-Tag tumors, hexokinase activity is already elevated during tumor development in vivo. When these tumors are cultured to derive βTC cell lines, the cells manifest an abnormal response to subphysiologic glucose levels during the initial passages. More commonly, the activation of hexokinase occurs during cell propagation in culture, perhaps to allow more efficient energy production from glucose oxidation, which is needed in actively proliferating cells. To determine whether the changes in hexokinase activity represent an adaptation of the entire cell population, or a selection of a subpopulation with increased hexokinase activity, we attempted to derive single-cell clonal lines from βTC6 cells at a passage that manifests glucose responsiveness in both the subphysiologic and physiologic concentration ranges. One of these clones—βTC6-F7—was characterized in detail.[19] These cells were found to maintain correct glucose responsiveness for more than 58 passages (longer than a year) in culture. βTC6-F7 cells expressed high glucokinase and low hexokinase activity, similar to that of normal islets. In addition, they expressed mRNA for the GLUT-2 glucose transporter isotype and no detectable GLUT-1 mRNA, as is characteristic of normal β-cells. These results demonstrate that transformed β-cells can stably maintain a highly differentiated phenotype during prolonged propagation in culture, including glucose responsiveness in the physiologic concentration range and the expression of specialized proteins in a pattern normally associated with differentiated nonproliferating β-cells in vivo. The results also suggest that the drift in glucose response characteristics observed in the nonclonal βTC lines results from a selection of abnormally regulated subpopulations, rather than from changes associated with the simultaneous adaptation of the entire population to growth in culture. Such cells may have a selective growth advantage owing to the elevated hexokinase activity. Remarkably, the transformed β-cells in the RIP-Tag tumors and cell lines do not manifest substantial changes in glucokinase activity.

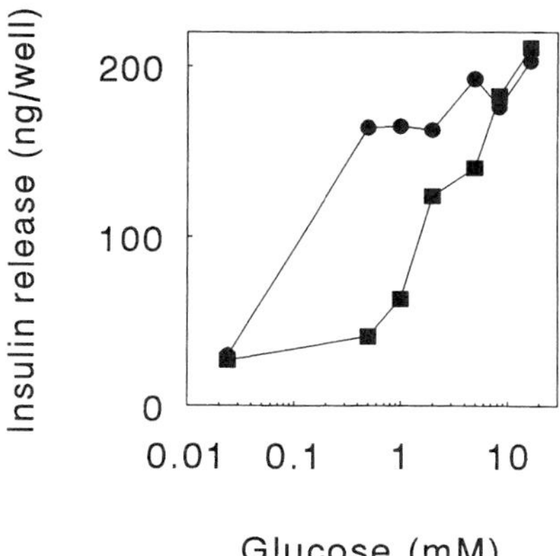

FIGURE 47-4. Effect of 2-deoxyglucose on insulin release from βTC3 cells. Insulin release was measured following 2-hour incubation in Krebs-Ringer buffer containing the indicated glucose concentration and 0.5 mM of isobutylmethylxanthine (IBMX), either in the absence (*circles*) or presence (*squares*) of 10 mM of 2-deoxyglucose.

These results suggest that cloning of β-cell lines at early passages may allow the selection of cells that maintain low hexokinase activity for prolonged periods. However, such low hexokinase activity may not be permanent. Therefore, gene targeting and antisense approaches may be needed to prevent cell lines from acquiring increased hexokinase expression.

Conditional Immortalization

When βTC cells are injected into syngeneic recipients, they develop noninvasive tumors at the site of injection. Because of these tumors (insulinomas), the recipient mice eventually die of hypoglycemia. An ideal β-cell line would be one that could be easily propagated in culture to allow generation of large numbers of transplantable cells and, in addition, would have the ability to withdraw from proliferation following transplantation. This is necessary to prevent uncontrolled expansion in vivo and may also enhance the differentiated properties of the cells.

We have attempted to adapt a genetic strategy for reversible induction of proliferation in β-cells. This approach employs the bacterial lac repressor to control the expression of Tag.[20] The repressor recognizes a short palindromic DNA sequence (operator) and binds to it, forming a complex that inhibits gene transcription. The lactose analogue isopropyl-thiogalactoside (IPTG) is capable of binding to the repressor and inactivating it, thereby opening the way for expression of the gene. The RIP-Tag construct was modified to include multiple copies of the lac operator sequence in the intron and 5′-untranslated region (RIP-Tag/op). Transgenic mice expressing this gene developed β-cell tumors similar to those of the original RIP-Tag mice, indicating that the operator sequences did not interfere with expression of the gene (Efrat et al., unpublished data, 1992). In parallel, the gene encoding the lac repressor (lacR) was placed under control of the insulin promoter (RIP-lacR) and microinjected into mouse embryos. A nuclear localization signal was included to target the repressor to the nucleus. RIP-lacR mice showed nuclear lacR immunoreactivity in the islets; they did not, however have a phenotype, as the mouse genome does not contain target sequences recognized by the repressor. In the next stage, the two transgenic lineages were crossed so as to generate double-transgenic mice that coexpress both genes in β-cells. Islets isolated from these mice were incubated in culture for 3 days in the presence or absence of IPTG and were stained with a Tag antiserum. As seen in Figure 47-5, Tag is expressed at high levels in most of the cells when the lacR is inactivated in the presence of IPTG. A small number of cells, however, seem to express Tag even in the absence of IPTG. This population may be responsible for the finding that insulinomas eventually develop in these double-transgenic mice. These results suggest that, for reasons unknown, the lacR regulation is sufficiently ''leaky'' in a small number of β-cells to allow tumor development. Tighter regulatory systems are, therefore, required for the development of a reversible immortalization approach in vivo, such as those employing the bacterial tetracycline repressor[21] to control Tag expression or Cre recombinase[22] to delete the Tag gene once a sufficient number of β-cells has been generated. Recently, successful reversible immortalization of murine β-cells has been achieved utilizing the bacterial tetracycline (tet) operon system to control Tag expression.[22a] In this system, transgenic mice were produced that express a fusion protein in β-cells composed of the tet repressor and a potent viral transactivator. A second transgenic line was produced that contained the Tag gene linked to tandem array of the tet operator sequences. In the double transgenic animals, the binding of the tet repressor to the tet operator activated Tag gene. A cell line (βTC-tet) created from an insulinoma from one of these mice grows in the absence of tet. In the presence of tet, the repressor protein is prevented from binding to the tet operator, Tag expression is blocked and the βTC-tet cells cease replicating. Upon removal of tet, replication resumes.

-IPTG

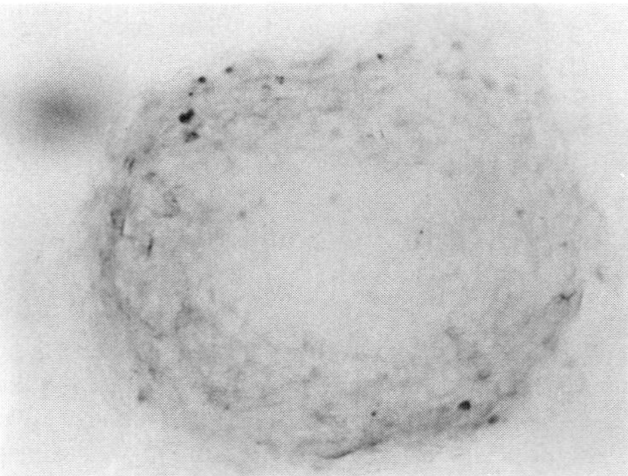

+IPTG

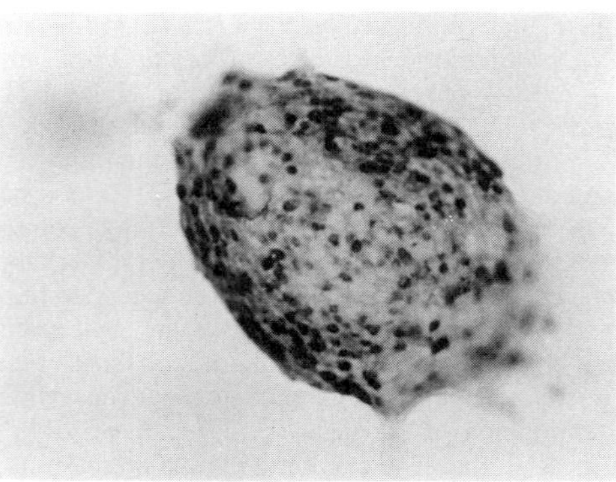

Figure 47-5. Inducible Tag expression in islets from double-transgenic RIP-Tag/op × RIP-lacR mice. Islets were isolated from the pancreas and incubated in culture for 3 days in the absence or presence of IPTG. They were then stained with antibodies to Tag. (Original magnification ×230.)

Altering β-Cell Immunogenicity

Substantial evidence suggests that cell surface class I major histocompatibility complex (MHC)–mediated antigen presentation is the major target in allograft rejection. By employing targeted gene disruption in mouse embryonic stem cells, two groups have generated mutant mice deficient in β_2-microglobulin, a protein that is required for the formation of the antigen-presenting complex between the class I MHC heavy chain and the antigen peptide.[23,24] Cells from mice homozygous for the mutation lack surface class I MHC molecules. Islets from these mice, transplanted under the renal capsule of allogeneic mice, manifested markedly increased survival compared with that of normal islets.[25,26] These results suggest that genetic manipulation of class I MHC antigen presentation may facilitate transplantation of allogeneic β-cells. This suggestion is further supported by recent studies in transgenic mice using viral immunosuppressive proteins. Human adenoviruses (Ads) code for several proteins that alter the host response to infected cells. One of these is the E3-region 19Kd glycoprotein (gp19) that binds to the heavy chain of the class I MHC protein and prevents its transport from the endoplasmic reticulum to the cell surface. The splicing within the E3-region is complex and results in the production of other proteins, in addition to gp19, that might have an effect on graft survival. Islets isolated from transgenic mice expressing the E3 region of the human adenovirus gene in β-cells survive when transplanted into allogeneic hosts.[26a] It should be noted that modification of class I MHC expression, even if successful in preventing rejection, may be inadequate protection against the autoimmune process characteristic of type I diabetes.

Engineering Non–β-Cells to Replace β-Cells

Several research groups have attempted to engineer non–β-cells to produce insulin. Such attempts are interesting cell biology studies with the potential for improving our understanding of insulin gene expression and insulin synthesis, processing, and secretion. From the standpoint of production of a cell line to treat diabetes, such experiments have both advantages and disadvantages. For instance, non–β-cells can avoid the autoimmune destructive process targeted against β-cells in type I diabetes. Furthermore, if an insulin-producing cell line could be developed from a non–β-cell type that was accessible by biopsy, it might be possible to create a cell line from each patient, thus avoiding the complications associated with rejection and autoimmune destruction. The concept behind this approach is that, as the various genes involved in the regulation of insulin synthesis, processing, and secretion are identified, they can be transfected into a non–β-cell, which eventually will be built into a surrogate β-cell. The major difficulty in this approach concerns the ability to reconstruct in a non–β-cell the highly regulated insulin secretion of the normal β-cell. Physicians who have utilized various open-loop systems to treat diabetic patients are well aware of the advantages of a closed-loop system, as provided by the normal β-cell. The reconstruction of correct glucose sensing and its potentiation by various incretins, however, as well as the coupling of these signals to insulin secretion in a non–β-cell, are formidable genetic engineering tasks. Nevertheless, some interesting early data have emerged.

The cDNA for insulin has been transfected into FAO cells, a hepatic cell line that manifests certain differentiated functions.[27] Such transfected cells synthesize some proinsulin and process some of it to insulin. The regulation of this insulin synthesis, however, is not analogous to that of the normal β-cell.

Another approach to the development of a surrogate β-cell is illustrated by the work of Newgard and colleagues.[28] They utilized the AtT-20 cell line, derived from pituitary corticotrophs, which has been stably transfected with human proinsulin cDNA. These cells synthesize and process proinsulin. Because they are derived from cells that possess the capacity for regulated secretion, they can be induced to increase insulin secretion in response to secretagogues. Interestingly, overexpression of GLUT-2 in these cells by gene transfection resulted in increased production of insulin and some increased secretion in response to glucose. The exact mechanism for this effect is not clear. Such cells produce far less insulin than βTC cells and are not properly regulated. They illustrate, however, the potential for generating a surrogate β-cell, although the current state of our knowledge precludes early success in this area.

Future Prospects

Based on the rate of scientific progress in the area of cell biology, immunology, and genetic engineering in the past 10 years, and assuming uninterrupted continuation of this rate, we believe that the development of genetically engineered β-cells for use in human transplantation is clearly achievable. It is likely that the efficiency of gene expression obtained with transgenic methodology will eventually be attained in cultured human islets, allowing the development of human β-cell lines that have the desired characteristics described in this chapter.

References

1. Hellestrom C. The life story of the pancreatic β cell. Diabetologia 1984;26:393
2. Chick WL, Warren S, Chute RN, et al. A transplantable insulinoma in the rat. Proc Natl Acad Sci USA 1977;74:628
3. Santerre RF, Cook RA, Crisel RMD, et al. Insulin synthesis in a clonal cell line of simian virus 40-transformed hamster pancreatic beta cells. Proc Natl Acad Sci USA 1981;78:4339
4. Hanahan D. Heritable formation of pancreatic B-cell tumours in transgenic mice expressing recombinant insulin simian virus 40 oncogenes. Nature 1985;315:115
5. Miyazaki J-I, Araki K, Yamato E, et al. Establishment of a pancreatic β cell line that retains glucose-inducible insulin secretion: Special reference to expression of glucose transporter isoforms. Endocrinology 1990;127:126
6. Hamaguchi K, Gaskins HR, Leiter EH. NIT-1, a pancreatic β-cell line established from a transgenic NOD/Lt mouse. Diabetes 1991;40:842
7. Efrat S, Linde S, Kofod H, et al. Beta-cell lines derived from transgenic mice expressing a hybrid insulin gene-oncogene. Proc Natl Acad Sci USA 1988; 85:9037
8. Radvanyi F, Christgau S, Baekkeskov S, et al. Pancreatic β cells cultured from individual preneoplastic foci in a multistage tumorigenesis pathway: A potentially general technique for isolating physiologically representative cell lines. Mol Cell Biol 1993;13:4223
9. D'Ambra R, Surana M, Efrat S, et al. Regulation of insulin secretion from B-cell lines derived from transgenic mice insulinomas resembles that of normal B-cells. Endocrinology 1990;126:2815
10. Meglasson MD, Matschinsky FM. Pancreatic islet glucose metabolism and regulation of insulin secretion. Diabetes Metab Rev 1986;2:163
11. Holz GG, Habener JF. Signal transduction crosstalk in the endocrine system: Pancreatic β cells and the glucose competence concept. Trends Biochem Sci 1992;17:388
12. Bell G, Kayano T, Buse JB, et al. Molecular biology of mammalian glucose transporters. Diabetes Care 1990;13:198
13. Thorens B, Charron MJ, Lodish HF. Molecular physiology of glucose transporters. Diabetes Care 1990;13:209
14. Meglasson MD, Matschinsky FM. New perspectives in pancreatic islet glucokinase. Am J Physiol 1984;246:E1
15. Efrat S, Tal M, Lodish HF. The pancreatic β-cell glucose sensor. Trends Biochem Sci 1994;19:535
16. Tal M, Thorens B, Surana M, et al. Glucose transporter isotype switch in T-antigen-transformed pancreatic β cells growing in culture and in mice. Mol Cell Biol 1992;12:422
17. Efrat S, Leiser M, Surana M, et al. Murine insulinoma cell line with normal glucose-regulated insulin secretion. Diabetes 1993;42:901
18. Asfari M, Janjic D, Meda P, et al. Establishment of 2-mercaptoethanol-dependent differentiated insulin-secreting cell lines. Endocrinology 1992;130:167
19. Knaack D, Fiore DM, Surana M, et al. Clonal insulinoma cell line which stably maintains correct glucose responsiveness. Diabetes 1994;43:1413
20. Deuschle U, Hipskind RA, Bujard H. RNA polymerase II transcription blocked by *Escherichia coli* lac repressor. Science 1990;248:480
21. Gossen M, Bujard H. Tight control of gene expression in mammalian cells by tetracycline-responsive promoters. Proc Natl Acad Sci USA 1992;89:5547
22. Gu H, Marth JD, Orban PC, et al. Deletion of a DNA polymerase β gene segment in T cells using cell type-specific gene targeting. Science 1994; 265:103

22a. Efrat S, Fusco-DeMane D, Lemberg H, Emran O, and Wang X. (1995) Conditional transformation of a pancreatic beta-cell line derived from transgenic mice expressing a tetracycline-regulated oncogene. Proc Natl Acad Sci USA 1992;3576–3580

23. Zijstra M, Li E, Sajjadi F, et al. Germ-line transmission of a disrupted β_2-microglobulin gene produced by homologous recombination in embryonic stem cells. Nature 1989;342:435
24. Koller BH, Smithies O. Inactivating the β_2-microglobulin locus in mouse embryonic stem cells by homologous recombination. Proc Natl Acad Sci USA 1989;86:8932
25. Markmann JF, Bassiri H, Desai NM, et al. Indefinite survival of MHC class I–deficient murine pancreatic islet allografts. Transplantation 1992;54:1085
26. Osorio RW, Ascher NL, Jaenisch R, et al. Major histocompatibility complex class I deficiency prolongs islet allograft survival. Diabetes 1993;42:1520

26a. Efrat S, Fejer G, Brownlee M, and Horwitz M. (1995) Prolonged survival of pancreatic islet allografts mediated by adenovirus immunoregulatory transgenes. Proc Natl Acad Sci USA 1992;6947–6951

27. Vollenweider F, Irminger JC, Gross DJ, et al. Processing of proinsulin by transfected hepatoma (FAO) cells. J Biol Chem 1992;267:14629
28. Newgard CB. Cellular engineering and gene therapy strategies for insulin replacement in diabetes. Diabetes 1994;43:341

Diabetes Mellitus, edited by Derek LeRoith, Simeon I. Taylor, and Jerrold M. Olefsky. Lippincott–Raven Publishers, Philadelphia

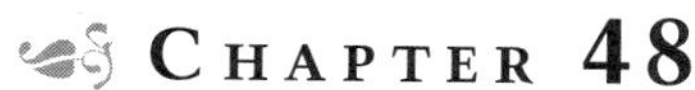

CHAPTER 48

Principles and Fundamentals of Glucose Monitoring

EBTISAM WILKINS, PLAMEN ATANASOV, AND DAVID S. SCHADE

Diabetes mellitus is a complex endocrine metabolic disorder that results from insulin deficiency or resistance, or both. This leads to hyperglycemia and tissue damage.[1] Recent long-term studies have demonstrated that if glucose levels can be tightly regulated, then diabetic complications can be significantly reduced.[2]

The desire to maintain normal glucose levels has led to the development of a series of glucose-sensing devices suitable for measuring glucose in physiologic fluids both in vivo and in vitro. These sensors are based on electrochemical principles and employ enzymes as biologic components for molecular recognition. Recently, several other methods and techniques have been proposed for glucose sensing.[3] For continuous long-term monitoring in vivo, however, the electrochemical biosensor is still the focus of much research.[4]

Several new techniques have evolved for glucose analysis in clinical practice,[5] as well as in biotechnology[6] and the food industry.[7] This wide field of applications has inspired much of the glucose sensor development and diversification during the last decade. The goal of normoglycemia in diabetic patients, however, remains a dominant force behind the research efforts of numerous investigators from different academic disciplines and industry. The studies in this field consist of three parts: (1) selection of the measuring principle and basic sensor development; (2) evaluation of the sensor in vitro and its refinement; (3) in vivo tests of the sensor performance in laboratory animals and, ultimately, in humans.

A variety of methods are currently used to analyze glucose concentration.[3,8] Many of these approaches are motivated by the need for automated, fast, and accurate clinical, hospital, and biomedical research applications. All of these methods may be evaluated according to criteria:

- Fast response—Changes in glucose concentration must be detected within 1–5 minutes, depending on the specific application.

- Accuracy—Glucose level must be measured with minimum errors due to the presence of interfering substances or changes in physiologic parameters (maximum deviation should not exceed 10 mg/dL).
- Sensitivity—The signal-to-noise ratio must be large, and a detectable signal must result from small (0.1 mM or approximately 2 mg/dL) changes in glucose concentration.
- Range—All glucose concentrations in the physiologic and pathophysiologic range (hypoglycemia and hyperglycemia) of 1 to 30 mM (20 to 600 mg/dL) must be measurable.
- Stability—Depending on the specific application, the signal due to glucose must not deviate more than ± 5% of its average value during the operational time of the measuring instrument.

The development of methods and techniques for glucose concentration measurement starts with the use of dedicated laboratory equipment requiring specially trained technicians, and evolves toward simplification and user-friendliness. For example, automated glucose analyzers have been developed for operation by nontechnical personnel. Miniature glucose monitors are popular for self-monitoring by patients.[3]

Glucose Measuring Principles

Based on the interaction between the patient's body and analytic devices, glucose measuring techniques can be classified into two main groups: invasive and noninvasive (Fig. 48-1). Invasive techniques involve intimate physical contact between the sensing part of the device and biologic tissues or fluids. During noninvasive measurement, the information is obtained without invasive intervention, using characteristic properties (spectral, optical, thermal, electromagnetic, etc.) of the analyte (glucose), which can be detected remotely.

Noninvasive Methods

For glucose concentration measurements and monitoring, the Near InfraRed (NIR) spectra of the analyte can be used.[9] The site of measurement is usually a finger or other accessible extremity. Devices based on this principle are fast, extremely convenient, and easy to use by semiskilled technicians. However, they are not particularly accurate, even in the normal physiologic range.[10] The noninvasiveness of the method prevents tissue damage, and the device can be used by many patients in various settings (e.g., office, outpatient clinic, home, etc.). Ultimately, these devices may be developed for self-monitoring (i.e., for use by the diabetic patient at home).

Currently, however, noninvasive devices based on NIR absorption measurements suffer from low sensitivity and, thus, low accuracy of measurement. From an analytic point of view, this method currently is an experimental technique rather than an exact analytic means of measurement. Poor selectivity of such devices has also been reported, probably caused by NIR absorption by other body substances.[11] These devices may also be affected by the personal characteristics of different patients at the measurement site (e.g., skin location, skin and tissue structure, and skin contamination by foreign substances).

Another type of noninvasive technique for glucose monitoring involves the direct analysis for glucose of physiologic fluids obtained from the patient, such as saliva, urine, sweat, or tears.[12] This approach combines the use of well-developed methods for clinical and analytic glucose concentration measurements with the advantages of noninvasiveness. There are several physiologic factors, however, such as diet, exercise, and dehydration, which can affect glucose levels in the aforementioned fluids. In general, there is a poor correlation between glucose concentration in the blood and in these fluids. Moreover, the lag time between blood and urine glucose concentration can be large enough to render such measurements problematic.

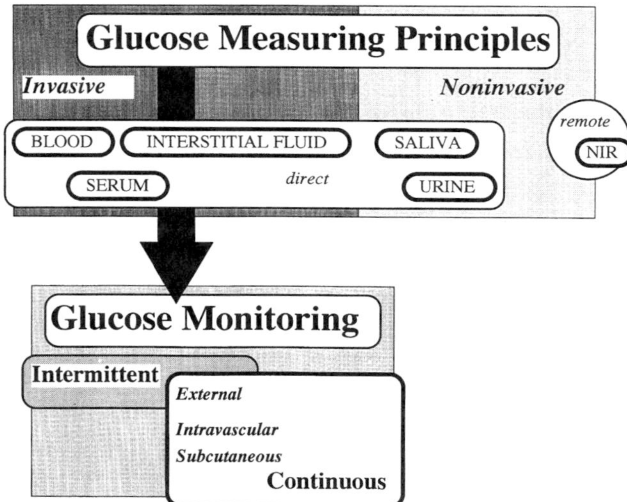

FIGURE 48-1. Glucose measuring and monitoring principles.

Invasive Methods

Currently, the use of invasive measurement methods is widespread, dominating the clinical and home glucose monitoring practice.[13] These techniques are classified according to the method by which samples are obtained and analyzed: that is, either by invasive insertion of a sensor or by puncturing tissues to obtain a sample. Most of the glucose measuring devices in routine use in hospitals, clinics, and at home involve equipment external to the patient's body.[3,13] In all cases, a sample of a physiologic fluid (blood, serum, interstitial fluid, etc.) is obtained by aspiration or by puncture, and glucose analysis is performed by the external measuring instrument.

Analytic techniques and devices for in vitro glucose measurements have a high level of accuracy (error <1%). Many of these routine methods are accepted as the standards by which new devices under development are compared.[8] They are available in a wide range of models and styles, from automated and computerized analytic machines for clinical laboratory use to pocket-sized devices for domestic use by the diabetic patient.[3] Patient management of diabetes mellitus currently relies on these methods to control the disease and, ultimately, to prevent complications.

Use of these in vitro methods for monitoring glucose is associated with two main disadvantages. First, as an invasive method, sampling even a minimal amount of blood on a regular daily basis is associated with the risk of infection, nerve and tissue damage, and/or patient discomfort. Second, in the case of dynamic changes of glucose concentration, very frequent or even continuous measurement of blood glucose is required.

Continuous Glucose Monitoring

Continuous glucose monitoring[3] would be beneficial for the intensive treatment of diabetes, the prevention of complications,[2] the provision of continuous data on glucose level,[13] as well as for glycemia research.[2] This monitoring could be external, as when samples of physiologic fluid are continuously withdrawn from the patient, or internal, as when the sensing device is in intermediate contact with fluid in vivo (see Fig. 48-1).

Since the pioneering reports on direct measurement of glucose concentration,[14,15] the ultimate goal has been the development of a device suitable for continuous monitoring in vivo.[16–18] The research has been inspired by the successful development of the artificial pancreas and the promising initial human trials using implantable insulin delivery systems (insulin pumps).[19,20] The motivation behind this effort was the hypothesis that the maintenance of normoglycemia could prevent complications secondary to diabetes mellitus. This hypothesis has been confirmed after years of clinical trials with patients living as normal a life as possible.[2] Thus, the implantable insulin pump, which uses a glucose sensor as a feedback system, can provide improvement of care and quality of life for millions of patients, as well as significant reductions in the cost of medical care.

Numerous studies have focused on the need for an implantable glucose sensor to close the loop for an insulin pump, simulating an artificial pancreas.[14,19–23] Devices with this function in mind can be classified into three groups, based on the size and site of application:[19]

1. Bedside units that are suitable for hospital or intensive care use
2. Wearable modules that are attached to the patient's body (arm, belt, waist, or leg)
3. Implantable devices

The bedside unit is a large, complex device, that is placed on a cart near the patient. Insulin infusion and blood extraction catheters link the patient to the device. A modified automated laboratory glucose analyzer with adequate speed or a miniature sensor system is used for continuous blood glucose monitoring at the required frequency and flow rates.[24] Combinations of this bedside insulin delivery system with miniature implantable sensors have also been described.[25]

Wearable units are presently used in research for short-term glucose monitoring and in the development of an implantable glucose sensor.[26–28] These employ direct coupling either with a sensor,[17] which is usually subcutaneously implanted,[20–23,26,27] or with a microdialysis sampling device used to supply the sensor with fluid through the skin.[29–31]

Implantable devices will ultimately be used in diabetic patients to maintain normoglycemia through internal insulin infusion, or as alarm devices for continuous monitoring of the patient's glucose level. They will serve as alternatives to the use of insulin injections and glucose self-monitoring strips or portable glucometers.[32–34]

Development of implantable insulin pumps is at a very advanced stage;[35–37] indeed, some units have been implanted for many years in vivo.[38] These implantable pumps, however, lack a continuously functioning implantable glucose sensor with long-term stability. At present, the pumps used in clinical trials deliver insulin following an external command from the physician or from the patient, or based on some programmed cycle that coincides with the patient's diet.[37] Closing the loop by means of a glucose sensor that can continuously monitor glucose level will provide feedback on the exact amount of insulin needed at any moment, and will convert these insulin delivery systems into a complete internal artificial pancreas.

Glucose Sensors

Glucose measuring devices (glucose sensors) can be categorized according to the physical principle underlying the transducer used[39] (Fig. 48-2):

- electrochemical
- piezoelectric
- thermoelectric
- acoustic
- optical

Electrochemical Sensors

In electrochemical sensors, the electrical signal is a direct consequence of some (chemical) process occurring at the transducer/analyte interface. Research is being conducted on several types of potentially implantable glucose sensors, including electrocatalytic sensors based on direct electro-oxidation of glucose on noble metal electrodes[40] and biosensors combining the selectivity of glucose-specific enzymes with the versatility and simplicity of electrochemical electrode systems.[4] Electrocatalytic sensors have specific problems associated with their low analyte selectivity. The general approach in overcoming these problems has been reviewed previously.[41] An approach used to achieve high selectivity is based on the molecular recognition principle, combining biologically active components (enzymes, antibodies, cells, tissues, or microorganisms) with some physical transducer. Biosensors used in or proposed for in vivo experiments are direct enzyme biosensors or affinity sensors based on enzyme-labeled immunoassays.[39,41] In both cases, biologic catalysts (enzymes) are used as a molecular recognition element in glucose sensing. Immunoassays make it possible to sense extremely low amounts of analyte. In diabetes-related studies, however, this is not absolutely necessary, because physiologic and pathophysiologic glucose concentrations are measurable using a less complicated direct enzyme assay.[39]

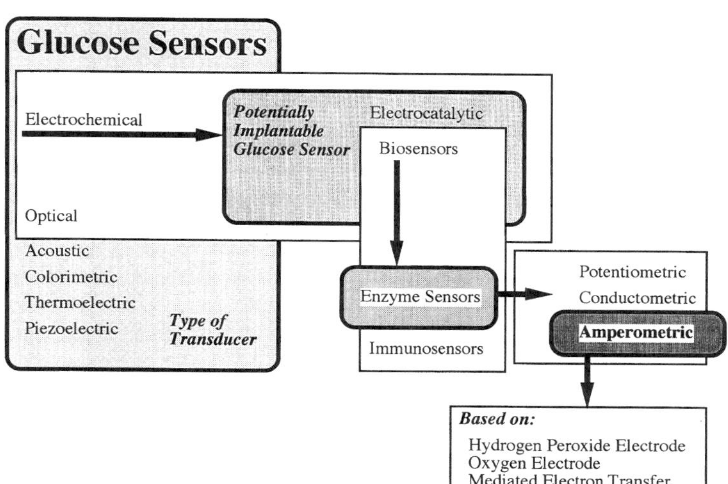

FIGURE 48-2. Types of glucose sensors.

Piezoelectric, Thermoelectric, and Acoustic Sensors

In piezoelectric, thermoelectric, and acoustic (surface acoustic wave, SAW) sensors used for glucose measurement, an enzyme-catalyzed reaction is used to create a measurable change in a physical parameter detected by the transducer. The development of these sensors is at an early laboratory stage.[39]

Optical Sensors

Optical sensors (especially optical biosensors), which are based on the fast-developing optoelectronic technique, may become an alternative means of glucose sensing in the future. These sensors measure changes in some optical parameter owing to enzyme reactions or antibody-antigen bonding at the transducer interface. Based on the main process used, they can be divided into two categories: enzyme optrodes and optical immunosensors.[39] Based on the nature of the monitored process, they are densitometric, refractometric, or colorimetric devices. At present, none of these meets the selectivity requirements to sense and accurately measure glucose in real physiologic fluids. Thus, the field is presently dominated by the electrochemical sensor owing to the relative simplicity of electrochemical measuring principles and the advanced state of development of this biosensor.

Electrochemical Glucose Biosensors

The main method for the construction of electrochemical glucose biosensors involves the use of enzyme electrodes in which the biologic component (enzyme) is incorporated as a part of the transducer design. Glucose biosensors are generally based on the enzyme glucose oxidase (GOD). This enzyme catalyzes the oxidation of β-D-glucose by molecular oxygen, producing gluconolactone and hydrogen peroxide.[42] It is a two-stage enzyme process. The process consists of enzymatic oxidation of glucose by the enzyme in which the cofactor flavin-adenine dinucleotide (FAD) is reduced to $FADH_2$ (reaction 1), followed by oxidation of the enzyme cofactor (regeneration of the biocatalyst) by molecular oxygen with formation of hydrogen peroxide (reaction 2):

$$\beta\text{-D-glucose} + \text{GOD(FAD)} \rightarrow \text{glucono-}\delta\text{-lactone} + \text{GOD(FADH}_2\text{)} \quad (1)$$

$$\text{GOD(FADH}_2\text{)} + O_2 \rightarrow \text{GOD(FAD)} + H_2O_2 \quad (2)$$

$$\text{glucono-}\delta\text{-lactone} + H_2O \rightarrow \text{gluconic acid} \quad (3)$$

The gluconolactone produced in reaction 1 is hydrolyzed (reaction 3) in aqueous media to gluconic acid (reaction 3), so the overall reaction is usually expressed as:

$$\beta\text{-D-glucose} + O_2 + H_2O \rightarrow \text{gluconic acid} + H_2O_2 \quad (4)$$

Electrochemical biosensors are constructed on the amperometric principle based on the oxidation or reduction of electrochemically active substances involved or produced in reactions 1–3.[43] Another possibility is to measure the changes in local pH resulting from the gluconic acid produced in reaction 3 at a potentiometric sensor, usually a coated-wire pH-selective electrode or an ion-selective field effect transistor (ISFET).[44] Changes in the electrical resistance during the overall process (reaction 4) are used as a basis for conductometric biosensors.[45] At present, the potentiometric and conductometric glucose biosensors proposed for in vivo monitoring have very limited applicability owing to numerous interfering processes caused by components of the physiologic environment (other than glucose).

Several potentiometric glucose sensors (coated-wire sensors) have been proposed for implantable use.[41] Coated-wire sensors are easy to fabricate and are suitable for miniaturization to diameters of 50 to 200 μm. They can be used in combination with a standard electrocardiographic (ECG) reference electrode.[29] The main disadvantage of these sensors is their low sensitivity. The signal of a potentiometric glucose sensor is based on the Nernst equation, which gives a logarithmic dependence of the potential change (signal) on analyte concentration.[39] This can be very useful when the amplitude of analyte concentration change is of several orders of magnitude (as in the case of pH measurements). In physiologic fluids, however, glucose concentration changes by no more than two orders of magnitude, so a sensor with a linear signal versus concentration proportionality is preferable to a logarithmic response.

The introduction of microelectronic techniques in sensor development through the use of ISFET as a basis for the sensor design is promising in the sense of miniaturization and integration of the transducer with some part of the associated electronic circuitry into a single chip.[44] Corrosion of the semiconductor material surface in saline (and in physiologic) solutions is presently a problem in using these devices for in vivo trials. This problem may be overcome through surface modification by passivation or by coating.[44] Being potentiometric measuring devices, biosensors based on enzyme FETs have the same general disadvantages as the coated-wire sensors.

It appears from the development of biosensors that the amperometric techniques are most useful. The preference for this concept for implantable applications is primarily attributable to the possibility of obtaining a signal that is linearly related to analyte concentration. The linearity of the sensor response is of great importance in the repeated recalibration over time of implantable glucose sensors.[24] Microprocessor evaluation of the nonlinear glucose calibration curve allows recalibration of the sensor in vivo if the nonlinear function is known.

If the limiting process in signal generation is enzymatic reactions (reactions 1 and 2), the dependence of the signal versus glucose concentration is nonlinear according to Michaelis-Menten kinetics. When the sensor operates in a diffusion-limited mode, linear proportionality between the signal and analyte concentration occurs.

The amperometric glucose biosensors are usually categorized into three different classes (sometimes called "generations") based on the mechanism of the electrochemical (charge transfer) reaction involved.[43] In the first class are biosensors involving glucose oxidation by GOD (reactions 1–3) in natural conditions.[46] In this case, the increase in hydrogen peroxide concentration or the decrease in oxygen concentration due to the reaction (reaction 4) is detected electrochemically, both being proportional to the glucose concentration. In the second class of amperometric glucose biosensors, low-molecular-weight compounds are used as mediators in the process of enzyme oxidation (reaction 2) and signal generation at the electrode surface.[25] The third class of amperometric biosensors is based on direct electron transfer between the enzyme and an electrode with special properties.[47]

Oxygen Electrode–based Glucose Biosensors

The oxygen-detecting electrode as a basic transducer for glucose monitoring was the first electrochemical method developed.[14,15] In this case, the amperometric signal is a result of the electrochemical reduction of oxygen on a cathodically polarized platinum electrode:

$$O_2 + 2H^+ + 2e^- \xrightarrow{Pt} H_2O_2 \quad (5)$$

$$H_2O_2 + 2H^+ + 2e^- \xrightarrow{Pt} 2H_2O \quad (6)$$

A linear dependence of the amperometric signal resulting from reactions 5 and 6 is obtained when the mass transfer of oxygen is the limiting process. Thus, the polarization of the platinum cathode is usually sufficient (usually from −0.6 to −0.9 V versus a reference electrode, Ag/AgCl). The enzyme-catalyzed reaction (reaction 4) is limited by glucose diffusion as well. This is achieved by use of a variety of glucose diffusion semipermeable membranes separating the enzyme layer from the testing solution.[15,28,48–50]

In oxygen electrode–based glucose biosensors, the signal output is the difference between the base oxygen level and the level attained as a result of oxygen depletion by the enzymatic reaction. In practice, a combination of identical oxygen detectors, with and without an active enzyme layer, is used so the signal output is the difference between the glucose-dependent current and the oxygen-dependent background current.[15] The oxygen electrode–based sensors have the advantage of requiring a cathodic potential with which only a few endogenous chemical species can interfere.[51–53] Also, the gas-permeable hydrophobic layer over the electrode prevents diffusion of electrochemical interferents to the electrode surface.[54] Despite these advantages, the oxygen electrode signal depends on the ambient oxygen concentration, which has to be monitored. This results in increased complexity in the construction of the sensors, as they require two electrodes, making miniaturization a difficult task.[51–53]

Hydrogen Peroxide Electrode–based Biosensors

For hydrogen peroxide electrode–based sensors, the signal is produced by the oxidation of hydrogen peroxide at a catalytic (usually platinum) anode at potentials from +0.6 to +0.8 V versus Ag/AgCl.[46]

$$H_2O_2 \xrightarrow{Pt} O_2 + H_2O + 2e^- \quad (7)$$

The most important advantages of the hydrogen peroxide electrode–based sensor are its ease of fabrication and the possibility of miniaturization. A linear dependence of the amperometric signal is obtained when the mass transfer of both electrochemically active species (hydrogen peroxide) and glucose are the limiting processes. This is achieved by use of a variety of diffusion membranes in the construction of the biosensor. Its main disadvantage is that it is characterized by poor electrochemical selectivity owing to electro-oxidation of species other than glucose present in physiologic fluids.[24,55,56] This problem can be overcome, to a large extent, by the use of semipermeable membranes with specific transport properties.[20,56,57] Dependence of the sensor signal on oxygen concentration resulting from the reaction (reaction 2) is another source of difficulty. The use of membranes or coatings with hydrophobic properties allows restriction of glucose flux, thus allowing an oxygen flux that exceeds that of glucose, thereby avoiding dependence of the signal on oxygen.

Amperometric Biosensors with Mediated Electron Transfer

In the second class of glucose sensors, oxygen as an electron acceptor (reaction 2) is substituted by an artificial mediator.[25] Ferrocene [dicyclopentadienyl iron, $Fe^{2+}(Cp)_2$] and its derivatives are the most commonly used mediators. In these sensors, instead of reaction 2, a process involving the mediator takes place:

$$GOD(FADH_2) + Fe^{3+}(Cp)_2 \rightarrow GOD(FAD) + Fe^{2+}(Cp)_2 \quad (8)$$

The oxidation of the ferrocene (signal-generating reaction) can be performed at potentials much lower (usually +0.15 to +0.25 V) than that of hydrogen peroxide (reaction 6), and it does not require catalytic or noble metal electrodes:

$$Fe^{2+}(Cp)_2 \xrightarrow{anode} Fe^{3+}(Cp)_2 \quad (9)$$

At such low potentials, the interference effect from other oxidizable compounds is minimal. As oxygen is not involved in the signal generation process, the sensor signal becomes independent of oxygen concentration.[58–60] Based on the independence of the signal on oxygen concentration and the diminished interference effect, the true glucose concentration in the subcutaneous tissue can be measured.[59,60]

The main problem associated with in vivo use of such sensors is mediator leakage and its toxicity. Immobilization of the mediator by adsorption on the electrode or entrapment in an inert polymer[58] or albumin matrix[59] are the solutions proposed for in vivo use. The possibility of lethal or serious side effects from the leaking mediator or damaged sensors limits the use of this system in in vivo experiments.

Amperometric Biosensors with Direct Electron Transfer

It has been shown that oxidation of glucose by the enzyme GOD at an electrode constructed of conducting organic salts (charge-transfer organic complexes with electron conductivity) does not depend on oxygen concentration.[47,61] The mechanisms of action of such biosensors are not yet clear. Direct electro-oxidation of $GOD(FADH_2)$ on the electrode surface instead of oxidation by molecular oxygen (reaction 2) is one of the proposed hypotheses:[61]

$$GOD(FADH_2) \xrightarrow{\text{organic salt}} GOD(FAD) + 2H^+ + 2e^- \quad (10)$$

In this reaction (10), direct electron transfer between the enzyme and the electrode is assumed. Biosensors based on this principle, the third class of biosensors, have low operating potential (usually +0.2 to +0.4 V) and have all the advantages of the mediated sensors. They are a typical example of a solid-state biosensor. There is no soluble or partially soluble compound involved in their construction. Sensors based on this principle have been tested successfully in monitoring brain glucose levels in rats.[62] However, intensive application of such biosensors in vivo is limited by the lack of knowledge of the biocompatibility of the new electrode materials involved.

Design Approaches

Implantable glucose sensors for feedback control of the insulin pumps are of two types: sensors for long-term implantation[16,48,63,64] and needle glucose biosensors.[20,57,65] The first type can be relatively large (being an integrated part of the pump itself) and thus is suitable for chronic implantation for as long as the life span of the pump. The miniature needle-sized type of sensor is suitable for subcutaneous monitoring of glucose at a site different from the site of the insulin pump, or in combination with a wearable artificial pancreas. The latter concept allows consecutive use of several sensors within the lifetime of the insulin pump. The problems associated with standardization of the sensors and their in vivo calibration are of critical importance.[65–68]

Development of the microdialysis technique and commercialization of microsampling devices have allowed a third approach to in vivo monitoring of glucose by coupling the biosensor with a wearable microdialysis device in an extracorporeal circulation loop.[29–31,69] The general advantage of such a method lies in the separation of the sampling and measuring processes.

Needle-Type Glucose Biosensor

Short-term studies have demonstrated the feasibility of an implanted glucose sensor–controlled insulin infusion system in achieving normoglycemia. Unfortunately, these studies have also demonstrated the major limitation of this type of sensor: the rapid deterioration of GOD. Despite much recent research effort, a long-term implantable glucose sensor is not yet a reality.

The general size of the needle-type glucose sensors is in the range of 16- to 28-gauge needles.[20,57,65] A sensor usually consists of three layers: (1) an inner selectively permeable membrane (which may or may not be present), (2) an enzyme layer containing GOD, and (3) an outer semipermeable membrane.[55,66] The sensor generally consists of a platinum working electrode (polarized as the anode) and a silver,[20] stainless steel,[66] Ag/AgCl, or platinum[55,68] counter-electrode.

Shichiri et al.[20] were the first to report success in miniaturizing a glucose sensor, introducing a needle enzyme electrode with an outer diameter of 1 mm. The sensor consisted of a platinum working electrode, a silver reference electrode, and an outer polyurethane membrane. The sensor had a short response time of 16 seconds and a linear concentration range of 27 mM of glucose. The sensor was implanted in dogs and had a lifetime of 4 days.[20] The sensor was later implanted subcutaneously in humans, and the sensor output showed a high correlation with blood glucose level.[66] Shichiri et al. also developed a telemetry system for integration with their glucose sensor for monitoring and control of an insulin delivery system.[27]

Vadgama et al.[65] presented a similar glucose sensor with an outer polyurethane membrane that extended the linear range of glucose concentration to 70 mM. The sensor also had a fast response time (60 seconds). These authors also evaluated the effect of varying the concentration of polyurethane in the outer membrane on the linearity of the sensor response.[65] Pfeiffer et al.[19] constructed a glucose sensor using standard stainless steel needles as a cathode and a sensor body. The sensor had a response time of 100 seconds and a lifetime of 6 days. The sensor was implanted subcutaneously in sheep. It was found that the delay in response between the sensor signal and the intravenous glucose level did not exceed 5 minutes.[70]

Moatti-Sirat et al.[71] recently proposed a new configuration in which the sensing element is located at the sides of the sensor body in the form of a cavity. The size is equivalent to that of a 26-gauge needle (outer diameter of 0.4 mm). The sensor has an Ag/AgCl reference electrode and a linear range of 15 mM of glucose. These researchers used an inner cellulose acetate membrane, which reduced the effect of interferents. This sensor was implanted in the subcutaneous tissue of rats and had a lifetime of 10 days.[55,71,72] This same group has also reported on the use of the same construction, but with lactate oxidase enzyme for lactate monitoring.[73]

Chen et al.[68] developed a needle glucose sensor that employs an inner Nafion membrane and an outer cellulose acetate membrane. This sensor has been reported to show diminished response to interferents, a response time of less than 30 seconds, and a lifetime of 25 days. Harrison et al.[56,57] also have used Nafion for the outer membrane in the development of their needle glucose sensor. A cross-sectional view of this miniature sensor, which is suitable for intravascular glucose monitoring and subcutaneous implantation, is shown in Figure 48-3.[56] They electrically deposited an inner poly(o-phenylenediamine) membrane on the working electrode.[57] They reported that this combination of inner and outer membranes produced high selectivity and diminished interference effects. The sensor was implanted subcutaneously in dogs and had a lifetime of 14 days.

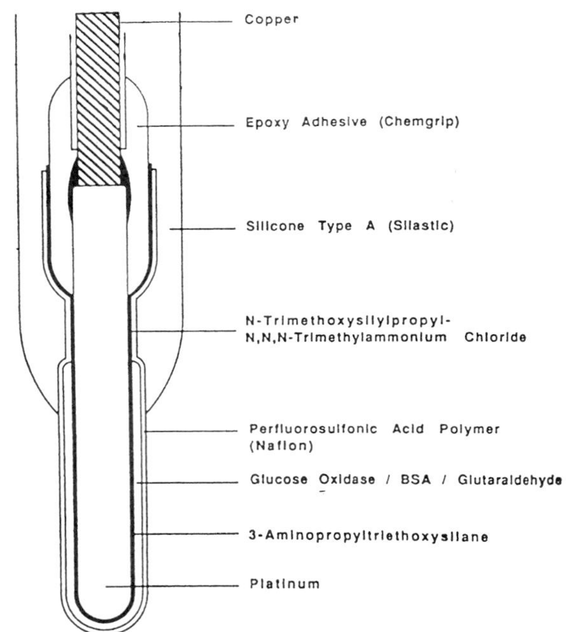

Figure 48-3. Cross-sectional view of an implantable enzyme electrode for glucose analysis in whole blood. (Reproduced with permission from Turner RFB, Harrison DJ, Rajotte RV, Baltes HP. A biocompatible for continuous in vivo glucose monitoring in whole blood. Sensors Actuators 1990;1:561.)

Difficulties associated with in vivo glucose monitoring in a site close to the pump implantation site (abdominal cavity) or in subcutaneous tissue can be avoided by extracting a subcutaneous dialysate and passing it through a small cell with the sensor in it. In this case, however, the microdialysis system and the sensor should be in a wearable unit. The experimental advantages of this technique are more controllable conditions and the ability to analyze the same sample with different methods.[30] There is a problem with biocompatibility of such techniques, however, as well as the possibility of infection during long-term microdialysis.

Some of the leading groups in implantable glucose biosensor development have turned to this concept of glucose monitoring.[69] There is much debate on the superiority of the microdialysis approach in comparison to in vivo monitoring with needle sensors.[74] Predicting the glycemia profile over time by using a combination of needle sensors and microdialysis sampling is reported to be very accurate (Fig. 48-4).[69] One advantage of the microdialysis technique is the ease of replacing the sensor in case of failure. The primary disadvantage of this approach is its use of additional equipment. Employing this technique with additional sophisticated equipment makes it impossible to integrate the measuring device (the sensor) and the acting device (the insulin pump) in one unit. The ultimate goal is to integrate the electromechanical analogue of the pancreas into one device.

Glucose Biosensors for Chronic Implantation

Chronically implantable glucose biosensors are usually designed as an integrated part of the implantable insulin delivery system (artificial pancreas).[19] Another application of such sensors is in an autonomously powered device (often using a radio transmitter), the prototype of a diabetic alarm system.[17,18] Figure 48-5 shows a schematic drawing of a sensor/transmitter system that was implanted and operated in a dog model for 3 months.[18] Devices based on oxygen and on hydrogen peroxide measuring principles have been described. For in vivo evaluation of such sensors, the usual choice is large animals, such as dogs or sheep. The most preferable site of implantation is usually the abdominal cavity, and the glucose level is measured in the intraperitoneal fluid.[81]

Calibration of the implantable sensor is achieved using two glucose levels (two-point calibration), which is satisfactory in the case of linear dependence of the sensor response.[82,83] In the development of the integrated implantable sensor, the critical issue is that of long-term operational stability of the sensor. Because the glucose biosensor will be a part of the implantable insulin delivery system, its lifetime must be at least as long as that of the other parts of the system. The lifetime of the biosensor is limited mainly by the

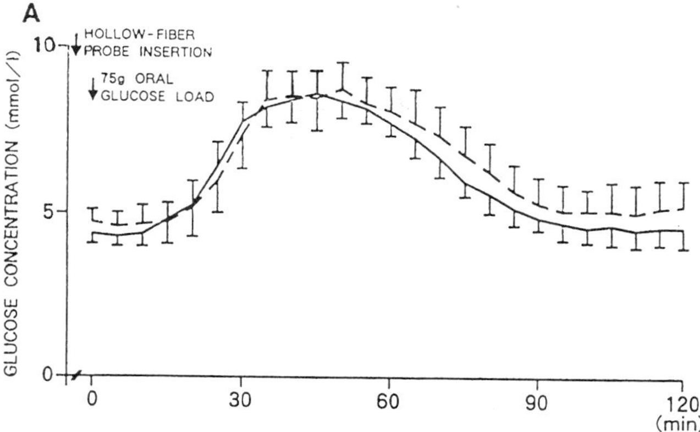

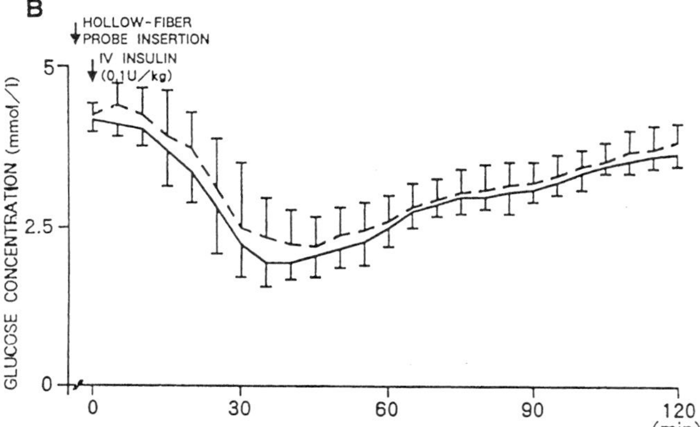

FIGURE 48-4. Continuous monitoring of subcutaneous tissue glucose concentrations measured by the extracorporeal glucose monitoring system with microdialysis sampling methods after a 75-g oral glucose load (*A*) and after intravenous insulin injection (0.1 U/kg) (*B*) in five healthy subjects. Subcutaneous tissue glucose concentrations (---) were compared with blood glucose concentration (——) measured by the glucose monitoring system (STG, Nikkiso). Results are analyzed at 5-minute intervals of the continuous monitoring records and expressed as means ± SE. (Reproduced with permission from Hashiguchi Y, Sakaida M, Nishida K, et al. Development of a miniaturized glucose monitoring system by combining a needle-type glucose sensor with microdialysis sampling method. Diabetes Care 1994;5:387.)

processes of enzyme deactivation.[75] The immobilization of the enzyme in gels, on membranes, or on inert dispersed carriers (usually carbon materials) can significantly increase its stability.[39] However, the lifetime of the biosensors with immobilized enzymes is still limited. An increase in the sensor lifetime has been achieved by using an optimized immobilized enzyme and protective layers.[75–78] Successful chronic implantation of such sensors in dogs for a period of 3 months has recently been reported.[17,18]

Rechargeable Glucose Biosensors

An alternative approach, developed at the University of New Mexico, makes it possible to extend sensor lifetime by in situ sensor refilling—replacing spent immobilized enzyme with fresh enzyme.[64] GOD is immobilized on dispersed carbon powder, which is then held in a liquid suspension. The construction of the biosensor is such that the spent immobilized enzyme can be removed from the sensor body and fresh enzyme suspension injected via a septum,

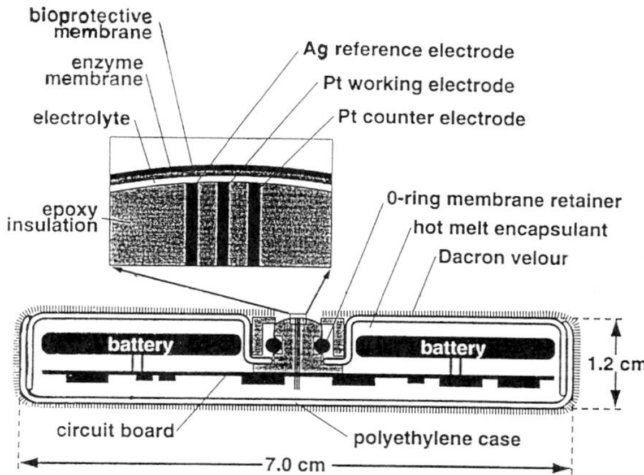

FIGURE 48-5. Section of sensor/transmitter with detail of membranes and sensor construction. (Reproduced with permission from Gilligan BJ, Scults MC, Rhodes RK, Updike SJ. Evaluation of a subcutaneous glucose sensor out to 3 months in a dog model. Diabetes Care 1994;17:882.)

without sensor disassembly. This concept facilitates recharging of the implanted sensor without surgical removal from the animal or patient.

Rechargeable sensors based on both hydrogen peroxide[79] and oxygen measuring principles[50] have been reported. Figure 48-6 shows a cross-sectional schematic view of the rechargeable glucose biosensors based on hydrogen peroxide (Fig. 48-6*A*) and oxygen measuring principles (Fig. 48-6*B*).

The glucose biosensor consists of two parts: an amperometric electrode system and an enzyme microbioreactor. A three-electrode amperometric scheme is used in both types of the biosensors: (1) a platinum working electrode, (2) an Ag/AgCl reference electrode,

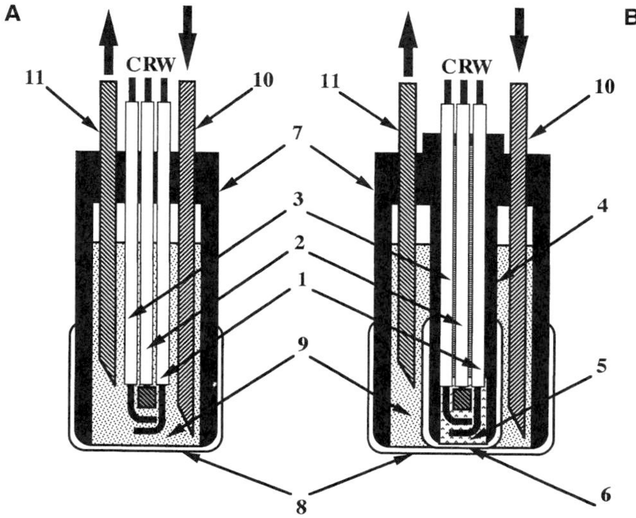

FIGURE 48-6. Schematic diagram of rechargeable glucose biosensors based on hydrogen peroxide (*A*) and oxygen-selective electrodes (*B*). The biosensor parts include the following: Pt working electrode (*1*); Ag/AgCl reference electrode (*2*); Pt auxiliary electrode (*3*); oxygen-selective electrode housing (*4*); gel electrolyte in the oxygen-selective electrode (*5*); oxygen permeable membrane (*6*); biosensor housing (*7*); glucose diffusion membrane (*8*); microbioreactor with enzyme suspension (*9*); inlet recharge tube (*10*), and exhaust discharge tube (*11*).

and (3) a counterelectrode. The working electrode is polarized +0.6 V for hydrogen peroxide oxidation, or −0.6 V for oxygen reduction versus the reference electrode.

In the oxygen measurement–based sensor (Fig. 48-6*B*), these three electrodes are symmetrically assembled and housed in a separate glass tube (4) and cemented by epoxy resin. At the face-end of the housing, a cavity is formed and filled with gelled electrolyte (5). An oxygen-permeable hydrophobic membrane (6) separates the three-electrode system and the enzyme microbioreactor.

In the hydrogen peroxide–based biosensor (Fig. 48-6*A*), the three-electrode amperometric system is directly inserted in the sensor housing (7), with the face-side closed by a glucose diffusion membrane (8). This enzyme-modified dispersed carbon is used to form a liquid suspension for refilling of the enzyme microbioreactor (9), or recharging of the sensor.[64] Two capillary plastic tubes—the inlet recharge tube (10) and the exhaust discharge tube (11)—are used for replacing spent enzyme from the microbioreactor without sensor disassembly.[50] This biosensor was integrated with a miniature potentiostat with a signal transmitter into a small, independently functioning device suitable for canine or other large animal implantation.[80] By combining two enzymes (in oxygen electrode–based biosensors)—GOD and catalase—the recharge cycle (time between biosensor refillings) can be extended up to 1 month as a result of the elimination of hydrogen peroxide as an enzyme deactivator. This glucose biosensor has been implanted and tested in vivo in a sheep.[80]

The capability of refilling an implanted glucose sensor by external means without its surgical removal represents a major advance in the development of a practical glucose sensor for diabetes control. Our use of enzyme, in the form of a liquid suspension of carbon powder with immobilized GOD on the powder, allows enzyme replacement (without surgery) by injection via a subcutaneous septum using a procedure similar to that developed for refilling of implantable insulin pumps.[35–37] This approach offers the possibility of constructing sensors that are suitable for implantation in the body and that have lifetimes greater than several months.

Conclusion

The development of glucose monitoring techniques and approaches during the last decade demonstrates the predomination of electrochemical measuring principles. Biosensors are still the main focus of research of most teams owing to their high selectivity for glucose determination. Different design approaches have been proposed and are currently under development in an attempt to overcome the problems associated with sensor reproducibility and limited lifespan. The approach that utilizes small replaceable (disposable) sensors, usually designed as a needle-type electrode, is most popular. The coupling of such a sensor with an insulin pump, usually wearable on the patient's body (arm), is a disadvantage because of the necessity of frequent subcutaneous needle insertions when the sensor is replaced.

The needle-sized glucose sensor appears to be most advantageous when used in combination with the microdialysis technique for subcutaneous liquid sampling. In this case, the problems of in situ biocompatibility of the sensor interface to the living tissue is avoided. Sensor replacement and other sensor manipulations are not associated with invasive interventions. This design, however, only allows the development of a wearable artificial pancreas.

The development of a chronically implantable glucose sensor is necessary to achieve an implantable insulin delivery system with internal feedback control. Enzyme immobilization techniques have allowed the construction of sensors with an in vivo lifetime of up to 3 months, which is much less than the lifetime of an implantable insulin pump. The approach involving replacement of the spent enzyme and recharging of the implanted sensor in situ is a promising new approach that may increase the life span of the system. The most promising nonelectrochemical approach for glucose monitoring is the remote transcutaneous NIR measurement. Although in an early stage of development, this method could provide a noninvasive method for glucose sensing.

Acknowledgments

The research on rechargeable glucose biosensors at the University of New Mexico is currently supported by a grant from the National Science Foundation and the Whitaker Foundation (Grant No. BCS - 9315118).

References

1. Symposium on Implantable Glucose Biosensors. Diabetes Care 1982;3:1–216
2. DCCT Research Group. Diabetes Control and Complications Trial (DCCT) update. Diabetes Care 1990;13:427
3. Page SR, Peacock I. Blood glucose monitoring: Does technology help? Diabetic Med 1993;10:793
4. Fischer U. Fundamentals of glucose sensors. Diabetic Med 1991;8:309
5. Pickup LC. Biosensors: A clinical perspective. Lancet 1985;2:817
6. Clarke DJ. Biosensors in process control. Phyl Trans R Soc London B Biol Sci 1987;B316:169
7. Karube I, Tamiya E. Biosensors in food industry. Food Biotechnol 1987;1:147
8. Pickup JC, Crook MA, Tutt P. Blood glucose and glycated haemoglobin measurement in hospital: Which method? Diabetic Med 1993;10:402
9. Kaiser N. Laser absorption spectroscopy with an ATR prism—Noninvasive *in vitro* determination of glucose. Horm Metab Res [suppl] 1979;8:30
10. Robinson MR, Eaton RP, Haaland DM, et al. Noninvasive glucose monitoring in diabetic patients: A preliminary evaluation. Clin Chem 1992;38:1618
11. Guilbault G. Noninvasive in vivo glucose measurements. Artif Organs 1988; 13:172
12. Karube I. Proceedings of the Third World Congress on Biosensors. New Orleans, LA, June 1–3, 1994
13. Vadgama P. Biosensors in clinical biochemistry. Ann Clin Biochem 1993; 30:337
14. Clark LC, Lyons C. Electrode system for continuous monitoring in cardiovascular surgery. Ann NY Acad Sci 1962;102:29
15. Updike SJ, Hicks GP. The enzyme electrode. Nature 1967;214:986
16. Clark LC, Noyes LK, Okane RBS, et al. Long-term implantation of voltammetric oxidase/peroxidase glucose sensors in rat peritoneum. Methods Enzymol 1988;137:68
17. Updike SJ, Scults MC, Rhodes RK, et al. Enzymatic blood glucose sensor: Improved long-term performance *in vitro* and *in vivo*. J Am Soc Artif Intern Organs 1994;40:157
18. Gilligan BJ, Scults MC, Rhodes RK, Updike SJ. Evaluation of a subcutaneous glucose sensor out to 3 months in a dog model. Diabetes Care 1994;17:882
19. Pfeiffer EF. On the way to automated (blood) glucose regulation in diabetes: The dark past, the grey present and the rosy future. Diabetologia 1987;30:51
20. Shichiri M, Kawamori R, Hakui N, et al. Closed loop glycemic control with a wearable artificial endocrine pancreas. Diabetes 1984;33:1200
21. Ito K, Ikeda S, Asai K, et al. Development of subcutaneous-type glucose sensor for implantable portable artificial pancreas. In: Schuetzle D, Hamerle R, Butles JW, eds. Fundamentals and Applications of Chemical Sensors. Washington, DC: Am Chem Soc;1986:271
22. Velho G, Reach G, Thevenot DR. The design and development of *in vivo* glucose sensor for an artificial endocrine pancreas. In: Turner APF, Karube I, Wilson GS, eds. Biosensors: Fundamentals and Applications. Oxford: Oxford University Press;1987:390
23. Abel P, Muller A, Fisher U. Experience with an implantable glucose sensor as a prerequisite of an artificial beta cell. Biomed Biochem Acta 1984;43:577
24. Reach G, Wilson GS. Can continuous glucose monitoring be used for the treatment of diabetes? Anal Chem 1992;64:381A
25. Cass AEG, Davis G, Francis GD, et al. Ferrocene mediated enzyme electrode for amperometric determination of glucose. Anal Chem 1984;56:667
26. Bruckel J, Zeir H, Kerner W, Pfeiffer EF. The Glucose Unitec Ulm—A portable monitor for continuous blood glucose measurement. Horm Metab Res 1990;22:382
27. Shichiri M, Asasawa N, Yamasaki Y, et al. Telemetry glucose monitoring device with needle glucose sensor: A useful tool for blood glucose monitoring in diabetic individuals. Diabetes Care 1986;9:298
28. Schmidt FJ, Aalders AL, Schoonen AJM, Doornebos H. Calibration of a wearable glucose sensor. Int J Artif Organs 1992;15:55
29. Meyerhoff C, Bischof F, Sternberg F, et al. On-line continuous monitoring of subcutaneous tissue glucose in men by combining portable glucosensor with microdialysis. Diabetologia 1992;35:1087
30. Moscone D, Mascini M. Microdialysis and glucose biosensor for *in vivo* monitoring. Ann Biol Clin 1992;50:223
31. Palmisano F, Centonze D, Gurrrieri A, Zombonin PG. An interference-free biosensor based on glucose oxidase electrochemically immobilized in a non-

conducting poly(pyrrole) film for continuous subcutaneous monitoring of glucose through microdialysis sampling. Biosensors Bioelectronics 1993; 8:393
32. Rebrin K, Fischer U, von Dorsche HH, et al. Subcutaneous glucose monitoring by means of electrochemical sensors: Fiction or reality? J Biomed Engin 1992;14:33
33. Reach G. Artificial or bioartificial systems for the totally automatic treatment of diabetes mellitus: The gap between the dream and the reality. Diabetes Nutr Metab 1989;2:165
34. Pickup JC. Glucose sensors and closed-loop insulin delivery. In: Pickup JC, ed. Biotechnology of Insulin Therapy. Oxford: Blackwell;1991:126
35. Waxman K, Turner D, Nguen T. Implantable Programable insulin pumps for the treatment of diabetes. Arch Surg 1992;127:1032
36. Buchwald H, Thomas TD. Implantable pumps: Recent progress and anticipated future advances. Trans Am Soc Artif Intern Organs 1992;38:772
37. Zoltobrocki M. Insulin delivery by implantable pumps. Horm Metab Res [suppl] 1992;26:140
38. Scavini M, Day PW, Eaton RP. Long-term implantation of a new programmable implantable insulin pump in two diabetic dogs. Artif Organs 1992;16(5): 518
39. Hall E. Biosensors. Oxford: Oxford University Press;1990
40. Lerner H, Giner J, Soeldner JS, Colton CK. Development of an implantable glucose sensor. Artif Organs 1981;5:743
41. Wilkins E. Towards implantable glucose sensors: A review. J Biomed Eng 1989;11:353
42. Weibel MK, Bright HJ. The glucose oxidase mechanism. J Biol Chem 1971;246:2743
43. Turner APF, Karube I, Wilson GS. Biosensors: Fundamentals and Applications. Oxford: Oxford University Press;1987
44. Lammbrechts M, Sansen W. Biosensors: Microelectrochemical Devices. Bristol: Institute of Physics Publishing;1992
45. Kell DB, Davey CL. Conductimetric and impedimetric devices. In: Cass AEG, ed. Biosensors: A Practical Approach. Oxford: Oxford University Press; 1990:125
46. Guilbault GG, Lubrano GJ. An enzyme electrode for amperometric determination of glucose and lactate. Anal Chim Acta 1973;64:439
47. Cenas NK, Kulys JJ. Biocatalytic oxidation of glucose on the conductive charge transfer complex. Bioelectrochem Bioenerget 1981;8:103
48. Gough DA, Leypoldt J, Armor JC. Progress towards a potentially implantable enzyme-based glucose sensor. Diabetes Care 1982;5:190
49. Koudelka M. Performance characteristics of a planar Clark-type oxygen sensor. Sensors Actuators 1986;9:249
50. Xie SL, Wilkins E, Atanasov P. Towards an implantable refillable glucose sensor based on oxygen electrode principles. Sensors Actuators B 1993;17:133
51. Atanasov P, Wilkins E. Development of a biosensor for glucose monitoring. Biotechnol Bioengin 1994;43:262
52. Urban G, Jobst G, Aschayer E, et al. Performance of integrated glucose and lactate thin-film microbiosensors for clinical analyzers. Sensors Actuators B 1994;18–19:592
53. Schalkhammer T, Lobmaier C, Ecker B, et al. Microfabricated glucose, lactate, glutamate and glutamine thin-film biosensors. Sensors Actuators B 1994; 18–19:587
54. Leypoldt J, Gough DA. Model of a two-substrate enzyme electrode for glucose. Anal Chem 1984;56:2896
55. Moatti-Sirat D, Velho G, Reach G. Evaluating *in vitro* and *in vivo* the interference of ascorbate and acetaminophen on glucose detection by a needle-type glucose sensor. Biosensors Bioelectronics 1992;7:345
56. Turner RFB, Harrison DJ, Rajotte RV, Baltes HP. A biocompatible glucose sensor for continuous *in vivo* glucose monitoring in whole blood. Sensors Actuators B 1990;1:561
57. Moussy F, Harrison DJ, O'Brien DW, Rajotte RV. Performance of subcutaneously implanted needle-type glucose sensor employing a novel trilayer coating. Anal Chem 1993;65:2072
58. Pickup JC, Show GW, Claremont JD. *In vivo* molecular sensing in diabetes mellitus: An implantable glucose sensor with direct electron transfer. Diabetologia 1989;32:213
59. Sakakida M, Ichinose K, Fukushima H, et al. Development of a ferrocene-mediated needle-type glucose sensor as a measure of true subcutaneous tissue glucose concentrations. Artif Organs Today 1992;2:145
60. Matthews DR, Bown E, Beck TW, et al. An amperometric needle-type glucose sensor tested in rats and man. Diabetic Med 1988;5:248
61. Albery WJ, Bartlett PN, Cracton D. Amperometric enzyme electrodes. Part 2: Conducting organic salt as electrode materials for the oxidation of glucose oxidase. J Electroanal Chem 1985;194:223
62. Boutelle MG, Stanford C, Fillenz M, et al. An amperometric enzyme electrode for continuous monitoring of brain glucose in freely moving rat. Neurosci Lett 1987;72:283
63. Johnson KW, Mastrotataro JJ, Howey BRL, et al. *In vivo* evaluation of an electroenzymatic glucose sensor implanted in subcutaneous tissue. Biosensors Bioelectronics 1992;7:709
64. Xie SL, Wilkins E. Performances of potentially implantable rechargeable glucose sensor *in vitro* at body temperature. Biomed Instrum Technol 1991;25:393
65. Vadgama P, Spoors J, Tang LX, Battersby C. The needle glucose electrode: *In vitro* performance and optimization for implantation. Biomed Biochem Acta 1989;48:935
66. Shichiri M, Kawamori R, Yamasaki Y. Needle-type Glucose Sensor. Methods Enzymol 1988;137:326
67. Ikeda S, Ito K, Ohkura K, et al. Artificial pancreas: Development of a new needle-type glucose sensor based on oxygen electrode with a new concept. Artif Organs Today 1991;1:303
68. Chen CY, Tamia E, Ishihara K, et al. A biocompatible needle-type glucose sensor based on platinum electroplated carbon electrode. Appl Biochem Biotech 1992;36:211
69. Hashiguchi Y, Sakaida M, Nishida K, et al. Development of a miniaturized glucose monitoring system by combining a needle-type glucose sensor with microdialysis sampling method. Diabetes Care 1994;5:387
70. Bruckel J, Kerner W, Zeir H, et al. *In vivo* measurement of subcutaneous glucose concentrations with an enzymatic glucose sensor and Wick method. Klin Wochenschr 1989;67:491
71. Moatti-Sirat D, Copron F, Poitout V, et al. Towards continuous glucose monitoring: *In vivo* evaluation of a miniaturized glucose sensor implanted for several days in rat subcutaneous tissue. Diabetologia 1992;35:224
72. Poitout V, Moatti-Sirat D, Reach G, et al. A glucose monitoring system for on-line estimation in man of blood glucose concentration using a miniaturized glucose sensor implanted in the subcutaneous tissue and a wearable control unit. Diabetologia 1993;36:658
73. Hu Y, Zhang Y, Wilson GS. A needle-type enzyme-based lactate sensor for *in vivo* monitoring. Anal Chim Acta 1993;281:503
74. Sternberg F, Meyerhoff C, Mennel FJ, et al. Comments on subcutaneous glucose monitoring. Diabetologia 1994;37:540
75. Gough DA. Issues related to *in vitro* operation of potentially implantable enzyme electrode glucose sensors. Horm Metab Res [suppl] 1988;20:30
76. Armor JC, Lucisano JY, McKean BD, Gough DA. Application of chronic intravascular blood glucose sensor in dogs. Diabetes 1990;39:1519
77. Bobbioni-Harsch E, Rohner-Jeanrenaud F, Koudelka M, et al. Lifespan of subcutaneous glucose sensors and the performances during glycemia changes in rats. J Biomed Engin 1993;15:547
78. Rebrin K, Fischer U, Woedtke TV, et al. Automated feed-back control of subcutaneous glucose concentration in diabetic dogs. Diabetologia 1989;32: 573
79. Wilkins E. A rechargeable glucose sensor—Long-term activity and performance. Biomed Instrum Technol 1993;27:325
80. Wilkins E, Atanasov P, Muggenburg BA. Integrated implantable device for long-term glucose monitoring. Biosensors Bioelectronics 1995;10:485
81. Schmidt FJ, Slutter WJ, Schoonen AJM. Glucose concentration in subcutaneous extracellular space. Diabetes Care 1993;16:695
82. Velho G, Froguel Ph, Thevenot DR, Reach G. *In vivo* calibration of a subcutaneous glucose sensor for determination of subcutaneous glucose kinetics. Diabetes Nutr Metab 1988;1:227
83. Velho G, Froguel Ph, Thevenot DR, Reach G. Strategies for calibrating a subcutaneous glucose sensor. Biomed Biochem Acta 1989;48:957

Part VI

Type II Diabetes

Diabetes Mellitus, edited by Derek LeRoith, Simeon I. Taylor, and Jerrold M. Olefsky. Lippincott–Raven Publishers, Philadelphia © 1996.

CHAPTER 49

Epidemiology of Non–Insulin-Dependent Diabetes

PETER H. BENNETT

Non–insulin-dependent diabetes (NIDDM) is the most common form of diabetes. Its complications primarily affect the vascular system and lead to excessive rates of coronary heart disease, renal disease and failure, retinopathy and blindness, and peripheral vascular disease, neuropathy, and amputation. These complications give rise to most of the morbidity and excess mortality associated with diabetes. In recent years, much has been learned about the epidemiology of NIDDM, particularly since the introduction of internationally accepted criteria for its diagnosis.[1] Population studies based on standardized methods and diagnosis have shown much variation in the frequency of the disease, and prospective studies have provided new insights into its associated risk factors and its pattern of development.

Prevalence of Non–Insulin-Dependent Diabetes

The prevalence of NIDDM varies enormously from population to population and throughout the world (Fig. 49-1).[2] The highest rates have been recorded in the Pima Indians, a Native American population living in the Southwest United States. Extraordinarily high rates are also found in the Micronesian population living in Nauru in the Central Pacific.

As can be seen in Figure 49-1, rates in different ethnic groups living in the same country may vary considerably. Rates differ in migrants as compared to persons remaining in their own country. In most instances, the rates in migrants are higher than in the indigenous population, and these increases reflect the effect of changing environment on the disease. In some populations, dramatic increases in the prevalence of diabetes have been observed over short periods of time. These increases in prevalence also appear to be related to rapidly changing lifestyles.

The overall pattern of diabetes prevalence throughout the world suggests that populations most likely to have high rates of the disease are those in rapidly developing countries and among the underprivileged persons in developed nations. It has been estimated that the number of persons with diabetes will be about 100 million by the year 2000.

In the United States, about 12 million people have NIDDM. The prevalence is highest among Native Americans, but African Americans and Hispanics (primarily Mexican Americans) have rates that exceed those recorded for the Caucasian population.[3,4] Although many Native American tribes have extraordinarily high rates of NIDDM, the Pima Indians of Arizona have the highest rate recorded anywhere in the world.[5] This tribe resides in the desert of south-central Arizona and is of particular interest because it has been studied longitudinally for some 30 years in an ongoing epidemiologic study.

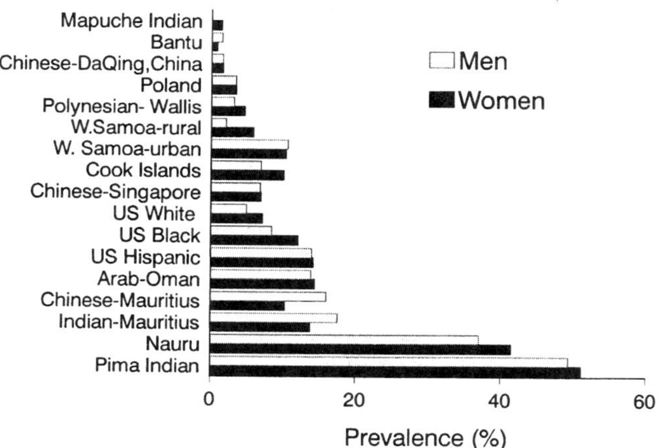

FIGURE 49-1. Prevalence of non–insulin-dependent diabetes mellitus in selected populations age-standardized to 30- to 64-year-old world population.

What Is Non–Insulin-Dependent Diabetes?

Non–insulin-dependent diabetes mellitus describes a number of types of diabetes, but only in a few of these has the underlying cause been defined. Rarely, NIDDM is associated with mutations of the insulin receptor or the glucokinase gene. It may be associated with other endocrinologic disorders, such as acromegaly and Cushing's syndrome, but these causes are rare. The extent to which most cases of NIDDM represent a single disease is uncertain. Nevertheless, although the prevalence of the disease varies considerably from one population to another, the disease has a distinctive epidemiology, with much of the variation in frequency being accounted for by known risk factors. Furthermore, consistent relationships with known risk factors prevail within populations, suggesting that most cases have a similar pathogenetic basis. Much of the information on the risk factors and knowledge of the pathogenesis has been derived from studies of high-frequency populations, such as the Pima Indians and Mexican Americans, but similar patterns are found in other racial groups and on other continents.[5]

NIDDM is often asymptomatic, so many cases remain undiagnosed. Even in countries with well-developed health care systems, such as the United States, there is typically one undiagnosed case for each diagnosed case in the population. In less developed countries, undiagnosed cases usually outnumber diagnosed ones. Consequently, population-based studies in which all individuals in representative samples of the population are tested are necessary for a clear understanding of NIDDM's epidemiology.

Genetic Factors

Non–insulin-dependent diabetes mellitus results from the interaction of genetic and environmental factors. The disease has long been recognized as showing familial aggregation, but the most convincing evidence of its genetic basis comes from studies of twins. Concordance rates for NIDDM in older identical twins range from about 50–90%—much higher than among similarly aged nonidentical twins, siblings, or other first-degree relatives.[6] However, although twin studies indicate genetic susceptibility to NIDDM, they provide no information as to whether it is caused by one or many genes, or what its mode of inheritance is.

Besides twin studies, other evidence of the importance of genetic determinants comes from studies of admixed populations and from populations of different genetic backgrounds living in similar environments. The prevalence of NIDDM in different ethnic groups living in the same communities varies considerably. Major differences were first described among the different ethnic groups residing in Hawaii, but differences in prevalence have subsequently been shown in many places and among diverse populations: for example, Asian Indians, Chinese, and Malays living in Singapore; Asian Indians and Melanesians in Fiji; Asian Indians and Europeans in Great Britain; and different ethnic groups in the United States.[2] More direct evidence of the importance of genetic susceptibility comes from populations residing in exactly the same environment but within which there is a genetic admixture. For example, among the population of the Gila River Indian Community in Arizona, the prevalence of NIDDM is twice as high in full-blooded Pima Indians as in non-Indians, and the prevalence among those of half-Pima, half–non-Indian ancestry is intermediate.[8]

Other less direct evidence of the importance of genetic susceptibility has emerged from studies of genetic markers. Associations between NIDDM and several genetic markers located on different chromosomes have been described. These associations vary from population to population, but such markers serve as indicators of genetic admixture. The association of NIDDM with these markers (which are not genetically *linked* with the disease) indicates that the level of susceptibility to NIDDM varies in different gene pools within populations.

Apart from the rare cases of NIDDM associated with abnormalities of the insulin receptor, mitochondrial mutations, or mutations of the glucokinase gene, the specific genetic basis for NIDDM remains unknown. Nevertheless, in populations such as the Pima Indians and Nauruans, segregation analyses suggest the operation of a major gene. Although these findings cannot be taken as evidence that NIDDM is caused by the same genes in all populations, they do provide a basis for specific searches for the chromosomal location of the putative susceptibility genes. Once it is possible to recognize individual genes that confer susceptibility to NIDDM, the mode of inheritance and the extent of genetic heterogeneity will be clarified.

Genetic susceptibility does appear to be a prerequisite for the development of NIDDM. There is much evidence, however, that the ultimate expression of the disease is largely determined by environmental factors.

Environmental Factors

The development of NIDDM is influenced by exposure to different environments. Some of the effect of environment can be assessed by comparing the frequency of the disease in migrants with that among persons who remain in the original environment, assuming that both groups share similar gene pools. For example, populations of Asian Indian origin are found in many parts of the world. The prevalence of NIDDM in those aged 15 years and older in India has been estimated to be about 2% in urban populations and about 1.5% in rural ones. Studies of similar age groups in expatriate Indian populations, however, show much higher rates of the disease.[7] For example, in Singapore, 9% of Asian Indians are reported to have NIDDM, compared with 5% in South Africa, and 13% in Fiji. Similar differences have been reported among Japanese migrants in Hawaii, where those aged 40 years and older had a disease prevalence of 12%, compared with 7% in Hiroshima, Japan.[9] Marked differences are also found among Chinese populations in different parts of the world.

A further example can be found in the Pacific, specifically in New Caledonia, where Polynesians from the island of Wallis (where the primary occupation is agriculture and the way of life very traditional) migrated in the 1970s to take advantage of the opportunities provided by the nickel industry. In 1980, the prevalence of diabetes among those aged 20 years and older in Wallis was 3%, compared with 12% in New Caledonia, even after adjustment for differences in obesity.[10] The prevalence in New Caledonia was six times higher in men and four times higher in women compared with that in Wallis. Thus, these differences in prevalence in migrant populations provide evidence of the importance of environmental factors as determinants of NIDDM.

Rapid changes have occurred in the prevalence of diabetes within certain populations. For example, among the Pima Indians, age-adjusted prevalence rates for diabetes increased more than 40% during the period between 1967 and 1977.[11] Although this increase could have been attributed to improved survival among diabetic patients, an increase in the incidence (the rate of development of new cases) of the disease was actually the major contributor. In 1967, the prevalence of diabetes among the Pima Indians was 10 times higher than in the U.S. population as a whole, yet some 30 years earlier, the prevalence of diagnosed diabetes was no greater among the Pima Indian population than among the general population. Such changes over the course of one or two generations can only be attributed to changes in the way of life; hence, they reflect the major influence of environmental factors on the expression of the disease.

A less dramatic, but substantial increase in the prevalence of NIDDM in the general U.S. population has also occurred. The prevalence of diagnosed diabetes in persons aged 18 to 74 years increased from about 1% in 1960 to 3.6% in 1980. This increase is partially attributable to a rise in the average age of the population and to the widespread use of automated methods for determining plasma glucose levels, a practice that has increased the likelihood of recognition of previously undiagnosed NIDDM. Moreover, some part of the increase since 1970 can probably be attributed to decreased mortality from diabetes and cardiovascular disease, both of which result in increased survival among diabetic patients. Since 1973, however, the age-specific incidence of NIDDM in the United States has been stable, suggesting that any increase in prevalence since that time is largely the result of demographic changes and decreasing mortality.[12]

Obesity

Obesity is a major determinant of the incidence of NIDDM, but in most populations, only a small proportion of obese persons develop the disease. Longitudinal studies among the Pima Indians have demonstrated that the likelihood of developing NIDDM results from an interaction between the effect of obesity in the offspring and a parental history of diabetes, which presumably reflects inherited susceptibility.[13] Among obese subjects with a diabetic parent, the incidence of NIDDM is many times higher than among equally obese persons whose parents do not have the disease. Among those who are not obese, however, the incidence of NIDDM is much lower, even if NIDDM has been diagnosed in one or both parents. Thus, even when genetic susceptibility is present, the expression of the disease is largely dependent on other factors.

Not only the presence but the distribution of obesity influences the risk of developing NIDDM. Upper body or central obesity is associated with an increased risk for developing NIDDM, as has been shown in many different ethnic and racial groups. Central obesity in many populations is also associated with an increased incidence of coronary heart disease, hyperinsulinemia, high serum triglyceride and low high-density lipoprotein (HDL) cholesterol levels, hypertension, and disturbances in the patterns of sex hormones. Hyperinsulinemia, or insulin resistance, appears to be a central feature of this cluster of abnormalities related to truncal or abdominal obesity.[14] Insulin resistance is a characteristic of patients with NIDDM, but also precedes and predicts the development of the disease.

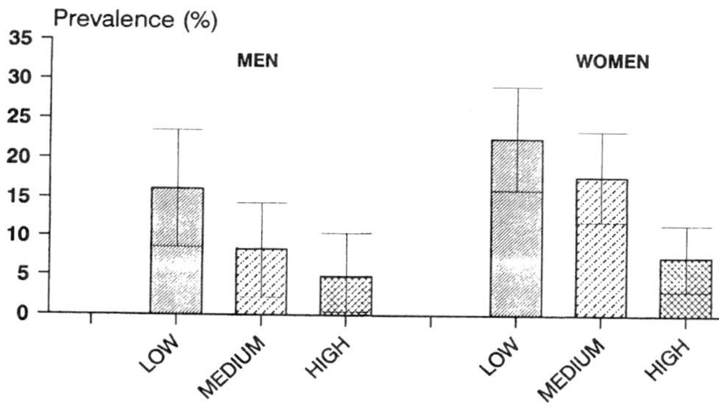

Figure 49-2. Age-adjusted prevalence of non–insulin-dependent diabetes mellitus (with 95% confidence intervals) according to tertiles of leisure activity in Pima Indians aged 15 to 36 years. (Reproduced with permission from Kriska AM, LaPorte RE, Pettitt DJ, et al. The association of physical activity with obesity, fat distribution, and glucose tolerance in Pima Indians. Diabetologia 1993;36:863.)

Differences in the extent or distribution of obesity, however, do not entirely account for differences in the prevalence of diabetes among or within populations, nor does obesity entirely account for differences in the prevalence of diabetes among migrants.[9] Thus, it has been necessary to search for other factors.

Physical Activity

A substantial body of evidence indicates that physical activity influences the incidence of NIDDM. Cross-sectional studies in populations of several ethnic groups show that the prevalence of diabetes among physically inactive persons is typically 2 to 3 times higher than among active subgroups of the same population.[15] This finding is illustrated in Figure 49-2, which shows that the prevalence of diabetes among Pima Indians in the lowest tertile of activity is 2.5 times that of persons who are in the most active third of the population.[15] Moreover, three prospective observational studies, involving primarily U.S. whites, have indicated that even modest physical activity is associated with a lower incidence of NIDDM.[16–18]

Other Environmental Factors

Differences in physical activity account for at least some of the variation in the prevalence of diabetes among populations of similar genetic background after adjustments are made for differences in obesity. Certainly, the lifestyle changes that occur in many migrant populations and in recently urbanized populations as they shift from a traditional to a more affluent or westernized environment are accompanied by an increase in obesity and a reduction in the average amount of physical activity. Increased obesity and reduced physical activity both favor the development of insulin resistance, which appears to be a critical component in the pathogenesis of NIDDM.

Another factor that may contribute to the development of insulin resistance is consumption of a diet containing a high percentage of calories from fat, decreased fiber content, and decreased unrefined carbohydrate content. Populations with a high prevalence of diabetes characteristically consume a diet that contains more fat, particularly saturated fat, than the one they ate when they followed a more traditional way of life.[19] Indeed, the pattern of changes that accompanies the shift from a traditional to a westernized environment, or from a rural to an urban environment, and the pattern of changes experienced by populations having rapid increases in the prevalence of diabetes include an increase in obesity, a reduction in physical activity, and an increase in the consumption of dietary fat.[20] Further, these dietary modifications and the changes associated with decreased physical activity appear to be additive, thus offering the hope that changes in lifestyle may lead to a reduction in the incidence of NIDDM.

Development of Non–Insulin-Dependent Diabetes

Insulin Resistance

Non–insulin-dependent diabetes mellitus is preceded by hyperinsulinemia and impaired glucose tolerance (IGT). Populations with a high risk of developing NIDDM, such as Pima Indians, Mexican Americans, Asian Indians, and Australian Aborigines, have higher circulating insulin levels at the time they have normal glucose tolerance than do populations in which the risk of NIDDM is much lower.[21,22] These findings suggest that insulin resistance is a characteristic that precedes the development of IGT and NIDDM.

Hyperinsulinemia, especially in the fasting state, represents an index of insulin resistance. Insulin resistance shows familial aggregation and is associated with both obesity and physical inactivity. For example, Mexican American and Pima Indian offspring of diabetic parents have higher insulin levels than do those without a family history of diabetes.[23,24] The development of IGT is predicted by the presence of hyperinsulinemia. IGT is a strong risk factor for NIDDM, as has been demonstrated in many populations,[25] and its presence can be regarded as a stage in the development of NIDDM.

Impaired Glucose Tolerance

An inverted U-shaped relationship between insulin level and degree of glycemia is found within populations.[14,26] As a group, subjects with IGT have high insulin levels, whereas persons with normal glucose tolerance have lower insulin levels, both fasting and following a glucose load, than do persons with IGT. Longitudinal epidemiologic studies have shown that hyperinsulinemia, even at a stage when glucose tolerance is within the normal range, is an important predictor of NIDDM. The natural history of the disease follows a sequence that parallels the cross-sectional relationships between insulin levels and glycemia.[26,27] Persons with normal glucose tolerance who ultimately develop NIDDM have increased insulin levels that subsequently reach a peak when these persons develop IGT. The increase in insulin level appears to be a compensatory response to increasing intracellular insulin resistance. This, in turn, leads to small increases in circulating glucose levels and a resultant increase in insulin secretion, as well as subsequent increases in both fasting and stimulated insulin levels. As insulin resistance worsens, glucose tolerance deteriorates and IGT eventually occurs.[26]

Decompensation to Diabetes

After IGT develops, decompensation to diabetes is associated with diminishing insulin responsiveness to secretagogues. The insulin response to secretagogues—particularly to glucose itself—diminishes, hyperglycemia worsens, and NIDDM appears. The reasons pancreatic β-cells become less responsive to the effects of ingested glucose are uncertain, but it is widely believed that glycemia itself may downregulate the glucose-sensing mechanisms in the β-cell (glucotoxicity), leading to diminished insulin secretion. Nevertheless, fasting insulin levels, which still reflect the underlying degree

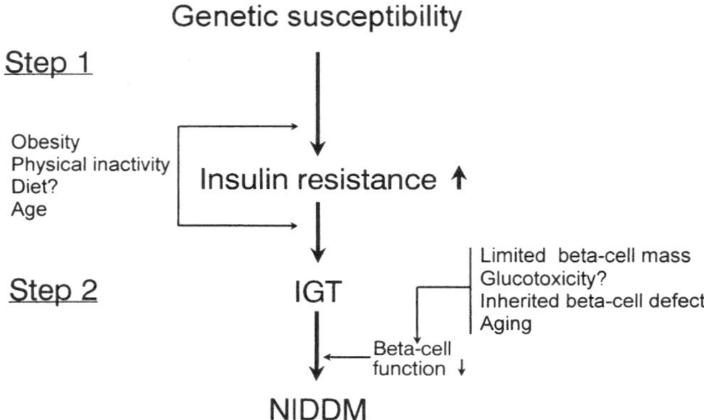

Figure 49-3. Major steps in the development of non–insulin-dependent diabetes mellitus. (Adapted with permission from Saad MF, Knowler WC, Pettitt DJ, et al. A two-step model for development of non–insulin-dependent diabetes. Am J Med 1991;90:229.)

of insulin resistance, remain high in recent-onset diabetes, although later in the course of the disease, even fasting insulin levels may diminish.

From longitudinal epidemiologic data on the Pima Indians, we have proposed a two-step model for the development of NIDDM,[28] as summarized in Figure 49-3. The first step consists of the development and worsening of insulin resistance up to the time of development of IGT. The second step occurs when β-cells fail to sense and respond normally to increasing degrees of hyperglycemia. Once β-cell failure occurs, increased hepatic glucose output—a direct result of insulin deficiency—occurs, and fasting hyperglycemia becomes established.

Other Pathogenetic Mechanisms in Non–Insulin-Dependent Diabetes

Whether there is a significant subgroup of patients with NIDDM for whom the initiating abnormality is insulin deficiency rather than insulin resistance is widely debated. At this time, no longitudinal studies have demonstrated that insulin insufficiency initiates the chain of events leading to NIDDM or occurs before the onset of IGT. Lack of insulin secretion, however, is the major abnormality in the chain of events that leads to insulin-dependent diabetes. In some patients with NIDDM, a less severe but primary β-cell lesion—rather than insulin resistance—seems likely to be the initiating event. Although rare, recently described genetic abnormalities of glucokinase that result in a diminished capacity for insulin secretion account for some cases of mild NIDDM.[29] There are also patients with mild degrees of autoimmune-related pancreatic β-cell destruction who develop NIDDM, which may later progress to insulin-dependent diabetes. Nevertheless, in most populations, insulin resistance is almost certainly the initiating abnormality in most cases of NIDDM.

Summary

In summary, NIDDM is a common disease that affects all races, but some much more than others. Its prevalence and incidence have increased in many populations, especially those in developing countries. The major environmental factors identified as contributing to this increase are obesity and reduced physical activity. The disease shows strong familial aggregation in all populations and is clearly the result of an interaction between genetic susceptibility and environmental factors. Most people with NIDDM have close relatives with the disease and most are obese when they develop it. Before NIDDM develops, insulin concentrations are high for the degree of glycemia and for the degree of obesity, reflecting an abnormal degree of insulin resistance. If insulin resistance worsens, glucose levels increase and insulin levels increase correspondingly. Eventually, glucose tolerance becomes impaired, and finally, the insulin response diminishes and NIDDM begins.

References

1. WHO Expert Committee on Diabetes Mellitus. Second Report. WHO Technical Report Series No. 646. Geneva: World Health Organization;1980:1
2. King H, Rewers M, WHO Ad Hoc Diabetes Reporting Group. Global estimates for prevalence of diabetes mellitus and impaired glucose tolerance in adults. Diabetes Care 1993;16:157
3. Harris MI, Hadden WC, Knowler WC, Bennett PH. Prevalence of diabetes and impaired glucose tolerance and plasma glucose levels in the U.S. population aged 20–74 years. Diabetes 1987;36:523
4. Flegal KM, Ezzati TM, Harris MI, et al. Prevalence of diabetes in Mexican Americans, Cubans and Puerto Ricans from the Hispanic Health and Nutrition Examination Survey, 1982–1984. Diabetes Care 1991;14:628
5. Knowler WC, Bennett PH, Hamman RF, Miller M. Diabetes incidence and prevalence in Pima Indians: A 19-fold greater incidence than in Rochester, Minnesota. Am J Epidemiol 1978;108:497
6. Zimmet PZ. Kelly West Lecture 1991. Challenges in diabetes epidemiology—From West to the rest. Diabetes Care 1992;15:232
7. Kaprio J, Tuomilehto J, Koskenvuo M, et al. Concordance for type 1 (insulin-dependent) and type 2 (non–insulin-dependent) diabetes mellitus in a population-based cohort of twins in Finland. Diabetologia 1992;35:1060
8. Knowler WC, Williams RC, Pettitt DJ, Steinberg AG. Gm3;5,13,14 and type 2 diabetes mellitus: An association in American Indians with genetic admixture. Am J Hum Genet 1988;43:520
9. Kawate R, Yamakido M, Nishimoto Y, et al. Diabetes mellitus and its vascular complications in Japanese migrants on the island of Hawaii. Diabetes Care 1979;2:161
10. Taylor R, Bennett P, Uili R, et al. Diabetes in Wallis Polynesians: A comparison of residents of Wallis Island and first generation migrants in Noumea, New Caledonia. Diabetes Res Clin Pract 1985;1:169
11. Bennett PH, Knowler WC. Increasing prevalence of diabetes in the Pima (American) Indians over a ten-year period. In: Waldhäusl WK, ed. Diabetes 1979: Proceedings of 10th Congress of the International Diabetes Federation. Amsterdam: Excerpta Medica;1979:507
12. Harris MI. Prevalence of non–insulin-dependent diabetes and impaired glucose tolerance. In: Harris MI, Hamman RF, eds. Diabetes in America. Diabetes Data Compiled 1984. NIH Publ. No. 85-1468. Washington, DC: US DHEW; 1985:VI1
13. Knowler WC, Pettitt DJ, Savage PJ, Bennett PH. Diabetes incidence in Pima Indians: Contributions of obesity and parental diabetes. Am J Epidemiol 1981; 113:144
14. DeFronzo RA, Ferrannini E. Insulin resistance: A multifaceted syndrome response for NIDDM, obesity, hypertension, dyslipidemia, and atherosclerotic cardiovascular disease. Diabetes Care 1991;14:173
15. Kriska AM, LaPorte RE, Pettitt DJ, et al. The association of physical activity with obesity, fat distribution and glucose tolerance in Pima Indians. Diabetologia 1993;36:863
16. Helmrich SP, Ragland DR, Leung RW, Paffenbarger RS. Physical activity and reduced occurrence of non–insulin-dependent diabetes mellitus. N Engl J Med 1991;325:147
17. Manson JE, Nathan DM, Krolewski AS, et al. A prospective study of exercise and incidence of diabetes among US male physicians. JAMA 1992;268:63
18. Manson JE, Rimm EB, Stampfer MJ, et al. Physical activity and incidence of non–insulin-dependent diabetes mellitus in women. Lancet 1991;338:774
19. Bennett PH, Knowler WC, Baird HR, et al. Diet and development of non–insulin-dependent diabetes mellitus: An epidemiological perspective. In: Pozza G, Micossi P, Catapano AL, Paoletti R, eds. Diet, Diabetes, and Atherosclerosis. New York: Raven Press;1984:109
20. O'Dea K. Marked improvement in carbohydrate and lipid metabolism in diabetic Australian Aborigines after temporary reversion to traditional lifestyle. Diabetes 1984;33:596
21. Aronoff SL, Bennett PH, Gorden P, et al. Unexplained hyperinsulinemia in normal and ''prediabetic'' Pima Indians compared with normal Caucasians. Diabetes 1977;26:827
22. Haffner SM, Stern MP, Hazuda HP, et al. Hyperinsulinemia in a population at high risk for non–insulin-dependent diabetes mellitus. N Engl J Med 1986; 315:220
23. Lillioja S, Mott DM, Zawadzki JK, et al. In vivo insulin action is familial characteristic in non-diabetic Pima Indians. Diabetes 1987;36:1329
24. Haffner SM, Stern MP, Hazuda HP, et al. Increased insulin concentrations in nondiabetic offspring of diabetic parents. N Engl J Med 1988;319:1297
25. Saad MF, Knowler WC, Pettitt DJ, et al. The natural history of impaired glucose tolerance in the Pima Indians. N Engl J Med 1988;319:1500
26. Lillioja S, Mott DM, Howard BV, et al. Impaired glucose tolerance as a

disorder of insulin action: Longitudinal and cross-sectional studies in Pima Indians. N Engl J Med 1988;318:1217

27. Saad MF, Pettitt DJ, Mott DM, et al. Sequential changes in serum insulin concentration during development of non–insulin-dependent diabetes. Lancet 1989;1:1356
28. Saad MF, Knowler WC, Pettitt DJ, et al. A two-step model for development of non–insulin-dependent diabetes. Am J Med 1991;90:229
29. Vionnet N, Stoffel M, Takeda J, et al. Nonsense mutation in glucokinase gene causes early-onset non–insulin-dependent diabetes mellitus. Nature 1992;356:721

Diabetes Mellitus, edited by Derek LeRoith, Simeon I. Taylor, and Jerrold M. Olefsky. Lippincott–Raven Publishers, Philadelphia © 1996.

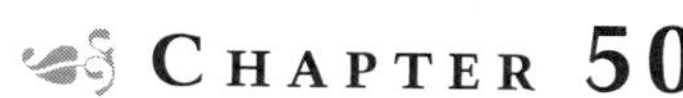

Chapter 50
Metabolic Abnormalities in the Development of Non–Insulin-Dependent Diabetes Mellitus

Clifton Bogardus

Diabetes mellitus is a common disease defined by fasting plasma hyperglycemia (≥140 mg/100 dL, 7.8 mM) and/or hyperglycemia (200 mg/100 dL, 11.1 mM) 2 hours after ingesting 75 g of glucose.[1,2] There are two major subclasses of diabetes mellitus: insulin-dependent (IDDM) and non–insulin-dependent (NIDDM). IDDM is distinguished from NIDDM by the patient's dependence on insulin for survival. In this chapter, all others who meet the glycemic criteria for diabetes mellitus and do not have malnutrition-related or gestational diabetes, or diabetes secondary to a known genetic defect (e.g., an insulin receptor mutation[3] or glucokinase mutation[4]), are considered to have NIDDM. IDDM results from an insulin deficiency that is caused by pathologic autoimmune mechanisms. As is apparent from its present definition, the etiology of NIDDM is unknown. However, considerable progress has been made in the last decade in defining the natural history of metabolic characteristics of persons who have, or who later develop, NIDDM. Those cross-sectional and prospective clinical data relevant to an understanding of the development of NIDDM from normal glucose tolerance are reviewed. As discussed, many investigators have reported similar data from different populations around the world. The consistency of the data is indicative of the reliability and universal applicability of the findings and the conclusions to be drawn from them.

Cross-Sectional Data

Obesity

It was a generally accepted clinical impression for centuries (see review in ref. 5) that fatter people were more likely to develop diabetes. Overwhelming evidence has accumulated to confirm the accuracy of this clinical impression. The association of obesity with NIDDM has been observed in comparisons of different populations and within populations. In 10 different populations from divergent areas of the world, West and Kalbfleisch[6] observed a remarkably strong correlation between population prevalences of NIDDM (what they referred to as maturity-onset diabetes) and mean percent of standard weight of the populations. Similar associations were found in several intrapopulation studies, beginning as early as 1921 in a study of the U.S. population conducted by Joslin,[7] and subsequently in other populations.[5] The strength of the association between obesity and NIDDM reported in these studies was probably even underestimated, as individuals with diabetes frequently lose weight, either as a result of the disease itself, or as part of their treatment.

In addition to being more obese than nondiabetics, persons with NIDDM have a more central distribution of body fat. As early as 1956, Vague[8] suggested that central obesity, or what he called "android obesity," was more common in people with diabetes than in nondiabetics. Feldman et al.,[9] using different measures of body fat distribution, confirmed these findings. In 1984, Hartz and colleagues[10] reported the results of a survey of more than 30,000 American women. The data revealed that the highest prevalence of diabetes occurred in women with the greatest proportion of body fat at the waist (as opposed to the hips), even in those with comparable degrees of obesity. In addition to these intrapopulation surveys, West reported that the Plains Indians of Oklahoma, a population with a high prevalence of NIDDM, had a more central distribution of body fat compared to Caucasians in the U.S. population, a group with a lower prevalence of NIDDM.[5]

Despite the large number of studies in which the degree of obesity of persons with NIDDM has been compared to that of nondiabetics, less data have been reported on the relationship between degree of obesity (and central obesity) and the extent of glycemia. These relationships in Pima Indians are shown in Figure 50-1. It is apparent that, on average, those with NIDDM are more obese, and more centrally obese, than nondiabetics. In addition, the most hyperglycemic diabetics are less obese than those with less severe diabetes. Glycemia is negatively correlated with degree of obesity expressed as percentage of body fat (determined by hydrodensitometry) in men and women with NIDDM. Moreover, glycemia is unrelated to the distribution of fat in diabetics. In contrast to these correlations in diabetics, in nondiabetics, glycemia is positively correlated with percent body fat and the distribution of fat.

Insulin Secretory Dysfunction

A definition of the cross-sectional relationship between glycemia and insulin secretory function began to evolve several years after the introduction of the insulin radioimmunoassay by Yalow and Berson.[11] Reaven and Miller[12] were the first to report an inverted U-shaped relationship between insulin and glucose responses to glucose ingestion in lean and obese people. Of their Caucasian

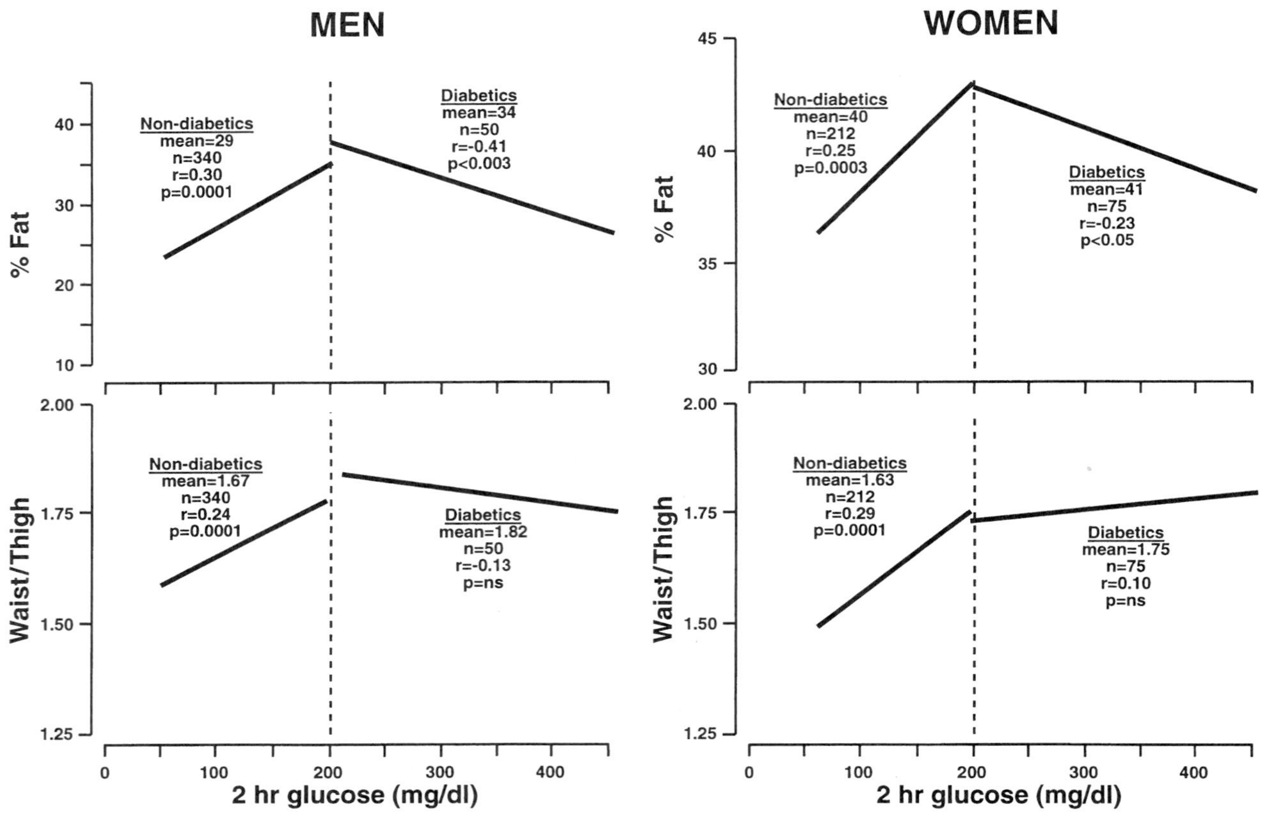

Figure 50-1. The relationship between percent body fat (% fat) and central distribution of fat (waist/thigh [WT] ratio) and the plasma glucose concentration 2 hours after ingestion of 75 g of glucose in Pima Indians. The % fat was estimated by hydrodensitometry and W/T ratio measured as the ratio of the waist circumference at the umbilicus (supine) and the thigh circumference at the gluteal fold (standing).

subjects, those with moderately impaired glucose tolerance, or with NIDDM and modest elevations of plasma glucose concentrations, had the highest insulin responses. Compared to this group, patients with NIDDM and more severe hyperglycemia had lower insulin responses, but the responses were not lower than those with normal glucose tolerance unless the hyperglycemia was extreme. This inverted U-shaped relationship of insulin and glucose response to oral glucose has subsequently been confirmed by other investigators in other Caucasian populations in Australia[13] and in the United States.[14]

Further clarification of the relationships between glycemia and insulin secretory function in humans came with the introduction of the IV glucose tolerance test. The insulin response to a bolus of intravenously injected glucose was found to be biphasic, and persons with NIDDM, even those with only mild fasting hyperglycemia and/or mild hyperglycemia following glucose ingestion, had a marked defect in first-phase response.[15] This lack of a first-phase response, or acute insulin response (AIR), in persons with NIDDM has been observed by many investigators.[15] Subsequent work indicated that a decreased AIR in persons with NIDDM occurred only with glucose, as opposed to other islet cell stimulants, such as arginine.[16] Halter et al.[17] pointed out, however, that the AIR was dependent on the prestimulus plasma glucose concentration. At similar prestimulus plasma glucose concentrations, persons with NIDDM had reduced AIRs in response to a variety of islet cell stimuli.[16] From these studies, it was clear that all persons with NIDDM, regardless of a measurable hyperinsulinemic response to oral glucose, had a detectable defect in insulin secretory function. In the past, the physiologic relevance of a reduced AIR to a nonphysiologic stimulus (intravenous glucose) has been questioned. It was recently reported, however, that the AIR is positively correlated with the insulin response 30 minutes after ingestion of glucose.[18] Moreover, results recently collected in nondiabetic Pima Indians indicate that the AIR is positively correlated with the insulin response 30 minutes after ingesting a mixed meal (Table 50-1). Because AIR is also positively correlated with insulin action, this relationship could be a result of insulin resistance. This is not the case, however. AIR is positively correlated with the plasma insulin concentration 30 minutes after a meal, independent of insulin resistance (see Table 50-1).

Table 50-1. Predicting the Plasma Insulin Concentration 30 Minutes After a Mixed Meal in Nondiabetic Pima Indians (N=296) Using Multiple Linear Regression

Models and Covariants	Standardized Beta*	P Value for Beta	Overall R^2	Overall P Value
(1) AIR[†]	0.285	0.0001	0.081	0.0001
(2) AIR	0.235	0.0001	–	–
M[‡]	−0.360	0.0001	0.209	0.0001

*Betas were standardized by standardizing the covariates to a mean of zero and a standard deviation of 1.

[†]Acute insulin response from 3 to 5 minutes after a bolus intravenous injection of 25 g of glucose.

[‡]Insulin-mediated glucose uptake rate at a plasma insulin concentration of ~130 μU/mL, as determined by the hyperinsulinemic, euglycemic clamp technique (see ref. 5 for methodology).

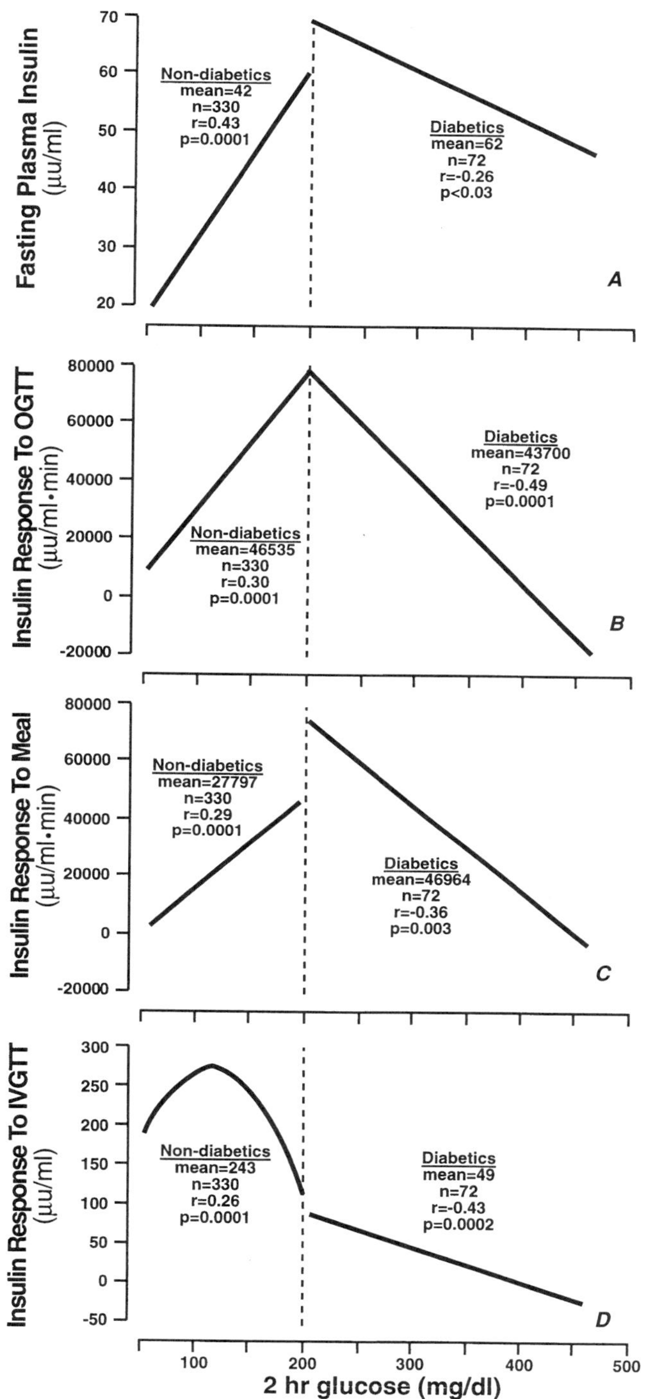

Figure 50-2. The relationships between fasting plasma insulin concentrations (*A*), the 3-hour insulin response to ingestion of 75 g of glucose (*B*), the 4-hour insulin response to ingestion of a standard mixed meal (*C*), and the acute insulin response to an intravenous glucose bolus and the plasma glucose concentration 2 hours after ingestion of 75 g of glucose (*D*). The best fitting, significant regression between the two variables is shown, determined separately in nondiabetics and diabetics. *OGTT*, oral glucose tolerance test; *IVGTT*, intravenous glucose tolerance test.

The cross-sectional relationships between AIR, fasting insulin concentration, and insulin responses to oral glucose and a mixed meal in Pima Indians are summarized in Figure 50-2. These data on 399 Pimas confirm the results collected in various Caucasian groups and demonstrate two additional features of the relationship between glycemia and insulin secretory function in man. Among those persons with untreated NIDDM, fasting insulin concentrations and the insulin responses to oral glucose and a mixed meal are negatively correlated with glycemia. In contrast to these negative relationships in persons with NIDDM, among nondiabetics, fasting insulin concentrations and insulin responses to oral glucose and a mixed meal are positively correlated with glycemia.

The cross-sectional relationship between AIR and glycemia in Pima Indians is quite different from the relationships of insulin responses with glycemic responses to oral nutrients. As in other populations, the AIR to intravenous glucose is absent in many persons with NIDDM,[15,16] including those with only slightly higher glucose levels than nondiabetics. Interestingly, and not yet reported in other groups (probably because of the fewer numbers of subjects studied), an inverted U relationship between AIR and glycemia has been noted among nondiabetics.

Insulin Resistance

Based on their pioneering studies of glucose responses to combined glucose ingestion and IV insulin infusion, Himsworth and Kerr[19] were the first to suggest (in the 1940s) that some people with diabetes mellitus were hyperglycemic because of resistance to the action of insulin to remove glucose from the blood rather than because of insulin deficiency. Their work was apparently largely ignored until Yalow and Berson[20] reported in 1960 that some people with NIDDM were hyperinsulinemic. In the ensuing decades, different investigators, using many different methods and studying various populations, have confirmed that insulin resistance is a consistent feature of the metabolic syndrome of NIDDM. Several groups of investigators[21–23] measured the rate of insulin-mediated glucose uptake of the forearm in subjects with and without NIDDM. If their results were corrected for the effect of hyperglycemia to increase glucose uptake, it was evident that those with NIDDM responded less well to insulin. Early evidence of insulin resistance of the whole body in persons with NIDDM was deduced from the fact that the rate of decline of the plasma glucose concentration in response to insulin infusion was decreased in persons with fasting hyperglycemia.[24] To avoid hypoglycemia during such tests, and to better quantitate the degree of insulin resistance, techniques were developed to evaluate whole body insulin action in nondiabetics and persons with NIDDM at similar and constant plasma insulin concentrations. Endogenous insulin secretion was inhibited using either a combination of epinephrine and propranolol[25] or somatostatin.[26] The plasma glycemic response to a constant infusion of insulin and glucose was then a measure of insulin action in the whole body. Using such techniques, Reaven and colleagues[25] and, later, Harano et al.,[26] confirmed that persons with NIDDM were more insulin-resistant than nondiabetics.

In 1979, DeFronzo, Tobin, and Andres[27] introduced another method to measure whole body insulin action in vivo: the glucose/insulin clamp technique. With this technique, whole body insulin action is quantitated as the rate of a variable glucose infusion required to maintain a constant plasma glucose concentration during a constant insulin infusion. Compared to nondiabetics, people with NIDDM were found by many investigators to be insulin-resistant.[14,28–32]

In recent years, the simple dichotomous studies of nondiabetics compared to subjects with NIDDM have been expanded to examine the relationship between glycemia and insulin action in vivo across the entire range of glycemia. The consistency of this relationship, as documented by different investigators in both lean and obese groups, is demonstrated in Figure 50-3. As indicated in the figure, and as reported in studies of the Pima Indians,[30] at physiologic plasma insulin concentrations, there is little or no correlation between glycemia and insulin action in vivo in persons with NIDDM, whereas in nondiabetics, these metabolic variables are negatively correlated.

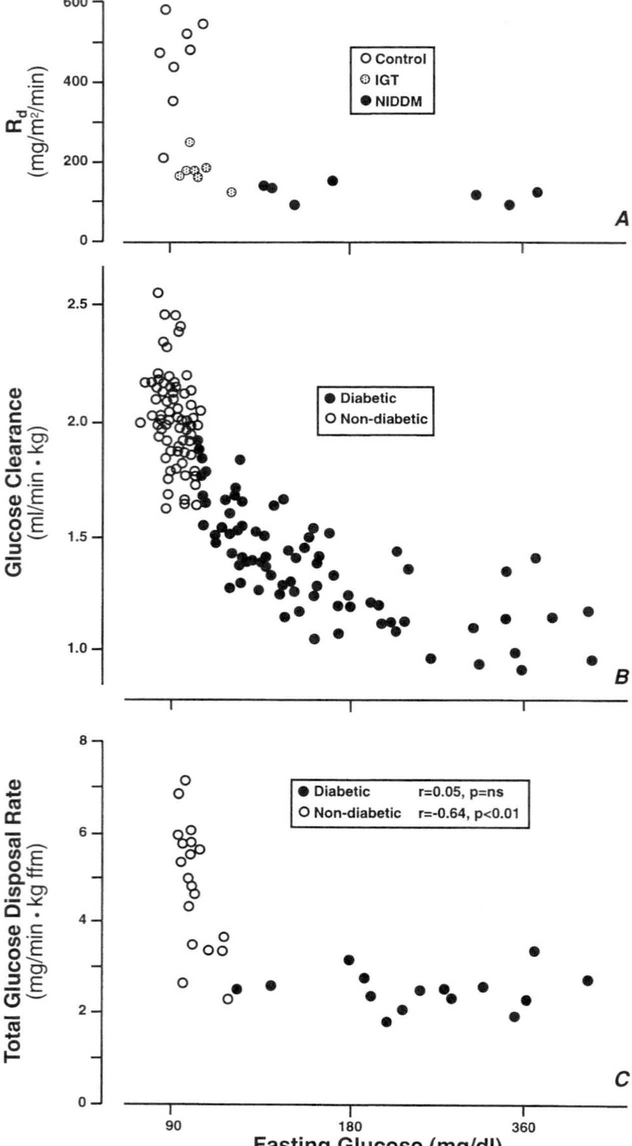

Figure 50-3. The relationship between insulin action in vivo and fasting plasma glucose concentrations in three different studies. Insulin action was estimated in each study using the hyperinsulinemic, euglycemic clamp technique at physiologic plasma insulin concentrations. *IGT*, impaired glucose tolerance. (Adapted with permission from Golay A, Chen Y-DI, Reaven GM. Effect of differences in glucose tolerance on insulin's ability to regulate carbohydrate and free-fatty acid metabolism in obese individuals. J Clin Endocrinal Metab 1986;62:1081–1088. © The Endocrine Society. [***A***]; DeFronzo RA. Lilly Lecture 1987. The triumvirate: B-cell muscle liver. A collusion responsible for NIDDM. Diabetes 1988;37:667–687 [***B***]; Bogardus C, Lillioja S, Howard B, et al. Relationships between insulin secretion, insulin action, and fasting plasma glucose concentration in nondiabetic and non–insulin-dependent diabetic subjects. J Clin Invest 1984;74:1238–1246 [***C***].)

Many investigators have also determined which of the insulin-sensitive tissue—liver, adipose tissue, and skeletal muscle—are insulin-resistant in persons with NIDDM. Decreased insulin action on glucose transport, on the activity of insulin receptor tyrosine kinase, and on other insulin-sensitive metabolic pathways has been found in isolated adipocytes and skeletal muscle tissue obtained from Caucasians[32–38] and Pima Indians with NIDDM.[39–45] Experiments in which the glucose/insulin clamp technique was combined with calorimetry and/or measures of arteriovenous differences in glucose across the leg[30,46,47] have indicated indirectly that persons with NIDDM are resistant to the action of insulin on skeletal muscle glycogenesis. In 1989, Schulman et al.[48] demonstrated directly that the rate of insulin-mediated glycogenesis, as determined by nuclear magnetic resonance, was reduced in persons with NIDDM compared to that in nondiabetics.

Caro et al.[32] obtained liver tissue by open biopsy during gastric bypass surgery in obese nondiabetics and obese persons with NIDDM. They reported decreased insulin-stimulated insulin receptor tyrosine kinase activity and decreased insulin-stimulated aminoisobutyric acid (AIB) uptake into isolated hepatocytes in diabetics as compared with nondiabetics. This in vitro evidence of hepatic insulin resistance in persons with NIDDM is consistent with the results of clinical experiments. During a glucose/insulin clamp procedure, the rate of hepatic glucose production can be quantitated using glucose tracers. Many studies have confirmed that there is a rightward shift in the insulin-dose responsive curve for suppression of hepatic glucose production in persons with NIDDM compared to controls.[29,31,49] At high plasma insulin concentrations, there is complete suppression of hepatic glucose production in diabetics and nondiabetics. At lower, more physiologic, plasma insulin concentrations, hepatic glucose production is fully suppressed in nondiabetic subjects, but incompletely suppressed in those with NIDDM, indicating hepatic insulin resistance in the latter group.

Obesity undoubtedly is a contributing cause of insulin resistance in persons with NIDDM. Recent data in Caucasians and Pima Indians, however, indicate that it is likely not the only cause of insulin resistance.[50,51] In both of these populations, obesity is not linearly correlated with the degree of obesity in nondiabetic subjects. Although in leaner to moderately obese subjects, obesity is negatively correlated with insulin action, at a percent body fat of about 30% in Pima Indians, and at an ideal body weight of greater than ~130% in Caucasians, obesity and insulin action in vivo are unrelated. Equally important, at any given percent body fat or body mass index, there is considerable variance in insulin action which is not attributable to obesity.[52] As predicted from these relationships in nondiabetics, in Pima Indians with NIDDM, who are generally obese and insulin-resistant, there is no negative correlation between degree of obesity and insulin action (data not shown).

Excess Hepatic Glucose Production

A major action of insulin in the liver is to suppress hepatic glucose production. It might be expected, therefore, that diabetics with hepatic insulin resistance would also have an excess rate of postabsorptive hepatic glucose production, especially those with fasting plasma insulin concentrations similar to, or below, that of nondiabetics (see earlier section on insulin secretory dysfunction). Most investigators, using either glucose tracer methodology or organ balance techniques, have reported excess rates of postabsorptive hepatic glucose production in persons with NIDDM compared to nondiabetics.[14,29,30] In several Caucasian groups and in Pima Indians, it has also consistently been found that the fasting plasma glucose concentration is positively correlated with the rate of fasting hepatic glucose production in persons with NIDDM, which is not the case in nondiabetics.[14,29,30]

Summary and Implications of Cross-Sectional Data

On average people with NIDDM, when compared to nondiabetics: (1) are more obese, particularly centrally; (2) have abnormal insulin secretory function; (3) are insulin-resistant in all three insulin-responsive tissues, and (4) have an excess rate of hepatic glucose production. These average metabolic characteristics of persons with NIDDM have been found so consistently by so many different investigators in divergent populations that they should be widely accepted without controversy.

There is more to be inferred from these cross-sectional data than just a comparison of diabetic and nondiabetic groups, however. Within the diabetic group, the degree of glycemia is positively correlated with the rate of hepatic glucose production and is negatively correlated with insulin responses. Glycemia is not correlated with the degree of insulin resistance in diabetics, and the most severely hyperglycemic diabetics are less obese than those who are less hyperglycemic. Thus, although persons with NIDDM are often obese and insulin-resistant, the metabolic characteristics that distinguish those who are most hyperglycemic from those who are less so are reduced insulin secretion and excess hepatic glucose production.

The relationships between obesity, insulin secretion, insulin resistance, and hepatic glucose production are considerably different in the nondiabetic population. In this group, increasing glycemia is not correlated with fasting rates of hepatic glucose production, but is positively correlated with increasing obesity, and central obesity, increasing severity of insulin resistance and increasing hyperinsulinemic responses to oral nutrients. Interestingly, there is an inverted U-shaped relationship between the AIR (to IV glucose) and glycemia in this group, which is similar to the relationship of insulin responses to oral nutrients and glycemia in the entire population of diabetics and nondiabetics.

It can be inferred from these data that, in nondiabetics, insulin resistance, owing entirely or partly to obesity and central obesity, is a contributing cause of increased glucose concentrations after glucose ingestion in this group. The contribution of abnormal secretory function to hyperglycemia in the nondiabetic population is less apparent. The nondiabetics who are most hyperglycemic have the highest insulin responses to ingestion of glucose and a mixed meal. Conversely, the same individuals have lower AIRs to an IV glucose stimulus compared to some nondiabetics who are less hyperglycemic. Because the AIR significantly predicts early insulin responses to a mixed meal, it can be inferred that the insulin response to a mixed meal would be even greater and the degree of hyperglycemia less if the AIR of the most hyperglycemic nondiabetics was as high as that in some of the less hyperglycemic nondiabetics. Thus, both insulin resistance and abnormal insulin secretory function contribute to hyperglycemia in the most hyperglycemic nondiabetics. Compared to the most glucose-tolerant subjects, nondiabetics with modest increases in glycemia have both higher insulin responses to ingested nutrients and higher AIRs. The modest increase in glycemia in these subjects, therefore, can be attributed to insulin resistance alone. Thus, variance in both insulin action and insulin secretory function, in varying degrees, account for the variance in glucose tolerance in nondiabetics.

Prospective Data

Large numbers of cross-sectional studies have firmly established the metabolic characteristics of persons with NIDDM compared to those of nondiabetics with impaired glucose tolerance or normal glucose tolerance. Several characteristics of persons with NIDDM are observed in nondiabetics, but it cannot be concluded which characteristic is a prediabetic abnormality. Such conclusions can only be drawn from prospective studies, in which nondiabetics are metabolically characterized and followed over time to determine who does and does not develop NIDDM. A major advance in the last decade has been the large number of prospective studies that have determined which metabolic abnormalities are prediabetic and which are not.

Obesity

Prospective studies of Caucasians in Norway,[53] Sweden,[54] Israel,[55,56] and the United States,[57–59] as well as in Mexican Americans in Texas[60] and in Pima Indians in Arizona,[61] have shown conclusively that obesity is a major risk factor for NIDDM. In addition, recent studies of Israelis and Pima Indians have indicated that duration of obesity, in addition to the degree of obesity, is a risk factor for NIDDM.[56,62] The risk for NIDDM in Pima Indians is twice as high in those who have been obese for 10 years or more compared to those who have been obese for less than 5 years.[62]

A central distribution of body fat is also a major risk factor for NIDDM, in addition to the effect of the degree of obesity per se. In Swedish men matched for body mass index, a central distribution of fat, as estimated by the ratio of waist to hip circumferences, was found to be a major risk factor for NIDDM.[63] In Pima Indians, central obesity, as estimated by the ratio of waist to thigh circumferences, was determined to be an additional risk factor for the disease.[64] Moreover, increased intra-abdominal fat in Japanese American men, estimated using computed tomography, was found to increase the risk of NIDDM.[65]

It is clear, however, that obesity is not the only major risk factor for NIDDM. Although many U.S. Caucasians are obese, only about 10% of the population has NIDDM. Among Caucasians,[57] as well as among Pima Indians,[61] parental diabetes is a major risk factor for NIDDM, independent of the effect of obesity. This parental effect on the risk of NIDDM must be related to other familial, probably genetic, metabolic abnormalities that affect insulin secretory function, insulin resistance, and/or hepatic glucose production.

Insulin Secretory Dysfunction

Three groups of investigators have reported the results of prospective studies in which early insulin secretory responses to IV glucose were measured in nondiabetic subjects who underwent follow-up for several years to determine who developed NIDDM. These studies included nondiabetics who had normal glucose tolerance (according to the criteria of the World Health Organization[1,2]), as well as nondiabetics who had abnormal or impaired glucose tolerance. Based on studies of a Swedish population, Efendic, Luft and Wajngot[66] concluded that ". . . subjects with an inappropriately low insulin response in relation to insulin sensitivity . . ." were prediabetic. Similarly, prospective studies of nondiabetic Pima Indians indicated that a relatively low AIR to IV glucose was a weak risk factor for NIDDM, but only when referenced to the degree of insulin resistance.[64] Lungdren et al.[67] also found a low AIR to be a predictor of NIDDM in Swedish women. They further observed that many women with a low response did not develop diabetes, and a few women with the highest insulin response developed diabetes, leading them to conclude that ". . . no safe level could be identified above which diabetes did not appear." This is similar to the results found among the Pimas, in which diabetes occurred in some persons with the highest insulin responses[64] (Fig. 50-4).

In contrast to the three studies of subjects with normal and impaired glucose tolerance, Warram et al.[68] and Martin et al.[69] conducted prospective studies of offspring of two parents with NIDDM who had normal glucose tolerance at the time of baseline examination. In their analyses, a low AIR was not predictive of NIDDM. This is different from the results in Pima Indians, in

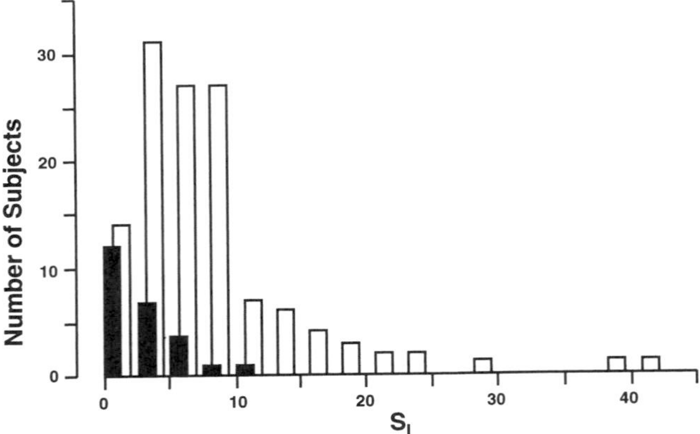

Figure **50-4.** Results of a prospective study of 155 offspring of parents with NIDDM attending the Joslin Clinic. □, Remained nondiabetic (n=126); ■, developed diabetes (n=25); S_I, insulin sensitivity as determined from the intravenous glucose tolerance test using the Bergman minimal model. (Adapted with permission from Martin BC, Waarom JH, Krolewski AS, et al. Role of glucose and insulin resistance in development of type 2 diabetes mellitus. Results of a 25-year follow-up study. Lancet 1992;340:925–929. © by The Lancet Ltd.)

whom a low AIR was still a weak predictor of NIDDM if the analyses were restricted to those who initially had normal glucose tolerance.[64]

There are several prospective studies of the predictive effect of insulin responses to glucose ingestion and of the late, or second-phase, insulin response to IV glucose. These can generally be divided into studies of subjects who originally had normal glucose tolerance or impaired glucose tolerance. In subjects with impaired glucose tolerance, a low insulin response 2 hours after glucose ingestion is predictive of NIDDM in French men,[70] Nauruans,[71] the Japanese population,[72] and Pima Indians.[73] In those with normal glucose tolerance, the converse is true; that is, a high, late insulin response is predictive of NIDDM in normal glucose-tolerant U.S. Caucasians,[68,69] Nauruans,[71] and Pima Indians.[73]

Insulin Resistance

As the fasting plasma insulin concentration is well correlated with the degree of insulin resistance in nondiabetics, it has, therefore, been used as a surrogate measure of whole body insulin action in many prospective studies. In several populations, including Caucasians in the U.S. and Sweden,[67] French men,[70] Mexican Americans,[60] Nauruans,[71] and Pima Indians,[73] a high fasting plasma insulin concentration has been found to be a major risk factor for NIDDM in persons with either normal glucose tolerance or impaired glucose tolerance, or both.

Confirmation of these findings implicating insulin resistance as a major risk factor for NIDDM has been reported in Caucasians[68,69] and Pima Indians,[64] in whom more accurate measurements of insulin action in the whole body were made. In the Caucasian study,[68,69] IV glucose tolerance tests were performed in the normal glucose-tolerant offspring of two parents with NIDDM; these subjects then underwent follow-up for approximately 15 years to determine diabetes status. Insulin action was estimated from the results of the IV glucose tolerance test using either the Kg (the rate of decline of the plasma glucose concentration)[68] or the Bergman minimal model.[69] Those subjects in the study who were most insulin-resistant had a several-fold increased risk of NIDDM (see Fig. 50-4).

In studies of Pima Indians, insulin action in vivo was measured using the hyperinsulinemic euglycemic clamp technique. Compared to the most insulin-sensitive Pimas (90th percentile), the most insulin-resistant Pimas (10th percentile) had a 30-fold greater risk of NIDDM after 6 years of follow-up (Fig. 50-5).[64]

Importantly, in both these studies, insulin resistance was a major risk factor for NIDDM in addition to the effect of obesity and, in the Pima study, in addition to the effect of central obesity.

Excess Hepatic Glucose Production

The rate of postabsorptive hepatic glucose production has been measured only in a prospective study of Pima Indians.[64] In that study, the rate of hepatic glucose production, measured after an overnight fast using glucose tracers, was not predictive of NIDDM. However, the extent of insulin-mediated suppression of hepatic

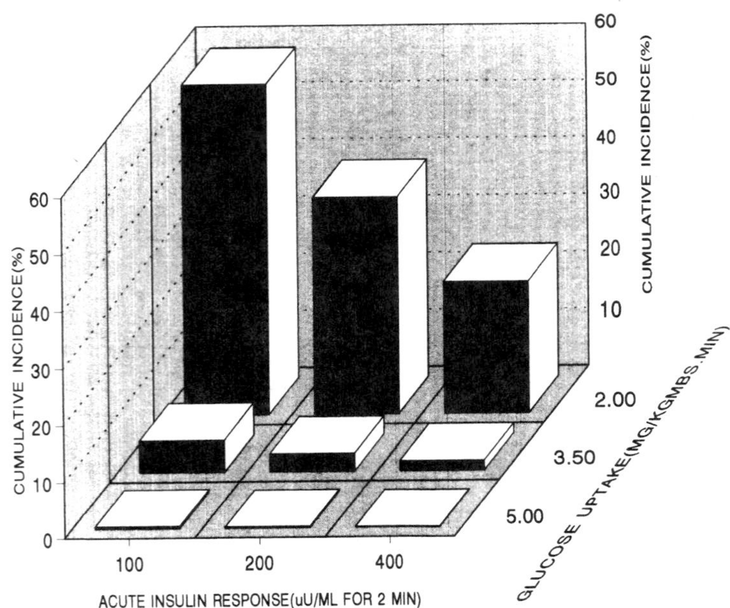

Figure **50-5.** The 6-year cumulative incidence of NIDDM (determined by proportional hazards analysis) by tertiles of insulin action in vivo and acute insulin response to glucose in 200 nondiabetic Pima Indians. KGMBS = kilograms of metabolic body size. (Reproduced with permission from Lillioja A, Mott DM, Spraul M, et al. Insulin resistance and insulin secretory dysfunction as precursor of non–insulin-dependent diabetes mellitus. Prospective studies of Pima Indians. N Engl J Med 1993;329:1988–92.)

glucose production, measured during use of a hyperinsulinemic clamp, was a weak predictor of NIDDM, indicating that hepatic insulin resistance was a weak risk factor for the disease.[64]

Summary and Implications of Prospective Data

Obesity is a major risk factor for NIDDM, and a central distribution of fat adds additional risk. Insulin resistance is another, independent, major risk factor. These data have been confirmed by different investigators in different populations and are found in nondiabetic subjects with normal glucose tolerance or impaired glucose tolerance, or both. There are no reports in which obesity and insulin resistance were found not to be predictive of NIDDM.

Based on data from different populations with impaired glucose tolerance, it has also been firmly established that reduced insulin secretion hours after glucose ingestion, or 10–60 minutes after IV glucose infusion, is predictive of NIDDM. Conversely, in those with normal glucose tolerance, a late hyperinsulinemic response is predictive. In addition, among normal glucose-tolerant subjects, a lower AIR is frequently, but not universally, predictive of NIDDM. Thus, a low AIR appears to be a weaker predictor than either obesity or insulin resistance.

Excess fasting hepatic glucose production was not predictive of NIDDM in the one study in which it was measured. Although this study needs to be repeated in other populations, the result is consistent with the cross-sectional observation that the rate of fasting hepatic glucose production is unrelated to the degree of glucose tolerance among nondiabetics.

Of the four metabolic characteristics of people with NIDDM—obesity, insulin resistance, insulin secretory dysfunction, and excess hepatic glucose production—all but the last of these are found among nondiabetics with some impairment of glucose tolerance, and each abnormality increases the risk of NIDDM. Among nondiabetics with normal glucose tolerance, obesity and insulin resistance are major risk factors; a relatively low AIR appears to be an additional, but much weaker risk factor.

Overall Summary and Conclusions

It is clear from cross-sectional data collected from many different populations that, compared to nondiabetics with normal glucose tolerance, nondiabetics with impaired glucose tolerance are more obese, more insulin-resistant, and more hyperinsulinemic in response to oral nutrients. They also have lower AIRs to IV glucose, and the physiologic relevance of this is supported by its correlation with early insulin responses after a mixed meal. Thus, except for excess fasting hepatic glucose production, nondiabetics with impaired glucose tolerance have all the abnormal characteristics of persons with NIDDM, although in differing severity and proportion. It is not surprising, therefore, that each of these metabolic defects—obesity, insulin resistance, and insulin secretory dysfunction—has been found to be uniformly predictive of NIDDM in nondiabetics with impaired glucose tolerance.

The available prospective data have also uniformly identified obesity and insulin resistance as major risk factors for NIDDM among nondiabetics with normal glucose tolerance. In three of four studies, abnormal insulin secretory function was also predictive of NIDDM, although in two of these three studies, it was a much weaker predictor than obesity and insulin resistance.

The general conclusion to be made from all these cross-sectional and prospective data is that obesity, insulin resistance, and insulin secretory dysfunction are metabolic abnormalities that can be identified in prediabetic subjects years before they develop NIDDM.

If these data are considered in the context of diabetes mellitus secondary to other causes, a generalized view of the risk of diabetes in various populations emerges. Assuming obesity affects diabetes risk only by affecting insulin action or insulin secretion, then the risk of diabetes can be viewed as a function of variations in insulin action and insulin secretion. In this scheme, several points are well established. When insulin secretion is reduced to zero as a result of destruction of β-cells by autoimmune mechanisms (as in insulin-dependent diabetes mellitus or by chronic pancreatitis, etc.), the lifetime risk of diabetes approaches 100%. In persons with the most severe degrees of insulin resistance (e.g., those with insulin receptor mutations), diabetes risk is extremely high,[74] and only those with the greatest insulin secretory responses will not develop the disease. Between these extremes lie the more common situations. The risk of diabetes increases approximately linearly, and only gradually, from high to low insulin secretory function, until the lowest levels of insulin secretion are reached, when diabetes risk increases more abruptly. The slope of the relationship between diabetes risk and insulin secretory function becomes steeper in those who are more insulin-resistant; that is, the risk of diabetes increases more geometrically relative to decreases in insulin action.

Relative to U.S. Caucasians, Pima Indians have greater insulin secretory responses,[75] but they have an increased risk of NIDDM owing to greater degrees of insulin resistance.[75] The Mexican American population has a risk that is intermediate between these two groups, and persons with glucokinase mutations[4] have an increased risk of diabetes secondary to a defect in insulin secretion. There is, of course, considerable overlap between these groups. For example, there are likely some Caucasians who are as insulin-resistant as the average Pima Indian, but because their insulin secretory function is not as high, they may actually have a greater risk of NIDDM than most Pimas. Similarly, there are Pimas with insulin secretory function similar to the average Caucasian, which, because of their increased insulin resistance, would increase their risk of NIDDM.

Although recent prospective data have clarified the relative roles of insulin resistance and insulin secretory function in diabetes risk, it remains unclear how these physiologic factors interact to result in NIDDM. It is easy to understand how diabetes develops in the absence of insulin secretion, but how does insulin resistance gradually result in the disease? Does insulin secretory function simply decrease with age? Preliminary data indicate that chronic mild hyperglycemia (which must occur with insulin resistance to increase insulin responses) gradually impairs β-cell function.[76] It has also been suggested that hyperglycemia can worsen insulin resistance.[14] The precise mechanisms of this "glucose toxicity" effect are unknown, however. It is also not known how a relatively lower AIR may increase the risk of NIDDM. Because a lower AIR may be associated with higher plasma glucose concentrations within 30 minutes after a meal, could its effect on diabetes risk also be attributable to a "glucose toxicity" effect? It has also been hypothesized that insulin oversecretion can result in insulin resistance and, eventually, in diabetes.[77] In this scheme, however, the mechanism of declining insulin secretion is entirely unclear.

The available cross-sectional and prospective data indicate that no simple metabolic defect is likely to explain the cause of NIDDM in large numbers of people, as previously hoped by many physicians and scientists. A complete understanding of the causes of NIDDM will require a better knowledge of the environmental and molecular genetic determinants of both insulin action and insulin secretory function and, equally importantly, a better knowledge of how they interact pathophysiologically over time.

References

1. WHO Expert Committee on Diabetes Mellitus: Second report. WHO Technical Report Series No. 646. Geneva: World Health Organization; 1980:9
2. WHO Study Group. Diabetes mellitus. WHO Technical Report Series No. 727. Geneva: World Health Organization; 1985:9
3. Taylor SI. Lilly Lecture. Molecular mechanisms of insulin resistance. Lessons from patients with mutations in the insulin-receptor gene. Diabetes 1992;41: 1473

4. Froguelle P, Zouali H, Bionnet N, et al. Familial hyperglycemia due to mutations in glucokinase: Definition of a new subtype of non–insulin-dependent (type 2) diabetes mellitus. N Engl J Med 1993;328:697
5. West KM. Epidemiology of Diabetes and Its Vascular Lesions. New York: Elsevier;1978
6. West KM, Kalbfleisch JM. Influence of nutritional factors on prevalence of diabetes. Diabetes 1971;20:99
7. Joslin EP. The prevention of diabetes mellitus. JAMA 1921;76:79
8. Vague J. The degree of masculine differentiation of obesities: A factor determining predisposition to diabetes, atherosclerosis, gout, and uric calculous disease. Am J Clin Nutr 1956;4:20
9. Feldman R, Sender AJ, Siegelaub AB. Difference in diabetic and nondiabetic fat distribution patterns by skinfold measurements. Diabetes 1969;18:478
10. Hartz AJ, Rupley DC, Rimm AA. The association of girth measurements with disease in 32,856 women. Am J Epidemol 1984;119:71
11. Yalow RS, Berson SA. Immunoassay of endogenous plasma insulin in man. J Clin Invest 1960;39:1157
12. Reaven G, Miller R. Study of the relationship between glucose and insulin responses to an oral glucose load in man. Diabetes 1968;17:560
13. Welborn TA, Stenhouse NS, Johnstone CG. Factors determining serum-insulin response in a population sample. Diabetologia 1969;5:263
14. DeFronzo RA. Lilly Lecture 1987. The triumvirate: B-cell, muscle liver. A collision responsible for NIDDM. Diabetes 1988;37:667
15. DeFronzo RA, Ferrannini E. The pathogenesis of non–insulin-dependent diabetes. An update. Medicine 1982;62(3):125
16. Porte D Jr. Banting Lecture 1990. B-cells in type II diabetes mellitus. Diabetes 1991;40:166
17. Halter JB, Graf RJ, Porte D Jr. Potentiation of insulin secretory responses by plasma glucose levels in man: Evidence that hyperglycemia in diabetes compensates for impaired glucose potentiation. J Clin Endocrinol Metab 1979;48:946
18. Yoneda H, Ikagami H, Yamamoto Y, et al. Analysis of early phase insulin responses in non-obese subjects with mild glucose intolerance. Diabetes Care 1992;15(11):1517
19. Himsworth HP, Kerr RB. Insulin-sensitive and insulin-insensitive types of diabetes mellitus. Clin Sci 1942;4:120
20. Yalow RS, Berson SA. Plasma insulin concentrations in nondiabetics and early diabetic subjects. Diabetes 1960;9:254
21. Butterfield WJH, Whichelow MJ. Peripheral glucose metabolism in control subjects and diabetic patients during glucose, glucose-insulin and insulin sensitivity tests. Diabetologia 1965;1:43
22. Jackson RA, Perry G, Rogers J, et al. Relationship between the basal glucose concentrations, glucose tolerance and forearm glucose uptake in maturity-onset diabetes. Diabetes 1973;22:751
23. Zierler KI, Rabinowitz D. Roles of insulin and growth hormone, based on studies of forearm metabolism in man. Medicine 1963;42:385
24. Alford FP, Martin FIP, Pearson MJ. The significance of interpretation of mildly abnormal oral glucose tolerance. Diabetologia 1971;7:173
25. Reaven GM, Farquhar JW. Steady state plasma insulin response to continuous glucose infusion in normal and diabetic subjects. Diabetes 1969;18:273
26. Harano Y, Ohgaku S, Hidaka H, et al. Glucose insulin and somatostatin infusion for the determination of insulin sensitivity. J Clin Endocrinol Metab 1977;45:1124
27. DeFronzo RA, Tobin JD, Andres R. Glucose clamp technique: A method for quantifying insulin secretion and resistance. Am J Physiol 1979;6:E214
28. Reaven GM. Role of insulin resistance in human disease. Diabetes 1988; 37:1595
29. Kolterman OG, Gray RS, Griffin J, et al. Receptor and post-receptor defects contribute to the insulin resistance in non–insulin-dependent diabetes mellitus. J Clin Invest 1981;68:957
30. Bogardus C, Lillioja S, Howard B, et al. Relationships between insulin secretion, insulin action and fasting plasma glucose concentration in nondiabetic and non–insulin-dependent diabetic subjects. J Clin Invest 1984;74:1238
31. Rizza RA, Mandarino LJ, Gerich JE. Mechanism and significance of insulin resistance in non–insulin-dependent diabetes mellitus. Diabetes 1981;30: 990
32. Caro JF, Dohm LG, Pories WJ, Sinha MK. Cellular alterations in liver, skeletal muscle, and adipose tissue responsible for insulin resistance in obesity and type II diabetes mellitus. Diabetes/Metab Rev 1989;5(8):665
33. Olefsky JM, Garvey WT, Henry RR, et al. Cellular mechanisms of insulin resistance in non–insulin-dependent (type II) diabetes. Am J Med 1988;85 (suppl 5A):86
34. Arner P, Pollare T, Lithell H, Livingston JN. Defective insulin receptor tyrosine kinase in human skeletal muscle in obesity and type 2 (non–insulin-dependent) diabetes mellitus. Diabetologia 1987;30:437
35. Obermaier-Kusser B, White MF, Pongratz DE, et al. A defective intramolecular autoactivation cascade may cause the reduced kinase activity of the skeletal muscle insulin receptor from patients with non–insulin-dependent diabetes mellitus. J Biol Chem 1989;264:9497
36. Thorburn AW, Gumbiner B, Bulacan F, et al. Multiple defects in glycogen synthase activity contribute to reduced glycogen synthesis in non–insulin-dependent diabetes mellitus. J Clin Invest 1991;87:489
37. Damsbo P, Vaag A, Hother-Nielson O, Beck-Nielsen H. Reduced glycogen synthase activity in skeletal muscle from obese patients with and without type 2 (non–insulin-dependent) diabetes mellitus. Diabetologia 1991;34:239
38. Wright KS. Beck-Nielsen H, Kolterman O, Mandarino LJ. Decreased activation of skeletal muscle glycogen synthase by mixed-meal ingestion in NIDDM. Diabetes 1988;37:436
39. Foley JE. Mechanism of impaired insulin action in isolated adipocytes from obese and diabetic subjects. Diabetes/Metab Rev 1988;4:487
40. Bogardus C, Lillioja S, Stone K, Mott DM. Correlation between muscle glycogen synthase activity and in vivo insulin action in man. J Clin Invest 1984;73:1185
41. Kida YA, Esposito-Del Puente A, Bogardus C, Mott DM. Insulin resistance is associated with reduced fasting and insulin-stimulated glycogen synthase phosphatase activity in human skeletal muscle. J Clin Invest 1990;85:476
42. Nyomba BL, Ossowski VM, Bogardus C, Mott DM. Insulin-sensitive tyrosine kinase: Relationship with in vivo insulin action in human. Am J Physiol 1990;250:E964
43. Kida Y, Nyomba BL, Bogardus C, Mott DM. Defective insulin response of cyclic adenosine monophosphate dependent protein kinase in insulin-resistant human. J Clin Invest 1991;87:673
44. Sommercorn J, Fields R, Raz I, Maeda R. Abnormal regulation of ribosomal protein S6 kinase in insulin skeletal muscle of insulin-resistant humans. J Clin Invest 1993;91:509
45. McGuire MC, Fields RM, Nyomba BL, et al. Abnormal regulation of protein tyrosine phosphatase activities in skeletal muscle of insulin-resistant humans. Diabetes 1991;40:939
46. DeFronzo RA, Gunnarsson R, Bjorkman O, et al. Effects of insulin on peripheral and splanchnic glucose metabolism in non–insulin-dependent (type II) diabetes mellitus. J Clin Invest 1985;76:149
47. Kelly DE, Mokaw M, Mandarino LJ. Intracellular defects in glucose metabolism in obese patients with NIDDM. Diabetes 1992;41:698
48. Shulman GI, Rothman DL, Jue T, et al. Quantitation of muscle glycogen synthesis in normal subjects and subjects with non–insulin-dependent diabetes by ^{13}C nuclear magnetic resonance spectroscopy. N Engl J Med 1989;322:223
49. Ferrannini E, Groop LC. Hepatic glucose production in insulin-resistant states. Diabetes Metab Rev 1989;5(8):711
50. Elbein SC, Ward WK, Bearch JC, Permutt MA. Familial NIDDM. Molecular-genetic analysis and assessment of insulin action and pancreatic β-cell function. Diabetes 1988;37:377
51. Lillioja S, Bogardus C. Obesity and insulin resistance: Lessons learned from the Pima Indians. Diabetes Metab Rev 1988;4(5):517
52. Lillioja S, Mott DM, Zawadzki JK, et al. In vivo insulin action is a familial characteristic in non-diabetic Pima Indians. Diabetes 1987;36:1329
53. Westlund K, Nicolaysen R. Ten year mortality and morbidity related to serum cholesterol. A follow-up of 3,751 men aged 40–49. Scand J Lab Clin Invest 1972;30(suppl)127:1
54. Ohlson L-O, Larsson B, Eriksson H, et al. Diabetes in Swedish middle-aged men: The study of men born in 1913 and 1923. Diabetologia 1987;30:386
55. Madelie JH, Herman JB, Goldbourt U, Papier CM. Variations in incidence of diabetes among 10,000 adult Israeli males and the factors related to their development. In: Levine R, Luft R, eds. Advances in Metabolic Disorders. New York: Academic Press; 1978:93
56. Modan M, Karasik A, Halkin H, et al. Effect of past and concurrent body mass index on prevalence of glucose intolerance and type 2 (non–insulin-dependent) diabetes and on insulin response. The Israeli study of glucose intolerance, obesity and hypertension. Diabetologia 1986;29:82
57. O'Sullivan JB, Mahan CM. Blood sugar levels, glycosuria, and body weight related to development of diabetes mellitus. JAMA 1965;194:587
58. Dunn JP, Ipsen J, Elsom KO, Ohtani M. Risk factors in coronary artery disease, hypertension and diabetes. Am J Med Sci 1970;259:309
59. Wilson PW, McGee DL, Kannel WB. Obesity, very low density lipoproteins, and glucose intolerance over fourteen years. The Framingham study. Am J Epidemiol 1981;114:697
60. Haffner SM, Stern MP, Mitchell BD, et al. Incidence of type II diabetes in Mexican-Americans predicted by fasting insulin and glucose levels, obesity and body fat distribution. Diabetes 1990;39:283
61. Knowler WC, Pettitt DJ, Saad MF, Bennett PH. Diabetes mellitus in the Pima Indians: Incidence risk factors and pathogenesis. Diabetes/Metab Rev 1990; 6(1):1
62. Everhart JE, Pettitt DJ, Slaine KR, Knowler WC. Duration of obesity is a risk factor for non–insulin-dependent diabetes mellitus. Diabetes 1992;41:235
63. Ohlson L-D, Larsson B, Svardsudd K, et al. The influence of body fat distribution on the incidence of diabetes mellitus. 13.5 years of follow-up of the participants in the study of men born in 1913. Diabetes 1985;34:1055
64. Lillioja S, Mott DM, Spraul M, et al. Insulin resistance and insulin secretory dysfunction as precursors of non–insulin-dependent diabetes mellitus. Prospective studies of Pima Indians. N Engl J Med 1993;329:1988
65. Bergstrom RW, Newell-Morris LL, Leonetti DL, et al. Association of elevated fasting C-peptides levels and increased abdominal fat distribution with development of NIDDM in Japanese-American men. Diabetes 1990;39:104
66. Efendic S, Luft R, Wajngot A. Aspects of the pathogenesis of type 2 diabetes. Endocr Rev 1984;5(3):395
67. Lundgren H, Bengtsson C, Blohmé G, et al. Fasting serum insulin concentration and early insulin response as risk determinants for developing diabetes. Diabetic Med 1990;7:407
68. Warram JH, Martin BC, Krolewski AS, et al. Slow glucose removal rate and hyperinsulinemia precede the development of type II diabetes in the offspring of diabetic parents. Ann Intern Med 1990;113:909
69. Martin BC, Warram JH, Krolewski AS, et al. Role of glucose and insulin resistance in development of type 2 diabetes mellitus. Results of a 25-year follow-up study. Lancet 1992;340:925

70. Charles MA, Fontbonne A, Thibult N, et al. Risk factors for NIDDM in white population: Paris prospective study. Diabetes 1991;40:796
71. Sicree RA, Zimmet PZ, King HOM, Coventry JS. Plasma insulin response among Nauruans: Prediction of deterioration in glucose tolerance over 6 years. Diabetes 1987;36:179
72. Kadowaki T, Miyake Y, Hagura R, et al. Risk factors for worsening to diabetes in subjects with impaired glucose tolerance. Diabetologia 1984;26:44
73. Saad MF, Knowler WC, Pettitt DJ, et al. A two-step model for development of non–insulin-dependent diabetes mellitus. Am J Med 1991;90:229
74. Taylor SI, Accili D, Imai Y. Perspectives in diabetes. Insulin resistance or insulin deficiency—which is the primary cause of NIDDM? Diabetes 1994;43:735
75. Lillioja S, Nyomba BL, Saad MF, et al. Exaggerated early insulin release and insulin resistance in a diabetes-prone population: A metabolic comparison of Pima Indians and Caucasians. J Clin Endocrinol Metab 1991;73:866
76. Leahy JL, Cooper HE, Deal DA, Weir GC. Chronic hyperglycemia is associated with impaired glucose influence on insulin secretion: A study in normal rats using chronic in vivo glucose infusions. J Clin Invest 1986;77:908
77. McGarry JD. Disordered metabolism in diabetes: Have we underemployed the fat component? J Cell Biochem 1994;558:29
78. Golay A, Chen Y-DI, Reaven GM. Effect of differences in glucose tolerance on insulin's ability to regulate carbohydrate and free-fatty acid metabolism in obese individuals. J Clin Endocrinol Metab 1986;62:1081

Diabetes Mellitus, edited by Derek LeRoith, Simeon I. Taylor, and Jerrold M. Olefsky. Lippincott–Raven Publishers, Philadelphia © 1996.

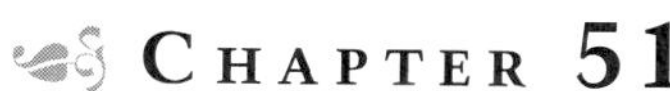

Chapter 51
Impaired Glucose Tolerance: Risk Factor or Diagnostic Category

Michael P. Stern

History and Definitions

The term impaired glucose tolerance (IGT) was introduced by the National Diabetes Data Group (NDDG) in 1979 as part of its new classification scheme and diagnostic criteria for diabetes and "other categories of glucose tolerance."[1] Later, the same term was adopted by the World Health Organization (WHO).[2] One of the principal motivations for the new criteria stemmed from the consensus that earlier glucose cutpoints for diabetes had been "set too low"[1]; that is, they labeled as diabetic those individuals who were at minimal risk of developing either the clinical syndrome of diabetes or its complications. Therefore, the higher plasma glucose cutpoints shown in Table 51-1 were recommended for the diagnosis of diabetes. Commenting on the category that they had labeled as IGT, the NDDG stated the following:

> While individuals in this class are not considered diabetic, they are at higher *risk* than the general population for the development of diabetes . . . to avoid the psychological and socioeconomic *stigma* of the term diabetes, these individuals are more appropriately designated as having IGT, and it is recommended that the terms chemical, borderline, subclinical, asymptomatic and latent diabetes . . . be abandoned."[1]*

The plasma glucose cutpoints recommended by the NDDG and the WHO for the diagnosis of both diabetes and IGT are presented in Table 51-1. The two sets of criteria are highly concordant for the diagnosis of diabetes. Ninety to 98% of the patients diagnosed as diabetic according to the WHO criteria will also be diagnosed as diabetic using the NDDG criteria.[3,4] The NDDG criteria, however, have two disadvantages compared to the WHO criteria: (1) for a diagnosis of diabetes or IGT, they require that an additional plasma glucose concentration intermediate between the fasting and the 2-hour value also exceed 200 mg/dL (11.1 mM), thereby necessitating an additional venipuncture; and (2) the criteria for classification as diabetic, IGT, and normal do not exhaust the universe of all possible combinations of plasma glucose values that can occur on an oral glucose tolerance test (OGTT); as a result, a "nondiagnostic" category was inadvertently created. Although this anomaly could easily have been avoided had one of the three diagnostic categories been defined by difference (as was done with the WHO criteria), the so-called "nondiagnostic" category has led to confusion, as some authors have treated it as if it were a legitimate category.[4] Because the WHO criteria are based on only two, rather than three, plasma glucose values, and because all OGTT results can be classified as either diabetic, IGT, or normal, they are generally preferred to the NDDG criteria.[5]

The precise details of how the OGTT should be performed, including enumeration of conditions and drugs that can lead to false-positive and other confounding results, are not reviewed here, as they are readily available in other authoritative documents.[1,2,6] It should be noted, however, that dietary preparation with a high-carbohydrate diet is not generally considered necessary for healthy, free-living subjects consuming unrestricted diets.[2,6]

An important point to be made about IGT is that individuals who carry this label are minimally, if at all, hyperglycemic under free-living conditions. This seeming paradox occurs because the plasma glucose response to the nonphysiologic glucose load that is used in the standard OGTT is much higher than the response to a calorically equivalent mixed meal. Reaven et al.[7] showed that, although subjects with "chemical diabetes" had abnormal glucose values in response to an oral glucose load (mean plasma glucose of approximately 200 mg/dL at 1 hour and 175 mg/dL at 2 hours), they had essentially normal values in response to a mixed meal. Among Pima Indians, 70% of the subjects with IGT had normal glycosylated hemoglobins, whereas this was true of only 15% of diabetics.[8] For the IGT group as a whole, glycosylated hemoglobin was only minimally higher than among normal individuals (5.86% versus 5.43%) and much lower than among diabetics (8.45%).[8]

*Italics added by this author.

Table 51-1. Summary of National Diabetes Data Group and World Health Organization Criteria for Classification of Categories of Glucose Intolerance

Plasma Glucose (md/dL)	NDDG			WHO		
	Normal	IGT	Diabetes	Normal	IGT	Diabetes
Fasting	<115	<140	≥140	<140	<140	≥140
1-Hour value	<200	≥200	≥200	—	—	—
2-Hour value	<140	140–199	≥200	<140	140–199	≥200

Thus, we should think of subjects with IGT as being euglycemic or nearly so under ordinary circumstances (i.e., when they are not being stressed with a large oral glucose load, such as occurs during OGTTs or during the consumption of large quantities of soft drinks).

Finally, it should be noted that, whereas the diagnostic criteria for IGT are essentially arbitrary, those for diabetes itself are not. Plasma glucose concentrations 2 hours after an oral glucose load have been found to be bimodally distributed in a number of populations at high risk for diabetes, such as Pima Indians, Micronesians from the Pacific Island of Nauru, and Mexican Americans.[9] In all populations in which bimodality has been demonstrated, the nadir between the two modes lies approximately at the cutpoints that the NDDG and WHO have recommended as the diagnostic criteria for diabetes.[9] (Actually, the nadir tends to be slightly higher than the NDDG and WHO cutpoints, which makes these cutpoints slightly more sensitive, but less specific, than the minimum misclassification cutpoints.[9]) Thus, it is reasonable to suggest that the first mode represents the normal population and the second mode represents the diabetic population. Although bimodality has thus far not been demonstrated in populations at low risk for diabetes, a plausible explanation is that there are too few diabetics in such populations to appear as a distinct mode, given the usual size of most data bases.[9,10] In any case, the presence of bimodality of the glucose distribution means that the definition of diabetes is not altogether arbitrary. The same cannot be said of IGT. As illustrated in Figure 51-1,[11] there is nothing in the distribution of plasma glucose values to indicate a cutpoint between IGT and normal glucose levels.

Having defined scientifically defensible criteria for diabetes, one may ask why the NDDG and WHO did not simply declare all individuals who do not meet these criteria to be normal. The remainder of this chapter is devoted to a critical examination of the rationale for defining an intermediate category of IGT.

Impaired Glucose Tolerance as a Risk Factor

The next two sections examine the evidence that IGT is a risk factor; first, for diabetes, and then, for cardiovascular disease. An important question will be: even if IGT is a risk factor for these conditions, is it the optimal method for identifying individuals at increased risk for these disorders?

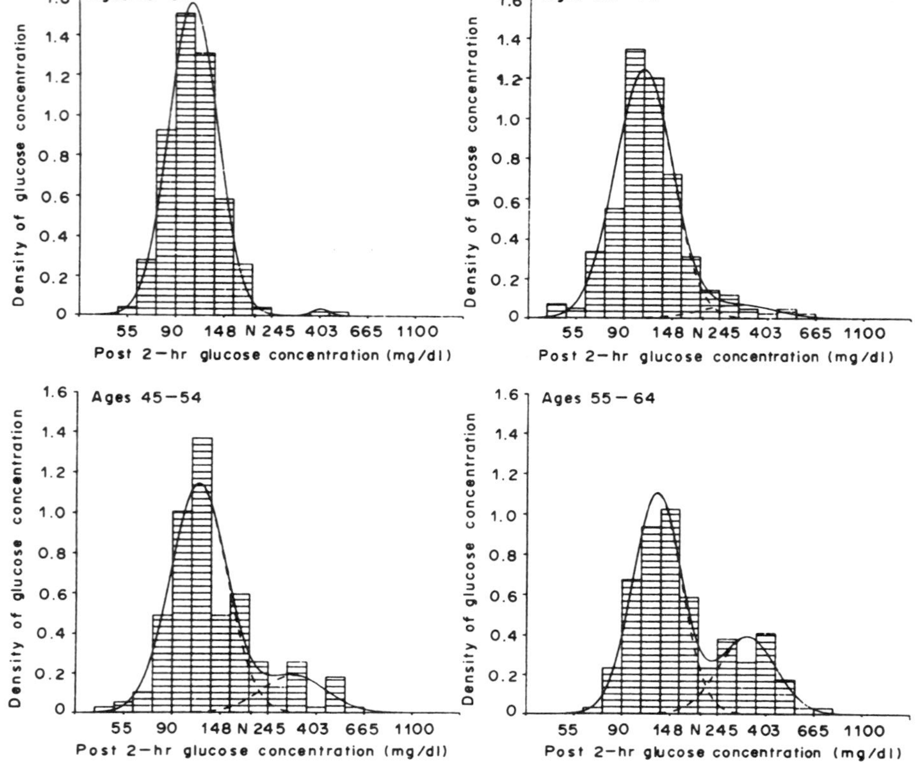

Figure 51-1. Plasma glucose distribution in Mexican Americans illustrating bimodality.[11] The nadir between the two modes is near the NDDG and WHO cutpoints and remains fairly constant with increasing age, although the number of subjects who cross into the second mode increases with increasing age. These distributions also illustrate the lack of any clear demarcation between IGT and NGT. (Reprinted from J Chron Dis 1985;38:5 with kind permission from Elsevier Science Ltd, The Boulevard, Langford Lane, Kidlington OX5 IGB, UK)

Impaired Glucose Tolerance as a Risk Factor for Diabetes

There is little question that IGT is a risk factor for the development of diabetes. This phenomenon has been documented using WHO criteria in numerous populations of diverse racial and ethnic backgrounds. In general, the relative risk of diabetes in subjects with IGT, compared to those with normal glucose tolerance (NGT), increases with the duration of the follow-up period. Thus, among Japanese Americans followed for 2.5 years, the relative risk of developing diabetes among those who had IGT at baseline was 4.2 times greater than among those who had NGT at baseline.[12] The corresponding relative risks were 6.3 among Pima Indians with an average follow-up period of 3.3 years,[13] 7.9 among elderly Finns with a follow-up period of 3.5 years,[14] and 8.04 among Mexican Americans with a follow-up period of 8-years.[15] Among Micronesians from the Pacific Island of Nauru, the rate of developing diabetes among individuals with IGT at baseline was 3.9 times greater than among those with NGT at baseline, a relative risk which, based on the preceding data, is somewhat lower than expected for a follow-up duration of 6 years.[16]

Given that IGT is a consistent risk factor for the future development of diabetes, we may, nevertheless, ask if this definition constitutes the optimal method of extracting the information implicit in the glucose tolerance data. It is a mathematical truism that more information is contained in the continuous distribution of a quantitative variable, such as glucose concentration, than is contained in a dichotomous separation of that distribution into high and low values. This is easily demonstrated in the case of IGT. It has been shown repeatedly that, among individuals classified as having either IGT or NGT, plasma glucose levels remain highly predictive of subsequent decompensation to diabetes. This proves that there is residual information in the plasma glucose concentrations themselves, even after classification of the subjects into IGT and NGT subgroups. Two early studies that demonstrated this phenomenon were the Whitehall Study[17] and the Bedford Study.[18] Using definitions of "borderline diabetes" that were similar, although not identical, to the WHO criteria for IGT, these studies showed that blood glucose concentration 2 hours after a 50-g oral glucose load was not only the strongest predictor of subsequent conversion to diabetes, but was independent of other risk factors, including age, body mass index, blood pressure, and triglyceride level. These findings have subsequently been confirmed in numerous studies in which the specific WHO criteria for IGT were used. Thus, among Nauruans with IGT, both fasting and 2-hour plasma glucose concentrations predicted worsening to diabetes.[19] Although body mass index was predictive in univariate analyses, only the glucose values remained statistically significant in multivariate analyses. Among Japanese patients with IGT who underwent follow-up study for 5–12 years, maximum body weight and fasting and 2-hour glucose levels were all independently related to worsening to diabetes in multivariate analyses.[20] Similar findings have been reported for Japanese Americans.[12] Among South African Indians studied for 4 years, fasting and 2-hour glucose values and body mass index were all predictive of conversion from IGT to diabetes in univariate analyses, but only the glucose values were predictive in multivariate analyses.[21] Among Hispanics from Colorado, fasting, 1-hour, and 2-hour plasma glucose values were all predictive of worsening to diabetes in subjects with IGT at baseline.[22]

A number of studies have demonstrated that there is also residual information contained in the glucose values of subjects with NGT. Figure 51-2 presents data on Caucasians studied in the Paris Prospective Study.[23] As shown in the figure, both among those with NGT and those with IGT at baseline, progressively higher fasting glucose levels were associated with progressively higher rates of developing diabetes during the ensuing 3 years. Similar results have been reported for Pima Indians.[13] As shown in Figure 51-3, the 5-year cumulative incidence of diabetes rose as a function of the 2-hour glucose values both in subjects with IGT and in those with NGT. The results shown in Figure 51-3 were adjusted for, and hence are independent of, age, sex, and body mass index. Finally, among Japanese American men who, at baseline, were classified as having NGT, all points on the baseline glucose tolerance curve were higher among those who, over the next 2.5 years, developed diabetes than among those who did not.[12] Even though only 3 of 75 individuals with NGT developed diabetes, their 60- and 90-minute serum glucose values relative to the values in those individuals who remained normal were statistically significantly elevated.

Given that residual information is contained in both the fasting and 2-hour glucose distributions after classification of subjects according to glucose tolerance (NGT and IGT), the question remains as to how this information can best be captured. One method is mathematical modeling. Using data from the San Antonio Heart Study, in which 2193 nondiabetic subjects who had undergone glucose tolerance testing at baseline were followed for 7–8 years, we developed a multiple logistic model to predict conversion to diabetes from the baseline fasting and 2-hour plasma glucose concentrations. The following model was obtained:

$$\ln(p/(1-p)) = -11.098 + 0.054(\text{FPG}) + 0.030(\text{2hrPG})$$

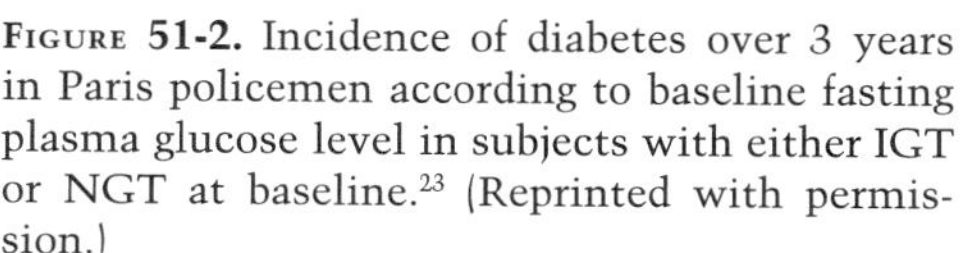

Figure 51-2. Incidence of diabetes over 3 years in Paris policemen according to baseline fasting plasma glucose level in subjects with either IGT or NGT at baseline.[23] (Reprinted with permission.)

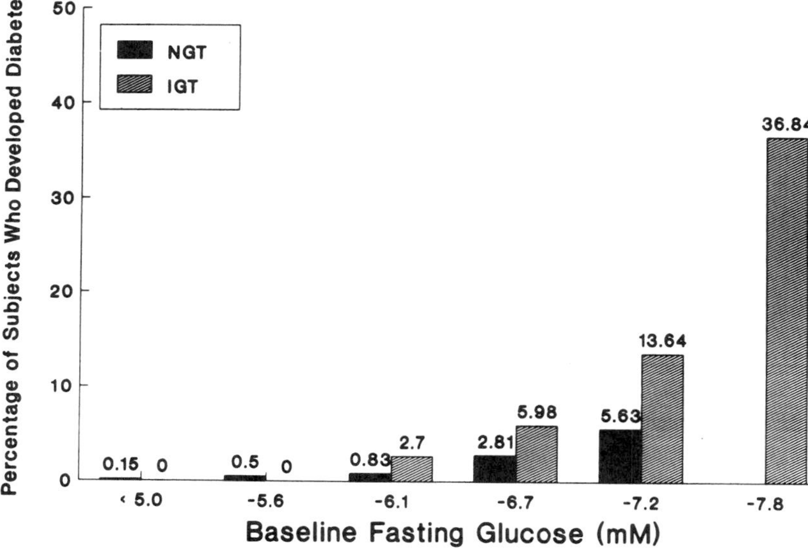

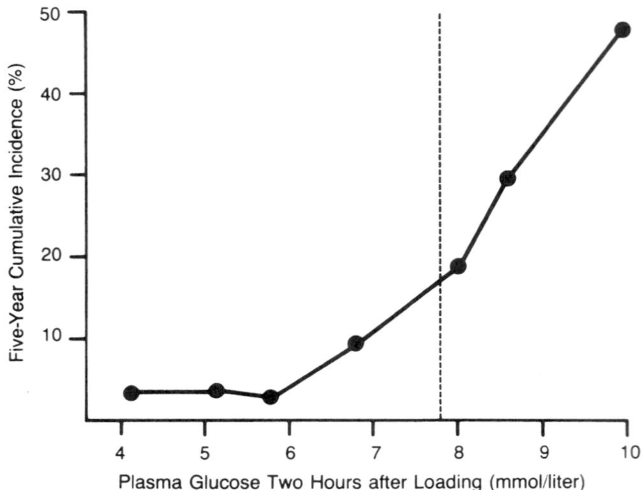

FIGURE 51-3. Incidence of diabetes over 5 years in Pima Indians as a function of 2-hour plasma glucose level at baseline. The dashed line represents the division between NGT and IGT.[13] (Reprinted with permission.)

where p represents the 7- to 8-year probability of developing diabetes, FPG is the fasting plasma glucose level (mg/dL), and 2hrPG is the plasma glucose level 2 hours after a standard oral glucose load (mg/dL).

This model can be used to predict the probability of developing diabetes over 7–8 years for any individual, based on fasting and 2-hour glucose concentrations. It is not immediately apparent that this approach is superior to classifying subjects as IGT or NGT. However, if we rank order the risk scores derived from this model for the 2193 subjects in the study (by inserting each individual's fasting and 2-hour glucose values and solving for p) and then compare the incidence of diabetes in those whose risk scores fall into the top 15.9% of the distribution with the incidence of diabetes in the rest of the population, we can compare the relative risk so obtained to the relative risk of the 15.9% of the population who meet WHO criteria for IGT. (Note that "high risk" was defined as the top 15.9% of the risk score distribution so as to correspond to the prevalence of IGT, which, in our data base, was 15.9%.) The 15.9% of subjects who have the highest risk scores have a 7.8-fold greater probability of developing diabetes than the rest of the population, whereas the 15.9% with IGT have only a 7.1-fold excess risk relative to those with NGT. Thus, even if we dichotomize the model-derived risk scores (not necessarily the optimal way to use them), they outperform IGT as a way to predict future diabetes. Moreover, there is no reason to limit the risk factors to glucose values. Obesity, lipids, and blood pressure are also predictive of diabetes.[15,24] Using a stepwise multiple logistic regression approach on a panel of 14 variables measured at baseline in the San Antonio Heart Study, we developed the following predictive model for the development of diabetes over 7–8 years:

$$\ln(p/(1-p)) = -13.907 + 0.565(\text{sex}) - 0.593(\text{ethnicity}) + 0.055(\text{BMI}) + 0.059(\text{FPG}) + 0.025(\text{2hrPG}) - 0.033(\text{HDL}) + 0.023(\text{SBP})$$

where p is the 7- to 8-year probability of developing diabetes, males are coded as 1 and females are coded as 2, Mexican Americans are coded as 1 and non-Hispanic whites are coded as 2, BMI is body mass index (kg/m^2), FPG is the fasting plasma glucose level (mg/dL), 2hrPG is the plasma glucose level 2 hours after a standard oral glucose load (mg/dL), HDL is high-density lipoprotein cholesterol (mg/dL), and SBP is the systolic blood pressure (mm Hg).

Individuals who fall into the top 15.9% of the risk scores on this model have a 9.7-fold excess risk of developing diabetes compared to the rest of the population whose risk scores are lower. Thus, this model not only outperforms IGT as a predictor of diabetes, it also outperforms the model based only on fasting and 2-hour glucose concentrations.

Impaired Glucose Tolerance as a Risk Factor for Cardiovascular Disease

Although diabetes itself is an unquestioned risk factor for cardiovascular disease,[25] studies of plasma glucose levels among nondiabetics have yielded mixed results. Whether analyzed as a continuous or categorical variable, some studies have found the effect of glucose levels on cardiovascular risk to be independent of other established cardiovascular risk factors, whereas others have not. Still other studies have failed to find even a univariate effect.

The classical studies of this problem are the Framingham Study, the Bedford Study, and the Tecumseh Study, although none of these studies used the modern WHO definition of IGT. In the Framingham Study,[26] casual blood glucose levels were found to be an independent risk factor for cardiovascular disease in nondiabetic women, but not in nondiabetic men. Although the effect in women was independent of other risk factors, these "other" risk factors included cholesterol, blood pressure, and cigarette smoking, but not triglyceride or HDL cholesterol concentrations, as the latter had not been measured at baseline. This limitation, to be discussed later in more detail, is a feature of most other studies that have reported an independent effect of glucose on cardiovascular risk. Thus, the 10-year follow-up of the Bedford Study population also showed an independent effect of "borderline diabetes" on coronary heart disease (CHD) mortality in women, but not in men,[27] and the results in women were independent of systolic blood pressure, obesity, and cigarette smoking. As in the Framingham Study, however, triglyceride and HDL cholesterol concentrations were not available for analysis. In the Tecumseh Study, an independent effect of blood glucose concentration, determined 1 hour after a 100-g glucose load, on cardiovascular risk was observed, but this time, the effect was stronger in men than in women.[28] As in the prior two studies, however, adjustments were made for cholesterol, blood pressure, and cigarette smoking, but not for triglyceride or HDL concentrations.

In 1979, the International Collaborative Group published a summary of nine studies of the effect of postload glucose values on CHD mortality.[29] In only three studies were substantial univariate effects of glucose documented, and none of the studies confirmed glucose as an independent CHD risk factor in multivariate analyses. Additional long-term follow-up results were subsequently published from three of the studies initially reviewed by the International Collaborative Group: the Whitehall Study, the Paris Prospective Study, and the Helsinki Policeman Study. In the Whitehall Study, nondiabetics showed a nonlinear association between blood glucose levels measured 2 hours after a 50-g oral glucose load and subsequent mortality from CHD or stroke.[30] There appeared to be a threshold for this effect that occurred when the 2-hour glucose value exceeded the 95th percentile for the population. This cutpoint corresponded to blood glucose values of 96 to 199 mg/dL, but because these values were obtained on capillary blood specimens following a 50-g, rather than the non-standard 75-g load, the results cannot readily be translated into the current IGT category. The effect of glucose level was independent of the standard cardiovascular risk factors, but, as in the previously cited studies, triglyceride and HDL concentrations were not available for analysis. Univariate effects on CHD mortality of both fasting and 2-hour glucose levels were reported in the Paris Prospective Study,[31] but these effects were found to be no longer statistically significant in multivariate analyses, which, in this case, included triglyceride and serum insulin concentrations. Although HDL concentrations at baseline were not available in this study, it is of interest that adjusting for insulin levels eliminated the independent effect of glucose. This finding

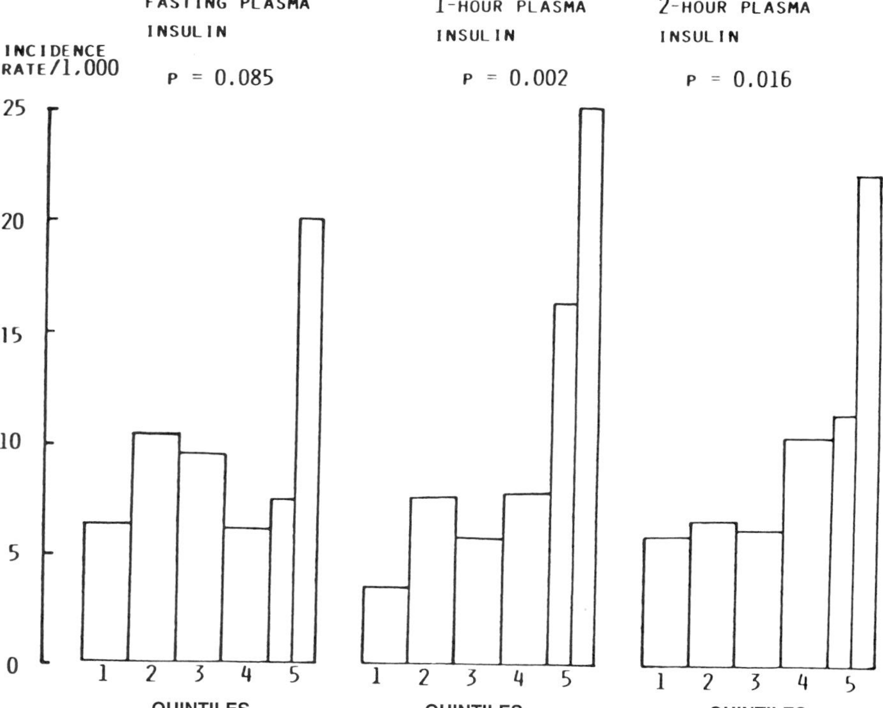

Figure 51-4. Incidence of diabetes over $9^1/_2$ years in Helsinki policemen according to quintile of fasting, 1-hour, and 2-hour blood glucose levels (top quintile divided into two deciles).[33]

may relate to the role played by the insulin resistance syndrome (IRS) as a cardiovascular risk factor, to be discussed later. The results of the Paris Prospective Study were similar whether glucose level was analyzed as a continuous variable or as IGT according to WHO criteria.[32] Subjects classified as having IGT at baseline had a 10-year CHD mortality intermediate between that of normal subjects and diabetics, but again, the effect was not independent of other risk factors. Figure 51-4 shows evidence of a threshold effect for the fasting and the 2-hour blood glucose concentrations (although the 1-hour effect appears more linear) on the $9^1/_2$-year incidence of coronary heart disease in the Helsinki Policemen Study.[33] Once again, the effect was not statistically significant in multivariate analyses. In the Rancho Bernardo Study of a retirement community in Southern California, a threshold effect was seen in women, but the effect in men appeared to be linear across the entire glucose range.[34] Again, these effects were independent of age, cholesterol level, systolic blood pressure, obesity, cigarette smoking, and estrogen use in women, but triglyceride, insulin, and HDL cholesterol concentrations were not analyzed.

These results need to be put in the context of IRS, initially described by Reaven in his 1988 Banting Lecture as "Syndrome X."[35] The features of this syndrome include, in addition to mild glucose intolerance, insulin resistance, hyperinsulinemia, dyslipidemia of the hypertrigliceridemia–low-HDL type, and hypertension. Although not part of Reaven's original description, most subjects with IRS also have excess adiposity and, in particular, excess visceral adiposity.[24] IRS is thought to be a risk factor for both type II diabetes and cardiovascular disease. Indeed, the multivariate predictive model for diabetes presented in the preceding section contains most of the elements of IRS. IRS has been reviewed in detail elsewhere.[24,25] For present purposes, it is sufficient to note that many of the elements of IRS are well-established cardiovascular risk factors (e.g., hypertension and low levels of HDL cholesterol). Moreover, IRS and, in particular, hypertriglyceridemia, are closely correlated with a shift in the spectrum of low-density lipoproteins (LDLs) toward smaller, denser particles.[24,25] Such particles are thought to be relatively more atherogenic,[36–38] perhaps as a result of their enhanced vulnerability to oxidation.[39] IRS is also associated with increased levels of plasminogen activator inhibitor-1 (PAI-1), which provide an additional mechanism by which this syndrome could lead to enhanced atherogenesis.[24,25] In any case, the mixed performance of IGT as a cardiovascular risk factor, summarized earlier, is compatible with the idea that it is but one feature of a comprehensive syndrome that contains other, more potent cardiovascular risk factors. As noted earlier, glucose levels are minimally, if at all, elevated in IGT under ordinary, free-living conditions,[7,8] making it unlikely that these minimal elevations are themselves directly involved in atherogenesis. Given the complex nature of the metabolic syndrome that precedes cardiovascular disease, one may question whether categorizing individuals as having IGT or not is the optimal means of identifying a group at increased risk for cardiovascular disease.

Limitations in the Use of Multivariate Predictive Models

Multivariate predictive models are theoretically superior to predictive models based on a single variable, as it is evident that more prognostic information is contained in multiple variables than in only one. Moreover, statistical techniques exist by which these variables can be combined in an optimal way. Nevertheless, there are several drawbacks to the use of these models.

First, a multiple logistic model requires that the user solve a logarithmic equation. Although this may have been a problem in the past, with the ubiquity of today's personal computers and the advent of programmable, hand-held calculators, solving these equations is hardly an insuperable obstacle. In fact, multivariate predictive models are already used in ordinary clinical practice and research settings. For example, the cardiovascular risk of noncardiac surgery is often assessed clinically by a multivariate point system that estimates the risk of postoperative mortality as a function of a number of prognostic indicators.[40,41] This index was developed using discriminant function analysis on 1001 patients.[40] Multivariate predictive models have also been used in research applications. For example, enrollment in the Multiple Risk Factor Intervention Trial was based on the top 15% (and, later, the top 10%) of risk scores derived from a multiple logistic model based on data from the Framingham Study.[42]

A more serious limitation of multivariate predictive models is that, although they are *theoretically* superior to invariate predicting, the magnitude of this superiority may not be sufficient to justify the greater complexity. Moreover, presently available predictive models are narrowly based. For example, the models for predicting diabetes that were presented earlier and published in greater detail elsewhere[15] have all been derived from the San Antonio Heart Study. Although similar models have been published from other studies, thus far, no effort has been made to validate models derived from one study in any of the other studies. In the field of cardiovascular epidemiology, by contrast, the Framingham model for predicting cardiovascular disease was cross-validated in the Peoples Gas Company Study.[43]

Unlike the multivariate predictive models, the predictive ability of IGT has been replicated in numerous studies. Thus, if one wishes to identify a group of individuals at increased risk for diabetes in a population not previously studied, selecting individuals with IGT will almost certainly identify such a group. By contrast, if one chooses a group defined by the San Antonio Heart Study model, one cannot be entirely confident of the generalizability of the model to the new population. Thus, despite its theoretical deficiencies, we are likely to see IGT used to identify groups at increased risk for diabetes for some time to come.

Impaired Glucose Tolerance as a Diagnostic Category

IGT is asymptomatic and unassociated with any manifest morbidity. Indeed, it is not even associated with significant hyperglycemia except when a nonphysiologic oral glucose load is administered.[7,8] Its sole significance lies in the fact that it predicts future diabetes and/or cardiovascular disease, although it may not constitute the optimal method for predicting either of these conditions. Nevertheless, some authors have tended to regard IGT as a diagnostic category. Is there any harm in this? I believe there is.

In many scientific papers, the results are presented separately for individuals with IGT and those with NGT. Indeed, journal reviewers sometimes ask that this be done. This approach has the potential of seriously distorting the interpretation of the results. For example, in a recent paper comparing two techniques for measuring insulin resistance—the insulin-modified frequently sampled IV glucose tolerance test (FSIVGTT) and the glucose clamp—the results were reported separately for NGT and IGT.[44] Although statistically significant, the correlations between the two techniques were rather low: r=0.53 in NGT subjects and r=0.48 in IGT subjects. If no further information had been provided, one might have been left with the impression that the two techniques were poorly correlated. Fortunately, the authors also presented the correlation for the NGT and IGT groups combined, which was 0.62. The reason the two previous correlations were lower is because when one truncates a continuous distribution—in this case, the glucose distribution—one reduces the ability to detect a correlation. If we concede that the division of the glucose distribution into NGT and IGT is arbitrary and without a solid, theoretical basis, we must conclude that the correlation of 0.62 is the more fair assessment of the degree of correlation between the two techniques for measuring insulin resistance.

Of course, there is no guarantee that an effect will necessarily be linear across the entire glucose range. For example, in Pima Indians with NGT, an elevated 2-hour serum insulin response was positively associated with 2-hour glucose levels measured 2–4 years later, whereas in those with IGT at baseline, these two variables were inversely related.[45] The authors interpreted these results as suggesting that, for subjects with NGT, insulin resistance (as reflected by a high 2-hour insulin response) is the principal risk factor for glucose deterioration, whereas among subjects with IGT, a low 2-hour insulin response was predictive of glucose deterioration. If a nonlinear effect is suspected, it is entirely appropriate to examine the effect separately in quantiles of the glucose distribution, although there is no necessary reason to assume that the IGT/NGT dichotomy represents the optimal quantization. Tertiles or quartiles, for example, may be just as appropriate or even superior. Moreover, it is by no means obligatory to quantize the data. Nonlinear effects can be modeled using continuous variables by introducing quadratic (i.e., squared) or interactive terms. For example, in the 6-year follow-up study of Nauruans,[16] diabetes risk was found to be a function of both serum insulin level 2 hours after an oral glucose load and the product of 2-hour glucose times 2-hour insulin. Thus:

$$\ln(p/(1-p)) = 1.6(2hrPG) + 0.151(2hrIns) - 0.0194(2hrG \times 2hrIns) + \text{intercept}$$

where p represents the 6-year probability of developing diabetes, 2hrPG is the plasma glucose concentration 2 hours after a standard oral glucose load (mM), 2hrIns is the serum insulin concentration 2 hours after a standard oral glucose load (μU/mL), and the intercept is −13.71 (for a 45-year-old male). This equation indicates that at low 2-hour glucose concentrations, the effect of insulin on risk is dominated by the second term in the equation, which is positive; that is, the risk rises with rising insulin concentration. As glucose levels rise, however, the third term assumes increasing importance and, since it is negative, at higher glucose levels, the risk begins to rise with *falling* insulin levels. Table 51-2 shows the predicted 6-year incidence of diabetes for various combinations of 2-hour glucose and insulin levels at baseline. When baseline glucose concentration is 7 mM or lower, insulin is a positive risk factor (rising incidences with rising 2-hour insulin levels). When baseline glucose is 8 mM or greater, declining insulin levels correlate with increased risk. Theoretically, this model, because it is data-driven, should have greater predictive value than one in which the effects of insulin are modeled separately for NGT and IGT.

A number of studies have reported the "prevalence" of IGT.[46,47] If IGT is a legitimate diagnostic category, there is nothing remarkable about estimating its prevalence. If, on the other hand, it is merely a risk factor, this practice is dubious. By combining IGT and diabetes itself, it is possible to come up with some alarmingly high estimates of "total" glucose intolerance. Thus, using WHO criteria, it has been reported that 18% of U.S. adults aged 20–74 years, and 41.5% of U.S. adults aged 65–74 years, have "glucose intolerance."[46] On a world-wide basis, a number of populations are said to have prevalences of "total" glucose intolerance in excess of 25% among individuals 30–64 years of age.[47] There is no doubt that type II diabetes is a serious public health problem in developed countries and a growing public health problem in developing countries.[48] These extraordinarily high prevalence fig-

TABLE 51-2. Interactive Effect of Varying Glucose and Insulin Concentrations on the 6-Year Incidence of Type II Diabetes in Nauruans

2-Hour Insulin Concentration at Baseline (μU/mL)	2-Hour Glucose Concentration at Baseline			
	6 mM	7 mM	8 mM	9 mM
50	0.08	0.14	0.24	0.37
75	0.18	0.20	0.22	0.25
100	0.34	0.27	0.70	0.15
125	0.55	0.35	0.19	0.09
150	0.76	0.44	0.17	0.05

ures, however, exaggerate the problem. Many of the people included in the total glucose intolerance category will never develop diabetes or suffer from its complications. Thus, Yudkin et al.[49] summarized 14 prospective studies of IGT, 7 of which used WHO or NDDG criteria, and noted that only 14–47% of patients (median, 28%) progressed to clinical diabetes over a follow-up period ranging from 2–17 years (median, 8 years). The remainder either remained stable with persistent IGT (20–51%; median, 29%) or reverted to normal (13–53%; median, 35%).

Reproducibility of Oral Glucose Tolerance Test Results

There is a large body of literature documenting the poor reproducibility of the results of OGTTs.[50–54] O'Sullivan et al. studied 52 women who underwent OGTTs in the third trimester of each of three pregnancies and 53 nonpregnant women who underwent three annual OGTTs.[51] For each group, these investigators partitioned the variance in blood glucose measurements into four components: interindividual variation; intraindividual variation; time effect; and laboratory variation. For both groups and for both the fasting and 1-hour values, intraindividual variation accounted for more than 50% of the overall variation (range of 54.5–68.0%), whereas interindividual variation accounted for 15–33.8%. Laboratory variation accounted for about 18% of the overall variation in fasting values, but only about 3% of the overall variation in 1-hour values. Olefsky and Reaven[53] administered two OGTTs 48 hours apart to 31 individuals and found that 9 of 31 replicate fasting values deviated by more than 10%, but none by more than 30%. The 1-hour values, by contrast were considerably more variable, with 22 of 31 replicate values deviating by more than 10% and 6 by more than 30%. Riccardi et al.[54] studied a group of 67 individuals who were classified as having IGT according to the criteria of the European Association for the Study of Diabetes, which are similar, although not identical, to the WHO criteria. A second test performed 2–4 months later revealed that only 56% continued to show IGT. Thirty-five percent were normal on the second test and 9% were reclassified as diabetic.

A number of reasons have been offered to explain the poor reproducibility of the OGTT, such as variations in gastric emptying time and in intestinal absorption.[55] There is evidence to suggest, however, that there is no significant difference in reproducibility between OGTTs and IV glucose tolerance tests (IVGTTs), implying that the variability of the OGTT is not solely or even primarily attributable to gastrointestinal function.[52]

It is important to realize that, despite the rather distressing degree of intraindividual variability, the *mean* values for a group of individuals is quite stable on repeat testing.[50,52,53] For example, in the study by McDonald et al.[50] the *mean* fasting blood glucose values in 334 men ranged from only 76.0–78.2 mg/dL on six independent surveys over the course of 1 year. Similarly, the mean 1-hour values ranged from 101.9–108.1 mg/dL, and the mean 2-hour values ranged from 84.7–88.1 mg/dL. As shown in Figure 51-5 the *mean* glucose values on the paired OGTTs in the study by Olefsky and Reaven[53] were virtually superimposable. By contrast, Swai et al.[56] noted a downward drift in the *mean* 2-hour glucose value when the test was repeated 1 week after an original survey in a Tanzanian population, most of whose members had not previously experienced venipuncture. Because of the study design, these investigators believed that this drift could not be explained by regression to the mean and attributed it instead to an acclimatization response similar to that which is seen with repeat blood pressure measurements.

Although the marked intraindividual variability of the OGTT makes it hazardous to use this test to forecast outcomes for individuals, the more satisfactory reproducibility of group mean values allows one to use the test to forecast outcomes for groups. It is this feature that accounts for the consistently high relative risk for developing diabetes among *groups* of individuals with IGT versus those with NGT, which, as noted above, is 4- to 8-fold higher than that of the NGT group, despite the poor reproducibility of the test at the level of the individual. It remains to be seen if risks scores based on multivariate models will be any more reproducible than IGT.

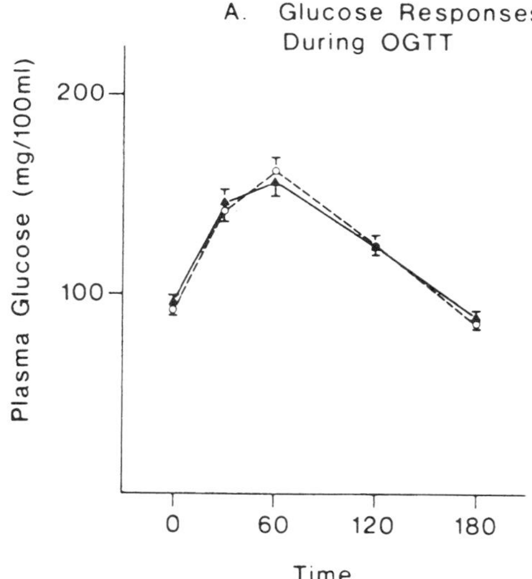

Figure 51-5. Mean glucose response to two identical OGTTs performed 48 hours apart in 31 subjects.[53] (Reprinted with permission.)

Summary and Conclusions

Whereas the NDDG and WHO cutpoints for the diagnosis of diabetes correspond roughly to the nadir of the bimodal glucose distribution and are, therefore, not wholly arbitrary, the cutpoints between NGT and IGT are arbitrary. Although subjects with IGT become hyperglycemic following large glucose loads, most of these individuals are minimally, if at all, hyperglycemic under ordinary circumstances. IGT is unquestionably a predictor of future diabetes, but it predicts less well than the glucose distributions themselves, and also less well than multivariate statistical models. Nevertheless, the role of IGT as a diabetes risk factor is well established, having been replicated many times. By contrast, model-based predicting, although theoretically superior, has not been extensively studied. Although poorly reproducible in individuals, IGT is consistently predictive for groups. Unlike the data on predicting diabetes, the data on IGT as a cardiovascular risk factor are mixed. IGT is part of a complex metabolic syndrome known as IRS, which contains many established and potential cardiovascular risk factors that probably explain the statistical association between IGT and cardiovascular disease.

Because most subjects with IGT do not progress to diabetes, and because many revert to normal, the practice of measuring the prevalence of IGT as if it were a diagnostic category is questionable. When combined with the prevalence of diabetes to produce a category of "total" glucose intolerance, exaggerated prevalence rates are obtained.

References

1. National Diabetes Data Group. Classification and diagnosis of diabetes mellitus and other categories of glucose intolerance. Diabetes 1979;28:1039

2. WHO Expert Committee on Diabetes Mellitus: Second report. WHO Technical Report Series No. 646. Geneva: World Health Organization;1980:9
3. Haffner SM, Stern MP, Mitchell BD, et al. Incidence of type II diabetes in Mexican Americans predicted by fasting insulin and glucose levels, obesity, and body-fat distribution. Diabetes 1990;39:283
4. Massari V, Eschwege E, Valleron AJ. Imprecision of new criteria for the oral glucose tolerance test. Diabetologia 1983;24:100
5. Harris MI, Hadden WC, Knowler WC, Bennett PH. International criteria for the diagnosis of diabetes and impaired glucose tolerance. Diabetes Care 1985; 8:562
6. American Diabetes Association. Office guide to diagnosis and classification of diabetes mellitus and other categories of glucose tolerance. Diabetes Care 1994;18(suppl 1):4
7. Reaven GM, Olefsky J, Farquhar JW. Does hyperglycemia or hyperinsulinaemia characterise the patient with chemical diabetes? Lancet 1972;1:1247
8. Little RR, England JD, Wiedmeyer H-M, et al. Relationship of glycosylated hemoglobin to oral glucose tolerance. Implications for diabetes screening. Diabetes 1988;37:60
9. Stern MP. Type II diabetes mellitus. Interface between clinical and epidemiological investigation. Diabetes Care 1988;11:119
10. Stern MP, Rosenthal M, Haffner SM. A new concept of impaired glucose tolerance: Relation to cardiovascular risk. Arteriosclerosis 1985;5:311
11. Rosenthal M, McMahan CA, Stern MP, et al. Evidence for bimodality of two-hour plasma glucose concentrations in Mexican Americans: Results from the San Antonio Heart Study. J Chron Dis 1985;38:5
12. Bergstrom RW, Newell-Morris LL, Leonetti DL, et al. Association of elevated fasting C-peptide level and increased intra-abdominal fat distribution with development of NIDDM in Japanese-American men. Diabetes 1990;39:104
13. Saad MF, Knowler WC, Pettitt DJ, et al. The natural history of impaired glucose tolerance in the Pima Indians. N Engl J Med 1988;319:1500
14. Mykkänen L, Kuusisto J, Pyörälä K, Laakso M. Cardiovascular disease risk factors as predictors of type 2 (non–insulin-dependent) diabetes mellitus in elderly subjects. Diabetologia 1993;36:553
15. Stern MP, Morales PA, Valdez RA, et al. Predicting diabetes: Moving beyond impaired glucose tolerance. Diabetes 1993;42:706
16. Sicree RA, Zimmet PZ, King HOM, Coventry JS. Plasma insulin response among Nauruans: Prediction of deterioration in glucose tolerance over 6 years. Diabetes 1987;36:179
17. Jarrett RJ, Keen H, McCartney P. The Whitehall Study: Ten-year follow-up report on men with impaired glucose tolerance with reference to worsening to diabetes and predictors of death. Diabetic Med 1984;1:279
18. Keen H, Jarrett RJ, McCartney P. The ten-year follow-up of the Bedford Survey (1962–1972): Glucose tolerance and diabetes. Diabetologia 1982;22:73
19. King H, Zimmet P, Raper LR, Balkau B. The natural history of impaired glucose tolerance in the Micronesian population of Nauru: A six-year follow-up study. Diabetologia 1984;26:39
20. Kadowaki T, Miyake Y, Hagura R, et al. Risk factors for worsening to diabetes in subjects with impaired glucose tolerance. Diabetologia 1984;26:44
21. Motala AA, Omar MAK, Gouws E. High risk of progression to NIDDM in South-African Indians with impaired glucose tolerance. Diabetes 1993;42: 556
22. Marshall JA, Shetterly S, Hoag S, Hamman RF. Dietary fat predicts conversion from impaired glucose tolerance to NIDDM: The San Luis Valley Diabetes Study. Diabetes Care 1994;17:50
23. Charles MA, Fontbonne A, Thibult N, et al. Risk factors for NIDDM in white population: Paris Prospective Study. Diabetes 1991;40:796
24. Stern MP. The insulin resistance syndrome. *In:* Alberti KGMM, DeFronzo RA, Zimmet P, eds. International Textbook of Diabetes Mellitus. 2nd ed. Chichester, England: John Wiley and Sons, Ltd. In press.
25. Stern MP. Type II diabetes and its macrovascular complications. *In:* Schwartz C, Born G, eds. New Horizons in Diabetes Mellitus and Cardiovascular Disease. London: Current Science;1995:1–10.
26. Wilson PWF, Cupples LA, Kannel WB. Is hyperglycemia associated with cardiovascular disease? The Framingham Study. Am Heart J 1991;121:586
27. Jarrett RJ, McCartney P, Keen H. The Bedford Survey: Ten-year mortality rates in newly diagnosed diabetics, borderline diabetics and normoglycaemic controls and risk indices for coronary heart disease in borderline diabetics. Diabetologia 1982;22:79
28. Butler WJ, Ostrander LD, Carman WJ, Lamphiear DE. Mortality from coronary heart disease in the Tecumseh Study: Long-term effect of diabetes mellitus, glucose tolerance and other risk factors. Am J Epidemiol 1985;121:541
29. Stamler R, Stamler J, eds. Asymptomatic hyperglycaemia and coronary heart disease. A series of papers by the International Collaborative Group, based on studies on fifteen populations. J Chron Dis 1979;32:683
30. Fuller JH, Shipley MJ, Rose G, et al. Mortality from coronary heart disease and stroke in relation to degree of glycemia: The Whitehall Study: Br Med J 1983;287:867
31. Fontbonne A, Charles MA, Thibult N, et al. Hyperinsulinaemia as a predictor of coronary heart disease mortality in a healthy population: The Paris Prospective Study, 15-year follow-up. Diabetologia 1991;34:356
32. Eschwège E, Richard JL, Thibult N, et al. Coronary heart disease mortality in relation with diabetes, blood glucose and plasma insulin levels: The Paris Prospective Study, ten years later. Horm Metab Res [Suppl] 1985;15:41
33. Pyörälä K, Laakso M, Uusitupa M. Diabetes and atherosclerosis: An epidemiologic view. Diabetes/Metab Rev 1987;3:463
34. Barrett-Conner E, Wingard DL, Criqui MH, Suarez L. Is borderline fasting hyperglycemia a risk factor for cardiovascular death? J Chron Dis 1984;37:773
35. Reaven GM. Banting Lecture 1988: Role of insulin resistance in human disease. Diabetes 1988;37:1595
36. Austin MA, Breslow JL, Hennekens CH, et al. Low-density lipoprotein subclass patterns and risk of myocardial infarction. JAMA 1988;260:1917
37. Campos H, Genest JJ, Blijlevens E, et al. Low-density lipoprotein particle size and coronary artery disease. Arteriosclerosis 1992;12:187
38. Crouse JR, Parks JS, Schey HM, Kahl FR. Studies of low-density lipoprotein molecular weight in human beings with coronary artery disease. J Lipid Res 1985;26:566
39. Tribble DL, Hull LG, Wood PD, Krauss RM. Variations in oxidative susceptibility among six low-density liopoprotein subfractions of different density and particle size. Atherosclerosis 1992;93:189
40. Goldman L, Caldera DL, Nussbaum SR, et al. Multifactorial index of cardiac risk in noncardiac surgical procedures. N Engl J Med 1977;297:845
41. Goldman L. Assessment of the patient with known or suspected ischaemic heart disease for non-cardiac surgery. Br J Anaesth 1988;61:38
42. Multiple Risk Factor Intervention Trial Research Group. Multiple Risk Factor Intervention Trial: Risk factor changes and mortality results. JAMA 1982;248: 1465
43. Stamler J, Epstein FH. Coronary heart disease: Risk factors as guides to preventive action. Prev Med 1972;1:27
44. Saad MF, Anderson RL, Laws A, et al. (for the Insulin Resistance Atherosclerosis Study). A comparison between the minimal model and the glucose clamp in the assessment of insulin sensitivity across the spectrum of glucose tolerance. Diabetes 1994;43:1114
45. Knowler WC, Bennett PH. Serum insulin concentrations predict changes in oral glucose tolerance. Diabetes 1983;32(suppl 1):46A
46. Harris MI, Hadden WC, Knowler WC, Bennett PH. Prevalence of diabetes and impaired glucose tolerance and plasma glucose levels in U.S. population aged 20-74 yr. Diabetes 1987;36:523
47. King H, Rewers M, WHO Ad Hoc Diabetes Reporting Group. Global estimates for prevalence of diabetes mellitus and impaired glucose tolerance in adults. Diabetes Care 1993;16:157
48. King H, Rewers M (on behalf of the WHO Ad Hoc Diabetes Reporting Group). Diabetes in adults is now a third world problem. Bull WHO 1991;69:643
49. Yudkin JS, Alberti KGMM, McLarty DG, Swai ABM. Impaired glucose tolerance: Is it a risk factor for diabetes or a diagnostic ragbag? Br Med J 1990;301:397
50. McDonald GW, Fisher GF, Burnham C. Reproducibility of the oral glucose tolerance test. Diabetes 1965;14:473
51. O'Sullivan JB, Mahan CM. Glucose tolerance test: Variability in pregnant and nonpregnant women. Am J Clin Nutr 1966;19:345
52. Ganda OP, Day JL, Soeldner JS, et al. Reproducibility and comparative analysis of repeated intravenous and oral glucose tolerance tests. Diabetes 1978;27: 715
53. Olefsky JM, Reaven GM. Insulin and glucose responses to identical oral glucose tolerance tests performed forty-eight hours apart. Diabetes 1974; 23:449
54. Riccardi G, Vaccaro O, Rivellese A, et al. Reproducibility of the new diagnostic criteria for impaired glucose tolerance. Am J Epidemiol 1985;121:422
55. Unger RH. The standard two-hour oral glucose tolerance test in the diagnosis of diabetes mellitus in subjects without fasting hyperglycemia. Ann Intern Med 1957;47:1138
56. Swai ABM, McLarty DG, Kitange HM, et al. Study in Tanzania of impaired glucose tolerance: Methodological myth? Diabetes 1991;40:516

Diabetes Mellitus, edited by Derek LeRoith, Simeon I. Taylor, and Jerrold M. Olefsky. Lippincott–Raven Publishers, Philadelphia © 1996.

Chapter 52
Obesity in Non–Insulin-Dependent Diabetes Mellitus

Henning Beck-Nielsen and Ole Hother-Nielsen

The number of subjects with non–insulin-dependent diabetes (NIDDM) seems to have increased epidemically over the past several years.[1,2] Therefore, diagnosis and treatment of the NIDDM syndrome presents a serious challenge, not only to clinicians, but also to scientists and politicians. In the Western world (i.e., Europe and the United States), 5–10% of the adult population older than 40 years of age suffers from the obese form of NIDDM,[2] and in other ethnic groups, the prevalence is even higher. In all populations, the increasing incidence seems to be related to the degree of wealth and urbanization.[1]

In the Western world, more than 80% of patients with NIDDM are obese, but only 10% of obese subjects are diabetic.[2] This means that obesity and NIDDM are not necessarily linked together, but rather, most obese subjects can resist the metabolic burden of Western civilization without developing diabetes, most likely because they do not possess the ''diabetogenes.'' However, the high prevalence of obesity in NIDDM patients indicates that obesity may be of pathophysiologic importance in subjects who are genetically prone to develop hyperglycemia.

Are all obese subjects at risk of developing NIDDM, or is the risk limited to a subgroup of obese subjects with specific characteristics? This question is the focus of this chapter, along with current views on the pathophysiology of obesity and NIDDM.

Estimation of Body Fat

Body weight comprises lean body mass and fat mass. Obesity and overweight are lay terms that denote increased body fat content above a defined normal, ideal, or standard range. Body mass is related to body height. Clinically, therefore, the degree of obesity is often expressed relative to height as body mass index (BMI), which is body weight, expressed in kilograms, divided by the square of height in meters (kg/m^2). Clearly, direct measurements of fat mass would be more appropriate. Body fat mass can be estimated indirectly by the impedance technique, by determining skinfold thickness, or by Dexascanning (i.e., dual photon absorptiometry).[3]

Fat tissue may distribute centrally around and, particularly, within the abdomen, or more peripherally, predominantly in subcutaneous sites. Because adipose tissue in the central and peripheral regions may behave differently in metabolic terms, evaluation of fat distribution may be important. A simple measure of fat distribution can be obtained from the waist/hip ratio—that is, the ratio of circumferential measurement at the waist (midway between the iliac crest and lowest rib) to that around the hips (at the level of the trochanters) or more precise by CT-scan. Normal values for BMI, % body fat, and waist/hip ratio are given in Table 52-1.

Table 52-1. Acceptable Values for Body Mass Index (BMI), Composition, and Waist/Hip Ratio in the General Population

	Men	Women
BMI (kg/m^2)	20–25	19–24
% Body fat	10–20	20–30
Waist/hip ratio	0.8–1.0	0.7–0.85

Energy Balance in Obesity

Obesity develops as a result of an imbalance between energy intake and energy expenditure in genetically prone subjects.[4] This imbalance results in an accumulation of triglyceride deposits.

A schematic flowchart of energy balance is shown in Fig. 52-1. This diagram illustrates that the size of energy stores depends on food intake and total energy expenditure, that is, basal metabolic rate (BMR), exercise, and thermogenesis (metabolic heat production). Therefore, an increase in energy stores can be caused both by overeating and by reduced energy expenditure.

In most subjects, obesity is attributable to overeating. In some cultures, obesity is a symbol of wealth; in others, it represents an ideal of beauty. In the Western culture, however, obesity does not symbolize wealth and beauty, but rather overeating, and concealed dietary fat seems to be an important etiologic factor. The role

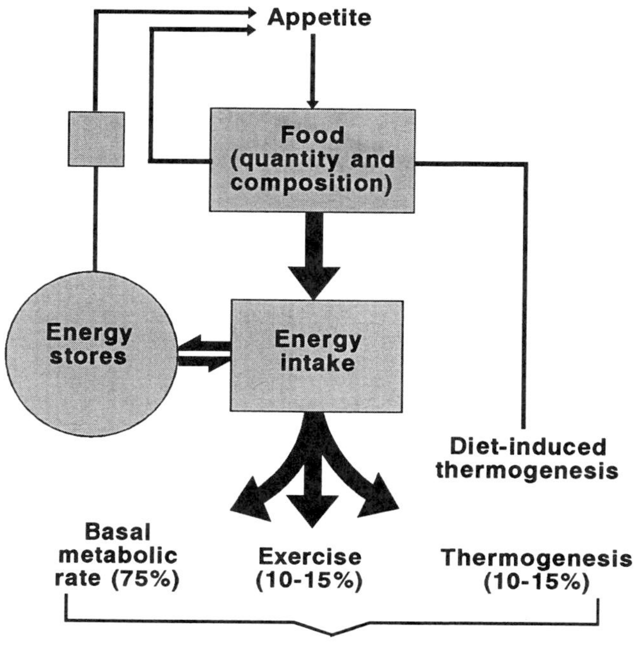

Figure 52-1. Schematic presentation of energy balance in humans.

of Leptin,[63] the new "obesity hormone," has to be researched. Theoretically, reduced production or insensitivity in the hypothalamus may result in overeating.

Additionally, reduced energy expenditure owing to low physical activity may cause obesity. Reduced thermogenesis in obese subjects,[5] especially in obese diabetics, seems less obvious as a primary pathophysiologic factor. In fact, reduced thermogenesis may be of secondary origin. Nevertheless, this factor may add to the development of obesity. Recent studies of postobese and preobese subjects indicate that low BMR may be an important factor contributing to the positive energy balance in many subjects. It has been hypothesized that reduced lipid oxidation could be the inherited defect resulting in low BMR, as both preobese and postobese subjects have elevated respiratory quotients (RQ) and obesity has been proven to be genetically determined with a heritability factor of 0.8.[6,7] A putative explanation for inheritance of reduced fat oxidation could be a missense mutation in the β3-adrenergic receptor gene, as recently found in Pima Indians, and African Americans, and Mexican Americans (in 13–31% of the population).[8] Reduced activity of this receptor, which is expressed mainly in omental fat, may lead to reduced lipolysis and, therefore, to reduced lipid oxidation and low BMR, with abdominal weight gain as an obvious consequence. This genetic defect may be one of several others of pathophysiologic importance in the development of obesity.

Reduced lipolysis and, consequently, reduced lipid oxidation in preobese subjects may lead to increased glucose oxidation (increased RQ) in skeletal muscles. This results in stimulation of glycogenolysis, which leads to depletion of glycogen stores in skeletal muscles. Because glycogen stores are subject to tight regulation, reduced glycogen stores may lead to increased appetite, as suggested by Flatt and coworkers.[9] Thus, a genetic defect in lipid oxidation may lead to elevated appetite and, consequently, to increased food (fat) intake and fat storage.

In prediabetic subjects, glucose storage may also be impaired owing to a genetic defect in glycogen storage, resulting in compensatory hyperinsulinemia.[10] Hyperinsulinemia may inhibit lipolysis and stimulate energy intake, thereby promoting fat deposition. Thus, several defects, including putative diabetogenic defects, may induce obesity.

When lipid stores expand during development of obesity this eventually results in elevation of lipolysis and, thus, in lipid oxidation rate. When lipid oxidation has increased to the level of dietary fat intake, a new steady state is achieved; body weight is maintained at a constant, but higher, level. The obese subject does not only increase fat mass, but also lean body mass, resulting in an elevated BMR.[11] Obesity, therefore, may be considered to be a balanced state characterized by enlarged fat deposits, increased lean body mass, increased BMR, and absolute or relative overeating.

Regulation of Energy Stores

In humans, energy is mainly stored as glycogen in skeletal muscles and liver, and as triglycerides in subcutaneous and intra-abdominal tissues.

Glycogen

Glycogen stores in skeletal muscles are important and, therefore, are subject to tight regulation.[9] They represent rapidly available energy for bursts of rapid muscle activity. Therefore, maintenance of adequate glycogen stores in skeletal muscle may have been important for survival during evolution.

Dysregulation of glycogen stores may play an important role in the development of both obesity and NIDDM. Homeostatic mechanisms compensating for abnormalities in glycogen metabolism may lead to both obesity and diabetes. Glycogen stores seem to be maintained at normal or near-normal levels. In obese subjects, hyperinsulinemia may compensate; in obese diabetic subjects, hyperglycemia may compensate for abnormalities in glycogen metabolism.

A metabolic scheme for the regulation of glycogen synthesis and breakdown is shown in Fig. 52-2.[12] The double regulation of glycogen synthase and phosphorylase activity by insulin and by changes in glucose-6-phosphate (G-6-P) concentrations (allosteric activation) and by glycogen concentrations (negative feedback on glycogen synthesis) is shown. A rise in G-6-P and insulin stimulates glycogen synthase activity but inhibits glycogen phosphorylase activity. Conversely, a rise in glycogen concentrations inhibits glycogen synthase activity while stimulating glycogen phosphorylase.

Glycogen metabolism is influenced by both plasma free fatty acid (FFA) and glucose values. Increased FFA values influence this system, not only by inhibition of glucose oxidation (substrate competition, Randle cycle), but also by inhibition of glycogenolysis and, therefore, of glycogen turnover, resulting in accumulation of glycogen and, eventually, reduced glucose storage.[12,13] Therefore, when glycogen breakdown is inhibited, both glycogen synthesis and glucose uptake will decrease. Because FFA availability (lipolysis) is elevated in proportion to adipose tissue mass, elevated lipolysis in obesity may induce insulin resistance with regard to glucose metabolism, resulting in hyperglycemia, which by mass action may increase glucose uptake in skeletal muscles, thereby elevating intracellular G-6-P concentration.[14] This may stimulate glycogen synthesis and inhibit glycogenolysis, resulting in maintenance of normal glycogen concentrations despite insulin resistance (reduced insulin-mediated glycogen synthesis) in NIDDM. This compensation for reduced glucose storage by hyperglycemia may link obesity to diabetes mellitus.[14]

Fat

Fat stores in subcutaneous tissue and intra-abdominally are not under the same tight regulation as glycogen stores. Fat stores in adipose tissue may expand in an almost unlimited manner during positive energy balance. With any surplus of energy intake, fat and, in extremes, also carbohydrate, will be stored as triglycerides in adipose tissue. These stores only stop increasing when energy expenditure balances the elevated energy intake.

The amount of triglyceride in these stores depends on the balance between lipogenesis and lipolysis. FFA used for lipogenesis in adipocytes is delivered by breakdown of triglyceride in lipoprotein particles in plasma; lipoprotein lipase (LPL) is the key enzyme regulating this process. In adipose tissue, LPL activity is stimulated by insulin, and insulin also stimulates intracellular reesterification of FFA.[15] In obese subjects, adipose tissue LPL activity has been found to be twofold to threefold higher than in lean subjects.[15] In contrast, LPL activity in skeletal muscles is inhibited by insulin.[16] This inhibition, however, is impaired in obese subjects. Indeed, in obese subjects with diabetes, insulin has been shown to enhance LPL activity.[17] These changes, in combination with elevated plasma FFA levels, may induce increased FFA uptake in skeletal muscles in obese subjects and, in particular, in obese subjects with diabetes. This results in elevation of both lipid oxidation and lipid storage in skeletal muscles. As suggested earlier, these abnormalities in lipid metabolism may impair glucose metabolism, thereby linking obesity to NIDDM.

Lipolysis in fat cells seem to be reduced in preobese and postobese subjects, indicating that this defect may play a pathophysiologic role in the development of obesity. The reduced lipolysis may be the genetic cause for the reduction in lipid oxidation seen in some preobese subjects. When obesity develops, however, lipolysis must increase in order to match the elevated fat intake. The etiology for this seems to be, at least in part, an increase in lipolysis in the individual adipocyte, but also is a consequence of the increased fat stores. When diabetes develops, however, insulin resistance

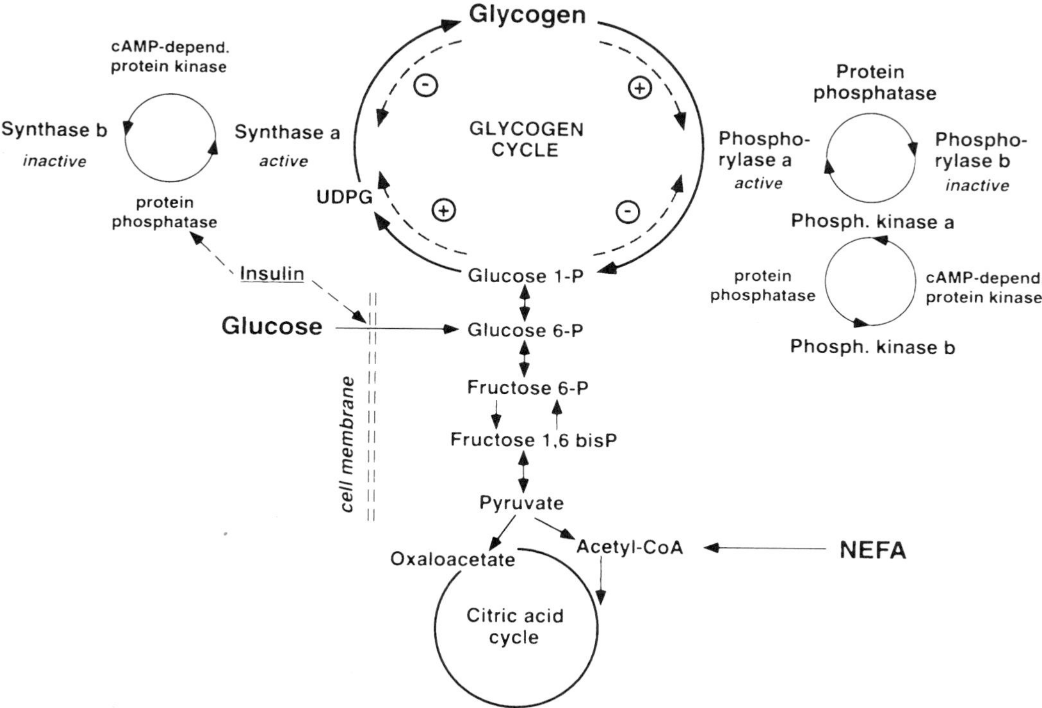

Figure 52-2. Glycogen homeostasis in skeletal muscles. Glycogen synthesis is favored by an increase in insulin values and in G-6-P concentration, resulting in stimulation of glycogen synthase and inhibition of glycogen phosphorylase. Intracellular accumulation of glycogen may itself inhibit glycogen synthesis and, consequently, glucose uptake as well. Hyperglycemia may compensate for a reduction in glucose uptake by simple mass action, resulting in an increase in glycogen synthesis and glycolysis. When glycogen synthesis and glucose oxidation are inhibited, as in obese diabetics, nonoxidative glycolysis may increase, resulting in elevated lactate production (increased Cori cycle activity). *Phosph. kinase,* phosphorylase kinase; NEFA, nonesterified fatty acid. (Reproduced with permission from Felber JP, Haesler E, Jequier E. Metabolic origin of insulin resistance in obesity with and without type 2 (non–insulin-dependent) diabetes mellitus. Diabetologia 1993;36: 1221.)

may also affect lipolysis in individual adipocytes, resulting in a further elevation of FFA values in plasma.[18] Therefore, induction of insulin resistance in fat cells may limit expansion of fat tissue.

Interplay Between Glucose and Fat Metabolism in Liver

Hepatic glucose uptake is normal in obese subjects with and without diabetes and, therefore, does not impair the glucose tolerance in these subjects.[19] Hepatic glucose production (HGP), by contrast, has an important role in the regulation of glucose homeostasis, in particular in the postabsorptive state. The basal HGP rate (postabsorptive state) is normal in obese nondiabetic subjects; assessment of basal glucose production in patients with NIDDM, however, has been flawed by methodologic problems.[20,21] More recent studies suggest that the basal glucose production rate is also normal or near-normal in patients with NIDDM,[20,22–24] despite the presence of both hyperinsulinemia and hyperglycemia, which would be expected to suppress HGP. Maintenance of normal rates of basal HGP could be attributable to increased gluconeogenetic activity in the liver, as the increased lipolytic activity in obese diabetics has been shown to stimulate gluconeogenesis.[25] The mechanism seems to be that the augmented intrahepatic oxidation of lipids results in a reduction of NAD and an elevation of acetyl-coenzyme A (CoA) and ATP concentrations, which causes a reduction of pyruvate dehydrogenase (PDH) activity and an increase in phosphoenolpyruvate carboxykinase (PEPCK) activity, the rate-limiting enzymes in glucose oxidation and gluconeogenesis, respectively. In other words, an increase in lipolysis and, consequently, in lipid oxidation in the liver may inhibit glucose oxidation and increase gluconeogenesis, resulting in maintenance of normal glucose production rates. The substrate for gluconeogenesis may be lactate supplied from the muscles (augmentation of the Cori cycle) and glycerol supplied from adipocytes, which also may add to the lactate supply.

Recent studies have suggested that HGP may be regulated indirectly from peripheral tissues by the substrate supply (e.g., FFA and gluconeogenic precursors). If this hypothesis is correct, then, the degree of insulin resistance in muscles and adipocytes may influence gluconeogenesis and, thus, HGP.[26] The liver may thus be able to produce exactly the amount of glucose needed to keep plasma glucose at the level necessary to compensate for the defects in peripheral glucose metabolism (i.e., insulin resistance).

Fat Distribution

In humans, lipid is stored either predominantly as intra-abdominal fat in the major omentum and in the retroperitoneal space, giving the subject an apple-shaped figure, or subcutaneously on the thighs and hips, resulting in a more pear-shaped figure.

Abdominal adiposity is associated with NIDDM, cardiovascular events, dyslipidemia and arterial hypertension (the insulin resistance syndrome). Therefore, central (abdominal) obesity has a worse prognosis than the more peripheral form of obesity.[27] The cause of intra-abdominal fat accumulation may be of both genetic and environmental origin. High androgen and cortisol values in women and reduced sex hormone–binding globulin (SHBG) values in men promote abdominal obesity.[28] Furthermore, this shape is enhanced by a high consumption of alcohol and tobacco, coupled with a sedentary lifestyle.[29] By contrast, the pear-shaped figure seems to be linked to an increase in estrogens. Because prognosis and metabolic complications differ markedly between these two forms of obesity, subclassification of obesity is clinically important. Therefore, waist/hip ratio is a clinically and prognostically important parameter (see Table 52-1).

Lipolytic activity in abdominal fat stores is considerably higher than in subcutaneous stores.[30] Therefore, because FFA release from abdominal fat deposits is elevated and is delivered directly to the liver through the portal vein, lipoprotein synthesis may be accelerated. In cases of stable body weight, increased lipolysis in abdominal fat must be accompanied by increased lipogenesis. This means that, in abdominal obesity, turnover of FFA and lipoproteins must be very rapid, which, in turn, means that rates of fat supply to endothelial cells, skeletal muscles, and liver must also be very rapid. This phenomenon may contribute to accelerated atherosclerosis and to the induction of insulin resistance in subjects with abdominal obesity.

Causal Relationship Between Obesity and Non–Insulin-Dependent Diabetes Mellitus

In a recent survey in Denmark, the prevalence of obesity in newly diagnosed patients with NIDDM was about 80%, whereas the prevalence of obesity in the background population of similar age was around 40%.[31] Comparable figures have been obtained in other industrialized countries.[32] NIDDM seems to follow the dispersal of wealth and, therefore, the degree of obesity in the society. In certain populations, such as the Pima Indians and Nauruans (inhabitants of an island in Micronesia), where the prevalence of obesity in the adult population approaches 80%, the prevalence of NIDDM is about 40%.[1,32] Thus, epidemiologic evidence suggests that there may be a causal relationship between obesity and development of NIDDM[33,34] (Fig. 52-3).

Obesity seems to precede NIDDM and may provoke diabetes in genetically predisposed subjects. This suggestion is supported by data from a recent Danish study of newly diagnosed patients with NIDDM in general medical practice.[31] The change in body weight from the age of 20 years and until clinical onset of diabetes in the 60s was evaluated from historical weight recalls. Most subjects who developed NIDDM in their 60s were slim at 20 years of age, but from then on, body weight steadily increased until 5–10 years before clinical onset of diabetes. Apparently, a critical BMI level of, on average, 30 kg/m^2 was necessary before hyperglycemia developed. This critical BMI level was higher in subjects developing diabetes at younger ages than in subjects developing diabetes at older ages. This phenomenon may relate to the physiologic decline in β-cell function that occurs with age. Thus, with increasing age, the ability to increase insulin secretion in response to obesity-induced insulin resistance may decrease. Subjects with very rapid weight gain between the age of 20–30 years have been found to have the highest risk for developing NIDDM.

Does prevention of obesity prevent development of NIDDM? This question is difficult to evaluate in human subjects. Experimental studies, however, can be conducted in laboratory animals in which control of food intake is possible. With age, Rhesus monkeys may develop a type of diabetes that seems to be quite similar to NIDDM in humans, both clinically and metabolically. These monkeys, therefore, have been used to study the pathophysiology of human NIDDM. Recently, it was shown that dietary restriction to prevent development of obesity provides an excellent model for evaluation of the primacy of various defects. Under laboratory conditions of ad libitum food availability, about 30–60% of the monkeys developed diabetes, whereas it was shown that prevention of obesity prevented development of NIDDM in all monkeys, in which body weight was stabilized at a mature adult level.[35] Nevertheless, several of these monkeys had defects in insulin action (i.e., reduced glycogen synthase activity in skeletal muscles). Apparently, however, the monkeys may live with this defect without developing diabetes as long as body weight is maintained at normal levels.[36] These observations emphasize the importance of obesity in the development of NIDDM in genetically predisposed individuals.

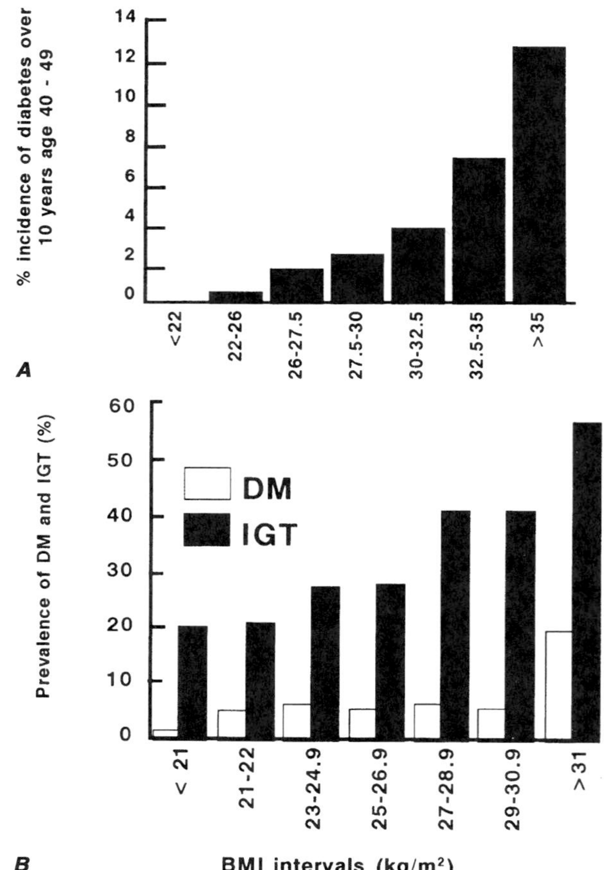

FIGURE 52-3. The likelihood of developing NIDDM increases with the degree of obesity (BMI). Data from Norwegian men (***A***)[33] and Israelis (***B***).[34] *DM,* diabetes mellitus; *IGT,* impaired glucose tolerance. (Reproduced with permission from Westlund K, Nicolaysen R. Ten-year mortality and morbidity related to serum cholesterol. A follow-up of 3751 men aged 40–49. Scand J Clin Lab Invest [Suppl] 1972;127:1; and Modan M, Karasik A, Halkin H, et al. Effect of past and concurrent body mass index on prevalence of glucose intolerance and type 2 (non–insulin-dependent) diabetes and on insulin response. The Israel study of glucose intolerance, obesity, and hypertension. Diabetologia 1986;29:82.)

The Role of Food Quality in Non–Insulin-Dependent Diabetes Mellitus

When people gain weight, they are consuming more energy than they are using. An important question, therefore, may be whether metabolic abnormalities associated with obesity are attributable to being overweight per se or, rather, to the overeating of fat. Apparently, fat-containing foodstuffs seem to be preferred by obese subjects. Several studies suggest that the quality of food plays a major

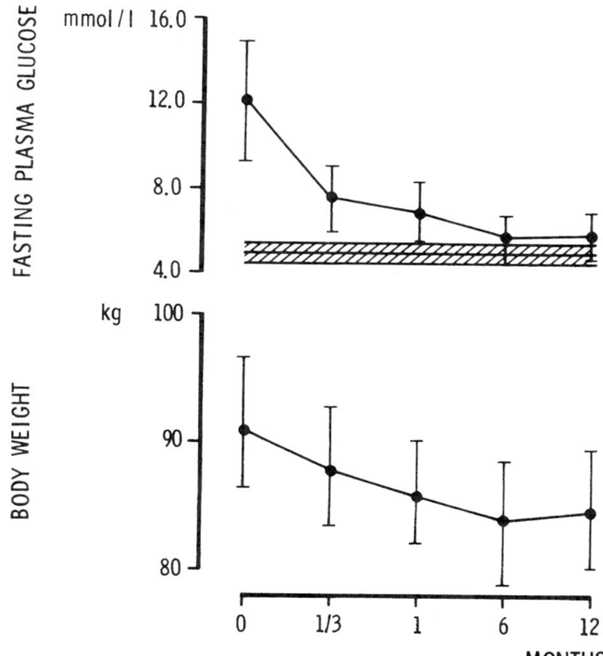

FIGURE 52-4. Normalization of fasting plasma glucose values, despite persistent obesity, in obese patients with NIDDM treated for 1 year with a hypocaloric (6000 kj) diet.[38] (Reproduced with permission from Beck-Nielsen H, Pedersen O, Sorensen NS. Effects of dietary changes on cellular insulin binding and in vivo insulin sensitivity. Metabolism 1980;29:482.)

role in the pathophysiology of diabetes. In Australia, a group of aboriginals with NIDDM were taken back to the desert to hunt for living. They were allowed to shoot kangaroos (kangaroo meat contains only 10% fat) and to catch fish. After 3 months, their diabetes almost disappeared although their weight loss was very modest.[37] A similar experience has been reported in several studies of dietary treatment in obese diabetics. We conducted follow-up studies of a group of obese diabetics for 1 year during treatment with diet only (i.e., a low-fat diet of about 6000 kJ) (Fig. 52-4).[38] Although these subjects were still obese after 1 year, their blood glucose values were normalized. This indicates that reduced energy intake and, in particular, reduced intake of saturated fat may improve glucose metabolism despite persistent obesity.

Recent data indicate that the amount of saturated fat in the diet is especially important, as overeating of saturated fat has been shown to induce insulin resistance and dyslipidemia.[39] In accordance with this, the prevalence of NIDDM has been found to be positively correlated to the % dietary energy derived from fat.[40] Saturated fat may induce insulin resistance by changing the phospholipid composition in the cell membranes, by changing insulin signaling, by inhibition of glycogen synthesis, or by other mechanisms.[41] Unsaturated fat, by contrast, may be less diabetogenic.[41] Although the importance of food quality is well documented, additional studies are needed to clarify the underlying mechanisms.

Insulin Resistance in Obesity and Diabetes

In most studies, insulin resistance is defined as reduced insulin-mediated glucose disposal (Rd) during application of a euglycemic hyperinsulinemic clamp.[42] According to this definition, obese subjects with and without diabetes are insulin-resistant in comparison to subjects of normal weight. Obese subjects with NIDDM, however, are more insulin-resistant than their nondiabetic counterparts (Fig. 52-5).[43] Insulin resistance in diabetic subjects may be inherited. In young, normal-weight, glucose-tolerant, first-degree relatives of patients with NIDDM, we found reduced insulin-mediated glucose disposal 2–3 decades before these subjects may develop frank diabetes.[10] This premise is supported by the finding of insulin resistance—characterized by a 40% reduction in insulin-mediated glucose storage—in the nondiabetic twins of monocygotic twin pairs, who were discordant for NIDDM.[44] Recently, in a prospective study of subjects predisposed to develop NIDDM, it was found that obesity impaired insulin action to a greater extent than in subjects without this genetic predisposition.[45] The effect of obesity was not only added to the degree of insulin resistance, but seemed to potentiate this abnormality. Thus, obesity seems to potentiate the effect of the "diabetogenes" on insulin action. This means that obesity seems to be more harmful to genetically predisposed subjects than to subjects without this predisposition.

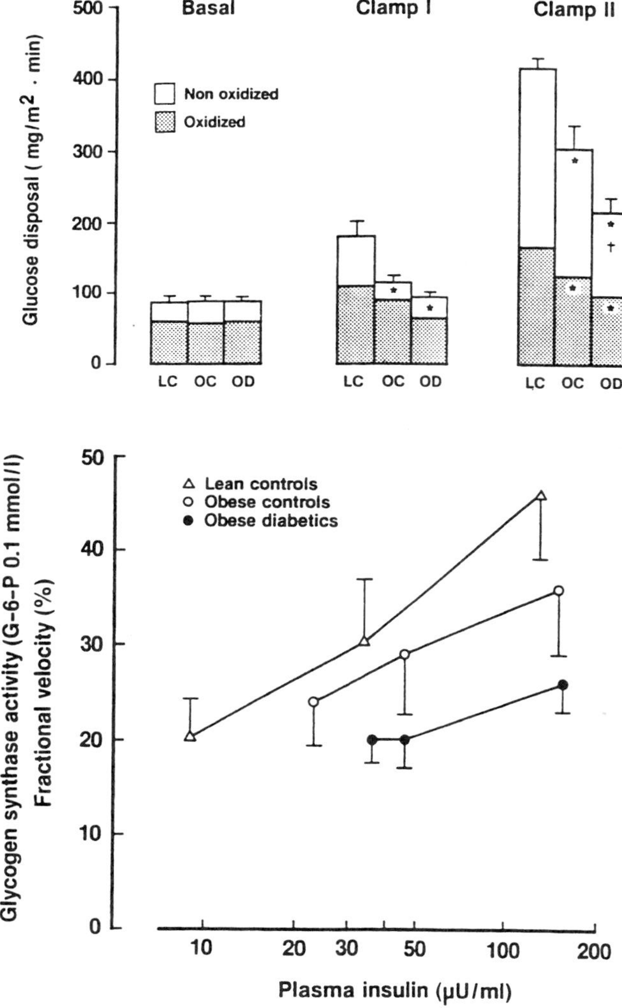

FIGURE 52-5. Glucose disposal and glycogen synthase activity as a function of plasma insulin values in lean, obese, and obese diabetic subjects during euglycemic hyperinsulinemic clamp studies.[43] *LC*, lean controls; *OC*, obese controls; *OD*, obese diabetics. (Reproduced with permission from Damsbo P, Vaag A, Hother-Nielsen O, Beck-Nielsen H. Reduced glycogen synthase activity in skeletal muscle from obese patients with and without type 2 (non–insulin-dependent) diabetes mellitus. Diabetologia 1991;34: 239.)

Inherited insulin resistance, however, is not the only reason for the reduced insulin action in obese diabetics. During weight gain, fasting plasma insulin, FFA, and glucose values increase. This may cause further impairment in insulin action, called ''metabolic'' or ''secondary'' insulin resistance. This insulin resistance will be greater in proportion to the degree of metabolic derangement.[43]

Whether obese subjects who do not develop NIDDM have inherited insulin resistance or only metabolic insulin resistance has been discussed. Until now, no data have supported the presence of inherited insulin resistance in nondiabetic obese subjects. Rather, it has been observed that some preobese subjects may have enhanced insulin sensitivity (increased glucose oxidation and glycogen synthesis), and some postobese patients may have normal insulin action.[4,6] Furthermore, insulin resistance in obese nondiabetic subjects seems to disappear completely after weight loss. Therefore, it is likely that only those obese subjects who will later develop NIDDM may have inherited insulin resistance. This premise is supported by the observation of Martin et al.[45] that early insulin resistance in normal-weight subjects has a high predictive value for development of diabetes 2–3 decades later.

Subjects with abdominal obesity are more insulin-resistant than subjects with peripheral obesity, and insulin-mediated glucose uptake (Rd) in peripheral tissues correlates negatively with the amount of intra-abdominal fat.[46] It is possible, therefore, that either the genetic insulin resistance may predispose an individual to abdominal obesity or that the metabolic burden of intra-abdominal fat is greater than that of subcutaneous fat. The latter possibility seems more likely, as the lipolytic activity in abdominal fat is higher than in subcutaneous fat, which may explain the increased insulin resistance.[30] Furthermore, subjects with abdominal obesity also have an increased number of white muscle fibers with fewer capillaries in skeletal muscles.[47] This phenotype characterized by abdominal obesity, therefore, may be determined by both genetic and environmental factors.

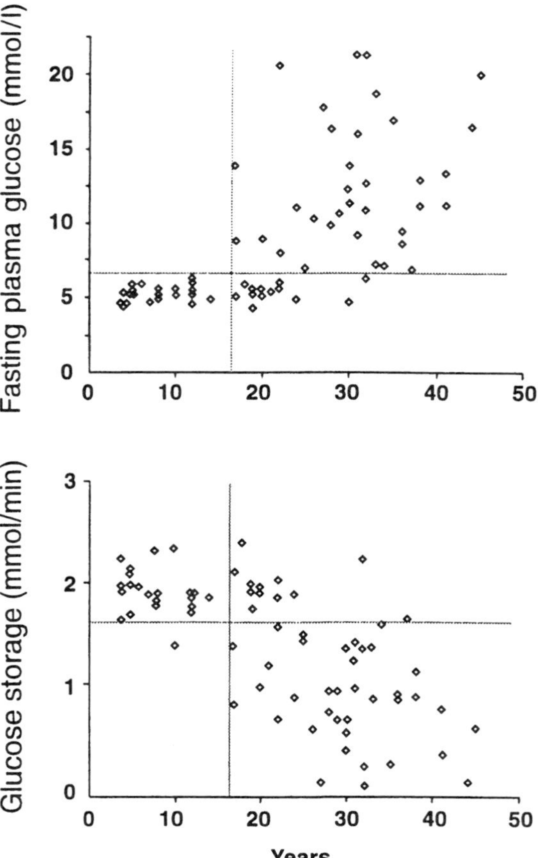

Figure 52-6. Time course for changes in fasting plasma glucose concentration and glucose storage during OGTT in obese subjects developing NIDDM. After about 17 years' observation, plasma glucose concentration started to increase, accompanied by a decline in glucose storage, thus linking these two events together.[12] (Reproduced with permission from Felber JP, Haesler E, Jequier E. Metabolic origin of insulin resistance in obesity with and without type 2 (non–insulin-dependent) diabetes mellitus. Diabetologia 1993;36:1221.)

Cellular Defects in Insulin Action in Skeletal Muscles of Obese Diabetics

In euglycemic hyperinsulinemic clamp studies, it has been shown that obese subjects with and without diabetes are insulin-resistant in both oxidative and nonoxidative pathways in skeletal muscles (see Fig. 52-5).[43] In obese diabetics, the insulin-mediated glycogen synthesis in skeletal muscles is severely impaired. This defect seems to be pathognomonic for obese diabetics, as fasting hyperglycemia first develops when the compensatory mechanisms (hyperinsulinemia) for glycogen storage break down, most likely as a result of impaired insulin secretion. A close relationship between fasting plasma glucose level and glucose storage after a meal has recently been demonstrated by Felber and coworkers (Fig. 52-6).[12] The mechanism underlying the defect in glycogen storage is a completely insulin-resistant enzyme—namely, glycogen synthase.[43] This defect in stimulation of glycogen synthase seems to be of genetic or at least of primary origin (primary to hyperglycemia), because it is present decades before the development of overt diabetes, as demonstrated in normal-weight, glucose-tolerant, first degree relatives of patients with NIDDM.[10] In these genetically predisposed subjects, glycogen content in skeletal muscles was found to be normal, most likely owing to a compensating effect of hyperinsulinaemia.

It is likely that the reduced glycogen synthase activity in obese diabetics is not only attributable to genetic defects, but also to metabolic abnormalities (e.g., increased lipid oxidation and triglyceride storage in skeletal muscles). It has been shown that this metabolic insulin resistance is not only additive, but seems to potentiate the genetic component, which may explain the marked differences observed between obese and obese diabetic subjects in terms of stimulation of glycogen synthase activity (see Fig. 52-5). The defect in insulin action in obese subjects may be of metabolic origin only (i.e., secondary to changes in fat metabolism). The mechanism by which increased fat oxidation and lipid storage in skeletal muscle may inhibit glycogen synthesis seems to be a negative feedback inhibition of glycogen synthase owing to an accumulation of glycogen (as outlined earlier).[12]

In all obese subjects, the reduced glucose oxidation and elevated lipid oxidation that occurs during insulin stimulation may be of secondary origin owing to increased FFA uptake in skeletal muscles, as suggested by Randle et al.[13] Because both insulin-mediated glycogen synthesis and glucose oxidation is reduced, and because glucose uptake is fairly normal, nonoxidative glycolysis must increase, as we and others recently demonstrated.[48,49] This may result in an increase in the Cori cycle, thereby adding to the substrate supply to the liver.

The cause of the primary defect in glycogen synthase activity in diabetic patients has been subjected to intense investigation. Whether it is a defect in the signal from the receptor to the enzyme, a defect in the enzyme itself, or a defect in its regulatory enzymes is still an open question. Recently, however, it was shown that, in cultured fibroblasts from patients with NIDDM, insulin stimulation of glycogen synthase was absent, despite normal activation of the insulin receptor tyrosine kinase.[50] This finding supports the view that the reduced glycogen synthase activity could be an inherited defect in obese diabetics. The glycogen synthase gene, therefore, may be an important candidate gene in NIDDM. Until now, however, mutations have been found in only a few families. Moreover, the protein amount of the enzyme and the transcript seem to be within normal range. Several polymorphisms of the glycogen synthase gene have been described, also in the promoter region, but most likely, they can only be considered to be markers for the disease.[51,52]

The signaling pathways from the receptor to glycogen synthase have been a focus during the last few years. Although these pathways have still not been completely elucidated, mutations in several proteins (e.g., in the insulin receptor and in insulin receptor substrate-1 [IRS-1]) have been described.[53] These mutations, however, may only explain insulin resistance in less than 5% of the patients with NIDDM. Interestingly, the IRS-1 mutation in codon 972, which only seems to be important in obese subjects, may be another example of a potentiating effect of obesity on genetic insulin resistance.

Much work must be done before all candidate genes are studied, and it cannot be excluded that we may not find any major defects in the DNA structure. It is possible that the reduced glycogen deposition and increased storage of fat may be caused by an evolutionary selection of "normal genes"—the so-called thrifty genotype.[54] According to this theory, genes favoring abdominal and intramuscular fat deposition may have conferred a survival advantage during evolution, allowing hunting and gathering people from primitive cultures to survive during periods of starvation. The cause or the consequence of this gene selection is reduced insulin-mediated glucose storage in skeletal muscles (i.e., insulin resistance). Thus, subjects with reduced insulin-mediated glycogen synthesis may have had improved chances to survive during evolution; that is, insulin resistance may have been a protective mechanism. In our time, however, in which overfeeding rather than starvation is a common problem, this tendency to store fat does not confer survival advantage, but rather results in obesity and NIDDM.

The "thrifty" genes have not yet been identified, but glycogen synthase is one good candidate. This premise is supported by the recent finding that the locus for development of diabetes in certain mice strains during fat feeding is linked to chromosome 7 or, more precisely, to the glycogen synthase locus.[55] Genes coding for reduced fat oxidation, proteins in the insulin signaling cascade, and peptides involved in appetite regulation are other candidates.

Insulin Secretion in Obesity

Hypersecretion of insulin is an early feature in nondiabetic obese subjects. This hypersecretion is necessary to compensate for metabolic insulin resistance secondary to obesity and overeating.[42] Primary hypersecretion of insulin as the cause of insulin resistance and obesity has been proposed, but never proven. Very recent data from insulin-resistant animals, however, have shown that expression of both the GLUT-2 gene and the glucokinase gene is increased, which may explain why hyperinsulinemia may develop despite normal or near-normal plasma glucose values.[56] These results confirm the compensation of insulin resistance by hyperinsulinemia, but the signal from the muscles to β-cells has not yet been identified.

Insulin secretion may decline in time in obese subjects who develop hyperglycemia.[57] The reason for this decline in β-cell function may be genetic in origin. In our twin studies, we found that insulin deficiency developed years before hyperglycemia in genetically predisposed subjects. This may indicate that, for genetic reasons, the β-cells in obese diabetics may be unable to compensate for insulin resistance in the long term.[44] Although declining β-cell function during development of NIDDM seems to be genetically determined, the genes responsible remain to be identified. In contrast, in maturity onset diabetes of the young (MODY), mutations in the glucokinase gene have been described, which may explain hyperglycemia in about 75% of the patients. Exogenous factors, such as "glucose toxicity" (or the "toxic" effects of hyperglycemia on β-cell function), may also be important in NIDDM, as may intracellular accumulation of amyloid. In NIDDM, the number of β-cells is only slightly reduced (by about 30%), whereas the functional β-cell capacity is markedly reduced (by more than ~80%), especially during the initial response.

Lipoproteins and Obesity

High FFA levels (especially from abdominal deposits with direct delivery to the liver), hyperinsulinemia, and hyperglycemia are all stimulators of very low-density lipoprotein (VLDL) production in the liver. Furthermore, hepatic insulin resistance may result in increased lipoprotein secretion. Turnover of plasma VLDL particles may be increased. The consequence may be elevation of plasma VLDL concentrations and reduction of plasma high-density lipoprotein (HDL) concentrations, an atherogenic lipoprotein profile that may play a role in the increased mortality from cardiovascular diseases in obese diabetics.[58]

Pathophysiologic Role of Obesity and β-Cell Defect in the Development of Non–Insulin-Dependent Diabetes Mellitus (and Macroangiopathy)

Insulin action and secretion are the two key players in the development of diabetes mellitus in obese subjects. These two variables seem to regulate glucose uptake and metabolism in skeletal muscles, together with glucose production in the liver (HGP).

To develop frank diabetes, defects in both variables are necessary; hyperglycemia first develops when insulin resistance cannot be compensated for by appropriate elevation of insulin secretion. It is important to emphasize that, as long as β-cell function is normal, even severe insulin resistance may not lead to frank diabetes mellitus.

The relationship between insulin action and secretion seems to follow the mathematical law of a hyperbola function, as illustrated in Fig. 52-7.[59] The two variables seem to compensate for each other in order to maintain normal glucose tolerance. Induction of insulin resistance (e.g., by obesity) is followed by a compensatory increase in insulin secretion. The product of the two variables seems to remain constant as long as glucose tolerance is normal:

$$\text{Insulin action} \times \text{insulin secretion} = k$$

Thus, k is a measure of the degree of glucose tolerance. In obese subjects with normal glucose tolerance, k is normal, despite marked variation in insulin action. One explanation is that the β-cells are able to compensate for even severe insulin resistance. Thus, the demand for β-cell capacity in obese subjects is much higher than in lean subjects. By contrast, obese diabetic subjects are characterized by low k values, as they are insulin-resistant but also insulin-deficient, absolutely or relatively, to the degree of insulin sensitivity (see Fig. 52-7). Thus, the obese subjects who develop diabetes are predisposed not only to insulin resistance, but also to development of insulin deficiency. The genetic defect in glycogen synthesis is present early in life, whereas the β-cell defect is first expressed later in life, a few years before the onset of hyperglycemia.

In frank diabetes mellitus in obese subjects, peripheral insulin resistance is compensated for by hyperglycemia. In the basal state, normal glucose production rates are necessary to maintain this compensating hyperglycemia. Elevated hepatic glyconeogenesis

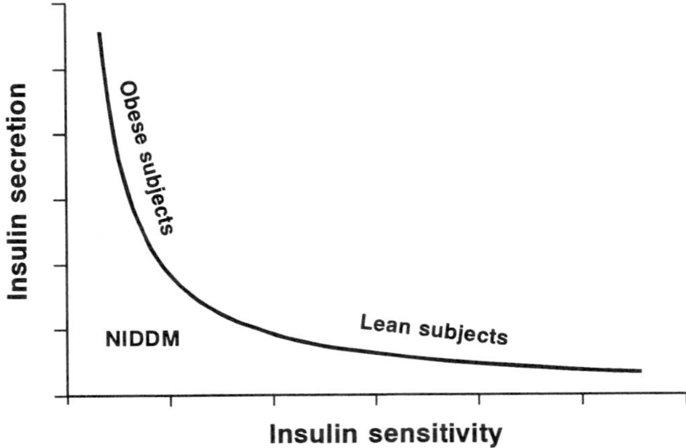

Figure 52-7. Relationship between insulin secretion and insulin sensitivity in lean and obese subjects. Subjects with NIDDM are characterized by both insulin resistance and insulin deficiency. (Modified with permission from Henriksen JE, Alford F, Handberg A, et al. Increased glucose effectiveness in normoglycemic but insulin-resistant relatives of patients with non–insulin-dependent diabetes mellitus. A novel compensatory mechanism. J Clin Invest 1994;94:1196.)

may be involved in this compensation. Also, hyperinsulinemia contributes to the compensation. Both fasting and postprandial plasma insulin concentrations are increased, although not to the level necessary for full compensation of the insulin resistance. These metabolic abnormalities do not only induce hyperglycemia, but also dyslipidemia (elevated VLDL and reduced HDL values), and 50–75% of these subjects develop arterial hypertension.

The mechanisms involved in the development of NIDDM in obese subjects are summarized in Figure 52-8.

NIDDM must be multigenetic, as insulin resistance, abdominal obesity, and the β-cell defect seem to be of genetic origin. The "thrifty gene" hypothesis may be the best explanation for the epidemic dispersal of NIDDM worldwide and, specifically, in developing countries. These genes are not yet characterized, but genes regulating glycogen synthesis, lipolysis, and appetite regulation are good candidates. β-Cell genes responsible for rapid exhaustion (glucose toxicity?) when exposed to obesity, and for development of intracellular amyloid depositions, seem to be present, but have not yet been described.

The "thrifty genes" result in increased fat storage, reduced glucose storage, and compensatory hyperinsulinemia. Consequently, genetically prone subjects will be brought into a positive fat balance. When the environmental factors induced by urbanization (i.e., overeating, specifically of saturated fat; a sedentary lifestyle with reduced VO_2 max; and increased consumption of alcohol and tobacco) are added to (or potentiate) the genetic defects, frank abdominal obesity may develop. This situation may further impair insulin action owing to the effect of increased lipolysis on glycogen synthesis and glucose oxidation. In susceptible subjects, the β-cells may not be able to cope with this challenge, and first-phase insulin secretion will start to decline, glucose tolerance will deteriorate, and states of impaired glucose tolerance will develop. In time, these derangements may deteriorate further, in particular when β-cells are damaged by hyperglycemia and amyloid deposition, and when insulin resistance is augmented by, for example, dyslipoproteinemia and arterial hypertension. Frank NIDDM then develops.

During this process, not only is hyperglycemia induced, but also macroangiopathy.[60] This macroangiopathy, therefore, cannot only be considered a complication of NIDDM, but rather a pathologic process developing in concert with an impairment in glucose tolerance. NIDDM or the insulin resistance syndrome, therefore,

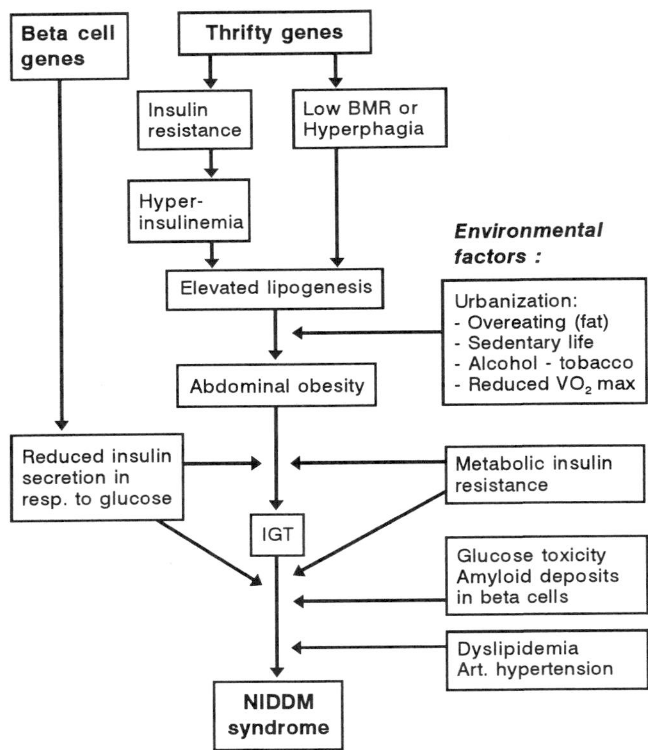

Figure 52-8. Flow chart for pathophysiologic development of obesity and NIDDM. resp., response; art., arterial.

must be considered a life-long disease in which frank hyperglycemia is a late event. By contrast, macroangiopathy, in particular that involving coronary arteries, and arterial hypertension may develop years in advance of the onset of diabetes.[42]

Based on the natural history of NIDDM, therefore, it is clear that prevention of the syndrome is necessary in order to avoid the increased mortality associated with macrovascular diseases.

Concluding Clinical Remarks

From this description, it appears that genetic variables are important in the development of both obesity and hyperglycemia in obese subjects. Characteristically, all obese subjects eat too much fat (in particular, saturated fat) and seem to prefer a sedentary lifestyle. Metabolism of these lipids interferes with glucose metabolism in the muscles and liver, may potentiate defects in insulin sensitivity, and may induce diabetes in subjects with genetic defects in insulin secretion. Furthermore, lipid accumulation in tissues, together with abnormalities in glucose and lipid metabolism, is responsible for the increase in morbidity and mortality from cardiovascular disease in these patients. Presently, therefore, the preferred mode of treatment and prevention is to reduce the intake of saturated fat, especially in genetically predisposed subjects, and to encourage physical activity with the aim of normal body weight.[61,62]

Dietary compliance and prevention of obesity, however, are difficult in practice. Further research, therefore, is needed on the pathophysiologic mechanisms leading to obesity and NIDDM. It is hoped that, in the future, we may be able to prevent these diseases by a treatment modality that interferes with the primary defects. Possibly, elimination of the inherited insulin resistance—for example, by pharmacologic or gene therapy—may reduce or eliminate the risk for development of NIDDM and may also do the same for obesity.

Summary

The following are the key points discussed in this chapter:

- The prevalence of NIDDM in the Western world is about 5–10% in subjects older than 40 years of age.
- Eighty percent of all subjects with NIDDM are obese, but only 10% of all obese subjects develop NIDDM.
- Most obese subjects are insulin-resistant (meaning that they have reduced insulin-mediated glucose storage in skeletal muscles) and hyperinsulinemic.
- Only obese subjects who are predisposed to defects in β-cell function will develop NIDDM.
- NIDDM in obese subjects is a multigenetic disease involving obesity genes (e.g., genes coding for reduced fat oxidation [reduced BMR]), diabetogenes (e.g., genes coding for reduced glycogen synthesis in skeletal muscles and for reduced β-cell response to glucose [insulin deficiency]), and β-cell genes (a defect which over time, renders an individual unable to maintain insulin hypersecretion so as to compensate for defects in insulin action).
- Obesity and increased intake of saturated fat potentiate the genetic insulin resistance and, therefore, may induce hyperglycemia in predisposed subjects.
- Most obese diabetics have abdominal obesity, increased fat turnover, and dyslipidemia.
- Subjects prone to develop NIDDM are characterized by insulin resistance, hyperinsulinemia, dyslipidemia, and arterial hypertension (and consequently, macroangiopathy) decades in advance of the onset of frank diabetes mellitus.
- Obese diabetics are subject to excess morbidity and mortality from cardiovascular diseases.
- The goal for future treatment is to prevent not only NIDDM, but also macroangiopathy.

References

1. Zimmet PZ. Kelly West Lecture 1991. Challenges in diabetes epidemiology—From West to the rest. Diabetes Care 1992;15:232
2. Harris MI, Hadden WC, Knowler WC, Bennett PH. Prevalence of diabetes and impaired glucose tolerance and plasma glucose levels in U.S. population aged 20–74 yr. Diabetes 1987;36:523
3. Pierson RNJ, Wang J, Heymsfield SB, et al. Measuring body fat: Calibrating the rulers. Intermethod comparisons in 389 normal Caucasian subjects. Am J Physiol 1991;261:E103
4. Astrup A, Raben A. Obesity: An inherited metabolic deficiency in the control of macronutrient balance? Eur J Clin Nutr 1992;46:611
5. Schutz Y, Bessard T, Jequier E. Diet-induced thermogenesis measured over a whole day in obese and nonobese women. Am J Clin Nutr 1984;40:542
6. Ravussin E, Swinburn BA. Pathophysiology of obesity. Lancet 1992;340:404
7. Stunkard AJ, Foch TT, Hrubec Z. A twin study of human obesity. JAMA 1986;256:51
8. Walston J, Silver K, Bogardus C, et al. Time of onset of non-insulin dependent diabetes mellitus and genetic variation in the β_3-adrenergic-receptor gene. N Engl J Med 1995;333:343
9. Flatt JP. Importance of nutrient balance in body weight regulation. Diabetes Metab Rev 1988;4:571
10. Vaag A, Henriksen JE, Beck-Nielsen H. Decreased insulin activation of glycogen synthase in skeletal muscles in young nonobese Caucasian first-degree relatives of patients with non–insulin-dependent diabetes mellitus. J Clin Invest 1992;89:782
11. Prentice AM, Black AE, Coward WA, et al. High levels of energy expenditure in obese women. Br Med J [Clin Res] 1986;292:983
12. Felber JP, Haesler E, Jequier E. Metabolic origin of insulin resistance in obesity with and without type 2 (non–insulin-dependent) diabetes mellitus. Diabetologia 1993;36:1221
13. Randle PJ, Garland PB, Hales CN, Newsholme EA. The glucose fatty-acid cycle. Its role in insulin sensitivity and the metabolic disturbances of diabetes mellitus. Lancet 1963;1:785
14. Vaag A, Damsbo P, Hother-Nielsen O, Beck-Nielsen H. Hyperglycaemia compensates for the defects in insulin-mediated glucose metabolism and in the activation of glycogen synthase in the skeletal muscle of patients with type 2 (non–insulin-dependent) diabetes mellitus. Diabetologia 1992;35:80
15. Ong JM, Kern PA. Effect of feeding and obesity on lipoprotein lipase activity, immunoreactive protein, and messenger RNA levels in human adipose tissue. J Clin Invest 1989;84:305
16. Kiens B, Lithell H, Mikines KJ, Richter EA. Effects of insulin and exercise on muscle lipoprotein lipase activity in man and its relation to insulin action. J Clin Invest 1989;84:1124
17. Pollare T, Vessby B, Lithell H. Lipoprotein lipase activity in skeletal muscle is related to insulin sensitivity. Arterioscler Thromb 1991;11:1192
18. Arner P, Bolinder J, Engfeldt P, Ostman J. The antilipolytic effect of insulin in human adipose tissue in obesity, diabetes mellitus, hyperinsulinemia, and starvation. Metabolism 1981;30:753
19. DeFronzo RA, Gunnarsson R, Bjorkman O, et al. Effects of insulin on peripheral and splanchnic glucose metabolism in non–insulin-dependent (type II) diabetes mellitus. J Clin Invest 1985;76:149
20. Hother-Nielsen O, Beck-Nielsen H. On the determination of basal glucose production rate in patients with type 2 (non–insulin-dependent) diabetes mellitus using primed-continuous 3-^{3}H-glucose infusion. Diabetologia 1990;33:603
21. Hother-Nielsen O, Beck-Nielsen H. Basal glucose metabolism in type 2 diabetes. A critical review. Diabetes Metab 1991;17:136
22. Hother-Nielsen O, Beck-Nielsen H. Insulin resistance, but normal basal rates of glucose production in patients with newly diagnosed mild diabetes mellitus. Acta Endocrinol (Copenh) 1991;124:637
23. Saad MF, Anderson RL, Laws A, et al. A comparison between the minimal model and the glucose clamp in the assessment of insulin sensitivity across the spectrum of glucose tolerance. Diabetes 1994;43:1114
24. Jeng CY, Sheu WH, Fuh MMT, et al. Relationship between hepatic glucose production and fasting plasma glucose concentration in patients with NIDDM. Diabetes 1994;43:1440
25. Consoli A, Nurjhan N, Capani F, Gerich J. Predominant role of gluconeogenesis in increased hepatic glucose production in NIDDM. Diabetes 1989;38:550
26. Vranic M. Banting Lecture: Glucose turnover. A key to understanding the pathogenesis of diabetes (indirect effects of insulin). Diabetes 1992;41:1188
27. Larsson B, Svardsudd K, Welin L, et al. Abdominal adipose tissue distribution, obesity, and risk of cardiovascular disease and death: 13-year follow up of participants in the study of men born in 1913. Br Med J [Clin Res] 1984;288:1401
28. Seidell JC, Bjorntorp P, Sjostrom L, et al. Visceral fat accumulation in men is positively associated with insulin, glucose, and C-peptide levels, but negatively with testosterone levels. Metabolism 1990;39:897
29. Bjorntorp P. Abdominal fat distribution and disease: An overview of epidemiological data. Ann Med 1992;24:15
30. Marin P, Andersson B, Ottosson M, et al. The morphology and metabolism of intraabdominal adipose tissue in men. Metabolism 1992;41:1242
31. Olivarius Nd, Andreasen AH. Weight history and its impact on risk factors and diabetic complications of newly diagnosed diabetic patients 40 years of age and over [Abstract]. Proceedings of the 15th IDF Congress, Kobe, Japan:1994:122
32. Bennett PH, Knowler WC, Rushforth NB, et al. The role of obesity in the development of diabetes in the Pima Indians. In: Vague J, Vague PH, eds. Diabetes and Obesity. Amsterdam, Oxford: Excerpta Medica;1979:117
33. Westlund K, Nicolaysen R. Ten-year mortality and morbidity related to serum cholesterol. A follow-up of 3751 men aged 40–49. Scand J Clin Lab Invest 1972;127(suppl):1
34. Modan M, Karasik A, Halkin H, et al. Effect of past and concurrent body mass index on prevalence of glucose intolerance and type 2 (non–insulin-dependent) diabetes and on insulin response. The Israel study of glucose intolerance, obesity and hypertension. Diabetologia 1986;29:82
35. Hansen BC, Bodkin NL. Primary prevention of diabetes mellitus by prevention of obesity in monkeys. Diabetes 1993;42:1809
36. Ortmeyer HK, Bodkin NL, Hansen BC. Chronic calorie restriction alters glycogen metabolism in rhesus monkeys. Obesity Res 1995; in press
37. O'Dea K. Cardiovascular disease risk factors in Australian aborigines. Clin Exp Pharmacol Physiol 1991;18:85
38. Beck-Nielsen H, Pedersen O, Sorensen NS. Effects of dietary changes on cellular insulin binding and in vivo insulin sensitivity. Metabolism 1980;29:482
39. Hunnicutt JW, Hardy RW, Williford J, McDonald JM. Saturated fatty acid-induced insulin resistance in rat adipocytes. Diabetes 1994;43:540
40. West KM. Epidemiology of diabetes and its macrovascular complications. Diabetes Care 1979;2:63
41. Storlien LH, Jenkins AB, Chisholm DJ, et al. Influence of dietary fat composition on development of insulin resistance in rats. Relationship to muscle triglyceride and omega-3 fatty acids in muscle phospholipid. Diabetes 1991;40:280
42. Beck-Nielsen H, Groop LC. Metabolic and genetic characterization of prediabetic states. Sequence of events leading to non–insulin-dependent diabetes mellitus. J Clin Invest 1994;94:1714
43. Damsbo P, Vaag A, Hother-Nielsen O, Beck-Nielsen H. Reduced glycogen synthase activity in skeletal muscle from obese patients with and without type 2 (non–insulin-dependent) diabetes mellitus. Diabetologia 1991;34:239
44. Vaag A, Henriksen JE, Madsbad S, et al. Insulin secretion, insulin action, and hepatic glucose production in identical twins discordant for non–insulin-dependent diabetes mellitus. J Clin Invest 1995;95:690
45. Martin BC, Warram JH, Krolewski AS, et al. Role of glucose and insulin resistance in development of type 2 diabetes mellitus: Results of a 25-year follow-up study. Lancet 1992;340:925

46. Carey D, Jenkins A, Campbell L, et al. Body fat distribution and insulin resistance: Measurements of central obesity by dual-energy x-ray absorptiometry (DEXA). Eur J Nucl Med 1994;21(suppl):S21
47. Wade AJ, Marbut MM, Round JM. Muscle fibre type and aetiology of obesity. Lancet 1990;335:805
48. Vaag A, Alford F, Lund Henriksen F, et al. Multiple defects in both hepatic and peripheral intracellular glucose processing contribute to the hyperglycaemia of NIDDM. Diabetologia 1995;38:326
49. Del Prato S, Bonadonna RC, Bonora E, et al. Characterization of cellular defects of insulin action on type 2 (non–insulin-dependent) diabetes mellitus. J Clin Invest 1993;91:484
50. Wells AM, Sutcliffe IC, Johnson AB, Taylor R. Abnormal activation of glycogen synthesis in fibroblasts from NIDDM subjects. Evidence for an abnormality specific to glucose metabolism. Diabetes 1993;42:583
51. Groop LC, Kankuri M, Schalin Jantti C, et al. Association between polymorphism of the glycogen synthase gene and non–insulin-dependent diabetes mellitus. N Engl J Med 1993;328:10
52. Zouali H, Velho G, Froguel P. Polymorphism of the glycogen synthase gene and non–insulin-dependent diabetes mellitus. N Engl J Med 1993;328:1568
53. Almind K, Bjorbaek C, Vestergaard H, et al. Amino acid polymorphisms of insulin receptor substrate-1 in non–insulin-dependent diabetes mellitus. Lancet 1993;342:828
54. Neal JV. Diabetes mellitus: A thrifty genotype rendered detrimental by "progress"? Am J Hum Genet 1962;14:353
55. Seldin MF, Mott D, Bhat D, et al. Glycogen synthase: A putative locus for diet-induced hyperglycemia. J Clin Invest 1994;94:269
56. Chen C, Hosokawa H, Bumbalo LM, Leahy JL. Mechanisms of compensatory hyperinsulinemia in normoglycemic insulin-resistant spontaneously hypertensive rats. Augmented enzymatic activity of glucokinase in beta-cells. J Clin Invest 1994;94:399
57. Porte DJ. Banting Lecture 1990. Beta-cells in type II diabetes mellitus. Diabetes 1991;40:166
58. Howard BV, Abbott WG, Beltz WF, et al. Integrated study of low-density lipoprotein metabolism and very low-density lipoprotein metabolism in non–insulin-dependent diabetes. Metabolism 1987;36:870
59. Henriksen JE, Alford F, Handberg A, et al. Increased glucose effectiveness in normoglycemic but insulin-resistant relatives of patients with non–insulin-dependent diabetes mellitus. A novel compensatory mechanism. J Clin Invest 1994;94:1196
60. Modan M, Halkin H, Almog S, et al. Hyperinsulinemia. A link between hypertension obesity and glucose intolerance. J Clin Invest 1985;75:809
61. Hadden DR, Blair AL, Wilson EA, et al. Natural history of diabetes presenting age 40–69 years: A prospective study of the influence of intensive dietary therapy. Q J Med 1986;59:579
62. Skarfors ET, Wegener TA, Lithell H, Selinus I. Physical training as treatment for type 2 (non–insulin-dependent) diabetes in elderly men. A feasibility study over 2 years. Diabetologia 1987;30:930
63. Halaas JL, Gajiwala KS, Maffei M, et al. Weight-reducing effects of the plasma protein encoded by the obese gene. Science 1995;269:543

Diabetes Mellitus, edited by Derek LeRoith, Simeon I. Taylor, and Jerrold M. Olefsky. Lippincott–Raven Publishers, Philadelphia © 1996.

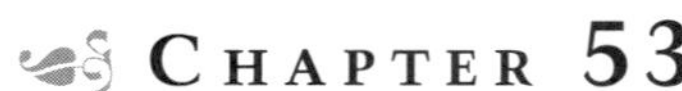

Chapter 53
Effects of Aging on Glucose Homeostasis

Jeffrey B. Halter

Diminished homeostatic control of glucose metabolism is a common characteristic related to aging, particularly in humans. Healthy older adults have higher glucose levels during oral glucose tolerance tests (OGTTs), as illustrated in Figure 53-1, as well as delayed glucose disappearance during IV glucose tolerance tests (IVGTTs), than do young healthy subjects.[1,2] Using either National Diabetes Data Group (NDDG) or World Health Organization (WHO) criteria for the OGTT, there is a high prevalence rate of both diabetes mellitus and impaired glucose tolerance among older humans in multiple, ethnically diverse populations. Data from the National Health and Nutrition Examination Survey conducted by the National Center for Health Statistics from 1976 to 1980 indicate that 15–20% of Americans 65–74 years old meet OGTT criteria for diabetes mellitus, and an additional 25% of the elderly population meet criteria for impaired glucose tolerance.[3] Not only does the prevalence of diabetes mellitus increase with age, but also the incidence rate of new cases increases in people older than the age of 65 years by 0.5–1% per year compared to <0.2% per year in individuals aged 25–44 years.[4]

Diminished glucose tolerance has been observed in some animal models of aging, but the findings are variable.[1] Many previous studies have not been done in trained animals with catheters and have sometimes not included a wide enough age range to separate changes of senescence from changes related to early development. Naturally occurring diabetes mellitus has been reported in rhesus monkeys with onset in mid- to late-life, including many metabolic characteristics that are similar to age-related human non–insulin dependent diabetes mellitus.[5]

The alterations of glucose metabolism with age may have important pathophysiologic consequences. In both animal models and humans, these age-related changes are associated with an accumulation of advanced glycosylation end products,[6,7] hypothesized to contribute to diabetes-related long-term complications.[8] Older adults with diabetes are clearly at risk for these complications.[9]

Effects of Aging on Carbohydrate Metabolism

Studies using radioisotopically labeled glucose or a combined IV and oral glucose clamp protocol have compared aspects of glucose kinetics following oral glucose ingestion in normal old and young people.[10–12] These studies suggest that glucose intolerance occurs in older people despite delayed absorption of oral glucose and delayed posthepatic glucose delivery. Increased hyperglycemia in older adults results from delayed suppression of hepatic glucose output and a decreased rate of peripheral glucose uptake following oral glucose ingestion.

Insulin Secretion

Studies of the effects of aging on insulin secretion in experimental animals and in humans suggest that aging is associated with subtle impairments of insulin secretion (see ref. 13 for review). However, there is considerable variability among the findings, probably because of the relatively small magnitude of the age effect, the variable sensitivity of measures of pancreatic β-cell function used, the use of different animal models, and the presence of multiple potentially confounding factors in human studies.

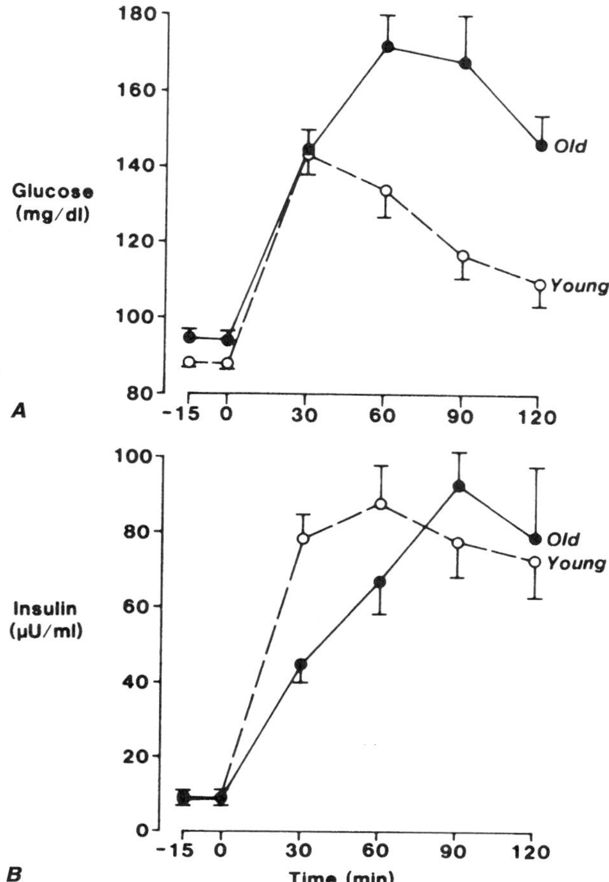

FIGURE 53-1. Plasma glucose (*A*) and insulin (*B*) levels before and after oral ingestion of 100 g of glucose in 18 healthy old (solid circles) and 18 young (open circles) subjects matched for relative body weight and socioeconomic group. Subjects were eating an ad lib diet which, in the older subjects, included approximately 10% fewer total calories and 15% fewer carbohydrate calories than the diet of their younger counterparts.[2]

Animal Studies

A decline in insulin output occurs in male Sprague-Dawley rats between the ages of 2–4 months and 12 months, with little further decline at greater age in these animals. The age effect appears to be most pronounced when small islets are studied, which is the predominant type of islet in younger animals. However, age-related obesity is prominent in this rat strain, making interpretation of studies in older animals difficult because of the potential impact of age-related obesity on insulin secretion. The Fischer 344 rat has been used more widely to study aging effects because obesity is less of a problem in this animal model. In this model, insulin secretion from whole perfused pancreas does not decline with age,[14,15] but an age-related decline is clear when insulin secretion is expressed as a rate per β-cell.[16]

The animal models present an opportunity to explore mechanisms for age-related changes. Studies of effects of aging on glucose oxidation by β-cells have yielded conflicting results.[13,15] Islets from aged animals demonstrate diminished margination of insulin secretion vesicles at the plasma membrane in response to glucose stimulation, as well as decreased production of cAMP via the adenyl cyclase system.[13] The effects of other islet hormones within the pancreatic islets on insulin secretion have also been considered. In particular, evidence has been presented for enhanced sensitivity of pancreatic β-cells to inhibition by somatostatin with aging.[17]

Studies of isolated islets have reported no age effect on levels of insulin mRNA.[18] Aging has more of an effect on secretion of preformed insulin than on newly synthesized insulin, although both pools appear to be affected.[13,18] Proinsulin synthesis is also reduced as a function of age during high glucose stimulation. These findings suggest multiple age-related alterations in the signal transduction and biosynthetic pathways leading to insulin secretion.

Human Studies

Levels of insulin in the fasting state and during OGTT or following a meal have been measured in many studies. These data are extremely difficult to interpret, however, because of their lack of sensitivity and specificity as quantitative measures of pancreatic β-cell function. Although delayed insulin response during OGTT has been observed in some studies (see Fig. 53-1), the OGTT data suggest overall that gross impairment of pancreatic β-cell function is not characteristic of normal human aging.[1] Use of the hyperglycemic glucose clamp technique has demonstrated little, if any, decrement in insulin secretory responses as a function of age in humans. When the hyperglycemic clamp procedure was combined with oral glucose ingestion to assess the contribution of enteric mediators, a possible increased β-cell sensitivity to gastric inhibitory polypeptide with age was suggested.[19] A number of studies have reported a small but consistent decrease in insulin clearance with age in humans.[1] Thus, circulating insulin levels may underestimate insulin secretory rates in older subjects, thereby tending to mask age-related differences.

When the use of C-peptide measurements, in combination with an assessment of C-peptide kinetics, has been applied to the study of insulin secretory responses of aging humans to meal ingestion or during a glucose infusion protocol designed to closely match circulating glucose levels, no age difference in absolute insulin secretion rate has been observed.[20] This study did suggest, however, a diminished relative insulin secretory response in the older subjects. Other researchers have found evidence for diminished insulin secretory rate with age during a prolonged IV glucose

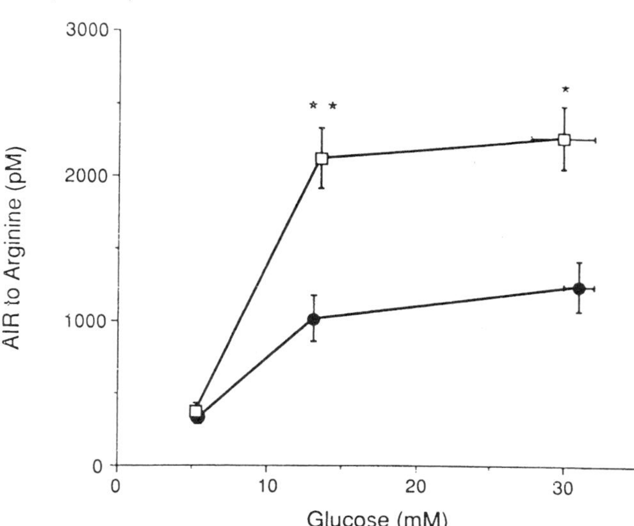

FIGURE 53-2. A comparison of the acute insulin response (AIR) to a bolus of 5 g of IV arginine as a function of the plasma glucose level in exercise-trained older subjects (solid circle; n=14) and exercise-trained younger subjects (open square; n=11). Short-term glucose infusions were used to achieve elevated circulating glucose levels in the subjects. For comparison of AIRs at similar glucose levels between old and young subjects, * =p<0.01; * * =p<0.005. Both subject groups had a similar sensitivity to insulin as measured during a frequently sampled IVGTT protocol.[24]

tolerance test protocol[21,22] or hyperglycemic clamp technique.[23] Another approach that has helped to identify age-related pancreatic β-cell functional deficits is to quantitate the potentiating effect of glucose on insulin secretory responses to a nonglucose stimulus, such as the amino acid arginine.[21,24]

A problem in the interpretation of studies of pancreatic β-cell function in aging has to do with the potential confounding effect of coexistent insulin resistance in elderly people. As described in more detail later in this chapter, a number of studies have provided evidence for the presence of insulin resistance in elderly humans. The normal physiologic feedback control mechanism for regulation of glucose homeostasis should result in hyperinsulinemia to compensate for the presence of insulin resistance if pancreatic β-cell function is completely normal. Thus, the finding of similar pancreatic β-cell responses to glucose challenge in old and young subjects may, in fact, represent a relative impairment if the older subjects are also insulin resistant. When older people were selected for study based on having a quantitative measure of insulin action similar to that of healthy young subjects, a clear decrease in pancreatic β-cell function was apparent in the older group,[24] as illustrated in Figure 53-2.

Insulin Action

Animal Studies

Many studies have provided evidence of resistance to the metabolic effects of insulin in aging animals (see ref. 1 for review). The interpretation of these findings, however, is an ongoing challenge. For example, many aging studies have been done in Wistar and Sprague-Dawley rats, which rapidly become obese as they get older. Thus, it has been particularly difficult to separate the effects of obesity from those of aging in the development of insulin resistance. Using a hyperinsulinemic euglycemic clamp approach, a shift to the right of the dose-response curve for both stimulation of glucose uptake and inhibition of hepatic glucose production as a function of insulin level has been demonstrated with increasing age for male Wistar rats.[25] Although these effects appear to be a continuous function of age, the largest effects occur in early life, with little further decline in insulin-stimulated glucose utilization between 4–6-month-old rats and older rats. Similarly, a decrease of insulin binding and receptor number occurs in early development in both fat and muscle cells, with little further change in insulin receptor number as a function of further aging.[25,26]

A progressive decline of insulin-mediated tyrosine kinase activity has been observed in skeletal muscle during the life span of the male Wistar rat,[27] and decreased insulin-mediated tyrosine kinase activity has been observed in muscle from 24-month-old female Fischer 344 rats compared to that in 2-month-old rats.[26] A decline in insulin-mediated autophosphorylation of the tyrosine kinase domain of the insulin receptor was also observed,[26,27] but only during early life development in the Wistar rats. Thus, the observed life span–related decline in insulin receptor–mediated tyrosine kinase activity does not appear to be explained by diminished autophosphorylation of the tyrosine kinase domain of the insulin receptor itself. Studies in fat cells of male Sprague-Dawley rats have demonstrated a decrease in insulin receptor recycling between the ages of 2 and 12 months, an effect that was unrelated to any decrease in insulin receptor binding.[28] This finding has not been extended, however, to rats of older age.

Human Studies

Studies using the hyperinsulinemic euglycemic clamp procedure in combination with radioisotope labelled glucose infusion have reported no age-related impairment of insulin-mediated suppression of hepatic glucose production in humans.[29,30] As illustrated in Figure 53-3, however, insulin-mediated total glucose disposal declines with age.[29,31,32] There is a shift to the right in the dose-response curve in older people for insulin effects on glucose utilization, as glucose utilization at maximally stimulating insulin levels appears to be relatively unaffected.[29,32] Studies of forearm glucose uptake during glucose infusions of varying rates to match glucose levels over time have also demonstrated diminished glucose utilization under conditions of comparable circulating glucose and insulin levels in older, as compared to younger, subjects.[33] Using the frequently sampled IVGTT, diminished sensitivity to insulin has also been demonstrated in aging humans.[21,34] A comprehensive analysis of several different modeling approaches to assessment of insulin action in a large cohort of healthy men has provided additional evidence for an age-related decline in tissue sensitivity to insulin.[35] Indirect calorimetry during use of a euglycemic insulin clamp has suggested that the age-related decline in glucose disposal in men, but not in women, is associated with a substantial decline in nonoxidative glucose metabolism, but not in oxidative glucose metabolism.[36] Because other studies demonstrating age-related insulin resistance in humans have been limited to male subjects, further work using more heterogeneous populations is clearly needed.

At the cellular level, studies of insulin binding to human adipocytes have yielded varying results, and studies of insulin binding in monocytes have not identified an age-related decline.[1] A decline in maximal glucose transport, as measured by 3-O-methyl glucose uptake, was observed in cells from elderly men, but there was no effect on the glucose level for half maximal transport.[37] These findings are consistent with in vivo observations in the same elderly subjects of comparably decreased glucose uptake over a range of glucose levels studied, despite constant insulin levels.[38] Overall, these findings suggest a reduction of glucose transport capacity in fat cells from elderly people rather than a reduction in the function of the glucose transport units.

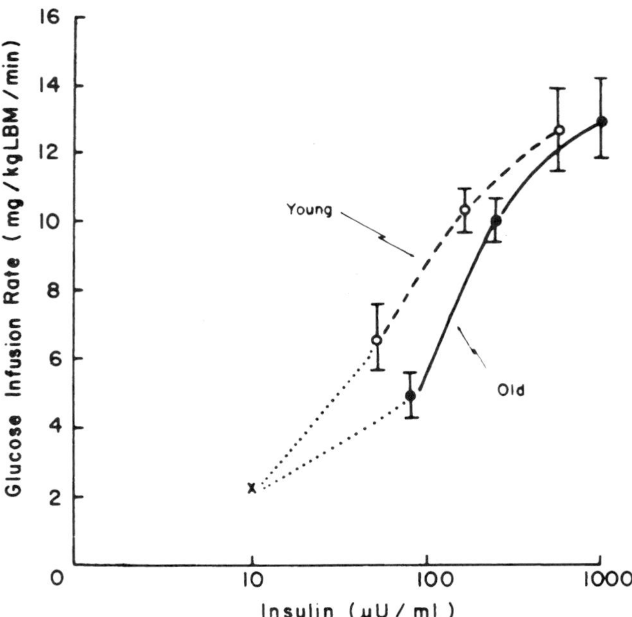

Figure 53-3. A comparison of dose-response curves for insulin levels achieved during a euglycemic clamp protocol versus the glucose infusion rate needed to maintain euglycemia in healthy, nonobese young (n=17) and old (n=10) subjects. The experimental data were extrapolated to known basal hepatic glucose production rates for young and old subjects. Glucose infusion rates were similar in young and old at the highest insulin level tested, but were significantly lower in the older subjects at the low insulin infusion rate. *LBM,* lean body mass.[32]

It is possible that an age-related impairment in a component of glucose uptake, occurring independently of insulin, could contribute to impaired glucose tolerance with aging. When somatostatin was used to suppress endogenous insulin secretion, and glucose utilization was measured during maintenance of a constant glucose level, glucose utilization was lower in elderly subjects than in young subjects at approximately normal fasting levels. When glucose levels were raised to approximately 11 mM, however, glucose utilization rates were similar in both young and old subjects.[39] These findings suggest that, at least at some physiologic glucose levels, non–insulin-mediated glucose uptake is reduced in elderly people. Estimation of glucose effectiveness using the frequently sampled IVGTT protocol, however, has shown no difference in values for elderly subjects compared to young persons.[21,34]

Glucose Transport

Changes in glucose transporter expression could contribute to diminished cellular glucose uptake in aging. Reduced amounts of GLUT 4 protein in membranes of both fat cells and gastrocnemius muscle were observed in 12- or 20-month-old Wistar or Sprague-Dawley rats compared with 1- to 2-month-old animals.[40–42] This decrease appears to be specific for the GLUT 4 transporter because measurements of GLUT 1 transporter protein showed no difference between groups.[41] Assessment of GLUT 4 mRNA has suggested that the age-related decrease in GLUT 4 protein is a result of decreased biosynthesis.[42] In addition, less translocation of GLUT 4 protein from the intracellular microsome fraction to the plasma membrane fraction was observed in cells from aged animals upon exposure to insulin.[41]

A decrease of GLUT 4 protein in muscle has also been observed in male Fischer 344 rats across the age range of 3–24 months,[43] but this effect was most apparent in exercise-trained animals, with only small changes observed with age in sedentary rats.[26,43] In a study of glucose uptake and GLUT 4 protein in several muscles from Long-Evans rats of varying age, however, age-related decreases in both glucose uptake and GLUT 4 protein were apparent when comparing 1- and 10-month-old animals, but no further decline was noted in 25-month-old animals.[44] These findings are most consistent with other work in experimental animals demonstrating changes in insulin action and glucose uptake primarily when comparing very young with mature rats, but little further effect when comparing aged with mature animals.

Effects of Other Hormones

Many hormones that influence glucose metabolism in vivo could contribute to age-related changes in glucose homeostasis. Glucagon secretion does not appear to be significantly influenced by aging in humans in the fasting state, following amino acid stimulation, or with suppression by insulin.[1] Older subjects, however, have been reported to have an increased hyperglycemic and hepatic glucose production response to glucagon infusion, suggesting enhanced hepatic sensitivity to glucagon in these subjects.[45] Growth hormone secretion declines, rather than increases, with age and so cannot be directly implicated in age-related glucose intolerance. Consistent with the decline of growth hormone secretion in the elderly, particularly during the night, is the observation of a lack of an early morning increase in glucose levels.[46,47] Human growth hormone administration has been tested in clinical trials for possible anabolic effects in elderly people. Such trials have shown small effects on fasting and postchallenge glucose levels.[48,49] Regulation of glucocorticoid production appears to be relatively unaffected by aging in humans.[50,51] There is little information available about the sensitivity of elderly animals or people to the hyperglycemic effects of glucocorticoids.

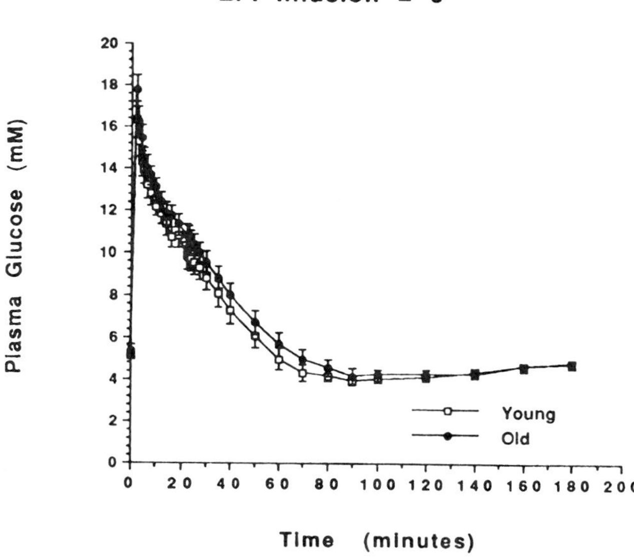

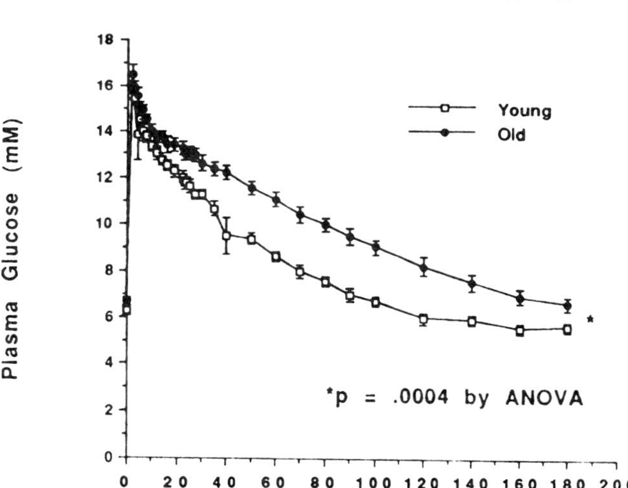

FIGURE 53-4. A comparison of plasma glucose levels during an IV GTT in healthy young (n=7) and old (n=7) subjects. The upper panel shows IVGTT results in the absence of an infusion of epinephrine (EPI). The lower panel shows the slower decline of glucose levels in the older subjects, compared to the younger subjects, during EPI infusion. The circulating EPI levels achieved were comparable in both subject groups during EPI infusion.[60]

The potential role of endogenous sympathetic nervous system activity in age-related glucose intolerance remains uncertain. Plasma norepinephrine levels and norepinephrine release are consistently increased in aging humans.[52,53] However, age-related glucose intolerance and insulin resistance are poorly correlated with the degree of elevation in norepinephrine levels.[34,54] Short-term suppression of sympathetic nervous system activity does not result in any consistent improvement in insulin action in older individuals.[55] Although a number of studies have demonstrated age-related decreases in the nonmetabolic effects of catecholamines (both β-adrenergic[56] and α-adrenergic[57]), no reduction in insulin secretory response to the β-adrenergic agonist isoproterenol was observed in healthy older people.[58] Decreased sensitivity to β-adrenergic stimulation, however, has been observed in the fat cells of older adults with impaired glucose tolerance or asymptomatic fasting hyperglycemia.[59]

As illustrated in Figure 53-4, during infusion of a dose of epinephrine that achieved circulating epinephrine levels comparable to those achieved during physiologic stress, significantly increased hyperglycemia was observed in older subjects, indicating an enhanced overall sensitivity to the hyperglycemic effects of epinephrine.[60] Epinephrine inhibition of the insulin secretion response to IV glucose and the effects of epinephrine on diminishing tissue sensitivity to insulin, however, were similar in old and young subjects. The primary difference observed between old and young subjects was a greater suppression in the old of the effectiveness of the glucose level to increase fractional glucose removal rate. Thus, although sympathetic nervous system activity and catecholamine release do not appear to be important in age-related changes of glucose metabolism in the normal resting state, enhanced sensitivity to the metabolic effects of catecholamines may contribute to increased hyperglycemia under stressful situations.

Confounding Factors

Because glucose metabolism is sensitive to a wide range of influences, it may be very difficult to define specifically the effects of aging that are independent of such other influences. As summarized in Figure 53-5, it is likely that there are primary changes in pancreatic β-cell function and, possibly, changes in insulin action with aging that contribute to age-related changes of glucose metabolism. Genetic factors may influence the expression of glucose intolerance with aging, although such genetic factors have not yet been defined. Studies that have attempted to control for the other variables affecting glucose metabolism have suggested that there is a residual decline in glucose tolerance with age, both in men and women, but that this age effect is relatively modest in magnitude. The following discussion addresses a number of the specific confounding factors that can influence glucose metabolism in aging.

Adiposity

Several studies in humans have attempted to control for the influence of adiposity by including a large sample size and multiple measurements of various aspects of body fat mass and distribution in order to control for age group differences statistically. Although all of these studies are not in full agreement, overall, they suggest that there is a persistent effect of aging on both glucose tolerance and insulin action that is independent of body fat mass and distribution in humans.[61–64] Older people who meet the criteria for normal glucose tolerance, however, have less adiposity, particularly central adiposity, and do not experience a detectable decrease in insulin sensitivity.[65,66] Increased adiposity in healthy elderly people is associated with increased free fatty acid levels, rates of lipolysis, and rates of lipid oxidation.[67] Thus, the availability of fatty acids for fuel metabolism could contribute directly to decreased glucose utilization in older adults.

Studies in experimental animals have been difficult to interpret. Many of the age-related metabolic alterations reported in studies of fat cells have occurred during the phase of rapid increase of body size in early development and are associated directly with increased fat cell size. In fact, age-related changes in glucose metabolism have been reported to be entirely explained by variations in fat cell size.[68]

Physical Activity

Aging-associated decreased mobility and diminished physical activity may also be important confounding factors in understanding the age-related changes of glucose homeostasis. Healthy older men with greater degrees of physical fitness have better glucose tolerance and less evidence of insulin resistance than do less active older men.[63,69,70] More physically fit elderly men also tend to have less body fat and less central adiposity. Although glucose intolerance appears to persist with age even when controlling for these factors, the age-related change is modest.[63,70] When insulin action was assessed using a glucose clamp protocol in healthy older men, the degree of physical fitness and of central adiposity were the

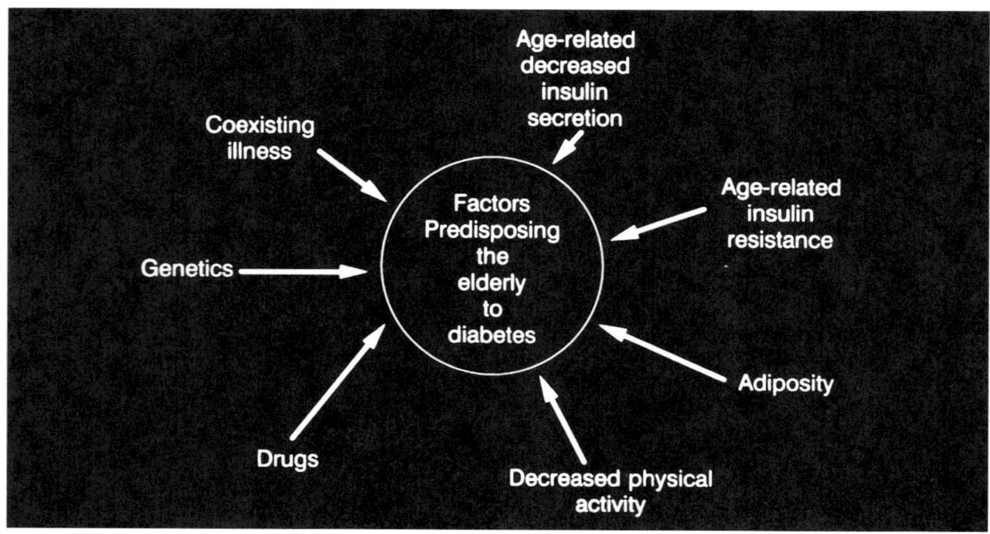

Figure 53-5. A summary of factors that may contribute to the high rate of diabetes mellitus and impaired glucose tolerance in elderly people.

most important predictors of the degree of insulin resistance observed, and age was not an independent predictor.[63] Physically fit older men have also been reported to have increased levels of muscle GLUT 4.[71]

Exercise training without concomitant weight reduction has had little effect on overall oral glucose tolerance in elderly men. A significant improvement in insulin action, measured either with a glucose clamp protocol or by computer modeling of IVGTT results, has been demonstrated, however, in older men following exercise training,[72–74] and muscle GLUT 4 has been found to increase.[74] The reduction in insulin resistance accompanying exercise training under these circumstances is associated with diminished pancreatic β-cell sensitivity to stimulation.[73] This compensatory effect on insulin secretion may explain why the improvement of insulin action associated with exercise training has not affected overall glucose tolerance.

Dietary Factors

Some studies have suggested that total caloric intake of older adults may be relatively low, and that carbohydrate intake, in particular, may be less compared to that in younger individuals.[1,2] Thus, it is possible that impaired glucose tolerance in aging may be due, in part, to diminished dietary carbohydrate intake. Conversely, excessive intake of calories leading to obesity is an important contributing factor to insulin resistance and impaired glucose tolerance in the older adult population. Circulating glucose levels and insulin levels are lower in lifelong diet-restricted rats and monkeys, as well.[75,76]

Studies in humans have addressed the effects of short-term alterations in dietary carbohydrate intake on aspects of age-related changes in glucose metabolism. Healthy elderly people demonstrate improved glucose tolerance, enhanced tissue sensitivity to insulin, and improved pancreatic β-cell function when ingesting an 85% carbohydrate diet for 3–5 days, as compared to an ad lib diet.[54] Studies of old and young subjects with comparable carbohydrate diet regimens have revealed that age differences in glucose tolerance, insulin secretion, and insulin action are reduced but still persistent.[2,54] Thus, dietary carbohydrate intake is an additional factor that can contribute to age-related changes of glucose metabolism.

Hypertension

Given the high prevalence rate of hypertension among elderly people, blood pressure may be an important variable when trying to understand age-related glucose intolerance. Among a population of elderly people in Rancho Bernardo, California, increased blood pressure was found to be associated with impaired glucose tolerance or NIDDM, independent of concomitant obesity or use of antihypertensive medications.[77] By contrast, in the predominantly Caucasian population of the Baltimore Longitudinal Study of Aging, little, if any, relationship between hyperinsulinemia and blood pressure was found after adjusting for other confounding variables.[78] Diminished insulin sensitivity has been documented in older hypertensive men using a glucose clamp protocol.[79]

As discussed previously, there is evidence that increased sympathetic nervous system activity, as well as insulin resistance and glucose intolerance, accompanies human aging. Careful analysis of these factors in a population of otherwise healthy men and women, however, has indicated that blood pressure and degree of adiposity are the best predictors of declining insulin action.[34] Neither age nor circulating norepinephrine levels contribute independently to the age-related decrease in insulin action. Similarly, among a group of older people, including those with mild hypertension, there is a close association between blood pressure and degree of adiposity as predictors of sensitivity to insulin, but no relationship to norepinephrine levels.[55]

An alternative hypothesis for the association between hypertension and insulin resistance in older people is the adverse long-term effect of hypertension on the small blood vessels.[80] The loss of function of such small blood vessels could result in impaired delivery of glucose to tissues and, thus, diminished insulin-mediated glucose utilization. Thus, this hypothesis postulates that insulin resistance is secondary to underlying long-term hypertension. The lack of association of insulin resistance with hypertension in some animal models and some human populations argues against this hypothesis, although it is possible that other genetic or physiologic regulatory factors may prevent the development of insulin resistance under these circumstances.

Table 53-1. Drugs That May Cause Hyperglycemia

Antihypertensives
Diuretics
β-Adrenergic blockers
α_2-Adrenergic agonists
? Ca^{++} channel blockers
Anti-inflammatory agents
Glucocorticoids
Nonsteroidal anti-inflammatory drugs
Stimulants
Adrenergic agonists
Caffeine
Nicotine
Others
Alcohol
Nicotinic acid
Oral contraceptives (estrogen/progesterone)
Phenytoin
Pentamidine

Drugs

A number of pharmacologic agents in common use have known effects on glucose metabolism. Because older adults are frequent users of pharmacologic agents, interpretation of alterations in glucose metabolism in such individuals must take into account the drugs they are using. Table 53-1 lists drugs that are known to affect glucose metabolism. Because of the association of hypertension with insulin resistance and glucose intolerance, as described previously, effects of antihypertensive agents on glucose metabolism have been of particular interest.[81] Nonpharmacologic drugs may also contribute to age-related glucose tolerance. For example, ingestion of modest amounts of alcohol has been found to cause insulin resistance and decreased glucose oxidation in elderly men.[82]

References

1. Halter JB. Aging and carbohydrate metabolism. In: Masoro EJ, ed. Handbook of Physiology. Volume on Aging. New York: Oxford University Press, Inc.; 1995:119
2. Chen M, Halter JB, Porte D Jr. The role of dietary carbohydrate in the decreased glucose tolerance of the elderly. J Am Geriatr Soc 1987;35:417
3. Harris MI, Hadden WC, Knowler WC, Bennett PH. Prevalence of diabetes and impaired glucose tolerance and plasma glucose levels in U.S. population aged 30–74 yr. Diabetes 1987;36:523
4. Herman WH, Sinnock P, Brenner E, et al. An epidemiologic model for diabetes mellitus: Incidence, prevalence, and mortality. Diabetes Care 1984;7:367
5. Bodkin ML, Metzger BL, Hansen BC. Hepatic glucose production and insulin sensitivity preceding diabetes in monkeys. Am J Physiol 1989;256(Endocrinol. Metab. 19):E676
6. Graf R, Halter JB, Porte D Jr. Glycosylated hemoglobin in normal subjects

and maturity-onset diabetics. Evidence for a saturable system in man. Diabetes 1978;27:834

7. Oimomi M, Maeda Y, Hata F, et al. A study of the age-related acceleration of glycation of tissue proteins in rats. J Gerontol Biol Sci 1988;43:B98
8. Brownlee M, Cerami A, Vlassara H. Advanced glycosylation endproducts in tissue and the biochemical basis of diabetic complications. N Engl J Med 1988;318:1315
9. Carter Center of Emory University. Closing the gap: The problem of diabetes mellitus in the United States. Diabetes Care 1985;8:391
10. Robert JJ, Cummins JC, Wolfe RR, et al. Quantitative aspects of glucose production and metabolism in health elderly subjects. Diabetes 1982;31:203
11. Jackson RA, Hawa MI, Roshania RD, et al. Influence of aging on hepatic and peripheral glucose metabolism in humans. Diabetes 1988;36:119
12. Tonino RP, Minaker KL, Rowe JW. Effect of age on systemic delivery of oral glucose in men. Diabetes Care 1989;12:394
13. Adelman R. Secretion of insulin during aging. J Am Geriatr Soc 1989;37:983
14. Starnes JW, Cheong E, Matschinsky FM. Hormone secretion by isolated perfused pancreas of aging Fischer 344 rats. Am J Physiol 1991;260 (Endocrinol. Metab.):E59
15. Ruhe RC, Curry DL, Herrmann S, McDonald RB. Age and gender effects on insulin secretion and glucose sensitivity of the endocrine pancreas. Am J Physiol 1992;262 (Reg Integrative Comp Physiol):R671
16. Reaven EP, Gold G, Reaven GM. Effect of age on glucose-stimulated insulin release by the β-cell of the rat. J Clin Invest 1979;64:591
17. Casad RC Jr, Adelman RC. Aging enhances inhibitory action of somatostatin in rat pancreas. Endocrinology 1992;130:2420
18. Wang SY, Halban PA, Rowe JW. Effect of aging on insulin synthesis and secretion: Differential effects on preproinsulin messenger RNA levels, proinsulin biosynthesis, and secretion of newly made and preformed insulin in the rat. J Clin Invest 1988;81:176
19. Elahi D, Andersen DK, Muller DC, et al. The enteric enhancement of glucose-stimulated insulin release: The role of GIP in aging, obesity, and non–insulin-dependent diabetes mellitus. Diabetes 1984;33:950
20. Gumbiner B, Polonsky KS, Beltz WF, et al. Effects of aging on insulin secretion. Diabetes 1989;38:1549
21. Chen M, Bergman RN, Pacini G, Porte D Jr. Pathogenesis of age-related glucose intolerance in man: Insulin resistance and decreased β-cell function. J Clin Endocrinol Metab 1985;60:13
22. Pacini G, Beccaro F, Valerio A, et al. Reduced β-cell secretion and insulin hepatic extraction in healthy elderly subjects. J Am Geriatr Soc 1990;38:1283
23. Bourney RE, Kohrt WM, Kirwan JP, et al. Relationship between glucose tolerance and glucose-stimulated insulin response in 65-year-olds. J Gerontol Med Sci 1993;48:M122
24. Kahn SE, Larson VG, Schwartz RS, et al. Exercise training delineates the importance of β-cell dysfunction to the glucose intolerance of human aging. J Clin Endocrinol Metab 1992;74:1336
25. Nishimura H, Kuzuya H, Okamoto M, et al. Change of insulin action with aging in conscious rats determined by euglycemic clamp. Am J Physiol 1988;254 (Endocrinol Metab 17):E92
26. Barnard RJ, Lawani LO, Martin DA, et al. Effects of maturation and aging on the skeletal muscle glucose transport system. Am J Physiol 1992;262 (Endocrinol Metab 25):E619
27. Kono S, Kuzuya H, Okamoto M, et al. Changes in insulin receptor kinase with aging in rat skeletal muscle and liver. Am J Physiol 1990;259 (Endocrinol Metab):E27
28. Trischitta V, Reaven GM. Evidence of a defect in insulin-receptor recycling in adipocytes from older rats. Am J Physiol 1988;254 (Endocrinol Metab 17):E39
29. Fink RI, Kolterman OG, Griffin J, Olefsky JM. Mechanisms of insulin resistance in aging. J Clin Invest 1983;71:1523
30. Meneilly GS, Minaker KL, Elahi D, Rowe JW. Insulin action in aging man: Evidence for tissue-specific differences at low physiologic insulin levels. J Gerontol 1987;42:196
31. DeFronzo RA. Glucose intolerance and aging: Evidence for tissue insensitivity to insulin. Diabetes 1979;28:1095
32. Rowe JW, Minaker KL, Pallotta JA, Flier JS. Characterization of the insulin resistance of aging. J Clin Invest 1983;71:1581
33. Jackson RA, Blix PM, Matthews JA, et al. Influences of aging on glucose homeostasis. J Clin Endocrinol Metab 1982;55:840
34. Supiano MA, Hogikyan RV, Morrow LA, et al. Aging and insulin sensitivity: Role of blood pressure and sympathetic nervous system activity. J Gerontol Med Sci 1993;48:M237
35. Walton C, Godsland IF, Proudler AJ, et al. Evaluation of four mathematical models of glucose and insulin dynamics with analysis of effects of age and obesity. Am J Physiol 1992;262 (Endocrinol Metab 25):E755
36. Franssila-Kallunki A, Schalin-Jantti C, Groop L. Effect of gender on insulin resistance associated with aging. Am J Physiol 1992;263 (Endocrinol Metab):E780
37. Fink RI, Kolterman OG, Kao M, Olefsky JM. The role of the glucose transport system in the postreceptor defect in insulin action associated with human aging. J Clin Endocrinol Metab 1984;58:721
38. Fink RI, Wallace P, Olefsky JM. Effects of aging on glucose-mediated glucose disposal and glucose transport. J Clin Invest 1986;77:2034
39. Meneilly GS, Elahi D, Minaker KL, et al. Impairment of noninsulin-mediated glucose disposal in the elderly. J Clin Endocrinol Metab 1989;63:566
40. Hissin PJ, Foley JE, Wardzala LJ, et al. Mechanism of insulin-resistant glucose transport activity in the enlarged adipose cell of the aged, obese rat. Relative depletion of intracellular glucose transport systems. J Clin Invest 1982; 70:780
41. Ezaki O, Fukuda N, Itakura H. Role of two types of glucose transporters in enlarged adipocytes from aged obese rats. Diabetes 1990;39:1543
42. Lin J-L, Asano T, Shibasaki Y, et al. Altered expression of glucose transporter isoforms with aging in rats—Selective decrease in GluT4 in the fat tissue and skeletal muscle. Diabetologia 1991;34:477
43. Kern M, Dolan PL, Mazzeo RS, et al. Effect of aging and exercise on GLUT-4 glucose transporters in muscle. Am J Physiol 1992;263 (Endocrinol Metab 26):E362
44. Gulve EA, Henriksen EJ, Rodnick KJ, et al. Glucose transporters and glucose transport in skeletal muscles of 1- to 25-mo-old rats. Am J Physiol 1993;264 (Endocrinol Metab 27):E319
45. Simonson DD, DeFronzo RA. Glucagon physiology and aging: Evidence for enhanced hepatic sensitivity. Diabetologia 1983;25:1
46. Meneilly GS, Elahi D, Minaker KL, Rowe JW. The dawn phenomenon does not occur in normal elderly subjects. J Clin Endocrinol Metab 1986;63:292
47. Rosenthal M, Argoud GM. Absence of the dawn glucose rise in nondiabetic men compared by age. J Gerontol Med Sci 1989;4:M57
48. Marcus R, Butterfield G, Holloway L, et al. Effects of short-term administration of recombinant human growth hormone to elderly people. J Clin Endocrinol Metab 1990;70:519
49. Rudman D, Feller AG, Nagraj HS, et al. Effects of human growth hormone in men over 60 years old. N Engl J Med 1990;323:1
50. Sherman B, Wysham C, Pfohl B. Age-related changes in the cicadian rhythm of plasma cortisol in man. J Clin Endocrinol Metab 1985;61:439
51. Waltman C, Blackman MR, Chrousos GP, et al. Spontaneous and glucocorticoid-inhibited adrenocorticotropic hormone and cortisol secretion are similar in healthy young and old men. J Clin Endocrinol Metab 1991;73:495
52. Linares OA, Halter JB. Sympathochromaffin system activity in the elderly. J Am Geriatr Soc 1987;35:448
53. Supiano MA, Linares OA, Smith MJ, Halter JB. Age-related differences in norepinephrine kinetics: Effect of posture and sodium-restricted diet. Am J Physiol 1990;259 (Endocrinol Metab 22):E422
54. Chen M, Halter JB, Porte D Jr. Plasma catecholamines, dietary carbohydrate, and glucose intolerance: A comparison between young and old men. J Clin Endocrinol Metab 1986;62:1193
55. Supiano MA, Hogikyan RV, Morrow LA, et al. Hypertension and insulin resistance: Role of sympathetic nervous system activity. Am J Physiol 1992;26 (Endocrinol Metab):E935
56. Scarpace PJ. Decreased receptor activation with age. Can it be explained by desensitization? J Am Geriatri Soc 1988;36:1067
57. Supiano MA, Hogikyan RV, et al. Regulation of venous alpha-adrenergic responses in older humans. Am J Physiol 1991;260 (Endocrinol Metab 23): E599
58. Morrow LA, Rosen SG, Halter JB. Beta-adrenergic regulation of insulin secretion in the elderly: Evidence of heterogeneity of beta-adrenergic responsiveness. J Gerontol Med Sci 1991;46:M108
59. Reynisdottir S, Ellerfeldt K, Warenberg H, et al. Multiple lipolysis defects in the insulin resistance (metabolic) syndrome. J Clin Invest 1994;93:2590
60. Morrow LA, Morganroth GS, Herman WH, et al. Effects of epinephrine on insulin secretion and action in humans. Interaction with aging. Diabetes 1993;42:307
61. Reaven GM, Chen N, Hollenbeck C, Chen Y-DI. Effect of age on glucose tolerance and glucose uptake in healthy individuals. J Am Geriatr Soc 1989;37:735
62. Busby MJ, Bellantoni MF, Tobin JD, et al. Glucose tolerance in women: The effects of age, body composition, and sex hormones. J Am Geriatr Soc 1992;40:497
63. Meyers DA, Goldberg AP, Beecker ML, et al. Relationship of obesity and physical fitness to cardiopulmonary and metabolic function in healthy older men. J Gerontol Med Sci 1991;46:M57
64. Shimokata H, Muller DC, Fleg JL, et al. Age as independent determinant of glucose tolerance. Diabetes 1991;40:44
65. Coon PJ, Rogus EM, Drinkwater D, et al. Role of body fat distribution in the decline in insulin sensitivity and glucose tolerance with age. J Clin Endocrinol Metab 1992;75:1125
66. Kohrt WM, Kirwan JP, Staten MA, et al. Insulin resistance in aging is related to abdominal obesity. Diabetes 1993;42:273
67. Bonadonna BC, Groop LC, Simonson DC, DeFronzo RA. Free fatty acid and glucose metabolism in human aging: Evidence for operation of the Randle cycle. Am J Physiol 1994;266 (Endocrinol Metab 29):E501
68. Lawrence JC Jr, Colvin J, Cartee GD, Holloszy JO. Effects of aging and exercise on insulin action in rat adipocytes are correlated with changes in fat cell volume. J Gerontol Biol Sci 1989;44:B88
69. Seals DR, Hagberg JM, Allen WK, et al. Glucose tolerance in young and older athletes and sedentary men. J Appl Physiol Respirat Environ Exercise Physiol 1984;56:1521
70. Wang JT, Ho LT, Tang KT, et al. Effect of habitual physical activity on age-related glucose intolerance. J Am Geriatr Soc 1989;37:203
71. Houmard JA, Egan PC, Neufer PD, et al. Elevated skeletal muscle glucose transporter levels in exercise-trained middle-aged men. Am J Physiol 1991;261 (Endocrinol Metab 24):E437
72. Tonino RP. Effect of physical training on the insulin resistance of aging. Am J Physiol 1989;256 (Endocrinol Metab 19):E352
73. Kahn SE, Larson VG, Beard JC, et al. Effect of exercise on insulin action,

glucose tolerance, and insulin secretion in aging. Am J Physiol 1990;258 (Endocrinol Metab):E937

74. Hughes VA, Fiatarone MA, Fielding RA, et al. Exercise increases muscle GLUT-4 levels and insulin action in subjects with impaired glucose tolerance. Am J Physiol 1993;264 (Endocrinol Metab 27):E855

75. Cutler RG, Davis BJ, Ingram DK, Roth GS. Plasma concentration of glucose, insulin, and percent glycosylated hemoglobin are unaltered by food restriction in rhesus and squirrel monkeys. J Gerontol Biol Sci 1992;47:B9

76. Masoro EJ, McCarter RJM, Katz MS, McMahan CA. Dietary restriction alters characteristics of glucose fuel use. J Gerontol Biol Sci 1992;47:B202

77. Reaven PD, Barrett-Connor EL, Browner DK. Abnormal glucose tolerance and hypertension. Diabetes Care 1990;13:119

78. Muller DC, Elahi D, Pratley RE, et al. An epidemiological test of the hyperinsulinemia-hypertension hypothesis. J Clin Endocrinol Metab 1993;76:544

79. Dengel DR, Pratley RE, Hagberg JM, Goldberg AP. Impaired insulin sensitivity and maximal responsiveness in older hypertensive men. Hypertension 1994;23:320

80. Julius S, Gudbrandsson T, Jamerson K, et al. The hemodynamic link between insulin resistance and hypertension. J Hypertens 1991;9:983

81. Lithell HOL. Effect of antihypertensive drugs on insulin, glucose, and lipid metabolism. Diabetes Care 1991;14:203

82. Boden G, Chen X, DeSantis R, et al. Effects of ethanol on carbohydrate metabolism in the elderly. Diabetes 1993;42:28

Diabetes Mellitus, edited by Derek LeRoith, Simeon I. Taylor, and Jerrold M. Olefsky. Lippincott–Raven Publishers, Philadelphia © 1996.

CHAPTER 54

Drug-Induced Diabetes

RICHARD J. COMI

A large number of pharmacologic agents perturb carbohydrate metabolism. Many of these drugs aggravate the hyperglycemic state of diabetes and require adjustment in diabetic therapeutic regimens. Recently, these agents have been comprehensively reviewed.[1,2] Fewer agents have been reported to cause new diabetes in previously nondiabetic persons. In this chapter, drug-induced diabetes is defined as the new development of a hyperglycemic state that meets the definition of diabetes and that is due to the ingestion of a drug.

Diabetes is defined by certain levels of blood glucose in the fasted state or after a defined oral glucose load. One reason for using defined numeric glucose criteria for the diagnosis is that there is a normal distribution of fasting and post–glucose load blood glucose levels in most populations (the Pima Indians are a notable exception in having a bimodal distribution of postprandial glucose levels).[3] This distribution of post–glucose load glycemia is depicted in Figure 54-1. The distribution of plasma glucose concentrations at 2 hours postchallenge is divided into three groups:

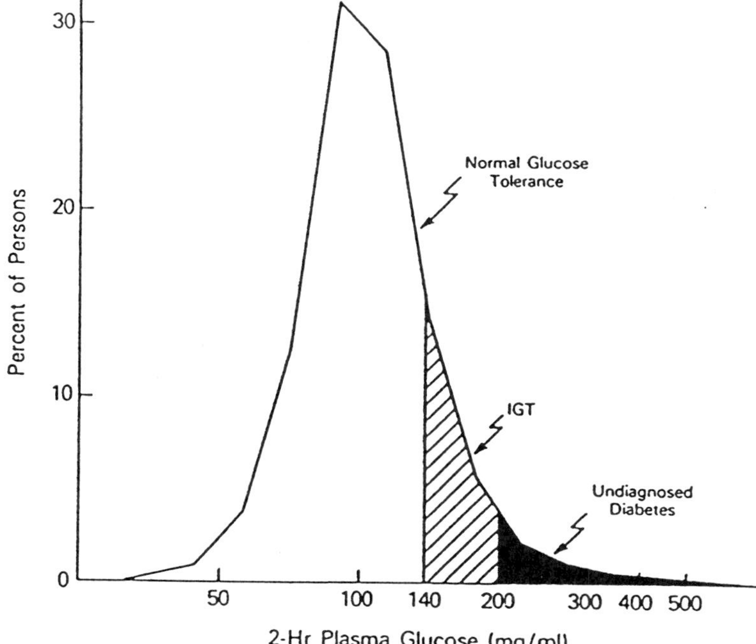

FIGURE 54-1. Percentage of persons in 0.1 log increments of venous plasma glucose 2 hours after a 75 g glucose challenge in the Second National Health and Nutrition Examination Survey, excluding those with previously diagnosed diabetes.

less than 140 mg/dL (7.8 mM), 141–200 mg/dL (7.8–11.1 mM), and greater than 200 mg/dL (11.1 mM). The last group is defined as having the disorder diabetes mellitus; the middle group is defined as "glucose intolerant" but not diabetic. A large proportion of the general U.S. population (11%) falls into the category glucose intolerant. If one imagines a medication that shifts a patient's position on this curve to the right, then that medication will shift a proportion of the population from the glucose-intolerant group to the diabetic group. Despite the rather large number of persons who are glucose intolerant and the large number of drugs known to worsen glucose tolerance, drug-induced diabetes is unusual. This suggests that only subpopulations of the glucose-intolerant population are actually at risk and might be prospectively identified or that other mechanisms might explain many of the cases. Both statements are likely to be true based on the reports reviewed in the rest of this chapter.

This chapter is organized according to the mechanism by which an agent induces diabetes. The first group of drugs interferes with insulin production or secretion; the second group blocks insulin action; and the third group interferes with both insulin secretion and action. The final group raises blood glucose using mechanisms independent of insulin's actions.

Table 54-1. Drugs That Induce Diabetes

Drugs That Cause Diabetes by Interfering with Insulin Production and Secretion
Vacor
Pentamidine
β-receptor antagonists
L-Asparaginase
Diphenylhydantoin
Diazoxide
Drugs That Cause Diabetes by Reducing the Effectiveness of Insulin in Regulating Metabolism
Steroids
Glucocorticoids
Megesterol acetate
β-Receptor agonists
Growth hormone
Drugs That Act on Both Insulin Secretion and Insulin Sensitivity
Thiazide diuretics
Cyclosporin
FK 506 (tacrolimus)
Treatments That Induce Diabetes by Increasing Nutrient Flux
Nicotinic acid
Total parenteral nutrition

Drugs That Cause Diabetes by Interfering with Insulin Production and Secretion

Several drugs and toxins are known to injure the β-cells of the pancreatic islet, which are the source of endogenous insulin (Table 54-1).

Vacor

The paradigm for this mechanism in humans is the toxic effects of the rodentcide *N*-3 pyridyl methyl *N′ p*-nitrophenyl (PNU, Vacor.)[4–6] Accidental or deliberate ingestion of this chemical causes rapid death of the insulin-producing islet β-cells. There are two phases to this process: first, insulin release from dying cells, which can be accompanied by hypoglycemia, and second, absolute insulin deficiency, which is accompanied by diabetes or diabetic ketoacidosis. This chemical appears to act by antagonizing the nucleotide niacinamide, an essential enzymatic cofactor. Early treatment with niacinamide is believed to be protective, although there is no case report documenting the efficacy of this therapy.[4,6]

Pentamidine

Pentamidine is an antiparasitic agent frequently used to treat infections with *Pneumocystis carinii* in patients with the acquired immune deficiency syndrome (AIDS) who are intolerant of trimethoprim-sulfa regimens. The mesylate, isethionate, and aerosolized forms have all been reported to induce dose- and duration-dependent cytolytic injury in the β-cell.[7–12] Up to 26% of patients treated with this agent experience hypoglycemia within 1 week due to acute cytolytic release of insulin. Following one or several courses of pentamidine therapy, hyperglycemia develops within 2 to 6 months in up to 19% of patients, most of whom have already experienced the hypoglycemic phase. Diabetic ketoacidosis has been reported.[13] Diabetes has not been reported in patients with AIDS treated with other antiparasitic agents, such as cotrimazole. The mechanism of injury is not known, although the histologic picture in the islet cells resembles that following Vacor ingestion.[9] Although diabetes may be temporary after one course of pentamidine, permanent diabetes is more common, especially after repeated courses of therapy.

L-Asparaginase

The antineoplastic agent L-asparaginase causes diabetes without injuring β-cells.[14–16] L-Asparaginase is an enzyme that metabolizes asparagine and limits the availability of this essential nutrient to leukemic cells. There are several case reports of diabetes and diabetic ketoacidosis in nondiabetic children treated with L-asparaginase. In these cases, there were very low levels of circulating insulin. L-Asparaginase does not directly metabolize the insulin molecule.[16] Instead, low levels of asparagine may impair insulin production because the insulin molecule contains three asparagine residues. Consistent with this hypothesis, diabetes usually resolves when treatment is withdrawn or completed.[14]

β-Antagonists

Antagonists to β-adrenergic receptors are commonly used medications known to impair insulin secretion, especially agents that are not selective for the β-1 receptor subtype. β-Receptor blockade inhibits insulin secretion by pancreatic islets in response to glucagon, glucose, or argenine. Several studies have linked chronic use of β-blockers with an increased risk for the development of diabetes. In two studies of men treated for hypertension, a community-based health survey in England over 9 years[17] and a 12-year follow-up of a cohort of Swedish men,[18] there was a relative risk of 6–6.1 compared to that of nonhypertensive control subjects. One abstract has even reported the new development of diabetes in 23/40 men with hypertension treated with propranolol for more than 6 months! These findings have not been confirmed in all studies, especially those using β-selective agents.[19] However, the risk of diabetes with the use of beta antagonists reported in most studies exceeds the known twofold increase in the risk of diabetes found in hypertensive populations.[20]

Propranolol therapy induced small increases in fasting glucose levels in 687 men treated in a Veterans Administration study for 48 months—from 99.6 mg/dL to 106 mg/dL.[21] In a 10-year study in Sweden, patients treated with hydrochlorothiazide plus propranolol showed an increase of 0.56 mM (10 mg/dL) compared to 0.18 mM (3.24 mg/dL) in patients treated with hydrochlorothiazide alone.[22] These data suggest that propranolol therapy may shift persons from the glucose intolerance to the frank diabetes portion of the curve shown in Figure 54-1. Because many factors, including age, weight, family history, and hypertension, play a role in the risk for diabetes, the true risk can only be assessed when these variables are controlled through a randomized study design. In a randomized trial comparing hydrochlorothiazide and propranolol (a nonselective β-blocker), oral glucose tolerance testing at 0, 1, and 6 years, did not show significantly different effect from β-blockade.[23] However, more and larger randomized trials will be needed to assess the true attributable risk of diabetes from β-blockade.

Diphenylhydantoin

Diphyenylhydantoin is a commonly used anticonvulsant that is known to inhibit insulin secretion.[24] In a randomized trial, 46 patients were treated with placebo or diphenylhydantoin for 3 years after myocardial infarction.[25] Oral glucose tolerance test results showed no difference between the groups, nor were they compared to baseline in either group at the end of the treatment period. However, the diphenylhydantoin group did show a small decrease in insulin secretion during the test, which suggested a compensatory increase in insulin sensitivity. Because there are numerous case reports of diphenylhydantoin-induced diabetes, it is likely that persons with other risk factors for diabetes, such as glucose intolerance and a limited ability to increase insulin sensitivity, may develop diabetes with this medication. Diabetes usually resolves once the medication is discontinued.

Diazoxide

Diazoxide is a vasodilator commonly used in the past for control of malignant hypertension. Parenteral diazoxide therapy inhibits insulin secretion, and there are reports of diabetic ketoacidosis in nondiabetic patients treated with multiple intravenous doses of diazoxide.[26,27] The mechanism is not known, but it is reversible on discontinuing the drug.

Drugs That Cause Diabetes by Reducing the Effectiveness of Insulin in Regulating Metabolism

Steroids

Glucocorticoids such as hydrocortisone, dexamethasone, prednisone, and methylprednisolone may induce diabetes. These drugs are used in a wide variety of disorders and in a wide range of doses. The actual incidence of diabetes induced by these agents is unknown because of these variations and because the most powerful influences on the risk of steroid-induced diabetes are likely to be the underlying metabolic and non-metabolic disorders of the patient.[28] This is underscored in data presented in a study from 1954, in which Fajans and Conn[29] proposed a combined cortisone glucose tolerance test to identify those at risk of developing diabetes. In the report, 50–62.5 mg of oral cortisone (12–15 mg of prednisone) were administered 8.5 and 2 hours before a glucose challenge. Of 37 persons with normal glucose tolerance, 1 developed diabetic glucose tolerance after the cortisone, an incidence of 2.7%. However, when 75 persons with normal glucose tolerance but a family history of diabetes were tested, 24% had a diabetic response to the glucose load. Thus, the presence of an asymptomatic underlying genetic risk or metabolic disorder (i.e., glucose intolerance) increased the risk of acute steroid-induced diabetes 10-fold.

Glucocorticoid-induced diabetes can be detected within hours of administration of the steroid.[29] Usually there is improvement in glucose tolerance with continued steroid use and a pathophysiologic state consistent with insulin resistance (increased endogenous insulin secretion).[30–32] The exact pathophysiology is controversial because several mechanisms are operating simultaneously.[30] Glucocorticoids encourage the breakdown of stored protein and fat stores, which causes an increased stream of free fatty acids and branched amino acids to the liver.[33] Steroids also induce increased cellular concentrations of gluconeogenic enzymes. The result of increased amounts of substrate for gluconeogenesis and increased amounts of the hepatic enzymatic machinery for gluconeogenesis is increased hepatic glucose output. Hepatic glucose output is usually regulated by insulin, but the effect of insulin is diminished in the presence of steroids. Glucose uptake by fat and muscle is reduced due to insulin resistance and direct steroid effects. Glucocorticoid therapy is a challenge to endogenous insulin secretion, and those who have limited reserves may become diabetic.

Megesterol acetate is a progestin steroid used to stimulate appetite and weight gain in patients with cachexia related to cancer and AIDS. There are two case reports of new-onset diabetes in patients with AIDS who were taking 80 mg of megesterol four times a day.[34,35] In one report, diabetes resolved when megesterol was discontinued but recurred upon rechallenge.[34] The mechanism has not been studied but is probably a combination of steroid-induced decreased sensitivity to insulin and increased caloric intake.

Oral contraceptives are steroid combinations that are known to increase average glucose concentrations in patients with and without diabetes by decreasing insulin sensitivity. However, in large epidemiologic studies, there is little evidence to link the use of modern low-dose estrogen or triphasic oral contraceptives to the development of diabetes. In the Nurses Health Study of 121,700 women over more than 15 years, current oral contraceptive use did not increase the risk of diabetes ($RR = 0.86$), and past use conferred a small increase in risk ($RR = 1.12$) that was not related to the dose or the duration of exposure.[36] It is prudent to monitor women who have already manifested a tendency toward diabetes in the presence of increased sex steroids, such as those with a history of gestational diabetes.

β-Agonists

Ironically, both β-antagonists and β-agonists have been implicated in causing diabetes, albeit through different mechanisms. β-Agonists mimic the effects of adrenergic members of the counter-regulatory hormone system in response to hypoglycemia. They cause insulin resistance, diminished glucose utilization, and increased glucose production. Stimulation of β-adrenergic receptors will increase hepatic glucose output and diminish insulin sensitivity. These agents do not confer an increased risk of diabetes when used topically for pulmonary disease. In the setting of pregnancy, however, in which insulin sensitivity is already reduced, the use of terbutaline to halt premature labor has been reported to result in an incidence of gestational diabetes of 12–33%.[37–39] Increased concentrations of blood glucose and insulin have been demonstrated after 5–7 days of oral or subcutaneous therapy, suggesting insulin resistance.[37] In a study of 91 women with preterm labor who were known to have normal glucose tolerance before terbutaline therapy, 11% of those treated with 30 mg/day of oral terbutaline developed gestational diabetes.[38] A control cohort of 634 similar women had an incidence of 6%. Interestingly, women treated with subcutaneous terbutaline, <3 mg/day, had an incidence of gestational diabetes of 5%. These data suggest a dose-response relationship. Alternatively, the oral route of administration may be more diabetogenic than the subcutaneous route of administration with this drug.

Growth Hormone

Another member of the counter-regulatory system with pharmacologic uses is growth hormone (GH). GH causes insulin resistance at a cellular site after the binding of insulin to its receptor. Since recombinant GH has become available, there has been increased use of the peptide to treat GH-deficient children and exploration of widening its uses for other causes of short stature, cardiac remodeling, and reduced muscle mass in the elderly. In the natural example of GH excess, acromegaly, diabetes is a prominent problem. There have been two case reports of diabetes that developed in GH-deficient children treated with GH and reversed after cessation of treatment.[40,41] In one, abnormalities of glucose tolerance remained after withdrawal of therapy.[40] Because juvenile-onset autoimmune diabetes (type I) is characterized by a progressive decrease in insulin secretory reserve, GH therapy may have unmasked relative insulin deficiency. It is likely that GH therapy will cause diabetes in susceptible persons and that the number of reported cases will increase if GH therapy is expanded to other patient groups.

Drugs That Act on Both Insulin Secretion and Insulin Sensitivity

Thiazides

Thiazide diuretics are commonly prescribed for control of hypertension that are often cited as causes of drug-induced diabetes. Many small, uncontrolled trials have shown an incidence of glucose intolerance in patients with hypertension treated with thiazides; in two studies, up to 22% of patients treated for 6 years had diabetes.[42,43] Bengtsson et al.[18] studied a population-based cohort of 1462 women over 10 years. The relative risk of an abnormal glucose tolerance test at the end of the study for persons with normal glucose tolerance at the start was 3.4–4.6 in those who were taking thiazide diuretics. Other investigators have not replicated these results; in a case-controlled study, Gurwitz et al.[44] found that the risk of developing diabetes was not increased by treatment with thiazides alone but was increased by treatment with more than one antihypertensive agent. The strongest evidence, however, would be that arising from a randomized intervention trial because hypertension itself increases the risk of developing diabetes by twofold or more.[20] Helgeland et al.[22] randomly assigned 785 men to either 50 mg of hydrochlorothiazide or placebo for 5 years and did not demonstrate a difference in fasting glucose values between the two groups at the beginning or end of the study. The European Working Group on Hypertension in the Elderly[45] randomly assigned 348 patients to 25 mg hydrochlorothiazide and 50 mg triamterene or placebo for up to 3 years. There was a large dropout rate in the study group, which may have biased the results. Although the blood glucose levels before and after challenge with glucose were increased by 13.2 and 30.2 mg/dL, respectively, no new cases of diabetes were noted in the treated group. Finally, two studies that compared thiazide therapy to propranolol therapy did not show an increased risk of diabetes after 6 years or 48 weeks of therapy in one regimen over the other.[21,23]

Acute administration of thiazide diuretics has been shown to cause a 27% decrease in endogenous insulin response to a hyperglycemic clamp protocol.[46] Gorden[47] had noted glucose intolerance and diminished serum insulin in association with potassium depleted states, and Heldren et al.[48] repeated the hyperglycemic clamp studies to show that the majority of the defect could be corrected by careful potassium repletion. Other data, however, have shown diminished insulin sensitivity after thiazide treatment and suggest that thiazide effects on carbohydrate metabolism may be more complex. In two studies, one a randomized double-blinded study, thiazide therapy increased plasma insulin and decreased the index of insulin sensitivity over a 12-week treatment period.[46,49]

In summary, thiazide diuretics are epidemiologically linked to an increased incidence of diabetes in hypertensive patients, but these data have not been supported by randomized, controlled trials. Potassium depletion due to thiazide diuretics exacerbates the problem. It is likely that new diabetes induced by thiazides is uncommon.

Cyclosporin

Cyclosporin A is a fungal metabolite used as an immunosuppressant to prevent the rejection of transplanted organs and to interfere with autoimmune processes. Cyclosporin interferes with the activation and proliferation of T cells by preventing the transcription of several genes, including those for interleukin-2 and c-myc. The incidence of diabetes in previously nondiabetic renal transplant recipients who receive cyclosporine has been reported to be 2–46%. Cyclosporine, however, is usually given in concert with glucocorticoids, which themselves are diabetogenic and may have an additive or synergistic effect.[1]

Koselj et al.[50] reported a retrospective series of 158 patients who received renal transplants and were treated with cyclosporine and steroids; 13.9% developed diabetes. In all series reported, diabetes develops within the first 2 months of therapy with cyclosporine, if at all, and requires insulin therapy for metabolic control. Yamamoto et al.[51] observed a greater incidence of diabetes in patients receiving cyclosporine and methylprednisolone (30%) than in patients who received azathiaprine and lower doses of steroids (7.5%). Ost et al.[52] studied intravenous glucose tolerance before and after transplantation in 19 renal transplant recipients who were taking cyclosporine and steroids and found a 53% incidence of newly abnormal glucose tolerance on therapy.[52] They compared this to an incidence of 7% in a group of 14 patients who were treated with azathiaprine and steroids. Boudreaux et al.[53] did not note an increased incidence of diabetes in patients treated with cyclosporine versus azathiaprine but did note a markedly enhanced development of diabetes in patients treated with cyclosporine, azathiaprine, and steroids (13.2% compared to 6.2%). They observed that older and heavier patients were much more at risk of developing diabetes (30% incidence) after transplantation than younger, lean patients.

The mechanism of cyclosporin-associated diabetes is a combination of inhibition of islet cell function and increased insulin resistance. In an early case report, a renal transplant recipient receiving cyclosporine developed diabetes and a decrease in C-peptide secretion simultaneously.[54] When cyclosporine treatment was decreased, C-peptide levels rose. Ost et al.,[52] however, reported that there was no change in C-peptide concentrations with cyclosporine treatment in patients who developed diabetes despite a decline in intravenous glucose tolerance, arguing for insulin resistance. In dog models, evidence for both mechanisms operating simultaneously has been demonstrated.[55]

FK 506

FK 506 (tacrolimus) is a macrolide used for immunosuppression that is more potent than cyclosporine but uses similar mechanisms of action. It appears to have a similar effect on carbohydrate metabolism, although few series have been reported. In a group of 24 renal transplant recipients receiving FK 506 and steroids, 4 developed diabetes. Two of the four experienced a remission when concomitant steroid therapy was stopped, leaving a final incidence of 8%—identical to that of a control group of 14 patients treated with cyclosporine and steroids.[56] In a recent comparison of FK 506 and cyclosporine for immunosuppression in liver transplant patients, the rate of hyperglycemia was similar (47% for FK 506 and 38% for cyclosporine), but twice as many nondiabetic patients developed diabetes in association with FK 506 compared to the cyclosporine group.[57]

Although there is no doubt that posttransplant recipients are at increased risk of developing diabetes compared to nontransplanted patients, no randomized trials of the agents used for immunosuppression have been performed to determine whether individual agents, certain combinations of agents, or allograft transplantation per se are responsible for this complication.

Treatments That Induce Diabetes by Increasing Nutrient Flux

Nicotinic Acid

Nicotinic acid is an effective therapy for dyslipidemias of very low and low density lipoproteins. Nicotinic acid therapy is associated with increased levels of blood glucose in both diabetic and nondiabetic patients, and uncontrolled hyperglycemia is a frequent reason for discontinuing therapy. Henkin et al.[58] reviewed 82 patients treated with nicotinic acid, including 17 heart transplant recipients. In the transplant recipients who had not previously had diabetes, there was a 33% incidence of new diabetes while on nicotinic acid. In the nontransplanted patients, the incidence of new-onset diabetes was 15%. The two groups differed in that the transplant patients were taking additional diabetogenic agents, such as steroids and cyclosporine, and the mean dose of nicotinic acid in the transplant patients (2.5 + 0.4 g/day) was nearly twice that of the nontransplant patients.

The mechanism for nicotinic acid–induced hyperglycemia is an increase in hepatic glucose output due to enhanced gluconeogenesis.[1] Actually, acute nicotinic acid administration results in a diminished flow of free fatty acids (FFA) to the liver and diminished gluconeogenesis. However, the effects of nicotinic acid after each dose are short-lived, and a rebound increase in FFA, by 50–100% over baseline, occurs.[59] This increased FFA flux to the liver results in increased oxidation of FFA by the liver and consumption of available cellular nicotinamide adenine dinucleotide. Ultimately, this decreased hepatocyte capacity for oxidation shifts metabolic activity to reductive pathways, such as glucose production. Kahn et al.[60] demonstrated a decline in both the responsiveness to insulin and the insulin sensitivity index in 11 patients treated for 2 weeks with nicotinic acid. Serum insulin levels rose, indicating an insulin-resistant state. Because of this mechanism, the use of long-acting nicotinic acid derivatives may avoid this hypergylcemic adverse effect.

Total Parenteral Nutrition

Total parenteral nutrition in the intensive care and non–intensive care settings is frequently associated with significant elevations in blood glucose concentrations. There are often inflammatory conditions or drugs that impair carbohydrate metabolism, such as steroids, in effect concurrently. No large studies have examined the frequency of diabetes induced by this therapy, which involves administration of high concentrations of glucose and FFA, but the physician must monitor these patients for the development of diabetes.

In summary, drug-induced diabetes occurs due to a variety of drugs and mechanisms. An underlying and often unsuspected abnormality in carbohydrate metabolism in the patient greatly increases the risk of developing drug-induced diabetes. In most cases, the drug induces a perturbation in metabolism that exceeds the patient's adaptive capacity. This suggests that sulfonylureas, which act primarily by enhancing endogenous insulin secretion, would not be expected to be effective therapy. In cases where the drug that induced diabetes must be continued, insulin therapy is the most efficacious approach. The new thiazolidinedione drugs, such as troglitazone and citaglazone, which increase insulin sensitivity in patients with glucose intolerance and diabetes, may be very useful in those circumstances where a drug-induced increase in insulin resistance has resulted in diabetes.[61]

References

1. Bressler P, DeFronzo RA. Drugs and diabetes. Diabetes Rev 1994;2:53–84
2. Pandit MK, Gustafson JBB, Minocha A, Peiris AN. Drug induced disorders of glucose tolerance. Ann Intern Med 1994;118:529–539
3. Harris M. Impaired glucose tolerance in the US population. Diabetes Care 1989;12:464–474
4. Pont A, Rulina JM, Bishop D, Peal R. Diabetes mellitus and neuropathy following vacor ingestion in man. Arch Intern Med 1979;139:185–187
5. Porte D. Carbohydrate intolerance during beta adrenergic blockade in hypertension. J Clin Invest 1967;46:86–94
6. Prosser PR, Karam JH. Diabetes mellitus following rodenticide ingestion in man. JAMA 1978;239:1148–1150
7. Bouchard P, Sai P, Reach G, et al. Diabetes mellitus following pentamidine induced hypoglycemia in humans. Diabetes 1982;31:40–45
8. Fisch A, Prazuk T, Malkin JE, et al. Diabetes mellitus in a patient with AIDS treated with pentamidine aerosol (letter). Br Med J 1990;301:875
9. Hauser L, Sheehan P, Simpkins H. Pancreatic pathology in pentamidine induced diabetes in acquired immunodeficiency. Hum Pathol 1991;22:926–929
10. Herchline TE, Plouffe JF, Pera MF. Diabetes mellitus presenting with ketoacidosis following pentamidine therapy in patients with AIDS. J Infect 1991;22:41–44
11. Pearson RD, Hewlett EL. Pentamidine for the treatment of *Pneumocystis carinii* and other protocol drugs. Ann Intern Med 1985;103:782–786
12. Peronne C, Bricaire F, Leport C, et al. Hypoglycemia and diabetes mellitus following parenteral pentamidine mesylate treatment in AIDS patients. Diabetic Med 1990;7:585–589
13. Lambertus MW, Murphy AR, Nagami P, Goetz MB. Diabetic ketoacidosis following pentamidine therapy in a patient with AIDS. West J Med 1988;149:602–604
14. Gillette PC, Hill LL, Sterling KA, Fernbach DJ. Transient diabetes mellitus secondary to L-asparaginase therapy in acute leukemia. J Pediatr 1972;81:109–111
15. Gailau S, Nussbaum A, Ohunma T, Freeman A. Diabetes in patients treated with asparaginase. Clin Pharmacol Ther 1971;12:487–490
16. Whitecar JP, Bodey GP, Hill CS, Samaan NA. Effect of L-asparaginase on carbohydrate metabolism. Metabolism 1970;19:581–586
17. Skarfors ET, Lithell HO, Selinas I, Aberg H. Do antihypertensive drugs precipitate diabetes in predisposed men? Br Med J 1989;298:1147–1152
18. Bengtsson C, Blohme G, Lapidus L, et al. Do antihypertensive drugs precipitate diabetes? Br Med J 1984;289:1495–1497
19. Vedin A, Wilhalmsson C, Bjorntorp P. Induction of diabetes and oral glucose tolerance tests during and after chronic beta blockade. Acta Med Scand 1975;575(suppl):1261–1263
20. Barret-Connor E, Criqui M, Klauber M, Holbrook M. Diabetes and hypertension in a community of older adults. Am J Epidemiol 1981;113:276–284
21. VA Cooperative Study Group on Aging. Comparison of propranolol and hydrochlorothiazide for the initial treatment of hypertension. II. Results of long term study. JAMA 1982;248:2004–2011
22. Helgeland A, Leren P, Fossi OP, et al. Serum glucose levels during long term observation of treated and untreated men with hypertension. The Oslo study. Am J Med 1984;76:802–805
23. Bergland G, Andersson O. Beta blocker or diuretics in hypertension? Six year follow-up of blood pressure and metabolic side effects. Lancet 1982;1:744–747
24. Kizer JS, Vargas-Cordon M, Brendel K, Bressler R. The in vivo inhibition of insulin secretion by diphenylhydantoin. J Clin Invest 1970;49:1942–1947
25. Perry-Keene DA, Larkin RG, Heyma P, et al. The effects of long term diphenylhydantoin on glucose tolerance and insulin secretion in a controlled trial. Clin Endocrinol 1980;12:575–580
26. DeBroe M, Mussche M, Ringoir S, Bosteels V. Oral diazoxide for malignant hypertension. Lancet 1972;1:1397
27. Updike SJ, Harrington AR. Acute diabetic ketoacidosis: A complication of intravenous diazoxide treatment for refractory hypertension. N Engl J Med 1969;280:768

28. Caldwell JR, Furst DE. The efficacy and safety of low-dose corticosteroids for rheumatoid arthritis. Semin Arthritis Rheum 1991;21:1–11
29. Fajans SS, Conn JW. An approach to the prediction of diabetes mellitus by modification of the glucose tolerance test with cortisone. Diabetes 1954; 3:296–304
30. Olefsky JM, Kimmerling G. Effects of glucocorticoids on carbohydrate metabolism. Am J Med Sci 1976;271:203–210
31. Shamoon H, Saamar V, Sherwin RS. The influence of acute physiological increments of cortisol on fuel metabolism and insulin binding to monocytes in normal humans. J Clin Endocrinol Metab 1980;50:495–501
32. Papagano G, Cavallo-Perin P, Cassader M, et al. An in vivo and in vitro study of the mechanism of prednisone induced insulin resistance in healthy subjects. J Clin Invest 1983;72:1814–1820
33. Zimmerman T, Haber F, Rodriguez N, et al. Contribution of insulin resistance to catabolic effect of prednisone on leucine metabolism. Diabetes 1989; 38:1238–1244
34. Henry K, Rathgaber S, Sullivan C, McCabe K. Diabetes mellitus induced by megesterol acetate in a patient with AIDS and cachexia. Ann Intern Med 1992;116:53–54
35. Panwalker A. Hyperglycemia induced by megesterol acetate (letter). Ann Intern Med 1992;116:878
36. Rimm E, Manson J, Stampfer M, et al. Oral contraceptive use and the risk of type 2 diabetes in a large population of women. Diabetologia 1992;35:967–972
37. Foley MR, Langdon MB, Gabbe SG, et al. Effect of prolonged oral terbutaline therapy on glucose tolerance in pregnancy. Am J Obstet Gynecol 1993; 168:100–105
38. Lindenbaum C, Ludmir J, Teplick FB, et al. Maternal glucose intolerance and the subcutaneous terbutaline pump. Am J Obstet Gynecol 1992;166:925–928
39. Regenstein A, Belluomini J, Katz M. Terbutaline tocolysis and glucose intolerance. Obstet Gynecol 1993;81:739–741
40. Botero D, Danon M, Brown R. Symptomatic non-insulin dependent diabetes during therapy with recombinant growth hormone. J Pediatr 1993;123: 590–592
41. Garg A. Hyperglycemia during replacement GH therapy. J Pediatr 1994;125: 329
42. Lewis PJ, Petrie A, Kohner EM, Doller CT. Determination of glucose tolerance in hypertensive patients on prolonged diuretic therapy. Lancet 1976;1:564–566
43. Murphy MB, Kohnen E, Lewis PJ, et al. Glucose intolerance in hypertensive patients treated with diuretics; a fourteen year follow-up. Lancet 1982;2: 1293–1295
44. Gurwitz JH, Bohn RL, Glynn RJ, et al. Antihypertensive drug therapy and the initiation of treatment for diabetes mellitus. Ann Intern Med 1992;118: 273–278
45. Amery A, Bulpitt C, Schaepdryver A, et al. Glucose tolerance during diuretic therapy. Results of a trial by the European Working Group on Hypertension in the Elderly. Lancet 1978;1:681–687
46. Rowe JD, Tobin JD, Rosa RM, Andus R. Effect of experimental potassium deficiency on glucose and insulin metabolism. Metabolism 1980;29:498–502
47. Gorden P. Glucose intolerance with hypokalemia. Diabetes 1973;22:544–551
48. Heldren JH, Elaki D, Andersen DK, et al. Prevention of glucose intolerance of thiazide diuretics by maintenance of body potassium. Diabetes 1983;32: 106–111
49. Plaunik FL, Rodriguez IS, Zanalle MT, Riberio AB. Hypokalemia, glucose intolerance and hyperinsulinemia during diuretic therapy. Hypertension 1992; 19(suppl):II26–II29
50. Koselj M, Koselj KM, Kveder R. Posttransplant diabetes mellitus in renal allograft recipients. Transplant Proc 1992;24:2756–2757
51. Yamamoto H, Azakawa S, Yamaguchi Y, et al. Effects of cyclosporine A and low dosage of steroids on posttransplant diabetes in kidney transplant recipients. Diabetes Care 1991;14:867–870
52. Ost L, Tyder G, Fehrman I. Impaired glucose tolerance in cyclosporine-prednisone treated renal graft recipients. Transplantation 1988;46:370–372
53. Boudreaux JP, McHugh L, Caanafax DM, et al. The impact of cyclosporine and combination immunosuppression on the incidence of posttransplant diabetes in renal allograft recipients. Transplantation 1987;44:376–381
54. Bending JJ, Ogg CS, Viberti GC. Diabetogenic effect of cyclosporin. Br Med J 1987;294:401
55. Wahlstrom HE, Akimoto R, Endres D, et al. Recovery and hypersecretion of insulin and reversal of insulin resistance after withdrawal of short term cyclosporine treatment. Transplantation 1992;53:1190–1195
56. Fung JJ, Alessiani M, AbuElmagad K, et al. Adverse effects associated with FK 506. Transplant Proc 1991;23:3105–3108
57. The U.S. Multicenter FK 506 Liver Study Group. A comparison of tacrolimus (FK 506) and cyclosporine for immunosuppression in liver transplantation. N Engl J Med 1994;331:1110–1115
58. Henkin Y, Oberman A, Hurst D, Segnest J. Niacin revisited: Clinical observations on an important but underutilized drug. Am J Med 1991;91:239–246
59. Pinter E, Patter C. Biphasic nature of blood glucose and free fatty acid changes following intravenous nicotinic acid in man. J Clin Endocrinol Metab 1967;27:430–443
60. Kahn S, Beard J, Schwartz M, et al. Increased beta cell secretory capacity as a mechanism for islet adaptation to nicotinic acid induced insulin resistance. Diabetes 1989;38:562–568
61. Nolan J, Ludvik B, Beerdsen P, et al. Improvement in glucose tolerance and insulin resistance in obese subjects treated with troglitazone. N Engl J Med 1994;331:1188–1193

Diabetes Mellitus, edited by Derek LeRoith, Simeon I. Taylor, and Jerrold M. Olefsky. Lippincott–Raven Publishers, Philadelphia © 1996.

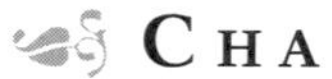

Chapter 55

Non–Insulin-Dependent Diabetes Mellitus Secondary to Other Endocrine Disorders

Michael Berelowitz and Eugene How Go

Diabetes mellitus that occurs in association with a variety of other disorders (endocrine or nonendocrine) is referred to as *secondary*. Endocrine causes of secondary diabetes occur in association with the therapeutic administration or excessive secretion of one of the counter-regulatory hormones—growth hormone, glucocorticoids, glucagon, or catecholamines. With cessation of hormone administration or removal of the source of overproduction, glucose homeostasis usually returns to normal. However, unmasking of a predisposition to non–insulin-dependent diabetes mellitus (NIDDM) may be the reason that secondary diabetes occurs in association with some but not all cases of the predisposing cause.

Endocrine conditions associated with secondary diabetes are listed in Table 55-1 and discussed below.

Acromegaly and Gigantism

Acromegaly in the adult and gigantism in the prepubertal child result from excessive autonomous secretion of growth hormone (GH). Autonomous GH excess usually arises from a somatotrope adenoma of the anterior pituitary or, more rarely, from somatotrope

TABLE 55-1. Endocrine Causes of Secondary NIDDM

Acromegaly or gigantism
Growth hormone administration
Cushing's syndrome and glucocorticoid therapy
Glucagonoma
Pheochromocytoma
Hyperthyroidism
Androgen excess
Hyperprolactinemia
Hyperaldosteronism
Carcinoid tumor

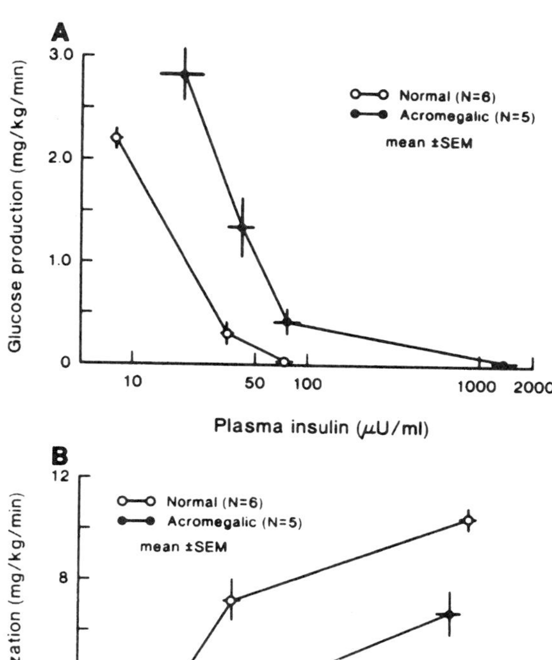

FIGURE 55-2. Dose-response curves for insulin on suppression of glucose production (**A**) and stimulation of glucose utilization (**B**) in normal subjects (○–○) and patients with acromegaly (●–●). (Reproduced from Hansen I, Tsalikian E, Beaufrere B, et al. Insulin resistance in acromegaly: Defects in both hepatic and extrahepatic insulin action. Am J Physiol 1986;250:E269.)

hyperplasia occurring as a result of eutopic or ectopic overproduction of GH releasing factor or (in one reported case) from ectopic GH secretion.[1] Clinical features characteristic of acromegaly or gigantism are due to the effect of long-standing excess of GH, either directly or indirectly, on cellular growth and tissue metabolism. Indirect effects of GH are mediated by insulin-like growth factor I (IGF-I; previously known as *somatomedin-C*), which is synthesized in the liver and many other tissues and circulates in plasma at levels determined by ambient GH.

GH influences the metabolism of carbohydrate, fats, and protein. Physiologically, GH can be considered a counter-regulatory hormone secreted under circumstances of decreased glucose availability (fasting, insulin-induced hypoglycemia).

GH has been described as diabetogenic and lipolytic; it also promotes protein anabolism.[2] Its effect on carbohydrate metabolism can be biphasic. Gh has an acute insulin-like effect and a chronic insulin-antagonistic effect. An early insulin-like effect of a physiologic dose of GH given to normal volunteers has been demonstrated in a study by McGorman et al.,[3] although other studies have not consistently confirmed this finding. An anti-insulin effect of GH was shown in GH-deficient children who demonstrated hypoglycemia with decreased hepatic glucose output, suggesting unopposed insulin actions; human growth hormone replacement therapy normalized the metabolic state.[4] Despite the ability of GH therapy in children with short stature to increase insulin secretion, glucose levels were not significantly altered,[5] suggesting induction of insulin resistance. Normal human volunteers demonstrate a right shift of the dose-response curve for insulin-stimulated glucose utilization and insulin-mediated suppression of glucose production in response to GH[6] (Fig. 55-1). Again, glucose levels were similar to those of control subjects, supporting the hypothesis of resistance to insulin action. Studies with acromegalic subjects have provided similar evidence of peripheral insulin resistance as well as elevated hepatic glucose output[7,8] (Fig. 55-2).

It is unclear which effects on carbohydrate, lipid, and protein metabolism are mediated by GH itself and which are mediated by IGF-I. Although GH stimulates IGF-I production, the level and activity of IGF-I are influenced by the different types of IGF binding proteins. Also, IGF-I can act on type I and type II, as well as on insulin receptors.[9] Studies on normal male volunteers by Turkalj et al.[10] showed that IGF-I given acutely resulted in an insulin-like effect, that is, increased glucose metabolism, decreased lipolysis, ketogenesis, and amino acid oxidation.

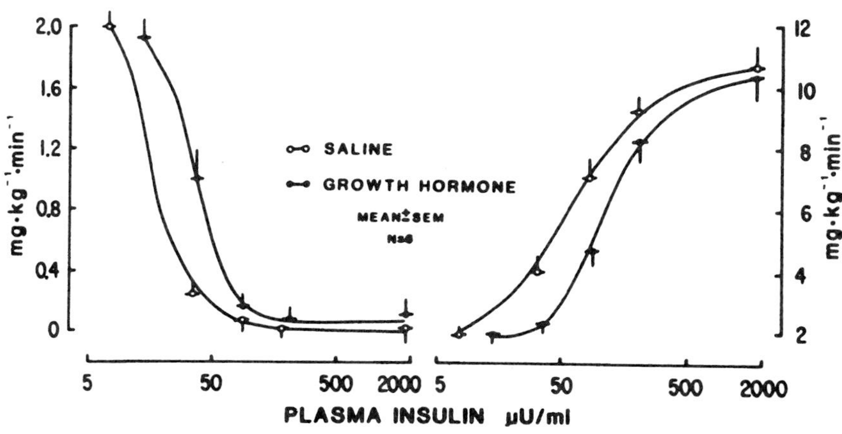

FIGURE 55-1. Dose-response curves for insulin on inhibition of glucose production and stimulation of glucose utilization in saline-treated control subjects (○–○) and growth hormone–treated (●–●) subjects. (Reproduced from Rizza R, Mandarino L, Gerich J. Effects of growth hormone on insulin action in man. Mechanism of insulin resistance, impaired suppression of glucose production, and impaired stimulation of glucose utilization. Diabetes 1982;31:663.)

Growth Hormone and Glucose Intolerance

The reported incidence of diabetes mellitus in patients with acromegaly varies from 13% to 32%,[11,12,18] whereas glucose intolerance has been reported in as many as 60% of cases.[13] Some of this variation may be explained by the severity of the acromegaly, and some is due to definitions of diabetes that differ among reports. Using the criteria of the National Diabetes Data Group,[14] a 36% incidence of impaired glucose tolerance and a 30% incidence of diabetes mellitus were reported in a series of 500 cases of acromegaly.[15]

A number of mechanisms have been implicated as potential causes of impaired glucose tolerance and diabetes mellitus in acromegaly. In normal subjects, GH causes impairment of insulin action within 2–12 hours, with no effect on glucose-mediated insulin secretion.[16] Decreased glucose uptake into forearm muscle occurs after GH infusion.[17] A number of studies demonstrate that this GH-induced insulin resistance in peripheral tissues, primarily muscle, is probably due to a postreceptor defect,[7,16,17] although some studies demonstrate a reduction in insulin receptor number.[18] An increase in hepatic glucose production has also been implicated as a cause of hyperglycemia,[8] perhaps influenced by the degree of hyperinsulinemia. Studies in acromegalics have revealed peripheral insulin resistance,[8] as well as elevated hepatic glucose output.[7] At the cellular level, a decrease in oxidative[8] and nonoxidative[17] glucose metabolism, elevated fatty acid levels with sparing of glucose metabolism by the Randle cycle,[8] and futile cycling of glucose play a role in the development of glucose intolerance and diabetes in acromegaly. Overt diabetes may result in the group of patients with the most limited insulin secretory capacity.

Therapy is primarily directed at the underlying cause of acromegaly. In a series reported by Nabarro,[19] slightly more than half of the patients cured of acromegaly demonstrated resolution of their diabetes, whereas some showed improvement and others no change at all. Improvement in glucose metabolism may take as long as 6–12 months, and may depend on the severity and duration of the diabetes mellitus and on recovery of pancreatic islet function.[19] Studies using octreotide for the treatment of acromegaly have shown no consistent effect on glucose metabolism. Improvement, worsening, or no change in glucose metabolism have been reported, and a few patients with normal glucose tolerance may develop impaired glucose tolerance, perhaps due to the effect of octreotide on insulin secretion.[20] It is therefore prudent to monitor glucose tolerance closely if octreotide is initiated in acromegalic patients.

As in patients with insulin-dependent diabetes mellitus (IDDM) and NIDDM, patients with acromegaly who have diabetes may develop complications, including retinopathy and neuropathy.

Cushing's Syndrome

Cushing's syndrome results from a chronic increase in circulating glucocorticoids. Endogenous glucocorticoid excess can result from adrenocorticotropic hormone overproduction (usually from a pituitary microadenoma or, less commonly, ectopic production by a nonpituitary tumor) or autonomous adrenocortical hyperfunction (adenoma, carcinoma, or nodular hyperplasia). Administration of exogenous glucocorticoids for therapeutic purposes is a frequent cause of Cushing's syndrome.

Glucocorticoids and Glucose Intolerance

Glucocorticoids act physiologically over the intermediate term as counter-regulatory hormones to insulin action. They can be viewed as primarily catabolic hormones promoting release of gluconeogenic precursors—amino acids, glycerol, and free fatty acids from muscle and adipose tissue and stimulating hepatic and renal gluconeogenesis through enzyme induction. They also decrease peripheral glucose uptake and clearance under basal and insulin-stimulated conditions accompanied by insulin resistance[21,22] (Fig. 55-3). In vitro this insulin resistance results in part from a decrease in insulin receptor affinity, but, more important, it results from a postreceptor defect[23] in insulin-stimulated glucose transport[24] leading to a decrease in glucose utilization that is also seen in vivo in normal subjects given glucocorticoid.[21,22]

Studies in patients with Cushing's syndrome with normal fasting plasma glucose concentrations reveal that the primary defect in glucose metabolism is one of impaired glucose disposal.[25] In vivo the effect of glucocorticoids to induce insulin resistance results in a compensatory increase in insulin secretion[26] that tends to inhibit hepatic glucose production, lipolysis, and muscle amino acid release and to promote muscle glucose uptake, thus achieving a new steady state.

The diabetogenic effect of glucocorticoids has been reported to be more pronounced in subjects defined as low insulin responders (to a glucose infusion test) compared to high insulin responders. Thus, those subjects with a low insulin secretory reserve failed to respond with an insulin response to dexamethasone during a hyperglycemic clamp, and demonstrated increased basal hepatic glucose production, total hepatic glucose output, and glucose cycling. Insulin release correlated negatively with the glucose area under the curve during an oral glucose tolerance test.[27] From these data and from previous studies, it would appear that non–insulin-dependent diabetes mellitus (NIDDM) will occur in states of glu-

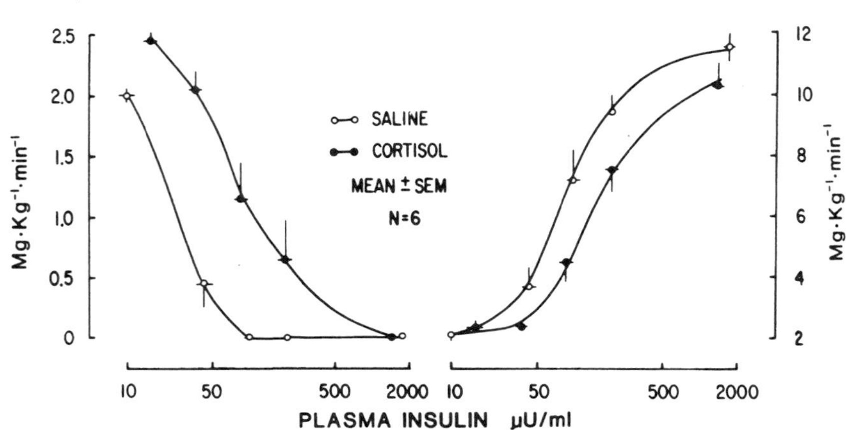

Figure 55-3. Dose-response curves for insulin on suppression of glucose production and stimulation of glucose utilization in saline-treated control subjects (○–○) and cortisol-treated (●–●) subjects. (Reproduced from Rizza RA, Mandarino LJ, Gerich JE. Cortisol-induced insulin resistance in man: Impaired suppression of glucose production and stimulation of glucose utilization due to a postreceptor defect of insulin action. J Clin Endocrinol Metab 1982;54:131.)

cocorticoid excess when insulin secretory compensation is inadequate.

Insulin metabolism may also be altered in patients with Cushing's syndrome who have been demonstrated to have a reduced serum insulin : C-peptide ratio.[25] These findings agree with studies in rat hepatocytes in which dexamethasone pretreatment has been shown to increase the rate of insulin degradation.[28] Abnormal glucose tolerance with insulin resistance and hyperinsulinemia occurs in 80–90% of patients with Cushing's syndrome. Overt diabetes mellitus has been reported as a common occurrence, with a frequency of up to 29%.[29] Just as the occurrence of NIDDM varies in different population groups, so may its expression vary in the particular Cushing's syndrome patient cadre studied.

Clinical predictors for the development of diabetes in patients treated with glucocorticoids include those factors considered risk factors for NIDDM—age, weight, and a family history of diabetes mellitus or gestational diabetes.

Complications of diabetes in patients with Cushing's syndrome include hyperosmolar nonketotic coma. Microvascular complications are very rare, confined to case reports that include a patient who developed proliferative retinopathy.[30]

Treatment of the cause of Cushing's syndrome results in reversal of the diabetic state in the majority of patients. Persistent diabetes is likely in those with more severe metabolic disturbance—perhaps those with the most limited insulin secretory reserve. Insulin therapy is considered the treatment of choice in patients with glucocorticoid-induced hyperglycemia, with the goals of metabolic normalization and prevention of a hyperosmolar state.

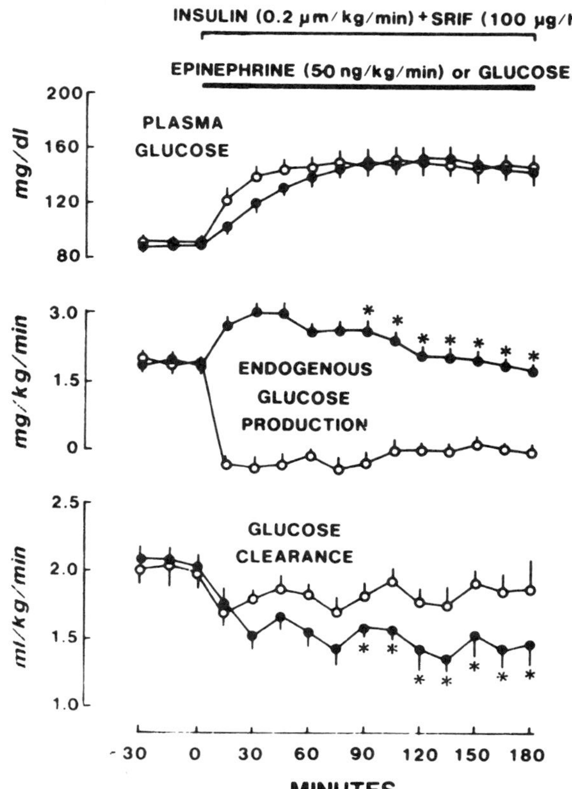

Figure 55-4. Effect of epinephrine infusion (●–●) or control infusion of glucose (○–○) on plasma glucose concentrations (top panel), endogenous glucose production (middle panel), and glucose clearance (lower panel) during insulin/somatostatin infusion designed to maintain plasma glucose insulin and glucagon concentrations. (Reproduced from Rizza RA, Cryer PE, Haymond MW, Gerich JE. Adrenergic mechanisms for the effects of epinephrine on glucose production and clearance in man. J Clin Invest 1980;65:682.)

Pheochromocytoma

Pheochromocytomas are tumors of neuroectodermal origin (benign in >90%) that secrete the catecholamines epinephrine, norepinephrine, and dopamine. They can be located anywhere within the sympathoadrenal system, with 90% in the adrenal medulla (~10% bilateral) and the remainder most commonly in the mediastinum, bladder, and organ of Zuckerkandl.[31] Disorders of glucose metabolism resulting from pheochromocytomas are common but are usually mild. In various series, glucose intolerance has been reported in up to 30% and mild fasting blood glucose elevation in 50%, with overt diabetes being unusual.[32]

Catecholamines and Glucose Intolerance

Catecholamines are normally secreted as an acute response to insulin-induced hypoglycemia and act to counter many of the metabolic effects of insulin. Their major physiologic effect is an increase in glucose production[33] (Fig. 55-4) through glycogenolysis in muscle and liver, increases in gluconeogenic precursor availability, and stimulation of gluconeogenesis and lipolysis.[34,35] At the same time, they inhibit insulin secretion, stimulate glucagon release, and inhibit glucose utilization.

Exogenously administered epinephrine and norepinephrine inhibit insulin secretion. This effect may be reversed by α-adrenergic blockade using phentolamine and is likely mediated by the α_2-adrenergic receptor.[36] β-Adrenergic catecholamine effects stimulate insulin secretion. In patients with pheochromocytoma, glucose-mediated insulin secretion is usually inhibited in the presence of endogenously elevated catecholamine levels and is reversed by α-blockade.[37] Insulin secretion in response to arginine, interestingly, is unaffected in pheochromocytoma patients, and responses are similar before and after tumor removal.[38] Glucagon secretion, in contrast, is reported to be increased in pheochromocytoma patients.[39] This may be explained by the β-adrenergic stimulation of glucagon secretion that has been well described in vivo and in vitro.[40] Authors have, however, reported normal[37] and even suppressed glucagon[38] levels, with lack of response to arginine in pheochromocytoma patients.[38] Glucagon secretion in these patients may therefore depend on which catecholamines are present and, in general, may play a small role in the observed glucose intolerance.

Catecholamines influence glucose metabolism in liver, muscle, and adipose tissue by direct receptor-mediated effects. Infusion of epinephrine results in sustained hyperglycemia.[41] This appears to result from an early (<30-minute) increase in glucose production that returns to near-basal levels by 180 minutes together with a sustained decrease in glucose clearance.[33] Glucagon does not appear to be involved in the mediation of this effect.[41] The increase in glucose production rate is mediated largely through β-adrenergic receptors via a cAMP-dependent mechanism; it occurs through an increase in muscle and liver glycogenolysis and stimulation of hepatic gluconeogenesis with an increased supply of substrates (lactate and products of increased lipolysis).

Peripheral glucose utilization is inhibited by a variety of mechanisms in pheochromocytoma, including a decrease in insulin concentration and induction of peripheral insulin resistance at the postreceptor level and through an increased free fatty acid concentration, probably through the Randle cycle.[33]

Pharmacologic treatment with combined α- and β-adrenergic blockade, using phentolamine or phenoxybenzamine plus propranolol, improves insulin secretion and glucose tolerance.

Tumor removal is the treatment of choice and results in normalization of glucose metabolism. In some cases, glucose intolerance may persist for several months after resection of the tumor due to a state of residual insulin resistance, which slowly returns to normal.[42]

Glucagonoma

The glucagonoma syndrome, due to a pancreatic islet glucagon-secreting tumor, is characterized by weight loss, glossitis, necrolytic migratory rash, normochromic normocytic anemia, and glucose intolerance.[43]

Glucagon and Glucose Intolerance

Glucagon under physiologic conditions acts as a counter-regulatory hormone primarily on the liver, where it acts via a G-protein–linked receptor to stimulate cAMP-dependent kinases to increase glycogenolysis and gluconeogenesis.

Studies in dogs demonstrate that the glucagon effect is time dependent, with glycogenolysis being the predominant effect early (<15 minutes) and then, as this attenuates, an increase in gluconeogenesis about 2 1/2 hours later.[44] The reason for the attenuation in glycogenolysis in the continued presence of glucagon is unclear but is probably not caused by depletion of glycogen stores.[44] Glucagon also acts on muscle and adipose tissue to promote the release of gluconeogenic precursors—amino acids and fatty acids. By these mechanisms, glucagon effectively helps to maintain the blood glucose concentration in the fasted state. The presence of insulin counteracts the effects of glucagon on adipose tissue and muscle.

In patients with glucagonoma, increased gluconeogenesis has been identified as the major cause of hyperglycemia.[45] Decreased circulating amino acid concentrations are present and account for the dermal and mucosal abnormalities.[46] High concentrations of glucagon may be associated with suppression of insulin secretion and, therefore, with relative insulin deficiency by a direct effect of glucagon (locally or via the circulation) on β-cell function and/or by glucagon stimulation of adrenal medullary epinephrine release, which may tend to inhibit insulin secretion and increase hepatic glucose production.[47] Insulin resistance does not appear to play a role in the pathogenesis of the glucose intolerance seen.

The glucagon-like peptides released from glucagonoma include native pancreatic glucagon, as well as a larger molecular weight species (~9000 d) that is present in the circulation in large amounts and that disappears from plasma after successful tumor resection.[48] Although its activity is less than that of native glucagon, its high circulating concentration may contribute to glucose intolerance in these patients.[48]

Glucose intolerance occurs almost universally in glucagonoma patients, who may demonstrate mild to severe hyperglycemia. Although glucagon has been implicated as ketogenic in insulin-deficient states, patients with glucagonoma generally do not become ketotic.[49]

Successful surgical resection results in cure of the diabetes,[50] but resection is not always possible because these tumors are frequently malignant, with secretory metastatic disease. Scanning with the labeled somatostatin analog octreotide may enable localization of the primary tumor and major metastatic deposits as a preliminary to successful surgical resection. Receptors for somatostatin on these tumors predict that they can be successfully treated with octreotide, with symptomatic and biochemical improvement but, to date, with no effect on tumor growth.[51] Other agents used for the treatment of islet-cell tumors, such as streptozotocin, have also been used, with lowering of serum glucagon concentrations and improvement in hyperglycemia.

Hyperthyroidism

Hyperthyroidism is seen commonly; thus, its coexistence with glucose intolerance and diabetes mellitus is not unexpected. Diabetes, however, is twice as prevalent in hyperthyroid patients as in the general population. Various surveys have placed the incidence of diabetes in hyperthyroid patients at 7–57%.[52–54] In patients with pre-existing diabetes, either insulin-dependent diabetes mellitus (IDDM) or non–insulin-dependent diabetes mellitus (NIDDM), the presence of hyperthyroidism renders blood glucose management more difficult.[55]

Thyroid Hormone and Glucose Intolerance

The underlying mechanism whereby hyperglycemia occurs in hyperthyroid patients remains unclear. Influences of thyroid hormone on insulin secretion and cellular metabolism have been implicated on the basis of in vitro and animal studies. In rats, thyroxine and triiodothyronine treatment inhibits the delayed phase of glucose-mediated insulin secretion—triiodothyronine being fivefold more potent than thyroxin.[56] The opposite is seen in response to antithyroid drugs. Mice (*ob/ob* strain) made hyperthyroid developed a decrease in pancreatic islet cell volume with a decrease in insulin content.[57]

In hyperthyroid states, gluconeogenic precursors (lactate and glycerol) are present in increased concentration in plasma. In rats, increased activity of mitochondrial glycerol phosphate oxidase increases the capacity for gluconeogenesis from glycerol.[58] It has also been shown in rats and pigs that hyperthyroidism leads to an increase in futile cycling of glucose, which could contribute to hyperglycemia.[59,60]

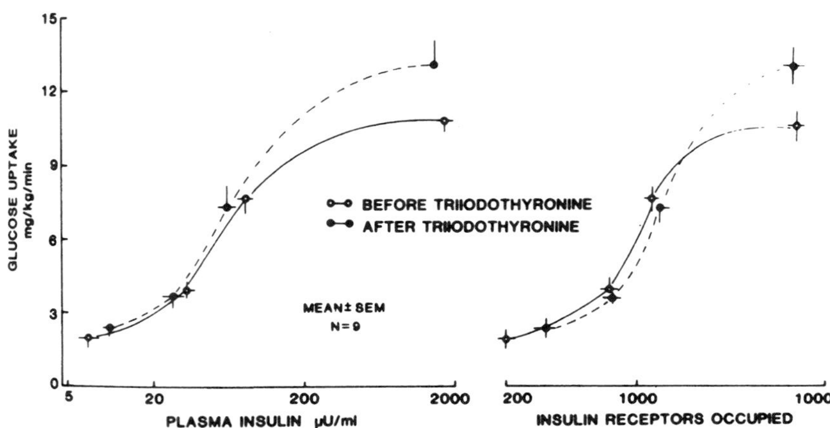

Figure 55-5. Stimulation of glucose uptake in relation to plasma insulin (left panel) or insulin receptor occupancy (right panel) in control (○–○) and triiodothyronine-treated (●–●) subjects. (Reproduced from Dimitriadis G, Baker B, Marsh H, et al. Effect of thyroid hormone excess on action, secretion, and metabolism of insulin in humans. Am J Physiol 1985;248:E593.)

Normal humans rendered thyrotoxic demonstrate an increase in hepatic glucose production rates and in gluconeogenesis[61] (Fig. 55-5). Increased activity of several enzymes that could be implicated in the increase in gluconeogenesis have been seen in response to thyroid hormone, including glucokinase, pyruvate carboxylase, phosphoenolpyruvate carboxykinase, and glucose-6-phosphatase.[62] Studies in hyperthyroid patients report impairment in insulin suppression of hepatic glucose production.

Effects of hyperthyroidism on peripheral insulin action in normal subjects are not clear. Some studies have suggested insulin resistance, whereas others have not. Similarly confusing results have been seen in thyrotoxic subjects, with some studies showing insulin resistance and another suggesting an increase in peripheral (forearm) glucose utilization.

Insulin levels may be affected by a reported effect of thyroid hormone to increase insulin's clearance. A role for glucagon in the hyperglycemia of thyrotoxicosis remains to be confirmed.

Treatment of hyperthyroidism with achievement of euthyroidism generally leads to improvement in or, in some cases, remission of glucose intolerance or diabetes.

Hyperandrogenism

An association between hyperandrogenism, the insulin resistance syndrome, and abdominal obesity has become a well-recognized clinical entity since the description of diabetes in a bearded woman by Achard and Thiers more than 80 years ago.[63]

Several studies have shown that elevated testosterone levels can contribute to progression of glucose intolerance and non–insulin-dependent diabetes mellitus (NIDDM). In a study involving 1400 women for 12 years in Gothenburg, Sweden, low sex hormone binding globulin levels were shown to be an independent risk factor for NIDDM development.[64] Low levels of this globulin were shown in the past to be correlated with elevated free testosterone levels.[65] NIDDM has been observed in patients with polycystic ovarian (PCO) disease with or without obesity. Whether hyperandrogenism in these situations leads to insulin resistance or whether elevated insulin levels in insulin-resistant subjects lead to increased androgen production remains an unsettled issue.

Androgens and Glucose Intolerance

Administration of excessive androgenic steroids to normal men or women, transsexual women,[66] and patients with aplastic anemia[67] can lead to insulin resistance. This insulin resistance has been ascribed to a variety of factors. In muscle of androgenized persons, an increase of insulin-insensitive type II, (particularly type IIB) fast twitch fibers has been observed at the expense of insulin-sensitive type I slow twitch fibers.[68] Similar morphometric findings followed testosterone treatment of rats, with resulting insulin resistance.[69] Metabolic differences in androgenized subjects could be explained by decreased muscle glycogen synthesis caused by decreased glycogen synthase activity in type IIB muscle fibers.[70] Capillary density declines in androgenized muscle, a change that has been postulated to be associated with a decline in endothelial insulin receptor sites and, thus, in diminished potential for transcapillary transfer of insulin to the extracellular space.[68,69] In one recent study, patients with PCO demonstrated decreased insulin receptor binding, decreased glucose disappearance following IV insulin administration, and decreased postbinding insulin degradative activity; all of this may suggest a postbinding defect in hyperandrogenized persons.[71] A decrease in adipocyte GLUT-4 glucose transporter content has been described in PCO patients, although this change was not observed in animal studies of testosterone effects.

The response of insulin resistance to therapy aimed at decreasing hyperandrogenism has been variable. Treatment of women with PCO using spironolactone (an antiandrogen) in one study and 17β estradiol in another resulted in a decrease in androgen concentration and an improvement in insulin sensitivity.[66] Likewise, leuprolide acetate (Lupron) treatment of patients with PCO and mild insulin resistance led to increased insulin sensitivity, an effect not seen in severely insulin-resistant subjects.[72]

In other studies, suppression of androgen levels has not been associated with improvement in insulin sensitivity. The question of causality in the relationship between insulin resistance and hyperandrogenism thus remains open and awaits elucidation.

References

1. Giovanni F, Arosio M, Bazzoni N. Ectopic acromegaly. In: Melmed S, ed. Acromegaly. Endocrinol Metab Clin North Am 1992;21:575
2. Casanueva FF. Physiology of growth hormone secretion and action. In: Melmed S, ed. Acromegaly. Endocrinol Metab Clin North Am 1992;21:483
3. McGorman LR, Rizza R, Gerich J. Physiological concentrations of growth hormone exert insulin-like and insulin antagonistic effects on both hepatic and extrahepatic tissues in man. J Clin Endocrinol Metab 1981;53:556
4. Bougneres PF, Artavia-Loria E, Ferre P, et al. Effects of hypopituitarism and growth hormone replacement therapy on production and utilization of glucose in childhood. J Clin Endocrinol Metab 1985;61:1152
5. Walker J, Chaussain JL, Bougneres PF. Growth hormone treatment of children with short stature increases insulin secretion but does not impair glucose disposal. J Clin Endocrinol Metab 1989;69:253
6. Rizza R, Mandarino L, Gerich J. Effects of growth hormone on insulin action in man. Mechanism of insulin resistance, impaired suppression of glucose production, and impaired stimulation of glucose utilization. Diabetes 1982; 31:663
7. Hansen I, Tsalikian E, Beaufrere B, et al. Insulin resistance in acromegaly: Defects in both hepatic and extrahepatic insulin action. Am J Physiol 1986; 250:E269
8. Moller N, Schmitz O, Jorgensen JOL, et al. Basal and insulin-stimulated substrate metabolism in patients with active acromegaly before and after adenomectomy. J Clin Endocrinol Metab 1992;74:1012
9. Kolaczynski JW, Caro JF. Insulin-like growth factor-1 therapy in diabetes: Physiologic basis, clinical benefits, and risks. Ann Intern Med 1994;120:47
10. Turkalj I, Keller U, Ninnis R, et al. Effect of increasing doses of recombinant human insulin-like growth factor-I on glucose, lipid and leucine metabolism in man. J Clin Endocrinol Metab 1992;75:1186
11. Wright AD, McLachlan MSF, Doyle FH, Frazer TR. Serum growth hormone levels and size of pituitary tumor in untreated acromegaly. Br Med J 1969; IV.582
12. Wass JAH, Cudworth AG, Bottazzo GF, et al. An assessment of glucose intolerance in acromegaly and its response to medical treatment. Clin Endocrinol 1980;12:53
13. Sonksen PH, Greenwood FC, Ellis JP, et al. Changes in carbohydrate tolerance in acromegaly with progress of the disease and in response to treatment. J Clin Endocrinol Metab 1967;27:1418
14. National Diabetes Data Group. Classification and diagnosis of diabetes mellitus and other categories of glucose intolerance. Diabetes 1979;28:1039
15. Ezzat S, Foster MJ, Berchtold P, et al. Acromegaly. Clinical and biochemical features in 500 patients. Medicine 1994;73:233
16. Bratusch-Marrain PR, Smith D, DeFronzo RA. The effects of growth hormone on glucose metabolism and insulin secretion in man. J Clin Endocrinol Metab 1982;55:973
17. Moller N, Butler PC, Antsiferov MA, Alberti KGMM. Effects of growth hormone on insulin sensitivity and forearm metabolism in normal man. Diabetologia 1989;32:105
18. Muggeo M, Saviolakis GA, Businaro V, et al. Insulin receptor on monocytes from patients with acromegaly and fasting hyperglycemia. J Clin Endocrinol Metab 1982;56:733
19. Nabarro JDN. Acromegaly. Clin Endocrinol 1987;26:481
20. Koop BL, Harris A, Ezzat S. Effect of octreotide on glucose tolerance in acromegaly. Eur J Endocrinol 1994;130:581
21. Shamoon H, Soman V, Sherwin R. The influence of acute physiological increments of cortisol on fuel metabolism and insulin binding to monocytes in normal humans. J Clin Endocrinol Metab 1980;50:495
22. Rizza RA, Mandarino LJ, Gerich JE. Cortisol-induced insulin resistance in man: Impaired suppression of glucose production and stimulation of glucose utilization due to a post-receptor defect of insulin action. J Clin Endocrinol Metab 1982;54:131
23. Yasuda K, Hines E III, Kitabchi A. Hypercortisolism and insulin resistance: Comparative effects of prednisone, hydrocortisone, and dexamethasone on insulin binding of human erythrocytes. J Clin Endocrinol Metab 1982;55:910
24. Carter-Su C, Okamoto K. Effect of insulin and glucocorticoids on glucose transporters in rat adipocytes. Am J Physiol 1987;252:E441
25. Bowes SB, Benn JJ, Scobie IN, et al. Glucose metabolism in patients with Cushing's syndrome. Clin Endocrinol 1991;34:311
26. Kitabchi AE, Jones GM, Duckworth WC. Effect of hydrocortisone and cortico-

tropin on glucose induced insulin and proinsulin secretion in man. J Clin Endocrinol Metab 1973;37:79
27. Wajngot A, Giacca A, Grill V, et al. The diabetogenic effects of glucocorticoids are more pronounced in low- than in high-insulin responders. Proc Natl Acad Sci USA 1992;89:6035
28. Caro JF, Amatruda JM. Glucocorticoid-induced insulin resistance. The importance of postbinding events in the regulation of insulin binding action and degradation in freshly isolated hepatocytes. J Biol Chem 1982;250:8389
29. Welbourn RB, Montgomery DAD, Kennedy TL. The natural history of treated Cushing's syndrome. Br J Surg 1971;58:1
30. Cassar J, Joplin GF, Kohner EM. Diabetic retinopathy in Cushing's disease. Postgrad Med J 1981;57:645
31. Gifford RW, Manger WM, Bravo EL. Pheochromocytoma. Endocrinol Metab Clin North Am 1994;23:387
32. Gifford RW, Kuale WF, Maher FT, et al. Clinical features, diagnosis and treatment of pheochromocytoma. Mayo Clin Proc 1964;39:281
33. Rizza RA, Cryer PE, Haymond MW, Gerich JE. Adrenergic mechanisms for the effects of epinephrine on glucose production and clearance in man. J Clin Invest 1980;65:682
34. Cherrington AD, Fuchs H, Stevenson RW, et al. Effect of epinephrine on glycogenolysis and gluconeogenesis in conscious overnight-fasted dogs. Am J Physiol 1984;247:E137
35. Stevenson RW, Steiner KE, Connolly CC, et al. Dose-related effects of epinephrine on glucose production in conscious dogs. Am J Physiol 1991; 260:E363
36. Metz SA, Halter JB, Robertson RP. Induction of defective insulin secretion and impaired glucose tolerance by clonidine. Selective attenuation of metabolic alpha-adrenergic pathways. Diabetes 1978;27:554
37. Turnbull DM, Johnston DG, Alberti KGMM, Hall R. Hormonal and metabolic studies in a patient with a pheochromocytoma. J Clin Endocrinol Metab 1980;51:930
38. Hamaji M. Pancreatic α- and β-cell function in pheochromocytoma. J Clin Endocrinol Metab 1979;49:322
39. Gerich JE, Karam JH, Forshham PH. Stimulation of glucagon secretion by epinephrine in man. J Clin Endocrinol Metab 1973;37:479
40. Schuit FC, Pipeleers DG. Differences in adrenergic recognition by pancreatic A and B cells. Science 1986;232:875
41. Gray DE, Lickley HLA, Vranic M. Physiologic effects of epinephrine on glucose turnover and plasma free fatty acid concentrations mediated independently of glucagon. Diabetes 1980;29:600
42. Nestler JE, McClanahan MA. Diabetes and adrenal disease. Baillieres Clin Endocrinol Metab 1992;6:829
43. Mallison CN, Bloom SR, Warin AP, et al. A glucagonoma syndrome. Lancet 1974;2:1
44. Cherrington AD, Williams PE, Shulman GI, Lacy WW. Differential time course of glucagon's effect of glycogenolysis and gluconeogenesis in the conscious dog. Diabetes 1981;30:180
45. Klein S, Jahoor F, Baba H, et al. In vivo assessment of the metabolic alterations in glucagonoma syndrome. Metabolism 1992;41:1171
46. Norton JA, Kahn CR, Schiebinger R, et al. Amino acid deficiency and the skin rash associated with glucagonoma. Ann Intern Med 1979;91:213
47. Unger RH. Glucagon physiology and pathophysiology. N Engl J Med 1971; 285:443
48. Danforth DN Jr, Triche T, Doppman J, et al. Elevated plasma proglucagon-like component with a glucagon secreting tumor effect of streptozotocin. N Engl J Med 1976;295:242
49. Jaspan JB, Rubenstein AH. Circulating glucagon plasma profiles and metabolism in health and disease. Diabetes 1977;26:887
50. Edney JA, Hoffman S, Thompson JS, Kessinger A. Glucagonoma syndrome is an underdiagnosed clinical entity. Am J Surg 1990;160:625
51. Jockenhovel F, Lederbogen S, Olbricht T, et al. The long-acting somatostatin analogue octreotide alleviates symptoms by reducing posttranslational conversion of prepro-glucagon to glucagon in a patient with malignant glucagonoma, but does not prevent tumor growth. Clin Invest 1994;72:127
52. Kreines K, Jeh M, Knowles HC Jr. Observation in hyperthyroidism of abnormal glucose tolerance and other traits related to diabetes mellitus. Diabetes 1965; 14:740
53. Doar JWH, Stamp TCB, Wynn V, Audhya TK. The effect of oral and intravenous glucose loading in thyrotoxicosis. Studies of plasma glucose, free fatty acid, plasma insulin and blood pyruvate levels. Diabetes 1969;18:633
54. Komiya I, Takasu N, Yamada T, et al. Studies on the association of NIDDM in Japanese patients with hyperthyroid disease. Horm Res 1992;38:264
55. Coopan R, Kozak GP. Hyperthyroidism and diabetes mellitus. Arch Intern Med 1980;140:370
56. Lenzen S. Dose-response studies in the inhibitory effect of thyroid hormones on insulin secretion in the rat. Metabolism 1978;27:81
57. Lenzen S, Kloppel G. Insulin secretion and the morphological and metabolic characteristics of pancreatic islets of hyperthyroid ob/ob mice. Endocrinology 1978;103:1546
58. Sestoft L. Metabolic aspects of calorigenic effect of thyroid hormone in mammals. Clin Endocrinol 1980;13:489
59. Huang MT, Landy HA. Effects of thyroid states on the cori cycle, glucose-alamine cycle and futile cycling of glucose metabolism in rats. Arch Biochem Biophys 1981;209:41
60. Muller MJ, Paschen U, Seitz HJ. Thyroid hormone regulation of glucose homeostasis in miniature pig. Endocrinology 1983;112:2025
61. Dimitriadis G, Baker B, Marsh H, et al. Effect of thyroid hormone excess on action, secretion, and metabolism of insulin in humans. Am J Physiol 1985;248:E593
62. Larsen PR, Ingbar SH. The Thyroid Gland. In: Wilson JD and Foster DW, eds. Williams Textbook of Endocrinology. 8th ed., Philadelphia: W.B. Saunders;1992:357
63. Achard C, Thiers J. Le Virilism Pilaire et Son Association a l'isufficiense Glycolytique (Diabete a Femmes de Barbe). Bull Acad Natl Med Paris 1921;86:51
64. Lindstedt G, Lunberg P, Lapidus L, et al. Low sex hormone-binding globulin concentration as independent risk factor for development of NIDDM. 12 year follow-up of population study of women in Gothenburg, Sweden. Diabetes 1991;40:123
65. Dunn JF, Nisula BC, Rodbard D. Transport of steroid hormones: Binding of 21 endogenous steroids to both testosterone-binding globulin and corticosteroid-binding globulin in human plasma. J Clin Endocrinol Metab 1981;53:58
66. Bjorntrop P. Hyperandrogenicity in women—a prediabetic condition? J Intern Med 1993;234:579
67. Woodard TL, Burghen GA, Kitabchi AE, William JA. Glucose intolerance and insulin resistance in aplastic anemia treated with oxymetholone. J Clin Endocrinol Metab 1981;53:905
68. Krotkiewski M, Bjorntorp P. Muscle tissue in obesity with different distribution of adipose tissue. Effects of physical training. Int J Obes 1986;10:331
69. Holmang A, Brzezinska Z, Bjorntrop P. Effects of hyperinsulinemia on muscle fiber composition and capillarization in rats. Diabetes 1993;42:1073
70. Saltin B, Henriksson J, Nygaard E, et al. Fiber types and metabolic potentials of skeletal muscle in sedentary man and endurance runners. Ann NY Acad Sci 1977;301:3
71. Buffington CK, Givens JR, Kitabchi AE. Enhanced adrenocortical activity as a contributing factor to diabetes in hyperandrogenic women. Metabolism 1994;43:584
72. Elkind-Hirsh KE, Valdes CT, Malinak LR. Insulin resistance improves in hyperandrogenic women treated with Lupron. Fertil Steril 1993;60:634

Diabetes Mellitus, edited by Derek LeRoith, Simeon I. Taylor, and Jerrold M. Olefsky. Lippincott–Raven Publishers, Philadelphia © 1996.

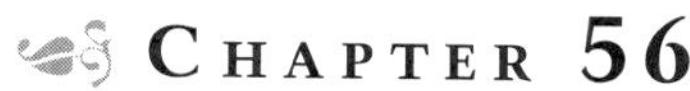

CHAPTER 56
Insulin Secretion in Non–Insulin-Dependent Diabetes Mellitus

GORDON C. WEIR AND SUSAN BONNER-WEIR

Finally, there is general agreement about essential contributions of both insulin resistance and β-cell failure to the pathogenesis of non–insulin-dependent diabetes mellitus (NIDDM).[1–3] The definition of NIDDM is phenotypic and helps little in categorizing the different varieties of this heterogeneous syndrome, but hopefully, genetic markers soon will lead the way to more rigorous classification. A common pathogenic pathway appears to exist for most people with NIDDM (Fig. 56-1). Genes play a major role, with those exerting control over insulin action, obesity, and the regulation of β-cell mass and function presumably being especially important. Environment also has a major impact, with the plentiful food and inactivity of affluent societies having a detrimental influence. Although definitions of insulin resistance must be arbitrary, the vast majority of persons destined to develop NIDDM are resistant. Nonetheless, most persons with insulin resistance never progress to diabetes, although it could be argued that they would if they lived long enough. Only those whose β-cells fail to compensate develop NIDDM. Therefore, even though hyperinsulinemia is almost always found in the prediabetic period, either absolute or relative insulin deficiency is always present when NIDDM finally appears.

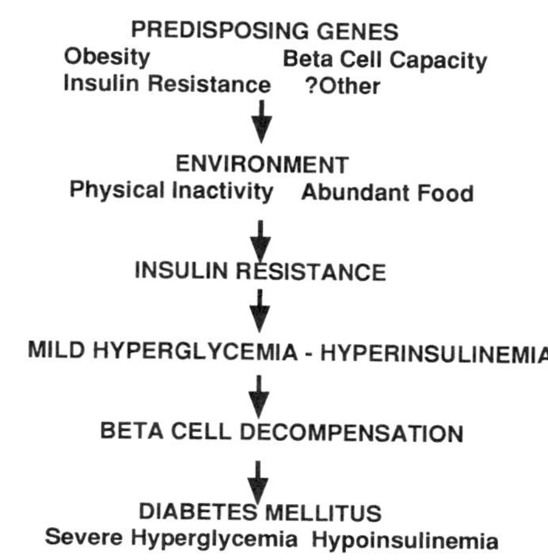

FIGURE 56-1. Sequence of events in the pathogenesis of NIDDM.

Heterogeneity Within NIDDM: Autoimmunity and Mutations of Insulin, Glucokinase, and Mitochondrial DNA

Although most seem to have a similar phenotype, it is important to search for the variants within this heterogeneous syndrome. For example, in some populations many patients diagnosed with non–insulin-dependent diabetes mellitus (NIDDM) have a syndrome called *latent autoimmune diabetes* in adults.[4] Autoimmune damage to β-cells can occur at any age and may be a slow-moving, incomplete process that can even become quiescent at some point. Indeed, a self-limited, asymptomatic, autoimmune process occurring in childhood might show up many years later as NIDDM. It is often forgotten that overweight persons are just as likely to develop autoimmune diseases as thin persons. In Scandinavia, over 10% of subjects with NIDDM have islet cell antibodies or antibodies to glutamic acid decarboxylase.[5,6] Such persons with antibody markers and HLA-DR4 or-DR3 haplotypes also will be more likely to require insulin therapy.[7,8] Because immune markers often disappear with time, more than 10%, perhaps even 20% or more, of patients with NIDDM in populations where autoimmune disease is common, such as Northern European countries, may have some contribution from immune β-cell destruction. In other groups with a high prevalence of NIDDM, such as Micronesians or Pima Indians, autoimmune destruction of β-cells must be very rare, judging from the lack of reports.

Several mutations of the proinsulin gene have been described, including insulin Chicago (Phe-B25-Leu), insulin Los Angeles (Phe-B24-Ser), and insulin Wakayama (Val-A3-Leu).[9] These mutations almost completely obliterate biologic activity. Only heterozygotes have been found, and some do not even have diabetes; this finding provides insight into the capacity of only one normal allele to provide sufficient insulin for decades. Other mutations lead to hyperproinsulinemia, which may also be associated with NIDDM[10]; these include Arg-C65-His and His-B10-Asp.

Maturity-onset diabetes of the young also is heterogeneous, and about half of the affected families have been found to have mutations of the glucokinase gene. Glucokinase is known to play a key role in regulating the rate of insulin secretion, and over 20 mutations have already been defined.[11–13] These subjects have mild diabetes, which usually does not require insulin treatment, and an altered set point for glucose-induced insulin secretion, as is predicted by a reduction of glucokinase activity.[13] Glucokinase is a critical enzyme for glucose handling by both β-cells and hepatocytes,[14] but the relative contributions of these two tissues to the hyperglycemia of maturity-onset diabetes of the young has not yet been clarified. Glucokinase mutations appear to account for less than 1% of the cases of NIDDM. Other families with maturity-onset diabetes of the young, who tend to have more severe insulin deficiency without insulin resistance and higher glucose concentrations, have an as yet unidentified gene defect somewhere on chromosome 20.[15]

Mutations of mitochondrial DNA can be associated with both insulin-dependent diabetes mellitus (IDDM) and NIDDM.[16] Mitochondrial DNA contains 16,569 base pairs, which code for 37 genes including those for 13 enzymes involved in oxidative phosphorylation. One mutation linked with diabetes is a substitution of guanidine for adenine at position 3243 of leucine tRNA, which leads to problems with the synthesis of mitochondrial proteins. These mutations are passed on by maternal transmission, and problems other than diabetes, including sensory hearing loss and the mitochondrial myopathy, encephalopathy lactic acidosis and stroke-like episodes (MELAS) syndrome, are often found. This form of diabetes, which is associated with insulin deficiency and probably not with insulin resistance, is rare and is usually diagnosed in the second or third decade. Oxidative metabolism of glucose is required for insulin secretion, so it is not surprising that such a mutation would cause problems. Much remains to be learned about the specific characteristics of insulin secretion in this syndrome and the pathologic events that befall the islets.

β-Cell Function in Established Non–Insulin-Dependent Diabetes Mellitus

Even though hyperinsulinemia is usually found in the state of impaired glucose tolerance (IGT), once non–insulin-dependent diabetes mellitus (NIDDM) develops, insulin secretion is deficient in either an absolute or a relative sense (Fig. 56-1). Proper matching of research subjects is needed to appreciate the relative quantities of insulin being secreted. For example, obesity is associated with insulin resistance, so obese persons with NIDDM may have higher plasma insulin concentrations than nondiabetic subjects of normal weight, but they will be found to be insulin deficient when matched with overweight nondiabetic controls.[17,18]

Fasting plasma insulin levels provide little information about insulin secretory capacity. In fact, they are a better indicator of the degree of insulin resistance and have been found to correlate very well with this characteristic. As is true in the nondiabetic state and the prediabetic state, even in NIDDM insulin levels are highest in persons with the most insulin resistance. In prospective studies, high fasting insulin concentrations have been found to be a risk factor for the development of NIDDM.[19,20]

Insulin responses to an oral glucose tolerance test can be misleading. In mild NIDDM, insulin responses at 60 to 120 minutes may be higher than those of normal controls, but this is caused by insulin resistance and the higher glucose concentrations seen at these time points. In contrast, the early insulin responses at 30 minutes are typically lower in NIDDM subjects; this leads to inefficient suppression of hepatic glucose output and partially accounts for the higher glucose levels found later in the oral glucose tolerance test.[21] To compare the insulin secretory capacity between persons, the degree of insulin resistance and the glucose concentrations used to challenge the β-cells both must be controlled.

Insulin responses to an intravenous glucose challenge are profoundly abnormal in diabetes. First-phase insulin responses are absent, and in some subjects a paradoxical fall in plasma insulin concentration is found.[3,22–25] A second phase of insulin release can be seen in all but the most severe cases of NIDDM, but when glucose levels and the degree of insulin resistance are taken into account, these second-phase responses are deficient. The loss of first-phase glucose-induced insulin secretion is specific for glucose because β-cells can respond to acute challenges by other secretogogues such as arginine, isoproterenol, secretin, and tolbutamide.

TABLE 56-1. Potentially Important β-Cell Defects in NIDDM

GLUT-2 reduction	Triglyceride accumulation
GLUT-2/glucokinase dysfunction	Long chain fatty acids
Glucokinase alteration	Malonyl CoA
Glucose cycling	Glycogen accumulation
Glucose-6-phosphatase increase	Insulin gene expression
Phosphofructokinase	Ion channel dysfunction
Lactate dehydrogenase	
Mitochondrial glycerol phosphate dehydrogenase	

It is interesting that the insulin responses to these agents are usually of the same magnitude as those seen in subjects without diabetes. However, when glucose concentrations are experimentally raised in nondiabètic subjects, their insulin responses to arginine and isoproterenol greatly exceed those of comparable persons with diabetes.[26]

Careful study of insulin secretory capacity suggests the presence of severe impairment in the diabetic state, even when β-cell mass is taken into account. For example, postmortem studies indicate that the β-cell mass in typical NIDDM is about 50% of normal, yet the insulin responses to maximal stimulation by a combination of arginine and glucose is only about 15% of that found in control subjects.[26] Therefore, NIDDM is characterized by both reduced β-cell mass and inefficient secretion from whatever β-cells remain.

Adverse Influence of Chronic Hyperglycemia on β-Cell Function

Some of the abnormalities of insulin secretion in non–insulin-dependent diabetes mellitus (NIDDM) may result from the adverse influence of the hyperglycemic environment. This phenomenon has been referred to as "glucose toxicity."[3,27] It has been difficult to determine the structural abnormalities induced by chronic hyperglycemia, but the functional defects have been easier to define. Probably the most clinically relevant and best demonstration of functional glucose toxicity in humans comes from the findings of a Japanese study that insulin secretion improved during challenges with meals or oral glucose after hyperglycemia was reduced by diet, sulfonylurea treatment, or insulin administration.[28]

Hyperglycemia is virtually always associated with a reduction of glucose-induced insulin secretion.[3,27] This abnormal secretion has been found in all forms of human diabetes including NIDDM and early insulin-dependent diabetes mellitus (IDDM), as well as in persons with failing pancreas transplants. Similar abnormalities have been found in primates, dogs, and many rodent models. The mechanisms responsible for these changes have still not yet been defined, but several biochemical alterations have emerged. Perhaps the most striking abnormality is the profound reduction in the β-cell glucose transporter GLUT-2 found in all rodent models of hyperglycemia.[27,29] Unfortunately, it is not known why GLUT-2 expression is reduced or whether it leads to a change in glucose-induced insulin secretion. Glucokinase plays a critical role in regulating the rate of insulin secretion,[14] and changes in the intrinsic activity of this enzyme are found in hyperglycemic states.[30] These changes may help explain the abnormal dose-response curves for glucose-induced insulin secretion in insulin-resistant states, but they do not fully explain the loss of response to glucose. There appear to be important functional interactions between GLUT-2 and glucokinase, but these remain to be clarified.[31] There also is interest in the possible impairment of glucose oxidation, which may be linked to reduced activity of the mitochondrial glycerol phosphate shuttle.[32] Other potential trouble spots include increased glucose cycling with conversion of glucose-6-phosphate to glucose, which may lead to inefficient glycolysis.[33]

Even though the abnormal insulin secretion of diabetes seems likely to be caused by a direct effect of hyperglycemia on β-cells, an alternative hypothesis suggests that elevated free fatty acid (FFA) levels are responsible.[34–36] Provision of FFA could provide a source for the synthesis of lipid mediators such as diacylglycerol, which have an important influence on insulin secretion. Malonyl CoA levels in β-cells, which are increased by high glucose concentrations, can inhibit fatty acid oxidation and thus make fatty acids more available for synthesis of lipid mediators.[37] It is possible that the increased FFA concentrations seen in insulin-resistant states, such as obesity, contribute to hyperinsulinemia and *increased* responsiveness to glucose, and that further elevation of FFA in diabetes then causes a *loss* of glucose-induced insulin secretion. Nevertheless, convincing correlations between FFA levels and these disparate characteristics of insulin secretion remain to be established.

Concept of β-Cell Set Point

The β-cell is remarkably efficient at keeping glucose levels within a very narrow range. Yet, the set point (the dose-response relationship between glucose concentration and the rate of insulin secretion) for glucose-induced insulin secretion can vary under certain conditions. One puzzle concerns the insulin resistance of obesity, whereby obese and normal-weight control subjects can have markedly different insulin secretion in spite of having identical glucose levels.[38] Perhaps there has been a shift in the dose-response curve so that more insulin can be secreted at a particular glucose level. Administration of glucocorticoids to normal subjects produces modest increases in fasting glucose concentrations, which must be thought of as imperfect compensation. Certainly these subjects have not reached a limitation in their capacity for insulin secretion; somehow the set point has been shifted, perhaps from a direct influence of glucocorticoid on β-cells. Glucokinase is though to be the ''glucose sensor'' of the β-cell because it is the rate-limiting step in glucose metabolism.[14] Evidence is emerging that changes in ambient glucose concentrations can alter the intrinsic activity of glucokinase and thus alter the set point of the β-cell.[30] Perhaps some interaction between glucokinase and GLUT-2 is responsible for this change, or perhaps lipid mediators exert an important influence. Interesting variations in the set point must somehow be occurring during the evolution of non–insulin-dependent diabetes mellitus (NIDDM).

β-Cell Function in Pre-Non–Insulin-Dependent Diabetes Mellitus

By the time non–insulin-dependent diabetes mellitus (NIDDM) is diagnosed, the critical events that caused the problem are blurred. If good enough tools were available, we might be able to understand why, when fasting plasma glucose value of 80 mg/dL (4.4 mM) deteriorates to 95 mg/dL (5.2 mM), there is further progression to impaired glucose tolerance (IGT), and why only some persons with IGT then develop NIDDM. Valuable studies have focused on persons at risk for developing NIDDM, such as the offspring of two parents with NIDDM,[39] Pima Indians[40] or first-degree relatives of patients with NIDDM.[41] In all of these studies, insulin resistance has been unequivocally shown to be a major risk factor. Although an impairment of insulin secretion to an intravenous glucose tolerance test was not found in the offspring study,[39] the Pima Indian study[40] and several prospective studies[4,19,20] have shown that impaired β-cell secretory responses to glucose were predictive of subsequent diabetes.

Although most studies focus on the factors that increase the risk of developing NIDDM, there are important protective characteristics. Obviously, not having diabetogenic genes is the best protection. Studies of the offspring of parents with NIDDM show that those who were insulin sensitive had a very low risk of developing diabetes.[42] Other factors that reduce the likelihood of developing diabetes are lack of obesity, particularly central obesity, and regular exercise. β-Cell functional capacity is also of critical importance, but there are no good ways to measure this in the prediabetic state.

The main problem with β-cells in NIDDM is that at some point, after many years of coping with insulin resistance, they fail to produce enough insulin. The production of insulin depends on the total output and character of secretion from individual β-cells and on the total number of β-cells, which because of the complexities of variable cell size is usually viewed simply as the β-cell mass. Although a variety of interesting and important secretory abnormalities are described in this chapter, we suspect that failure

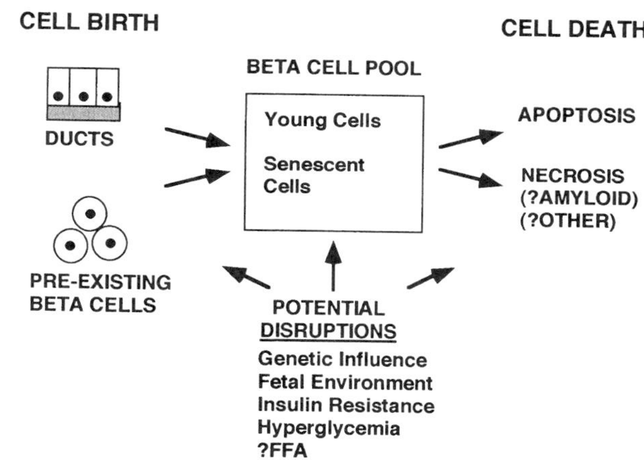

Figure 56-2. Regulation of β-cell mass and function. Sites of potential disruption associated with diabetes.

to maintain an adequate β-cell mass is the crux of the problem in NIDDM (Fig. 56-2). The as yet unidentified genes responsible for β-cell birth and death may play a key role. If the major problem is with growth capacity, then the failure to find any evidence of this from secretory studies done in the stage of pre-NIDDM is hardly surprising. In fact, it might even be expected that in subjects with pre-NIDDM, perfectly normal plasma glucose levels would be associated with normal insulin responses to an array of secretory challenges.

Problems with Understanding Low and High Insulin Responses

The concept of low and high insulin responses to a glucose challenge has led to much confusion. In some situations, a low insulin response could be perfectly normal; in others, it could be a sign of β-cell malfunction. For example, a thin, physically trained person with genetic insulin sensitivity and a fasting glucose level of 80 mg/dL (4.4 mM) will be expected to have a very low insulin response to a glucose challenge. Yet in spite of this low insulin response, such a person could have a β-cell capacity that could cope with severe insulin resistance for a lifetime. In this situation, the acute insulin response probably has no predictive value. A similar problem may be found in a young, sedentary person with genetic insulin resistance who also has a fasting glucose level of 4.4 mM. A high secretory response to glucose should be expected, but this response should provide no insight into whether β-cell function will deteriorate 20 years later.

In spite of this formulation, some studies of subjects at high risk of developing diabetes find that those who go on to develop diabetes have some reduction of their insulin responses to glucose.[20] Perhaps these prediabetic persons have a genetic problem with one of the steps in the pathway for glucose-induced insulin secretion, which is manifest by a low response, and that somehow this leads to β-cell failure in midlife, especially if aggravated by insulin resistance. On the other hand, perhaps the pathways of glucose-induced insulin secretion are perfectly normal but the β-cells are subject to glucose toxicity, which can occur with glucose levels that are only modestly elevated. An important study of adults with variable fasting glucose levels indicates that glucose-induced insulin secretion is abolished once a level of 115 mg/dL (6.3 mM) is reached and that some impairment can occur at lower levels, such as 100 mg/dL (5.5 mM).[25] This is in agreement with the finding of reduced insulin responses to intravenous glucose tolerance tests in subjects with pre–insulin-dependent diabetes mellitus (pre-IDDM) who have glucose levels that are ''normal'' at about 95–110 mg/dL[43] but probably higher than the 80–90 mg/dL they might have had before the autoimmune process began. Studies using various rodent models also indicate that deranged insulin secretion can be found with elevations of glucose concentrations that are difficult to distinguish from normal.[27] Some of the important questions that emerge from this discussion are as follows:

1. What is a truly normal glucose level, and how can it be defined?
2. Are there genetic differences in glucose levels that might be demonstrated in childhood?
3. If metabolic homeostasis is stressed by autoimmune loss of β-cells or by insulin resistance, and glucose levels start to rise, when does an impairment of secretion from glucose toxicity appear?
4. Are there genetic differences in susceptibility to glucose toxicity?
5. Are those who are more susceptible to an impairment of glucose-induced insulin secretion more likely to have further deterioration in function and go on to develop NIDDM?

Circulating Proinsulin-Like Peptides

Although the cleavage of proinsulin to insulin and C peptide is very efficient, about 2–4% of the secreted insulin immunoreactivity consists of proinsulin and proinsulin-related peptides. Because the clearance of these peptides is so much slower than that of insulin, they account for 10–40% of circulating immunoreactivity. About one-third of this is accounted for by intact proinsulin and two-thirds by des 32–33 split proinsulin; only small amounts of 65–66 split proinsulin are detectable.[44] For years it has been known that the ratio of circulating proinsulin-related peptides to insulin is increased in non–insulin-dependent diabetes mellitus (NIDDM).[45] Several studies have found this ratio to be positively correlated with the severity of hyperglycemia.[46] In the state of impaired glucose tolerance (IGT), modest elevations in the ratio have been found in some population groups.[47] Failure to appreciate the contribution of the proinsulin-related peptides has led to overestimation of insulin levels in NIDDM, but this is less of an issue in IGT, where hyperinsulinemia is most severe. Because these peptides have less than 5% of the biologic activity of insulin, their contribution to glucose homeostasis is probably minimal. There has been interest in determining whether disproportionately elevated proinsulin levels could be useful markers for progression to diabetes in high-risk groups. Even though abnormalities sometimes can be found in IGT and pre–insulin-dependent diabetes mellitus (pre-IDDM),[47,48] the changes are probably not consistent enough to be very useful. The mechanisms responsible for the abnormal ratios have not been defined, but when rodent β-cells are experimentally exposed to chronic hyperglycemia, this increases the ratio of proinsulin-related peptides to insulin secreted directly from β-cells.[49] Although complex alterations in the cleavage events of β-cells may be taking place, the explanation simply could be that increased secretory demand from hyperglycemia leads to depletion of mature granules and release of available immature granules in which conversion is incomplete.[45]

Pulsatile Insulin Secretion

Insulin secretion is pulsatile, with a periodicity of about 10–13 minutes, and these fluctuations are synchronized with oscillations in plasma glucose levels.[50] In addition, less frequent large-amplitude pulses of insulin secretion have been described, which occur 10–15 times per day and with greater frequency after meals.[51] The mechanisms responsible for the rapid oscillations are not known, but they are found with insulin secretion from the perfused canine pancreas when glucose levels are held constant.[52] Although metabolic coordination has been postulated,[53] it seems more likely that there is a pancreatic neural network that provides a functional linkage between islets.[54] Both the short- and long-term pulsations are disrupted in non–insulin-dependent diabetes mellitus (NIDDM), and even in the less severe state of impaired glucose tolerance (IGT).[55,56] It remains to be seen if abnormalities can be found before IGT develops and if such abnormalities will turn out to have any predictive value for the development of NIDDM. There are also interesting questions about the effects of these pulsations on insulin action. When insulin is administered in a pulsatile fashion, hepatic glucose output is more efficiently suppressed than when delivery is continuous.[57] Because the variations of insulin (and glucagon) concentrations in the portal vein are substantial, the possibility of their having an important influence on hepatic metabolism is attractive. The oscillations of insulin levels in arterial plasma are more modest, and there must be further dampening when insulin leaves the vasculature to reach muscle or fat cells. Thus, the influence of pulsatile insulin secretion on peripheral metabolism may be inconsequential.

Islet Pathology in Non–Insulin-Dependent Diabetes Mellitus

β-Cell Mass

The amount of β-cell mass is tightly regulated, being maintained at about 1% of the weight of the pancreas in adults. Several large autopsy studies provide evidence that the β-cell mass in non–insulin-dependent diabetes mellitus (NIDDM) is about 50% of normal. It is surprising that 50% would not be enough to maintain normoglycemic, but, as discussed earlier, these cells do not seem capable of secreting as much insulin as normal β-cells. Therefore, persons with NIDDM have lost the capacity to maintain a normal β-cell mass and have abnormal function from whatever β-cells are left.

Regulation of the β-cell mass is a more dynamic process than is generally realized. It has not been possible to learn much about the replicative capacity of human β-cells, but much work has been carried out in rodents.[58] The turnover of β-cells in adult humans is certainly lower than in rodents, but the general mechanisms for regulating the β-cell mass should be similar. There is evidence of new islet formation during autoimmune destruction in insulin-dependent diabetes mellitus (IDDM) and in patients with liver disease. Data also exist indicating that the β-cell mass is increased in the insulin-resistant state of obesity, although more studies on this question are needed. In adult rats there is a constant rate of β-cell replication, with a basal birth rate of about 2–3% per day; this rate can increase fivefold or more after partial pancreatectomy or during intravenous infusions of glucose. Not only can cell number increase (hyperplasia), but β-cell size can expand (hypertrophy) when confronted by glucose stimulation. New β-cells are derived from two sources: mitosis of existing β-cells and protodifferentiated precursor cells found in pancreatic ducts. It is estimated that in rodents the entire β-cell mass can turn over in a month or less. Moreover, if the β-cell mass is stable, the birth rate must be equaled by the death rate. The process of apoptosis (''programmed cell death'') has been documented to occur in β-cells. Nonapoptotic types of cell death, such as necrosis, also must occur. Presumably, β-cells, like other cell types, have the capacity for only a certain number of divisions. Perhaps this is genetically determined and influenced by hyperglycemia; the age at which stimulation takes place also could have an influence. It is highly likely that the β-cell mass varies during adult life in humans, expanding to meet the demands of the Western lifestyle and contracting with food restriction and regular exercise.

Some individuals reach a point where the β-cell mass can no longer be maintained and diabetes develops. Such a limitation is poorly understood, but rats with restricted protein intake early in life have less capacity for β-cell replenishment and are more susceptible to diabetes.[59] Follow-up studies of a male population with low birth weight found a greater likelihood of developing impaired glucose tolerance (IGT) and NIDDM late in life.[60] Another related finding was that the risk of developing NIDDM is greater for the offspring of diabetic mothers than for the offspring of diabetic fathers.[61] Maternal diabetes often leads to an unfavorable intrauterine environment, which could interfere with normal islet development and therefore compromise the capacity for compensation later in life. Many other factors might adversely influence the capacity of β-cells for long-term compensation. Some possibilities include a self-limited bout of autoimmune destruction, a period of obesity, exposure to a β-cell toxin, a viral infection of islets, or an episode of malnutrition.

Amyloid Deposition in Islets

Amyloid deposits in the islets of persons with diabetes were first described in 1900, but only in 1986 was the peptide that forms this amorphous material identified.[62,63] This peptide is called *islet-amyloid polypeptide (IAPP)* or *amylin* and consists of 37 amino acids. The sequence between positions 20 and 29, with position 25 being particularly important, determines the ability of this peptide to form amyloid. Because of these structural requirements, amyloid deposits are found in primates and cats but not in many other species. Production of IAPP is restricted to β-cells, and its content is only about 1% that of insulin, with this ratio being reflected in the amount secreted.[60]

There is no known functional role for IAPP, but various pharmacologic effects have been demonstrated. There is no persuasive evidence that secreted IAPP has any physiologic effect on peripheral tissues, particularly because the circulating levels are so low. Little attention has been paid to whether IAPP could exert some local effect through the islet-acinar portal circulation, somehow influencing the downstream non–β-cells of the islet or acinar cells. The suggestion that IAPP contributes to the insulin resistance of non–insulin-dependent diabetes mellitus (NIDDM) has received little support. Perhaps it has some chaperone function within insulin secretory granules to facilitate proinsulin processing. The mechanisms responsible for its deposition in many, but not all, of the islets of persons with NIDDM are unknown. It is not found often in the islets of nondiabetic individuals with insulin resistance. Perhaps there are clues in the finding of large amounts of amyloid in some insulinomas and in the islets of a patient with diabetes associated with extreme insulin resistance.[64] These are conditions, along with NIDDM, in which the ratio of secreted proinsulin-related peptides to insulin is increased. The question of whether amyloid has a detrimental influence on islet function is important in light of recent studies showing that human IAPP fibrils have a very toxic effect on both rat and human islets.[65] The amyloid deposits in islets seem to begin as small niduses that then enlarge. Perhaps patches of amyloid kill only the few adjacent β-cells with which they have direct contact, allowing survival of most of the cells of an islet. Such a process, occurring over years, could lead to a gradual but critical decline in β-cell mass. This formulation suggests that extracellular amyloid deposits cause the most damage, but a role for intracellular formation of amyloid with destruction has not been excluded.

Summary

Even though insulin resistance plays a critical role in the pathogenesis of non–insulin-dependent diabetes mellitus (NIDDM), β-cell failure—either failure to compensate or failure in an absolute sense—is a sine qua non for the development of the diabetic state. Much is known about the altered characteristics of insulin secretion in NIDDM, but the actual causes of β-cell failure are still poorly understood. There are three separate problem areas that need attention. First, there must be genes that determine the capacity of β-cells to produce insulin in the face of decades of insulin resistance. These genes could be responsible for the determinants of the β-cell mass, for insulin synthesis, or for the complex machinery of insulin secretion. Second, the adaptation of β-cells to both the prediabetic and diabetic states is very complex and must have a detrimental influence on insulin secretion. Third, there may be other factors associated with the diabetic state that lead to β-cell destruction; accumulation of amyloid in islets is an especially important candidate.

Therapeutic approaches to NIDDM could be targeted to or dependent on β-cell function. Agents that enhance insulin action—insulin sensitizers—could have a major impact because a substantial amount of β-cell capacity can still be present after many years of diabetes, even if insulin therapy is employed. It is not uncommon to see patients with long-standing NIDDM, who lose large amounts of weight either voluntarily or because of illness, with glucose values in the normal range. Drugs that enhance insulin secretion through pathways different from those affected by sulfonylureas might be useful. Preliminary studies with GLP-1 provide an example of one such approach.[66] The development of agents that could stimulate β-cell growth remains a hope for the future. Gene therapy might be exploited in some manner. Islet transplantation for NIDDM should be a viable option at some point. A search for drugs that could prevent amyloid formation or dissolve existing deposits should be undertaken.

References

1. Yki-Jarvinen H. Pathogenesis of non–insulin-dependent diabetes mellitus. Lancet 1994;343:91–94
2. Beck-Nielsen H, Groop LC. Metabolic and genetic characterization of prediabetic states. J Clin Invest 1994;94:1714–1721
3. Weir GC, Leahy JL. Pathogenesis of non–insulin-dependent (type II) diabetes mellitus. In: Joslin's Diabetes Mellitus. 13th ed. Kahn CR, Weir GE, eds. Philadelphia: Lea and Febiger;1994:240–264
4. Montana E, Bonner-Weir S, Weir GC. Transplanted beta cell response to increased metabolic demand. J Clin Invest 1994;93:1577–1582
5. Groop LC, Bottazzo GF. Genetic susceptibility to non–insulin-dependent diabetes mellitus. Diabetes 1986;35:237–241
6. Froguel P, Zouali H, Vionnet N, et al. Familial hyperglycemia due to mutations in the glucokinase gene. N Engl J Med 1993;328:697–702
7. Tuomilehto-Wolf E, Tuomilehto J, Hitman GA, et al. Genetic susceptibility to non–insulin-dependent diabetes mellitus and glucose intolerance are located in HLA region. Br Med J 1993;307:155–159
8. Groop LC, Groop PH, Koskimies S. Relationship between β-cell function and HLA antigens in patients with type 2 (non–insulin-dependent) diabetes. Diabetologia 1986;29:757–760
9. Steiner DF, Tager HS, Chan SJ, et al. Lessons learned from molecular biology of insulin-gene mutations. Diabetes Care 1990;13:600–609
10. Oohashi H, Ohgawara H, Nanjo K, et al. Familial hyperproinsulinemia associated with NIDDM. Diabetes Care 1993;16:1340–1346
11. Bell GI, Froguel P, Nishi S, et al. Mutations of the human glucokinase gene and diabetes mellitus. Trends Endocrinol Metab 1993;4:86–90
12. Tuomi T, Groop LC, Zimmet P, et al. Antibodies to glutamic acid decarboxylase (GAD) identify latent IDDM in patients with onset of diabetes after the age of 35 years. Diabetes 1993;42:359–362
13. Byrne MM, Sturis J, Clement K, et al. Insulin secretory abnormalities in subjects with hyperglycemia due to glucokinase mutations. J Clin Invest 1994; 93:1120–1130
14. Matschinsky F, Liang Y, Kesavan P, et al. Glucokinase as pancreatic β-cell glucose sensor and diabetes gene. J Clin Invest 1993;92:2092–2098
15. Bell GI, Xiang K-S, Newman MV, et al. Gene for non–insulin-dependent diabetes mellitus (maturity-onset diabetes of the young subtype) is linked to DNA polymorphism on human chromosome 20q. Proc Natl Acad Sci USA 1991;88:1484–1488
16. Kadowaki T, Kadowaki H, Mori Y, et al. A subtype of diabetes mellitus associated with a mutation of mitochondrial DNA. N Engl J Med 1994; 330:962–967
17. Perley M, Kipnis DM. Plasma insulin responses to glucose and tolbutamide of normal weight and obese diabetic and non-diabetic subjects. Diabetes 1966;15:867–874
18. Perley MJ, Kipnis DM. Plasma insulin responses to oral and intravenous

glucose: Studies in normal and diabetic subjects. J Clin Invest 1967;46: 1954–1962
19. Lundgren H, Bengtsson C, Blohme G, et al. Fasting serum Insulin concentration and early insulin response as risk determinants for developing diabetes. Diabetic Med 1990;7:407–413
20. Skarfors ET, Selenus KI, Lithell HO. Risk factors for developing non–insulin-dependent diabetes mellitus: A 10 year follow-up of men in Uppsala. Br Med J 1991;303:755–760
21. Mitrakoku A, Kelley D, Mokan M, et al. Role of suppression of glucose production and diminished early insulin release in impaired glucose tolerance. N Engl J Med 1992;326:22–29
22. Porte D Jr, Kahn SE. Hyperproinsulinemia and amyloid in NIDDM: Clues to etiology of β-cell dysfunction. Diabetes 1989;38:1333–1336
23. Leahy JL. Natural history of β-cell dysfunction in NIDDM. Diabetes Care 1983;13:992–1010
24. Metz SA, Halter JB, Robertson RP. Paradoxical inhibition of insulin secretion by glucose in human diabetes mellitus. J Clin Endocrinol Metab 1979;48: 827–835
25. Brunzell JD, Robertson RP, Lerner RL, et al. Relationships between fasting plasma glucose levels and insulin secretion during intravenous glucose tolerance tests. J Clin Endocrinol Metab 1976;42:222–229
26. Ward WK, Bolgiano DC, McKnight B, et al. Diminished β-cell secretory capacity in patients with noninsulin-dependent diabetes mellitus. J Clin Invest 1984;74:1318–1328
27. Leahy JL, Bonner-Weir S, Weir GC. β-Cell dysfunction induced by chronic hyperglycemia: Current ideas on mechanism of impaired glucose-induced insulin secretion. Diabetes Care 1992;15:442–455
28. Kosaka K, Kuzuya T, Akanuma Y, Hagura R. Increase in insulin response after treatment of overt maturity-onset diabetes is independent of the mode of treatment. Diabetologia 1980;18:23–28
29. Ogawa Y, Noma Y, Davalli AM, et al. Loss of glucose-induced insulin secretion and GLUT2 expression in transplanted β-cells. Diabetes 1995;44: 75–79
30. Chen C, Hosokawa H, Bumbalo LM, Leahy JL. Regulatory effects of glucose on the catalytic activity and cellular content of glucokinase in the pancreatic β-cell. J Clin Invest 1994;94:1616–1620
31. Ferber S, BeltrandelRio H, Johnson JH, et al. GLUT-2 gene transfer into insulinoma cells confers both low and high affinity glucose-stimulated insulin release. J Biol Chem 1994;269:11523–11529
32. Ostenson CG, Abdel-Halim SM, Rasschaert J, et al. Deficient activity of FAD-linked glycerophosphate dehydrogenase in islets of GK rats. Diabetologia 1993;36:722–726
33. Khan A, Ostenson CG, Berggren S. Glucocorticoid increases glucose cycling and inhibits insulin release in pancreatic islets of ob/ob mice. Am J Physiol 1992;263:E663–E666
34. Lee Y, Hirose H, Ohneda M, et al. β-Cell lipotoxicity in the pathogenesis of non–insulin-dependent diabetes mellitus of obese rats: Impairment in adipocyte-β-cell relationships. Proc Natl Acad Sci USA 1994;91:10878–10882
35. Zhou Y-P, Grill VE. Long-term exposure of rat pancreatic islets to fatty acids inhibits glucose-induced insulin secretion and biosynthesis through a glucose fatty acid cycle. J Clin Invest 1994;93:870–876
36. Sako Y, Grill VE. A 48-hour lipid infusion in the rat time-dependently inhibits glucose-induced insulin secretion and β-cell oxidation through a process likely coupled to fatty acid oxidation. Endocrinology 1990;127:1580–1589
37. Prentki M, Vischer S, Glennon MC, et al. Malonyl-coA and long chain acyl-coA esters as metabolic coupling factors in nutrient-induced insulin secretion. J Biol Chem 1992;267:5802–5810
38. Polonsky KS, Given BD, Hirsch L, et al. Quantitative study of insulin secretion and clearance in normal and obese subjects. J Clin Invest 1988;81:435–441
39. Martin BC, Warram JH, Krolewski AS, et al. Role of glucose and insulin resistance in development of type 2 diabetes mellitus: Results of a 25-year follow-up study. Lancet 1995;340:925–930
40. Lillioja S, Mott DM, Spraul M, et al. Insulin resistance and insulin secretory dysfunction as precursors of non–insulin-dependent diabetes mellitus. N Engl J Med 1993;329:1988–1992
41. Henriksen JE, Alford F, Handberg A, et al. Increased glucose effectiveness in normoglycemic but insulin-resistant relatives of patients with non–insulin-dependent diabetes mellitus. J Clin Invest 1994;94:1196–1204
42. Warram JH, Martin BC, Krolewski AS, et al. Slow glucose removal rate and hyperinsulinemia precede the development of type II diabetes in the offspring of diabetic parents. Ann Intern Med 1990;113:909–915
43. Bleich D, Jackson RA, Soeldner JS, Eisenbarth GS. Analysis of metabolic progression to type I diabetes in ICA+ relatives of patients with type I diabetes. Diabetes Care 1990;13:111–118
44. Temple RC, Carrington CA, Luzio SD, et al. Insulin deficiency in non–insulin-dependent diabetes. Lancet 1989;1:293–295
45. Rhodes CJ, Alarcon C. What beta cell defect could lead to hyperproinsulinemia in NIDDM? Diabetes 1994;43:511–517
46. Yoshioka N, Kuzuya T, Matsuda A, et al. Serum proinsulin levels at fasting and after oral glucose load in patients with type 2 (non–insulin-dependent) diabetes mellitus. Diabetologia 1988;31:355–360
47. Haffner SM, Mykkanen L, Valdez RA, et al. Disproportionately increased proinsulin levels are associated with the insulin resistance syndrome. J Clin Endocrinol Metab 1994;79:1806–1810
48. Roder ME, Knip M, Hartling SG, et al. Disproportionately elevated proinsulin levels precede the onset of insulin-dependent diabetes mellitus in siblings with low first phase insulin responses. J Clin Endocrinol Metab 1995;79:1570–1575
49. Leahy JL, Halban PA, Weir GC. Relative hypersecretion of proinsulin in rat model of NIDDM. Diabetes 1991;40:985–989
50. Lang DA, Matthews DR, Peta J, Turner RC. Cyclic oscillations of basal plasma glucose and insulin concentrations in human beings. N Engl J Med 1979; 301:1023–1027
51. Polonsky KS, Given BD, VanCauter E. Twenty-four-hour profiles and pulsatile patterns of insulin section in normal and obese subjects. J Clin Invest 1988; 81:442–448
52. Stagner J, Samols E, Weir GC. Sustained oscillations of insulin, glucagon and somatostatin from the isolated canine pancreas during exposure to a constant glucose concentration. J Clin Invest 1980;65:939–942
53. Chou H-F, Ipp E. Pulsatile insulin secretion in isolated rat islets. Diabetes 1990;39:112–117
54. Perksen N, Munn S, Ferguson D, et al. Coordinate pulsatile insulin secretion by chronic intraportally transplanted islets in the isolated perfused rat liver. J Clin Invest 1994;92:219–227
55. Lang DA, Matthews DR, Burnett M, Turner RC. Brief, irregular oscillations of basal plasma insulin and glucose concentrations in diabetic man. Diabetes 1981;30:435–439
56. O'Rahilly S, Turner RC, Matthews DR. Impaired pulsatile secretion of insulin in relatives of patients with non–insulin-dependent diabetes mellitus. N Engl J Med 1988;318:1225–1230
57. Bratusch-Marrain PR, Komjati M, Waldhausl WK. Efficacy of pulsatile versus continuous insulin administration on hepatic glucose production and glucose utilization in type I diabetic humans. Diabetes 1986;35:922–926
58. Bonner-Weir S. Regulation of pancreatic β-cell mass in vivo. Recent Prog Horm Res 1994;49:91–104
59. Swenne IO, Borg LAH, Crace CJ, Landstrom S. Persistent reduction of pancreatic β-cell mass after a limited period of protein-energy malnutrition in the young rat. Diabetologia 1992;35:939–945
60. Hales CN, Barker DJP. Type 2 (non–insulin-dependent) diabetes mellitus: The thrifty phenotype hypothesis. Diabetologia 1992;35:595–601
61. Thomas F, Balkau B, Vauzelle-Kervroedan F, et al. Maternal effect and familial aggregation in NIDDM. The CODIAB study. Diabetes 1994;43:63–67
62. Westermark P, Wernstedt C, Wilander E, et al. Amyloid fibrils in human insulinoma and islets of Langerhans of the diabetic cat are derived from a neuropeptide-like protein also present in normal islet cells. Proc Natl Acad Sci USA 1987;84:8628–8632
63. Cooper GJS, Willis AC, Clark A, et al. Purification and characterization of a peptide from amyloid-rich pancreases of type 2 diabetic patients. Proc Natl Acad Sci 1987;84:8628–8632
64. O'Brien TD, Rizza RA, Carney JA, Butler PC. Islet amyloidosis in a patient with chronic massive insulin resistance due to antiinsulin receptor antibodies. J Clin Endocrinol Metab 1994;79:290–292
65. Lorenzo A, Bronwyn R, Weir GC, Yanker BA. Pancreatic islet cell toxicity of amylin associated with type-2 diabetes mellitus. Nature 1994;368:756–760
66. Gutniack M, Orskov C, Holst JJ, et al. Antidiabetogenic effect of glucagon-like peptide-1 (7–36) amide in normal subjects and patients with diabetes mellitus. N Engl J Med 1992;326:1316–1322

Diabetes Mellitus, edited by Derek LeRoith, Simeon I. Taylor, and Jerrold M. Olefsky. Lippincott–Raven Publishers, Philadelphia © 1996.

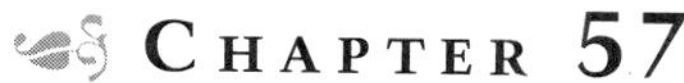

Chapter 57

Insulin Resistance and Its Consequences: Non–Insulin-Dependent Diabetes Mellitus and Coronary Heart Disease

Gerald M. Reaven

Introduction

The goal of this chapter is to summarize the evidence that the ability of insulin to stimulate glucose uptake varies widely from person to person, and that these differences, and how the person attempts to compensate for them, are of fundamental importance in the development and clinical course of what are often designated as diseases of Western civilization. The basic premise underlying this presentation is that non–insulin-dependent diabetes mellitus (NIDDM) results from a failure on the part of the pancreatic β-cell to compensate adequately for the defect in insulin action in insulin-resistant persons. However, the ability to maintain the degree of compensatory hyperinsulinemia necessary to prevent loss of glucose tolerance in insulin-resistant persons does not represent an unqualified homeostatic victory. In contrast, evidence will be presented supporting the view that the *combination* of insulin resistance and compensatory hyperinsulinemia predisposes to the development of coronary heart disease (CHD). In other words, irrespective of the degree of β-cell compensation, the more insulin-resistant the person, the more perilous the outlook.

Before proceeding further, two general principles should be addressed that underlie the subsequent presentation. First, no attempt will be made to address the molecular mechanism, or mechanisms, responsible for insulin resistance in various insulin-sensitive tissues. Second, only data obtained from studies of human beings will be considered. Although these decisions may detract to some extent from the completeness of this presentation, these relevant topics will be addressed in other chapters in this text.

Non–Insulin-Dependent Diabetes Mellitus

Muscle

The ability of insulin to stimulate in vivo glucose disposal has been extensively studied for more than 25 years, and there is abundant evidence that this action of insulin is markedly decreased in patients with non–insulin-dependent diabetes mellitus (NIDDM).[1–3] Since the major site of glucose disposal in these infusion studies is the muscle,[4] it seems reasonable to conclude that the vast majority of patients with NIDDM have a defect in insulin-stimulated glucose disposal by muscle. It should be emphasized that this abnormality in insulin action on muscle in patients with NIDDM does not depend on whether or not the patient is obese.[1–3,5]

The fact that resistance to insulin-mediated glucose disposal by muscle is present in most patients with NIDDM suggests that this abnormality is responsible for the development of hyperglycemia in these persons. Although this is an appealing hypothesis, available data make it highly unlikely. The major problem is that resistance to insulin-mediated glucose disposal by muscle is not limited to patients with NIDDM. For example, muscle insulin resistance is a common finding in nondiabetic subjects with impaired glucose tolerance.[3,6,7] Resistance to insulin-mediated glucose disposal by muscle can also be demonstrated in nondiabetic first-degree relatives of patients with NIDDM.[8,9] Finally, significant differences in the ability of insulin to stimulate glucose disposal by muscle are present in persons with normal glucose tolerance.[10,11] Indeed, in a significant number of these persons, the magnitude of the defect in insulin-mediated glucose disposal approximates that of patients with NIDDM.[10,11] The implications of these observations can be easily seen by inspection of the data in Figure 57-1, in which the relationship between insulin-stimulated glucose disposal by muscle and fasting plasma glucose concentration was defined in 50 nonobese persons. It is obvious from these data that there was not a simple relationship between insulin resistance and fasting plasma glucose concentration, and that a relatively normal fasting plasma glucose concentration could be maintained by persons who were essentially as insulin resistant as patients with frank NIDDM. In addition, once fasting hyperglycemia supervened, significantly higher fasting plasma glucose concentrations were seen with relatively small decreases in insulin-mediated glucose disposal. Consequently, it seems reasonable to conclude that resistance to insulin-mediated muscle glucose uptake by muscle is present in the great majority of persons with glucose intolerance, but that this defect,

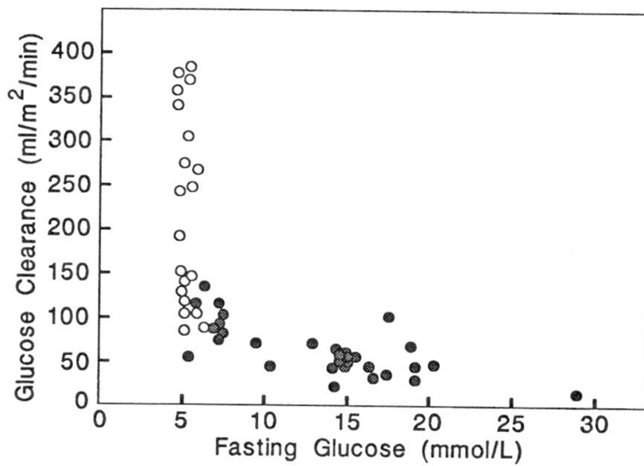

Figure 57-1. The relationship between fasting plasma glucose concentration and glucose metabolic clearance rates observed during hyperinsulinemic, glucose clamp studies in 20 nondiabetic subjects (○) and 30 patients with NIDDM (●). The clamp studies were performed over a 120-minute period, with a steady-state plasma insulin concentration of approximately 100 μU/mL.

by itself, accounts neither for the development of significant hyperglycemia in patients with NIDDM nor for the severity of fasting hyperglycemia in these persons.

β-Cell

As emphasized above, muscle insulin resistance can be demonstrated in a significant number of persons with normal glucose tolerance, and the ability of these persons to maintain glucose homeostasis appears to be due to their ability to sustain a state of chronic hyperinsulinemia. By inference, it seems most likely that non–insulin-dependent diabetes mellitus (NIDDM) with significant fasting hyperglycemia will develop only when insulin-resistant subjects are incapable of secreting enough insulin to compensate for the defect in cellular insulin action. This possibility has received experimental support from both cross-sectional and longitudinal studies,[12–18] and there is considerable evidence that patients with NIDDM and significant hyperglycemia are characterized by the combination of muscle resistance to insulin-mediated glucose uptake and an insulin secretory response of insufficient magnitude to overcome the abnormality in insulin action.

Although this controversy has been going on for approximately 30 years, strong opinions continue to be expressed as to whether insulin resistance or insulin deficiency is the basic defect in patients with NIDDM. In this context, it is often stated that patients with NIDDM are all insulin deficient, either in absolute or relative terms. If euglycemia is assumed to be the natural state, and that it is the function of the pancreatic β-cell to accomplish this, the development of hyperglycemia, by definition, means that β-cell failure has taken place. However, to understand why hyperglycemia develops in patients with NIDDM, and the relative roles played by defects in insulin action and insulin secretion in the pathophysiology of this syndrome, it is necessary to focus on the changes in these two variables that characterize these patients. More specifically, it is necessary to explain why hyperglycemia supervenes when insulin-resistant persons are no longer able to maintain a state of compensatory hyperinsulinemia.

Before attempting to define the role of insulin secretion in the pathophysiology of NIDDM, attention must be given to the method used to measure plasma insulin concentration. Conventional immunoassays used to measure plasma insulin concentration do not distinguish between insulin and proinsulin, and it has been suggested recently that all patients with NIDDM are insulin deficient in absolute terms when specific insulin assays are used.[19] In support of this view is the evidence that the concentration of proinsulin in the plasma is higher in patients with NIDDM and tends to be related to the magnitude of hyperglycemia.[20,21] On the other hand, the fact that patients with NIDDM and significant hyperglycemia secrete relatively more proinsulin does not mean that these patients are *hypoinsulinemic* in absolute terms. Figure 57-2 illustrates ambient concentrations of glucose, total immunoreactive insulin, C peptide, and proinsulin in obese and nonobese persons

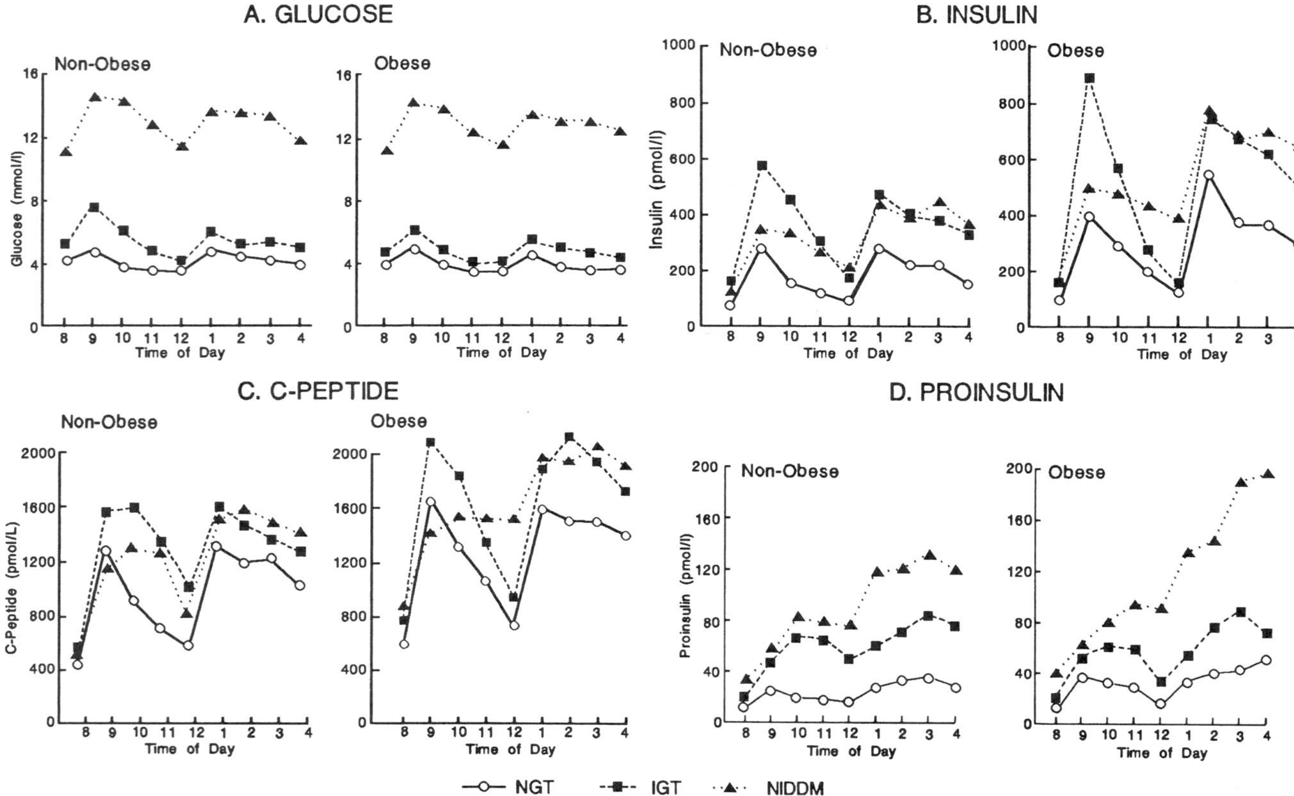

Figure 57-2. Plasma glucose (***A***), immunoreactive insulin (***B***), C peptide (***C***), and proinsulin (***D***) concentrations in subjects with normal glucose tolerance (NGT, ○), IGT (■), and NIDDM (▲) from 8 A.M. to 4 P.M. Statistical significance of the data is as follows: **A** (glucose), $p < 0.001$, NIDDM vs. IGT and NGT; $p < 0.01$, IGT vs. NGT; **B** (insulin), $p < 0.002$, NGT vs. IGT and NIDDM; **C** (C peptide), $p < 0.002$, NGT vs. IGT and NIDDM; **D** (proinsulin), $p < 0.001$, NIDDM vs. NGT; $p < 0.002$, IGT vs. NGT. (Reproduced with permission from The Endocrine Society and the authors from Reaven GM. Plasma insulin, C peptide, and proinsulin concentrations in obese and non-obese individuals with varying degrees of glucose tolerance. J Clin Endocrinol Metab 1993;76:44.)

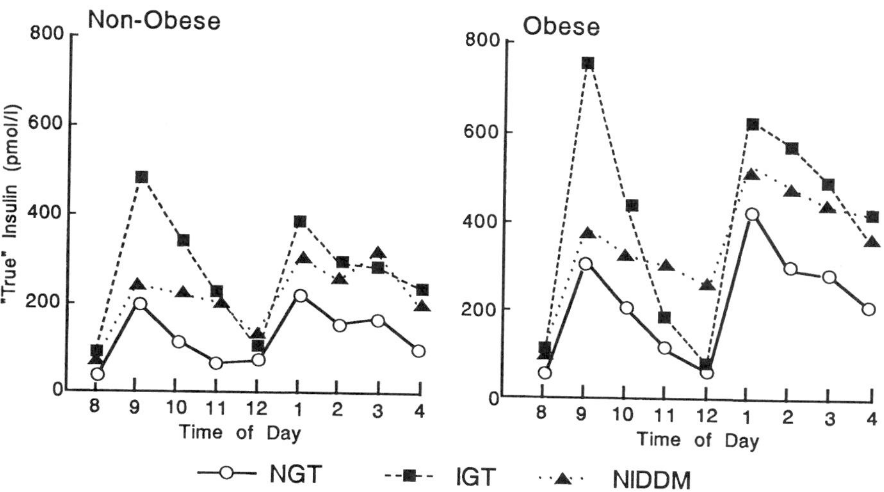

Figure 57-3. True plasma insulin concentrations in subjects with NGT (○), IGT (■), and NIDDM (▲) from 8 A.M. to 4 P.M. Statistical significance of the data is as follows: $p < 0.002$, IGT vs. NGT; $p < 0.02$, NIDDM vs. NGT; $p < 0.05$, IGT vs. NIDDM. (Reproduced with permission from The Endocrine Society and the authors from Reaven GM. Plasma insulin, C peptide, and proinsulin concentrations in obese and non-obese individuals with varying degrees of glucose tolerance. J Clin Endocrinol Metab 1993;76:44.)

with varying degrees of glucose tolerance.[22] These data illustrate hourly determinations from 8 A.M. to 4 P.M. of the four variables, before and after meals (breakfast at 8 A.M. and lunch at noon). These results show that persons with impaired glucose tolerance (IGT) have the highest day-long insulin and C-peptide concentrations, and that values for both of these variables are comparable in normal persons and hyperglycemic patients with NIDDM. The results in Figure 57-2 also demonstrate that hyperglycemic patients with NIDDM have higher plasma proinsulin concentrations than the other two groups, providing support for the view that these persons secrete relatively more proinsulin. It should be emphasized, however, that the molar plasma concentrations of proinsulin are much lower than the molar concentrations of total immunoreactive insulin. It should also be noted that there is a progressive increase in proinsulin concentrations throughout the day, reflecting the relatively slow plasma clearance of proinsulin. Absolute day-long concentrations of "true" insulin are shown in Figure 57-3, and these data show that hyperglycemic patients with NIDDM are not hypoinsulinemic in absolute terms compared to persons with normal glucose tolerance. Furthermore, the highest day-long insulin levels are seen in persons with IGT. These results confirm the fact that conventional measurements of immunoreactive insulin also measure proinsulin, and that the higher the ambient glucose concentration, the higher the day-long plasma proinsulin concentration. However, they also clearly indicate that true insulin concentrations are not lower than normal in persons with varying degrees of glucose tolerance, and that even patients with NIDDM and significant hyperglycemia have true insulin concentrations that are similar to those of glucose-tolerant persons. In other words, patients with glucose intolerance, irrespective of the magnitude of hyperglycemia, are not absolutely insulin deficient.

Two additional points must be made from the data in Figures 57-2 and 57-3. First, the fact that absolute concentrations of insulin are similar in normal persons and hyperglycemic patients with NIDDM does not mean that the β-cells of these patients are normal. Given their degree of hyperglycemia, it could be argued that they should be secreting large amounts of insulin in an effort to restore their plasma glucose concentration to normal levels. Second, it is essential that a distinction be made between the ability of the pancreas to overcome the insulin resistance in patients with NIDDM and maintain euglycemia and the absolute circulating levels of insulin in patients with this syndrome. It is this latter variable that plays the central role in the pathophysiology of NIDDM.

It should be emphasized that the conclusion that patients with NIDDM are not *hypoinsulinemic* in absolute terms is based on measurements that were performed throughout the day in response to conventional mixed meals. It can also be seen from the data in Figures 57-2 and 57-3, as well as in the results of previous reports,[20,21] that fasting true insulin levels are not decreased in patients with NIDDM. Indeed, the conclusion that patients with NIDDM are hypoinsulinemic when insulin-specific assays are used has been derived from measurements made within the first 60 minutes after a pure oral glucose challenge.[19] Thus, both the timing and the insulinogenic stimulus were quite different from those used to collect the data in Figures 57-2 and 57-3. In fact, a similar conclusion about a decreased plasma insulin response within the first 60 minutes after a pure glucose load in patients with NIDDM and fasting hyperglycemia does not require a special insulin assay.[12]

Adipose Tissue

The results in Figure 57-3 show that day-long plasma true insulin levels were comparable in magnitude in normal subjects and patients with non–insulin-dependent diabetes mellitus (NIDDM) and severe fasting hyperglycemia. It can also be seen, however, that these patients had lower true insulin concentration than did the subjects with impaired glucose tolerance (IGT), and that the relatively small difference in true insulin levels between subjects with IGT and patients with NIDDM was associated with a much greater difference in plasma glucose concentrations. Similar cross-sectional data, published almost 30 years ago,[12] first called attention to this relationship, and it was described as representing a horseshoe. On the basis of this relationship, it was suggested that the initial defect in patients with NIDDM was resistance to insulin-mediated glucose disposal and that, if the pancreas could respond to this abnormality by maintaining a state of compensatory hyperinsulinemia, gross decompensation of glucose tolerance could be prevented. Many[13–16,23–27] studies published since the initial description of the horseshoe relationship between plasma glucose and insulin concentrations have validated this original observation.

If it is assumed that significant fasting hyperglycemia develops only when the β-cells of patients with NIDDM cannot overcome the muscle resistance to insulin-mediated glucose disposal, it is necessary to define the consequences of this decline in insulin secretory capacity to understand the pathophysiology of NIDDM. Because the data in Figure 57-3 demonstrate that dramatic changes in the level of glycemia are associated with relatively minor quantitative differences in day-long insulin concentrations, it is necessary to ask: What metabolic events that occur as the result of the observed differences in circulating insulin level could account for the development of this degree of hyperglycemia? In this context, the data shown in Figure 57-4 raise the possibility that resistance to

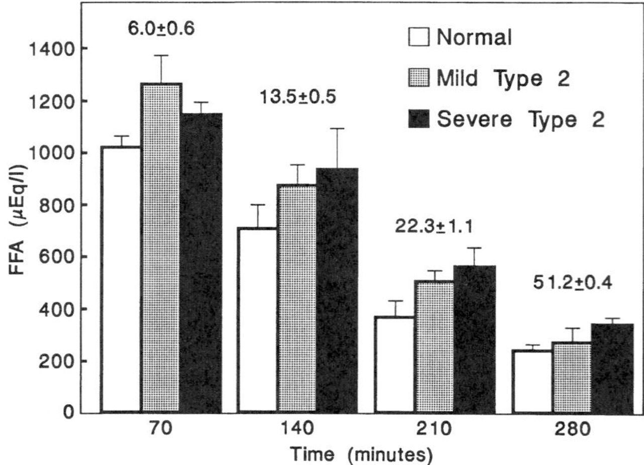

Figure 57-4. Mean ± SE plasma FFA concentrations in normal persons (□) and patients with either mild (⊞, fasting plasma glucose concentrations <175 mg/dL) or severe (■, fasting plasma glucose concentration >250 mg/dL) NIDDM in response to progressive increases in steady-state plasma insulin concentration. The study lasted for 280 minutes, with insulin infused at different rates during each 70-minute period. Plasma glucose concentration was kept constant throughout, and FFA concentration at the end of each 70-minute period is shown. Mean ± SE steady-state plasma insulin concentration achieved during each 70-minute period is shown at the top of each set of three bars. (Reproduced with permission from Reaven GM. Role of insulin resistance in human disease. Diabetes 1988;37:1495.)

insulin regulation at the level of the adipose tissue may offer a reasonable explanation. The study that led to the results shown in Figure 57-4 involved determining plasma free fatty acid (FFA) concentrations in response to the sequential infusion of increasing amounts of insulin while endogenous insulin secretion was blocked by somatostatin. These data show that plasma FFA concentrations fell dramatically as insulin levels were increased from ~5 to 50 μU/mL, and that plasma FFA plasma concentrations were half-maximally suppressed at a plasma insulin concentration of ~20 μU/mL.[28] In other words, adipose tissue is very insulin sensitive, and small changes in plasma insulin concentration can have profound effects on plasma FFA concentrations. Although plasma FFA concentrations were suppressed as insulin concentrations were increased in normal subjects, as well as in patients with NIDDM, the absolute concentrations were always higher in the diabetic subjects. It has also been shown that ambient plasma FFA concentrations are higher than normal in patients with NIDDM, that is, their adipose tissue is also insulin resistant.[29–31] Furthermore, the greater the increase in plasma FFA concentration, the higher the plasma glucose concentration.[31]

Based on the above considerations, it is postulated that the increase in plasma FFA concentration that occurs when insulin-resistant persons cannot maintain a state of compensatory hyperinsulinemia is primarily responsible for the development of significant hyperglycemia in patients with NIDDM. This could occur for the following reasons. In the first place, evidence has been published showing that an increase in plasma FFA concentration will decrease insulin-stimulated glucose uptake.[32] In addition, and suggested as being of much greater importance, is the fact that an increase in FFA flux to the liver, secondary to higher plasma FFA concentrations, will stimulate gluconeogenesis, presumably as the result of increased FFA oxidation by the liver. The biochemical mechanisms that link hepatic FFA oxidation and gluconeogenesis have recently been the subject of a thoughtful review, and there is abundant evidence in support of the view that hepatic FFA oxidation and gluconeogenesis are closely linked.[33] Because insulin-mediated glucose uptake is dramatically reduced in patients with NIDDM, stimulation of hepatic glucose production, secondary to high plasma FFA concentration, would be expected to increase greatly the plasma glucose concentration. Furthermore, as the plasma FFA and glucose concentrations increase, β-cell secretory function will be further compromised. In the case of hyperglycemia, the deleterious effect of "glucotoxicity" on insulin secretion is well recognized.[34] What may be less well appreciated are relatively recent data suggesting that chronic increases in FFA concentration, as distinct from acute elevations, also inhibit the β-cell response to glucose.[35,36] Thus, the increase in FFA concentration associated with a small decline in insulin secretion will further decrease glucose uptake by muscle, increase hepatic FFA oxidation, and stimulate gluconeogenesis; the resultant plasma elevations of FFA and glucose concentration may further compromise β-cell function.

Hepatic Glucose Production

Perhaps the most controversial issue concerning the pathogenesis of hyperglycemia in patients with non–insulin-dependent diabetes mellitus (NIDDM) is the role of the liver. It has been suggested that fasting hyperglycemia in patients with NIDDM is directly related to an absolute increase in hepatic glucose production (HGP). The data that have led to this general opinion have been derived largely from studies in which HGP was estimated by isotopic techniques over a relatively short time period,[37–43] and artifacts associated with these unsteady-state conditions are likely to have led to falsely high values for this variable. This issue has been discussed in some detail in previous publications[44–48] and cannot be fully addressed in this presentation. Suffice it to say that the majority of previous studies in which HGP was measured in patients with NIDDM involved the use of tritiated glucose, took place over a 2-hour period, and, given the expanded glucose pool size in these patients with NIDDM, isotopic steady-state conditions were not reached in this time period. The equations used in an attempt to compensate for this are inadequate,[45,46] leading to falsely high values for HGP. In addition, the greater the magnitude of fasting hyperglycemia, the more HGP will be overestimated. In other words, the relationship between fasting plasma glucose concentration and HGP was a self-fulfiling prophecy.

The results in Figure 57-5 present an entirely different view of the relationship between HGP and fasting plasma glucose (FPG) concentration, one that emerges when tracer techniques that do not overestimate HGP are used. In this study,[48] the relationship between FPG and HGP was examined in 18 normal volunteers and 33 patients with NIDDM, using an isotopic approach to assess HGP that is not confounded by glucose pool size. The patients with NIDDM were divided into three groups: DM-1 (FPG < 10 mM), DM-2 (FPG > 10 < 13 mM), and DM-3 (FPG > 13 mM). Figure 57-5 displays the mean FPG and HGP values for the four groups of subjects, and it can be seen that although the FPG values increased progressively from normal subjects to the DM-3 group, this was not true of the measurements of HGP. Indeed, HGP was not increased above normal in the DM-1 group (FPG < 10 mM) and was increased by only approximately 30% in the patients with the highest FPG (>13.0 mM). These results differ substantially in two fundamental respects from the vast majority of previous studies: (1) HGP in patients with the most severe degree of fasting hyperglycemia was only 30% higher than normal values, not increased by twofold to threefold; (2) fasting hyperglycemia in patients with NIDDM cannot be considered to be solely a function of an absolute increase in HGP. Data essentially similar to ours have been published by Hother-Nielsen and Beck-Nielsen,[47] who concluded that HGP is not higher than normal in even the most severely

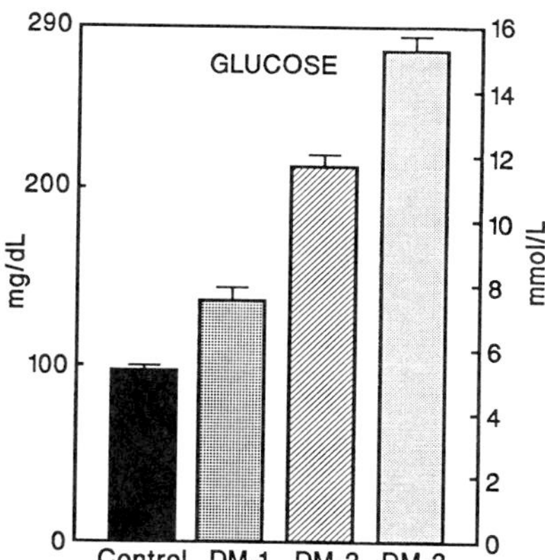

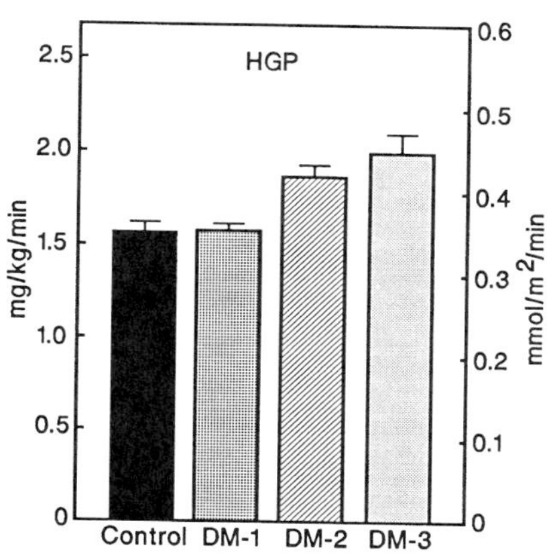

Figure 57-5. Fasting plasma glucose concentration and HGP in control subjects ($n = 11$) and three groups of patients with NIDDM (DM-1, DM-2, and DM-3). The patients with NIDDM were divided into three groups of 11 each on the basis of their fasting plasma glucose concentration: DM-1, <180 mg/dL; DM-2, 180–250 mg/dL; and DM-3, >250 mg/dL. (Reproduced with permission from Jeng C-Y, Sheu WH-H, Fuh MM-T, et al. Relationship between hepatic glucose production and fasting glucose concentrations in patients with non–insulin-dependent diabetes mellitus. Diabetes 1994;43:140.)

hyperglycemic patients with NIDDM. Their data are somewhat different from ours, most likely due to the fact that more patients with very high FPG concentrations were included in our study than in theirs. On the other hand, the point to emphasize from the results of their study and ours is that when efforts are made to correct the methodologic problems inherent in quantifying HGP under non–steady-state conditions, HGP rates in most patients with NIDDM, in absolute terms, are comparable to those in normal persons.

The implication of these findings raises an important issue concerning the role of the liver in the pathogenesis of hyperglycemia in patients with NIDDM. At the simplest level, the observation that absolute values for HGP are similar in normal subjects and hyperglycemic patients with NIDDM does not mean that the liver is acting normally in these persons. For example, it could be argued that the liver in patients with NIDDM is not responding appropriately; for example, HGP is not suppressed by the hyperglycemia. The behavior of the liver in this situation in analogous to β-cell function in these same patients. More specifically, the β-cell is abnormal in that it cannot secrete enough insulin to maintain euglycemia in hyperglycemic patients with NIDDM. In a comparable fashion, the liver is abnormal in that HGP is not suppressed in hyperglycemic patients with NIDDM.

Summary

Resistance to insulin-mediated glucose disposal by muscle can be seen in a significant proportion of glucose-tolerant individuals and in nondiabetic first-degree relatives of patients with non–insulin-dependent diabetes mellitus (NIDDM), as well as in true prediabetes, that is, nondiabetic persons who subsequently develop NIDDM. As long as insulin-resistant persons are capable of increasing their insulin secretory response, gross decompensation of glucose homeostasis can be prevented. When the insulin secretory response declines to the point at which circulating plasma free fatty acid (FFA) levels become significantly elevated, the plasma glucose concentration increases precipitously, presumably due to the fact that hepatic glucose production (HGP) is no longer normally suppressible. Thus, hyperglycemia occurs in NIDDM when the liver continues to secrete normal amounts of glucose into a greatly expanded plasma glucose pool. The advantage to the patient in this situation is presumably the ability to maintain normal absolute rates of peripheral glucose disposal; the loss is the long-term consequence of chronic hyperglycemia. Philosophically, it seems that the ability to maintain glucose utilization was more crucial in evolutionary terms than the maintenance of normal plasma glucose concentration.

Syndrome X

As discussed at the outset, a defect in insulin-mediated glucose disposal of a magnitude comparable to that seen in glucose-intolerant persons is present in a substantial proportion of the normal, nondiabetic population. The fact that these persons are able to compensate for this abnormality by secreting enough insulin to overcome the insulin resistance dose not mean that this state of chronic hyperinsulinemia is benign. In this section, an effort will be made to summarize the pathophysiologic consequence of insulin resistance and/or chronic hyperinsulinemia in nondiabetic persons.

Manifestation of Syndrome X

Hypertension

Patients with high blood pressure are glucose intolerant and hyperinsulinemic when compared to a matched group of persons with normal blood pressure,[3,49] and as many as 50% of an unselected population with hypertension may show these changes.[50] Existence of glucose intolerance and hyperinsulinemia in patients with high blood pressure suggests that resistance to insulin-stimulated glucose uptake may be present in these persons, and this possibility has now been established.[3,49] Furthermore, hyperinsulinemia and insulin resistance are present in both obese and nonobese patients with hypertension and can still be detected when antihypertensive treatment has effectively controlled blood pressure.[3,49]

Since insulin resistance and hyperinsulinemia occur commonly in patients with hypertension, the possibility arises that these changes may play a role in regulation of blood pressure. For example, hyperinsulinemia can both enhance renal sodium retention and increase sympathetic nervous system activity, events that would certainly tend to increase blood pressure.[49] In this chapter, it is not possible to address fully the potential role of insulin resistance and hyperinsulinemia in the regulation of blood pressure, but it may be useful to review briefly some of the major issues. In support of the view that changes in insulin metabolism may modulate blood pressure is the observation that as many as 50% of patients with essential hypertension appear to be insulin resistant and hyperinsulinemic.[50] Furthermore, abnormalities of insulin metabolism can be discerned in normotensive first-degree relatives of patients with high blood pressure[51,52] but not in patients with secondary forms of hypertension.[53] Two major arguments, however, have been advanced against the view that insulin resistance and hyperinsulinemia are involved in blood pressure regulation. The first stems from the observation that acute hyperinsulinemia in human beings leads to vasodilation, and blood pressure does not increase.[54] In addition, blood pressure does not change when insulin is infused into dogs for periods of up to 2 weeks.[55] On the other hand, blood pressure does increase when rats are infused with insulin.[56] Furthermore, blood pressure has been shown to fall when the insulin dose is decreased in obese, hypertensive patients with non–insulin-dependent diabetes mellitus (NIDDM)[57] and to increase when insulin treatment is initiated in patients with NIDDM whose disease is poorly controlled by oral agents.[58]

The second major argument relates to the fact that a relationship between insulin level and blood pressure cannot always be seen in population studies. For example, a recent report has shown that blood pressure and insulin concentration were significantly correlated in whites, but in neither Afro-Americans nor Pima Indians.[59] On the other hand, hypertensive Afro-Americans are insulin resistant and hyperinsulinemic when compared to Afro-Americans with normal blood pressure,[60,61] raising questions as to the significance of the lack of a relationship between blood pressure and insulin described in Afro-Americans in epidemiologic studies.

Dyslipidemia

Triglyceride

The importance of resistance to insulin-stimulated glucose uptake and hyperinsulinemia in the regulation of lipoprotein metabolism has recently been reviewed,[62] and there is considerable evidence that resistance to insulin-stimulated glucose uptake leads to a compensatory increase in plasma insulin concentration, enhanced hepatic very low density (VLDL)-triglyceride (TG) secretion, and hypertriglyceridemia. In persons who retain insulin secretory function, particularly nondiabetics, there is a relatively linear relationship between measures of insulin resistance and plasma insulin concentration,[10,11] that is, the higher the insulin resistance, the greater the magnitude of hyperinsulinemia. In addition, statistically significant correlations exist between resistance to insulin-stimulated glucose uptake, plasma insulin concentration, VLDL-TG secretion rate, and plasma TG concentration in both normotriglyceridemic and hypertriglyceridemic persons.[63,64] Furthermore, experimental manipulations that modify insulin action and/or plasma insulin concentration lead to predictable changes in VLDL-TG secretion rate and plasma TG concentration. For example, weight loss is associated with a commensurate decrease in resistance to insulin-mediated glucose disposal, plasma insulin concentration, hepatic VLDL-TG secretion, and plasma TG concentration.[65] In contrast, feeding patients a high-carbohydrate diet leads to day-long increases in both plasma insulin and TG concentration, and the increment in plasma TG concentration is significantly correlated with the degree of carbohydrate-induced hyperinsulinemia.[66]

Given these considerations, it seems likely that resistance to insulin-mediated glucose disposal and compensatory hyperinsulinemia lead to hypertriglyceridemia in a variety of situations. Once the plasma VLDL-TG pool size increases, a variety of associated abnormalities in plasma lipoprotein metabolism are also present. Whether these changes are simply a function of the increase in plasma TG concentration is not clear, but the possibility exists that at least some of them are directly related to insulin resistance and/or compensatory hyperinsulinemia. Indeed, the link between all of these related phenomena cannot be defined precisely at this time.

High Density Lipoprotein Cholesterol

The best-established association with hypertriglyceridemia is between a high plasma triglyceride (TG) concentration and a low high density lipoprotein (HDL)-cholesterol concentration; there are also associations between high plasma TG and low HDL-cholesterol concentrations and hyperinsulinemia.[67,68] One explanation for the inverse relationship between a high TG concentration and a low HDL-cholesterol concentration relates to the activity of cholesteryl ester transfer protein promoting the movement of cholesteryl ester from HDL to very low density lipoprotein (VLDL).[69] Thus, the higher VLDL-TG level, the greater the loss of cholesteryl ester from HDL and the lower the plasma HDL-cholesterol concentration. It also appears that a low HDL-cholesterol concentration is associated with an increase in the fractional catabolic rate of apoprotein A-I.[70] Given evidence that apoprotein A-I fractional catabolic rate is increased in states of hyperinsulinemia,[71,72] it is possible that insulin resistance and/or compensatory hyperinsulinemia also directly modulate HDL-cholesterol concentrations via this mechanism as well.

Low Density Lipoprotein-Particle Diameter

There is now substantial evidence[73–75] indicating that individuals with smaller low density lipoprotein (LDL) particles are at increased risk of developing coronary heart disease (CHD). Analysis of LDL particle size distributions[74,75] has identified distinct LDL subclasses and has shown that LDL in most persons can be characterized by a predominance of larger LDL (diameter usually > 255 Å, subclass pattern A) or smaller LDL (diameter ≤ 255 Å, subclass pattern B) particles. Persons with subclass pattern B have been shown to have higher plasma triglyceride (TG) concentrations and lower high density lipoprotein (HDL)-cholesterol concentrations.[74,75] Because similar changes in plasma TG and HDL-cholesterol concentrations are associated with resistance to insulin-mediated glucose uptake and/or hyperinsulinemia,[3,62–68] it seemed likely that subclass pattern B was also associated with insulin resistance. We have recently published the results of a study of 100 normal persons demonstrating that those with small, dense LDL particles (pattern B) were relatively insulin resistant, glucose intolerant, hyperinsulinemic, hypertensive, hypertriglyceridemic and had a lower HDL-cholesterol concentration.[76] These observations support the view that this change in LDL composition should be added to the cluster of abnormalities previously defined as constituting Syndrome X.

Postprandial Lipemia

The higher the fasting triglyceride (TG) concentration, the greater the degree of postprandial lipemia.[77] Since insulin resistance and/or compensatory hyperinsulinemia are highly correlated with the development of hypertriglyceridemia,[3,62–68] it is likely that increases in the magnitude of postprandial lipemia will be present in insulin-resistant subjects. Indeed, there is evidence that postprandial lipemia is accentuated in subjects with obesity or non–insulin-dependent diabetes mellitus (NIDDM),[78–80] states in which resistance to insulin-mediated glucose disposal is known to occur. It is not completely clear at this moment if the relationship between insulin resistance and/or compensatory hyperinsulinemia and an increase in the degree of postprandial lipemia is entirely secondary to changes in fasting plasma TG concentration. For example, postprandial lipemia is exaggerated in patients with NIDDM when compared to nondiabetic persons matched for fasting plasma TG concentrations, and the higher the plasma insulin response to meals, the greater the degree of postprandial lipemia.[80] Obviously, this issue needs further study. However, the fact that there is not complete understanding of the link between insulin resistance and postprandial lipemia should not prevent us from adding an increase in postprandial lipemia to the features that comprise Syndrome X.

Plasminogen Activator Inhibitor 1

Plasminogen activator inhibitor (PAI-1) concentrations are higher in patients with coronary heart disease (CHD), and it has been suggested that this change may be a primary risk factor for myocardial infarction in younger men.[81,82] The relationship between CHD and PAI-1 is presumably a function of the observation that plasma PAI-1 and fibrinolysis are inversely related, that is, and increase in PAI-1 concentration is associated with decreased fibrinolysis.

Plasminogen activator inhibitor (PAI-1) concentrations also appear to be higher in patients with hypertriglyceridemia,[81,82] NIDDM,[83] or hypertension.[84] Given the association between PAI-1 and the other features of Syndrome X, it seemed possible that PAI-1 concentrations were related to insulin resistance and/or compensatory hyperinsulinemia.[83] Perhaps the best evidence in this context is the conclusion from the European Concerted Action on Thrombosis and Disabilities Angina Pectoris Study of 1500 patients with angina pectoris that PAI-1 concentrations were significantly associated with hyperinsulinemia, hypertriglyceridemia, and hypertension.[85] Consequently, there are significant data showing that an increase in PAI-1 concentrations might appropriately be said to belong to Syndrome X. Because there is a very close relationship between PAI-1 and plasma TG concentrations, however, the nature of the relationship between insulin resistance and/or compensatory hyperinsulinemia and PAI-1 concentrations requires further definition.

Hyperuricemia

Since increases in serum uric acid concentration are commonly seen in association with glucose intolerance, dyslipidemia, and hypertension, it seemed reasonable to see if uric acid concentration also varied as a function of insulin resistance and/or hyperinsulinemia. Such a study was performed in normal volunteers,[86] which demonstrated that significant correlations existed between serum uric acid concentration and both insulin resistance and the plasma insulin response to an oral glucose challenge. These relationships persisted when differences in age, sex, body mass index, and ratio of waist-to-hip girth were taken into account. Of interest was the observation that both resistance to insulin-mediated glucose uptake and the plasma insulin response were inversely correlated with the urinary clearance of uric acid, suggesting that the link between insulin metabolism and hyperuricemia was the renal handling of uric acid. It has also been shown that healthy volunteers with asymptomatic hyperuricemia have higher plasma insulin responses to oral glucose, higher plasma triglyceride (TG) and lower high density lipoprotein (HDL)-cholesterol concentrations, and higher blood pressure when compared to a well-matched group of volunteers with normal serum uric acid concentrations.[87] Thus, hyperuricemia appears to be a member of the cluster of abnormalities comprising Syndrome X.

Syndrome X, Obesity, and Physical Activity

Obesity per se can lead to a decrease in insulin-mediated glucose uptake, whereas weight loss in obese persons is associated with enhanced in vivo insulin action.[65] However, obesity is not the only environmental change that can modulate insulin resistance; the level of habitual physical activity seems to be as potent as obesity in this regard.[88,89] Furthermore, it is known that exercise training can enhance insulin sensitivity, lower plasma triglyceride (TG) and insulin concentrations, lower blood pressure, and increase high density lipoprotein (HDL)-cholesterol concentrations.[90,91] The fact that obesity and habitual activity can modify the presentation of Syndrome X, however, does not mean that the various manifestations of Syndrome X are determined solely by these environmental variables. For example, in nondiabetic volunteers of European and Native American backgrounds, it was shown that less than 50% of the total variance in insulin-stimulated glucose uptake could be attributed to the combined effects of differences in age, maximal oxygen consumption, and obesity.[89] Age had relatively little effect, and the relative impact of differences in maximal oxygen consumption was at least as great as that due to variations in body weight. Because all of the clinical features of Syndrome X can develop independently of obesity, sedentary activity, and so on, some of the terms used to describe Syndrome X—the ''deadly quartet''[92] or the ''GHO syndrome'' (glucose intolerance, hypertension, and obesity)[93]—are misleading in that they imply that obesity is an essential attribute of the system complex being described. Perhaps the clearest demonstration of this point can be seen in the results of a recently published study in which 32 obese and 32 nonobese subjects were selected on the basis of their hyperinsulinemic or normoinsulinemic state.[94] None of the subjects had diabetes, and their insulin responses can be seen in Figure 57-6. The results in Figure 57-7 demonstrate that plasma TG levels were higher and HDL-cholesterol levels lower in the hyperinsulinemic subjects, *irrespective* of the degree of obesity. Furthermore, both systolic and diastolic blood pressure were increased to a similar degree in the obese and nonobese persons selected because they were hyperinsulinemic.

The fact that the changes comprising Syndrome X can occur to a similar degree in both obese and nonobese, hyperinsulinemic (and presumably insulin-resistant) subjects is not meant to diminish the impact that variations in weight and/or regional fat distribution and level of physical activity have on resistance to insulin-mediated glucose disposal. Indeed, the changes associated with Syndrome

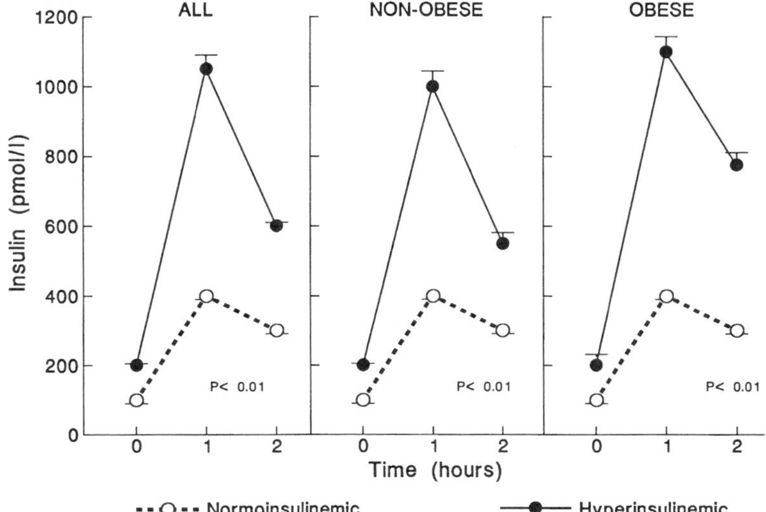

FIGURE 57-6. Mean (± th SE) plasma insulin concentration in 32 hyperinsulinemic (●) and 32 normoinsulinemic (○) persons before and after a 75-g oral glucose challenge. The left panel presents the comparison in the entire population; the middle and right panels depict the results in the nonobese and obese groups, respectively. (Reproduced with permission from the Journal of Internal Medicine from Zavaroni I. Hyperinsulinemia, obesity and Syndrome X. J Intern Med 1994;235:51.)

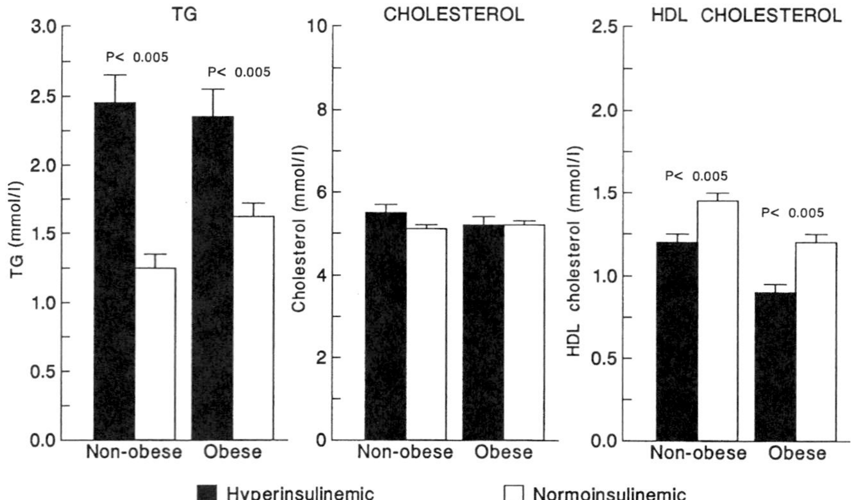

FIGURE 57-7. Mean (± th SE) fasting plasma TG, cholesterol, and HDL-cholesterol concentrations in 32 hyperinsulinemic (■) and 32 normoinsulinemic (□) persons further subdivided into either 16 nonobese or 16 obese hyperinsulinemic or normoinsulinemic subjects. (Reproduced with permission from the Journal of Internal Medicine from Reaven GM. Hyperinsulinemia, obesity and Syndrome X. J Intern Med 1994;235:51.)

X are accentuated when persons become heavier and/or less active. On the other hand, it is necessary to emphasize that insulin resistance, and the consequent manifestations of this defect, do not depend on obesity or a sedentary lifestyle.

Relationship Between Syndrome X and Coronary Heart Disease

Perhaps the best way to begin this section is to address the matter of two syndromes called X. In 1967, Kemp suggested that the term *Syndrome X* be used to describe patients with symptoms and electrocardiographic evidence of coronary heart disease (CHD) in the absence of a positive coronary angiogram.[95] The term *microvascular angina* has tended to replace *Syndrome X* in the cardiologic literature, reflecting the growing belief that patients can have CHD as the result of impaired perfusion of the microvasculature of the heart without evidence of significant macrovascular atherosclerosis.[96] Thus, although the cardiologic and metabolic forms of Syndrome X appeared to be related to CHD, the two syndromes were not known to share other characteristics. However, Dean et al.[97] have shown that nondiabetic patients with microvascular angina had higher plasma insulin responses to an oral glucose load than did a control population and were also dyslipidemic. More recently, we quantified insulin-mediated glucose disposal, plasma glucose and insulin responses to oral glucose, and various measures of lipoprotein metabolism in patients with the clinical diagnosis of microvascular angina.[98] The results of these studies demonstrated that patients with the clinical diagnosis of microvascular angina were significantly more insulin resistant and had higher insulin levels than did the control population. In addition, they had higher plasma triglyceride (TG) and lower high density lipoprotein (HDL)-cholesterol levels. Evidence that patients with microvascular angina are resistant to insulin-mediated glucose uptake was also presented in a recent publication from Denmark.[99] Thus, there is evidence that patients with the clinical diagnosis of microvascular angina (the cardiologic version of Syndrome X) are, as a group, resistant to insulin-mediated glucose uptake, glucose intolerant, hyperinsulinemic, and dyslipidemic, with high plasma TG and low HDL-cholesterol concentrations. Because these changes in glucose, insulin, and lipid metabolism define the endocrinologic version of Syndrome X, it seems most likely that we are really describing one syndrome, a metabolic one, which is associated with ischemic heart disease, involving both the macrovasculature and the microvasculature of the heart.

If we now consider the abnormalities that comprise Syndrome X, the possible relationships between these changes and CHD are easy to define. Although hypercholesterolemia is often the major focus when the pathogenesis of CHD is discussed, the abnormalities subsumed under the general heading of Syndrome X appear to play a major role in the etiology of CHD.[100] CHD is recognized as a major cause of morbidity and mortality in patients with NIDDM, but there is evidence that the risk of CHD is also increased in persons with normal glucose tolerance who have the highest plasma glucose concentration after a glucose load.[101–103] Although hyperinsulinemia may maintain glucose tolerance in persons who have a defect in insulin-stimulated glucose uptake, endogenous hyperinsulinemia has been shown to be associated with an increased risk of CHD.[102,104]

The importance of hypertriglyceridemia as a risk factor for CHD is often minimized in publications from the United States,[105,106] but this has not been the case in Europe.[107,108] This issue has recently been reviewed in detail,[109] and an important role for hypertriglyceridemia in the genesis of CHD cannot be easily dismissed. The combination of high plasma TG and low HDL-cholesterol concentrations as an important risk factor for CHD has been emphasized by the results of recent epidemiologic studies,[110,111] and there is abundant evidence that a low plasma HDL-cholesterol concentration increases the risk of CHD in nondiabetics.[112] Finally, hypertriglyceridemic subjects tend to have both smaller, denser LDL particles[73–76] and an accentuation of their degree of postprandial lipemia,[77] changes that would also increase the risk of CHD.[73–75,113,114]

The importance of hypertension as a CHD risk factor is well recognized, making somewhat confusing the evidence that little or no reduction in CHD was demonstrated when blood pressure was lowered in clinical trials.[115] A possible explanation for this finding is that no attention was directed in these trials to the abnormalities in carbohydrate and lipoprotein metabolism now known to be associated with high blood pressure,[49] which increase the risk of CHD. As a corollary, it seems likely that the presence of these changes in patients with high blood pressure contributes significantly to their risk of CHD.

An increase in plasminogen activator inhibitor 1 (PAI-1) also appears to be a risk factor for CHD,[81,82,85] presumably due to a defect in the fibrinolytic system. On the other hand, metabolic risk factors for CHD known to be associated with an increase in PAI-1 (e.g., hyperinsulinemia, hypertriglyceridemia, and a low HDL-cholesterol concentration) were not routinely measured in the studies linking the fibrinolytic system to CHD, and it is possible that they also contributed to the development of ischemic heart disease.

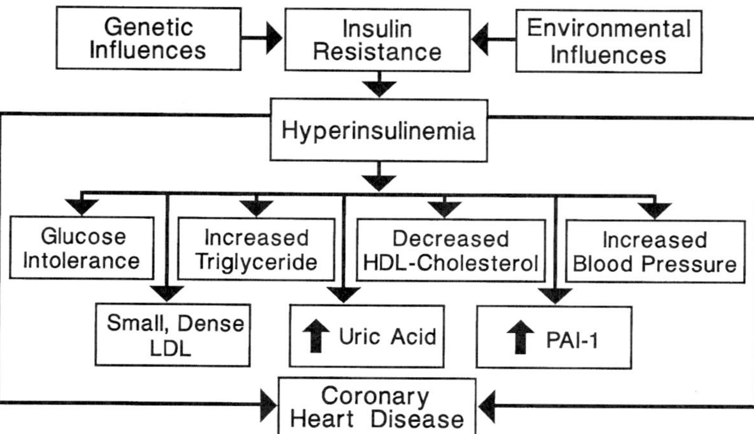

FIGURE 57-8. A schematic description of the putative relationships between resistance to insulin-mediated glucose disposal, compensatory hyperinsulinemia, the multiple consequences that ensue from the defect in insulin action and comprise Syndrome X, and CHD.

Summary

The cluster of abnormalities that make up the current version of Syndrome X are shown in Figure 57-8. It can be seen from this formulation that resistance to insulin-mediated glucose disposal and compensatory hyperinsulinemia are viewed as the central defects. Arguments may continue as to why resistance to insulin-mediated glucose disposal occurs, but there is general agreement that this defect will lead to an effort by the β-cell to secrete more insulin to prevent decompensation of glucose homeostasis. Normal or near-normal glucose tolerance can be maintained if insulin-resistant persons are able to maintain a state of chronic hyperinsulinemia. Unfortunately, the consequences of this "victory" are likely to include various abnormalities of lipoprotein metabolism, high blood pressure, and an increase in PAI-1 activity, hyperuricemia, and CHD. Given these considerations, it seems reasonable to suggest that the various facets of Syndrome X are involved to a substantial degree in the cause and clinical course of CHD.

Conclusion

Perhaps the most important generalization that should be made at the end of this chapter is that the ability of insulin to stimulate glucose uptake varies widely from person to person. In an effort to maintain an ambient plasma glucose concentration between approximately 80 to 140 mg/dL, the pancreatic β-cell will attempt to secrete whatever amount of insulin is required to accomplish this goal. The more resistant a normal person is to insulin-mediated glucose disposal, the greater the degree of compensatory hyperinsulinemia needed to maintain normal glucose tolerance. If the β-cell cannot sustain this philanthropic effort, plasma glucose concentrations begin to rise. The degree to which glucose homeostasis decompensates will, to some extent, be a function of the magnitude of insulin resistance but, much more crucially, it will reflect the relative decline in insulin secretory response. Once the plasma glucose concentration begins to increase and the plasma insulin to decrease, a series of other events take place, largely involving the liver and adipose tissue, that further conspire to accentuate the degree of fasting hyperglycemia.

Although the pathophysiologic consequences of the combination of insulin resistance and failing β-cell secretory function are clearly disastrous, the ability of insulin-resistant persons to remain normal or near-normal glucose tolerance by secreting large amounts of insulin is hardly benign. As described in detail, this combination of events greatly increases the likelihood that such persons will develop hypertension, become dyslipidemic, and have abnormalities of fibrinolytic function, all of which increase the risk of CHD.

Based on the above considerations, it seems reasonable to suggest that resistance to insulin-mediated glucose disposal, and the manner in which the organism responds to this defect, play major roles in the pathogenesis and clinical course of what are often referred to as diseases of Western civilization.

References

1. Ginsberg H, Kimmerling G, Olefsky JM, Reaven GM. Demonstration of insulin resistance in untreated adult onset diabetic subjects with fasting hyperglycemia. J Clin Invest 1975;55:454
2. Reaven GM. Insulin resistance in noninsulin-dependent diabetes mellitus. Does it exist and can it be measured? Am J Med 1983;74:3
3. Reaven GM. Role of insulin resistance in human disease. Diabetes 1988; 37:1495
4. DeFronzo RA, Gunnarsson R, Bjorkman O, et al. Effects of insulin on peripheral and splanchnic glucose metabolism in non–insulin dependent diabetes mellitus. J Clin Invest 1985;76:149
5. Hollenbeck CB, Chen Y-DI, Reaven GM. A comparison of the relative effects of obesity and non–insulin-dependent diabetes mellitus on *in vivo* insulin-stimulated glucose utilization. Diabetes 1984;33:622
6. Shen S-W, Reaven GM, Farquhar JW. Comparison of impedance to insulin mediated glucose uptake in normal and diabetic subjects. J Clin Invest 1970; 49:2151
7. Ginsberg H, Olefsky JM, Reaven GM. Further evidence that insulin resistance exists in patients with chemical diabetes. Diabetes 1974;23:674
8. Laws A, Stefanick ML, Reaven GM. Insulin resistance and hypertriglyceridemia in nondiabetic relatives of patients with noninsulin-dependent diabetes mellitus. J Clin Endocrinol Metab 1989;69:343
9. Ho LT, Chang ZY, Wang JT, et al. Insulin insensitivity in offspring of parents with type 2 diabetes mellitus. Diabetic Med 1990;7:31
10. Hollenbeck CB, Reaven GM. Variations in insulin-stimulated glucose uptake in healthy individuals with normal glucose tolerance. J Clin Endocrinol Metab 1987;64:1169
11. Reaven GM, Brand RJ, Chen Y-DI, et al. Insulin resistance and insulin secretion are determinants of oral glucose tolerance in normal individuals. Diabetes 1993;42:1324
12. Reaven G, Miller R. Study of the relationship between glucose and insulin responses to an oral glucose load in man. Diabetes 1968;17:560
13. Sicree RA, Zimmet PZ, King HOM, Coventry JS. Plasma insulin response among Nauruans: Prediction of deterioration in glucose tolerance over 6 yr. Diabetes 1987;36:179
14. Reaven GM, Hollenbeck CB, Chen Y-DI. Relationship between glucose tolerance, insulin secretion, and insulin action in non-obese individuals with varying degrees of glucose tolerance. Diabetologia 1989;32:52
15. Saad MF, Pettit DJ, Mott DM, et al. Sequential changes in serum insulin concentration during development of non–insulin-dependent diabetes. Lancet 1989;1:1356
16. Haffner SM, Stern MP, Mitchell BD, et al. Incidence of type II diabetes in Mexican Americans predicted by fasting insulin and glucose levels, obesity, and body-fat distribution. Diabetes 1990;39:283
17. Warram JH, Martin BC, Krolewski AS, et al. Slow glucose removal rate and hyperinsulinemia precede the development of type II diabetes in the offspring of the diabetic parents. Ann Intern Med 1990;113:909

18. Lillioja S, Mott DM, Spraul M, et al. Insulin resistance and insulin secretory dysfunction as precursors of non–insulin-dependent diabetes mellitus. N Engl J Med 1993;329:1988
19. Temple RC, Carrington CA, Luzio SD, et al. Insulin deficiency in non–insulin-dependent diabetes. Lancet 1989;1:293
20. Yoshioka N, Kuzuya T, Matsuda A, et al. Serum proinsulin levels at fasting and after oral glucose load in patients with type 2 (non–insulin-dependent) diabetes mellitus. Diabetologia 1988;31:355
21. Saad MF, Kahn SE, Nelson RG, et al. Disproportionately elevated proinsulin in Pima Indians with noninsulin-dependent diabetes mellitus. J Clin Endocrinol Metab 1990;70:1247
22. Reaven GM, Chen Y-DI, Hollenbeck CB, et al. Plasma insulin, C-peptide, and proinsulin concentrations in obese and non-obese individuals with varying degrees of glucose tolerance. J Clin Endocrinol Metab 1993;76:44
23. Chiles R, Tzagournis M. Excessive serum insulin response to oral glucose in obesity and mild diabetes. Diabetes 1970;19:458
24. Savage PJ, Dippe SE, Bennett PH, et al. Hyperinsulinemia and hypoinsulinemia: Insulin responses to oral carbohydrate over a wide spectrum of glucose tolerance. Diabetes 1975;25:362
25. Zimmet P, Whitehouse S, Alford F, Chisholm D. The relationship of insulin response to a glucose stimulus over a wide range of glucose tolerance. Diabetologia 1976;15:23
26. Reaven GM, Miller RG. An attempt to define the nature of chemical diabetes using a multidimensional analysis. Diabetologia 1979;16:17
27. Defronzo RA. The triumvirate: β-Cell, muscle, liver: A collusion response for NIDDM. Diabetes 1988;37:667
28. Swislocki ALM, Chen Y-DI, Golay A, et al. Insulin suppression of plasma-free fatty acid concentration in normal individuals and patients with type 2 (non–insulin-dependent) diabetes. Diabetologia 1987;30:622
29. Fraze E, Donner CC, Swislocki ALM, et al. Ambient plasma free fatty acid concentrations in noninsulin-dependent diabetes mellitus: Evidence for insulin resistance. J Clin Endocrinol Metab 1985;61:807
30. Chen Y-DI, Golay A, Swislocki ALM, Reaven GM. Resistance to insulin suppression of plasma free fatty acid concentrations and insulin stimulation of glucose uptake in noninsulin-dependent diabetes mellitus. J Clin Endocrinol Metab 1987;64:17
31. Golay A, Swislocki ALM, Chen Y-DI, Reaven GM. Relationships between plasma-free fatty acid concentration, endogenous glucose production, and fasting hyperglycemia in normal and non–insulin-dependent diabetic individuals. Metabolism 1987;36:692
32. Bonadonna RC, Groop LC, Zych K, et al. Dose-dependent effect of insulin on plasma free fatty acid turnover oxidation in humans. Am J Physiol 1990; 259:E736
33. Foley JE. Rationale and application of fatty acid oxidation inhibitors in treatment of diabetes mellitus. Diabetes Care 1992;15:773
34. Leahy JL, Cooper HE, Deal DA, Weir GC. Chronic hyperglycemia is associated with impaired glucose influence on insulin secretion. J Clin Invest 1986;77:908
35. Sako Y, Grill VE. A 48-hour lipid infusion in the rat time-dependently inhibits glucose-induced insulin secretion and β cell oxidation through a process likely coupled to fatty acid oxidation. Endocrinology 1990;127:1580
36. Zhou Y-P, Grill VE. Long-term exposure of rat pancreatic islets to fatty acids inhibits glucose-induced insulin secretion and biosynthesis through a glucose fatty acid cycle. J Clin Invest 1994;93:870
37. Kolterman OG, Gray RS, Griffin J, et al. Receptor and postreceptor defects contribute to the insulin resistance in non–insulin-dependent diabetes mellitus. J Clin Invest 1981;68:957
38. DeFronzo RA, Simonson D, Ferrannini E. Hepatic and peripheral insulin resistance: A common feature of type 2 (non–insulin-dependent) and type 1 (insulin dependent) diabetes mellitus. Diabetologia 1982;23:313
39. Nankervis A, Proietto J, Aitken P, et al. Differential effects of insulin therapy on hepatic and peripheral insulin sensitivity in type 2 (non–insulin-dependent) diabetes. Diabetologia 1982;23:320
40. Best J, Judzewitsch R, Pfeifer M, et al. The effect of chronic sulfonylurea therapy on hepatic glucose production in non-insulin dependent diabetes. Diabetes 1982;31:333
41. Bogardus C, Lillioja S, Howard BV, et al. Relationships between insulin secretion, insulin action and fasting plasma glucose concentration in nondiabetic and non-insulin dependent diabetic subjects. J Clin Invest 1984;74:1238
42. Firth RG, Bell PM, Marsh HM, et al. Postprandial hyperglycemia in patients with noninsulin-dependent diabetes mellitus. Role of hepatic and extrahepatic tissues. J Clin Invest 1986;77:1525
43. Campbell PJ, Mandarino LJ, Gerich JE. Quantification of the relative impairment in actions of insulin on hepatic glucose production and peripheral glucose uptake in non–insulin-dependent diabetes mellitus. Metabolism 1988;37:15
44. Chen Y-DI, Jeng C-Y, Hollenbeck CB, et al. Relationship between plasma glucose and insulin concentration, glucose production, and glucose disposal in normal subjects and patients with non–insulin-dependent diabetes. J Clin Invest 1988;82:21
45. Chen Y-DI, Swislocki ALM, Jeng C-Y, et al. Effect of time on measurement of hepatic glucose production. J Clin Endocrinol Metab 1988;67:1084
46. Hother-Nielsen O, Beck-Nielsen H. On the determination of basal glucose production rate in patients with Type 2 (non–insulin-dependent) diabetes mellitus using primed-continuous 3-^{3}H-glucose infusion. Diabetologia 1990; 33:603
47. Hother-Nielsen O, Beck-Nielsen H. Insulin resistance, but normal basal rates of glucose production in patients with newly diagnosed mild diabetes mellitus. Acta Endocrinol (Copenh) 1991;124:637
48. Jeng C-Y, Sheu WH-H, Fuh MM-T, et al. Relationship between hepatic glucose production and fasting plasma glucose concentration in patients with non-insulin-dependent diabetes mellitus. Diabetes 1994;43:1440
49. Reaven GM. Insulin resistance, hyperinsulinemia, hypertriglyceridemia, and hypertension: Parallels between human disease and rodent models. Diabetes Care 1991;14:195
50. Zavaroni I, Mazza S, Dall'Aglio E, et al. Prevalence of hyperinsulinaemia in patients with high blood pressure. J Intern Med 1992;231:235
51. Ferrari P, Weidmann P, Shaw S, et al. Altered insulin sensitivity, hyperinsulinemia, and dyslipidemia in individuals with a hypertensive parent. Am J Med 1991;91:589
52. Facchini F, Chen Y-DI, Clinkingbeard C, et al. Insulin resistance, hyperinsulinemia, and dyslipidemia in nonobese individuals with a family history of hypertension. Am J Hypertens 1992;5:694
53. Shamiss A, Carroll J, Rosenthal T. Insulin resistance in secondary hypertension. Am J Hypertens 1992;5:26
54. Anderson EA, Mark AL. The vasodilator action of insulin: Implications for the insulin hypothesis of hypertension. Hypertension 1993;21:136
55. Hall JE, Brands MW, Kivlighn SD, et al. Chronic hyperinsulinemia and blood pressure. Hypertension 1990;15:519
56. Brands MW, Hildebrandt DA, Mizelle HL, Hall JE. Sustained hyperinsulinemia increases arterial pressure in conscious rats. Am J Physiol 1991; 260:R764
57. Tedde R, Sechi LA, Marigliano A, et al. Antihypertensive effect of insulin reduction in diabetic-hypertensive patients. Am J Hypertens 1989;2:163
58. Randeree HA, Omar MAK, Motala AA, Seedat MA. Effect of insulin therapy on blood pressure in NIDDM patients with secondary failure. Diabetes Care 1992;15:1258
59. Saad M, Lillioja S, Myomba BL, et al. Racial differences in the relation between blood pressure and insulin resistance. N Engl J Med 1991;324:733
60. Falkner B, Hulman S, Tennenbaum J, Kushner H. Insulin resistance and blood pressure in young black men. Hypertension 1990;16:706
61. Falkner B, Hulman S, Kushner H. Insulin-stimulated glucose utilization and borderline hypertension in young adult blacks. Hypertension 1993;22:18
62. Reaven GM, Chen Y-DI. Role of insulin in regulation of lipoprotein metabolism in diabetes. Diabetes/Metab Rev 1988;4:639
63. Tobey TA, Greenfield M, Kraemer F, Reaven GM. Relationship between insulin resistance, insulin secretion, very low density lipoprotein kinetics and plasma triglyceride levels in normotriglyceridemic man. Metabolism 1981; 30:165
64. Olefsky JM, Farquhar JW, Reaven GM. Reappraisal of the role of insulin in hypertriglyceridemia. Am J Med 1974;57:551
65. Olefsky JM, Reaven GM, Farquhar JW. Effects of weight reduction on obesity: Studies of carbohydrate and lipid metabolism. J Clin Invest 1974; 53:64
66. Reaven GM, Lerner RL, Stern MP, Farquhar JW. Role of insulin in endogenous hypertriglyceridemia. J Clin Invest 1967;46:1756
67. Zavaroni I, Dall'Aglio E, Alpi O, et al. Evidence for an independent relationship between plasma insulin and concentration of high density lipoprotein cholesterol and triglyceride. Atherosclerosis 1985;55:259
68. Laws A, King AC, Haskell WL, Reaven GM. Relation of fasting plasma insulin concentration to high density lipoprotein cholesterol and triglyceride concentrations in men. Arterio Thromb 1991;11:1636
69. Swenson TL. The role of the cholesteryl ester transfer protein in lipoprotein metabolism. Diab/Metab Rev 1991;7:139
70. Brinton EA, Eisenberg S, Breslow JL. Human HDL cholesterol levels are determined by ApoA-I fractional catabolic rate, which correlates inversely with estimates of HDL particle size. Arterio Thromb 1994;14:707
71. Golay A, Zech L, Shi M-Z, et al. High density lipoprotein (HDL) metabolism in noninsulin-dependent diabetes mellitus: Measurement of HDL turnover using tritiated HDL. J Clin Endocrinol Metab 1987;65:512
72. Chen Y-DI, Sheu WH-H, Swislocki ALM, Reaven GM. High density lipoprotein turnover in patients with hypertension. Hypertension 1991;17:386
73. Crouse JR, Parks JS, Schey HM. Studies of low density lipoprotein molecular weight in human beings with coronary artery disease. J Lipid Res 1985;26:566
74. Austin MA, Breslow JL, Hennekens CH, et al. Low-density lipoprotein subclass patterns and risk of myocardial infarction. JAMA 1988;260:1917
75. Austin MA, King M-C, Vranizan KM, Krauss RM. Atherogenic lipoprotein phenotype: A proposed genetic marker for coronary heart disease risk. Circulation 1990;82:495
76. Reaven GM, Chen Y-DI, Jeppesen J, et al. Insulin resistance and hyperinsulinemia in individuals with small, dense, low density lipoprotein particles. J Clin Invest 1993;92:141
77. Wilson DE, Chan I, Buchi KN, Horton SC. Postchallenge plasma lipoprotein retinoids: Chylomicron remnants in endogenous hypertriglyceridemia. Metabolism 1985;34:551
78. Lewis GF, O'Meara NM, Soltys PA, et al. Postprandial lipoprotein metabolism in normal and obese subjects: Comparison after the vitamin A fat-loading test. J Clin Endocrinol Metab 1990;71:1041
79. Lewis GF, O'Meara NM, Soltys PA, et al. Fasting hypertriglyceridemia in noninsulin-dependent diabetes mellitus is an important predictor of postprandial lipid and lipoprotein abnormalities. J Clin Endocrinol Metab 1991;72:934
80. Chen Y-DI, Swami S, Skowronski R, et al. Differences in postprandial lipemia

between patients with normal glucose tolerance and non–insulin-dependent diabetes mellitus. J Clin Endocrinol Metab 1993;72:172
81. Hamsten A, Wiman B, Defaire U, Blomback M. Increased plasma level of a rapid inhibitor of tissue plasminogen activator in young survivors of myocardial infarction. N Engl J Med 1985;313:1557
82. Mehta J, Mehta P, Lawson D, Saldeen T. Plasma tissue plasminogen activator inhibitor levels in coronary artery disease: Correlation with age and serum triglyceride concentrations. J Am Coll Cardiol 1987;9:263
83. Juhan-Vague I, Alessi MC, Vague P. Increased plasma plasminogen activator inhibitor 1 levels. A possible link between insulin resistance and atherothrombosis. Diabetologia 1991;34:457
84. Landin K, Tengvory L, Smith U. Elevated fibrinogen and plasminogen activator (PAI-I) in hypertension are related to metabolic risk factors for cardiovascular disease. J Intern Med 1990;227:273
85. Juhan-Vague I, Thompson SG, Jespersen J, on Behalf of the ECAT Angina Pectoris Study Group. Involvement of the hemostatic system in the insulin resistance syndrome. Arterioscler Thromb 1993;13:1865
86. Facchini F, Chen Y-DI, Hollenbeck CB, Reaven GM. Relationship between resistance to insulin-mediated glucose uptake, urinary uric acid clearance, and plasma uric acid concentration. JAMA 1991;266:3008
87. Zavaroni I, Mazza S, Fantuzzi M, et al. Changes in insulin and lipid metabolism in males with asymptomatic hyperuricaemia. J Intern Med 1993;234:24
88. Rosenthal M, Haskell WL, Solomon R, et al. Demonstration of a relationship between level of physical training and insulin-stimulated glucose utilization in normal humans. Diabetes 1983;32:408
89. Bogardus C, Lillioja S, Mott DM, et al. Relationship between degree of obesity and in vivo insulin action in man. Am J Physiol 1985;248 (Endocrinol Metab 11):E286
90. Krotkiewski M, Mandroukas K, Sjostrom L, et al. Effects of long-term physical training on body fat, metabolism, and blood pressure in obesity. Metabolism 1979;28:650
91. Schwartz RS. The independent effects of dietary weight loss and aerobic training on high density lipoproteins and apolipoprotein A-I concentrations in obese men. Metabolism 1987;36:165
92. Kaplan NM. The deadly quartet. Upper-body obesity, glucose intolerance, hypertriglyceridemia, and hypertension. Arch Intern Med 1989;149:1514
93. Modan M, Halkin H, Almog S, et al. Hyperinsulinemia: A link between hypertension, obesity and glucose intolerance. Hypertension 1985;75:809
94. Zavaroni I, Bonini L, Fantuzzi M, et al. Hyperinsulinaemia, obesity, and syndrome X. J Intern Med 1994;235:51
95. Kemp HG, Elliott WC, Gorlin R. The anginal syndrome with normal coronary arteriography. Trans Assoc Am Physicians 1967;80:59
96. Cannon RO, Epstein SE. "Microvascular angina" as a cause of chest pain with angiographically normal coronary arteries. Am J Cardiol 1988;61:1338
97. Dean JD, Jones CJH, Hutchison SJ, et al. Hyperinsulinenaemia and microvascular angina ("Syndrome X"). Lancet 1992;337:456
98. Fuh MM-T, Jeng C-Y, Young MM-S, et al. Insulin resistance, glucose intolerance, and hyperinsulinemia in patients with microvascular angina. Metabolism 1993;42:1090
99. Botker HR, Moller N, Ovesen P, et al. Insulin resistance in microvascular angina (Syndrome X). Lancet 1993;342:136
100. Reaven GM, Laws A. Coronary heart disease in the absence of hypercholesterolaemia. J Intern Med 1990;228:415
101. Fuller JH, Shipley MJ, Rose G, et al. Coronary-heart-disease risk and impaired glucose tolerance. Lancet 1980;i:1373
102. Pyörälä K. Relationship of glucose tolerance and plasma insulin to the incidence of coronary heart disease: Results from two populations studies in Finland. Diabetes Care 1979;2:131
103. Vaccaro O, Ruth KJ, Stamler J. Relationship of postload plasma glucose to mortality with 19-yr follow-up. Diabetes Care 1992;13:1328
104. Ducimetiere P, Eschwege E, Papoz L, et al. Relationship of plasma insulin levels to the incidence of myocardial infarction and coronary heart disease mortality in a middle-aged population. Diabetologia 1980;19:205
105. Hulley SB, Rosenman RH, Bawol RD, Brand RJ. Epidemiology as a guide to clinical decisions. The association between triglyceride and coronary heart disease. N Engl J Med 1980;302:1383
106. Criqui MH, Heiss G, Cohn R, et al. Plasma triglyceride level and mortality from coronary heart disease. N Engl J Med 1993;328:1220
107. Cambien F, Jaqueson A, Richard JL, et al. Is the level of serum triglyceride a significant predictor of coronary death in "normocholesterolemic" subjects? The Paris Prospective Study. Am J Epidemiol 1986;124:624
108. McKeigue PM, Marmot MG, Syndercombe Court YD, et al. Diabetes, hyperinsulinemia, and coronary risk factors in Bangladeshis in East London. Br Heart J 1988;60:390
109. Reaven GM. Are triglycerides important as a risk factor for coronary disease? Heart Dis Stroke 1993;2:44
110. Manninen V, Tenkanen L, Koskinen P, et al. Joint effects of serum triglyceride and LDL cholesterol and HDL cholesterol concentrations on coronary heart disease risk in the Helsinki heart study: Implications for treatment. Circulation 1992;85:37
111. Assmann G, Schulte H. Relation of high-density lipoprotein cholesterol and triglycerides to incidence of atherosclerotic coronary artery disease (the PROCAM experience). Am J Cardiol 1992;70:733
112. Castelli WP, Doyle JT, Gordon T, et al. HDL cholesterol and other lipids in coronary heart disease. Circulation 1977;55:767
113. Patsch JR, Miesenböck G, Hopferwieser T, et al. Relation of triglyceride metabolism and coronary artery disease: Studies in the postprandial state. Arteriosc1 Thromb 1992;12:1336
114. Karpe F, Bard JM, Steiner G, et al. HDLs and alimentary lipemia: Studies in men with previous myocardial infarction at young age. Arteriosc1 Thromb 1993;13:11
115. Collins R, Peto R, MacMahon S, et al. Blood pressure, stroke, and coronary heart disease. Part 2, Short-term reduction in blood pressure: Overview of randomized drug trials in their epidemiological context. Lancet 1990;335:827

Diabetes Mellitus, edited by Derek LeRoith, Simeon I. Taylor, and Jerrold M. Olefsky. Lippincott–Raven Publishers, Philadelphia © 1996.

Chapter 58

Biochemical Defects of Insulin Action in Humans

José F. Caro

Introduction

Type II diabetes is characterized by abnormalities in insulin secretion, as well as other endocrine pancreas functions, and abnormalities in insulin action. This chapter will focus on the multiple cellular defects of insulin action present in most patients with type II diabetes. However, it is not certain at this time which of the defects demonstrated so far, if any, are (1) primary and the immediate consequence of the putative genetic abnormality of type II diabetes; (2) secondary to the metabolic abnormalities of the disease, that is, hyperglycemia, hyperinsulinemia, elevated free fatty acids, and so on; or (3) secondary to other processes, that is, physical inactivity, obesity, age, and so on.

Many reasons for this uncertainty exist: (1) Although an explosion of information on normal insulin action has occurred over the last decade, the picture is still incomplete. (2) Type II diabetes is not a single disease but rather a collection of diseases having hyperglycemia as their final common pathway. Several such diseases have been discovered. However, in over 90% of the cases, the etiology of type II diabetes remains unknown. (3) The onset of the process that leads to type II diabetes precedes its diagnosis by decades, but in some cases there is no progression or return to a normal state. (4) Finally, there is wide variation in the precision and experimental pitfalls of the in vivo and in vitro techniques used to examine the endocrine pancreas and insulin action in different tissues in humans. Therefore, what is thought to be normal today might prove to be abnormal with the refinement or development of new methodologies.

Having recognized the difficulties in extrapolating from static and fragmentary experiments of insulin action to considerations of the etiology of type II diabetes in humans, we will first review the cellular abnormalities present in subjects with the full metabolic syndrome. These data should provide the biochemical mechanism(s) of the pathophysiology of type II diabetes. Second, we will review experiments on subjects with impaired glucose tolerance and first-degree relatives with normal glucose tolerance, collectively called *prediabetics*. These data, although incomplete, should provide the biochemical mechanism(s) for the progression of the disease. Finally, we will review and speculate on cellular abnormalities that might play a role in the etiology of type II diabetes.

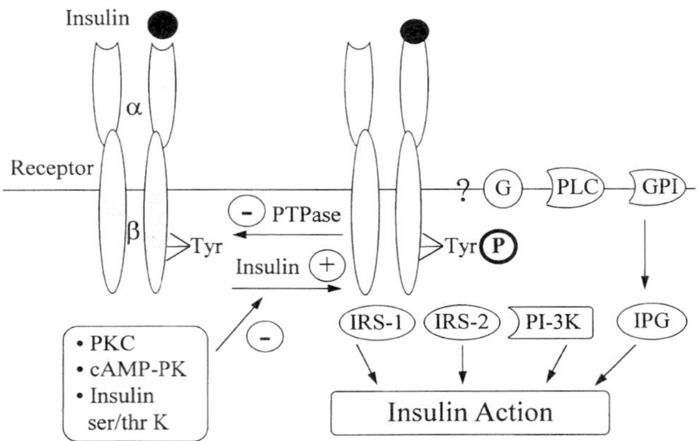

FIGURE 58-1. A simplified scheme of insulin action. The pathways and molecules are briefly described in the text.

Biochemical Defects of Insulin Action in Type II Diabetes: Cellular Pathophysiology

Defects in insulin action result in tissue insulin resistance. Insulin resistance is a metabolic state in which physiologic concentrations of insulin produce a less than normal biologic response. This is a universal finding in type II diabetes that could be due to (1) abnormal insulin molecules; (2) incomplete conversion of proinsulin to insulin; (3) elevated levels of growth hormone, cortisol, glucagon, or catecholamines; (4) the presence of insulin or insulin receptor antibodies; (5) decreased capillary density or the failure of insulin to facilitate its own delivery by increasing blood flow; (6) impaired transcapillary passage from the intravascular compartment to the interstitial compartment; or (7) insulin resistance at the cellular level.

Although any of these factors may contribute to insulin resistance in some patients and are discussed in other chapters, the major cause of insulin resistance in the majority of patients with type II diabetes is at the cellular level. The development of methods to isolate insulin-responsive hepatocytes,[1] muscle fibers,[2] and adipocytes[3] from patients has enabled investigators to prove clearly that the biologic responses of insulin at submaximal and maximal concentrations are attenuated in type II diabetes.

The major metabolic consequence of insulin resistance is hyperglycemia caused both by the failure of insulin to inhibit glucose production by the liver and by the failure to increase glucose utilization by peripheral tissues. We will focus here on the cellular abnormalities that may explain insulin resistance and the biochemical defects that lead to hyperglycemia.

Mechanism(s) of Insulin Resistance

Brief Overview of Normal Insulin Action

To understand the cellular and molecular mechanism(s) leading to insulin resistance, it is useful to review the general concept of insulin's mechanism of action.[4] Figure 58-1 is an extremely simplified diagram of cellular insulin action in a target cell. The reader is referred to Chapters 12–26 for a comprehensive analysis of insulin action.

The first step in insulin's cellular action involves binding to its cell surface receptor. The insulin receptor is composed of two extracellular α-subunits that contain the insulin-binding site and two transmembrane β-subunits that contain the insulin-regulated tyrosine protein kinase. The α-subunits are linked to the β-subunits and to each other by disulfide bonds. The β-subunit has an ATP-binding domain and autophosphorylation sites at the juxtamembrane, regulatory, and COOH terminus regions. Insulin binds to the α-subunit of one of the αβ-dimers and stimulates the transphosphorylation of the adjacent, covalently linked β-subunit. Autophosphorylation of all three tyrosine residues in the regulatory region stimulates kinase activity 10–20-fold. The dephosphorylation by protein–tyrosine phosphatase of individual receptor phosphotyrosyl residues in the kinase regulatory domain and other sites can serve as a switch-off mechanism. Furthermore, the insulin receptor is phosphorylated on serine and threonine residues in the basal state and in response to stimulation by phorbol esters, cAMP analogues, and insulin itself. Sometimes serine phosphorylation decreases insulin-stimulated tyrosine kinase (IRTK) activity. Therefore, the combination of ligand binding, tyrosine autophosphorylation, serine/threonine phosphorylation, and protein–tyrosine phosphatase activity provides four levels of control of the IRTK activity that are sensitive to intracellular message events and extracellular events that may be altered in type II diabetes.

A major substrate of the IRTK is the cytoplasmic protein insulin receptor substrate 1 (IRS-1). Tyrosine phosphorylation of IRS-1 results in its interaction with proteins that have Src homology with two domains: phosphatidylinositol 3′-kinase (PI3k) and growth receptor binding protein 2, which becomes functionally activated. It has been recently demonstrated that IRS-1 and PI3K serves to couple the insulin receptor to the glucose transport system.[5] Also, growth receptor binding protein 2 couples IRS-1 through a serine-phosphorylation cascade to the glycogen synthesis system. Furthermore, mice homozygous for target disruption of the IRS-1 gene[6,7] demonstrate the existence of both IRS-1–dependent and IRS-1–independent pathways for signal transduction of insulin. Insulin-stimulated glucose transport is IRS-1 dependent. Also, additional high molecular weight substrates of the insulin receptor kinase such as IRS-2 have now been cloned and will be shown to play an important role in insulin action. Therefore, it is possible that insulin has overlapping and parallel signaling pathways.

There is evidence that insulin binding to its receptor also activates a pertussis toxin–sensitive, heterotrimeric G-protein. One of the consequences of this interaction is the activation of a phospholipase and the cleavage from lipid and proteinated glycosylphosphatidyl inositol species diacylglycerol (DAG) and inositol phosphoglycan mediators.[8] The inositol phosphoglycan insulin mediators function allosterically in the kinase/phosphatase network cascade to control the enzyme phosphorylation state—for example, to inhibit adenylate cyclase and cAMP-dependent protein kinase and to activate pyruvate dehydrogenase and glycogen synthesis phosphoprotein phosphatases.[8] However, although this work started over two decades ago, the structure of these mediators remains unknown.

In summary, although the picture of insulin action is far from complete, it allows us to start asking questions regarding the defects in type II diabetes.

The Insulin Receptor α-Subunit in Type II Diabetes

The earliest studies using circulating blood cells indicated decreased binding of insulin to the insulin receptor α-subunit in type II diabetes. More recent studies in humans, however, only demonstrate a decrease in insulin binding in adipose tissue that is not due to obesity per se.[9] In human liver[1] and human skeletal muscle,[10] no additional decrease in insulin binding in type II diabetes can be observed that is due to factors other than obesity. Furthermore, in lean patients with type II diabetes, there is no decrease in insulin binding in liver[11] or muscle.[12]

Therefore, the available data allow us to conclude that post–insulin-binding defect(s) must be responsible for insulin resistance in type II diabetes.

The Insulin Receptor β-Subunit in Type II Diabetes

Figure 58-2 demonstrates the first proximal post–insulin-binding defect discovered in type II diabetes.[1] In these experiments, insulin receptors from human liver were isolated, and basal and insulin-stimulated tyrosine kinase (IRTK) was determined in lean and obese control subjects and in obese subjects with type II diabetes. Basal kinase activity was similar in the three groups of subjects. As shown in Figure 58-2, however, whereas insulin stimulated the insulin receptor kinase in lean and obese control subjects, it had a smaller effect on the liver insulin receptor from subjects with type II diabetes. When the insulin-stimulated protein kinase activity of insulin receptors was plotted against the amount of bound insulin, for a given amount of insulin bound the receptors from the subjects with type II diabetes were severalfold less responsive to the hormone than those from the two control groups. To study this process using a more physiologic system, a procedure was developed for preparation of human liver plasma membranes containing functional insulin receptor kinase.[13] Using this system, the ability of insulin to stimulated β-subunit autophosphorylation and tyrosine phosphorylation of endogenous substrates was found to be markedly abnormal in type II diabetes.[13] All studies of type II diabetes in humans have demonstrated similar defects of the insulin receptor β-subunit in skeletal muscle,[10,12,14–17] adipocytes,[18–20] and circulating blood cells,[21,22] regardless of whether the studies were performed in vitro in a cell-free system,[1] in vitro in an intact cell system,[20] or on the most physiologic activation by insulin in vivo followed by tissue biopsy and receptor isolation.[16,17] The decreased IRTK in diabetes is caused entirely by a decrease in the Vmax of the enzyme and not by changes in insulin-binding affinity or the capacity of the Km values for ATP.[12] Also, the receptors show a decreased level of tris-phosphorylation of the regulatory region, which is closely related to the decreased kinase activity.[12] Furthermore, studies have demonstrated that this kinase defect is associated with an increased proportion of receptors that are kinase inactive.[23] This is an important observation because kinase-negative receptors themselves are inactive and may inhibit the function of the normal receptors, behaving as a dominant negative modulator.[21]

Because obesity is also associated with insulin resistance and is present in the majority of patients with type II diabetes, it was also of interest to study IRTK in this disease. Figure 58-2 demonstrates that liver IRTK is normal in obesity.[1] Similar data have been generated in adipocytes[18] and in human skeletal muscle when

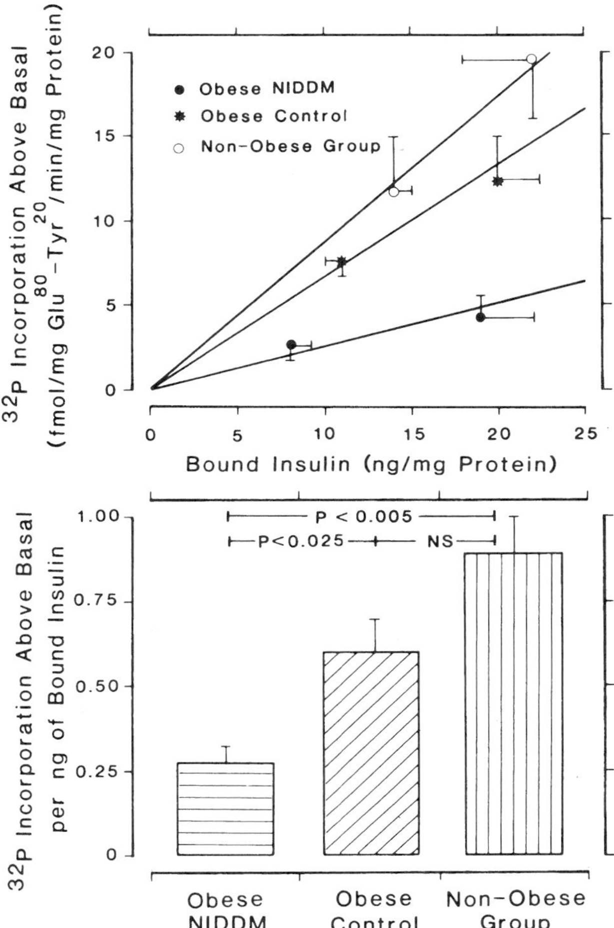

Figure 58-2. Insulin-stimulated insulin receptor kinase activity in human liver (upper panel). The insulin receptor kinase data are plotted against the bound insulin (lower panel). The same data are normalized by nanograms of insulin specifically bound to the insulin receptor. (Reproduced with permission from Caro JF, Ittoop O, Pories WJ, et al. Studies of the mechanism of insulin resistance in the liver from humans with noninsulin-dependent diabetes. J Clin Invest 1986;78:249.)

studied in vivo,[16,17] but not when studied in a cell-free system, where a decrease equal to that of diabetes is observed.[10,15]

Therefore, the available data allow one to conclude that the ability of insulin to stimulate the IRTK of the β-subunit is markedly altered in type II diabetes and is a possible mechanism for insulin resistance.

Mechanism(s) of Altered Insulin Receptor Tyrosine Kinase

Because type II diabetes has a strong genetic component, it is important to ask whether the insulin-stimulated tyrosine kinase (IRTK) defect is either a primary causative factor accounting for the disease or an abnormality secondary to the metabolic process of the disease. In other words, is the insulin receptor gene a diabetogene? The accumulated data argue against this possibility: (1) In twin studies, a decrease in IRTK was found in one twin affected with type II diabetes, but kinase activity was normal in the nonaffected twin.[24] (2) IRTK is normal in cultured fibroblasts from patients with type II diabetes propagated in tissue cultures removed from the in vivo milieu.[25] (3) When obese patients with type II diabetes are induced to lose weight, the hyperglycemia is markedly improved and IRTK function reverts to normal.[26] (4) Finally, and most important, are the results of direct studies analyzing the insulin receptor gene in type II diabetes. The sequence of exons 16 through 22, which contained the cytoplasmic domain of the β-subunit in seven patients with type II diabetes, was entirely normal.[27] Other studies using molecular scanning approaches to screen a large number of patients for mutations have revealed that the degree of genetic variation in the insulin receptor is exceedingly small in type II diabetes, on the order of 1–2%.[28] Thus, if the insulin receptor (IR) is not a diabetogene, why is insulin receptor kinase resistant to insulin in type II diabetes?

Several possibilities exist to explain the IRTK defect in diabetes, but none are entirely proven: (1) Protein-tyrosine phosphatase may be elevated and inactivate the IRTK, as depicted in Figure 58-1. Skeletal muscle biopsy specimens from Pima Native Americans demonstrated elevated phosphotyrosine phosphatase (PTPase) activity, and the failure of insulin to decrease this activity, in comparison with insulin-sensitive control subjects.[29] A similar study in a different patient population, however, demonstrated decreased PTPase activity.[30] These conflicting data clearly show the need for future work in this important area. (2) Serine/threonine kinases may be abnormal and inactivate the IRTK, as depicted in Figure 58-1. One of the candidates is protein kinase C (PKC). PKC has been implicated in the development of insulin resistance and inactivation of IRTK in a variety of isolated cells and tissue systems.[31] Furthermore, inhibitors of PKC prevent glucose-induced insulin resistance in rat fat cells.[32] There are several reasons why PKC might be increased in type II diabetes: (1) Glucose-induced increases in diacylglycerol (DAG) and membrane PKC have been demonstrated in several cell lines.[33] (2) Phosphatidylinositol-4,5-bisphosphate–specific phospholipase C activity is increased in liver plasma membranes in type II diabetes.[34] The resulting increase in DAG would result in activation of PKC. In fact, the increase in PKC in human liver in type II diabetes has recently been proven, and the data are shown in Figure 58-3.[35] It is, however, not yet proven if serine/threonine phosphorylation of the insulin receptor is indeed increased in type II diabetes. However, phorbol myristate acetate (PMA)-mediated inhibition of IRTK and an increase in

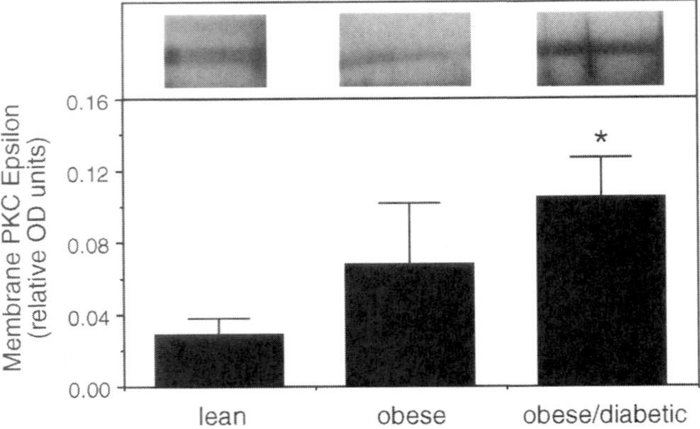

Figure 58-3. Immunodetection of membrane-associated PKC in liver from lean, obese, and obese/diabetic patients. Representative bands for each patient group are illustrated above the bar graph. The band density was measured by scanning densitometry in reference to the amount of isozyme present in the mouse brain control. Values represent the mean SEM for five patients in each group. $p = 0.05$ compared to the amount of isozyme in the lean group. (Reproduced with permission from Considine RV, Nyce MR, Allen LE, et al. Protein kinase C is increased in the liver of humans and rats with non–insulin-dependent diabetes mellitus: An alteration not due to hyperglycemia. J Clin Invest 1995;95:2938.)

insulin resistance have been demonstrated in cells expressing a truncated insulin receptor lacking the major PKC phosphorylation site.[36] Another serine/threonine kinase candidate could be one of the recently described family members of the insulin-stimulated serine/threonine kinases.[37] Overfeeding in the sand rat induces hyperinsulinemia, insulin resistance, and a dramatic decrease in IRTK activity in both liver and muscle,[38] a phenomenon previously demonstrated in vitro. In this regard, insulin may also be responsible for the increase in PKC.[39] Finally, cAMP-dependent protein kinases have the potential to inactivate IRTK,[4] and a twofold increase in Gs protein concentration has been shown in the liver of patients with type II diabetes.[40]

Therefore, the available data allow us to conclude that the altered IRTK is not due to a mutation of the receptor; that improvement of insulin action reverses the defect; and that the cause of this defect remains unknown.

Probes to Bypass the Insulin-Stimulated Tyrosine Kinase Defect(s)

If, in type II diabetes, the insulin-stimulated tyrosine kinase (IRTK) defect is the major and only abnormality in the insulin signaling pathway, compounds that stimulate insulin action, either without interacting with the insulin receptors or without stimulating IRTK, should exert a greater effect than insulin.

Human skeletal muscle has insulin-like growth factor 1 (*IGF1*)[41,42] and *IGF2* receptors.[43] Both *IGF1* and *IGF2* stimulate glucose transport through interactions with the *IGF1* receptor, as demonstrated using blocking antibodies to the insulin, *IGF1*, and *IGF2* receptors, respectively.[42,43] Furthermore, in type II diabetes, *IGF2* binding and *IGF1*-stimulated tyrosine kinase of the *IGF1* receptors are normal.[41,42] Human muscle fibers of patients with type II diabetes, however, are equally resistant to both insulin and *IGF1*, indicating that an abnormality distal to the IRTK must be present in these patients.[42]

This experimental paradigm could not be used in other tissues because in adipocytes, even though *IGF1*[44] and *IGF2* receptors[45] are present, both hormones stimulate glucose transport by interacting with the insulin receptor. Also, in the human liver, the concentration of *IGF1* receptor is extremely low.[46] Therefore, a monoclonal antibody to the insulin receptor that stimulates glucose transport in adipocytes without any detectable IRTK stimulation was used to bypass the IRTK defect.[47] Here also, adipocytes from patients with type II diabetes were resistant to both insulin and the insulin receptor antibody.[48]

Therefore, the available data strongly suggest that, in addition to the IRTK defect, other abnormalities distal to the receptor must be present in type II diabetes.

In Search of the Proximal Post–Insulin Receptor Defect(s)

The most proximal of the possible post–insulin receptor defect is the insulin receptor substrate 1 (IRS-1). Data from the first experiments investigating insulin-stimulated tyrosine kinase (IRTK) and IRS-1 in adipocytes from control subjects, obese subjects, and subjects with type II diabetes can be seen in Figure 58-4.[20] Decreased insulin-stimulated β-subunit autophosphorylation was found to occur in type II diabetes, but the ability to phosphorylate IRS-1 was normal.[22] Because the amount of autophosphorylated β-subunit is decreased, however, it is evident that the total amount of phosphorylated IRS-1 is decreased in the cells from patients with type II diabetes.

In skeletal muscle, obese subjects with insulin resistance demonstrate a moderate decrease in insulin receptor (IR), IRS-1, and phosphatidylinositol 3′-kinase (PI3K) proteins. However, whereas the decrease in IR and IRS-1 phosphorylation was similar, the

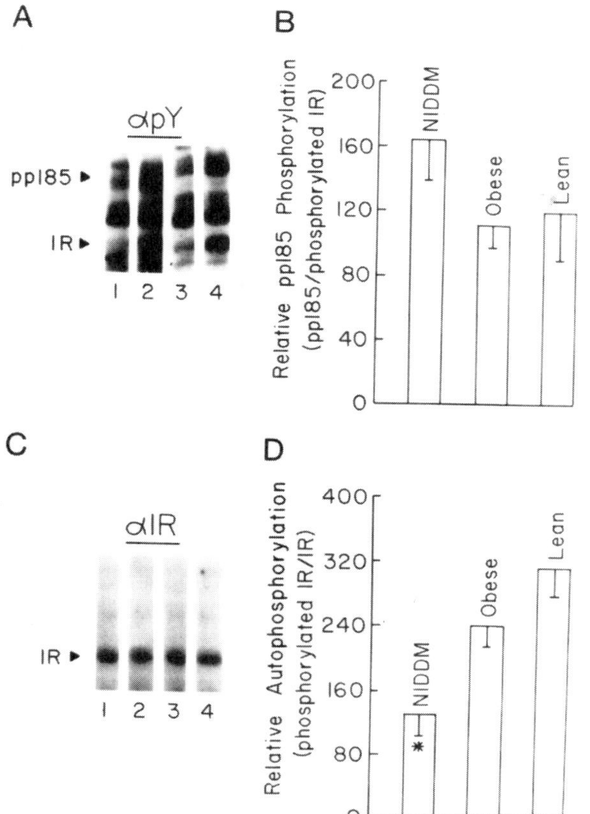

FIGURE 58-4. Insulin-stimulated phosphorylation of IRS-I and pp185 in adipocytes from type II diabetes mellitus (non–insulin-dependent diabetes mellitus, NIDDM) obese, and lean subjects. (*A*) A representative autoradiograph. Adipocytes from NIDDM patients (lanes 1 and 2) and obese (lanes 3 and 4) subjects incubated with (lanes 2 and 4) or without (lanes 1 and 3) insulin were solubilized and immunoblotted with antiphosphotyrosine antibody. (*B*) To estimate coupling efficiency between insulin-receptor activation and IRS-I phosphorylation, autoradiographs of antiphosphotyrosine immunoblots from cells treated with 10 ng/mL insulin for 5 minutes were subjected to scanning densitometry, and the ratio of phosphorylated pp185 to phosphorylated IR β-subunit was expressed as relative densitometry units. There is no statistically significant difference between cells from NIDDM ($n = 8$), obese ($n = 8$), and lean ($n = 3$) subjects in efficiency of pp185 phosphorylation. (*C*) Representative autoradiograph. Cells from NIDDM with (lanes 2, 3, and 4) or without (lane 1) insulin were solubilized and immunoblotted with anti–IR antibody. (*D*) To estimate the efficiency of IR autophosphorylation, the ratio of phosphorylated β-subunit from antiphosphotyrosine immunoblots to total β-subunit in gel lanes from anti-IR immunoblots is expressed as relative densitometry units. Insulin-stimulated receptor autophosphorylation is significantly lower ($p < 0.02$) in cells from NIDDM subjects vs. obese or lean, nondiabetic subjects. (Reproduced with permission from Thies RS, Molina JM, Ciaraldi TP, et al. Insulin-receptor autophosphorylation and endogenous substrate phosphorylation in human adipocytes from control, obese, and NIDDM subjects. Diabetes 1990;39:250.)

insulin stimulation of PI3K activity was markedly reduced in insulin resistance (10-fold vs. 30-fold stimulation in control subjects).[49] These are important findings because it is clear now that IRS-1 and PI3K are essential components in the insulin signaling of glucose transport.[15] Furthermore, a number of variant sequences in the IRS-1 gene have been reported to be prevalent among patients with type II diabetes.[50]

Therefore, the available data point out that although the search for proximal postreceptor defects in type II diabetes has just begun, it has already provided substantial information. Because several dozen already cloned proteins are believed to participate in insulin signaling, this should prove to be an exciting and productive area of clinical investigation.

Alternative Insulin Signaling Defects

On phosphorylation, the receptor undergoes a conformational change that could result in noncovalent interaction with other signaling molecules. It is possible that in some cases these interactions could occur even in the presence of markedly reduced insulin-stimulated tyrosine kinase (IRTK) activity. One of these interactions is with some classes of G-proteins.[51,52] In human liver plasma membranes, insulin stimulates guanosine diphosphate (GDP) release from G-proteins[53] and inhibits pertussis toxin–catalyzed adenine diphosphate (ADP) ribosylation of G_i.[40] Furthermore, GTPγs inhibits the affinity of insulin for its receptor.[54] The functional "cross-talk" between the insulin receptor (IR) and G-proteins is altered in the liver of patients with type II diabetes,[40] as seen in Figure 58-5. This defect was not intrinsic to G_i because Mg^{2+} and GTPγs inhibited pertussis toxin–catalyzed ADP ribosylation in both diabetic and nondiabetic patients. Furthermore, $G_{i3\alpha}$ protein concentration was normal in diabetes patients and $Gi_{1-2\alpha}$ was decreased by only 40% compared to the obese control subjects but normal compared to the lean control subjects. Finally, this cross-talk appeared not to involve IRTK. It is not clear, however, to which of the multiple insulin-signaling pathways the IR is functionally coupled by G-proteins and to which of the G-proteins.

It is possible that the IR is coupled to a specific phospholipase C (PLC) that cleaves glycosyl-phosphatidylinositol (GPI) into

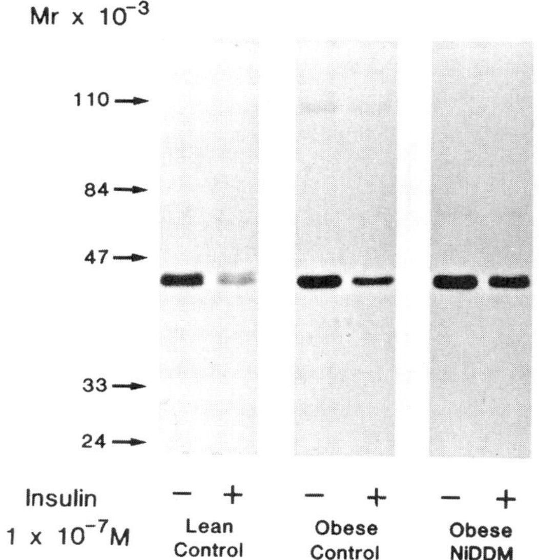

FIGURE 58-5. Effect of insulin on pertussis toxin–catalyzed ADP ribosylation of G_i in lean, obese, and diabetic patients. Representative autoradiograph of pertussis-catalyzed ADP ribosylation of G_i in the presence and absence of insulin in lean controls, obese controls, and obese diabetic patients. (Reproduced with permission from Caro JF, Raju MS, Caro M, et al. Guanine nucleotide binding regulatory protein in liver from obese humans with and without type II diabetes: Evidence for altered "cross-talk" between the insulin receptor and Gi-protein. J Cell Biochem 1994;54:309.)

inositol phosphoglycan (IPG) and diacylglycerol (DAG).[8] Different species of IPG mediators have been described; one of these species contains D-chiroinositol and galactosamine. The significance of chiroinositol is heightened by the recent finding of low concentrations in the urine and skeletal muscle in type II diabetes and by the failure of insulin to increase its concentration in comparison with normal controls.[8] Administration of D-chiroinositol or IPG mediators has a moderately hypoglycemic effect in monkeys with type II diabetes and other animal models of type II diabetes.[8]

Therefore, the available data allow us to conclude that other signaling abnormalities exist in type II diabetes in addition to the better-understood pathway of reversibly tyrosine-phosphorylated substrates of the insulin receptor. In many ways, it is better to recognize that not only one thing is abnormal, even at the risk of reaching the point where everything is believed to be abnormal. Time will eventually allow us to fit the covalent and allosteric puzzle pieces together in order to see clearly the key cellular defects of insulin signaling in type II diabetes.

Cellular Basis for Hyperglycemia

With the recognition that insulin resistance may cause alterations in the metabolism of sugars, lipids, proteins, and ions due to abnormalities in gene transcription, enzyme regulation, transport, and protein translocation, this section focuses on the cellular basis of hyperglycemia because it is the clinical hallmark of type II diabetes.

Hyperglycemia is, in a general sense, caused by decreased glucose utilization by tissues or an increased glucose supply by the liver or the diet. Some of the processes that lead to hyperglycemia are insulin dependent and others are insulin independent. We will not debate here which of these processes is more important because once the type II diabetes syndrome is established, multiple derangements are present. Instead, we will present the cellular abnormalities that may be responsible for the decrease in glucose utilization and the increase in glucose production.

Defects in Insulin-Stimulated Glucose Utilization

Postprandially, insulin promotes glucose uptake, metabolism, and storage in muscle, adipose cells, and other tissues, with skeletal muscle being quantitatively the most important. Since the Km of the GLUT-4 transporter isoform (2–10 mM) is in the range of physiologic glucose concentrations, this transport can be nearly saturated in vivo, making transport rate limiting for glucose metabolism. Therefore, much effort has been spent studying glucose transport in type II diabetes.

Glucose Transport and Transporters

Defects in submaximal and maximal insulin-stimulated glucose transport in type II diabetes were first demonstrated in vitro utilizing isolated adipocytes.[9] This abnormality could be caused by a decrease in the ability of insulin to signal the translocation of GLUT-4 to the plasma membrane; a decrease in the intrinsic activity of GLUT-4; a decrease in the GLUT-4 protein; or a combination of defects.

GLUT-4 protein and mRNA were determined in adipose tissue from patients with type II diabetes and lean and obese controls[55] to attempt to separate those possibilities; the data are presented in Figure 58-6. Relative to lean controls, GLUT-4 protein was decreased 40% in obese controls and 85% in diabetic patients, with a similar decrease in GLUT-4 mRNA. Such changes in GLUT-4 protein and GLUT-4 translocation correspond to glucose transport rates in intact cells. These studies were confirmed, although the changes in GLUT-4 in obesity were less severe.[56] The demonstration of decreased insulin stimulation of glucose transport in skeletal

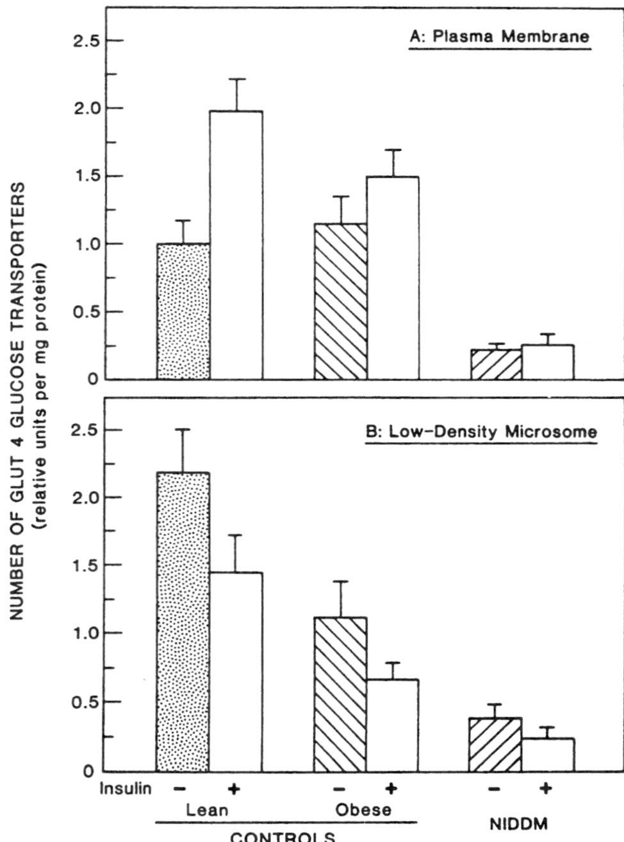

FIGURE 58-6. Effects of NIDDM and obesity on GLUT-4 glucose transporters in adipocyte membrane subfractions. Adipocytes were isolated from lean, obese, and NIDDM subjects, incubated in the absence and presence of insulin (100 ng/mL), and subjected to differential ultracentrifugation for preparation of plasma membrane and low-density microsome subfractions. Membrane proteins were subjected to immunoblot analysis using antibodies specific for GLUT-4, and GLUT-4 was quantitated using autoradiography and densitometry. The data represent the mean SE of eight lean controls, six obese controls, and seven NIDDM subjects. (Reproduced with permission from Garvey WT, Maianu L, Hueckstead TP, et al. Pretranslational suppression of a glucose transporter protein causes insulin resistance in adipocytes from patients with non–insulin-dependent diabetes mellitus and obesity. J Clin Invest 1991;87:1072.)

muscle had to wait for the development of an in vitro human muscle preparation suitable for metabolic studies. In this system, severe insulin resistance was demonstrated in obese subjects with or without type II diabetes.[2] Of particular interest is the demonstration that, in skeletal muscle, neither GLUT-4 protein nor GLUT-4 mRNA concentration correlated with the degree of glycemic control, fasting plasma glucose or insulin concentration, diabetes duration, body mass index, gender, or age.[57] These data, which represent the first determination of GLUT-4 in any tissue in humans, are shown in Figure 58-7. That the GLUT-4 protein concentration is normal in the skeletal muscle in type II diabetes has been confirmed by all laboratories.[57–60] Only one study has shown a 23% decrease in obesity but no significant difference in diabetes.[59]

The previous studies, however, were cross-sectional and revealed a considerable range of values for glucose transporter levels even among the lean controls. Hence, longitudinal studies were

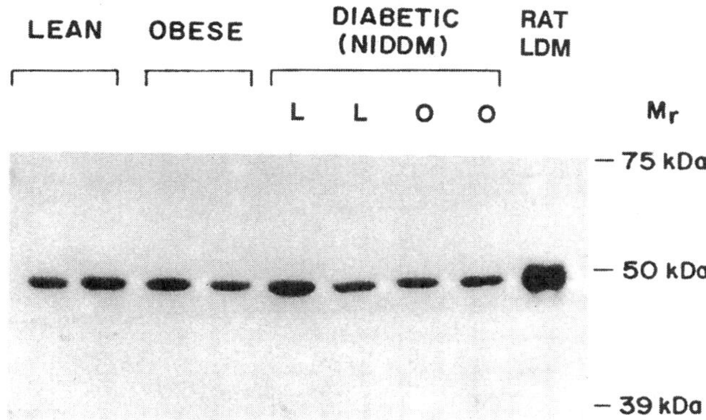

FIGURE 58-7. Immunoblots showing the relative abundance of GLUT-4 protein in skeletal muscle (vastus lateralis) of lean and obese control subjects and lean (L) and obese (O) diabetic subjects. Anti-GLUT-4 COOH-terminal peptide antiserum was used; 125 μg human muscle membrane protein was loaded on each lane with 30 μg rat adipose cell low-density microsomes for comparison of molecular weight (M_r). Blots represent three separate Western blots on 22 subjects (7 lean control subjects, 6 obese control subjects, and 9 patients with NIDDM). (Reproduced with permission from Pedersen O, Bak JF, Andersen H, et al. Evidence against altered expression of GLUT1 or GLUT 4 in skeletal muscle of patients with obesity or NIDDM. Diabetes 1990;39:865.)

needed to determine whether individual GLUT-4 levels can be modulated by therapeutic interventions such as weight reduction. The results of the first longitudinal study are shown in Figure 58-8.[62] Loss of 36% of the initial body weight (body mass index 45.8 ± 2.5 to 30 ± 2.1) for 1 year resulted in a threefold increase in insulin-stimulated glucose disposal in vivo, a twofold increase in insulin-stimulated glucose transport in vitro, and no change in GLUT-4 protein concentration.[62] Thus, there is no doubt that, even within individual subjects, there is no correlation between GLUT-4 protein and glucose transport. This is not to say that GLUT-4 cannot be regulated by other interventions. For example, physical training increases muscle GLUT-4 protein to the same extent in matched subjects with and without type II diabetes.[62,63] Also, sulfonylureas increase the GLUT-4 protein content in type II diabetes.[64]

Based on the previous studies, the mechanism of decreased glucose transport in the skeletal muscle in type II diabetes must be either a defect in GLUT-4 intrinsic activity or a defect in signaling of translocation to the membrane. A defect in intrinsic activity could be a structural defect in the protein itself. Is GLUT-4 a diabetogene? To answer this question, the primary sequence of the GLUT-4 gene in a series of typical type II diabetes patients was determined,[65] followed by large-scale molecular scanning studies.[66] From these studies, it can be concluded that genetic variations in the GLUT-4 sequence are exceedingly uncommon (less than 1–2%) in type II diabetes. Furthermore, the 5′ untranslated region and the promoter region of GLUT-4 have been found to be unaltered in type II diabetes.[67] It has been difficult to demonstrate GLUT-4 translocation in skeletal muscle in humans,[68] although GLUT-4 has been found to be decreased in muscle membranes in patients with type II diabetes.[69] Therefore, it is very likely that the defect in glucose transport is entirely due to a defect in insulin signaling. First, hypoxia stimulates glucose transport normally in human muscle fibers from patients with diabetes[70]; second, the serine/threonine phosphatase inhibitor okadiac acid and the tyrosine phosphatase inhibitors phenylarsine oxide and vanadate restore insulin-stimulated glucose transport.[71] Thus, the glucose transport effector system is intact, and the defect in insulin signaling may be within the phosporylation cascade.

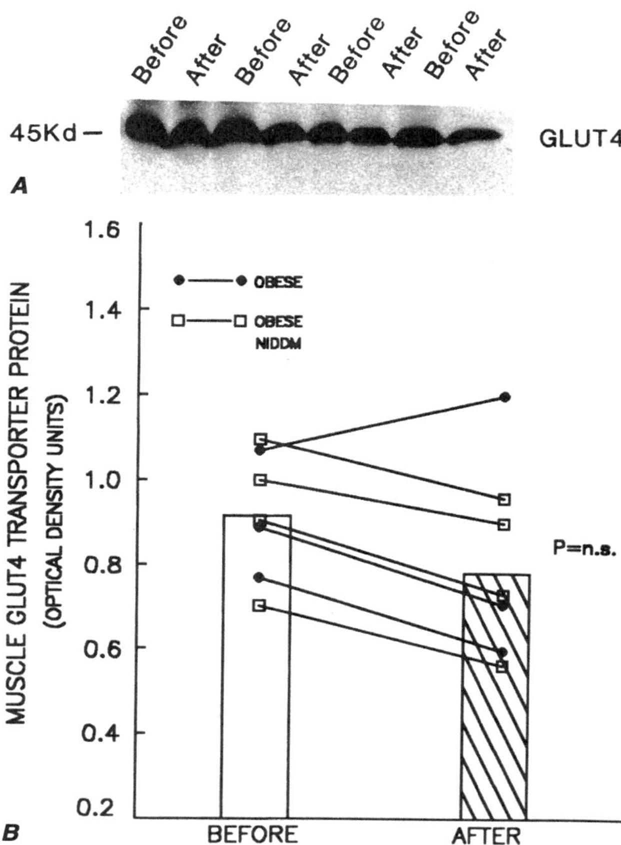

FIGURE 58-8. Effect of weight loss on immunodetection of GLUT-4 glucose transporters in human skeletal muscle. (**A**) Muscle biopsy specimens were obtained from vastus lateralis muscle before and after weight loss and from crude membranes. Identical quantities of protein (50 μg) were applied to each lane, subjected to SDS-PAGE, transferred to nitrocellulose, and immunoblotted using affinity-purified polyclonal antibody to the COOH-terminal portion (30 amino acids) of GLUT-4 transporter protein. The figure represents an autoradiogram from a typical experimental. (**B**) Quantification by scanning densitometry of individual and group mean GLUT-4 transporters obtained before (□) and after (■) weight loss. (Reproduced with permission from Friedman FE, Dohm GL, Elton CW, et al. Restoration of insulin responsiveness in skeletal muscle of morbidly obese patients after weight loss. J Clin Invest 1992;89:701.)

Therefore, the available data support the hypothesis that insulin-stimulated glucose transport is a major defect in type II diabetes. Whereas in adipose tissue it is caused by both a decrease in GLUT-4 and insulin signaling, in skeletal muscle the defect appears to result entirely from insulin signaling.

Glucose Metabolism

After transport of glucose into skeletal muscle, the glucose molecule can be converted into glycogen, or it can undergo glycolysis and be released as lactate or oxidized in the Krebs cycle. Incorporation of glucose into glycogen is regulated by the enzyme glycogen synthase, and entry of glucose carbon into the Krebs cycle for oxidation is regulated by the pyruvate dehydrogenase multienzyme complex. We will avoid the debate over which process is more important in type II diabetes. Both enzymes are activated in vivo by insulin in normal humans, and the activation of both enzymes is abnormal in type II diabetes.[72]

In the majority of metabolic studies, skeletal muscle glucose oxidation and nonoxidative glucose storage (glycogen synthesis) have been derived from estimates using indirect calorimetry and overall isotopic glucose disposal in subjects with euglycemia.[73] Although limb balance techniques more closely approximate muscle metabolism than do whole body measurement, the contribution of plasma free fatty acids, changes in muscle blood flow, and responses of skin and adipose tissue require assumptions for quantification.[74] These pathways can be investigated more precisely in vitro using an incubated muscle preparation.[75] Therefore, basal and insulin-stimulated glucose oxidation, glycogen formation, and nonoxidative glycolysis (lactate and amino acid release) were studied under controlled in vitro conditions in human muscle fibers from patients with and without type II diabetes. Using 5 mM glucose in the absence of insulin, there were no alterations in diabetes. However, whereas physiologic concentrations of insulin stimulated the four metabolic pathways of glucose in normal subjects, patients with type II diabetes were equally resistant to insulin in regard to these four pathways. When muscle of subjects with type II diabetes was incubated with 20 mM glucose, insulin responsiveness increased significantly for glycogen formation, glucose oxidation, and nonoxidative glycolysis to levels similar to those of the control at 5 mM glucose. These in vitro studies are to those in vivo studies who found that maintaining fasting hyperglycemia normalized insulin-stimulated glucose disposal across the leg of nonobese diabetics.[76] It has been shown, however, that when normal subjects are studied with 12 mM glucose, the maximal insulin-stimulated glucose disposal rate is increased 6-fold, whereas the increase in diabetics is only 2.8-fold above the basal level.[77] Thus, a defect in glucose transport exists in diabetes.

It is clear, however, that in vivo, 70–85% of glucose taken up by muscle is metabolized nonoxidatively. Using nuclear magnetic reasonance spectroscopy, it was demonstrated that reduced muscle glycogen formation could account for nearly all of the reduced glucose disposal in type II diabetes.[78] These findings have led to detailed studies of glucogen synthesis in humans.[79] Glycogen synthase (GS) activity is regulated by phosphorylation and dephosphorylation. A number of serine-specific kinases phosphorylate glycogen synthase at different residues, and at least two phosphatases regulate the dephosphorylation. Dephosphorylation converts the enzyme from a glucose-6-phosphate–dependent form to a glucose-6-phosphate–independent form. Insulin activates the enzyme by activating glycogen synthase phosphatase and inhibiting one of the glycogen synthase kinases, cAMP-dependent kinase. The inhibition of cAMP-dependent kinase appears to lower the phosphorylation of glycogen synthase phosphatase inhibitor I, leading to activation of glycogen synthase phosphatase. It is well proven that the insulin effect on glycogen synthase in skeletal muscle of type II diabetic patients is reduced.[80] Elevated cAMP-dependent protein kinase activity and resistance of insulin to inhibition of this kinase have been reported in diabetes.[81] This elevated kinase activity could contribute to reduced glycogen synthase activity as a result of the deactivation of type 1 protein phosphatase. In fact, lower type 1 protein phosphatase concentration and resistance of insulin to stimulation of its activity have been demonstrated in diabetes, which could explain in part the reduced insulin-stimulated glycogen synthase concentration.[82] The fact that activation of the enzyme by glucose-6-phosphate is normal however, suggests that no defect in the enzyme itself exists.[80] Nevertheless, the observation in cultured fibroblasts from type II diabetes patients that insulin failed to stimulate GS, despite having normal insulin-stimulated tyrosine kinase (IRTK), led to the belief the GS might be a diabetogene.[83] However, as was the case for the insulin receptor and GLUT-4, molecular analysis of the GS promoter and coding regions in type II diabetes has not yielded positive results.[63,84] Therefore, alterations in insulin-stimulated glycogen synthase are likely to be caused entirely by defects in insulin signaling. Furthermore, a more recent nuclear magnetic resonance spectroscopy study demonstrated that the lower concentration of glucose-6-phosphate in subjects with type II diabetes, despite a decreased rate of nonoxidative glucose metabolism, is consistent with a defect in muscle glucose transport or phosphorylation, reducing the rate of muscle glycogen synthesis.[85]

Therefore, insulin regulation of the different pathways of intercellular glucose metabolism is abnormal in the skeletal muscle in type II diabetes. There are no biochemical data supporting a selective defect; in particular, GS is not a diabetogene.

Increased Hepatic Glucose Production

The liver overproduces glucose in the basal state, primarily because of increased gluconeogenesis.[86] Exaggerated hormonal stimulation is provided by increased glucagon concentrations in combination with hepatic insulin resistance. The increased gluconeogenic precursor flow ensures adequate substrate availability. Finally, elevated free fatty acid concentrations provide the necessary source of intracellular energy, via fatty acid oxidation, to drive the gluconeogenic process. In spite of this logical sequence of events learned from in vivo studies in humans, controversy exists over whether or not hepatic glucose production is abnormal in type II diabetes. This controversy reflects the deficiencies and pitfalls in methodology used to study liver metabolism in vivo.

In vitro studies using freshly isolated hepatocytes from patients with type II diabetes have demonstrated insulin resistance at submaximal and maximal insulin concentrations.[1] More recently, the adaptation to human liver of a tissue slice technique has allowed us to study the liver in vitro, eliminating the time and requirements of proteolytic enzymes normally employed in cell isolation. Furthermore, tissue slicing provides stability of the differentiated state based on cell-cell and cell-matrix interaction, and therefore a higher level of biologic organization. Using this system in liver biopsy specimens from patients with the full-blown syndrome of type II diabetes with fasting glucose concentrations above 180 mg/dL, the following data were generated: (1) In the absence of neoglucogenic substrates and hormones, glucose production, mainly reflecting glycogenolysis, was identical to that of the controls. Furthermore, glycogen content was normal. (2) In the presence of lactate/pyruvate (10/1 mM) and without hormones, the gluconeogenic component of hepatic glucose production (HGP) was increased in diabetes (29 vs. 13 μg glucose per milligram of liver per minute in controls). (3) In the presence of insulin (1×10^{-7} M), gluconeogenesis was still higher in diabetes (14 vs. 5 μg glucose per milligram of liver per minute in controls). (4) Glucagon (1×10^{-7} M) increased gluconeogenesis equally in both groups (84 vs. 92 μg glucose per milligram of liver per minute in controls), which could be inhibited by insulin (1×10^{-7} M) by 31% in diabetes versus 48% in controls (C. Mateo, J. Serrano, and J.F. Caro, unpublished data). It is clear from these data that the efficiency of conversion of substrates into glucose is increased in type II diabetes and that the balance between insulin and glucagon action is altered. The biochemical mechanism(s), however, is (are) not entirely clear. The activity of none of the three gluconeogenic enzymes—phosphoenolpyruvate carboxikinase, fructose 1,6-diphosphatase, and glucose-6-phosphatase—was increased as expected. The activity of phosphofructokinase and pyruvate kinase, as well as the concentration of fructose 2,6-bisphosphate, were all normal in the livers of patients with type II diabetes (J.F. Caro and G.L. Dohm, unpublished data). Also, GLUT-2 protein and mRNA concentration of the liver/pancreas glucose transporter was normal in type II diabetes. In contrast, glucokinase activity was markedly decreased in the livers of patients with type II diabetes mellitus.[87] Glucokinase mRNA is increased by insulin and decreased by glucagon; the latter effect overrides the insulin effect and is independent of the ambient glucose concentration.[88] Thus, insulin resistance with a normal glucagon effect in diabetes is consistent with the changes observed in glucokinase activity.[87] Because increased substrate flux through glucokinase is required for glucose-induced inhibition of HGP, defective hepatic glucokinase may impair the ability of hyperglycemia to inhibit HGP in diabetes.[89]

Therefore, the available data allow us to conclude that insulin action and HGP are decidedly abnormal in type II diabetes. In fact, elevated HGP in the presence of high fasting plasma glucose concentrations, or normal HGP in the presence of high fasting plasma glucose concentrations, or even normal HGP in the presence of normal fasting plasma glucose but elevated plasma insulin concentrations are all different degrees of abnormal liver metabolism in type II diabetes.

Biochemical Defects of Insulin Action in Prediabetes: The Basis for Disease Progression

Study of insulin action at the cellular level in subjects with prediabetes is important because, in a large prospective study of the offspring of two parents with type II diabetes, insulin resistance and hyperinsulinemia were the most powerful predictors of future development of type II diabetes.[90] Accordingly, biochemical studies of insulin action in prediabetes serve three purposes: (1) They tell us about the defects found in type II diabetes that may be unrelated to hyperglycemia or insulin deficiency. This is because, in every patient with established diabetes, regardless of the type, it is possible to trace a vicious cycle that include insulin resistance, insulin deficiency, and hyperglycemia. (2) Regarding the defects found in type II diabetes, they tell us which are the earliest and which are secondary. This information will provide an understanding of disease progression and the basis for prevention. (3) Most important, these studies provide a guide to the search for the diabetogene(s).

Is the insulin receptor altered? A defect in insulin-stimulated tyrosine kinase activity of the insulin receptor in skeletal muscle in prediabetes has been demonstrated.[91] Other tissues have not been studied, but it can be predicted that the adipose tissue insulin-stimulated tyrosine kinase (IRTK) is normal because the defects found in type II diabetes are reversible after weight loss and improvement of glycemic control.[26] If indeed it can be demonstrated that IRTK is defective only in skeletal muscle, these studies at the very least would point out the site where this presumably functional abnormality is established first.[92] None of the other events related to receptor tyrosine kinase activity have yet been studied in prediabetes. Also, none of the alternative insulin signaling pathways, with the exception of demonstrating low chiroinositol production in some relative of patients with type II diabetes,[8] have been investigated.

Is glucose disposal altered in prediabetes? Insulin-stimulated glucose disposal is altered in prediabetes.[92] The ability of glucose to regulate its own uptake independently of insulin varies from low[93] to high.[94] GLUT-4 protein and mRNA are decreased in the adipose tissue.[55] GLUT-4 protein is normal, and GLUT-4 mRNA is increased in the skeletal muscle.[95] The acute regulation of GLUT-4 mRNA by insulin is altered in the skeletal muscle in prediabetes as well as in diabetes.[95]

Insulin stimulation of glycogen synthesis is abnormal in prediabetes.[96] Glucose oxidation, however, is normal at high insulin concentrations but decreased at low insulin concentrations.[73] Furthermore, the pyruvate dehydrogenase multienzyme complex has not been studied at the cellular level.

HGP has been demonstrated to be normal in prediabetes in all studies[73,96,97] except one.[98] It should be recognized, however, that the persons studied were hyperinsulinemic. Also, insulin normally suppresses HGP in prediabetes; however, the insulin concentration used to suppress glucose production was near maximal. Therefore, whether a defect in suppression of HGP could be revealed with a smaller increase in the plasma insulin concentration requires further investigation. Furthermore, the liver has not been studied in vitro in prediabetes.

Therefore, the sparse, fragmentary data available from studies in prediabetes allow us to conclude the following: (1) There are too many defects, and they are not due to hyperglycemia. In fact, the metabolic profile of early type II diabetes is fully established in prediabetes,[73] that is, impaired insulin-mediated nonoxidative and oxidative glucose disposal in muscle; impaired inhibition of lipolysis in adipose tissue; and normal HGP in the presence of increased portal insulin concentration. (2) The most severe defect is insulin stimulation of glycogen synthesis, in skeletal muscle. In fact, at submaximal insulin concentrations, this pathway of insulin action is totally refractory to insulin. Thus, it is possible that this defect is also one of the earliest. (3) A caveat for most of the biochemical studies reported so far is the difficulty in defining a prediabetic population when in fact diabetes has not developed or a normal population when in fact it is not certain if any member of the population will develop diabetes. Nevertheless, this work has been informative, and it should proceed to detailed and further studies of muscle, adipose tissue, and liver at the cellular level.

Biochemical Defects That Cause Type II Diabetes: The Diabetogene(s)

Type II diabetes comprises a group of genetic diseases of slow, progressive pathogenesis; the environment plays a key role in its ultimate clinical expression. Although it is generally believed today that insulin resistance to nonoxidative glucose disposal in skeletal muscle is the earliest biochemical detectable defect, it is true that other investigators have reported abnormalities in insulin secretion preceding any defect in insulin action.[50] The reality is that the technical expertise and beliefs of the investigator, in part, determine the likelihood of finding a defect. There is no longitudinal study in which the most powerful techniques used to study the endocrine pancreas have been combined with the most sophisticated techniques of insulin action in liver and peripheral tissues. Perhaps that study will never be done because of the expense and time required. It is likely that by the time the expert physiologists in insulin action and secretion agree on a common protocol, the diabetogene(s) will have been cloned by the molecular biologists. It is imperative, however, that the search for the diabetogene is done with the recognition that in type II diabetes many things go wrong, and that the phenotype of the prediabetic state is incompletely known, so that many other things might also be wrong. We know that in a very small group of patients with type II diabetes the diabetogene has been identified. It is either a pure defect in insulin secretion—that is, mutations in the insulin molecule altering its bioactivity[99]; mutations in glucokinase, altering the glucose-sensing mechanisms[100]; mutations in mitochondrial DNA altering insulin secretion[101]; or a pure defect in insulin action, that is, mutation of the insulin receptors[50] or mutations of insulin receptor substrate 1 (IRS-1).[50] The description of the diabetogene(s) responsible for the majority of cases of type II diabetes, however, will have to wait for the second or third edition of this book to be printed. The gene defect may be a structural region in any of the known signaling or secretory mechanisms of insulin. The mutation can also be in any of the transacting genes that regulate the structural regions. Alternatively, the diabetogene may be a new protein, such as Ras-associated with diabetes, recently described to be overexpressed in type II diabetes,[102] or perhaps the system that regulates membrane fluidity in all cells,[103] or something else totally unexpected at this time. The solution might also be even more difficult because diabetogenes of insulin action and insulin secretion might be found that interact with each other and with the environment.

It is clear that the length of the three parts of this chapter is inversely related to the accumulated data. In fact, in terms of its relationship to the common form of type II diabetes, this last section could have been summarized by a simple question mark. It is certain, however, that the primary cause of diabetes will be found, and that this discovery will not be the end but rather the beginning of rational approaches to prevent, treat, and someday even cure type II diabetes.

References

1. Caro JF, Ittoop O, Pories WJ, et al. Studies of the mechanism of insulin resistance in the liver from humans with noninsulin-dependent diabetes. J Clin Invest 1986;78:249
2. Dohm GL, Tapscott EB, Pories WJ, et al. An in vitro human muscle preparation suitable for metabolic studies. J Clin Invest 1988;82:486
3. Ciaraldi TP, Kolterman OG, Scarlett JA, et al. Role of the glucose transport system in the post-receptor defect of non-insulin dependent diabetes mellitus. Diabetes 1982;31:1016
4. White MF, Kahn CR. The insulin signaling system. J Biol Chem 1994;269:1
5. Quon MJ, Butte AJ, Zarnowski MJ, et al. Insulin receptor substrate 1 mediates the stimulatory effect of insulin on GLUT4 translocation in transfected rat adipose cells. J Biol Chem 1994;269:27920
6. Tamemoto H, Kadowaki T, Tobe K, et al. Insulin resistance and growth retardation in mice lacking insulin receptor substrate-1. Nature 1994;372:182
7. Araki E, Lipes MA, Patti ME, et al. Alternative pathway of insulin signalling mice with targeted disruption of the IRS-1 gene. Nature 1994;372:186
8. Larner J. Multiple pathways in insulin signaling—fitting the covalent and allosteric puzzle pieces together. Endocrine J 1994;2:167
9. Olefsky JM. Insulin resistance and insulin action. Diabetes 1981;30:148
10. Caro JF, Sinha MK, Raju SM, et al. Insulin receptor kinase in human skeletal muscle from obese subjects with and without noninsulin dependent diabetes. J Clin Invest 1987;79:1330
11. Arner P, Einarsson K, Backman L, et al. Studies of liver insulin receptors in non-obese and obese human subjects. J Clin Invest 1983;72:1729
12. Obermaier-Kusser B, White MF, Pongratz DE, et al. A defective intramolecular autoactivation cascade may cause the reduced kinase activity of the skeletal muscle insulin receptor from patients with non–insulin-dependent diabetes mellitus. J Biol Chem 1989;264:9497
13. Caro JF, Shafer JA, Taylor SI, et al. Insulin stimulated protein phosphorylation in human plasma liver membranes: Detection of endogenous or plasma membrane associated substrates for insulin receptor kinase. Biochem Biophys Res Commun 1987;149:1008
14. Maegawa H, Shigeta Y, Egawa K, Kobayashi M. Impaired autophosphorylation of insulin receptors from abdominal skeletal muscles in nonobese subjects with NIDDM. Diabetes 1991;40:815
15. Arner P, Pollare T, Lithell H, Livingston JN. Defective insulin receptor tyrosine kinase in human skeletal muscle in obesity and Type 2 (non–insulin-dependent) diabetes mellitus. Diabetologia 1987;30:437
16. Nyomba BL, Ossowski VM, Bogardus C, Mott DM. Insulin-sensitive tyrosine kinase: Relationship with in vivo insulin action in humans. Am J Physiol 1990;258:E964
17. Nolan JJ, Freidenberg G, Henry R, et al. Role of human skeletal muscle insulin receptor kinase in the in vivo insulin resistance of noninsulin-dependent diabetes mellitus and obesity. J Clin Endocrinol Metab 1994;78:471
18. Freidenberg GR, Henry RR, Klein HH, et al. Decreased kinase activity of insulin receptors from adipocytes of non–insulin-dependent diabetic subjects. J Clin Invest 1987;79:240
19. Sinha MK, Pories WJ, Flickinger EG, et al. Insulin-receptor kinase activity of adipose tissue from morbidly obese humans with and without NIDDM. Diabetes 1987;36:620
20. Thies RS, Molina JM, Ciaraldi TP, et al. Insulin-receptor autophosphorylation and endogenous substrate phosphorylation in human adipocytes from control, obese, and NIDDM subjects. Diabetes 1990;39:250
21. Comi RJ, Grunberger G, Gorden P. Relationship of insulin binding and insulin-stimulated tyrosine kinase activity is altered in type II diabetes. J Clin Invest 1987;79:453
22. Santos RF, Palmieri MG, Wajchenberg BL, Azhar S. Insulin-receptor tyrosine kinase activity is decreased in erythrocytes from non-obese patients with NIDDM. Horm Metab Res 1994;26:283
23. Brillon DJ, Freidenberg GR, Henry RR, Olefsky JM. Mechanism of defective insulin receptor kinase activity in NIDDM: Evidence for two receptor populations. Diabetes 1989;38:397
24. Kahn CR. Insulin actions, diabetogenes, and the cause of type II diabetes. Diabetes 1994;43:1066
25. Freidenberg GR, Reichart D, Olefsky JM. Insulin receptor kinase activity is not reduced in fibroblasts from subjects with non-insulin dependent diabetes mellitus (NIDDM) (abstract). Clin Res 1990;38:119A
26. Freidenberg GR, Reichart D, Olefsky JM, Henry RR. Reversibility of defective adipocyte insulin receptor kinase activity in non–insulin dependent diabetes mellitus. J Clin Invest 1988;82:1398
27. Kusari J, Berma US, Buse JB, et al. Analysis of the gene sequences of the insulin receptor and the insulin sensitive glucose transporter (Glut-4) in patients with common type non–insulin dependent diabetes mellitus. J Clin Invest 1991;88:1323
28. O'Rahilly S, Choi WH, Patel P, et al. Detection of mutations in insulin-receptor gene in NIDDM patients by analysis of single-stranded conformation polymorphisms. Diabetes 1991;40:777
29. Kusari J, Kenner KA, Suh KI, et al. Skeletal muscle protein tyrosine phosphatase activity and tyrosine phosphatase 1B protein content are associated with insulin action and resistance. J Clin Invest 1994;93:1156
30. McGuire MC, Fields RM, Nyomba BL, et al. Abnormal regulation of protein tyrosine phosphatase activities in skeletal muscle of insulin-resistant humans. Diabetes 1991;40:939
31. Considine RV, Caro JF. Protein Kinase C: Mediator or inhibitor of insulin action? J Cell Biochem 1993;52:8
32. Muller HK, Kellerer M, Ermel B, et al. Prevention of protein kinase C inhibitors of glucose-induced insulin receptor tyrosine kinase resistance in rat fat cells. Diabetes 1991;40:1440
33. Inoguchi T, Battan R, Handler E, et al. Preferential elevation of protein kinase C isoform β11 and diacylglycerol levels in the aorta and heart of diabetic rats: Differential reversibility to glycemic control by islet cell transplantation. Proc Natl Acad Sci USA 1992;89:11059
34. Thakker JK, DiMarchi R, MacDonald K, Caro JF. Effect of insulin and insulin-like growth factors I and II on phosphatidylinositol and phosphatidylinositol 4,5-bisphosphate breakdown in liver from humans with and without type II diabetes. J Biol Chem 1989;264:7169
35. Considine RV, Nyce MR, Allen LE, et al. Protein kinase C is increased in the liver of humans and rats with non–insulin-dependent diabetes mellitus: An alteration not due to hyperglycemia. J Clin Invest 1995;95:2938
36. Anderson CM, Olefsky JM. Phorbol ester–mediated protein kinase C interaction with wild-type and COOH-terminal truncated insulin receptors. J Biol Chem 1991;266:21760
37. Boulton TJ, Nye SH, Robbins DJ. ERKs: A family of protein-serine/threonine kinases that are activated and tyrosine phosphorylated in response to insulin and NGF. Cell 1991;65:663
38. Kanety H, Moshe S, Shafrir E, et al. Hyperinsulinemia induces a reversible impairment in insulin receptor function leading to diabetes in the sand rat model of non–insulin-dependent diabetes mellitus. Proc Natl Acad Sci USA 1994;91:1853
39. Ishizuka T, Cooper DR, Hernandez H, et al. Effects of insulin on diacylglycerol–protein kinase C signaling in rat diaphragm and soleus muscles and relationship to glucose transport. Diabetes 1990;39:181
40. Caro JF, Raju MS, Caro M, et al. Guanine nucleotide binding regulatory protein in liver from obese humans with and without type II diabetes: Evidence for altered "cross-talk" between the insulin receptor and G_i-protein. J Cell Biochem 1994;54:309
41. Livingston N, Pollare T, Lithell H, Arner P. Characterization of insulin-like growth factor I receptor in skeletal muscles of normal and insulin resistant subjects. Diabetologia 1988;31:871
42. Dohm, GL, Elton CW, Raju MS, et al. IGF-I-stimulated transport in human skeletal muscle and IGF-I resistance in obesity and NIDDM. Diabetes 1990;39:1028
43. Burguera B, Elton CW, Caro JF, et al. Stimulation of glucose uptake by insulin-like growth factor II in human muscle is not mediated by the insulin-like growth factor II/mannose 6-phosphate receptor. Biochem J 1994;300:781
44. Sinha MK, Buchanan C, Leggett N, et al. Mechanism of IGF-I-stimulated glucose transport in human adipocytes. Diabetes 1989;38:1217
45. Sinha MK, Buchanan C, Raineri-Maldonado C, et al. IGF-II receptors and IGF-II stimulated glucose transport in human fat cells. Am J Physiol 1990; 258:E534
46. Caro JF, Poulos J, Ittoop O, et al. Insulin-like growth factor I binding in hepatocytes from human liver, human hepatoma, and regenerating and fetal rat liver. J Clin Invest 1988;81:976
47. Forsayeth JR, Caro JF, Sinha MK, et al. Monocloncal antibodies to the human insulin receptor that activate glucose transport but not insulin receptor kinase activity. Proc Natl Acad Sci USA 1987;84:3448
48. Sinha MK, Buchanan C, Raineri-Maldonado C, et al. Regulation of glucose transport by insulin and monoclonal insulin receptor antibodies in adipocytes of patients with NIDDM. Adv Diabet 1990;3:149
49. Goodyear L, Giorgino F, Sherman LA, et al. Insulin receptor phosphorylation, IRS-1 phosphorylation, and phosphatidylinositol 3-kinase activity are decreased in intact skeletal muscle strips from obese subjects. J Clin Invest 1995;95(5):2195
50. Taylor SI, Accili D, Imai Y. Insulin resistance or insulin deficiency: Which is the primary cause of NIDDM? Diabetes 1994;43:735
51. Houslay MD, Pyne NJ, Kilgour E, et al. Insulin, cyclic nucleotide metabolism and the G-protein system. Horm Cell Regul 1989;176:31
52. Rothenberg PL, Kahn CR. Insulin inhibits pertussis toxin–catalyzed ADP-ribosylation of G-proteins. J Biol Chem 1988;263:15546
53. Ravindra R, Caro JF. Insulin stimulates GDP release from G proteins in the rat and human liver plasma. J Cell Biochem 1993;53:181
54. Poulos JE, Madigan T, Serrano J, et al. The effects of GYPγs on insulin binding to human liver plasma membranes. Horm Metab Res 1995;27:253
55. Garvey WT, Maianu L, Huecksteadt TP, et al. Pretranslational suppression of a glucose transporter protein causes insulin resistance in adipocytes from patients with non–insulin-dependent diabetes mellitus and obesity. J Clin Invest 1991;87:1072

56. Sinha MK, Raineri-Maldonado C, Buchanan C, et al. Adipose tissue glucose transporters in NIDDM. Diabetes 1991;40:472
57. Pedersen O, Bak JF, Andersen PH, et al. Evidence against altered expression of GLUT1 or GLUT4 in skeletal muscle of patients with obesity or NIDDM. Diabetes 1990;39:865
58. Garvey WT, Maianu L, Hancock JA, et al. Gene expression of GLUT4 in skeletal muscle from insulin-resistant patients with obesity, IgT, GDM, and NIDDM. Diabetes 1992;41:465
59. Dohm GL, Elton CW, Friedman JE, et al. Decreased expression of glucose transporter in muscle from insulin-resistant patients. Am J Physiol 1991; 23:E459
60. Andersen PH, Lund S, Vestergaard H, et al. Expression of the major insulin regulatable glucose transporter (GLUT4) in skeletal muscle of noninsulin-dependent diabetic patients and healthy subjects before and after insulin infusion. J Clin Endocrinol Metab 1993;77:27
61. Eriksson J, Koranyi L, Bourey R, et al. Insulin resistance in type 2 (non–insulin-dependent) diabetic patients and their relatives is not associated with a defect in the expression of the insulin-responsive glucose transporter (GLUT4) gene in human skeletal muscle. Diabetologia 1992;35:143
62. Friedman JE, Dohm GL, Elton CW, et al. Restoration of insulin responsiveness in skeletal muscle of morbidly obese patients after weight loss. J Clin Invest 1992;89:701
63. Dela F, Ploug T, Handberg A, et al. Physical training increases muscle GLUT4 protein and mRNA in patients with NIDDM. Diabetes 1994;43:862
64. Schmitz O, Lund S, Bak JF, et al. Effects of glipizide on glucose metabolism and muscle content of the insulin-regulatable glucose transporter (GLUT4) and glycogen synthase activity during hyperglycemia in type II diabetic patients. Acta Diabetol 1994;31:31
65. Kusari J, Verma US, Buse JB, et al. Analysis of the gene sequences of the insulin receptor and the insulin-sensitive glucose transporter (GLUT-4) in patients with common-type non–insulin-dependent diabetes mellitus. J Clin Invest 1991;88:1323
66. Choi WH, O'Rahilly S, Rees A, et al. Molecular scanning of the insulin-responsive glucose transporter (GLUT4) gene in patients with non-insulin dependent diabetes mellitus. Diabetes 1991;40:1712
67. Bjorbaek C, Echwald SM, Hubricht P, et al. Genetic variants in promoters and coding regions of the muscle glycogen synthase and the insulin-responsive GLUT4 Genes in NIDDM. Diabetes 1994;43:976
68. Lund S, Vestergaard H, Andersen PH, et al. GLUT-4 content in plasma membrane of muscle from patients with non–insulin-dependent diabetes mellitus. Am J Physiol 1993;265:E889
69. Vogt B, Mühlbacher C, Carrascosa J, et al. Subcellular distribution of GLUT4 in the skeletal muscle of lean Type 2 (non–insulin-dependent) diabetic patients in the basal state. Diabetologia 1992;35:456
70. Azevedo JL, Carey JO, Pories WJ, et al. Hypoxia stimulates glucose transport in insulin resistant human skeletal muscle. Diabetes 1995;44(6):695
71. Carey JO, Azevedo JL, Morris PG, et al. Okadaic acid, vanadate, and phenylarsine oxide stimulate 2-deoxyglucose transport in insulin-resistant human skeletal muscle. Diabetes 1995;44(6):682
72. Mandarino LJ. Regulation of skeletal muscle pyruvate dehydrogenase and glycogen synthase in man. Diabetes/Metab Rev 1989;5:475
73. Gulli G, Ferrannini E, Stern M, et al. The metabolic profile of NIDDM is fully established in glucose-tolerant offspring of two Mexican-American NIDDM parents. Diabetes 1992;11:1575
74. Laakso M, Edelman SV, Brechtel G, Baron AD. Impaired insulin-mediated skeletal muscle blood flow in patients with NIDDM. Diabetes 1992;41:1076
75. Friedman JE, Caro JF, Pories WJ, et al. Glucose metabolism in incubated human muscle: Effect of obesity and non–insulin-dependent diabetes mellitus. Metabolism 1994;43:1047
76. Kelley DE, Mandarino JL. Hyperglycemia normalizes insulin-stimulated skeletal muscle glucose oxidation and storage in noninsulin-dependent diabetes mellitus. J Clin Invest 1990;86:1999
77. Henry RR, Thorburn AW, Beerdsen P, et al. Dose-response characteristics of impaired glucose oxidation in noninsulin-dependent diabetes mellitus. Am J Physiol 1991;261:E132
78. Shulman GI, Rothman DL, Jue T, et al. Quantitation of muscle glycogen synthesis in normal subjects and subjects with non–insulin-dependent diabetes by ^{13}C nuclear magnetic resonance spectroscopy. N Engl J Med 1990; 322:223
79. Häring HU, Mehnert H. Pathogenesis of type 2 (non–insulin-dependent) diabetes mellitus: Candidates for a signal transmitter defect causing insulin resistance of the skeletal muscle. Diabetologia 1993;36:176
80. Damsbo P, Vaag A, Hother-Nielsen O, Beck-Nielsen H. Reduced glycogen synthase activity in skeletal muscle from obese patients with and without type 2 (non–insulin-dependent) diabetes mellitus. Diabetologia 1991;34:239
81. Kida Y, Nyomba BL, Bogardus C, Mott DM. Defective insulin response of cyclic adenosine monophosphate–dependent kinase in insulin-resistant humans. J Clin Invest 1991;87:673
82. Kida Y, Raz I, Maeda R, et al. Defective insulin response of phosphorylase phosphatase in insulin resistant humans. J Clin Invest 1992;89:610
83. Wells AM, Sutcliffe IC, Johnson AB, Taylor R. Abnormal activation of glycogen synthesis in fibroblasts for NIDDM subjects. Evidence for an abnormality specific to glucose metabolism. Diabetes 1993;42:583
84. Vestergaard H, Lund S, Larsen FS, et al. Glycogen synthase and phosphofructokinase protein and mRNA levels in skeletal muscle from insulin-resistant patients with non–insulin-dependent diabetes mellitus. J Clin Invest 1993; 91:2342
85. Rothman DL, Shulman RG, Shulman GI. ^{31}P nuclear magnetic resonance measurements of muscle glucose-6-phosphate. J Clin Invest 1992;89:1069
86. Consoli A, Nurjahan N, Reilly JJ, et al. Mechanism of increased gluconeogenesis in noninsulin-dependent diabetes mellitus. J Clin Invest 1990;86: 2038
87. Caro JF, Triester S, Patel VK, et al. Liver glucokinase: Decreased activity in patients with type II diabetes. Horm Metab Res 1995;27:18
88. Granner DK, O'Brien RM. Molecular physiology and genetics of NIDDM. Diabetes Care 1992;15:369
89. Rossetti L, Giaccari A, Barzilai N, et al. Mechanism by which hyperglycemia inhibits hepatic glucose production in conscious rats. J Clin Invest 1993; 92:1126
90. Martin B, Warram JH, Krolewski AS, et al. Role of glucose and insulin resistance in development of type 2 diabetes mellitus: Results of a 25-year follow-study. Lancet 1992;340:925
91. Handberg A, Vaag A, Vinten J, Beck-Nielsen H. Decreased tyrosine kinase activity in partially purified insulin receptors from muscle of young, non-obese first degree relatives of patients with Type 2 (non–insulin-dependent) diabetes mellitus. Diabetologia 1993;36:668
92. Beck-Nielsen H, Groop LC. Metabolic and genetic characterization of prediabetes states. J Clin Invest 1994;94:1714
93. Warram JH, Martin BC, Krolewski AS, et al. Slow glucose removal rate and hyperinsulinemia precede the development of type II diabetes in the offspring of diabetic parents. Ann Intern Med 1990;113:909
94. Henriksen JE, Alford F, Handberg A, et al. Increased glucose effectiveness in normoglycemic but insulin-resistant relatives of patients with non–insulin-dependent diabetes mellitus. J Clin Invest 1994;94:1196
95. Schalin-Jäntti C, Yki-Järvinen H, Koranyi L, et al. Effect of insulin on GLUT-4 mRNA and protein concentrations in skeletal muscle of patients with NIDDM and their first-degree relatives. Diabetologia 1994;37:401
96. Vaag A, Henriksen JE, Beck-Nielsen H. Decreased insulin activation of glycogen synthase in skeletal muscles in young nonobese caucasian first-degree relatives of patients with non–insulin-dependent diabetes mellitus. J Clin Invest 1992;89:782
97. Eriksson J, Franssila-Kallunki A, Ekstrand A, et al. Early metabolic defects in persons at increased risk for non-insulin dependent diabetes mellitus. N Engl J Med 1989;321:337
98. Osei K. Increased basal glucose production and utilization in nondiabetic first-degree relatives of patients with NIDDM. Diabetes 1990;39:597
99. Steiner DF, Tager HS, Chan SJ, et al. Lessons learned from molecular biology of insulin-gene mutations. Diabetes Care 1990;13:600
100. Permutt MA, Chiu KC, Tanizawa Y. Glucokinase and NIDDM, a candidate gene that paid off. Diabetes 1992;41:1367
101. Ballinger S, Shoffner JM, Hedaya EV, et al. Maternally transmitted diabetes and deafness associated with a 10.4-kb mitochondrial DNA deletion. Nature Genet 1992;1:11
102. Reynet C, Kahn CR. Rad: A member of the ras family overexpressed in muscle of type II diabetic humans. Science 1993;262:1441
103. Borkman M, Storlien LH, Pan DA, et al. The relation between insulin sensitivity and the fatty-acid composition of skeletal-muscle phospholipids. N Engl J Med 1993;4:238

Diabetes Mellitus, edited by Derek LeRoith, Simeon I. Taylor, and Jerrold M. Olefsky. Lippincott–Raven Publishers, Philadelphia © 1996.

CHAPTER 59

Glucose Transporters and Pathophysiologic States

E. DALE ABEL, PETER R. SHEPHERD, AND BARBARA B. KAHN

Introduction

The effect of insulin to acutely stimulate glucose uptake into muscle and adipose tissue is essential for normal glucose homeostasis. A major pathologic feature of obesity, non–insulin-dependent diabetes (NIDDM), and, to a lesser extent, insulin-dependent diabetes mellitus (IDDM), is resistance to this effect of insulin, which has been demonstrated both in vivo using nuclear magnetic resonance[1] and forearm perfusion with indirect calorimetry,[2,3] and in vitro in isolated adipocytes[4] and muscle strips.[5,6] Furthermore, glucose transport is the rate-limiting step for glucose utilization in muscle at most physiologic glucose and insulin levels,[7–9] as well as in NIDDM,[1,2] IDDM,[3] and insulin-deficient diabetes in rats.[10] Thus, defects in the insulin-stimulated glucose transport system are likely to be a major cause of peripheral insulin resistance.

Glucose transport into muscle and adipose cells occurs by facilitated diffusion mediated by six homologous proteins encoded by distinct but closely related genes (GLUT-1-5 and GLUT-7). This family includes a homologous pseudogene (GLUT-6 or GLUT-3P1).[11,12] In tissues with insulin-sensitive glucose transport (i.e., muscle and adipose cells), GLUT-4 is the predominant isoform. The large stimulatory effect of insulin in these tissues results from the unique targeting of GLUT-4. In the absence of insulin, GLUT-4 is sequestered in intracellular vesicles; in response to insulin and other stimuli, these vesicles translocate to the plasma membrane (Fig. 59-1). Many studies have addressed the role of glucose transporters in insulin-resistant and other pathophysiologic states. This chapter will review molecular mechanisms that could potentially account for altered glucose transport in both human and animal models of insulin resistance and enhanced insulin responsiveness. One of the salient themes is that the regulation of glucose transporter gene expression is tissue specific, with much greater changes in expression in adipocytes than in muscle in altered metabolic states.

Cellular Mechanisms for Stimulation of Glucose Transport: Potential Molecular Defects in Insulin-Resistant States

The stimulatory effect of insulin on glucose transport involves a series of cellular events (Fig. 59-1). Dysregulation of any of these steps could result in insulin resistance. The binding of insulin to its receptor generates intracellular signals that regulate GLUT-4 gene transcription and protein levels, stimulate transporter translocation, and modulate the intrinsic activity of the transporter. The nature of the signaling intermediates that mediate these processes is under intense investigation. It is likely that distinct abnormalities in signaling account for insulin-resistant glucose transport in some pathologic states. The recent identification of some of the upstream regulatory elements of the GLUT-4 gene[13] should increase our understanding of the mechanisms by which the changes in GLUT-4 expression occur in altered metabolic states. Evidence indicates, however, that insulin resistance in many pathophysiologic states probably results from alterations in GLUT-4 vesicle translocation, fusion with the plasma membrane, or intrinsic activity rather than from changes in GLUT-4 gene expression.

A uniquely important characteristic of GLUT-4 is its targeting to specific intracellular vesicles distinct from that of GLUT-1.[14] Studies utilizing GLUT-1/GLUT-4 chimeras suggest that specific domains are important for targeting the transporters to their respective vesicles.[15] The recent identification of proteins such as a novel aminopeptidase, GP160 or VP165, which is also localized exclusively in GLUT-4 vesicles,[16,17] should add to our understanding of the factors involved in GLUT-4 targeting. There is no evidence to date to implicate altered GLUT-4 targeting as a contributor to altered glucose transport in pathophysiologic states. Translocation of GLUT-4-containing vesicles to the plasma membrane is the major step leading to the increase in transport in response to a variety of stimuli, including insulin, exercise, hypoxia, other growth factors such as IGF1, and in vitro activation of guanine triphosphate binding proteins.[18] Colocalization of the small guanine triphosphate binding protein rab4 with the GLUT-4 vesicle and identification of insulin-stimulated translocation of rab4 from low-density microsomes to the cytosol, with the same time course as that of GLUT-4 translocation to the plasma membrane,[19,20] may lead to insights into the vesicle translocation and fusion process.

Translocation time course studies show that after insulin stimulation there is a delay between the arrival of GLUT-4-containing vesicles at the plasma membrane and an increase in glucose transport.[21] This implies that the docking and/or fusion of these vesicles with the plasma membrane may be a regulated step in glucose transport or that the transporters have to be activated once they are inserted in the plasma membrane (Fig. 59-1). Evidence to support this hypothesis includes the observation that isoproterenol-induced reduction in glucose transport in adipocytes is associated with no alteration in the total amount of plasma membrane–bound immunodetectable GLUT-4. There is, however, a reduction in the ability of the exofacial bis-mannose photolabel ATB-BMPA to label GLUT-4 at the plasma membrane, implying that the GLUT-4 is not in the correct orientation to bind the photolabel or to transport glucose.[22] Such a mechanism may have physiologic relevance in the counter-regulatory effects of epinephrine on glucose transport into muscle. With epinephrine exposure, glucose transport decreases despite an apparently paradoxic stimulation by epinephrine of GLUT-4 translocation to the plasma membrane.[23] This example further demonstrates the potential for hormonal/metabolic regulation of GLUT-4 availability to glucose.

Several lines of evidence support the concept that the glucose transporter intrinsic activity can be modulated once transporters are appropriately inserted in the plasma membrane, and that such alterations may contribute to insulin resistance in some states, such as in muscle of rats after high-fat feeding.[24] The mechanisms by which changes in intrinsic activity occur are not known. In 3T3-L1 adipocytes, protein synthesis inhibitors result in a rapid increase in glucose transport with no change in the plasma membrane levels of glucose transporters,[25] implicating a role for a rapidly turning

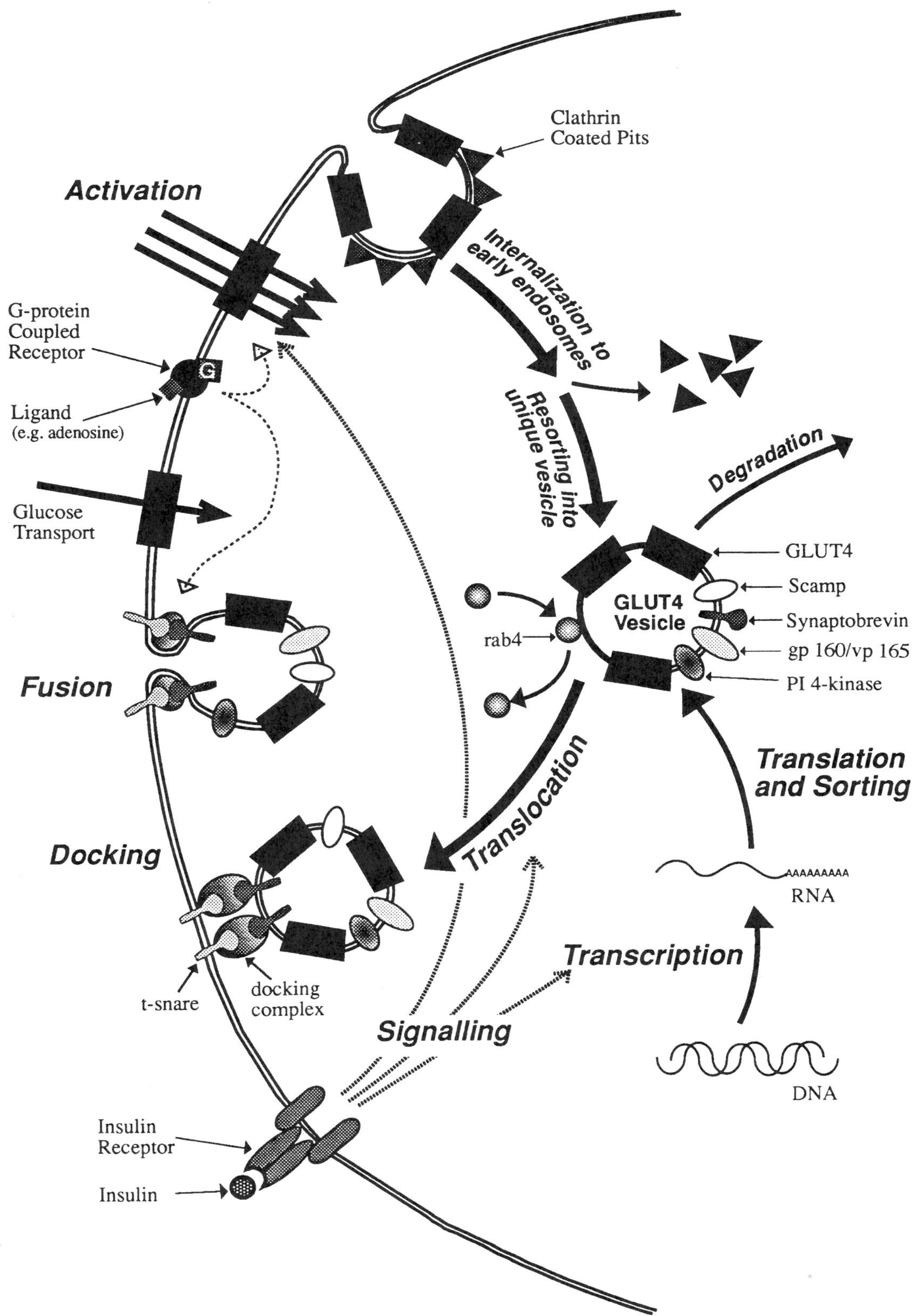

FIGURE 59-1. Sequence of events involved in insulin stimulation of glucose transport in muscle and adipose cells: (1) In the absence of insulin, the GLUT-4 glucose transporter resides within the cell. Other proteins associated with GLUT-4 vesicles include synaptobrevin (VAMP), GP160/VP165, PI4-kinase, rab4, and SCAMPS. (2) When insulin binds to its receptor in the plasma membrane, it initiates a cascade of signals affecting transcription, translocation, and possibly activation of the glucose transporter. (3) Rab4 dissociates from the vesicle, and the vesicle translocates to the plasma membrane, where it docks and fuses, and glucose transport is activated. (4) GLUT-4 vesicles are endocytosed and recycle through endosomes. (Adapted with permission from Shepherd PR, Kahn BB. Expression of the GLUT4 glucose transporter in diabetes. In: Draznin B, LeRoith D, eds. Molecular Biology of Diabetes, Vol II. Totowa, NJ: Humana Press; 1994:535–536.)

over protein in the regulation of intrinsic activity. The observation that vanadate, a phosphatase inhibitor, increases intrinsic activity in rat muscle plasma membrane vesicles[26] suggests that phosphorylation of cellular proteins, but not necessarily of GLUT-4, also may play a role in the regulation of intrinsic activity. Finally, kinetic data indicate that glucose transporters are constantly recycling between the plasma membrane and the intracellular pool and that insulin increases the rate of exocytosis.[21,27] This represents another potentially regulated step in glucose transport, and insulin resistance could result from a relative increase in endocytosis versus exocytosis.

Role of Glucose Transporters in Diabetes, Obesity, and Other Insulin-Resistant States in Humans

Muscle is the major site of insulin-stimulated glucose disposal in vivo,[28] and in normal subjects GLUT-4 levels in muscle in the basal state correlate positively with whole body insulin-stimulated glucose disposal.[29] Therefore, mutations in GLUT-4 or reductions in GLUT-4 levels in muscle could be expected to result in insulin resistance due to reduction in insulin-stimulated glucose disposal.

Potential Mutations in the GLUT-4 Gene

Investigations of the possibility that mutations in GLUT-4 could contribute to insulin resistance have revealed only one alteration affecting amino acid sequence: a single nucleotide change that results in the substitution of an isoleucine for valine at codon 383. The Ile[383] GLUT-4 allele is present in a small (1–3%) fraction of the population and does not appear to segregate with NIDDM.[30,31] Single stranded conformational polymorphism (SSCP) and direct sequencing analysis of the GLUT-4 promoter region revealed three genetic variants in 30 NIDDM patients. These variants, however, had no impact on GLUT-4 expression in skeletal muscle.[32] Initial reports of a restriction fragment length polymorphism of the GLUT-1 locus that segregated with NIDDM[33] have not been substantiated.[34]

Regulation of GLUT-4 Gene Expression

Obesity and diabetes do not appear to be associated with altered GLUT-4 protein levels in any of the human skeletal muscle groups investigated (Table 59-1). GLUT-4 protein levels were found to be similar to age- and weight-matched control subjects in membranes prepared from vastus lateralis muscle in obese,[35,36] NIDDM,[35,36] and IDDM[37] subjects and also in quadriceps femoris muscle of IDDM subjects[38] and gastrocnemius muscle of NIDDM subjects.[39] One study reported a small decrease in GLUT-4 levels in rectus abdominus muscle in massively obese nondiabetic and NIDDM subjects.[40] Weight reduction, however, did not reverse this small reduction in spite of improved glucose disposal, indicating that this small decrease did not explain the insulin resistance of obesity or NIDDM.[6] In other insulin-resistant states such as gestational diabetes mellitus,[36] uremia,[41] and pseudoacromegaly,[42] muscle GLUT-4 content is also unchanged.

Because GLUT-4 concentrations vary widely in muscles of normal humans[35,36,37] and those with obesity[35,36] and diabetes,[35,36,37,43] small differences between groups could be obscured by intergroup variation. Hence longitudinal studies of the same subjects before and after a therapeutic intervention are important. In the studies mentioned above, where gastric bypass led to weight reduction,[6] as well as in studies where sulfonylurea therapy improved glycemic control in NIDDM subjects,[44] improved whole body glucose disposal was not accompanied by any changes in muscle GLUT-4 content. Although there is little evidence to support the role of altered GLUT-4 levels in muscle in the basal state, recent studies have suggested that the in vivo regulation by insulin of this transporter may be deranged in NIDDM and IDDM.[45,46] In normal subjects, euglycemic hyperinsulinemia for up to 4 hours resulted in an increase in GLUT-4 mRNA and a decrease in GLUT-4 protein concentration in skeletal muscle. These changes did not occur in the diabetic subjects.[45,46] However, in IDDM subjects after pancreas transplantation, chronic hyperinsulinemia is associated with 45% lower muscle GLUT-4 content compared to nondiabetic control subjects in the face of markedly increased plasma insulin concentrations.[47] This could represent adaptative regulation to prevent hypoglycemia.

Defects in GLUT-4 Translocation

Although GLUT-4 expression is normal in muscles of obese and diabetic subjects, it is possible that defects exist in translocation of the glucose transporters that would contribute to the insulin-resistant glucose disposal in muscle. Investigations of translocation in human muscle are limited by the large amount of tissue required and the relatively small (1.4–2-fold) degree of GLUT-4 translocation in human muscle.[48] One attempt to measure plasma membrane GLUT-4 content in normal and NIDDM subjects after a hyperinsulinemic clamp failed to reveal any difference between the two

Table 59-1. Regulation of GLUT-4 Expression in Humans

Condition	Muscle	Fat	References
Type I diabetes (IDDM)	↔	ND	37, 38
Type II diabetes (NIDDM)	↔	↓	4, 35, 36, 39
Obesity	↔	↓	4, 35, 36, 40
Gestational diabetes	↔	↔ or ↓	36, 51
Aging	↓	ND	111
Uremia	↔	ND	41
Polycystic ovary syndrome	ND	↓	50
Pseudoacromegaly	↔	ND	42
Exercise (normal subjects, impaired glucose tolerance, NIDDM)	↑	ND	54–56
Sulfonylurea therapy	↔	ND	44
Weight loss	↔	ND	6

ND = no data.
Source: Adapted from ref. 24.

groups. These investigators were also unable to detect any significant increase in plasma membrane transporter content between the baseline muscle biopsy specimen and that obtained after the hyperinsulinemic clamp in both diabetics and controls.[49] Another study found that basal plasma membrane GLUT-4 content was lower in gastrocnemius muscle from amputated limbs from NIDDM patients even though GLUT-4 levels in the whole muscle were similar in the control and NIDDM subjects.[39] Because these specimens were obtained at amputation, these observations may be confounded by underlying ischemia, infection, drugs, and counter-regulatory hormone concentrations.

Studies in Human Adipose Cells

In contrast to muscle, GLUT-4 levels are markedly downregulated in adipose cells in obese human subjects,[4] and this reduction is more pronounced in obese subjects with impaired glucose tolerance or overt NIDDM.[4] GLUT-4 levels are also decreased in adipocytes from lean and obese patients with polycystic ovarian syndrome when compared with age- and weight-matched controls.[50] Insulin-stimulated recruitment of GLUT-4 to the plasma membrane is impaired in adipocytes isolated from gestational diabetics, due to changes in expression or subcellular localization of GLUT-4.[51] Because fat is thought to play only a minor role in insulin-stimulated glucose disposal,[52] however, the impact of changes in GLUT-4 content or function on in vivo insulin resistance is unclear.

Ameliorative Effects of Exercise

Exercise is one of the few states in which GLUT-4 content can be modulated in human muscle. Exercise increases insulin sensitivity in normal and NIDDM subjects independently of changes in body composition.[53,54] In middle-aged men with normal glucose tolerance, subjects with impaired glucose tolerance, and subjects with NIDDM,[54–56] exercise is associated with increases in muscle GLUT-4 content and in vivo glucose uptake. The increment in in vivo insulin sensitivity was accounted for by the increase in GLUT-4 in the study of middle-aged men,[55] but in those with impaired glucose tolerance, insulin sensitivity increased by 11% despite a 60% increase in skeletal muscle GLUT-4 content.[54] This suggests either that GLUT-4 regulation by exercise is fiber specific, so that the net impact on in vivo glucose uptake is less than the increase in GLUT-4 observed in the muscle sampled; that the increased transporters are not present in or recruited to the plasma membrane; or that factors in addition to GLUT-4 content regulate muscle glucose uptake. An increase in GLUT-4 content could not fully account for the enhanced in vivo glucose uptake observed in athletes by Andersen et al.,[57] and no correlation was found between insulin-mediated glucose uptake and GLUT-4 levels in muscle after a hyperinsulinemic clamp. These data suggest that exercise-induced improvements in insulin sensitivity are only partially explained by increases in GLUT-4 expression.

Glucose Transporters in Animal Models of Obesity, Diabetes, and Insulin Resistance

Genetic Models Associated with Hyperinsulinemia

Obese and Spontaneously Diabetic Monkeys

Rhesus monkeys spontaneously developing obesity and diabetes have been used as a model for human NIDDM and have allowed the identification of stages in the development of NIDDM.[58] Hyper-secretion of insulin in response to a glucose challenge is the first detectable defect in the development of diabetes, followed by more obvious peripheral insulin resistance that precedes any deficiency in insulin secretion. This sequence further emphasizes the potential importance of impaired glucose transport in the pathophysiology of diabetes. Preliminary studies of the levels of GLUT-4 glucose transporter protein in postnuclear membranes show no decrease in obese or diabetic monkeys (J.E. Weinreb et al., unpublished observation). No studies of glucose transporter translocation or function, however, have been reported in this model.

Zucker Rats

Zucker rats carry the autosomal recessive *fa* gene, which in homozygotes causes obesity and progressive insulin resistance. Preweaned Zucker (*fa/fa*) rats (21d) reveal hyperresponsive insulin-stimulated glucose uptake in diaphragm muscle that progressively declines, so that by 31 days it is similar to that of lean controls. By 70 days of age, however, glucose uptake in diaphragm muscle is impaired, heralding the development of insulin resistance.[59] These changes are not associated with any change in GLUT-4 mRNA or protein in muscle.[59] At a time when this insulin-resistant glucose uptake develops in skeletal muscle, heart, and brown adipose tissue, insulin-stimulated glucose disposal remains elevated in white fat.[60] Thus, hyper-responsive glucose transport in isolated adipocytes from young Zucker rats persists longer than in muscle, but insulin-resistant glucose uptake in adipocytes eventually ensues in older animals.[61] Unlike muscle, in adipocytes of young obese Zucker rats, the insulin hyper-responsiveness corresponds to an increase in GLUT-4 protein levels compared with that of lean littermates[61] (Fig. 59-2*A*). Older Zucker (*fa/fa*) obese rats exhibit insulin resistance and reduced insulin-stimulated glucose utilization in adipocytes and all muscle groups.[60,62,63] Levels of GLUT-4 in muscle are the same between lean and obese Zucker rats[63] even as they age (Fig. 59-2*B*). In contrast, by 20 weeks of age, the increase in adipocyte GLUT-4 content seen in young Zucker rats is reversed to levels below those of lean controls (Fig. 59-2*A*), in parallel with the reversal of hyper-responsive, insulin-stimulated glucose transport.[61] These changes are summarized in Table 59-2.

Although not confirmed by all groups,[64] the major cause of insulin resistance in muscle appears to be a defect in translocation of GLUT-4 to the plasma membrane,[65,66] as the intrinsic activity[65] and overall level of GLUT-4 in muscle are the same in lean and obese Zucker rats.[62,63,66] The translocation defect appears to be confined to translocation signaled by insulin because exercise-stimulated glucose transport in muscle is normal in obese Zucker rats.[66] Interestingly, expression of the α-subunit of the heterotrimeric G-protein G_s is significantly reduced in the cardiac myocytes of Zucker rats, whereas expression of GLUT-4 remains normal,[67] raising the question of whether G-proteins could be involved in the signaling defect.

The potential involvement of glucocorticoids in the insulin resistance of obese Zucker rats is suggested by elevated corticosterone concentrations in this model.[68,69] Lowering of corticosterone concentrations by adrenalectomy lowers insulin concentrations[69] and partially restores the translocation of GLUT-4 in muscle.[68] Chronic vanadate treatment normalizes insulin concentrations in obese Zucker rats without changing fasting glucose concentrations.[62] This is accompanied by increased glucose utilization in muscle without altering GLUT-4 expression. These effects are not seen when insulin concentrations are lowered by streptozotocin treatment,[63] which results in a rise in blood glucose to diabetic levels. Thus the insulin concentration alone is not the major determinant of in vivo insulin sensitivity in the Zucker rat.

The phenotype of the *fa* gene depends on the genetic background on which it is expressed. Males of the ZDF strain of the *fa/fa* rat (ZDF/*drt-fa*) have obesity and insulin resistance similar to that of *fa/fa* rats but are prone to develop overt diabetes associated

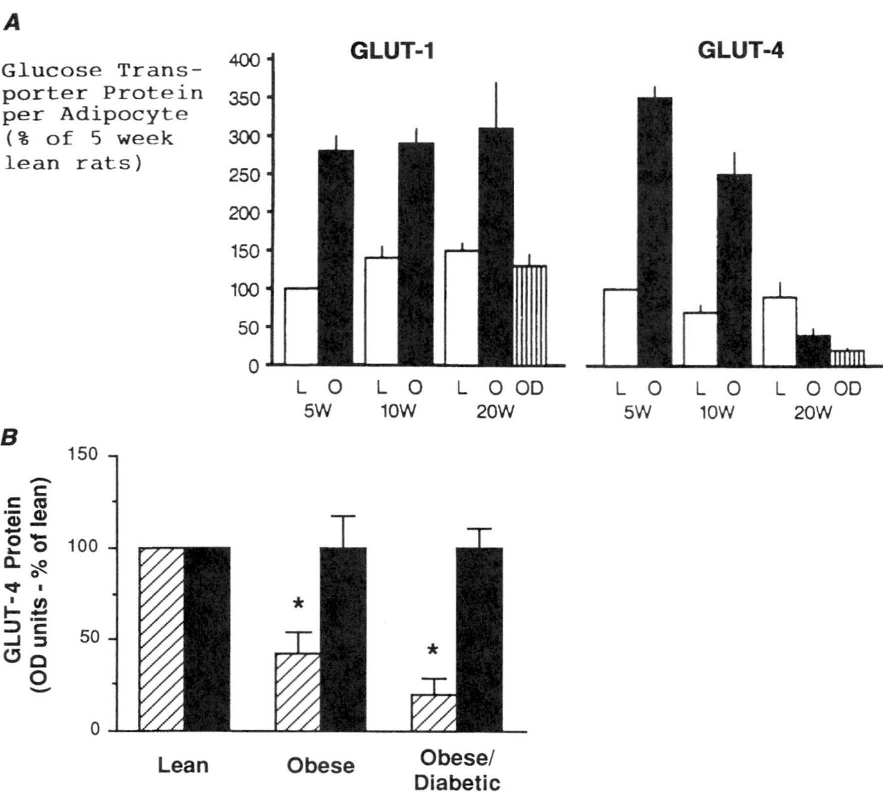

FIGURE 59-2. Altered glucose transporter expression in insulin-resistant Zucker (*fa/fa*) rats. (***A***) Increased levels of GLUT-1 and GLUT-4 protein in adipose cells of young (5-week and 10-week) obese Zucker rats but decreased GLUT-4 levels in older (20-week) obese (O) and obese/diabetic (OD) Zucker rats compared to lean controls (L). Obese/diabetic Zucker rats were rendered diabetic with streptozotocin injection and were analyzed 36 hours after diabetes induction. GLUT-4 protein levels were determined by scanning densitometry of autoradiograms of Western blots and are expressed per adipocyte. Values in obese rats are expressed as a percentage of the values in 5-week lean Zucker rats. Results are mean S ± SEM of four separate experiments. (Panel A is reproduced with permission from ref. 61.) (***B***) Tissue-specific regulation of GLUT-4 protein levels in skeletal muscle (black) and adipose cells (shaded) from 20-week Zucker rats. GLUT-4 protein levels were determined by scanning densitometry of autoradiograms of Western blots. Results are means ± SEM. *Difference from control at $p \leq 0.05$. (Panel B is reproduced with permission from Kahn BB, Pedersen O. Suppression of Glut 4 expression in skeletal muscle of rats that are obese from high fat feeding but not from high carbohydrate feeding or genetic obesity. Endocrinology 1993;132:13.)

with a reduced capacity to secrete insulin. In these obese diabetic rats, GLUT-4 protein levels are significantly reduced in skeletal muscle and adipose tissue.[70,71] Reduction of hyperglycemia, by decreasing absorption of glucose in the gut with acarbose, results in normalization of GLUT-4 levels and a significant increase in insulin secretion.[71] Transfer of the *fa* gene to a Wistar rat background also result in obesity and overt diabetes, although GLUT-4 mRNA levels in muscle are unchanged from those of lean controls.[72]

Db/db Diabetic Mouse

The *db* gene is inherited as an autosomal recessive trait that confers obesity associated with hyperglycemia and hyperinsulinemia in homozygotes. Insulin-stimulated glucose transport into skeletal muscle is impaired in *db/db* mice,[73] but in young (5-week-old) mice, GLUT-4 protein concentrations in skeletal muscle and adipose tissue are similar between obese diabetics and lean controls.[74] Defects in glucose transporter translocation or intrinsic activity have not been investigated in this model. As in myocytes from obese Zucker rats, however, concentrations of the regulatory α-subunits of the heterotrimeric receptor G-proteins G_s and G_i are reduced in adipocytes of obese *db/db* mice.[75]

Ob/ob Obese Mouse

Like the *db* gene, the *ob* gene is inherited in an autosomal recessive manner, and *ob/ob* mice have an obese insulin-resistant phenotype similar to that of the *db/db* mice, with less severe hyperglycemia. The *ob* gene has recently been cloned. It is expressed solely in fat and encodes a secreted protein.[76] Dysfunctional insulin-stimulated glucose transport appears to play a primary role in the development of insulin resistance in *ob/ob* mice.[77] Glucose transporter expression and function, however, have not been characterized in this model. As in the *db/db* model, defects in G-protein action have been noted.[75] Similarities with the hyperinsulinemic but normoglycemic Zucker model are also seen, as *ob/ob* mice have elevated levels of glucocorticoids,[78] and adrenalectomy[79] or vanadate treatment[80] reduces peripheral insulin resistance in *ob/ob* mice.

Table 59-2. GLUT-4 Protein Levels in Animal Models of Insulin Resistance

Animal Model	Fasting Insulin	Fasting Glucose	GLUT-4 in Muscle	GLUT-4 in Fat	References
Obese (*fa/fa*) Zucker rat					
Young	↑	↔	↔	↑↑	59–61
Old	↑↑	↔	↔	↓↓	60–63
Diabetic (ZDF/drt) Zucker rat	↑	↑↑	↓↓	↓↓	70, 71
db/db mice	↑	↑	↔	↔	74
KK/AY	↑↑	↑	↓↓	↓↓	90
A^{vy}/a	↑↑	↑	↓↓	↓↓	70
Brown fat ablation	↑↑	↑	↔	ND	87–89
Spontaneously hypertensive rat	↑	↔	↔	ND	85
Aged rat	↑	↔	↓↓	↓↓	109, 112, 113
Gold thioglucose obesity	↑↑	↑	↔	↓↓	94
Ventromedial hypothalamus obesity	↑	↔	↔	↑, then ↔*	93
Neuropeptide Y injection	↑	↔	↔	↑†	95
Streptozotocin diabetes	↓	↑↑	↔ or ↓	↓↓	124–127
High-fat feeding	↑‡	↓ or ↔	↓ or ↔	↓↓	61, 118, 120, 121
Dexamethasone treatment	↑	↑	↔	ND	104

ND = no data.
*One week versus 6 weeks.
†After 1 week.
‡Plasma insulin concentration is elevated in the fasting state but decreased in the fed state.
Source: Adapted from ref. 18.

Rodent Hypertension

Hypertension is associated with insulin resistance in humans.[81] The spontaneously hypertensive rat has been used to study the mechanism of this insulin resistance. Some investigators have taken normal glycemia but elevated insulin levels as an indication of insulin resistance in these animals.[82] This conclusion is controversial, however, because insulin-stimulated glucose disposal, as measured by hyperinsulinemic-euglycemic clamp, showed increased sensitivity and normal maximal responsiveness in one study[83] and decreased responsiveness in another study using different conditions.[84] Insulin receptor tyrosine kinase activity, GLUT-4 protein content and GLUT-4 translocation are apparently normal in muscle of spontaneously hypertensive rats.[85] Isolated adipocytes from hypertensive rats, however, have lower basal and insulin-stimulated glucose transport capacity, possibly indicating a reduction in transporter number or intrinsic activity.[82] This contrasts with observations in another rodent model of hypertension, the Milan rat. These mice do not exhibit in vivo insulin resistance, however a profound decrease in muscle GLUT-4 content, with normal adipocyte GLUT-4 content has been observed.[86] Thus, whether genetic models of rodent hypertension will prove to be useful for the study of the association of insulin resistance and hypertension in humans remains to be determined.

Other Genetic Rodent Models of Obesity and Diabetes

Glucose transporters have been studied in several other genetic models of obesity exhibiting hyperinsulinemia and hyperglycemia. Transgenic mice with genetic ablation of brown adipose tissue have marked obesity and insulin resistance.[87] Impaired glucose transport is associated with normal GLUT-4 levels in skeletal muscle, and precedes the down-regulation of GLUT-4 observed in adipocytes.[88,89] In contrast, GLUT-4 levels are reduced in fat, quadriceps, and soleus muscles in the KK/A^{Y} obese mouse,[90] in soleus and heart in the A^{vy}/a viable yellow mouse,[70] and in all membrane fractions of hind limb muscle homogenates in the SHR/N-cp obese rat[91] and the LA/N-cp rat.[92]

Experimental Models Associated with Hyperinsulinemia

Experimentally Induced Obesity

Obesity can be experimentally induced by surgical[93] or gold thioglucose–induced lesions[94] of the ventromedial hypothalamus, by intraventricular injection of neuropeptide Y,[95] or by systemic neonatal injection of monosodium glutamate.[96] Gold thioglucose treatment or neuropeptide Y administration induces obesity associated with marked hyperinsulinemia and mild hyperglycemia.[94] No difference is seen between the skeletal muscle GLUT-4 content of obese and control animals, although there is a significant decrease in GLUT-4 levels in brown and white adipose tissue.[94] Changes in adipose cell GLUT-4 content has also been temporally linked to changes in glucose metabolism during the process of developing obesity in rats with surgically induced ventromedial hypothalamus lesions[93] or after neuropeptide Y injection.[95] After 1 week, ventromedial hypothalamus–lesioned rats are slightly obese but have normal plasma insulin and glucose concentrations.[93] After 1 week of neuropeptide Y infusion, hyperphagia, weight gain, and hyperinsulinemia occur, with insulin-resistant glucose transport in skeletal muscle.[95] In both models, adipose tissue is hyper-responsive to insulin in this initial phase, and this correlates with increased GLUT-4 protein levels in adipocytes.[93,95] By 6 weeks after ventromedial hypothalamus lesioning, the plasma insulin levels are markedly elevated, indicating insulin resistance.[93] The hyper-responsiveness in adipose tissue disappears, and GLUT-4 levels in fat fall to the level of controls. One group[97] has reported that GLUT-4 translocation is intact in fat of animals with hypothalamic obesity induced by monosodium glutamate or gold thioglucose. In contrast to other groups, they also reported a 40% reduction in cardiac and skeletal muscle GLUT-4 content in all membrane fractions.[96]

Hyperinsulinemia Caused by Insulin Infusion

Insulin infusion in the rat results in hyperinsulinemia and hypoglycemia and is associated with insulin resistance in several muscle groups, although insulin responsiveness in fat may actually be increased.[98,99] GLUT-4 protein levels are elevated in adipocytes in parallel with the hyper-responsiveness of this tissue. This effect in fat in vivo contrasts with the effect of insulin in vitro in 3T3-L1 adipocytes where downregulation of GLUT-4 expression is seen.[100] The link between GLUT-4 and insulin resistance in skeletal muscle is unclear, however, as GLUT-4 protein content is elevated in soleus muscle of insulin-infused hypoglycemic Sprague-Dawley rats[101] but is unchanged in diaphragm and lowered in tibialis muscles of insulin-infused, normoglycemic lean Zucker rats.[102] These discrepancies may reflect differences in the fiber types of the muscles studied or a difference in the genetic background of the animals. Theoretically, hypoglycemia or the counter-regulatory hormone response elicited by the hypoglycemia could affect GLUT-4 expression in muscle of the Sprague-Dawley rat model, but there are no data to support this possibility.

Hyperglycemia Caused by Glucose Infusion

Glucose infusion induces a state of insulin resistance in humans[9] and a state of hyperinsulinemia and hyperglycemia in rats. Glucose infusion does not change GLUT-4 protein content in rat muscle despite an increase in GLUT-4 mRNA.[103] This suggests that GLUT-4 levels are subject to post-transcriptional/pretranslational regulation. The insulin-resistant glucose transport in muscle observed in this model is probably mediated through changes in GLUT-4 translocation or intrinsic activity.

Glucocorticoid Excess

Many genetic rodent models of obesity and insulin resistance exhibit elevated levels of glucocorticoids.[68,69,77] The treatment of normal animals with pharmacologic doses of glucocorticoids can also induce hyperinsulinemia and hyperglycemia.[104,105] Levels of GLUT-4 are not changed in skeletal muscle of dexamethasone-treated animals, however, indicating that in this model alterations in muscle GLUT-4 content are not the primary mechanism for insulin resistance.[104] Incubation of isolated adipocytes with dexamethasone results in rapid redistribution of glucose transporters from the plasma membrane to the intracellular pool.[106] Such a translocation defect may be involved in dexamethasone-induced insulin resistance in vivo. Interestingly, a recent report indicates that glucocorticoid treatment lowers tyrosine phosphorylation of the insulin receptor and its substrate, IRS-1.[105] However, the link between this defect in substrate phosphorylation and resistance to insulin-stimulated glucose disposal is not known.

Growth Hormone Excess

Chronic exposure to elevated concentrations of growth hormone in vivo results in insulin resistance, manifested by marked hyperinsulinemia and mild hyperglycemia.[107] Adipocytes chronically exposed to growth hormone in vitro have lowered capacity to transport glucose.[108] This is caused by downregulation of GLUT-1.[108] In a transgenic model of growth hormone overexpression, GLUT-4 expression was perturbed, with GLUT-4 mRNA being decreased in skeletal muscle, whereas in fat, GLUT-4 mRNA was significantly increased.[107] GLUT-4 protein content was not investigated in this study, so the functional significance of these findings remains in doubt, especially because GLUT-4 mRNA and protein abundance have been shown to change in opposite directions in other insulin-resistant states.[103,109]

The importance of normal growth hormone concentrations in the regulation of glucose transporter number in the plasma membrane is suggested by experiments showing that restoration of growth hormone concentrations, but not insulin, IGF-1, or IGF-2 concentrations, could reverse the increase in basal glucose transport seen in isolated adipocytes from hypophysectomized mice.[110]

Animal Models of Aging

Aging is associated with mild insulin resistance and hyperinsulinemia.[111] Although GLUT-4 protein levels are greatly decreased in both muscle and fat of aged rats, the mechanisms for this decrease differ in the two tissues. In fat the decline in GLUT-4 protein parallels a fall in mRNA, whereas in muscle the decline in protein is associated with increasing mRNA, implying decreased translational efficiency or protein stability.[109] The decrease in GLUT-4 content in skeletal muscle is fiber specific, with decreases reported in the heart[112] and epitrochlearis[113] but not in the flexor digitorum brevis.[113] The decrement in muscle glucose transport has also been shown to be greater than can be accounted for by changes in GLUT-4 content.[113] In adipocytes of older rats, subcellular distribution and translocation of GLUT-4 are intact, suggesting that the insulin resistance can be accounted for by the decreased concentrations of the transporter in this tissue.[114] A potential role for diminished recruitability/intrinsic activity in adipocytes has, however, been recently described.[115] Aging is not associated with any changes in GLUT-1 abundance in adipocytes. There is a redistribution of the GLUT-1 transporter, with increased abundance in the plasma membrane in the basal state.[114] GLUT-1 levels in the plasma membrane are not increased further by insulin treatment, suggesting additional dysregulation in GLUT-1 transporter subcellular trafficking.[114,116]

Hypoinsulinemic Models

Diet-Induced Obesity

High concentrations of fatty acids have been implicated as a cause of insulin resistance in humans.[117] In animal models, high-fat feeding causes obesity associated with marked insulin resistance and hypoinsulinemia in the fed state compared with the condition of animals fed a high-carbohydrate diet.[118] The magnitude of the insulin resistance depends on the fatty acid composition of the lipid and correlates with the triglyceride content of skeletal muscle.[119] There appear to be multiple mechanisms by which high-fat feeding results in insulin resistance. A high-fat diet (50–80% of total calories from fat) results in significant reductions of GLUT-4 mRNA and protein in adipose tissue.[120] Very high dietary fat content (80%) for prolonged periods also causes downregulation of GLUT-4 expression in skeletal muscle.[61] Translocation of GLUT-4 in muscle remains intact, but the normal increase in GLUT-4 intrinsic activity in response to insulin or exercise is blunted compared with animals made obese by high-carbohydrate feeding.[121] This accounts for the decrease in glucose transport in plasma membrane vesicles from the muscles of rats on a modestly high-fat diet.[121] In vitro evidence for altered intrinsic activity is seen in the effect of sodium oleate to increase basal glucose uptake in isolated adipocytes without changing GLUT-4 or GLUT-1 levels or subcellular distribution.[122] High-fat feeding results in alterations in membrane lipid composition, which could affect transporter translocation, docking and fusion with the plasma membrane, or activation. The change in lipid composition is also hypothesized to alter membrane phosphoinositide composition, which could alter the signal transduction mediated by phosphoinositol derivatives.[119]

In spite of insulin resistance, the decrease in GLUT-4 is not seen in all types of diet-induced obesity. Obesity induced by overfeeding a mixture of carbohydrate, fat, and protein results in increased fat mass, normal insulin concentrations, and normoglycemia.[120] Basal glucose transport is elevated in adipocytes from these animals, but the maximal rate of transport stimulated by insulin is unaltered. Compared with chow-fed lean control rats, GLUT-4 protein levels are unchanged in fat or skeletal muscle,[63,120] and transporter translocation and activation by insulin and exercise remain intact.[121]

Experimentally Induced Diabetes

Pancreatectomy[123] or chemical destruction of the pancreatic β-cells with streptozotocin[124] results in hypoinsulinemia, hyperglycemia, and secondary insulin resistance caused by a glucose transport defect.[123] In vivo glucose uptake is impaired within 24 hours as a result of impaired whole body glycolysis. This is followed by impaired suppression of hepatic glucose output by day 3 and impaired insulin-stimulated 2 deoxy-glucose (2DG) uptake into muscle by day 7.[125] GLUT-4 levels in white and brown adipose tissue are markedly downregulated within 48 hours.[124] In skeletal muscle, however, impaired glucose transport precedes significant alterations in muscle GLUT-4 content.[125] Furthermore, the degree of downregulation of GLUT-4 is quantitatively much greater in fat (more than fivefold by 3 days)[126] versus a 20% decrease in muscle GLUT-4 content by 14 days (Fig. 59-3).[125] Within muscle groups there are differences in the degree of downregulation of GLUT-4, with concentrations falling earliest in heart, then in red muscle, and finally in white muscle.[127] The decrease in muscle GLUT-4 content does not necessarily correspond to transport measurements, which may actually increase in white muscle (vastus lateralis) despite diminished GLUT-4 content[128] (Table 59-3). Fiber-specific differences in GLUT-4 content may reflect in part fiber-specific differences in GLUT-4 transcriptional regulation.[129] After 7 days of streptozotocin diabetes, GLUT-4 transcription is reduced by 35% and mRNA levels by 50% in red muscle, with no change in gene transcription and mRNA levels, which may be unchanged or increased in white muscle.[129] Importantly, although decreased

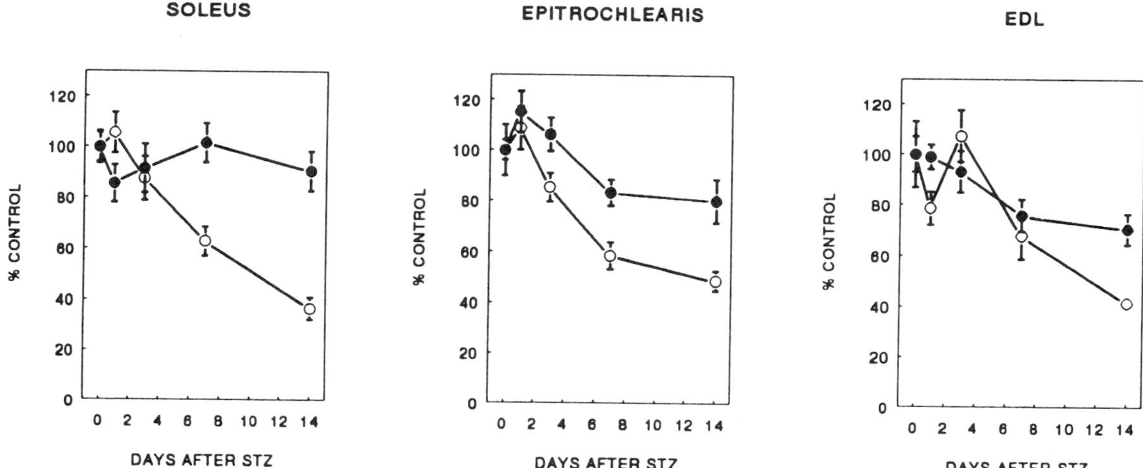

Figure 59-3. Time courses of changes in GLUT-4 protein content (●) and insulin-stimulated glucose uptake in vivo (○) in soleus, epitrochlearis, and EDL muscles 0–14 days after STZ (streptozotocin injection). Each point represents means ± SE for six to eight experiments, expressed as a percentage of the average value of the control. There is no significant change in soleus muscle GLUT-4 content at 14 days ($p = 0.56$ by ANOVA). At 7 days GLUT-4 protein levels are not reduced in any of the three muscles, but at 14 days GLUT-4 protein levels are reduced by 20% and 30% in the epitrochlearis and EDL, respectively ($p < 0.05$). On days 7 and 14, in vivo glucose uptake is reduced by 37 ± 6% and 63 ± 4%, respectively, in soleus ($p < 0.01$) and by 41 ± 5% and 51 ± 4% in epitrochlearis. In EDL, glucose uptake is decreased by 58 ± 3% at 14 days. There is no correlation between GLUT-4 protein content and maximal in vivo glucose uptake in soleus and EDL. In epihochlearis a weak relationship ($r^2 = 0.24$, $p < 0.01$) exists between GLUT-4 content and glucose uptake. (Reproduced with permission from Youn J, Kim J, Buchanan T. Time courses of changes in hepatic and skeletal muscle insulin action and GLUT4 protein in skeletal muscle after STZ injection. Diabetes 1994;43:546.)

Table 59-3. Discordance Between Glucose Transport and GLUT-4 and GLUT-1 Content in Specific Muscles After 12–16 Weeks of Streptozotocin Diabetes

Muscle	Fiber Type	GLUT-4	GLUT-1	In Vivo Glucose Uptake
Soleus	I	↓ 30%	(↔)	↓ 60%
Plantaris and red gastrocnemius	IIa + IIb	↓ 45%	(↔)	↔
White gastrocnemius	IIb	↓ 55%	↔	↑ 100%
Diaphragm	Ia + IIa + IIb	↓ 40%	↔	↓ 60%
Heart	—	↓ 70%	↓ 60%	↓ 75%

Source: Adapted from ref. 128.

transporter number is likely to play an important role in the maintenance of the insulin-resistant state, the initial defect probably involves impaired exposure of plasma membrane transporters to the extracellular milieu or decreased intrinsic activity.

In streptozotocin-induced diabetic rats, normalization of blood sugar with insulin treatment is associated with rapid restoration of insulin responsiveness and glucose transporter levels in fat and muscle.[124,130] Normalizing blood sugar levels with phlorizin, however, which blocks renal tubular reabsorption of glucose, thus enhancing glucose excretion, restores insulin responsiveness in isolated adipocytes without increasing GLUT-4 concentrations in the plasma membrane.[123] This suggests that alterations in blood glucose concentrations affect glucose transporter intrinsic activity. Interesting clues to signaling mechanisms that may be involved in the divergent effects of insulin- and phlorizin-induced restoration of insulin responsiveness are provided by studies of the 185-kd insulin receptor substrate IRS-1,[131] and GLUT-4 phosphorylation[130] in streptozotocin-induced diabetic rats. In muscle of streptozotocin-induced diabetic rats, insulin-stimulated phosphorylation of IRS-1 was impaired. This impairment was corrected by restoration of glucose concentrations with insulin treatment, which increased intrinsic activity and restores glucose transporter expression, but not when glucose concentrations were restored by phlorizin treatment, which only affects glucose transporter intrinsic activity. This implies that IRS-1 could be involved in signaling of glucose transporter transcription and translation but that it may not be associated with alterations in intrinsic activity.[131] Increased phosphorylation of the GLUT-4 transporter is seen in diabetic animals and is associated with diminished cytosolic phosphoserine phosphatase activity. Insulin treatment restores transporter phosphorylation to normal but phlorizin does not, implying that phosphorylation is not involved in regulation of the intrinsic activity of the transporter.[130]

Fasting

Fasting produces hypoinsulinemia and insulin resistance in fat.[132] Insulin-resistant glucose uptake into muscle in vivo is seen in anesthetized fasted rats but is milder (L. Rossetti personal communication) in chronically catheterized, awake rats. In brown and white adipose tissue and heart, GLUT-4 protein levels are significantly reduced, although GLUT-1 levels are unchanged.[127,133] In skeletal muscle, however, fasting results in a paradoxic increase in the abundance of both GLUT-1 and GLUT-4 despite insulin-resistant glucose uptake in the same model.[101,127,133] In adipocytes, fewer transporters are recruited to the plasma membrane as a result of the depleted intracellular pool.[133] In muscle, however, the translocation is actually increased.[134] Refeeding results in normalization of GLUT-4 content in skeletal muscle and a significant increase in GLUT-4 levels above control in fat.[133] There is a marked increase in glucose utilization by brown adipose tissue and muscle on refeeding, and these changes precede any change in GLUT-4 mRNA.[135] These data therefore indicate that the in vivo insulin resistance associated with fasting results largely from changes in the activation, fusion state, or intrinsic activity of the transporter.

Alteration of Glucose Transporters in Transgenic Models

Transgenic mice overexpressing glucose transporters have been created using either the native promoter or a heterologous promoter to target the expression to a single tissue. Transgenic mice expressing the 5′ untranslated region of the human GLUT-4 gene coupled to a reporter gene show expression limited to muscle and fat, identical to that of the endogenous mouse GLUT-4 gene.[13] The regulatory elements that confer this tissue specificity, as well as hormonal and metabolic regulation of the transgene, reside within 2.4 kb of the transcription initiation site.[13] Overexpression of the GLUT-4 gene product driven by its homologous promoter results in increased systemic glucose clearance and insulin-mediated glucose utilization in muscle in vivo. There is a marked increase in compensatory lipid mobilization and muscle glycogenolysis to maintain substrate availability in order to counteract fasting hypoglycemia.[136,137] Expression of this transgene in a mouse that is prone to insulin resistance and diabetes (C57BL/KsJ *db/db*) results in alleviation of the insulin resistance and in markedly enhanced glycemic control.[138] Overexpression of the human GLUT-4 gene selectively in fat using the aP2 promoter results in enhanced in vivo glucose disposal and hyperplastic obesity.[139] The number of GLUT-4 transporters is increased in plasma membranes of isolated adipocytes from these transgenic mice even in the absence of insulin.[139,140] This results in marked increases in basal and insulin-stimulated glucose transport in vitro, as well as enhanced whole body glucose tolerance.[140,141] This model demonstrates that the number of GLUT-4 transporters is rate limiting for glucose transport by adipose tissue and that increasing glucose transport into fat can enhance whole body glucose disposal.

Mice with genetic ablation of the GLUT-4 gene exhibit surprisingly normal ambient blood glucose concentrations despite glucose intolerance and significant insulin resistance. They are growth retarded and exhibit a diminished life span. They develop cardiac hypertrophy, heart failure and severely reduced adipose tissue. This model suggests that GLUT-4 is essential for normal cardiac function. Whether the decrease in adipocyte mass occurs as a result of loss of GLUT-4 or is secondary either to increased lipolysis or to the effect of chronic illness in these mice with heart failure is unclear. Skeletal muscle glucose uptake was not directly measured.[142] Further characterization of these animals will be necessary in order to determine the nature of the compensatory mechanisms which are responsible for relatively minor alterations in glucose homeostasis.[143]

Overexpression of the human GLUT-1 transporter in skeletal muscle using the myosin light chain promoter is associated with increased basal glucose transport and muscle glycogen synthesis in vitro, as well as enhanced glucose tolerance.[144,145] Insulin-mediated glucose uptake in vivo is impaired, however, as is the ability of insulin, IGF-1, hypoxia, and muscle contraction to increase glucose transport into skeletal muscle in vitro.[146] This model therefore suggests that increased basal glucose flux can inhibit the activation of glucose transport by stimuli that mediate this through GLUT-4 translocation and activation.

Other Models

Exercise-Induced Alterations in Insulin Sensitivity

Muscle contraction and insulin appear to stimulate GLUT-4 translocation by different mechanisms[147] and some data suggest that these two stimuli mobilize distinct pools of GLUT-4–containing vesicles.[148] In addition to acute effects of muscle contraction on glucose transporter translocation and intrinsic activity, chronic exercise training increases insulin sensitivity in animals.[149] The beneficial effects of chronic exercise training are associated with significant increases in GLUT-4 levels in muscle and fat in normal[149] and insulin-resistant rats[150] and are more pronounced in younger animals.[151] The elevated GLUT-4 levels in skeletal muscle persist for several days after cessation of training even after glucose transport rates return to baseline.[149,152] There are fiber-specific differences in GLUT-4 content, as well as insulin-stimulated and contraction-mediated increases in glucoses transport.[150,152] This is exemplified by studies in endurance-trained Zucker rats in which the increase in GLUT-4 content in the plantaris muscle with exercise corresponds with increased insulin- and contraction-stimulated glucose transport. In contrast, in soleus muscle, an increase in GLUT-4 content is associated with an increase in contraction-stimulated glucose transport, whereas insulin-stimulated glucose transport remains unchanged from baseline.[150] In skeletal muscle, chronic exercise training produces a marked increase in GLUT-4 protein in the plasma membrane in the basal state and after insulin stimulation.[153] The increase in GLUT-4 content in skeletal muscle is associated with increased hexokinase II activity and glycogen synthesis.[153] Intrinsic activity is unchanged,[150] in contrast to the situation of white adipocytes, in which intrinsic activity might also be increased by exercise.[115] The changes in glucose clearance rates seen with chronic exercise training are at least partially explained by the increased numbers of transporters in the plasma membrane. The presence of additional factors is suggested by the reduction of transport with cessation of training despite persistent elevations of GLUT-4.

Physical Inactivity and Denervation

Physical inactivity in rats results in in vivo insulin resistance.[154] This insulin-resistant state is associated with decreased GLUT-4 concentrations in gastrocnemius and quadriceps muscles.[154] Soleus muscle, however, shows hyper-responsive, insulin-stimulated glucose uptake, which is associated with increased levels of GLUT-4.[155] These data indicate that the effect of physical inactivity on regulating glucose transporter expression varies with fiber type.

Denervation of muscle results in insulin resistance that is dependent on muscle fiber type but is not associated with defects in activation of the insulin receptor.[156] GLUT-4 protein levels are progressively downregulated in muscle after denervation, which can be reversed with electrical stimulation in the absence of contraction.[155,157] As is also seen in streptozotocin diabetes, however, insulin resistance develops before the decline in GLUT-4 content,[155] indicating that the decrease in GLUT-4 content alone cannot explain the onset of the insulin-resistant state.

Oral Antidiabetic Agents

A number of established and potential therapeutic agents act in part by improving insulin sensitivity. The possibility that these effects are mediated through changes in GLUT-4 concentration or function has been investigated. The sulphonylurea glimepiride increases GLUT-4 translocation and decreases its phosphorylation in cultured rat adipocytes.[158] The biguanide metformin reverses the downregulation of GLUT-4 translocation to the plasma membrane, as observed in adipocytes cultured in the presence of insulin.[159] In vivo administration of metformin to *fa/fa* Zucker rats is associated with increased insulin-stimulated glucose transport in adipocytes, increased translocation of GLUT-4 and GLUT-1 to the plasma membrane, and increased intrinsic activity of the transporters.[160] In the same model, metformin treatment improved in vivo glucose transport without altering GLUT-4 abundance in muscle.[161] Application of metformin to cultured L6 myocytes in vivo increased glucose transport without changing GLUT-4 abundance or translocation. The increased transport was accounted for by increased translocation of GLUT-1 to the plasma membrane of metformin-treated cells.[162] Data in humans are sparse, but increased GLUT-1 expression has been noted in fibroblasts obtained from diabetics after metformin treatment.[162]

The thiazolidinedione pioglitazone increases the expression of GLUT-1 and GLUT-4 in 3T3F442A cells through stabilization of the mRNA transcript[163] and enhances the differentiation of 3T3L1 adipocytes by accelerating the rate at which metabolically important genes such as GLUT-4, lipoprotein lipase, and glucose-6-phosphate dehydrogenase become activated.[164] In vivo administration of pioglitazone reverses dexamethasone-induced insulin resistance in rats without changing GLUT-4 levels in skeletal muscle.[165] The specific mechanism by which thiazolidinediones modulate glucose uptake in vivo remains to be elucidated. Vanadate induces GLUT-4 translocation in rat adipocytes in vitro[166] and increases GLUT-4 intrinsic activity in sarcolemmal vesicles.[26] In vivo vanadate increases glucose utilization in the muscle of *fa/fa* rats without changing GLUT-4 expression.[62] In addition to its effect on muscle glucose transport, vanadate exhibits multiple metabolic effects in vivo, which counteract the dysregulated glucose homeostasis in experimental diabetes (streptozotocin induced). These effects include inhibition of the diabetes-induced upregulation of phosphoenolpyruvate-carboxykinase, tyrosine aminotransferase, and hydroxymethylglutaryl (HMG) coA reductase. Hepatic GLUT-2 levels are decreased, and the downregulation of glucokinase and pyruvate kinase is reversed.[167]

Thyroid Hormone

Thyroid hormone plays an important role in the upregulation of GLUT-4 and the downregulation of GLUT-1, which occur shortly after birth.[168] Treatment of normal rats with thyroid hormone is associated with increased basal and insulin-stimulated glucose uptake in skeletal muscle. GLUT-4 content is increased in these muscles, which accounts for the enhanced insulin-mediated glucose uptake but not the basal uptake.[169] GLUT-4 levels in the plasma membrane of both muscle and adipocytes from hyperthyroid rats are greatly elevated in the basal state but are normal in the insulin-stimulated state, indicating a dysregulation in GLUT-4 distribution.[170,171] Conversely, hypothyroid rats show reduced GLUT-4 content in muscle. Hypothyroidism is associated with increased GLUT-1 content in rat heart.[172] GLUT-4 levels in heart, however, are not altered by either hypothyroidism or hyperthyroidism despite increased cardiac glucose uptake in the hyperthyroid animals.[172]

Cold Exposure

Cold exposure increases metabolic activity and glucose transport rate acutely in brown fat without changing GLUT-4 levels. With chronic exposure, GLUT-4 protein levels increase in brown fat, although a similar rise is not seen in muscle. This effect is abolished by sympathectomy.[173,174]

Tumor Necrosis Factor

The cytokine tumor necrosis factor-α (TNFα) has been recently proposed to play a role in the insulin resistance of obesity and NIDDM.[175] Infusion of TNFα causes insulin resistance in rats.[176] TNFα expression is elevated in the adipose tissue of multiple experimental models of obesity. Neutralization of TNFα in one such model, the Zucker (*fa/fa*) rat, results in improved insulin sensitivity.[175] TNFα mediates insulin resistance at multiple levels and appears to act primarily as a potent inhibitor of the insulin-stimulated tyrosine phosphorylation on the β-subunit of the insulin receptor and of IRS-1. TNFα has been shown to downregulate GLUT-4 mRNA levels in adipocyte and myocyte cultures. In fat cells, this effect occurs in the context of downregulation of the expression of several fat-specific genes, such as aP2 and adipsin, indicating that the effect is not entirely specific. Furthermore, TNFα can dramatically inhibit insulin-stimulated glucose transport in adipocytes at doses that have no effect on the cellular content of GLUT-4. Muscle levels of GLUT-4 are not downregulated in animal models of obesity in which TNFα expression is increased, and neutralization of TNFα in these models has no effect on GLUT-4 mRNA expression despite improvements in insulin sensitivity. Current evidence therefore suggests that the effect of TNFα on glucose transport is mediated by its effects on the proximal insulin-signaling pathway.[175]

Summary

Alterations in insulin responsiveness in vivo result from changes in GLUT-4 gene expression, as well as changes in the function of the GLUT-4 protein. GLUT-4 expression undergoes tissue-specific regulation in insulin-resistant states; in many models, greater changes in glucose transporter gene expression are seen in adipose cells than in muscle. Both ambient insulin and ambient glucose concentrations affect GLUT-4, but in different ways. GLUT-4 protein levels are not altered in muscle or fat by glucose infusion or in fat by restoration of elevated glucose concentrations to normal in diabetic rats with phlorizin. In contrast, GLUT-4 content is depressed in both the muscle and fat of hypoinsulinemic animal models of diabetes, and GLUT-4 is restored to normal by insulin treatment. Whereas insulin treatment of normal animals increases GLUT-4 expression in fat, insulin-resistant animals with endogenous hyperinsulinemia and euglycemia do not show major alterations in GLUT-4 protein content in skeletal muscle, the most important site of insulin-stimulated glucose disposal. In contrast, in adipose tissue from these models, GLUT-4 content may be reduced or increased, and these alterations in GLUT-4 tend to parallel changes in insulin responsiveness in isolated adipocytes. The quantitative contribution of adipocyte glucose transport to in vivo glucose disposal is thought to be small. Therefore, downregulation of the GLUT-4 content in adipose tissue may contribute minimally to whole-body insulin resistance. However, recent data in transgenic mice overexpressing GLUT-4 exclusively in fat indicate that under certain circumstances, adipose tissue may play an important role in in vivo glucose disposal.

Defects in insulin-stimulated translocation of glucose transporters in muscle may play a role in some models of insulin resistance, such as the Zucker rat, but are unlikely to be the primary mechanism causing insulin resistance in all models. With high-fat feeding, impaired activation of GLUT-4 intrinsic activity is the major cause of insulin-resistant glucose transport in muscle. In states such as fasting and streptozotocin diabetes, in vivo circulating or local factors appear to impair the action of GLUT-4 in muscle, either by interfering with membrane docking/fusion or by decreasing transporter intrinsic activity. Glucose transporter intrinsic activity can also be altered in adipose cells—for example, with phlorizin treatment of diabetic rats or refeeding of fasted rats.

Whereas glucose transporter levels are altered in fat in many insulin-resistant models, glucose transporter levels in muscle are largely unaffected. Even in states in which transporter expression is reduced in muscle, this does not appear to be the primary lesion responsible for the onset of insulin resistance, as resistance develops before glucose transporter content decreases. Once glucose transporter levels are lowered, however, the reductions are likely to influence the progression and severity of the insulin-resistant state. Even though impairment of GLUT-4 expression may not be the primary lesion in most insulin-resistant states, increased GLUT-4 abundance in muscle during exercise training are associated with increased in vivo insulin responsiveness. Therefore, future approaches to overcoming insulin resistance may involve efforts to augment GLUT-4 expression in muscle, as well as attempts to modulate currently unknown factors involved in GLUT-4 translocation, fusion with the plasma membrane, and activation.

References

1. Rothman DL, Shulman RG, Shulman GI. 31P nuclear magnetic resonance measurements of muscle glucose-6-phosphate. J Clin Invest 1992;89:1069
2. Butler P, Kryshak E, Marsh M, Rizza R. Effect of insulin on oxidation of intracellularly and extracellularly derived glucose in patients with NIDDM: Evidence for primary defect in glucose transport and/or phosphorylation but not oxidation. Diabetes 1990;39:1373
3. Yki-Jarvinen H, Sahlin K, Ren JM, Koivisto VA. Localization of rate-limiting defect for glucose disposal in skeletal muscle of insulin-resistant type I diabetic patients. Diabetes 1990;39:157
4. Garvey WT, Maianu L, Huecksteadt TP, et al. Pretranslational suppression of a glucose transporter protein causes insulin resistance in adipocytes from patients with non–insulin-dependent diabetes mellitus and obesity. J Clin Invest 1991;87:1072
5. Dohm GL, Tapscott EB, Pories WJ, et al. An in vitro human muscle preparation suitable for metabolic studies. J Clin Invest 1988;82:486
6. Friedman J, Dohm G, Leggett-Frazier N, et al. Restoration of insulin responsiveness in skeletal muscle of morbidly obese patients after weight loss. Effect on muscle glucose transport and glucose transporter. J Clin Invest 1992;89:701
7. Fink R, Wallace P, Brechtel G, Olefsky J. Evidence that glucose transport is rate limiting for in vivo glucose uptake. Metabolism 1992;41:897
8. Katz A, Nyomba B, Bogardus C. No accumulation of glucose in human skeletal muscle during euglycemic hyperinsulinemia. Am J Physiol 1988;255:E942
9. Yki-Jarvinen H, Helve E, Koivisot V. Hyperglycemia decreases glucose uptake in type I diabetes. Diabetes 1987;36:892
10. Ziel F, Venkatesan N, Davidson M. Glucose transport is rate limiting for skeletal muscle glucose metabolism in normal and streptozotocin induced diabetic rats. Diabetes 1988;37:885
11. Waddell ID, Zomerschoe AG, Voice MW, Burchell A. Cloning and expression of a hepatic microsomal glucose transporter protein. Biochem J 1992;286:173
12. Bell GI, Kayano T, Buse JB, et al. Molecular biology of mammalian glucose transporters. Diabetes Care 1990;13:198
13. Olson A, Liu M, Moye-Rowley W, et al. Hormonal/metabolic regulation of the human GLUT4/muscle-fat facilitative glucose transporter gene in transgenic mice. J Biol Chem 1993;268:9839
14. Zorzano A, Wilkinson W, Kotliar N, et al. Insulin-regulated glucose uptake in rat adipocytes is mediated by two transporter isoforms present in at least two vesicle populations. J Biol Chem 1989;264:12358
15. James D, Piper R. Mini-review on the cellular mechanisms of disease. J Cell Biol 1994;126:1123
16. Kandror K, Pilch P. gp160, a tissue-specific marker for insulin-activated glucose transport. Proc Natl Acad Sci USA 1994;91:8017
17. Mastick CC, Aebersold R, Lienhard GE. Characterisation of a major protein in GLUT4 vesicles. J Biol Chem 1994;269:6089
18. Shepherd P, Kahn B. Cellular defects in glucose transport: Lessons from

animal models and implications for human insulin resistance. In: Moller DE, ed. Insulin Resistance. London, Wiley;1993:253–300
19. Cormont M, Tanti JF, Zahraoui A, et al. Insulin and okadaic acid induce rab4 redistribution in adipocytes. J Biol Chem 1993;268:19491
20. Ricort JM, Tanti JF, et al. Parallel changes in GLUT4 and Rab4 movements in two insulin resistant states. FEBS Lett 1994;347:42
21. Clark A, Holman G, Kozka I. Determination of the rates of appearance and loss of glucose transporters at the cell surface of rat adipose cells. Biochem J 1991;278:235
22. Vannucci SJ, Nishimura H, Satoh S, et al. Cell surface accessibility of Glut 4 glucose transporters in insulin stimulated rat adipose cells. Modulation by isoprenaline and adenosine. Biochem J 1992;(288):325
23. Bonen A, Megeney L, McCarthy S, et al. Epinephrine administration stimulates GLUT4 translocation but reduces glucose transport in muscle. Biochem Biophys Res Commun 1992;187:685
24. Shepherd PR, Kahn BB. Expression of the GLUT4 glucose transporter in diabetes. In Draznin B, LeRoith D, eds. Molecular Biology of Diabetes, Vol. II. Totowa, NJ: Humana Press;1994:535–536
25. Clancy B, Harrison S, Buxton J, Czech M. Protein synthesis inhibitors activate glucose transport without increasing plasma membrane glucose transporters in 3T3-L1 adipocytes. J Biol Chem 1991;266:10122
26. Okumura N, Shimazu T. Vanadate stimulates D-glucose transport into sarcolemmal vesicles from rat skeletal muscles. J Biochem 1992;112:107
27. Jhun B, Rampal A, Liu H, et al. Effects of insulin on steady state kinetics of GLUT4 subcellular distribution in rat adipocytes. Evidence of constitutive GLUT4 recycling. J Biol Chem 1992;267:17710
28. DeFronzo RA, Jacot E, Jequier E, et al. The effect of insulin on the disposal of intravenous glucose. Diabetes 1981;30:1000
29. Koranyi L, Bourey R, Vuorinen-Markkola H, et al. Level of skeletal muscle glucose transporter protein correlates with insulin stimulated whole body glucose disposal in man. Diabetologia 1991;34:763
30. Kusari J, Verma US, Buse JB, et al. Analysis of the gene sequences of the insulin receptor and the insulin-sensitive glucose transporter (GLUT4) in patients with common-type non–insulin-dependent diabetes mellitus. J Clin Invest 1991;88:1323
31. Choi W-H, O'Rahilly S, Buse JB, et al. Molecular scanning of insulin-responsive glucose transporter (GLUT4) gene in NIDDM subjects. Diabetes 1991;40:1712
32. Bjorbaek C, Echwald S, Hubricht P, et al. Genetic variants in promoters and coding regions of the muscle glycogen synthase and the insulin-responsive GLUT4 genes in NIDDM. Diabetes 1994;43:976
33. Baroni M, Oelbaum R, Pozzilli P, et al. Polymorphisms at the GLUT1 (HepG2) and GLUT4 (muscle/adipocyte) glucose transporter genes and non–insulin-dependent diabetes mellitus (NIDDM). Hum Genet 1992;88:557
34. Baroni MG, Alcolado JC, Gragnoli C, et al. Affected sib pair analysis of the GLUT1 glucose transporter gene locus in non–insulin-dependent-diabetes mellitus (NIDDM): Evidence for no linkage. Hum Genet 1994;93:675
35. Pedersen O, Bak JF, Andersen PH, et al. Evidence against altered expression of Glut 1 or Glut 4 in skeletal muscle of patients with obesity or NIDDM. Diabetes 1990;39:865
36. Garvey WT, Maianu L, Hancock JA, et al. Gene expression of Glut 4 in skeletal muscle from insulin resistant patients with obesity, IGT, GDM, and NIDDM. Diabetes 1992;41:465
37. Kahn BB, Rosen AS, Bak JS, et al. Expression of Glut 1 and Glut 4 glucose transporters in skeletal muscle of humans with insulin dependent diabetes mellitus: Regulatory effects of metabolic factors. J Clin Endocrinol Metab 1992;74:1101
38. Koivisto V, Bourey R, Vuorinen-Markkola H, Koranyi L. Exercise reduces muscle glucose transport protein (GLUT-4) mRNA in type 1 diabetic patients. J Appl Physiol 1993;74:1755
39. Vogt B, Muhlbacher C, Carrascosa J, et al. Subcellular distribution of GLUT 4 in the skeletal muscle of lean type 2 (non–insulin-dependent) diabetic patients in the basal state. Diabetologia 1992;35:456
40. Dohm GL, Elton CW, Friedman JE, et al. Decreased expression of glucose transporter in muscle from insulin-resistant patient. Am J Physiol 1991; 260:E459
41. Friedman J, Dohm G, Elton C, et al. Muscle insulin resistance in uremic humans: Glucose transport, glucose transporters and insulin receptors. Am J Physiol 1991;261:E87
42. Flier J, Moller D, Moses A, et al. Insulin-mediated pseudoacromegaly: Clinical and biochemical characterization of a syndrome of selective insulin resistance. J Clin Endocrinol Metab 1993;76:1533
43. Garvey WT. Glucose transport and NIDDM. Diabetes Care 1992;15:396
44. Vestergaard H, Weinreb JE, Rosen AS, et al. Sylfonylurea therapy improves glucose disposal without changing skeletal muscle GLUT4 levels in NIDDM subjects: A longitudinal study. J Clin Endocrinol Metab 1995;80:270
45. Andersen P, Lund S, Vestergaard H, et al. Expression of the major insulin regulatable glucose transporter (GLUT4) in skeletal muscle of noninsulin-dependent diabetic patients and healthy subjects before and after insulin infusion. J Clin Endocrinol Metab 1993;77:27
46. Yki-Jarvinen H, Vuorinen-Markkola H, Koranyi L, et al. Defect in insulin action on expression of the muscle/adipose tissue glucose transporter gene in skeletal muscle of type 1 diabetic patients. J Clin Endocrinol Metab 1992;75:795
47. Elahi D, McAloon-Dyke M, Clark B, et al. Sequential evaluation of islet cell responses to glucose in the transplanted pancreas in humans. Am J Surg 1993;165:15
48. Guma A, Zierath J, Wallberg-Henriksson H, Klip A. Insulin induces translocation of GLUT-4 glucose transporters in human skeletal muscle. Am J Physiol 1995;268:E613
49. Lund S, Vestergaard H, Andersen P, et al. GLUT-4 content in plasma membrane of muscle from patients with non–insulin-dependent diabetes mellitus. Am J Physiol 1993;265:E889
50. Rosenbaum D, Haber RS, Dunaif A. Insulin resistance in polycystic ovary syndrome: Decreased expression of GLUT4 glucose transporters in adipocytes. Am J Physiol 1993;264:E197
51. Garvey WT, Maianu L, Zhu JH, et al. Multiple defects in the adipocyte glucose transport system cause cellular insulin resistance in gestational diabetes. Heterogeneity in the number and a novel abnormality in subcellular localization of GLUT4 glucose transporters. Diabetes 1993;42:1773
52. Marin P, Rebuffe-Scrive M, Smith U, Bjorntorp P. Glucose uptake in human adipose tissue. Metabolism 1987;36:1154
53. Houmard JA, Egan PC, Neufer PD, et al. Elevated skeletal muscle glucose transporter levels in exercise-trained middle-aged man. Am J Physiol 1991;261:E437
54. Hughes V, Fiatarone M, Fielding R, et al. Exercise increases muscle GLUT-4 levels and insulin action in subject with impaired glucose tolerance. Am J Physiol 1993;264:E855
55. Houmard J, Shinebarger M, Dolan P, et al. Exercise training increases GLUT-4 protein concentration in previously sedentary middle-aged men. Am J Physiol 1993;264:E896
56. Dela F, Ploug T, Handberg A, et al. Physical training increases muscle GLU4 protein and mRNA in patients with NIDDM. Diabetes 1994;43:862
57. Andersen P, Lund S, Schmitz O, et al. Increased insulin-stimulated glucose uptake in athletes: The importance of GLUT4 mRNA, GLUT4 protein and fibre type composition of skeletal muscle. Acta Physiol Scand 1993;149: 393
58. Bodkin N, Metzger B, Hansen B. Hepatic glucose production and insulin sensitivity preceding diabetes in monkeys. Am J Physiol 1989;256: E676
59. Zarjevski N, Doyle P, Jeanrenaud B. Muscle insulin resistance may not be a primary etiological factor in the genetically obese *fa/fa* rat. Endocrinology 1992;130:1564
60. Penicaud L, Ferre P, Terretaz J, et al. Development of obesity in Zucker rats. Diabetes 1987;36:626
61. Pedersen O, Kahn CR, Kahn BB. Divergent regulation of the Glut 1 and Glut 4 glucose transporters in isolated adipocytes from Zucker rats. J Clin Invest 1992;89:1964
62. Brichard S, Assimacopoulos-Jeannet F, Jeanrenaud B. Vanadate treatment markedly increases glucose utilization in muscle of insulin-resistant *fa/fa* rats without modifying glucose transporter expression. Endocrinology 1992;131: 311
63. Kahn BB, Pedersen O. Suppression of Glut 4 expression in skeletal muscle of rats that are obese from high fat feeding but not from high carbohydrate feeding or genetic obesity. Endocrinology 1993;132:13
64. Galante P, Scholz MER, Rett K, et al. Insulin-induced translocation of GLUT4 in skeletal muscle of insulin-resistant Zucker rats. Diabetologia 1994;37:3
65. King P, Horton E, Hirshman M, Horton E. Insulin resistance in obese Zucker rat (*fa/fa*) skeletal muscle is associated with a failure of glucose transporter translocation. J Clin Invest 1992;90:1568
66. Brozinick JT, Etgen GJ, Yaspelkis BB, Ivy JL. Contraction activated glucose uptake is normal in insulin resistant muscle of the obese Zucker rat. J Appl Physiol 1992;73:382
67. Petersen S, Russ M, Reinauer H, Eckel J. Inverse regulation of glucose transporter Glut4 and G-protein Gs mRNA expression in cardiac myocytes of insulin resistant rats. FEBS Lett 1991;286:1
68. Betts J, Valyou PM, Hirshman M, et al. Adrenalectomy and glucose metabolism in the obese (*fa/fa*) Zucker rat. Diabetes 1991;41:152A
69. Stubbs M, York DA. Central glucocorticoid regulation of parasympathetic drive to pancreatic β-cells in the obese *fa/fa* rat. Int J Obes 1991;15:547
70. Slieker L, Sundell K, Heath W, et al. Glucose transporter levels in tissues of spontaneously diabetic Zucker *fa/fa* rat (ZDF/drt) and viable yellow mouse (*Avy/a*). Diabetes 1992;41:187
71. Friedman J, Venti J, Peterson R, Dohm G. Altered expression of muscle glucose transporter GLUT4 in diabetic fatty Zucker rats (ZDF/Drt-fa). Am J Physiol 1991;261:E782
72. Yamamoto T, Fukumoto H, Koh G, et al. Liver and muscle fat type glucose transporter gene expression in obese and diabetic rats. Biochem Biophys Res Commun 1991;175:995
73. Chan T, Tatoyan A. Glucose transport in the perfused hindquarters of lean and obese hyperglycemic (*db/db*) mice: Effect of insulin and electrical stimulation. Biochem Biophys Acta 1984;798:325
74. Koranyi L, James D, Muekler M, Permutt MA. Glucose transporter levels in spontaneously obese (*db/db*) insulin resistant mice. J Clin Invest 1990; 85:962
75. Begin-Heick N. Adenylate cyclase in lean and obese (*ob/ob*) mouse epididymal white adipocytes. Can J Biochem 1980;58:1033
76. Zhang Y, Proenca R, Maffei M, et al. Positional cloning of the mouse obese gene and its human homologue. Nature 1994;372:425
77. Grundleger M, Godbole V, Thenen S. Age related development of insulin

resistance of soleus muscle in genetically obese (*ob/ob*) mice. Am J Physiol 1980;239:E363

78. McGinnis R, Walker J, Margules D. Genetically obese (*ob/ob*) mice are hypersensitive to glucocorticoid stimulation of feeding but dramatically resist glucocorticoid induced weight loss. Life Sci 1987;40:1561
79. Ohshima K, Shargill N, Chan T, Bray G. Adrenalectomy reverses insulin resistance in muscle from obese (*ob/ob*) mice. Am J Physiol 1984;246: E193
80. Brichard S, Bailey C, Henquin J. Marked improvement of glucoses homeostasis in diabetic *ob/ob* mice given oral vandate. Diabetes 1990;39:1326–1332
81. Lachaal M, Jung C. Insulin resistance in hypertension. Mol Cell Biochem 1992;109:119
82. Reaven G, Chang H, Hoffman B, Azhar S. Resistance to insulin stimulated glucose uptake in adipocytes isolated from spontaneously hypertensive rats. Diabetes 1989;38:1155
83. Frontoni S, Haywood J, DeFronzo R, Rossetti L. In vivo insulin action in genetic models of hypertension. Am J Physiol 1992;262:E191
84. Mondon C, Reaven G. Evidence of abnormalities of insulin metabolism in rats with spontaneous hypertension. Metabolism 1988;37:303
85. Bader S, Scholz R, Kellerer M, et al. Normal insulin receptor tyrosine kinase activity and glucose transporter (GLUT4) levels in skeletal muscle of hyperinsulinaemic hypertensive rats. Diabetologia 1992;35:712
86. Campbell IW, Dominiczak AF, Livingstone C, Gould GW. Analysis of the glucose transporter compliment of metabolically important tissues from the Milan hypertensive rat. Biochem Biophys Res Commun 1995;211:780
87. Lowell BB, Susulic V, Hamann A, et al. Development of obesity in transgenic mice after genetic ablation of brown adipose tissue. Nature 1993;366:740
88. Hamann A, Berecke H, Le Marchand-Brustel Y, et al. Characterization of insulin resistance and NIDDM in transgenic mice with reduced brown fat. Diabetes 1995;44:1266
89. Frevert EU, Hamann A, Lowell BB, Flier JS, Kahn BB. Decreased insulin action precedes down regulation of Glut4 in adipocytes in a novel transgenic model of obesity and NIDDM. Diabetes 1995;44(1):38A
90. Hofmann C, Lorenz K, Colca J. Glucose transporter deficiency in diabetic animals is corrected by treatment with the oral antihyperglycemic agent pioglitizone. Endocrinology 1991;129:1915
91. Marette A, Atgie C, Liu Z, et al. Differential regulation of GLUT1 and GLUT4 glucose transporters in skeletal muscle of a new model of type II diabetes. The obese SHR/N-cp rat. Diabetes 1993;42:1195
92. Kern M, Mondon C, Butte J, Azhar S. Glucose transporter (GLUT 4) content and insulin receptor kinase activity in muscles of the LA/N-cp rat. Horm Metab Res 1994;26:129
93. Cousin B, Agou K, Leturque A, et al. Molecular and metabolic changes in white adipose tissue of the rat during development of ventromedial hypothalamic obesity. Eur J Biochem 1992;207:377
94. Marchand-Brustel Y, Olichon-Berthe C, Gremeaux T, et al. Glucose transporter in insulin sensitive tissues of lean and obese mice: Effect of thermogenic agent BRL26830A. Endocrinology 1990;127:2687
95. Zarjevski N, Cusin I, Vettor R, et al. Intracerebroventricular administration of neuropeptide Y to normal rats has divergent effects on glucose utilization by adipose tissue and skeletal muscle. Diabetes 1994;43:764
96. Machado U, Shimizu Y, Saito M. Decreased glucose transporter (GLUT 4) content in insulin-sensitive tissues of obese aurothioglucose- and monosodium glutamate–treated mice. Horm Metab Res 1993;25:462
97. Machado U, Shimizu I, Saito M. Reduced content and preserved translocation of glucose transporter (GLUT 4) in white adipose tissue of obese mice. Physiol Behav 1994;55:621
98. Cusin I, Terrattaz J, Rohner-Jeanrenaud F, Jeanrenaud B. Metabolic consequences of hyperinsulinaemia imposed on normal rats on glucose handling by white adipose tissue, muscles and liver. Biochem J 1990;267:99
99. Kahn BB, Cushman SW. Mechanism for markedly hyperresponsive insulin-stimulated glucose transport activity in adipose cells from insulin-treated streptozotocin diabetic rats. J Biol Chem 1987;262:5118
100. Flores-Riveros J, McLenithan J, Ezaki O, Lane M. Insulin down-regulates expression of the insulin-responsive glucose transporter (GLUT4) gene: Effects on transcription and mRNA turnover. Proc Natl Acad Sci USA 1993;90:512
101. Bourey R, Koranyi L, James D, et al. Effects of altered glucose homeostasis on glucose transporter expression in skeletal muscle of the rat. J Clin Invest 1990;86:542
102. Cusin I, Terrattaz J, Rohner-Jeanrenaud F, et al. Hyperinsulinemia increases the amount of GLUT4 mRNA in white adipose tissue and decreases it in muscle: A clue for increased fat depot and insulin resistance. Endocrinology 1990;127:3246
103. Hager SR, Pastorek D, Jochen AL, Meier D. Divergence between GLUT4 mRNA and protein abundance in skeletal muscle of insulin resistant rats. Biochem Biophys Res Commun 1991;181:240
104. Haber R, Weinstein S. Role of glucose transporters in glucocorticoid-induced insulin resistance: GLUT4 isoform in rat skeletal muscle is not decreased by dexamethasone. Diabetes 1992;41:728
105. Giogino F, Almahfouz A, Goodyear LJ, Smith RJ. Glucocorticoid regulation of insulin receptor and substrate IRS-1 tyrosine phosphorylation in rat skeletal muscle in vivo. J Clin Invest 1993;91:2020
106. Carter-Su C, Okamoto K. Effect of insulin and glucocorticoids on glucose transport in rat adipocytes. Am J Physiol 1987;252:E441
107. McGrane M, Yun J, Moorman A, et al. Metabolic effects of developmental, tissue, and cell specific expression of chimeric phosphoenolpyruvate carboxykinase (GTP)/bovine growth hormone gene in transgenic mice. J Biol Chem 1990;265:22371
108. Tai P, Liao J, Chen E, et al. Differential regulation of two glucose transporters by chronic growth hormone treatment of cultured 3T3-F442A adipose cells. J Biol Chem 1990;265:21828
109. Oka Y, Asano T, Lin J, et al. Expression of glucose transporter isoforms with aging. Gerontology 1992;38:3
110. Schoenle E, Zapf J, Froesch E. Regulation of rat adipocyte glucose transport by growth hormone: No mediation by insulin-like growth factors. Endocrinology 1983;112:384
111. Houmard J, Weidner M, Dolan P, et al. GLUT-4 protein concentration in human skeletal muscle is negatively related to chronological age. Diabetes 1995;44:555
112. Cartee G. Myocardial GLUT-4 glucose transporter protein levels of rats decline with advancing age. J Gerontol 1993;48:B168
113. Gulve E, Henriksen E, Rodnick K, et al. Glucose transporters and glucose transport in skeletal muscles of 1- to 25-mo-old rats. Am J Physiol 1993; 264:E319
114. Ezaki O, Fukuda N, Itakura H. Role of two types of glucose transporters in enlarged adipocytes from aged and obese rats. Diabetes 1990;39:1543
115. Stallknecht B, Andersen P, Vinten J, et al. Effect of physical training on glucose transporter protein and mRNA levels in rat adipocytes. Am J Physiol 1993;265:E128
116. Matthaei S, Benecke H, Klein H, et al. Potential mechanism of insulin resistance in aging: Impaired insulin stimulated glucose transport due to a depletion of the intracellular pool of glucose transporters in Fischer rat adipocytes. J Endocrinol 1990;126:99
117. Johnson AB, Argyraki M, Thow JC, et al. Effect of increased free fatty acid supply on glucose metabolism and skeletal muscle glycogen synthase activity in normal man. Clin Sci 1992;82:219
118. Kraegen E, James D, Storlein L, et al. In vivo insulin resistance in individual peripheral tissues of the high fat fed rat: Assessment by euglycemic clamp plus deoxyglucose administration. Diabetologia 1986;29:192
119. Storlien L, Jenkins A, Chisholm D, et al. Influence of dietary rat composition on development of insulin resistance in rats: Relationship to muscle triglyceride and omega 3 fatty acids in muscle phospholipid. Diabetes 1991;40: 280
120. Pedersen O, Kahn CR, Flier JS, Kahn BB. High fat feeding causes insulin resistance and a marked decrease in the expression of glucose transporters (Glut 4) in fat cells of rats. Endocrinology 1991;129:771
121. Rosholt M, King P, Horton E. High-fat diet reduces glucose transporter responses to both insulin and exercise. Am J Physiol 1994;266:R95
122. Murer E, Boden G, Gyda M, Deluca F. Effects of oleate and insulin on glucose uptake, oxidation, and glucose transporter proteins in rat adipocytes. Diabetes 1992;41:1063
123. Kahn BB, Shulman GI, Defronzo RA, et al. Normalization of blood glucose in diabetic rats with phlorizin treatment reverse insulin-resistant glucose transport in adipose cells without restoring glucose transporter gene expression. J Clin Invest 1991;87:561
124. Kahn BB, Rossetti L, Lodish HF, Charron MJ. Decreased in vivo glucose uptake but normal expression of Glut 1 and Glut 4 in skeletal muscle of diabetic rats. J Clin Invest 1991;87:2197
125. Youn J, Kim J, Buchanan T. Time courses of changes in hepatic and skeletal muscle insulin action and GLUT4 protein in skeletal muscle after STZ injection. Diabetes 1994;43:564
126. Sivitz W, DeSautel S, Lee E, Pessin J. Time-dependent regulation of rat adipose tissue glucose transporter (GLUT4) mRNA and protein by insulin in streptozocin-diabetic and normal rats. Metabolism 1992;41:1267
127. Camps M, Castello A, Munoz P, et al. Effect of diabetes and fasting on GLUT-4 (muscle/fat) glucose-transporter expression in insulin-sensitive tissues. Heterogeneous response in heart, red and white muscle. Biochem J 1992;282:765
128. Kainulainen H, Breiner M, Schurmann A, et al. In vivo glucose uptake and glucose transporter proteins GLUT1 and GLUT4 in heart and various types of skeletal muscle from streptozotocin-diabetic rats. Biochim Biophys Acta 1994;1225:275
129. Neufer P, Carey J, Dohm G. Transcriptional regulation of the gene for glucose transporter GLUT4 in skeletal muscle. Effects of diabetes and fasting. J Biol Chem 1993;268:13824
130. Begum N, Draznin B. Effect of streptozotocin-induced diabetes on GLUT-4 phosphorylation in rat adipocytes. J Clin Invest 1992;90:1254
131. Giorgino F, Chen J, Smith R. Changes in tyrosine phosphorylation of insulin receptors and a 170,000 molecular weight nonreceptor protein in vivo in skeletal muscle of streptozotocin induced diabetic rats: Effects of insulin and glucose. Endocrinology 1992;130:1433
132. Penicaud L, Kandé J, Magnen JL, Girard JR. Insulin action during fasting and refeeding in rat determined by euglycemic clamp. Am J Physiol 1985; 249:E514
133. Charron MJ, Kahn BB. Divergent molecular mechanisms for insulin-resistant glucose transport in muscle and adipose cells in vivo. J Biol Chem 1990; 265:7994
134. Kahn BB, Rosen AS. Increased insulin stimulated recruitment of GLUT4 to the plasma membrane in skeletal muscle of fasted rats. Diabetes 1992;41:12A

135. Smith D, Bloom S, Sugden M, Holness M. Glucose transporter expression and glucose utilization in skeletal muscle and brown adipose tissue during starvation and re-feeding. Biochem J 1992;282:231
136. Liu ML, Gibbs EM, McCoid SC, et al. Transgenic mice expressing the human GLUT4/muscle-fat facilitative transporter protein exhibit efficient glycemic control. Proc Natl Acad Sci USA 1993;90:11346
137. Treadway J, Hargrove D, Nardone N, et al. Enhanced peripheral glucose utilization in transgenic mice expressing the human GLUT-4 gene. J Biol Chem 1994;269:29956
138. Gibbs E, Stock J, McCoid S, et al. Glycemic improvement in diabetic (*db/db*) mice by overexpression of the human insulin-regulatable glucose transporter GLUT-4. J Clin Invest 1995;95:1512
139. Shepherd PR, Gnudi L, Tozzo E, et al. Adipose cell hyperplasia and enhanced glucose disposal in transgenic mice overexpressing GLUT4 selectively in adipose tissue. J Biol Chem 1993;268:22243
140. Tozzo E, Gnudi L, Bliss LL, Kahn BB. Overexpression of GLUT4 driven by a heterologous promoter is maintained in streptozotocin diabetic mice and prevents insulin resistance in isolated adipocytes. Diabetes 1994;43(suppl 1):14A
141. Gnudi L, Tozzo E, Shepherd PR, et al. High level overexpression of GLUT4 driven by an adipose-specific promoter is maintained in transgenic mice on a high fat diet, but does not prevent impaired glucose tolerance. Endocrinology 1995;136:995
142. Katz EB, Stenbit AE, Hatton K, et al. Cardiac and adipose tissue abnormalities but not diabetes in mice deficient in GLUT-4. Nature 1995;377:151
143. Mueckler M, Holman G. Homeostasis without a GLUT. Nature 1995;377:100
144. Marshall BA, Ren JM, Johnson DW, et al. Germline manipulation of glucose homeostasis via alteration of glucose transporter levels in skeletal muscle. J Biol Chem 1993;268:18442
145. Ren JM, Marshall BA, Gulve EA, et al. Evidence from transgenic mice that glucose transport is rate-limiting for glycogen deposition and glycolysis in skeletal muscle. J Biol Chem 1993;268:16113
146. Gulve EA, Ren JM, Marshall BA, et al. Glucose transport activity in skeletal muscles from transgenic mice overexpressing GLUT1. Increased basal transport is associated with a defective response to diverse stimuli that activate GLUT4. J Biol Chem 1994;269:18366
147. Lund S, Holman GD, Schmitz O, Pedersen O. Contraction stimulates translocation of glucose transporter GLUT-4 in skeletal muscle through a mechanism distinct from that of insulin. Proc Natl Acad Sci USA 1995;92:5817
148. Brozinick J, Etgen GJ, Yaspelkis BB 3rd, Ivy J. The effects of muscle contraction and insulin on glucose-transporter translocation in rat skeletal muscle. Biochem J 1994;297:539
149. Goodyear L, Hirshman M, Valyou P, Horton E. Glucose transporter number, function, and subcellular distribution in rat skeletal muscle after exercise training. Diabetes 1992;41:1091
150. Brozinick JJ, Etgen G, Yaspelkis BB 3rd, Ivy J. Effects of exercise training on muscle GLUT-4 protein content and translocation in obese Zucker rats. Am J Physiol 1993;265:E419
151. Kern M, Dolan PL, Mazzeo RS, et al. Effect of aging and exercise on GLUT-4 glucose transporters in muscle. Am J Physiol 1992;263:E362
152. Etgen GJ, Brozinick JJ, Hy K, Ivy J. Effects of exercise training on skeletal muscle glucose uptake and transport. Am J Physiol 1993;264:C727
153. Ren J, Semenkovich C, Gulve E, et al. Exercise induces rapid increases in GLUT4 expression, glucose transport capacity, and insulin-stimulated glycogen storage in muscle. J Biol Chem 1994;269:14396
154. Fushiki T, Kano T, Inoue K, Sugimoto E. Decrease in muscle glucose transporter number in chronic physical inactivity. Am J Physiol 1991;260:E403
155. Henriksen E, Rodnick K, Mondon C, et al. Effect of denervation or unweighting on GLUT4 protein in rat soleus muscle. J Appl Physiol 1991;70:2322
156. Burant C, Treutelaar M, Buse M. In vitro and in vivo activation of the insulin receptor tyrosine kinase in control and denervated skeletal muscle. J Biol Chem 1986;261:8985
157. Etgen GJ, Farrar R, Ivy J. Effect of chronic electrical stimulation on GLUT-4 protein content in fast-twitch muscle. Am J Physiol 1993;264:R816
158. Muller G, Wied S. The sulfonylurea drug, glimepiride, stimulates glucose transport, glucose transporter translocation, and dephosphorylation in insulin-resistant rat adipocytes in vitro. Diabetes 1993;42:1852
159. Kozka I, Holman G. Metformin blocks downregulation of cell surface GLUT4 caused by chronic insulin treatment of rat adipocytes. Diabetes 1993;42:1159
160. Matthaei S, Reibold J, Hamann A, et al. In vivo metformin treatment ameliorates insulin resistance: Evidence for potentiation of insulin-induced translocation and increased functional activity of glucose transporters in obese (*fa/fa*) Zucker rat adipocytes. Endocrinology 1993;133:304
161. Handberg A, Kayser L, Hoyer P, et al. Metformin ameliorates diabetes but does not normalize the decreased GLUT 4 content in skeletal muscle of obese (*fa/fa*) Zucker rats. Diabetologia 1993;36:481
162. Hundal H, Ramlal T, Reyes R, et al. Cellular mechanism of metformin action involves glucose transporter translocation from an intracellular pool to the plasma membrane in L6 muscle cells. Endocrinology 1992;131:1165
163. Sandouk T, Reda D, Hofmann C. The antidiabetic agent pioglitazone increases expression of glucose transporters in 3T3-F442A cells by increasing messenger ribonucleic acid transcript stability. Endocrinology 1993;133:352
164. Kletzien R, Clarke S, Ulrich R. Enhancement of adipocyte differentiation by an insulin-sensitizing agent. Mol Pharmacol 1992;41:393
165. Weinstein S, Holand A, O'Boyle E, Haber R. Effects of thiazolidinediones on glucocorticoid-induced insulin resistance and GLUT4 glucose transporter expression in rat skeletal muscle. Metabolism 1993;42:1365
166. Paquet M, Romanek R, Sargeant R. Vanadate induces the recruitment of GLUT-4 glucose transporter to the plasma membrane of rat adipocytes. Mol Cell Biochem 1992;109:149
167. Valera A, Rodriguez-Gil J, Bosch F. Vanadate treatment restores the expression of genes from key enzymes in the glucose and ketone bodies metabolism in the liver of diabetic rats. J Clin Invest 1993;92:4
168. Castello A, Rodriguez-Manzaneque J, Camps M, et al. Perinatal hypothyroidism impairs the normal transition of GLUT4 and GLUT1 glucose transporters from fetal to neonatal levels in heart and brown adipose tissue. Evidence for tissue-specific regulation of GLUT4 expression by thyroid hormone. J Biol Chem 1994;269:5905
169. Weinstein S, O'Boyle E, Haber R. Thyroid hormone increases basal and insulin-stimulated glucose transport in skeletal muscle. Diabetes 1994;43:1185
170. Weinstein S, Watts J, Haber R. Thyroid hormone increases muscle/fat glucose transporter gene expression in rat skeletal muscle. Endocrinology 1991;129:455
171. Casla A, Rovira A, Wells J, Dohm G. Increased glucose transporter (GLUT4) protein expression in hyperthyroidism. Biochem Biophys Res Commun 1990;171:182
172. Weinstein W, Haber R. Differential regulation of glucose transporter isoforms by thyroid hormone in rat heart. Biochim Biophys Acta 1992;136:302
173. Shimizu Y, Nikami H, Tsukazaki K, et al. Increased expression of glucose transporter GLUT-4 in brown adipose tissue of fasted rats after cold exposure. Am J Physiol 1993;264:E890
174. Takahashi A, Shimazu T, Maruyama Y. Importance of sympathetic nerves for the stimulatory effect of cold exposure on glucose utilization in brown adipose tissue. Jpn J Physiol 1992;42:653
175. Hotamisligil G, Spiegelman B. Perspective in diabetes: Tumor necrosis factor α: A key component of the obesity-diabetes link. Diabetes 1994;43:1271
176. Lang C, Dobrescu C, Bagby G. Tumor necrosis factor impairs insulin action on peripheral glucose disposal and hepatic glucose output. Endocrinology 1992;130:43

Diabetes Mellitus, edited by Derek LeRoith, Simeon I. Taylor, and Jerrold M. Olefsky. Lippincott–Raven Publishers, Philadelphia © 1996.

Chapter 60

Glucose "Toxicity": Effect of Chronic Hyperglycemia on Insulin Action

Luciano Rossetti

Introduction

The value of glycemic control in the prevention and amelioration of the microvascular complications of insulin-dependent diabetes mellitus (IDDM) is now well established in prospective clinical trials.[1–8] A considerable amount of epidemiologic and animal data also support the link between chronic hyperglycemia and long-term microvascular complications of diabetes mellitus, including retinopathy, neuropathy, and nephropathy.[9–14] In addition to causing microvascular complications, hyperglycemia may contribute to macrovascular disease[15] and impaired cellular immunity[16,17] in diabetes mellitus.

Recently, it has become clear that chronic hyperglycemia also has a deleterious effect on both insulin secretion[18–23] and insulin action,[24,25] a concept referred to as *glucose toxicity.*[18,26,27] In this regard, chronic hyperglycemia not only represents a hallmark of diabetes mellitus but is itself a self-perpetuating regulatory factor that contributes to poor metabolic control.

In this chapter, I shall focus on the effect of chronic hyperglycemia on insulin action. The ensuing discussion will review our current understanding of the pathophysiology, biochemistry, and clinical significance of glucose-induced insulin resistance. The deleterious effects of hyperglycemia on insulin secretion and microvascular complications are discussed in Chapters 10, 55, and 94, respectively.

Hyperglycemia and Tissue Sensitivity to Insulin

Skeletal muscle insulin resistance is present in conventionally treated insulin-dependent diabetes mellitus (IDDM)[28,29] and in non–insulin-dependent diabetes mellitus (NIDDM).[30–34] In the former, the defect in insulin action is thought to be multifactorial and at least in part inherited,[35–42] whereas in the latter, it is likely to be acquired.[29] In an editorial, Unger and Grundy[18] suggested that chronic hyperglycemia may be partly responsible for the defect in insulin-mediated glucose disposal in persons with IDDM and NIDDM. Preliminary evidence in support of this hypothesis was derived from several observations in animals and humans:

1. Insulin resistance in IDDM is a consequence of poor metabolic control.
2. Tight metabolic control leads to some improvement in insulin sensitivity.
3. Defects in insulin secretion lead to the development of insulin resistance.

1. *In IDDM, insulin sensitivity appears to be a consequence of poor metabolic control and is well correlated with the glycosylated hemoglobin concentration.*[43–49] Patients with moderately and poorly controlled IDDM have some peripheral (skeletal muscle) insulin resistance.[28,29,43–49] Insulin sensitivity is normal during remission, however,[44–47,49] suggesting that insulin resistance in IDDM is an acquired and reversible defect. Yki-Jarvinen et al.,[29] in a comprehensive analysis of insulin resistance in patients with IDDM, found a significant correlation between the degree of insulin resistance and the glycosylated hemoglobin concentration.

2. *Near-normal glycemic control in diabetic persons, however it is achieved (diet, insulin therapy, sulfonylureas), leads to some improvement in insulin sensitivity.*[44–47,49–70] If hyperglycemia contributes to the insulin resistance observed in human diabetes mellitus, one would expect that normalization of the plasma glucose profile, regardless of the means, would lead to an improvement in tissue sensitivity. Several studies have shown a significant improvement in insulin sensitivity in diabetic patients following institution of intensified insulin therapy.[44–47,49–58] Using the insulin clamp technique, a number of investigators have examined the effect of diet (weight loss),[63–67] sulfonylureas,[68–72] and insulin therapy[50,53–57,73,74] on insulin action in persons with IDDM and NIDDM. Strict glycemic control with insulin in patients with IDDM[44–47,49] uniformly improved insulin sensitivity, whereas a similar degree of glycemic control had a less consistent effect on improving insulin action in patients with NIDDM.[50–74] Furthermore, in patients with NIDDM, only partial reversal of insulin resistance was seen.[26] At first, one might interpret these results in patients with NIDDM as evidence against the glucose toxicity hypothesis. It should be remembered, however, that a primary abnormality that is inherited in NIDDM is insulin resistance,[35–42] and that the defect in insulin action becomes maximally manifest early in the natural history of NIDDM.[38–42] Thus, even when another severely insulin-resistant state, such as obesity, is superimposed on type II diabetes, the insulin resistance is only slightly greater than that with diabetes alone or obesity alone.[75] Therefore, if one were to superimpose the insulin resistance due to glucose toxicity on the insulin resistance of obesity and on that inherited in NIDDM, one would not expect much of an additional deterioration in insulin action. Thus, normalization of the plasma glucose concentration and removal of glucose toxicity would not be expected to produce a major improvement in insulin sensitivity. Conversely, in IDDM in humans and in experimental animal models of diabetes—where the insulin resistance is likely to be entirely acquired—glycemic control, however achieved, would be expected to lead to an improvement in insulin-mediated glucose disposal.

From the above studies, however, it cannot be ascertained whether it is the insulin replacement per se, the correction of the hyperglycemia, or the normalization of other nonglucose (lipid, amino acid/protein, etc.) metabolic abnormalities that is responsible for the improvement in insulin action. In addition, chronic, sustained hyperinsulinemia has been shown to downregulate insulin receptor number and to result in an impairment in postreceptor events that regulate insulin-mediated glucose disposal.[76,77] This may explain, in part, why intensified insulin treatment in persons with NIDDM fails to correct completely the defect in insulin action.[50–74]

3. *In several animal models, an initial defect in insulin secretion leads to the development of insulin resistance.*[24,78–84] In fact, in animal models, a primary reduction in β-cell mass, and the consequent moderate to severe hypoinsulinemia and hyperglycemia, lead to impaired insulin action in vivo[24,78–82] and at the cellular level in vitro.[81–85] In particular, skeletal muscle insulin resistance has been clearly demonstrated in rodents and dogs made diabetic by pharmacologic (streptozotocin, alloxan) or surgical reduction of the β-cell mass.[24,78–82] After 90% partial pancreatectomy in rats, a moderate increase in the fed plasma glucose concentrations to ~300 mg/dL induced a 30% decrease in the ability of insulin to promote peripheral glucose disposal.[24,81,82] Because fasting plasma insulin and free fatty acid concentrations were similar to control concentrations in this model, it could be argued that the insulin resistance was at least partially due to the sustained increase in the plasma glucose concentrations.[81,82]

It is not clear, however, whether insulin deficiency or some other metabolic derangement that occurs as a result of the insulinopenia is responsible for defects in insulin action. A similar argument can be made concerning the beneficial effects of weight loss, sulfonylureas, and insulin therapy on tissue sensitivity to insulin.

A more rigorous test of the *glucose toxicity* hypothesis was provided by studies in which either:

1. Experimentally induced, prolonged hyperglycemia led to peripheral insulin resistance in persons with IDDM and in normal animals and
2. Lowering the plasma glucose concentration in diabetic animals without altering the concentrations of circulating hormones and other substrates normalized tissue sensitivity to insulin.

1. *Prolonged hyperglycemia resulted in peripheral insulin resistance in persons with IDDM and in normal animals.*[86–92] If the above findings have relevance to the development of insulin resistance in humans, one would expect that sustained physiologic hyperglycemia should lead to the development of insulin resistance. In fact, if the deleterious effect of hyperglycemia on muscle insulin sensitivity is a universal biologic phenomenon, then it should be reproducible in vivo by the induction of sustained hyperglycemia in humans and animals. Indeed, severe reduction in insulin-mediated muscle glucose uptake after prolonged elevation of the glucose concentrations has been shown in intact rats and in perfused hindquarters. In particular, Hager et al.[86] showed that 72-hour glucose infusions in healthy rats caused sustained hyperglycemia and hyperinsulinemia and the onset of severe skeletal muscle insulin resistance. Richter and colleagues,[87–89] in a series of studies, induced defective insulin stimulation of hindlimb glucose uptake and glycogen synthesis after prolonged exposure to glucose and insulin. Considerable evidence suggests that this glucose-induced desensitization of muscle glucose uptake may operate in humans as well. This question has been examined in persons with well-controlled IDDM after prolonged (24–48-hour) experimental hyperglycemia.[90–92] In particular, Vuorinen-Markkola et al.[91] studied patients with IDDM who were receiving chronic subcutaneous insulin infusion therapy. Subjects participated in two euglycemic insulin clamp procedures. During the first study, the plasma glucose concentration was maintained at the basal level (128 ± 7 mg/dL) for 24 hours before the insulin clamp; before the second study, the plasma glucose concentration was elevated to 360 ± 5 mg/dL for 24 hours. As can be seen in Figure 60-1, as little as 24 hours of hyperglycemia was sufficient to induce a 35% decline in the rate of insulin-mediated glucose disposal. Similar results were obtained by Fowellin et al.[92] Thus, moderate whole-body and skeletal muscle insulin resistance were induced within 24 hours of hyperglycemia, with moderate impairment of both glucose uptake and nonoxidative glucose disposal.

2. *Lowering the plasma glucose concentration in diabetic animals without altering circulating hormone and substrate concentrations (other than glucose) normalized tissue sensitivity to insulin.* There is one agent that fulfills these requirements—phlorizin. Phlorizin is a potent inhibitor of renal tubular glucose transport and blocks proximal tubular glucose reabsorption when the plasma glucose concentration is increased above the basal level. Thus, it leads to normalization of the plasma glucose concentration without causing hypoglycemia or altering plasma insulin, amino acid, free fatty acid, or other substrate/hormone concentrations.[24,93,94] Furthermore, in the doses employed in the present study, phlorizin has no effect on gut or muscle glucose transport.

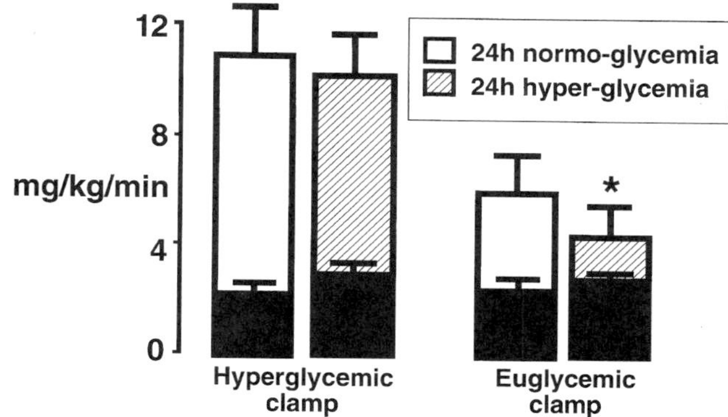

Figure 60-1. Rates of total (whole bar) and oxidative (solid area of the bar) tissue glucose uptake during hyperglycemic and euglycemic clamp studies in IDDM patients after 24 hours of normoglycemia or hyperglycemia. During the euglycemic clamp studies, the rates of glucose disposal were significantly lower after 24 hours of hyperglycemia. This decrease was entirely accounted for by a severe impairment in nonoxidative glucose disposal (open or gray areas of the bars). (Reproduced by permission from the American Diabetes Association from Vuorinen-Markkola H, Koivitso VA, Yki-Jarvinen H. Mechanisms of hyperglycemia-induced insulin resistance in whole body and skeletal muscle of type 1 diabetic patients. Diabetes 1992;41:571.)

In a diabetic animal model of NIDDM, we provided experimental proof that hyperglycemia per se plays a central role in the development of insulin resistance after insulin deficiency.[24] Four groups of chronically catheterized, awake, unstressed rats were studied: group 1—sham-operated controls; group 2—90% surgically pancreatectomized rats; group 3—90% pancreatectomized rats treated with phlorizin to normalize the plasma glucose profile; group 4—diabetic rats treated with phlorizin for 6 weeks and restudied 2 weeks after discontinuation of the drug. Groups 1–3 were studied 6 weeks after pancreatectomy or sham pancreatectomy. The pancreatectomized rats had mild fasting hyperglycemia and an abnormal meal tolerance test compared with the control rats.[24] Insulin secretion in response to the mixed meal was markedly impaired in the diabetic group. Phlorizin treatment normalized the fasting plasma glucose concentration and the postmeal glucose profile without causing any change in plasma insulin or other hormone/substrate concentrations. When the phlorizin was discontinued, glucose intolerance returned and the plasma insulin response remained markedly deficient.

If hyperglycemia per se is an important regulator of insulin action in vivo, the diabetic animals should be insulin resistant, and phlorizin would be expected to improve the defect in insulin-mediated glucose disposal even though insulin secretion remained markedly deficient. To examine this question, we performed euglycemic insulin clamp studies in conscious rats. As can be seen in Figure 60-2, this is precisely what was observed. Not only was insulin sensitivity improved in phlorizin-treated diabetic rats, it was completely eliminated. As further proof of the deleterious effect of hyperglycemia on insulin-mediated glucose disposal, discontinuation of phlorizin therapy was associated with a return of the insulin resistance. Because phlorizin failed to enhance insulin sensitivity in sham-operated rats,[24] the improvement in insulin action in diabetic rats cannot be attributed to a nonspecific effect of phlorizin.

Our results also demonstrated an inverse relationship between the defect in total body (primarily muscle) glucose uptake and the plasma glucose concentration during the meal tolerance test.[24] Thus, correction of hyperglycemia with phlorizin resulted in the complete normalization of tissue sensitivity to insulin in diabetic rats with no change in basal or meal-stimulated insulin levels.[24,93,94] Furthermore, the close inverse relationship between the postmeal plasma glucose concentrations and the insulin-mediated glucose uptake during insulin clamp studies suggests the presence of a link between severity of hyperglycemia and degree of peripheral insulin resistance.[24]

Although correction of hyperglycemia with phlorizin is capable of normalizing meal tolerance and total body insulin-mediated glucose disposal in diabetic animals, one cannot conclude a priori that the intracellular pathways of glucose metabolism are intact. To examine this question, we contrasted the effects of vanadate (an insulinomimetic agent) and phlorizin on whole body and muscle glucose metabolism in 90% pancreatectomized rats.[94] As previously described,[24] diabetic rats manifested a 30% reduction in whole body tissue sensitivity to insulin, which was corrected completely by phlorizin treatment. A similar improvement was observed with vanadate (Fig. 60-3). Phlorizin, however, unlike vanadate, did not correct the severe impairment in muscle glycogen synthesis (Fig. 60-3). Consistent with this result, the maximum oxygen uptake of muscle glycogen synthase was reduced in diabetic rats and returned to normal with vanadate but not with phlorizin.[94] These results indicate that correction of hyperglycemia in diabetic rats normalizes the defect in glucose transport but does not improve the intracellular abnormality in glycogen synthesis. Thus, the glucose toxicity effect in muscle appears to be directed specifically against the glucose transport system.

In summary, a variety of experimental designs, using both in vivo and in vitro techniques, have demonstrated that chronic physiologic hyperglycemia is capable of inducing a state of insulin resistance.

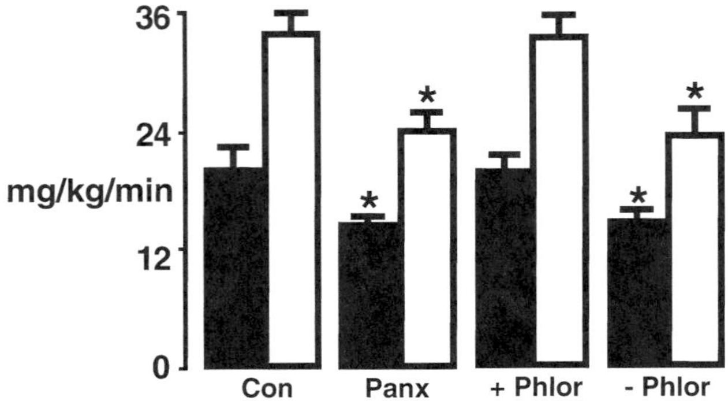

FIGURE 60-2. Rates of whole body insulin-mediated tissue glucose uptake during +80 μU/mL (solid bars) and +160 μU/mL (open bars) euglycemic insulin clamp studies performed in four groups of awake, unstressed, chronically catheterized rats: sham-operated controls (Con), partially (90%) pancreatectomized diabetic rats (Panx), and partially pancreatectomized diabetic rats treated with phlorizin for 6 weeks (+ Phlor) and again after discontinuation of the phlorizin for 2 weeks (− Phlor). *$p < 0.01$ vs. Con. (Reproduced by permission from the American Society for Clinical Investigation from Rossetti L, Smith D, Shulman GI, et al. Correction of hyperglycemia with phlorizin normalizes tissue sensitivity to insulin in diabetic rats. J Clin Invest 1987;79:1510.)

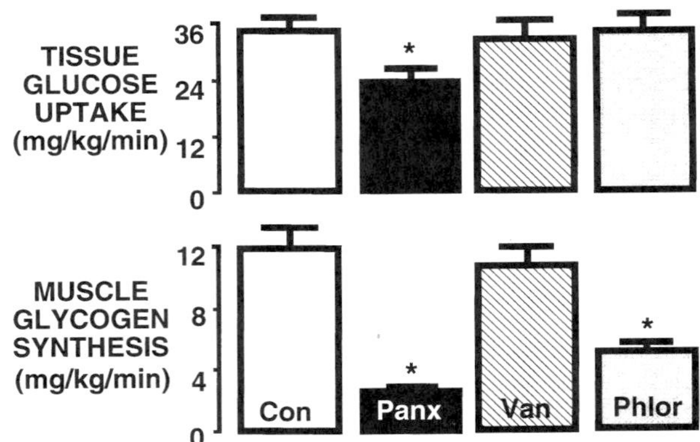

FIGURE 60-3. Rates of whole body insulin-mediated tissue glucose uptake (upper panel) and of muscle glycogen synthesis (lower panel) during +700 μU/mL euglycemic insulin clamp studies performed in four groups of awake, unstressed, chronically catheterized rats: sham-operated controls (Con; open bar), partially (90%) pancreatectomized diabetic rats (Panx; solid bar), partially pancreatectomized diabetic rats treated with vanadate for 4 weeks (Van; crosshatched bar), and partially pancreatectomized diabetic rats treated with phlorizin for 4 weeks (Phlor; gray bar). *$p < 0.01$ vs. Con. (Reproduced by permission of the American Society for Clinical Investigation from Rossetti L, Laughlin MR. Correction of chronic hyperglycemia with vanadate, but not with phlorizin, normalizes in vivo glycogen repletion and in vitro glycogen synthase activity in diabetic skeletal muscle. J Clin Invest 1989; 84:892.)

Biochemical Mechanism(s) of Glucose Toxicity

Glucose-Induced Desensitization of Glucose Uptake

At the cellular level, diabetes in both animals[85,95–97] and humans[98,99] is associated with a reduction in insulin-stimulated glucose transport activity in muscle and adipose cells. Glucose transport in isolated cell systems is substrate, that is, glucose, regulated.[100–107] In vitro, glucose starvation of fibroblasts,[100] 3T3-L1 preadipocytes,[101] and cultured, intact muscle cells[102] results in increased basal and insulin-stimulated glucose transport, whereas hyperglycemia leads to downregulation of glucose transport activity.[101,103] Garvey et al.[103] demonstrated the synergistic effect of insulin and glucose in causing desensitization of the glucose transport system in primary cultures of adipose cells. Thus, incubation of muscle cells and adipocytes with a high medium glucose concentration (10–20 mM) leads to a progressive decline in glucose transport activity, loss of cytochalasin B binding activity in both plasma and low-density microsomal membrane fractions, and the development of insulin resistance.[100–104] Conversely, glucose starvation leads to upregulation of the glucose transport system in cultured muscle cells, adipocytes, and fibroblasts.[100,104–107] The studies of Sasson and Cerasi[102] and Sasson et al.[104] are particularly relevant to the preceding discussion. When rat soleus muscle or myocytes were incubated for 24 hours in a high medium glucose concentration, a progressive decline in insulin-mediated glucose transport was demonstrated. This effect of hyperglycemia was both dose- and time-dependent and fully reversible.[102]

Because several characteristics of the glucose transport system—for example, responsiveness to insulin, abundance of glucose transporter species—may be altered in cultured cells, however, caution should be used in extrapolating these results to skeletal muscle in the intact organism. To define the mechanism(s) responsible for the insulin resistance observed after chronic hyperglycemia in partially pancreatectomized diabetic rats, we measured 3-O-methylglucose transport in isolated adipose cells 6 weeks after pancreatectomy.[85] In vivo, 3–4 weeks of normalization of the plasma glucose profile with phlorizin restored insulin-stimulated 3-O-methylglucose transport in adipose cells to normal levels in diabetic rats[85]; these changes paralleled the normalization of whole body insulin-mediated glucose uptake.[24,85,94] Our results indicate that insulin-stimulated glucose transport is diminished in diabetic rats and that the defect in glucose transport is restored to normal with phlorizin treatment. Moreover, the improvement in glucose transport activity was closely correlated with the improvement in in vivo insulin sensitivity.

In summary, strong experimental support for a secondary form of insulin resistance after sustained elevation of the extracellular glucose concentrations is available in both humans and animals in vivo and in a variety of isolated cell systems. Although decreased glucose uptake is a common endpoint in all experimental settings, the potential role of a sustained elevation in hexose-phosphate concentrations at the onset and during the evolution of the desensitization process has recently been proposed. In particular, it is intriguing that the onset of glucose toxicity at the level of glucose transport/phosphorylation is accelerated by the concomitant presence of high insulin concentrations. This may indicate that enhanced glucose disposal rather than high glucose concentration per se is the primary cause of the downregulation of glucose uptake. An early defect in intracellular glucose disposal—caused by different mechanisms, depending on the experimental setting (e.g., glycogen "saturation" in the prolonged glucose infusion studies and hypoinsulinemia in diabetic animal models)—may also exacerbate the deleterious effects of high glucose and insulin concentrations by amplifying the glucose-induced "signal." Because defective skeletal muscle glycogen synthase activity is a common feature of both diabetic and nondiabetic models of glucose toxicity, it will be particularly important to examine whether defective insulin action on muscle glycolysis, glycogenolysis, and/or glycogen synthesis, as well as the consequent increase in hexose-phosphate concentrations, can contribute to the onset and development of the desensitization process.

Time-Dependent Changes in Insulin Action: Onset and Reversal of "Glucose Toxicity"

It is conceivable that the acquisition of defects in glucose metabolism, and in particular in insulin-mediated glucose uptake after a sustained increase in extracellular glucose concentrations, proceeds in a sequential manner. Several investigators have attempted to address this important issue in culture cells, perfused organ systems, and intact animals and humans. Traxinger and Marshall[108] examined the time required for the development of desensitization of the glucose transport system and for its recovery in primary culture of adipose cells exposed to high glucose and insulin concentrations. They described a strong correlation between rates of recovery and desensitization in this cell system with an average time required for half-maximal effect ($t_{1/2}$) of 3 hours for the induction of insulin resistance and of 3.3 hours for the recovery of insulin responsiveness. Marshall et al.[109] also proposed that the desensitization of the glucose transport system, mediated by the glucosamine pathway, develops through an early stage characterized by impaired translocation of glucose transporters in response to insulin and later effects on glucose transporters gene expression. In perfused rat hindquarters, Hansen, Richter, and colleagues[87–89] examined the time course of the glucose-induced decrease in insulin responsiveness. The appearance of insulin resistance in this system was extremely rapid (<2 hours). This resistance was related to the glucose concentration in a dose-dependent manner, and its extent was enhanced by a concomitant elevation in the perfusate insulin concentration. Importantly, glucose-mediated desensitization of hindquarter glucose uptake occurred even in the absence of insulin and of a significant decline in glycogen synthase activity, suggesting a primary effect on the glucose transport system.[87]

Unfortunately, extrapolation of these in vitro data to the in vivo condition may be misleading. In fact, the disposition of glucose in response to insulin stimulation under these experimental conditions is often characterized by a marked decrease in insulin's action on oxidative pathways and an enhanced disposal in anaerobic glycolysis.[110,111] Additionally, in cultured cell systems, the relative role of the various glucose transporters species involved in the response to insulin may differ from those operating in vivo. The above limitations are particularly relevant when examining the time courses and the relative contributions of different metabolic/biochemical alterations to the glucose-induced desensitization.

Some information on the development of peripheral insulin resistance in diabetic animal models is also available. It is important to note that the time course of the onset of insulin resistance and the underlying molecular mechanism(s) have often been shown to be divergent in different insulin target tissues; in particular, discrepancies were apparent between adipose cells and skeletal muscle.[112,113] In adipose cells, decreased GLUT-4 mRNA and protein have been consistently reported as early as 3 days following streptozocin-induced diabetes in rats.[113–117] Near-normalization of the plasma glucose concentration by phlorizin treatment, however, was equally ineffective in restoring GLUT-4 mRNA concentrations to normal after 3 days[118] and after 3 weeks,[85] suggesting that the decrease in GLUT-4 gene expression in these diabetic models was the result of insulin deficiency rather than chronic hyperglycemia. In skeletal muscle, we reported a severe impairment in insulin-mediated glucose uptake but normal skeletal muscle GLUT-4 protein 7 days after the induction of insulinopenic diabetes by streptozocin.[113] Decreased skeletal muscle GLUT-4 protein was shown only 14 days poststreptozocin.[113,119] Although the latter study did not distinguish between the consequences of hyperglycemia, hypoinsulinemia, and other associated metabolic alterations, it underscores the sequential appearance of biochemical and molecular defects in insulin-sensitive tissues. Dimitrakoudis et al.[120] showed a significant increase in GLUT-4 protein in a skeletal muscle plasma membrane fraction only 2 days after normalization of the fasting plasma glucose concentration by phlorizin in streptozocin diabetic rats. It is not known, however, whether reversal of a hyperglycemic state of such short duration had any beneficial effect on insulin stimulation of skeletal muscle glucose uptake. Finally, moderate impairment in insulin-mediated glucose uptake (18–24% decrease) was demonstrated in persons with insulin-dependent diabetes mellitus (IDDM) after just 24 hours of sustained hyperglycemia.[90–92]

In summary, large variations have been reported in the time course of the onset of metabolic defects after sustained elevation of the glucose concentration. These differences are mostly due to the selection of the experimental system and perhaps to the concomitant insulin levels. In vivo, although decreased insulin stimulation of glucose uptake is an early effect of severely insulinopenic diabetes, there is no information on the time interval required for its reversal after correction of hyperglycemia. Definition of the progressive appearance and reversal of glucose-induced metabolic alterations appears to be germane to the understanding of the mechanism(s) of glucose-induced insulin resistance that are operating in vivo. For example, if an early defect in intracellular glucose disposal precedes the onset of defective insulin-mediated glucose uptake, it may suggest that an interplay between increased glucose availability (hyperglycemia) and defective disposal though insulin-sensitive pathways is a plausible explanation for the in vivo expression of glucose-induced insulin resistance. It is particularly important to examine whether defective insulin action on muscle glycogenolysis, and the consequent increase in hexose-phosphate concentrations, precede the onset of desensitization of the glucose transport system.

Recent studies have attempted to define the mechanism(s) by which prolonged glucose and insulin infusions lead to decreased insulin-mediated glucose uptake in skeletal muscle. Hager et al.[86] demonstrated severe downregulation in skeletal muscle insulin-stimulated glucose uptake in 72-hour glucose-infused rats in the absence of any alteration in insulin binding. Similarly, Hansen et al.[89] induced marked skeletal muscle insulin resistance in glucose-infused hindquarters in the absence of a detectable alteration in muscle insulin receptor tyrosine kinase activity. Consistent with these observations, we could not demonstrate any alteration in muscle and liver insulin receptor tyrosine kinase activity in insulin-resistant diabetic rats, and found no change after normalization of plasma glucose concentrations and insulin-mediated glucose disposal by phlorizin treatment.[121] In vitro studies in primary culture of adipose cells demonstrated complete dissociation between the insulin effect on glucose uptake (decreased) and on protein metabolism (stimulated) after 7-hour incubations with glucose, insulin, and amino acids.[122,123] Together these studies appear to suggest that the glucose-induced desensitization of muscle glucose uptake should be attributed to factors other than impaired *early* insulin signal transduction.

A common interpretive problem with these in vivo studies is the difficulty in discerning the relative role (primary or secondary) of the marked downregulation of glucose transport and glycogen synthase activity in the sequence of events that leads to desensitization of the glucose transport system. Recently, Hansen et al.[89] argued for the primary role of the glucose transport defect because both skeletal muscle free glucose and glucose-6-phosphate concentrations were not increased in the glucose-infused hindquarters compared to the control study. Similarly, Vuorinen-Markkola et al.[91] showed a marked decrease in insulin action on skeletal muscle glucose uptake and glycogen storage in persons with IDDM infused with glucose for 24 hours in the absence of any detectable increase in free glucose and glucose-6-phosphate concentrations in muscle biopsy specimens. Using a completely different experimental approach—the reversal of glucose-induced insulin resistance in phlorizin-treated diabetic rats—we reached a similar conclusion.[85,94] In fact, although surgical reduction of the β-cell mass and the consequent hypoinsulinemia and hyperglycemia caused the onset of defects in both skeletal muscle glucose transport/phosphorylation and glycogen synthase activity, normalization of the plasma glucose concentration by phlorizin treatment restored insulin-mediated glucose uptake to normal without improving the decreased maximum velocity of skeletal muscle glycogen synthase.[94] We recently reported that 3–4 weeks of normalization of the plasma glucose profile with phlorizin restores insulin-stimulated 3-O-methylglucose transport in adipose cells to normal levels in diabetic rats.[85] These effects on glucose transport activity occurred in the absence of alterations in the expression of the two types of glucose transporters present in adipose cells—GLUT-4 and GLUT-1—or in their translocation to the plasma membrane in response to insulin. Thus, we suggested that it may result from changes in glucose transporters' functional activity. Similarly, we were unable to demonstrate any recovery of GLUT-4 protein and mRNA in skeletal muscle of diabetic rats chronically treated with phlorizin (B.B. Kahn and L. Rossetti, unpublished observation). Consistent with our finding, Sivitz et al.[118] reported no change in GLUT-4 mRNA in adipose cells from streptozocin diabetic rats following near-normalization of the plasma glucose concentration by phlorizin treatment and concluded that "the relative glycemic state does not influence GLUT-4 mRNA expression in vivo." Importantly, Dimitrakoudis et al.[120] reported that in phlorizin-treated streptozocin diabetic rats, although GLUT-4 protein in skeletal muscle tends to return toward normal concentrations in the plasma membrane fraction, it does not change in the intracellular pool. Although this study did not examine the effect of insulin stimulation on GLUT-4 translocation, it suggests that increased translocation of GLUT-4 to the plasma membrane is a potential mechanism for the improved skeletal muscle glucose uptake after correction of hyperglycemia by phlorizin treatment.

Thus, defective insulin stimulation of the glucose transport system has been proposed as the major cellular manifestation of prolonged hyperglycemia. Although glucose-mediated alterations in the concentration of GLUT-4 protein have not been firmly established, defects in glucose transporters' translocation and/or in "functional activity" have been proposed.

The "Glucosamine Hypothesis"

Using primary cultures of adipose cells, Marshall and colleagues[124] suggested that desensitization of the glucose transport system in cells incubated with high concentrations of glucose and insulin required the metabolism of glucose/hexose phosphates in a quantitatively minor pathway of intracellular glucose utilization, that is, the hexosamine biosynthesis pathway (Fig. 60-4), which is initiated by the conversion of fructose-6-phosphate to glucosamine-6-phosphate by the enzyme glutamine:fructose-6-phosphate amidotransferase. They first showed that insulin had a permissive effect on glucose-induced desensitization that was independent of changes in insulin receptor binding.[83,103] The authors suggested that it may act by promoting glucose uptake and metabolism, and that the latter was indispensable for the development of glucose-induced desensitization. The potential role of the hexosamine biosynthesis pathway was suggested by the observation that, in addition to glucose and insulin, the amino acid glutamine (a donor of amido groups that is needed for glutamine:fructose-6-phosphate amidotransferase activity) was also required for the onset of desensitiza-

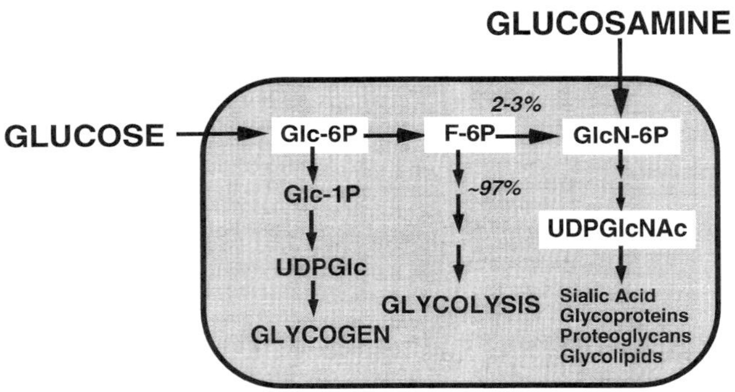

Figure 60-4. Schematic representation of the common steps in the intracellular metabolism of glucose and glucosamine. In skeletal muscle and adipose cells, glucose enters the cells through the action of glucose transporters (mostly GLUT-4 in the presence of insulin) and is then rapidly phosphorylated to glucose-6-phosphate (Glc-6P) by the action of hexokinases with a low Michaelis constant. The great majority of Glc-6P is metabolized through glycogen synthesis, glycolysis, and a pentose phosphate shunt (not shown). Approximately 1–3% of the incoming glucose, however, is used to form glucosamine-6-phosphate (GlcN-6P) via the action of the enzyme glutamine:fructose-6-phosphate amidotransferase. Glucosamine is also transported via the glucose transporter system and then directly enters the hexosamine biosynthetic pathway at the level of GlcN-6P. Further metabolism of GlcN-6P ultimately leads to the formation of uridine diphosphate *n*-acetyl glucosamine (UDPGlcNAc), the precursor for the formation of sialic acid and oligosaccharide side chains of proteins and lipids. (Reproduced by permission from the American Society for Clinical Investigation from Rossetti L, Hawkins M, Chen W, et al. In vivo glucosamine infusion induces insulin resistance in normoglycemic but not in hyperglycemic conscious rats. J Clin Invest 1995;96:132–140.)

tion in primary culture of adipose cells.[125] Strong evidence for this "hexosamine hypothesis" was provided by experiments inducing desensitization of the glucose transport system after prolonged incubations with glucosamine (GlcN) in the absence of glucose and the prevention of desensitization in the presence of glucose and insulin by the inhibition of glutamine:fructose-6-phosphate amidotransferase.[124] Further experimental support for this hypothesis comes from recent studies indicating that the metabolism of glucose through the hexosamine biosynthesis pathway may mediate some of insulin's effects on pyruvate kinase[126] and glycogen synthase.[127,128] Thus, in these isolated cell systems, hyperactivity of the hexosamine biosynthesis pathway per se caused, and its inhibition prevented, the development of desensitization of the glucose transport system. Whether this negative feedback system is operating in the skeletal muscle of intact animals is not known at present.

In summary, some evidence supports the notion that the hexosamine biosynthesis pathway functions as a regulatory pathway capable of desensitizing the glucose transport system to insulin in adipose tissue and skeletal muscle. This would represent an attractive *unifying hypothesis* for the presence of defective insulin action on glucose uptake in insulin-resistant states. In fact, increased routing of glucose carbons through the GlcN pathway could result from a sustained elevation in intracellular fructose-6-phosphate concentrations caused by increased glucose availability and/or decreased disposal through alternative major pathways, that is, glycolysis and/or glycogen synthesis. Thus, the mechanism by which hyperglycemia causes the impairment of insulin-stimulated glucose transport may unveil a more fundamental feedback control mechanism that downregulates cellular glucose uptake in response to a sustained increase in the intracellular availability of hexose phosphates. If such a regulatory pathway is operating in skeletal muscle in vivo and is capable of desensitizing the glucose transport system to insulin, it may help to explain the universal presence of defective insulin action on glucose transport/phosphorylation in insulin-resistant states.

Thus, we wished to investigate whether the hexosamine biosynthetic pathway may function as a regulatory pathway capable of desensitizing the glucose transport system to insulin in skeletal muscle in vivo. For this purpose, we examined whether the glucose-induced desensitization of insulin-mediated glucose uptake can be induced in the absence of sustained hyperglycemia via increased exogenous availability of glucosamine (GlcN)/glucosamine-6-phosphate, and whether this effect is modulated by concomitant chronic hyperglycemia. We monitored glucose uptake, glycolysis, and glycogen synthesis during insulin clamp studies in 6-hour fasted, conscious rats in the presence of a sustained (7-hour) increase in GlcN availability.[129]

The glucosamine hypothesis, as proposed by Marshall and colleagues, is based on the observation that approximately 1–3% of the glucose metabolized in insulin-sensitive tissues is through the GlcN biosynthetic pathway (see Fig. 60-4). Because the glucose concentrations required to induce insulin resistance in short-term studies is ~20 mM and because the affinity of GlcN for the glucose transport system is approximately fourfold lower than that of glucose, it may be calculated that extracellular GlcN concentrations of 0.8–2.4 mM may be required to simulate the glucose flux through the GlcN pathway under conditions that cause maximal desensitization of the glucose transport system to insulin stimulation. Similarly, the initial glucose flux during glucose "desensitization protocols" (high glucose + high insulin) is ~420 μmol/kg/min, of which 8 μmol/kg/min (~2%) may enter the GlcN pathway. Taking into account the lower affinity of GlcN versus glucose for the glucose transport system, it may be calculated that the infusion of GlcN at a rate of ~32 μmol/kg/min may be required to reproduce the flux of glucose to GlcN-6-P during glucose-induced insulin resistance. Based on these estimates, we increased the plasma GlcN concentration to ~1.2 mM by infusing GlcN at a rate of 30 μmol/kg/min. These circulating concentrations of GlcN closely approximate the concentrations of GlcN (1 mM for 5 hours) required for maximal desensitization of the glucose transport system in isolated adipose cells,[124] but they are lower than the GlcN concentration (10 mM for 60–180 minutes) that induced decreased insulin-mediated glucose transport in isolated muscle.[127]

The effect of GlcN infusions on insulin-mediated glucose uptake and metabolism (Figs. 60-5 and 60-6) was then examined.[129] Plasma GlcN concentrations were increased to ~1.2 mM during prolonged *eu*glycemic hyperinsulinemic clamp studies. The infusion of GlcN was associated with a time-dependent decline in the rates of glucose uptake and glycogen synthesis during these studies.[129] After approximately 5 hours, GlcN infusion caused a ~32% decrease in insulin-mediated glucose uptake, despite no impairment of muscle glycogen synthase kinetics and no increase in glucose-6-phosphate concentrations. Both glycogen synthesis and glycolysis were significantly impaired during the second clamp study compared with the first or with saline control studies (Fig. 60-6). Though glycolysis was significantly decreased (by 22%), however, the decline in glycogen synthesis was more severe and accounted for ~80% of the decreased rate of disappearance of glucose (Rd). In additional studies, we established that the GlcN-induced decrease in Rd reached a maximal effect by 5 hours and that the time required for a half-maximal effect of the amino sugar

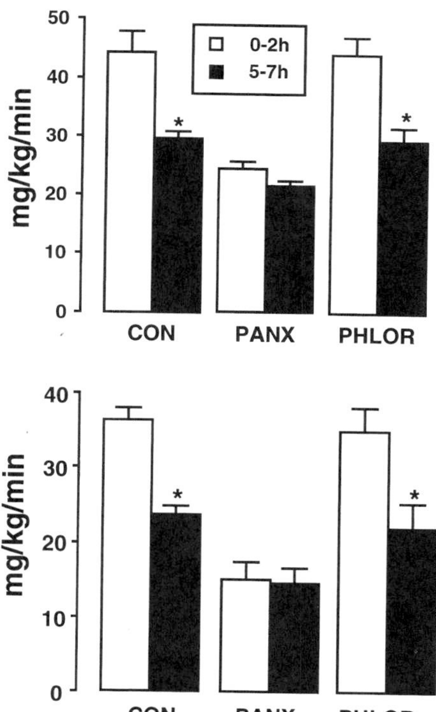

Figure 60-5. Rates of glucose disappearance (upper panel) and of glucose fusion (lower panel) in control rats (CON), 90% pancreatectomized diabetic rats (PANX), and phlorizin-treated diabetic rats (PHLOR) in the presence of similar concentrations of glucosamine. Results were obtained during identical insulin clamp studies performed during the first 2 hours and the last 2 hours of the 7 hours glucosamine infusion. *$p < 0.01$ 5–7 hours vs. 0–2 hours. (Reproduced by permission from the American Society for Clinical Investigation from Rossetti L, Hawkins M, Chen W, et al. In vivo glucosamine infusion induces insulin resistance in normoglycemic but not in hyperglycemic conscious rats. J Clin Invest 1995;96:132–140.)

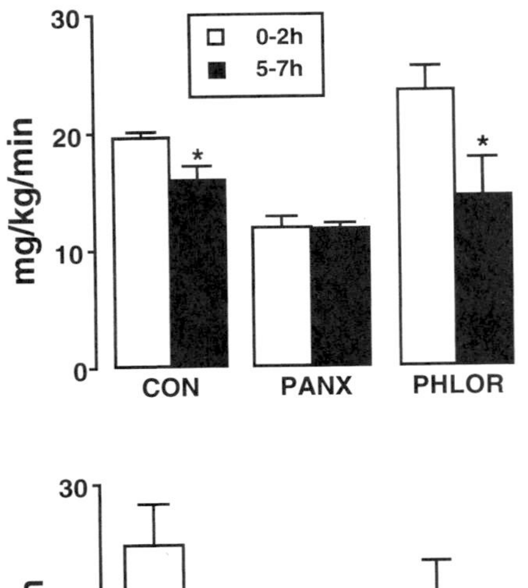

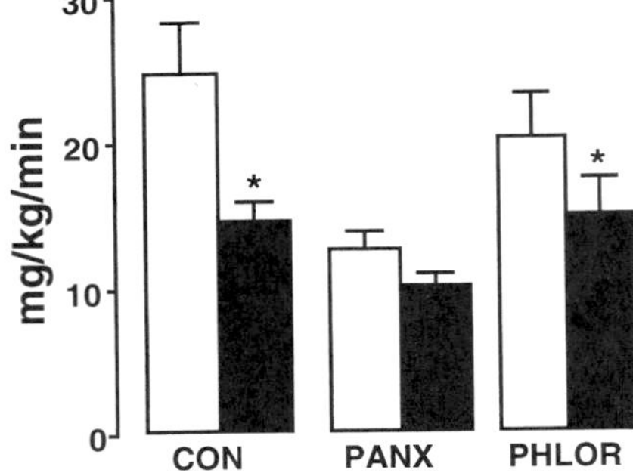

FIGURE 60-6. Rates of glycolysis (upper panel) and of glycogen synthesis (lower panel) in control rats (CON), 90% pancreatectomized diabetic rats (PANX), and phlorizin-treated diabetic rats (PHLOR) in the presence of similar concentrations of glucosamine. Results were obtained during identical insulin clamp studies performed during the first 2 hours and the last 2 hours of the 7-hour glucosamine infusion. $*p < 0.01$ 5–7 hours vs. 0–2 hours. (Reproduced by permission from the American Society for Clinical Investigation from Rossetti L, Hawkins M, Chen W, et al. In vivo glucosamine infusion induces insulin resistance in normoglycemic but not in hyperglycemic conscious rats. J Clin Invest 1995;96:132–140.)

on Rd was about 3 hours.[129] The proportionally greater decrease in glycogen synthesis suggests that a step beyond glucose transport/phosphorylation was also involved in the GlcN-induced insulin resistance. Because muscle glycogen synthase was normally activated by insulin, it is likely that the marked decrease in muscle uridine diphosphate glucose concentrations contributed to the impairment of glycogen synthesis (Fig. 60-7). Thus, increased GlcN availability can induce peripheral insulin resistance in vivo in conscious *nondiabetic* rats in the absence of prolonged exposure to high glucose and insulin concentrations.

Can the increased routing of glucose in the GlcN pathway cause further desensitization of glucose uptake in diabetic rats? We reasoned that if the impaired insulin action on skeletal muscle glucose uptake in diabetic rats is due to a chronic increase in the flux of glucose carbons through the GlcN pathway, the short-term effects of GlcN infusion on insulin-mediated glucose uptake may be blunted in chronically hyperglycemic diabetic rats versus nondiabetic rats. Similarly, we hypothesized that the ability of GlcN infusions to generate peripheral insulin resistance may be restored in diabetic rats by normalizing the plasma glucose concentration with phlorizin. Thus, we examined the short-term regulation of glucose uptake and intracellular glucose disposal by the enhanced carbon flux through the GlcN pathway in chronically hyperglycemic diabetic rats and in phlorizin-treated diabetic rats.[129] GlcN infusions generated similar plasma GlcN and muscle uridine diphosphate GlcNAc concentrations in all groups. Peripheral glucose uptake, glycolysis, and glycogen synthesis, however, were not significantly affected by increased GlcN availability in diabetic rats (Figs. 60-5 and 60-6). Long-term normalization of the plasma glucose concentrations by phlorizin treatment restored insulin-mediated glucose uptake, but not glycogen synthesis, to normal in diabetic rats. Correction of hyperglycemia also restored the marked effects of the GlcN infusion on insulin-mediated glucose uptake, glycolysis, and glycogen synthesis (Figs. 60-5 and 60-6). This alteration in glucose fluxes occurred in the absence of significant changes in the kinetics of muscle glycogen synthase and hexokinase and in the concentration of glucose-6-phosphate.[129]

Because a sustained increase in the availability of GlcN caused a marked impairment in glucose uptake, glycogen synthesis, and glycolysis in the absence of significant elevations in muscle glucose-6-phosphate concentrations, GlcN is likely to act at an early step of glucose uptake. Although most previous studies point to an impairment in glucose transport system as the major mechanism of action, an alteration in the phosphorylation of glucose cannot be excluded.

The above studies demonstrate that increased GlcN availability in vivo impairs insulin's ability to stimulate glucose uptake and glycogen synthesis in normoglycemic but not in chronically hyperglycemic conscious rats. These observations indicate that increased flux through the GlcN pathway can generate marked insulin resistance in skeletal muscle in vivo, and that this effect is not additive to the insulin resistance induced by chronic hyperglycemia. Because the ability of prolonged GlcN infusions to induce peripheral insulin resistance is lost in diabetic rats and is restored in phlorizin-treated diabetic rats, the deleterious effects of chronic hyperglycemia and GlcN infusions on peripheral insulin resistance do not appear to be additive, and they may act on a common pathway. This supports the hypothesis that increased flux through the GlcN pathway in skeletal muscle may play an important role in glucose-induced insulin resistance in vivo.

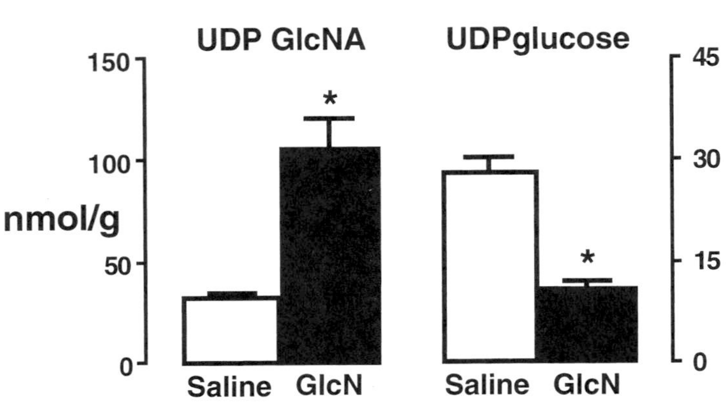

FIGURE 60-7. Skeletal muscle concentrations of uridine diphosphate-*n*-acetyl-glucosamine (UDP GlcNA) and UDP-glucose at the end of insulin clamp studies in combination with saline and glucosamine (GlcN) infusions. (Reproduced by permission from the American Society for Clinical Investigation from Rossetti L, Hawkins M, Chen W, et al. In vivo glucosamine infusion induces insulin resistance in normoglycemic but not in hyperglycemic conscious rats. J Clin Invest 1995;96:132–140.)

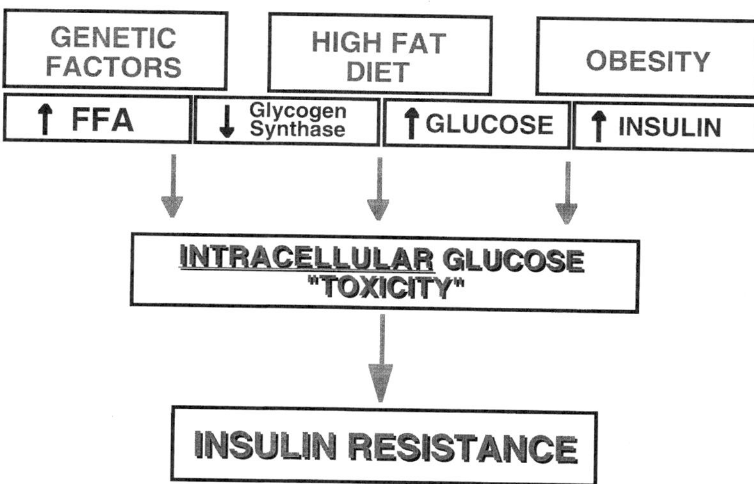

Figure 60-8. Unifying hypothesis for the pathogenesis of insulin resistance in NIDDM. Genetic and/or acquired alterations in carbohydrate metabolism may generate decreased insulin-mediated uptake of glucose in skeletal muscle via a common biochemical mechanism. In fact, a primary cause of either moderate glucose intolerance (e.g., a β-cell and/or hepatic defect) or a primary impairment in a major pathway of intracellular glucose disposal (e.g., glycogen synthesis and/or glycolysis) may cause a sustained elevation in intracellular hexose phosphates concentrations (*intracellular* glucose toxicity) and the increased routing of glucose carbons through the GlcN pathway due to increased glucose availability (high insulin and/or glucose) and/or decreased disposal through alternative major pathways, that is, glycolysis (e.g., high free fatty acid [FFA] and glycogen concentration) synthesis.

"Intracellular Glucose Toxicity": Implications for Non–Insulin-Dependent Diabetes Mellitus

Over the past several years, evidence has been provided for the multifactorial origin of insulin resistance in non–insulin-dependent diabetes mellitus (NIDDM). Despite some unique features, however, there are some biochemical/metabolic characteristics that are common to the majority of persons once the syndrome of insulin resistance is fully expressed. In particular, the impaired ability of insulin to promote skeletal muscle glucose uptake is a common endpoint of these conditions that ultimately requires the impairment of insulin action on glucose transport and/or phosphorylation.

We and others have suggested that the similarity of all insulin-resistant syndromes, regardless of their primary cause, may be due to the deleterious effects of chronic hyperglycemia per se on insulin action, in particular on skeletal muscle glucose transport. The latter hypothesis may explain the evolution of syndromes of insulin resistance that are associated with some degree of hyperglycemia. Several authors, however, have reported that peripheral insulin resistance may be a feature of persons with normal glucose tolerance as well. In particular, defects in insulin action on skeletal muscle glucose transport/phosphorylation and on glucose oxidation, ''glucose storage,'' and glycogen synthase have been shown in these persons. Although a common primary defect in insulin activation of both skeletal muscle glucose transport and glycogen synthase remains a viable hypothesis, the variety of pathophysiologic conditions (e.g., nondiabetic siblings of diabetic parents, obesity, hypertension) and of ethnic backgrounds (e.g., European and American Caucasians, Pima Indians, Mexican-Americans) appears to indicate that the primary genetic and/or acquired defect(s) is likely to be different both between and within groups.

A potential explanation is that a primary cause of either moderate glucose intolerance (e.g., a β-cell and/or a hepatic defect) or a primary impairment in a major pathway of intracellular glucose disposal (e.g., glycogen synthesis and/or glycolysis) may underlie the full expression of the insulin resistance syndrome through a common mechanism.

Marshall's observation that desensitization of the glucose transport system in cells incubated with high concentrations of glucose and insulin requires the metabolism of glucose in a quantitatively small pathway of glucose disposal, the glucosamine pathway, and our recent report in conscious rats[129] provide evidence that this regulatory pathway is operating in skeletal muscle in vivo and is capable of desensitizing the glucose transport system to insulin. Thus, a *unifying hypothesis* for the universal presence of defective insulin action on glucose transport/phosphorylation in insulin-resistant states may be advanced. In fact, increased routing of glucose carbons through the GlcN pathway could result from a sustained elevation in intracellular fructose-6-phosphate concentrations caused by increased glucose availability and/or decreased disposal through alternative major pathways, that is, glycolysis and glycogen synthesis (Fig. 60-8).

Thus, the mechanism by which hyperglycemia leads to impaired insulin action on glucose transport/phosphorylation may shed light on a more fundamental ''feedback control system'' that downregulates cellular glucose uptake in response to a sustained increase in the intracellular availability of hexose phosphates.

References

1. The Diabetes Control and Complications Trial Research Group. The effect of intensive treatment of diabetes on the development and progression of long-term complications in insulin-dependent diabetes mellitus. N Engl J Med 1993;329:977
2. Reichard P, Nilsson B-Y, Rosenqvist U. The effect of long-term intensified insulin treatment on the development of microvascular complications of diabetes mellitus. N Engl J Med 1993;329:304
3. Job D, Eshwege E, Guyot-Argenton C, et al. Effect of multiple daily insulin injection on the course of retinopathy. Diabetes 1976;25:463
4. Lauritzen T, Frost-Larsen K, Larsen HW, Deckert T. Steno Study Group: Two year experience with continuous subcutaneous insulin infusion in relation to retinopathy and neuropathy. Diabetes 1985;34(suppl 3):74
5. Deckert T, Lauritzen T, Parving H, Christensen JS. Steno Study Group: Effect of two years of strict metabolic control on kidney function in long-term insulin dependent-diabetics. Diabetic Nephropathy 1983;2:6
6. Feldt-Rasmussen B, Mathiesen ER, Deckert T. Effect of two years of strict metabolic control on progression of incipient nephropathy in insulin-dependent diabetes. Lancet 1986;2:1300
7. Dahl-Jorgensen K, Brichmann-Hanssen O, Hanssen KF, et al. Effect of near normoglycemia for two years on progression of early diabetic retinopathy, nephropathy, and neuropathy: The Oslo study. Br Med J 1986;293:1194
8. Rosenstock J, Friberg T, Raskin P. The effect of glycemic control on the microvascular complications in patients with type I diabetes mellitus. Am J Med 1986;81:1012
9. Raskin P, Pietri A, Unger R, Shannon WA. The effect of diabetic control on skeletal muscle capillary basement membrane width in patients with type I diabetes mellitus. N Engl J Med 1983;309:1546
10. Krolewski AS, Canessa M, Warram JH, et al. Predisposition to hypertension and susceptibility to renal disease in insulin-dependent diabetes mellitus. N Engl J Med 1988;319:140
11. Engerman R, Bloodworth JMB, Nelson S. Relationship of microvascular disease in diabetes to metabolic control. Diabetes 1977;26:760
12. Mauer SM, Steffes MW, Sutherland DER, et al. Studies of the rate of regression of the glomerular lesions in diabetic rats treated with pancreatic islet transplantation. Diabetes 1975;24:280
13. Johnsson SL. Retinopathy and nephropathy in diabetes mellitus: Comparison of the effect of two forms of treatment. Diabetes 1960;9:1
14. Pirart J. Diabetes mellitus and its degenerative complications: A prospective study of 4,400 patients observed between 1947 and 1973. Diabetes Metab 1977;3:97
15. Eschwege E, Richard JL, Thibult N, et al. Coronary heart diseased mortality in relation with diabetes, blood glucose and plasma insulin levels: The Paris Prospective Study, ten years later. Horm Metab Res 1985;15(suppl):41

16. Hostetter MK. Handicaps to host defenses. Effect of hyperglycemia on C3 and *Candida albicans*. Diabetes 1990;39:271
17. Rayfield EJ, Ault MJ, Keusch GT, et al. Infection and diabetes: The case for glucose control. Am J Med 1982;72:439
18. Unger RH, Grundy S. Hyperglycaemia as an inducer as well as a consequence of impaired islet cell function and insulin resistance: Implications for the management of diabetes. Diabetologia 1985;28:119
19. Bonner-Weir S, Trent DF, Weir GC. Partial pancreatectomy in the rat and subsequent defect in glucose-induced insulin release. J Clin Invest 1983; 71:1544
20. Rossetti L, Shulman GI, Zawalich W, DeFronzo RA. Effect of chronic hyperglycemia on in vivo insulin secretion in partially pancreatectomized rats. J Clin Invest 1987;80:1037
21. Leahy JL, Cooper HE, Weir GC. Chronic hyperglycemia is associated with impaired glucose influence on insulin secretion. J Clin Invest 1986;77: 908
22. Leahy JL, Bonner-Weir S, Weir GC. Minimal chronic hyperglycemia is a critical determinant of impaired insulin secretion after an incomplete pancreatectomy. J Clin Invest 1988;81:1407
23. Robertson RP. Type II diabetes, glucose "non-sense," and islet cell desensitization. Diabetes 1989;38:1501
24. Rossetti L, Smith D, Shulman GI, et al. Correction of hyperglycemia with phlorizin normalizes tissue sensitivity to insulin in diabetic rats. J Clin Invest 1987;79:1510
25. Yki-Jarvinen H, Helve E, Koivisto VA. Hyperglycemia decreases glucose uptake in type I diabetes. Diabetes 1987;36:892
26. Rossetti L, Giaccari A, DeFronzo RA. Glucose toxicity. Diabetes Care 1990;13:610
27. Yki-Jarvinen H. Glucose toxicity. Endocrine Rev 1992;13:415
28. DeFronzo RA, Hendler R, Simonson D. Insulin resistance is a prominent feature of insulin dependent diabetes. Diabetes 1982;31:795
29. Yki-Jarvinen, Koivisto VA. Natural history of insulin resistance in type I diabetes. N Engl J Med 1986;315:224
30. Himsworth HP, Kerr RB. Insulin-sensitive types of diabetes mellitus. Clin Sci 1942;4:120
31. DeFronzo RA, Diebert D, Hendler R, Felig P. Insulin sensitivity and insulin binding in maturity onset diabetes. J Clin Invest 1979;63:939
32. Kolterman OG, Gray RS, Griffin J, et al. Receptor and postreceptor defects contribute to the insulin resistance in noninsulin-dependent diabetes mellitus. J Clin Invest 1981;68:957
33. Rizza RA, Mandarino LJ, Gerich JE. Mechanism and significance of insulin resistance in noninsulin-dependent diabetes mellitus. Diabetes 1981;30: 990
34. DeFronzo RA, Gunnarsson R, Bjorkman O, et al. Effects of insulin on peripheral and splanchnic glucose metabolism in noninsulin dependent (type II) diabetes mellitus. J Clin Invest 1985;76:149
35. Kobberling J, Tillil H. Empirical risk figures for first-degree relatives of non-insulin-dependent diabetics. In: Kobberling J, Tsttersal R, eds. The Genetics of Diabetes Mellitus. London: Academic Press;1982:201–210
36. Newman B, Selby JV, King MC, et al. Concordance for type 2 (non–insulin-dependent) diabetes mellitus in male twins. Diabetologia 1987;30:763
37. Barner AH, Eff C, Leslie RD, Pyke DA. Diabetes in identical twins: A study of 2 pairs. Diabetologia 1981;20:87
38. Lillioja S, Mott DM, Zawadzki JK, et al. In vivo insulin action is a familial characteristic in nondiabetic Pima Indians. Diabetes 1987;36:1329
39. Lillioja S, Bogardus C. Obesity and insulin resistance: Lessons learned from the Pima Indians. Diabetes/Metab Rev 1988;4:515
40. Eriksson J, Franssila-Kallunki A, Edstrand A, et al. Early metabolic defects in persons at increased risk of non–insulin-dependent diabetes mellitus. N Engl J Med 1989;321:337
41. Vaag A, Henriksen JE, Beck-Nielsen H. Decreased insulin activation of glycogen synthase in skeletal muscle in young nonobese Caucasian first-degree relatives of patients with non–insulin-dependent diabetes mellitus. J Clin Invest 1992;89:782
42. Gulli G, Ferrannini E, Stern M, et al. The metabolic profile of NIDDM is fully established in glucose-tolerant offspring of two Mexican-American NIDDM parents. Diabetes 1992;41:1575
43. DeFronzo RA, Simonson D, Ferrannini E. Hepatic and peripheral insulin resistance. A common feature of insulin-independent and non insulin-dependent diabetes. Diabetologia 1982;23:313
44. Beck-Nielsen H, Richelsen B, Hasling C, et al. Improved in vivo insulin effect during continuous subcutaneous insulin infusion in patients with IDDM. Diabetes 1984;33:832
45. Yki-Jarvinen H, Koivisto VA. Continuous subcutaneous insulin infusion therapy decreases insulin resistance in type I diabetes. J Clin Endocrinol Metab 1984;58:659
46. Yki-Jarvinen H, Koivisto VA. Insulin sensitivity in newly diagnosed type I diabetics after ketoacidosis and after three months of insulin therapy. J Clin Endocrinol Metab 1984;59:371
47. Lager I, Lonnroth P, Von Schenck H, Smith U. Reversal of insulin resistance in type I diabetes after treatment with continuous subcutaneous insulin infusion. Br Med J 1983;287:1001
48. Kurszynska YT, Petranyi G, Home PD, et al. Muscle enzyme activity and insulin sensitivity in type I (insulin-dependent) diabetes mellitus. Diabetologia 1986;29:699
49. Gray RS, Cowan P, Duncan LJP, Clarke BF. Reversal of insulin resistance in type I diabetes following initiation of insulin treatment. Diabetic Med 1986;3:18
50. Garvey WT, Olefsky JM, Griffin J, et al. The effect of insulin treatment on insulin secretion and insulin action in type II diabetes mellitus. Diabetes 1985;34:222
51. Foley J, Kashiwagi A, Verso MA, et al. Improvement in in vitro insulin action after one month of insulin therapy in obese noninsulin-dependent diabetics. J Clin Invest 1983;72:1901
52. Nankervis A, Proietto J, Aitken P, et al. Differential effects of insulin therapy on hepatic and peripheral insulin sensitivity in type 2 (non–insulin-dependent) diabetes. Diabetologia 1982;23:320
53. Greenfield M, Lardinois C, Doberne L, Vreman H. Metabolic effects of intensive insulin therapy in patients with non–insulin-dependent diabetes (NIDDM). Diabetes 1982;31(suppl 2):58A
54. Andrews WJ, Vasquez B, Nagulesparan M, et al. Insulin therapy in obese, non–insulin-dependent diabetes induces improvements in insulin action and secretion that are maintained for two weeks after insulin withdrawal. Diabetes 1984;33:634
55. Scarlett JA, Garvey RS, Griffin J, et al. Insulin treatment reverses the insulin resistance of type II diabetes mellitus. Diabetes Care 1982;5:353
56. Gormley MJJ, Hadden DR, Woods R, et al. One month's insulin treatment of type II diabetes: The early and medium-term effects following insulin withdrawal. Metabolism 1986;35:1029
57. Hidaka H, Nagulesparan M, Klimes I, et al. Improvement of insulin secretion but not insulin resistance after short term control of plasma glucose in obese type II diabetics. J Clin Endocrinol Metab 1982;54:217
58. Scarlett JA, Kolterman OG, Ciaraldi TP, et al. Insulin treatment reverses the postreceptor defect in adipocyte 3-O-methylglucose transport in type II diabetes mellitus. J Clin Endocrinol Metab 1983;56:1195
59. Savage PJ, Bennion LO, Flock EV, et al. Diet-induced improvement of abnormalities in insulin and glucagon secretion and in insulin receptor binding in diabetes mellitus. J Clin Endocrinol Metab 1979;48:999
60. Henry RR, Scheaffer L, Olefsky JM. Glycemic effects of intensive caloric restriction and isocaloric refeeding in noninsulin-dependent diabetes mellitus. J Clin Endocrinol Metab 1985;61:917
61. Henry RR, Wiest-Kent TA, Scheaffer L, et al. Metabolic consequences of very-low-calorie diet therapy in obese non–insulin-dependent diabetic and nondiabetic subjects. Diabetes 1986;35:155
62. Nagulesparan N, Savage PJ, Bennion LJ, et al. Diminished effect of caloric restriction on control of hyperglycemia with increasing duration of type II diabetes mellitus. J Clin Endocrinol Metab 1981;53:560
63. Henry RR, Wallace P, Olefsky JM. Effects of weight loss on mechanisms of hyperglycemia in obese non–insulin-dependent diabetes mellitus. Diabetes 1986;35:990
64. Beck-Nielsen H, Pedersen O, Sorensen NS. Effects of dietary changes on cellular insulin binding and in vivo insulin sensitivity. Metabolism 1980; 29:482
65. Laakso M, Uusitupa M, Takala J, et al. Effects of hypocaloric diet and insulin therapy on metabolic control and mechanisms of hyperglycemia in obese non–insulin-dependent diabetic subjects. Metabolism 1988;37:1092
66. Zawadski JK, Bogardus C, Foley JE. Insulin action in obese non–insulin-dependent diabetics and in their isolated adipocytes before and after weight loss. Diabetes 1987;36:227
67. Walshe K, Andrews WJ, Sheridan B, et al. Three months energy restricted diet does not induce peripheral insulin resistance in new diagnosed non–insulin dependent diabetics. Horm Metab Res 1987;19:197
68. Kolterman OG, Grag RS, Shapiro G, et al. The acute and chronic effects of sulfonylurea therapy in type II diabetes. Diabetes 1984;33:346
69. Firth RG, Bell PM, Rizza RA. Effects of tolazamide and exogenous insulin on insulin action in patients with non–insulin-dependent diabetes mellitus. N Engl J Med 1986;314:1280
70. Mandarino LJ, Gerich JE. Prolonged sulfonylurea administration decreases insulin resistance and increases insulin secretion in non–insulin-dependent diabetes mellitus: Evidence for improved insulin action at a postreceptor site in hepatic as well as extrahepatic tissues. Diabetes Care 1984;7(suppl 1):89
71. Simonson DC, Ferrannini E, Bevilacqua S, et al. Mechanism of improvement in glucose metabolism after chronic glyburide therapy. Diabetes 1984;33: 838
72. Groop L, Schalin C, Franssila-Kalolunki A, et al. Characteristics of non–insulin dependent diabetic patients with secondary failure to oral antidiabetic therapy. Am J Med 1989;87:183
73. Castillo M, Scheen AJ, Paolisso G, Lefebvre PJ. The addition of glipizide to insulin therapy in type II diabetic patients with secondary failure to sulfonylureas is useful only in the presence of a significant residual insulin secretion. Acta Endocrinol 1987;116:364
74. Yki-Jarvinen H, Nikkila E, Eero H, Taskinen MR. Clinical benefits and mechanisms of a sustained response to intermittent insulin therapy in type 2 diabetic patients with secondary drug failure. Am J Med 1988;84:185
75. Hollenbeck CB, Chen Y-DI, Reaven GM. A comparison of the relative effects of obesity and non–insulin-dependent diabetes mellitus on in vivo insulin-stimulated glucose utilization. Diabetes 1984;33:622
76. Garvey WT, Olefsky JM, Marshall S. Insulin receptor down-regulation is linked to an insulin-induced postreceptor defect in the glucose transport system in rat adipoctyes. J Clin Invest 1985;76:22
77. Rizza RA, Mandarino LJ, Genest J, et al. Production of insulin resistance by hyperinsulinemia in man. Diabetologia 1985;28:70

78. Reaven GM, Sageman WS, Swenson RS. Development of insulin resistance in normal dogs following alloxan-induced insulin deficiency. Diabetologia 1977;13:459
79. Dall'Aglio E, Chang H, Hollenbeck CB, et al. In vivo and in vitro resistance to maximal insulin stimulated glucose disposal in insulin deficiency. Am J Physiol 1985;249:E312
80. Bevilacqua S, Barrett EJ, Smith D, et al. Hepatic and peripheral insulin resistance following streptozotocin-induced insulin deficiency in the dog. Metabolism 1985;34:817
81. Rossetti L, Giaccari A. Relative contribution of glycogen synthesis and glycolysis to insulin-mediated glucose uptake. A dose-response euglycemic clamp study in normal and diabetic rats. J Clin Invest 1990;85:1785
82. Rossetti L, Hu M. Skeletal muscle glycogenolysis is more sensitive to insulin than is glucose transport/phosphorylation. Relation to the insulin-induced inhibition of hepatic glucose production. J Clin Invest 1993;92:2963
83. Levy J, Gavin J III, Fausto A, et al. Impaired insulin action in rats with non-insulin dependent diabetes. Diabetes 1984;33:901
84. Kruszynska YT, Home PD. Liver and muscle insulin sensitivity, glycogen concentration, and glycogen synthase activity in a rat model of non–insulin dependent diabetes. Diabetologia 1988;31:304
85. Kahn BB, Shulman GI, DeFronzo RA, et al. Normalization of blood glucose in diabetic rats with phlorizin treatment reverses insulin resistant glucose transport in adipose cells without restoring glucose transporter gene expression. J Clin Invest 1991;87:561
86. Hager SR, Jochen AL, Kalkhoff RK. Insulin resistance in normal rats infused with glucose for 72h. Am J Physiol 1991;260:E353
87. Richter EA, Hansen BF, Hansen SA. Glucose-induced insulin resistance of skeletal muscle glucose transport and uptake. Biochem J 1988;252:733
88. Richter EA, Hansen SA, Hansen BF. Mechanisms limiting glycogen storage in muscle during prolonged insulin stimulation. Am J Physiol 1988; 255:E621
89. Hansen BF, Hansen SA, Ploug T, et al. Effects of glucose and insulin on development of impaired insulin action in muscle. Am J Physiol 1992; 262:E440
90. Yki-Jarvinen H, Helve E, Koivisto VA. Hyperglycemia decreases glucose uptake in type 1 diabetes. Diabetes 1987;36:892
91. Vuorinen-Markkola H, Koivisto VA, Yki-Jarvinen H. Mechanisms of hyperglycemia-induced insulin resistance in whole body and skeletal muscle of type 1 diabetic patients. Diabetes 1992;41:571
92. Fowelin J, Attvall S, Von Schenck H, et al. Effect of prolonged hyperglycemia on growth hormone levels and insulin sensitivity in insulin-dependent diabetes mellitus. Metabolism 1993;42:387
93. Rossetti L, Shulman GI, Zawalich W, DeFronzo RA. Effect of chronic hyperglycemia on in vivo insulin secretion in partially pancreatectomized rats. J Clin Invest 1987;80:1037
94. Rossetti L, Laughlin MR. Correction of chronic hyperglycemia with vanadate, but not with phlorizin, normalizes in vivo glycogen repletion and in vitro glycogen synthase activity in diabetic skeletal muscle. J Clin Invest 1989; 84:892
95. Karnieli E, Hissin PJ, Simpson IA, et al. A possible mechanism of insulin resistance in the rat adipose cell in streptozotocin-induced diabetes mellitus. Depletion of intracellular glucose transport systems. J Clin Invest 1981; 68:811
96. Kasuga MY, Akanuma Y, Iwamoto K, Kosaka K. Insulin binding and glucose metabolism in adipocytes from streptozotocin-diabetic rats. Am J Physiol 1978;235:E175
97. Kobayashi M, Olefsky JM. Effects of streptozotocin-induced diabetes on insulin binding, glucose transport, and intracellular glucose metabolism in isolated rat adipocytes. Diabetes 1979;28:87
98. Dohm GL, Tapscott EB, Pories WJ, et al. An in vitro human muscle preparation suitable for metabolic studies. Decreased insulin stimulation of glucose transport in muscle from morbidly obese and diabetic subjects. J Clin Invest 1988;82:486
99. Garvey WT, Huecksteadt TP, Matthaei S, Olefsky JM. Role of glucose transporters in the cellular insulin resistance of type II non–insulin-dependent diabetes mellitus. J Clin Invest 1988;81:1528
100. Haspal HC, Vilk EW, Birnbaum MT, et al. Glucose deprivation and hexose transporter polypeptides of murine fibroblasts. J Biol Chem 1986;261:6778
101. Van Putten JPM, Krans HMJ. Glucose as a regulator of insulin-sensitive hexose uptake in 3T3 adipocytes. J Biol Chem 1985;260:7996
102. Sasson S, Cerasi E. Substrate regulation of the glucose transport system in rat skeletal muscle. J Biol Chem 1986;261:16827
103. Garvey WT, Olefsky JM, Matthaei S, Marshall S. Glucose and insulin coregulate the glucose transport system in primary cultured adipocytes. A new mechanism of insulin resistance. J Biol Chem 1987;262:189
104. Sasson S, Edelson D, Cerasi E. In vitro autoregulation of glucose utilization in rat soleus muscle. Diabetes 1987;36:1041
105. Kletzien RF, Perdue JF. Induction of sugar transport in chick embryo fibroblasts by hexose starvation: Evidence for transcriptional regulation of transport. J Biol Chem 1985;250:593
106. Ullrey D, Gammon BMT, Kalckar HM. Uptake patterns and transport enhancements in cultures of hamster cells deprived of carbohydrates. Arch Biochem Biophys 1975;167:410
107. Ullrey DB, Kalckar HM. The nature of regulation of hexose transport in cultured mammalian fibroblasts: Aerobic "repressive" control by D-glucosamine. Arch Biochem Biophys 1981;209:168
108. Traxinger RR, Marshall S. Recovery of maximal insulin responsiveness after induction of insulin resistance. J Biol Chem 1989;264:8156
109. Marshall S, Garvey WT, Traxinger RR. New insights into the metabolic regulation of insulin action and insulin resistance: Role of glucose and amino acids. FASEB J 1991;5:3031
110. Crettaz M, Prentky M, Zaninetti D, Jeanrenaud B. Insulin resistance in soleus muscle from obese Zucker rats. Biochem J 1980;186:525
111. Berger M, Hagg SA, Goodman MN, Rudermann NB. Glucose metabolism in perfused skeletal muscle. Biochem J 1976;158:191
112. Charron MJ, Kahn BB. Divergent molecular mechanisms for insulin resistant glucose transport in muscle and adipose cells in vivo. J Biol Chem 1990; 265:7994
113. Kahn BB, Rossetti L, Lodish HF, Charron MJ. Decreased in vivo glucose uptake but normal expression of GLUT1 and GLUT4 in skeletal muscle. J Clin Invest 1991;87:2197
114. Garvey WT, Huecksteadt TP, Birnbaum MT. Pretranslational suppression of an insulin-responsive glucose transporter in rats with diabetes mellitus. Science (Wash DC) 1989;245:60
115. Sivitz WI, DeSautel SL, Kayano T, et al. Regulation of glucose transporter messenger RNA in insulin-deficient states. Nature (Lond) 1989;340:72
116. Berger JC, Biswas P, Vicario P, et al. Decreased expression of the insulin-responsive glucose transporter in diabetes and fasting. Nature (Lond) 1989;340:70
117. Kahn BB, Charron MJ, Lodish HF, et al. Differential regulation of two glucose transporters in adipose cells from diabetic and insulin treated diabetic rats. J Clin Invest 1989;84:404
118. Sivitz WI, DeSautel SL, Kayano T, et al. Regulation of glucose transporter messenger RNA levels in rat adipose tissue by insulin. Mol Endocrinol 1990;4:583
119. Kahn BB, Flier JS. Regulation of glucose transporter gene expression in vivo and in vitro glucose. Diabetes Care 1991;87:561
120. Dimitrakoudis D, Ramlal T, Rastogi S, et al. Glycemia regulates the glucose transporter number in the plasma membrane of the rat skeletal muscle. Biochem J 1992;284:341
121. Cordera R, Andraghetti G, DeFronzo RA, Rossetti L. Effect of in vivo vanadate treatment on insulin receptor tyrosine kinase activity in partially pancreatectomized diabetic rats. Endocrinology 1990;126:2177
122. Marshall S, Monzon R. Amino acid regulation of insulin action in isolated adipocytes. J Biol Chem 1989;264:2037
123. Marshall S. Kinetics of insulin action on protein synthesis in isolated adipocytes. Ability of glucose to selectively desensitize the glucose transport system without altering insulin stimulation of protein synthesis. J Biol Chem 1989;264:2029
124. Marshall S, Bacote V, Traxinger RR. Discovery of a metabolic pathway mediating desensitization of the glucose transport system: Role of hexosamine biosynthesis in the induction of insulin resistance. J Biol Chem 1992; 266:4706
125. Traxinger RR, Marshall S. Role of amino acids in modulating glucose-induced desensitization of the glucose transport system. J Biol Chem 1989;264: 20910
126. Traxinger RR, Marshall S. Insulin regulation of pyruvate kinase activity in isolated adipocytes. Crucial role of glucose and the hexosamine biosynthesis pathway in the expression of insulin action. J Biol Chem 1992;267: 9718
127. Robinson KA, Sens DA, Buse MG. Pre-exposure to glucosamine induces insulin resistance of glucose transport and glycogen synthesis in isolated rat skeletal muscles. Diabetes 1993;42:1333
128. Crook ED, Daniels MC, Smith TM, McClain DA. Regulation of insulin-stimulated glycogen synthase activity by overexpression of glutamine:fructose-6-phosphate amidotransferase in rat-1 fibroblasts. Diabetes 1993;42: 1289
129. Rossetti L, Hawkins M, Chen W, et al. In vivo glucosamine infusion induces insulin resistance in normoglycemic but not in hyperglycemic conscious rats. J Clin Invest 1995;96:132

Diabetes Mellitus, edited by Derek LeRoith, Simeon I. Taylor, and Jerrold M. Olefsky. Lippincott–Raven Publishers, Philadelphia © 1996.

Chapter 61
TNFα and the Insulin Resistance of Obesity

Gökhan S. Hotamisligil and Bruce M. Spiegelman

The close association between obesity and diabetes has been recognized since before the time of Christ.[1] Because insulin resistance is a ubiquitous correlate of obesity and a central component of non–insulin-dependent diabetes mellitus (NIDDM), it is generally believed that insulin resistance is a key physiologic component that links these disorders.[2–4] How an expanded adipose mass can result in a defect in systemic insulin action has been difficult to understand. New data have emerged over the last few years indicating that the potent cytokine tumor necrosis factor-α (TNFα) may be a very important molecule that is produced by fat cells in obesity and interferes with insulin action.[5,6] This chapter will provide a brief overview of TNFα's signaling mechanisms and review recent data concerning the role of this molecule in obesity-linked insulin resistance and other related disorders.

Tumor Necrosis Factor-α

Tumor necrosis factor-α (TNFα), along with its close relative lymphotoxin-α (LTα, also called TNFβ), was first isolated as the active principal causing tumor necrosis in bacterially infected animals.[7,8] Subsequently, TNFα was purified as the mediator of hypertriglyceridemia and wasting (cachexia) in parasitically infected animals.[9] It is now recognized that TNFα defines a family of effectors among cytokines that modulate many immune functions.[10] TNFα is encoded by a single gene within the major histocompatibility complex on human chromosome 6 and mouse chromosome 17, and lies next to LTα and a recently characterized member, LTβ.[10] The protein product can exist as a 26-kd membrane-bound monomer or as a secreted trimer of 17 kd subunits.[11] Although the functional significance of these two forms is not entirely clear, inhibition of the processing of the 26-kd form can block many of the effects of TNFα. Like many other cytokines, TNFα has diverse functions in both the immune and extraimmune systems. Examples include the induction of apoptotic cell death, lysis of tumor cells, stimulation of thymocyte growth, induction of the production of other cytokines such as granulocyte monocyte-colony stimulating factor (GM-CSF) and interleukin-1, and regulation of cell differentiation.[10,12,13] Understanding the biologic function(s) of TNFα in normal physiology and development has been quite complicated. Recently, the generation of mice with targeted mutations at the TNFα and LTα loci has illustrated the importance of these molecules during development.[14,15] The *LTα*-as well as the *LTα-TNFα* double mutants exhibited abnormal development of peripheral lymphoid organs and altered immune responses.[14,15] These animal models (along with a TNFα-deficient mouse that is yet to be developed) will assist the elucidation of the full spectrum of TNFα and LTα activities.

In pathophysiologic states, elevated TNFα production has been associated with septic shock, rheumatoid arthritis, graft-versus-host disease, inflammatory bowel diseases, and various other disorders.[16] TNFα also has profound effects on whole body lipid metabolism.[17] In vivo, TNFα administration causes an increase in serum triglyceride and very low density lipoprotein concentrations in rats and humans.[17] This hyperlipidemia is thought to be the result of increased hepatic lipogenesis and lipolysis rather than decreased peripheral clearance.[18] In addition to TNFα, interleukin-1 and interferonγ also stimulate hepatic fatty acid synthesis in rodents.[17,18] Previous studies have associated TNFα expression with catabolic states (such as cancer and infection) leading to a wasting syndrome termed *cachexia*.[12,19] This effect of TNFα has been recently reviewed[5] and will be briefly discussed below. TNFα and a number of other cytokines (e.g., TNFβ, interleukin-1 and interferonγ) also affect glucose homeostasis in various tissues.[17,18]

With respect to adipocytes, where most of our own work has been done, previous work has shown that TNFα causes suppression of most lipogenic enzymes, including lipoprotein lipases, and induces "dedifferentiation" of adipocytes when used in fairly high doses.[20] This effect potentially involves the activation of phospholipase A2 and the generation of arachidonic acid metabolites.[21] At lower doses (≤100 pM), however, changes in gene expression are more specific (e.g., suppression of GLUT-4 and adipsin expression) and occur in the absence of general alterations in the adipocyte phenotype.[6,22] These changes in gene expression patterns have been postulated to involve regulation of the transcription factor CAAT/Enhancer Binding Protein (C/EBP-α).[23] The interference with insulin action by TNFα, discussed below, also occurs at doses that are insufficient to cause generalized suppression of adipocyte gene expression.

Tumor Necrosis Factor Receptors and Signaling

Tumor necrosis factor-α, (TNFα), like most peptide effectors, is believed to function through transmembrane receptors. There are two identified receptors for TNF: TNF-R1 (p55 in the rodent, p60 in humans) and TNF-R2 (p75 in the rodent, p80 in humans).[10,24] TNF-R1 and TNF-R2 are also encoded by single genes on human chromosomes 12p13 and 1p36 and on mouse chromosomes 6 and 4, respectively.[25,26] The receptors are coexpressed in virtually all cells, albeit in different ratios. Both of these receptors can bind to TNFα and lymphotoxin-α (LTα), and they are both active in signaling TNF responses.[10,24] The TNF receptors exist as monomers on the cell surface but undergo ligand-induced multimerization, which is believed to be critical for signaling. In addition, both receptors can be released from the cell surface through proteolytic cleavage and exist in soluble form. As might be expected for ligands binding overlapping receptors, there is a great deal of overlap of function between TNFα and TNFβ. The two receptors for TNF, however, share almost no homology outside of the ligand binding domain, suggesting that they signal for different biologic functions.[10,24,27] Recently, mice carrying targeted mutations of both *TNF-R1,* and *TNF-R2* have been generated.[28,29,30] The *TNF-R1*-deficient mice were resistant to endotoxin-induced shock but exhibited susceptibility to *Listeria monocytogenes*.[28,29] The *TNF-R2*-deficient mice had a minimal phenotype in terms of altered immune responses to infection and endotoxin but displayed dramatic decreases in TNF-induced tissue necrosis.[30] None of these genetic models exhibit any developmental abnormality.

The TNF receptors also belong to a larger family of receptors comprising at least 12 members, including TNF-receptor related protein, which has been shown to bind preferentially LTβ (or LTα-β heterotrimers), as well as the nerve growth factor NGF and Fas receptors.[10] One interesting feature of this family is that their intracellular domains do not immediately suggest a biochemical function; they apparently do not act directly as ligand-stimulated protein kinases. On the other hand, TNFα is known to initiate a cascade of signal transduction that includes the activation of protein kinases and phosphoprotein phosphatases.[13] Multiple protein kinases are activated by TNFα, including protein kinase A and C, mitogen activated protein, and kinases p38, p42, p44, and p54.[31–34] A number of novel kinases have also been defined in TNFα-stimulated cells, including an hsp27 kinase, a β-casein kinase, and a ceramide-activated protein kinase.[35,36] In addition to the activation of various kinases, TNFα regulates phosphoprotein phosphatase activities during the early phases of its signal transduction cascades. Recent evidence suggests that the sphingomyelin pathway is a critical component in the initiation of these TNFα-induced phosphorylation/dephosphorylation cascades, employing ceramide as a second messenger.[37]

Further downstream responses include the activation of certain transcription factors, such as nuclear factor-κB, the AP-1 family of transcription factors (c-*fos* and c-*jun*), interferon regulatory factor-1 (IRF-1), and IRF-2.[13] Recently, a novel class of accessory molecules has been identified as associated molecules (TNF receptor associated factor-1 and TRAF-2) with the cytoplasmic domain of TNF-R2.[38] Finally, a long list of genes (e.g., TNFα itself and other cytokines, growth factors, and hormones, cell adhesion molecules, and inflammatory mediators) are regulated by TNFα through the activity of one or more of these transcription factors.[13,39] Apparently TNFα's ability to cause a bewildering array of biochemical changes in a wide variety of cells is attributable to its utilization of multiple signaling pathways through its cell surface receptors.

Mediators of Insulin Resistance in Non–Insulin-Dependent Diabetes Mellitus

The biochemical basis of insulin resistance in non–insulin-dependent diabetes mellitus (NIDDM) has been the subject of many studies. Although the quantitative regulation of the insulin-sensitive glucose transporters (GLUT-4) and insulin receptors themselves may contribute to this disorder, these two factors are probably inadequate to explain the extent of insulin resistance.[3,40] Studies on postreceptor defects in NIDDM have recently focused on the intrinsic catalytic activity of the insulin receptor (IR) and on downstream signaling events. A reduction in tyrosine phosphorylation of both the IR and insulin receptor substrate-1 (IRS-1) has been noted in animal and human NIDDM.[41,42] Importantly, this appears to occur in all of the major insulin-sensitive tissues: muscle, fat, and liver. In addition, it has been recently demonstrated that stimulation of PI-3′-kinase activity by insulin is also decreased in rodent models of obesity and insulin resistance, confirming defects in further downstream events in IR signaling in this disease.[43,44] It is now clear that decreases in the intrinsic tyrosine kinase activity of the IR, as well as defects in downstream elements in IR signaling, are important components of this disease.

Because 70–80% of all patients with NIDDM are obese, a central question in understanding NIDDM is how obesity can bring about resistance to insulin in the key tissues. Previously, much attention focused on various lipids that are commonly elevated in obesity, such as free fatty acids (FFA). It has been hypothesized that elevated concentrations of FFA can have adverse effects on glucose metabolism due to increased uptake and intracellular oxidation of fatty acids.[45] In support of this hypothesis, administration of FFA to normal persons induces a mild state of insulin resistance, as determined by insulin clamps.[46] In addition, fatty acid treatment of cultured cells suppresses insulin action.[47] There is no conclusive evidence, however, supporting a major pathophysiologic role for FFA in NIDDM. Similarly, the role of hormonal antagonists or inhibitory molecules in insulin resistance of obesity is not yet clear.

Expression of Tumor Necrosis Factor-α in Adipose Tissue

Recent data have indicated a role for tumor necrosis factor-α (TNFα) in linking obesity with the insulin resistance of non–insulin-dependent diabetes mellitus (NIDDM).[6,22,48,49] Earlier studies on an endogenous pathway of complement activation from adipose tissues of obese animals had suggested the possible presence of a cytokine in this tissue.[50] It was subsequently shown that adipose tissue of the obese-diabetic (*db/db*) mouse produced significantly higher levels of TNFα mRNA and protein compared to the lean mouse.[22] This elevated TNFα expression in fat appears to be a common, if not a universal, correlate of obesity attended by significant insulin resistance. In addition to the *db/db* mouse, overexpression is seen in *ob/ob, tub/tub,* and KKAγ mice and in the Zucker *fa/fa* rat (Fig. 61-1).[22,51] Besides these natural genetic models, elevated TNFα mRNA expression has also been observed in a transgenic model of obesity/insulin resistance created by ablation of brown adipose tissue via a bacterial toxin gene driven by the uncoupling protein promoter.[52] In contrast, significant overexpression of TNFα mRNA is not observed in the monosodium glutamate-injection mouse model, which at the early stages induces mild obesity with little or no insulin resistance.[22] Similarly, the streptozotocin-injected rat, a model of type I diabetes with β-cell loss and hyperglycemia but no obesity, does not show elevated TNFα gene expression.

Interestingly, those animals that demonstrated TNFα mRNA expression from the fat tissues did not show evidence of altered expression of other cytokines, such as TNFβ, interleukin-1, or interferon-γ. In other physiologic contexts, such as in infection, several cytokines are often coexpressed.[12,13] This observation suggested that the regulation of cytokine cascades in adipose tissue during rodent obesity may differ from that in other cell types such as immune cells.

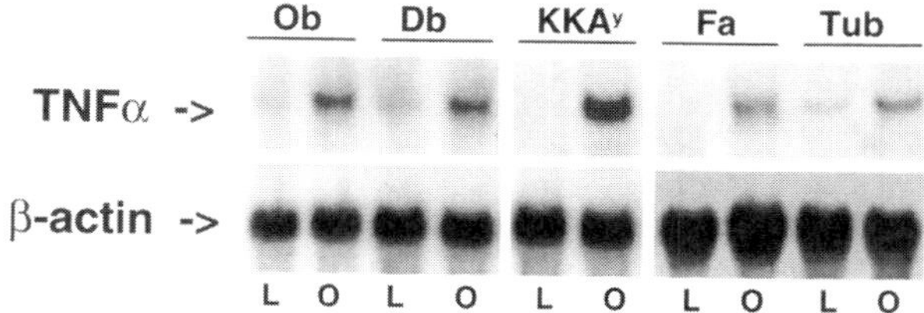

FIGURE 61-1. Adipose expression of TNFα mRNA in different rodent models of genetic obesity. Total RNA (20 μg) from epididymal fat pads of different animal models was subjected to Northern blot analysis, as described.[22] All animals are males; *ob/ob, db/db, tub/tub* and KKA^y obese mice and their lean controls were 12 to 13 weeks old, and *fa/fa* rats and their lean controls were 7 to 8 weeks old. L = lean; O = obese. The animal models are indicated above the lanes. β-Actin mRNA is shown as a control for the loading and integrity of the RNA.

Role of Tumor Necrosis Factor-α in the Insulin Resistance of Non–Insulin-Dependent Diabetes Mellitus and Other Diseases

The role of abnormal tumor necrosis factor-α (TNFα) expression in the obese-diabetic rodents (*fa/fa* rats) was investigated by neutralization of TNFα in vivo with a soluble TNF receptor-immunoglobulin G (TNFR-IgG) fusion protein. Following TNFα neutralization, obese rats were notably more sensitive to insulin, as measured by a two-step hyperinsulinemic-euglycemic clamp.[22] This increase in insulin sensitivity was attributable to a two- to threefold increase in insulin-stimulated peripheral glucose uptake, whereas hepatic glucose output remained unaffected. Although an effect on hepatic insulin responsiveness cannot be ruled out definitively, it was not readily apparent from these experiments. The increase in insulin sensitivity after TNFα neutralization represents a substantial improvement, but not a complete reversal, because the absolute levels of insulin-stimulated glucose disposal in the obese animals do not reach those seen in their lean littermates. Additional experimental systems will be necessary to determine the full extent of this cytokine's role in obesity-linked insulin resistance at relevant sites of insulin action.

Other studies have also suggested a role for TNFα in other insulin resistance states in vivo. Insulin resistance frequently develops during the course of certain cancers, infections, and trauma, such as burn injuries.[17,53–55] Several studies have demonstrated elevated production of TNFα in naturally occurring and experimentally induced sepsis and burn injury.[12,56] Similarly, in certain cancers, a correlation has been observed between TNFα production and insulin resistance.[57] A causal relationship between abnormal cytokine production and insulin resistance in these pathologic states, however, has not yet been established. In addition to these correlative studies, it has been reported that administration of TNFα to humans induces a state of hyperinsulinemia without hyperglycemia, indicating reduced insulin sensitivity.[58] Finally, chronic infusion of TNFα into normal rats led to the development of severe hepatic and peripheral insulin resistance, as determined by hyperinsulinemic-euglycemic clamp studies.[59]

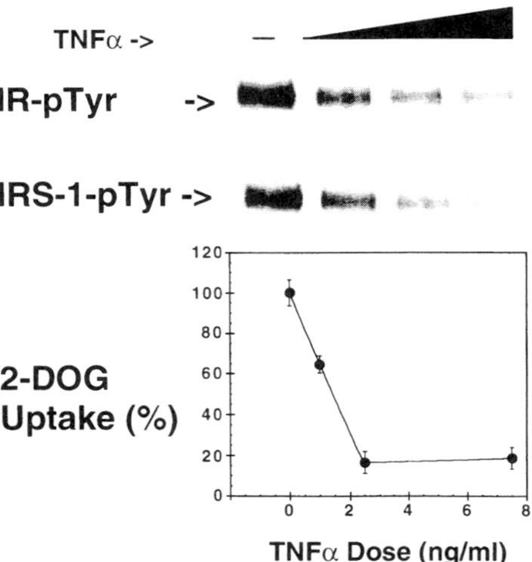

Figure 61-2. Effect of TNFα on insulin-stimulated tyrosine phosphorylation of the IR and IRS-1 (above) and insulin-stimulated glucose transport (below) in cultured 3T3-L1 adipocytes. The extent of insulin-stimulated tyrosine phosphorylation was determined by immunoprecipitation of IR and IRS-1 (from protein extracts from cells treated for 5 days with 0, 1, 2.5, and 7.5 ng/mL TNFα and stimulated with 100 ng/mL insulin) with anti-IR or anti-IRS-1 antibodies, followed by immunoblotting with anti-phosphotyrosine antibody. The half-maximal inhibition of insulin-stimulated tyrosine phosphorylation of IR and IRS-1 was achieved at a 2.0 ± 0.5 ng/mL TNFα concentration. Insulin-stimulated glucose transport assays were performed in parallel, as described.[48] The half-maximal inhibition of insulin-stimulated glucose transport was achieved at a 1.5 ± 0.5 ng/mL TNFα concentration.

Mechanisms of Tumor Necrosis Factor–α-Induced Insulin Resistance

The observed effects of tumor necrosis factor-α (TNFα) on insulin action in vivo may result from a direct effect of this cytokine on insulin-sensitive cells or indirectly, via substances produced by other cells or tissues in response to TNFα. Indeed, these possibilities are not mutually exclusive. In animals infused with TNFα and rendered insulin resistant, elevated levels of the stress hormones glucocorticoids and epinephrine are observed.[59] Both of these hormones have been shown to cause insulin resistance in model cultured cells and whole organisms.[3] Catecholamines are known to generate intracellular cyclic AMP, which leads to the activation of protein kinase A, an enzyme that has been shown to inhibit the protein kinase activity of the IR.[60] Moreover, it has been reported that α-adrenergic blockade can protect, at least in part, from TNFα-induced insulin resistance in rats.[61] Nevertheless, the evidence for an indirect effect of TNF via other hormones is largely circumstantial.

On the other hand, treatment of insulin-sensitive cells with TNFα can clearly alter the catalytic activity of the IR. In adipocytes, TNFα treatment leads to moderate reduction (20–50%) of insulin-stimulated IR autophosphorylation and a more pronounced effect on IRS-1 phosphorylation (Fig. 61-2).[48] Although certain doses of TNFα can reduce the absolute level of IRs, doses of up to 200 pM have little apparent effect on the number of receptors or their insulin binding, but these doses reduce their intrinsic catalytic activity.[48] The actual defect induced by TNFα in these studies is likely to be at or near the IR itself. Partially purified receptors isolated from TNFα-treated cells show reduced autophosphorylation and phosphorylation of exogenously added recombinant IRS-1.[48] This suggests that the IR itself is modified or that TNFα promotes the production of an inhibitor of the receptor that is associated with these preparations. Recently, we have shown that TNFα induces serine phosphorylation of IRS-1 in cultured adipocytes and this modified IRS-1 inhibits the IR tyrosine kinase activity in vitro. TNFα-induced inhibition of IR signaling is also dependent upon the presence of IRS-1 in intact cells. Myeloid 32D cells, which lack endogenous IRS-1, are resistant to the effect of TNFα on IR tyrosine phosphorylation. When IRS-1 is expressed ectopically in these cells, insulin-stimulated IR autophosphorylation becomes very sensitive to inhibition by TNFα. In addition, an inhibitory form of IRS-1 is also observed in muscle and fat tissues of obese *fa/fa* rats. These results not only provided biochemical and genetic evidence for a novel mechanism by which TNFα induces insulin resistance, but also demonstrated an unexpected role for IRS-1 in the termination of the IR signaling.[62]

Sensitivity to TNFα is also seen in insulin signaling in liver-derived cells.[63] Treatment with TNFα inhibits insulin-stimulated autophosphorylation of the IR, as well as phosphorylation of IRS-1 in hepatoma cells, without affecting cell surface insulin-binding activity.[62] However, the detailed analysis of the mechanism by which TNFα acutely decreases the insulin-stimulated tyrosine phosphorylation of IR and IRS-1 in hepatoma cells has not yet been performed. Whether the operative mechanisms in these cells are similar to adipocytes remains to be determined.

Studies have also suggested other potential targets for direct actions of TNFα on insulin-sensitive cells. For example, TNFα has been shown to downregulate GLUT-4 mRNA concentrations in cultured adipocytes.[22,23] Because downregulation of GLUT-4 expression has also been observed in adipose tissues of obese animals and humans, it could be postulated that overexpression of TNFα in fat tissue may play a role in defective gene expression in obesity. In fat cells, however, this effect occurs in the context of downregulation of expression of several fat-specific genes, such as aP2 or adipsin.[22,23] Finally, TNFα dramatically inhibits insulin-stimulated glucose transport at doses that have no effect on the cellular content of GLUT-4 protein.[48] Therefore, the mechanism of TNFα-induced insulin resistance in cultured cells is unlikely to exist primarily at the level of gross cellular content of GLUT-4.

In an attempt to evaluate these several possible mechanisms by which TNFα might regulate insulin action in vivo, we again neutralized TNFα in Zucker *fa/fa* rats using the soluble TNFR-IgG fusion protein and analyzed the expression of GLUT-4 mRNA and the number and catalytic activity of the IRs. Neutralization of TNFα had no obvious effect on GLUT-4 mRNA levels.[49] The tyrosine phosphorylation of the IR and IRS-1, however, was dramatically increased in response to acute insulin injection after TNFα neutralization.[49] This effect was observed in fat and muscle, but no effect was visible in the liver. No changes in absolute levels of the IR or IRS-1 protein were observed after TNFR-IgG injection, indicating that the effect of this agent was on specific quantities of tyrosine phosphorylation per protein molecule. Indeed, each animal receiving the neutralizing agent showed increased tyrosine phosphorylation, and in some cases, the levels approached the insulin-stimulated phosphorylation of IR or IRS-1 observed in lean controls. This amelioration of phosphorylation cascades was observable only in the obese animals, and was not seen on TNFR-IgG injection into lean controls.[49] Because TNFα overexpression is observed only in the obese, this strongly suggests that the agent improved insulin sensitivity via neutralization of TNFα rather than through some other process unrelated to TNFα.

Importantly, the effects of these improvements in insulin-stimulated tyrosine phosphorylation appear to be of sufficient magnitude to cause improvements in the pathophysiology of NIDDM. TNFα neutralization in *fa/fa* rats resulted in a dramatic improvement in the marked hyperinsulinemia, with this parameter being reduced to near the control (lean) levels. In addition, the elevated FFA levels of the obese animals were greatly reduced by these treatments.[49] Presumably, the simultaneous improvements shown in these metabolic parameters all reflect improvements in the sensitivity to insulin.

Tumor Necrosis Factor-α Expression in Human Obesity

Because tumor necrosis factor-α (TNFα) expression in rodent obesity is a common feature of many model systems, there is considerable interest in the possibility that the fat tissues of obese human populations may overexpress TNFα and induce insulin resistance. In recent studies, abdominal fat tissues from obese persons were found to overexpress TNFα mRNA and protein compared to age- and sex-matched lean controls.[64,65] The relative level of TNFα mRNA in adipose tissue was in strong correlation with the degree of obesity and fasting plasma insulin concentrations but in negative correlation with the adipose tissue lipoprotein lipase activity.[64,65] Furthermore, dietary treatment of obesity that produces improved insulin sensitivity results in a significant decrease in TNFα expression in fat tissue. Finally, recent studies have shown a genetic linkage between a polymorphism in the TNFα locus and body mass index in Pima Indians.[66] These observations suggest that abnormal TNFα expression in obesity may be an important pathophysiologic element in human disease. Additional studies will be necessary to evaluate the detailed metabolic parameters in subtypes of obesity and non–insulin-dependent diabetes mellitus (NIDDM) and their relation to TNFα expression in fat tissue.

A Model for the Role of Tumor Necrosis Factor-α in Obesity/Diabetes

The data described above, derived from animal studies and cultured cell systems, allow the description of a new model that places tumor necrosis factor-α (TNFα) centrally in the insulin resistance of obesity-linked diabetes (Fig. 61-3). TNFα is synthesized and secreted by the adipocytes in the obese state.[6,22,51] The mRNA and

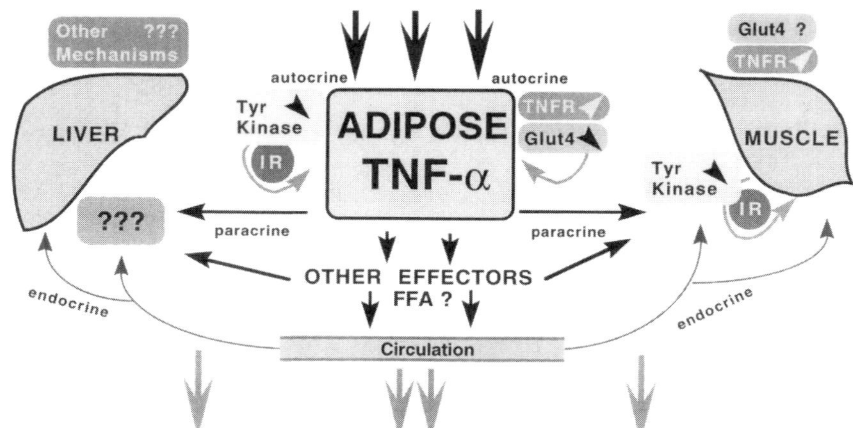

FIGURE 61-3. Model for the role of TNFα in obesity-linked insulin resistance. This model, discussed in the text, suggests that TNFα expression in fat tissue is induced in obesity and causes insulin resistance by interfering with IR tyrosine kinase activity in fat and muscle tissues. Effects on liver are not clear at this time. The action of TNFα on fat and muscle appears to be through autocrine/paracrine routes; however, it is not clear whether these actions are direct or indirect. An endocrine effect is also possible through the access of secondary mediators such as FFA to the systemic circulation. Other abnormalities that might potentially be induced by TNFα such as regulation of mRNA levels of GLUT-4 in fat (decrease) and TNFR in fat and muscle (increase), are also shown.

protein concentrations are elevated on a per unit RNA, protein, or per cell basis compared to lean animals. In addition, there is a greater adipose mass in the obese, often including more fat cells, so this would be expected to have an additional amplifying effect on total body TNFα expression.

A key question is whether TNFα acts directly or indirectly to suppress insulin function in fat and muscle. Both tissues express mRNA for both of the characterized TNF receptors, types 1 and 2.[51] Because TNFα mRNA and protein are produced by adipose tissue, and because exogenous TNFα has been shown to suppress insulin action in adipocytes, it is reasonable to suppose that this cytokine acts directly in fat cells via an autocrine loop.[6,48,49,62]

The basis of TNFα's actions on muscle cells is less clear. Although an endocrine effect via circulating TNFα could influence muscle, the plasma concentrations of TNFα are low in the animal models of obesity/non–insulin-dependent diabetes mellitus (NIDDM) that have been studied to date. Although obese *db/db* mice have both a greater incidence of detectable TNFα in the plasma and higher average circulating concentrations compared to control mice, the absolute concentrations observed (20–200 pg/mL) are well below those required to suppress insulin action in cultured cell systems.[22] Furthermore, in preliminary studies, obese humans did not appear to have detectable levels of circulating TNFα.[64,65,67] Although these measurements may not be accurate, because TNFα is quite difficult to measure in assays of serum or plasma due to the presence of interfering binding proteins, a direct endocrine role for TNFα appears to be somewhat unlikely in NIDDM. On the other hand, TNFα could act directly on muscle cells via a paracrine mechanism because muscle tissue and fibers are often associated with a significant amount of adipose tissue. If obesity tends to increase the number of adipose cells around or within muscle tissue, as has been noted, it is likely that a paracrine effect of TNFα on muscle may be increased. Thus, in addition to the effects of obesity on the relative increases in specific TNFα mRNA expression and increases in total body adipose content, obesity may also play a third role: bringing fat cells into closer proximity with muscle.

Finally, the possibility must be considered that TNFα acts directly on adipose cells to cause the production of other molecules that act directly on muscle. TNFα neutralization causes a decrease in the concentrations of circulating FFA, presumably because of a reduction in adipose lypolysis as a consequence of improved insulin action.[49] As discussed above, fatty acids have been implicated as a potential causal agent in insulin resistance, so this lipid, alone or in combination with TNFα, could inhibit insulin action on muscle. Further studies will be necessary to determine the role of fatty acids or additional novel mediators that may be involved in TNFα-induced insulin resistance in muscle tissue.

Neutralization studies of TNFα done in obese/diabetic animals to date have not shown an effect on hepatic glucose output or insulin-stimulated phosphorylation cascades in liver.[22,49] On the other hand, TNFα infusion in normal rats causes insulin resistance, including an effect on liver.[59] Moreover, TNFα can influence insulin signaling in cultured hepatoma cells.[62] Thus, whether and to what extent TNFα contributes to insulin resistance in the liver in NIDDM is unclear.

Future Prospects and Problems

Molecular Mechanisms of Tumor Necrosis Factor-α–Mediated Insulin Resistance and Tumor Necrosis Factor Signaling

The detailed molecular mechanisms inhibiting insulin signaling by tumor necrosis factor-α (TNFα) will be important to delineate. Although the insulin receptor substrate-1 (IRS-1) is covalently modified by serine phosphorylation in cultured cells treated with TNFα, the enzyme(s) responsible for this increased serine phosphorylation are not yet characterized.[62] The exact phosphorylation sites on IRS-1 are also not known. It is possible that the TNFα-induced inhibition of the IR tyrosine kinase activity is due to an inhibitory molecule and/or a tyrosine phosphatase associated with IRS-1. If such a protein or activity is observed on TNFα treatment, it will be important to purify and characterize these molecules. Finally, it is of interest to understand whether TNFα is utilizing a physiologic serine/threonine based regulatory pathway which attenuates the insulin receptor signaling. Previous studies have shown that covalent modification of IR through serine and threonine phosphorylation is correlated with reduced tyrosine kinase activity.[68,69] It has also been demonstrated that ocadaic acid-induced serine/threonine phosphorylation of IRS-1 can interfere with insulin action by preventing insulin-stimulated tyrosine phosphorylation of IRS-1.[70] However, the physiologic relevance of these observations has not been clear. Obviously, an understanding of the signal transduction pathways that interfere with insulin action may be of broad significance in NIDDM, whether or not TNFα is the physiological effector in man.

In addition to the induction of defects at or near the insulin receptor, it will be important to understand the upstream signals deriving from TNFα and its receptors. As noted above, TNFα has two identified receptors. Studies so far have shown that the majority of the biologic actions of TNFα can be mediated through TNF-R1, and very few activities have been assigned to TNF-R2.[24,27] Interestingly, it has been shown that TNF-R2 mRNA levels are increased in obesity (G.S. Hotamisligil and B.M. Spiegelman, unpublished observations) and regulated in fat and muscle by diet and drug treatments that are known to modulate insulin sensitivity.[51] Although the relative roles of the two TNF receptors in the inhibition of insulin receptor signaling are not yet clear, they are likely to provide important insights into the cross-talk between these two receptor systems.

β-Cell Function and Tumor Necrosis Factor-α

As stated above, insulin resistance is an early and central component in non–insulin-dependent diabetes mellitus (NIDDM), but persistent fasting hyperglycemia must also involve a defect in insulin secretion. Although there is no a priori reason why the mechanisms of insulin resistance and insulin secretion should be linked, it may be worth considering whether tumor necrosis factor-α (TNFα) may contribute to β-cell dysfunction in NIDDM. In this regard, several cytokines, including TNFα, have been shown to interfere with insulin secretion by β-cells in response to glucose.[71] Moreover, TNFα alters the human leukocyte antigen class II antigen expression and has toxic effects on human β-cells.[72] Severe inflammatory changes in islets have also been observed in transgenic animals expressing TNFα and TNFβ in pancreatic islet cells.[73] Whether TNFα or other cytokines play such a role in NIDDM is entirely unknown at present but represents an interesting area for future study.

Induction of Tumor Necrosis Factor-α Expression in Obesity

Another important question is the nature of the physiologic factors that cause adipose tissue to elevate the expression of tumor necrosis factor-α (TNFα) in obesity. Because this occurs in many different models of obesity, it is highly unlikely that it represents a proximal step in the action of an obesity gene. More likely, some common metabolic event in the early development of the obese state leads to the production of an inducing signal. At the cellular level, it is possible that the enlargement of fat cells themselves to an "obese" size triggers this change in gene expression. Alternatively, a hormone or hormones dysregulated in obesity, such as insulin, insulin like growth factor-1 (IGF-1), or glucocorticoids, may play an important role. Finally, as obesity often correlates with elevated lipoprotein concentrations or altered lipid profiles, it is conceivable that such molecules may play an important role in TNFα induction. However, it is not yet clear whether the obesity-linked induction of TNFα is via transcriptional or post-transcriptional mechanisms.

Tumor Necrosis Factor-α, Cachexia, and Obesity

Tumor necrosis factor-α (TNFα) expression has previously been associated with cachexia, a wasting disorder involving both muscle and fat tissues.[12,19] How can the association with obesity be reconciled with a role for TNFα in cachexia? It is entirely possible that obesity-related TNFα expression by fat cells also affects obesity itself. In fact, the degree of insulin resistance in humans has been shown to correlate negatively with further weight gain, so it is possible that TNFα expression is a compensatory mechanism to limit fat development.[74] The negative correlation of TNFα expression levels and lipoprotein lipase activity of adipose tissue in human obesity also supports this possibility.[65] On the other hand, recent data suggest that aberrant TNFα production plays a role in cachexia primarily when it occurs in the context of a mixture of cytokines or other substances secreted by tumors.[5] In addition, when TNFα has been associated with cachexia, there have been significant circulating levels (>200 ng/mL) of this cytokine. In contrast, we have observed little or no expression of other cytokines in addition to TNFα in models of obesity-diabetes, and circulating concentrations of TNFα in these models are very low when they are detectable.[6,22,64,65] Furthermore, obesity is often associated with other hormonal abnormalities, including elevated glucocorticoid and insulin concentrations, which can alter the response to TNFα. Previous reports have also suggested that the site of expression is an important determinant of the metabolic responses to TNFα.[75] In this context, TNFα expressed from fat tissue may induce a divergent spectrum of biologic responses through an autocrine/paracrine mode of action. Considering that TNFα has been shown to be a growth factor for cultured preadipocytes, and to increase vascular permeability and induce angiogenesis, it could be postulated that TNFα may contribute to the development of obesity.[75,76] Experimental manipulation of TNFα in fat via transgenic studies should be illuminating in this regard.

Human Disease and Therapeutics

If fat-derived tumor necrosis factor-α (TNFα) is playing an important role in inducing insulin resistance in patients with non–insulin-dependent diabetes mellitus (NIDDM), it may be worthwhile to speculate on the possible therapeutic implications. First, there is good evidence from a variety of studies that agents that improve insulin sensitivity may be of great value in the treatment of NIDDM.[77] The most obvious therapeutic approach in the context discussed here would be to neutralize TNFα with an antibody or "immunoadhesin" such as the soluble TNFR-IgG fusion.[22,49] Although such reagents would presumably require injection, they are quite stable in the bloodstream and would require only infrequent administration. Of course, chronic long-term neutralization of TNFα could ultimately compromise the beneficial tropic functions of this cytokine in the immune system, such as the ability to fight certain infections and the stimulation of thymocyte growth.[10,27–29] This problem could be circumvented by appropriate dosing of a neutralizing agent if less TNFα is necessary to produce TNF's beneficial effects than its deleterious ones. Alternatively, it may ultimately be possible to separate these effects at the level of the receptors by the creation of receptor-specific antagonists. Finally, because insulin resistance appears to be linked to inappropriate adipose-specific expression of TNFα, the development of drugs that specifically modulate this process could, in theory, have the desired degree of specificity. Whether any of these classes of agents can be used to treat human NIDDM remains to be determined.

References

1. Kahn CR. Insulin action, diabetogenes, and the cause of type II diabetes. Diabetes 1994;43:1066
2. Moller DE, Flier JS. Insulin resistance: Mechanisms, syndromes, and implications. N Engl J Med 1992;325:938
3. Olefsky JM, Molina JM. Insulin resistance in man. In: Rifkin H, Porte DJ, eds. Diabetes Mellitus. New York: Elsevier;1990:121–153
4. Taylor SI, Accili D, Imai Y. Insulin resistance or insulin deficiency. Which is the primary cause of NIDDM? Diabetes 1994;43:735
5. Spiegelman BM, Hotamisligil GS. Through thick and thin: Wasting, obesity, and TNF-α. Cell 1993;73:625
6. Hotamisligil GS, Spiegelman BM. TNFα: A key component of obesity-diabetes link. Diabetes 1994;43:1271
7. Gray PW, Aggarwal BB, Benton CV, et al. Cloning and expression of cDNA for human lymphotoxin, a lymphokine with tumor necrosis activity. Nature 1984;312:721
8. Pennica D, Nedwin GE, Hayflick JS, et al. Human tumor necrosis factor: Precursor structure, expression and homology to lymphotoxin. Nature 1984; 312:724
9. Beutler B, Greenwald D, Hulmes JD, et al. Identity of tumor necrosis factor and the macrophage secreted factor cachectin. Nature 1985;316:552
10. Smith CA, Farrah T, Goodwin RG. The TNF receptor superfamily of cellular and viral proteins: Activation, costimulation and death. Cell 1994;76:959
11. Aggarwal BB, Vilcek J. Protein and gene structure of TNF-α and TNF-β. In: Aggarwal BB, Vilcek J, eds. Tumor Necrosis Factors. Structure, Function and Mechanism of Action. New York: Marcel Dekker;1992a:239–589
12. Beutler B, Cerami A. The biology of cachectin/TNF-α primary mediator of the host response. Ann Rev Immunol 1989;7:625
13. Vilcek J, Lee TH. Tumor necrosis factor, new insights into the molecular mechanisms of its actions. J Biol Chem 1991;266:7313
14. De Togni P, Goellner J, Ruddle NH, et al. Abnormal development of peripheral lymphoid organs in mice deficient in lymphotoxin. Science 1994;264:703
15. Eugster HP, Muller M, Car BD, et al. TNFα and LTα double knockout mice: Definitive answers to old questions? Eur Cytokine Network 1994;5:146
16. Aggarwal BB, Vilcek J. Biological actions of TNF. In: Aggarwal BB, Vilcek J, eds. Tumor Necrosis Factors. Structure, Function and Mechanism of Action. New York: Marcel Dekker;1992:239–589
17. Grunfeld C, Feingold KR. Metabolic disturbances and wasting in the acquired immunodeficiency syndrome. N Engl J Med 1992;327:329
18. Feingold KR, Grunfeld C. Role of cytokines in inducing hyperlipidemia. Diabetes 1992;41(suppl 2):97
19. Oliff A, Defeo Jones D, Boyer M, et al. Tumors secreting human TNF/cachectin induce cachexia in mice. Cell 1987;50:555
20. Torti FM, Dieckmann B, Beutler B, et al. A macrophage factor inhibits adipocyte gene expression: An in vitro model of cachexia. Science 1985;229: 867
21. Reid TR, Torti FM, Ringold G. Evidence for two mechanisms by which tumor necrosis factor kills cells. J Biol Chem 1989;262:4583
22. Hotamisligil GS, Shargill NS, Spiegelman BM. Adipose expression of tumor necrosis factor-alpha: Direct role in obesity-linked insulin resistance. Science 1993;259:87
23. Stephens JM, Pekala PH. Transcriptional repression of the GLUT4 and C/EBP genes in 3T3-L1 adipocytes by tumor necrosis factor-alpha. J Biol Chem 1991;266:21839
24. Tartaglia LA, Goeddel DV. Two TNF receptors. Immunol Today 1992;13: 151
25. Baker E, Chen LZ, Smith CA, et al. Chromosomal location of the human tumor necrosis factor receptor genes. Cytogenet Cell Genet 1991;57:117
26. Goodwin RG, Anderson D, Jerzy R, et al. Molecular cloning and expression of the type 1 and type 2 murine receptors for tumor necrosis factor. Mol Cell Biol 1991;11:3020
27. Tartaglia LA, Weber RF, Figari IS, et al. The two different receptors for tumor necrosis factor mediate distinct cellular responses. Proc Natl Acad Sci USA 1991;88:9292
28. Rothe J, Lesslauer W, Lotscher H, et al. Mice lacking the tumour necrosis factor receptor 1 are resistant to TNF-mediated toxicity but highly susceptible to infection by *Listeria monocytogenes*. Nature 1993;364:798
29. Pfeffer K, Matsuyama T, Kundig TM, et al. Mice deficient for the 55 kd tu-

mor necrosis factor receptor are resistant to endotoxic shock, yet succumb to *L. monocytogenes* infection. Cell 1993;73:457
30. Erickson SL, de Sauvage FJ, Carver-Moore K, et al. Decreased sensitivity to tumor necrosis factor but normal T cell development in TNF receptor-2-deficient mice. Nature 1994;372:560
31. Zhang Y, Lin J-X, Yip YK, Vilcek K. Enhancement of cAMP levels and of protein kinase activity by tumor necrosis factor and interleukin 1 in human fibroblasts: Role in the induction of interleukin 6. Proc Natl Acad Sci USA 1988;85:6802
32. Han J, Lee JD, Bibbs L, Ulevitch RJ. A MAP kinase targeted by endotoxin and hyperosmolarity in mammalian cells. Science 1994;265:808
33. Vietor I, Schwenger P, Li W, et al. Tumor necrosis factor–induced activation and increased tyrosine phosphorylation of mitogen-activated (MAP) kinase in human fibroblasts. J Biol Chem 1993;268:18994
34. Kyriakis JM, Banerjee P, Nikolakaki E, et al. The stress-activated protein kinase subfamily of c-jun kinases. Nature 1994;369:156
35. Liu J, Mathias S, Yang Z, Kolesnick RN. Renaturation and tumor necrosis factor-α stimulation of a 97-kDa ceramide-activated protein kinase. J Biol Chem 1994;269:3047
36. Gueston F, Freshney N, Waller RJ, et al. Interleukin-1 and tumor necrosis factor stimulate two novel protein kinases that phosphorylate the heat shock protein hsp27 and β-casein. J Biol Chem 1993;268:4236
37. Kolesnick R, Golde DW. The sphingomyelin pathway in tumor necrosis factor and interleukin-1 signaling. Cell 1994;77:325
38. Rothe M, Wong SC, Henzel WJ, Goeddel DV. A novel family of putative signal transducers associated with cytoplasmic domain of the 75 kDa tumor necrosis factor receptor. Cell 1994;78:681
39. Kronke M, Schutze S, Scheurich P, Pfizenmaier K. TNF signal transduction and TNF-responsive genes. Immunol Ser 1992;56:189
40. Shepherd PR, Kahn BB. Cellular defects in glucose transport: Lessons from animal models and implications for human insulin resistance. In: Moller DE, ed. Insulin resistance. West Sussex: Wiley;1993:253–300
41. Saad MJA, Araki E, Miralpeix M, et al. Regulation of insulin receptor substrate-1 in liver and muscle of animal models of insulin resistance. J Clin Invest 1992;90:1839
42. Thies RS, Molina JM, Ciaraldi TP, et al. Insulin-receptor autophosphorylation and endogenous substrate phosphorylation in human adipocytes from control, obese, and NIDDM subjects. Diabetes 1990;39:250
43. Folli F, Saad MJ, Backer JM, Kahn CR. Insulin stimulation of phosphatidylinositol 3-kinase activity and association with insulin receptor substrate 1 in liver and muscle of the intact rat. J Biol Chem 1992;267:22171
44. Heydrick SJ, Jullien D, Gautier N, et al. Defect in skeletal muscle phosphatidylinositol-3′-kinase in obese insulin-resistant mice. J Clin Invest 1993;91:1358
45. Randle PJ, Garland PB, Hales LN, Newsholme EA. The glucose fatty acid cycle, its role in insulin sensitivity and the metabolic disturbances of diabetes mellitus. Lancet 1963;i:785
46. Ferrannini E, Barret EJ, Bevilacqua S, De Fronzo RA. Effect of fatty acids on glucose production and utilization in man. J Clin Invest 1983;72:1737
47. Svedberg J, Bjorntorp P, Smith U, Lonnroth P. Free-fatty acid inhibition of insulin binding, degradation, and action in isolated rat hepatocytes. Diabetes 1990;39:570
48. Hotamisligil GS, Murray DL, Choy LN, Spiegelman BM. TNF-α inhibits signaling from insulin receptor. Proc Natl Acad Sci USA 1994;91:4854
49. Hotamisligil GS, Budavari A, Murray DL, Spiegelman BM. Reduced tyrosine kinase activity of the insulin receptor in obesity-diabetes: Central role of tumor necrosis factor-α. J Clin Invest 1994;94:1543
50. Choy LN, Rosen BS, Spiegelman BM. Adipsin and an endogenous pathway of complement from adipose cells. J Biol Chem 1992;267:12736
51. Hofmann C, Lorenz K, Braithwaite SS, et al. Altered gene expression for tumor necrosis factor-α and its receptors during drug and dietary modulation of insulin resistance. Endocrinology 1994;134:264
52. Lowel BB, Susulic SV, Hamann A, et al. Development of obesity in transgenic mice after genetic ablation of brown adipose tissue. Nature 1993;366:740
53. Copeland GP, Leinster SJ, Davis JC, Hipkin LJ. Insulin resistance in patients with colorectal cancer. Br J Surg 1987;74:1031
54. Frayn KN. Effects of burn injury on insulin secretion and on sensitivity to insulin in the rat in vivo. Eur J Clin Invest 1975;5:331
55. Clowes GHJ, ODonnel TF, Blackburn GL, Maki TN. Energy metabolism and proteolysis in traumatized and septic man. Surg Clin North Am 1976;56:1169
56. Marano MA, Moldawer LL, Fong Y, et al. Cachectin/TNF production in experimental burns and *Pseudomonas* infection. Arch Surg 1988;123:1383
57. McCall JL, Tuckey JA, Parry BR. Serum tumor necrosis factor alpha and insulin resistance in gastrointestinal cancer. Br J Surg 1992;79:1361
58. Van Der Poll T, Romijn JA, Endert E, et al. Tumor necrosis factor mimics the metabolic response to acute infection in healthy humans. Am J Physiol 1991;261:E457
59. Lang CH, Dobrescu C, Bagby DJ. Tumor necrosis factor impairs insulin action on peripheral glucose disposal and hepatic glucose output. Endocrinology 1992;130:43
60. White MF, Kahn CR. The insulin signaling system. J Biol Chem 1994;269:1
61. Bagby GJ, Lang CH, Skrepnik N, Spitzer JJ. Attenuation of glucose metabolic changes resulting from TNF-α administration by adrenergic blockade. Am J Physiol 1992;262:R628
62. Hotamisligil GS, Peraldi P, Budavari A, et al. IRS-1 mediated inhibition of insulin receptor tyrosine kinase in TNF-α- and obesity-induced insulin resistance. Science, in press
63. Feinstein R, Kanety H, Papa MZ, et al. Tumor necrosis factor-α suppresses insulin-induced tyrosine phosphorylation of insulin receptor and its substrates. J Biol Chem 1993;268:26055
64. Hotamisligil GS, Arner P, Caro JF, et al. Increased adipose expression of tumor necrosis factor-α in human obesity and insulin resistance. J Clin Invest 1995;95:2409
65. Kern PA, Saghizadeh M, Ong JM, et al. The expression of tumor necrosis factor in adipose tissue: regulation by obesity, weight loss, and relationship to lipoprotein lipase. J Clin Invest 1995;95:2111
66. Norman RA, Bogardus C, Ravussin E. Linkage between obesity and a marker near the tumor necrosis factor-α locus in Pima Indians. J Clin Invest 1995; 96:158
67. Boeck MA, Chen C, Cunningham-Rundles S. Altered immune function in a morbidly obese pediatric population. Ann NY Acad Sci 1993;699:252
68. Takayama S, White MF, Lauris V, Kahn CR. Phorbol esters modulate insulin receptor phosphorylation and insulin action in cultured hepatoma cells. Proc Natl Acad Sci USA 1988;81:7797
69. Stadtmauer L, Rosen OM. Increasing the cAMP content of IM-9 cells alters the phosphorylation state and protein kinase activity of the insulin receptor. J Biol Chem 1986;261:3402
70. Tanti JF, Gremeaux T, Van Obberghen E, Marchand-Brustel Y. Serine/threonine phosphorylation of insulin receptor substrate 1 modulates insulin receptor signaling. J Biol Chem 1994;269:6051
71. Corbett JA, Sweetland MA, Wang JL, et al. Nitric oxide mediates cytokine-induced inhibition of insulin secretion by human islets of Langerhans. Proc Natl Acad Sci USA 1993;90:1731
72. Pujol-Borrell R, Todd I, Doshi M, et al. HLA class II induction in human islet cells by interferon-gamma plus tumour necrosis factor or lymphotoxin. Nature 1987;326:304
73. Picarella DE, Kratz A, Li CB, et al. Transgenic tumor necrosis factor alpha production in pancreatic islets leads to insulinitis, not diabetes. Distinct patterns of inflammation in TNF-alpha and TNF-beta transgenic mice. J Immunol 1993;150:4136
74. Swinburn BA, Nyomba BL, Saad MF, et al. Insulin resistance associated with lower rates of weight gain in Pima Indians. J Clin Invest 1991;88: 168
75. Tracey KJ, Cerami A. Pleitrophic effects of TNF in infection and neoplasia: Beneficial, inflammatory, catabolic, or injurious. In: Aggarwal BB, Vilcek J, eds. Tumor Necrosis Factors. New York: Marcel Dekker;1992:431–452
76. Vilcek J, Palombella VJ, Henriksen-DeStefano D, et al. Fibroblast growth enhancing activity of tumor necrosis factor and its relationship to other polypeptide growth factors. J Exp Med 1986;163:632
77. Nolan JJ, Ludvik B, Beerdsen P, et al. Improvement in glucose tolerance and insulin resistance in obese subjects treated with troglitazone. N Engl J Med 1994;331:1188

Diabetes Mellitus, edited by Derek LeRoith, Simeon I. Taylor, and Jerrold M. Olefsky. Lippincott–Raven Publishers, Philadelphia © 1996.

Chapter 62

Positional Cloning Strategies to Identify Causal Genes for Non–Insulin-Dependent Diabetes Mellitus

Stephen S. Rich

Diabetes mellitus represents a group of disorders that have in common an elevated blood glucose concentration associated with a relatively or absolutely insufficient insulin secretory response and with varying degrees of insulin resistance. The clinical manifestations of diabetes range from asymptomatic glucose intolerance to an acute event of ketoacidosis. Chronic complications of diabetes, including nephropathy, retinopathy, neuropathy, and accelerated atherosclerosis, often accompany the disease. Although *diabetes mellitus* is often used as a single clinical term, its pathogenesis is likely the reflection of a heterogeneous group of disorders that share glucose intolerance as a primary characteristic.

The World Health Organization has established four major classes of diabetes, defining insulin-dependent diabetes mellitus (IDDM, or type I), non–insulin-dependent diabetes mellitus (NIDDM, or type II), malnutrition-related diabetes mellitus, and other types associated with other clinical conditions and syndromes.[1] For IDDM and NIDDM, both genetic and environmental risk factors play an important role in the underlying pathogenesis of disease susceptibility and progression to overt glucose intolerance.[2] Significant progress has been made recently that has increased our basic understanding of the genetic factors that contribute to susceptibility to IDDM. The genes that contribute to IDDM susceptibility, once limited to the human leukocyte antigen region on the short arm of human chromosome 6,[3–5] and later to a locus on the short arm of chromosome 11,[6–8] now include loci on the long arm of chromosome 11,[9–11] the long arm of chromosome 6,[9] the long arm of chromosome 15,[11] and the long arm of chromosome 2.[12] The use of the positional cloning strategy to uncover IDDM susceptibility genes points to the power of the approach and provides hope that similar progress can be made in the identification of NIDDM susceptibility genes. This chapter will focus on the evidence that genes play a role in NIDDM, outline the strategies for gene localization, and discuss the prospects for positional cloning in discovering NIDDM susceptibility genes.

Genetic Factors in Susceptibility to Non–Insulin-Dependent Diabetes Mellitus

There is considerable direct and indirect evidence that genetic factors play an important role in susceptibility to non–insulin-dependent diabetes mellitus (NIDDM). Direct evidence comes from the identification of mutations in specific genes (such as the insulin receptor) that result in a diabetic phenotype.[13] Indirect evidence comes from the assessment of familial aggregation and statistical genetic modeling that supports patterns of NIDDM in populations and families that is consistent with a genetic effect.

Population Prevalence

Large variation in the prevalence of non–insulin-dependent diabetes mellitus (NIDDM) has been observed among ethnically diverse populations. Very low prevalence rates (approaching 0% for both men and women) have been demonstrated in Melanesians from Papua, New Guinea.[14] The Pima Indians of Arizona are reported to have among the highest prevalence rates.[15] These rates (33% in men, 37% in women) are approximately a 10-fold increase over those seen in the general U.S. population.[16] Although the prevalence in persons over the age of 18 years is 6.6%, it increases with age and is higher in nonwhite Americans, particularly Hispanics and blacks.[17,18]

Studies of admixed populations have provided other evidence for the role of genes in susceptibility to NIDDM. It has been observed that the age-adjusted prevalence of NIDDM among Pima Indians varies directly with the degree of non-Indian admixture[19]; in full-blooded Pima Indians, the prevalence of NIDDM is nearly twice that observed in non-Indians, and those with half-Indian ancestry are intermediate in prevalence. Similar results have been reported from Nauru,[20] where persons of partial Nauruan ancestry have a lower prevalence of NIDDM than those of full Nauruan heritage. These differences relate to the importance of genetic factors in NIDDM susceptibility, since the members of the closed community would minimize environmental variability in risk level.

Twin Studies

Twin studies represent an approach to resolving the role of genetic and environmental risk factors in defining disease susceptibility. Monozygotic (MZ) twins, who have identical genotypes, show almost complete concordance for non–insulin-dependent diabetes mellitus (NIDDM).[21] The concordance in dizygotic (DZ) twins (who share, on average, one-half of their genes) is much less than that observed in MZ twins and approaches the risk for siblings, suggesting that environmental factors that are unique to a rearing environment are not sufficiently important in providing susceptibility. The high MZ concordance rate relative to the DZ rate clearly indicates the important contribution of genes to NIDDM susceptibility.

Family Studies

Molecular studies of rare mutations in the coding regions of candidate genes have shown the importance of specific genes to the diabetes phenotype. Mutations in the insulin receptor locus on chromosome 19 have been shown to result in cases of diabetes.[13] Genes that are involved in the suspected pathogenesis of diabetes, such as the insulin receptor, represent attractive candidates, as do the glucokinase locus (MODY, chromosome 7[22]) and a series of mitochondrial mutations.[23,24] Unfortunately, most cases of non–insulin-dependent diabetes mellitus (NIDDM) in the population cannot be attributed to these candidate genes, either by sequencing the entire coding region or by evaluating single base pair changes in candidates. Thus, although molecular studies that focus on the role of rare mutations support the existence of genetic factors that produce some cases of NIDDM, the existing pattern of familial aggregation in the general population suggests a more pervasive role for genetic factors.

As noted above, concordance in monozygotic (MZ) twins approaches 100% over a lifetime, consistent with the importance of genetic factors in NIDDM susceptibility. Among first-degree relatives of an NIDDM proband there is a 30% risk of NIDDM, compared with the population prevalence of approximately 5%.[2] Among specific ethnic populations, the rates of NIDDM appear higher, as do the risks to relatives. Thus, among the Pima Indians, the population risk approaches 50%, yet the risk to offspring from a mating with one diabetic parent is increased 2.3 times; the risk to offspring of two diabetic parents is increased 3.9 times.

Both population data and familial aggregation studies support the role of genetic factors, yet no clear underlying model to explain genetic susceptibility has been presented. In the Pima Indians, commingling analysis provided results of bi- and trimodality of insulin values, consistent with a single major gene.[25] Segregation analysis of fasting blood glucose values[26] and insulin concentrations[27] has suggested the presence of a single major locus governing the inheritance of this intermediate phenotype of NIDDM. On the other hand, studies of candidate genes with inheritance of NIDDM have been equivocal or negative.[28,29] Thus, although there is clear and consistent evidence of genetic factors contributing to NIDDM susceptibility, there has been limited success in identifying specific genes that provide a significant population risk of NIDDM. These results are consistent with the existence of multiple genetic factors that play a role in NIDDM susceptibility and serves as the rationale for initiating a search for NIDDM susceptibility genes.[30]

Table 62-1. A Sampling of Disease Genes Identified by Positional Cloning

Disease	Location	Symbol (ref)
Duchenne muscular dystrophy	X	DMD*
Retinoblastoma	13	RB†
Cystic fibrosis	7	CFTR‡
Neurofibromatosis type I	9	NF1§
Fragile X syndrome	X	FRAX‖
Myotonic dystrophy	19	DM¶
Norrie syndrome	X	ND#
Menkes disease	X	MNK**
Huntington's disease	4	HD††
Spinocerebellar ataxia 1	6	SCA1‡‡

*Monaco AP, Neve RL, Colletti-Feener C, Bertelson CJ, Kurnit DM, Kunkel LM. Isolation of candidate cDNAs for portions of the Duchenne muscular dystrophy gene. Nature 1986;323:646.
†Friend SH, Bernards R, Rogelj S, et al. A human DNA segment with properties of the gene that predisposes to retinoblastoma and osteosarcoma. Nature 1986;323:643.
‡Riordan JR, Rommens JM, Kerem B-S, et al. Identification of the cystic fibrosis gene: Cloning and characterization of complementary DNA. Science 1989;245:1066.
§Wallace MR, Marchuk DA, Andersen LB, et al. Type I neurofibromatosis gene: Identification of a large transcript disrupted in three NF1 patients. Science 1990; 249:181.
‖Fu Y-H, Kuhl DPA, Pizzuti A, et al. Variation of the CGG repeat at the fragile X site results in genetic instability: Resolution of the Sherman paradox. Cell 1992;67:1047.
¶Aslanidis C, Jansen G, Amemiya C, et al. Cloning of the essential myotonic dystrophy region and mapping of the putative defect. Nature 1992;355:548.
#Berger W, Meindl A, van de Pol TJR, et al. Isolation of a candidate gene for Norrie disease by positional cloning. Nat Genet 1992;1:199.
**Chelly J, Tumer Z, Tonnesen T, et al. Isolation of a candidate gene for Menkes disease that encodes a potential heavy metal binding protein. Nat Genet 1993;3:14.
††Huntington's Disease Cooperative Research Group. A novel gene containing a trinucleotide repeat that is expanded and unstable on Huntington's disease chromosomes. Cell 1993;72:971.
‡‡Orr HT, Chung M, Banfi S, et al. Expansion of an unstable trinucleotide CAG repeat in spinocerebellar ataxia type 1. Nat Genet 1993;4:221.

Positional Cloning

The accumulated evidence suggests that non–insulin-dependent diabetes mellitus (NIDDM) is determined in part by the action of several genes, some of which may have a large effect. The current strategy of choice to isolate and characterize NIDDM susceptibility genes is by positional cloning.[31] Positional cloning, also known as *reverse genetics,* is a strategy used to identify a disease gene based on its chromosomal location without knowing the biochemical function of its product. Since the early 1980s, this strategy has led to the cloning of many disease genes (Table 62-1).

Positional cloning starts with the assignment of a disease gene (locus) to a chromosomal location and subsequently to a region of a chromosome. This can be achieved by two basic approaches in screening—use of candidate genes and/or anonymous DNA markers. The candidate gene approach assumes that the candidate plays an important role in the etiology of the disease; this assumed disease-locus relationship then serves as *a priori* evidence that determines where the search should begin. The anonymous marker approach to a genome search uses highly polymorphic markers that are distributed throughout the genome. In both cases, the evidence for assignment is gathered through analyses by linkage analysis using lod scores,[32] identity-by-descent, or identity-by-state methods.[33]

Lod score (linkage) analysis assumes that the risk for the trait in question (NIDDM) is transmitted according to a known genetic model. For NIDDM, this fact is not known with certainty. Under an assumed genetic transmission model, linkage of a genetic marker (or candidate gene, such as the insulin receptor) with NIDDM tests the cosegregation at meiosis of the marker locus with the trait locus. The proportion of crossing-over events (recombinants) observed in transmission of the trait with the genetic marker estimates the recombination fraction (θ), which is related to the genetic distance (in centimorgans, cM)—which, in turn, is related to physical distance (in kilobases, kb). In a linear genetic model, the smaller the recombination fraction, the closer together the loci. Clearly, the detection of recombinants not only requires specification of the genetic model (misclassification of the model infers recombination) but also polymorphic genetic markers in parents.

Statistical analysis of linkage is based on the maximum likelihood approach of hypothesis testing, in which the likelihood ratio statistic is formed. This ratio consists of (1) the likelihood of the family data (observing a series of recombinant and nonrecombinant events under the assumed transmission model) at a recombination fraction θ relative to (2) the likelihood of the family data when the trait (NIDDM) is not linked to the marker (the recombination fraction is 50%, or $\theta = 0.5$). This odds ratio, or likelihood function, relates the maximum support for linkage between the trait (NIDDM) and the genetic marker at the observed recombination fraction, compared to the situation in which the marker is not linked to the trait. The logarithm of the odds ratio is termed the *lod score* and is a useful summary of all information on linkage. A lod score of 3 or more has been traditionally viewed as strong evidence for linkage (1000:1 odds), whereas a lod score of -2 or less (100:1 odds) has been taken as evidence against linkage at some recombination fraction θ.

Identity by descent occurs if the allele in two siblings arose from the replication of one allele in a previous generation (the same allele transmitted to both offspring from the parent). Identity by state occurs when the alleles are the same but their origin is from different parents. An important assumption in the use of these methods is that the genetic marker locus is sufficiently polymorphic to allow identification of the four parental genotypes, even if these genotypes are not available (both parents deceased, for example). A genetic marker with 10 alleles (1, 2, . . . , 10) could be used in a study of affected sibling pairs in the anticipation that the sharing of marker alleles can be determined with precision. For example, two siblings with NIDDM, one carrying the 1 and 3 alleles and the other carrying the 2 and 4 alleles, would be classified as sharing no alleles, either identity by descent or identity by state. In another sibling pair, one could carry the 2 and 5 alleles at the marker, and the other could carry the 5 and 7 alleles. In this case, without the benefit of parental marker data, it is unclear whether the 5 allele arose from one parent transmitting that allele to both offspring (sibs sharing one allele, identity by descent) or each parent transmitting a 5 allele to a different offspring (sibs sharing one allele, identity by state).

For many of the genes that have been cloned (see Table 62-1), the assignment was greatly facilitated by the discovery of either a chromosomal abnormality or X-linked inheritance. The exceptions (cystic fibrosis, myotonic dystrophy, Huntington's disease, spinocerebellar ataxia 1) were the result of genome searches with polymorphic markers. It should be noted that in the case of spinocerebellar ataxia 1, the search was accomplished initially with protein polymorphisms and linkage was established with human leukocyte antigen, a highly polymorphic marker.

Once a chromosomal assignment is made for a disease locus, the next step is to reduce the size of the region to one that can be managed by physical mapping methods. It is estimated that there are 50,000 to 100,000 genes in the human genome. This means that there are, on average, 16 to 34 genes in a one megabase (1 Mb) area, assuming equal distribution of genes. A candidate region with a size of 1–2 Mb (roughly equivalent to 1–2 cM, or 1–2% recombination on the scale of genetic distance) would therefore be ideal for the isolation of candidate genes.

At a time when there were not many polymorphic markers in the human genome and cloning capacity was limited to DNA fragments in the range of 50 kb or less, chromosome jumping was also employed to reduce the size of a candidate region.[34] The goal of chromosome jumping was to clone only the ends of DNA fragments with a size in the hundreds of kilobases, so that the clones could be used to "jump" from one point to another on a chromosome. As the human genome has become saturated with informative markers, however, the analysis of markers mapped to the candidate region with respect to marker-disease recombinants can reduce the size of the region.[35] This definition of a minimal critical region relies on identifying true recombinants and on detecting the markers that have no apparent recombination with the disease.

The distance determined by linkage analysis is a genetic distance measured by the frequency of recombination observed in pedigrees and converted, using a mapping function, to centiMorgans. Although 1 cM is roughly equivalent to 1 million base pairs (1 Mb), the frequency of recombination varies considerably from one region to another and often differs between the genders. Thus, the physical distance between adjacent genetic markers needs to be determined by pulse-field gel electrophoresis, allowing resolution of large DNA fragments ranging from 20 kb to 5 Mb. In addition to determining physical distance, pulse-field gel electrophoresis analysis provides additional information for the isolation of candidate genes, because most of the restriction enzymes used in pulse-field gel electrophoresis recognize DNA sequences with CG-dinucleotide. This dinucleotide is relatively rare in the human genome but frequently appears at the 5′-end of several genes.[36] A CpG or HTF (*H*paII *t*iny *f*ragment) island or a clustering of restriction enzyme sites on a pulse-field gel electrophoresis map may indicate the possible presence of genes in the neighboring region.

The development of yeast artificial chromosomes (YACs) as a cloning tool has greatly advanced positional cloning because it allows cloning of DNA fragments ranging in size from 50 kb to 1 Mb.[37] The YAC vector is derived from a plasmid vector, pBR322, and contains two additional elements. The first type of sequences, including ARS, CEN4, and TEL, are essential for DNA replication in a yeast cell, proper chromosome segregation into daughter cells in the cell cycle, and maintenance of stability of an artificial chromosome. The TRP1, URA3, and SUP4 sequences allow nutritional and color selections of a recombinant clone. The YAC clones can be screened for markers in the candidate region by polymerase chain reaction (PCR) analysis, facilitating the collection of overlapping YAC clones (YAC contig) that forms an essential resource for sequence analysis of the candidate region.

Once a disease locus is positioned within a YAC contig of 1–2 Mb, several methods can be employed in the search for candidate genes. DNA sequences can be subcloned and used as a probe to hybridize to a "zoo blot," a Southern blot containing DNA from several different species. As most important genes are conserved throughout evolution, cross-hybridization to DNA from another species is an indication that a sequence may be contained in an expressed gene. The gene for cystic fibrosis (CFTR, cystic fibrosis transmembrane conductance regulator) was identified due to the presence of a CpG island at its 5′-end and its cross-hybridization to DNA from other species.[38]

Another method used to search for candidate genes is to use a YAC directly as a probe to screen a cDNA library. This method was used in the isolation of the neurofibromatosis type I gene.[39] Another method used cloned sequences from the candidate region that were immobilized onto a matrix for selection of clones from cDNA libraries of choice.[40] Transcribed sequences can also be recovered based on the presence of consensus sequences of splice sites. The cloning vectors used in this approach are designed so that the spliced message can be amplified by reverse transcriptase polymerase chain reaction and subcloned (or propagated) as a retrovirus for further selection and manipulation (exon amplification[41] and exon trapping,[42] respectively). The IT-5 and three other genes discovered in the Huntington's disease search were identified using exon amplification.[43]

Once a candidate gene is identified, the next step is to determine if the gene is the disease locus of interest. Several criteria can be used in this process. First, the gene should be expressed in the tissues affected by the disease. Second, sequence changes should be detected in affected subjects but not in unaffected subjects. Sequence analysis should be able to resolve normal polymorphism and silent mutations from disease mutation by examining a panel of normal and affected persons and by translating a nucleic acid sequence into an amino acid sequence.

To prove ultimately that a candidate gene is the disease gene is perhaps a more formidable task than the process of fine mapping. Expression of a wild-type gene in an affected cell line should be able to complement the defect. For diseases that result in a decrease of dosage, antisense oligonucleotides can be used to block gene expression. Transgenic animals can be established to assess the function of the gene in vivo, so that the appearance of a disease phenotype in a transgenic animal provides evidence that the candidate is the disease gene.

Identifying Non–Insulin-Dependent Diabetes Mellitus Susceptibility Genes

The strategies outlined above for launching a search for non–insulin-dependent diabetes mellitus (NIDDM) susceptibility genes are conceptually straightforward. The diseases that have been successfully identified by the positional cloning approach, however, have, to date, been monogenic, with clear Mendelian inheritance. To consider the prospects for mapping, cloning, and sequencing NIDDM genes, it should be recalled that NIDDM does not exhibit clear Mendelian inheritance and that the expression of diabetes may reflect the joint contribution of multiple genetic risk factors in a permissive (environmentally susceptible) host.

To consider the optimal design(s) for a search for NIDDM genes, several parameters of importance are needed, including (1) the lifetime cumulative incidence (or prevalence) of NIDDM; (2) the estimates for monozygotic (MZ) and dizygotic (DZ) twin concordance for NIDDM; and (3) the risk to siblings (or other relatives) of an NIDDM proband. Other information that may influence the study design is whether the risks to relatives appear greater when the proband has NIDDM diagnosed at a younger age and the amount of subclinical disease in relatives of persons with NIDDM.

Strategies for mapping NIDDM genes also must reflect the age distribution of NIDDM. Because NIDDM is a disease that has the majority of clinical diagnoses after 50 years of age, the availability of parents is limited. This suggests that few extended families will be available for study, and that the primary material for genetic study will be sibships and their offspring (many of whom are too young to express the diabetes phenotype). With newly identified NIDDM probands of young age at onset, many families can be identified with multiple siblings affected with NIDDM and at least one parent living and available for study. Thus, the majority of clinical material will consist of (incomplete) nuclear families.

Whether anonymous DNA markers or candidate genes are used, the purpose of the NIDDM search is to determine the optimal number of "experimental units" (families, sibships, and their composition) and the saturation level of the genetic map to identify NIDDM genes. Because pedigree material is limited and the mode of inheritance of NIDDM is not known with certainty, the mapping methods that appear most applicable are those based on affected relative pairs.[44,45] These methods rely on the proportion of alleles at a genetic marker locus that are shared by the affected relatives. Using affected relatives also avoids some of the problems of model-dependent analysis (lod scores) in that no genetic model needs to be specified and information from unaffected relatives is not used in the test statistic. In a complex disease such as NIDDM, family members may be unaffected because of failure to be at risk genetically (no disease genes), or they can be at risk genetically but have a low environmental risk (good diet and exercise habits).

The increase in interest in the affected relative pair methods (including affected sib pairs) has accompanied the discovery of multitudes of highly polymorphic marker loci based on simple tandem repeat polymorphisms.[46] In this fashion, affected relatives are genotyped with highly polymorphic markers and scored for the number of marker alleles that they have in common (none, one, or two). This distribution is then compared with that expected under the null hypothesis of "no linkage," depending on the probability that pairs of relatives share no, one, or two alleles identical by state. Previous work has demonstrated that for studies of affected sib pairs, the critical statistic that guides the number of pairs needed for reasonable power is the ratio of the risk of NIDDM in siblings to the risk in the general population.[33] Estimates made from previous studies have suggested that this ratio may range from 2 to 6, depending on the population and the age at onset of probands. Given a series of assumptions, it has been estimated that 200 affected sib pairs would be needed to provide 80% power to detect a single disease locus that increases the sibling risk by a factor of 2 with a 10-cM map. This suggests that if NIDDM is caused by several genes that act in additive fashion, we may be able to identify several with ratios in the 2.0 range; however, if NIDDM is caused by genes that act in multiplicative fashion (the effects are multiplied together), the search may be quite difficult.

Recent experience with IDDM has generated significant optimism in the search for NIDDM genes.[8,10–12] IDDM, in contrast to NIDDM, is one-tenth as common (0.5% prevalence), and has a lower MZ twin concordance (approaching 50%) and a lower risk to siblings of an IDDM proband (8%). The ratio of sibling risk to prevalence, however, is much greater (about 16), and two major contributing loci have already been identified: the human major histocompatibility complex on 6p (human leukocyte antigen) and the insulin gene region on 11p. After a genome search using highly polymorphic markers in a series of affected sibling pair families, several IDDM susceptibility genes of moderate effect have been identified using the sib pair strategy—linkage to chromosome 11q (IDDM4) near the FGF3 region and linkage to chromosome 6q (IDDM5) near the Estrogen Receptor region. In different populations, some degree of heterogeneity with respect to human leukocyte antigen genotype was observed, suggesting complex inheritance and population-specific genetic architecture.[8,11] In the case of NIDDM, the same may be true, but it is also complicated by problems with diagnostic criteria, etiologic heterogeneity, and environmental confounding. Nevertheless, this is the first clear demonstration of mapping of complex disease loci and provides reason for optimism. It should be noted, however, that the search for the individual genes and how they interact to determine susceptibility remains a distant goal.

Summary Remarks

The transmission of non–insulin-dependent diabetes mellitus (NIDDM) susceptibility is complex, and represents the joint contribution of genetic and environmental risk. The strategy of positional cloning has been highly successful in identifying a number of single-gene disorders that exhibit clear Mendelian patterns of inheritance. Positional cloning of NIDDM may be helped by the expansion of molecular genetic tools and highly informative markers, but it may also be hindered by the complexity of the disease itself. Recent developments in analytic and experimental genetics have renewed enthusiasm for the use of identity by descent (state) methods that utilize affected relatives (sib pairs) rather than pedigrees as a fundamental tool of gene mapping. Given the relative position of NIDDM susceptibility genes, major steps in understanding the roles of the identified genes in defining genetic susceptibility, as well as function, lie ahead.

References

1. Diabetes mellitus: Report of a WHO Study Group. World Health Organization Technical Report Series 1985;727:1
2. Warram JH, Rich SS, Krolewski AS. Epidemiology and genetics of diabetes mellitus. In: Kahn CR, Weir GC, eds. Joslin's Diabetes Mellitus. Philadelphia: Lea & Febiger; 1994:201
3. Cudworth AG, Woodrow JC. Evidence for HL-A linked genes in "juvenile" diabetes mellitus. Br Med J 1975;2:133
4. Barbosa J, King R, Noreen H, Yunis EJ. The histocompatibility system in juvenile, insulin-dependent diabetes multiplex kindreds. J Clin Invest 1977;60:989
5. Christy M, Green A, Christau B, et al. Studies of the HLA system and insulin-dependent diabetes mellitus. Diabetes Care 1979;2:209
6. Owerbach D, Nerup J. Restriction fragment length polymorphism of the insulin gene in diabetes mellitus. Diabetes 1982;31:275
7. Bell GI, Horita S, Karam JH. A polymorphic locus near the human insulin gene is associated with insulin-dependent diabetes mellitus. Diabetes 1984;33:176
8. Lucassen AM, Julier C, Beressi JP, et al. Susceptibility to insulin dependent diabetes mellitus maps to a 4.1 kb segment of DNA spanning the insulin gene and associated VNTR. Nat Genet 1993;4:305
9. Davies JL, Kawaguchi Y, Bennett ST, et al. A genome-wide search for human type 1 diabetes susceptibility genes. Nature 1994;371:130
10. Hashimoto L, Habita C, Beressi JP, et al. Genetic mapping of a susceptibility locus for insulin-dependent diabetes mellitus on chromosome 11q. Nature 1994;371:161
11. Field LL, Tobias R, Magnus T. A locus on chromosome 15q26 (IDDM3) produces susceptibility to insulin-dependent diabetes mellitus. Nat Genet 1994;8:189
12. Owerbach D, Gabbay KH. The HOXD8 locus (2q31) is linked to Type I diabetes mellitus: Interaction with chromosome 6 and 11 diabetes susceptibility genes. Diabetes 1995;44:132
13. Taylor SI, Kadowaki T, Kadowaki H, et al. Mutations in insulin-receptor gene in insulin-resistant patients. Diabetes Care 1990;13:257
14. King H, Zimmet P. Trends in the prevalence and incidence of diabetes: Non–insulin-dependent diabetes mellitus. World Health Statistics Q 1988;41:190

15. Knowler WC, Pettitt DJ, Saad MF, Bennett PH. Diabetes mellitus in the Pima Indians: Incidence, risk factors and pathogenesis. Diabetes/Metab Rev 1990;6:1
16. Harris MI, Hadden WC, Knowler WC, Bennett PH. Prevalence of diabetes and impaired glucose tolerance and plasma glucose levels in U.S. population aged 20–74 yr. Diabetes 1987;36:523
17. Flegal KM, Ezzati TM, Harris MI, et al. Prevalence of diabetes in Mexican Americans, Cubans, and Puerto Ricans from the Hispanic Health and Nutrition Examination Survey, 1982–1984. Diabetes Care 1991;14:628
18. Harris MI. Noninsulin-dependent diabetes in black and white Americans. Diabetes/Metab Rev 1990;6:71
19. Knowler WC, Williams RC, Pettitt DJ, Steinberg AG. Gm 3; 5, 13, 14 and type 2 diabetes mellitus: An association in American Indians with genetic admixture. Am J Hum Genet 1988;43:520
20. Serjeantson SW, Owerbach D, Zimmet P, et al. Genetics of diabetes in Nauru: Effects of foreign admixture, HLA antigens and the insulin-gene-linked polymorphism. Diabetologia 1983;25:13
21. Newman B, Selby JV, King MC, et al. Concordance for type 2 (non–insulin-dependent) diabetes mellitus in male twins. Diabetologia 1987;30:763
22. Vionnet N, Stoffel M, Takeda J, et al. Nonsense mutation in the glucokinase gene causes early-onset non–insulin-dependent diabetes mellitus. Nature 1992;356:721
23. Ballinger SW, Shoffner JM, Hedaya EV, et al. Maternally transmitted diabetes and deafness associated with a 10.4 kb mitochondrial DNA deletion. Nat Genet 1992;1:11
24. van den Ouweland JM, Lemkes HH, Ruitenbeek W, et al. Mutation in mitochondrial tRNA(Leu)(URR) gene in a large pedigree with maternally transmitted type II diabetes mellitus and deafness. Nat Genet 1992;1:368
25. Bogardus C, Lillioja S, Nyomba BL, et al. Distribution of in vivo insulin action in Pima Indians as mixture of three normal distributions. Diabetes 1989;38:1423
26. Williams WR, Morton NE, Rao DC, et al. Family resemblance for fasting blood glucose in a population of Japanese Americans. Clin Genet 1983;23:287
27. Iselius L, Lindsten J, Morton NE, et al. Evidence for an autosomal recessive gene regulating the persistence of the insulin response to glucose in man. Clin Genet 1982;22:180
28. Raben N, Barbetti F, Cama A, et al. Normal coding sequence of insulin gene in Pima Indians and Nauruans, two groups with highest prevalence of Type II diabetes. Diabetes 1991;40:118
29. Choi WH, O'Rahilly S, Buse JB, et al. Molecular scanning of insulin-responsive glucose transporter (GLUT4) gene in NIDDM subjects. Diabetes 1991;40:1712
30. Rich SS. Mapping genes in diabetes: Genetic epidemiological perspective. Diabetes 1990;39:1315
31. Collins FS. Positional cloning: Let's not call it reverse genetics anymore. Nat Genet 1992;1:3
32. Lathrop GM, Lalouel JM, Julier C, Ott J. Strategies for multilocus linkage analysis in humans. Proc Natl Acad Sci USA 1984;81:3443
33. Risch N. Linkage strategies for genetically complex traits. I. Multilocus models. Am J Hum Genet 1990;46:222
34. Poustka A, Pohl TM, Barlow DP, et al. Construction and use of human chromosome jumping libraries from NotI-digested DNA. Nature 1987;325:353
35. Weissenbach J, Gyapay G, Dib C, et al. A second-generation linkage map of the human genome. Nature 1992;359:794
36. Lindsay S, Bird AP. Use of restriction enzymes to detect potential gene sequences in mammalian DNA. Nature 1987;327:336
37. Burke DT, Carle GF, Olson MV. Cloning of large segment of exogenous DNA into yeast by means of artificial chromosome vectors. Science 1987;236:806
38. Rommens JM, Iannuzzi MC, Kerem B-S, et al. Identification of the cystic fibrosis gene: Chromosome walking and jumping. Science 1989;245:1059
39. Wallace MR, Marchuk DA, Andersen LB, et al. Type I neurofibromatosis gene: Identification of a large transcript disrupted in three NF1 patients. Science 1990;249:181
40. Lovett M, Kere J, Hinton LM. Direct selection: A method for the isolation of cDNA encoded by large genomic regions. Proc Natl Acad Sci USA 1991;88:9628
41. Buckler AJ, Chang DD, Graw SL, et al. Exon amplification: A strategy to isolate mammalian genes based on RNA splicing. Proc Natl Acad Sci USA 1991;88:4005
42. Duyk GM, Kim S, Myers RM, Cox DR. Exon trapping: A genetic screen to identify candidate transcribed sequences in cloned mammalian genomic DNA. Proc Natl Acad Sci USA 1990;87:8995
43. Huntington's Disease Cooperative Research Group. A novel gene containing a trinucleotide repeat that is expanded and unstable on Huntington's disease chromosomes. Cell 1993;72:971
44. Green JR, Woodrow JC. Sibling method for detecting HLA-linked genes in disease. Tissue Antigens 1977;9:31
45. Suarez BK, Rice J, Reich T. The generalized sib pair IBD distribution: Its use in the detection of linkage. Ann Hum Genet 1978;42:87
46. Weber JL, May PE. Abundant class of human DNA polymorphisms which can be typed using the polymerase chain reaction. Am J Hum Genet 1989;44:388

Diabetes Mellitus, edited by Derek LeRoith, Simeon I. Taylor, and Jerrold M. Olefsky. Lippincott–Raven Publishers, Philadelphia © 1996.

Chapter 63

Candidate Genes for Non–Insulin-Dependent Diabetes Mellitus

Alan R. Shuldiner and Kristi D. Silver

Introduction

Genetics of Typical Non–Insulin-Dependent Diabetes Mellitus

Although the contribution of heredity is well recognized, progress toward an understanding of the genetic basis of non–insulin-dependent diabetes mellitus (NIDDM) has been largely restricted to a few distinct rare monogenic syndromes with predictable modes of inheritance.[1–4] For example, autosomal recessive syndromes of extreme insulin resistance such as leprechaunism are the result of mutations in the insulin receptor gene.[5,6] Autosomal dominant maturity onset diabetes of the young (MODY) is often caused by mutations in the glucokinase (MODY2) gene on chromosome 7,[7,8] whereas in other families, linkage to regions on chromosomes 20q (MODY1)[9] and 12q (MODY3)[10] has been demonstrated. A few families have been identified with insulin gene mutations (so-called insulinopathies).[11,12] Others have described a rare subphenotype of NIDDM characterized by maternal inheritance of diabetes and deafness that is caused by mutations in mitochondrial DNA.[13–15]

Thus, in only a small minority of patients with diabetes can we expect a tight link between a single gene, a clinical syndrome, and straightforward inheritance patterns (e.g., glucokinase-MODY-autosomal dominant; insulin receptor-leprechaunism-autosomal recessive). In the large majority of patients with typical NIDDM,

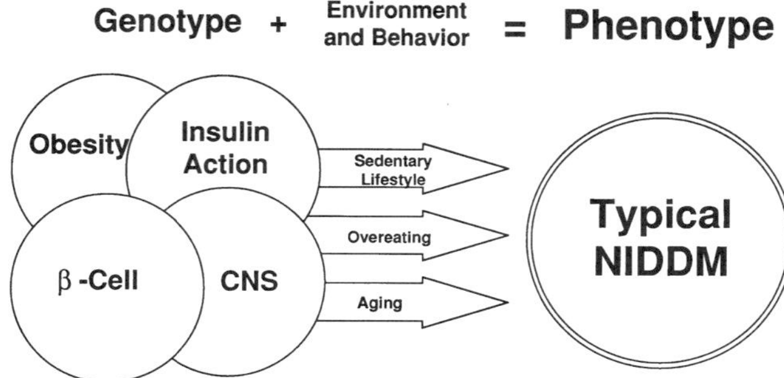

Figure 63-1. Schematic of the genetics of NIDDM in which several genes interact with each other and with environmental and behavioral influences to result in the disease. CNS = central nervous system.

we expect to find genetic influences that are very strong but not definable in simple mendelian terms, clinical syndromes that are heterogeneous even within a single family, and substantial environmental influences. It is reasonable to hypothesize (in accord with majority expectation) that the common forms of NIDDM are the result of a pool of mutant genes, each of which contributes modestly and conspires with environment and aging to manifest the disease. Individually, these genes are more accurately termed susceptibility genes and are likely to be those involved in insulin action, insulin secretion, obesity/energy expenditure, and central nervous system (CNS) regulation of satiety and appetite behavior (Fig. 63-1). Identifying these genes and defining their relative contributions is difficult but highly relevant to the disease as well as its cause, prevention, and treatment.

Approaches to Elucidating Non–Insulin-Dependent Diabetes Mellitus Susceptibility Genes: Positional Cloning and Candidate Genes

There are two general approaches to elucidating genetic defects that cause or predispose to disease: candidate genes (also known as forward genetics) and positional cloning (also known as reverse genetics.)[16] Positioning cloning makes no *a priori* assumptions about the underlying biochemical abnormality or genetic defect and uses polymorphic markers dispersed throughout the genome to search for specific chromosomal regions that are inherited more often in affected members of pedigrees than in unaffected members (linkage analysis).[16–18] Once a specific chromosomal region is localized, physical mapping of the locus is performed to identify the disease gene, which is then analyzed further for specific mutations. The disease gene may very well be one not previously known and may require additional studies to determine the function of its gene product and how the specific defect leads to its pathophysiologic consequences.

Although it is reasonably straightforward for highly penetrant monogenic diseases, positional cloning/linkage analysis is much more difficult for complex disorders such as NIDDM in which the genetic basis is likely to be heterogeneous in the population and several genes in the same individual/family each contribute modestly. The problem is further complicated with NIDDM because the disease manifests itself later in life as a result of environmental and/or other influences. Nonetheless, this approach has been adapted for the study of complex disorders, particularly in populations that are well defined and relatively genetically homogeneous. A detailed review of positional cloning strategies for the identification of NIDDM susceptibility genes is beyond the scope of this chapter.

Over the last three decades, the genetic basis for many monogenic diseases (e.g., sickle cell anemia) has been elucidated through the use of candidate gene approaches. With this approach, based upon the role of a given protein in a biochemical pathway thought to be involved in the disease, molecular biologic methods are applied to elucidate specific mutations in the gene. Whereas early studies relied on cumbersome and time-consuming cloning and sequencing strategies, newer methods, including the use of the polymerase chain reaction (PCR), have significantly increased the ease and power of screening for and identifying mutations in specific candidate genes.

Candidate gene approaches are now being applied to polygenic and heterogeneous genetic disorders such as asthma, hypertension, Alzheimer's disease, and NIDDM. In this chapter, we will review (1) the theory of candidate gene approaches, including its advantages and disadvantages, (2) the methods that are currently being employed to screen for mutations, (3) progress to date on several candidate genes for NIDDM, and (4) future applications of this approach to elucidate NIDDM susceptibility genes. Several candidate genes are reviewed, including insulin, glycogen synthase, glucagon receptor, intestinal fatty acid binding protein, glucose transporters, and others. Of particular interest is the β_3-adrenergic receptor gene as a candidate for several features of the insulin resistance syndrome (so-called syndrome X), which also will be reviewed in detail. The insulin receptor, insulin receptor substrate-1 (IRS-1), glucokinase, and mitochondrial DNA-encoded genes are not covered because they are discussed separately in other chapters.

Candidate Genes: Theory of the Method and Experimental Approaches

Once a gene is identified as a candidate for a disease, several approaches may be applied to determine whether it is indeed defective. The most straightforward approach is to use traditional strategies to clone and sequence the gene of interest from several individuals with the disease and to compare the obtained sequence with that of the normal sequence. Several individuals (at least 50–100 alleles) are required to analyze complex disorders such as NIDDM, since a mutation in a given gene may be responsible for the disease in only a subset of patients. Further, the gene of interest must be studied in several distinct ethnic groups, since it is likely that diabetes susceptibility genes differ among ethnic populations. In addition to studying coding regions, other functionally important regions of the gene should be studied, including exon-intron splice junctions and regulatory regions. Identifying mutations in regulatory regions is difficult because for most genes all regulatory regions are not known and may be many kilobases upstream or downstream from the coding region. In addition, these regions tend to be polymorphic. Minimally, the immediate 5′-flanking region of the gene should be screened.

Given the fact that some candidate genes are quite large and that many subjects need to be studied, the use of traditional (manual) cloning and sequencing strategies is not practical in most laboratories. However, with the advent of PCR and high throughput automated DNA sequencing, this approach has become a viable option for some with access to this equipment.

More rapid and higher throughput alternatives to sequence analysis to screen for mutations in candidate genes include electrophoretic methods in which variations in nucleotide sequences may be detected. These methods include denaturing gradient gel electrophoresis (DGGE),[19] temperature gradient gel electrophoresis (TGGE),[20] single-stranded conformational polymorphism (SSCP)[21] analysis, and heteroduplex (HD) analysis.[22] These approaches generally involve the amplification of a segment of the candidate gene (usually a few hundred base pairs in length) by PCR, followed by gel electrophoresis under special conditions. Altered mobility through the gel when compared with the normal sequence may indicate sequence variation, which may then be confirmed by DNA sequence analysis. SSCP is an easy, rapid, and highly sensitive method for screening for point mutations as well as small insertions and deletions and for these reasons has become the method of choice for most applications.[21,23,24] The above methods (including traditional cloning and sequence analysis) do not detect heterozygotes for large deletions or duplications, since the normal allele is amplified and detected as normal. To detect large deletions and duplications, restriction fragment length polymorphism (RFLP)/Southern blot analysis or gene dosage-PCR[25] must be performed.

An alternative to searching directly for mutations in candidate genes is to use polymorphic markers in or near the candidate gene to determine whether specific alleles segregate with diabetes (or other pertinent phenotypes) in pedigrees, are shared more often in affected pairs of siblings, or are present at a higher frequency in subjects with diabetes than in those without diabetes in the population. This approach is advantageous since it is rapid. A positive result is used as evidence that a yet to be identified functional mutation in the candidate gene is present and responsible for the phenotype, which is then confirmed using sequence analysis or one of the screening methods described above. However, it is also possible that a previously unsuspected gene that is in linkage disequilibrium with the polymorphic marker is the disease-causing locus.

Generally, polymorphic markers are not useful if negative (indeterminant) results are obtained. False-negative results may occur if the polymorphic marker is too far from the candidate gene and thus recombination occurs frequently. Further, as described above, a negative result may be obtained even if diabetes is caused by a mutation in a candidate gene that is present in a relatively small subset of subjects or families in the study group (so-called genetic heterogeneity) or if a particular gene, rather than being a major determinant of the phenotype, plays a more modest role. Thus, polymorphic markers are best used in large pedigrees in populations that are relatively genetically homogeneous.

Candidate Genes for Non–Insulin-Dependent Diabetes Mellitus

Recent insights into the molecular mechanisms of insulin signaling and insulin secretion and into the pathophysiologic changes in these and other pathways thought to be responsible for diabetes have resulted in an explosion in the number of potential candidate genes for NIDDM.[26–28] Almost as quickly as new molecules are identified in these pathways, their genes are studied as candidates for diabetes. With only a few exceptions, these studies have produced negative findings. However, owing to the relatively small number of subjects studied, usually in a single ethnic population and limited in scope to coding regions or a small number of nearby polymorphic markers, these negative studies must not be overinterpreted. In this chapter, we focus primarily on a few candidate genes for which genetic variants (and in some cases functional mutations) have actually been identified.

The Insulin Gene

Insulin is the product of a single copy gene located on human chromosome 11p15.[29] The mature mRNA is 446 nucleotides in length (excluding the poly A tail) and is encoded by three exons.[29] Translation results in preproinsulin, a 105 amino acid precursor composed of a signal (pre) peptide, B-chain, connecting piece, and A-chain.[30] Post-translational processing, which includes cleavage of the signal peptide and formation of three disulfide bonds (one within the A-chain and two between the A- and B-chains), results in proinsulin. Subsequent proteolytic excision of the two pairs of dibasic amino acids that flank the connecting piece results in mature insulin and the C peptide.[30]

Since the cloning of the human insulin gene in 1980, insulin has been a candidate gene for NIDDM. Early studies used cumbersome RFLP/Southern blot analysis to determine if specific alleles were associated with or linked to NIDDM. In particular, a region in the 5′ flank of the insulin gene with three alleles differing by the number of tandem repeats (designated class I, II, and III alleles) has been studied extensively.[31–36] Taken together, these studies suggest that the insulin gene is not a major susceptibility locus for NIDDM. Interestingly, recent studies indicate that the longer class III allele is linked to insulin-dependent diabetes mellitus (IDDM) and has been designated the IDDM-2 locus.[37] Since a subset of subjects with NIDDM may have a form of IDDM in which autoimmune β-cell destruction is more insidious and of later onset,[38] IDDM-2 may also play a role in this subset of subjects with NIDDM. Further studies will be required to address this hypothesis more directly.

Rare families have been identified as having circulating insulin or proinsulin molecules with abnormal biochemical properties sometimes associated with glucose intolerance or diabetes.[30,39] Mutations in the insulin gene were identified in several of these families and include Val92Leu (Insulin Wakayama, A-chain)[40]; Phe48Ser (Insulin Los Angeles, B-chain)[41]; Phe49Leu (Insulin Chicago, B-chain)[42]; His34Asp (Proinsulin Providence, B-chain)[43]; Arg65His (Proinsulin Tokyo/Denver/Boston, connecting piece)[44]; Arg65Leu (Proinsulin Kyoto, connecting piece)[45]; and Arg65Pro (Proinsulin Oxford, connecting piece).[46] Several investigators have searched for these and other coding region mutations in subjects with typical NIDDM and have concluded that they are quite rare.[47–49]

Recently, Olansky and coworkers[50] identified an eight base pair (bp) insertion at position -315 of the insulin promoter. The insertion was associated with NIDDM in African Americans and Mauritius Creoles. In African Americans, 5% of those with NIDDM were heterozygous for the insertion, whereas only 1% of subjects without NIDDM had the insertion.[50] The insertion was not present in 40 Pima Indians or 35 caucasians from St. Louis. The eight bp insertion was associated with decreased promoter activity in vitro, suggesting functional significance.[50] Larger population- and family-based studies are required to further define the importance of this variant in the insulin promoter to NIDDM in these and other populations.

The Glucagon Receptor Gene

Glucagon is one of the insulin counter-regulatory hormones that controls hepatic glucose production and is also involved in the regulation of insulin secretion by islet β-cells. Some subjects with NIDDM have elevated circulating levels of glucagon, suggesting that abnormalities in glucagon secretion and/or signaling may play a pathophysiologic role in the disease. The glucagon receptor is a seven membrane spanning receptor that is linked to guanine nucleotide binding (G) proteins. Binding of glucagon to its receptor results in activation of adenylyl cyclase and intracellular accumulation of cAMP.

The glucagon receptor gene is located on chromosome 17q25 and contains 13 exons spanning about 5.5 kilobases.[51] Using SSCP analysis, Hager and colleagues[52] identified a missense mutation (Gly40Ser) in the glucagon receptor gene. In French caucasians, the frequency of the mutation was 10/216 (4.6%) in subjects with NIDDM and 0/159 in subjects without NIDDM or a family history of NIDDM ($P = 0.015$). The Gly40Ser mutation was also linked to NIDDM in French families, particularly when subjects with impaired glucose tolerance and fasting hyperglycemia were also considered affected. When studied in BHK cells in vitro, the Gly40Ser glucagon receptor had an approximately threefold higher binding affinity for glucagon than the wild-type receptor, suggesting that the mutation results in a functional change.[52] How a mutant receptor with increased binding affinity produces increased susceptibility to NIDDM is unclear. More in-depth functional studies, including those of expression/biosynthesis, intracellular signaling, desensitization, and downregulation are required to elucidate the functional importance of this mutation. In addition, genetic studies in other cohorts and populations are necessary.

The Intestinal Fatty Acid Binding Protein Gene

Initially using positional cloning approaches, Prochazka and coworkers[53] identified a region on chromosome 4q that was linked to insulin resistance in Pima Indians. Although insulin resistance is a predictor of NIDDM, this locus was not linked to NIDDM itself. Among the several genes known to be encoded within this chromosomal region was the intestinal fatty acid binding protein (IFABP). Molecular scanning of IFABP by SSCP uncovered a missense mutation (Ala54Thr).[54] The Ala54Thr mutation is frequent in Pima Indians with an allele frequency of 0.29; 9% of the population is homozygous for the mutation, 42% are heterozygous for the mutation, and 49% lack the mutation. Subjects with the mutation had higher fasting insulin values and decreased glucose uptake during a euglycemic hyperinsulinemic clamp, indicating greater insulin resistance.[54] They also had higher rates of fat oxidation. This mutation appears to be either autosomal dominant or codominant, since heterozygotes are affected.

Ala54Thr IFABP was expressed in vitro and found to bind long chain fatty acids with twofold greater affinity than the wild-type receptor.[55] Further, in Caco 2 cells, Ala54Thr IFABP had an increased ability to transport fatty acids.[55] These studies provide evidence that Ala54Thr IFABP may cause increased absorption and oxidation of dietary free fatty acids, which may in turn lead to insulin resistance.

Further evidence that the IFABP is a likely susceptibility gene for NIDDM comes from a study of caucasian populations from the United Kingdom, Finland, and Wales in which a polymorphic microsatellite marker near the IFABP gene was used.[56] When each of the populations was analyzed separately, there was a nonsignificant trend for the IFABP A_3 allele to be more frequent in subjects with NIDDM. When results from the three populations were combined, this trend became statistically significant ($P = 0.027$).[56] There were no differences in fasting glucose or insulin levels in subjects with the IFABP A_3 allele.

The Glycogen Synthase Gene

Glycogen synthase is the key enzyme that regulates the synthesis and storage of glycogen from glucose in muscle and liver.[27,57] Insulin stimulates glycogen synthesis by activating a type 1 protein phosphatase that converts the inactive phosphorylated enzyme into its dephosphorylated active form. Recent studies indicate that a decrease in the ability of insulin to stimulate glycogen synthesis is a very early defect in the progression to hyperglycemia and NIDDM.[58,59]

The glycogen synthase gene is located on chromosome 19q13.3 and encodes a 737 amino acid protein.[60] Groop and coworkers,[61] using a glycogen synthase cDNA probe and RFLP/Southern blot analysis, identified two polymorphic alleles in Finnish caucasians, designated A_1 and A_2. The glycogen synthase A_2 allele was found in 32 of 107 (30%) subjects with NIDDM compared with only 14 of 164 (8%) subjects without NIDDM ($P < 0.001$). Subjects with the glycogen synthase A_2 allele had decreased glycogen synthesis during a euglycemic-hyperinsulinemic clamp, although the concentrations of glycogen synthase in muscle were not significantly different.[61] Subjects with the glycogen synthase A_2 allele also had a stronger family history of NIDDM and were more likely to be hypertensive. Sequence analysis revealed that the polymorphism was caused by a substitution of thymidine for cytidine in an intron, which created a new XbaI site. Thus, while possibly providing a marker for NIDDM in Finns, this nucleotide substitution is unlikely to have functional consequences. It is possible that the glycogen synthase A_2 allele is in linkage disequilibrium with a putative functionally important mutation on the same gene or a nearby gene.

An increase in the frequency of the glycogen synthase A_2 allele in subjects with NIDDM could not be demonstrated in French caucasians,[62] Japanese,[63] or Swedes living in Western Finland,[64] nor could linkage be demonstrated in pedigrees or sib pairs in Mormon families from Utah,[65] again highlighting the need to study several different populations. These seemingly discordant results may be caused by differences in the phenotypic expression of the putative mutation, depending on genetic background, absence of the putative mutation in French, Japanese, and Swedes (genetic heterogeneity), or a spurious positive association in Finns owing to stratification (admixture) bias or other factors.[66]

Vestergaard and coworkers[67] used SSCP to study the coding region of the glycogen synthase gene in eight caucasian subjects with NIDDM and found no polymorphisms. These studies were limited because of the small number of subjects and the fact that they screened cDNA (and not genomic DNA). Thus, heterozygous mutations resulting in poor transcription, defective RNA processing, or accelerated mRNA degradation would result in decreased or absent mutant mRNA and could therefore be missed. Indeed, the investigators found a 39% reduction in glycogen synthase mRNA levels in muscle from subjects with NIDDM.[67] Clearly, further studies are warranted to rigorously examine the role of the glycogen synthase gene in insulin resistance and NIDDM.

Genes for Glucose Transporters

The facilitative glucose transporter proteins are a family of five structurally related proteins with 52–65% amino acid identity (Table 63-1).[68,69] These proteins span the membrane 12 times with the amino- and carboxy-terminals facing the cytoplasm. Each of the glucose transporters has a specific pattern of tissue distribution (Table 63-1). Although all of the glucose transporters are reasonable

TABLE 63-1. Summary of Glucose Transporters

Name	Chromosome	Length (Amino Acids)	Tissue Distribution (Major Sites)
GLUT-1	1p33	492	Brain, peripheral nerves, choroid plexus, epithelium, red blood cells
GLUT-2	3q26.1-26.3	524	β-Cell, liver, kidney, small intestine
GLUT-3	12p13	496	Brain, placenta, kidney, small intestine
GLUT-4	17p13	509	Muscle, adipose tissue
GLUT-5	1p32-22	501	Small intestine, sperm, adipose tissue, kidney

candidates for glucose intolerance and NIDDM, GLUT-2 and GLUT-4 have received the most attention. GLUT-4 is expressed in muscle and adipose tissue, two of the major target tissues for insulin. Stimulation with insulin results in a rapid 20- to 30-fold increase in the Y_{max} of facilitative glucose transport, which is mediated by an increase in the intrinsic activity of the transporter as well as translocation of transporters to the cell surface.[70] GLUT-2 is expressed in the β-cell and is involved in the transport and sensing of glucose, which ultimately results in insulin synthesis and secretion.[71]

The Glucose Transporter-4 (GLUT-4) Gene

Encoded by 11 exons spanning approximately 30 kilobases, the GLUT-4 gene has been studied as a candidate for NIDDM by several groups. Studies utilizing RFLP/Southern blot analysis have failed to show linkage or association with NIDDM.[72,73] Molecular scanning approaches using sequence analysis or SSCP have uncovered a conservative missense mutation (Ile383Val) in the fifth extracellular loop.[74,75] Ile383Val was found to be very rare and was not associated with NIDDM. Although this mutation is not likely to be involved in NIDDM, screening for other mutations in additional subjects, particularly in the promoter region, is necessary to further define the importance of the GLUT-4 gene in NIDDM.

The Glucose Transporter-2 (GLUT-2) Gene

Several studies have used RFLP/Southern blot analysis to investigate the GLUT-2 gene in NIDDM.[76–78] Except for a study by Alcolado and coworkers,[78] all findings have been negative. In a study of Pima Indians, Janssen and coworkers[79] used a microsatellite polymorphism near the GLUT-2 locus. In sib pair analysis for quantitative traits, they found linkage with borderline statistical significance to acute insulin release as determined by intravenous glucose tolerance tests (a familial trait and a predictor of NIDDM in Pima Indians).[79] The marker was not linked to NIDDM. SSCP of the coding region in 40 Pima subjects with NIDDM revealed a missense mutation (Thr110Ile) in the second transmembrane domain. In the 796 subjects subsequently studied, 3 were homozygous for the Thr110Ile mutation, 38 were heterozygous for the mutation, and 755 lacked the mutation (allele frequency = 0.03). Although the number of subjects with the mutation was small, there was no clear association with acute insulin release or NIDDM. Expression of the Thr110Ile mutation in *Xenopus* oocytes failed to reveal a functional defect in the uptake of 2-deoxyglucose, suggesting that it is a polymorphism without major relevance to NIDDM.[80]

The GLUT-2 gene was also studied in 48 African-Americans who had gestational diabetes and subsequently developed NIDDM.[81] SSCP revealed several nucleotide substitutions; all were silent or in introns except two: Thr110Ile and Val197Ile. Thr110Ile was found to be much more common in African Americans than in Pima Indians.[81] In the 48 African-American subjects with NIDDM, 8 were homozygous for the Thr110Ile mutation, 22 were heterozygous for the mutation, and 18 were homozygous for the normal allele (allele frequency = 0.40). The frequency of the Thr110Ile mutation did not differ significantly between subjects with NIDDM and 52 nondiabetic control subjects. Val197Ile, a substitution in the fifth transmembrane loop, was found in one subject with NIDDM and none of 52 nondiabetic control subjects. Expression of the Val197Ile mutation in *Xenopus* oocytes revealed that this seemingly conservative substitution completely abolished glucose transport.[80] Thus although this mutation appears to be rare, it may be causally involved in the pathogenesis of NIDDM in a small subset of patients.

In a study of Japanese subjects with NIDDM, the Thr110Ile substitution was present in 4 of 48 subjects with NIDDM and 3 of 48 nondiabetic controls.[82] Two novel substitutions—Val101Ile and Gly519Glu—were rare, and neither was associated with NIDDM.[82]

The β_3-Adrenergic Receptor Gene

The marked susceptibility of populations to NIDDM has been hypothesized to be caused by a putative "thrifty genotype."[83] In traditional populations subjected to periods of feast and famine, evolution favored enhanced food intake as well as efficiency in energy storage and utilization. However, in an environment of assured access to a diet abundant in refined carbohydrates and fats and a more sedentary lifestyle, this "thrifty genotype" becomes disadvantageous, leading to insulin resistance, hyperinsulinemia, β-cell dysfunction, and NIDDM.[83] These thrifty genes are likely to overlap with genes that predispose to obesity, which is a known risk factor for the development of NIDDM.[84,85] As in NIDDM, family and twin studies support an important genetic component to obesity.[86,87]

In humans, resting metabolic rate is a familial trait, and a low resting metabolic rate is a risk factor for weight gain and obesity.[88,89] In rodents, resting metabolic rate is regulated by the sympathetic nervous system and acts through modulation of thermogenesis in brown adipose tissue.[90,91] Although adult humans do not have anatomically distinct depots of brown adipose tissue, the identification of human uncoupling protein, a marker widely regarded as being specific for brown adipose tissue, suggests that modulation of thermogenesis by the sympathetic nervous system may also be important in human adipose tissue.[92]

Table 63-2. Allele Frequencies and Predicted Prevalences of Trp64Arg β3AR in Several Populations

Population	Allele Frequency	Predicted Prevalence (%)		
		Trp64Arg Homozygotes	Trp64Arg Heterozygotes	Normal Homozygotes
Pima Indians	0.31	9.6	42.8	47.6
Japanese	0.20	4.0	32.0	64.0
Mexican Americans	0.13	1.7	22.6	75.7
African Americans	0.12	1.4	21.2	77.4
Caucasians				
Finland	0.11	1.2	19.6	79.2
France	0.10	1.0	18.0	81.0
Baltimore	0.08	0.6	14.8	84.6
Samoans	0.06	0.4	11.2	88.8
Nauruans	0.00	0	0	100

Table 63-3. Prevalence and Age of Onset of Non–Insulin-Dependent Diabetes Mellitus by β3AR Genotype in Pima Indians

Genotype	Diabetes Onset Any Age (%)	Mean Age of Onset ±SEM	Diabetes Onset Prior to Age 25 (%)
Trp64Arg homozygotes	41/57 (72%)	35.9 ± 1.6*	5/57 (9)†
Heterozygotes	173/290 (60%)	40.2 ± 0.8	10/290 (3)
Normal homozygotes	176/295 (60%)	40.9 ± 0.8	9/295 (3)

*Significantly different by analysis of variance ($P = 0.022$).
†$P = 0.06$ Trp64Arg homozygotes vs. normal homozygotes; $P = 0.05$ Trp64Arg homozygotes vs. normal homozygotes and heterozygotes combined (odds ratio 2.9; 95% confidence limits 0.9–8.6).

The β_3-adrenergic receptor (β3AR) is a seven membrane spanning guanine nucleotide binding (G) protein coupled receptor that is localized in adipose tissue.[93–95] Stimulation by β-agonists (or the sympathetic nervous system) activates adenylyl cyclase, which increases intracellular cAMP concentrations and results in increased lipolysis and thermogenesis. Using SSCP analysis, Walston and coworkers[96] identified a missense mutation at the junction between the first transmembrane domain and the first intracellular loop. Tryptophan, normally present at codon 64, was replaced by arginine (Trp64Arg).[96] Initially identified in Pima Indians, the mutation was also prevalent in Mexican Americans and African Americans, two other minority populations at increased risk for NIDDM and obesity, as well as in caucasians (Table 63-2). Interestingly, the mutation was detected in Samoans but was absent in Nauruans, two genetic isolates of the South Pacific with high rates of NIDDM and obesity (Table 63-2).

In Pima Indians, subjects homozygous for the Trp64Arg β3AR mutation tended to have a higher prevalence of NIDDM, although this was not statistically significant (Table 63-3).[96] Subjects homozygous for the mutation had a significantly earlier onset of NIDDM than those who lacked it (Table 63-3). They also tended to have lower resting metabolic rates and increased body mass indices (Figure 63-2).[96]

The mutation has subsequently been studied in diabetic and nondiabetic Mexican Americans,[97] Finnish caucasians,[98] Japanese,[99] and nondiabetic morbidly obese French caucasians[100] (Table 63-4). There were no differences in the frequency of the Trp64Arg mutation between subjects with NIDDM and non-diabetic controls in Mexican Americans, Finnish caucasians or Japanese. However, as in Pima Indians, Mexican Americans[97] and Finnish caucasians[98] with the Trp64Arg mutation had a significantly earlier onset of NIDDM (see Table 63-4). Further, in Mexican Americans,[97] Finnish caucasians[98] and Japanese,[99] nondiabetic subjects with the mutation had higher plasma insulin levels during a 2-hour glucose tolerance test.[98] Finnish caucasians with the mutation had direct evidence of greater insulin resistance as measured by the hyperinsulinemic-euglycemic clamp technique.[98] Both Mexican Americans and Finnish caucasians with the Trp64Arg mutation had similar body mass indices when compared with those without the mutation. However, in both groups those with the Trp64Arg mutation (particularly females) had higher waist-to-hip ratios, suggesting a central distribution of fat, as well as higher diastolic blood pressures. In Japanese,[99] the Trp64Arg mutation was significantly associated with greater body mass index. In morbidly obese non-diabetic French caucasians,[100] those with the mutation gained significantly more weight over time, and were significantly heavier at the time of examination. These findings suggest a role for the mutation in promoting positive energy balance, which results in increased capacity to gain weight.

Although the major findings in the five cohorts described above are consistent with each other, a few differences suggest that genetic background influences the phenotypic expression of the Trp64Arg β3AR mutation both quantitatively (gene dose) and qualitatively. For example, in Pima Indians the mutation in its homozygous form was associated with an earlier onset of NIDDM, whereas Pima Indians who were heterozygous for the mutation were minimally if at all affected. By contrast, the mutation, even in its heterozygous form, was associated with an earlier onset of NIDDM in both Mexican Americans and Finnish caucasians. In Japanese, no relationship to age of onset of NIDDM was evident in either Trp64Arg heterozygotes or homozygotes. Furthermore, the mutation was associated with a central distribution of fat (i.e., increased waist-to-hip ratio) in Finnish women and possibly in Mexican-American women but not in men or in Pima Indians of either gender. The relationship between insulin resistance and the mutation was most marked in Mexican Americans, Finnish caucasians, and Japanese, and was absent or negligible in Pima Indians.

The mechanism(s) whereby this mutation increases susceptibility to features of the insulin resistance syndrome (so called syndrome X) is currently unknown. We hypothesize that the Trp64Arg substitution results in a receptor with defective signaling properties that causes decreased lipolysis and thermogenesis, predominantly in visceral adipose tissue (the major site of β3AR expression). This leads to preferential deposition of fat viscerally, which in turn, through mechanisms that are not fully understood, leads to the remainder of the syndrome, including insulin resistance and increased blood pressure.

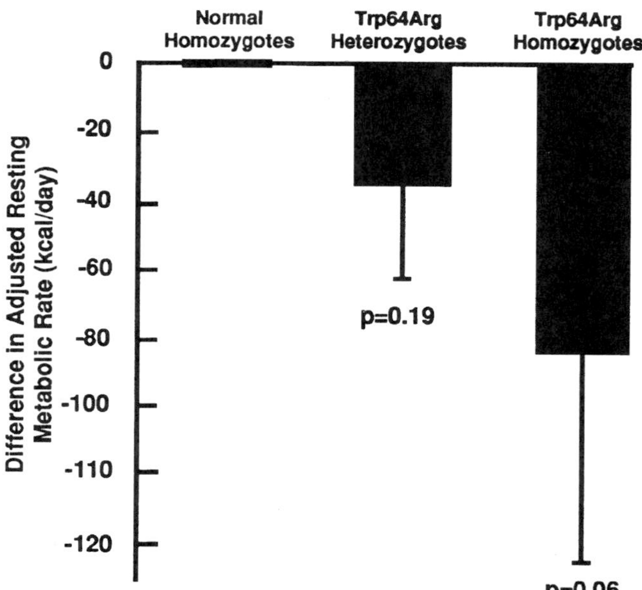

Figure 63-2. Difference in resting metabolic rate by β3AR genotype. Data are corrected for fat-free mass, fat mass, and gender, known covariates of resting metabolic rate. ($p = 0.14$ by analysis of covariance).

TABLE 63-4. Summary of Association Studies of Trp64Arg β3AR in Five Distinct Populations

Trait	Pima Indians (n = 642)	Mexican Americans (n = 62)	Finnish Caucasians (n = 335)	Japanese (n = 350)	French Caucasians (n = 185)
Ascertainment criteria	Diabetic and nondiabetic	Diabetic and nondiabetic	Diabetic and nondiabetic	Diabetic and nondiabetic	Obese and nonobese
Decreased energy expenditure	Borderline	Not done	Not done	Not done	Not done
Increased body mass index	Trend	Trend	Trend	*Significant*	*Significant*
Weight gain	Not done	Not done	Not done	Not done	*Significant*
Earlier onset of NIDDM	*Significant*	*Significant*	*Significant*	None	Not done
Hyperinsulinemia/ insulin resistance	Trend	*Significant*	*Significant*	*Significant*	Not done
Increased diastolic blood pressure	Trend	Borderline	*Significant*	Trend	Not done

$p < 0.05$—*Significant*; $p = 0.06$ to 0.10—borderline; $p > 0.11$—Trend.

In summary, the Trp64Arg β3AR increases susceptibility to several features of the insulin resistance syndrome including hyperinsulemia/insulin resistance, central obesity, and hypertension as well as an earlier (accelerated) onset of NIDDM.[96–100] Although it does not have a major influence on these traits, it is relatively common in diverse populations and is among the first mutations to be identified to influence the typical (polygenic) forms of NIDDM and obesity in humans.

The Hexokinase II Gene

Hexokinases are a family of four enzymes that catalyze the first step in glucose metabolism, namely, phosphorylation of glucose to form glucose-6-phosphate. Glucokinase (hexokinase IV) is specifically expressed in the pancreatic islet and liver and is important for glucose sensing by β-cells. Although mutations in the glucokinase gene have been identified in some subjects with autosomal dominant MODY,[7,8,101] these mutations are very rare or absent in typical NIDDM.[102,103]

Recently human hexokinase II, which is the dominant hexokinase isoform in insulin-responsive peripheral tissues, has been investigated as a candidate for NIDDM. The gene is about 50 kilobases in length and is encoded by 18 exons.[104] Three separate reports in which SSCP analysis was used in a total of approximately 100 subjects with NIDDM revealed several missense mutations: Gln142His, Leu148Phe, Ala314Val, Arg353Cys, Arg497Gln, Arg775Gln, and Arg844Lys.[105–107] Follow-up screening in larger cohorts revealed that all of these mutations except Gln142His were rare. In the two studies in which Gln142His was detected,[105,106] it was present in approximately 18% of all subjects. In both studies, the frequency of the mutation was no greater in subjects with NIDDM than in those without NIDDM.

Other Candidate Genes

In this section, we present early data on several candidate genes for which a limited number of studies have been performed. Clearly, before excluding their roles as NIDDM susceptibility genes, further studies are required.

The ob Gene

The recent cloning of the gene responsible for extreme obesity and diabetes in the C57BL/6J *ob*/*ob* mouse has sparked great interest in determining its potential role in human obesity and NIDDM.[108] The *ob* gene was initially identified by positional cloning in this inbred mouse strain.[108] It encodes a 167 amino acid protein that is produced and secreted by adipocytes and is believed to act in the hypothalamus as a satiety signal, thus closing the feedback loop between appetite behavior and fat (energy) storage.[107] Two distinct strains of *ob*/*ob* mice were found to be homozygous for different mutations in the *ob* gene (one a nonsense mutation and the other a deletion), thus leading to the complete absence of a functional gene product.

The human *ob* gene is 84% similar to its mouse homolog.[108] Recently, Considine and colleagues[109] have sequenced the coding region of the *ob* gene in ten human subjects (five with obesity and five without obesity) and did not find any nucleotide substitutions. *Ob* mRNA levels in fat tissue correlated with body mass index; those with the highest body mass indices had the highest levels of *ob* mRNA.[109] Others have similarly reported increased expression of *ob* in humans with obesity.[110,111] These data provide evidence against a primary (genetic) role of the *ob* gene in typical forms of human obesity with NIDDM.

The Prohormone Convertase-2 Gene

Proinsulin is converted to insulin by the concerted action of three enzymes: prohormone convertase-2 (PC2), which cleaves at the junction between the connecting piece and the A-chain; prohormone convertase-3 (PC3), which cleaves at the junction between the B-chain and the connecting piece; and carboxypeptidase, which trims the two remaining dibasic amino acids at the carboxy-terminus of the B-chain.[112,113] Subjects with NIDDM have higher circulating concentrations of proinsulin and partially cleaved proinsulin products, and thus genes encoding these processing enzymes are reasonable candidate genes for NIDDM.[114,115] Indeed, the *fa*/*fa* mouse, a monogenic mouse model of obesity and diabetes, has been shown to be caused by a mutation in the carboxypeptidase E gene.[116]

PC2 consists of 12 exons that span a region of more than 130 kilobases on chromosome 20p11.2[117] Recently Yoshida and coworkers[118] identified a microsatellite polymorphism with seven alleles (designated A_1 to A_7) within intron 2 of the PC2 gene. The frequency of the PC2 A_1 allele was 0.11 in subjects with NIDDM compared with 0.04 in subjects without diabetes ($P = 0.068$). Diabetic subjects with and without the PC2 A_1 allele were no different with respect to their clinical characteristics, in particular fasting insulin and proinsulin levels. SSCP analysis of the coding region failed to detect any mutation in subjects with the PC2 A_1 allele. Interestingly, one of the 60 subjects screened (who had a

PC2 A_3/A_3 genotype) was found to have a G→T substitution two base pairs before the ATG initiation codon. At the present time, the significance of this variant is unclear.

Tumor Necrosis Factor-α

Tumor necrosis factor-α (TNF-α) is a cytokine that is overexpressed in adipocytes of obese subjects and is thought to be a cause of insulin resistance in muscle and adipose tissue.[119] Its gene is located on chromosome 6p21.3 and is composed of four exons.[120] Norman and coworkers[121] studied this locus in Pima Indians using a microsatellite polymorphism within 10 kilobases of the TNF-α locus. They demonstrated linkage with body mass index in 304 sib pairs ($P = 0.002$). There was no evidence for linkage of this locus with measurements of insulin sensitivity or with resting metabolic rate. Linkage could not be demonstrated in a larger cohort of 874 sib pairs. SSCP of 20 obese and 20 nonobese Pima Indians identified a single nucleotide substitution in the promoter region that was not linked to obesity. Further studies are required to define the potential importance of the TNF-α locus in NIDDM and obesity.

The Islet-1 Gene

Islet-1 (Isl-1), located on chromosome 5q, is a member of the LIM/homeodomain family of transcription factors.[122] Isl-1 binds to the enhancer region of the insulin gene and may be involved in the regulation of insulin gene transcription. In studies of St. Louis African-Americans and Nigerians using a closely linked informative microsatellite polymorphism, no evidence for association of any of the alleles could be demonstrated.[123] Evidence for linkage could be rejected in 15 families with MODY previously shown not to be caused by glucokinase gene mutations.[123]

The Islet Amyloid Polypeptide Gene

Islet amyloid polypeptide (IAPP) is a 37 amino acid polypeptide with homology to the calcitonin family.[124] Studies have demonstrated that subjects with NIDDM have excessive IAPP in islets as well as in circulating blood, suggesting that it may play a role in β-cell dysfunction and/or insulin resistance.[125–127] The IAPP gene is located on chromosome 12 and encodes an 89 amino acid precursor.[128] A single study using a PvuII RFLP in four British pedigrees as well as 88 unrelated subjects with NIDDM and 67 nondiabetic controls failed to show linkage or association of this IAPP RFLP with NIDDM.[129]

The Glucagon-like Peptide Receptor Gene

Secretion of glucagon-like peptide-1 (GLP-1) by L cells in the proximal small intestine is stimulated by ingestion of a meal.[130,131] GLP-1 binds to receptors on β-cells and through stimulation of adenylyl cyclase increases insulin biosynthesis and secretion.[132,133] The GLP-1 receptor gene is located on chromosome 6p and encodes a 463 amino acid membrane-associated receptor.[134,135] Recently, Tanizawa and coworkers[134] hypothesized that genetic defects in the GLP-1 receptor may contribute to impaired glucose-stimulated insulin secretion in NIDDM. Two informative microsatellite polymorphisms were used to study unrelated African-American subjects, 95 with NIDDM and 93 without NIDDM, as well as 16 Utah Mormon pedigrees. No evidence for association or linkage could be demonstrated in these two populations.[134]

The Ras Associated with Diabetes Gene

The ras associated with diabetes (*rad*) gene was identified by substraction cloning and is overexpressed in muscle of subjects with NIDDM.[135] The function of *rad* is currently unknown. The *rad* gene is located on chromosome 16q22. Recently Doria and coworkers[136] identified a microsatellite polymorphism near the *rad* locus and suggested that some rare alleles may be more common in subjects with NIDDM than in nondiabetic controls. Further studies are necessary to determine the relevance of this locus to insulin resistance and NIDDM.

Conclusions and Future Prospects

NIDDM is a complex genetic disorder that is both polygenic and heterogeneous. It is likely that mutations in some genes will be distinct for a given population, whereas others may occur more broadly in several populations. Furthermore, the phenotypic expression of a given mutation may vary markedly between populations (and even within individuals of the same population), depending on genetic background and differences in environment and behavior. Some of the genes that increase susceptibility to NIDDM are likely to overlap with those that increase susceptibility to obesity. Although monogenic rodent models of NIDDM and obesity such as the *ob/ob* mouse and the *fa/fa* mouse appear to simulate the human phenotype, their applicability to the genetic basis of human NIDDM remains to be determined.

Several groups have ascertained and phenotypically characterized cohorts and families for genetic studies. Both candidate gene and positional cloning approaches are being used. Because of the inherent difficulties in elucidating susceptibility genes for polygenic and heterogeneous diseases such as NIDDM, early positive results for any gene or locus must be regarded with suspicion until their authenticity is supported by studies in the same or other populations and/or until evidence for a functional defect in the mutant gene product is demonstrated. Despite these difficulties and caveats, the next several years will be exciting in the search for NIDDM susceptibility genes. With these new discoveries, fundamental insights into the molecular basis of NIDDM will lead to improved early diagnostics and to the development of novel interventions (pharmacologic as well as the prospect of gene therapy) for the prevention, delay, and treatment of NIDDM.

References

1. Harris MI, Hadden WC, Knowler WC. Prevalence of diabetes and impaired glucose tolerance and plasma levels in U.S. populations aged 20–74 years. Diabetes 1987;36:523
2. Rich SS. Mapping genes in diabetes. Genetic epidemiological perspective. Diabetes 1990;39:1315
3. Rotter JL, Vadheim CM, Rimoin DL. Genetics of diabetes mellitus. In: Rifkin H, Porte D Jr, eds. Diabetes Mellitus: Theory and Practice. Amsterdam: Elsevier; 1990:378–413
4. Barnett AH, Eff C, Leslie RDG, et al. Diabetes in identical twins: A study in 200 pairs. Diabetolgia 1981;20:78
5. Taylor SI, Cama A, Accili D, et al. Mutations in the insulin receptor gene. Endocrine Rev 1992;13:566
6. Moller DE, Cohen O, Yamaguchi Y, et al. Prevalence of mutations in the insulin receptor gene in patients with type A syndrome of insulin resistance. Diabetes 1994;43:247
7. Vionnet N, Stoffel M, Takeda J, et al. Nonsense mutation in the glucokinase gene causes early-onset non–insulin-dependent diabetes mellitus. Nature 1992;356:721
8. Froguel P, Zouali H, Vionnet N, et al. Familial hyperglycemia due to mutations in glucokinase. Definition of a subtype of diabetes mellitus. N Engl J Med 1993;328:697
9. Bell GI, Xiang KS, Newman MV, et al. Gene for non–insulin-dependent diabetes mellitus (maturity-onset diabetes of the young subtype) is linked to DNA polymorphism on human chromosome 20q. Proc Natl Acad Sci USA 1991;88:1484
10. Vaxillaire M, Boccio V, Philippi A, et al. A gene for maturity onset diabetes of the young (MODY) maps to chromosome 12q. Nat Genet 1995;9:418
11. Steiner DF, Tager HS, Chan SJ, et al. Lessons learned from molecular biology of insulin-gene mutations. Diabetes Care 1990;13:600
12. Tager H, Given B, Baldwin D, et al. A structurally abnormal insulin causing human diabetes. Nature 1979;281:122

13. Gerbitz KD. Does the mitochondrial DNA play a role in the pathogenesis of diabetes? Diabetologia 1992;35:1181
14. Kadowaki T, Kadowaki H, Mori Y, et al. A subtype of diabetes mellitus associated with a mutation of mitochondrial DNA. N Engl J Med 1994; 330:962
15. Reardon W, Ross RJ, Sweeney MG, et al. Diabetes mellitus associated with a pathogenic point mutation in mitochondrial DNA. Lancet 1992;340:1376
16. Collins FS. Positional cloning: Let's not call it reverse anymore. Nat Gen 1992;1:3
17. Ott J. In: Analysis of Human Genetic Linkage. Baltimore: Johns Hopkins University Press; 1991:1–302
18. Blackwelder WC, Elston RC. Power and robustness of sib pair linkage tests and extension to larger sibships. Comm Stat Theory Method 1992;11:449
19. Meyers RM, Lumelsky N, Lerman LS, Maniatis T. Detection of single base substitutions in total genomic DNA. Nature 1985;313:495
20. Henco K, Harders J, Wiese U, Riesner D. Temperature gradient gel electrophoresis (TGGE) for the detection of polymorphic DNA and RNA. Methods Mol Biol 1994;31:211
21. Orita M, Suzuki T, Sekiya T, et al. Rapid and sensitive detection of point mutations and DNA polymorphisms using the polymerase chain reaction. Genomics 1989;5:874
22. Keen JD, Lester C, Inglehearn A, et al. Rapid detection of single base mismatches at heteroduplexes on Hydrolinks gels. Trends Genet 1991;7:5
23. O'Rahilly S, Choi WH, Patel P, et al. Detection of mutations in insulin-receptor gene in NIDDM patients by analysis of single-stranded conformational polymorphisms. Diabetes 1991;40:777
24. Sheffield VC, Beck JS, Kwitel AE, et al. The sensitivity of single-stand conformation polymorphism analysis for the detection of single base substitutions. Genomics 1993;19:325
25. Celi FS, Cohen MM, Antonarakis S, et al. Determination of gene dosage by a quantitative adaptation of the polymerase chain reaction (gd-PCR): Rapid detection of deletions and duplications of gene sequences. Genomics 1994; 21:304
26. Kahn CR. Insulin action, diabetogenes, and the cause of type II diabetes. Diabetes 1994;43:1066
27. Defronzo RA. The triumvirate: β-cell, muscle, liver: A collusion responsible for NIDDM. Diabetes 1988;37:667
28. Haring HU, Mehnert H. Pathogenesis of type 2 (non–insulin-dependent) diabetes mellitus: Candidates for a signal transmitter defect causing insulin resistance of the skeletal muscle. Diabetologia 1993;36:176
29. Bell GI, Pictet RL, Rutter WJ, et al. Sequence of the human insulin gene. Nature 1980;284:26
30. Steiner DF, Bell GI, Tager HS. Chemistry and biosynthesis of pancreatic protein hormones. In: De Groot LH, ed. Endocrinology. 2nd ed, vol 2. Philadelphia: WB Saunders; 1989:75
31. Owerbach D, Nerup J. Restriction fragment length polymorphism of the insulin gene in diabetes mellitus. Diabetes 1982;31:275
32. Rotwein PS, Chirgwin J, Province M, et al. Polymorphism in the 5′ flanking region of the human insulin gene: A genetic marker for non–insulin-dependent diabetes mellitus. N Engl J Med 1983;308:65
33. Bell GI, Horita S, Karam JH. A polymorphic locus near the human insulin gene is associated with insulin-dependent diabetes mellitus. Diabetes 1984;33:176
34. Hitman GA, Jowett NI, Williams LG, et al. Polymorphisms in the 5′-flanking region of the insulin gene and non–insulin-dependent diabetes. Clin Sci 1984;66:383
35. Knowler WC, Pettitt DJ, Vasquez B, et al. Polymorphism in the 5′-flanking region of the human insulin gene. J Clin Invest 1984;74:2129
36. Elbein S, Rotwein P, Permutt MA, et al. Lack of association of the polymorphic locus in the 5′-flanking region of the human insulin gene and diabetes in American blacks. Diabetes 1985;34:433
37. Rich SS. Positional cloning works: Identification of genes that cause NIDDM. Diabetes 1995;44:139
38. Niskanen LK, Tuomi T, Karajalainen J, et al. GAD antibodies in NIDDM. The one-year follow-up from the diagnosis. Diabetes Care 1995;12:1557
39. Steiner DF, Tager HS, Chan SJ, et al. Lessons learned from molecular biology of insulin-gene mutations. Diabetes Care 1990;13:600
40. Nanjo K, Sanke T, Miyano M, et al. Diabetes due to secretion of a structurally abnormal insulin (insulin Wakayama). Clinical and functional characteristics of [Leu A3] insulin. J Clin Invest 1986;77:514
41. Shoelson SE, Polonsky KS, Zeidler A, et al. Human insulin B24 (Phe→Ser). Secretion and metabolic clearance of the abnormal insulin in man and in a dog model. J Clin Invest 1984;73:1351
42. Given BD, Mako ME, Tager HS, et al. Diabetes due to secretion of an abnormal insulin. N Engl J Med 1980;302:129
43. Gruppuso PA, Gorden P, Kahn CR, et al. Familial hypoproinsulinemia due to a proposed defect in conversion of proinsulin to insulin. N Engl J Med 1984;311:629
44. Robbins DC, Blix PM, Rubenstein AH, et al. A human proinsulin variant at arginine 65. Nature 1981;291:679
45. Yano H, Kitano N, Morimoto M, et al. A novel point mutation in the human insulin gene giving rise to hyperproinsulinemia (proinsulin Kyoto). J Clin Invest 1993;89:1902
46. Warren-Perry MG, Mussett S, Morris R, et al. A novel point mutation in the insulin gene giving rise to hyperproinsulinemia (Abstract). Diabetes 1995; 44(Suppl 1):162A
47. Raben N, Barbetti F, Cama A, et al. Normal coding sequence of insulin gene in Pima Indians and Nauruans. Diabetes 1991;40:118
48. Kishimoto M, Sakura H, Hayashi K, et al. Detection of mutations in the human insulin gene by single strand conformation polymorphisms. J Clin Endocrinol Metab 1991;74:1027
49. Olansky L, Janssen R, Welling C, Permutt MA. Variability of the insulin gene in American blacks with NIDDM. Analysis by single-strand conformational polymorphisms. Diabetes 1992;41:742
50. Olansky L, Janssen R, Welling C, et al. Variability of the insulin gene in American blacks with NIDDM. J Clin Invest 1992;89:1596
51. Lok S, Kuijper JL, Jelinek W, et al. The human glucagon receptor encoding gene: Structure, cDNA sequence and chromosomal localization. Gene 1994;140:203
52. Hager J, Hansen L, Vaisse C, et al. A missense mutation in the glucagon receptor gene is associated with non–insulin-dependent diabetes mellitus. Nat Gen 1995;9:299
53. Prochazka M, Lillioja S, Tait JF, et al. Linkage of chromosomal markers on 4q with a putative gene determining maximal insulin action in Pima Indians. Diabetes 1993;42:514
54. Baier LJ, Sacchettini JC, Knowler WC, et al. An amino acid substitution in the human intestinal fatty acid binding protein is associated with increased fatty acid binding, increased fat oxidation, and insulin resistance. J Clin Invest 1995;95:1281
55. Baier LJ, Sacchettini JC. An amino acid substitution in the human intestinal fatty acid binding protein alters the rate of transport of fatty acids across intestinal-like cells. (Abstract) Diabetes 1995;44(Suppl 1):41A
56. Humphreys P, McCarthy M, Tuomilehto J, et al. Chromosome 4q locus associated with insulin resistance in Pima Indians. Diabetes 1994;43:800
57. Groop LC, Bonadonn RC, DelPrato S, et al. Glucose and free fatty acid metabolism in non–insulin-dependent diabetes mellitus: Evidence for multiple sites of insulin resistance. J Clin Invest 1989;84:205
58. Eriksson J, Franssila-Kallunki A, Ekstrand A, et al. Early metabolic defects in persons at increased risk for non–insulin-dependent diabetes mellitus. N Engl J Med 1987;321:337
59. Vaag A, Henrikson JE, Beck-Nielsen H. Decreased insulin activation of glycogen synthase in skeletal muscles in young nonobese caucasian first-degree relatives of patients with non–insulin-dependent diabetes mellitus. J Clin Invest 1992;89:782
60. Lehto M, Stoffel M, Groop L, et al. Assignment of the gene encoding glycogen synthase (GYS) to human chromosome 19, band q13.3. Genomics 1993; 15;460
61. Groop LC, Kankura M, Schalin-Jantti C, et al. Association between polymorphism of the glycogen synthase gene and non–insulin-dependent diabetes mellitus. N Engl J Med 1993;328:10
62. Zouali H, Velho G, Froguel P. Polymorphism of the glycogen synthase gene and non–insulin-dependent diabetes mellitus. N Engl J Med 1993;328:1568
63. Kadowaki T, Kadowaki H, Yazaki Y. Polymorphism of the glycogen synthase gene and non–insulin-dependent dabetes mellitus. N Engl J Med 1993;328: 1568
64. Groop L, Schalin-Jantti C, Lehto M. Polymorphism of the glycogen synthase gene and non–insulin-dependent diabetes mellitus. N Engl J Med 1993; 328:1569
65. Elbein SC, Hoffman M, Ridinger D, et al. Description of a second microsatellite marker and linkage analysis of the muscle glycogen synthase locus in familial NIDDM. Diabetes 1994;43:1061
66. Cox NJ, Bell GI. Disease associations. Chance, artifact, or susceptibility genes? Diabetes 1989;38:947
67. Vestergaard H, Bjorback C, Anderson PH, et al. Impaired expression of glycogen synthase mRNA in skeletal muscle of NIDDM patients. Diabetes 1991;40:1740
68. Mueckler M. Family of glucose-transporter genes: Implications for glucose homeostasis and diabetes. Diabetes 1990;39:6
69. Mueckler M. Facilitative glucose transporters. Eur J Biochem 1994;219:713
70. Holman GD, Cushman SW. Subcellular localization and trafficking of the GLUT4 glucose transporter isoform in insulin-response cells. Bioessays 1994;16:753
71. Fukumoto H, Seino S, Imura H, et al. Sequence, tissue distribution and chromosomal localization of mRNA encoding a human glucose transporter-like protein. Proc Natl Acad Sci USA 1988;85:5434
72. Matsutani A, Koranyi L, Cox N, et al. Polymorphisms of GLUT2 and GLUT4 genes. Use in evaluation of genetic susceptibility to NIDDM in blacks. Diabetes 1990;39:1534
73. Baroni MG, Oelbaum RS, Pozzilli P, et al. Polymorphisms at the GLUT1 (HepG2) and GLUT4 (muscle/adipocyte) glucose transporter genes and non–insulin-dependent diabetes mellitus (NIDDM). Hum Genet 1992;88:557
74. Choi WH, O'Rahilly S, Buse JB, et al. Molecular scanning of insulin-responsive glucose transporter (GLUT4) gene in NIDDM subjects. Diabetes 1991; 40:1712
75. Kusari J, Verma US, Buse JB, et al. Analysis of the gene sequences of the insulin receptor and the insulin-sensitive glucose transporter (GLUT-4) in patients with common-type non–insulin-dependent diabetes mellitus. J Clin Invest 1991;88:1323
76. Patel P, Bell GI, Cook JTE, et al. Multiple restriction fragment length polymorphisms at the GLUT2 locus: GLUT2 haplotypes for genetic analysis of type 2 (non–insulin-dependent) diabetes mellitus. Diabetologia 1991;34:817
77. Baroni MG, Alcolado JC, Pozzilli P, et al. Polymorphisms at the GLUT2

(beta-cell/liver) glucose transporter gene and non–insulin-dependent diabetes mellitus (NIDDM): Analysis in affected pedigree members. Clin Genet 1992;41:229
78. Alcolado JC, Baroni MG, Li SR. Association between a restriction fragment length polymorphism at the liver/islet cell (Glut 2) glucose transporter and familial type 2 (non–insulin-dependent) diabetes mellitus. Diabetologia 1991;34:734
79. Janssen RC, Bogardus C, Takeda J, et al. Linkage analysis of acute insulin secretion with GLUT2 and glucokinase in Pima Indians and the identification of a missense mutation in GLUT2. Diabetes 1994;43:558
80. Mueckler M, Kruse M, Strube M, et al. A mutation of the GLUT2 glucose transporter gene of a diabetic patient abolishes transport activity. J Biol Chem 1994;269:17765
81. Tanizawa Y, Riggs AC, Chiu KC, et al. Variability of the pancreatic islet beta cell/liver (GLUT2) glucose transporter gene in NIDDM patients. Diabetologia 1994;37:420
82. Shimada E, Makino H, Iwaoka H, et al. Identification of two novel amino acid polymorphisms in beta-cell/liver (GLUT2) glucose transporter in Japanese subjects. Diabetologia 1995;38:211
83. Neel JV. The thrifty genotype revisited. In: Kobberling J, Tattersall R, eds. The Genetics of Diabetes Mellitus. Proceedings of the Serono Symposium, London: Academic Press;1982:283–293
84. Barrett-Connor E. Epidemiology, obesity, and non–insulin-dependent diabetes mellitus. Epidemiol Rev. 1989;11:172
85. Knowler W, Pettitt D, Saad M, et al. Obesity in the Pima Indians: Its magnitude and relationship with diabetes. Am J Clin Nutr 1991;53:1543
86. Stunkard A, Foch T, Hrubec Z. A twin study of human obesity. JAMA 1986;256:51
87. Bouchard C, Despres J, Tremblay A. Genetics of obesity and human energy metabolism. Proc Nutr Soc 1991;50:139
88. Bouchard C, Tremblay A, Nadeau A, et al. Genetic effect in resting and exercise metabolic rates. Metabolism 1989;38:364
89. Ravussin E, Lillioja M, Knowler WC, et al. Reduced rate of energy expenditure as a risk factor for body weight gain. N Engl J Med 1988;318:467
90. Himms-Hagen J. Brown adipose tissue thermogenesis: Interdisciplinary studies. FASEB J 1990;4:2890
91. Landsberg L, Young JB. The role of the sympathoadrenal system in modulating energy expenditure. Clin Endocrinol Metab 1984;13:475
92. Cassard A-M, Bouillaud F, Mattel M-G, et al. Human uncoupling protein gene: Structure, comparison with rat gene, and assignment to the long arm of chromosome 4. J Cell Biochem 1990;43:255
93. Emorine LJ, Marullo S, Briend-Sutren M-M, et al. Molecular characterization of the human β_3-adrenergic receptor. Science 1990;245:1118
94. Emorine L, Feve B, Pairault J, et al. The human β_3-adrenergic receptor: Relationship with atypical receptors. Am J Clin Nutr 1992;55:215S
95. Krief S, Lonnquist F, Raimbault S, et al. Tissue distribution of β_3-adrenergic receptor mRNA in man. J Clin Invest 1993;91:344
96. Walston J, Silver K, Bogardus C, et al. Earlier onset of non–insulin-dependent diabetes mellitus in subjects with a mutation in the β3-adrenergic receptor gene. N Engl J Med 1995;333:337
97. Silver K, Walston J, Sorkin JD, et al. TRP64ARG β3-adrenergic receptor in Mexican Americans accelerates the onset of diabetes and associates with features of syndrome X. Submitted for publication
98. Widen E, Lehto M, Kanninen T, et al. Association of a polymorphism in the β3-adrenergic receptor gene with features of the insulin resistance syndrome in Finns. N Engl J Med 1995;333:348
99. Kadowaki H, Kazuki Y, Iwamoto K, et al. A mutation in the β_3-adrenergic receptor gene is associated with obesity and hyperinsulinemia in Japanese subjects. Biochem Biophys Res Commun 1995;215:555
100. Clement K, Vaisse C, Manning BS-J, et al. A mutation in the β3-adrenergic receptor and increased capacity to gain weight in patients with morbid obesity. N Engl J Med 1995;333:352
101. Permutt MA, Chiu KC, Tanizawa Y. Glucokinase and NIDDM: A candidate gene that paid off. Diabetes 1992;41:1357
102. Elbein SC, Hoffman M, Chiu K, et al. Linkage analysis of the glucokinase locus in familial type 2 (non–insulin-dependent) diabetic pedigrees. Diabetologia 1993;36:141
103. Zouali H, Vaxillaire M, Lesage S, et al. Linkage analysis and molecular scanning of glucokinase gene in NIDDM families. Diabetes 1993;42:1238
104. Printz RL, Ardehali H, Koch S, Granner DK. Human hexokinase II mRNA and gene structure. Diabetes 1995;44:290
105. Vidal-Puig A, Printz RL, Stratton IM, et al. Analysis of the hexokinase II gene in subjects with insulin resistance and NIDDM and detection of a Gln^{142}→His substitution. Diabetes 1995;44:340
106. Echwald SM, Bjorbaek C, Hansen T, et al. Identification of four amino acid substitutions in hexokinase II and studies of relationships to NIDDM, glucose effectiveness and insulin sensitivity. Diabetes 1995;44:347
107. Laakso M, Malkki M, Debb SS. Amino acid substitutions in hexokinase II among patients with NIDDM. Diabetes 1995;44:330
108. Zhang Y, Proenca R, Maffei M, et al. Positional cloning of the mouse gene and its human homologue. Nature 1994;372:425
109. Considine RV, Cosidine EL, Williams CJ, et al. Evidence against either a premature stop codon or the absence of obese gene mRNA in human obesity. J Clin Invest 1995;95:2986
110. Maffei M, Halaas J, Ravussin E, et al. Leptin levels in human and rodent: Measurement of plasma leptin and ob RNA in obese and weight-reduced subjects. Nature Medicine 1995;11:1155
111. Lonnqvist F, Arner P, Nordfors L, Schalling M. Overexpression of the obese (*ob*) gene in adipose tissue of human obese subjects. Nature 1995;9:950
112. Smeekens SP, Steiner DF. Post-translational proteolysis in polypeptide hormone biosynthesis. Ann Rev Physiol 1982;44:625
113. Smeekens SP, Avruch AS, LaMendol J, et al. Identification of a cDNA encoding a second putative prohormone convertase related to PC2 in AtT20 cells and islets of Langerhans. Proc Natl Acad Sci USA 1991;88:340
114. Yoshioka N, Kuzuya T, Taniguuchi M, Iwamoto Y. Serum proinsulin levels at fasting and after oral glucose load in patients with type II (non–insulin-dependent) diabetes mellitus. Diabetologia 1988;31:355
115. Rhodes CJ, Alarcon C. What β-cell defect could lead to hyperproinsulinemia in NIDDM? Some clues from recent advances made in understanding the proinsulin-processing mechanism. Diabetes 1994;43:51
116. Naggert JK, Fricker LD, Varlamov O, et al. Hyperproinsulinaemia in obese fat/fat mice associated with a carboxypeptidase E mutation which reduces enzyme activity. Nature Genetics 1995;10:135
117. Ohagi S, LaMendola J, BeBeau MM, et al. Identification and analysis of the gene encoding human PC2, a prohormone covertase expressed in neuroendocrine tissues. Proc Natl Acad Sci USA 1992;89:4977
118. Yoshida H, Ohagi S, Sanke T, et al. Association of the prohormone convertase 2 gene (PCSK2) on chromosome 20 with NIDDM in Japanese subjects. Diabetes 1995;44:389
119. Hotamisligil GS, Shargill NS, Spiegelman BM. Adipose expression of tumor necrosis factor-α: Direct role in obesity-linked insulin resistance. Science 1993;259:87
120. Nedospasov SA, Udalova IA, Kuprash DV, Turetskaya RL. DNA sequence polymorphism at the human tumor necrosis factor (TNF) locus. Numerous TNF/lymphotoxin alleles tagged by two closely linked microsatellites in the upstream region of the lymphotoxin (TNF-beta) gene. J Immunol 1991;147:1053
121. Norman RA, Bogardus C, Ravussin E. Linkage between obesity and a marker near the tumor necrosis factor-α locus in Pima Indians. J Clin Invest 1995;96:158
122. Karlsson O, Thor S, Norbert T, et al. Insulin gene enhancer binding protein Isl-1 is a member of a novel class of proteins containing both a homeo- and Cys-His domain. Nature 1990;334:879
123. Tanizawa Y, Riggs AC, Dagogo-Jack S, et al. Isolation of the human LIM/homeodomain gene islet-1 and identification of a simple sequence repeat. Diabetes 1994;43:935
124. Sanke T, Bell GI, Sample C, et al. An islet amyloid peptide is derived from an 89-amino-acid precursor by proteolytic processing. J Biol Chem 1988; 263:17243
125. Clark A, Cooper GJS, Lewis CE, et al. Islet amyloid formed from diabetes-associated peptide may be pathogenic in type 2 diabetes. Lancet 1987;2:231
126. Clark A, Saad MF, Nezzer T, et al. Islet amyloid in diabetic and non-diabetic Pima Indians. Diabetologia 1990;33:285
127. Clark A. Islet amyloid and type 2 diabetes. Diab Med 1989;6:561
128. Mosselman S, Hoppener JWM, Zandberg J, et al. Islet amyloid polypeptide: Identification and chromosomal localization of the human gene. FEBS Lett 1988;239:227
129. Cook J, Patel PP, Clark A, et al. Non-linkage of the islet amyloid polypeptide gene with type 2 (non–insulin-dependent) diabetes mellitus. Diabetologia 1991;34:103
130. Orskov C. Glucagon-like peptide-1, a new hormone of the entero-insular axis. Diabetologia 1992;35:701
131. Nauck MA, Heimesaat MM, Orskov C, et al. Preserved incretin activity of glucagon-like peptide 1 [7-36] but not of synthetic human gastric inhibitory polypeptide in patients with type-2 diabetes mellitus. J Clin Invest 1993; 91:301
132. Drucker DJ, Philippe J, Mojsov S, et al. Glucagon-like peptide-1 stimulates insulin gene expression and increases cyclic AMP levels in a rat islet cell line. Proc Natl Acad Sci USA 1987;84:3434
133. Orskov C, Jeppesen J, Madsbad S, Holst JJ. Proglucagon products in plasma of non–insulin-dependent diabetics and nondiabetic controls in the fasting state and after oral glucose and intravenous arginine. J Clin Invest 1991; 87:415
134. Tanizawa Y, Riggs AC, Elbein SC, et al. Human glucagon-like peptide-1 receptor gene in NIDDM: Identification and use of simple sequence repeat polymorphisms in genetic analysis. Diabetes 1994;3:752
135. Thorens B. Expression cloning of the pancreatic β-cell receptor for the glucoincretin hormone glucagon-like peptide-1. Proc Natl Acad Sci USA 1992; 89:8641
136. Doria A, Caldwell JS, Ji L, et al. Trinucleotide repeats at the rad locus: Allele distributions in NIDDM and mapping to a 3-cM region on chromosome 16q. Diabetes 1995;44:243

Diabetes Mellitus, edited by Derek LeRoith, Simeon I. Taylor, and Jerrold M. Olefsky. Lippincott–Raven Publishers, Philadelphia © 1996.

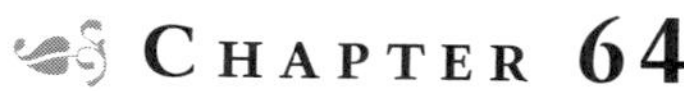

Chapter 64

Mutations in the Genes Encoding the Insulin Receptor and Insulin Receptor Substrate-1

Simeon I. Taylor and Domenico Accili

Introduction

The insulin receptor is an oligomeric glycoprotein that is located on the surface of cells and mediates the first step in insulin action.[1,2] Binding of insulin to the extracellular domain activates the receptor tyrosine kinase, thereby initiating the biologic responses within the target cell. Thus, the receptor serves a crucial role in mediating insulin action. Consequently, defects in the function of the insulin receptor function cause insulin resistance. For example, mutations in the insulin receptor gene have been shown to cause several genetic syndromes associated with insulin resistance (leprechaunism, type A insulin resistance, and the Rabson-Mendenhall syndrome).[1,2] In addition to elucidating the molecular mechanisms of disease in these syndromes, identification of these mutations has provided insight into the structure-function relationships of the insulin receptor.

Mutations in the Insulin Receptor Gene

Classification of Mutations in the Insulin Receptor Gene

The first steps in biosynthesis of the insulin receptor include transcription of the gene, processing of the transcript, and transport of the mature mRNA out of the nucleus (Fig. 64-1). Thereafter, the mRNA is translated by ribosomes located on the rough endoplasmic reticulum. As the proreceptor is transported through the endoplasmic reticulum and Golgi apparatus, it undergoes post-translational processing (i.e., formation of disulfide bonds, proteolytic cleavage, *N*-linked and *O*-linked glycosylation, and acylation). After the insulin receptor is inserted in the plasma membrane, it is available to bind insulin. When insulin binds to the extracellular domain of the receptor, this activates the tyrosine kinase that is necessary to mediate most (if not all) of insulin's biologic actions. In addition, insulin binding accelerates endocytosis of receptors. Thereafter, two alternative fates are available to internalized receptors: (1) recycling back to the plasma membrane for reutilization or (2) transport to lysosomes for intracellular degradation. Mutations in the insulin receptor gene have been demonstrated to cause insulin resistance by interfering with any of these steps required for normal function of the receptor.[1-3]

Class 1A. Mutations That Decrease the Number of Insulin Receptors Without Altering Receptor Structure

Mutations that decrease the level of insulin receptor mRNA cause insulin resistance by decreasing the number of insulin receptors on the cell surface. For example, a deletion of the entire insulin receptor gene was identified in a patient with leprechaunism.[4] This patient, who was born into a consanguineous pedigree, was homozygous for this deletion mutation.

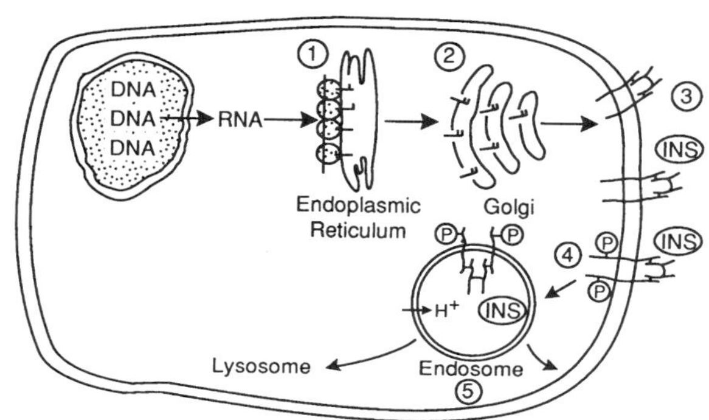

Class of Mutation	Synthesis	Transport to Plasma Membrane	Insulin Binding	Trans-membrane Signaling	Endocytosis, Recycling, Degradation
1	→ ×				
2	→	→ ×			
3	→	→	→ ×		
4	→	→	→	→ ×	
5	→	→	→	→	→ ×

Figure 64-1. Classification of mutations in insulin receptor gene. A summary of the major steps in the life of an insulin receptor.[1,2] First, the gene is transcribed and the RNA is spliced. The mature mRNA is transported from the nucleus to the cytosol, where it is translated by ribosomes on the rough endoplasmic reticulum. The receptor is transported through the endoplasmic reticulum and Golgi, in which organelles it undergoes multiple post-translational modifications. Eventually, the mature receptor is inserted in the plasma membrane. Insulin binds to the receptor on the cell surface. As a result, the receptor undergoes autophosphorylation and becomes activated as a tyrosine kinase. The interaction of insulin with its receptor initiates the various responses of the target cell to insulin. In addition, insulin binding triggers receptor endocytosis. The acid pH in the endosome dissociates insulin from its receptor. Subsequent to receptor internalization, the receptor is either transported to lysosomes for degradation or recycled back to the plasma membrane for reutilization. The five major classes of genetic defects in receptor function are summarized in the table. This classification scheme is an adaptation of the classification originally proposed by Brown and Goldstein[96] for genetic defects in the function of the low-density lipoprotein receptor.

Several other types of mutations lead to a decrease in the level of insulin receptor mRNA. For example, several patients have been identified in whose cells there is a decreased level of mRNA despite the fact that the deduced amino acid sequence of the insulin receptor was determined to be normal. The prototype of this type of mutation was identified in a patient with leprechaunism (leprechaun/Minn-1) who inherited this mutant allele from her mother.[5,6] In the patient's cells, the mutant allele was paired with a second mutant allele (inherited from the father) that contained a nonsense mutation at codon 897. In contrast, in the mother's cells, the mutant allele was paired with a normal allele of the insulin receptor gene. The two alleles in the mother's cells could be distinguished because they contained two different codons (GAC versus GAT) encoding Asp^{234}. This biochemical marker permitted quantitation of the mRNA derived from each allele. The mutant allele (containing GAT at codon 234) was expressed at ≈10% of the level of the normal allele (containing GAC at codon 234) despite the fact that both alleles were present in the same nucleus and exposed to the same array of trans-acting factors. This observation provides indirect evidence that the allele containing GAT at codon 234 has a *cis*-acting mutation that decreases the level of insulin receptor mRNA. This putative mutation has not yet been defined precisely or identified directly. Similar evidence has suggested the existence of unidentified *cis*-acting mutations that decrease the level of insulin receptor mRNA in other patients.[7–9]

Class 1B. Mutations That Encode Nonfunctional Truncated Receptors

Some mutations introduce premature chain termination codons that lead to truncation of the receptor in its extracellular domain (Fig. 64-2). Consequently, these truncated receptors lack the transmembrane anchor and the entire intracellular domain. Lacking a transmembrane domain, the truncated receptors are not expressed on the cell surface and are presumed to be completely nonfunctional (i.e., null alleles). This class of mutations includes nonsense mutations at codons 121, 133, 372, 672, 786, and 897.[5,8,10–13] Similarly, when there is a deletion (or insertion) of a sequence that is not an integral multiple of 3 base pairs, this leads to a shift in the reading frame, which introduces a premature chain termination codon downstream from the site of the actual mutation.[14–19] In addition to truncating the receptor protein, most (but not all) premature chain termination codons also exert a *cis*-acting effect to decrease the level of insulin receptor mRNA.[1–3,5]

Class 1C. Mutations Encoding Receptors That Are Truncated in the Intracellular Domain

At least two mutant alleles have been reported to have premature termination codons in the region of the gene encoding the cytoplasmic domain of the receptor (see Fig. 64-2). One allele contained a nonsense mutation replacing the codon for Arg^{1000} with a chain termination codon.[11,20] This mutation exerted a *cis*-acting effect to decrease the level of insulin receptor mRNA. In another mutant allele, an *ALU-ALU* recombination was identified that resulted in deletion of exons 18–22 in addition to the 3′-half of exon 17.[21] This deletion mutation appeared not to alter the level of insulin receptor mRNA. However, both mutant alleles are predicted to encode truncated receptors containing a normal extracellular domain but only a short fragment of the intracellular domain lacking most of the tyrosine kinase domain. These truncated receptors have the potential to be expressed on the cell surface. Indeed, transfection of cDNA encoding truncated receptors lacking most or all of the intracellular domain leads to expression of insulin binding sites on the cell surface. Nevertheless, it appears likely that these truncated receptors would be impaired in their ability to mediate most (if not all) of the biologic actions of insulin.[22]

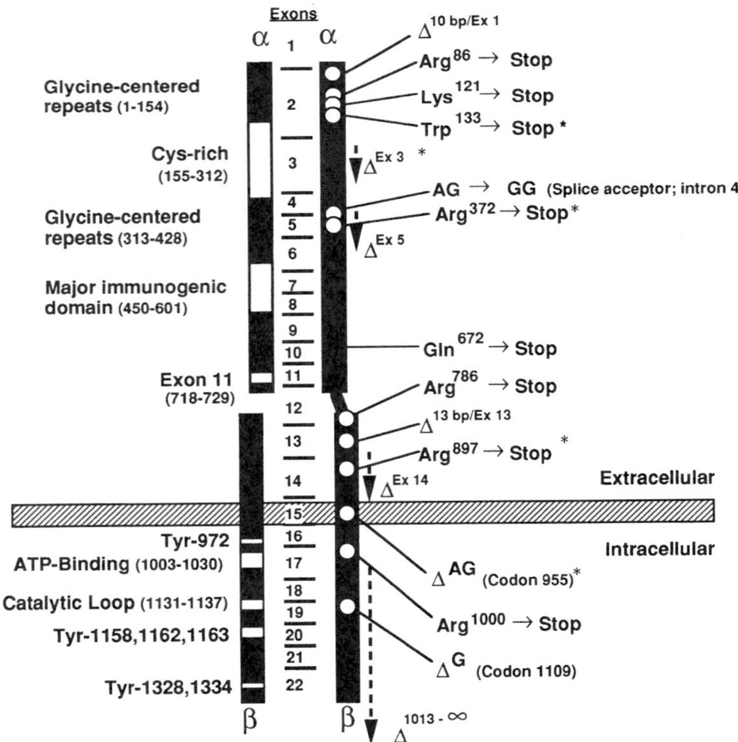

FIGURE 64-2. Class 1—premature chain termination mutations in the insulin receptor gene in insulin-resistant patients. Key structural landmarks of the insulin receptor are identified at the left, and the exons are indicated in the middle. The locations of all of the reported premature chain termination mutations are indicated in the right half of the receptor.[1-3] These include nonsense mutations, deletions (indicated by the Greek letter Δ), and a mutation at a splice acceptor site at the junction of intron 4 and exon 5.

Class 2. Mutations That Impair Intracellular Transport to the Plasma Membrane

Mutations in this class decrease the number of receptors in the plasma membrane by impairing the transport of receptors through the endoplasmic reticulum and Golgi apparatus to the plasma membrane (Fig. 64-3). Apparently, these mutations, most of which have been identified in the extracellular domain, interfere with the folding of the receptor into its normal conformation.

The insulin receptor is synthesized by post-translational processing of a precursor molecule with M_r = 190,000.[1,2,23,24] This post-translational processing takes place in the endoplasmic reticulum and Golgi apparatus.[1,2] The major steps in biosynthesis are summarized below. The proreceptor undergoes cotranslational *N*-linked glycosylation. Then the proreceptor folds into a conformation that is competent to bind insulin—a step that is catalyzed by BiP, a chaperonin located in the endoplasmic reticulum. Intrasubunit disulfide bonds are formed in a process catalyzed by protein disulfide isomerase. The proreceptor assembles into a dimer at some point in the biosynthetic process, possibly while the proreceptor still resides in the endoplasmic reticulum. Subsequent to dimerization, the proreceptor undergoes proteolytic cleavage into α- and β-subunits. Thereafter, the high mannose form of *N*-linked oligosaccharide is processed into the complex form of *N*-linked oligosaccharide, an event that leads to a decrease in the electrophoretic mobility in sodium dodecyl sulfate-polyacrylamide gels. Finally, the receptor undergoes two additional post-translational processing steps (*O*-linked glycosylation and acylation); the precise timing of these two steps has not been elucidated.

The Phe^{382} → Val mutation is among the best characterized of the mutations that impair transport of receptors to the cell surface.[25–27] When cells are labeled by incubation in the presence of [^{35}S]methionine, the *VAL**382 mutant proreceptor can be coimmunoprecipitated by monoclonal antibody to BiP.[27] In contrast, the normal insulin receptor is not coimmunoprecipitated by anti-BiP antibody under the same circumstances. Although it seems likely that the normal receptor binds transiently to BiP, only the mutant receptor forms a stable complex with BiP. The failure of BiP to release the *VAL**382 mutant proreceptor leads to retention of the mutant proreceptor molecules within the endoplasmic reticulum. A minority of the receptors (approximately 10–20%) appear to undergo normal post-translational processing and are eventually transported to the plasma membrane.[25,27] However, the biosynthetic block inhibits the majority of the receptors from undergoing the steps of normal post-translational processing: dimerization, proteolytic cleavage into subunits, and terminal processing of the *N*-linked oligosaccharide. In the case of the *VAL**382 mutant receptor, the mutation leads to a defect that impairs the ability of the receptor tyrosine kinase to be activated by insulin.[26,28] However, the defect in tyrosine kinase activity is not typical of all mutations that impair the ability of the receptor to be transported to the plasma membrane. For example, the *LYS**15 mutation decreases the affinity of insulin binding.[11,29] However, the *ARG**209 mutant receptor binds insulin normally and retains the ability of the tyrosine kinase to be activated by insulin binding.[11,30]

There are several other examples of mutations in class 2 (see Fig. 64-3): Val^{28} → Ala; Gly^{31} → Arg; Arg^{86} → Pro; Pro^{193} → Leu; Leu^{233} → Pro; Gly^{366} → Arg; Trp^{412} → Ser; and Ala^{1135} → Glu.[4,31–39] In addition to point mutations, there are two reported mutations[12,40] leading to the deletion of a single amino acid residue from the N-terminal half of the extracellular domain of the receptor: Lys^{121} or Asn^{281}. Although the effects of these mutations have not been established by transfection studies, their location suggests that they may impair post-translational processing and transport of the receptor to the cell surface (see Fig. 64-3).

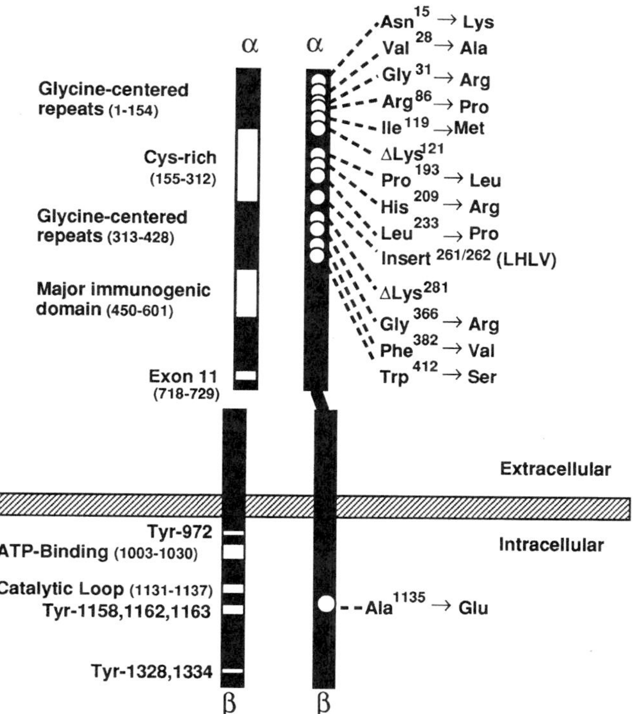

FIGURE 64-3. Class 2—mutations that impair post-translational processing and intracellular transport of the receptor to the plasma membrane. Key structural landmarks of the insulin receptor are identified at the left. The locations of all of the reported class 2 mutations are indicated in the right half of the receptor.[1–3]

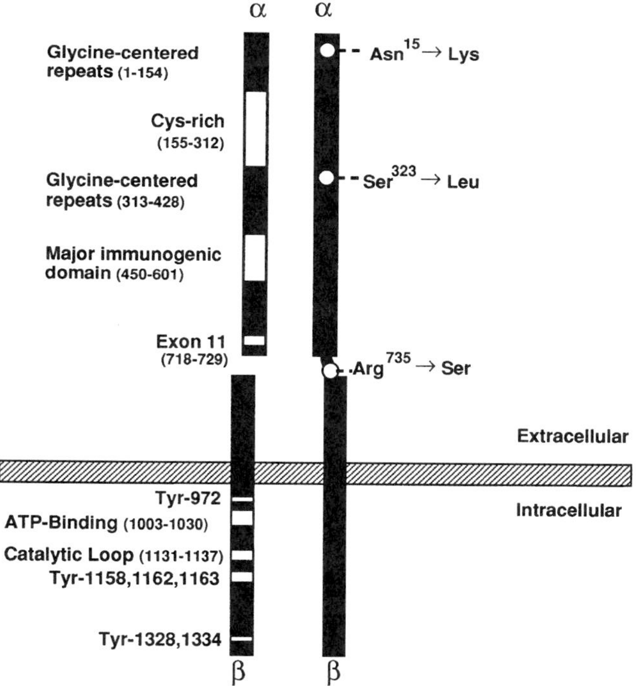

FIGURE 64-4. Class 3—mutations that decrease the affinity of insulin binding. Key structural landmarks of the insulin receptor are identified at the left. The locations of all of the reported class 3 mutations are indicated in the right half of the receptor.[1–3]

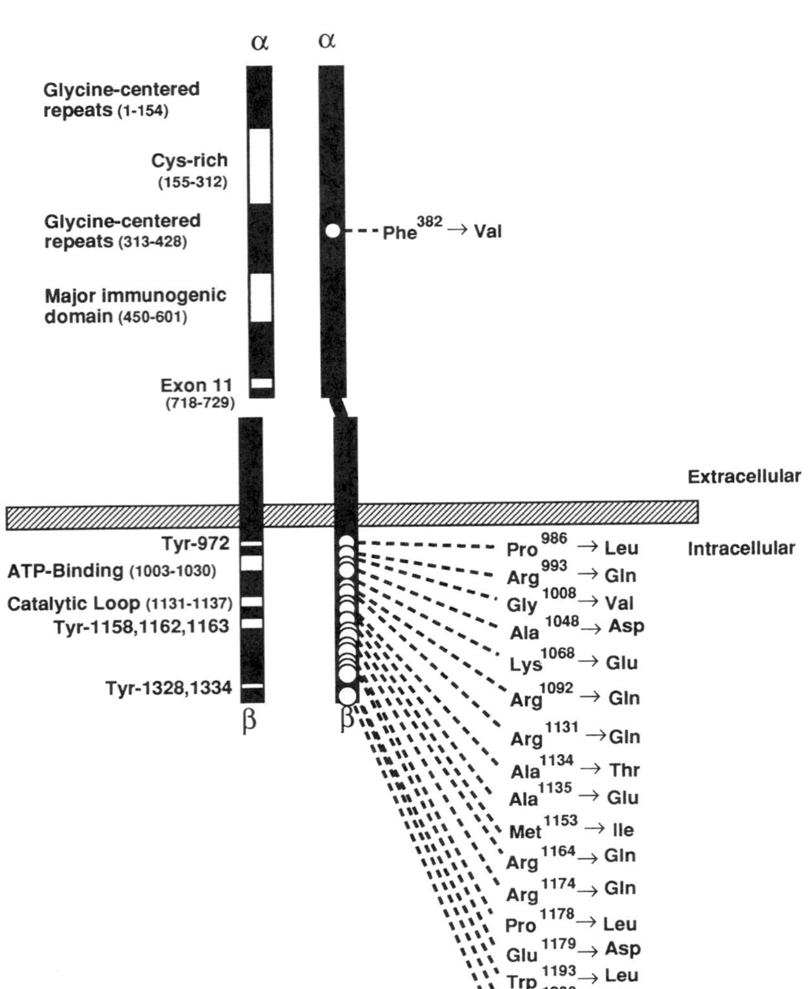

Figure 64-5. Class 4—mutations that inhibit receptor tyrosine kinase activity. Key structural landmarks of the insulin receptor are identified at the left. The locations of all of the reported class 4 mutations are indicated in the right half of the receptor.[1–3]

At least two mutations impair post-translational processing of the receptor, even though the mutations map outside of the α-subunit. For example, substitution of Ser for Arg^{735}, the last amino acid in the Arg-Lys-Arg-Arg sequence in the proteolytic cleavage site between the α- and β-subunits,[41–44] inhibits proteolytic processing of the proreceptor into separate subunits. However, the *SER**735 mutation does not inhibit the transport of the receptor to the cell surface.[41–44] The *GLU**1135 mutation inhibits both proteolytic cleavage of the proreceptor and transport of the receptor to the plasma membrane, although this mutation is located in the tyrosine kinase domain rather than the extracellular domain. These two mutant alleles are discussed further under the sections on class 3 (*SER**735 allele) and class 4 (*GLU**1135 allele) mutations.

Class 3. Mutations That Decrease the Affinity of Insulin Binding

Several mutations have been described that decrease the affinity of the receptor to bind insulin (Fig. 64-4). As described above, the *SER**735 mutation in the proteolytic cleavage site inhibits proteolytic processing of the mutant proreceptor into α- and β-subunits.[41–44] Although the uncleaved *SER**735 mutant proreceptor is expressed on the cell surface, the *SER**735 mutation has the potential to decrease the affinity of insulin binding. Interestingly, the effects of the *SER**735 mutation depend upon the context of the nearby amino acid sequence.[45,46] Exon 11 of the insulin receptor gene is a variably spliced sequence that encodes the C-terminal 12 amino acid residues of the α-subunit. In the uncleaved proreceptor isoform lacking these 12 amino acids (Ex 11$^-$), the *SER**735 mutation leads to a marked (≈50-fold) decrease in the affinity of insulin binding. In contrast, the *SER**735 mutation has a much smaller effect (≈3-fold) to decrease the affinity with which insulin binds to the proreceptor isoform containing the 12 amino acids encoded by exon 11 (Ex 11$^+$).

The *LYS**15 mutation leads to a fivefold decrease in the affinity of insulin binding,[29] an observation that is consistent with the conclusion that the amino acid sequence encoded by exon 2 of the insulin receptor gene constitutes a domain that contributes to high-affinity binding of insulin.[47–49] Furthermore, the *LYS**15 mutation resembles other missense mutations in the *N*-terminal half of the insulin receptor in that it impairs post-translational processing and transport of receptors to the plasma membrane (class 2 mutation). Thus, the *LYS**15 mutation inhibits insulin binding by two mechanisms: (1) by decreasing the number of receptors on the cell surface, and (2) by decreasing the affinity of insulin binding.

Recently, two other mutations (Arg^{86} → Pro and Ser^{323} → Leu) have been reported to decrease the affinity of insulin binding.[33,50,51] Indeed, when the mutant receptors were expressed by transfection of mutant cDNA in cultured cells, there was no detectable binding of ^{125}I insulin binding to the *PRO**86 and *LEU**323 mutant receptors.[33,50]

Class 4. Mutations That Inhibit Receptor Tyrosine Kinase Activity

Binding of insulin to the insulin receptor leads to phosphorylation of at least six tyrosine residues in the intracellular domain.[1,52] Phosphorylation of Tyr^{1158}, Tyr^{1162}, and Tyr^{1163} results in activation of the receptor tyrosine kinase. The activated receptor tyrosine kinase phosphorylates tyrosine residues in various protein substrates within the cell.[53,54] Several lines of evidence demonstrate that activation of the receptor tyrosine kinase plays a necessary role in the mechanism whereby the receptor mediates insulin action. Among the most convincing pieces of evidence is the observation that mutations that abolish the tyrosine kinase of the insulin receptor cause insulin resistance in vivo.[1-3,55]

Several of the mutations that inhibit receptor tyrosine kinase map to amino acid sequence motifs that are crucial for the catalytic activity of the receptor. One such mutation ($Gly^{1008} \rightarrow$ Val) was identified in the ATP binding site—specifically, at the position of the third conserved glycine residue in the Gly-Xaa-Gly-Xaa-Xaa-Gly motif.[55] Several mutations were identified in the "catalytic loop" (Arg-Asp-Leu-Xaa_1-Xaa_2-Xaa_3-Asn; amino acid residues 1131–1137) located approximately 100 amino acid residues downstream from the ATP binding site. Based upon x-ray crystallographic studies of cAMP-dependent protein kinase, this highly conserved sequence motif has been demonstrated to contain amino acid residues that catalyze the phosphotransferase reaction and determine the substrate specificity for the phosphorylation site. One mutation ($Arg^{1131} \rightarrow$ Gln)[56] was identified at the first arginine residue that appears to be universally conserved in all protein kinases.[57] Two additional mutations have been identified in the Xaa_1-Xaa_2-Xaa_3 sequence in the catalytic loop: $Ala^{1134} \rightarrow$ Thr[58,59] and $Ala^{1135} \rightarrow$ Glu.[39] In most receptor tyrosine kinases, this tripeptide sequence (Xaa_1-Xaa_2-Xaa_3) is Arg-Ala-Ala, completely different from the Lys-Pro-Glu sequence in the cAMP-dependent protein kinase. All three mutations in the catalytic loop inhibit receptor tyrosine kinase activity. Furthermore, the *GLU**1135 mutation is also associated with a defect in post-translational processing and intracellular transport of receptors to the plasma membrane.[39] Consequently, unlike most mutations in the tyrosine kinase domain, the *GLU**1135 mutation leads to a decrease in the number of insulin receptors on the surface of the patient's cells in vivo.[60]

Numerous mutations have been identified at other positions within the tyrosine kinase domain (Fig. 64-5): $Ala^{1048} \rightarrow$ Asp, $Lys^{1068} \rightarrow$ Glu, $Arg^{1092} \rightarrow$ Gln, $Met^{1153} \rightarrow$ Ile, $Arg^{1164} \rightarrow$ Gln, $Arg^{1174} \rightarrow$ Gln, $Pro^{1178} \rightarrow$ Leu, $Glu^{1179} \rightarrow$ Asp, $Trp^{1193} \rightarrow$ Leu, and $Trp^{1200} \rightarrow$ Ser.[51,59,61-72] As shown in an x-ray crystallographic study, these mutations are scattered widely throughout the three-dimensional structure of the isolated recombinant insulin receptor tyrosine kinase domain.[73] Although the precise role of many of these amino acid residues in enzyme function is not known, most of the normal amino acid residues are conserved in all three members of the insulin receptor family (i.e., the insulin receptor, the type 1 insulin-like growth factor receptor, and the insulin receptor–related receptor). In fact, some of these amino acid residues are conserved in other receptor tyrosine kinases as well. This suggests that they serve an important role in the function of tyrosine kinase.

In addition, three mutations have been identified in the cytoplasmic domain of the receptor in regions that lie outside the tyrosine kinase domain. Two mutations are located in the juxtamembrane domain ($Pro^{986} \rightarrow$ Leu and $Arg^{993} \rightarrow$ Gln),[74,75] and one mutation is located in the C-terminal domain ($Arg^{1351} \rightarrow$ Gln).[51]

Because all of the patients with mutations in the tyrosine kinase domain of the insulin receptor were resistant to the action of insulin in lowering the level of glucose in plasma, this fact supports the hypothesis that the receptor tyrosine kinase is required for the metabolic actions of insulin in vivo. Furthermore, when the mutant receptors were expressed by transfection of cDNA in tissue culture cells, these mutations in the tyrosine kinase domain inhibited the ability of the receptor to mediate the mitogenic action of insulin in vitro. Moreover, mutations in the tyrosine kinase domain inhibit endocytosis of the mutant receptors,[1,22,76,77] a phenomenon that provides the major mechanism responsible for clearance of insulin from the plasma. Thus, mutations in the tyrosine kinase domain are associated with an increase in the level of insulin in plasma,[78] caused, at least in part, by the defect in the clearance of insulin. In addition, kinase-deficient mutant receptors are resistant to insulin-induced downregulation because insulin-stimulated endocytosis is the mechanism of homologous downregulation. This explains an early observation that, despite the presence of elevated levels of insulin in patients' plasma, they tend to have normal numbers of insulin receptors on the surface of their target cells.[60] Nevertheless, at least in the case of the *GLU**1135 mutation in the tyrosine kinase domain, the number of receptors was decreased on the surface of the patient's cells in vivo.[60] However, the diminished number of mutant receptors on the cell surface was not caused by downregulation but rather by an impairment in post-translational processing and intracellular transport to the cell surface.[39]

Mutations in the tyrosine kinase domain appear to cause insulin resistance in a dominant fashion, unlike many mutations in other domains of the insulin receptor. Much evidence suggests that the dominant negative effect results from the heterotetrameric ($\alpha_2\beta_2$) structure of the receptor.[1,79,80] It has been hypothesized that three forms of the oligomeric receptor exist in the cells of a patient who is heterozygous for the mutation: $\alpha_2\beta_2$, $\alpha_2\beta\beta_{mut}$, and $\alpha_2(\beta_{mut})_2$ (Fig. 64-6). The biochemistry of hybrid receptors has been studied extensively in the case of the *ALA**1030 mutant receptor, a site-directed mutant with an inactive tyrosine kinase.[79,80] The hybrid mutant receptor has abnormal tyrosine kinase activity. Although the normal half receptor can transphosphorylate the mutant half receptor in the presence of insulin, this transphosphorylation does not activate the mutant tyrosine kinase domain. Because the mutant tyrosine kinase does not phosphorylate the normal tyrosine kinase domain, insulin binding does not stimulate the activity of the hybrid receptor to phosphorylate other proteins. Nevertheless, because it was not possible to detect the formation of hybrid receptors in

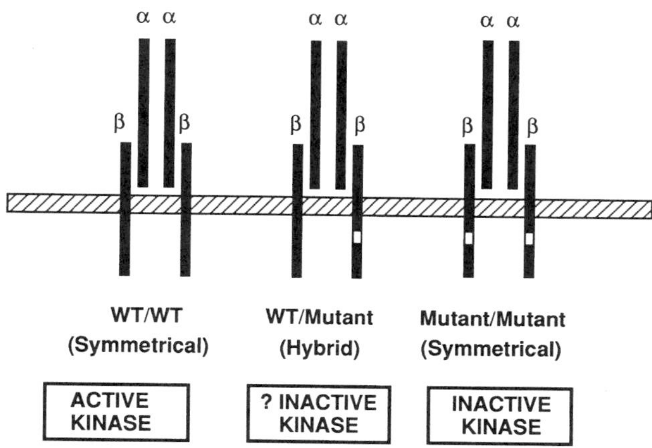

Figure 64-6. Hybrid forms of receptors in heterozygous patients. In a patient who is heterozygous for a mutation in one allele of the insulin receptor gene, at least three forms of heterotetramers can be formed: symmetric wild-type molecules [$\alpha_2\beta_2$]; symmetric mutant receptors [$\alpha_2(\beta_{mut})_2$]; and hybrid receptors [$\alpha_2\beta\beta_{mut}$]. If the mutation inactivates the receptor tyrosine kinase, then the symmetric $\alpha_2(\beta_{mut})_2$ molecule would have an inactive receptor tyrosine kinase. Moreover, available data suggest that the hybrid $\alpha_2\beta\beta_{mut}$ molecule is inactive as a tyrosine kinase.[79,80] If the mutation does not affect the efficiency of oligomerization, the various forms of the receptor would exist in a ratio of 1:2:1 [$\alpha_2\beta_2 : \alpha_2\beta\beta_{mut} : \alpha_2(\beta_{mut})_2$]. Accordingly, it would be predicted that heterozygosity for a single mutant allele would result in a 75% decrease in receptor tyrosine kinase activity.[1-3,79,80]

studies of *ILE**1153 mutant receptors,[81] it is possible that other molecular mechanisms may contribute to the dominant negative effect of mutations in the tyrosine kinase domain.

Class 5. Mutations That Accelerate Degradation of Receptors

Insulin stimulates internalization of receptors into endosomes. Because endosomes have proton pumps in their membranes, the lumina of the endosomes acquire a pH of approximately 5.5. Acid pH inside the endosome accelerates the dissociation of insulin from its receptor.[82] After internalization, both the receptor and the ligand partition between two pathways: recycling back to the plasma membrane or degradation within the lysosome. Two mutations have been reported to impair the ability of acid pH to dissociate the insulin-receptor complex (Fig. 64-7). The $Lys^{460} \rightarrow$ Glu substitution was the first mutation to be shown to cause this type of defect.[10,82,83] After [^{125}I]insulin binds to the wild-type receptor, approximately 20% of the [^{125}I]insulin dissociates from the receptor in 5 minutes at pH 8. Decreasing the pH to 5.5 leads to a three- to fourfold increase in the dissociation rate. However, [^{125}I]insulin dissociates two- to threefold more slowly from the *GLU**460 mutant receptor at all values of pH. Furthermore, in either the presence or absence of insulin (10^{-5} M), the *GLU**460 mutant receptor is degraded more rapidly than the wild-type receptors expressed in transfected cells. This accelerated rate of degradation for the recombinant *GLU**460 mutant receptor is consistent with previous observations that the half-life of cell surface receptors is shorter (1.5 versus 6 h) in Epstein-Barr virus–transformed lymphoblasts from the patient with the *GLU**460 mutation than in lymphoblasts from normal subjects.[84] Furthermore, the accelerated rate of receptor degradation probably provides a mechanism to explain the 85% decrease in the number of insulin receptors on the surface of the patient's circulating monocytes in vivo.[85]

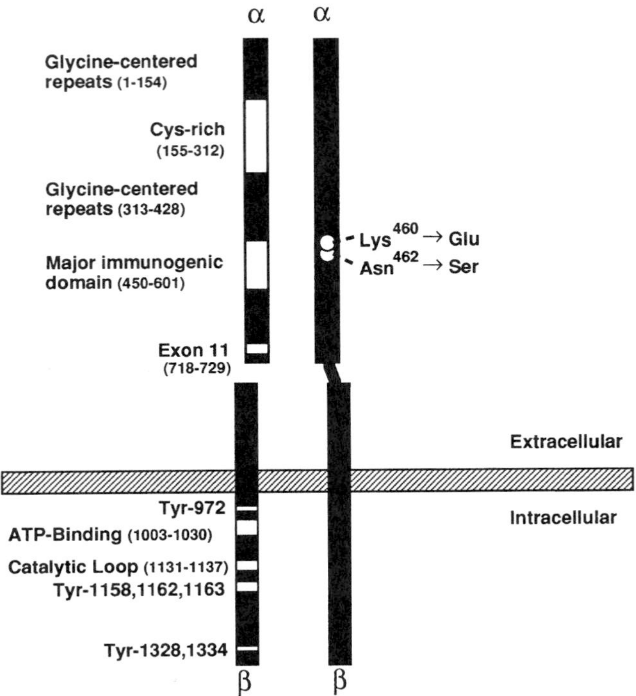

Figure 64-7. Class 5—mutations that accelerate receptor degradation. Key structural landmarks of the insulin receptor are identified at the left. The locations of all of the reported class 5 mutations are indicated in the right half of the receptor.[1-3]

A similar (although less severe) defect in the ability of pH to accelerate dissociation of insulin from the receptor has been described with another mutation (the $Asn^{462} \rightarrow$ Ser mutation) located just two amino acids away from the site of the GLU*460 mutation.[11,18] Although the rate of receptor degradation has not been measured for the recombinant *SER**462 mutant receptor expressed in transfected cells, insulin receptors on the surface of Epstein-Barr virus lymphoblasts from the patient with the *SER**462 mutation are degraded more rapidly ($t_{1/2} \approx 2.8$ h versus 6 h for cells from normal subjects).[84] In addition, there was a marked reduction in the number of insulin receptors expressed on the surface of the patient's circulating monocytes.[60]

Prevalence of Mutations in the Insulin Receptor Gene

Data available at present do not allow for a reliable estimate of the prevalence of mutations in the insulin receptor gene. Nevertheless, it is possible to estimate a minimum prevalence based upon the incidence of leprechaunism.[1,2] If it is assumed that one child with leprechaunism is born in the United States each year, this implies an incidence of ≈ 1:4,000,000/year. Furthermore, if the existence of a Hardy-Weinberg equilibrium is assumed, the prevalence of mutant alleles in the gene pool is ≈ 1:2000. As we have discussed in detail elsewhere,[1,2] the real prevalence of mutant alleles is likely to be greater than this estimate of 1:2000. For example, many mutations in the insulin receptor gene cause less severe clinical syndromes (e.g., type A insulin resistance or Rabson-Mendenhall syndrome). These less severe mutations have not been included in the estimate based on the incidence of the syndrome of leprechaunism. Furthermore, it is unlikely that a true Hardy-Weinberg equilibrium exists. For example, inasmuch as heterozygosity for a mutant allele may predispose to the development of hyperandrogenism in females, this may decrease the fertility of these heterozygous carriers. This fact also suggests that 1:2000 is likely to be an underestimate of the prevalence of mutant alleles of the insulin receptor gene. Finally, a minimum estimate of 1:2000 for the frequency of mutant alleles in the gene pool corresponds to a prevalence of heterozygous carriers of at least 1:1000 in the general population. Because it is likely that mutations in the insulin receptor gene predispose to insulin resistance, it is also likely that the prevalence of mutant alleles of the insulin receptor gene may be considerably greater than 1:1000 among patients with noninsulin-dependent diabetes mellitus. In fact, the limited data that are available are consistent with the conclusion that ≈ 1% of patients with noninsulin-dependent diabetes mellitus are heterozygous for mutant alleles of the insulin receptor gene. One study has suggested that the allele encoding the *MET**985 receptor has a tenfold higher prevalence among Dutch patients with noninsulin-dependent diabetes mellitus as compared to among normal controls (prevalence of 5% versus 0.5%) (J.A. Maassen, personal communication). Although these epidemiologic data suggest that the $Val^{985} \rightarrow$ Met substitution may impair receptor function, direct studies of the recombinant *MET**985 receptor have not demonstrated any functional abnormalities.[59,62]

Correlation of Genotype with Phenotype

Most of the mutations have been identified in patients with relatively uncommon clinical syndromes associated with extreme insulin resistance. Patients with leprechaunism, the syndrome associated with the most severe degree of insulin resistance, generally have two mutant alleles of the insulin receptor gene. For example, one patient with leprechaunism has been reported to be homozygous for a deletion of the entire insulin receptor gene.[4] In contrast, patients who are heterozygous for a single mutant allele are less severely affected. Some mutant alleles (especially mutations in the tyrosine kinase domain) cause disease by either dominant or co-dominant mechanisms. For example, heterozygous patients have been reported to have either type A insulin resistance (i.e., insulin resistance in association with acanthosis nigricans and hyperandrogenism) or noninsulin-dependent diabetes mellitus.[1–3] Furthermore, some mutant alleles are recessive with respect to clinical phenotype so that heterozygotes do not have clinically apparent disease.[1–3,10,25,86]

Despite the fact that the genotype at the insulin receptor locus appears to be a major determinant of the phenotype, this does not provide a complete explanation of the patient's clinical status. It is likely that environmental and behavioral factors (e.g., diet and exercise) may affect the clinical phenotype. Furthermore, it is likely that other genes (in addition to the major disease locus) also impact upon the patient's clinical syndrome.[1,2,87]

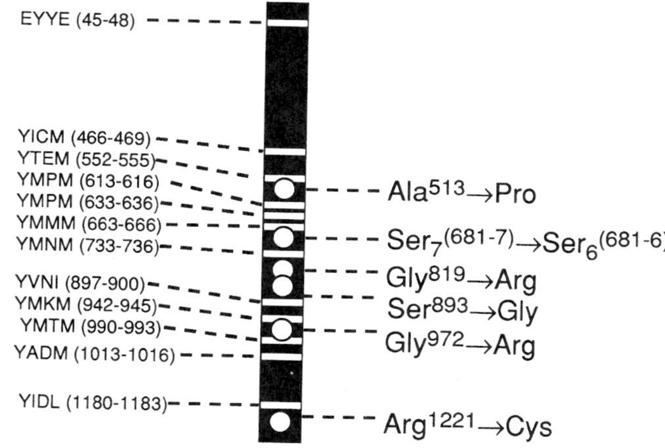

Figure 64-8. Variant sequences of IRS-1. In this cartoon of IRS-1, tyrosine phosphorylation sites are indicated on the left; observed amino acid substitutions in IRS-1 are indicated on the right.

Mutations in the Gene Encoding Insulin Receptor Substrate-1

Recent studies have provided considerable insight into postreceptor mechanisms in the biochemical pathway of insulin action.[53,54] Insulin binding to its receptor activates the receptor tyrosine kinase, which phosphorylates multiple tyrosine residues on several intracellular proteins, including insulin receptor substrate-1 (*IRS-1*) (see Chapter 16). Several proteins containing SH2 domains bind to phosphotyrosine residues on IRS-1:[53,54] for example, growth factor receptor binding protein-2 (GRB-2), the p85 regulatory subunit of phosphatidyl inositol 3-kinase, and the Syp phosphotyrosine protein phosphatase. This leads to activation of several enzymes that may be responsible for mediating insulin action within the target cell. Thus, binding of p85 leads to activation of the p110 catalytic subunit of phosphatidyl inositol 3-kinase. Binding of GRB-2 leads to activation of mSOS (mammalian son-of-sevenless homolog), a guanine nucleotide exchange factor for Ras. This, in turn, leads to activation of Ras with consequent activation of the mitogen-activated protein (MAP) kinase cascade. Two additional lines of evidence support the hypothesis that IRS-1 plays a role in mediating the metabolic actions of insulin in target cells. First, mice that are homozygous for null alleles of the *IRS-1* gene exhibit some degree of insulin resistance.[88,89] However, despite the fact that these mice are insulin-resistant, they are not entirely unresponsive to insulin. Accordingly, it has been concluded that insulin action is not entirely dependent upon phosphorylation of IRS-1.[88,89] Second, if IRS-1 is ablated in normal cells, this leads to an impairment in insulin action. For example, when an antisense ribozyme directed against IRS-1 mRNA was expressed in primary cultures of rat adipocytes, it led to a rightward shift in the dose-response curve for the effect of insulin to stimulate translocation of GLUT-4 glucose transporters to the plasma membrane.[90]

Because of the important role of IRS-1 in current models of insulin action, several laboratories investigated the possibility that mutations in the *IRS-1* gene might cause insulin resistance. When patients with noninsulin-dependent diabetes mellitus were screened for the presence of mutations in the *IRS-1* gene, at least five nonconservative substitutions at conserved amino residues were identified in the *IRS-1* gene (Fig. 64-8): $Ala^{513} \rightarrow$ Pro, $Gly^{819} \rightarrow$ Arg, $Ser^{893} \rightarrow$ Gly, $Gly^{972} \rightarrow$ Arg, and $Arg^{1221} \rightarrow$ Cys.[91–93] With the exception of the *GLY**893 mutation, all of these amino acid variants have been reported to have increased prevalence in patients with noninsulin-dependent diabetes mellitus.[91,92] However, some investigations did not confirm the observation of increased prevalence of variant sequences of IRS-1 among patients with noninsulin-dependent diabetes mellitus. For example, several laboratories have reported that the *ARG**972 substitution has the same prevalence in the normal population as among patients with noninsulin-dependent diabetes mellitus.[93–95] Thus, this issue remains controversial.

Furthermore, biochemical studies of the mutant IRS-1 molecules have not yet been reported. Thus, it is not known with certainty whether these amino acid variants are polymorphisms that impair the function of IRS-1. Nevertheless, these provocative observations provide an attractive hypothesis to explain the genetic basis of insulin resistance in some patients with noninsulin-dependent diabetes mellitus.[91,92]

Summary

Insulin resistance contributes significantly to the pathogenesis of noninsulin-dependent diabetes mellitus. Furthermore, genetic factors contribute to the development of insulin resistance. However, the disease genes have not been identified in the majority of patients with noninsulin-dependent diabetes mellitus. This problem has been investigated by screening for mutations in genes encoding proteins that function in the pathway of insulin action. The insulin receptor, which mediates the first step in insulin action, is a logical candidate to be a locus for mutations causing genetic forms of insulin-resistant diabetes. Indeed, >50 mutant alleles of the insulin receptor gene have been identified—mostly in patients with rare syndromes (e.g., leprechaunism, Rabson-Mendenhall syndrome, type A insulin resistance). However, some mutations have been identified in patients with the common form of noninsulin-dependent diabetes mellitus. Mutations in the insulin receptor gene can be grouped into several classes: (1) mutations that decrease the number of insulin receptors expressed on the cell surface, and (2) mutations that impair receptor function by decreasing the affinity of insulin binding or by inhibiting receptor tyrosine kinase activity. Because receptor tyrosine kinase is necessary to mediate insulin action, it is logical to screen for mutations in genes encoding proteins that are phosphorylated by the insulin receptor. At least five variant amino-acid sequences have been identified in the *IRS-1* gene. Although the findings are controversial, the prevalence of variant sequences has been reported to be increased among patients with noninsulin-dependent diabetes mellitus. Studies are under way to determine whether these variant sequences impair the function of *IRS-1*.

References

1. Taylor SI, Cama A, Accili D, et al. Mutations in the insulin receptor gene. Endocr Rev 1992;13:566
2. Taylor SI. Lilly Lecture: Molecular mechanisms of insulin resistance. Lessons

from patients with mutations in the insulin-receptor gene. Diabetes 1992; 41:1473
3. Taylor SI, Wertheimer E, Accili D, et al. Mutations in the insulin receptor gene: Update 1994. In: Underwood LE, eds. Endocrine Reviews Monographs. 2. The Endocrine Pancreas. Bethesda, Md: The Endocrine Society; 1994:58–65
4. Wertheimer E, Lu SP, Backeljauw PF, et al. Homozygous deletion of the human insulin receptor gene. Nature Genetics 1993;5:71
5. Kadowaki T, Kadowaki H, Taylor SI. A nonsense mutation causing decreased levels of insulin receptor mRNA: Detection by a simplified technique for direct sequencing of genomic DNA amplified by the polymerase chain reaction. Proc Natl Acad Sci USA 1990;87:658
6. Taylor S, Samuels B, Roth J, et al. Decreased insulin binding in cultured lymphocytes from two patients with extreme insulin resistance. J Clin Endocrinol Metab 1982;54:919
7. Imano E, Kadowaki H, Kadowaki T, et al. Two patients with insulin resistance due to decreased levels of insulin receptor mRNA. Diabetes 1991;40:548
8. Longo N, Langley SD, Griffin LD, Elsas LJ II. Reduced mRNA and a nonsense mutation in the insulin receptor gene produce heritable insulin resistance. Am J Hum Genet 1992;50:998
9. Suzuki Y, Hatanaka Y, Taira M, et al. Insulin resistance associated with decreased levels of insulin-receptor messenger ribonucleic acid: Evidence of a de novo mutation in the maternal allele. J Clin Endocrinol Metab 1995;80:1214
10. Kadowaki T, Bevins CL, Cama A, et al. Two mutant alleles of the insulin receptor gene in a patient with extreme insulin resistance. Science 1988; 240:787
11. Kadowaki T, Kadowaki H, Rechler MM, et al. Five mutant alleles of the insulin receptor gene in patients with genetic forms of insulin resistance. J Clin Invest 1990;86:254
12. Jospe N, Zhu R, Livingston JN, Furlanetto RW. Heterozygous deletion of 3 base-pairs resulting in the deletion of lysine-121 in the insulin receptor α-subunit from a patient with leprechaunism. Diabetes 1993;42(suppl 1):63A (abstract 202)
13. Jospe N, Kaplowitz PB. Homozygous mutation in the insulin receptor β-subunit of a patient with leprechaunism altering arginine 786 to a stop codon. Program & Abstracts of the 75th Annual Meeting of The Endocrine Society. Las Vegas;1993:453 (abstract 1609)
14. Shimada F, Taira M, Suzuki Y, et al. Insulin-resistant diabetes associated with partial deletion of insulin-receptor gene. Lancet 1990;335:1179
15. Wertheimer E, Litvin Y, Ebstein RP, et al. Deletion of exon 3 of the insulin receptor gene in a kindred with a familial form of insulin resistance. J Clin Endocrinol Metab 1994;78:1153
16. Matsuura N, Tonoki H, Okuno A, Fujieda K. A case of leprechaunism: Its insulin-receptor gene analysis. Diabetes 1991;40(suppl 1):113A (abstract 450)
17. Kadowaki H, Kadowaki T, Takahashi Y, et al. Three mutant alleles of the insulin receptor gene: Identification of a common mutation in two phenotypically distinct syndromes with insulin resistance. Diabetes 1992;41(suppl 1): 185A (abstract 646)
18. Cama A, Sierra ML, Kadowaki T, et al. Two mutant alleles of the insulin receptor gene in a family with a genetic form of insulin resistance: A 10 base pair deletion in exon 1 and a mutation substituting serine for asparagine-462. Hum Genet 1995;95:174
19. Hone J, Accili D, Sinclair L, Taylor SI. Homozygosity for a null allele of the insulin receptor gene in a patient with leprechaunism. Clin Res 1993;41:599A
20. Kusari J, Verma US, Buse JB, et al. Analysis of the gene sequences of the insulin receptor and the insulin-sensitive glucose transporter (GLUT-4) in patients with common-type non-insulin-dependent diabetes mellitus. J Clin Invest 1991;88:1323
21. Taira M, Taira M, Hashimoto N, et al. Human diabetes associated with a deletion of the tyrosine kinase domain of the insulin receptor. Science 1989;245:63
22. Haft CR, Taylor SI. Deletion of 343 amino acids from the carboxyl-terminus of the β-subunit of the insulin receptor inhibits insulin signalling. Biochemistry 1994;33:9143
23. Ullrich A, Bell JR, Chen EY, et al. Human insulin receptor and its relationship to the tyrosine kinase family of oncogenes. Nature 1985;313:756
24. Ebina Y, Ellis L, Jarnagin K, et al. The human insulin receptor cDNA: The structural basis for hormone-activated transmembrane signalling. Cell 1985; 40:747
25. Accili D, Frapier C, Mosthaf L, et al. A mutation in the insulin receptor gene that impairs transport of the receptor to the plasma membrane and causes insulin-resistant diabetes. EMBO J 1989;8:2509
26. Accili D, Mosthaf L, Ullrich A, Taylor SI. A mutation in the extracellular domain of the insulin receptor impairs the ability of insulin to stimulate receptor autophosphorylation. J Biol Chem 1991;266:434
27. Accili D, Kadowaki T, Kadowaki H, et al. Immunoglobulin heavy chain-binding protein binds to misfolded mutant insulin receptors with mutations in the extracellular domain. J Biol Chem 1992;267:586
28. Lebrun C, Baron V, Kaliman P, et al. Antibodies to the extracellular receptor domain restore the hormone-insensitive kinase and conformation of the mutant receptor valine 382. J Biol Chem 1993;268:11272
29. Kadowaki T, Kadowaki H, Accili D, Taylor SI. Substitution of lysine for asparagine at position 15 in the alpha-subunit of the human insulin receptor. A mutation that impairs a transport of receptors to the cell surface and decreases the affinity of insulin binding. J Biol Chem 1990;265:19143
30. Kadowaki T, Kadowaki H, Accili D, et al. Substitution of arginine for histidine at position 209 in the alpha-subunit of the human insulin receptor. A mutation that impairs receptor dimerization and transport of receptors to the cell surface. J Biol Chem 1991;266:21224
31. Barbetti F, Gejman PV, Taylor SI, et al. Detection of mutations in insulin receptor gene by denaturing gradient gel electrophoresis. Diabetes 1992;41:408
32. van der Vorm ER, van der Zon GCM, Möller W, et al. An Arg for Gly substitution at position 31 in the insulin receptor, linked to insulin resistance, inhibits receptor processing and transport. J Biol Chem 1992;267:66
33. Longo N, Langley SD, Griffin LD, Elsas LJ. Activation of glucose transport by a natural mutation in the human insulin receptor. Proc Natl Acad Sci USA 1993;90:60
34. Carrera P, Cordera R, Ferrari M, et al. Substitution of Leu for Pro-193 in the insulin receptor in a patient with a genetic form of severe insulin resistance. Hum Mol Genet 1993;2:1437
35. Takata Y, Egawa K, Iwanishi M, et al. Insulin resistance due to the impaired processing of the mutant insulin receptor [Leu^{193}]. Diabetes 1993;42(suppl 1):217A (abstract 693)
36. Klinkhamer M, Groen NA, van der Zon GCM, et al. A leucine-to-proline mutation in the insulin receptor in a family with insulin resistance. EMBO J 1989;8:2503
37. Maassen JA, Van der Vorm ER, Van der Zon GCM, et al. A leucine to proline mutation at position 233 in the insulin receptor inhibits cleavage of the proreceptor and transport to the cell surface. Biochemistry 1991;30:10778
38. Van der Vorm ER, Van der Zorn GCM, Kielkopf-Renner S, et al. A mutation in the α-chain of the insulin receptor at codon 412 associated with decreased insulin binding and leprechaunism. Exp Clin Endocrinol 1993;101(suppl 2):357
39. Cama A, Sierra ML, Quon MJ, et al. Substitution of glutamic acid for alanine-1135 in the putative "catalytic loop" of the tyrosine kinase domain of the human insulin receptor: A mutation that impairs proteolytic processing into subunits and inhibits receptor tyrosine kinase activity. J Biol Chem 1993; 268:8060
40. Caron M, Sert Langeron C, Desbois C, et al. Insulin and IGF1 receptor defects in two sisters with leprechaunism. Exp Clin Endocrinol 1993;101(suppl 2):38
41. Yoshimasa Y, Seino S, Whittaker J, et al. Insulin-resistant diabetes due to a point mutation that prevents insulin proreceptor processing. Science 1988; 240:784
42. Kakehi T, Hisatomi A, Kuzuya H, et al. Defective processing of insulin receptor precursor in cultured lymphocytes from a patient with extreme insulin resistance. J Clin Invest 1988;81:2020
43. Kobayashi M, Sasaoka T, Takata Y, et al. Insulin resistance by unprocessed insulin proreceptors point mutation at the cleavage site. Biochem Biophys Res Commun 1988;153:657
44. Kobayashi M, Sasaoka T, Takata Y, et al. Insulin resistance by uncleaved insulin proreceptor. Emergence of binding site by trypsin. Diabetes 1988; 37:653
45. Yoshimasa Y, Paul JI, Whittaker J, Steiner DF. Effects of amino acid replacements within the tetrabasic cleavage site on the processing of the human insulin receptor precursor expressed in Chinese hamster ovary cells. J Biol Chem 1990;265:17230
46. Pashmforoush M, Yoshimasa Y, Steiner DF. Exon 11 enhances insulin binding affinity and tyrosine kinase activity of the human insulin proreceptor. J Biol Chem 1994;269:32639
47. Kjeldsen T, Andersen AS, Wiberg FC, et al. The ligand specificities of the insulin receptor and the insulin-like growth factor I receptor reside in different regions of a common binding site. Proc Natl Acad Sci USA 1991;88:4404
48. Andersen AS, Kjeldsen T, Wiberg FC, et al. Changing the insulin receptor to possess insulin-like growth factor I ligand specificity. Biochemistry 1990; 29:7363
49. Schumacher R, Mosthaf L, Schlessinger J, et al. Insulin and insulin-like growth factor-1 binding specificity is determined by distinct regions of their cognate receptors. J Biol Chem 1991;266:19288
50. Roach P, Zick Y, Accili D, et al. A novel human insulin receptor gene mutation uniquely inhibits insulin binding without impairing post-translational processing. Diabetes 1994;43:1096
51. Krook A, Kumar S, Laing I, et al. Molecular scanning of the insulin receptor gene in syndromes of insulin resistance. Diabetes 1994;43:357
52. Feener EP, Backer JM, King GL, et al. Insulin stimulates serine and tyrosine phosphorylation in the juxtamembrane region of the insulin receptor. J Biol Chem 1993;268:11256
53. Myers MJ, White MF. The new elements of insulin signaling. Insulin receptor substrate-1 and proteins with SH2 domains. Diabetes 1993;42:643
54. Quon MJ, Butte AJ, Taylor SI. Insulin signal transduction pathways. Trends Endocrinol Metab 1994;5:369
55. Odawara M, Kadowaki T, Yamamoto R, et al. Human diabetes associated with a mutation in the tyrosine kinase domain of the insulin receptor. Science 1989;245:66
56. Kishimoto M, Hashiramoto M, Yonezawa K, et al. Substitution of glutamine for arginine 1131. A newly identified mutation in the catalytic loop of the tyrosine kinase domain of the human insulin receptor. J Biol Chem 1994; 269:11349
57. Hanks SK, Quinn AM, Hunter T. The protein kinase family: Conserved features and deduced phylogeny of the catalytic domains. Science 1988;241:42
58. Moller DE, Yokota A, White M, et al. A naturally occurring mutation of insulin receptor Ala^{1134} impairs tyrosine kinase function and is associated with dominantly inherited insulin resistance. J Biol Chem 1990;265:14979
59. Moller DE, Benecke H, Flier JS. Biologic activities of naturally occurring

human insulin receptor mutations. Evidence that metabolic effects of insulin can be mediated by a kinase-deficient insulin receptor mutant. J Biol Chem 1991;266:10995
60. Bar RS, Muggeo M, Kahn CR, et al. Characterization of insulin receptors in patients with the syndromes of insulin resistance and acanthosis nigricans. Diabetologia 1980;18:209
61. Haruta T, Takata Y, Iwanishi M, et al. Ala1048 → Asp mutation in the kinase domain of insulin receptor causes defective kinase activity and insulin resistance. Diabetes 1993;42:1837
62. O'Rahilly S, Choi WH, Patel P, et al. Detection of mutations in insulin-receptor gene in NIDDM patients by analysis of single-stranded conformation polymorphisms. Diabetes 1991;40:777
63. Takahashi Y, Kadowaki H, Momomura K, et al. Identification of a homozygous mutation of the insulin receptor gene decreasing tyrosine kinase activity in a patient with leprechaunism. Diabetes 1993;42(suppl 1):63A (abstract 203)
64. Cama A, Sierra ML, Ottini L, et al. A mutation in the tyrosine kinase domain of the insulin receptor associated with insulin resistance in an obese woman. J Clin Endocrinol Metab 1991;73:894
65. Cama A, Quon MJ, Sierra ML, Taylor SI. Substitution of isoleucine for methionine at position 1153 in the beta-subunit of the human insulin receptor. A mutation that impairs receptor tyrosine kinase activity, receptor endocytosis, and insulin action. J Biol Chem 1992;267:8383
66. Cocozza S, Porcellini A, Riccardi G, et al. NIDDM associated with mutation in tyrosine kinase domain of insulin receptor gene. Diabetes 1992;41:521
67. Moller DE, Cohen O, Yamaguchi Y, et al. Prevalence of mutations in the insulin receptor gene in subjects with features of the type A syndrome of insulin resistance. Diabetes 1994;43:247
68. Kim H, Kadowaki H, Sakura H, et al. Detection of mutations in the insulin receptor gene in patients with insulin resistance by analysis of single stranded conformational polymorphisms. Diabetologia 1992;35:261
69. Imamura T, Takata Y, Iwanishi M, Kobayashi M. A kinase defective insulin receptor (Asp^{1179}) causes decreased number of receptors in a patient with type A insulin resistant syndrome. Diabetes 1993;42(suppl 1):218A (abstract 698)
70. Iwanishi M, Haruta T, Takata Y, et al. A mutation (Trp1193 → Leu1193) in the tyrosine kinase domain of the insulin receptor associated with type A syndrome of insulin resistance. Diabetologia 1993;36:414
71. Moller DE, Flier JS. Detection of an alteration in the insulin-receptor gene in a patient with insulin resistance, acanthosis nigricans, and the polycystic ovary syndrome (type A insulin resistance). N Engl J Med 1988;319:1526
72. Moller DE, Yokota A, Ginsberg-Fellner F, Flier JS. Functional properties of a naturally occurring Trp^{1200} → Ser^{1200} mutation of the insulin receptor. Mol Endocrinol 1990;4:1183
73. Hubbard SR, Wei L, Ellis L, Hendrickson WA. Crystal structure of the tyrosine kinase domain of the human insulin receptor. Nature 1994;372:746
74. Kadowaki T, Kadowaki H, Ando A, et al. Two mutant alleles of the insulin receptor gene in insulin resistant patients. Program and Abstracts of 73rd Annual Meeting of The Endocrine Society. Washington DC:1991:310 (abstract 1119)
75. Kusari J, Takata Y, Hatada E, et al. Insulin resistance and diabetes due to different mutations in the tyrosine kinase domain of both insulin receptor gene alleles. J Biol Chem 1991;266:5260
76. Carpentier JL, Paccaud JP, Gorden P, et al. Insulin-induced surface redistribution regulates internalization of the insulin receptor and requires its autophosphorylation. Proc Natl Acad Sci USA 1992;89:162
77. Carpentier JL, Paccaud JP, Backer J, et al. Two steps of insulin receptor internalization depend on different domains of the beta-subunit (published erratum appears in J Cell Biol 1993;123:1047). J Cell Biol 1993;122:1243
78. Flier JS, Minaker KL, Landsberg L, et al. Impaired in vivo insulin clearance in patients with severe target-cell resistance to insulin. Diabetes 1982;31:132
79. Treadway JL, Morrison BD, Soos MA, et al. Transdominant inhibition of tyrosine kinase activity in mutant insulin/insulin-like growth factor I hybrid receptors. Proc Natl Acad Sci USA 1991;88:214
80. Frattali AL, Treadway JL, Pessin JE. Transmembrane signaling by the human insulin receptor kinase. Relationship between intramolecular beta subunit trans- and cis-autophosphorylation and substrate kinase activation. J Biol Chem 1992;267:19521
81. Levy-Toledano R, Caro LHP, Accili D, Taylor SI. Investigation of mechanism of dominant negative effect of mutations in tyrosine kinase domain of insulin receptor. Clin Res 1993;41:131A (abstract)
82. Kadowaki H, Kadowaki T, Cama A, et al. Mutagenesis of lysine 460 in the human insulin receptor. Effects upon receptor recycling and cooperative interactions among binding sites. J Biol Chem 1990;265:21285
83. Taylor SI, Roth J, Blizzard RM, Elders MJ. Qualitative abnormalities in insulin binding in a patient with extreme insulin resistance: Decreased sensitivity to alterations in temperature and pH. Proc Natl Acad Sci USA 1981;78:7157
84. McElduff A, Hedo JA, Taylor SI, et al. Insulin receptor degradation is accelerated in cultured lymphocytes from patients with genetic syndromes of extreme insulin resistance. J Clin Invest 1984;74:1366
85. Taylor SI, Marcus Samuels B, Ryan Young J, et al. Genetics of the insulin receptor defect in a patient with extreme insulin resistance. J Clin Endocrinol Metab 1986;62:1130
86. Taouis M, Levy-Toledano R, Roach P, et al. Rescue and activation of binding-deficient insulin receptor: Evidence for intermolecular transphosphorylation. J Biol Chem 1994;269:27762
87. Taylor S. Prenatal screening for mutations in the insulin receptor gene. How reliably does genotype predict phenotype? J Clin Endocrinol Metab 1995; 80:1493
88. Tamemoto H, Kadowaki T, Tobe K, et al. Insulin resistance and growth retardation in mice lacking insulin receptor substrate-1. Nature 1994;372:182
89. Araki E, Lipes MA, Patti ME, et al. Alternative pathway of insulin signalling in mice with targeted disruption of the IRS-1 gene. Nature 1994;372:186
90. Quon MJ, Butte AJ, Zarnowski MJ, et al. Insulin receptor substrate 1 mediates the stimulatory effect of insulin on GLUT4 translocation in transfected rat adipose cells. J Biol Chem 1994;269:27920
91. Almind K, Bjørbaek C, Vestergaard H, et al. Aminoacid polymorphisms of insulin receptor substrate-1 in non-insulin-dependent diabetes mellitus. Lancet 1993;342:828
92. Imai Y, Fusco A, Suzuki Y, et al. Variant sequences of insulin receptor substrate-1 in patients with noninsulin-dependent diabetes mellitus. J Clin Endocrinol Metab 1994;79:1655
93. Laakso M, Malkki M, Kekalainen P, et al. Insulin receptor substrate-1 variants in non-insulin-dependent diabetes. J Clin Invest 1994;94:1141
94. Hager J, Zouali H, Velho G, Froguel P. Insulin receptor substrate (IRS-1) gene polymorphisms in French NIDDM families [letter]. Lancet 1993;342:1430
95. Shimokawa K, Kadowaki H, Sakura H, et al. Molecular scanning of the glycogen synthase and insulin receptor substrate-1 genes in Japanese subjects with non-insulin-dependent diabetes mellitus. Biochem Biophys Res Commun 1994;202:463
96. Brown MS, Goldstein JL. A receptor-mediated pathway for cholesterol homeostasis. Science 1986;232:34

Diabetes Mellitus, edited by Derek LeRoith, Simeon I. Taylor, and Jerrold M. Olefsky. Lippincott–Raven Publishers, Philadelphia © 1996.

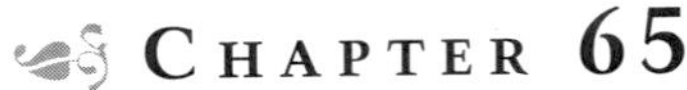

Chapter 65
Clinical Syndromes Associated with Insulin Resistance

David E. Moller

Introduction

A wide variety of common and rare clinical syndromes are associated with the presence of insulin resistance and a related increase in the prevalence of noninsulin-dependent diabetes mellitus (NIDDM) (Table 65-1). Thus, patients with diabetes mellitus who appear to require extraordinarily high doses of insulin represent only a small fraction of patients with insulin resistance. Obesity (and abdominal adiposity in particular) is strongly associated with the presence of mild to moderate degrees of insulin resistance (see Chapter 52).

Table 65-1. Clinical Syndromes Associated with Insulin Resistance

States of Mild to Moderate Insulin Resistance
Obesity
NIDDM (and to a minor degree in IDDM)
Atherosclerotic cardiovascular disease
Essential hypertension?
Polycystic ovary syndrome
Other endocrinopathies:
Cushing's syndrome
Acromegaly
Thyrotoxicosis
Catecholamine excess (pheochromocytoma)
Glucagon excess (glucagonoma)
Insulinoma
Other abnormal physiologic states:
Uremia
Cirrhosis
Sepsis
Ketoacidosis
Starvation
Other severe illness
Normal physiologic states:
Puberty
Fasting
Pregnancy
Advancing age
Rare congenital disorders:
Myotonic dystrophy
Friedreich's ataxia
States of Severe Insulin Resistance
Congenital:
Leprechaunism
Rabson-Mendenhall syndrome
Lipodystrophies
Type A syndrome and variants
Alström's syndrome
Acquired:
Type B syndrome (anti-insulin receptor antibodies)
Lipodystrophies

Importantly, patients with "typical" NIDDM, even independent of obesity, manifest similar impairment in insulin sensitivity (see Chapter 55). To a substantial extent, the insulin resistance associated with common diabetes may be secondary to hyperglycemia per se (or other aspects of the altered metabolic milieu), since improved insulin sensitivity accompanies attempts to normalize blood glucose levels.

Obviously, there is substantial insulin resistance in the context of other endocrinopathies that are also associated with NIDDM, such as states of growth hormone (e.g., acromegaly), glucocorticoid (e.g., Cushing's syndrome), or catecholamine (e.g., pheochromocytoma) excess.[1] Given that hyperinsulinemia may result in insulin receptor downregulation (and possibly postreceptor desensitization), it is worth noting that resistance to exogenous insulin can even be demonstrated in patients with insulinomas.[2] A number of serious medical conditions are known to be accompanied by the presence of insulin resistance. These include uremia and hepatic cirrhosis.[3,4] Normal aging, puberty, pregnancy, and fasting are complex physiologic states that are also reported to result in diminished insulin sensitivity. Finally, there is a large body of emerging data demonstrating that insulin resistance is often associated with essential hypertension, atherosclerotic cardiovascular disease, and dyslipidemias, although a causative role for insulin resistance in contributing to these disorders has not been firmly established.[5,6] In most of these conditions and disorders, the precise molecular mechanism(s) that bring about insulin resistance remain to be defined.

This chapter is devoted to a discussion of the clinical syndromes of severe insulin resistance. The discovery of a wide variety of insulin receptor mutations in certain patients with these syndromes has provided us with the first defined genetic locus capable of causing inherited insulin resistance (see Chapter 62). Since not all syndromes of severe insulin resistance are caused by mutant insulin receptors, patients with congenital syndromes of severe insulin resistance will continue to serve as valuable resources in the search for new signaling molecules that play a role in mediating the cellular effects of insulin. Thus, future studies in this area are likely to have implications for our understanding of more common forms of insulin resistance, such as NIDDM and obesity.

General Clinical Features of Severe Insulin Resistance

Several clinical features are commonly noted in patients with otherwise distinct syndromes of severe insulin resistance. It is convenient to view clinical sequelae of insulin resistance as potential consequences of insufficient insulin action (as with growth retardation) or as "paradoxical" effects of insulin excess (as with ovarian hyperandrogenism or accelerated growth). Since insulin-deficient states (insulin-dependent diabetes mellitus, IDDM) are not associated with these latter findings, an important component of the clinical phenotype of many patients with these syndromes may

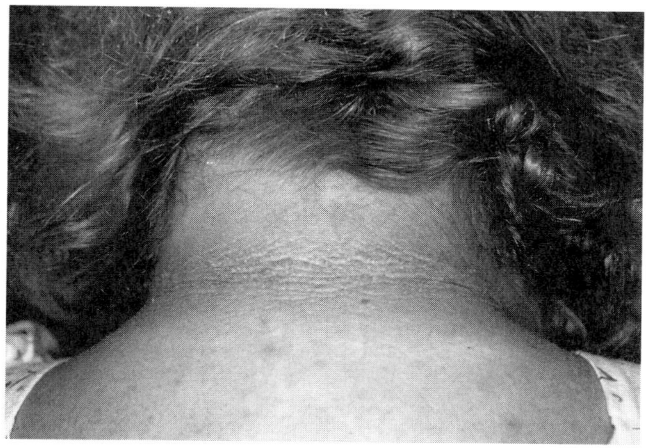

Figure 65-1. Acanthosis nigricans. The nape of the neck of a 26-year-old female with the type A syndrome is shown. Moderate to severe acanthosis nigricans is evident. (Reproduced with permission from Moller DE, ed. Insulin Resistance. New York: John Wiley & Sons;1993.)

result from the adverse consequences of hyperinsulinemia, which occurs in compensation for impairment of insulin-regulated glucose metabolism.

Acanthosis Nigricans

Acanthosis nigricans is a skin lesion that is nearly universally present in patients with syndromes of severe insulin resistance,[7,8] and has also been described in patients with modest degrees of insulin resistance such as those with obesity, Cushing's syndrome, and acromegaly.[8] Elevated plasma insulin levels and mild acanthosis nigricans were also found in 5–13% of hispanic and African-American school children, suggesting that substantial degrees of insulin resistance are very common among these ethnic groups.[9] Clinically, skin lesions appear as hyperpigmented, hyperkeratotic plaques that may also be characterized by a velvety texture (Fig. 65-1). Thickened papillomatous patches may also occur.[10] Acanthosis nigricans usually is found at certain sites, including the axillae, nape of the neck, antecubital and popliteal fossae, or other skinfold locations. Examination of skin biopsies reveals prominent hyperkeratosis and epidermal papillomatosis with a modest increase in melanocyte number and melanin deposition.[10] Staining with colloidal iron has revealed prominent infiltration of the dermis with glycosaminoglycans (mostly hyaluronic acid).[8]

The mechanism(s) that underlie the development of acanthosis nigricans remain obscure. The interaction of elevated insulin levels with other growth factor receptors such as the IGF-1 receptor is a commonly held theory.[11] However, acanthosis nigricans is usually absent in patients with acromegaly (in whom IGF-1 levels are generally high) and may improve in severely insulin-resistant patients receiving exogenous IGF-1 therapy.

Ovarian Hyperandrogenism and the Relation Between Insulin Resistance and the Polycystic Ovary Syndrome

Ovarian hyperandrogenism is a very frequent finding in postpubertal females with severe insulin resistance.[12,13] Precocious pseudopuberty along with elevated androgen levels has also been seen in many affected females and even in neonates with the syndrome of leprechaunism. The affected ovaries show stromal hyperplasia, cysts, and hyperthecosis, which are essentially indistinguishable from findings in patients with common polycystic ovary syndrome (PCOS).[12] Indeed, it is now widely appreciated that at least a certain fraction of women with "typical" PCOS have significant degrees of insulin resistance. Importantly, hyperandrogenism and hyperinsulinemia are positively correlated in women with PCOS, independent of obesity.[12,13] In addition, the skin lesion of acanthosis nigricans is fairly common among women undergoing evaluation for hyperandrogenism.[14] Dunaif and coworkers have shown that histologic evidence of cutaneous acanthosis was a nearly universal finding in obese women with typical features of PCOS.[15] In these subjects, the severity of acanthosis nigricans was correlated with the degree of impaired insulin-mediated glucose disposal.

A general consensus has emerged concerning the potential role of insulin resistance (and hyperinsulinemia) in causing or contributing to the development of PCOS. In several kindreds with insulin receptor mutations, it is clear that the extreme insulin resistance per se is sufficient to cause full-blown PCOS in affected postpubertal females (see Chapter 62). Since effective treatment of the hyperandrogenism fails to improve insulin resistance in women with PCOS, it appears that elevated androgen levels do not substantially contribute to reduced insulin sensitivity.[16] In contrast, infusion of exogenous insulin into patients with PCOS has been associated with variable increases in androgen levels.[12] Since human ovarian cells express both insulin and IGF-1 receptors and both ligands can stimulate steroidogenesis,[17] it is logical to conclude that hyperinsulinemia might promote ovarian hyperandrogenism via interactions with insulin receptors (in the absence of mutations) or with IGF-1 receptors.

The molecular basis for insulin resistance in women with common forms of PCOS remains obscure. Patients with the so-called *h*yper*a*ndrogenism *i*nsulin *r*esistance *a*canthosis *n*igricans (HAIRAN) syndrome represent a group of generally obese women with PCOS and moderate to severe insulin resistance. Mutations of the insulin receptor gene appear to be very infrequent in subjects with this clinical profile.[18] Recent data suggest that certain insulin-resistant women with PCOS may have a primary defect affecting insulin receptor-mediated cellular signaling (independent of receptor mutations) as well as a potential decrease in the expression of GLUT-4 glucose transporters.[13] Alternatively, there may be defects affecting signaling pathways that link the receptor to activation of glucose transport.[19]

Abnormal Glucose Tolerance

It is surprising to note that many patients affected by the congenital syndromes of severe insulin resistance do not display overt diabetes mellitus but rather may exhibit only mildly impaired glucose tolerance. This fact argues strongly in favor of an absolute requirement for (acquired or genetic) defects in insulin secretion in the pathogenesis of typical NIDDM. In cases where the molecular defect is known (e.g., a defined insulin receptor mutation), a unique opportunity to prospectively study the effects of a "pure" defect in insulin action may be afforded. Although some patients with inherited syndromes of severe insulin resistance have overt diabetes that is unresponsive to exogenous insulin, a more common scenario is initial presentation with normal or mildly impaired glucose tolerance followed by slow progression toward frank diabetes. Paradoxical episodes of hypoglycemia have been reported in patients with leprechaunism (see below) and occasionally in other cases of congenital severe insulin resistance. The mechanism(s) responsible for hypoglycemia in such cases is uncertain. It is plausible to consider that in some cases, extreme compensatory hypersecretion of insulin and impaired insulin clearance may result in discordant prolongation of an insulin effect in the postprandial setting.

Patients with the type B syndrome of insulin resistance, which is mediated by antibodies to the insulin receptor, often exhibit overt diabetes that is resistant to therapy with high doses of exogenous insulin. Alternatively, they may have mild or extreme hypoglycemia, depending upon the extent to which the autoantibodies exert insulinomimetic effects (see below). Individual patients may even exhibit fasting hypoglycemia and postprandial hyperglycemia simultaneously (D. Moller and J. Flier, unpublished data, 1987).

Leprechaunism and the Rabson-Mendenhall Syndrome

Leprechaunism is a very rare congenital syndrome of extreme insulin resistance characterized by marked intrauterine and postnatal growth retardation, diminished subcutaneous adipose tissue, acanthosis nigricans, failure to thrive, and early death.[20] Other skin abnormalities may include hypertrichosis, pachyderma, and prominent rugae around body orifices.[21] Physical features also typically include an unusual facial appearance (Fig. 65-2) with large ears, globular eyes, and micrognathia.[22] Penile enlargement in male infants or clitoromegaly and enlarged cystic ovaries in females have been observed.[22] Impaired glucose tolerance or overt diabetes often associated with fasting hypoglycemia is characteristic, and massive hyperinsulinemia is universal. The prognosis in cases of leprechaunism is very poor, since very few children survive beyond the first year of life.

Several older studies of cells derived from patients with leprechaunism implicated severe inherited defects involving the insulin receptor. Thus, markedly reduced insulin receptor affinity and/or number was previously observed.[22,23] Additional defects in receptor autophosphorylation or kinase activity, beyond that expected for the diminished level of insulin binding, have also been demonstrated.[23] Impairment of insulin-mediated DNA synthesis, cell growth, and protein synthesis in cells from patients with leprechaunism has been observed and may be relevant to the clinical feature of growth retardation.

In recent years, insulin receptor mutations have been identified in several patients with this disorder (see Chapter 62). Since parental consanguinity was often noted, leprechaunism was perceived as an autosomal recessive condition. Indeed, both alleles of the receptor gene are affected in all cases reported thus far. Given that at least three reported cases were associated with homozygosity for insulin receptor null alleles, it is apparent that leprechaunism is the direct consequence of total or near total absence of functional insulin receptors. The possible involvement of other growth factor receptors in the pathogenesis of leprechaunism remains a puzzling phenomenon. Since potential defects involving the epidermal growth factor (EGF) and IGF-1 receptors have been noted,[23] it remains possible that primary defects involving these receptors may exist, although secondary alterations that occur as a consequence of a marked deficit in insulin action represent a more likely explanation.

Both Rabson[24] and Mendenhall[25] described cases of a related rare syndrome of extreme insulin resistance. Subjects with the Rabson-Mendenhall syndrome have several clinical features seen in other syndromes of severe insulin resistance, including acanthosis nigricans, phallic enlargement, and precocious pseudopuberty.[24] Markedly abnormal dentition, thick and rapidly growing scalp hair, and thickened nails are also characteristic features of the syndrome.[24,25] Hyperplasia of the pineal gland is an unusual feature of this syndrome that was noted in several reported cases.[24–26] The prognosis for this rare syndrome is poor because diabetes may develop in childhood and be extremely difficult to control even with huge doses of insulin.[27]

Rabson-Mendenhall syndrome has been shown to be associated with genetic defects involving both alleles of the insulin receptor gene. However, unlike most cases of leprechaunism, mutations may not completely abolish all insulin action mediated by the insulin receptor. The etiology of the pineal hyperplasia is unknown.

The Type A Syndrome and Variants

The term type A insulin resistance is used to describe patients with essentially normal growth and development who have severe insulin resistance, acanthosis nigricans, and (in postpubertal females) ovarian hyperandrogenism, often with signs of virilization.[28] In contrast to this apparently inherited disorder, the type B syndrome is one in which acquired autoantibodies to the insulin receptor may result in a similar clinical phenotype (see below). Studies of several patients with the type A syndrome were notable for apparent primary insulin receptor defects (e.g., diminished insulin binding or impaired receptor function).[28,29] Subsequently, a number of point mutations involving one or both alleles of the insulin receptor gene have been demonstrated to cause dominant or recessively inherited forms of the type A syndrome (see Chapter 62).

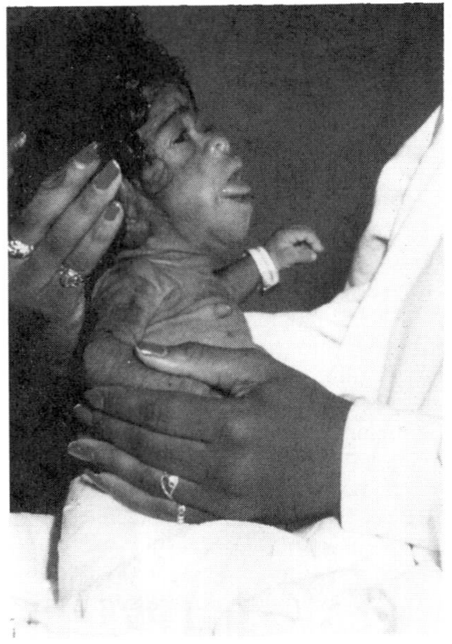

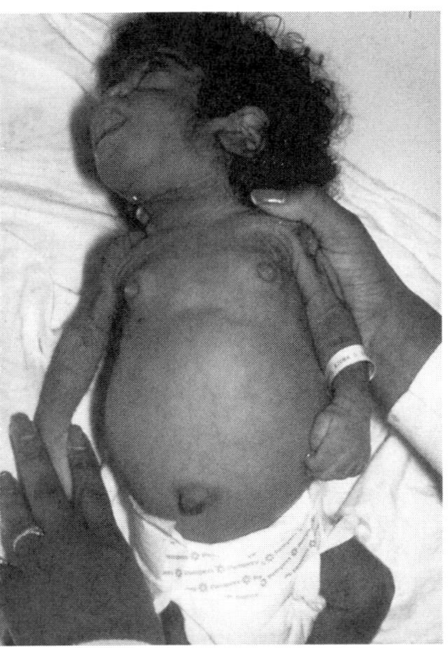

FIGURE 65-2. Leprechaunism. This infant has several features of leprechaunism including dysmorphic facies, acanthosis nigricans, hypertrichosis and hirsutism, breast enlargement, abdominal distention, and lipoatrophy. (Photographs were kindly provided by Louis J. Elsas II, Emory University, Atlanta, GA. Reproduced with permission from Moller DE, ed. Insulin Resistance. New York: John Wiley & Sons;1993.)

The term type C insulin resistance was previously used to describe patients with similar features in whom no obvious biochemical defects at the level of the insulin receptor were detected.[30] This term should be avoided, since some patients with apparently normal insulin binding or receptor tyrosine kinase activity could still harbor functionally significant mutations that affect receptor-mediated cellular signaling. Furthermore, the phenotype of patients with and without mutations in the insulin receptor gene may be indistinguishable.[18] Clinical descriptions of patients with the so-called HAIRAN syndrome[31] overlap largely with features described for patients with the type A syndrome, except that initially described patients with the type A syndrome were extremely insulin resistant and did not include obese subjects.[28] Since scrutiny of other family members reveals that males may also be affected by severe insulin resistance and acanthosis nigricans, type A insulin resistance is the preferred term to describe patients with congenital forms of insulin resistance and acanthosis nigricans (with females being affected by ovarian hyperandrogenism) but in whom no other obvious phenotypic changes (such as growth retardation or lipodystrophy) are evident.

It is clear that clinical features of the type A syndrome represent a continuum ranging from mild to severe. Thus, patients may be variably affected by acanthosis nigricans or impairment of glucose tolerance. In females, the consequences of ovarian hyperandrogenism may include oligomenorrhea or amenorrhea, anovulation, hirsutism, acne, and in some cases marked masculinization.[31] Uncommon clinical features may include hypertrichosis[32] and muscle cramps.[33]

In addition to substantial impairment of in vivo insulin-mediated glucose disposal and impaired suppression of hepatic glucose output, a reduction of in vivo insulin clearance has been demonstrated in some patients,[34] providing an additional mechanism for marked degrees of hyperinsulinemia. As noted above, a minority of patients with clinical features of the type A syndrome have underlying defects in the insulin receptor gene. Apart from unknown genetic defects that are likely to affect molecules mediating postreceptor insulin signaling, an insulin receptor kinase-inhibitor has been detected in cultured dermal fibroblasts derived from several patients with features of the type A syndrome.[35] This inhibitor has recently been identified at the molecular level.[35a]

Several patients with features of the type A syndrome have also been reported to have clinical signs of acromegaly (e.g., acral hypertrophy, coarsened features) in the absence of elevated growth hormone or IGF-1 levels.[36–38] Some of the patients with "pseudoacromegaly" or "acromegaloidism" are also afflicted with severe muscle cramps.[33] Accelerated linear growth and obesity may also occur. The association of physical changes similar to those of acromegaly with severe insulin resistance may involve the interaction of insulin at markedly elevated levels with IGF-1 receptors, thereby resulting in an IGF-1-like effect. We described a case in which resistance to insulin-mediated glucose uptake/disposal was present but insulin was able to normally stimulate other biologic effects.[38] Thus, "selective resistance" to the glucose-lowering effects of insulin could result in hyperinsulinemia that can excessively promote anabolic biologic effects.

Insulin Resistance and Lipodystrophy

Patients with severe insulin resistance occasionally manifest complete or partial absence of adipose tissue.[39–41] As shown in Table 65-2, the lipodystrophies are distinct syndromes that can be classified according to the anatomic distribution of affected fat depots or according to whether or not the disorder is genetic (and the mode of inheritance). Generalized forms of lipodystrophy with insulin-resistant diabetes are also referred to as "lipoatrophic diabetes."[41] Other lipodystrophies occur in which lipoatrophy is confined to specific regions of the body. Subcutaneous fat present elsewhere may be either normal or hypertrophied. Depending on the degree of insulin resistance, patients with lipodystrophic syndromes also tend to display general features of severe insulin resistance (e.g., acanthosis nigricans and ovarian hyperandrogenism). In general, variable degrees of hyperlipidemia and hepatic disease can occur in patients with apparently different lipodystrophic syndromes. The pathophysiology of these syndromes remains largely unexplained, since no specific gene(s) or molecular mechanism(s) have been reported to date. Although these syndromes are indeed rare, defining their causes is likely to provide new insights into the biology of adipose tissue differentiation and function and the pathogenesis of common obesity.

Table 65-2. Classification of the Lipodystrophic Syndromes

Congenital Lipodystrophies

1. Congenital generalized lipodystrophy* (Berardinelli-Seip syndrome)
   Autosomal recessive; total lipoatrophy
2. Partial congenital lipodystrophy (face-sparing lipodystrophy, Kobberling-Dunnigan syndrome)
   X-linked dominant; onset of partial lipodystrophy after birth; variable lipoatrophy with sparing (or hypertrophy) of facial adipose tissue
3. Mandibuloacral dysplasia
   Lipodystrophy and insulin resistance with skeletal abnormalities

"Acquired" Lipodystrophies

1. Acquired generalized lipodystrophy* (Lawrence syndrome)
   Sporadic; female preponderance; +/− antecedent infection
2. Generalized lipodystrophy associated with tumors of the diencephalon
3. Cephalothoracic lipodystrophy
   Sporadic; female preponderance; lipoatrophy of face and upper trunk; associated with C_3 nephritic factor and mesangiocapillary glomerulonephritis

*Both syndromes referred to as "lipoatrophic diabetes."

Congenital (Inherited) Lipodystrophies

Congenital generalized lipodystrophy is a rare autosomal recessive disorder characterized by apparent total lipoatrophy.[42] This disease is also known as the Berardinelli-Seip syndrome. There is a high incidence of parental consanguinity, and the generalized absence of adipose tissue is usually noted soon after birth (Fig. 65-3). Extreme hyperlipidemia is a common feature, with predominantly elevated plasma triglycerides, which may contribute to the development of acute pancreatitis. Hepatomegaly secondary to fat infiltration is also a common occurrence that can lead to cell necrosis and fibrotic change.[41] Impaired glucose tolerance with marked insulin resistance may lead to overt diabetes[43]; hence the name "lipoatrophic diabetes."[41] Intellectual and psychomotor disabilities are occasionally also noted.[42] It remains unclear whether this disorder results from impaired fat cell triglyceride deposition (either a biosynthetic defect or an absence of differentiated adipocytes) or from accelerated lipolysis.[44,45] It appears most likely that severe insulin resistance is a secondary consequence of the markedly altered metabolic milieu. Thus, insulin receptor mutations have not been detected in a number of cases where they were searched for.[18,46]

Face-sparing lipodystrophy is a familial syndrome also known as partial congenital lipodystrophy or the Kobberling-Dunnigan syndrome.[47,48] This rare disorder often shows an inheritance pattern that is suggestive of X-linked dominance.[48] Partial lipoatrophy appears to begin in childhood or early adolescence, sparing the face and sometimes truncal fat. The face may assume an obese, plethoric appearance. Severe insulin resistance is often present, although hyperlipidemia is not as marked as in generalized lipodystrophy. In the majority of cases, essential hypertension is also

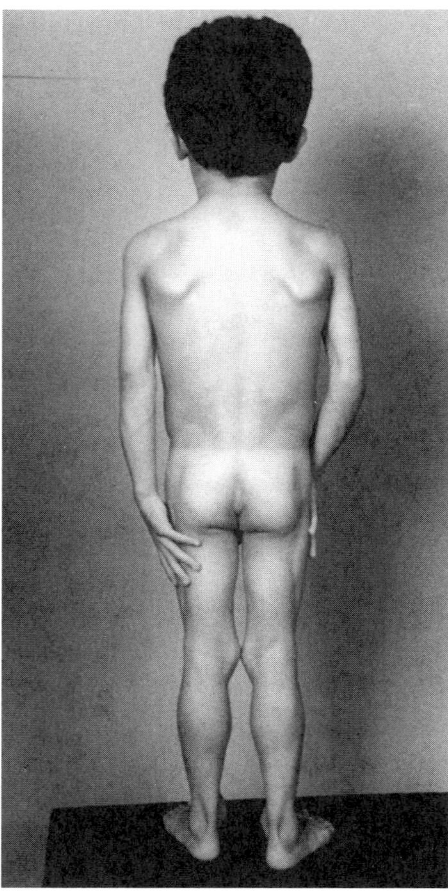

Figure 65-3. Congenital generalized lipodystrophy. This 7-year-old male demonstrates apparent total lipoatrophy despite adequate nutrition. Marked hepatomegaly (not shown) was also evident. (Photograph provided by Jeffrey S. Flier, Beth Israel Hospital, Boston, MA. Reproduced with permission from Moller DE, ed. Insulin Resistance. New York: John Wiley & Sons;1993.)

evident.[47] The pathophysiology of this unusual disorder remains completely obscure, although one group of investigators suggested that regional variations in sympathetic nervous system tone might promote accelerated regional lipolysis.[49]

Mandibuloacral dysplasia is a term used to describe several unusual cases of lipoatrophy and insulin resistance that were also associated with a variety of skeletal and morphologic abnormalities.[50,51] Thus, progressive osteolysis of the mandible and clavicles and joint contractures were noted in these patients.[50] Since several pairs of siblings have been similarly affected, the syndrome is presumed to be inherited. Despite marked hyperinsulinemia, patients have been reported to have little or no acanthosis nigricans. One case was associated with impaired signaling by insulin *and other growth factors*,[52] suggesting a generalized cellular defect in growth factor–mediated signaling (which might also explain the paucity of acanthosis nigricans).

"Acquired" Lipodystrophies

Patients with *acquired generalized lipodystrophy* have apparently normal fat mass and distribution at birth but subsequently develop atrophy of all their adipose tissue.[41] This syndrome is sometimes referred to as the Lawrence syndrome.[41,53] Females are more frequently affected, and there is no apparent familial tendency.[41] In many cases, an antecedent infection has been implicated as part of the cause.[40] The clinical features are very similar to those seen in patients with congenital generalized lipodystrophy, although the hyperlipidemia may be even more severe and result in eruptive xanthomas.[42] Since fat biopsies have reportedly shown changes resembling panniculitis,[40] destruction of adipose tissue has been implicated. Rare patients with tumors in the diencephalon have also been reported to develop acquired generalized lipodystrophy.[54] The mechanism of this unusual association is obscure.

Cephalothoracic lipodystrophy (also known as partial progressive lipodystrophy) is another uncommon acquired form of lipodystrophy in which the face and upper trunk are affected by lipoatrophy, sparing the rest of the body.[55] This sporadic disorder also affects females more often and may occur acutely after an infection. Signs of severe insulin resistance are uncommon, as is diabetes, although some patients are hyperinsulinemic.[56] This form of lipodystrophy is specifically associated with the presence of abnormal complement activation, the presence in serum of C_3 nephritic factor, and mesangiocapillary glomerulonephritis.[57] Interestingly, another connection between adipose tissue and the complement system was made by the discovery of adipsin—a secreted fat cell product—which is also a component of the alternative complement pathway (factor D).[58] The mechanism by which this form of lipodystrophy and complement disturbances may be related remains obscure.

Other Rare Inherited Disorders Associated with Insulin Resistance

Several other rare inherited disorders with heterogeneous phenotypic features are associated with moderate to severe degrees of insulin resistance. *Alström's syndrome* is an autosomal recessive syndrome of severe insulin resistance that is associated with retinal pigment degeneration, sensorineural deafness, obesity, and hypogonadism.[59] The pigmentary retinopathy differs from typical retinitis pigmentosa because classic "bony spicules" are absent. Hearing loss is variable, but diabetes mellitus and renal dysfunction caused by glomerulosclerosis are common features.[59]

Myotonic dystrophy is a dominantly inherited neurologic disorder that has been reported to be associated with modest degrees of insulin resistance.[60] Interestingly, this rare disease is apparently caused by mutations affecting the gene encoding a novel cellular protein kinase, raising the possibility that this new enzyme may participate in insulin-mediated cellular signal transmission.[61] *Friedreich's ataxia* is a rare, recessively inherited neurologic disorder with an increased incidence of impaired glucose tolerance or NIDDM. Modest hyperinsulinemia associated with a mild defect in monocyte insulin binding has been observed.[62]

Autoimmune Insulin Resistance

The Type B Syndrome

The term type B syndrome refers to insulin resistance caused by the presence of (acquired) autoantibodies directed against the insulin receptor.[28,63] Thus, this disorder is similar to Grave's disease or myasthenia gravis, which are caused by autoantibodies to the thyroid-stimulating hormone or acetylcholine receptors, respectively. The type B syndrome affects females predominantly, with a mean age of onset of 44 years.[64] Most patients display one or more features of a systemic autoimmune disorder. Mild abnormalities may include only leukopenia, elevated erythrocyte sedimentation rate, proteinuria, or high titers of anti-DNA antibodies.[64–66] Alternatively, the syndrome is associated with defined diseases, including systemic lupus erythematosus, Sjögren's syndrome, primary biliary cirrhosis, and idiopathic thrombocytopenic purpura.[64,65,67]

Affected patients are frequently noted to have acanthosis nigricans, and ovarian hyperandrogenism has also been reported in female patients.[64] As noted above, abnormal glucose homeostasis is a prominent feature, with both hyperglycemia and hypoglycemia (particularly fasting) being commonly noted. In the context of hyperglycemia, extreme resistance to exogenous insulin has been documented with little or no response to greater than 1000 U of insulin.[64] In contrast, severe hypoglycemia occurs rarely but can require large amounts of parenteral glucose to treat effectively.[67] In some cases, the clinical course is notable for remissions and recurrences with alternating periods of marked hyperglycemia and hypoglycemia.[68] Treatment aimed at curtailing the production of autoantibodies is occasionally required. Both glucocorticoids and other immunosuppressive agents have been successfully used to chronically normalize glucose levels.[64,67]

The mechanism of the type B syndrome is fairly well characterized. Spontaneously occurring polyclonal (usually IgG) antibodies usually bind to the extracellular domain of the receptor. A frequently targeted epitope appears to be present within residues 450–601.[69] The autoantibodies have several different effects: (1) they may compete with insulin for binding (by blocking the binding site and/or by steric inhibition); (2) the receptor-antibody complex can be internalized and degraded, leading to accelerated receptor degradation; (3) antibodies may (variably) activate the receptor, causing insulin-like effects and potentially leading to postreceptor desensitization to insulin.[63,64,66,70] These effects account for the fact that acute insulin-like effects are typically seen in vitro, whereas chronic incubation of cells with antiserum results in desensitization to subsequent insulin stimulation.[64] Most cases can be diagnosed by the ability of patient serum to inhibit in vitro insulin binding, although in some cases,[66] patient serum fails to block insulin binding, and the antibodies can only be detected by their ability to immunoprecipitate insulin receptor protein.

Ataxia-telangiectasia is a rare recessive syndrome associated with cerebellar ataxia, telangiectasias, and recurrent respiratory tract infections. Patients with this disorder have frequently been reported to display insulin-resistant glucose intolerance. The presence of IgM autoantibodies directed against the insulin receptor has been reported in these patients,[71] suggesting that insulin resistance in the context of ataxia-telangiectasia may be a variant of the type B syndrome.

Autoimmune Insulin Syndrome

In rare individuals, especially those with other autoimmune disorders, spontaneously occurring autoantibodies to insulin may develop.[64] These antibodies are not a true cause of insulin resistance because they do not affect target cell insulin sensitivity. Such antibodies are a defined cause of hypoglycemia known as the *autoimmune insulin syndrome*. This syndrome has specifically been associated with autoimmune thyroid disease and treatment with antithyroid drugs.[64] The antibodies appear to function by sequestering insulin within the circulation, where it may later be released in the postprandial setting.

Insulin Antibodies in Diabetic Patients Taking Insulin

With the advent of recombinant human insulin and improved insulin purity, the development of clinically significant high-titer anti-insulin antibodies in patients with diabetes requiring insulin is now rarely encountered. However, extreme resistance to exogenous insulin can still occur, especially in the context of associated cutaneous insulin-allergic symptoms. The use of alternative insulin formulations, including sulfated insulin, may be helpful.[72]

References

1. Flier JS, Moses AC. Diabetes in acromegaly and other endocrine disorders. In: DeGroot LJ, ed. Endocrinology. Philadelphia: WB Saunders; 1989:1389–1399
2. Marangou AG, Weber KM, Boston RC, et al. Metabolic consequences of prolonged hyperinsulinemia in humans. Evidence for induction of insulin insensitivity. Diabetes 1986;35:1383
3. Hager SR. Insulin resistance of uremia. Am J Kidney Dis 1989;14:272
4. Carallo-Perin P, Cassader M, Bozzo C, et al. Mechanism of insulin resistance in humăn liver cirrhosis. J Clin Invest 1985;75:1659
5. Smith U. Insulin resistance and hypertension. In: Moller DE, ed. Insulin Resistance. New York: John Wiley & Sons; 1993
6. Stout RW. Insulin resistance, hyperlipidemia and atherosclerosis. In: Moller DE, ed. Insulin Resistance. New York: John Wiley & Sons; 1993
7. Plourde PV, Marks JG, Hammond JM. Acanthosis nigricans and insulin resistance. J Am Acad Dermatol 1984;10:887
8. Matsuoka LY, Wortsman J, Gavin JR, Goldman J. Spectrum of endocrine abnormalities associated with acanthosis nigricans. Am J Med 1987;83:719
9. Stuart CA, Pate CJ, Peters EJ. Prevalence of acanthosis nigricans in an unselected population. Am J Med 1989;87:269
10. Rogers DL. Acanthosis nigricans. Semin Dermatol 1991;10:160
11. Cruz PD, Hud JA. Excess insulin binding to insulin-like growth factor receptors: Proposed mechanism for acanthosis nigricans. J Invest Dermatol 1992;98:82S
12. Barbieri RL, Smith S, Ryan KJ. The role of hyperinsulinemia in the pathogenesis of ovarian hyperandrogenism. Fertil Steril 1988;50:197
13. Dunaif A. Insulin resistance and ovarian dysfunction. In: Moller DE, ed. Insulin Resistance. New York: John Wiley & Sons; 1993
14. Flier JS, Eastman RC, Minaker KL, et al. Acanthosis nigricans in obese women with hyperandrogenism: Characterization of an insulin-resistant state distinct from the type A and B syndromes. Diabetes 1985;34:101
15. Dunaif A, Green G, Phelps RG, et al. Acanthosis nigricans, insulin action, and hyperandrogenism: Clinical, histological, and biochemical findings. J Clin Endocrinol Metab 1991;73:590
16. Dunaif A, Green G, Futterweit W, Dobrjansky A. Suppression of hyperandrogenism does not improve peripheral or hepatic insulin resistance in the polycystic ovary syndrome. J Clin Endocrinol Metab 1990;70:699
17. Poretsky L. On the paradox of insulin-induced hyperandrogenism in insulin-resistant states. Endocr Rev 1991;12:3
18. Moller DE, Cohen O, Yamaguchi Y, et al. Prevalence of mutations in the insulin receptor gene in subjects with features of the type A syndrome of insulin resistance. Diabetes 1994;43:247
19. Ciaraldi TP, El-Roeiy A, Madar Z, et al. Cellular mechanisms of insulin resistance in polycystic ovarian syndrome. J Clin Endocrinol Metab 1992; 75:577
20. Donohue WL, Uchida I. Leprechaunism: A euphemism for a rare familial disorder. J Pediatr 1954;45:505
21. Elders MJ, Schedewie HK, Olefsky J, et al. Endocrine-metabolic relationships in patients with leprechaunism. J Natl Med Assoc 1982;74:1195
22. Elsas LJ, Endo F, Priest JH, Strumlauf E. Leprechaunism: An inherited defect in insulin-receptor interaction. In: Wapnir RA, ed. Congenital Metabolic Disease: Diagnosis and Treatment. New York: Marcel Dekker; 1985:301–334
23. Sethu-Kumar Reddy S, Lauris V, Kahn CR. Insulin receptor function in fibroblasts from patients with leprechaunism: Differential alterations in binding, autophosphorylation, kinase activity, and receptor-mediated internalization. J Clin Invest 1988;82:1359
24. Rabson SM, Mendenhall EN. Familial hypertrophy of pineal body, hyperplasia of adrenal cortex and diabetes mellitus: Report of 3 cases. Am J Clin Pathol 1956;26:283
25. Mendenhall EN. Tumor of the pineal body with high insulin resistance. J Indiana Med Assoc 1950;43:32
26. West RJ, Lloyd JK, Turner WML. Familial insulin-resistant diabetes, multiple somatic anomalies, and pineal hyperplasia. Arch Dis Child 1975;50:703
27. West RJ, Leonard JV. Familial insulin resistance with pineal hyperplasia: Metabolic studies and effect of hypophysectomy. Arch Dis Child 1980;55:619
28. Kahn CR, Flier JS, Bar RS, et al. The syndromes of insulin resistance and acanthosis nigricans: Insulin receptor disorders in man. N Engl J Med 1976; 294:739
29. Bar RS, Muggeo M, Kahn CR, et al. Characterization of insulin receptors in patients with the syndromes of insulin resistance and acanthosis nigricans. Diabetologia 1980;18:209
30. Nakamura F, Taira M, Hashmoto N, et al. Familial type C syndrome of insulin resistance and short stature with possible autosomal dominant transmission. Endocrinol Jpn 1989;36:349
31. Barbieri RL. Clinical aspects of the hyperandrogenism-insulin resistance-acanthosis nigricans syndrome. Semin Reprod Endocrinol 1994;12:26
32. Grigorescu F, Herzberg V, King G, et al. Defects in insulin binding and autophosphorylation of erythrocyte insulin receptors in patients with syndromes of severe insulin resistance and their parents. J Clin Endocrinol Metab 1987;64:549
33. Flier JS, Young JB, Landsberg L. Familial insulin resistance with acanthosis nigricans, acral hypertrophy and muscle cramps: A new syndrome. N Engl J Med 1980;390:970
34. Flier JS, Minaker KL, Landsberg L, et al. Impaired in vivo insulin clearance in patients with severe target cell resistance of insulin. Diabetes 1982;31:132

35. Maddux BA, Sbraccia P, Reaven GM, et al. Inhibitors of insulin receptor tyrosine kinase in fibroblasts from diverse patients with impaired insulin action: Evidence for a novel mechanism of postreceptor insulin resistance. J Clin Endocrinol Metab 1993;77:73
35a. Maddux BA, Sbraccia P, Kumakura S, et al. Membrane glycoprotein PC-1 and insulin resistance in non–insulin-dependent diabetes mellitus. Nature 1995;373:448
36. Holdaway IM, Frengley PA, Graham FM, Wong M. Insulin resistance with acanthosis nigricans and acral hypertrophy. NZ Med J 1984;97:286
37. Low L, Chernausek SD, Sperling MA. Acromegaloid patients with type A insulin resistance: Parallel defects in insulin and insulin-like growth factor-1 receptors and biological responses in cultured fibroblasts. J Clin Endocrinol Metab 1989;69:329
38. Flier JS, Moller DE, Moses AC, et al. Insulin-mediated pseudoacromegaly: Clinical and biochemical characterization of a syndrome of selective insulin resistance. J Clin Endocrinol Metab 1993;6:1533
39. Senior B, Gellis SS. The syndromes of total and partial lipodystrophy. Pediatrics 1964;33:593
40. Kobberling J. Genetic syndromes associated with lipoatrophic diabetes. In: Creutzfeldt J, Kobberling J, Neel JV, eds. The Genetics of Diabetes Mellitus. New York: Springer Verlag;1976:147–154
41. Rossini AA. Lipoatrophic diabetes. In: Marble A, Krall LP, Bradley RF, et al., eds. Joslin's Diabetes Mellitus. Philadelphia: Lea & Febiger;1985:834–842
42. Seip M. Generalized lipodystrophy. Ergebnisse der Inneren Medizin und Kinderheilkunde. Heidelberg: Springer-Verlag;1971:XXXI:59–69
43. Oseid S. Studies in congenital generalized lipodystrophy (Seip-Berardinelli syndrome). I. Development of diabetes. Acta Endocrinol 1973;72:475
44. Boucher BJ, Cohen RD, France MW, Mason SA. Plasma free fatty acid turnover in total lipodystrophy. Clin Endocrinol 1973;4:83
45. Berg SW, Jersild RA, Powell RC. Studies of lipid synthesis and release. J Lab Clin Med 1970;76:1005
46. Van der Vorm ER, Kupers A, Bonenkamp JW, et al. Patients with lipodystrophic diabetes mellitus of the Seip-Berardinelli type, express normal insulin receptors. Diabetologia 1993;36:172-174
47. Dunnigan MG, Cochrane M, Kelly A, Scott JW. Familial lipoatrophic diabetes with dominant transmission. Q J Med 1974;49:33
48. Kobberling J, Dunnigan MG. Familial partial lipodystrophy: Two types of an X linked dominant syndrome, lethal in the hemizygous state. J Med Genet 1986;23:120
49. Davidson MB, Young RT. Metabolic studies in partial lipodystrophy of the lower trunk and extremities. Diabetologia 1975;11:561
50. Tenconi R, Miotti F, Miotti A, et al. Another Italian family with mandibuloacral dysplasia: Why does it seem more frequent in Italy? Am J Med Genet 1986;24:357
51. Freidenberg G, Jones M, Hall B, et al. A new syndrome of insulin resistance, diabetes mellitus, and mandibuloacral dysplasia. Clin Res 1989;37:192A
52. Hoepffner HJ, Dreyer M, Reimers U, et al. A new familial syndrome with impaired function of three related growth factor receptors. Hum Genet 1989;83:209
53. Lawrence RD. Lipodystrophy and hepatomegaly with diabetes, lipaemia, and other metabolic disturbances. A case throwing new light on the action of insulin. Lancet 1946;1:724
54. Seip M. Lipodystrophy and gigantism with associated endocrine manifestations. A new diencephalic syndrome? Acta Paediatrica 1959;48:555
55. Barraquer FL. Pathogenesis of progressive cephalothoracic lipodystrophy. J Nerv Ment Dis 1949;109:193
56. Boucher BJ, Cohen RD, Rankel RJ, et al. Partial and total lipodystrophy: Changes in circulating sugar, free fatty acids, insulin and growth hormone following the administration of glucose and insulin. Clin Endocrinol 1973; 2:111
57. Sissons JGP, West RJ, Fallows J. The complement abnormalities of lipodystrophy. N Engl J Med 1976;294:461
58. Rosen BS, Cook KS, Yaglom J, et al. Adipsin and complement factor D activity: An immune-related defect in obesity. Science 1989;244:1483
59. Charles SJ, Moore AT, Yates JRW, et al. Alstroms syndrome: Further evidence of autosomal recessive inheritance and endocrinological dysfunction. J Med Genet 1990;27:590
60. Tevaarwerk GJ, Hudson AJ. Carbohydrate metabolism and insulin resistance in myotonia dystrophica. J Clin Endocrinol Metab 1977;44:491
61. Brook JD, McCurrach ME, Harley HG, et al. Molecular basis of myotonic dystrophy: Expansion of trinucleotide (CTG) repeat at the 3′ end of a transcript encoding a protein kinase family member. Cell 1992;68:799
62. Khan RJ, Andermann E, Fantus IG. Glucose intolerance in Friedreich's ataxia: Association with insulin resistance and decreased insulin binding. Metabolism 1986;35:1017
63. Flier JS, Kahn CR, Roth J, Bar RS. Antibodies that impair insulin receptor binding in an unusual diabetic syndrome with severe insulin resistance. Science 1975;190:63
64. Gorden P, Collier E, Roach P. Autoimmune mechanisms of insulin resistance and hypoglycemia. In: Moller DE, ed. Insulin Resistance. New York: John Wiley;1993:123–141
65. Tsokos GC, Gorden P, Antonovych T, et al. Lupus nephritis and other autoimmune features in patients with diabetes mellitus due to autoantibody to insulin receptors. Ann Int Med 1985;102:176
66. Taylor SI, Barbetti F, Accili D, et al. Syndromes of autoimmunity and hypoglycemia: Autoantibodies directed against insulin and its receptor. Endocrinol Metab Clin North Am 1989;18:123
67. Moller DE, Ratner RE, Borenstein DG, Taylor SI. Autoantibodies to the insulin receptor as a cause of autoimmune hypoglycemia in systemic lupus erythematosus. Am J Med 1988;84:334
68. Flier JS, Bar RS, Muggeo M, et al. The evolving clinical course of patients with insulin receptor autoantibodies: Spontaneous remission or receptor proliferation with hypoglycemia. J Clin Endocrinol Metab 1978;47:985
69. Zhang B, Roth RA. A region of the insulin receptor important for ligand binding (residues 450–601) is recognized by patient's autoimmune antibodies and inhibitory monoclonal antibodies. Proc Natl Acad Sci USA 1991;88:9858
70. Flier JS, Kahn CR, Roth J. Receptors, antireceptor antibodies and mechanisms of insulin resistance. N Engl J Med 1979;300:413
71. Bar RS, Levis WR, Rechler MM, et al. Extreme insulin resistance in ataxia telangiectasia: Defect in affinity of insulin receptors. N Engl J Med 1978; 298:1164
72. Flier JS, Poretsky L. Insulin allergy and insulin resistance. In: Lichtenstein LM, Fauci AS, eds. Current Therapy in Allergy, Immunology and Rheumatology. Philadelphia: BC Decker Inc.;1985:135–140

Diabetes Mellitus, edited by Derek LeRoith, Simeon I. Taylor, and Jerrold M. Olefsky. Lippincott–Raven Publishers, Philadelphia © 1996.

Chapter 66

Maternally Inherited Diabetes and Deafness: A New Subtype of Diabetes Mellitus

Takashi Kadowaki

Introduction

Mitochondrial genes are plausible candidates for causing diabetes mellitus because the mitochondrion appears to play a crucial role in insulin secretion from pancreatic β-cells in response to glucose and other nutrients. ATP, mainly produced through oxidative phosphorylation, closes the ATP-sensitive potassium channel, depolarizes the β-cell membrane, and opens the voltage-dependent calcium channel. The influx of Ca^{++} stimulates insulin secretion.[1] Therefore, a defect in oxidative phosphorylation might produce a defect in insulin secretion and create a predisposition for diabetes mellitus. In fact, an A to G mutation in the transfer ribonucleic acid $(RNA)^{LEU(UUR)}$ gene at position 3243 (3243 mutation) has been identified in patients with diabetes and deafness. Hallmarks of diabetic patients with the 3243 mutation are the maternal inheritance and sensorineural hearing loss of variable severity. Thus, the terminology of maternally inherited diabetes and deafness (MIDD) seems appropriate for this subtype of diabetes. Significantly, at present MIDD may be the most prevalent subtype of diabetes with a defined genetic defect. In this chapter, the molecular biology of the mitochondrial genome and genetics and the clinical characteristics, and pathophysiology of this subtype of diabetes mellitus are described.

Mitochondrial Genome[2–4]

Eukaryotic cells contain one copy of nuclear DNA and several thousand copies of mitochondrial (mt) DNA. The mt genome, whose sequence was published in 1981, is a 16,569 base pair circular, double-stranded DNA molecule encoding 13 subunits of the respiratory chain complexes, 22 transfer RNAs (tRNAs) and 2 ribosomal RNAs (rRNAs) (Fig. 66-1). The mt genome shows extreme compactness with almost no intervening sequences between coding regions. Mitochondria have their own replication, transcription, and translation apparatus. The noncoding on displacement (D) loop region is the site for the control of both replication and transcription. mtDNA replication is bidirectional but asynchronous and proceeds from two origins, one for the guanine-rich heavy (H) strand and one for the cysteine-rich light (L) strand. mtDNA transcription proceeds symmetrically in opposite directions from the two promoters located in the D loop and generates polytranscripts. The long polycistronic RNAs are subsequently processed by endonucleolytic cleavage, resulting in the individual ribosomal, messenger, and transfer RNAs. H-strand transcription generates an excess of rRNA transcripts over messenger RNA (mRNAs), which is accomplished by specific binding of a transcription termination factor near the 16S rRNA gene.

Another unique feature of mtDNA is its maternal transmission. mtDNA molecules are predominantly maternally inherited, as the sperm cell makes a negligible contribution to the maternal oocytes. This means that mtDNA is transmitted solely by mothers to all of their offspring, and only the daughters will transmit their mtDNA to the next generation.[5] Furthermore, each cell contains hundreds of mitochondria, and each mitochondrion contains two to ten copies of mtDNA. Patients have variable proportions of mutant and normal mtDNA (heteroplasmy) in different tissues. A change in phenotype becomes apparent only when the proportion of the mutant mtDNA exceeds a certain level (threshold effect). Organs and tissues such as muscle, brain, and heart with high energy requirements are affected most frequently, but endocrinopathies and diabetes are also common occurrences. Because mitochondria are randomly distributed to the daughter cells, the proportion of these different mtDNAs can change widely during a number of cell divisions.

Finally, the mtDNA has very high mutation rate for the following reasons: (1) mtDNA evolves faster than nuclear DNA. (2) Moreover, mtDNA is more exposed to chemical attack than nuclear DNA because the mtDNA is not protected by histones. (3) Furthermore, the mtDNA lacks sufficient DNA repair mechanisms. (4) Finally, oxygen radicals that are formed along the mitochondrial chain as byproducts of respiration may especially attack the mtDNA. This high susceptibility of mtDNA to mutational events makes the mt genome highly vulnerable. Given that mtDNA is highly organized and consists almost exclusively of coding regions, these mutations inevitably lead to defects in mitochondrial function and disease.

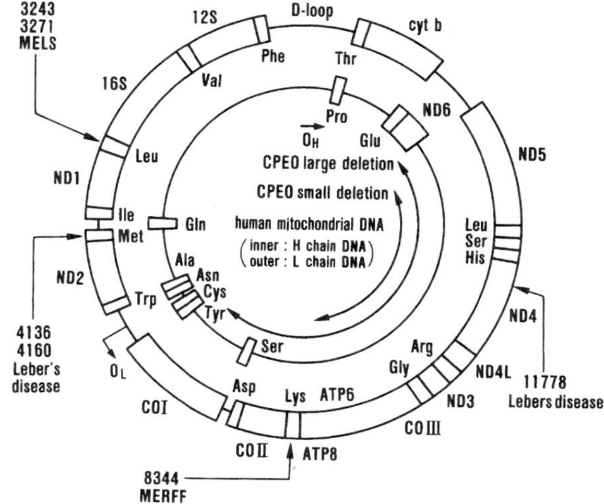

Figure 66-1. Map of the human mitochondrial genome. The mtDNA encompasses 16,569 base pairs with numbering starting at OH and proceeding counterclockwise around the circular map. The outer and inner strands are the H strand and L strand, respectively. Dark regions are rRNA and polypeptide genes. The tRNA genes are indicated by the letter of their cognate amino acid. OH, OL, PH, and PL are origins of replication and promoters for the H and L strands, respectively. D loop, displacement loop.

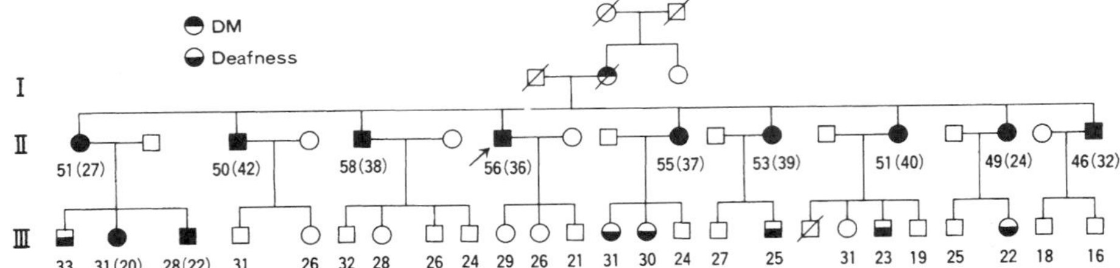

FIGURE 66-2. Pedigree of maternally inherited diabetes and deafness associated with the 3243 mutation.

Alterations of mtDNA Are Associated with Disease[6,7]

It has only recently been recognized that mutations in the mitochondrial genome are associated with human disease, particularly those affecting organs with high energy requirements such as brain, skeletal muscle, and heart. Thus, large deletions or insertions are found in mitochondrial DNA from patients with chronic progressive external ophthalmoplegia or the Kearns-Sayre syndrome. Several point mutations were described in large pedigrees of the maternally inherited Leber's hereditary opticus neuropathy, in myoclonus epilepsy with ragged red fibers, and in myoencephalopathy with lactic acidosis and stroke-like episodes. The clinical phenotype of an individual with a mutation is related to the nature of the mtDNA mutation and has also been suggested to be related to the proportion of mutant mtDNA in the various organs and tissues, each with their own energetic thresholds for oxidative phosphorylation. This complex situation makes it more difficult to observe a clear correlation between genotypes and phenotypes in patients with mt disease.

Identification of Maternally Inherited Diabetes and Deafness

In 1992, van den Ouweland and colleagues showed a G for A substitution in heteroplasmic form at position 3243 in the mitochondrial DNA encoded tRNA (leu, UUR) gene (3243 mutation) in a family in which diabetes and deafness are inherited via maternal transmission[8] (Fig. 66-2). In this family, all nine children of a mother with diabetes exhibited diabetes and deafness of variable severity. When the third generation was examined, diabetes and deafness were present only in children from the maternal lineage. This pattern of inheritance is highly suggestive of maternal inheritance, which is a hallmark of mitochondrial diseases.

Independent support of the theory that alterations in mitochondrial DNA can be the cause of diabetes came from the findings by the group of Wallace that duplications and deletions in mitochondrial DNA are also associated with diabetes and deafness.[9,10]

Initially, diabetes associated with mtDNA mutations was considered a rare form. However, subsequent studies revealed that the prevalence of diabetes (and deafness) associated with a particular 3243 mutation may be much greater than was originally suspected.[11–28] Indeed, the 3243 mutation may be the most prevalent single mutation-causing human disease.

TABLE 66-1. Characteristics of Diabetes Mellitus Associated with the 3243 bp Mutation

1. Often maternally transmitted
2. Variable clinical phenotypes including NIDDM, slowly progressive IDDM, or IDDM
3. Patient often young at onset; infrequent obesity
4. Tendency toward progression
5. Impaired endogenous insulin secretion; often treated with insulin
6. Often associated with sensory hearing disturbance

Clinical Characteristics of Patients with 3243 Mutation

Most patients with diabetes associated with the 3243 mutation (Table 66-1) present with the clinical syndrome of non–insulin-dependent diabetes mellitus (NIDDM), although some have insulin-dependent diabetes mellitus (IDDM), that is, ketosis-prone unless treated with insulin. Age of onset is quite variable, ranging from childhood to 60 years of age. Approximately 50% of patients with diabetes associated with the 3243 mutation have a maternal history of diabetes, and some of them also have siblings with the same subtype of diabetes. Although a minor portion of this subtype of diabetes represents acute onset diabetes, which requires insulin treatment, most of the patients show disease of gradual onset and can be treated by diet alone or oral hypoglycemic agents, at least initially. However, many show a progressive decrease in insulin secretory capacity and exacerbation of glucose intolerance, and they eventually need insulin to control their glycemia. Based upon these clinical courses, sometimes patients with this subtype of diabetes can be diagnosed as having secondary sulfonylurea failure or slowly progressive IDDM (SPIDDM). Autoantibodies against islets such as ICA and CAD are usually negative. However, in three patients with the 3243 mutation, low titers of ICA have been identified. Insulin deficiency is a hallmark of this subtype of diabetes. Thus, urinary C-peptide excretion is usually low and sometimes below 20 μg/day. However, unlike in typical IDDM, there is nearly always some residual C-peptide excretion. Diabetic complications such as retinopathy, neuropathy, and nephropathy are often seen, especially in patients in whom glycemic control is poor. It remains unclear whether MIDD patients are more susceptible to diabetic complications when glycemic control is matched with common NIDDM patients. Patients with MIDD often exhibit signs and symptoms of involvement of other organs such as deafness, cardiomyopathy and electrocardiographic changes, neuromuscular problems, and proteinuria, yet rarely show the syndrome of myoencephalopathy with lactic acidosis and stroke-like episodes.

TABLE 66-2. Diagnostic Criteria of Maternally Inherited Diabetes and Deafness

1. Diabetes
2. Maternal inheritance
3. Deafness
4. tRNALeu(UUR) (3243) A→G (3243 base pair mutation)

Definite: 1 + 4 (frequently associated with 2, 3, and a–e)
Probable: 1 + 2 + 2 out of a–e (definite when 4 is confirmed)
1 + 3 + 1 out of a–e (definite when 4 is confirmed)
1 + 2 + 3 (definite when 4 is confirmed)

Suggestive Findings
a. Progressive insulin secretory defect
b. Early onset (<25 yr)
c. Absence of obesity
d. Multiorgan disorder (e.g., electrocardiographic abnormality, neuromuscular signs, proteinuria.)
e. Elevated serum lactate or lactate:pyruvate ratio

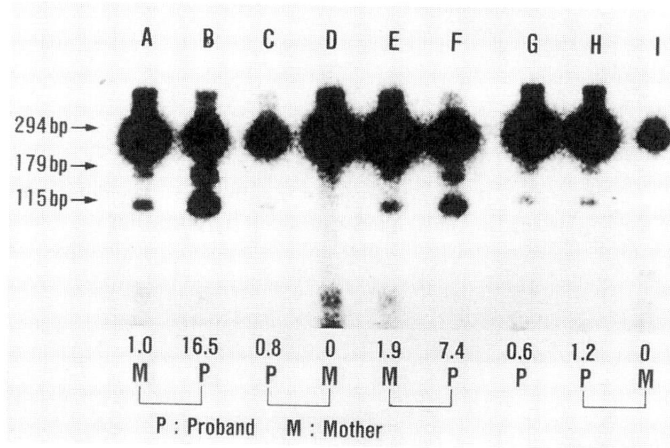

Figure 66-3. Identification of the 3243 mutation using ^{32}P radiolabeled primer. ^{32}P labeled polymerase chain reaction products (294 base pairs) are digested with Apa 1. The presence of mutant mtDNA results in the formation of 182 and 112 base pair fragments.

Diagnosis

Diagnosis of MIDD (Table 66-2) can first be made by major clinical characteristics, that is, diabetes mellitus with maternal inheritance and deafness. Findings such as progressive insulin secretory defects, early onset, absence of obesity, multiorgan disorders, and elevated serum lactate levels are also helpful in the clinical diagnosis. Nevertheless, the final diagnosis should be reserved until the presence of the 3243 mutation is confirmed by molecular diagnosis (Fig. 66-3). There are major pitfalls in the molecular diagnosis of MIDD related to the issue of sensitivity. First, the use of ^{32}P-labeled primer rather than just ethidium bromide staining is required to detect 3243 mutation with low heteroplasmy using peripheral blood leukocytes. Second, if possible and appropriate, other tissues such as muscle and mucosal cells should also be used, since they generally contain higher ratios of mutant mtDNA, especially when the 3243 mutation cannot be detected in patients with all the clinical hallmarks of MIDD. When diabetes is associated with maternal inheritance and deafness but not with the 3243 mutation, duplications, deletions, and other point mutations of mtDNA may be identified. When diabetes is associated with certain clinical characteristics fulfilling the criteria of myoclonus epilepsy with ragged red fibers or the Kearns-Sayre syndrome, a mutation in tRNA^{Lys} 8344 or deletions may be identified. Finally, there are reports describing some patients with Wolfram's syndrome as having mtDNA deletions.[30–36]

Table 66-3. Prevalence of the 3243 Base Pair Mutation

Characteristics of Mutation		Prevalence of 3243 Base Pair
Group I	IDDM/family history (+)	5.5% (3/55)
Group II	NIDDM/family history (+)	2.0% (2/100)
Group III	NIDDM onset <40 yr/ family history (+)	2.4% (5/209)
Group IV	Randomly selected diabetes mellitus	0.9% (5/550)
Group V	Normal glucose tolerance/ family history (−)	0.0% (0/250)

Incidence

A number of diabetic patients with the 3243 mutation have been documented during the short period since the first pedigree with this mutation was reported in 1992. The occurrence of this mutation in diabetic patients has been reported in both randomly selected cohorts and selected cohorts with some clinical characteristics such as a family history of diabetes, young age of onset, the presence of sensory hearing disturbance, insulin treatment, gestational diabetes, and association with myoencephalopathy with lactic acidosis and stroke-like episodes (see Table 66-3).

Pathophysiology of Maternally Inherited Diabetes and Deafness[38–44]

Cells and organs from MIDD contain varying ratios of mutant and WT mtDNA (heteroplasmy), thus making the understanding of the pathogenic mechanism quite complicated. Recently, a method has been developed based upon the transfer of mitochondria from cells of patients with a mitochondrial disease to a human cell line completely lacking mtDNA (^{0}). In this way, stable cell lines can be created that contain various proportions of mutant mtDNA and even cell lines in which nearly all the mtDNA is mutated. Using this method, marked defects in mitochondrial protein synthesis and cell respiration were observed in transformants containing 80–100% mutant DNA either from patients with myoencephalopathy with lactic acidosis and stroke-like episodes or more recently from MIDD patients. It was shown that this mutation is recessive, as defects in mitochondrial function could be rescued by a small proportion of wild-type mtDNAs (>1.0%). In addition, several clonal cell lines containing mixtures of WT and mutant mtDNAs were found to undergo a rapid shift of their genotype toward the pure mutant type in the course of continuous culturing, most likely by the preferential replication of mutant DNA molecules over wild-type molecules.

The 3243 mutation was originally identified in heteroplasmic form in patients with the syndrome of myoencephalopathy with lactic acidosis and stroke-like episodes.[37] It is noteworthy that in the families we studied some of the patients who had the mutation had diabetes (and deafness) without this syndrome and other family members with the mutation had the syndrome without diabetes. Thus, it may be reasonable to conclude that MIDD is not just a mild form of myoencephalopathy with lactic acidosis and stroke-like episodes. Rather, they are two clinically distinct entities with some overlapping. It is tempting to speculate that the fraction of the abnormal mitochondria with the 3243 mutation is relatively high in those tissues implicated in glucose homeostasis such as pancreatic islet cells, liver cells, and skeletal muscle cells in MIDD, whereas it is relatively abundant in nerve and muscle tissues in myoencephalopathy with lactic acidosis and stroke-like episodes. We have extensively studied insulin secretory capacity assessed by the oral glucose tolerance test, the glucagon test, and C-peptide excretion in MIDD. Most if not all patients with MIDD have impaired insulin secretion. The insulin secretory defect probably plays an important role in the pathogenesis of diabetes considering the fact that many patients have decreased insulin secretion even before the development of or at the initial stage of diabetes, and exacerbation of poor diabetes control was almost always accompanied by progressive reduction of endogenous insulin secretory capacity. Euglycemic clamp studies of a very limited number of MIDD patients revealed normal glucose uptake primarily by the muscle. In findings consistent with our results, Reardon and coworkers[11] described two patients with this mutation who had poor insulin secretory responses to glucose. In contrast, van den Ouweland and associates[26] reported that insulin secretion was apparently normal in affected patients, suggesting the pathogenic importance of peripheral insulin resistance. Although it seems likely that the mechanism whereby this mutation causes diabetes can be heteroge-

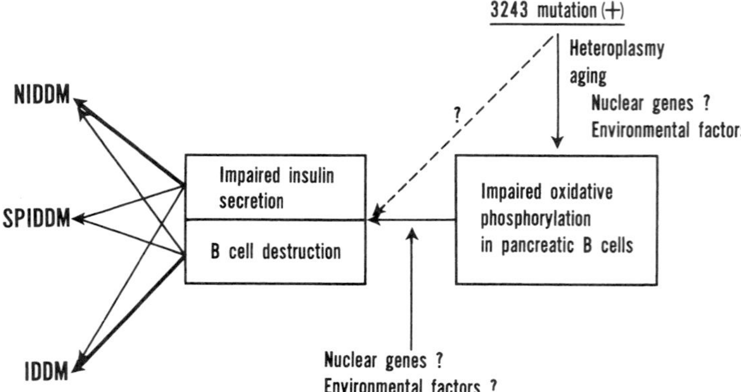

FIGURE 66-4. Pathogenesis of insulin secretory defect and diabetes owing to 3243 mutation (hypothesis).

neous, the vast majority of patients with MIDD have varied degrees of insulin secretory defects.

How might this mutation cause dysfunction of pancreatic β-cells? The 3243 mutation appears to result in a defect in the pathway of glucose metabolism (oxidative phosphorylation) in the pancreatic β-cells that causes a defect in ATP production and insulin secretion (functional defect). Moreover, the presence of MIDD patients who show either secondary failure of sulfonylurea therapy or a clinical phenotype of SPIDDM strongly suggests that a reduction of β-cell mass may also be implicated in the defect in insulin secretion in MIDD patients. In fact, we have recently had the opportunity to carry out a pathohistologic analysis of several autopsy pancreata samples with the 3243 mutation in patients with myoencephalopathy with lactic acidosis and stroke-like episodes. We not only confirmed the presence of the 3243 mutation in the pancreas (in one case in islets) but also observed (1) atrophy of the islets of Langerhans, (2) a reduction in β-cell number, and (3) an occasional reduction in α-cell number. These data are consistent with the hypothesis that the 3243 mutation in the pancreatic β-cells may be associated with a reduction in β-cell mass. Similarly, small islets, together with a relative paucity of β-cells, have also been reported in the pancreas from a patient with Kearns-Sayre syndrome and diabetes requiring insulin therapy. Whether this was caused by autoimmune destruction, or apoptosis, or some other mechanism such as interference with replication remains to be clarified.

Whatever the mechanisms are, as depicted in Figure 66-4, the 3243 mutation may cause impaired insulin secretion by two major mechanisms: (1) impairment of glucose metabolism and glucose signaling in the β-cells, and (2) reduction in β-cell mass. Depending on the severity and predominance of the two major mechanisms, clinical phenotypes may exhibit a wide range of variability from NIDDM and SPIDDM to IDDM.

Acknowledgments

I am indebted to Drs. Hiroko Kadowaki, Kazuki Yasuda, Hiroshi Sakura, Shun-ichi Otabe, Yasumichi Mori, Kazuyuki Tobe, and Yoshio Yazaki for valuable comments in writing this chapter.

References

1. Ashcroft E, Ashcroft S. Mechanisms of insulin secretion. In: Ashcroft F, Ashcroft S, eds. Insulin: Molecular Biology to Toxicology. Oxford: Oxford University Press; 97–150
2. Anderson S, Bankier AT, Barrell BG, et al. Sequence and organization of the human mitochondrial genome. Nature (Lond) 1981;290:457
3. Attardi G, Schatz G. Biogenesis of mitochondria. Annu Rev Cell Biol 1988;4:289
4. Clayton DA. Replication and transcription of vertebrate mitochondrial DNA. Annu Rev Cell Biol 1991;7:453
5. Giles RE, Blanc H, Cann HM, Wallace DC. Maternal inheritance of human mitochondrial DNA. Proc Natl Acad Sci USA 1980;77:6715
6. Wallace DC. Mitochondrial genetics—a paradigm for aging and degenerative diseases. Science 1992;256:628
7. Wallace DC. Diseases of the mitochondrial DNA. Annu Rev Biochem 1992; 61:1175
8. van den Ouweland JMW, Lemkes HHPJ, Ruitenbeck W, et al. Mutation in mitochondrial $tRNA^{Leu(UUR)}$ gene in a large pedigree with maternally transmitted type II diabetes mellitus and deafness. Nature Genet 1992;1:368
9. Ballinger SW, Shoffner JM, Hedaya EV, et al. Maternally transmitted diabetes and deafness associated with a 10.4 kb deletion. Nature Genet 1992;1:11
10. Ballinger SW, Shoffner JM, Gebhart S, et al. Mitochondrial diabetes revisited [letter]. Net Genet 1994;7:458
11. Reardon W, Ross RJM, Sweeney MG, et al. Diabetes mellitus associated with a pathogenic point mutation in mitochondrial DNA. Lancet 1992;340:1376
12. Kadowaki H, Tobe K, Mori Y, et al. Mitochondrial gene mutation and insulin-deficient type of diabetes mellitus. Lancet 1993;341:893
13. Katagiri H, Asano T, Yamanouchi T, et al. Glucokinase-defective NIDDM. Lancet 1993;341:961
14. Awata T, Matsumoto T, Iwamoto Y, et al. Japanese case of diabetes mellitus and deafness with mutation in mitochondrial $tRNA^{Leu(UUR)}$ gene. Lancet 1993;341:1291
15. Oka Y, Katagiri H, Yazaki Y, et al. Mitochondrial gene mutation in islet-cell-antibody-positive patients who were initially non-insulin-dependent diabetes. Lancet 1993;342:527
16. Vionnet N, Passa P, Froguel P. Prevalence of mitochondrial gene mutations in families with diabetes-mellitus. Lancet 1993;342:1429
17. Schulz JB, Klockgether T, Dichgans J, et al. Mitochondrial gene mutations and diabetes mellitus. Lancet 1993;341:438
18. Remes AM, Majamaa K, Herva R, Hassinen IE. Adult-onset diabetes mellitus and neurosensory hearing loss in maternal relatives of MELAS patients in a family with the $tRNA^{Leu(UUR)}$ mutation. Neurology 1993;43:1015
19. Onishi H, Inoue K, Osaka H, et al. Mitochondrial myopathy, encephalopathy, lactic acidosis and stroke-like episodes (MELAS) and diabetes mellitus: Molecular genetic analysis and family study. J Neurol Sci 1993;114:205
20. Kadowaki T, Kadowaki H, Mori Y, et al. A subtype of diabetes mellitus associated with a mutation of mitochondrial DNA. N Engl J Med 1994;330:962
21. Katagiri II, Asano T, Ishibarar H, et al. Mitochondrial diabetes mellitus: Prevalence and clinical characterization of diabetes due to mitochondrial $tRNA^{Leu(UUR)}$ gene mutation in Japanese patients. Diabetologia 1994;37:504
22. Suzuki S, Hinokio Y, Hirai S, et al. Pancreatic beta-cell secretory defect associated with mitochondrial point mutation of the tRNALeu(UUR) gene: A study in seven families with mitochondrial encephalomyopathy, lactic acidosis and stroke-like episodes (MELAS). Diabetologia 1994;37:818
23. Otabe S, Sakura H, Shimokawa K, et al. The high prevalence of diabetic patients with a mutation in the mitochondrial gene in Japan. J Clin Endocrinol Metab 1994;79:768
24. Kishimoto M, Hashiramoto M, Araki S, et al. Diabetes mellitus carrying a mutation in the mitochondrial tRNALeu(UUR) gene. Diabetologia 1995;37: 193
25. Sue CM, Holmes Walker DJ, et al. Mitochondrial gene mutations and diabetes mellitus. Lancet 1993;341:437
26. van den Ouweland JMW, Lemkes HHPJ, Trembath RC, et al. Maternally inherited diabetes and deafness is a distinct subtype of diabetes and associates with a single point mutation in the mitochondrial $tRNA^{Leu(UUR)}$ gene. Diabetes 1994;43:746
27. Gerbitz KD, Paprotta A, Jacsch M, et al. Diabetes mellitus is one of the heterogeneous phenotypic features of a mitochondrial DNA point mutation within the transfer $RNA^{Leu(UUR)}$ gene. FEBS Lett 1993;321:194
28. Odawara M, Sasaki K, Yamasha K. Prevalence and clinical characterization

of Japanese diabetes mellitus with an A to G mutation at nucleotide 3243 of the mitochondrial tRNALeu(UUR) gene. J Clin Endocrinol Metab 1995;80:1290
29. Yanagisawa K, Uchigata Y, Sanaka M, et al. Mutation in the mitochondrial tRNA[Leu] at position 3243 and spontaneous abortions in Japanese women attending a clinic for diabetic pregnancy. Diabetologia 1995;38:809
30. Suzuki S, Hinokio Y, Hirai S, et al. Diabetes with mitochondrial gene tRNA[LYS] mutation. Diabetes Care 1994;17:1428
31. Holt IJ, Harding AE, Morgan-Hughes JA. Deletions of muscle mitochondrial DNA in patients with mitochondrial myopathies. Nature (Lond) 1988;331:717
32. Dunbar DR, Moonie PA, Swingler RJ, et al. Maternally transmitted partial direct tandem duplication of mitochondrial DNA associated with diabetes mellitus. Hum Mol Genet 1993;2:1619
33. Rötig A, Cormier V, Chatelain P, et al. Deletion of mitochondrial DNA in a case of early-onset diabetes mellitus, optic atrophy, and deafness (Wolfram syndrome, MIM 222300). J Clin Invest 1993;91:1095
34. Rötig A, Bessis J-L, Romero N, et al. Maternally inherited duplication of the mitochondrial genome in a syndrome of proximal tubulopathy, diabetes mellitus, and cerebellar ataxia. Am J Hum Genet 1992;50:364
35. Shoffner JM, Lott MT, Lezza AMS, et al. Myoclonic epilepsy and ragged-red fiber disease (MERRF) is associated with a mitochondrial tRNAlys mutation. Cell 1990;61:931
36. Tanabe Y, Miyamoto S, Kinoshita Y, et al. Diabetes mellitus in Kearns-Sayre syndrome. Eur Neurol 1988;28:34
37. Goto Y, Nonaka I, Horai S. A mutation in the tRNA[Leu(UUR)] gene associated with the MELAS subgroup of mitochondrial encephalomyopathies. Nature 1990;348:651
38. King MP, Koga Y, Davidson M, Schon EA. Defects in mitochondrial protein synthesis and respiratory chain activity segregate with the tRNA[Leu(UUR)] mutation associated with mitochondrial transcription termination by a point mutation associated with the MELAS subgroup of mitochondrial encephalomyopathies. Nature (Lond) 1991;351:236
39. Hess JF, Parisi MA, Bennett JL, Clayton DA. Implement of mitochondrial transcription termination by a point mutation associated with the MELAS subgroup of mitochondrial encephalomyopathies. Nature (Lond) 1991;351:236
40. Chomyn A, Martinuzzi A, Yoneda M, et al. MELAS mutation in mt DNA binding site for transcription termination factor causes defects in protein synthesis and in respiration but no change in levels of upstream and downstream mature transcripts. Proc Natl Acad Sci USA 1992;89:4221
41. Bindoff LA, Howell N, Pulton J, et al. Abnormal RNA processing associated with a novel transfer RNA mutation in mitochondrial DNA—a potential disease mechanism. J Biol Chem 1993;268:19559
42. Poulton J, O'Rahilly S, Morten KJ, Clark A. Mitochondrial DNA, diabetes and pancreatic pathology in Kearns-Sayre syndrome. Diabetologia 1995;38:868
43. Gerbitz K-D. Does the mitochondrial DNA play a role in the pathogenesis of diabetes? Diabetologia 1992;35:1181
44. Alcolado JC, Alcolado R. Importance of maternal history of non-insulin dependent diabetic patients. Br Med J 1991;302:1178

Diabetes Mellitus, edited by Derek LeRoith, Simeon I. Taylor, and Jerrold M. Olefsky. Lippincott–Raven Publishers, Philadelphia © 1996.

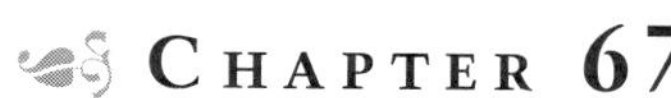

Chapter 67

Primate Animal Models of Non–Insulin-Dependent Diabetes Mellitus

Barbara Hansen

The extraordinary similarity of spontaneous non–insulin-dependent diabetes (NIDDM) in monkeys to that in humans, together with the unique advantages of constant and identifiable environmental features and a shorter life span for monkeys, has made possible many insights into the human condition through the study of nonhuman primates. For example, the rapid 10- to 14-minute periodicity in the secretion of insulin under basal conditions was first discovered in monkeys and later identified in humans, and in both species the deterioration of this oscillatory secretory pattern has been identified under early diabetic conditions. Further, longitudinal studies of monkeys have provided the clearest vision of the natural history and the earliest phases in the development of NIDDM,[1] and such studies have provided the basis for a long-term successful trial to prevent NIDDM in monkeys through the prevention of obesity.[2] A diabetes prevention program is now under way in human subjects, and the outcomes, predicted on the basis of the nonhuman primate data, are likely to be directly related to the success in obtaining a minimal but important degree of weight reduction and the sustaining of that weight loss by continued calorie restraint.[3] Finally, nonhuman primates have provided and continue to provide unique opportunities to examine the basic physiologic, biochemical, and molecular bases of insulin resistance, obesity, diabetes, and the associated metabolic syndrome.

Definition of Non–Insulin-Dependent Diabetes Mellitus in Monkeys

Obesity-associated NIDDM (type II or type 2) develops spontaneously during adulthood in nonhuman primates, and both the form of this diabetes and its associated metabolic disorders provide ample evidence that this is the same disease that most commonly develops in humans.[1,4–7] The use of either the National Diabetes Data Group's (NDDG)[8] or the World Health Organization's (WHO)[9] definitions of impaired glucose tolerance and overt NIDDM provides an accurate but very conservative description of diabetes in nonhuman primates. Since normal young lean monkeys typically have fasting glucose levels that are about 20 mg/dL lower than those found in similarly normal humans, it is possible that the "onset" of NIDDM could be defined by somewhat lower thresholds than those currently accepted for application to humans in clinical settings.

In monkeys, the availability of data from prospective longitudinal studies makes it possible to identify those animals that are progressing toward the overt disease well before these traditional diagnostic thresholds are reached. Examination of the prodrome leading to overt diabetes in monkeys provides many lessons for application to the evaluation and clinical management of diabetes in humans.

The subsequent sections consider the current state of understanding of obesity-associated NIDDM in nonhuman primates as well as of the metabolic or insulin resistance syndrome and examine the effects of long-term efforts that have successfully prevented the development of the disease. The relevance of these prevention studies to the worldwide epidemic of diabetes is clear.

Comparison of Non–Insulin-Dependent Diabetes Mellitus in Humans and Monkeys

Over the past 20 years, numerous cases of the spontaneous occurrence of NIDDM in nonhuman primates have been reported. Species in which adult-onset diabetes has been clearly documented include *Macaca mulatta* (rhesus monkey), *Papio hamadryas* (sacred baboon), *Macaca nemestrina* (pig-tailed macaque monkey), *Macaca fascicularis* (cynomolgus or crab-eating macaque), *Sanguinis oedipus* (tamarin), *Saimiri sciureus* (squirrel monkey), *Pan troglodytes* (chimpanzee), and many others as reviewed previously.[7] These case reports as well as the data derived from the reported longitudinal studies of middle-aged and aging rhesus monkeys are sufficient to identify the common features of this disease as it is manifest in nonhuman primates.[10–12] The complications of NIDDM that have been identified in nonhuman primates include retinopathy,[13] nephropathy,[14] and neuropathy.[15] Gestational diabetes has also been reported in nonhuman primates.[16] NIDDM develops spontaneously not only in laboratory housed nonhuman primates but also in free-ranging monkeys.[17,18] Table 67-1 identifies the usual clinical features and the frequently associated risk factors for NIDDM in monkeys; these are clearly the same as those found in the most common form of diabetes in humans.

Although direct comparison of the prevalence of diabetes in nonhuman primates with that in humans is difficult, we would estimate that among rhesus monkeys maintained under ad libitum feeding conditions in the protective environment of a laboratory and with optimal health care, possibly 50% would become diabetic at some point in their lives. In a group of longitudinally studied rhesus monkeys, we identified the earliest age of onset as 10 years, and the oldest monkey to become diabetic while under study was 29 years old. (The age of onset was defined using the human NDDG or WHO criteria or the age at which fasting glucose levels remained above 140 mg/dL.) We have found that in monkeys, as in various human populations, the prevalence of NIDDM increases with age. Figure 67-1 provides our best estimate of the prevalence of diabetes in monkeys compared with published reports of various human populations.[19,20]

Table 67-1. Clinical Features of Non–Insulin-Dependent Diabetes in Monkeys (*Macaca mulatta*)

Obesity with central distribution
"Middle age" adult onset
Polyphagia
Polydipsia
Polyuria with glycosuria
Hyperglycemia
Proteinuria
Hypertriglyceridemia
Reduced high-density lipoprotein cholesterol
Hypertension
Complications including neuropathy, nephropathy, and retinopathy

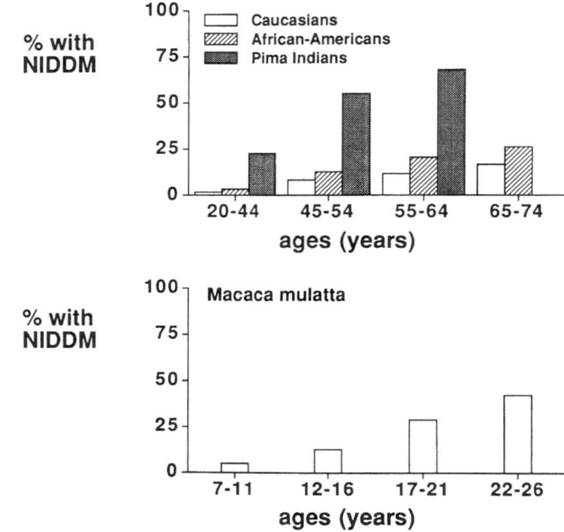

Figure 67-1. Estimates of the prevalence of NIDDM in several human populations and in rhesus monkeys (Data compiled from references 56–58 and personal unpublished laboratory data.)

The Structure of Insulin and the Insulin Receptor in Monkeys

As shown in Table 67-2, monkeys have significantly higher circulating insulin levels than humans. This four- to ten-fold increase is not caused by an insulin molecule difference, since the sequence of monkey insulin has been previously shown to be identical to that of human insulin.[21] Monkey proinsulin has been shown to have a single amino acid substitution in the C-peptide portion, but this does not interfere with the C-peptide assay.[22] We have also not found a disproportionate amount of proinsulin in the circulation of monkeys.

The insulin receptor structure and/or postreceptor factors could be involved in the relatively higher insulin resistance in monkeys, as suggested by the relative hyperinsulinemia compared to humans. In the search for the molecular basis of this apparent insulin resistance, we examined the coding region of the insulin receptor gene.[23] As expected, the rhesus insulin receptor gene was found to be highly similar to the human gene, with 98% nucleotide identity and 99% amino acid identity. Nine sites within the receptor gene showed predicted amino acid changes, and these were distributed throughout the receptor. All were conservative changes except for two, a 3 base deletion plus an amino acid substitution between exons 14 and 15 ($Leu^{921}Asp^{922} \rightarrow Tyr^{921}$) and a serine to proline substitution ($Ser^{991} \rightarrow Pro^{991}$). To date neither of these differences has been reported as a mutation in an insulin-resistant patient.

Table 67-2. Comparison of Commonly Observed Fasting Plasma Insulin Levels in Rhesus Monkeys and Humans

	Fasting Insulin (μU/mL)	
	Human	Rhesus
Normal (lean)	1–7	20–70
Obese	10–50	50–500
Diabetic	0–40	2–400

To determine whether either of these mutations could be responsible for the relative insulin resistance of monkeys, site-directed mutagenesis of the wild-type human insulin receptor cDNA was used to introduce these two nonconservative changes, individually and combined, and these cDNAs were stably expressed in NIH3T3 cells. Binding affinities for insulin, basal receptor autophosphorylation, and insulin-stimulated receptor autophosphorylation were not different between the cell lines with the mutated or wild type cDNA.[24] Thus, these two amino acid differences do not appear to be responsible for the relative insulin resistance in monkeys compared with humans.

The insulin receptor mRNA of monkeys, like that of humans, undergoes alternative splicing of exon 11 in the C-terminal α-subunit domain to produce two isoforms. The presence (exon 11+) or absence (exon 11−) of this 12 amino acid residue could play a role in insulin resistance since the exon 11+ isoform binds with twofold lower affinity than the exon 11− isoform. Interestingly, in hyperinsulinemic normoglycemic prediabetic monkeys and in hyperinsulinemic early mild diabetic monkeys the higher affinity exon 11− isoform was expressed in increased percentage in muscle relative to both normal insulinemic and severely diabetic (normoinsulinemic) monkeys.[25] These studies may provide reconciliation of the discrepant views reported for human exon 11 expression in diabetes, since the relative expression levels are normal or increased in diabetes and nondiabetic controls differ depending upon whether or not they are hyperinsulinemic.

Other studies to examine the insulin receptor function in skeletal muscle of monkeys have not identified diabetes-related differences in the expression of IRS-1 or Rad (C.R. Kahn and M. Patti, personal communication 1995), although Rad had previously been identified as a member of the Ras family, which was found to be overexpressed in muscle of diabetic humans.[26] Furthermore, total GLUT-4 glucose transporter was not reduced in diabetic monkeys (personal communication, B. Kahn 1994), a finding consistent with studies in humans. GLUT-4 expression levels may in fact be somewhat increased in prediabetic and diabetic monkeys.[27] Expression of GLUT-5, the facilitative fructose-glucose transporter, showed a significant increase in prediabetic monkeys and returned to normal in overtly diabetic monkeys.[27,28] Defects in insulin action on glycogen synthase and glycogen phosphorylase activity have been identified in monkeys and in humans (see below). The search continues to identify the postreceptor defects associated with insulin resistance and diabetes in monkeys as well as in humans and to identify the genes or gene markers for such defects.

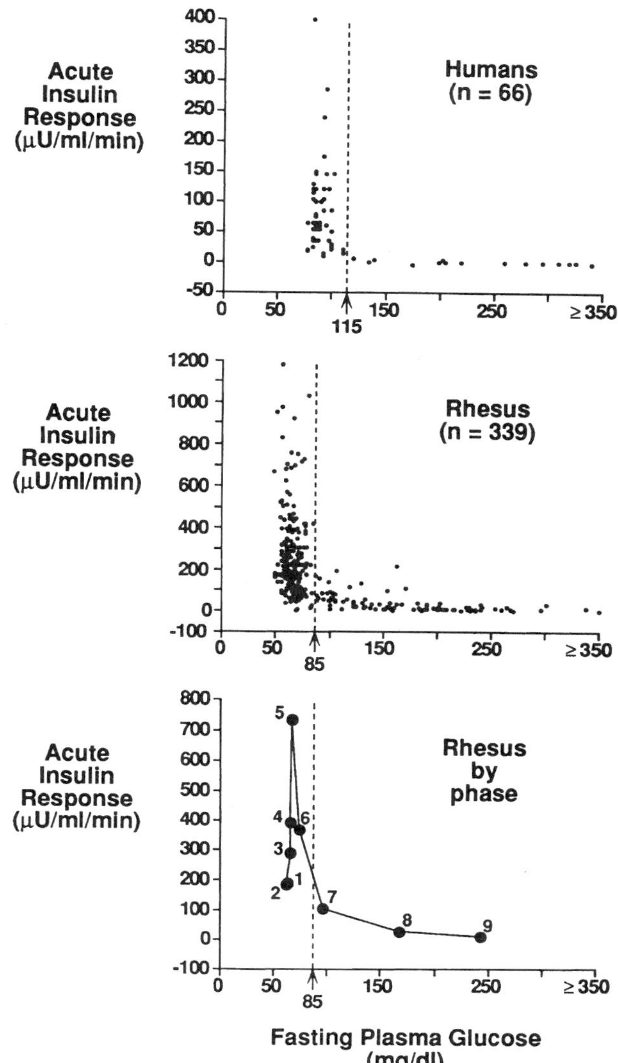

Figure 67-2. Relationship between fasting plasma glucose and the acute insulin response to intravenous glucose in humans and in monkeys. Lower panel shows graphically the longitudinal sequence across time of changes in both variables. In the top panel the vertical line at 115 mg/dL and in the other two panels the lines at 85 mg/dL indicate the fasting glucose levels in humans and monkeys, respectively, above which the acute insulin response to glucose is essentially absent. (Top panel redrawn with permission from Brunzell JD, Robertson RP, Lerner RL, et al. Relationships between fasting plasma glucose levels and insulin secretion during intravenous glucose tolerance tests. J Clin Endocrinol Metab 1976;42:222. Middle panel: extensive data added to and revised from published data.[33])

The Dynamics of Fasting Glucose Levels and Early β-Cell Responses to Glucose

Since the development of the insulin assay, numerous investigators have contemplated the enigmatic relationship between fasting plasma glucose levels and both fasting and glucose-stimulated insulin levels.[29-31] We have examined the changes in these features prospectively and longitudinally in monkeys and have noted the exceedingly early appearance of both fasting hyperinsulinemia and β-cell hyper-responsiveness.[5]

More recently attention has been focused on the possibility that elevated glucose levels or glucose toxicity might be responsible for the falling phase or deterioration in β-cell response. In Figure 67-2 data previously published for humans[29] have been redrawn for comparison with the data from rhesus monkeys.[5] Several features should be noted. First, the fasting plasma glucose levels of 65 to 70 mg/dL in normal monkeys (numbered 1 and 2 in the lower panel of the figure) are comparable to fasting glucose levels of 85 to 90 mg/dL in humans. Second, both the basal insulin levels and the insulin responses to glucose are significantly higher in monkeys across the entire range compared with humans. Nevertheless, the pattern of progression, clearly documented in the bottom panel for monkeys, appears to be the same for humans. Also, consistently, the threshold for increasing fasting glucose level, above which the acute response of the β-cell to glucose is absent, is 115 mg/dL in humans and 85 mg/dL in monkeys. It would thus be appropriate to define the diabetes-onset threshold for monkeys at 120 mg/dL. Note, however, that for consistency we have retained the more conservative definition, as noted above, and used the human diagnostic threshold of 140 mg/dL.

Once a monkey's fasting glucose level rises above 85 mg/dL, it is clearly en route to diabetes and the same is undoubtedly true for humans at the threshold of 115 mg/dL (provided that the blood sample has been obtained under optimal conditions to ensure a consistent duration of fasting and basal sampling conditions).

Pancreatic β-Cell Dysfunction: A Late Event Immediately Preceding Overt Diabetes

Despite recent suggestions that defects in β-cell function are among the earliest events identified in individuals with increased familial predisposition to diabetes,[32] data from longitudinal studies of monkeys clearly show that reduced first- and second-phase insulin secretion are late developments in the prodrome to diabetes, occurring only in the immediate prediabetic or early diabetic state.[5] The discrepancies between the inferences drawn from studies of humans, such as the one noted above, and the results in monkeys appear to be due to the cross-sectional nature of those human studies and to the selection of a ''matched'' control group that was probably immediately adjacent to the prediabetic group in the continuum leading to diabetes and therefore not statistically differentiated one from the other.

The Natural History of the Prodrome of Overt Diabetes

It should be remembered that the definition of diabetes in humans is one which was developed by consensus to provide for comparability of different groups in diagnosis and treatment. The definition even today is not based on causal mechanisms but rather serves to identify a treatment-prescribing threshold. More clinicians are beginning to recognize that the 140 mg/dL threshold may be higher than necessary for the start of treatment and that lower thresholds for intervention may indeed be in the patient's best interest. The question is, when can an individual be defined with a fair degree of accuracy to have diabetes? Although social and financial issues may argue for a conservative or delayed diagnosis, treatment or mitigation may be more effective if instituted earlier. What can nonhuman primates tell us about the longitudinal trajectory and the potential for intervention at various phases along the progression of the disease?

The life span of the rhesus monkey is about one-third that of humans, and the peak age of onset of diabetes in the monkey appears to be about 18 years old compared to about 45–50 years of age in humans. Thus, longitudinal studies of the development of diabetes are far easier to complete in monkeys. Furthermore, the environment is held constant, essentially for a lifetime, including provision of a constant diet and constant lifestyle, thus greatly facilitating the examination of longitudinal data under consistent conditions and stable protocols.

In 1985 we reported the results of a then 6-year study of rhesus monkeys in which 26 animals had shown progression toward or developed overt diabetes using the human criteria.[33] That study showed that the progressive development of hyperglycemia took place 3 to 5 years after the initial observation of β-cell hyperresponsiveness and that the loss of first-phase insulin release was a very late occurrence, immediately preceding gradual reduction in fasting insulin toward normal levels and reduction in insulin responsiveness to subnormal levels at the time the final phase of overt diabetes was reached. We concluded then that the apparent heterogeneity in the features of early or pre-NIDDM patients is actually a result of the multiple distinct phases in the longitudinal development of the disease in humans. Evidence did not suggest either incipient hyperglycemia or deficient insulin secretion as the initial event but showed β-cell hyper-responsiveness to a glucose stimulus as preceding other abnormalities.[33]

In the 10 years since that report additional details have been identified, but the basic process and the prodrome to diabetes have been confirmed again and again in monkeys.[1,5,34] The cumulative evidence from longitudinal studies of various groups of humans, particularly those at high risk for the development of the disease, appears to be entirely consistent with the nonhuman primate-delineated progression. Furthermore, earlier cross-sectional data on groups of human subjects were suggestive of the same progressive processes.[30] Indeed, the report in Pima Indians of a bimodal distribution of fasting glucose[35] is precisely what would be expected if this group, as subsequently shown, moved through the same progressive process, with any one individual spending only a brief time in the transitional phase of elevated glucose levels in the 115–140 mg/dL range prior to the development of overt diabetes.

We originally defined eight phases in the continuum from lean young normal to overt diabetes[1] and have subsequently modified this to include a ninth phase (the latter useful in separating advanced severe diabetes from the early mild or moderate diabetes [phase eight]). The longitudinal progression for each of eight variables is shown in Figure 67-3.

Phase one represents the most normal condition and is limited to young (<9 year old) monkeys with normal glucose, normal glucose tolerance, and normal fasting plasma insulin levels. Phase two includes normoglycemic and normoinsulinemic monkeys over the age of 9 years. They may be lean or somewhat obese, but in all diabetes-related respects they are normal. Phase three monkeys are in transition to hyperinsulinemia (defined retrospectively after a monkey reaches a statistically significant rise in fasting insulin level above the levels of lean young normal monkeys). Phase four monkeys are obese and hyperinsulinemic, with normoglycemia and normal glucose tolerance. Phase five constitutes progressive hyperinsulinemia and progressive β-cell hyperresponsiveness (increasing acute insulin response to glucose). In phase six, the highest levels of fasting plasma insulin are observed concomitant with a decline in acute insulin release—although on average it is still well above normal levels of response. Although on average glucose tolerance falls gradually throughout the progression to diabetes, both inter- and intra-animal variability make it difficult to discern the fall in tolerance within an individual until about phase seven. Phase seven provides the first statistically significant reduction in glucose tolerance (glucose disappearance rate as measured by the intravenous glucose tolerance test). During phase seven the acute insulin response to glucose declines toward negligible and the fasting plasma glucose shows its first statistically significant rise. Progressively and gradually, such monkeys move toward phase eight. We have defined phase eight as that point and beyond when a monkey reaches the NDDG definition for obesity-associated type II NIDDM, with fasting plasma glucose levels consistently above 140 mg/dL.[8] Phase nine monkeys are severely diabetic and if untreated have glucose levels >220 mg/dL, elevated hepatic glucose production,[4] and normal or somewhat subnormal insulin levels.

Hypertriglyceridemia and reduced high-density lipoprotein cholesterol concentrations develop gradually across the phases, but both become most evident as diabetes becomes overt. Hypertension develops in prediabetic and diabetic animals, but no direct association with these phases could be discerned.

The development of the conceptual approach (in which the phase of progression can be defined for any monkey at any time) was essential to the ability to pool data across monkeys during the progressive process. The reason for this is that monkeys, like humans, begin their progression toward overt diabetes at varying adult ages and progress at varying rates. Ultimately they develop diabetes which varies in severity or at least in the rate of progression of the disease to a severe state (not all reach severe diabetes before death). In the past, humans on this continuum have most often been grouped as normal, obese hyperinsulinemic, impaired glucose tolerant, and diabetic. It is clear, however, that clinical studies in

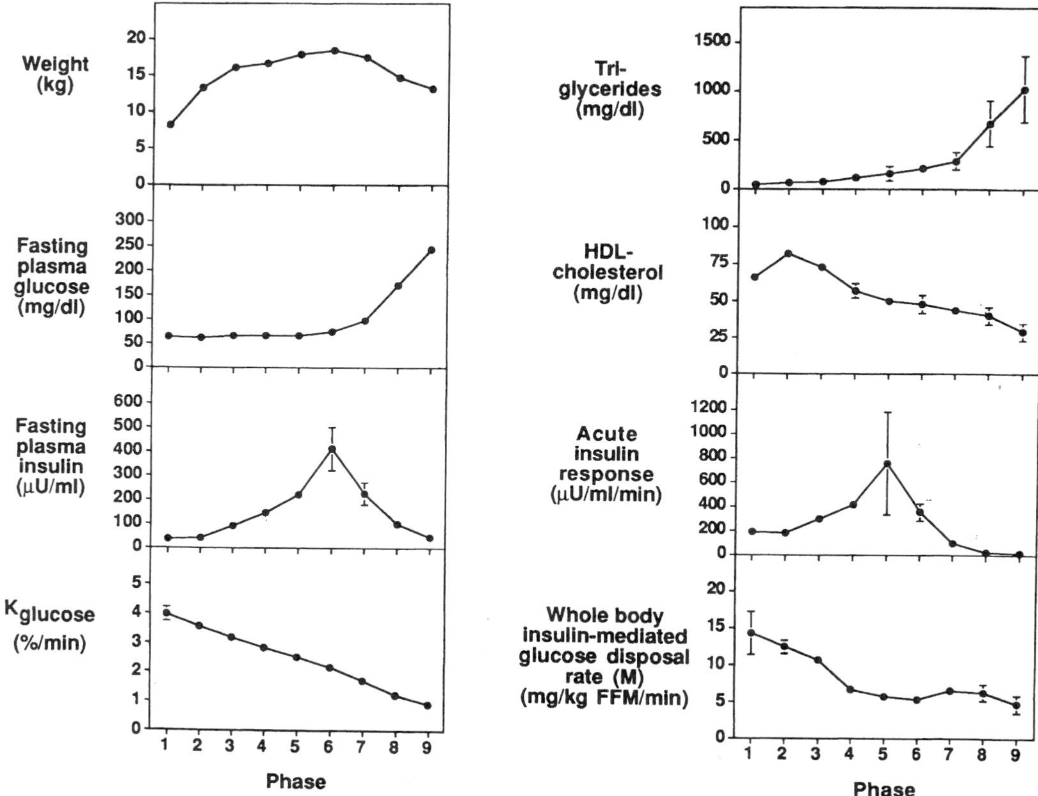

FIGURE 67-3. Nine phases in the continuum progressing from lean young normal monkeys (phase one) to severe diabetes (phase 2). (See text for details of the intervening phases.)

humans would greatly benefit from a finer gradation of stages or phases in the progression of disease so as to examine mechanisms in more homogenous subgroups. These criteria are likely to be very similar to those we have used to "phase" the development of disease in monkeys. We prefer the term "phase" to "stage" because phase better represents the very continuous nature of this progressive set of processes.

As Granner and O'Brien have noted,[36] the molecular physiology and genetics of NIDDM will become much clearer when appropriate identification of criteria for defining the temporal sequence of events in the pathophysiology of diabetes is accomplished for humans as has been done for monkeys. This becomes increasingly possible as long trains of in vivo data become available for within subject analysis of the sequence of events. Anything less will continue to result in murky interpretations of the presence of absence of various defects, as failure to phase produces unnecessary and inappropriate heterogeneity in data and makes interpretation suspect. We have used our understanding of the phases in the progression to diabetes to consider the likely genetics of NIDDM and the possible contributions of major and minor genes.

The Genes for Non–Insulin-Dependent Diabetes Mellitus: An Age-of-Onset Gene Modifying a Major Gene Effect?

As might be evident from the wide range of age of onset of NIDDM in both humans and monkeys, there is clearly a strong age-of-onset gene that interacts with the major diabetes gene(s). There is no evidence in monkeys to support any environmental factor as the determinant of age of onset (other than calorie availability). Those individuals programmed for the latest age of onset are clearly the least likely to have an informative family history. (Parents' diabetes status could be unknown at time of death, especially some 50+ years ago; or they may have died too early for the gene to be fully expressed, resulting in overt NIDDM; or they were more frequently underdiagnosed—probably by even more than the present estimates of 50% of cases undiagnosed.

Some have suggested that this wide range of age of onset for NIDDM is evidence for heterogeneity in the underlying disease itself, or, alternatively, is evidence for a differential impact of environmental factors in different individuals. Neither of these positions appears to be substantially supported by the nonhuman primate data. While allowing that both factors—different environments and genetic heterogeneity—may contribute in small ways to the so-called heterogeneity of NIDDM, we are convinced by all of the primate data that there is a basic unified mechanism of defective regulation that is likely to be held in common by upward of 90% of all individuals with NIDDM.

This is somewhat contrary to the multiple gene position most commonly assumed at this time, when so many candidate genes have been examined and either ruled out or believed to account for only a tiny segment of the diabetic population.

Where Shall We Look for the Major Gene for Non–Insulin-Dependent Diabetes Mellitus?

What is it about our studies of nonhuman primates and our evaluation of the published studies of humans that has led us to predict a major gene effect underlying the vast majority of NIDDM? Where is that defect likely to be located and what is its primary effect?

The longitudinal picture of the development of diabetes in monkeys seems to have extraordinary consistency across animals that have been studied long enough and frequently enough to be able to discern a sequence of biologic changes.

That pattern has almost invariably been shown to be initiated with an increase in basal circulating plasma insulin level and an increase in β-cell responsiveness to glucose. Thus, one could conclude that the β-cell defect comes first, but in contrast to the report of Pimenta and coworkers[32] mentioned earlier and of others who have focused on the already obese subject, this defect is *not* a deterioration in β-cell function or structure (e.g., amyloid deposition) but is instead an exaggerated hyperfunctionality! The decline of insulin output in response to glucose has been well recognized for most of the 30 years since the insulin assay was developed. Yet today few focus on the early cause of the exaggerated insulin output. In part, this may arise from the presumption that the rise in insulin is a result of compensation for growing insulin resistance at the periphery. Several lines of evidence from nonhuman primates (and these are not in disagreement with the available data from humans) argue against that scenario. First, although in intermittent longitudinal data it is exceedingly difficult to discern the moment at which plasma insulin levels begin to rise or the β-cell hyper-responsiveness to glucose begins, both are clearly very early events.[33] What, in turn, might make the β-cell hypersensitive? The time course of the exaggerated response (1 to 3 minutes after intravenous glucose load) makes it unlikely that failure of the periphery to take up glucose or resistance of muscle to the action of insulin could be feeding back upon the β-cell to produce the altered response.

It is clear that this exaggerated response takes place when plasma glucose levels are entirely normal and when glucose tolerance is fully normal. These, the likely means by which a peripheral insulin sensitivity defect could feed back to increase β-cell function, are quite simply normal. Increasing insulin levels themselves, if altering β-cell function, would be likely to reduce, not increase β-cell output.

What Controls the Exaggerated β-Cell Output?

What other controls of β-cell function could be amiss at the earliest identifiable point in the progression toward diabetes? Noninsulin hormones to which the β-cell is sensitive could be increased or decreased; however, to date, no changes in either regulatory or counter-regulatory hormones have been observed at this early phase. Neural input to the β-cell seems to be a highly probable candidate for early involvement in determining the tonic β-cell output and for altering its sensitivity to stimuli.

Jeanrenaud and colleagues have pointed to the central nervous system as a likely culprit in the dysregulation of the pancreatic β-cell.[37] Indeed, long ago it was noted that ventromedial lesions of the hypothalamus in rodents and in primates resulted in immediate release of the β-cell from its tonic inhibition, producing immediate hyperinsulinemia and β-cell hyper-responsiveness. Hyperinsulinemia, in turn, has been shown to result in the increase in body weight and obesity that are hallmarks of ventromedial lesions of the hypothalamus. Whether the same factors are operative in the earliest phases of NIDDM is not yet know, however, these arguments provide evidence in favor of a central neural origin for the earliest phases of altered β-cell function.

Why Does the β-Cell Fail?

What causes the β-cell failure without which diabetes does not ensue?[38]

A number of hypotheses have been considered. β-cells, in their heightened "revved-up" state after a prolonged period, might simply "exhaust" themselves. This β-cell exhaustion theory would suggest that the higher the insulin levels and the longer they are elevated, the more likely it is that β-cell failure will develop. This proposition finds some support across both human and monkey data sets. Primate data do not, however, support a simple exhaustion hypothesis, since those that develop greater degrees of hyperinsulinemia do not develop diabetes earlier. Certainly, however, those with longstanding hyperinsulinemia are more likely to develop diabetes than those with recent-onset hyperinsulinemia. This, however, reflects the fact that diabetes usually develops slowly over a long period of time. Unfortunately, in cross-sectional data with humans it is very difficult to differentiate those individuals who are in the insulinemia-increasing phases from those in the insulinemia-declining phases and therefore it is difficult to examine the β-cell exhaustion hypothesis. Longitudinal data certainly help in this respect, as shown in the data of Saad and colleagues[39] wherein trains of data or segments from different individuals could be pieced together to show the entire progressive process in Pima Indians. They showed the progression in this group to be very similar to what occurred in the longitudinal studies published 10 years ago in nonhuman primates[2] and in an ongoing series of updates as summarized earlier in Figure 67-3.

The tipping over "Starling's curve of the pancreas" was identified in monkeys[33] and was labeled by DeFronzo[38] who was able to discern in mostly cross-sectional data from humans many of the same sequential features. What, indeed, is responsible for the tipping over or falling off of both basal fasting insulin levels and insulin output in response to glucose? The glucose sensor of the β-cell provides an interesting candidate for an induced or late-onset defect. To date, however, evidence is scant for a major role of defective β-cell glucose sensors in the declining β-cell function.

Islet-Associated Polypeptide and β-Cell Dysfunction

Hyalinization of the islets of Langerhans has long been recognized as characteristic of diabetes.[40] Since the purification and characterization of the 37 amino acid peptide that forms the amyloid fibrils of the amyloid deposits,[41] the possibility that this islet-associated polypeptide (IAPP, amylin) might be involved in the pathogenesis of NIDDM has been vigorously examined. In monkeys with the physiologic characteristics of prediabetes, immunoreactive IAPP was found radially arranged in some islets; however, amyloid occupied less than 30% of the islet mass.[42] In a cross-sectional study of physiologically characterized monkeys, the islet size was larger in prediabetic and diabetic monkeys and the mean β-cell area per islet was increased in the hyperinsulinemic prediabetic monkeys but reduced in the diabetic monkeys.[43] Small deposits of amyloid were identified in 7 of 13 monkeys over the age of 15, and in the 6 who were clearly prediabetic, amyloid occupied up to 45% of the islet space. In these monkeys there were, however, significant numbers of functioning β-cells, judging by the high circulating insulin levels. Eight out of eight diabetic animals had amyloid present in the islets, with the amyloid occupying between 37 and 81% of the islet area. Thus, IAPP appears to play a role in the deterioration of β-cell function, is present to some degree before the development of overt diabetes, and could play a physiologic role in the loss of β-cell function in the prodrome to diabetes. Nevertheless, gross destruction of the β-cell mass does not appear to account for the declining insulin levels and absent insulin response. Efforts to understand the physiologic role of circulating IAPP, possible local effects, and the pathophysiologic role of IAPP deposition continue.

In Vivo Insulin Resistance and Defects in Insulin Action

The euglycemic hyperinsulinemic clamp procedure has been used to examine the whole-body insulin-mediated defects in glucose uptake in diabetes and in its prodrome. In monkeys, as in humans, in the latter stages of the disease, when impaired glucose tolerance was present, the progression to overt diabetes resulted in little further change in the already significantly impaired insulin-stimulated glucose uptake rate; however, the hepatic glucose production rate began to increase.[4] Thus, in more severe diabetes, insulin failed to suppress hepatic glucose production, even under supramaximal insulin stimulation. Resistance to the action of insulin at the liver has thus been clearly demonstrated; however, no evidence points to this as an early defect, and it is most likely a consequence of other diabetes-related disorders.

Table 67-3 summarizes the apparent defects in insulin secretion and in insulin action that have been identified in monkeys.

The apparent resistance to insulin at the periphery (assumed to be principally at the skeletal muscle because of the predominant role of muscle in glucose uptake under insulin-stimulated conditions) is the target of much investigation at the cellular, biochemical, and molecular levels. Reduced glycogen formation and glycogen synthase activity have been clearly demonstrated in both humans with diabetes[44] and in monkeys with diabetes.[45] Basal glycogen synthase activity was reduced in hyperinsulinemic monkeys,[46] and insulin stimulation produced a lower increase in activity compared to normals.[45] This later defect was evident during the same period that β-cell response to glucose was highly exaggerated (see Fig. 67-3).[45] As shown in Figure 67-4, there was a significant relationship between whole-body insulin-mediated glucose uptake as determined by the euglycemic hyperinsulinemic clamp and the effect of insulin on activating glycogen synthase in muscle biopsies obtained before and during the clamp.[45]

In diabetic monkeys, basal synthase levels returned to normal from the lower levels during the hyperinsulinemic phase; however, insulin failed to activate glycogen synthase and muscle glycogen levels were reduced. Insulin-resistant and diabetic monkeys also had higher muscle glucose-6-phosphate concentrations compared with normal monkeys.[46]

Table 67-3. Insulin Sensitivity and Insulin Secretory Defects in Non–Insulin-Dependent Diabetes Mellitus in Monkeys (*Macaca mulatta*)

Impaired Insulin Action
Reduced glucose oxidation (adipocyte)
Decreased lipid synthesis (adipocyte)
Reduced insulin binding (adipocyte)
Reduced whole body glucose uptake
Failure to suppress hepatic glucose production (late)
Reduced in vivo activation of glycogen synthase in muscle and adipose tissue
Increased muscle glucose-6-phosphate
Defects in Insulin Secretion
Insulin molecule normal and identical to human
Hyperinsulinemia (early)
β-Cell hyper-responsiveness to glucose (increased acute insulin release) (early)
β-Cell unresponsiveness to glucose (late)
Dysregulation of the oscillatory control of basal insulin secretion
Amyloid deposition (IAPP, amylin) (late)
β-Cell number depletion (late)
Insulin clearance reduced only during hyperinsulinemia

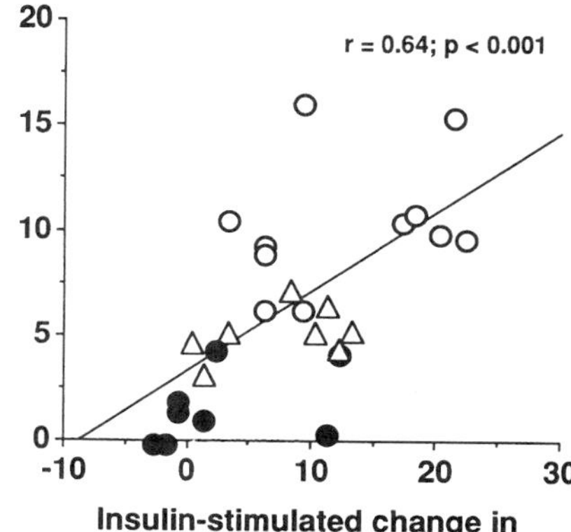

Figure 67-4. The relationship between whole-body insulin-mediated glucose disposal rate (M rate) and the insulin-stimulated change in skeletal muscle glycogen synthase fractional velocity in normal (*open circles*), hyperinsulinemic prediabetic (*triangles*), and diabetic (*closed circles*) monkeys. FFM = Fat free mass. (Redrawn with permission from Ortmeyer HK, Bodkin NL, Hansen BC. Insulin-mediated glycogen synthase activity in muscle of spontaneously insulin-resistant and diabetic rhesus monkeys. Am J Physiol 1993;266:R552.)

These observations made the glycogen synthase gene a prime candidate for involvement in skeletal muscle insulin resistance. However, despite early positive suggestive evidence, a mutation in the glycogen synthase gene does not appear to be involved in the defect in glycogen synthesis.[47] Other biochemical and genetic bases are being sought to explain the impaired activation of glycogen synthase by insulin.[48]

Prevention of Obesity Prevents Non–Insulin-Dependent Diabetes Mellitus and Alters Insulin Action and Glycogen Metabolism

In a long-term study of the effects of chronic calorie restriction on monkeys, a group of adult monkeys, upon reaching the age of approximately 10 years (equivalent to about 25 years in humans), were placed on a protocol in which their caloric intake was restricted to that required to maintain normal body weight and to prevent weight gain and obesity. This study, which has been ongoing for more than 10 years, has shown that in preventing obesity, we have prevented the development of overt NIDDM in these monkeys.[1] They are now at a point when about half of the ad libitum fed monkeys would be obese and diabetic; yet, none of the restricted animals has shown any hyperglycemia or glucose intolerance.[1] Insulin sensitivity, as measured by the euglycemic hyperinsulinemic clamp, has been shown to be significantly better in these animals than in an age-matched ad libitum fed comparison group.[49] Interestingly, the chronic calorie restriction process (even though it acts to maintain adult body weight and excellent health) has uncovered substantial effects on glycogen metabolism and possible inherent defects within some of the restricted animals.[50]

Comparison of the group of calorie-restricted monkeys to three other ad libitum fed groups, a normal group, an insulin-resistant group, and a group with overt NIDDM is shown in Figure 67-5, using data compiled from several studies.[45,46,50,51]

Basal glycogen synthase activity was significantly higher in the calorie-restricted group than in the others. Insulin, which clearly

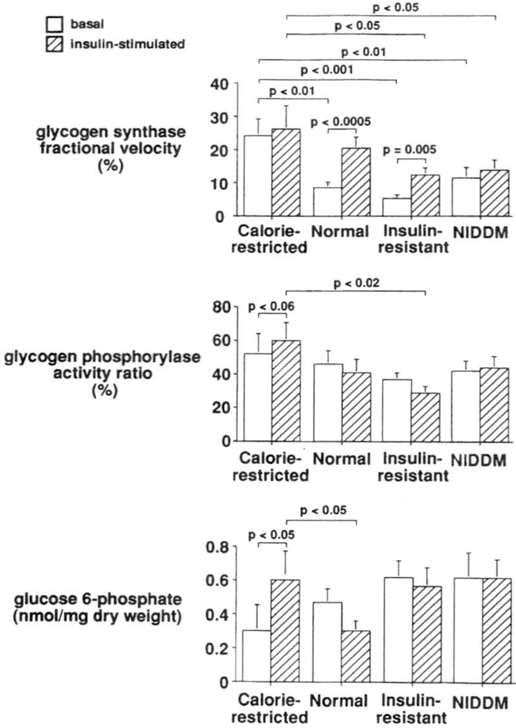

FIGURE 67-5. Comparison of basal (*solid bars*) and insulin-stimulated (*hatched bars*) glycogen synthase fractional velocity, glycogen phosphorylase activity ratio, and glucose-6-phosphate concentration in muscle of four groups of monkeys. Chronically calorie-restricted nonobese adult monkeys are compared with normal adult monkeys, insulin-resistant monkeys, and monkeys with NIDDM. (Data compiled from Ortmeyer et al.[45,46,50,51])

increased glycogen synthase activity in the normal group, had less effect on the insulin-resistant group and no effect on the NIDDM group or the calorie-restricted group. Insulin tended to inhibit glycogen phosphorylase activity in the normal and insulin-resistant groups, had no effect on the NIDDM group, and tended to stimulate glycogen phosphorylase activity in the calorie-restricted group. Finally, as shown in the bottom panel of Figure 67-5, whereas the normal group showed a decrease in glucose-6-phosphate concentration with insulin stimulation (in accord with the stimulation of glycogen synthase activation), the calorie-restricted group, already in a state with maximally active glycogen synthase, showed a significant increase in insulin-stimulated glucose-6-phosphate concentration, probably owing to the failure of glucose to move to glycogen. It is clear from these studies that the process of preventing obesity, and thereby of preventing the progression to overt diabetes results in major changes in the glycogen storage pathway. An improvement in insulin-stimulated glycogen synthase activity was also found in a study in which obese NIDDM patients were weight reduced.[52] These metabolic effects require further study to determine whether, as we hypothesize, the weight reduction and calorie restriction processes have in fact uncovered an inherent defect in the insulin-stimulated glycogen synthesis pathway.[50]

Also intriguing are the recent findings in normal rhesus monkeys that the intravenous administration of D-chiroinositol can increase glycogen synthase fractional velocity and decrease the glycogen phosphorylase activity ratio compared to maximal insulin stimulation.[53] Since D-chiroinositol has been found to be reduced in the urine of both humans and monkeys with NIDDM,[54] this suggests a possible role for altered inositol metabolism in diabetes. D-chiroinositol has been postulated to be a component of one of the mediators of insulin action in the glucose metabolism pathway.[55] Structuring and synthesis of this mediator will permit further examination of its putative role in the mechanisms of insulin resistance and NIDDM.

Summary

Nonhuman primates have contributed significantly to our understanding of NIDDM, and continued longitudinal study of this diabetes-prone species will help to identify candidate genes for the defects underlying insulin resistance and NIDDM. The diabetes developed by rhesus monkeys appears to be the same disease found in the large majority of obese type II diabetic patients. Indeed, all of the same complications of diabetes develop with sustained disease, and prevention of both the complications and the disease itself has been shown to be possible in nonhuman primates and is a goal of future therapy in humans.

References

1. Hansen BC, Bodkin NL. Heterogeneity of insulin responses: Phases in the continuum leading to non-insulin-dependent diabetes mellitus. Diabetologia 1986;29:713
2. Hansen BC, Bodkin NL. Primary prevention of diabetes mellitus by prevention of obesity in monkeys. Diabetes 1993;42:1809
3. Hansen BC, Ortmeyer HK, Bodkin NL. Prevention of obesity in middle-aged monkeys: Food intake during body weight clamp. Obes Res 1995;3:199
4. Bodkin NL, Metzger BL, Hansen BC. Hepatic glucose production and insulin sensitivity preceding diabetes in monkeys. Am J Physiol 1989;256 (Endocrinol Metab 19):E676
5. Hansen BC, Bodkin NL. β-Cell hyperresponsiveness: Earliest event in development of diabetes in monkeys. Am J Physiol 1990;259 (Regul Integrative Comp Physiol 28):R612
6. Hansen BC, Bodkin NL, Jen K-LC, Ortmeyer HK. Primate models of diabetes. In: Rifkin H, Colwell JA, et al., eds. Diabetes. Amsterdam: Elsevier Science; 1991:587
7. Hansen BC, Ortmeyer HK, Bodkin NL. Obesity, insulin-resistance and non-insulin-dependent diabetes in aging monkeys: Implications for NIDDM in humans. In: Shafrir E, Renold AE, eds. Frontiers in Diabetes Research: Lessons from Animal Diabetes V London: Smith-Gordon; 1994:93–105
8. National Diabetes Data Group: Classification and diagnosis of diabetes mellitus and other categories of glucose intolerance. Diabetes 1979;28:139
9. World Health Organization Expert Committee: Second report on diabetes mellitus. WHO Technical Report Series No. 646, Geneva, 1980
10. DiGiacomo RF, Myers RE, Baez LR. Diabetes mellitus in a rhesus monkey *(Macaca mulatta):* A case report and literature review. Lab Anim Sci 1971; 21:572
11. Hamilton CL, Ciaccia P. The course of development of glucose intolerance in the monkey (Macaca mulatta). J Med Primatol 1978;7:165
12. Kirk JH, Casey HW, Harwell JF. Diabetes mellitus in two rhesus monkeys. Lab Anim Sci 1972;22:245
13. Laver NM, Robison WG Jr, Hansen BC. Demonstration of retinal histopathologic conditions in spontaneously diabetic monkeys (abstract). Am J Clin Pathol 1993;99:349
14. Kopp JB, Marinos NJ, Bodkin NL. Increased laminin in nodular glomerulosclerosis affecting rhesus monkeys with non-insulin dependent diabetes mellitus (NIDDM) (abstract). J Am Soc Nephrol 1990;1:551A
15. Cornblath DR, Hillman MA, Striffler JS, et al. Peripheral neuropathy in diabetic monkeys. Diabetes 1989;38:1365
16. Kessler MJ, CF Howard J, London WT. Gestational diabetes mellitus and impaired glucose tolerance in an aged *Macaca mulatta.* J Med Primatol 1985;14:237
17. Howard CF Jr, Kessler MJ, Schwartz S. Carbohydrate impairment and insulin secretory abnormalities among *Macaca mulatta* from Cayo Santiago. Am J Prim 1986;11:147
18. Dunair A, Tattersall I. Prevalence of glucose intolerance in free-ranging *Macaca fascicularis* of Mauritius. Am J Prim 1987;13:435
19. Harris MI, Hadden WC, Knowler WC, Bennett PH. Prevalence of diabetes and impaired glucose tolerance and plasma glucose levels in U.S. populations aged 20–74 yr. Diabetes 1987;36:523
20. Knowler WC, Pettit DJ, Saad MF, Bennett PH. Diabetes mellitus in the Pima Indians: Incidence, risk factors and pathogenesis. Diabet Metab Rev 1990;6:1
21. Naithani VK, Steffens GJ, Tager HS. Isolation and amino-acid sequence determination of monkey insulin and proinsulin. Hoppe-Seyler's Z Physiol Chem 1984;365:571
22. Koerker DJ, Goodner CJ, Hansen BC, et al. Synchronous sustained oscillations

of C-peptide and insulin in the plasma of fasting monkeys. Endocrinology 1978;102:1649

23. Huang Z, Hansen BC, Shuldiner AR. Characterization of the insulin receptor gene in the rhesus monkey, a diabetes-prone species. Exp Clin Endocrinol 1993;101:358
24. Fan Z, Kole H, Bernier M, et al. Molecular mechanism of insulin resistance in the spontaneously obese and diabetic rhesus monkey: Site directed mutagenesis of the insulin receptor (abstract). The Endocrine Society 1995;77:180
25. Huang Z, Bodkin NL, Ortmeyer HK, et al. Hyperinsulinemia is associated with altered insulin receptor mRNA splicing in muscle of the spontaneously obese diabetic rhesus monkey. J Clin Invest 1994;94:1289
26. Reynet C, Kahn CR. Rad: A member of the Ras family overexpressed in muscle of type II diabetic humans. Science 1993;262:1441
27. Gibbs EM, McCoid SC, Ortmeyer HK. Altered expression of the facilitative fructose/glucose transporter (GLUT 5) in the development of diabetes. Exp Clin Endocrinol 1993;101:214
28. Shepherd PR, Gibbs EM, Wesslau C, et al. Human small intestine facilitative fructose/glucose transporter (GLUT5) is also present in insulin-responsive tissues and brain. Diabetes 1992;41:1360
29. Brunzell JD, Robertson RP, Lerner RL, et al. Relationships between fasting plasma glucose levels and insulin secretion during intravenous glucose tolerance tests. J Clin Endocrinol Metab 1976;42:222
30. Reaven GM, Olefsky JM. Relationship between heterogeneity of insulin responses and insulin resistance in normal subjects and patients with chemical diabetes. Diabetologia 1977;13:201
31. Welborn TA, Rubenstein AH, Haslam R, Fraser R. Normal insulin response to glucose. Lancet 1966;i:280
32. Pimenta W, Korytkowski M, Mitrakou A, Jenssen T. Pancreatic beta-cell dysfunction as the primary genetic lesion in NIDDM. JAMA 1995;273:1855
33. Hansen BC, Bodkin NL. Beta cell hyperresponsiveness to glucose precedes both fasting hyperinsulinemia and reduced glucose tolerance (abstract). Diabetes 1985;34(suppl 1):8A
34. Hansen BC, Striffler JS, Bodkin NL. Decreased hepatic insulin extraction precedes overt noninsulin dependent (type 2) diabetes in obese monkeys. Obes Res 1993;1:252
35. Bennett PH, Knowler WC, Pettitt WC, et al. Longitudinal studies of the development of diabetes in the Pima Indians. In: Eschwege E, ed. Advances in Diabetes Epidemiology. Amsterdam: Elsevier;1982:65–74
36. Granner DK, O'Brien RM. Molecular physiology and genetics of NIDDM. Diabetes Care 1992;15:369
37. Jeanrenaud B, Halimi S, van de Werve G. Neuro-endocrine disorders seen as triggers of the triad: Obesity—insulin resistance—abnormal glucose tolerance. Diabet Metab Rev 1985;1:261
38. DeFronzo RA. The triumvirate: β-Cell, muscle, liver—a collusion responsible for NIDDM. Diabetes 1988;37:667
39. Saad MF, Knowler WC, Pettit DJ, et al. Sequential changes in serum insulin concentration during the development of non-insulin-dependent diabetes. Lancet 1989;i:1356
40. Bell ET. Hyalinization in the islets of Langerhans in diabetes mellitus. Diabetes 1952;1:341
41. Cooper GJS, Willis AC, Clark A, et al. Purification and characterization of a peptide from amyloid-rich pancreas of type 2 diabetic patients. Proc Natl Acad Sci USA 1987;84:8628
42. Clark A, Morris JF, Scott LA, et al. Intracellular formation of amyloid fibrils in β-cells of human insulinoma and pre-diabetic monkey islets. In: Natvis JB, ed. Amyloid and Amyloidosis. Amsterdam: Kluwer;1991:453–456
43. de Koning EJP, Bodkin NL, Hansen BC, Clark A. Diabetes in *Macaca mulatta* monkeys is characterized by severe islet amyloidosis and reduction in β-cell population. Diabetologia 1993;36:378
44. Thorburn AW, Gumbiner B, Bulacan F, et al. Multiple defects in muscle glycogen synthase activity contribute to reduced glycogen synthesis in non-insulin-dependent diabetes. J Clin Invest 1991;87:489
45. Ortmeyer HK, Bodkin NL, Hansen BC. Insulin-mediated glycogen synthase activity in muscle of spontaneously insulin-resistant and diabetic rhesus monkeys. Am J Physiol 1993;266 (Regul Integrative Comp Physiol 34):R552
46. Ortmeyer HK, Bodkin NL, Hansen BC. Relationship of skeletal muscle glucose-6-phosphate to glucose disposal rate and glycogen synthase activity in insulin-resistant and non-insulin-dependent diabetic rhesus monkeys. Diabetologia 1994;37:127
47. Elbein SC, Hoffman M, Ridinger D, et al. Description of a second microsatellite marker and linkage analysis of the muscle glycogen synthase locus in familial NIDDM. Diabetes 1994;43:1061
48. Hansen BC. Genetics of insulin action. In: Ferrannini E, ed. Insulin Resistance and Disease. London: Bailliere's Clinical Endocrinology and Metabolism; 1993:1033–1061
49. Bodkin NL, Ortmeyer HK, Hansen BC. Long-term dietary restriction in older-aged rhesus monkeys: Effects on insulin resistance. J Gerontol 1995;50A:B142
50. Ortmeyer HK, Bodkin NL, Hansen BC. Chronic caloric restriction alters glycogen metabolism in rhesus monkeys. Obes Res 1994;2:549
51. Ortmeyer HK, Bodkin NL, Hansen BC. In vivo insulin inactivates muscle phosphorylase in normal monkeys with high activation of glycogen synthase (abstract). FASEB J 1994;8:A55
52. Bak JF, Moller N, Schmitz O, et al. In vivo insulin action and muscle glycogen synthase activity in type 2 (non-insulin-dependent) diabetes mellitus: Effects of diet treatment. Diabetologia 1992;35:777
53. Ortmeyer HK, Bodkin NL, Hansen BC, Larner J. In vivo D-chiroinositol activates skeletal muscle glycogen synthase and inactivates glycogen phosphorylase in rhesus monkeys. J Nutr Biochem 1995;6:499
54. Kennington AS, Hill CR, Craig J, et al. Low urinary *chiro*-inositol excretion in non-insulin-dependent diabetes mellitus. N Engl J Med 1990;323:373
55. Larner J, Huang LC, Schwartz CFW. Rat liver insulin mediator which stimulates pyruvate dehydrogenase phosphatase contains galactosamine and d-chiroinositol. Biochem Biophys Res Commun 1988;151:1416
56. Anderson AB. Pinitol from sugar pine stump wood. Ind Engin Chem 1953; 45:593
57. Bocek RM, Beatty CH. Glycogen synthetase and phosphorylase in red and white muscle of rat and rhesus monkey. J Histochem Cytochem 1966;14:549
58. Craig J, Larner J. Influence of epinephrine and insulin on uridine diphosphate glucose and glucan transferase and phosphorylase in muscle. Nature 1964; 202:971

Diabetes Mellitus, edited by Derek LeRoith, Simeon I. Taylor, and Jerrold M. Olefsky. Lippincott–Raven Publishers, Philadelphia © 1996.

CHAPTER 68

Rodent Genetic Models for Obesity and Non–Insulin-Dependent Diabetes Mellitus

FRED T. FIEDOREK, JR.

Insights into the Corresponding Human Syndromes Through Shared Pathophysiology and Comparative Mammalian Genetics

The development and detailed examination of suitable animal models of obesity and diabetes have long been major research priorities to aid in our understanding of the corresponding human disorders. Rodent obesity syndromes induced by toxins such as gold thioglucose or caused by precise surgical lesions in the ventromedial hypothalamus as well as numerous genetic models of obesity have been extensively characterized.[1] Diabetes induced by chemicals such as alloxan and streptozocin,[2] diabetes secondary to partial pancreatectomy,[3] and rodent genetic models analogous to non–insulin-dependent diabetes mellitus (NIDDM) and insulin-dependent diabetes mellitus (IDDM) have also been examined.[4] Experimental studies of these models have helped delineate the metabolic pathophysiology underlying obesity and NIDDM over the past three to four decades since there are inherent difficulties in obtaining biopsies of important target organs such as pancreatic islets, muscle, and adipose tissues from human patients. The availability and genetic uniformity of rodent genetic models, in particular, has enabled countless investigators to gain reproducible and increasingly sophisticated experimental insights into disease mechanisms of obesity and NIDDM as the sciences of physiology, biochemistry, and modern molecular genetics and cellular biology have advanced. Many concepts discussed in Sections I (Insulin Secretion), II (Insulin Action), and VI (Type II Diabetes) of this text were formulated using cells, tissues, and other in vivo and ex vivo systems derived from genetic animal models. Similarly, our understanding of diabetic therapeutics and complications discussed in Sections VII (Type II Diabetes: Therapeutics) and X (Complications: Mechanisms) have also relied heavily on the use of genetic animal models.

Unfortunately, our knowledge of the specific genetic determinants responsible for the etiology of human and rodent forms of NIDDM and obesity lags behind insights gained into metabolic pathophysiology. Numerous epidemiologic surveys and twin studies have firmly established the contribution of both dietary-environmental triggers and genetic susceptibility determinants as etiologic factors for human obesity and NIDDM[5] (reviewed in Chapter 61). Although such genetic clues are abundant and unmistakable, the molecular lesions conferring the inherited susceptibility for these syndromes are unknown. Much of the difficulty inherent in identifying human diabetes and obesity genes is because of the heterogeneous and polygenic nature of these increasingly prevalent disorders.[6] Successful medical detective work in this area has depended heavily on the identification of specific inheritance patterns or unusual phenotypic features that distinguish some patients and their families from so-called garden variety NIDDM and obesity. As reviewed in several chapters in Section VI (Type II Diabetes) of this text, mutations in candidate genes, including insulin, glucokinase, the insulin receptor, and mitochondrial tRNA genes, have been identified as primary lesions causing well-defined subtypes of diabetes or related syndromes such as leprechaunism.[7,8] However, even these known gene defects probably account collectively for less than 1–2% of all NIDDM cases. Likewise, specific forms of dysmorphic, early-onset obesity such as the Prader-Willi and Bardet-Biedl syndromes have been identified and genetically mapped to specific human chromosomal sites.[9–11] At present, the identification of the primary mutations and/or imprinting defects responsible for such rare autosomal genetic syndromes is being intensively investigated.[9,12] It remains to be seen whether defects in the genes responsible for these rare monogenic syndromes will also contribute major gene effects to the more common forms of human obesity and/or NIDDM.

The prospect of gaining an understanding of the complex genetics underlying human obesity and NIDDM provides the impetus for mapping and studying genes in the rodent genetic models of these disorders. Such insights will probably rely on molecular methods that can exploit the increasingly detailed homologies that exist between the genetic maps of human chromosomes and those of model organisms such as the mouse and laboratory rat.[13] Although the mouse has traditionally been viewed as the model organism of mammalian genetics and the rat as a more accessible model for physiologic studies for many decades, newer methods based on the polymerase chain reaction (PCR) are enabling gene mapping approaches to be applied to both species, even though the diversity of available inbred rat strains is more limited. Through such comparative mammalian genomic analysis, genes responsible for hypertension, IDDM, and cancer are also being pursued in humans and rodent genetic models.[14]

There are several advantages in using rodent genetic models to study human multifactorial and polygenic disorders such as obesity and NIDDM. Obviously, programmed breeding of affected individuals to dissect systematically the genes involved cannot be undertaken in human studies. Since disease heterogeneity represents a major obstacle in human genetic studies, especially of complex genetic disorders like obesity and NIDDM, the availability of several distinct autosomal and polygenic inbred rodent genetic models to provide unlimited numbers of genetically identical subjects for analysis is an advantage. In addition, uncontrollable environmental factors constitute a major difficulty in studying multifactorial human disorders, but such potential confounders can either be minimized in rodent models maintained on uniform diets and controlled environments or specifically manipulated to examine gene-environment interactions. Finally, hypotheses regarding candidate genes can be directly tested in rodents either through meiotic mapping and positional cloning in previously identified genetic models or through complementation experiments using transgenic and/or gene targeting methods in order to generate potential disease models from wild-type mice.[15,16]

The best known rodent genetic models of obesity and NIDDM include the recessive *ob/ob* and *db/db* mouse models, the dominant yellow obese $A^{y}/+$ and $A^{vy}/+$ mouse models, and the recessive *fa/fa* rat model. Recently, the primary genetic lesions responsible for three mutant models have been elucidated using positional cloning and candidate gene analysis approaches. It is anticipated that further study of the proteins mutated in these models will provide new insights into the neuroendocrine mechanisms of body weight maintenance, appetite-satiety regulation, and energy substrate metabolism. It remains to be determined whether the human homologues for these newly identified genes will also harbor mutations and/or allelic variants that confer major gene effects in human obesity and/or NIDDM. In addition to these now classic autosomal mutants, several polygenic models have been developed either through selective breeding programs to select unique inbred strains exhibiting stable NIDDM and/or obesity phenotypes or through the imposition of dietary stressors on standard inbred rodent strains that have been propagated in the absence of any selective pressure. The genetic susceptibility determinants for these polygenic, multifactorial models are unknown at present. Newer genetic approaches such as quantitative trait locus mapping made possible by polymerase chain reaction genotyping techniques may help to discern genes contributing to polygenic rodent models of obesity and NIDDM.[14,17]

This chapter details the historical origins and genotypic aspects of these rodent models. Both monogenic and polygenic rodent models of obesity and NIDDM are described with an emphasis on in vivo phenotypic features that are analogous to clinical parameters frequently assessed in humans. A summary of the developmental progression of body weights and gradings of the severity of glycemia, insulinemia, and lipidemia for each genetic model is included in order to provide the best context for comparing individual rodent genetic models to more heterogeneous human disorders. Even in rodents, such quantitative phenotypes span a wide range that corresponds to varying grades of obesity and often logarithmic differences in circulating hormone or substrate levels. From a historical point of view, such phenotypic measures formed the basis for considering differing rodent genetic obesity-NIDDM models as better or worse paradigms of the comparable human disorders. These fundamental phenotypic traits are now regaining relevance as emerging methods for quantitative genetic analysis are being applied both to complex inherited diseases in humans and rodent models of these diseases.[14]

Monogenic Models of Obesity: Candidates for Major Gene Effects in Humans

The monogenic rodent obesities map to defined autosomal loci (Table 68-1) and differ in their overall severity (Figure 68-1). The fundamental phenotype(s) for these discrete mutations include obesity of varying degrees and onset, hyperinsulinemia, some demonstration of hyperglycemia (either transient or sustained), and more variable hyperlipidemia. Thus, many mutant rodent models exhibit a ''syndrome X'' spectrum of altered metabolic parameters commonly associated with human obesity. The most severe autosomal recessive rodent models also demonstrate marked hyperphagia, thermoregulatory defects, hypogonadism, and functional sterility. Such neuroendocrine features are not typical in the common forms of human obesity but are apparent in rare childhood disorders exhibiting Mendelian patterns of inheritance such as Prader-Willi, Bardet-Biedl, and other severe obesity syndromes.[5] Many of these monogenic rodent obesity models have been studied for decades and have been discussed extensively in past reviews.[1,18–20]

This section concentrates on phenotypic aspects of these monogenic models that are most related to the clinical human phenotypes of obesity and diabetes. To as great an extent as possible, the major phenotypic features evident in the original background genomes carrying the relevant mutations are emphasized. Unique phenotypic features exhibited by particular inbred strains in the presence of a mutant allele and/or dietary or environmental factors are also highlighted. These important secondary aspects of the monogenic obesity-diabetes syndromes in rodents are likely attributable to modifying genes that contribute substantially to variability of the phenotypes described in the extensive literature on these mutant models. Such modifying genes may also be determinants for the polygenic and multifactorial models discussed later in this chapter. Finally, newer molecular genetic advances that have elucidated the primary lesions in three of the monogenic obesity models are also discussed in detail.

Obese (*ob*) Recessive Obesity Mouse Model

The obese (*ob*) mutation is an autosomal recessive locus that maps to mouse chromosome 6 and consists of two known alleles designated ob^{J} and ob^{2J}. Both alleles arose spontaneously at The Jackson Laboratories (JAX) mouse colonies. The original ob^{J} mutant arose over 40 years ago in a noninbred stock.[21] It has since been maintained as a congenic C57BL/6J strain; most published experimental studies have been performed on inbred offspring of this original allele. Since *ob/ob* mice are functionally sterile, the mutation has been propagated since its initial characterization by mating known *ob/+* heterozygotes.

The fundamental phenotype of C57BL/6J *ob/ob* mice includes profound early-onset obesity, hyperphagia, extreme insulin resistance, and mild hyperglycemia which typically does not progress to frank diabetes (reviewed in references 1, 19, and 22). Although frank obesity cannot be discerned visually before 4 weeks of age, impaired thermogenesis following exposure to a cold environment is detectable as early as 10 days of age,[23] and an increase in carcass lipid content determined by whole body ashing techniques is apparent by 3 weeks of age.[24] Unequivocal obesity develops rapidly following weaning and coincides with behavioral changes also evident in human obesity such as relative inactivity[25] and hyperphagia with a dietary preference for more fat-derived calories relative to carbohydrate or protein.[26] However, neither of these behavioral changes can entirely account for the development of obesity, since *ob/ob* mice show no decrease in locomotor activity prior to the development of obesity[25] and both pair-fed and pair-gained *ob/ob* mice still show three- to fourfold increases in percent body adiposity.[22,27] C57BL/6J *ob/ob* adiposity peaks with maturity at triglyceride contents of 52%.[28] Even when ob/ob mice are placed on severe dietary restriction (2 g of food intake/day for 4 months) and drop their weights to 24 g, they still possess 20% body fat, whereas control *ob/+* mice consume approximately 5 g per day, attain a weight of 35 g, and possess only 12% body fat.[29] Final body weights of *ob/ob* mice on unrestricted intakes typically reach 60–75 g by 6–9 months of age and remain relatively stable thereafter (see Fig. 68-1). Extreme cases can attain weights up to 90 g late in life.[19] Marked hyperplasia and hypertrophy of adipose cells underlie the expansion of numerous adipose tissue depots in *ob/ob* mice.[30]

Obese (*ob/ob*) mice also show profound hyperinsulinemia in both fasting and fed states.[31] Serum insulin levels rise progressively beginning at 3–4 weeks of age, eventually reaching 50-fold the corresponding values in control littermates.[32] Marked insulin resistance is most dramatically demonstrated by the ability of *ob/ob* mice to survive insulin injections up to doses of 400 U/kg with no decline in blood glucose values, whereas insulin doses of 20 U/kg cause lethal hypoglycemia in control mice.[26] The impairment of insulin action in *ob/ob* mice has also been documented at multiple cellular and biochemical levels in essentially all insulin-responsive tissues using a variety of in vivo and ex vivo experimental approaches (reviewed in reference 33). Despite this profound insulin resistance, severe diabetes is not characteristic of C57BL/6J *ob/ob* mice. Mild to moderate hyperglycemia, particularly in the fed state or in response to a glucose challenge that is proportional to the weight of the animal, is apparent.[24,34,35] However, it is important to note that most investigators studying glucose intolerance in rodents have used glucose loads that are proportional to body weight varying from 1–5 mg/g body weight and that are administered by a variety of routes. In contrast, standardization of routine

Table 68-1. Rodent Genetic Models of Non–Insulin-Dependent Diabetes Mellitus

Single Gene Models of Obesity

Name	Allele Symbol(s)	Inheritance Mode	Rodent-Human Mapping
Yellow	A^{y}, A^{vy}, A^{sy}, A^{iy}	AD	MMU 2—20q13
Obese	*ob*, ob^{2J}	AR	MMU 6—7q31
Fat	*fat*	AR	MMU 8—16q22-24
Diabetes	*db*, db^{2J}, db^{3J}, db^{ad}, db^{Pas}, db^{5J}	AR	MMU 4—1p31
Tubby	*tub*	AR	MMU 7—11p
Fatty	*fa*	AR	RNO 5—1p31
Corpulent	fa^{cp}	AR	RNO 5—1p31

Name	Inbred Strains	Gene Defect(s)	Modifier Loci
Yellow	C57BL/6J, C3H/HeJ	*Asp* (*Raly*)	?
Obese	C57BL/6J, C57BL/KsJ, SM/Ckc-Dac	*Ob* (“leptin”)	ESTs, ? others
Fat	HRS/J, C57BL/KsJ	*Cpe*	?
Diabetes	C57BL/KsJ, C57BL/6J, others	?	ESTs, ? others
Tubby	C57BL/6J	?	?
Fatty	Zucker (ZDF), Wistar-Kyoto (WKY)	?	?
Corpulent	SHR/N, LA/N, WKY/N	?	?

Polygenic Models of Obesity

Obese Strain	Inheritance Mode	Stressors	QTLs
NZO mice	SIB	None	?
KK mice	SIB	None	?
C57BL/6J × *Mus spretus*	BC (heterozygotes)	HF/HCh diet	MMU 6, 7
AKR/J mice	IB	HF diet	MMU 4, 11, 15
Multiple rat strains	CCIB	HF or “cafeteria” diets	?

Polygenic Models of NIDDM

NIDDM Strain	Inheritance Mode	Stressors	QTLs
C57BL/6J mice	IB	HF/HSC diet	MMU 7
C57BL/KsJ mice	IB	Obesity (*db* or *ob*)	ESTs, ? others
KK mice	SIB	High-calorie diet	?
GK rats	SIB	None	? Gene imprinting
OTELF rats	IB	None	?

oral glucose intolerance testing in humans employs the administration of a fixed 75-g glucose load. Thus, by the variable criteria used for rodents, *ob/ob* mice can exhibit marked glucose intolerance to either an oral 5 mg/g or intravenous 1 mg/g glucose load[35] or to intraperitoneal glucose loads of 2–4 mg/g body weight[36,37] and mild glucose intolerance to an oral 3.6 mg/g glucose challenge administered after an overnight fast.[37] However, no differences in glucose excursions following administration of a fixed 100-mg oral glucose load in the fasted state are evident between *ob/ob* mice and lean littermates.[35] Detailed longitudinal analysis of C57BL/6J *ob/ob* mice shows that glucose tolerance curves in response to weight-adjusted (2.5 mg/g) intraperitoneal doses of glucose administered to nonfasted mice peak in severity in *ob/ob* mice ranging between 40–50 g in size and improve in *ob/ob* mice larger than 60 g in size.[36] Thus, the mild degree of glucose intolerance apparent in *ob/ob* mice does not worsen in contrast to the progression of hyperglycemia evident in either C57BL/KsJ *db/db* mice or NZO mice, as discussed more fully below.[22,36] It is also interesting to note that these intraperitoneal glucose tolerance curves are similar in magnitude to glucose excursions others have seen in the C57BL/6J strain not bearing the *ob* mutation.[38] Thus, C57BL/6J *ob/ob* mice may not exhibit marked hyperglycemia relative to the underlying hyperglycemia-prone genetic background of the C57BL/6J strain.[39] (See later discussion of potential polygenic determinants of hyperglycemia and other quantitative parameters related to NIDDM and obesity.) The imposition of more rigid criteria for the definition of glucose intolerance in humans may partially account for why only 10–20% of obese human subjects are defined as developing NIDDM despite the existence of marked insulin resistance in both of these overlapping disorders. As in human obesity/NIDDM, dietary caloric restriction in *ob/ob* mice can ameliorate hyperinsulinemia and normalize glucose intolerance[31] even if it does not correct the underlying inherited tendency for *ob/ob* mice to partition energy stores into adipose tissue.

The *ob/ob* metabolic phenotype also includes two- to threefold elevations of fasting triglyceride and cholesterol levels[40–42] and more striking three- to fourfold elevations in serum corticosterone concentrations.[43] As described earlier, the familiar syndrome X grouping of metabolic parameters also includes hyperlipidemia, but human obesity is not associated with elevated corticosteroid levels.[44] Homozygous *ob/ob* mutants of both sexes are typically infertile, but this reproductive dysfunction is probably not intrinsic to the ob mutation itself, since *ob/ob* males can mate successfully after austere dietary restriction is imposed to keep adult weights at 26–30 g.[45] *Ob/ob* females show more complete hypogonadotropic infertility, perhaps because of deleterious effects of the *ob* mutation on the female hypothalamic-pituitary axis. However, since ovulation induced with gonadotropin injections and transplantation of *ob/ob* ovaries can yield viable *ob/ob* progeny, ovarian function per se is not affected by the *ob* mutation.[46]

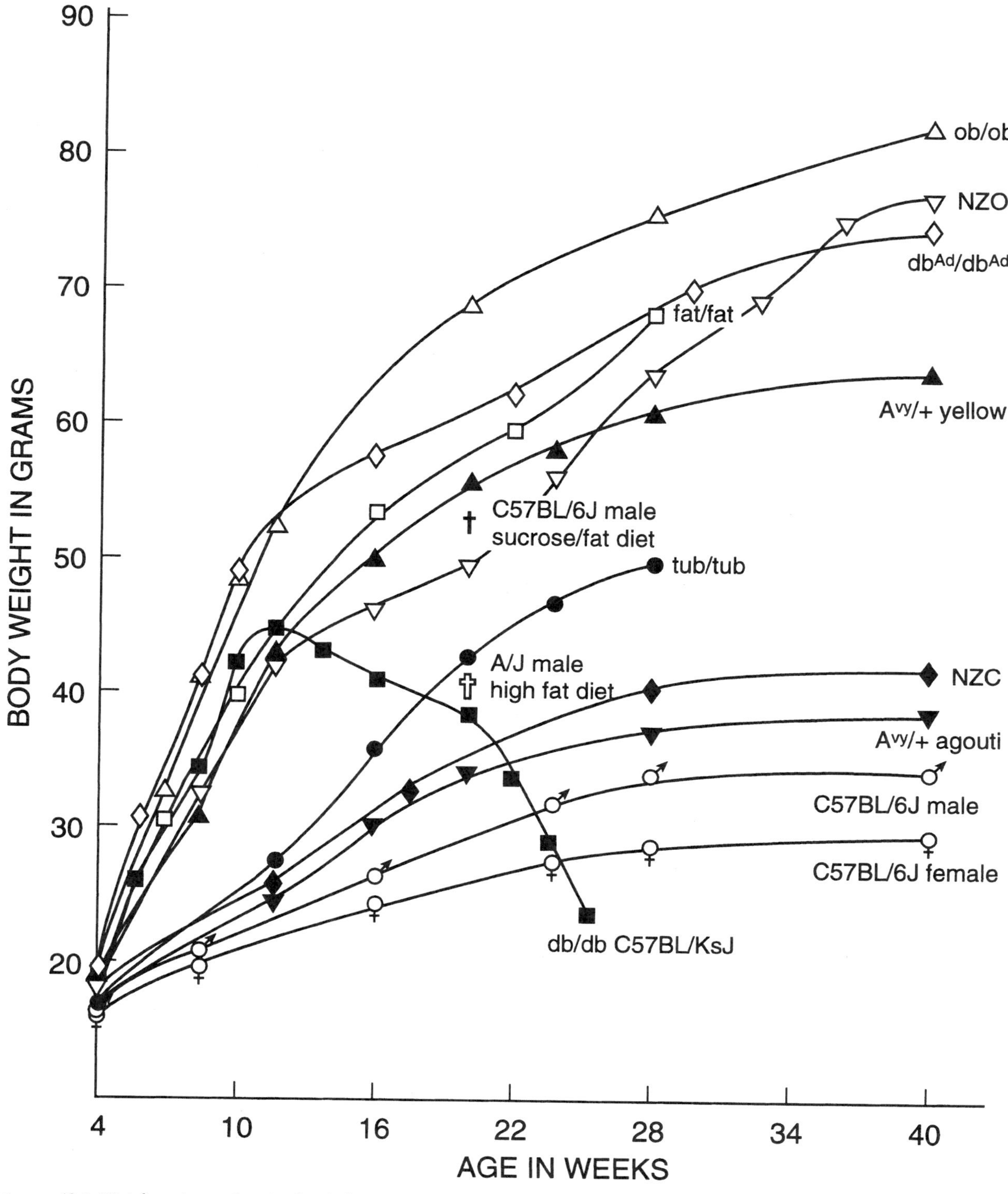

Figure 68-1. Weight gain as a longitudinal phenotype in mouse obesity models. The developmental progression of body weight versus age is shown for several monogenic and polygenic mouse models of obesity as well as for four different control mouse strains exhibiting the approximate range for a normal progression of body weight in mice in the absence of obesity gene(s) or any dietary pressure. Each weight curve is labeled with the corresponding mutation-inbred strain as described in the text. Most monogenic obesity models can be compared with control data for the C57BL/6J male and female mice. The NZO polygenic obesity model contrasts with its control, the NZC strain. The yellow obese $A^{vy}/+$ model with full ectopic expression of the agouti gene should be compared with the pseudo-agouti $A^{vy}/+$ mouse that fails to express the agouti gene in all tissues because of epigenetic inactivation. Also indicated by crosses are the attained weights at 20 weeks of age following 16 weeks of either a sucrose–high-fat diet or a high-fat diet alone in C57BL/6J and A/J male mice, two standard inbred strains of mice susceptible to dietary obesity. These data were compiled from references 31, 38, 45, 52, 54, 77, 127, 133, 134, and 137.

Refined meiotic mapping of the *ob* mutation in back-crosses generated from such *ob/ob* ovarian transplants positioned *ob* to proximal mouse chromosome 6.[47] Using positional cloning approaches, the mouse *ob* gene as well as its human homologue have recently been cloned by Friedman and colleagues.[48] The mouse *ob* cDNA encodes small protein 167 amino acids in length and includes a predicted signal sequence and a long ~3700 base pair 3′ untranslated region. The *ob* translation product is processed in vitro from an 18 kd precursor to a mature 16 kd form.[48] In rodents *ob* is expressed exclusively in white adipose tissue and the mature ob protein is probably secreted either as a circulating satiety hormone that directly signals the accumulation of adipose depots in order to coordinate body weight homeostasis or as a local paracrine factor that functions indirectly in a similar manner. Such a notion fits with prior hypotheses based on classic parabiosis experiments performed by Coleman and colleagues using *ob/ob, db/db,* and wild-type mice that suggested that abnormal energy balance in these mouse mutants involved defects in an interacting ligand-receptor physiologic control system.[22,49] The only two known alleles (ob^J and ob^{2J}) for the mouse ob mutation have been examined at the molecular level. The original ob^J gene carries a C → T substitution in codon 105Arg yielding a premature TGA stop codon that probably results in the production of a nonfunctional ob protein. The *ob* mRNA transcript is overproduced 20-fold in ob^J/ob^J mice, suggesting that the level of expression is induced in a failed attempt to signal the size of adipose depots in the whole organism, since the secreted ob peptide is inactive.[48] The second ob^{2J} mutation maintained in the SM/Ckc-Dac mouse strain leads to the absence of any detectable *ob* mRNA in adipose tissue. This mutation is also associated with a *Bgl*II restriction fragment length polymorphism mapping upstream of the *ob* gene transcription start site, and it presumably results from an unidentified genomic mutation, possibly in the promoter of the *ob* gene, which results in the complete absence of *ob* gene expression by adipose tissue.[48] A human *OB* gene homologue has also been cloned based on its DNA sequence conservation with the mouse cDNA.[48] Future studies of *OB* will undoubtedly focus on its role in the development and complex genetics of human obesity and its potential role as a treatment for human obesity.

Diabetes (*db*) Recessive Obesity Mouse Model

Like obese (*ob*), diabetes (*db*) is also an autosomal recessive mutation that results in an extreme, early-onset obesity syndrome. The original db^J allele occurred spontaneously in the mid-1960s on the C57BL/KsJ inbred strain at JAX,[50] but numerous allelic mutations (db^{2J}, db^{3J}, db^{4J}, db^{Ad}, and db^{Pas}) mapping to the same mouse chromosome 4 locus have occurred in other inbred strains maintained at JAX and other breeding facilities.[51] In fact, the first mutation at the *db* locus occurred on a mixed genetic background in England and was initially termed Adipose (*Ad*).[52] Genetic complementation with *db* alleles later established that both mutations involved the identical genetic locus and the designation *Ad* was changed to db^{Ad}.[22] Therefore, the *db* gene is likely to be a highly mutable locus, possibly in several species, since the autosomal recessive rat *fa* gene (discussed in more detail in the later section on the Fatty Rat Models of Obesity) probably represents the homologue of the mouse *db* gene based on conserved synteny of their chromosomal map positions in these two species.[53]

The original db^J mutant allele carried by the C57BL/KsJ strain forms the basis for most of the published literature on the *db* model.[50] The phenotypic characterization in this inbred strain led early workers to coin *db* (for diabetes) as the symbol for this mutant model, since the animals exhibit hyperglycemia >300 mg/dL in the fed state by 6 weeks of age, which increases in severity over time.[54] Like human patients with uncontrolled NIDDM, C57BL/KsJ *db/db* mice experience polydipsia, polyuria, and glycosuria during their hyperglycemic stage but they still gain weight during the first 3 months of life if fed ad libitim. Hyperinsulinemia is evident as early as 10 days of age and remains six- to tenfold elevated until 3–4 months of age in the C57BL/KsJ strain and indefinitely in other strains.[4,22,55] Prior to and for 6–10 weeks after the onset of frank diabetes, *db/db* mice on the C57BL/KsJ as well as other genetic backgrounds consistently show increases in overall adiposity,[22] thermoregulatory defects,[56,57] and functional sterility.[58] C57BL/KsJ *db/db* mice plateau at ~42% triglyceride content before both adipose and lean tissue wasting develops with the onset of worsening diabetes and frank ketosis.[28] It is now apparent that the *db* mutation, like *ob,* results primarily in a profound and progressive obesity syndrome that is essentially identical to the C57BL/6J *ob/ob* phenotype described above in severity and the early time course of its development.[22] The unique distinguishing feature of the original db^J mutation on the C57BL/KsJ genetic background is marked hyperglycemia accompanied by pancreatic islet atrophy with eventual ketosis and death by 6–8 months of age. Other than this progressive hyperglycemia-ketosis, only a few other metabolic differences exist between either *db* or *ob* mutant phenotypes expressed by the C57BL/KsJ strain and other inbred strains. Not surprisingly, hypertriglyceridemia and hypercholesterolemia are also more severe in C57BL/KsJ *db/db* mice relative to those with other genetic backgrounds.[42] In addition, the expansion of the adipose tissue mass in *db/db* mice during the first 3–4 months of life primarily shows hypertrophy of adipocytes,[30] although some obese females homozygous for the *dbPas* allele show hyperplasia as well.[51] Attained weights and overall body mass indexes can be slightly higher for females relative to males in genetic backgrounds other than C57BL/KsJ that allow fat accretion to progress.[51,52]

As described briefly in the section on the Obese Recessive Obesity Mouse Model above, *db* and *ob* are hypothesized to encode interacting gene products (perhaps as ligand and receptor) in a putative biochemical pathway involving control of appetite and satiety. The most compelling support for this notion was provided by classic parabiosis experiments performed by Coleman and colleagues in the 1960s.[22,59] Parabiosis is the chronic surgical union of two animals resulting in a continuous plasma exchange typically equivalent to 1–2% of one animal's blood volume passing in each direction per minute.[60] Similar parabiosis studies performed on Zucker *fa/fa* rats and rats with discrete lesions within the hypothalamus argue that a satiety-energy metabolism sensor feedback loop is likely to involve an integrated system of afferent signals, perhaps including circulating hormonal signals such as the ob peptide as well as central nervous system-brain stem response proteins and perhaps peripheral nerve (i.e., vagal or sympathetic) efferent signal proteins.[49]

The spontaneous appearance of the db^{2J} mutation in the C57BL/6J inbred strain and complementation breeding experiments of this and other *db* alleles onto both the C57BL/KsJ and C57BL/6J strains firmly established that modifier genes in the inbred background of different strains contribute significantly to diabetes metabolic phenotypes of varying severities.[22,61] Obesity without severe hyperglycemia is apparent on all inbred genetic backgrounds examined except for the C57BL/KsJ and C3H.SW/J strains.[4,51,62] The progression from hyperglycemia along with the maintainence of hyperinsulinemia at 3–4 months of age to eventual islet failure without autoimmunity in C57BL/KsJ *db/db* mice has been likened to the pancreatic β-cell exhaustion hypothesized to occur over time during the pathogenesis of NIDDM in humans (possibly secondary to direct glucose toxicity in genetically susceptible individuals).[63,64] Recent studies have implicated the induction of the estrogen sulfotransferase (*EST*) gene, possibly by elevated corticosterone levels caused by the *db* (or *ob*) gene, as a key factor in the severe hyperglycemia that develops in C57BL/KsJ *db/db* mice. *EST* induction leads to more complete inactivation of circulating estrogens. Since levels of circulating androgens remain unaffected, the more virilized metabolic milieu that occurs in female as well as male mice appears to contribute to hyperglycemia as a pleiotropic consequence of either the *db* or *ob* obesity mutation.[65] A similar virilized endocrine environment has been commonly noted in some human female patients with NIDDM.[66]

Although *EST* mRNA induction is evident in obese C57BL/KsJ *db/db* mice, it is not clear if the *EST* gene itself is an actual modifier locus conferring the allelic hyperglycemia differences apparent between C57BL/KsJ and other inbred strains. The C57BL/6J and C57BL/KsJ substrains diverged around 1950.[67] Modern molecular genotyping using polymerase chain reaction–based DNA microsatellite markers and a variety of proviral markers indicates that the C57BL/KsJ strain probably arose from a genetic contamination of C57BL/6J mice by inadvertent DBA/2J mouse strain genetic admixture at the time the original C57BL/KsJ strain was established.[68,69] The modifier gene or genes in the C57BL/KsJ inbred background that presumably confer these impressive differences in EST induction and glucose intolerance in the presence of an obesity mutation may have either spontaneously mutated in the short time since this divergence or been fixed in a susceptible combination of C57BL/6J and DBA/2J alleles. Overall, it is clear that both a mutant obesity allele (either *db* or *ob*) and the inbred strain genome interact to yield distinct or overlapping metabolic phenotypes. This fortuitous experiment of nature in a mouse breeding colony originating about 1950 supports evolving concepts of obesity and NIDDM in humans as complex, overlapping genetic disorders with subtle genetic changes in several loci probably contributing to a large but continuous gradient of phenotypic differences (see Concluding Section of this chapter). It is also interesting (and also perhaps a daunting harbinger for future analysis of the complex genetics of human NIDDM) that a sex steroid metabolizing gene or its unknown transcriptional activators can now be considered candidate genes for determining inherited susceptibility to developing glucose intolerance in this rodent genetic obesity/NIDDM model, even though they would not be considered logical candidates a priori based on involvement in fuel metabolism, insulin secretion, or insulin action.

Although the *db* gene itself remains unknown, it has been further localized to a defined middle region of mouse chromosome 4 while its expected human homologue maps to chromosome 1p32-34.[70,71] The anticipated cloning of the *db* gene should identify a gene product that interacts with the ob protein either directly or indirectly through intervening physiologic signals. Future molecular genetic analysis should also reveal why the *db/fa* genetic locus has been so susceptible to recurrent mutations in both mice and rats and whether gene defects in the human gene homologue contribute to human obesity.

Yellow (A^y) Dominant Obesity Mouse Model

The yellow mouse models of obesity consist of four allelic mutations that map coincident to the well-studied agouti coat color locus on distal mouse chromosome 2 (lethal yellow A^y, viable yellow A^{vy}, siena yellow A^{sy}, and intermediate yellow A^{iy}; see Table 68-1). Besides conferring a yellow coat color as an autosomal dominant trait, these mutations lead to other pleiotropic effects including moderate to severe obesity, increased somatic growth, and increased susceptibility to mammary, hepatic, and bladder tumors.[72] The A^y mutation is an old mutation of obscure origin that was maintained and propagated for decades dating back before 1900 by naturalists and pet devotees referred to as the "mouse fancy." Current A^y/+ stocks have been inbred and maintained at JAX and other animal facilities primarily on the C57BL/6J inbred strain. The A^{iy} mutation arose spontaneously in the same C57BL/6J genetic background, whereas the A^{vy} and A^{sy} mutations arose in inbred C3H/HeJ mouse colonies.[73] The A^y mutation causes embryonic lethality when homozygous. In contrast, the other yellow agouti alleles are all viable in the homozygous state or when hemizygous with A^y.[74]

All dominant yellow agouti alleles confer obesity of comparable degree in either the heterozygous or homozygous state.[73,75] The A^y and A^{vy} mutant yellow obese phenotypes have been extensively characterized over the past four decades.[42,73,76,77] In contrast, only allelism tests and preliminary physiologic studies have been performed on the A^{iy} and A^{sy} mutants[75] prior to recent molecular genetic experiments elucidating the nature of all these mutations (see below). Both male and female A^y/+ and A^{vy}/+ mutant mice develop a moderate obesity phenotype with onset during puberty (8–12 weeks) and attain ~50–60 g peak weights at 28–30 weeks of age.[76,77] Unlike other rodent monogenic obesities, yellow obese mice also show increases in linear growth parameters.[73,78] Nonetheless, the carcass fat content of mature yellow obese mice still reaches ~26% adiposity compared with 6–8% values in control mice.[28] Thus, yellow obesity is more gradual and ultimately less severe than the autosomal recessive C57BL/KsJ *db/db* or C57BL/6J *ob/ob* models. The adiposity of yellow obese mice is hypertrophic rather than hyperplastic.[30] Final weights of yellow obese mice can be augmented by 10–15 g on a high-fat diet, and aging mice may show a mild reduction in overall weight.[76]

Like *db/db* and *ob/ob* mice, yellow obese mice are more hyperphagic and inactive than control littermates, but the degree of hyperphagia and inactivity alone fails to account for their fourfold greater carcass lipid content.[73] Early parabiosis experiments showed no effect of the A^y mutation on body weight or fat content of either parabiont partner.[79] Interestingly, a correlation of the intensity of the yellow coat coloration with the severity of obesity and related metabolic parameters such as plasma insulin levels has long been noted.[77] A developmental time course of the A^y and A^{vy} yellow obese syndrome phenotype on C57BL/6J and C3H/HeJ background strains is shown in comparison to other rodent mutant obese models in Figure 68-1.

Hyperinsulinemia develops in yellow mice parallel to obesity, with initial rises apparent at 6 weeks and four- to tenfold elevations by 8–10 weeks; males typically show higher insulin values than females.[73] Blood glucose values may be mildly elevated in fed animals but are normal after fasting.[76] Impaired glucose tolerance testing in response to 1 mg/g glucose challenge is evident indicating that yellow obese mice are more similar to the C57BL/6J *ob/ob* model, since glucose intolerance is dependent on weight-related glucose loads and severe diabetes does not develop. Hyperglycemia and mild serum cholesterol and triglyceride elevations also tend to be worse in males for unknown reasons.[42,72] Interestingly, when the A^{vy} mutation was bred onto the C57BL/KsJ genetic strain background, diabetes was not evident,[80] although severe hyperglycemia can be readily induced by glucocorticoid administration.[81] Thus, when hyperglycemia does occur, it may also relate more to inbred strain genetic modifiers (such the inducibility of EST activity described for C57BL/KsJ *db* mutations) than to the yellow agouti mutations per se. Obviously, A^y/+ heterozygous mice are not sterile, but they do exhibit decreased fertility and subtle abnormalities of gonadal function[82] and temperature regulation,[83] implying some degree of functional hypothalamic impairment.

The yellow obese (A^y) model was the first rodent obesity mutation to be characterized at the molecular level.[84,85] Positional cloning of the normal agouti coat color gene and characterization of the A^y obesity mutation were aided by the fortuitous identification of a radiation-induced translocation mutant that was discerned as an altered coat color (but nonobese) phenotype.[86] The agouti protein encoded by wild-type (A/+) mice is expressed almost exclusively in neonatal skin; its regulated expression leads to the deposition of a subapical band of pheomelanin in individual coat hairs. It is a highly basic protein, 15–16 kd in predicted size, containing multiple cysteine residues and bearing a putative signal sequence characteristic of secreted proteins.[84,85] The normal developmental expression of the agouti protein in mice with the A/+ genotype is responsible for producing the brown and black agouti coat coloration of many inbred and most feral mouse strains. Homozygous *a/a* mice do not produce a subapical band of pheomelanin in individual coat hairs, allowing many other coat color phenotypes encoded by distinct genetic loci to become penetrant.[87]

Ectopic and persistent expression of the agouti protein in the skin and multiple additional tissues occurs in all dominant agouti mutants and appears to be primarily responsible for the yellow coat colors and other pleiotropic phenotypic effects such as obesity and increased susceptibility to developing certain tumors.[84,85] However, dysregulated agouti expression is not all or none, since interesting gradations of coat coloration termed "mottled" or "pseudoagouti" patterns can occur in either $A^{y}/+$ or $A^{vy}/+$ mice.[87] The attenuation of coat color intensity and associated phenotypic effects may be mediated by epigenetic modifications possibly involving genomic imprinting determined by parental origin and/or modifier genes carried by the background strain genome.[73,88] Studies of the penetrance of various phenotypes in obese mottled and lean pseudoagouti A^{vy}/a mice indicate that higher levels of ectopic expression of the agouti protein are likely required for the development of obesity and associated metabolic phenotypes than are necessary for the increased susceptibility to lung and liver tumor formation, since pseudoagouti mice are not obese but show an increased tumor incidence even though agouti expression is not detectable by Northern RNA analysis.[73] At the molecular level, aberrant agouti expression in the A^{y} mutant occurs as a consequence of a large deletion leading to the replacement of the normal agouti gene promoter with that of another gene (an RNA binding protein termed Raly), which is normally constitutively active in all tissues. Disruption of the normal *Raly* gene in the A^{y} deletion allele is responsible for its homozygous lethality.[89,90] In the A^{vy} and A^{iy} alleles, dysregulated ectopic expression of the agouti protein arises as a result of the insertion of viral intracisternal A particles (IAP) 5′ of the normal agouti gene without affecting *Raly* expression; hence, these other yellow obese mutations are not lethal when homozygous.[91] The variable expressivity of the agouti gene in pseudoagouti or mottled $A^{vy}/+$ and $A^{iy}/+$ mice previously described probably occurs as a consequence of epigenetic inactivation of the IAP long terminal repeat promoter in these yellow obese alleles.[91] Regardless, it is now clear that all dominant yellow mutations (including the above IAP alleles, A^{sy}, and two newly described mutations) involve gain-of-function mutations in the agouti gene promoter whereby either a transposable viral element or an endogenous housekeeping gene promoter such as the *Raly* promoter assumes control of normal tissue- and time-specific agouti expression.[92,93]

A human homologue for agouti (also termed ASP for "agouti signaling protein") has recently been identified and cloned based on sequence similarity to the mouse gene.[94,95] Its precise physical genetic map position on chromosome 20q excludes it as a candidate gene for the MODY 1 locus (see Chapter 63 of this text). The function of the agouti homologue in humans is currently unknown. Human *ASP* is less restricted in its expression, showing highest mRNA signals in testis, ovary, and heart and detectable transcript in kidney, liver, and foreskin.[95] Overexpression of both the mouse and human agouti gene in transgenic mice recapitulates the yellow obese phenotype seen in the pre-existing dominant agouti mutations and supports the prevailing hypothesis that aberrant agouti protein production is pathogenic.[95,96] It is interesting to note that hyperglycemia in transgenic yellow obese mice is also more severe in males.[96] Despite the identification of the conserved agouti protein and characterization of several spontaneous and engineered agouti mutations, the precise mechanism whereby its inappropriate expression leads to obesity is not known. Recent biochemical studies suggest that the agouti protein may act as a paracrine antagonist of melanocyte stimulating hormone (MSH) receptor isotypes leading either to physiologic or pathologic phenotypes or both. Thus, an agouti coat pattern develops when MSH receptor inhibition by agouti protein occurs normally within the hair follicle in a time-restricted manner, but obesity and other metabolic effects may develop if agouti inhibits melanocortin-4 receptor (MC4-R) signaling at sites outside the hair follicle.[97] Another recent study has suggested that agouti protein production at ectopic sites induces increases in intracellular free calcium concentrations that ultimately lead to the pleiotropic phenotypes evident in $A^{vy}/+$ mice and other dominant yellow mutants.[98] Future work to elucidate the role of agouti protein in the pathogenesis of obesity and associated phenotypes in rodent genetic models will probably attempt to restrict overexpression of the agouti protein to defined target tissues using tissue-specific transgene constructs. In humans, major questions to be addressed include the role of specific agouti protein/melanocortin receptor isoforms in the genetics and pathogenesis of inherited obesity and NIDDM.

Zucker and Wistar Fatty (*fa*) and Corpulent (fa^{cp}) Recessive Obesity Rat Models

The original fatty (*fa*) mutation in rats arose spontaneously over three decades ago in an outbred stock of rats (the 13 M strain) maintained in the Zucker laboratory at Stow, Massachusetts.[99] Another spontaneous obesity mutation variously termed the Koletsky obese rat or corpulent (*cp*) rat arose among matings between Wistar/Kyoto (WKY) spontaneously hypertensive (SH) rats and Sprague-Dawley rats.[100] The Koletsky obese hypertensive rat has been shown to be an allele of the original fatty mutation.[101] Although the background strain genetics of the fatty (*fa*) rat and its alleles has been complicated by breeding in both outbred and inbred strains, physiologic studies for the *fa/fa* mutants have been even more extensive than for many of the autosomal murine obesity models, particularly since the larger size of the rat makes it better suited for some types of physiologic studies relevant for diabetes and obesity.[102] Many of the physiologic and biochemical features characterizing the allelic *fa* mutations have been extensively reviewed.[103–105] Accordingly, this discussion of the *fa* mutant obesity model focuses on basic metabolic parameters potentially relevant to quantitative genetic analysis.

As described briefly above, the *fa* mutation probably represents a rat homologue of the mouse *db* mutation based on conservation of genetic map positions in these two species.[53] Like *db/db* mice, homozygous *fa/fa* mutants of both sexes are functionally infertile requiring mating of *fa/+* heterozygotes to generated affected animals.[103] The fundamental phenotype of *fa/fa* rats also includes many features similar to those of the mouse *db* and *ob* autosomal recessive models such as early-onset obesity, hyperphagia, and severe insulin resistance. Although *fa/fa* offspring cannot be discerned visually until 5 weeks of age, lower rectal temperatures and reduced oxygen consumption rates following exposure to a cold environment are apparent much earlier.[106,107] Marked hypercellularity and hypertrophy of adipose depots was noted by Hirsch and colleagues for the Zucker fatty rat even before comparable analyses were undertaken in obese mice.[108] *Fa/fa* rats also exhibit feeding behavior abnormalities like *ob/ob* and *db/db* mice, including hyperphagia conspicuous both during the day and at night,[109] a macronutrient preference for more fat-derived calories,[110] and the failure of pair feeding with control rats to arrest the development of obesity.[111] Adiposity in Zucker *fa/fa* rats peaks with maturity at triglyceride contents over 50%.[108,111,112] Final body weights for fatty rats exhibit more sexual dimorphism than do the autosomal mouse obesity mutations, with females reaching 650–750 g and males 800–900 g on unrestricted intakes by 10 months of age (Fig. 68-2).[99,100,113] *Fa/fa* rats exhibit only minimal elevations in serum corticosterone concentrations, but stressful stimuli can lead to an exaggerated release.[114]

Unlike their *db* mouse homologues,[53] Zucker *fa/fa* homozygotes do not develop clear-cut hyperglycemia or impaired glucose tolerance, although increased serum insulin levels are detectable at 3 weeks of age and remain elevated throughout life.[112,115] Marked insulin resistance has been demonstrated by performing insulin clamps in the allelic *fatty* models.[116,117] Impairment of insulin action in *fa/fa* rats, more severe in muscle than in adipose tissue, may in part explain abnormal nutrient partitioning leading to obesity in

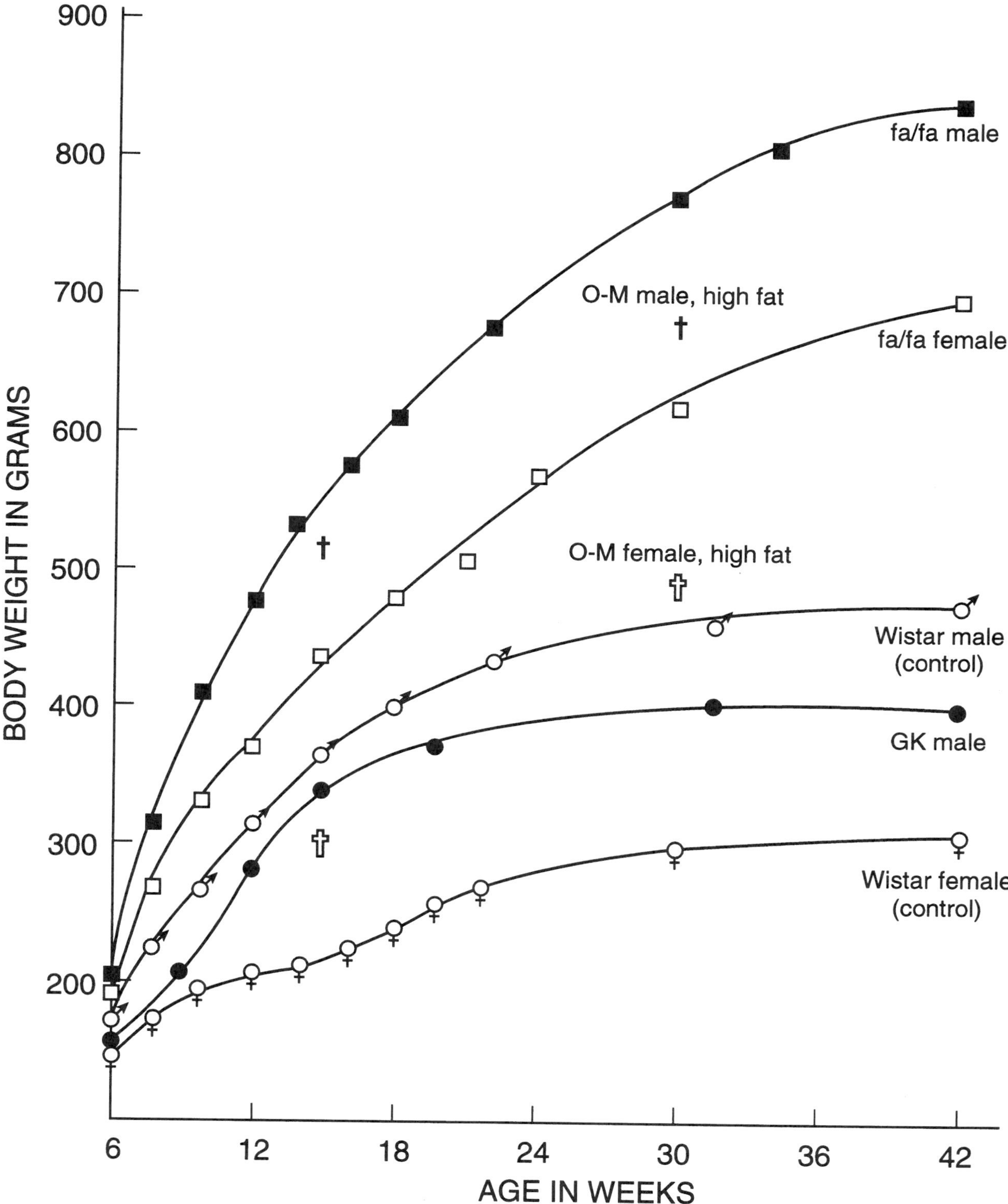

FIGURE 68-2. Weight gain as a longitudinal phenotype in rat obesity models. The developmental progression of body weight versus age is shown for males and females of monogenic and polygenic rat models of obesity and NIDDM and for the Wistar strain, a representative control strain exhibiting a normal progression of body weight in rats in the absence of an obesity gene or any dietary pressure. Each weight curve is labeled with the corresponding mutation-inbred strain as described in the text. Also indicated by crosses are the weights attained on a high fat diet at 15 and 30 weeks of age in male and female Osborne-Mendel (O-M) rats, a rat strain susceptible to dietary obesity. These data were compiled from references 99, 100, 112, 113, and 154.

the *fatty* rat model.[118] The original *fa* mutation has been transferred to a normotensive WKY rat strain to produce a more hyperglycemic rat obesity model.[119] In addition, the *fa* or fa^{cp} mutation carried by other rat strain genetic backgrounds such as the LA/N or SHR/N strains results in mild degrees of both glucose intolerance and hypertension.[120] As for most mouse obesity models, the mild degree of glucose intolerance evident in most alleles of the *fa* mutation depends on weight-proportional glucose loads.[112,121,122] The Wistar *fatty* rat exhibits severe hyperglycemia comparable to the C57BL/KsJ *db/db* mouse with fed glucose levels over 300 mg/dL.[119] Interestingly, only males show glucose-intolerant phenotypes in both the Wistar *fatty* rat and other strains with milder NIDDM features.[119,122,123] It is not known if these gender-related differences are secondary to the higher weights and body mass indexes of male rats bearing the *fa* mutation or whether virilizing metabolic factors such as are seen with EST induction in the mouse C57BL/KsJ strain are involved in male-specific hyperglycemia.

The *fa/fa* metabolic phenotype in essentially all strains also includes two- to threefold elevations of cholesterol levels and striking six- to fifteenfold elevations of triglycerides on standard diets.[124] These lipoprotein abnormalities represent a major difference between this monogenic rat model and the autosomal mouse obesity phenotypes that require the administration of an atherogenic diet for severe vascular lesions to develop.[125] The presence of lipid abnormalities as well as obesity, insulin resistance, hypertension, and progressive atherosclerosis has established the recessive *fa* and fa^{cp} allelic mutations as important animal models of the interrelated syndrome X spectrum of phenotypes.[120,126]

Fat (*fat*) and Tubby (*tub*) Recessive Mouse Obesity

Although these two recessive mouse models of obesity arose spontaneously at JAX many years ago, they have been phenotypically characterized and definitively mapped to two different mouse autosomes only recently.[127] The *fat* mutation dates back to 1973 and originated in the HRS/J inbred strain, whereas the *tub* mutation appeared in a C57BL/6J breeding stock.[127] *Fat* maps to midproximal mouse chromosome 8 and *tub* maps to distal mouse chromosome 7 near the *Hbb* (hemoglobin β-chain complex) and *Ins2* (insulin 2) genetic loci.[128]

The obesity phenotype of *fat/fat* mice develops slowly with an onset at 6–8 weeks of age like the yellow obese mutants, but final weights of *fat/fat* mice ultimately reach 60–70 g, which is comparable in severity to the obesity conferred by the *ob* mutation. Adult weights are lower and the rate of progression to obesity is slower in *tub/tub* mice (see Fig. 68-1). Interestingly, adipose depots throughout the body are uniformly increased in size in both *fat/fat* and *tub/tub* mice in contrast to the massive adipose organ enlargement, primarily of inguinal and axial adipose depots, in *ob/ob* and *db/db* mice.[127] These differences in mutant obesity phenotypes are unexplained but may relate to the underlying mutations themselves or to varying metabolic aspects of the mutant phenotypes. For example, the *ob* and *db* mutants both exhibit moderate increases in adrenal steroid levels, which may in part explain qualitative differences in adipose distribution.[43] Marked and early (~4 weeks of age) hyperinsulinemia in *fat/fat* mutants is similar to that in *db/db* and *ob/ob* mutants on the C57BL/6J strain, and mild transient hyperglycemia is apparent. *Tub/tub* mice show only moderate hyperinsulinemia and exhibit no glucose intolerance. When the fat mutation was bred onto the C57BL/KsJ genetic strain background, diabetes was not evident. *Tubby* and *fat* homozygotes also exhibit reduced fertility, but matings can yield litters before severe obesity develops.[127]

Unlike *ob/ob* and *db/db* mice that show extreme insulin resistance, obese *fat/fat* mice were found to be very sensitive to exogenous insulin administration. This key observation and refined meiotic mapping of the *fat* mutation coincident with the locus for the carboxypeptidase E (*Cpe*) gene has established this positional candidate gene as the site of the mutation responsible for this obesity model.[129] A single Ser202Pro substitution in a highly conserved amino acid residue of the encoded carboxypeptidase E (CPE) protein eliminates all enzymatic activity for this hormone processing enzyme, leading to the secretion of inactive proinsulin rather than mature and biologically active insulin in *fat* homozygotes.[129] This failure in insulin processing alone is probably not directly responsible for the development of the obesity phenotype in *fat/fat* mice. Rather, since CPE is expressed in the pituitary, brain, and other neuroendocrine tissues, the failure of the mutant CPE in *fat/fat* mice to process other neuropeptides or hormones involved in the control of energy metabolism, satiety, and nutrient partitioning is likely to be critical. Future work will undoubtedly focus on what specific protein substrate for CPE is rendered inactive and consequently pathogenic. The mutated tub gene product is currently unknown.

Adipose (*Ad*) Semidominant Mouse Obesity

The mouse Adipose (*Ad*) model of adult obesity arose spontaneously in the late 1970s in randomly bred crosses among a colony of wild mice trapped in Cambridge, England (designated as the PBI strain) and an inbred mouse chromosome 7 marker stock.[130] (The *Ad* model is distinct from the recessive *ad* mutation, which was subsequently found to be allelic to *db*; this mutant allele is now designated db^{ad} to distinguish it from *Ad*.) *Ad* led to a rather mild obesity phenotype that originally was thought to be semidominant in penetrance since *Ad*/+ mice developed moderate obesity by 4–6 months of age and obesity was more severe in *Ad/Ad* homozygotes. Moderate hyperinsulinemia without glucose intolerance was also evident.[131] This model of mild obesity was fortuitously mapped genetically to mouse chromosome 7 by virtue of markers carried by one of the progeniter strains. However, *Ad* has not been mapped more precisely or studied extensively, and its designation as a true automosomal mutation should be considered uncertain. The *Ad* model may in fact represent a form of hybrid genetic obesity arising from a cross of feral and domesticated inbred mouse strains. Similar polygenic models, including the BSB model of obesity that recently has been characterized in progeny of a C57BL/6J X *Mus spretus* intercross,[132] are described in more detail in the following section. Because of this uncertainty, *Ad* has not been listed here with the other more established monogenic models of obesity.

Polygenic Models of Obesity and Diabetes: Quantitative Trait Loci and Susceptibility Genes

The polygenic rodent models differ from the single gene mutations discussed above because they represent inbred genetic strains that are obese and/or diabetic owing to multiple interacting genes rather than a single mutant gene transmitted in a discernible Mendelian inheritance pattern. Nevertheless, the series of experiments conducted by Coleman, Leiter, and colleagues on the *db* and *ob* autosomal obesity alleles carried by the C57BL/6J and C57BL/KsJ inbred strains have shown that mutant metabolic phenotypes are influenced by other genes as well as by environmental factors.[19,22,54,61,62,65] Thus, the distinction between monogenic and polygenic disease models is useful, but it can be ambiguous. Important modifier genes alter the phenotypes of the classic autosomal obesity mutations, and major genes may emerge from ongoing analysis of polygenic models. In many ways the polygenic rodent models may mimic more closely than do the monogenic rodent models the complex genetics involved in the more common and multifactorial forms of human NIDDM and obesity.

There are several polygenic rodent models of both obesity and NIDDM. Many rodent models of obesity and NIDDM have been progressively generated (over decades in some cases) using selective inbreeding of obesity-prone and hyperglycemia-prone offspring. In addition, although weight parameters are similar among most inbred strains of mice fed conventional diets[133] and those not bearing major autosomal mutations such as *ob*, quantitative obesity parameters do exhibit significant variance when assessed after prolonged feeding of high fat and/or high simple carbohydrate diets in several strains of rodents.[134] Although an environmental stressor is required, the susceptibility to such dietary-induced obesity is likely to be conferred by unknown genetic determinants. More recently, it has become clear that several standard inbred strains of mice also exhibit consistent differences in parameters of glycemia and insulinemia.[38,39] These differences can be augmented through intercrosses and back-crosses of unrelated strains of mice in order to elicit a hybrid form of obesity and associated metabolic parameters, which depends on the random assortment of obesity-predisposing genes from both parental strains in the right combination to yield striking obesity phenotypes.[132,135] Thus, many genetic differences in inbred strains of rodents are present, even though quantitative traits underlying an obesity and/or hyperglycemic phenotype have not been selected by directed breeding schemes. This section reviews the phenotypic characteristics of several of these multifactorial models and discusses progress and anticipates future trends to decipher the underlying obesity-NIDDM susceptibility polygenes likely to be involved.

Rodent Models with Selectively Inbred Obesity and/or NIDDM Phenotypes: The New Zealand Obese (NZO) Polygenic Obesity, KK Polygenic NIDDM, and Goto-Kakisaki (GK) and Otsuka Long-Evans Tokushima Fatty (OLETF) Polygenic NIDDM Models

The New Zealand obese (NZO) model was developed in the 1970s using selective inbreeding for progressively heavier progeny,[136] and these animals have been maintained as randomly bred and more strictly inbreeding colonies by several investigators up to the present time. The late onset of obesity in NZO mice diverges from the weights of NZC control mice beginning at 4–6 months of age; they ultimately attain final body weights of 60–80 g at 10–12 months of age.[19,36,137] Adipose tissue enlargement is uniformly distributed and caused by hypertrophy of adipocytes.[19] Unlike many autosomal mouse obesity models with severe insulin resistance, NZO mice remain only mildly insulin-resistant, having shown four to five times greater resistance to insulin-induced convulsions relevant to control mice in pre-radioimmunoassay studies in the 1960s[138] and two- to fourfold elevations in fasting plasma insulin levels compared with controls in a more recent study.[138] Although hyperglycemia has been described in fed NZO mice, with males worse than females, glucose intolerance is also mild and dependent on weight-proportional glucose challenges.[36,139] NZO mice do not show any infertility,[19] and other obesity-associated metabolic parameters have not been evaluated. Although a polygenic inheritance for NZO obesity has been hypothesized, no quantitative trait loci genetic analyses of the NZO model have been conducted to date. Another earlier polygenic model of obesity, the Paul Bailey Brown (PBB) strain,[139] may no longer be available.

The KK mouse (for the *K* group of mouse strains from the *K*asukabe habitat) is a *Mus musculus* strain established in Japan in the late 1950s as part of a selective breeding program for large body size.[140] Compared to other genetic models, KK mice develop a milder phenotype of obesity, reaching peak adult weights of ~50 g.[141] Subsequent phenotypic analysis of KK mice revealed four- to tenfold elevations in plasma insulin levels and mild to moderate hyperglycemia, particularly on high-calorie diets and after 3–4 months of age.[141,142] Hyperglycemia progresses in severity in obese, aging mice, as is typical for human NIDDM.[141,143] Glucose tolerance testing of KK mice with weight-proportional 2 mg/g intraperitoneal or oral glucose challenges results in profiles with blood glucose values remaining elevated between 400 and 500 mg/dL for 2 hours[142,143] (Fig. 68-3). This degree of glucose intolerance is more pronounced than testing in *ob/ob* C57BL/6J and NZO mice shows, but it is not as severe as the progressive glycemia and ketonemia evident in *db/db* C57BL/KsJ mice (see Fig. 68-3). KK mice apparently do not exhibit fertility problems; cholesterol and triglyceride levels have not been reported. Continued inbreeding of the original strain in Japan during the 1970s eventually led to the normalization of hyperglycemia for unclear reasons.[19,141] However, hyperglycemia and even frank diabetes phenotypes are still apparent in overfed animals and have been re-established genetically using a variety of breeding strategies, including transferring the A^y mutation onto the KK strain and hybrid breeding with C57BL/6J mice creating the Toronto KK (T-KK) hybrid.[19,142] The genetic integrity of diabetic KK mouse colonies is uncertain at present, since such hybrid breeding may have been employed to generate a consistent diabetes phenotype. Consequently, it may prove difficult to perform quantitative trait loci mapping of potential NIDDM susceptibility genes in KK mice.

As discussed in the introduction, inbred genetic strains have not been as routinely generated and maintained for rats as for mice. A few lines of rats generated in Japan, in particular the GK and OLETF rat strains, are notable exceptions and are proving to be useful genetic models for NIDDM.[143,144] The Goto-Kakisaki (GK) rat is a stable genetic model of NIDDM that was generated through selective breeding of Wistar rats using oral glucose intolerance as the selection criterion.[144] The GK rat begins to develop fed hyperglycemia as early as 8 days of life, and fasting hyperglycemia and glucose intolerance to a 2 mg/g intraperitoneal glucose tolerance test is evident by 2 months of age.[145] The GK rat has recently been characterized extensively by several investigators for pancreatic islet dysfunction and other accessible parameters of metabolic NIDDM pathophysiology.[146–149] In addition, breeding studies with this strain are beginning to provide insights into the complex genetics of NIDDM susceptibility genes in rats, including findings possibly consistent either with disturbances of maternal metabolism or with parental imprinting effects.[145,150]

Unlike other NIDDM models in rats and mice, the OTELF rat appeared spontaneously in a colony of outbred Long-Evans rats in the late 1980s.[151] Like KK mice and GK rats, OTELF rats develop moderate and persistent glucose intolerance profiles with glucose values greater than 20–25 mM for up to 2 hours following a 2-mg/g oral glucose challenge beginning at 24 weeks of age (see Figure 68-3).[145] The ability to perform more extensive phenotyping of obesity, NIDDM, and related metabolic phenotypes in rats (given their larger size compared to mice) may render feasible the genetic analysis of several quantitative traits related to obesity or NIDDM in such polygenic models. Future work on the GK and OTELF rat strains should continue to provide useful insights potentially applicable to the genetics of human NIDDM.

Rodent Obesity and NIDDM Models in Inbred Strains Exposed to a Dietary Stressor: Osborne-Mendel and "Cafeteria" Rats and AKR/J and C57BL/6J Mice

In addition to the selectively inbred polygenic models of obesity-NIDDM described above, several extant rodent strains have been described that exhibit obesity and/or hyperglycemia on either a

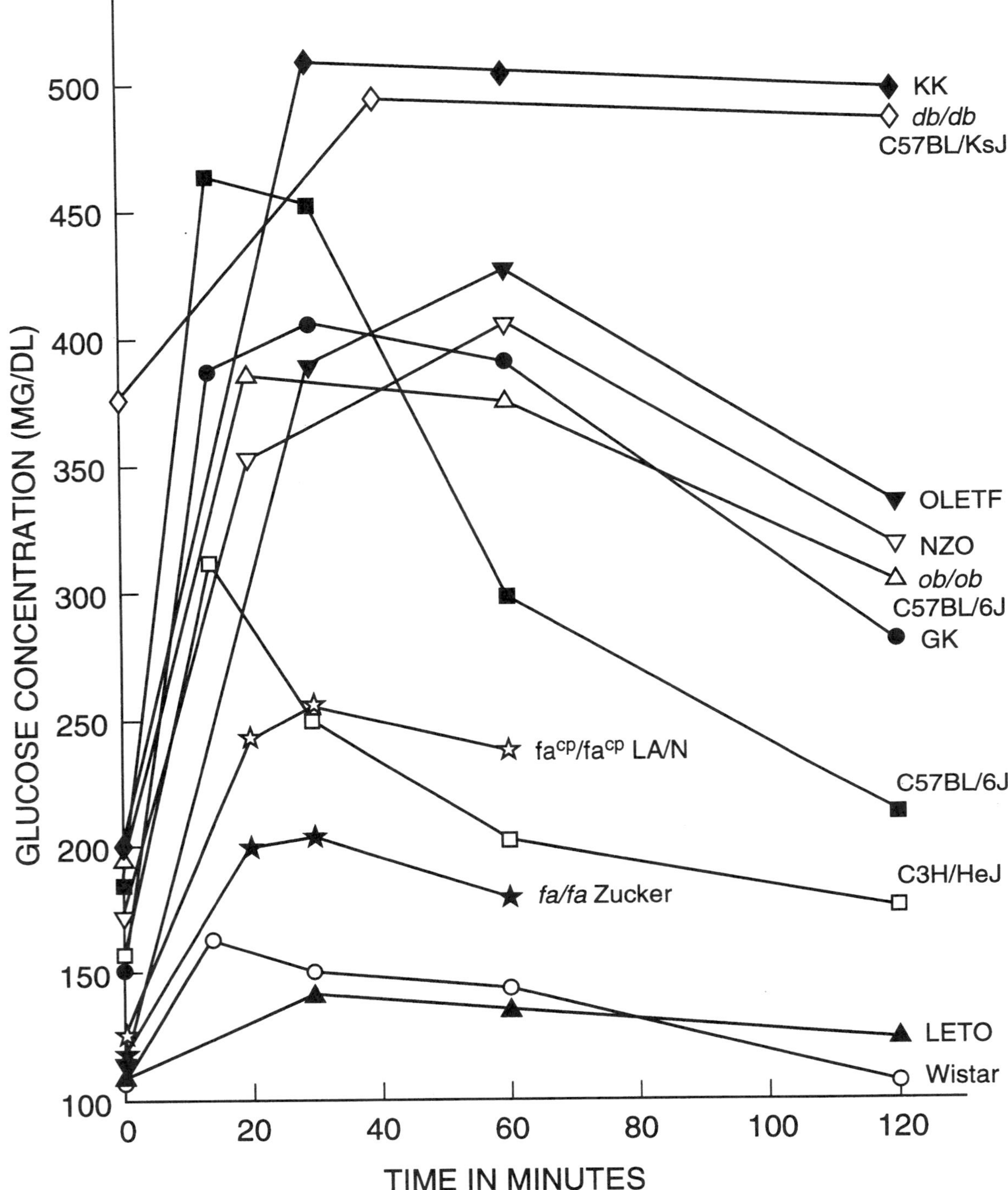

Figure 68-3. Relative glucose intolerance phenotype severities for rodent genetic NIDDM models. The relative severities of glucose tolerance testing in a variety of mouse and rat genetic models of NIDDM are shown. Each glucose tolerance curve is labeled with the corresponding mutation and/or strain as described in the text. The Wistar strain provides a glucose tolerance curve for a representative control rat strain. The LETO strain is the specific control strain from which the glucose intolerant OLETF strain was derived. The C3H/HeJ and C57BL/6J strains are inbred mouse strains that exhibit the extremes of glucose tolerance testing in the absence of obesity genes or a diabetogenic diet. Glucose tolerance differences conferred by either the *ob* or *db* recessive obesity genes are contrasted for the diabetes-susceptible C57BL/KsJ strain and the more resistant C57BL/6J strain. Similarly, the allelic fatty mutations may also lead to differences in relative glucose tolerance when carried by the LA/N or Zucker strains. The polygenic GK, NZO, and KK models of NIDDM are described in the text. Testing for each strain involved the administration of either oral or intraperitoneal glucose loads that were proportional to total body weight (1–2 mg/g). The data depicted in this figure have been compiled from references 35, 36, 116, 117, 119, 120, 121, 122, 123, 138, 142, 143, 144, 145, and 151.

high-fat diet or a palatable, so-called cafeteria diet.[152] The putative obesity genes that contribute to these diet-induced phenotypes should be considered susceptibility genes that require the imposition of a high-risk diet for their full expression. Pioneering work on diet-induced obesity was performed over four decades ago in nearly inbred strains of mice. Dietary fat led to a mild obesity phenotype in the early C3H and A mouse strains but not in C57BL/6J or I mice.[153] Subsequent work on diet-induced obesity was done by Schemmel and coworkers in seven different rat strains.[154] The most severely affected strain is the Osborne-Mendel rat, whereas S5B/P1 rats proved resistant to diet-induced obesity.[155] These seven rat strains were maintained as closed but not fully inbred colonies when these early studies were performed; therefore the genetic analysis of dietary obesity susceptibility genes in rats may depend on the generation and crossing of stable inbred lines.

More recently, several investigators have re-examined dietary obesity in inbred mouse strains and capitalized on their diversity and genetic uniformity to do more in-depth genetic analyses of dietary-induced phenotypes. West and colleagues have investigated the development of obesity in nine different inbred strains of mice fed a high-fat percentage diet.[133] As seen in earlier work in both mouse and rat strains described above, there was a segregation of dietary obesity phenotypes among these different strains. The AKR/J strain of mice has proved to be the most susceptible to dietary obesity, attaining ~23% body fat on a high-fat diet, whereas the SWR strain, like the S5B/P1 rat strain, is resistant to the development of dietary obesity, developing only ~7% body lipid composition.[133] Even though the obesity phenotypes in these models are less severe than in other monogenic and polygenic mouse models of obesity, further quantitative genetic analysis, including intercross and back-cross breeding of the AKR/J strain with the SWR/J strain, has been informative. A total of three different quantitative trait loci have been discerned in these genetic studies that contribute approximately 40% of the variance to the obesity seen in the AKR/J strain.[155,156] These quantitative trait loci have been designated *Dob1, Dob2,* and *Dob3* (for dietary obesity) and map to mouse chromosomes 4, 9, and 15, respectively. Further work to define possible allelic differences between the AKR/J and SWR/J strains at candidate gene loci near these quantitative trait loci is under way.

Using a similar approach, the C57BL/6J strain has also been shown to harbor potential hyperglycemia and obesity susceptibility genes when placed on sucrose drinking water or a high-fat–high-carbohydrate combination diet.[38,39,157] Initial studies of glucose intolerance in the C57BL/6J strain, including recombinant inbred genetic analysis using BXH lines, uncovered no major gene effect determining hyperglycemia in C57BL/6J mice.[38] Using different recombinant inbred lines (BXA and AXB), a potential quantitative trait locus for diet-induced hyperglycemia has been discerned in genetic analysis of the C57BL/6J strain that maps to mouse chromosome 7 at a location near the glycogen synthase gene.[158] Further work to define possible allelic differences at this locus or other nearby loci will be necessary to determine the identity of the putative hyperglycemia susceptibility gene at this chromosomal position.

In all of the above examples using extant strains in both mice and rats, the designation of obesity or hyperglycemia is made according to a quantitative trait threshold. Nonetheless, severe obesity phenotypes or full-fledged diabetes do not seem to be present in most inbred mouse or rodent strains examined. Rather, the quantitative traits of percent adiposity, impaired glucose tolerance, and/or hyperinsulinemia have all been examined as proxies for the full expression of NIDDM. Because plasma parameters such as hyperglycemia and insulin levels tend to be less reproducible than body weight and length parameters, which determine obesity in a quantitative way, it may prove difficult to perform detailed quantitative trait locus analysis of subphenotypes for diabetes. Careful sampling, particularly in newer rat strains such as the GK and OTELF rat models with NIDDM traits selected through programmed breeding may yield more reproducible results that can be analyzed using quantitative trait loci techniques. Like these polygenic rodent models, human populations appear to develop obesity as a result of an underlying genetic susceptibility plus the imposition of dietary and environmental stressors, such as inactivity or a high-fat diet. It remains to be determined whether the same susceptibility genes are involved in the development of dietary obesity and NIDDM phenotypes in rodents and human populations.

Polygenic Models of Obesity Caused by Interacting Genes Among Hybrid Crosses: BSB Obesity and Wellesley Hybrid Obesity

A final polygenic model of obesity and associated metabolic phenotypes has been examined recently by Warden and colleagues.[132] This model, termed BSB hybrid obesity, emerged somewhat fortuitously during the course of detailed genetic analysis of cholesterol metabolism differences in an interspecific back-cross between *Mus spretus* and the inbred C57BL/6J *Mus musculus* strain.[132,136,159] Although C57BL/6J parents and F_1(C57BL/6J × *Mus spretus*) offspring cluster at ~12% carcass lipid compositions and *Mus spretus* parents are even leaner, the individual F_1 × C57BL/6J back-cross progeny (BSB) varied widely from 1–50% carcass lipid. Quantitative trait loci genetic analysis of obesity parameters in these hybrid mice has identified four distinct loci designated *Mob1* through *Mob4* (for multigenic obesity) segregating in this cross and mapping to mouse chromosomes 6, 7, 12, and 15.[132,136] Future work on the BSB obesity model will undoubtedly attempt to identify and analyze candidate genes near these chromosomal sites for allelic differences. Overall, the BSB hybrid model of obesity and hypercholesterolemia is reminiscent of earlier hybrid mouse obesities such as the Wellesley obesity model.[18] The Wellesley polygenic model was noted over three decades ago in an F_1 intercross of lean C3H and I strain mice. Adult F_1 mice achieved weights of up to 50 g. Similar phenotypes of variable hybrid obesity with final weights up to 60 g have appeared in intercrossed and back-crossed progeny of 129/J and C57BL/6J mice bred to achieve background genetic uniformity following gene targeting experiments conducted at our institution (Fiedorek F, Bronson S, Maeda N, unpublished observations 1995). Thus, hybrid forms of polygenic obesity owing to heterosis (i.e., hybrid vigor) genetic interactions may be quite common among cross-breeding rodent strains. By analogy, such genetic influences leading to an increased prevalence of obesity in societies with plentiful diets may also be acting in the "melting pots" that are evident among human populations.[160]

Future Prospects and Limitations of Rodent Genetic Models

Dramatic advances in human molecular genetics and positional cloning methods over the past 10 years have allowed even rare human clinical material to be exploited. Human disease genes causing Duchenne's muscular dystrophy, cystic fibrosis, and many other disorders have been identified. The genes responsible for the rare Prader-Willi and Bardet-Biedl obesity syndromes will ultimately be discovered as well, but no such "easy" solutions may be available for common and complex inherited disorders like obesity and NIDDM. Newer sib pair genetic methods that do not rely on strict inheritance patterns and that take into account quantitative phenotypic variance are being developed for common polygenic human disorders.[14] Nonetheless, numerous potential confounders of the polygenic analysis of multifactorial inherited disorders in human populations exist. Such factors include the genetic interactions among heterogeneous (i.e., hybrid) human populations and the ready availability of "cafeteria" diets for people (as well as rodents). Indeed, for both obesity and NIDDM, penetrance in a susceptible individual and incidence in a population are increased by such nongenetic factors as a sedentary lifestyle and a high-fat diet. These Western societal influences coupled with the potential evolutionary advantage bestowed by obesity and diabetes susceptibility polygenes[160] apparently have conspired to create an ''epidemic-like'' prevalence of both obesity and NIDDM over the past several decades.[161] The genetic analysis and ultimate identification of ubiquitous obesity and NIDDM susceptibility genes amid changing diets and environments and in the presence of genetic admixture represent a major challenge for diabetes researchers and physicians. These factors can be controlled in genetic studies of mutant and inbred rodents.

Understanding the genetic determinants of these many rodent disease models should help illuminate genetic aspects of human NIDDM and obesity just as insights into pathophysiology have been made through their past examination. The monogenic and polygenic rodent genetic models discussed here offer particular virtues for the analysis of multifactorial inheritance involved in more common forms of obesity and NIDDM in humans. Mutations in major autosomal rodent obesity genes, allelic modifying genes that are responsible for phenotypic differences conferred by the same autosomal mutation in various inbred genetic strains, and other unknown obesity-diabetes susceptibility genes currently being defined by quantitative trait loci mapping should account for nearly all of the observed genetic variability for rodent obesity-NIDDM phenotypes.* Similarly, the susceptibility to obesity and NIDDM in humans is also hypothesized to involve interacting major and minor gene effects (see Chapters 61 and 62).

Although pathophysiology is shared between humans and rodents, it remains to be seen whether gene defects responsible for obesity and NIDDM also will be shared. The power of comparative mammalian genetics allows homologous genomic comparisons to be made, but the physiology, biochemistry, and developmental time course of disorders such as obesity and diabetes in mice and rats can be very different from those in human disease.[162] For example, mice show greater elevations of high-density lipoprotein cholesterol relative to low-density lipoprotein cholesterol because they do not possess the cholesterol ester transfer protein.[163] Nonetheless, the possibility of performing genetic analyses on uniform genetic rodent models of obesity and NIDDM should provide insights even if the exact disease genes are not shared. Such causative gene diversity appears to be the case in comparison of susceptibility to IDDM in humans and non-obese diabetes in mice.[164] Ultimately, the most important NIDDM and obesity disease genes may be shown to harbor relatively common allelic variations significant enough to contribute major gene effects responsible for human diabetes and obesity susceptibility much as *ApoE-4* allelic variants are hypothesized at present to contribute substantially to the susceptibility to late onset forms of Alzheimer's disease.[165] It is hoped that a better genetic understanding of the interrelated syndromes of obesity and NIDDM in both rodents and humans will bring about improved treatment approaches for these common disorders.

**Author's note*: In the course of the publication of this chapter, expression cloning of the leptin receptor and its tentative identification as the *db* gene product based on its chromosomal map position was accomplished.[166] In addition, quantitative trait analysis of the GK rat NIDDM model identified independent genetic loci contributing to the glucose intolerance phenotype of this rat strain.[167,168]

References

1. Bray GA, York DA. Hypothalamic and genetic obesity in experimental animals: An autonomic and endocrine hypothesis. Physiol Rev 1979;59:719
2. Wilson GL, Leiter EH. Streptozotocin interactions with pancreatic beta cells and the induction of insulin-dependent diabetes. Curr Top Microbiol Immunol 1990;156:27
3. Weir GC, Leahy JL, Bonner-Weir S. Experimental reduction of B-cell mass: Implications for the pathogenesis of diabetes. Diabetes Metab Rev 1986;2:125
4. Leiter EH. The genetics of diabetes susceptibility in mice. FASEB J 1989; 3:2231
5. Bouchard C, Perusse L. Heredity and body fat. Annu Rev Nutr 1988;8:259
6. King RA, Rotter JI, Motulsky AG, eds. The Genetic Basis of Common Disease. New York: Oxford University Press;1992
7. Taylor SI, Accili D, Imai Y. Insulin resistance or insulin deficiency: Which is the primary cause of NIDDM? Diabetes 1994;43:735
8. Matschinsky F, Liang Y, Kesavan P, et al. Glucokinase as pancreatic beta cell glucose sensor and diabetes gene. J Clin Invest 1993;92:2092
9. Nicholls RD. Genomic imprinting and candidate genes in the Prader-Willi and Angelman syndromes. Curr Opin Genet Dev 1993;3:445
10. Kwitek-Black AE, Carmi R, Duyk GM, et al. Linkage of Bardet-Biedl syndrome to chromosome 16q and evidence for non-allelic genetic heterogeneity. Nat Genet 1993;5:392
11. Leppert M, Baird L, Anderson KL, et al. Bardet-Biedl syndrome is linked to DNA markers on chromosome 11q and is genetically heterogeneous. Nat Genet 1994;7:108
12. Carmi R, Rokhlina T, Kwitek-Black AE, et al. Use of a DNA pooling strategy to identify a human obesity syndrome locus on chromosome 15. Hum Mol Genet 1995;4:9
13. O'Brien SJ, Womack JE, Lyons LA, et al. Anchored reference loci for comparative genome mapping in mammals. Nat Genet 1993;3:103
14. Lander ES, Schork NJ. Genetic dissection of complex traits. Science 1994; 265:2037
15. Lowell BB, S-Susulic V, Hamann A, et al. Development of obesity in transgenic mice after genetic ablation of brown adipose tissue. Nature 1993; 366:740
16. Tecott LH, Sun LM, Akana SF, et al. Eating disorder and epilepsy in mice lacking 5-HT2c serotonin receptors. Nature 1995;374:542
17. Tanksley SD. Mapping polygenes. Annu Rev Genet 1993;27:205
18. Bray GA, York DA. Genetically transmitted obesity in rodents. Physiol Rev 1971;51:598
19. Herberg L, Coleman DL. Laboratory animals exhibiting obesity and diabetes syndromes. Metabolism 1977;26:59
20. Johnson PR, Greenwood MR, Horwitz BA, Stern JS. Animal models of obesity: Genetic aspects. Annu Rev Nutr 1991;11:325
21. Ingalls AM, Dickie MM, Snell GD. Obese, a new mutation in the mouse. J Hered 1950;41:317
22. Coleman DL. Obese and diabetes: Two mutant genes causing diabetes-obesity syndromes in mice. Diabetologia 1978;14:141
23. Trayhurn P, Thurley PL, James WPT. Thermogenic defect in pre-obese *ob/ob* mice. Nature 1977;266:60
24. Dubec PU. The development of obesity, hyperinsulinemia, and hyperglycemia in *ob/ob* mice. Metabolism 1976;25:1567
25. Yen TTT, Acton JM. Locomotor activity of various types of genetically obese mice. Proc Soc Exp Biol Med 1972;140:647
26. Mayer J, Dickie MM, Bates MW, Vitale JJ. Free selection of nutrients by hereditarily obese mice. Science 1951;113:745
27. Dubec PU. Effects of limited food intake on the obese-hyperglycemic syndrome. Am J Physiol 1976;230:1474
28. Yen TT, Allan JA, Yu PL, et al. Triacylglycerol contents and *in vivo* lipogenesis of *ob/ob*, *db/db*, and A^{vy}/a mice. Biochim Biophys Acta 1976;441:213
29. Alonzo LG, Maren TH. Effect of food restriction on body composition of hereditary obese mice. Am J Physiol 1955;183:284
30. Johnson PR, Hirsch J. Cellurity of adipose depots in six strains of genetically obese mice. J Lipid Res 1972;13:2
31. Genuth SM, Przybylski RB, Rosenberg DM. Insulin resistance in genetically obese, hyperglycemic mice. Endocrinology 1971;88:1230
32. Genuth SM. Hyperinsulinism in mice with genetically determined obesity. Endocrinology 1969;84:386
33. Bailey CJ, Flatt PR. Islet defects and insulin resistance in models of obese non-insulin-dependent diabetes. Diabetes Metab Rev 1993;9:43S
34. Mayer J, Bates MW, Dickie MM. Hereditary diabetes in genetically obese mice. Science 1951;113:746
35. Chlouverakis C, Dade EF, Batt RAL. Glucose tolerance and time sequence of adiposity, hyperinsulinemia and hyperglycemia in obese-hyperglycemic mice (*obob*). Metabolism 1970;19:687
36. Herberg L, Major E, Henigs U, et al. Differences in the development of the obese-hyperglycemic syndrome in *obob* and NZO mice. Diabetologia 1970; 6:292
37. Beloff-Chain A, Freund N, Rookledge KA. Blood glucose and serum insulin levels in lean and genetically obese mice. Horm Metab Res 1974;7:374
38. Kaku K, Fiedorek FT Jr, Province M, Permutt MA. Genetic analysis of glucose tolerance in inbred mouse strains. Evidence for polygenic control. Diabetes 1988;37:707
39. Surwit RS, Kuhn CM, Cochrane C, et al. Diet-induced type II diabetes in C57BL/6J mice. Diabetes 1988;37:1163
40. Mayer J, Jones AK. Hypercholesterolemia in the hereditary obese-hyperglycemic syndrome of mice. Am J Physiol 1953;175:339
41. Zomzely C, Mayer J. Levels of serum cholesterol in obese mice. Nature 1958;182:1738
42. Nishina PM, Lowe S, Wang J, Paigen B. Characterization of plasma lipids in genetically obese mice: The mutants obese, diabetes, fat, tubby, and lethal yellow. Metabolism 1994;43:549

43. Naester P. Function of the adrenal cortex in obese-hyperglycemic mice (gene symbol *ob*). Diabetologia 1974;10:449
44. Kopelman PG. Hormones and obesity: Baillières Clin Endocrinol Metab 1994;8:549
45. Lane PW, Dickie MM. Fertile, obese male mice: Relative sterility in obese males corrected by dietary restriction. J Hered 1954;45:56
46. Runner MN, Gates A. Sterile, obese mothers. J Hered 1954;45:51
47. Friedman JM, Leibel RL, Siegel DS, et al. Molecular mapping of the mouse *ob* mutation. Genomics 1991;11:1054
48. Zhang Y, Proenca R, Maffei M, et al. Positional cloning of the mouse obese gene and its human homologue. Nature 1994;372:425
49. Weigle DS. Appetite and the regulation of body composition. FASEB J 1994;8:302
50. Hummel KP, Dickie MM, Coleman DL. Diabetes, a new mutation in the mouse. Science 1966;153:1127
51. Aubert R, Herzog J, Camus MC, et al. Description of a new model of genetic obesity: The db^{Pas} mouse. J Nutrition 1985;115:327
52. Falconer DS, Isaacson JH. Adipose, a new inherited obesity of the mouse. J Hered 1959;50:290
53. Truett GE, Bahary N, Friedman JM, Leibel RL. Rat obesity gene fatty (*fa*) maps to chromosome 5: Evidence for homology with the mouse gene diabetes (*db*). Proc Natl Acad Sci USA 1991;88:7806
54. Coleman DL, Hummel KP. Studies with the mutation, diabetes, in the mouse. Diabetologia 1967;3:238
55. Coleman DL, Hummel KP. Hyperinsulinemia in pre-weaning diabetes (*db*) mice. Diabetologia 1974;10:607
56. Yen TTT, Fuller RW, Pearson DV. The response of "obese" (*ob*/*ob*) and "diabetic" (*db*/*db*) mice to treatments that influence body temperature. Comp Biochem Physiol 1974;49A:377
57. Coleman DL. Thermogenesis in diabetes-obesity syndromes in mutant mice. Diabetologia 1982;22:205
58. Batt RAL, Harrison GA. The reproductive system of the adipose mouse. J Heredity 1963;54:135
59. Coleman DL, Hummel KP. Effects of parabiosis of normal with genetically diabetic mice. Am J Physiol 1969;217:1298
60. Finerty JC. Parabiosis in physiological studies. Physiol Rev 1952;32:277
61. Hummel KP, Coleman DL, Lane PW. The influence of genetic background on expression of mutations at the diabetes locus in the mouse: I. C57BL/KsJ and C57BL/6J strains. Biochem Genet 1972;7:1
62. Leiter EH, Chapman HD. Obesity-induced diabetes (diabesity) in C57BL/KsJ mice produces aberrant trans-regulation of sex steroid sulfotransferase genes. J Clin Invest 1994;93:2007
63. Wyse BM, Dulin WE. The influence of age and dietary conditions on diabetes in the db mouse. Diabetologia 1970;6:268
64. DeFronzo RA, Bonadonna RC, Ferrannini E. Pathogenesis of NIDDM. A balanced overview. Diabetes Care 1992;15:318
65. Leiter EH, Chapman HD, Falany CN. Synergism of obesity genes with hepatic steroid sulfotransferases to mediate diabetes in mice. Diabetes 1991; 40:1360
66. Bjorntorp P. Androgens, the metabolic syndrome, and non-insulin-dependent diabetes mellitus. Ann NY Acad Sci 1993;15:242
67. Bailey DW. Sources of subline divergence and their relative importance for sublines of six major inbred strains of mice. In: Morse HC III, ed. Origins of Inbred Mice. New York: Academic Press;1978:197–215
68. Naggert JK, Mu J-L, Frankel W, et al. Genomic analysis of the C57BL/Ks strain. Mamm Genome 1995;6:131
69. Lueders KK. Differences in intracisternal A-particle and GLN proviral loci suggest a genetic contribution from a DBA/2-like strain in generation of the C57BL-Ks strain. Mamm Genome 1995;6:134
70. Bahary N, Leibel RL, Joseph L, Friedman JM. Molecular mapping of the mouse *db* mutation. Proc Natl Acad Sci USA 1990;87:8642
71. Abbott CM, Blank R, Eppig JT, et al. Encyclopedia of the mouse genome III. Mouse chromosome 4. Mamm Genome 1993;3:S58
72. Wolff GL, Roberts DW, Galbraith DB. Prenatal determination of obesity, tumor susceptibility, and coat color pattern in viable yellow (A^{vy}/a) mice. The yellow mouse syndrome. J Hered 1986;77:151
73. Yen TT, Gill AM, Frigeri LG, et al. Obesity, diabetes, and neoplasia in yellow A^{vy}/-mice: Ectopic expression of the agouti gene. FASEB J 1994;8:479
74. Green MC. Catalog of mutant genes and polymorphic loci. In: Lyon MF, Searle AG, eds. Genetic Variants and Strains of the Laboratory Mouse, 2nd ed. Oxford: Oxford University Press;1989:17–20
75. Dickie MM. Mutations at the agouti locus in the mouse. J Hered 1969;60:20
76. Carpenter KJ, Mayer J. Physiologic observations on yellow obesity in the mouse. Am J Physiol 1958;193:499
77. Wolff GW. Body composition and coat color correlation in different phenotypes of "viable yellow" mice. Science 1965;147:1145
78. Heston W, Vlahakis G. Influence of the A^y gene on mammary gland tumours, hepatomas, and normal growth. J Natl Cancer Inst 1961;40:1161
79. Wolff GL. Growth of inbred yellow (A^ya) and non-yellow (*aa*) mice in parabiosis. Genetics 1963;48:1041
80. Coleman DL. Antiobesity effects of etiocholanotones in diabetes (*db*), viable yellow (A^{vy}), and normal mice. Endocrinology 1985;117:2279
81. Gill AM, Leiter EH, Powell JG, et al. Dexamethasone-induced hyperglycemia in obese A^{vy}/a (viable yellow) female mice entails preferential induction of a hepatic estrogen sulfotransferase. Diabetes 1994;43:999
82. Kasten FH. Comparative histological studies of endocrine glands of yellow (A^ya) and non-agouti (*aa*) mice in relation to problems of hereditary obesity. Science 1952;115:647
83. Turner ML. Hereditary obesity and temperature regulation. Am J Physiol 1948;152:197
84. Bultman SJ, Michaud EJ, Woychik RP. Molecular characterization of the mouse agouti locus. Cell 1992;71:1195
85. Miller MW, Duhl DM, Vrieling H, et al. Cloning of the mouse agouti gene predicts a secreted protein ubiquitously expressed in mice carrying the lethal yellow mutation. Genes Dev 1993;7:454
86. Bultman SJ, Russell LB, Gutierrez EGA, Woychik RP. Molecular characterization of a region of DNA associated with mutations at the agouti locus in the mouse. Proc Natl Acad Sci USA 1991;88:8062
87. Silvers WK. The agouti and extension series of alleles, umbrous, and sable. In: The Coat Colors of Mice. New York: Springer-Verlag;1979:1–44
88. Wolff GL. Influence of maternal phenotype on metabolic differentiation of agouti locus mutants in the mouse. Genetics 1978;88:529
89. Michaud EJ, Bultman SJ, Stubbs LJ, Woychik RP. The embryonic lethality of homozygous lethal yellow mice (A^y/A^y) is associated with the disruption of a novel RNA-binding protein. Genes Dev 1993;7:1203
90. Duhl DM, Stevens ME, Vrieling H, et al. Pleiotropic effects of the mouse lethal yellow (A^y) mutation explained by deletion of a maternally expressed gene and the simultaneous production of agouti fusion RNAs. Development 1994;120:1695
91. Duhl DM, Vrieling H, Miller KA, et al. Neomorphic *agouti* mutations in obese yellow mice. Nature Genetics 1994;8:59
92. Michaud EJ, van-Vugt MJ, Bultman SJ, et al. Differential expression of a new dominant agouti allele (A^{iapy}) is correlated with methylation state and is influenced by parental lineage. Genes Dev 1994;8:1463
93. Manne J, Argeson AC, Siracusa LD. Mechanisms for the pleiotropic effects of the agouti gene. Proc Natl Acad Sci USA 1995;92:4721
94. Kwon HY, Bultman SJ, Loffler C, et al. Molecular structure and chromosomal mapping of the human homolog of the agouti gene. Proc Natl Acad Sci USA 1994;91:9760
95. Wilson BD, Ollmann MM, Kang L, et al. Structure and function of ASP, the human homolog of the mouse agouti gene. Hum Mol Genet 1995;4:223
96. Klebig ML, Wilkinson JE, Geisler JG, Woychik RP. Ectopic expression of the agouti gene in transgenic mice causes obesity, features of type II diabetes, and yellow fur. Proc Natl Acad Sci USA 1995;92:4728
97. Lu D, Willard D, Patel IR, et al. Agouti protein is an antagonist of the melanocyte-stimulating-hormone receptor. Nature 1994;371:799
98. Zemel MB, Kim JH, Woychik RP, et al. Agouti regulation of intracellular calcium: Role in the insulin resistance of viable yellow mice. Proc Natl Acad Sci USA 1995;92:4733
99. Zucker LM, Zucker TF. Fatty, a new mutation in the rat. J Hered 1961;52:275
100. Koletsky S. Pathologic findings and laboratory data in a new strain of obese hypertensive rats. Am J Pathol 1976:129
101. Yen TT, Shaw WN, Yu P-L. Genetics of obesity in Zucker rats and Koletsky rats. Heredity 1977;38:373
102. Kraegen EW, James DE, Bennett SP, Chisholm DJ. *In vivo* insulin sensitivity in the rat determined by euglycemic clamp. Am J Physiol 1983;245:E1
103. Bray GA. The Zucker-fatty rat: A review. Fed Proc 1977;36:148
104. Argiles JM. The obese Zucker rat: A choice for fat metabolism 1968–1988: Twenty years of research on the insights of the Zucker mutation. Prog Lipid Res 1989;28:53
105. Kurtz TW, Morris RC, Pershadsingh HA. The Zucker fatty rat as a genetic model of obesity and hypertension. Hypertension 1989;13:896
106. Godbole V, York DA, Bloxham DP. Developmental changes in the fatty (*fafa*) rat: Evidence for defective thermogenesis preceding the hyperlipogenesis and hyperinsulinaemia. Diabetologia 1978;15:41
107. Berce PJ, Moore BJ, Horwitz BA, Stern JS. Metabolism at thermoneutrality and in the cold is reduced in the neonatal preobese Zucker fatty (*fa*/*fa*) rat. J Nutr 1986;116:2478
108. Johnson PR, Zucker LM, Cruce JAF, Hirsch J. Cellularity of adipose depots in the genetically obese Zucker rat. J Lipid Res 1971;12:706
109. Bray GA, York DA. Studies on food intake of genetically obese rats. Am J Physiol 1972;223:176
110. Castonguay TW, Hartman WJ, Fitzpatrick EA, Stern JS. Dietary self-selection and the Zucker rat. J Nutr 1982;112:796
111. Bray GA, York DA, Swerdloff RS. Genetic obesity in rats. I. The effects of food restriction on body composition and hypothalamic function. Metabolism 1973;22:435
112. Zucker LM, Antoniades HN. Insulin and obesity in the Zucker genetically obese rat "fatty." Endocrinology 1972;90:1320
113. Nguyen-Yamamoto L, Deal CL, Finkelstein JA, Van Vliet G. Hormonal control of growth in the genetically obese Zucker rat. I. Linear growth, plasma insulin-like growth factor-I (IGF-I) and IGF-binding proteins. Endocrinology 1984;134:1382
114. Guillaume-Gentil C, Rohner-Jeanrenaud F, Abramo F, et al. Abnormal regulation of the hypothalamo-pituitary-adrenal axis in the genetically obese *fa*/*fa* rat. Endocrinology 1990;126:1873
115. York DA, Steinke J, Bray GA. Hyperinsulinemia and insulin resistance in genetically obese rats. Metabolism 1972;21:277
116. Terrettaz J, Jeanrenaud B. In vivo and peripheral insulin resistance in genetically obese (*fa*/*fa*) rats. Endocrinology 1985;112:1346
117. Russell JC, Graham S, Hameed M. Abnormal insulin and glucose metabolism in the JCR:LA-corpulent rat. Metabolism 1994;43:538

118. Penicaud L, Ferre P, Terretaz J, et al. Development of obesity in Zucker rats. Early insulin resistance in muscles but normal sensitivity in white adipose tissue. Diabetes 1987;36:626
119. Ikeda H, Shino A, Matsuo T. A new genetically obese-hyperglycemic rat (Wistar fatty). Diabetes 1981;30:1045
120. Amy RM, Dolphin PJ, Pederson RA, Russell JC. Atherogenesis in two strains of obese rats. The fatty Zucker and LA/N-corpulent. Atherosclerosis 1988; 69:199
121. Ionescu E, Sauter JF, Jeanrenaud B. Abnormal oral glucose tolerance in genetically obese *(fa/fa)* rats. Am J Physiol 1985;248:E500
122. Russell JC, Ahuja SK, Manickavel V, et al. Insulin resistance and impaired glucose tolerance in the atherosclerosis-prone LA/N corpulent rat. Arteriosclerosis 1987;7:620
123. Kava RA, West DB, Lukasik VA, Greenwood MRC. Sexual dimorphism of hyperglycemia and glucose tolerance in Wistar fatty rats. Diabetes 1989;38: 159
124. Barry WS, Bray GA. Plasma triglycerides in genetically obese rats. Metabolism 1969;18:833
125. Nishina PM, Naggert JK, Verstuyft J, Paigen B. Atherosclerosis in genetically obese mice: The mutants obese, diabetes, fat, tubby, and lethal yellow. Metabolism 1994;43:554
126. Dolphin PJ, Stewart B, Amy RM, Russell JC. Serum lipids and lipoproteins in the atherosclerosis prone LA/N corpulent rat. Biochim Biophys Acta 1987;919:140
127. Coleman DL, Eicher EM. Fat *(fat)* and tubby *(tub)*: Two autosomal recessive mutations causing obesity syndromes in the mouse. J Hered 1990;81: 424
128. Jones JM, Meisler MH, Seldin MF, et al. Localization of insulin-2 *(Ins-2)* and the obesity mutant tubby *(tub)* to distinct regions of mouse chromosome 7. Genomics 1992;14:197
129. Naggert JK, Fricker LD, Varlamov O, et al. Hyperproinsulinaemia in obese *fat/fat* mice associated with a carboxypeptidase E mutation which reduces enzyme activity. Nature Genetics 1995;10:135
130. Wallace ME, MacSwiney FM. An inherited mild middle-aged adiposity in wild mice. J Hygiene 1979;82:309
131. Trayhurn P, James WPT. Studies on the body composition, fat distribution and fat cell size and number of 'Ad,' a new obese mutant mouse. Br J Nutr 1979;41:211
132. Warden CH, Fisler JS, Pace MJ, et al. Coincidence of genetic loci for plasma cholesterol levels and obesity in a multifactorial mouse model. J Clin Invest 1993;92:773
133. The Jackson Laboratories product literature: Comparative ages and weights of JAX mice. 1992:14–16
134. West DB, Boozer CN, Moody DL, Atkinson RL. Dietary obesity in nine inbred mouse strains. Am J Physiol 1992;262:R1025
135. Warden CH, Fisler JS, Shoemaker SM, et al. Identification of four chromosomal loci determining obesity in a multifactorial mouse model. J Clin Invest 1995;95:1545
136. Bielschowsky M, Goodall CM. Origin of inbred NZ mouse strains. Cancer Res 1970;30:834
137. Crofford OB, Davis CK Jr. Growth characteristics, glucose tolerance and insulin sensitivity of New Zealand obese mice. Metabolism 1965:271
138. Veroni MC, Proietto J, Larkins RG. Evolution of insulin resistance in New Zealand obese mice. Diabetes 1991;40:1480
139. Hunt CE, Lindsey JR, Walkley SU. Animal models of diabetes and obesity, including the PBB/Ld mouse. Fed Proc 1976;35:1206
140. Ikeda H. KK mouse. Diabetes Res Clin Pract 1994;24:S313
141. Dulin WE, Wyse BM. Diabetes in the KK mouse. Diabetologia 1970;6:317
142. Reddi AS, Camerini-Davalos RA. Hereditary diabetes in the KK mouse: An overview. Adv Exp Med Biol 1988;246:7
143. Goto Y, Suzuki K, Ono T, et al. Development of diabetes in the non-obese NIDDM rat (GK rat). Adv Exp Med Biol 1988;246:29
144. Kawano K, Hirashima T, Mori S, et al. Spontaneous long-term hyperglycemic rat with diabetic complications. Otsuka Long-Evans Tokushima Fatty (OLETF) strain. Diabetes 1992;41:1422
145. Abdel-Halim SM, Guenifi A, Luthman H, et al. Impact of diabetic inheritance on glucose tolerance and insulin secretion in spontaneously diabetic GK-Wistar rats. Diabetes 1994;43:281
146. Portha B, Serradas P, Bailbe D, et al. Beta-cell insensitivity to glucose in the GK rat, a spontaneous nonobese model for type II diabetes. Diabetes 1991;40:486
147. Ohneda M, Johnson JH, Inman LR, et al. GLUT2 expression and function in beta-cells of GK rats with NIDDM. Dissociation between reductions in glucose transport and glucose-stimulated insulin secretion. Diabetes 1993; 42:1065
148. Tsuura Y, Ishida H, Okamoto Y, et al. Glucose sensitivity of ATP-sensitive K+ channels is impaired in beta-cells of the GK rat. A new genetic model of NIDDM. Diabetes 1993;42:1446
149. Hughes SJ, Suzuki K, Goto Y. The role of islet secretory function in the development of diabetes in the GK Wistar rat. Diabetologia 1994;37:863
150. Gauguier D, Nelson I, Bernard C, et al. Higher maternal than paternal inheritance of diabetes in GK rats. Diabetes 1994;43:220
151. Kawano K, Hirashima T, Mori S, Natori T. OLETF (Otsuka Long-Evans Tokushima Fatty) rat: A new NIDDM rat strain. Diabetes Res Clin Pract 1994;24:S317
152. Sclafani A. Dietary obesity models. In: Bjorntorp P, Brodoff BN, eds. Obesity. Philadelphia: JB Lippincott;1992:241–248
153. Fenton PF, Carr CJ. The nutrition of the mouse: XI. Response of four strains to diets differing in fat content, 1951
154. Schemmel R, Mickelsen O, Gill JL. Dietary obesity in rats: Body weight and body fat accretion in seven strains of rats. J Nutr 1970;100:1041
155. West DB, Waguespack J, York B, et al. Genetics of dietary obesity in AKR/J × SWR/J mice: Segregation of the trait and identification of a linked locus on chromosome 4. Mamm Genome 1994;5:546
156. West DB, Goudey-Lefevre J, York B, Truett GE. Dietary obesity linked to genetic loci on chromosomes 9 and 15 in a polygenic mouse model. J Clin Invest 1994;94:1410
157. Surwit RS, Seldin MF, Kuhn CM, et al. Control of expression of insulin resistance and hyperglycemia by different genetic factors in diabetic C57BL/6J mice. Diabetes 1991;40:82
158. Seldin MF, Mott D, Bhat D, et al. Glycogen synthase: A putative locus for diet-induced hyperglycemia. J Clin Invest 1994;94:269
159. Fisler JS, Warden CH, Pace MJ, Lusis AJ. BSB: A new mouse model of multigenic obesity. Obesity Res 1993;1:271
160. Neel JV. Diabetes mellitus: A "thrifty" genotype rendered detrimental by "progress?" Am J Hum Genet 1962;14:353
161. Kuczmaarski RJ, Flegal KM, Campbell SM, Johnson CL. Increasing prevalence of overweight among US adults. JAMA 1994;272:205
162. Erickson RP. Why isn't a mouse more like a man? Trends Genet 1989;5:1–3
163. Agellon LB, Walsh A, Hayek T, et al. Reduced high density lipoprotein cholesterol in human cholesteryl ester transfer protein transgenic mice. J Biol Chem 1991;266:10796
164. Risch N, Ghosh S, Todd JA. Statistical evaluation of multiple-locus linkage data in experimental species and its relevance to human studies: Application to nonobese diabetic (NOD) mouse and human insulin-dependent diabetes mellitus (IDDM). Am J Hum Genet 1993;53:702
165. Corder EH, Saunders AM, Strittmatter WJ, et al. Gene dose of apolipoprotein E type 4 allele and the risk of Alzheimer's disease in late onset families. Science 1993;921:261
166. Tartaglia LA, Dembski M, Weng X, et al. Identification and expression cloning of a leptin receptor, OB-R. Cell 1995;83:1263
167. Gall, J, Li L-S, Glaser A, et al. Genetic analysis of non-insulin dependent diabetes mellitus in the GK rat. Nat Genet 1996;12:31
168. Gaugier D, Froguel P, Parent V, et al. Chromosomal mapping of genetic loci associated with non-insulin dependent diabetes in the GK rat. Nat Genet 1996;12:38

Part VII

Type II Diabetes: Therapeutics

Diabetes Mellitus, edited by Derek LeRoith, Simeon I. Taylor, and Jerrold M. Olefsky. Lippincott–Raven Publishers, Philadelphia © 1996.

CHAPTER 69

Prevention Strategies for Non–Insulin-Dependent Diabetes Mellitus: An Economic Perspective

RICHARD C. EASTMAN, JONATHAN C. JAVITT, WILLIAM H. HERMAN, ERIK J. DASBACH, AND MAUREEN I. HARRIS

Introduction

Measures targeted at reducing the long-term sequelae of chronic disease have been classified as primary, secondary, and tertiary prevention.[1] Primary prevention is intervention prior to the onset of the disease, secondary intervention is intervention after onset of the disease but before the development of complications, and tertiary intervention is intervention after the development of complications but before progression to end-stage sequelae. Laser photocoagulation, administration of angiotensin–converting enzyme inhibitors, and preventive foot care are tertiary interventions that have been shown to reduce the risk of severe vision loss, end-stage renal disease (ESRD), and lower extremity amputation in patients with diabetes. These interventions take place after the development of proliferative retinopathy or macular edema, macroproteinuria, and distal sensorimotor neuropathy. Diabetes treatment with the goal of normoglycemia is a secondary intervention that delays development of microvascular complications and slows the rate of disease progression.[2] Similar benefit of near-normoglycemia is expected in NIDDM and IDDM.[2,2a,2b,2c]

At the present time no interventions have been proved to prevent the development of diabetes, but large-scale trials are under way to test primary prevention strategies for both insulin-dependent diabetes mellitus (IDDM) and non–insulin-dependent diabetes mellitus (NIDDM). If it is proved effective, the cost-effectiveness of primary prevention will be compared with that of established therapies, and decisions may have to be made about allocation of resources. Thus, efforts to establish the scientific basis for primary prevention of diabetes must consider the economic implications.

Cost-effectiveness analysis is one way of comparing diverse treatments of disease. It takes into account both the efficacy of the intervention and the costs of treatment. Increasingly, cost-effectiveness is considered when allocating limited resources for health care. The analysis is usually done after clinical trials have established the efficacy of an intervention, when the costs and effects are known. It can also be used to examine the economic feasibility of an intervention that is as yet unproved and then be taken into consideration in allocating research resources for a particular program. This chapter analyzes the potential cost-effectiveness of various interventions on the natural history of NIDDM from a health and economic point of view and the potential role that primary prevention of diabetes may play in the future.

Principles of Cost-Effectiveness Analysis

Cost-effectiveness is expressed as a ratio of the cost and effectiveness of treatment.[3] The elements of the numerator are the direct costs of medical care (C_{Rx}), the direct costs of side effects of treatment (C_{SE}), the cost of treating complications of the disease (C_{Morb}), and the cost of treating diseases that occur as a result of the effect of the intervention on life expectancy ($C_{Rx\Delta LE}$).

The incremental cost of a preventive treatment is expressed in the following equation:

$$\Delta C = \Delta C_{Rx} + \Delta C_{SE} - \Delta C_{Morb} + \Delta C_{RxLE}$$ [3]

C_{Morb} is entered as a negative value representing the savings attributable to reduced complications of the disease process.

A commonly used unit of measure of effectiveness (E) is the quality-adjusted life-year (QALY). Cost-effectiveness can also be expressed in terms of years free of complications or other measures of disease. The QALY incorporates the effects of the intervention on life expectancy (life-years, Y), quality of life (Y_{Morb}), and the side effects of treatment (Y_{SE}). The difference in effectiveness between interventions is expressed as follows:

$$\Delta E = \Delta Y + \Delta Y_{Morb} - \Delta Y_{SE}$$ [3]

Y_{Morb} is entered as a positive value representing the improvement in quality of life owing to reduction in complications.

Cost-effectiveness is always relative to an established intervention. When comparing new with established interventions, the incremental cost-effectiveness, or the cost per unit of effectiveness gained (ΔCost/ΔEffectiveness), is the critical variable.[4]

Discounting of costs and effectiveness to present value is an important aspect of cost-effectiveness analysis.[3] Costs and benefits occurring in the future are discounted back to present value to adjust for differences in the temporal accrual of costs and effects. For example, one dollar (present value) invested at an interest rate of 5%/year for 10 years will have a future value of $1 \times (1 + 0.05)^{10}$ or $1.53. Conversely, $1.53 of future costs or savings is discounted to a present value of one dollar. The relationship between present and future value and interest and discount rates is shown below:

$$\text{Future Value} = \text{Present Value} \times (1 + \text{Interest Rate})^{\text{Years}}, \text{ and}$$
$$\text{Present Value} = \text{Future Value}/((1 + \text{Discount Rate})^{\text{Years}}).$$

It is important to note that discounting is independent of inflation. Economic analyses are best conducted in constant dollars, adjusting for inflation.[4] Discounting can have profound effects on the results of cost-effectiveness analysis. In general, the higher the discount rate, the greater the reduction of cost-effectiveness when dollars are spent in the present, when present value is high, and saved in the future, when present value is low. Discount rates of 7%/year are considered conservative, and rates of 3–5 are often used in cost-effectiveness analysis.[4] Effectiveness is discounted in the same manner as costs in order for the cost-effectiveness ratio to be meaningful.[3]

Modeling of Disease Outcomes

A model of the disease under study is an important ingredient of cost-effectiveness analysis of prevention of chronic disease outcomes. Modeling is particularly important when clinical trials are not feasible, such as in lifelong effect of diabetes treatment on complications. For example, analysis of cost-effectiveness of intervening in the course of retinopathy and diabetic nephropathy has been based on disease models.[5,6]

In models of diabetes, the rate of development of complications and mortality rates are based on epidemiologic studies. Progression through the model can be accomplished by allocating patients who are alive to the outcome based on simple probabilities (deterministic model) or using simulation techniques (Monte Carlo model).[7]

Disease progression is modeled in a cohort of patients of arbitrary size who are at risk for developing diabetes. Patients are allocated to disease outcomes based on the annual risk of developing diabetes or its complications. Thus, in a deterministic model, if the risk of developing background diabetic retinopathy is 5% per year, 5% of the patients alive in any year are allocated to that outcome. In a Monte Carlo simulation model, in contrast, each patient is modeled separately. An outcome is considered to have occurred if the patient is alive and a randomly drawn number is less than or equal to the annual risk of the complication. Multiple patients are simulated and the results accumulated. Deterministic models have been used to model primary and secondary interventions for diabetes and Monte Carlo models to model retinopathy and nephropathy.[5,6,8]

For the example under discussion, a model developed previously to analyze comprehensive treatment of NIDDM was adapted to simulate primary prevention. The model randomly selects individuals from a cohort with an age range of 15–61. Gender assignment is by random number, with 45% of the subjects male and 55% female. The average age of the cohort at entry into the model is 41 years. This cohort was selected to be representative of about 428,000 individuals estimated to develop NIDDM in this age range in the United States each year.[5,9] In the present model, patients are free of diabetes at the time of entry into the model. The rate of progression to diabetes is stipulated in the model parameters, and for the present analysis was 10%/year. Modeling progression to diabetes allows simulation of primary prevention of diabetes in addition to secondary and tertiary interventions in patients who have already developed the disease. The population modeled in the present analysis is at high risk of developing diabetes, such as occurs in Pima Indians with the most severe degree[10] of impaired glucose tolerance (based on glucose levels).

The model uses Monte Carlo techniques to allocate patients to disease states and mortality. For each microvascular complication, a series of health states is modeled (Fig. 69-1). The risks of progressing to each health state are based on epidemiologic studies (Table 69-1). Briefly, progression to background retinopathy and other retinopathy states is based on the Wisconsin Epidemiologic Study of Diabetic Retinopathy (WESDR)[5,11] (Table 69-1). Progression to microalbuminuria is based on prevalence data from WESDR and therefore may underestimate the true cumulative incidence.[12] Progression to macroproteinuria and ESRD was modeled from cumulative incidence data from the Rochester Epidemiology Project.[13,14] Development of distal sensorimotor neuropathy and progression to lower extremity amputation are based on data from the Rochester Diabetic Neuropathy and the Rochester Epidemiology Project.[15,16] Development of neuropathy is a condition for progressing to lower extremity amputation.

Mortality rates are based on retinopathy status and duration of diabetes and were developed by Javitt and coworkers from WESDR and other sources.[5,11] Patients who do not develop retinopathy but who do develop microalbuminuria or macroproteinuria are assigned the same mortality risk as patients with background retinopathy and macular edema, since mortality rates are similar for both.[17] Patients who become blind are assigned the same risk as patients with proliferative retinopathy, since the mortality rates also are similar for both of these complications. Prior to development of diabetes, patients are at risk for age-specific mortality, using U.S. Life Table rates for men and women.[18]

Four intervention programs were modeled: standard care, recommended care, comprehensive care, and primary prevention. The standard care model uses the risk functions developed from the epidemiologic data and assumes that the probability of being screened for retinopathy each year is 50%.[19] In the recommended care model the annual probability of screening for retinopathy is increased to 1.0. The model also assumes that all patients receive preventive foot care education and that this reduces the risk of lower extremity amputation by 50%/year.[20–23] Finally, the model assumes that angiotensin–converting enzyme inhibitors are administered to those with macroproteinuria, reducing the annual risk of progression from macroproteinuria to ESRD by 50%.[24]

The comprehensive care model adds to the recommended care model the effects of treatment with the goal of normoglycemia and assumes that near-normoglycemia has the same affect on microvascular complications in NIDDM that was observed in IDDM in the Diabetes Control and Complications Trial[2] (see Table 69-1). This assumption is consistent with observational data and clinical trials in NIDDM.[2a,2b] Secondary analysis of the DCCT data showing similar treatment effect under standard and comprehensive treatment also supports this assumption.[2c] No effect of intensive treatment on progression of macroproteinuria to ESRD or of neuropathy to lower extremity amputation is assumed in the model.

Primary prevention was simulated by reducing diabetes incidence from 20–80%. The primary prevention model uses the same risk functions as the comprehensive care model after development of diabetes (see Table 69-1). Implicit in the model is the assumption that delaying onset of diabetes will delay onset of microvascular complications.

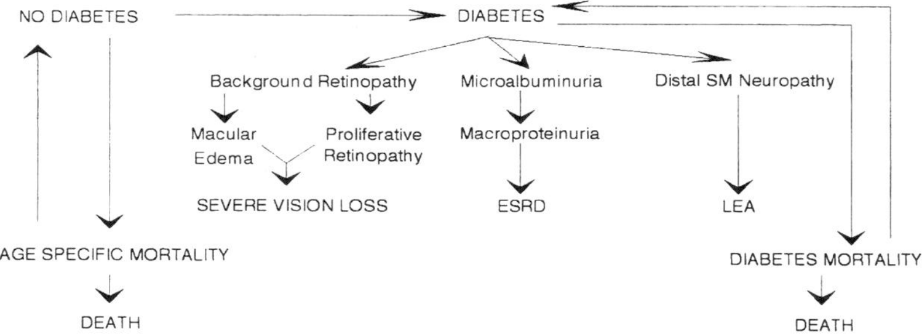

FIGURE 69-1. Structure of the Monte Carlo model of NIDDM. Patients enter the model with no diabetes and are at risk for developing diabetes and for age-specific mortality. If diabetes develops, mortality risk is diabetes-specific. Once diabetes develops, progression to retinopathy, nephropathy, and neuropathy complications and end-stage sequelae may occur spontaneously, until end-stage sequelae (severe vision loss, ESRD, lower extremity amputation) or death occurs.

TABLE 69-1. Assumptions Used in the Standard, Recommended, and Comprehensive Care Models

Hazard Rates	Standard Care Model		Recommended Care Model	Comprehensive Care Model*
Mortality risk/year				
nb Diabetes	age risk			
No retinopathy	(0.005 + 2*age-risk)/2		Same as standard care	Same as standard care
Background retinopathy	(0.06 + 2*age-risk)/2			
Macular edema	(0.076 + 2*age-risk)/2			
Proliferative retinopathy	(0.092 + 5*age-risk)/2			
Background retinopathy risk	1–4 yr	0.073/yr	Same as standard care	0.24 *Standard care rates
	5–9 yr	0.129/yr		
	10–14 yr	0.116/yr		
	15+ yr	0.113/yr		
Macular edema risk	1–4 yr	0.047/yr	Same as standard care	0.74 *Standard care rates
	5–9 yr	0.095/yr		
	10–14 yr	0.092/yr		
	15+ yr	0.113/yr		
Proliferative retinopathy risk	1–4 yr	0.003/yr	Same as standard care	0.53 *Standard care rates
	5–9 yr	0.009/yr		
	10–14 yr	0.010/yr		
	15+ yr	0.026/yr		
Dilated eye examination	0.50/yr		1.0/yr	1.0/yr
Progression of proliferative retinopathy to blindness				
Untreated	0.088/yr			
Panretinal photocoagulation	0.0148/yr		Same as standard care	Same as standard care
Progression of macular edema to blindness				
Untreated	0.05/yr			
Focal photocoagulation	0.033/yr		Same as standard care	Same as standard care
Progression to microalbuminuria	1–2 yr	0.0266/yr	Same as standard care	0.44 *Standard care rates
	3–6 yr	0.0531/yr		
	7–10 yr	0.0354/yr		
	11+ yr	0.0292/yr		
Progression to macroalbuminuria	1–4 yr	0/yr	Same as standard care	0.44 *Standard care rates
	5+ yr	0.1572/yr		
Progression to ESRD	1–11 yr	0.0042/yr	0.5 *Standard care rate	Same as recommended care rate
	12–20 yr	0.0385/yr		
	21+ yr	0.074		
Progression to diabetic neuropathy	0.017/yr		Same as standard care	0.31 *Standard care rate
Progression to lower extremity amputation	1–8 yr	0.0280/yr	0.5 *Standard care rate	Same as recommended care
	9–13 yr	0.0350/yr		
	14–19 yr	0.0467/yr		
	20+ yr	0.14/yr		

*The recommended care model and the risk reductions owing to treatment with the goal of normoglycemia constitute the comprehensive care model.

Model Outcomes

Diabetes develops in 78.5% of individuals modeled under standard, recommended, and comprehensive care (Table 69-2 and Fig. 69-2). Under standard and recommended care the cumulative incidences of retinopathy, nephropathy, and neuropathy are essentially identical, with small variations caused by the random occurrence of events in the models (Table 69-2 and Fig. 69-3).[3] Progression to blindness is reduced under recommended care because patients are screened annually and therefore receive more timely treatment that is associated with lower rates of progression to blindness after photocoagulation. Progression to ESRD and lower extremity amputation are reduced because of the effect of the angiotensin–converting enzyme inhibitors after development of macroproteinuria and because preventive foot care education is given (Fig. 69-4).

In the comprehensive care model, the cumulative incidence of all microvascular complications is reduced because of the effects of near-normoglycemia on the rates of development and progression of complications (Table 69-2 and Fig. 69-3). With comprehensive care cumulative incidence of end-stage sequelae is further reduced in comparison with recommended care because there are fewer patients with retinopathy, nephropathy, and neuropathy (Fig. 69-3).

Primary prevention reduces complications by delaying onset of diabetes; the rates of progression of complications are identical to those rates under comprehensive care (see Tables 69-1, 69-2 and Figs. 69-2, 69-3, and 69-4). The reduction in development of early complications results in a similar reduction of end-stage sequelae. For example, a 60% reduction in diabetes risk reduces the cumulative incidence of diabetes from 78.5% under comprehensive care to 52.4%. This is associated with a 40% decrease in cumulative incidence of blindness, ESRD, and lower extremity amputation (see Table 69-2).

The different interventions modeled also affected survival differently, although cumulative mortality was the same in all models, with no patients predicted to survive beyond 60 years after

TABLE 69-2. Projected Cumulative Incidence of Complications under Standard, Recommended, and Comprehensive Care and Primary Prevention

	Standard Care	Recommended Care	Comprehensive Care	Primary Prevention			
Risk Reduction from Primary Prevention	0	0	0	20%	40%	60%	80%
Annual Diabetes Risk	10%	10%	10%	8%	6%	4%	2%
Diabetes	78.5%	78.5%	78.5%	72.1%	63.8%	52.4%	32.9%
Nonproliferative retinopathy	46.7%	46.7%	20.4%	17.9%	15.8%	12.6%	7.7%
Macular edema	23.0%	23.2%	8.3%	7.1%	6.2%	4.8%	2.8%
Proliferative retinopathy	6.5%	6.6%	1.8%	1.5%	1.3%	1.1%	0.7%
Blindness	7.6%	5.9%	1.9%	1.6%	1.4%	1.1%	0.7%
Microalbuminuria	25.6%	25.4%	13.4%	12.2%	10.5%	8.7%	5.2%
Macroproteinuria	16.0%	15.6%	5.6%	4.8%	4.4%	3.7%	2.2%
ESRD	4.0%	2.4%	1.0%	0.9%	0.8%	0.6%	0.4%
Symptomatic distal neuropathy	12.2%	12.2%	4.4%	4.0%	3.4%	2.7%	1.7%
First lower extremity amputation	4.8%	3.0%	1.3%	1.0%	0.8%	0.6%	0.4%

entry into the model. Survival times are identical under standard and recommended care because the interventions under recommended care do not affect the development of retinopathy and nephropathy, which determine mortality risk (Fig. 69-5). Under comprehensive care the survival curve is shifted slightly to the right because fewer of these patients develop macular edema, proliferative retinopathy, blindness, microalbuminuria, and macroproteinuria which are associated with higher mortality rates (see Table 69-1 and Fig. 69-5). Primary prevention has the greatest effect on the survival curve, shifting it farther to the right (Fig. 69-5). This is because prior to development of diabetes, age-specific mortality rates are used, which are lower than diabetes-specific mortality rates.

Cost Analysis

The costs in the model include those of treatment of diabetes and of screening, work-up, and treatment of complications. A societal perspective is used in the present analysis and thus the costs to the federal government of disability for blindness and ESRD are included (Table 69-3). In the primary prevention model, there are additional costs for screening for individuals at high risk of developing diabetes and for intervention to prevent diabetes.

Under primary prevention, all individuals entering the model incur the costs of screening and annual intervention costs to prevent diabetes. The cost of screening for individuals at risk for developing

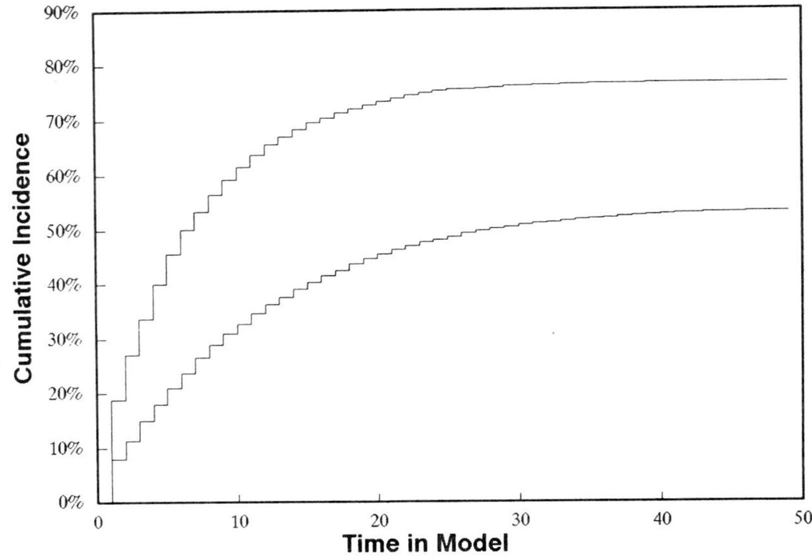

FIGURE 69-2. Model projections of development of diabetes in individuals at high risk for NIDDM. The upper curve is under standard, recommended, or comprehensive care, where the annual risk of developing diabetes is 10%/year. The lower curve is under primary prevention with a 60% reduction in risk of diabetes (annual risk reduced from 10% to 4%/year).

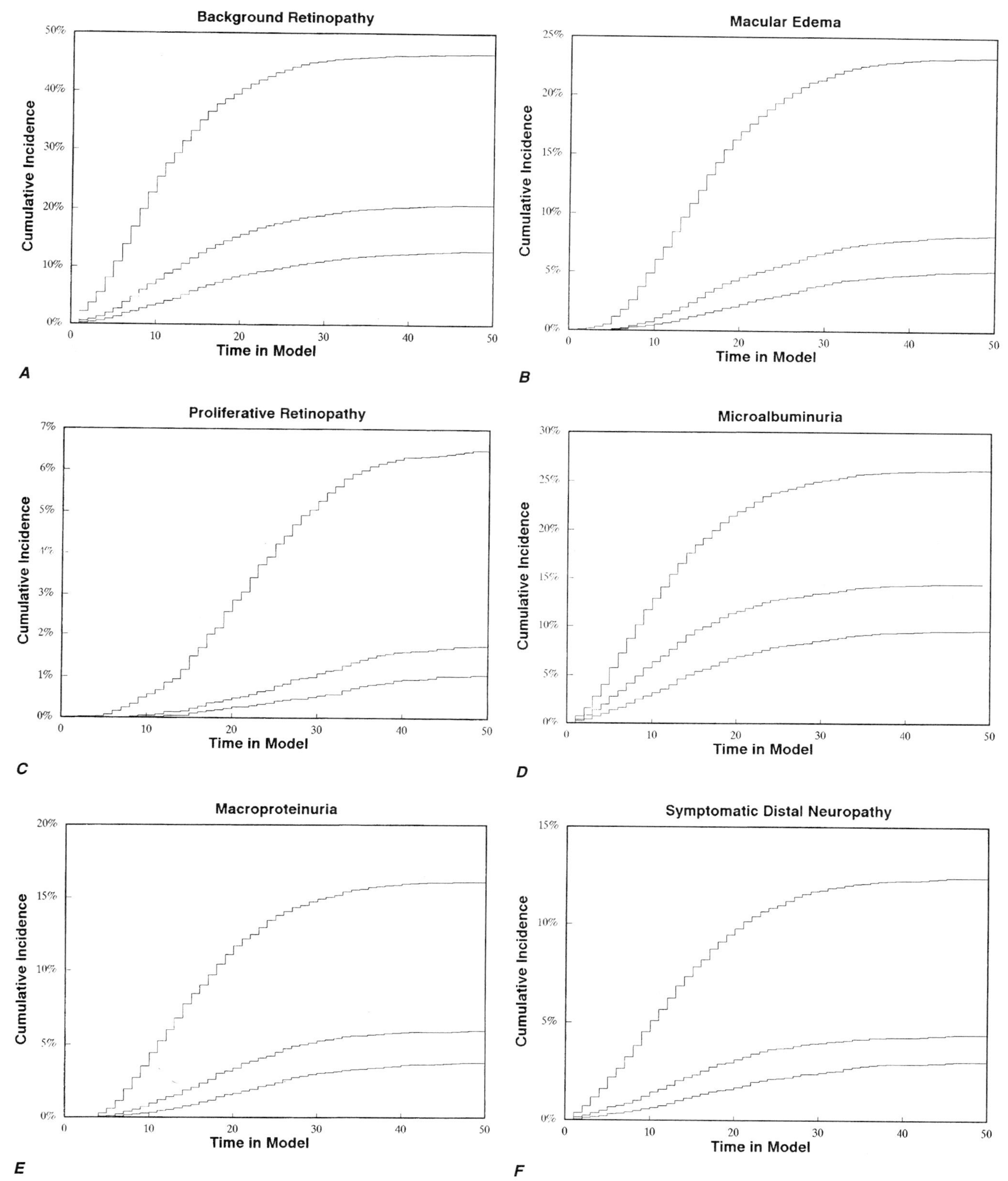

Figure 69-3. Development of microvascular and neuropathic complications of diabetes. For each panel (a–f), the upper curve is under standard or recommended care, the middle curve under comprehensive care, and the lower curve under primary prevention with 60% reduction in annual risk of diabetes, followed by comprehensive care after onset of diabetes.

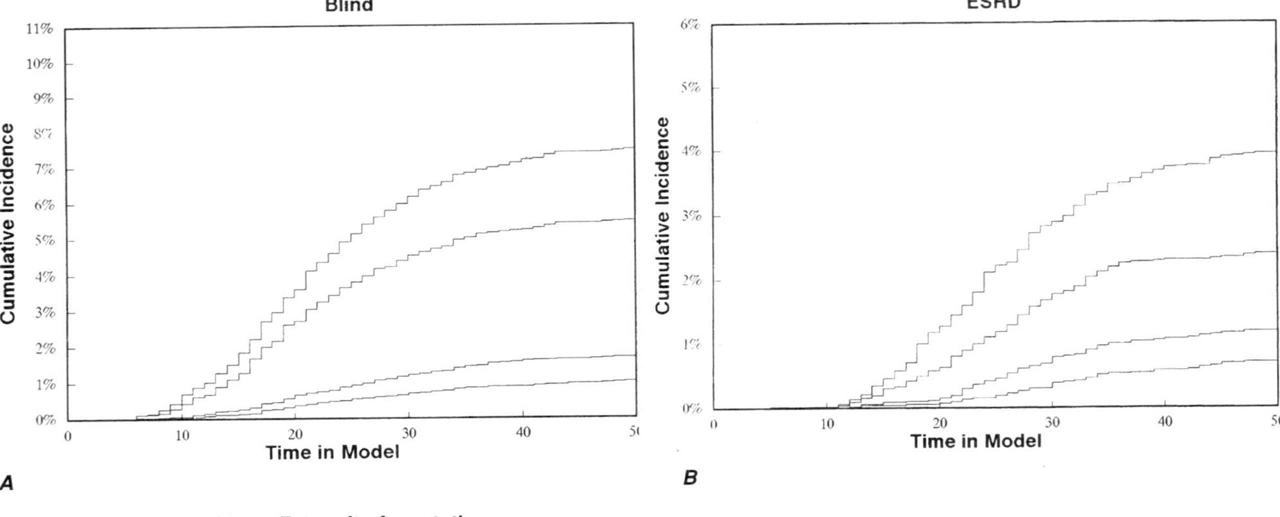

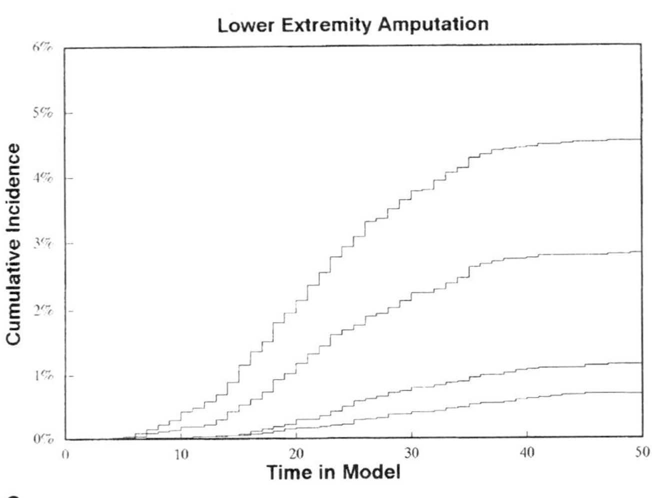

FIGURE 69-4. End-stage sequelae of microvascular complications of diabetes. For each panel (a–c) the sequence of curves is (from topmost curve to bottom curve) standard care (top), recommended care, comprehensive care, and primary prevention with 60% reduction in annual risk of diabetes (bottom curve). Cumulative incidence is given as the percentage of individuals in the entire cohort (including those who do and those who do not develop diabetes).

TABLE 69-3. Costs of Screening, Treatment, and Disability Incorporated in the Model

Dilated eye examination[5]	$62
Photocoagulation[5]	$1960, $42/yr additional follow-up costs
Disability benefit for legal blindness[5]	$14,962/yr until age 65, $38/yr after age 65
Treatment of end-stage renal disease[26]	$44,901/yr
Lower extremity amputation[26]	$9,434, $100/yr additional follow-up costs
Treatment with angiotensin-converting enzyme inhibitor[26]	$666/yr
Evaluation for neuropathy[26]	$266
Renal evaluation for proteinuria[26]	$1119
Standard diabetes treatment	$670/yr
Diabetes treatment with the goal of normoglycemia	$2450/yr
Screening for impaired glucose tolerance	$2000/patient found with more severe impaired glucose tolerance

*Cumulative incidence is expressed as a percentage of the population at risk for diabetes.

diabetes was estimated from the frequency of impaired glucose tolerance in the population from the National Health and Education Survey.[25] Costs of glucose determinations, oral glucose solution, and patient counseling are about $100 per person screened. The screening yield is 1 patient at high risk per 20 patients screened, and the population at risk is about half of all patients with impaired glucose tolerance.

The average cost of standard care for NIDDM was estimated from data provided by the Centers for Disease Control and Prevention (CDC) on cost of office visits, oral agent therapy, and insulin therapy.[26,27] These costs were applied to the proportion of patients using restricted diets, oral agents, and insulin treatment and to the frequency of office visits and glucose monitoring of patients who were and were not taking insulin from population-based surveys.[28,28a,28b]

The costs of screening for retinopathy, photocoagulation, and blindness are those used by Javitt and coworkers.[5] The costs of neurologic and renal evaluations, treatment with angiotension-converting enzyme inhibitors, lower extremity amputation, and renal failure were provided by the CDC.[26] The expenditure for blindness disability is reduced to $38 per year at age 65 when Social Security benefits begin. (see Table 69-3). Renal replacement treatment is given to all patients who develop renal insufficiency. Cost effects caused by changes in life expectancy ($\Delta C_{Rx\Delta LE}$) are not modeled, and the costs of side effects of treatment (ΔC_{SE}) are assumed to be negligible.

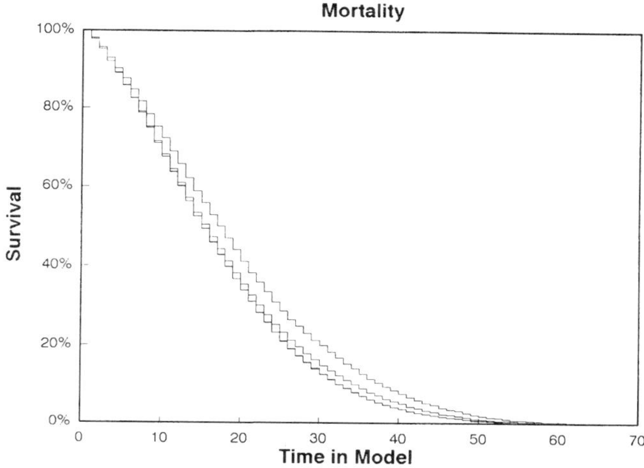

FIGURE 69-5. Survival under different intervention models. The lowermost curve is under standard and recommended care, the middle curve under comprehensive care, and the upper curve under primary prevention with 60% reduction in annual risk of diabetes.

The discounted (5%/year) present value of standard care is $8827/person/lifetime (Table 69-4). Under recommended care the cost of metabolic management of disease is identical to standard care, and the costs associated with eye disease, renal disease, and neuropathy are less. The net effect is a reduction in total cost to $7595/person/lifetime. The cost of eye disease incorporates the higher cost of screening for retinopathy, which is performed annually rather than every 2 years under standard care on average. Similarly, the cost of renal disease incorporates the expense of treating with angiotensin-converting enzyme inhibitors after development of macroproteinuria. The relatively low cost of neuropathy complications is attributable to the effect of discounting on complications occurring in the future.

Under comprehensive care, the total cost increases to $13,572/person at risk for diabetes/lifetime. The costs of medical management of hyperglycemia increase three- to fourfold over the costs under standard and recommended care. This is offset by reductions in the cost of eye, renal, and neuropathic complications by approximately 60%.

In the primary prevention model, the greatest reduction in risk was associated with the lowest total cost (see Table 69-4). Eighty percent reduction in risk of diabetes incurred the greatest prevention costs but reduced the cost of treatment of diabetes by about 60% compared with comprehensive care and reduced the costs of complications by three- to fourfold. In contrast, primary prevention that reduced diabetes risk by only 20% was associated with the greatest cost.

Cost-Effectiveness Analysis

The effectiveness of the different intervention models is expressed in terms of QALY and person-years free of end-stage sequelae. Life-years predicted by the models are adjusted for quality of life using adjustments referred to as utilities. For instance, the utility of being blind is 0.69, indicating that a year of life with blindness is valued at 69% of a year of life with normal vision. Utilities of 0.32 for end-stage renal disease,[30] and 0.7 for lower extremity amputation[26] are also used in the model. When multiple events occur in the same patient in the same year, the utility resulting in the greatest decrease in quality of life is used. For example, the utility for being blind and having ESRD and lower extremity amputation is 0.32, which is the utility of having ESRD alone. Quality-adjusted life-years are discounted to present value at a rate of 5%/year.[3]

Quality-adjusted life-years increase from 9.57 under standard care to 10.75 with primary prevention (80% reduction of risk of diabetes) (see Table 69-4). Compared with standard care, recommended care is cost-saving. Compared with recommended care, the incremental cost-effectiveness of comprehensive care is $29,177/QALY gained (see Table 69-4). The incremental cost-effectiveness of primary prevention was $42,135/QALY gained with the least reduction in diabetes risk (20%) and $2039 with the greatest reduction in risk.

The standard care model predicts that a cohort of 428,000 patients entering the model would experience 169,974 years of blindness, 121,670 years of ESRD, and 171,994 years with lower

TABLE 69-4. Effects of the Model Assumptions on the Cost and Effectiveness of Care in Different Intervention Models of Non–Insulin-Dependent Diabetes Mellitus Treatment*

	Standard Care	Recommended Care	Comprehensive Care	Primary Prevention			
Risk Reduction from Primary Prevention / Annual Diabetes Risk	0 / 10%	0 / 10%	0 / 10%	20% / 8%	40% / 6%	60% / 4%	80% / 2%
Cost of metabolic management	$3144	$3146	$11,890	$10,224	$8588	$6537	$3756
Cost of eye disease	$2291	$2024	$787	$621	$500	$400	$226
Cost of renal disease	$3215	$2313	$853	$720	$615	$451	$271
Cost of neuropathy/lower extremity amputation	$177	$111	$42	$34	$25	$17	$10
Cost of primary prevention	0	0	0	$7800	$8677	$9765	$11,229
Total costs	$8827	$7595	$13,572	$19,399	$18,404	$17,170	$15,492
QALY	9.57	9.61	9.81	9.95	10.16	10.42	10.75
Incremental costs		($1231)	$5977	$5827	$4832	$3598	$1920
Incremental QALY		0.03	0.20	0.14	0.35	0.61	0.94
Incremental cost/QALY gained		($36,035)	$29,177	$42,135	$13,740	$5924	$2039

*Costs and effects are discounted to present value at a rate of 5%/year. Incremental cost-effectiveness for each intervention is the difference in cost/difference in QALY. For recommended care, the comparison is with standard care. For comprehensive care, the comparison is with recommended care. For the primary prevention models with 20–80% reduction in risk of diabetes, the comparison is with comprehensive care.

TABLE 69-5. Person-Years of End-Stage Sequelae of Microvascular Complications of Diabetes under Different Intervention Models*

	Standard Care	Recommended Care	Comprehensive Care	Primary Prevention			
Risk Reduction from							
Primary Prevention	0	0	0	20%	40%	60%	80%
Annual Diabetes Risk	10%	10%	10%	8%	6%	4%	2%
Person-years of blindness	169,974	143,846	42,177	33,013	27,368	23,135	14,283
Person-years of ESRD	121,670	79,382	34,541	27,240	25,872	20,184	11,632
Person-years with lower extremity amputation	171,994	110,393	49,325	40,839	30,832	20,569	12,530
Person-years saved							
Blindness		26,128	101,669	9164	14,809	19,042	27,894
ESRD		42,288	44,841	7301	8669	14,357	22,909
Lower extremity amputation		61,601	61,068	8486	18,493	28,756	36,795

*Person-years saved under recommended care are in comparison with standard care, and person-years saved under comprehensive care are in comparison with recommended care. Under primary prevention, person-years saved are in comparison with comprehensive care in all interventions modeled.

extremity amputation (Table 69-5). Recommended care saved 26,128–61,601 person-years with these complications. Comprehensive care increased the person-years of blindness saved by almost fourfold. Comprehensive care doubled the person-years saved with ESRD and lower extremity amputation under recommended care. Even with optimal care, the cohort would experience 34,541–49,325 person-years with each complication. The least effective primary prevention model, with 20% reduction in diabetes risk, saved an additional 7301–9164 person-years with end-stage sequelae compared with comprehensive care and the most effective model saved 22,909–36,795 person-years in those with complications.

Sensitivity Analysis

Sensitivity analysis in the context of cost-effectiveness analysis refers to the process of varying critical parameters in the model to determine the effect on the results. In the present analysis, the cost-effectiveness of primary prevention with a 60% reduction in risk of developing diabetes was compared with cost-effectiveness comprehensive care and the results expressed as the incremental cost-effectiveness (Table 69-6).

Under the assumptions in the base case, with an annual risk of diabetes of 10%/year, the incremental cost-effectiveness of primary prevention is $5924/QALY gained (see Tables 69-4, and 69-6). Reducing the annual risk of diabetes to 5%/year and 2.5%/year increased the cost to $14,312 and $29,131/QALY gained, respectively. The model was most sensitive to the cost of primary prevention, where doubling the cost of prevention increased the cost to $24,970/QALY. The model is relatively insensitive to the cost of screening for impaired glucose tolerance because this is not a recurring cost. The model is also insensitive to the costs of complications because of their low rate under comprehensive care and primary prevention. This is also reflected by the insensitivity of the model to the quality of life adjustments, where eliminating this adjustment increased the cost to only $6189/QALY. In contrast, the incremental cost-effectiveness of comprehensive care compared with recommended care is much more sensitive to the cost of complications.

Finally, the model is sensitive to patient compliance with the interventions. Reducing patient compliance by 50% increased the cost\QALY gained by more than eightfold.

What Can Be Learned from This Analysis?

This analysis emphasizes, from an economic point of view, the importance of retinopathy screening and preventive foot care education and the potential for angiotensin–converting enzyme inhibitors for reducing the morbidity and cost of diabetes. This is manifested by the reductions in blindness, ESRD, and lower extremity amputation under recommended care when compared with standard care and by the net cost-saving achieved with recommended care (see Table 69-4 and Fig. 69-3). Implementing these interventions should

TABLE 69-6. Sensitivity Analysis of Different Intervention Models for Non–Insulin-Dependent Diabetes Mellitus*

Model Assumptions	Incremental Cost per QALY
Base case	$5924
Risk of diabetes	
2.5%/yr	$29,131
5%/yr	$14,312
Cost of screening	
Half ($1000)	$4924
Double ($4000)	$9924
Cost of primary prevention	
Half ($500)	($1091)
Double ($2000)	$24,970
Cost of end-stage complications	
Blindness = $1911 per year	$6613
ESRD = $0 per year	$6482
Blindness, ESRD, lower extremity amputation = $0	$7098
Disease state utilities	
Utility decrement = 0 per state	$6189
Discount rate	
10%	$12,840
0%	$139
Compliance	
50%	$50,669
25%	$84,508

*Costs and incremental cost-effectiveness of primary prevention with 60% reduction in risk of progressing to diabetes compared with comprehensive care. All costs, savings, and life-years are discounted to present value at a discount rate of 5% year.

be the first priority of providers seeking to improve the health of their patients. Currently in the U.S. most patients do not receive optimal eye screening and preventive foot care, and since the recommendations for use of angiotension–converting enzyme inhibitors in NIDDM have been made recently, it is unlikely that these agents are currently in widespread use.[31] Implementation of current recommendations for high blood pressure treatment, treatment of dyslipidemia, and smoking cessation are integral to the concept of recommended care.

Once recommended care is implemented, adding the goal of normoglycemia under comprehensive care also has the potential to greatly reduce morbidity from microvascular complications. The incremental cost-effectiveness is $29,177/QALY gained. Based on a review of previous analyses and guidelines, Laupacis and coworkers have shown that interventions with incremental cost-effectiveness less than $20,000/QALY are strongly recommended for adoption by the health care system and are usually widely implemented.[32] Interventions whose incremental cost-effectiveness falls between $20,000 and $100,000/QALY are usually provided routinely, although the availability of some may be limited.[32] The cost-effectiveness of comprehensive care falls in the range of $20,000 to $30,000, suggesting that the health-care system will widely apply this service.

The expenditure for treatment with the goal of normoglycemia ($2450/patient/year) assumed in the model is about half the amount expended for the clinical care of patients in the experimental group of the Diabetes Control and Complication trial (DCCT) who were treated with the goal of normoglycemia and for similar intensity of services at other centers.[26,33] It remains to be proved whether treatment of NIDDM with the goal of normoglycemia can achieve similar risk reductions for microvascular complications for this expenditure. Several caveats are worth noting.

Patients with NIDDM may be well controlled on diet or oral agents, alone or in combination with insulin. The cost of treatment may vary considerably, depending on the intensity of services needed. Based on current reimbursement levels and the frequency distribution of diet, oral agents, and insulin treatment in the U.S. population of patients with NIDDM, an expenditure of $2450/person/year would pay for six office visits/year, self–blood glucose monitoring four times/day, and four doses of oral hypoglycemic agents daily or 100 U of insulin given daily in three injections.[28,28a,28b] This intensity of services may be sufficient to achieve near-normoglycemia in many patients. Thus, in the United Kingdom Prospective Diabetes Study, standard treatment achieved a hemoglobin A_1c similar to intensive treatment in the DDCT, and patients treated with the goal of normoglycemia utilized blood glucose monitoring and office visits less than intensively treated patients in the DCCT.[2,34,34a]

This analysis also demonstrates that comprehensive care, although effective in reducing complications, does not eliminate the morbidity of NIDDM. Primary prevention has the potential to further reduce morbidity. For example, a 60% reduction in the annual risk of diabetes, followed by comprehensive care after diabetes onset, would save an additional 23,135 person-years of blindness, 20,184 person-years of ESRD, and 20,569 person-years with lower extremity amputation in the cohort modeled. Reducing the lifetime exposure to hyperglycemia by delaying onset of diabetes and treating with the goal of normoglycemia if diabetes develops are rational approaches to reducing morbidity from the disease.

The incremental cost-effectiveness of primary prevention compared with comprehensive care is $5925/QALY gained. The underlying cost assumptions are that individuals at high risk can be identified at a screening cost of $2000/person identified and that the risk of progression to diabetes can be reduced from 10%/year to 4%/year, a 60% reduction in risk at a cost of $1000/yr. Using the cutoffs developed by Laupacis, interventions that reduced risk by only 20% would probably be adopted by the health care system, since the cost-effectiveness of a 20% reduction in risk is $42,135/QALY (see Table 69-4).[32] If intervention reduced the risk of diabetes by 40–60%, the cost-effectiveness would be between $5924/QALY and $13,740/QALY and the intervention would be strongly recommended. Primary prevention is also cost-effective for individuals whose risk of diabetes is 2.5%/year, similar to the risk in the general population of individuals with impaired glucose tolerance (see Table 69-6). Two critical questions, then, are whether low-cost interventions are likely to reduce the risk of developing diabetes and whether screening strategies can be developed that identify individuals at increased risk for developing diabetes.

Prospects for Primary Prevention of Non–Insulin-Dependent Diabetes Mellitus

It seems likely that individuals at high risk for developing diabetes can be identified by screening. Demographic factors, racial-ethnic origin, history of gestational diabetes mellitus, sensitivity to glucose and insulin, and glucose tolerance status are known to influence the risk of developing diabetes.[35–40] In well-studied populations, the risk of progression to diabetes is related to the duration and severity of impaired glucose tolerance.[10] Rates of progression to diabetes from impaired glucose tolerance in the range of 10%/year are likely to be observed in those with more severe impaired glucose tolerance in certain racial and ethnic groups at high risk for diabetes, and in women with a history of gestational diabetes.

Impaired glucose tolerance is common in the U.S. population, supporting the feasibility of screening for high risk of progression to diabetes.[25] The prevalence of impaired glucose tolerance increases from 11% in the general population age 20–74 years to 24% in those 40–74 years of age with a family history of diabetes and a body weight higher than 120% of normal.[8] Applying more stringent screening criteria increases the specificity of screening but inevitably decreases sensitivity. Thus, only 16% of all patients with impaired glucose tolerance are identified by screening individuals 40–74 years of age with a family history of diabetes and weight higher than 120% of desirable.[8] More specific and sensitive screening tools need to be developed.

Are low-cost interventions likely to prevent progression to NIDDM? Epidemiologic studies show an inverse relationship between development of diabetes and moderate exercise.[41–43] Interventions leading to weight loss or prevention of weight gain, reduction in dietary fat, increase in complex carbohydrates, and increased exercise are lifestyle changes that reduce insulin resistance and have potential for preventing NIDDM.[1] It is encouraging that Chinese investigators recently completed a trial of primary prevention of NIDDM in individuals over the age of 20 with impaired glucose tolerance on two glucose tolerance tests. Modest exercise, diet, and diet and exercise combined reduced the risk of developing diabetes by about 40%.[44] This emphasizes the feasibility of preventing NIDDM in populations in which the overall incidence is low, as in China and the United States.

In addition to lifestyle changes, various pharmacologic agents have been tested as preventive treatments in small clinical trials, but the results are inconclusive.[45–48] The cost of pharmacologic agents is probably in the range of the costs assumed in this analysis. Clearly, clinical trials testing different intervention strategies for NIDDM prevention are in order and have been recommended by an expert panel on Diabetes Prevention convened by the World Health Organization.[1] Such trials are under way in the United Kingdom and France, and a multicenter trial is being supported by the National Institute of Diabetes and Digestive and Kidney Diseases.

References

1. WHO Study Group on Prevention of Diabetes Mellitus. Prevention of Diabetes Mellitus. WHO Geneva: World Health Organization; 1994 Technical Report Series

2. The Diabetes Control and Complications Trial Research Group. The effect of intensive treatment of diabetes on the development and progression of long-term complications in insulin-dependent diabetes mellitus. N Engl J Med 1993;329:977

2a. Klein R. Hyperglycemia and microvascular and macrovascular disease in diabetes. Diabetes Care 1995;2:258

2b. Ohkubo Y, Kishikawa H, Araki E, et al. Intensive insulin therapy prevents the progression of diabetic microvascular complications in Japanese patients with non-insulin-dependent diabetes mellitus: a randomized prospective 6-year study. Diabetes Res Clin Pract 1995;28:103

2c. The Diabetes Control and Complications Trial Research Group. The relationship of glycemic exposure (HbA1c) to the risk of development and progression of retinopathy in the diabetes control and complications trial. Diabetes 1995;44:968

3. Weinstein MC, Stason WB. Foundations of cost-effectiveness for health and medical practices. N Engl J Med 1977;296:716

4. Eisenberg JM. Clinical economics. A guide to the economic analysis of clinical practices. JAMA 1989;262:2879

5. Javitt JC, Aiello LP, Chiang Y, et al. Preventive eye care in people with diabetes is cost-saving to the federal government: Implications for health-care reform. Diabetes Care 1994;17:909

6. Siegel JE, Krolewski AS, Warram JH, Weinstein MC. Cost-effectiveness of screening and early treatment of nephropathy in patients with insulin-dependent diabetes mellitus. J Am Soc Nephrol 1992;3:S111

7. Canner JK, Chiang Y-P, Javitt JC. A Monte Carlo based simulation network model for a chronic progressive disease: The case of diabetic retinopathy. Proceedings of Winter Simulation Conference 1992;25:1041

8. Eastman RC, Siebert CS, Harris M, Gorden P. Clinical review 51:Implications of the Diabetes Control and Complications Trial. J Clin Endocrinol Metab 1993; 77:1105

9. Everhart J, Knowler WC, Bennet PH. Incidence and risk factors for noninsulin-dependent diabetes. NIH Publication No. 85-148. In: National Diabetes Data Group, ed. Diabetes in America. Bethesda, MD: Department of Health and Human Services, Public Health Service, National Institutes of Health; 1985; VI, 1–31

10. Saad MF, Knowler WC, Pettitt DJ, et al. The natural history of impaired glucose tolerance in the Pima Indians. N Engl J Med 1988;319:1500

11. Klein R, Klein BEK, Moss SE, et al. The Wisconsin Epidemiologic Study of Diabetic Retinopathy. X. Four-year incidence and progression of diabetic retinopathy when age at diagnosis is 30 years or more. Arch Ophthalmol 1989;107:244

12. Klein R, Klein BEK, Moss SE. Prevalence of microalbuminuria in older-onset diabetes. Diabetes Care 1993;16:1325

13. Humphrey LL, Ballard DJ, Frohnert PP, et al. Chronic renal failure in non-insulin-dependent diabetes mellitus. Ann Int Med 1989;111:788

14. Ballard DJ, Humphrey LL, Melton J III, et al. Epidemiology of persistent proteinuria in type II diabetes mellitus. Diabetes 1988;37:405

15. Dyck PJ, Kratz KM, Karnes JL, et al. The prevalence by staged severity of various types of diabetic neuropathy, retinopathy, and nephropathy in a population-based cohort: The Rochester Diabetic Neuropathy Study. Neurology 1993;43:817

16. Humphrey LL, Palumbo PJ, Butters MA, et al. The contribution of non-insulin-dependent diabetes to lower-extremity amputation in the community. Arch Intern Med 1994;154:885

17. Klein R, Moss SE, Klein BEK, DeMets DL. Relation of ocular and systemic factors to survival in diabetes. Arch Intern Med 1989;149:266

18. US Department of Health and Human Services. Public Health Service. National Center for Health Statistics, vol II, sec. 6. Vital Statistics of the US, 1984: Life Tables. Hyattsville, MD;1987

19. Brechner RJ, Cowie CC, Howie LJ, et al. Ophthalmic examination among adults with diagnosed diabetes mellitus. JAMA 1993;270:1714

20. Barth R, Campbell LV, Allen S, et al. Intensive education improves knowledge, compliance, and foot problems in type 2 diabetes. Diabetic Med 1991;8:111

21. Malone JM, Snyder M, Anderson G, et al. Prevention of amputation by diabetic education. Am J Surg 1989;158:520

22. Bild DE, Selby JV, Sinnock P, et al. Lower-extremity amputation in people with diabetes. Epidemiology and prevention. Diabetes Care 1989;12:24

23. Division of Diabetes Translation. The prevention and treatment of complications of diabetes mellitus. Atlanta, GA: Department of Health and Human Services, Public Health Service, Centers for Disease Control;1991

24. Lewis EJ, Hunsicker LG, Bain RP, Rohde RD. The Collaborative Study Group. The effect of angiotensin-converting-enzyme inhibition on diabetic nephropathy. N Engl J Med 1993;329:1456

25. Harris MI, Hadden WC, Knowler WC, Bennett PH. Prevalence of diabetes and impaired glucose tolerance and plasma glucose levels in the U.S. population. Diabetes 1987;36:523

26. Herman W. Personal communication, 1994

27. The Diabetes Control and Complications Trial Research Group. Resource utilization and costs of care in the Diabetes Control and Complications Trial. Diabetes Care 1995;18:1468

28. Harris MI, Eastman RC, Siebert C. The DCCT and medical care for diabetes in the U.S. Diabetes Care 1994;17:761

28a. Janes GR. Ambulatory medical care for diabetes. National Diabetes Data Group, eds. In: Diabetes in America. Bethesda, MD: National Institute of Diabetes and Digestive and Kidney Diseases, National Institutes of Health; 1995;541–552

28b. Javitt JC, Aiello LP, Chiang Y, et al. Preventive eye care in people with diabetes is cost-saving to the federal government: Implications for health-care reform. Diabetes Care 1994;17:909

29. Dasbach EJ, Fryback DG, Thornbury JR. Health utility preference differences (abstract). Med Decis Making 1992;12:4

30. Sackett DL, Torrance GW. The utility of different health states as perceived by the general public. J Chronic Dis 1978;11:697

31. Striker GE. Report on a workshop to develop management recommendations for the prevention of progression in chronic renal disease. Nephrol Dial Transplant 1995;10:290

32. Laupacis A, Feeny D, Detsky AS, Tugwell PX. How attractive does a new technology have to be to warrant adoption and utilization? Tentative guidelines for using clinical and economic evaluations. Can Med Assoc J 1992;146:473

33. Etzwiler D. Personal communication. 1994

34. UK Prospective Diabetes Study Group. UK Prospective Diabetes Study (UKPDS). Diabetologia 1991;34:877

34a. U.K. Prospective Diabetes Study 16. Overview of 6 years' therapy of type II diabetes: A progressive disease. Diabetes 1995;44:1249

35. NDDG, National Diabetes Data Group. Classification and diagnosis of diabetes mellitus and other categories of glucose intolerance. Diabetes 1979;1039

36. Harris MI, Hadden WC, Knowler WC, Bennett PH. International criteria for diagnosis of diabetes and impaired glucose tolerance. Diabetes Care 1985; 8:562

37. Yudkin JS, Alberti KGMM, Mclarty DG, Swai ABM. Impaired glucose tolerance. Br Med J 1990;301:397

38. Knowler WC, Pettitt DJ, Saad MF, Bennett PH. Diabetes mellitus in the Pima Indians: Incidence, risk factors, and pathogenesis. Diabetes Metab Rev 1990; 6:1

39. Martin BC, Warram JH, Krowlewski AS, et al. Role of glucose and insulin resistance in development of type 2 diabetes mellitus: Results of a 25 year follow-up study. Lancet 1992;340:925

40. Eriksson KF, Lindgarde F. Impaired glucose tolerance in a middle-aged male urban population: A new approach for identifying high risk cases. Diabetologia 1990;33:526

41. Helmrich SP, Ragland DR, Leung RW, Paffengarger RS Jr. Physical activity and reduced occurrence of non-insulin dependent diabetes mellitus. N Engl J Med 1991;325:147

42. Manson JE, Rimm EB, Stampfer MJ, et al. Physical activity and incidence of non-insulin-dependent diabetes mellitus in women. Lancet 1991;338:774

43. Manson JE, Nathan DM, Krowlewski AS, et al. A prospective study of exercise and incidence of diabetes among U.S. male physicians. JAMA 1992;268: 63

44. Pan X, Guangwei L, Yinghua H, et al. Effect of dietary and/or exercise interventions on incidence of diabetes in 530 subjects with IGT. The Da-Qing IGT and diabetes study IOF Federation Congress Program 1994;439 (Abstract)

45. Sartor G, Schersten B, Carlstrom S, et al. Ten-year follow-up of subjects with impaired glucose tolerance. Prevention of diabetes by tolbutamide and diet regulation. Diabetes 1980;29:41

46. Eriksson KF, Lindgarge F. Prevention of type 2 (non-insulin-dependent) diabetes mellitus by diet and physical exercise: The 6-year Malmo feasibility study. Diabetologia 1991;34:891

47. Melander A, Bitzen P, Sartor G, et al. Will sulfonylurea treatment of impaired glucose tolerance delay development and complications of NIDDM? Diabetes Care 1990;13:53

48. Jarrett RJ, Keen H, Fuller H, McCartney M. Worsening to diabetes in men with impaired glucose tolerance (''borderline diabetes''). Diabetologia 1979;16:25

Diabetes Mellitus, edited by Derek LeRoith, Simeon I. Taylor, and Jerrold M. Olefsky. Lippincott–Raven Publishers, Philadelphia © 1996.

CHAPTER 70

Dietary Therapy in Non–Insulin-Dependent Diabetes Mellitus: Spreading the Nutrient Load

DAVID J.A. JENKINS AND ALEXANDRA L. JENKINS

Introduction

What new approaches are warranted in nutritional care in diabetes, and is there still any value in carbohydrate foods? Current dietary advice for the management of diabetes provides guidelines[1,2] that in general do not differ from what would be considered prudent advice for the general public.[3–5] Where dyslipidemia exists, National Cholesterol Education Program (NCEP) guidelines are acknowledged as the authority.[6] In other respects, defined target levels for specific nutrients (proportion of total fat versus carbohydrate) are avoided.

Based on the Diabetes Control and Complications Trial (DCCT) data in type I diabetes,[7] it is assumed that good glycemic control will also help to prevent complications, especially microvascular complications, in type II diabetes.[2] Loss of excess body weight continues to be a goal for type II diabetes patients to improve blood glucose control and serum lipid profiles.[2] Furthermore, in view of the three- to fourfold increased risk of coronary heart disease (CHD) that accompanies diabetes,[8] additional strategies are sought to normalize a constellation of CHD risk factors (Table 70-1), including serum lipids and, where possible, clotting factors.

On the fat side of the equation, reduced body fat[9–11] and possibly increased intakes of w-9 monounsaturated fats (oleic acid)[12,13] or vegetable w-3 polyunsaturated fats (α-linolenic acid)[14] may improve glycemic control and correct some or many of the established risk factors for CHD.

The carbohydrate side of the dietary prescription is more controversial. Viscous soluble fiber is considered to have a very small effect on reducing serum cholesterol levels,[1,2] whereas fructose may raise low-density lipoprotein cholesterol by comparison with starch,[15–17] despite its glycemic advantage.[18,19] In other respects carbohydrate foods in general and specific types of starchy foods in particular have not been seen as conferring any benefits in the dietary management of diabetes.[2] This view, however, can be contested, especially since meal frequency or reducing the rate of nutrient delivery (e.g., slowing carbohydrate absorption) has been acknowledged as having a potential advantage in the management of diabetes.[2] Certain types of carbohydrate foods are also slowly absorbed. It is now over 10 years since Werner Creutzfeldt suggested that slowing absorption was a new therapeutic principle of scientific interest.[20] This chapter attempts to trace some of the science and document the implications of slowing absorption in terms of the dietary therapy of non–insulin-dependent diabetes mellitus (NIDDM) related to carbohydrate foods.

TABLE 70-1. Some Factors of Concern in Relation to Coronary Heart Disease in Non–Insulin-Dependent Diabetes Mellitus

1. Low high-density lipoproteins (high triglycerides).
2. Modified low-density lipoproteins (glycosylated, oxidized, acetylated).
3. Raised blood pressure.
4. Raised uric acid levels (a primary factor or simply an indicator of other abnormalities?).
5. Raised serum free fatty acid levels.
6. Raised insulin levels.
7. Raised factors VII, VIII, fibrinogen, and plasminogen activator inhibitor and low tissue plasminogen activator levels.

Spreading the Nutrient Load

There are a number of ways in which the absorption time for carbohydrate foods can be prolonged and the nutrient load can be spread over time (Table 70-2). The effects attributed to slowing absorption (Table 70-3) are many and relate to a range of metabolic abnormalities seen in type II diabetes associated with macro- and microvascular complications. Not every benefit has been associated with each method of slowing absorption. For this reason the food frequency paradigm is used to illustrate the general principle, since it is associated with most metabolic effects and is perhaps the cleanest model. This model eliminates the potentially confounding differences in macro- and micronutrients between test and control treatments.

"Sipping" versus "Gulping:" Prolonging Glucose Absorption

In its simplest form the metabolic effects of absorption rate can be assessed by either taking glucose as a bolus or sipping it at an even rate over an extended period of time. When 50 g of glucose were taken in solution by healthy volunteers either as a bolus over 5 minutes or sipped at an even rate over 3 hours, major differences were seen in the insulin response (Fig. 70-1).[21] After sipping, the peak blood glucose level was reduced, although the incremental blood glucose area was not significantly different between treatments. However, the insulin area was reduced by 54%. A corresponding reduction was seen in plasma C-peptide levels on sipping compared with bolus ingestion, whereas free fatty acid and

TABLE 70-2. Factors Contributing to Spreading the Nutrient Load

1. Increased food frequency (nibbling versus gorging).
2. Viscous soluble fibers (e.g., guar, pectin, β-glucan, psyllium).
3. Low glycemic index foods (dried legumes, barley, pasta).
4. Enzyme inhibitors of absorption (e.g., glucosidase inhibitors).

TABLE 70-3. Possible Effects of Prolonging Absorption Time of Carbohydrate

1. Flatter postprandial glucose profile.
2. Lower mean insulin levels postprandially and over the day.
3. Reduced incretion response (e.g., gastric inhibitory polypeptide).
4. Diminished 24-hour urinary C-peptide output.
5. Prolonged suppression of plasma free fatty acids.
6. Reduced urinary catecholamine output.
7. Reduced day-long total and low-density lipoprotein cholesterol levels.
8. Reduced hepatic cholesterol synthesis.
9. Lower serum apolipoprotein B levels.
10. Lower serum uric acid levels.
11. Increased urinary uric acid excretion.

branched-chain amino acid levels fell similarly on both treatments despite the lower insulin levels on sipping (see Fig. 70-1).[21] Furthermore, sipping appeared to avert the need for a counter-regulatory response seen at 180 minutes after the glucose bolus, since blood glucose levels showed no undershoot (see Fig. 70-1).[21] Associated with the blood glucose undershoot after the glucose bolus was an increase in serum growth hormone and urinary catecholamine excretion. At the same time there was a rebound rise in free fatty acid levels and higher levels of branched-chain amino acids than seen after sipping. An intravenous glucose tolerance test given at 4 hours (and therefore performed against either suppressed free fatty acid levels [postsipping] or high free fatty acid levels [postbolus]) confirmed the more rapid glucose disappearance (K_G) after sipping, suggesting less resistance to glucose uptake (Fig. 70-2).[21]

The implications of this study are that provision of carbohydrate at a reduced rate over a longer period of time reduces the need for insulin. This effect may relate to altered free fatty acid metabolism. Adipose tissue hormone–sensitive lipase is sensitive to insulin at levels that are below those required for cellular uptake of glucose.[22] The small increase in insulin secretion above baseline after nibbling is nevertheless sufficient to suppress free fatty acid release. Assuming that raised serum free fatty acid levels inhibit glucose uptake and utilization,[23] the low levels of insulin acting over a prolonged period of time may be all that is required to prevent the rise in glucose in peripheral blood, provided that the glucose is absorbed sufficiently slowly from the gut. Further evidence for increased sensitivity to insulin after sipping is provided by the lower levels and more prolonged suppression of the insulin-sensitive branched-chain amino acids—leucine, isoleucine, and valine—which like glucose are cleared by muscle under the action of insulin. The inhibitory effect of free fatty acids on glucose utilization is supported by the lower mean K_G value seen following intravenous glucose at 4 hours after the glucose bolus. At this time, free fatty acid levels were elevated by comparison with the postsipping free fatty acid level.

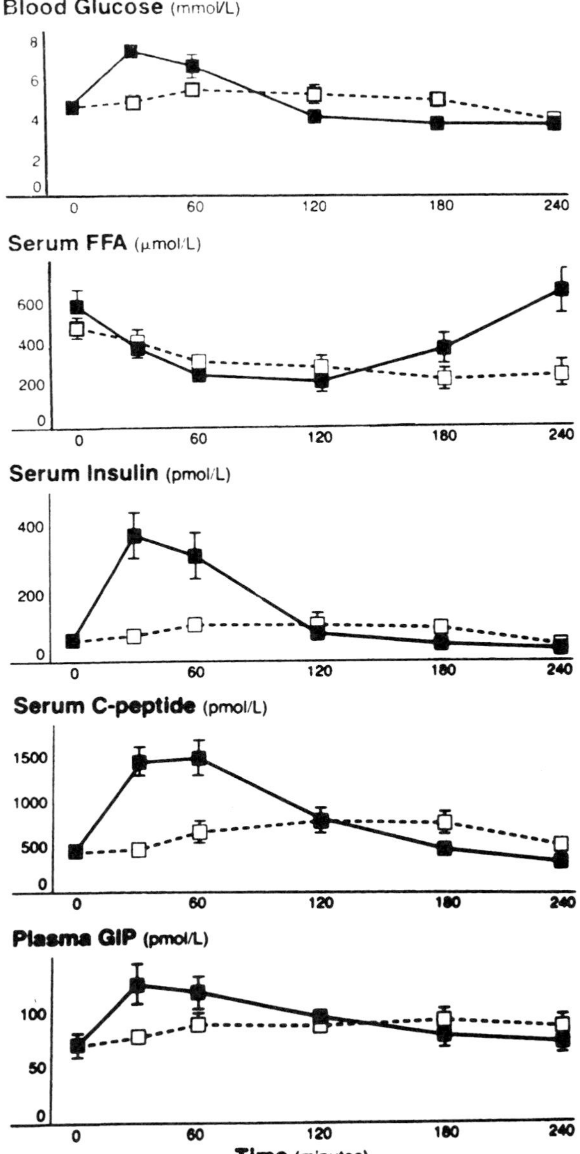

FIGURE 70-1. Mean (±SE) blood glucose; serum free fatty acid (FFA), insulin and C-peptide; and plasma gastric inhibitory polypeptide (GIP) after taking glucose solution as a bolus over 5 minutes (50 g in 700 mL water) at time 0 (□) or sipping same solution over 0–3.5 hours at an even rate (■).

Sipping in Diabetes

The principle of prolonging absorption also appears to have an application in type II diabetes. Figure 70-3 shows data derived from a physician volunteer with NIDDM who took 240 g of glucose over a 12-hour period of observation, either in bolus form at four hourly intervals (with 80 g of glucose taken on each occasion) or sipped at an even rate over the entire 12-hour period.[24] As indicated (Fig. 70-3), on sipping glucose levels declined progressively over the day. Mean insulin levels and total urinary glucose output were both reduced on sipping compared with bolus administration. With sipping the respiratory quotient rose progressively through the day, as opposed to the saw-tooth pattern which was seen on bolus administration, with each rise in respiratory quotient corresponding to a bolus.[24] The reduced requirement for insulin secretion and the diminished urinary glucose losses are the potential advantages seen with spreading the nutrient load. The mechanisms involved in the improved carbohydrate tolerance are likely to be the same as for nondiabetic subjects.

Second Meal Effect

Another illustration of the meal frequency phenomenon relates to the second meal effect or the effect that one meal may have on the next. Early on it was recognized that one carbohydrate load may facilitate the disposal of the next (the Staub-Traugott ef-

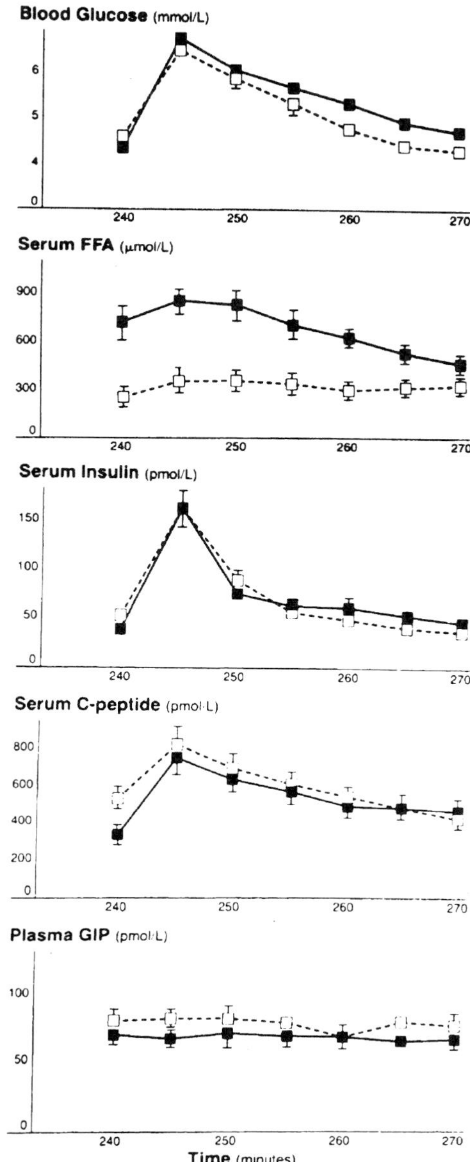

Figure 70-2. Mean (±SE) blood glucose; serum free fatty acid (FFA), insulin and C-peptide; and plasma gastric inhibitory polypeptide (GIP) after taking 5 g intravenous glucose ■, postglucose bolus; □, postsipping.

fect).[25,26] This does not appear to be the case if the first meal is a low carbohydrate meal by virtue of being low in total calories or high in fat.[27,28] However, those meals that result in prolonged suppression of free fatty acid levels appear to result in an improved glucose tolerance to the second meal. Studies in which viscous fiber (guar gum) was used to prolong absorption also demonstrated the improved "second meal" glucose tolerance and prolonged suppression of free fatty acid levels accompanied by the prolonged suppression of 3-hydroxybutyrate (3-OHB) (Fig. 70-4).[29] Similar effects on glucose tolerance have been seen when conventional foods have been fed as a meal or nibbled over a 4-hour period prior to a (second meal) test meal challenge.[27]

It has been claimed that the second meal effect and the Staub-Traugott phenomenon referred to above are not related phenomena.[30] It is also true that the fat and protein may be major determinants of the glycemic response.[31–33] However, there still appears to be sufficient evidence to implicate free fatty acid metabolism in addition to alterations in counter-regulatory hormones,[34] which in the postprandial period may also promote glycogenolysis and glucose mobilization.

Of even greater interest is the concept that blood glucose levels do not necessarily relate to the flux of glucose through the system. Thus tracer studies have demonstrated that, although glucose absorption after an 80 g glucose tolerance test (GTT) continues at a high rate for approximately a 3-hour period, the glycemia only lasts for 90 minutes or less in healthy subjects. Thus during the latter part of the GTT, the rate of peripheral tissue uptake equals or exceeds the rate of glucose absorption. By inference the glucose rise following a second meal (taken while glucose is still being absorbed from the first meal and thus free fatty acid levels are suppressed) should meet less "resistance," that is, should cause less rise in peripheral blood glucose level. Hence the "improved" second meal glucose tolerance and the advantage of increased meal frequency ("nibbling versus gorging").

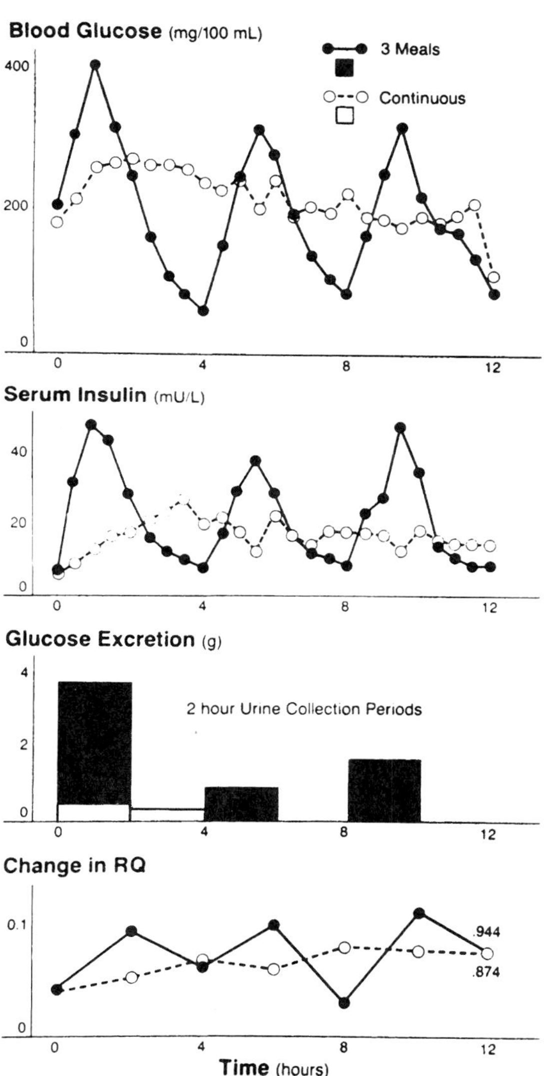

Figure 70-3. Blood glucose, insulin, and respiratory quotient (RQ) response and 2-hour urinary glucose loss, measured over 12 hours, are shown in a diabetic patient controlled on diet. On one occasion 80 g of glucose in solution was taken at 0, 4, and 8 hours, ●--●; and on another occasion 5 g glucose in solution was taken every 15 minutes by continuous sipping, ○--○.

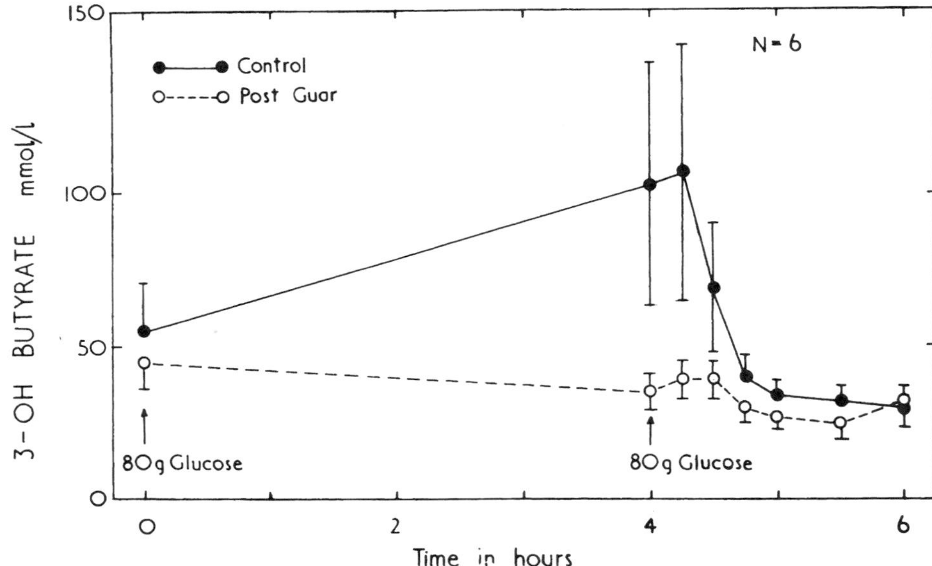

Figure 70-4. Mean (±SE) blood 3-hydroxybutyrate after two 80 g glucose loads taken 4 hours apart. In one instance, the first glucose load was mixed with guar gum (postguar) and no guar was added in the other instance (control). No guar was added to the second glucose load in either instance.

Nibbling Versus Gorging: Metabolic Effects of Altered Food Frequency

Interest in the health implications of altered food frequency dates back at least as far as Sanctorius in the late 16 and early 17 centuries. His observations were encapsulated in one of his axioms: "He who eats but once a day destroys himself whether he eats little or a lot." However, it was not until the early 1930s that Ellis applied the principle to the management of diabetes. He showed that hospitalized type I and possibly some type II diabetics could be managed more effectively with better glycemic control and less insulin if they were provided with small but frequent amounts of glucose and insulin throughout the day.[35] However, it remained for Fabry in the late 1950s and 1960s to make the claim, based on a prospective study of 1359 men over 60 years old in Prague, that increased meal frequency was associated with reduced CHD, diabetes, and obesity.[36] At that time his observations sparked considerable interest in the effects of meal frequency in improving glucose tolerance,[37] lowering serum cholesterol levels,[38–39] and favorably influencing adipose tissue enzyme levels that promote fatty acid mobilization rather than storage.[40]

More recently studies were carried out in normal volunteers who were placed in an extreme model of increased food frequency at 17 meals daily (one meal per hour for 16 hours) compared to a three-meal per day schedule for 2 weeks in a randomized crossover design.[41] The day profiles at the end of each period (Fig. 70-5)[41] indicated a flatter blood glucose profile on nibbling, although the incremental glucose area (above time zero) was not different between the two groups. However, both mean insulin and C-peptide levels over the day were lower on nibbling, confirming the previous observation in which "sipping" was used to "spread the nutrient load." Nevertheless the difference in free fatty acids and 3-OHB levels over the day did not reach significance between treatments (Fig. 70-5), nor were the branched-chain amino acid levels (not shown) significantly different between treatments.

Food Frequency and Diabetes

Single-day feeding studies have also been carried out in type II diabetes showing an advantage with increased meal frequency.[42,43] Studies of 13 hourly feedings compared with four meals during the 10 hours of observation (Fig. 70-6) showed both lower mean glycemia and insulinemia and a flatter gastric inhibitory polypeptide profile.[42] In addition, 24-hour urinary C-peptide output was reduced. However, again as with the nondiabetic volunteers, no significant difference was seen in the free fatty acid, 3-OHB, or branched-chain amino acid responses. Other studies have produced similar results.[43]

Studies dating back over the past 30 years noted reductions in total cholesterol levels with increased meal frequency.[38,39] More recently studies have demonstrated that the reduction was in low-density lipoprotein cholesterol when three meals were compared with 9 or 17 meals daily for 8 and 2 weeks respectively,[41,44,48] using both metabolic and ad libitum diets. After 17 meals daily, lower levels of apolipoprotein B were also demonstrated (Fig. 70-7).[41] Population studies of middle-aged and older volunteers have confirmed that total cholesterol levels were lower in those who ate more frequent meals daily.[46] In addition, mean plasma lipid levels over the course of the day were lower with greater meal frequency.[47] Stable isotope studies indicate that cholesterol synthesis was reduced at greater meal frequency,[48] and studies using urinary mevalonic acid excretion as a water-soluble marker of cholesterol synthesis indicated that the change in cholesterol levels also related to the change in urinary mevalonic acid output.[47] The reduction in cholesterol synthesis has been attributed to the lower insulin levels observed, since insulin is known to stimulate 3-hydroxy-3-methylglutaryl coenzyme A reductase activity, a rate-limiting enzyme in cholesterol synthesis.[49] A further possible reason for the reduction in serum cholesterol level on nibbling is the increased loss of bile acids that would result from the increased frequency of cycling of bile acids through the gut with each snack. The resulting increased losses of the cholesterol molecule as bile acids would again promote the cholesterol-lowering effect of increased meal frequency.

Last, serum uric acid levels were reduced and urinary uric acid excretion was increased with increased food frequency.[47] As with the reduction in serum cholesterol levels, the effect of lower insulin levels was invoked as an explanation.[47] It was suggested that insulin promoted renal reabsorption of uric acid, and this idea has been discussed in the context of hyperinsulinemic states.[50]

Additional physiologic effects of food frequency have been explored that are relevant to diabetes. In humans, acute studies of the effects of meal frequency have demonstrated a reduced thermogenic response to increased meal frequency. Thus no reason is provided for the metabolic benefits in weight management suggested to accrue from nibbling.[51] However, assessment of satiety in acute studies suggests that satiety fluctuates less over

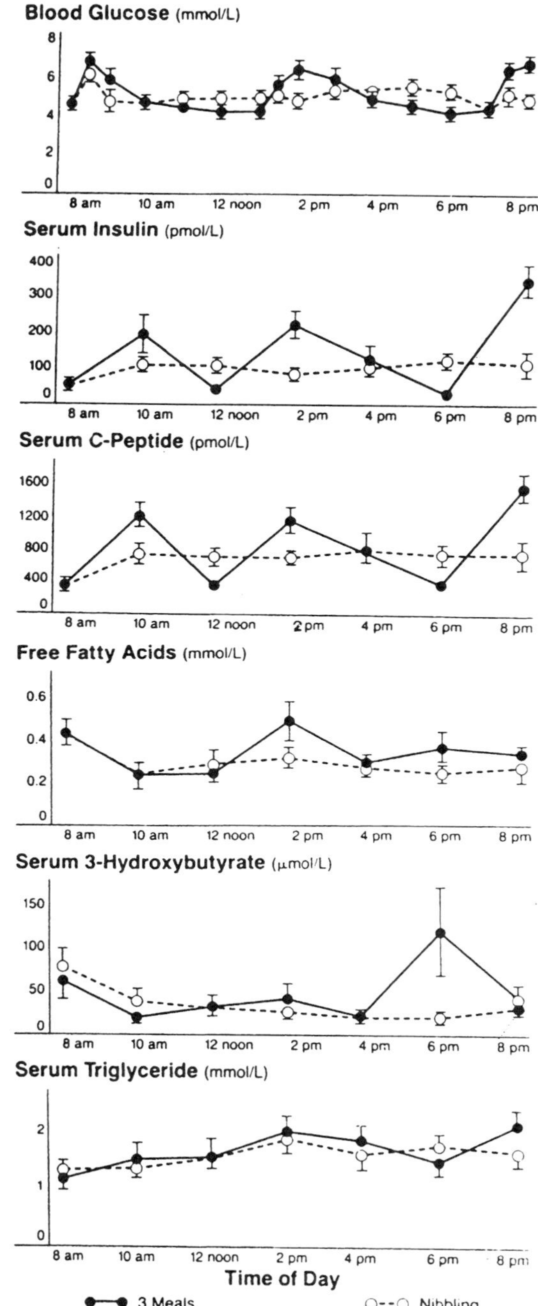

FIGURE 70-5. Mean (±SE) blood glucose levels and serum concentrations of insulin, C-peptide, free fatty acids, 3-hydroxybutyrate, and triglyceride in seven men on day 13 of nibbling and 3-meal diets. During the nibbling diet, meals were eaten hourly from 8 AM onward, and during the three-meal diet at 8 AM, 1 PM, and 7 PM.

the day and thus does not dip down into the "hunger" range.[42] Until now the all-important long-term studies have not been undertaken to determine whether in the long term fewer calories are consumed. Until then there remains the concern that snacking may increase the body weight of those who most need to lose weight. Nevertheless, irrespective of whether increased meal frequency as such is broadly applicable in practice, the demonstration that it can improve certain aspects of lipid and carbohydrate metabolism makes it a valuable model for other methods of "spreading the nutrient load."

Viscous Dietary Fibers

Viscous gums, gels, and mucilages depending on their viscosity, have also been shown to reduce the rate of absorption of sugars, and to flatten the postprandial glycemia and the serum insulin response.[52] These fibers have also been shown to reduce low-density lipoprotein cholesterol and apolipoprotein B levels.[53–58] The so-called particulate insoluble fibers such as wheat bran increase fecal bulk but have little effect on postglycemia[52] or other metabolic events.

The lack of enthusiasm in using viscous fibers in the treatment of diabetes stems from the relative difficulty in making palatable formulations for long-term use. This has limited the number and size of the studies undertaken. Initial test meal studies in diabetics appeared promising.[59] However, in the 1980s, the results of studies did not indicate a clear improvement in glycemic control.[60] As a result, recent guidelines have considered soluble fibers to play no role in glycemic control.[1,2] However, a number of new studies have appeared, suggesting a possible role for soluble viscous fibers in the treatment and prevention of diabetes complications. These include studies of guar gum in healthy men that demonstrated reduced low-density lipoprotein cholesterol and blood pressure and increased urinary sodium loss.[61] In diabetes, in parallel test and control studies in NIDDM, hemoglobin AIc (HbAIc) levels were reduced in those taking the test fiber (guar) but not in the controls, and a similar picture of reduction in the test situation was seen in relation to low-density lipoprotein cholesterol and the low-density lipoprotein: high-density lipoprotein cholesterol ratio.[62] Furthermore, long-term studies of guar lasting 48 weeks in NIDDM volunteers showed a mean reduction in HbAIc on guar, which rose significantly on cessation of guar supplementation.[63] These studies do not demonstrate the gold standard of improved glycemic control in which HbAIc is shown to fall in long-term randomized cross-over design studies.[60] However, this goal is often difficult to achieve even for approaches advocated for the treatment of diabetes (e.g., monounsaturated fats[13]) and for which there is considerable support.[2] Use of viscous fibers in the treatment of diabetes therefore continues to be of interest but requires further work to maximize the palatability and effectiveness of preparations for trial purposes.

Glycemic Index

The original impetus to classify foods using a glycemic index was to provide a ranking of the rates at which different starchy foods were digested.[64,65] It had been well documented that different starchy foods produced different glycemic effects.[66] It was hoped that selection of foods with lower glycemic indices would contribute to prolonging the absorption of nutrients, thereby improving the glycemic profile[67,68] and reducing insulin requirement and fasting lipids.[69]

Nevertheless, certain acute (up to one day) mixed meal studies during the middle to late 1980s suggested that a glycemic index classification of foods had no clinical utility.[70–72] However, since the late 1980s, when the effects of high and low glycemic index diets were compared, reports have documented improved glycemic control in both types I and II diabetes judged by serum fructosamine or HbAIc levels in studies of 2 weeks to 2 months' duration.[73–78] In some cases, changes in blood measurements have been noted despite relatively small differences in glycemic index between test and control diets. Furthermore, some studies also noted reductions

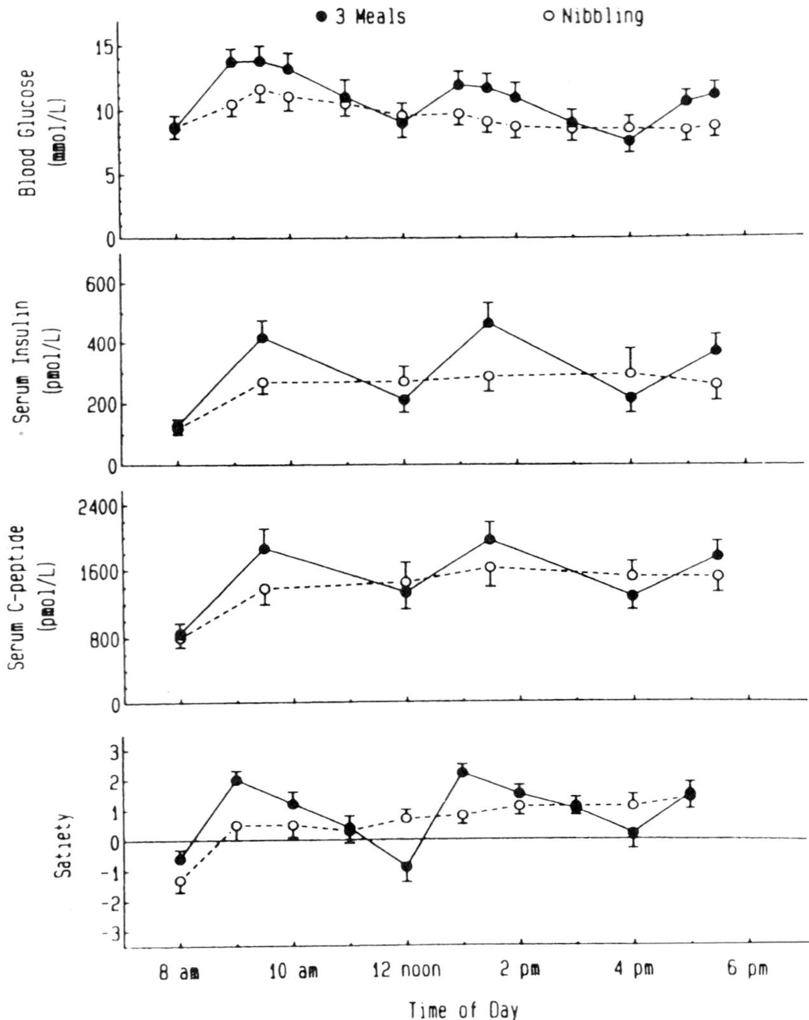

Figure 70-6. Mean satiety and concentrations of blood glucose (in 11 volunteers) and serum insulin and C-peptide (in 8 and 9 volunteers, respectively) over the course of 1 day on a nibbling (○) or three-meal diet (●).

in serum lipids.[73–77,79] The changes are therefore similar to those seen with viscous fiber, despite the absence of these fibers in some of the low glycemic index diets.

Enzyme Inhibitors

Alpha-glucosidase inhibitors such as acarbose, which reduce the rate of absorption of starch, sucrose, and to a lesser extent maltose,[80] have recently been shown in a large multicenter trial to result in a significant reduction in HbAlc in type II diabetes.[81] Changes in serum lipids were not observed. Nevertheless, findings of this nature provide additional encouragement that spreading the nutrient load, in addition to altering the amount and nature of the nutrients, may one day have a role in modifying glycemia in the management of diabetes.

Conclusion

A relatively new general approach to the dietary therapy of non–insulin-dependent diabetes mellitus is a conscious attempt to try to spread the nutrient load or lengthen the absorption time. This approach covers the effects of altered meal frequency, viscous dietary fibers, low glycemic index foods, and inhibitors of carbohydrate absorption. In its simplest form it is illustrated by studies of altered meal frequency (nibbling versus gorging). Reducing the size and increasing the frequency of carbohydrate feedings, either by sipping glucose or nibbling meals, has been shown acutely to result in lower mean blood glucose and insulin levels over the day in normal volunteers and type II diabetics and reduced 24-hour urinary C-peptide losses. In the longer term in nondiabetic subjects fasting and postprandial total and low-density lipoprotein cholesterol levels are reduced, together with fasting apolipoprotein B and serum uric acid levels, as risk factors for CHD. These and other physiologic effects make slowing carbohydrate absorption (lente carbohydrate) a potentially useful therapeutic modality.

The mechanism for the glycemic advantage of prolonging absorption may relate to the more efficient uptake and metabolism of glucose over time, possibly in part secondary to prolonged suppression of free fatty acid levels. The lower insulin levels observed may confer additional advantages in reducing the hepatic drive to cholesterol synthesis and reducing uric acid reabsorption by the kidney. Risk factors for CHD (cholesterol and uric acid levels) may therefore be reduced. Furthermore, increased bile acid losses via the colon may contribute to lower cholesterol levels. This effect may be the result of increased enterohepatic cycling of bile with increased meal frequency or of reduced ileal bile acid retrieval due to entrapment by viscous fibers. The metabolic effects of these nutritional maneuvers will further increase the value of spreading the nutrient load in order to reduce the risk of complications in diabetes.

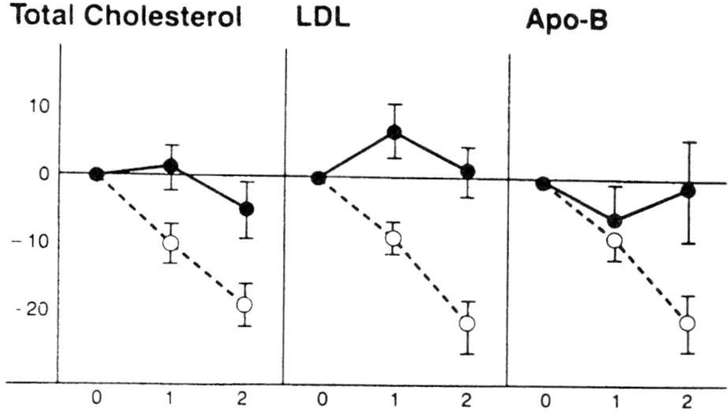

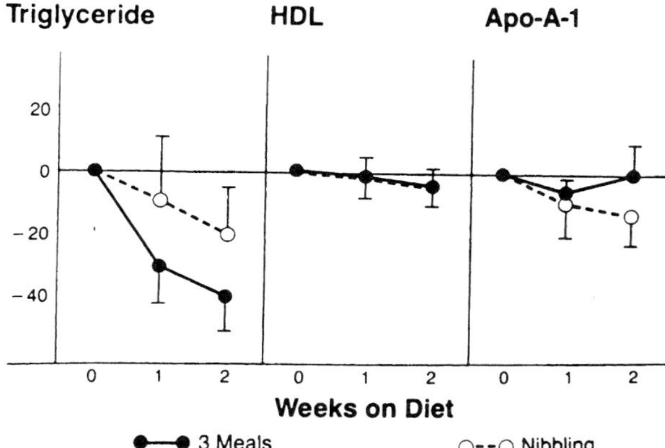

Figure 70-7. Mean (±SE) percentage change from time zero in serum lipid and apolipoprotein (Apo) concentrations in seven men during the nibbling diet and the three-meal diet.

References

1. American Diabetes Association. Nutrition recommendations and principles for people with diabetes mellitus. Diabetes Care 1994;17:519
2. Franz MJ, Horton ES, Bantle JP, et al. Nutrition principles for the management of diabetes and related complications. Diabetes Care 1994;17:490
3. US Department of Agriculture, US Department of Health and Human Services. Nutrition and Your Health: Dietary Guidelines for Americans, 3rd ed. Hyattsville, MD: USDA's Human Nutrition Information Service;1990
4. US Department of Agriculture. The Food Guide Pyramid. Hyattsville, MD: USDA's Human Nutrition Information Service;1992
5. Willett WC. Diet and health: What should we eat? Science 1994;264:532
6. Expert Panel on Detection, Evaluation, and Treatment of High Blood Cholesterol in Adults. Summary of the Second Report of the National Cholesterol Education Program (NCEP) Expert Panel on Detection, Evaluation, and Treatment of High Blood Cholesterol in Adults (Adult Treatment Panel II). JAMA 1993;269:3015
7. The Diabetes Control and Complications Trial Research Group. The effect of intensive treatment of diabetes on the development and progression of long-term complications in insulin treated diabetes mellitus. N Engl J Med 1993; 329:977
8. Stamler J, Vaccaro O, Neaton JD, Wentworth D, for the Multiple Risk Factor Intervention Trial Research Group: Diabetes, other risk factors, and 12-year cardiovascular mortality for men screened in the Multiple Risk Factor Intervention Trial. Diabetes Care 1993;16:434
9. Olefsky JM, Ciaraldi TP, Kolterman OG. Mechanisms of insulin resistance in non-insulin dependent (type II) diabetes. Am J Med 1985;79:12
10. Henry RR, Wallace P, Olefsky JM. Effects of weight loss on mechanisms of hyperglycaemia in obese non insulin dependent diabetes mellitus. Diabetes 1986;35:990
11. Golay A, Felber JP, Dusmet M, et al. Effect of weight loss on glucose disposal in obese and non-obese diabetes patients. Int J Obes 1985;9:181
12. Garg A, Bonanome A, Grundy SM, et al. Comparison of a high-carbohydrate diet with high-monosaturated-fat diet in patients with non-insulin-dependent diabetes mellitus. N Engl J Med 1988;91:829
13. Garg A, Bantle JP, Henry KR, et al. Effects of varying carbohydrate content of diet in patients with non-insulin-dependent diabetes mellitus. JAMA 1994;271:1421
14. de Lorgeril M, Renaul S, Mamelle N, et al. Mediterranean alpha-linolenic acid-rich diet in secondary prevention of coronary heart disease. Lancet 1994; 343:1454
15. Bantle JP, Laine CW, Thomas JW. Metabolic effects of dietary fructose and sucrose in types I and II diabetic subjects. JAMA 1986;256:3241
16. Bantle JP, Swanson JE, Thomas W, Laine DC. Metabolic effects of dietary fructose in diabetic subjects. Diabetes Care 1992;15:1468
17. Swanson JE, Laine DC, Thomas W, Bantle JP. Metabolic effects of dietary fructose in healthy subjects. Am J Clin Nutr 1992;55:851
18. Crapo PA, Kolterman OG, Henry RR. Metabolic consequence of two-week fructose feeding in diabetic subjects. Diabetes Care 1986;9:111
19. Thorburn AW, Crapo PA, Beltz WF, et al. Lipid metabolism in non-insulin-dependent diabetes: Effects of long-term treatment with fructose-supplemented mixed meals. Am J Clin Nutr 1989;50:1015
20. Creutzfeldt W. Introduction. In: Creutzfeldt W, Folsch UR, eds. Delaying Absorption As a Therapeutic Principle in Metabolic Diseases. New York: Thieme-Stratton;1983:1
21. Jenkins DJA, Wolever TMS, Ocana AM, et al. Metabolic effects of reducing rate of glucose ingestion by single bolus versus continuous sipping. Diabetes 1990;39:775
22. Jungas RL, Ball GE. Studies on the metabolism of adipose tissue XII. The effects of insulin and epinephrine on fatty acid and glycerol production in the presence and absence of glucose. Biochemistry 1963;2:383
23. Randle PJ, Garland PB, Hales CN, Newsholme GA. The glucose-fatty acid cycle: Its role in insulin sensitivity and the metabolic disturbances of diabetes mellitus. Lancet 1963;1:785
24. Jenkins DJA, Wolever TMS, Taylor RH, et al. Reply to letter by Abraira and Lawrence. Am J Clin Nutr 1983;37:153
25. Staub H. Untersuchenuber den Zuckerstoffwechsel des Menschen. I. Mitteilung. Z Klin Med 1921;91:44
26. Traugott K. Uber das Verhalten des Blutzuckerspiegels bei wiederholten und verschiedener Art enteraler zuckerzurzufuhr und dessen Bedeutung fur die leberfunktion. Klin Wochensch 1922;1:892
27. Jenkins DJA, Wolever TMS, Taylor RH, et al. Slow release dietary carbohydrate improves second meal tolerance. Am J Clin Nutr 1982;35:1339
28. Collier GR, Wolever TMS, Jenkins DJA. Concurrent ingestion of fat and reduction in starch content impairs carbohydrate tolerance to subsequent meals. Am J Clin Nutr 1987;45:963
29. Jenkins DJA, Wolever TMS, Nineburn R, et al. Improved glucose tolerance four hours after taking guar with glucose. Diabetologia 1980;19:21
30. Abraira C, Lawrence AM. Dietary Carbohydrate and second meal glycemic response. Am J Clin Nutr 1983;37:152
31. Nuttall FQ, Mooradinn AD, Gannon MC, et al. Effect of protein ingestion on glucose and insulin response to a standardized oral glucose load. Diabetes Care 1984;7:465
32. Collier G, O'Dea K. The effect of coingestion of fat on the glucose, insulin and gastric inhibitory polypeptide responses to carbohydrate and protein. Am J Clin Nutr 1983;37:941
33. Estrich D, Ravnick A, Schlierf G, et al. Effects of co-ingestion of fat and protein upon carbohydrate induced hyperglycaemia. Diabetes 1967;16:232
34. Gerich JE. Glucose counter regulation and its impact on diabetes mellitus. Diabetes 1988;37:1608
35. Ellis A. Increased carbohydrate tolerance in diabetes following hourly administration of glucose and insulin over long periods. Q J Med 1934;27:137
36. Fabry P, Tepperman J. Meal frequency—a possible factor in human pathology. Am J Clin Nutr 1970;25:1059
37. Gwinup G, Byron R, Roush W, et al. Effect of nibbling versus gorging on glucose tolerance. Lancet 1963;2:165
38. Cohn C. Feeding patterns and some aspects of cholesterol metabolism. Fed Proc 1964;23:76
39. Jagannathan SN, Connell WF, Beveridge JMR. Effect of gourmandizing and semicontinuous eating of equicaloric amounts of formula type high-fat diets on plasma cholesterol and triglyceride levels in human volunteer subjects. Am J Clin Nutr 1964;15:90
40. Bray GA. Lipogenesis in human adipose tissue: Some effects of nibbling and gorging. J Clin Invest 1972;51:537
41. Jenkins DJA, Wolever TMS, Vuksan V, et al. "Nibbling versus gorging:" Metabolic advantages of increased meal frequency. N Engl J Med 1989; 321:929
42. Jenkins DJA, Ocana A, Jenkins A, et al. Metabolic advantages of spreading the nutrient load: Effects of increased meal frequency in non-insulin-dependent diabetes. Am J Clin Nutr 1992;55:461
43. Bertelsen J, Christiansen C, Thomsen C, et al. Effect of meal frequency on blood glucose, insulin, and free fatty acids in NIDDM subjects. Diabetes Care 1993;16:3
44. Arnold LM, Ball MJ, Duncan AW, Mann J. Effect of isoenergetic intake of three or nine meals on plasma lipoproteins and glucose metabolism. Am J Clin Nutr 1993;57:446
45. McGrath SA, Gibney MJ. Effects of altered frequency of eating on plasma lipids of free-living healthy males on normal self-selected diets. Eur J Nutr 1994;48:402
46. Edelstein SL, Barrett-Connor EL, Wingard DL, Cohn BA. Increased meal frequency associated with decreased cholesterol concentrations; Rancho & Bernardo, CA, 1984–1987. Am J Clin Nutr 1992;55:664
47. Jenkins DJA, Khan A, Jenkins AL, et al. The effect of nibbling versus gorging on cardiovascular risk factors: Serum uric acid and blood lipids. Metabolism 1995;44:549

48. Jones PJH, Leitch CA, Pederson RA. Meal frequency effects of plasma hormone concentrations and cholesterol synthesis in humans. Am J Clin Nutr 1993;57:868
49. Lakshmanan MR, Nepokroeff CM, Ness GC, et al. Stimulation by insulin of rat liver beta-hydroxy-beta-methylglutaryl coenzyme-A reductase and cholesterol-synthesizing activities. Biochem Biophys Res Commun 1973;50:704
50. Faschini F, Chen YDI, Hollenbeck CB, Reaven GM. Relationship between insulin resistance to insulin-mediated glucose uptake, urinary uric acid clearance and plasma uric acid concentration. JAMA 1991;266:3008
51. Tai MM, Eastillo P, Pi-Sunyer FX. Meal size and frequency: Effect on the thermic effects of food. Am J Clin Nutr 1991;54:783
52. Jenkins DJA, Wolever TMS, Leeds AR, et al. Dietary fibres, fibre analogues and glucose tolerance: Importance of viscosity. Br Med J 1978;1:1392
53. Jenkins DJA, Reynolds D, Leeds AR, et al. Hypocholesterolemic action of dietary fiber unrelated to fecal bulking effect. AM J Clin Nutr 1979;32:2430
54. Anderson JW, Zettwoch N, Feldman T, et al. Cholesterol lowering effects of psyllium hydrophilic mucilloid for hypercholesterolemic men. Arch Intern Med 1988;148:292
55. Anderson JW, Gastaform NJ. Hypocholesterolemic effects of oat and bean products. Am J Clin Nutr 1988;48:749
56. Kay RM, Truswell AS. Effect of citrus pectin on blood lipids and fecal steroid excretion in men. Am J Clin Nutr 1977;30:171
57. Miettenen TA, Tarpila S. Effect of pectin on serum cholesterol, fecal bile acids and biliary lipids in normolipidaemic and hyperlipidaemic individuals. Clin Chim Acta 1979;79:471
58. Jenkins DJA, Wolever TMS, Rao AV, et al. Effect on blood lipids of very high intakes of fiber in diets low in saturated fat and cholesterol. N Eng J Med 1993;329:21
59. Jenkins DJA, Leeds AR, Gaosull MA, et al. Unabsorbable carbohydrates and diabetes: Decreased post prandial hyperglycemia. Lancet 1976;2:172
60. Nuttall FQ. Dietary fiber in the management of diabetes. Diabetes 1993;42:503
61. Landin K, Holm G, Tengborn L, Smith V. Guar gum improves insulin sensitivity, blood lipids, blood pressure, and fibrinolysis in healthy men. Am J Clin Nutr 1992;56:1061
62. Vuorinen-Markkola H, Sinisalo M, Koivisto VA. Guar gum in insulin dependent diabetes. Effect on glycemic control and serum lipoproteins. Am J Clin Nutr 1992;56:1056
63. Groop P-H, Aro A, Stenman S, Groop L. Long term effects of guar gum in subjects with non-insulin dependent diabetes mellitus. Am J Clin Nutr 1993;58:513
64. Jenkins DJA, Wolever TMS, Taylor RH, et al. Glycemic index of foods: A physiological basis for carbohydrate exchange. Am J Clin Nutr 1981;34:362
65. Jenkins DJA, Wolever TMS, Taylor RH, et al. Rate of digestion of foods and postporandial glycemia in normal and diabetic subjects. Br Med J 1980; 2:14
66. Crapo PA, Reaven G, Olefsky J. Post-prandial plasma glucose and insulin responses to different complex carbohydrates. Diabetes 1977;26:1178
67. Bornet FRJ, Costagliole D, Rizkalla SW, et al. Insulinemic and glycemic indexes of six starch-rich foods taken alone and in a mixed meal by type 2 diabetes. Am J Clin Nutr 1987;45:588
68. Collier GR, Wolever TMS, Wong GS, Josse RG. Prediction of glycemic response to mixed meals in non-insulin dependent diabetic subjects. Am J Clin Nutr 1986;44:349
69. Jenkins DJA, Wolever TMS, Kalmusky J, et al. Low glycemic index diet in hyperlipidemia: Use of traditional starchy foods. Am J Clin Nutr 1987;46:66
70. Hollenbeck CB, Coulston AM, Reaven GM. Comparison of plasma glucose and insulin responses to mixed meals of high, intermediate and low-glycemic potential. Diabetes Care 1988;11:323
71. Laine DC, Thomas W, Levitt MD, Bantle JP. Comparison of predictive capabilities of diabetic exchange lists and glycemic index of foods. Diabetes Care 1987;19:387
72. Nuttall FQ, Mooradian AD, DeMarais R, Parker S. The glycemic effect of different meals approximately isocaloric and similar in protein, carbohydrate and fat content as calculated using the ADA exchange lists. Diabetes Care 1983;6:432
73. Jenkins DJA, Wolever TMS, Buckley G, et al. Low glycemic-index starchy foods in the diabetic diet. Am J Clin Nutr 1988;48:248
74. Wolever TMS, Jenkins DJA, Vuksan V, et al. Beneficial effect of low-glycemic index diet in overweight NIDDM subjects. Diabetes Care 1992;15:562
75. Wolever TMS, Jenkins DJA, Vuksan V, et al. Beneficial effect of a low glycemic index diet in type 2 diabetes. Diabetic Med 1992;9:451
76. Fontvieille AM, Acosta M, Rizkalla SW, et al. A moderate switch from high to low glycemic index foods for 3 weeks improves the metabolic control of type 1 (IDDM) diabetic subjects. Diabetes Nutr Metab 1988;1:139
77. Fontvieille AM, Rizkalla SW, Penfornis A, et al. The use of low glycemic index foods improves metabolic control of diabetic patients over five weeks. Diabetic Med 1992;9:444
78. Brand JC, Calagiuri S, Crossman S, et al. Low-glycemic index foods improve long-term glycemic control in NIDDM. Diabetes Care 1991;14:95
79. Jenkins DJA, Wolever TMS, Kalmusky J, et al. Low-glycemic index diet in hyperlipidemia: Use of traditional starchy foods. Am J Clin Nutr 1987;46:66
80. Jenkins DJA, Taylor RH, Goff DV, et al. Scope and specificity of acarbose in slowing carbohydrate absorption in men. Diabetes 1978;27:563
81. Chiasson JL, Josse RG, Hunt JA, et al. Efficacy of acarbose in the treatment of patients with non-insulin-dependent diabetes mellitus. A multicenter controlled clinical trial. Ann Intern Med 1994;121:928

Diabetes Mellitus, edited by Derek LeRoith, Simeon I. Taylor, and Jerrold M. Olefsky. Lippincott–Raven Publishers, Philadelphia © 1996.

CHAPTER 71

Exercise in Patients with Non–Insulin-Dependent Diabetes Mellitus

EDWARD S. HORTON

Introduction

Regular physical exercise was recognized in ancient times as an important part of the treatment of diabetes mellitus[1] and was frequently prescribed during the preinsulin era for patients who would now be diagnosed as having non–insulin-dependent diabetes mellitus (NIDDM). In 1919, Allen et al.[2] demonstrated that exercise lowers the blood glucose concentration and transiently improves glucose tolerance in persons with diabetes, and in 1926, Lawrence[3] observed that exercise potentiates the hypoglycemic effect of injected insulin. As the use of insulin became widespread, it was soon recognized that regular exercise decreased insulin requirements and was associated with an increased risk of hypoglycemic reactions. In recent years, much has been learned about the role of insulin and other hormones in the regulation of metabolic fuels during and after exercise, and the role of exercise in the treatment of IDDM has been reexamined (See Chapter 42). Although exercise may create significant problems in blood glucose regulation in insulin-treated patients, it plays an important therapeutic role in the management of NIDDM and is often prescribed, along with diet and oral hypoglycemic agents, for this purpose. Furthermore, there is now strong evidence that regular physical exercise protects against the development of NIDDM in high-risk populations, supporting the recommendation that increased physical activity, along with the prevention or treatment of obesity by dietary restriction, is an important component of lifestyle modification for persons with impaired glucose tolerance, a history of gestational diabetes, or a family history of NIDDM. When exercise is to be used as a preventive or therapeutic intervention in NIDDM, its effectiveness and the associated risks must be taken into consideration. In this chapter, current knowledge of the benefits, risks, and metabolic effects of exercise in NIDDM will be reviewed.

Benefits of Exercise in Non–Insulin-Dependent Diabetes Mellitus

Many benefits of regular physical exercise have been identified for patients with non–insulin-dependent diabetes mellitus (NIDDM) (Table 71-1). Whereas exercise in normal persons has little impact on blood glucose concentrations, moderate-intensity exercise in patients with NIDDM is usually associated with a decrease in blood glucose toward normal. This reaction may be used by patients to help regulate blood glucose concentration on a day-to-day basis and may be a mechanism by which regular physical exercise results in improved long-term diabetic control.[4] In addition to the acute blood glucose–lowering effect of exercise, it has been recognized for many years that physical training is associated with lower fasting and postprandial insulin concentrations and increased insulin sensitivity.[5,6] Because NIDDM is characterized by insulin resistance in skeletal muscle, adipose tissue, and the liver,[7,8] there has been considerable interest in the use of physical training as a means of improving insulin sensitivity and thus ameliorating one of the major abnormalities of NIDDM.

A third benefit of regular exercise is a reduction in cardiovascular risk factors through improvement of the lipid profile and reduction of hypertension. It is now well documented that physical training is associated with a lowering of serum triglyceride concentrations, particularly very-low-density lipoproteins, and an increase in high density lipoprotein-2 (HDL_2) cholesterol.[9] There is also a slight decrease in low density lipoprotein (LDL) cholesterol with training.[10] Recent studies on the mechanism by which physical training results in lower very low density lipoprotein (VLDL) and increased HDL_2 concentrations have shown that physically trained skeletal muscle has increased lipoprotein lipase activity compared with untrained muscle. This results in greater extraction of circulating VLDL and increased release of HDL_2 resulting from a transfer of VLDL surface proteins to HDL_3 particles.[11] This improvement in the lipid profile with physical training is observed with running a minimum of 10–12 miles per week and increases in a dose-response fashion up to distances of approximately 40 miles per week.[12] Lower levels of physical activity have little or no effect on lipid profiles.

Another effect of physical training is improvement in mild to moderate hypertension. This occurs independently of weight loss or changes in body composition and can result in a decrease in both systolic and diastolic blood pressure of 5 to 10 mmHg.[13,14] Although the mechanism for this effect is not known, it is correlated with a decrease in serum insulin and triglyceride concentrations[15] and may be related to reversing an effect of chronic hyperinsulinemia on renal sodium retention.

In addition to improvement in cardiovascular risk factors, regular physical exercise may be an effective adjunct to diet for weight reduction. Combined with caloric restriction, exercise has been shown to result in greater loss of adipose tissue mass and relative preservation of lean body mass.[15,16] In some studies, however, particularly with very low calorie diets, exercise may not have a significant effect beyond that of diet alone.[17,18]

Finally, physical training of patients with NIDDM results in the same general benefits as in nondiabetic persons. These include increased cardiovascular fitness and physical working capacity. In addition, there may be psychological benefits, including an enhanced sense of well-being and an improved quality of life.

Table 71-1. Benefits of Regular Exercise for Patients with Non–Insulin-Dependent Diabetes Mellitus

1. Lower blood glucose concentrations during and after exercise
2. Lower basal and postprandial insulin concentrations
3. Improved insulin sensitivity
4. Lower glycosylated hemoglobin levels
5. Improved lipid profile
   - Decreased triglycerides
   - Slightly decreased LDL cholesterol
   - Increased HDL cholesterol
6. Improvement in mild to moderate hypertension
7. Increased energy expenditure
   - Adjunct to diet for weight reduction
   - Increased fat loss
   - Preservation of lean body mass
8. Cardiovascular conditioning
9. Increased strength and flexibility
10. Improved sense of well-being and enhanced quality of life

Risks of Exercise in Non–Insulin-Dependent Diabetes Mellitus

In addition to the benefits of exercise, a number of significant risks for patients with non–insulin-dependent diabetes mellitus (NIDDM) have been recognized (Table 71-2). In patients taking insulin or oral hypoglycemic agents, exercise may result in symptomatic hypoglycemia either during or after exercise. In insulin-treated patients, the increased risk of hypoglycemia may persist for up to 24 hours after prolonged, strenuous exercise.[19] In addition, extremely strenuous exercise of short duration may result in a rapid increase in blood glucose concentration that lasts for several hours after the exercise is stopped.[20] Another risk of exercise in persons with NIDDM is exacerbation of underlying cardiovascular disease that may not have been diagnosed previously. This includes the development of angina pectoris, myocardial infarction, or cardiac arrhythmias. Therefore, adults with NIDDM should have a tho-

Table 71-2. Risks of Exercise for Patients with Non–Insulin-Dependent Diabetes Mellitus

1. Hypoglycemia if treated with insulin or sulfonylureas
   - Exercise-induced hypoglycemia
   - Late-onset postexercise hypoglycemia
2. Hyperglycemia after very strenuous exercise
3. Precipitation or exacerbation of cardiovascular disease
   - Angina pectoris
   - Myocardia infarction
   - Arrhythmias
   - Sudden death
4. Worsening of long-term complications of diabetes
   - Proliferative retinopathy
     - Vitreous hemorrhage
     - Retinal detachment
   - Nephropathy
     - Increased proteinuria
   - Peripheral neuropathy
     - Soft tissue and joint injuries
   - Autonomic neuropathy
     - Decreased cardiovascular response to exercise
     - Decreased maximum aerobic capacity
     - Impaired response to dehydration
     - Postural hypotension

rough cardiac evaluation before beginning an exercise program. Degenerative joint disease is more common in obese persons and may be exacerbated by weight-bearing exercising. Also, patients with sensory neuropathy may experience joint and soft tissue injuries while participating in exercise.

A number of other complications of diabetes may be aggravated by exercise, and patients with NIDDM should be screened for these before being advised to undertake an exercise program. The most important complication is proliferative retinopathy, in which exercise may result in retinal or vitreous hemorrhage. Extremely strenuous exercise or exercise associated with Valsalva-like maneuvers are particularly dangerous and should be avoided by patients with proliferative retinopathy. Also, exercise resulting in jarring or rapid head motion may precipitate hemorrhage or retinal detachment. Physical exercise is associated with increased proteinuria in patients with diabetic nephropathy.[21,22] This is probably the result of changes in renal hemodynamics associated with exercise and is unlikely to have any effect on the progression of renal disease. As mentioned above, peripheral neuropathy increases the risk of soft tissue and joint injuries, and may be a contraindication to certain types of exercise such as running, jogging, or similar activities in which localized trauma may occur. If autonomic neuropathy is present, the capacity for high-intensity exercise may be impaired due to decreased maximum heart rate and aerobic capacity. In addition, there may be an impaired response to dehydration and problems with postural hypotension. With proper planning and selection of exercise, most of these complications can be avoided, although in some circumstances physical exercise programs may be contraindicated for the patient with NIDDM.

Exercise and Insulin Sensitivity

A possible role for physical exercise as a means of treating the insulin resistance associated with obesity and non–insulin dependent diabetes mellitus (NIDDM) was first suggested by Bjorntorp et al.[23] in the early 1970s. They observed that physically active middle-aged men had significantly lower fasting insulin concentrations and lower insulin responses to oral glucose compared with untrained men of the same age and body weight.[5] This finding suggested that regular physical activity is associated with increased insulin sensitivity and led the investigators to study the effects of 12 weeks of physical training on glucose tolerance and insulin responses in a group of obese patients with normal glucose tolerance but insulin resistance. After the period of physical training there was no change in the blood glucose responses, but insulin concentrations were significantly lower, both with fasting and after glucose administration.[6] Subsequently, numerous investigators demonstrated increased insulin sensitivity and responsiveness in physically trained subjects using a variety of techniques. For example, both normal control subjects and patients with NIDDM have been shown to have a 30–35% increase in insulin-stimulated glucose disposal after physical training when studied by the hyperinsulinemic-euglycemic clamp technique.[7,24] This increase in insulin sensitivity correlates closely with the training-induced increase in maximum aerobic capacity[25,26] and is due primarily to increased glucose uptake in skeletal muscle, because no changes have been observed in hepatic glucose production rates.

It was soon learned, however, that the increase in insulin sensitivity and responsiveness associated with physical conditioning is rapidly lost when exercise is discontinued. Burstein et al.[27] found that much of the effect is lost within 60 hours, and others have demonstrated that the effect is no longer present after 5–7 days without exercise. In a study by Bogardus et al.[17] comparing the effects of a very low calorie diet with the same diet plus a physical training program on weight loss and blood glucose regulation in NIDDM, the physically trained group had a significant increase in insulin-stimulated glucose disposal rates, whereas the group treated by diet alone had no change after 3 months of treatment. The increase in insulin-stimulated glucose disposal in the group treated by diet and physical training was due entirely to an increase in nonoxidative glucose disposal, presumably reflecting increased glycogen synthesis. In this study, the glucose clamp procedures were done 5–7 days after the last exercise session and therefore appear to demonstrate a true effect of physical training rather than a carryover effect from the last bout of exercise.

In more recent studies, Mikines et al.[28] have shown that a single bout of exercise increases the sensitivity and responsiveness of insulin-stimulated glucose uptake in untrained persons. This effect lasts for at least 2 days but is not observed after 5 days. In addition, physically trained subjects have increased insulin action when studied 15 hours after their last training session compared with untrained subjects. When studied 5 days after the last training session, insulin responsiveness remains increased compared with untrained subjects, suggesting that there is a long-term adaptive increase in whole body responsiveness to insulin with training.[29] Although the mechanism is not yet known, it may be related to increased capillary density in skeletal muscle, an increase in oxidative capacity of skeletal muscle, or other adaptations to training, such as increased skeletal muscle GLUT-4 content.[30]

Despite the increase in insulin-stimulated glucose uptake that can be demonstrated for at least 5–7 days after cessation of exercise in previously trained subjects, patients with NIDDM generally do not show improved fasting blood glucose homeostasis. Some investigators, however, have observed that physical training is associated with lower glycosylated hemoglobin concentrations.[4] The current interpretation is that this may be the cumulative result of decreased blood glucose concentrations associated with repeated bouts of exercise rather than a specific effect of physical training. Because it is known that exercise usually results in a fall of blood glucose concentrations toward normal in hyperglycemic patients with NIDDM, and because increased insulin-stimulated glucose disposal can be observed for many hours after a single bout of exercise,[31] it is likely that regular exercise 4–7 days a week may result in lower average blood glucose and glycohemoglobin concentrations without a significant effect on fasting blood glucose or on the glucose response to meals. Thus, the net effect of exercise repeated on a regular basis would be to improve long-term blood glucose control in patients with NIDDM.

Exercise in the Prevention of Non–Insulin-Dependent Diabetes Mellitus

Although the pathogenesis of non–insulin-dependent diabetes mellitus (NIDDM) is not fully understood, it is clear that at least three factors are important: a genetic predisposition to the disease; a decrease in the action of insulin in insulin-sensitive tissues, including adipose tissue, skeletal muscle, and the liver; and a defect in pancreatic β-cell function.[32] Conditions associated with the development of insulin resistance greatly increase the risk of NIDDM. Chief among these are obesity and advancing age. More recently, it has been recognized that hypertension may be associated with resistance to insulin and hyperinsulinemia.[33] So, too, may be the increase in plasma of very low density (VLDL) lipoprotein and the decrease in high density lipoprotein (HDL) cholesterol that are characteristic of patients with NIDDM. Thus, insulin resistance and hyperinsulinemia may have a critical role in the pathogenesis of the constellation of metabolic abnormalities that occur frequently in patients with NIDDM—namely, obesity, hyperlipidemia, and hypertension. Conversely, interventions that prevent or reverse insulin resistance through alterations in lifestyle, such as increased physical activity and the prevention of obesity, may have a substantial protective effect.

A role for physical conditioning in the prevention of NIDDM has long been suspected on the basis of population and cross-sectional studies. In a recent review by Kriska et al.[34] a large number of epidemiologic studies are summarized, supporting the concept that changes in diet and decreased physical activity in large populations are frequently associated with an increased prevalence of NIDDM. For example, Kawate et al.[35] compared Japanese living in Hiroshima with those who had migrated to Hawaii. Despite a similar genetic background, the prevalence of diabetes was nearly two times greater in the Japanese living in Hawaii than in those living in Hiroshima. This was correlated with a decreased frequency of moderate to heavy occupational physical activity in the Japanese Hawaiians, a finding that held true for both men and women. Many other studies have been done to determine the effects of urbanization of various populations on health status. Most such studies have found that those living in urban environments are less physically active than their rural cousins and that they have much more diabetes and obesity.[36–40]

In various populations, it has now been demonstrated that physical inactivity and abdominal obesity are significant risk factors for the development of NIDDM.[41] Only recently, however, have prospective studies demonstrated that increased physical activity, independent of other risk factors such as obesity, hypertension, and a family history of NIDDM, has a protective effect.[42–45]

In 1991, Helmrich et al.[43] presented convincing evidence from a long-term study of the development of chronic disease in former college students (the University of Pennsylvania Alumni Health Study) that there was an inverse relation between energy expenditure in leisure-time physical activity and the development of NIDDM during the subsequent 15 years.

Several key findings emerged from this prospective study of men who responded to detailed health questionnaires in 1962 and again in 1976. During this period, 3.4% of the men reported that diabetes mellitus had developed, with the age at the time of diagnosis ranging from 45 to 68 years. Significant risk factors included a parental history of diabetes, older age, a history of hypertension, the presence of obesity as measured by the body mass index, and low levels of leisure-time physical activity. The protective effect of physical activity was independent of the other risk factors and was particularly strong among men who participated in vigorous sports, although participation in less vigorous activities was also protective. The occurrence of NIDDM decreased by 6% for each increment of 500 kcal per week expended in physical activity in the whole study group. Two-thirds of the newly diagnosed cases of diabetes occurred among men who had the high-risk characteristics of obesity, hypertension, and a parental history of diabetes. In this subgroup, habitual physical activity had the greatest protective effect, reducing the incidence of diabetes by 24% from the highest activity group to the lowest. These findings strongly support the position that persons who are at substantial risk for NIDDM should be encouraged to maintain a high level of daily physical activity.

More recently, Manson et al.[44] reported the results of a prospective study of 87,253 female registered nurses aged 39–54, whose health status was followed for 8 years. Nondiabetic women were asked initially about their regular physical activity status, using a survey that included these questions: "At least once a week, do you engage in any regular activity similar to brisk walking, jogging, bicycling, etc., long enough to work up a sweat?" "If yes, how many times per week?" "What activity is this?" Activity levels estimated from questions about the frequency of sweat-inducing bouts of exercise per week have been found to correlate well with other assessments of physical activity status[46–48] and with measures of resting heart rate, obesity, and HDL cholesterol concentrations.[46,47] Women who engaged in vigorous physical activity at least once a week (enough to work up a sweat) had significantly less risk of developing NIDDM during the 8-year follow-up period than did those who exercised less often and less vigorously. No significant dose-response relationship was observed between the number of episodes of vigorous exercise per week and the decreased risk of developing diabetes, but the protective effect of exercise was found to be independent of the effects of age, family history of diabetes, body mass index, and duration of follow-up.

In another prospective study of 21,171 U.S. male physicians aged 40–84, who were followed for up to 5 years, a similar protective effect of vigorous exercise at least once a week was also demonstrated.[45] In this study, however, a significant effect of frequency of exercise was also found, the age-adjusted relative risk of developing NIDDM decreasing from 0.77 for vigorous exercise once weekly to 0.62 for two to four times weekly and to 0.58 for five or more times weekly. As in the Nurses Health Study, corrections for other known risk factors for NIDDM did not affect the conclusion that regular, vigorous exercise at least once per week has an independent protective effect against the development of NIDDM.

Although the mechanism of the protective effect of regular exercise is not addressed in these studies, the large body of literature demonstrating that physical training is associated with lower plasma insulin concentrations and increased sensitivity to insulin in skeletal muscle and adipose tissue strongly suggests that this may be a critical factor. The other critical factor in preventing NIDDM is, of course, the prevention or treatment of obesity through dietary restriction and increased energy expenditure. It can also be expected that increased physical exercise and the prevention of obesity will substantially lower the incidence of hypertension and hyperlipidemia, particularly in persons with insulin resistance, hyperinsulinemia, or both, and in those with NIDDM. Regular physical activity is an important component of a healthy lifestyle for everyone, but it may be particularly important for those at increased risk of chronic diseases such as NIDDM, hypertension, and hyperlipidemia.

Guidelines for Exercise in Non–Insulin-Dependent Diabetes Mellitus

Before starting an exercise program, all patients with non–insulin-dependent diabetes mellitus (NIDDM) should have a complete history and physical examination, with particular attention to identifying any long-term complications of diabetes that may affect exercise safety or tolerance. An exercise stress test is recommended for all persons >35 years of age who intend to start a program of moderate or vigorous exercise.[49] This test will help identify previously undiagnosed ischemic heart disease and abnormal blood pressure responses to exercise. A dilated retinal examination to identify proliferative retinopathy, renal function tests including screening for microalbuminuria, and a neurologic examination to determine peripheral and/or autonomic neuropathy should also be performed. If abnormalities are present, exercises of the appropriate type and intensity should be selected to avoid a significant risk of worsening complications. In general, an exercise program should consist of moderate-intensity aerobic exercises that can be sustained for 30 minutes or longer and do not result in a sustained heart rate in excess of 60–70% of the person's predetermined maximum heart rate. If the patient does not have proliferative retinopathy or hypertension, some resistance training or high-intensity exercises may also be well tolerated.

Each exercise session should begin with a warm up of low-intensity aerobic exercise and stretching for 5–10 minutes to prevent musculoskeletal injuries. The moderate- to high-intensity exercise phase should last for at least 30 minutes, with longer durations as tolerated by the level of physical conditioning. The patient should monitor his or her heart rate periodically during exercise to ensure that it is in the target range. Finally, each exercise session should conclude with a 5–10-minute cool-down phase to reduce the risk of postexercise cardiovascular and musculoskeletal complications.

Activities such as walking, stretching, and slow, rhythmic exercises are appropriate.

To produce a significant increase in cardiovascular fitness, to achieve improved insulin sensitivity and glycemic control, and to utilize exercise as an adjunct to diet in order to lose or maintain reduced body weight, patients should exercise at least 3 days a week, although 5–7 days a week is preferable. Individual or group activities are appropriate, and many patients find variety to be important in sustaining interest. For persons who are new to exercise or who have significant complications of diabetes, supervised exercise programs may be beneficial. Most patients, however, do not require formal supervision once the initial assessment is completed and an appropriate exercise program is established. Although blood glucose regulation during exercise in NIDDM differs from normal in several ways, elevated blood glucose concentrations usually fall toward normal with moderate-intensity exercise and exercise-induced hypoglycemia is rare. Exceptions to this may occur in patients taking insulin or sulfonylureas but not metformin. In patients treated by diet alone, there is no need to provide supplemental feedings before, during, or after exercise, except when exercise is exceptionally vigorous or of long duration. Persons treated with sulfonylureas or insulin may need supplemental feedings to prevent hypoglycemia, and insulin doses may be decreased to avoid hypoglycemia.

Summary

It is now clear that regular physical exercise plays an important role in both the prevention and treatment of non–insulin-dependent diabetes mellitus (NIDDM). The benefits of exercise are many and include increased energy expenditure, which, combined with dietary restriction, leads to decreased body fat, increased insulin sensitivity, improved long-term glycemic control, improved lipid profiles, lower blood pressure, and increased cardiovascular fitness. On the other hand, persons with NIDDM often find it difficult to exercise and are at increased risk for injury or exacerbation of underlying diseases or diabetic complications. Before starting an exercise program, all patients with NIDDM should have a complete history and physical examination, with particular attention to evaluation of cardiovascular disease, medications that may affect glycemic control during or after exercise, and diabetic complications including retinopathy, nephropathy, and neuropathy. Exercise programs should be designed to start slowly, build up gradually, and emphasize moderate-intensity exercise performed at least three times a week and preferably five to seven times a week for best results.

References

1. Sushruta SCS. Vaidya Jadavaji Trikamji Acharia. Bombay: Sagar; 1938
2. Allen FM, Stillan E, Fitz R. Total dietary regulation in the treatment of diabetes. In: Exercise. New York: Rockefeller Institute; 1919:monograph 11, chap. 5
3. Lawrence RH. The effects of exercise on insulin action in diabetes. Br Med J 1926;1:648
4. Schneider SH, Amoroso LF, Khachsdurian AK, Ruderman NB. Studies on the mechanism of improved glucose control during exercise in type 2 (non–insulin-dependent) diabetes. Diabetologist 1984;26:355
5. Bjorntorp P, Fahlen M, Grimby G, et al. Carbohydrate and lipid metabolism in middle aged physically well-trained men. Metabolism 1972;21:1037
6. Bjorntorp P, de Jonge K, Sjostrom L, Sullivan L. The effect of physical training on insulin production in obesity. Metabolism 1970;19:631
7. DeFronzo RA, Ferrannini E, Koivisto V. New concepts in the pathogenesis and treatment of non–insulin dependent diabetes mellitus. Am J Med 1983;74:52
8. DeFronzo RA. Lilly lecture 1987. The triumvirate: B-cell, muscle, liver—a collusion responsible for NIDDM. Diabetes 1988;37:667
9. Huttunen JK, Lansimies E, Voutilainen E, et al. Effect of moderate physical exercise on serum lipoproteins. Circulation 1979;60:1220
10. Haskell WL. The influence of exercise training on plasma lipids and lipoproteins in health and disease. Acta Med Scand 1986(suppl);711:25
11. Kiens B, Lithell H. Lipoprotein metabolism influenced by training induced changes in human skeletal muscle. J Clin Invest 1989;83:558
12. Rotkis TC, Cote R, Coyle E, et al. Relationship between high density lipoprotein cholesterol and weekly running mileage. J Cardiac Rehab 1982;2:109
13. Boyer J, Kasch F. Exercise therapy in hypertensive men. JAMA 1970;211:1668
14. Choquette G, Ferguson R. Blood pressure reduction in borderline hypertensives following physical training. Can Med Assoc J 1973;108:699
15. Krotkiewski M, Mandroukis K, Sjostrom L, et al. Effects of long-term physical training on body fat, metabolism and blood pressure in obesity. Metabolism 1979;28:650
16. Hill JO, Sparling PB, Shields TW, et al. Effects of exercise and food restriction on body composition and metabolic rate in obese women. Am J Clin Nutr 1987;46:622
17. Bogardus C, Ravussin E, Robbins DC, et al. Effects of physical training and diet therapy on carbohydrate metabolism in patients with glucose intolerance and non–insulin-dependent diabetes mellitus. Diabetes 1984;33:311
18. Warwick PM, Garrow JS. The effect of addition of exercise to a regimen of dietary restriction on weight loss, nitrogen balance, resting metabolic rate and spontaneous physical activity in three obese women in a metabolic ward. Int J Obesity 1981;5:25
19. MacDonald MJ. Post-exercise late-onset hypoglycemia in insulin-dependent diabetic patients. Diabetes Care 1987;10:584
20. Mitchell TH, Abraham G, Schiffrin A, et al. Hyperglycemia after intense exercise in IDDM subjects during continuous subcutaneous insulin infusion. Diabetes Care 1988;11:311
21. Mogensen CE, Vittinghus E. Urinary albumin excretion during exercise in juvenile diabetes. Scand J Clin Lab Invest 1975;35:295
22. Viberti GC, Jarrett RJ, McCartney M, Keen H. Increased glomerular permeability to albumin induced by exercise in diabetic subjects. Diabetologia 1978;14:293
23. Bjorntorp P, de Jong K, Sjostrom L, Sullivan L. Physical training in human obesity. II. Effects of plasma insulin in glucose intolerant subjects without marked hyperinsulinemia. Scand J Clin Lab Invest 1973;32:42
24. Sato Y, Iguchi A, Sakamoto N. Biochemical determination of training effects using insulin clamp technique. Horm Metab Res 1984;16:483
25. Yki-Jarvinen H, Kovisto VA. Effects of body composition on insulin sensitivity. Diabetes 1983;32:965
26. Rosenthal M, Haskell WL, Solomon R, et al. Demonstration of a relationship between level of physical training and insulin-stimulated glucose utilization in normal humans. Diabetes 1983;32:408
27. Burstein R, Polychronakos C, Toeus CJ, et al. Acute reversal of the enhanced insulin action in trained athletes. Diabetes 1985;34:756
28. Mikines KJ, Sonne B, Farrell PA, et al. Effect of physical exercise on sensitivity and responsiveness to insulin in humans. Am J Physiol 1988;254 (Endocrinol Metab 17):E248
29. Mikines KJ, Sonne B, Tronier B, Galbo H. Effects of acute exercise and detraining on insulin action in trained men. J Appl Physiol 1989;66:704
30. Goodyear LJ, Hirshman MF, Horton ED, Horton ES. Effect of exercise training and chronic glyburide treatment on glucose homeostasis in diabetic rats. J Appl Physiol 1992;72:143
31. Devlin JT, Horton ES. Effects of prior high-intensity exercise on glucose metabolism in normal and insulin-resistant men. Diabetes 1985;34:973
32. DeFronzo RA. The triumvirate: B-cell, muscle, liver, a collusion responsible for NIDDM. Diabetes 1988;37:667
33. Modan M, Halkin H, Almog S, et al. Hyperinsulinemia: A link between hypertension, obesity and glucose intolerance. J Clin Invest 1985;75:809
34. Kriska AM, Blair SN, Pereira MA. The potential role of physical activity in the prevention of non–insulin dependent diabetes mellitus: The epidemiological evidence. Exerc Sports Sci Rev 1991;22:121
35. Kawate R, Yamakido M, Nishimoto Y, et al. Diabetes mellitus and its vascular complications in Japanese migrants on the island of Hawaii. Diabetes Care 1979;2:161
36. Cruz-Vidal M, Costas R, Garcia-Palmieri M, et al. Factors related to diabetes mellitus in Puerto Rican men. Diabetes 1979;28:300
37. King H, Zimmet P, Raper L, Balkau B. Risk factors for diabetes in three Pacific populations. Am J Epidemiol 1984;119:396
38. Zimmet PZ, Faauiso S, Ainuu S, et al. The prevalence of diabetes in the rural and urban Polynesian population of Western Samoa. Diabetes 1981;30:45
39. Zimmet PZ, Taylor R, Ram P, et al. Prevalence of diabetes and impaired glucose tolerance in the biracial population of Fiji: A rural-urban comparison. Am J Epidemiol 1983;118:673
40. King H, Taylor R, Zimmet P, et al. Non–insulin-dependent diabetes in a newly independent Pacific nation: The republic of Kiribati. Diabetes Care 1984;7:409
41. Dowse GK, Zimmet PZ, Gareeboo H, et al. Abdominal obesity and physical activity are risk factors for NIDDM and impaired glucose tolerance in Indian, Creole, and Chinese Mauritians. Diabetes Care 1991;14:271
42. Frisch RE, Wyshak G, Albright TE, et al. Lower prevalence of diabetes in female former college athletes compared with nonathletes. Diabetes 1986;35:1101
43. Helmrich SP, Ragland DR, Leung RW, Paffenbarger RS. Physical activity and reduced occurrence of non–insulin-dependent diabetes mellitus. N Engl J Med 1991;325:147
44. Manson JE, Rimm EB, Stampfer MJ, et al. Physical activity and incidence of non–insulin dependent diabetes mellitus in women. Lancet 1991;338:774

45. Manson JE, Nathan DM, Krolewski AS, et al. A prospective study of exercise and incidence of diabetes among U.S. male physicians. JAMA 1992;268:63
46. Washburn RA, Adams LL, Haile GT. Physical activity assessment for epidemiologic research: The utility of two simplified approaches. Prev Med 1987;16:636
47. Washburn RA, Goldfield SRW, Smith KW, McKinlay JB. The validity of self-reported exercise-induced sweating as a measure of physical activity. Am J Epidemiol 1990;132:107
48. Paffenbarger RS Jr, Wing AL, Hyde RT. Physical activity as an index of heart attack risk in college alumni. Am J Epidemiol 1978;108:161
49. American College of Sports Medicine. Guidelines for Exercise Testing and Prescription. 4th ed. Philadelphia; Lea & Febiger;1991:5–9

Diabetes Mellitus, edited by Derek LeRoith, Simeon I. Taylor, and Jerrold M. Olefsky. Lippincott–Raven Publishers, Philadelphia © 1996.

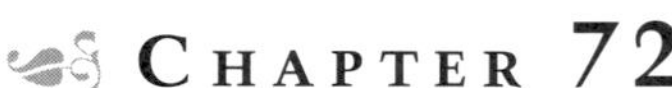

Chapter 72
α-Glucosidase Inhibitors in the Treatment of Diabetes

John M. Amatruda

Introduction

The goal of effective antidiabetic therapy is to approximate as closely as possible normal blood sugar fluctuations and glycated hemoglobin levels while avoiding serious hypoglycemia. This approach has recently been reinforced by the results of the Diabetes Control and Complications Trial (DCCT),[1] as well as the Stockholm trial[2] performed in patients with insulin-dependent diabetes mellitus (IDDM). The translation of the results of the DCCT trial to medical practice in the community, however, has been difficult because of the lack of patient acceptance of the stringent regimens required and the unwillingness of physicians to implement intensive treatment.

The goals for non–insulin-dependent diabetes mellitus (NIDDM) are similar to those for IDDM because the causes of microvascular complications are thought to be similar[3] and because the development and progression of retinopathy are related to the level of glycemic control in IDDM[1,2] and NIDDM.[4] Treatment options in patients with NIDDM must be viewed differently, however, because macrovascular disease is the major cause of mortality in NIDDM; is prevalent in undiagnosed and newly diagnosed NIDDM; and is associated with a metabolic syndrome characterized by central obesity, insulin resistance, hyperinsulinemia, hypertension, and dyslipedemia.[5–7] In addition, the consequences of tight control in NIDDM can be serious. Hypoglycemia in patients with NIDDM who are elderly and have significant cardiovascular disease is potentially lethal. Mortality rates of 7.5–14% related to hypoglycemia have been reported in the elderly.[8–10]

There are other problems with current therapies for NIDDM. Sulfonylureas, in addition to being the most common cause of hypoglycemia, are associated with high rates of primary and secondary failure, and can cause weight gain and hyperinsulinemia. Hyperinsulinemia, in turn, may be related to the increased risk of atherosclerosis in patients with NIDDM.[6] The use of metformin is somewhat limited by its known association with lactic acidosis in patients with impaired renal function and by restrictions on usage of the drug in the elderly and in patients with cardiac disease. Although metformin does not cause weight gain or hyperinsulinemia, sulfonylureas and insulin are associated with both of these adverse effects. With these issues in mind, it would be useful to have a therapeutic agent that could be used in patients with new-onset diabetes and in elderly patients without causing hypoglycemia or weight gain; would be effective in patients who are primary or secondary failures on sulfonylureas; does not cause hypoglycemia; can be used in patients with moderate abnormalities of renal function and in the elderly; works by a different mechanism and so is additive to existing treatment regimens; works primarily on postprandial hyperglycemia; and lowers insulin concentrations.

It is generally accepted that the first-line therapy for NIDDM is diet and weight loss. Diet is also an important adjunct to insulin therapy in IDDM in attempting to avoid large excursions in postprandial blood sugar. All of those who treat patients with diabetes, however, appreciate that dietary compliance is poor for most patients. Reduction of postprandial glucose through the use of soluble fiber as an adjunct to diet has not been widely accepted because of the large amounts necessary, the lack of palatability, the unpredictable effects, and the unpleasant side effects. A new alternative is the α-glucosidase inhibitor acarbose, which lowers postprandial glucose and insulin by retarding the digestion of carbohydrates in the small intestine, thereby delaying glucose absorption and smoothing postprandial increases in plasma glucose.[11]

Starch is digested to oligosaccharides by amylase and further digested by membrane-bound α-glucosidases (glucoamylase, isomaltase, maltase) to glucose.[11] Sucrose is similarly broken down by membrane-bound sucrase (an α-glucosidase) to glucose and fructose. Acarbose, the first commercially available α-glucosidase inhibitor, is approved for the treatment of diabetes in 57 countries. Acarbose is a pseudotetrasaccharide (Fig. 72-1) of microbial origin that competitively inhibits both amylase and membrane-

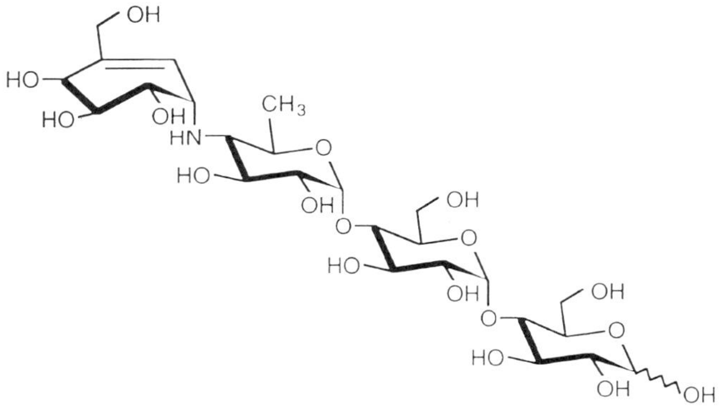

Figure 72-1. Structural formula for acarbose.

TABLE 72-1.* Inhibition of Intestinal α-Glucosidases: K_i Values (Mol^{-1}) of Acarbose, Miglitol, and Emiglitate (α-Glucosidases from Porcine Intestinal Mucosa)

	Sucrase	Maltase	Isomaltase
Acarbose	1.3×10^{-7}	1.1×10^{-6}	Very weak
Miglitol	1.4×10^{-7}	3.5×10^{-7}	5.7×10^{-8}
Emiglitate	3.9×10^{-8}	1.9×10^{-7}	3.2×10^{-7}

*Data adapted with permission from Bischoff H. Pharmacology of α-glucosidase inhibition. Eur J Clin Invest 1994(suppl 3);3:24

bound α-glucosidases with approximately equal affinity (Table 72-1). As a consequence of the ingestion of acarbose with meals, carbohydrate digestion is delayed, resulting in a significant decrease in the postprandial rise in plasma glucose after a mixed carbohydrate load.[11] Carbohydrate not digested in the upper part of the small bowel reaches the ileum, where further digestion and absorption occur. Because acarbose does not interfere with the sodium-dependent glucose transporter, the absorption of glucose is not affected. Nor does acarbose inhibit β-glucosidases such as lactase. Thus, lactose is digested normally.

Under normal circumstances, complex carbohydrate is digested in the proximal small bowel and little complex carbohydrate reaches the distal small bowel. As a result, there is usually little α-glucosidase activity in the ileum. If doses of acarbose are used initially that block all proximal α-glucosidase activity, carbohydrate malabsorption will result because of the delivery of complex carbohydrate to the colon, with resulting flatulence or even diarrhea. The initiation of therapy with small doses and slow titration upward ("start low, go slow") minimizes these side effects. Also, with continued use, these symptoms improve or disappear.[11–15] In animal studies it has been demonstrated that the competitive inhibition of proximal α-glucosidases by acarbose and the subsequent delivery of complex carbohydrate to the ileum results in the induction of ileal α-glucosidases.[16] Once induced distally, there is no further malabsorption of carbohydrate and carbohydrate digestion is only delayed. Similar results are achieved with high-fiber diets.[11] This delay in carbohydrate digestion results in a blunting of the postprandial peaks of blood glucose and insulin after meals and a smoothing of the daily glucose and insulin profiles.[12,17] The distal induction of α-glucosidases has led to the therapeutic strategy of starting patients on a low dose of acarbose, allowing 4 to 6 weeks for enzyme induction distally, and then gradually increasing the dose to avoid side effects.

The colon is capable of processing large quantities of carbohydrate without fecal loss of carbohydrate. Therapeutic doses of acarbose do not cause malabsorption. Clinical studies clearly demonstrate, however, that acarbose does not cause weight gain, unlike sulfonylurea and insulin therapy, and will largely prevent the weight gain caused by sulfonylureas when used in combination with acarbose.[18] The lack of weight gain in conjunction with improved glycemic control is most likely related to the decrease in postprandial insulin concentrations associated with acarbose, in contrast to the increase in insulin concentrations associated with sulfonylurea treatment. Animal data have demonstrated that the reduced postprandial hyperinsulinemia associated with acarbose use results in decreased hepatic and adipose tissue lipogenesis compared to the use of a sulfonylurea. Furthermore, combined administration of acarbose with a sulfonylurea prevents the sulfonylurea-induced increase in lipogenesis and triglyceride concentrations.[11]

Other α-glucosidase inhibitors in development include the deoxynojirimycin derivatives miglitol, voglibose, and emiglitate.[11] These α-glucosidase inhibitors are more potent than acarbose, are not active against α-amylase, and are extensively absorbed in the small intestine. Acarbose is only minimally absorbed (1–2%) systemically in its parent form. Miglitol is the best studied of the three deoxynojirimycin derivatives and appears to have an efficacy and a side effect profile similar to those of acarbose.[19] Little data are available for voglibose, which is currently marketed in Japan. Emiglitate has the potential to be a longer-acting inhibitor. Animal data have shown reduced postprandial glucose and insulin concentrations when a carbohydrate load is administered 4 and 17 hours after a small dose of emiglitate.[11] Although there are little data on alternative dosing regimens, all other α-glucosidase inhibitors are administered three times a day with meals.

The effects of acarbose on the complications of diabetes have been extensively studied in animals. Decreases in nonenzymatic glycation have been demonstrated with decreases in glycated hemoglobin (HbA1C) of 2–3% in both NIDDM and IDDM models of diabetes. This results in decreased gylcation of glomerular basement membranes; decreased advanced glycosylation end product formation in connective tissue; prevention of renal hypertrophy; decreased immunoglobulin deposition and thickening of the glomerular mesangium; decreased glomerular sclerosis; decreased cataract formation; and prevention of neuropathy and retinopathy.[11,20–21] Increased concentrations of GLUT-4 in muscle are also observed.[22]

The mitigation of neuronal injury has been demonstrated by Sima and Chakrabarti.[21] In an IDDM model of diabetes, these investigators showed that control of postprandial plasma glucose with acarbose prevents the development of peripheral and autonomic neuropathy. This was accompanied by partial or complete prevention of the histologic changes observed in diabetic neuropathy.

Whether these improvements are related to a reduction in total integrated glucose concentration over 24 hours or to a specific effect of reducing postprandial glucose is unknown. Recent studies, however, suggest that aldose reductase activity and mRNA concentrations are stimulated by glucose concentrations in the postprandial range.[23,24] Also, the K_m of aldose reductase is high.[25] Because of the high glucose concentrations required for enzyme induction and activity, one can postulate a specific role for the postprandial excursions in the development of complications related to increased polyol pathway activity.[21] Decreases in postprandial insulin concentrations are thought to be responsible for the reductions in hepatic and adipose tissue lipogenesis, reduced postprandial increases in lipids, and decreased VLDL concentrations observed in animals.[11]

Is the therapeutic profile of α-glucosidase inhibitors useful, and how could such a therapeutic profile be used to greatest advantage in patients with NIDDM and IDDM? To answer these questions, it is important to put the importance of new therapeutic advances in the treatment of NIDDM in perspective and to emphasize the stepped or combination approach to therapy.[5] This approach has been used for many years to successfully treat patients with hypertension. Monotherapy with any known agent frequently does not control plasma glucose adequately, especially now that the results of the DCCT trial suggest that complications are linearly related to serum glycated hemoglobin levels. As a result, drugs that act through different mechanisms, are additive in effect to existing therapies, and do not promote hypoglycemia or weight gain are important additions to treatment.

Acarbose and other α-glucosidase inhibitors may prove to be most useful as monotherapy in patients with impaired glucose tolerance or in patients with new-onset diabetes, in the elderly, and as part of a stepped or combination therapy program in which additive effects are needed. Also, acarbose may be useful in the treatment of IDDM to reduce postprandial excursions of blood sugar. Clinical studies with acarbose have demonstrated these advantages.

Several published studies have demonstrated that acarbose at doses of 50–200 mg tid reduces fasting (~1.8 mM) and postprandial (~3.5 mM) glucose concentrations, as well as postprandial insulin (~30%) and fasting and postprandial triglyceride concentrations.[12,18,26–33] HbA1C reductions are variable and in most studies range from a mean of approximately 0.6% to approximately 1.5%. In some studies, marked interindividual variation is seen.[27] In several large double-blind, placebo-controlled clinical trials performed by Bayer in the United States, average reductions in HbA1C of approximately 0.7% to 1% are seen, with reductions in fasting and postprandial glucose and insulin concentrations similar to those reported in published studies.[18,19] In large clinical trials, however, reductions in mean fasting triglyceride concentrations were not observed. This could be related to the mixed population studied.

Several published studies have also demonstrated the antihyperglycemic effects of acarbose in patients with IDDM.[34–39] In patients who are placed on an artificial pancreas (Biostator), a reduction in total insulin requirements of approximately 40% occurs.[35,40] Acarbose has also been shown to decrease nocturnal hypoglycemia in patients with IDDM because of its ability to retard carbohydrate absorption.[41]

In patients with alimentary hypoglycemia secondary to rapid gastric emptying and in reactive hypoglycemia either isolated or associated with impaired glucose tolerance, acarbose prevents hypoglycemia after a sucrose load.[42] As expected from its mechanism of action, acarbose also has beneficial effects in patients with impaired glucose tolerance leading to decreased glucose and insulin concentrations after sucrose loading and, after 4 months of treatment, to improved meal tolerance, increased insulin sensitivity, and reduced blood pressure.[43] Because impaired glucose tolerance manifests itself primarily as postprandial hyperglycemia, acarbose may be an ideal drug to treat this condition. Acarbose lowers postprandial insulin, as well as glucose, and may also preserve pancreatic function, thereby preventing NIDDM. Because macrovascular disease is already present in many patients with impaired glucose tolerance and because postprandial insulin concentrations are related to cardiovascular disease,[5,7,26] one can speculate that acarbose may be useful in the prevention of peripheral arterial insufficiency, stroke, and myocardial infarction.

In combination with sulfonylureas and metformin, acarbose is additive, leading to additional mean reductions in HbA1C of approximately 0.8%.[18,33,44] In addition, acarbose reduces the increase in insulin concentrations and prevents the weight gain seen with sulfonylurea treatment.[18] In patients with IDDM, acarbose either reduces insulin requirements or HbA1C concentrations, depending on the goals of treatment. Thus acarbose can be used with all existing pharmacologic agents used to treat NIDDM to produce an additive effect on glycemia control.

Unlike sulfonylureas and metformin, there is no evidence of secondary failure with acarbose. In addition, acarbose does not cause hypoglycemia.

In postmarketing surveillance studies,[45] acarbose has been shown to decrease fasting and postprandial glucose as well as HbA1C concentrations by approximately 1–2% in all subgroups of patients, both as monotherapy and as adjunctive treatment to sulfonylureas and insulin. These are not controlled clinical trials, although they provide an estimation of performance in the real world. Under these circumstances, acarbose is highly efficacious.

In summary, α-glucosidase inhibition by acarbose is a novel antihyperglycemic therapeutic principle that lowers primarily postprandial glucose and insulin concentrations without causing hypoglycemia. Acarbose is effective in all subsets of patients, including those with impaired glucose tolerance (IGT), those on diet alone, and those on diet plus sulfonylureas, metformin, or insulin. Acarbose's effects are added to those of all existing agents. Acarbose has also been shown to decrease postprandial glucose concentrations as well as insulin requirements in patients with IDDM. There is no evidence of secondary failure with acarbose.

There is reason to believe that a reduction of postprandial glucose and insulin concentrations might retard the development of the long-term complications of diabetes.[5,21,26] Except for the fetuses of pregnant women whose macrosomia is related to postprandial concentrations of glucose but not fasting glucose,[46] however, the contribution of postprandial glucose to complications has been directly demonstrated only in animals.[21] A recent study demonstrated that adjustment of insulin therapy in women with gestational diabetes based on postprandial rather than preprandial glucose led to improved glycemic control and decreased the risk of neonatal hypoglycemia, macrosomia and caesarean delivery.[47] Assuming that the results and conclusions of the DCCT apply to NIDDM, a reduction in HbA1C by acarbose of 0.7–1%, as shown in controlled clinical trials, or 1–2%, as shown in noncontrolled studies and surveys, should substantially reduce the incidence of long-term complications.[1]

The side effects of acarbose at doses used clinically are limited to the gastrointestinal tract and include abdominal pain, flatulence, soft stools, and occasionally diarrhea. These side effects can be prevented or markedly reduced by initiating therapy with low doses and titrating slowly to the therapeutic range, thereby preventing carbohydrate malabsorption and allowing sufficient time for the ileal induction of α-glucosidases.[11–15,18,19,33,45,48] Gastrointestinal side effects have also been shown to improve with time.[11–15] In some studies employing high doses (200–300 mg three times a day [tid]), an increased incidence of significant but reversible elevations in transaminase concentrations have been seen. These transaminase elevations were not associated with any other laboratory or clinical evidence of hepatic dysfunction.[15] In international post-marketing experience with acarbose in over 500,000 patients, 19 cases of serum transaminase elevations >500 U/L (12 of which were associated with jaundice) have been reported. Fifteen of the 19 cases received 100 mg tid or greater, and 13 of the 16 patients for whom weight was recorded weighed <60 kg. In the 18 cases where follow-up was recorded, hepatic abnormalities improved or resolved upon discontinuation of acarbose. The maximum recommended dosage for patients ≤60 kg is 50 mg tid and for patients >60 kg is 100 mg tid.

Experience indicates that patients with high-starch diets and diets low in simple sugars achieve the greatest benefit with the fewest side effects.[49]

Table 72-2 lists the potential indications for acarbose and the advantages of acarbose. It is likely that acarbose will be most useful

Table 72-2. Potential Indications for and Advantages of Acarbose

Indication	Advantages of Acarbose
Impaired Glucose Tolerance	Effect primarily on postprandial glucose concentration Reduces insulin concentrations and spares pancreatic insulin reserve Improves insulin sensitivity Decreases blood pressure ? Prevents conversion to NIDDM ? Prevents or delays macrovascular disease
New-onset NIDDM	Reduces postprandial glucose and insulin concentrations ? Preserves pancreatic insulin reserve No hypoglycemia No evidence of secondary failure ? Delays or prevents macrovascular disease
Established NIDDM	No hypoglycemia No evidence of secondary failure Novel mechanism—additive to effects of sulfonylurea, metformin, and insulin Lowers insulin concentrations Does not cause weight gain Prevents weight gain due to sulfonylureas
NIDDM in the elderly	Antihyperglycemia No hypoglycemia Side effects on the bowel may be seen as useful

with new-onset NIDDM, in patients with established NIDDM with a fasting plasma glucose concentration <200 mg%, as adjunctive therapy, and in elderly NIDDM patients. Studies are currently underway to further define acarbose's role in reducing postprandial glucose concentrations and regular insulin requirements in patients with IDDM, as well as its role in preventing diabetes in patients with impaired glucose tolerance. Because of acarbose's unique mechanism of action, it will be an important addition to a stepwise and combination approach to the treatment of NIDDM.[5]

References

1. The Diabetes Control and Complications Trial Research Group. The effect of intensive treatment of diabetes on the development of long-term complications in insulin-dependent diabetes. N Engl J Med 1993;329:977
2. Reichard P, Nilsson BY, Rosenquist U. Retardation of the development of the microvascular complications after long term intensified insulin treatment: The Stockholm Diabetes Intervention Study. N Engl J Med 1993;329:304
3. American Diabetes Association. Position statement: Implications of the Diabetes Control and Complications Trial. Diabetes 1993;42:1555
4. Klein R, Klein BEK, Mors SE. Epidemiology of proliferative diabetic retinopathy. Diabetes Care 1992;15:1875
5. Lebovitz HE. Stepwise and combination drug therapy for the treatment of NIDDM. Diabetes Care 1994;17:1542
6. Colwell JA. DCCT Findings: Applicability and implications for NIDDM. Diabetes Rev 1994;2:277
7. Harris MI. Undiagnosed NIDDM: Clinical and public health issues. Diabetes Care 1993;16:642
8. Seltzer HS. Drug induced hypoglycemia. Endocrinol Metab Clin North Am 1989;8:163
9. Asplund K, Wiholm BE, Lithner F. Glyburide-associated hypoglycemia: A report of 57 cases. Diabetologia 1983;24:412
10. Brodows RG. Benefits and risks with glyburide and glipizide in elderly NIDDM patients. Diabetes Care 1992;15:75
11. Bischoff H. Pharmacology of α-glucosidase inhibition. Eur J Clin Invest 1994(suppl 3);3:24
12. Balfour JA, McTavish D. Acarbose: An update of its pharmacology and therapeutic use in diabetes mellitus. Drugs 1993;46:1025
13. Hotta N, Kakuta H, Sano T, et al. Long-term effect of acarbose on glycemic control in non–insulin-dependent diabetes mellitus: A placebo-controlled double-blind study. Diabetic Med 1993;10:134
14. Hanefeld M, Fischer S, Schulze J, et al. Therapeutic potentials of acarbose as first-line drug in NIDDM insufficiently treated with diet alone. Diabetes Care 1991;14:732
15. Hollander P. Safety profile of acarbose, an α-glucosidase inhibitor. Drugs 1992;44(suppl 2):47
16. Lee SM, Bustamante SA, Koldovsky O. The effect of alpha-glucosidase inhibition on intestinal disaccharidase activity in normal and diabetic mice. Metabolism 1983;32:793
17. Hillebrand I, Boehme K, Frank G, et al. The effects of the α-glucosidase inhibitor Bay g 5421 (acarbose) on meal-stimulated elevation of circulating glucose, insulin and triglyceride levels in man. Res Exp Med 1979;175:81
18. Coniff RF, Shapiro J, Seaton TB, Bray GA. Multicenter, placebo-controlled trial comparing acarbose (BAY g 5421) with placebo, tolbutamide, and tolbutamide-plus-acarbose in non–insulin-dependent diabetes mellitus. Am J Med 1995;98:443
19. Johnston PS, Coniff RF, Hoogwerf BJ, et al. Effects of the carbohydrase inhibitor miglitol in sulfonylurea-treated NIDDM patients. Diabetes Care 1994;17:20
20. Lee SM. The effect of chronic α-glycosidase inhibition on diabetic nephropathy in the *db/db* mouse. Diabetes 1982;31:249
21. Sima AAF, Chakrabarti S. Long-term suppression of postprandial hyperglycaemia with acarbose retards the development of neuropathies in the *BB/W*-rat. Diabetologia 1992;35:325
22. Friedman JE, De Vente JE, Peterson RG, Dohm GL. Altered expression of muscle glucose transporter GLUT-4 in diabetic fatty Zucker rats (*ZDF/Drt-fa*). Am J Physiol 1991;261:E782
23. Ohtaka M, Tawata M, Hosaka Y, Onaya T. Glucose modulation of aldose reductase mRNA expression and its activity in cultured calf pulmonary artery endothelial cells. Diabetologia 1992;35:730
24. Ghahary A, Luo J, Gong Y, et al. Increased renal aldose reductase activity, immunoreactivity, and mRNA in streptozocin-induced diabetic rats. Diabetes 1993;38:1067
25. Pottinger PK. A study of three enzymes acting on glucose in the lens of different species. Biochem J 1967;104:663
26. Hoffmann J, Spengler M. Efficacy of 24-week monotherapy with acarbose, glibenclamide, or placebo in NIDDM patients. Diabetes Care 1994;17:561
27. Reaven GM, Lardinois CK, Greenfield MS, et al. Effect of acarbose on carbohydrate and lipid metabolism in NIDDM patients poorly controlled by sulfonylureas. Diabetes Care 1990;3(suppl 3):32
28. Zavaroni I, Reaven GM. Inhibition of carbohydrate-induced hypertriglyceridemia by a disaccharidase inhibitor. Metabolism 1981;30:417
29. Jenney A, Proietto J, O'Dea K, et al. Low-dose acarbose improves glycemic control in NIDDM patients without changes in insulin sensitivity. Diabetes Care 1993;16:499
30. Santeusanio F, Ventura MM, Contadini P, et al. Efficacy and safety of two different dosages of acarbose in non–insulin dependent diabetic patients treated by diet alone. Diab Nutr Metab 1993;6:147
31. Baron AD, Eckel RH, Schmeiser L, Kolterman OG. The effect of short-term α-glucosidase inhibition on carbohydrate and lipid metabolism in type II (noninsulin-dependent) diabetes. Metabolism 1987;36:409
32. Willms B, Sachse G, Unger H. Treatment of diabetes with a glycosidehydrolase inhibitor (acarbose, BAY g 5421). Front Hormone Res 1980;7:276
33. Chiasson JL, Josse RG, Hunt JA, et al. The effectiveness of acarbose in the treatment of patients with NIDDM. A multi-center Canadian trial. Ann Intern Med 1994;121:928
34. Raptis S, Dimtriadis G, Hadjidakis D. Acarbose treatment in insulin-dependent (type I) diabetes mellitus. Int Symp Acarbose West Berlin; November 1987
35. Tattersall R. Alpha-glucosidase inhibition as an adjunct to the treatment of type I diabetes. Diabetic Med 1993;10:688
36. Dimitriadis GD, Tessari P, Vay LW Go, Gerich JE. α-Glucosidase inhibition improves postprandial hyperglycemia and decreases insulin requirements in insulin-dependent diabetes mellitus. Metabolism 1985;34:261
37. LeCavalier L, Halet P, Chiasson JL. The effects of sucrose meal on insulin requirement in IDDM and its modulation by acarbose. Diabete Metab 1986;12:156
38. Dimitriadis G, Hatziagellaki E, Alexopoulos E, et al. Effects of α-glucosidase inhibition on meal glucose tolerance and timing of insulin administration in patients with type I diabetes mellitus. Diabetes Care 1991;15:393
39. Marena S, Tagliaferro V, Cavallero G, et al. Double-blind crossover study of acarbose in type I diabetic patients. Diabetic Med 1991;8:674
40. Dimitriadis G, Karaiskos C, Raptis S. Effects of prolonged (6 months) α-glucosidase inhibition on blood glucose control and insulin requirement in patients with insulin-dependent diabetes mellitus. Horm Metab Res 1986;18:253
41. McCulloch DK, Kurtz AB, Tattersall RB. A new approach to the treatment of nocturnal hypoglycemia using alpha-glucosidase inhibition. Diabetes Care 1983;6:483
42. Lefebvre PJ, Scheen AJ. The use of acarbose in the prevention and treatment of hypoglycemia. Eur J Clin Invest 1994;24(suppl 3):40
43. Chiasson JL, Josse RG, Leiter LA, et al. Can we prevent the development of non–insulin-dependent diabetes mellitus? Diabetes 1994;43:62A
44. Scheen AJ, Castillo MJ, Lefebvre PJ. Combination of oral antidiabetic drugs and insulin in the treatment of non–insulin-dependent diabetes. Acta Clin Belg 1993;48:259
45. Spengler M, Cagatay M. Evaluation of efficacy and tolerability of acarbose by postmarketing surveillance. Diab Stoffw 1992;1:218
46. Combs CA, Gunderson E, Kitzmiller JL, et al. Relationship of fetal macrosomia to maternal postprandial glucose control during pregnancy. Diabetes Care 1992;15:1251
47. DeVeciana M, Major CA, Morgan MA, et al. Postprandial versus preprandial blood glucose monitoring in women with gestational diabetes mellitus requiring insulin therapy. N Engl J Med 1995;333:1237
48. May C. Efficacy and tolerability of stepwise increasing dosage of acarbose in patients with non–insulin-dependent diabetes mellitus (NIDDM) treated with sulfonylureas. Diab Stoffw 1995;4:3
49. Toeller M. Dietary treatment and α-glucosidase inhibitors in NIDDM. Diab Nutr Metab 1990;3(suppl 1):43

Diabetes Mellitus, edited by Derek LeRoith, Simeon I. Taylor, and Jerrold M. Olefsky. Lippincott–Raven Publishers, Philadelphia © 1996.

Chapter 73

Intensive Insulin Therapy for Patients with Type II Diabetes

Steven V. Edelman and Robert R. Henry

Introduction

The benefits of normalizing glycosylated hemoglobin in patients with type I diabetes mellitus have been clearly demonstrated by the results of the Diabetes Control and Complications Trial (DCCT). The DCCT proved conclusively that intensive diabetes management with normoglycemia delays the onset and significantly retards the progression of microvascular complications. The results were so compelling that the study was terminated early, and a new standard of care was established for patients with this form of diabetes. It remains to be proved, however, whether tight glucose control with insulin therapy will be equally beneficial for patients with type II diabetes.

The prevalence of microvascular as well as macrovascular disease is substantial in patients with type II diabetes. As in type I diabetes, the pathophysiologic basis for vascular disease is related to the presence of uncontrolled hyperglycemia. Type II diabetes mellitus, however, is also associated with insulin resistance, hyperinsulinemia, and several other metabolic abnormalities including obesity, hypertension, and dyslipidemia, which may contribute to the development of accelerated vascular disease. These pathophysiologic and metabolic differences between the two forms of diabetes, combined with a lack of adequate long-term clinical trials with insulin therapy, make recommendations of therapeutic strategies to achieve normal glycemic control in type II diabetes less than clear-cut. Furthermore, there is no widely accepted, standard form of insulin therapy for patients with this form of diabetes.

The area of major concern when insulin therapy is used to achieve tight glucose control in type II diabetes is the well-recognized association of hyperinsulinemia with weight gain and accelerated atherosclerosis. Although the links between these complications and hyperinsulinemia do not necessarily indicate a cause-and-effect relationship, it is the general consensus that therapeutic interventions other than exogenous insulin should be thoroughly attempted first. In addition, when diet, exercise, and oral antidiabetic agents fail to control glycemia, then the lowest possible dose of insulin should be used to minimize peripheral hyperinsulinemia and the possible consequences of this form of therapy.

It is now recommended that the glycemic objective for patients with type II diabetes should be similar to that for type I diabetes: to normalize glycemia and glycosylated hemoglobin concentrations. This chapter discusses the different insulin therapeutic regimens available to normalize glycemia and glycosylated hemoglobin in patients with type II diabetes mellitus, and to review their application, possible benefits, and adverse effects.

Pathophysiology of Type II Diabetes: Relationship to Insulin Therapy

Of the estimated 5–10 million Americans diagnosed with type II diabetes, 80–90% are obese and the remainder are lean.[1] The genesis of hyperglycemia in type II diabetes involves a triad of abnormalities: excessive hepatic glucose production, impaired pancreatic insulin secretion, and peripheral resistance to insulin action occurring principally in liver and muscle tissue.[2] The severity of these abnormalities and their contribution to the degree of hyperglycemia can vary considerably, causing heterogeneity in the metabolic expression of the diabetic state. Such differences are best exemplified by the lean and obese varieties of type II diabetes, which have the same underlying pathophysiologic basis but differ in the extent to which each abnormality contributes to the development of the hyperglycemic state.

In lean type II diabetics, impaired insulin secretion is the predominant defect; insulin resistance tends to be less severe than in the obese variety.[3] On the other hand, insulin resistance and hyperinsulinemia are the classical abnormalities of obese persons with type II diabetes.[3] In this form of diabetes, insulin secretion is often excessive compared to the nondiabetic situation but is still insufficient to overcome the insulin resistance that is present. It is important to understand and appreciate these fundamental differences when considering insulin therapy of type II diabetes. Based on this knowledge, it can usually be predicted with considerable certainty that lean type II diabetic subjects, in whom insulin resistance is mild or moderate in severity, will require considerably less insulin to control their hyperglycemia than their obese counterparts. In contrast, large doses of exogenous insulin are the rule in the obese form of this disorder when euglycemia is desired.[4]

Several other aspects of the pathophysiology of hyperglycemia in type II diabetes deserve comment when insulin therapy is used to achieve normalization of glycemia and the glycosylated hemoglobin. The classic glycemic profile of type II diabetes consists of elevated basal or fasting glucose concentrations on which postprandial glycemic excursions are superimposed.[1] Clearly, the basal rate of hepatic glucose production is the primary determinant of the fasting plasma glucose concentration in type II diabetes.[5] Postprandial hyperglycemia is determined, in large part, by peripheral glucose utilization and the severity of insulin resistance. In type II diabetes, however, hepatic glucose output is more sensitive to suppression by insulin than is stimulation of glucose uptake, which usually requires the presence of high pharmacologic concentrations of circulating insulin.[6] This is particularly important when striving to achieve normoglycemia in the obese form of type II diabetes, in which exogenous insulin acts primarily to suppress excessive hepatic glucose output rather than to stimulate peripheral glucose uptake.[7] Because the degree of peripheral insulinemia has been directly linked to the development of weight gain during tight metabolic control,[1,7–10] one should consider using only the amount of exogenous insulin that is necessary to suppress hepatic glucose output and achieve normal fasting glucose concentrations. Using more insulin to overcome peripheral insulin resistance may expose patients not only to excessive weight gain but also to the risks of hypoglycemia and possibly to an increased incidence of cardiovascular disease, with minimal, if any, improvement in glycemic control.

The need for large amounts of exogenous insulin in obese type II diabetes also raises the question of the most appropriate methods of insulin delivery. Under normal circumstances, insulin is secreted from the pancreas into the portal vein. On reaching the liver, a large first-pass extraction of portal insulin occurs.[11] When insulin is injected subcutaneously, absorption occurs directly into the peripheral circulation, without the initial effects of hepatic extraction. Therefore, the tissues are exposed to greater hyperinsulinemia than if insulin was provided by the portal route. Furthermore, because the primary target of exogenous insulin is the liver, type II diabetes may be uniquely suited to delivery of insulin via the portal vein. Such a situation occurs when insulin is delivered intraperitoneally and the majority of insulin is absorbed into the portal circulation.[12] Intraperitoneal insulin delivery systems, discussed later, hold considerable promise in type II diabetes because of the more physiologic delivery of insulin and because of their ability to inhibit hepatic glucose output selectively, with less peripheral insulinemia than occurs with subcutaneous insulin injections.

Intensive Management Goals

The ultimate goals of management in patients with type II diabetes do not differ from those of type I diabetes. Preventing the acute and chronic complications of diabetes is a primary concern. The main clinical and metabolic parameters used to monitor diabetes management include the glycosylated hemoglobin, fasting and postprandial glucose values, lipoprotein analysis, blood pressure, and body weight (Table 73-1).

In most persons, glycosylated hemoglobin should be within three standard deviations from the mean or within one percentage point above the upper range of normal. This translates into a fasting plasma glucose concentration of 70 to 120 mg/dL and a 2-hour postprandial glucose concentration consistently below 180 mg/dL. In addition to glycemic control, there are several other parameters that should be systematically followed in patients with type II diabetes. Systolic and diastolic blood pressure should be below 135 and 85 mmHg, respectively, and efforts should be made to have the patient approach or maintain ideal body weight. Triglyceride concentrations, which often parallel glycemic control, should be below 200 mg/dL and high density lipoprotein (HDL) cholesterol above 35 mg/dL.[13] Efforts should be made to keep low-density lipoprotein cholesterol below 130 mg/dL, and if there is any evidence of coronary artery disease, a low density lipoprotein (LDL) cholesterol concentration below 100 mg/dL is advised.[14]

Table 73-1. Metabolic Goals of Effective Management

1. Glycosylated hemoglobin
   a. Within one percentage point above the upper range of normal
   b. Within three standard deviations from the mean
2. Fasting blood glucose concentration between 70 and 120 mg/dL
3. Two-hour postprandial blood glucose concentration less than 180 mg/dL
4. Systolic/diastolic blood pressure less than 135/85 mmHg*
5. Approach or maintain ideal body weight
6. Lipoprotein goals†
   a. Triglycerides less than 200 mg/dL
   b. HDL cholesterol greater than 35 mg/dL
   c. LDL cholesterol less than 100 mg/dL
   d. Total cholesterol—may be misleading in patients with type II diabetes (see text)

*Goals for blood pressure control are different if the patient has evidence of ischemic heart disease.
†Current NCEP guidelines.[14]

The total cholesterol value should be interpreted with caution in patients with type II diabetes, because it may be misleading and can result in an underestimation of the cardiovascular risk status.[13] The classic dyslipidemia of patients with insulin resistance consists in part of low HDL cholesterol and normal or low LDL cholesterol, which may be mainly small and dense or protein rich.[15] Because the HDL and LDL cholesterol concentrations contribute to the total cholesterol concentration, it is not unusual to have a desirable total cholesterol below 200 mg/dL and a very abnormal lipoprotein profile composition. This abnormal lipoprotein composition consists of very low density lipoprotein (VLDL) cholesterol and chylomicron remnants, increased intermediate density lipoprotein cholesterol, small dense or protein-rich LDL, and reduced and possibly abnormal HDL cholesterol.[16] These lipoprotein abnormalities are discussed in detail later and are considered to increase the coronary artery risk significantly by contributing to the high rate of cardiovascular morbidity and mortality seen in persons with type II diabetes.[17–20]

Successful insulin management requires an educated and motivated patient, as well as the participation of a multidisciplinary health care team. The cost:benefit ratio of achieving the desired goals of intensive management has not yet been determined for patients with type II diabetes. Intensive insulin therapy requires a substantial input of physician and support staff time, which has a significant economic impact on the health care system.[21] Therefore, data from future careful clinical trials comparing the outcomes of different therapeutic strategies are warranted before widespread pursuit of such goals can be justified in patients with type II diabetes.

Tools Used to Monitor Glycemic Control

In addition to a reliable laboratory to measure metabolic parameters, home glucose monitoring (HGM) is currently one of the most important tools for monitoring glycemic control and adjusting therapeutic regimens. An educated patient can also use HGM data to make day-to-day adjustments in the insulin regimen, as well as to avoid episodes of severe hypoglycemia. The feasibility of self-adjustment of insulin doses using algorithms has been a subject of considerable debate.[22] Patients often become frustrated and may discontinue HGM when accumulated results are repeatedly not acted on. When patients are properly educated on how to perform and evaluate HGM results and how to use an insulin algorithm, daily glycemic control tends to improve because the patient has a better sense of self-control by participating in his or her own care.[6]

The proper recommended times for HGM should be tailored to the type of insulin regimen used and the timing of insulin injections, as well as insulin pharmacokinetics in terms of initial peak and duration of action. HGM should normally coincide with the peak action of a particular type of insulin, such as 1–3 hours after regular insulin and 6–8 hours after NPH or Lente insulin, in order to evaluate the efficacy of the dose and to avoid hypoglycemia. One must also pay close attention to the amount and timing of meals and periods of exercise when advising the best times to test blood glucose during the day.

A convenient, ambulatory, reliable, continuous real-time glucose sensor would greatly increase our ability to manage patients with diabetes. More realistically, a premeal and 2-hour postmeal, bedtime, and occasional 3:00 A.M. blood glucose values (approximate time of the early morning glucose nadir) will enable the physician to monitor glycemic control adequately in most patients. Once a patient is stabilized on a particular insulin regimen, a reduction in HGM frequency may be feasible, with intermittent periods of more intensive monitoring.

It is crucial that patients know how to evaluate their HGM results.[22] Daily variations in eating and exercise habits, as well as inexplicable changes in insulin sensitivity over both long- and

Table 73-2. Techniques Used to Adjust for Premeal Hyperglycemia

1. *Nonpharmacologic*
   a. Increase the time interval between insulin injection and consumption of the meal
   b. Consume less than the usual number of calories
   c. Eliminate or replace foods containing refined carbohydrates and those having a high glycemic index, such as fruit exchanges
   d. Spread the calories over an extended period of time
   e. Do mild exercise after a meal
2. *Pharmacologic*
   a. Increase the amount of fast acting insulin via an algorithm
   b. If a consistent trend is identified, make the appropriate long-term adjustment in insulin dose to prevent hyperglycemia at that time

short-term periods, make daily adjustments of insulin doses by the patient invaluable for improving and maintaining glycemic control. Not only are algorithms required to make appropriate day-to-day changes in insulin dosing, but they can also be effectively utilized to guide long-term adjustments based on consistent glycemic trends. Thus, HGM values can be used to help the patient recognize abnormal excursions in glucose values, apply insulin algorithms to make short-term insulin adjustments, avoid the development of severe hypoglycemia, and adjust dietary and exercise regimens appropriately on a day-to-day basis.

In addition to adjusting the dose of insulin to be given, a number of nonpharmacologic tools can be used to control excessive glucose levels (Table 73-2). For example, one can increase the time interval between the insulin injection and mealtime to allow sufficient time for insulin to become active before a meal challenge. Consuming fewer calories, eliminating foods that cause rapid increases in blood glucose, spreading the calories over an extended period of time, and exercising lightly after meals are additional effective nonpharmacologic methods that can be used in concert with HGM values to reduce daily glycemic excursions (see Table 73-2). If the blood glucose concentration is consistently elevated at a particular time, then prospective long-term adjustments must be made to avoid the need to "chase" high blood glucose concentrations with extra insulin on a regular basis. Figure 73-1 demonstrates one of the insulin algorithm forms utilized in our clinic that exemplify these pharmacologic and nonpharmacologic tools.

Intensive Insulin Strategies

Insulin therapy should be reserved for patients who have failed on an adequate trial of diet, exercise, and oral antidiabetic agents. This stepwise approach is currently advocated by both the American and European Diabetes Associations.[21] Effective analysis and interpretation of studies on the efficacy and safety of insulin regimens in type II diabetes are limited due to the wide diversity of the various study protocols. Additional problems in comparing these studies are the heterogeneity of type II diabetes, patient selection, natural history of the clinical course, differences in current and prior therapeutic patient interventions, and lack of control of dietary and exercise variables. Many different insulin regimens are recommended, although it is not clear from the literature which regimen is best. The following section will focus on the different insulin regimens commonly used to normalize glucose concentrations and glycosylated hemoglobin in patients with type II diabetes mellitus.

In the United States, it is estimated that approximately 25% of all patients with type II diabetes mellitus are treated with some form of insulin compared to only 10% in Europe.[21] One reason for this discrepancy may be that other nonsulfonylureas and oral antidiabetic agents are available in Europe, including the biguanide metformin and the carbohydrate absorption inhibitors miglitol and acarbose.[23] There are also likely to be differences in the therapeutic preference of physicians and in their criteria for starting insulin therapy.

Based on the natural history of type II diabetes, many patients will eventually require therapy with insulin.[1] The period of time before insulin is necessary is highly variable and is based on numerous factors. The most important proposed explanation is β-cell exhaustion resulting in relative endogenous insulinopenia.[24–27] This leads to progressive loss of compensatory hyperinsulinemia, which is required to achieve and maintain a sufficient degree of glycemic control, especially in patients on oral hypoglycemic agents (Fig. 73-2). In other cases, obesity, pregnancy, or a variety of medications, as well as several illnesses, may exacerbate the insulin-resistant state and transform a patient previously well controlled on oral agents into one requiring insulin. Such factors often play an important role in determining when a patient no longer responds adequately to diet, exercise, and oral antidiabetic agents.

In addition to the natural history of type II diabetes, there is heterogeneity in the pathophysiology of type II diabetes mellitus that may influence when patients require insulin. Some patients with the diagnosis of type II diabetes may actually have a condition more closely related to insulin-dependent or type I diabetes with

Name________________________ Date__________________

Provider______________________ Phone__________________

Time between injection and meal in minutes	Blood glucose value (mg/dl)	Breakfast	Lunch	Dinner	Bedtime	Bedtime snack size
5-15	<80					large
30	81-150					medium
30-45	151-200					small
45-60	201-250					none
60	251-300					none
60+	301-350					none
60+	351-400					none
60+	401-450					none
60+	451+					none

AM long acting insulin dose________

PM long acting insulin dose________ ▫ Take before dinner ▫ Take at bedtime

Figure 73-1. Algorithm form used for patients receiving intensive insulin therapy. As the premeal blood glucose value rises, the amount of regular insulin recommended also increases and is adjusted based on postprandial glucose values. The time between the insulin injection and the meal should also be increased as the premeal blood glucose value rises, thus improving postprandial glucose values. Regular insulin can be given at lunch and at bedtime for extreme hyperglycemia. If the patient consistently (3 days in a row) requires higher regular insulin doses at a particular time, the appropriate long-term adjustments should be made.

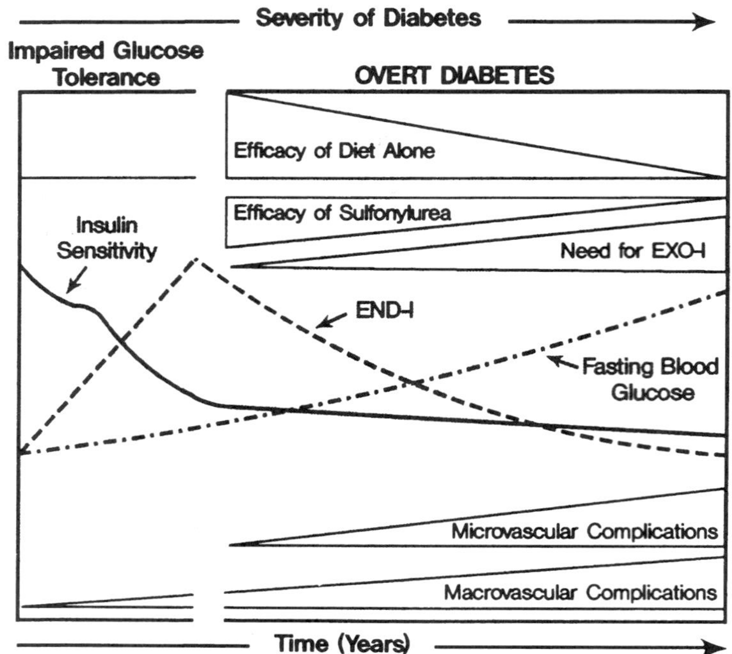

Figure 73-2. Theoretical time course of the natural history of the metabolic and clinical characteristics of patients with type II diabetes. At some point, estimated to be several years before the diagnosis of overt diabetes, insulin sensitivity decreases and endogenous insulin secretion increases. Eventually, the postprandial (not shown) and fasting blood glucose values will rise and the diagnosis of overt diabetes is made. Over time, the effectiveness of diet alone or with sulfonylureas diminishes and the need for exogenous insulin therapy increases. This clinical time course depends, in part, on the degree of endogenous insulin secretory ability and the severity of insulin resistance. The incidence of macrovascular complications is associated with hyperinsulinemia, and is commonly found before the diagnosis of overt diabetes. The development of microvascular complications is related to the duration and severity of the hyperglycemic state. (Reproduced with permission from the American Diabetes Association from ref. 1.)

severe insulinopenia. Many of these patients have been shown to have islet cell antibody positivity or antibodies to glutamic acid decarboxylase, with a decreased C-peptide response to glucagon stimulation and a propensity for primary oral medication failure.[28] There are also wide geographic and racial differences that may influence the need for insulin therapy.[29,30] For example, Asian patients with type II diabetes tend to be thinner, diagnosed with diabetes at an earlier age, fail oral hypoglycemic agents much sooner, and more sensitive to insulin therapy than the classic centrally obese patient in the United States and some parts of Europe (Edelman S, Henry RR, unpublished data, 1995).

Insulin therapy can improve or correct many of the metabolic abnormalities present in patients with type II diabetes mellitus. Insulin administration significantly reduces glucose concentrations by suppressing hepatic glucose production,[31] increasing postprandial glucose utilization,[1] and improving the abnormal lipoprotein composition commonly seen in patients with insulin resistance.[10] Insulin therapy may also decrease or eliminate the effects of glucose toxicity by reducing hyperglycemia to improve insulin sensitivity and β-cell secretory function[32,33] (see Fig. 73-2). The beneficial as well as the potentially adverse effects of intensive insulin therapy will be discussed in greater detail in a later section.

Application of Intensive Insulin Therapy

The goals of therapy should be individually tailored. Candidates for intensive management should be motivated, compliant, and educable, without other medical conditions and physical limitations that preclude accurate and reliable home glucose monitoring (HGM) and insulin administration. In addition, caution is advised in patients who are aged or have hypoglycemic unawareness. Other limitations to achieving normoglycemia may include high titers of insulin antibodies, especially in patients with a prior history of intermittent use of insulin of animal origin. The site of insulin injection may also change the pharmacokinetics, and absorption can be highly variable, especially if lipohypertrophy is present. The periumbilical area has been shown to be one of the most desirable areas to inject insulin because of the rapid and consistent absorption kinetics observed at this location.[21]

Before starting insulin therapy, the patient should be well educated in the techniques of HGM, proper insulin administration, and self-adjustment of the insulin dose, if appropriate, as well as knowledgeable about dietary and exercise strategies. The patient and family members also need to be informed about hypoglycemia prevention, recognition, and treatment. Initial and ongoing education by a diabetes management team is crucial for long-term success and safety.

Combination Therapy

Combination therapy usually refers to the use of oral antidiabetic agents together with a single injection of intermediate-acting insulin at bedtime. Several other combinations of these two forms of therapy have also been reported.[34–46] For many of the reasons mentioned earlier, analysis of prior studies to evaluate the efficacy and safety of combination therapy is difficult. Several review articles using meta-analysis have concluded that combination therapy results in only modest improvements in glucose control and considerably to the medical costs of diabetes management compared to insulin therapy alone. Because of heterogeneity in type II diabetes together with variability in the design and clinical situations of previous studies, however, use of meta-analysis may be inappropriate for making generalized statements regarding this form of therapy.[37] Based on several recent reports, the use of combination therapy has been quite successful in selected patients.[8,36–39]

The rationale for using an evening insulin strategy is based on the pathophysiology of fasting hyperglycemia in type II diabetes. Combination therapy is based on the assumption that if evening insulin lowers the fasting glucose concentration to normal, then daytime sulfonylureas will be more effective in controlling postprandial hyperglycemia and maintaining euglycemia throughout the day. Metabolic profiles of type II diabetes have clearly demonstrated that fasting blood glucose contributes more to daytime hyperglycemia than do postprandial changes.[38] In addition, the fasting blood glucose concentration is highly correlated with the degree of hepatic glucose production during the early morning hours.[4] Hepatic glucose output is directly decreased by insulin[10] and indirectly inhibited by the ability of insulin to reduce adipose tissue lipolysis, with lower concentrations of free fatty acids and gluconeogenesis.[47] Bedtime intermediate-acting insulin also has its peak action coinciding with the onset of the dawn phenomenon (early morning resistance to insulin due to diurnal variations in growth hormone and possibly to norepinephrine levels), which usually occurs between 3 and 7 A.M. Bedtime insulin also increases the morning serum insulin concentration and may assist in reducing the postbreakfast glucose in addition to the fasting value (Table 73-3).

Patient selection is very important when considering combination therapy. The question of whether a patient is still responding in a satisfactory manner to oral antidiabetic agents such as sulfonylureas is of primary importance. Patients have a higher likelihood of success using daytime sulfonylureas and bedtime insulin if they are obese, have had overt diabetes for less than 10–15 years, are diagnosed with type II diabetes after the age of 35, do not have fasting blood glucose values consistently over 250–300 mg/dL, and have evidence of endogenous insulin secretory ability. Although standard measurement conditions and C-peptide concentrations have not been established for this clinical situation, a fasting (≥0.2 nmol/L) or glucagon-stimulated (>0.40 nmol/L) C-peptide value indicates some degree of endogenous insulin secretory ability.[48,49] Patients with type II diabetes diagnosed before the age of 35 more often have atypical forms of diabetes. Patients with diabetes for more than 10–15 years tend to have a greater chance of β-cell exhaustion and thus to be less responsive to oral hypoglycemic agents.

Thin patients are more likely to be hypoinsulinemic and often respond inadequately to oral sulfonylureas, which leads to combination therapy failure. In addition, when the fasting glucose concentration becomes markedly elevated, this is often associated with a concomitant decrease in endogenous insulin secretory ability, which renders oral agents ineffective (see Table 73-3). Studies demonstrating the most favorable outcome from combination therapy have utilized patients who still had some response to sulfonylureas or had evidence of significant endogenous secretory ability. The actual number of patients who might fit into this category, and possibly respond to combination therapy is unknown, but is estimated to be between 20% and 40% of all patients failing with maximum doses of sulfonylureas as the sole therapy.

TABLE 73-3. Combination Therapy

1. *Metabolic Benefits of Bedtime Intermediate-Acting Insulin*
    1. Reduces the fasting and postprandial blood glucose values
    2. Suppresses hepatic glucose production directly
    3. Reduces free fatty acid levels, which suppresses hepatic glucose output indirectly
    4. Counteracts the dawn phenomenon
2. *Practical Benefits*
    1. Minimal education needed
    2. No need to learn how to mix different insulins
    3. Easily started on an outpatient basis
    4. Compliance may be better with one injection than with two or more
    5. Psychological acceptance of the needle is good
    6. Reduces the total amount of exogenous insulin needed compared to a two- or three-shot-per-day regimen.
3. *Patient Selection Guidelines**
    1. Diabetes for less than 10–15 years
    2. Normal weight or overweight
    3. Diagnosed with diabetes after age 35
    4. Fasting blood glucose concentration consistently less than 250 mg/dL
    5. Adequate C-peptide response to glucagon stimulation

*These are general guidelines not currently substantiated by clinical trials. Individual responses are variable.

Yki-Jarvinen et al.[8] recently compared combination therapy with a two- and four-injection-a-day regimen in patients with type II diabetes. After 3 months, all treatment groups had similar reductions in mean diurnal glucose concentrations and glycosylated hemoglobin (Fig. 73-3). The group treated with combination oral agents and bedtime NPH insulin, however, had the lowest mean diurnal serum free insulin concentrations and had the least weight gain (1.2 ± 0.5 kg) of any group (see Fig. 73-3). In this study, patients were selected who were receiving submaximal doses of glyburide (12.5 mg/day), glipizide (20 mg/day), and metformin (~1.4 g/day), with fasting blood glucose concentrations in the range of 225 mg/dL and mean fasting serum C-peptide values of 0.66 nM. There was no evidence of severe hypoglycemia with combination therapy, and patient acceptance was excellent. Several other recent publications also support the additional efficacy and safety of combination therapy in patients inadequately controlled by oral hypoglycemic agents alone.[36,38,39,43,46]

There are also a number of practical reasons why combination therapy may be beneficial (see Table 73-3). The patient does not need to learn how to mix different types of insulin, hospitalization is not required, and patient compliance and acceptance are better with a single injection than with multiple injections of insulin. Combination therapy also requires a lower total dose of exogenous insulin than a full two- or three-injection-a-day regimen. This usually contributes to less weight gain and peripheral hyperinsulinemia. Calculation of the initial bedtime dose of intermediate-acting insulin can be based on clinical judgment or various formulas based on the fasting blood glucose concentration or body weight. For example, one can divide the average fasting blood glucose (mg/dL) by 18 or divide the body weight in kilograms by 10 to calculate the initial dose of NPH or Lente insulin to be started at bedtime (modified from ref. 10). One can also safely start 5–10 units of intermediate-acting insulin for thin patients and 10–15 units for obese patients at bedtime as an initial estimated dose. In either case, the dose is increased in 2–5-unit increments every 3–4 days until the morning fasting blood glucose concentration is consistently in the range of 70–140 mg/dL.

The best time to give the evening injection of intermediate-acting insulin is between 10 P.M. and midnight. Many reliable patients can make their own adjustments using home glucose monitoring (HGM). Figure 73-4 is a patient self-instruction sheet for bedtime insulin adjustments. Once the fasting blood glucose concentrations are consistently in a desirable range, the prelunch, predinner, and bedtime blood sugar values must be monitored to determine if the oral hypoglycemic agents are maintaining day-long glycemia.

Based on the results of HGM, combination therapy can be altered to reduce hyperglycemia at identified times during the day. For example, a common situation seen with daytime sulfonylurea and bedtime intermediate-acting insulin therapy is an improvement in the fasting, prelunch, and predinner blood sugar values, although the postdinner blood glucose concentration remains excessively high (over 200 mg/dL). In this clinical situation, an injection of premixed regular and intermediate-acting insulin (i.e., 70/30 insulin) before dinner instead of a bedtime dose of intermediate-acting insulin may be more efficacious. This regimen will often improve the postdinner blood glucose values because the premixed insulin contains rapidly acting regular insulin yet still allows overnight glucose control secondary to the intermediate-acting component. With this regimen, however, one must be more cautious about early morning hypoglycemia because the intermediate-acting insulin given before dinner will exert its peak effect earlier. In our experience, this has not been a major clinical problem in patients with type II diabetes compared to those with type I diabetes mellitus.

It is recommended that after the addition of evening insulin, patients continue to take their maximal dose of oral antidiabetic agent. If the daytime blood glucose concentrations start to become excessively low, the dose of oral medication must be reduced. This situation is not uncommon because glucose toxicity may be reduced

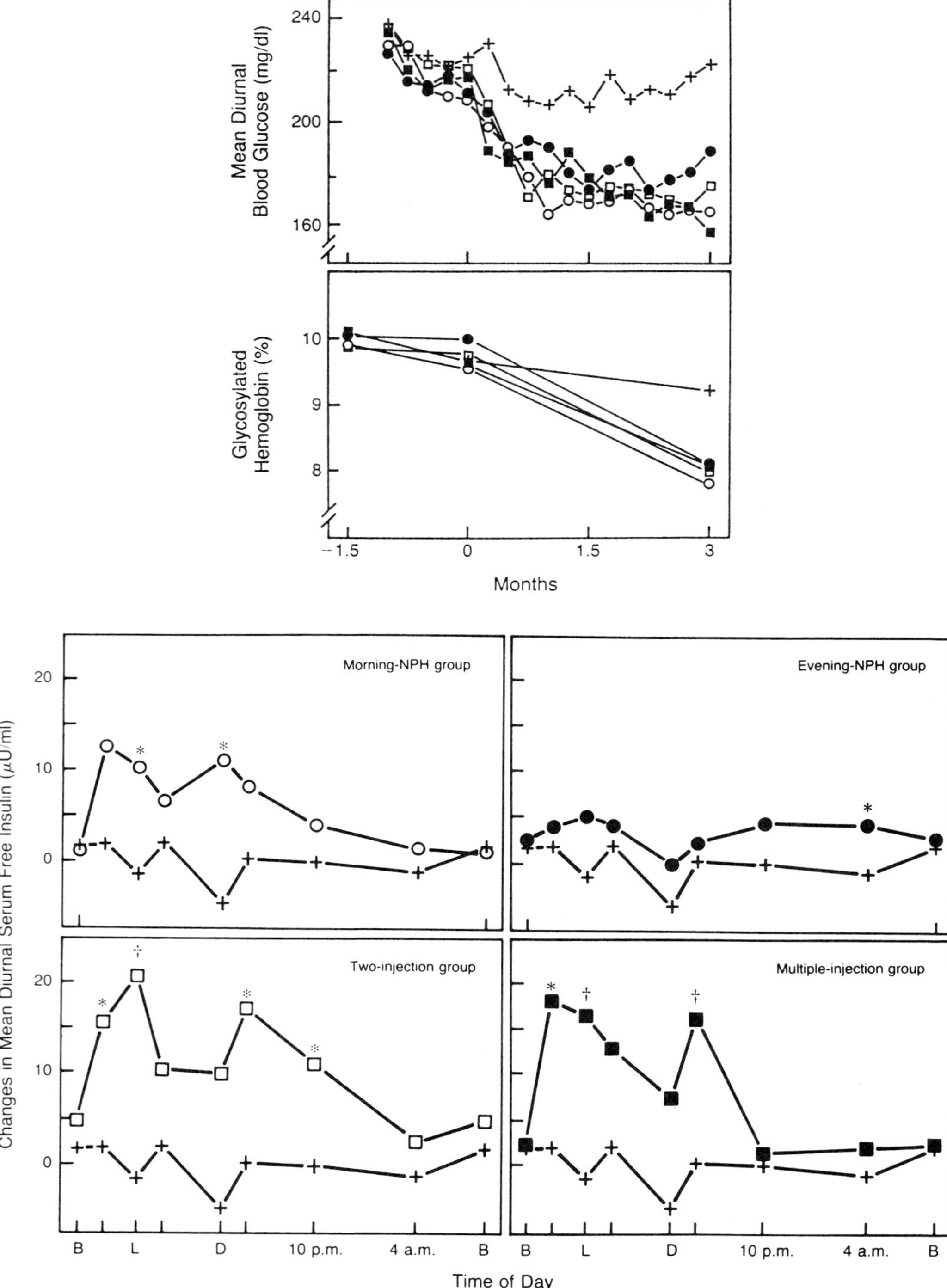

Figure 73-3. Glycemic control (upper two panels) and mean diurnal serum free insulin concentrations after 3 months of insulin therapy in each treatment group compared with the control group (lower panels). The curves for mean diurnal blood glucose concentrations and the mean glycosylated hemoglobin values were not significantly different between the four treatment groups; the control group (+), the morning-NPH combination group (E), the evening-NPH combination group (J), the two-injection group (W), and the multiple-injection group (B). The increment in the mean diurnal serum free insulin concentration, however, was 50–65% smaller in the evening-NPH combination group than in the other insulin treatment groups. The asterisks (*) ($p < 0.05$) and daggers (†) ($p < 0.01$) indicate a significant change in the serum free insulin concentration in the insulin treatment group shown compared with the control group. B = breakfast; L = lunch; D = dinner. See text. (From ref. 8.)

1. Begin with a dose of ______ units of NPH insulin administered just before bedtime.
2. If the prebreakfast blood sugar is greater than 140 mg/dL for 3 days in a row, then increase the evening NPH insulin dose by ______ units.
3. If the prebreakfast blood sugar is less than 100 mg/dL for 2 days in a row, then decrease the evening NPH insulin by ______ units.
4. Remember not to increase the insulin dose more frequently than every 3 days.
5. If you have any questions, please call me at

____

6. Provider's name: ______________________

____
Physician/Nurse Practitioner

Figure 73-4. Patient self-adjustment form for evening insulin therapy. Reliable patients properly educated in HGM techniques can safely and efficiently adjust insulin doses at home based on HGM results. Patient self-adjustment allows normoglycemia to be achieved more rapidly and reduces the physician and staff workload.

due to improved glucose control, leading to enhanced sensitivity to both oral agents and insulin. If the prelunch and predinner blood glucose concentrations remain excessively high on combination therapy, the oral antidiabetic agent is likely not contributing significantly to glycemic control throughout the day. In this situation, a more conventional two-injection-a-day regimen should be employed, discontinuing the oral antidiabetic agent.

In summary, combination therapy can be a simple and effective means of normalizing glycemia and glycosylated hemoglobin concentrations in selected patients with type II diabetes mellitus who fail with oral antidiabetic agents. The most common type of patient in whom combination therapy can succeed is the one who fails sulfonylurea therapy but has some evidence of responsiveness to oral agents. Bedtime intermediate-acting insulin is given and progressively increased to normalize the fasting blood glucose concentration. When the fasting blood glucose is brought under control, the success of combination therapy depends on the ability of the daytime oral antidiabetic agents to maintain euglycemia. If this cannot be achieved, then the oral hypoglycemic agents should be stopped and conventional insulin regimens employed.

Multiple-Injection Regimens

One of the most common insulin regimens utilized in type II diabetes mellitus is the split-mixed regimen consisting of a prebreakfast and predinner dose of an intermediate- and a fast-acting insulin. This split-mixed two-injection-a-day regimen is often inadequate for patients with type I diabetes mellitus and results in persistent early morning hypoglycemia and fasting hyperglycemia. Such problems do not appear to occur as frequently in type II diabetes. This is likely due to pathophysiologic differences, particularly in endogenous insulin secretory ability, insulin resistance, and counter-regulatory mechanisms in type I and type II diabetes.

In a recent clinical trial in type II diabetes, day-long glycemia and glycosylated hemoglobin were essentially normalized by 6 months of intensive treatment with a split-mixed insulin regimen.[7] In this study, 14 typical obese patients with type II diabetes mellitus (age, 59 ± 2 years; duration of diabetes, 7 ± 2 years; body mass index 31 ± 2 kg/M^2; fasting blood glucose concentration 283 ± 13 mg/dL) failing therapy with oral antidiabetic agents were intensively managed with prebreakfast and predinner NPH and regular insulin over a 6-month period. The insulin dose was adjusted based on four-times-a-day home glucose monitoring (HGM) results. Glycemic control was rapidly achieved within 1 month and was maintained for the duration of the study.

The average total insulin dose needed to maintain glycemic control approached 100 units per day, with approximately 50% of the total dose required before breakfast and 50% before dinner. The ratio of NPH to regular was 75%:25%. There was a very low incidence of hypoglycemic reactions, which decreased as the study progressed, and no reactions were severe or required assistance. Patient compliance and sense of well-being were excellent. Near-normalization of the glycosylated hemoglobin, however, produced some adverse effects in these patients. The mean serum insulin concentration obtained during 24-hour metabolic profile studies increased from 308 ± 80 pmol/L at baseline to 510 ± 102 pmol/L ($p < 0.05$) at completion of the 6-month study. The exacerbation of hyperinsulinemia by exogenous insulin therapy was strongly correlated with weight gain throughout the study. Despite biweekly visits with the study dietitian and instructions to reduce the daily caloric intake, a mean weight gain of approximately 9 kg occurred (Fig. 73-5). Interestingly, the total daily insulin dose was 86 ± 13 units at 1 month and 100 ± 24 units at 6 months despite minimal additional improvement in glycemic control during that period. Most of the improvement in glycemic control was due to suppression of basal hepatic glucose production (from 628 ± 44 to 350 ± 17 μmol · M^{-2} · min^{-1}, $p < 0.001$), with a more modest but significant improvement in peripheral glucose uptake (from 1418 ± 156 to 1657 ± 128 μmol · M^{-2} · min^{-1}, $p < 0.05$), as determined by the glucose clamp technique (Fig. 73-6).

This study emphasizes a number of important aspects of intensive glucose control of obese patients with type II diabetes failing sulfonylurea therapy. First, the average daily dose of insulin needed to control such patients may approximate 1 unit per kilogram of

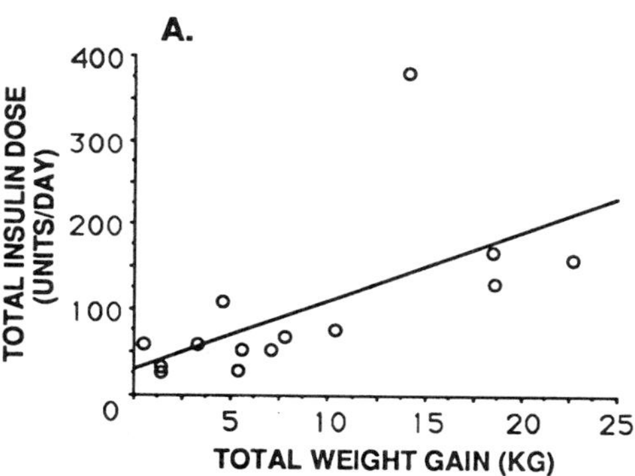

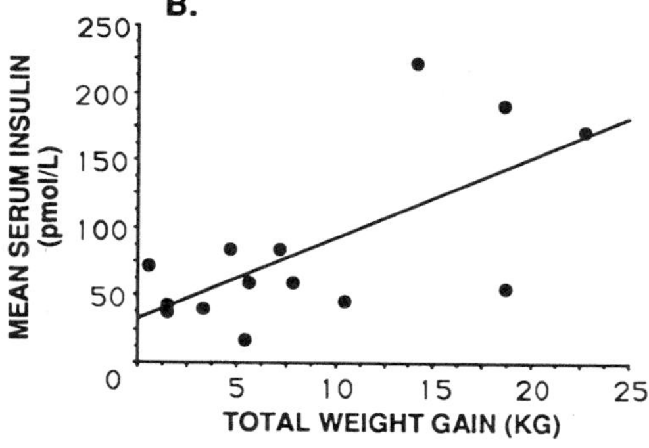

Figure 73-5. Correlation of total weight gain with total insulin dose (**A**) and mean serum insulin level (**B**) after 6 months of intensive insulin treatment. *A*: $r = 0.62$, $p < 0.02$; *B*: $r = 0.67$, $p < 0.01$; see text. (Reproduced with permission from the American Diabetes Association from ref. 6.)

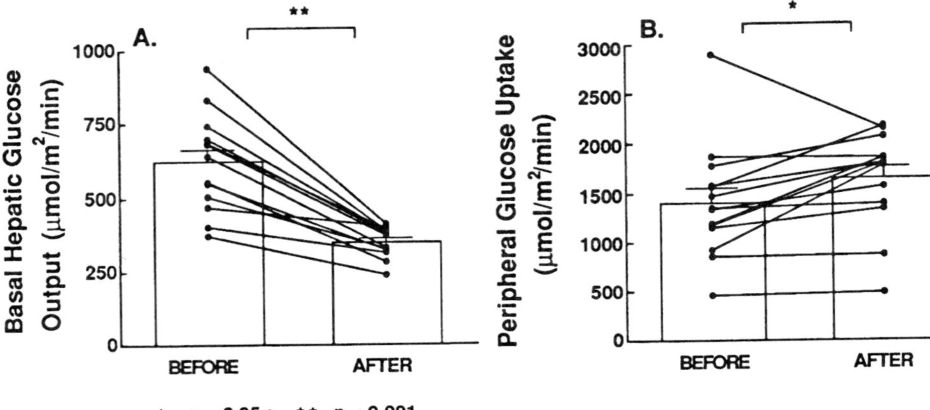

FIGURE 73-6. Individual and mean levels of basal hepatic glucose output (**A**) and peripheral glucose uptake (**B**) before and after 6 months of intensive insulin therapy with a split-mixed regimen; see text. (Reproduced with permission from the American Diabetes Association from ref. 6.)

body weight. Second, the total daily insulin requirement can be split equally between the prebreakfast and predinner injections. Third, the split-mixed regimen in patients with type II diabetes is usually devoid of the common problems seen with this regimen in type I diabetes, particularly early morning hypoglycemia and fasting (preprandial) hyperglycemia. Fourth, both severe and mild hypoglycemic events are much less frequent in patients with type II diabetes mellitus compared to patients with type I diabetes undergoing intensive insulin therapy. And finally, weight gain with peripheral hyperinsulinemia occurs, which may contribute to metabolic and vascular complications.

A similar but larger 3-month clinical trial recently compared a split-mixed combination with a multiple-injection regimen consisting of premeal regular and bedtime NPH insulin injections.[8] Both the split-mixed and multiple-injection regimen treatment groups achieved equivalent and near-normal glycosylated hemoglobin values. These therapies, however, were associated with weight gain of 0.8 ± 0.05 and 2.9 ± 0.05 kg, a 39% and 36% increase in mean diurnal serum free insulin levels and a total daily insulin dose of 43 and 45 units, respectively (see Fig. 73-3). The authors demonstrated that the change in body weight was negatively correlated with the change in glycosylated hemoglobin values and positively correlated with the mean diurnal serum free insulin values. The differences between these two studies with regard to total insulin requirements, mean insulin concentrations, and weight gain are probably due primarily to differences in patient characteristics. Patients in the latter study were leaner (body mass index 29 versus 31 kg/M^2), had lower baseline fasting blood glucose values (225 versus 283 mg/dL), and reduced baseline mean diurnal serum free insulin values (138 versus 308 pmol), and were previously treated with submaximal doses of sulfonylureas compared to the patients in the former study. In addition, the latter study was conducted over a shorter (3- vs. 6-month) period. Despite these differences, both studies clearly demonstrate the efficacy of various insulin regimens and the adverse consequences of such therapy.

Lindstrom et al.[9] measured 24-hour free insulin, proinsulin, and glucose values in 10 patients with type II diabetes mellitus. Split-mixed or multiple-injection insulin regimens were used in a randomized crossover fashion with 8-week treatment periods. These investigators reported that the two- and four-dose insulin regimens achieved similar glycemic control, although both led to significant increases in fasting insulin concentrations and a doubling of the 24-hour area under the curve for free insulin. The four-injection-a-day regimen also caused higher postprandial insulin concentrations at breakfast and dinner compared to the twice-a-day regimen. Serum proinsulin concentrations were significantly suppressed with exogenous insulin therapy compared to those of patients with type II diabetes treated with oral sulfonylureas. The biologic significance of this finding is unclear but may have relevance because proinsulin has been implicated as an atherosclerotic growth factor.[9] The conclusions of this study and others are similar: There is no added benefit of a four-dose insulin regimen over a conventional split-mixed regimen in patients with type II diabetes failing oral antidiabetic agents.[1,4,10]

In another recent long-term clinical trial, a split-mixed two-injection-a-day regimen was used to intensively treat 102 nonobese type II diabetic patients for 5 years.[50] The study group demonstrated a progressive decline in postprandial blood glucose and glycosylated hemoglobin values during the treatment period. As in other similar studies, continuous weight gain was seen over the 5-year period (from 24.5 to 28.9 kg), despite no reported change in caloric consumption and no change in total insulin dose after 2.5 years. Patient compliance was excellent, with an 85% completion rate, and no severe hypoglycemic reactions were reported. As in other studies, excellent glycemic control was achieved with intensive split-dose insulin without significant hypoglycemia, but at the expense of progressive weight gain.

In most cases, single-injection therapy with an intermediate- or long-acting insulin has been shown to be inadequate in normalizing glycosylated hemoglobin and maintaining 24-hour euglycemia in type II diabetes. In the United Kingdom Prospective Diabetes Study, however, normalization of glycosylated hemoglobin was achieved using a single injection of ultra Lente insulin, and fasting blood glucose concentrations were below 108 mg/dL.[51,52] One of the most important factors explaining this study's success with a simple one-injection-a-day regimen is that patients were newly diagnosed with type II diabetes. These patients were quite different from the participants of other studies, whose duration of type II diabetes was much longer and who had previously failed therapy with oral antidiabetic medications.

The VA Cooperative Study on Glycemic Control and Complications in Type II Diabetes Trial was designed to address many of the questions that the Diabetes Control and Complications Trial (DCCT) answered for type I diabetes.[53,54] In this 27-month feasibility trial, 150 patients with type II diabetes mellitus (~60 years of age, duration of diabetes ~8 years, body mass index ~32 kg/M^2) were randomized to either standard or intensive therapy. The patients in the intensively treated group all started in Phase I, which consisted of an evening injection of insulin alone. If normalization of the glycosylated hemoglobin was not achieved with this therapy, they were advanced in a stepwise fashion through three other phases until target glycemic control was reached. Phase II consisted of combination therapy with daytime glipizide and bedtime intermediate-acting insulin. Phase III included a split-mixed regimen of regular and intermediate-acting insulin injections twice a day, and Phase IV consisted of three or more daily injections of insulin. At the end of the trial, 12%, 24%, 30%, and 34% of the patients ended up in the Phase I, II, III, and IV groups, respectively. The average final insulin dose in these groups was 60.1 ± 38.1, 64.0 ± 41.9, 116.2 ± 68.6, and 133.0 ± 79.9 units per day, respectively. Surpris-

Table 73-4. Conservative Stepwise Approach to Initiating a Split-Mixed Regimen in Type II Diabetes*

1. First Goal—Fasting CBG 4.5–6.5 mM
   - Initial dose of NPH insulin 0.2 unit/kg before dinner
   - Change dose of evening NPH insulin based on subsequent fasting CBG as follows: >9.5 mM—increase by 0.5 unit/kg; 6.5–9.5 mM—increase by 0.05 unit/kg; 4.5–6.5 mM—no change in dose; <4.5 mM—decrease by 0.1 unit/kg
2. Second Goal—Presupper CBG 4.5–6.5 mM
   - Initial dose of NPG insulin before breakfast and criteria for adjustment identical to first goal, except based on subsequent presupper CBG
   - Proceed to third goal only after first and second goals are achieved
3. Third Goal—Postprandial (2-Hour) CBG <9.5 mM (After Breakfast and Supper)
   - Change each dose of regular insulin based on subsequent postprandial (2-hour) CBG as follows: >9.5 mM—increase by 0.025 unit/kg; 6.5–9.5 mM—no change in dose; 4.5–6.5 mM—decrease by 0.025 unit/kg; <4.5 mM—decrease by 0.05 unit/kg
   - All injections are given subcutaneously in the preumbilical region 30 minutes before breakfast and dinner

CBG = capillary blood glucose.
*Reproduced with permission from the American Diabetes Association.

ingly, the authors did not report significant weight gain in any of the treatment groups. Differences in micro- and macrovascular events were unavailable at the time this chapter was written.

There are several acceptable methods for initiating insulin therapy in type II diabetes. A conservative yet effective strategy utilizing a stepwise approach to institute a split-mixed regimen was employed successfully and safely by Henry et al.[6] (Table 73-4). A simple alternative method for initiating a split-mixed regimen in obese patients uses 70/30 premixed insulin with an initial total daily dose (0.4–0.8 units/kg) equally split between the prebreakfast and predinner meals. Adjustments are made based on home glucose monitoring (HGM) results, which may dictate the need to increase or decrease the ratio of intermediate- to regular-acting insulin. For morbidly obese patients, the insulin requirements rise almost exponentially as the percentage of ideal body weight increases above 150%.[55] In contrast, caution should be used when starting to use insulin with thin patients with type II diabetes, especially premixed insulins with fixed doses of regular insulin (total daily dose 0.2–0.5 units/kg). This group tends to be more sensitive to the glucose-lowering effects of insulin and thus more prone to severe hypoglycemia. If a multiple-insulin-injection regimen or subcutaneous insulin pump therapy is to be initiated, ultra Lente should be used to provide a steady basal rate of insulin bioavailability. This component should constitute approximately 50–60% of the total daily insulin requirement. Premeal boluses of regular insulin are also given, with adjustment based on the 2-hour postprandial blood glucose measurements.

In summary, it is apparent from review of the available literature that there is no one perfect insulin regimen that can be used in all cases of type II diabetes. In a subgroup of patients who fail to respond to maximum doses of sulfonylureas, combination therapy can be beneficial and easy to administer; it also reduces the need for large doses of exogenous insulin. Once a patient demonstrates unresponsiveness to combination therapy, however, a more conventional insulin regimen should be employed. When failure to respond to combination therapy occurs, a split-mixed regimen of intermediate- and regular-acting insulin given before breakfast and before dinner is usually preferred. Insulin adjustments are based on HGM, and premixed insulins are easy to administer and effective.

Particular attention should be directed to minimizing the weight gain seen with intensive insulin therapy. Obese patients who fail to respond to combination therapy usually require large amounts of insulin and are susceptible to weight gain, which may make therapeutic success more difficult. Normalizing glycosylated hemoglobin with a particular regimen depends on numerous variables, including the severity of insulin resistance, the extent and type of obesity, prior failure with oral hypoglycemic agents, preceding degree of glucose control, and other complicating medical conditions. Furthermore, the success of a particular insulin regimen is influenced by the severity of glucose toxicity. Prolonged hyperglycemia reduces β-cell secretory ability and worsens peripheral insulin resistance.[32,33] Thus, the metabolic success of these different insulin regimens can be highly variable.

External Subcutaneous Insulin Infusion Pumps

Continuous subcutaneous insulin infusion (CSII) pumps have been used primarily for patients with type I diabetes. At present, there is a paucity of clinical trials using CSII in type II diabetes. Although some studies demonstrate metabolic benefits of CSII in type II diabetes, all are limited by a relatively short period of evaluation and a small number of heterogeneous subjects. Interpretation of these studies is further confounded by the random assignment of subjects to dissimilar conventional insulin regimens, making comparison between studies difficult.

Jennings et al.[56] randomized 20 type II diabetic subjects (median age 61 years, duration of diabetes 6 years, and percentage of ideal body weight 120%) to either CSII or twice daily injections of regular and NPH insulin for 4 months. Glycemic control improved in both groups, although there was a 30% reduction in the glycosylated hemoglobin in the CSII-treated group and only a 17% reduction in the twice daily injection–treated group. There were no significant differences between the two groups in median daily insulin requirement (0.58 vs. 0.65 units/kg), weight gained (4.5 vs. 4.2 kg), prevalence of mild hypoglycemic reactions, or patient acceptance. There were also no episodes of severe hypoglycemia. The patients treated with CSII had no infusion site infections or mechanical problems leading to metabolic decompensation. In addition, in the CSII group, 58% of the total daily insulin requirement was given as a basal infusion, with the remainder as premeal bolus injections using insulin algorithms.

Garvey et al.[57] studied the effect of intensive insulin therapy on insulin secretion and insulin action before and after 3 weeks of CSII therapy in 14 patients with type II diabetes (age 50 ± 3 years, duration of diabetes 7.8 ± 2.1 years, and 119% ideal body weight). In 3 weeks of therapy, the mean fasting plasma blood glucose and glycosylated hemoglobin values fell 46% and 38%, respectively. The mean daily insulin dose stabilized at approximately 110 units/day, which resulted in mean serum insulin levels ranging between 414 ± 78 and 852 ± 126 pmol/L during meal tolerance testing. Metabolic studies utilizing the hyperinsulinemic glucose clamp technique were performed before and 1 week after CSII therapy. These authors reported that CSII therapy induced a 74% increase in the insulin-stimulated glucose disposal rate and a 45% reduction in hepatic glucose output to mean levels similar to those of normal subjects. Mean 24-hour serum profiles demonstrated significant improvement in both endogenous insulin and C-peptide secretion (Fig. 73-7). In addition, CSII therapy significantly improved the second-phase insulin response to an IV glucose challenge, although the first-phase insulin response remained abnormal and unchanged. Glazer et al.[58] reported similar improvements in β-cell function after only 16 days of CSII therapy in 12 patients with type II diabetes failing maximum doses of sulfonylureas and biguanide therapy. It is interesting to note that six of the patients in this study were successfully treated with oral antidiabetic agents alone for at least 2 years after this short period of intensive insulin therapy with CSII.

In summary, CSII pump therapy has not been fully evaluated in patients with type II diabetes. From the limited number of studies available, it is apparent that CSII therapy can safely improve

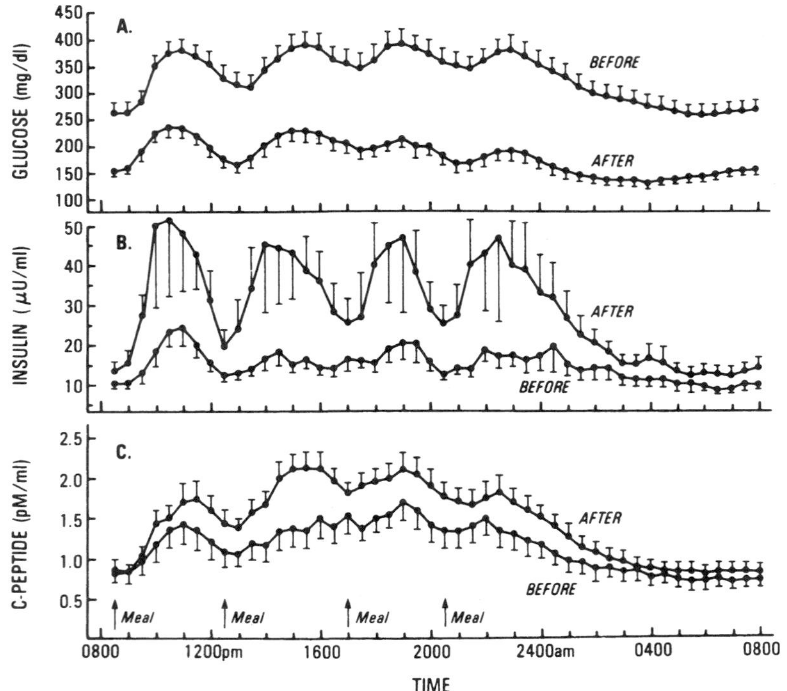

Figure 73-7. Mean 24-hour profile of integrated concentrations of glucose (**A**), insulin (**B**), and C-peptide (**C**) in 14 patients with type II diabetes mellitus before and after 3 weeks of intensive treatment with continuous subcutaneous insulin infusion pumps (see text). (Reproduced with permission from the American Diabetes Association from ref. 58.)

glycemic control and β cell function in a relatively short period of time. Like other forms of intensive subcutaneous insulin therapy, however, CSII therapy induces weight gain and exacerbates peripheral hyperinsulinemia. As it now stands, CSII may be particularly useful in treating patients with type II diabetes who do not respond satisfactorily to more conventional insulin treatment strategies.

Implantable Intraperitoneal Insulin Infusion Pumps

Implantable programmable variable-rate pumps with intraperitoneal insulin delivery are currently being evaluated in patients with type I and type II diabetes (Fig. 73-8). Studies of type I diabetes have been going on for the past 5 years. Preliminary reports indicate that excellent glucose control can be safely achieved, equal to that seen with CSII therapy, but with fewer glycemic excursions and subsequently fewer hypoglycemic reactions.[59]

The implantable insulin pump is surgically placed below the subcutaneous fat just above the rectus sheath in the abdominal area. The operation is short (approximately 30 minutes) and can be done under local, general, or high spinal anesthesia. The catheter is placed through the rectus sheath and floats freely in the peritoneal cavity. The major advantage of implantable over subcutaneous infusion pumps is the more physiologic absorption of delivered insulin. The majority of insulin delivered into the peritoneal cavity drains to the liver via the portal vein, where hepatic extraction, similar to the normal situation, occurs before the insulin is delivered to the systemic circulation. This more physiologic form of insulin delivery has several distinct advantages. First, intraperitoneal insulin is more rapidly and predictably absorbed than subcutaneous insulin, with direct effects on the liver.[11,12] Second, due to the effect of hepatic extraction, peritoneal administration may result in lower peripheral insulin concentration than an equivalent subcutaneous dose of insulin.[60]

The Department of Veterans Affairs Cooperative Studies Center has recently concluded a 1-year randomized feasibility trial (344A) in 113 patients with type II diabetes with prior failure to respond to other insulin regimens.[11,12,60,61] This study compared the effects of intensive metabolic control achieved using the implantable programmable pump with intraperitoneal insulin delivery to multiple daily subcutaneous insulin injections. Although the study results have yet to be completely analyzed, several interesting metabolic trends have already been observed.

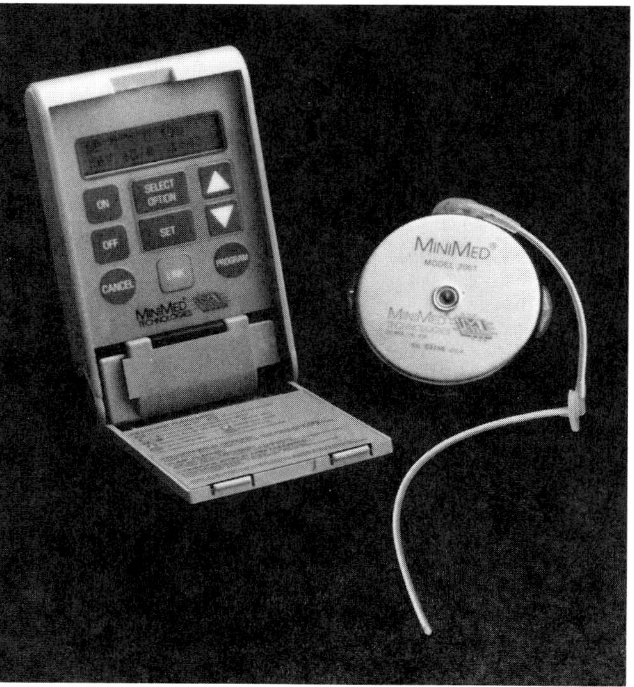

Figure 73-8. Photograph of an implantable programmable insulin pump with the patient controller. The pump is placed under the subcutaneous fat above the rectus sheath, and the distal half of the catheter is placed freely in the peritoneal cavity. The central inverted cone area is for insulin refills; see text. (Reproduced with permission of the MiniMed Company.)

Table 73-5. Veterans Affairs 344A Implantable Insulin Pump (IIP) Versus Multiple Daily Injection (MDI) Study: Preliminary Results ($n = 102$) After 12 Months of Therapy

	IIP	MDI	*p* Value (Between Groups)
Mean HbAlc	7.19 ± 0.98%	7.40 ± 0.96%	$p < 0.083$*
Mean 4×/day HGM	141 ± 28 mg/dL	145 ± 34 mg/dL	NS†
Mean SD of daily HGM	35 ± 11 mg/dL	44 ± 17 mg/dL	$p < 0.0001$
Weight (kg) change from baseline	−0.56 ± 5.61	3.20 ± 5.51	$p < 0.0015$
Hypoglycemia			
Definitely mild	2.37	7.16	Events/patient year
Suspected mild	7.33	21.1	Events/patient year
Definitely severe	.0098	.0785	Events/patient year
Suspected severe	.0256	.0975	Events/patient year

*Wilcoxon rank sum, baseline HbAlc, IIP 8.8 ± 1.2%, MDI 8.91.3%.
†Baseline mean 4×/day HGM IIP 185 ± 31 mg/dL, MDI 189 ± 35 mg/dL.
Source: Data reproduced with permission from the American Diabetes Association from refs. 61 and 62. See text.

Preliminary results demonstrate comparable improvement in glycemic control and glycosylated hemoglobin to near-normal values in both groups. The implantable insulin pump group, however, has demonstrated greater improvement in daily blood glucose excursions, as well as a reduced incidence of definite and suspected mild and severe hypoglycemic reactions compared to the multiple daily injection group[61] (Table 73-5). Furthermore, significant differences in other metabolic parameters such as body mass index, peripheral insulin concentration, and C-peptide concentration during meal tolerance tests were observed between the two treatment groups.[60] Quality of life surveys have shown improvement in both groups, with the implantable programmable pump patients scoring significantly higher despite the more invasive nature of the treatment. If these early results are borne out, implantable insulin pumps with intraperitoneal insulin delivery may prove to have several major physiologic advantages over subcutaneous insulin delivery systems that may have important implications for the future treatment of type II diabetes.

Insulin Analogs

DNA technology has allowed the development of several insulin analogs that appear to have favorable pharmacokinetic properties compared to currently available fast-acting insulin preparations.[63] Amino acids can be added to human insulin, resulting in monomeric or dimeric analogs.[1] These analogs, when given subcutaneously and immediately before a meal, have a more rapid and predictable onset of action and disappearance rate. These characteristics may markedly reduce the development of postprandial hyperglycemia, prolonged hyperinsulinemia, and delayed hypoglycemia. In addition, regional differences in the rate of subcutaneous insulin absorption from various injection sites may be minimized. With these analogs, the inconvenience of timing injections of currently available insulin preparations to at least 30 minutes before eating may no longer be necessary. Nasal and aerosolized insulins, which also have better pharmacokinetic properties than subcutaneous insulin, are currently being developed.[63,64] Although these forms of rapidly absorbed insulin would negate the need for injections, the existence of inconsistent and variable absorption and bioavailability characteristics, as well as a lack of long-term safety data, has limited their widespread application in treating patients with type II diabetes.

Human Insulin-Like Growth Factor

Human insulin-like growth factor I (IGF-I), which can be produced using recombinant DNA technology, may also have practical and physiologic advantages in treating patients with type II diabetes (see Chapter 92). Published clinical studies in humans are limited and of short duration, although Phase III clinical trials are currently ongoing.[65–70] IGF-I, when given to patients with type II diabetes for 5 days, has been shown to improve fasting and postprandial glycemia and to decrease triglyceride values.[68] In addition, the postprandial insulin and C-peptide areas under the curve are reported to be significantly lower, as is the proinsulin:insulin ratio. Furthermore, IGF-I has been shown to suppress insulin secretion and improve insulin sensitivity.[65] The risk of hypoglycemia in type II diabetes has also been reported to be significantly lower than with conventional insulin therapy.[69] Based on these initial reports, it has been suggested that IGF-I therapy may have a role in treating severely insulin-resistant patients unresponsive to currently available forms of insulin therapy.

Potential adverse effects of IGF-I include symptomatic complaints of jaw tenderness, arthralgias, and edema. Progression of diabetic microvascular complications and macrovascular disease may be accelerated due to IGF-I-mediated proliferation of endothelial and smooth muscle cells.[66] IGF-I may also have growth-promoting effects on various carcinomas.[65] Although early studies are promising, the safety and efficacy of IGF-I require further investigation with longer clinical trials before it can be considered for widespread use.

Benefits of Normoglycemia

The benefits of normoglycemia go far beyond delaying or preventing the classic vascular and other chronic complications that occur in patients with diabetes. One must also consider the numerous acute and subacute complications of hyperglycemia that contribute to a decrease in the quality of daily life.[31] Improved glycemic control may have more widespread benefits, such as reducing glycosylated end products, improving lipoprotein concentration and composition, and reducing the propensity for thrombotic events.[71] The Diabetes Control and Complications Trial (DCCT) has clearly defined the benefits and risks of intensive glycemic control in patients with type I diabetes.[73] One must be cautious in extrapolating the results of the DCCT to patients with type II diabetes, however, due to the lack of long-term clinical trials. The UK Prospective Diabetes Study is the only large (>5000 patients), long-term (approximately 10 years) clinical trial currently in progress. This study was designed to determine whether improved glycemic control can reduce micro- and macrovascular complications in patients with type II diabetes.[51,52] The results, when released, may alter current recommendations for intensive therapy in patients with type II diabetes.

Insulin therapy has been shown to improve some of the abnormal atherothrombotic macrovascular risk factors present in type II diabetes. The insulin-resistant state is clearly associated with the classic dyslipidemia commonly seen in patients with type II diabetes mellitus.[13,15,17–19,73,74] Any form of therapy that reduces hyperglycemia, including diet, exercise, oral antidiabetic agents, and exogenous insulin insulin, usually improves the dyslipidemia of type II diabetes. These therapies work primarily by reducing free fatty acid and glucose concentrations, which are substrates for triglyceride production.[75]

Despite the development of hyperinsulinemia, insulin therapy has also been shown to induce antiatherogenic changes in the lipoprotein composition of patients with type II diabetes. This results not only from improved glycemic control, but also from stimulating lipoprotein lipase activity.[40,76] Intensive insulin therapy may also reduce the amount of protein-rich or small dense low density lipoprotein (LDL) cholesterol particles, as well as glycosylation and oxidation of lipoproteins, which could have favorable effects on the cardiovascular risk profile.[15,17,20] Although lipid concentrations tend to improve, triglyceride concentrations seldom normalize completely with insulin therapy, and the use of pharmacologic therapy such as gemfibrozil may be needed.[75]

In summary, the potential benefits of normoglycemia in patients with type II diabetes are numerous. As hyperglycemia is diminished, many acute complications such as excessive thirst, nocturia, sleep disturbances, poor wound healing, and general lack of well-being improve. Because the pathophysiologic basis for microvascular complications appears to be similar in type I and type II diabetes and is significantly influenced by hyperglycemia, a decline in the incidence and severity of retinopathy, nephropathy, and neuropathy may be expected with improved long-term glycemic control. Intensive insulin therapy also improves lipid parameters and other risk factors, which may lead to reduced development of macrovascular disease.

Insulin Therapy and Weight Gain

More than a decade ago, several studies focused attention on the risk factors associated with differences in body fat distribution. Evidence linking central or abdominal obesity with hyperinsulinemia and cardiovascular disease is extensive.[77–79] Not only has hyperinsulinemia been found to occur more frequently in centrally obese persons, but this obese subpopulation is also at increased risk of cardiovascular disease.[80]

Whether hyperinsulinemia induces central fat deposition or is a consequence of abdominal obesity is still a matter of debate, with experimental evidence in support of both hypotheses.[81] Regardless of the nature of the relationship, however, attention must focus on the association between hyperinsulinemia and obesity, and the potential atherogenicity of both when considering the institution of insulin therapy in type II diabetes. Insulin therapy is a successful treatment strategy for patients with type II diabetes unable to achieve glycemic control through diet, exercise, and oral antidiabetic agents. Unfortunately, the lowering of blood glucose concentrations to normal usually requires large doses of exogenous insulin, resulting in hyperinsulinemia with weight gain.

Several of the previously cited studies have demonstrated that treatment of type II diabetes with exogenous insulin results in an average increase in pretreatment body weight of 3–9%, depending on the length of the study and the intensity of glucose control.[4,5,8,50] Henry et al.[6] reported an average weight gain after 6 months of insulin therapy of 9.3% of the patient's pretreatment body weight (8.7 ± 1.9 kg per patient). Although additional metabolic improvements were minimal after the first month of intensive insulin therapy, more than 50% of the weight gain occurred during the subsequent 5-month period as the insulin dose was progressively increased to completely normalize the glycosylated hemoglobin. This study, as well as others, has shown that weight gain is directly associated with peripheral serum insulin levels and the total exogenous insulin dose[1,4,7–10] (see Fig. 73-5). The weight gained resulting from exogenous insulin therapy has been shown to consist of approximately two-thirds adipose tissue and one-third lean body mass.[82]

In addition to exogenous insulin therapy, there are many other variables that may indirectly influence the degree of weight gain in type II diabetes. Pretreatment obesity plays a major role in weight gain; obese subjects require more insulin to achieve glycemic control and, as a result, become more hyperinsulinemic. Increased appetite[83] and reduced thermogenesis[84] induced by insulin may contribute to this common clinical situation, which can cause both the obese and hyperinsulinemic states to become self-perpetuating. β-cell exhaustion, glucose toxicity, and the severity of insulin resistance may also play a role in determining the ultimate insulin dose and thus the propensity for weight gain. The retention of calories previously lost as glycosuria lessens with improved control and contributes to weight gain. Excessive caloric consumption may be a response to, or a fear of, hypoglycemia that can also contribute to excessive weight gain.

Development of weight gain during exogenous insulin therapy is a serious clinical problem. The degree of obesity usually dictates the amount of exogenous insulin required to achieve normal glycemia and thus the propensity for weight gain. Excessive weight gain can be minimized by utilizing the lowest possible dose of insulin to achieve the desired glycemic goals and by educating the patient regarding diet, exercise, and the proper caloric response to hypoglycemia.

Hypoglycemia

Intensive insulin therapy brings with it an increased risk of hypoglycemic reactions. Severe hypoglycemia is usually defined as the inability to self-treat, with a need for assistance from others to properly administer therapy.[21] Most studies in the literature report on the incidence of severe, rather than mild, hypoglycemia because severe hypoglycemia is a more objective and definitive finding that does not tend to be over-reported. It is also important to recognize that neuroglycopenia can masquerade as a neurologic or cardiovascular event and thus can be unrecognized and under-reported.[85]

The development of severe hypoglycemia depends on numerous variables that make evaluation of risk factors and comparison of different study results difficult. The duration of diabetes and insulin therapy, the degree of glycemic control, and a history of prior severe hypoglycemic reactions have all been associated with a higher incidence of severe hypoglycemic reactions.[1] Additional causal factors in hypoglycemia include overinsulinization, underfeeding, strenuous unplanned exercise, excessive alcohol intake, and unawareness of hypoglycemia.

The risk of severe hypoglycemia in insulin-requiring type II diabetic patients has consistently been reported to be significantly reduced compared to the risk in type I diabetic patients undergoing intensive insulin therapy.[7,53,54,86,87,89] The Diabetes Control and Complications Trial (DCCT) and the Stockholm Diabetes Intervention Study recently reported a rate of 0.62 and 1.10 severe reactions per patient year in intensively treated type I diabetic subjects, respectively.[72,88] Other studies examining the adverse effects of intensive insulin therapy in patients with type I diabetes report rates as high as 1.7 severe reactions per patient year.[85] In the intensive insulin trial of type II diabetes reported by Henry et al.,[7] there were no severe reactions and a low incidence of mild self-treated hypoglycemic reactions that actually decreased as the 6-month study progressed. Similarly, the 344A Veterans Administration Cooperative Study of type II diabetes reported a very low rate (0.0156 and 0.0096) of severe hypoglycemic events per patient after 1 year of intensive treatment with multiple daily injections and intraperitoneal insulin pumps, respectively[61] (see Table 73-5). These and other studies of intensive insulin therapy confirm that the risk of severe hypoglycemic reactions in type II diabetes is low and is several orders of magnitude less than in patients with type I diabetes.

The wide range of reported incidences is partially due to the differences in the characteristics of the study groups and in the definitions of severe hypoglycemia utilized. The lower incidence of severe hypoglycemia in type II diabetes, however, may be best explained by the presence of insulin resistance, which is often quite severe.[24] It is interesting to note that an inverse relationship has been reported between body mass index and the incidence of hypoglycemia in type II diabetes,[89] suggesting that the obese, insulin-resistant state may protect against the development of insulin-induced hypoglycemia. Other investigators have hypothesized that patients with type II diabetes may not be fundamentally different but may have less hypoglycemia, principally because they tend to receive less aggressive diabetes therapy and have been treated with insulin for a shorter period of time than patients with type I diabetes.[85] Regardless of the reasons, it appears that aggressive insulin therapy in type II diabetes is less prone to severe hypoglycemia than in type I diabetes.

Summary

Type II diabetes is a common disorder often accompanied by numerous metabolic abnormalities and organ-specific complications. Improved glycemia may delay or prevent the development of microvascular disease and reduce many or all of the acute and subacute complications that worsen the quality of daily life. Exogenous insulin is usually the last line of treatment used to normalize glycosylated hemoglobin in patients with type II diabetes who have failed other therapeutic modalities. Not all patients are candidates for aggressive insulin management; therefore, the goals of therapy should be tailored to the individual. Candidates for intensive management should be motivated, compliant, and educable, without other medical conditions and physical limitations that would preclude accurate and reliable home glucose monitoring (HGM) and insulin administration.

In selected patients, combination therapy with insulin and oral antidiabetic medications can be an effective method for normalizing glycemia without the need for rigorous insulin regimens. The most common clinical situation in which combination therapy can be successful occurs in patients who are failing sulfonylurea therapy but who show evidence of some responsiveness to oral agents. Bedtime intermediate-acting insulin is administered and progressively increased until the fasting blood glucose concentration is normalized. Additional benefits of combination therapy include ease of administration, excellent patient compliance and safety, and lower exogenous insulin requirements with less peripheral hyperinsulinemia. If combination therapy is not successful, a split-mixed regimen of an intermediate- and a regular-acting insulin equally divided between the prebreakfast and predinner periods is advised.

Insulin adjustments are based on HGM, and premixed insulins such as 70/30 are effective and easy to administer. A single-injection regimen is usually not effective in controlling day-long glycemia, and there are no proven advantages to multiple daily injections over the split-mixed regimen in type II diabetes. Continuous subcutaneous insulin infusion pumps can be particularly useful in treating patients with type II diabetes mellitus who do not respond satisfactorily to more conventional treatment strategies. Intraperitoneal insulin delivery systems hold considerable promise in type II diabetes because of their more physiologic delivery of insulin and their ability to selectively inhibit hepatic glucose production, with less peripheral insulinemia than with subcutaneous insulin injections.

We believe that the glycemic objectives for patients with type II diabetes should be similar to those for patients with type I diabetes, namely, to normalize glycemia and glycosylated hemoglobin without causing undue weight gain or hypoglycemia or adversely affecting the quality of daily life. This is best achieved in a multidisciplinary setting using complementary therapeutic modalities that include a combination of diet, exercise, and pharmacologic therapy. Emphasis should be placed on diet and exercise initially, and throughout the course of management as well, since even modest success with these therapies will enhance the glycemic response to both oral antidiabetic agents and insulin, if they are also required.

References

1. Galloway JA. Treatment of NIDDM with insulin agonists or substitutes. Diabetes Care 1990;13:1209
2. DeFronzo RA. Insulin resistance, hyperinsulinemia, and coronary artery disease: A complex metabolic web. J Cardiovasc Pharm 1992;20(suppl 11):S1
3. Caro JF. Insulin resistance in obese and nonobese man (Clinical Review 26). J Clin Endocrinol Metab 1991;73:691
4. Genuth S. Insulin use in NIDDM. Diabetes Care 1990;13:1240
5. Rizza R, Mandarino L, Gerich J. Dose-response characteristics for effects of insulin on production and utilization of glucose in man. Am J Physiol 1981; 240:630
6. Floyd JC, Funnell MM, Kazi I, Templeton C. Feasibility of adjustment of insulin dose by insulin-requiring type II diabetic patients. Diabetes Care 1990;13:386
7. Henry RR, Gumbiner B, Ditzler T, et al. Intensive conventional insulin therapy for type II diabetes. Metabolic effects during a 6 month outpatient trial. Diabetes Care 1993;16:21
8. Yki-Jarvinen H, Kauppila M, Kujansuu E, et al. Comparison of insulin regimens in patients with non–insulin-dependent diabetes mellitus. N Engl J Med 1992;327:1426
9. Lindstrom TH, Arnqvist HJ, von Schenck HH. Effect of conventional and intensified insulin therapy on free-insulin profiles and glycemic control in NIDDM. Diabetes Care 1992;15:27
10. Turner RC, Holman RR. Insulin use in NIDDM. Rationale based on pathophysiology of disease. Diabetes Care 1990;13:1011
11. Duckworth WC, Saudek CD, Henry RR, Veterans Affairs Study Group. Perspectives in diabetes. Why intraperitoneal delivery of insulin with implantable pumps in NIDDM? Diabetes 1992;41:657
12. Saudek CD, Duckworth WC, Veterans Affairs Study Group. The Department of Veterans Affairs Implanted Insulin Pump Study. Diabetes Care 1992;15:567
13. NIH Consensus Development Conference on Triglyceride, High Density Lipoprotein, and Coronary Heart Disease. Held February 26–28, 1992, Bethesda, MD. JAMA 1993;269(4):505
14. Expert Panel on Detection, Evaluation, and Treatment of High Blood Cholesterol in Adults. Summary of the second report of the National Cholesterol Education Program (NCEP) expert panel on detection, evaluation, and treatment of high blood cholesterol in adults (Adult Treatment Panel II). JAMA 1993;269:3015
15. Brunzell JD, Chait A. Lipoprotein pathophysiology and treatment. In: Rifkin H, Porte D, eds. Ellenberg and Rifkinn's Diabetes Mellitus: Theory and Practice. New York: Elsevier;1990:756
16. Howard BV, Howard WJ. The pathophysiology and treatment of lipid disorders in diabetes mellitus. In: Kahn CR, Weir GC, eds. Joslin's Diabetes Mellitus. Philadelphia: Lea & Febiger;1994:372–396
17. Bierman EL. Atherogenesis in diabetes. Arterioscler Thromb 1992;12:393
18. Donahue RP, Ochard TJ. Diabetes mellitus and macrovascular complications: An epidemiological perspective. Diabetes Care 1993;15:1141
19. Lopes-Virella MF, Klein RL, Lyons TJ, et al. Glycosylation of low-density lipoprotein enhances cholesteryl ester synthesis in human monocyte-derived macrophages. Diabetes 1988;37:550
20. Duell PB, Oram JF, Bierman EL. Nonenzymatic glycosylation of HDL and impaired HDL-receptor-mediated cholesterol efflux. Diabetes 1991;40:377
21. American Diabetes Association 1992–1993. Clinical Practice Recommendations American Diabetes Association 1992–1993. Diabetes Care 1993; 16(suppl 2):1
22. Davidson MB. Futility of self-monitoring of blood glucose without algorithms for adjusting insulin doses. Diabetes Care 1986;9:209

23. Bressler R, Johnson D. New pharmacological approaches to therapy of NIDDM. Diabetes Care 1992;15:792
24. Moses AC, Abrahamson MJ. Therapeutic approaches to insulin resistance. In: Moller DE, ed. Insulin Resistance. Chichester, UK: Wiley;1993:385–410
25. DeFronzo RA, Ferrannini E. Insulin resistance. A multifaceted syndrome responsible for NIDDM, obesity, hypertension, dyslipidemia, and atherosclerotic cardiovascular disease. Diabetes Care 1991;14:173
26. Groop LC, Widen E, Ferrannini EL. Insulin resistance and insulin deficiency in the pathogenesis of type 2 (non–insulin-dependent) diabetes mellitus: Errors of metabolism or of methods? Diabetologia 1993;36:1326
27. Lillioja S, Mott DM, Spraul M, et al. Insulin resistance and insulin secretory dysfunction as precursors of non–insulin-dependent diabetes mellitus. N Engl J Med 1993;329:1988
28. Tuomi T, Groop LC, Zimmet PZ, et al. Antibodies to glutamic acid decarboxylase reveal latent autoimmune diabetes mellitus in adults with a non–insulin-dependent onset of disease. Diabetes 1993;42:359
29. World Health Organization. Diabetes mellitus: Report of a WHO study group (Tech Rep Ser No 727). Geneva: World Health Organization;1985
30. National Institute of Health. Publication No 95-1468. In: Harris M, ed. Diabetes in America, 2 ed. Bethesda, MD: National Institute of Health;1995:85–116
31. Henry RR, Edelman SV. Advances in treatment of type II diabetes mellitus in the elderly. Geriatrics 1992;47:24
32. Ferrannini E, Stern MP, Galvan AQ, et al. Impact of associated conditions on glycemic control of NIDDM patients. Diabetes Care 1992;15:508
33. Rossetti L, Giaccari A, DeFronzo RA. Glucose toxicity. Diabetes Care 1990; 13:610
34. Bailey TS, Mezitis NHE. Combination therapy with insulin and sulfonylureas for type II diabetes. Diabetes Care 1990;13:687
35. Lebovitz HE, Pasmantier R. Combination insulin-sulfonylurea therapy. Diabetes Care 1990;12:667
36. Groop LC, Widen E, Ekstrand A, et al. Morning or bedtime NPH insulin combined with sulfonurea in treatment of NIDDM. Diabetes Care 1992;15:831
37. Pugh JA, Wagner ML, Sawyer J, et al. Is combination sulfonylurea and insulin therapy useful in NIDDM patients? A metaanalysis. Diabetes Care 1992; 15:953
38. Riddle MC. Evening insulin strategy. Diabetes Care 1990;13:676
39. Taskinen M-R, Sane T, Helve E, et al. Bedtime insulin for suppression of overnight free-fatty acid, blood glucose, and glucose production in NIDDM. Diabetes 1989;38:580
40. Pasmantier R, Chaiken RL, Hirsch SR, Lebovitz HE. Metabolic effects of combination glipizide and human proinsulin treatment in NIDDM. Diabetes Care 1990;13(Suppl 3):42
41. Groop LC, Groop P-H, Stenman S. Combined insulin-sulfonylurea therapy in treatment of NIDDM. Diabetes Care 1990;13(Suppl 3):47
42. Karlander SG, Gutniak MKM, Efendic S. Effects of combination therapy with glyburide and insulin on serum lipid levels in NIDDM patients with secondary sulfonylurea failure. Diabetes Care 1991;14:963
43. Mezitis NHE, Heshka S, Saitas V, et al. Combination therapy for NIDDM with biosynthetic human insulin and glyburide. Diabetes Care 1992;15: 265
44. Vigneri R, Trischitta V, Italia S, et al. Treatment of NIDDM patients with secondary failure to glyburide: Comparison of the addition of either metformin or bedtime NPH insulin to glyburide. Diabetes Metab 1991;17:232
45. Raskin P. Combination therapy in NIDDM. N Engl J Med 1992;327:1453
46. Marks JB. Combination glyburide and insulin treatment in secondary sulfonylurea failure. Clin Diabetes 1994;12:21
47. Koivisto VA. Insulin therapy in Type II diabetes. Diabetes Care 1993;16 (suppl 3):29
48. Polonsky KS, Rubenstein AH. C-peptide as a measure of the secretion and hepatic extraction of insulin. Pitfalls and limitations. Diabetes 1984;33:486
49. Greco AC, Caputo S, Bertoli A, Ghirlanda G. The beta cell function in NIDDM patients with secondary failure: A three year follow-up of combined oral hypoglycemic and insulin therapy. Horm Metab Res 1992;24:280
50. Kudlacek S, Schernthaner G. The effect of insulin treatment on HbAlc, body weight and lipids in type 2 diabetic patients with secondary failure to sulfonylureas. A five year follow-up study. Horm Metab Res 1992;24:478
51. A multicenter study: U.K. Prospective Diabetes Study. II. Reduction in HbA_{1c} with basal insulin supplement, sulfonylurea, or biguanide therapy in maturity-onset diabetes. Diabetes 1985;34:793
52. Prospective Diabetes Study Group: Prospective Diabetes Study (UKPDS). II. Study design, progress and performance. Diabetologia 1991;34:877–890
53. Abraira C, Johnson N, Colwell J, et al. VA Cooperative Study on glycemic control and complications in type II diabetes (VACSCM). Diabetes Care 1995; 18:1113
54. Abraira C, Johnson N, Colwell JA, and the VA CSDM Group. A successful feasibility trial: The VA Cooperative Study on Control and Complications in Diabetes Mellitus Type II (CSDM) (abstract). Diabetes 1993;42(Suppl 1): 147A #459
55. Turner RC, Phillips MA, Ward EA. Ultralente based insulin regimens—clinical applications, advantages and disadvantages. Acta Med Scand 1983;671 (suppl):75
56. Jennings AM, Lewis KS, Murdoch S, et al. Randomized trial comparing continuous subcutaneous insulin infusion and conventional insulin therapy in type II diabetic patients poorly controlled with sulfonylureas. Diabetes Care 1991;14:738
57. Garvey WT, Olefsky JM, Griffin J, et al. The effect of insulin treatment on insulin secretion and insulin action in type II diabetes mellitus. Diabetes 1985;34:222
58. Glaser B, Leibovich G, Nesher R, et al. Improved beta-cell function after intensive insulin treatment in severe non–insulin-dependent diabetes. Acta Endocrinol 1988;118:365
59. Selam JL, Raccah D, Jean-Didier N, et al. Large-scale multicenter evaluation of a programmable implantable insulin pump in type I diabetes. Diabetes 1991;40(suppl 1):424A
60. Veterans Affairs Study Group, Chicago, IL: Veterans Affairs Implantable Insulin Pump (IIP) Study: Comparison of effects of implantable pumps and multiple insulin injections on metabolic and physiological parameters (abstract). Diabetes 1994;43(suppl 1):61A #195
61. Veterans Affairs Study Group, Veterans Affairs Medical Center Hines IL: Veterans Affairs Implantable Insulin Pump (IIP) Study: Mean glycemia and hypoglycemia (abstract). Diabetes 1994;43(suppl 1):61A #193
62. Brange J, Owens DR, Kang S, Volund A. Monermic insulins and their experimental clinical implications. Diabetes Care 1990;13:923
63. Laube BL, Georgopoulos A, Adams GK. Preliminary studies of the efficacy of insulin aerosol delivered by oral inhalation in diabetic patients. JAMA 1993;269:2106
64. Moses AC, Flier JS. Nasal insulin: An approach to periprandial control of blood glucose. In: Larkins RG, Zimmet PZ, Chisholm DJ, eds. Diabetes 1988; Amsterdam: Elsevier;1989:81–84
65. Bondy CA, Underwood LE, Clemmons DR, et al. Clinical uses of insulin-like growth factor I. Ann Intern Med 1994;120:593
66. Kolaczynski JW, Caro JF. Insulin-like growth factor-1 therapy in diabetes: Physiologic basic, clinical benefits, and risks. Ann Intern Med 1994;120:47
67. Guler H-P, Zapf J, Froesch ER. Short-term metabolic effects of recombinant human insulin-like growth factor I in healthy adults. N Engl J Med 1987; 317:137
68. Zenobi PD, Jaeggi-Groisman SE, Riesen WF, et al. Insulin-like growth factor-1 improves glucose and lipid metabolism in type 2 diabetes mellitus. J Clin Invest 1992;90:2234
69. Walker JL, Ginalska-Malinowska M, Romer TE, et al. Effects of the infusion of insulin-like growth factor I in a child with growth hormone insensitivity syndrome (laron dwarfism). N Engl J Med 1991;21:1483
70. Kolaczynski JW, Caro JF. Insulin-like growth factor-1 therapy in diabetes: Physiologic basis, clinical benefits, and risks. Ann Intern Med 1994;120:47
71. Brownlee M. Glycation products and the pathogenesis of diabetic complications. Diabetes Care 1992;15:1835
72. The Diabetes Control and Complications Trial Research Group: The effect of intensive treatment of diabetes on the development and progression of long-term complications in insulin-dependent diabetes mellitus. N Engl J Med 1993;329:977
73. Stern MP, Patterson JK, Haffner SM, et al. Lack of awareness and treatment of hyperlipidemia in type II diabetes in a community survey. JAMA 1989;262:360
74. Fontbonne A, Eschwege E, Cambien F, et al. Hypertriglyceridemia as a risk factor for coronary heart disease mortality in subjects with impaired glucose tolerance or diabetes. Diabetologia 1989;32:300
75. Garg A, Grundy SM. Management of dyslipidemia in NIDDM. Diabetes Care 1990;13:153
76. Dunn FL, Raskin P, Bilheimer DW, Grundy SM. The effect of diabetic control on very low-density lipoprotein-triglyceride metabolism in patients with type II diabetes mellitus and marked hypertriglyceridemia. Metabolism 1984;33:117
77. Stern MP, Haffner SM. Body fat distribution and hyperinsulinemia as risk factors for diabetes and cardiovascular disease. Arteriosclerosis 1986;6:123
78. Haffner SM, Fong D, Hazuda HP, et al. Hyperinsulinemia, upper body adiposity, and cardiovascular risk factors in non-diabetics. Metabolism 1988;37:338
79. Stout RW. Insulin resistance, hyperinsulinemia, dyslipidemia and atherosclerosis. In: Moller DE, ed. Insulin Resistance. Chichester, UK: Wiley; 1993: 355–383
80. Karam JH, Grodsky GM, Gorsham PH. Excessive insulin response to glucose in obese subjects as measured by immunochemical assay. Diabetes 1963;12:197
81. Stolar MW. Atherosclerosis in diabetes: The role of hyperinsulinemia. Metabolism 1988;37(suppl 1):1
82. Group L, Widen E, Franssila-Kalunki A, et al. Different effects of insulin and oral anti-diabetic agents on glucose and energy metabolism in type 2 diabetes mellitus. Diabetologia 1989;32:599
83. Flier JS. Obesity and lipoprotein disorders. In: Kahn RC, Weir GC, eds. Joslin's Diabetes Mellitus. Philadelphia: Lea & Febiger;1994:351–356
84. Bray GA. Basic mechanisms and very low calorie diets. In: Blackburn GL, Bray GA, eds. Management of Obesity by Severe Caloric Restriction. Littleton, Mass: PSG;1995:129–169
85. MacLeod KM, Hepburn DA, Frier BM. Frequency and morbidity of severe hypoglycaemia in insulin-treated diabetic patients. Diab Med 1993;10:238
86. Hepburn DA, MacLeod KM, Frier BM. Frequency of symptomatology of hypoglycaemia in patients with type 2 diabetes treated with insulin (abstract). Diabetic Medicine 1992;9(suppl 1):47A
87. Halter J, Anderson L, Herman W, et al. Intensive treatment safely improves glycemic control of elderly patients with diabetes mellitus (abstract). Diabetes 1993;42(suppl 1):146A #456
88. Reichard P, Pihl M. Mortality and treatment side-effects during long-term intensified conventional insulin treatment in the Stockholm Diabetes Intervention Study. Diabetes 1994;43:313
89. Casparie AF, Elving LD. Severe hypoglycemia in diabetic patients: Frequency, causes, prevention. Diabetes Care 1985;8:141

Diabetes Mellitus, edited by Derek LeRoith, Simeon I. Taylor, and Jerrold M. Olefsky. Lippincott–Raven Publishers, Philadelphia © 1996.

Chapter 74

New Therapies for Non–Insulin-Dependent Diabetes Mellitus: Thiazolidinediones

Randall W. Whitcomb, Alan R. Saltiel, and Dean H. Lockwood

Introduction

To date, the treatment of non–insulin-dependent diabetes mellitus (NIDDM) has involved the use of insulin and/or insulin secretagogues such as sulfonylureas and/or biguanides such as metformin. Although these agents have been efficacious to a degree, they do not deal directly with the underlying pathology of insulin-resistance.

The thiazolidinediones represent a novel drug class that may directly decrease insulin resistance by enhancing insulin action in skeletal muscle, liver, and adipose tissue. One of these compounds, troglitazone, has progressed to late-stage clinical development. Others, such as pioglitazone and ciglitazone, have yielded a side effect profile that has made them unacceptable for long-term human studies.

The structures of some thiazolidinedione compounds are shown in Figure 74-1. All of these compounds contain a substituted thiazolidinedione structure, with modifications selected to improve their pharmacologic effects. Some of these modifications have significantly enhanced the bioactivity of these compounds, although it is not known whether their increased potency results from changes in bioavailability, metabolism, or mechanistic efficacy. Troglitazone was designed to combine the insulin-sensitizing activity of the thiazolidinedione class with a potent lipid peroxide–lowering activity. Lipid peroxides have been suggested as one of the major causative factors of atherosclerosis and their concentrations are frequently elevated in diabetics, suggesting that troglitazone might be an especially effective agent for NIDDM.

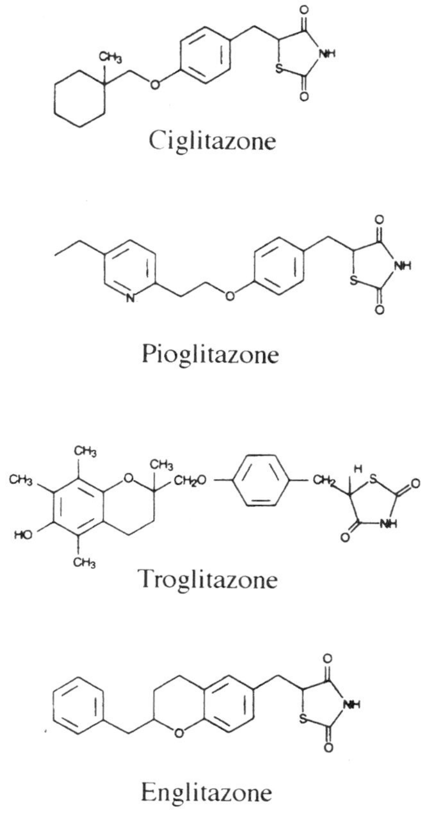

Ciglitazone

Pioglitazone

Troglitazone

Englitazone

Figure 74-1. Structures of some thiazolidinedione insulin-sensitizing agents.

Thiazolidinediones Improve Insulin Sensitivity in Animal Models of Diabetes

Thiazolidinediones appear to enhance insulin action without directly stimulating insulin secretion in pancreatic β-cells. As such, these drugs have been used to assess the impact of lowering insulin resistance on a wide variety of pathophysiologic processes. These agents markedly decrease plasma glucose, insulin, and triglyceride concentrations in genetically insulin-resistant animals, including the KKA, *ob/ob*, and *db/db* mice, the Zucker *fa/fa* rat, and others.[1,2] The antihyperglycemic activity of some thiazolidinediones has also been demonstrated in nongenetic insulin-resistance models, including both the fructose-fed and high fat diet–adapted rat.[3,4] In contrast, plasma glucose concentrations are unaffected by these drugs in the insulin-deficient streptozotocin diabetic rat unless administered with concomitant doses of insulin. The thiazolidinediones, however, improve insulin sensitivity in these animals, as determined by increased glucose infusion and decreased hepatic glucose output in euglycemic clamp studies.[5] Plasma glucose is similarly unaffected in normal animals, although thiazolidinediones can enhance insulin action in these animals, resulting in lower plasma insulin and lipid concentrations.[6] These observations highlight the distinguishing feature of these insulin-sensitizing agents: the apparent lack of hypoglycemic activity in euglycemic animals, despite the potent sensitization of insulin action. This property differentiates thiazolidinediones from other current therapies for non–insulin-dependent diabetes mellitus (NIDDM), including insulin itself and insulin secretagogues such as sulfonylureas, which have considerable hypoglycemic activity.

To assess the mechanism of insulin sensitization in diabetic animal models, both glucose disposal and hepatic glucose output have been studied by the euglycemic hyperinsulinemic clamp technique after administration of the drugs.[3,7,8] In general, improvements in insulin sensitivity induced by thiazolidinediones require several days of treatment, suggesting that transcriptional modifications are involved in the actions of these drugs (see below). A number of metabolic processes have been evaluated in tissues from animals exposed to these agents. Chronic treatment of obese Zucker rats with troglitazone (unpublished) or pioglitazone[9] led to increased sensitivity and responsiveness of insulin-induced glucose uptake in isolated adipocytes. In Wistar fatty rats, pioglitazone produced an increase in insulin-stimulated glycogen synthesis and glycolysis assayed in isolated soleus muscle.[10] Similar improvements in glucose uptake were observed with englitazone in obese Zucker rats.[7] Additionally, the thiazolidinediones dramatically reduce hepatic glucose output in a number of diabetic models. These effects appear to result from a decreased rate of gluconeogenesis in the liver.[11]

In addition to the profound effects of thiazolidinediones on glucose homeostasis, these agents exert lipid-lowering effects in diabetic and nondiabetic animals. Hypertriglyceridemia may be an important risk factor for atherosclerosis, especially in NIDDM patients. Plasma triglyceride and free fatty acid concentrations are markedly reduced in a number of diabetic rodent models by treatment with thiazolidinediones.[2–4,6,7,12,13] These effects are observed in both insulin-resistant and insulin-deficient animals, suggesting that the triglyceride-lowering actions of these drugs may not be related to the sensitization of insulin action. Thiazolidinediones also regulate cholesterol concentrations, as well as lipoprotein profiles in rodents. Although total plasma cholesterol does not respond dramatically to these agents, increased high density lipoprotein cholesterol and decreased low density and very low density lipoprotein cholesterol has been observed, along with some changes in circulating lipoproteins.[14]

The triglyceride-lowering effects of troglitazone result from inhibition of triglyceride synthesis in the liver, as well as increased clearance in the periphery.[2] The mechanism by which troglitazone reduces hepatic triglyceride secretion in either diabetic or normal rats is not clear. This effect might result from a direct action on the liver or perhaps may result indirectly from the reduction in plasma insulin and free fatty acid concentrations. Interestingly, although thiazolidinediones have no effect on plasma glucose in streptozotocin-treated rats, plasma triglyceride concentrations are significantly reduced. Moreover, treatment of obese Zucker rats with streptozotocin to block insulin production prevented the reduction of hepatic triglyceride synthesis by troglitazone without inhibiting triglyceride clearance. Troglitazone also increased post–heparin lipoprotein lipase activity in both streptozotocin-treated and untreated Zucker rats (unpublished). Thus, it appears that the decrease in triglyceride concentrations induced by thiazolidinediones involves both reduced synthesis and enhanced clearance, perhaps due to separate biochemical mechanisms on the liver and the periphery.

Although thiazolidinediones in general do not directly modulate insulin secretion in islet cells, the amelioration of insulin resistance might produce insulin-sparing effects, restoring the responsiveness of desensitized islets to external stimuli. Troglitazone produced marked regranulation of pancreatic islets in severely diabetic *db/db* mice, restoring cellular insulin content.[15] Although the precise mechanism of this effect is not known, it is likely to be a reflection of decreases in plasma glucose concentration. Indeed, glucose toxicity is thought to be responsible for attenuating glucose-dependent insulin secretion in some cases. Thus, the regranulation of islets in *db/db* mice may represent one of several effects of these drugs that are exerted indirectly through amelioration of glucose toxicity.

Thiazolidinediones May Improve the Insulin Resistance Syndrome

Insulin resistance is thought to be closely associated with a collection of metabolic abnormalities known as *insulin resistance syndrome*, or *syndrome X*, whose manifestations include glucose intolerance, dislipidemia, vascular disease, obesity, and hypertension.[16] Although it is not known whether insulin resistance is a causative factor for any or all of the symptoms associated with this syndrome, these abnormalities are also found in many animal models. In some of these cases, hypertension may result from hyperinsulinemia, perhaps due to increased sodium retention. Because of the profound insulin-lowering effects of thiazolidinediones, these agents have been tested for their hypotensive effects. Troglitazone reduced hypertension in obese Zucker rats[17] and high fructose–fed rats.[3] Pioglitazone was shown to suppress hypertension in Dahl salt-sensitive rats[18] and obese insulin-resistant rhesus monkeys.[19] The biochemical basis for the reduction in hypertension associated with insulin resistance is not known but may reflect increased renal sodium excretion, increased glomerular filtration rates, or inhibition of renal arterial smooth muscle cell proliferation. It is possible, however, that correction of hypertension in these animal models may not be related to insulin sensitization.

In Vitro Studies on Thiazolidinediones

Assessments of the molecular mechanisms underlying the actions of thiazolidinediones have been difficult in animal models. Because glucose and lipid metabolism is regulated by complex feedback systems, molecular changes induced by drugs or hormones are rapidly counteracted. Such homeostatic loops are generally not present in tissue culture cells, offering an opportunity to study specific responses to defined stimuli. Three such cell lines—the 3T3-L1 mouse fibroblast, which can differentiate into insulin-responsive adipocytes; HepG2, a human hepatoma cell line; and L-6 rat myocytes—have been used as model systems to evaluate the effects of thiazolidinediones on fat, liver, and muscle to probe the molecular actions of these drugs.

The cellular actions of insulin are characterized by a wide variety of effects initiated by the tyrosine kinase activity of the receptor. Although the precise mechanisms involved in the regulation of intermediary metabolism by insulin are not precisely understood, there are several candidate pathways that involve a complex series of protein phosphorylations.[20] The effects of thiazolidinediones on these pathways have been extensively evaluated and appear not to primarily involve mobilization of early signaling events in insulin action.

Pioglitazone, troglitazone, and BRL49653 increase dramatically the number of fibroblasts and the rate at which they are converted to adipocytes.[21–23] This effect is absolutely dependent on insulin, perhaps accounting for the observed increase in adiposity of rodents treated with these drugs. Thiazolidinediones also significantly increase both the basal and insulin-stimulated uptake of glucose in 3T3-L1 cells, as well as in L6 myocytes.[24–27] These effects may account for the increased glucose disposal produced by the drug in animal models and human clamp studies. Increased glucose transport correlates with enhanced expression of the transporters GLUT-1 and GLUT-4. More detailed studies in 3T3-L1 cells have suggested that increases in glucose transporter expression are not the result of a direct effect of thiazolidinediones on expression of these genes, but may reflect induction of another gene product that, in turn, regulates transporter expression. Additional studies suggest that the cellular effects of thiazolidinediones are likely to reflect an early transcriptional event in fat cell differentiation that requires a target already present in preadipocytes. One interesting candidate for such a target was recently identified as the fatty acid activated receptor, a member of the nuclear steroid/thyroid hormone superfamily that apparently interacts with fatty acids to regulate transcription.[28] Although the precise role of this factor in the biologic actions of thiazolidinediones remains to be established, the fatty acid activated receptor is a promising candidate for a thiazolidinedione "receptor." A hypothetical model showing how it might sensitize the actions of insulin is depicted in Figure 74-2.

In addition to enhancing glucose disposal, troglitazone facilitates insulin-dependent inhibition of hepatic glucose output, presumably due to attenuation of gluconeogenesis and/or activation of glycolysis.[29] Gene expression studies were performed in HepG2

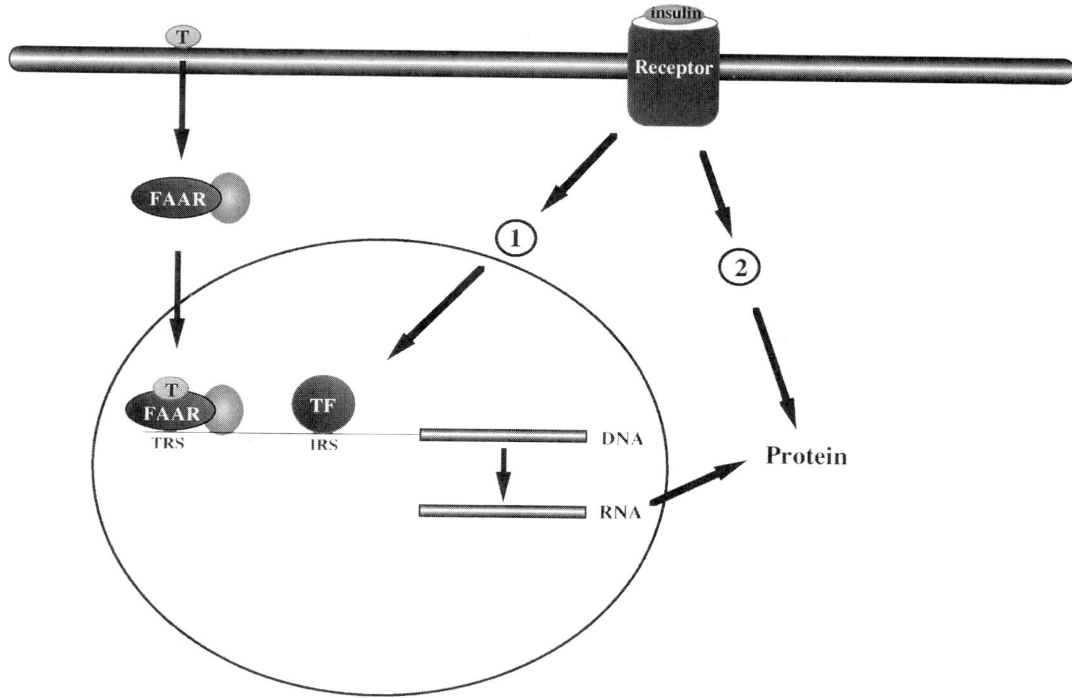

FIGURE 74-2. A hypothetical model for the mechanism of insulin sensitization by thiazolidinediones. A model is depicted for two mechanisms by which thiazolidinediones (T) might sensitize cells via transcriptional regulation. These agents may interact with a new class of nuclear receptors, called fatty acid activated receptors (FAAR), which interact with fatty acids to induce fat cell differentiation. This interaction, which may occur in the cytoplasm, can induce the binding of FAAR to specific DNA sequences (TRS) in thiazolidinedione-responsive genes. This DNA binding may involve the dimerization of FAAR with itself or a with a related transcription factor. In one hypothetical model, FAAR can regulate genes, such as lipoprotein lipase, that are themselves insulin responsive via separate insulin-regulated transcription factors (TF), resulting in enhanced transcriptional activity. Alternatively, thiazolidinediones may exert insulin-mimetic effects by interacting with sites that overlap with insulin-response sequences (IRS), as may be the case with the glucokinase promoter. In the second example, FAAR may induce the expression of genes that encode for proteins that are targets of insulin action, such as the glucose transporters.

and H35 cells transfected with the promoters for known insulin-responsive genes, such as glucokinase and PEPCK. Although the PEPCK promoter was unresponsive to the compound in H35 cells, troglitazone rapidly stimulated transcription of the glucokinase gene in HepG2 cells at doses as low as 1 nM, even in the absence of insulin (Li WW, Leff T, unpublished data, 1995). The effects of insulin and troglitazone were not additive, and a submaximal dose of the drug increased the insulin sensitivity. Comparison of the troglitazone-responsive promoter in the glucokinase gene to genes responding in fat cells may lead to a more complete understanding of the precise molecular mechanisms of the drug, particularly regarding the role of nuclear receptors such as the fatty acid activated receptor.

The manifestation of insulin resistance in humans as well as animal models is a complex phenomenon that may reflect multiple underlying metabolic abnormalities. Because the cellular basis for these phenomena remains largely unexplained, it has been difficult to study insulin resistance in tissue culture models. In addition to the genetically endowed insulin resistance that precedes the development of non–insulin-dependent diabetes mellitus (NIDDM), there is a secondary resistance that appears to be associated with hyperglycemia and that may be related to the resistance observed in insulin-dependent diabetes mellitus (IDDM). A number of studies have shown that insulin receptor tyrosine phosphorylation is significantly reduced in diabetic subjects.[30] Moreover, fibroblasts exposed to high ambient glucose concentrations exhibit reduced receptor tyrosine phosphorylation, which might be mediated through an inhibitory serine phosphorylation of the receptor.[31] Troglitazone restored the hyperglycemia-induced reduction of receptor phosphorylation in diabetic rats[32] and was shown to prevent the glucose-induced inhibition of insulin receptor tyrosine phosphorylation in cultured cells after only a 20-minute preincubation period.[33] Although this effect of the drug may not be relevant to its insulin-sensitizing effects in normoglycemic paradigms, it may contribute in some way to the antihyperglycemic actions of the drug. Moreover, the rapid onset of this effect on receptor phosphorylation suggests that it may be mechanistically distinct from the transcriptional effects described above.

Use of Troglitazone in Non–Insulin-Dependent Diabetes Mellitus

Initial studies with troglitazone indicate that this agent is efficacious in treating patients with non–insulin-dependent diabetes mellitus (NIDDM).[34] The initial studies carried out in Japan indicate that decreases in glucose, hemoglobin A_{1c}, and triglycerides occur in a dose-dependent fashion.[35] Longer-term studies (up to 1 year) have indicated that troglitazone's effect on these parameters is maintained. A recent study published by Suter et al.,[36] using detailed euglycemic clamp techniques, has elucidated the mechanism in part of the glucose-lowering effect of troglitazone in NIDDM patients. In this study, 11 subjects were treated with 400 mg/day of troglitazone for 6 to 12 weeks. Eight of these subjects showed a clinically significant response to the drug, and three patients had basically no response. The fasting plasma glucose concentration fell from 12.5 to 10.7 mmol/L in the total group; the responders demonstrated a more dramatic fall, from 12.7 to 8.3 mmol/L. Glucose disposal rates during the glucose clamp study were increased in all subjects after troglitazone treatment, with mean increases of 63% and 41% in the total group and in the responders, respectively, using both physiologic and high-dose insulin clamp settings. Basal hepatic glucose production fell by 17% in the total group and by 28% in the responders. More striking was the response of glucose and insulin following glucose challenge, either with a standard oral glucose tolerance test or with a meal tolerance test. The area under the oral glucose tolerance test glucose curve improved by 17% in the total group and by 29% in the responder group (Fig. 74-3). The area under the meal tolerance test glucose curve improved by 38% and 52%, respectively, in the total and responder groups. Meal tolerance test levels of insulin, free fatty acids, and glucagon were significantly lower after treatment. The high density lipoprotein cholesterol and total triglyceride concentrations were also positively affected, with an increase in high density lipoprotein of 4 mg/dL and a decrease in triglycerides of 40 mg/dL after treatment with the drug. The authors concluded that troglitazone improved insulin resistance, as well as reducing insulinemia and hepatic glucose production, with a very positive impact on both fasting and postprandial glycemia in NIDDM patients.

More recently, a large multicenter clinical trial has been carried out in NIDDM patients.[37] A 12-week placebo-controlled study in which patients were randomized to four doses of troglitazone or placebo was performed in 792 NIDDM patients with hemoglobin A_{1c} concentrations ranging between 7% and 11%. Decreases in glucose concentrations compared to placebo were 40, 48, 49, and 60 mg/dL in the 200-, 400-, 600-, and 800-mg groups, respectively. Insulin concentrations fell approximately 20% in the 400-, 600-, and 800-mg groups but did not fall significantly in the 200-mg group. It is noteworthy that fasting glucose concentrations continued to fall at 12 weeks of treatment. There was no change in the weight of patients during this study.

Further analysis of the glycemic response data indicates that there is a subgroup of patients who have a suboptimal response to troglitazone. These patients have minimal β-cell function, as characterized by a C-peptide concentration <1.5mg/mL. This is consistent with other animal and human data indicating that a minimal level of endogenous insulin is required for troglitazone to act. Further long-term studies will be necessary to characterize fully and perhaps predict more accurately which patients will respond in a clinically meaningful manner to troglitazone.

Fasting serum lipid profiles showed an increase in high density lipoprotein cholesterol, a decrease in triglycerides, and a dose-dependent decrease in free fatty acids during the study. As both triglycerides and circulating free fatty acids did decrease, this suggests that troglitazone may have a direct effect on lipolysis in adipose tissue. Whether this is due to insulin's regulation of lipoprotein lipase or to an effect on other lipolytic enzymes via troglitazone's insulin-enhancing actions will require further study.

The prevalence and nature of treatment-emergent adverse events were similar for placebo- and troglitazone-treated patients, including adverse events related to the hepatic, cardiac, hematologic, and digestive systems. The most frequent adverse events were a 4% incidence of dizziness in the troglitazone group compared with 2% in the placebo group and a 2% incidence of nausea in the troglitazone group compared with 0% in the placebo group. A total of 76% of the patients completed the study. Six percent of the patients in both the drug and placebo groups dropped out of the study because of an adverse event. Thirteen percent

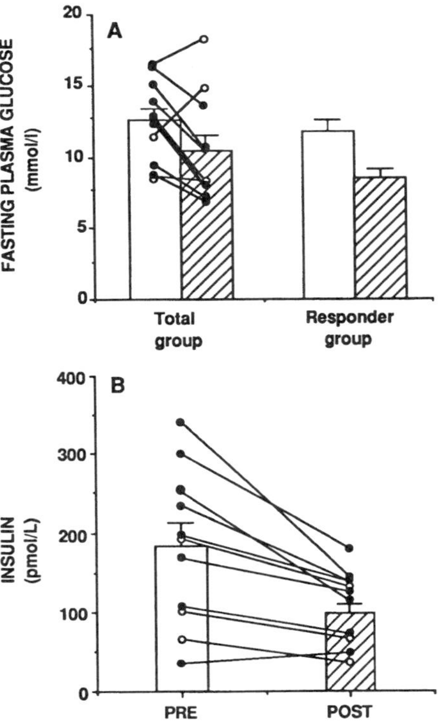

FIGURE 74-3. *A,* Mean ± standard error fasting glucose values before (open bars) and during (hatched bars) CS-045 treatment in total group and responder group ($p < 0.005$). ●, Nonresponders; ○, responders. *B,* Mean ± SE fasting insulin levels before (open bar) and during (hatched bar) CS-045 treatment. Individual data are plotted, and each subject's data before and during study are connected by lines. (Reproduced with permission from Yoshioku J, Nishiama H, Shiroki T, et al. Antihypertensive effects of CS-045 treatment in obese Zucker rats. Metabolism 1993;42:75–80).

dropped out because of lack of efficacy. A disproportionate number of dropouts was caused by lack of efficacy in the placebo group. These preliminary studies suggest that troglitazone will be an agent with multiple positive clinical effects in treating NIDDM patients.

Use of Troglitazone in Impaired Glucose Tolerance

As previously discussed, troglitazone improves insulin resistance in multiple disease states. There is recent evidence that patients with impaired glucose tolerance and insulin resistance progress to non–insulin-dependent diabetes mellitus (NIDDM) at a rate of up to 5% per year, thus representing an important risk factor for developing NIDDM.[38,39] Independent of this progression to NIDDM, however, is an increased incidence of cardiovascular disease that has been associated with impaired glucose tolerance.[40] As insulin resistance appears to be the primary disorder in persons with impaired glucose tolerance, a drug such as troglitazone, which improves insulin sensitivity, could be efficacious in treating impaired glucose tolerance and, theoretically, in preventing the progression of impaired glucose tolerance to NIDDM.

Recent data published by Nolan et al.[41] demonstrate that persons with impaired glucose tolerance have an increased rate of glucose disposal and of insulin sensitivity following 12 weeks of

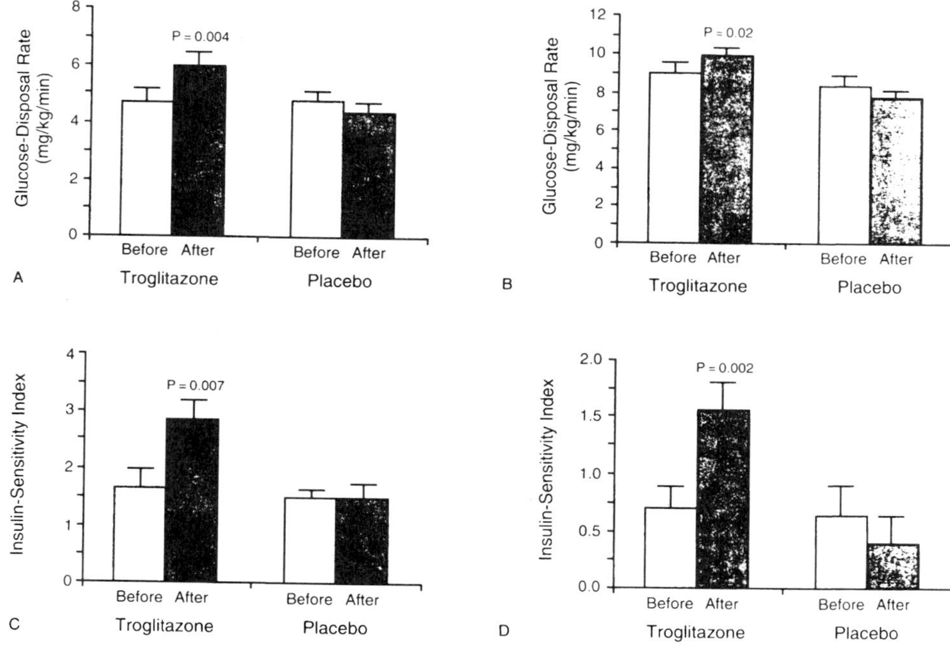

Figure 74-4. Measurements of insulin resistance before and after the administration of troglitazone or placebo for 12 weeks in obese subjects without diabetes. Values are means ± standard error. ***A*** shows the results of studies with the euglycemic-hyperinsulinemic clamp in which insulin was infused at a rate of 40 mU per square meter per minute. ***B*** shows the results of studies with the euglycemic-hyperinsulinemic clamp in which insulin was infused at a rate of 300 mU per square meter per minute. ***C*** shows the values for the insulin-sensitivity index as calculated from basal values and values measured during the studies with the euglycemic-hyperinsulinemic clamp in which insulin was infused at a rate of 40 mU per square meter per minute. ***D*** shows the values for the insulin-sensitivity index as calculated from the results of intravenous glucose-tolerance tests. (Reproduced with permission from Bowen L, Steven PP, Stevenson R, Shulman CI. The effect of CP-68772, a thiazolidine derivative, on insulin sensitivity in lean and obese Zucker rats. Metabolism 1993;40:1025–1030.)

treatment with troglitazone at a dose of 400 mg/day (Fig. 74-4). Both fasting and glucose-stimulated insulin concentrations decreased in these persons. In addition, they showed a significant decrease in both systolic and diastolic blood pressure after treatment with troglitazone.

An additional larger study involving 54 patients with impaired glucose tolerance has substantiated these findings.[42] The patients in this study were required to meet World Health Organization criteria for impaired glucose tolerance, as evidenced by 2-hour glucose concentration >140 mg/dL after a standard 75-g glucose challenge. After 6 weeks of treatment with either placebo or 400 mg troglitazone, 75% of the patients treated with troglitazone had converted to a normal glucose tolerance pattern compared with 38% of those receiving placebo. By 12 weeks, the conversion rates had increased to 80% of the patients receiving troglitazone and 48% of those receiving placebo, with a statistically significant decrease in the area under the curve of both insulin (Fig. 74-5) and glucose (Fig. 74-6) responses after an oral glucose tolerance test. Although there was no significant change in either low density or high density lipoprotein cholesterol, there was a significant decrease in fasting triglycerides in patients treated with troglitazone.

The ability of troglitazone to improve insulin resistance, lower plasma insulin concentrations, and normalize glucose tolerance in subjects with impaired glucose tolerance may have implications for the prevention of NIDDM in such persons. Longer-term treatment of persons with impaired glucose tolerance with troglitazone will be necessary to substantiate these preliminary findings.

Potential Use of Troglitazone in Polycystic Ovarian Syndrome

The estimated prevalence of polycystic ovaries is 10% in women of reproductive age.[43] Up to 50% of women with polycystic ovaries also have the metabolic findings of insulin resistance, hyperandrogenism, and acanthosis nigricans.[44,45] Polycystic ovarian syndrome (PCOS) is another example of the manifestations of insulin resistance—in this instance, in premenopausal women.

The histology of the ovary is abnormal in PCOS. This is caused by an abnormal hormonal environment in which continuous luteinizing hormone secretion leads to thecal and stromal hyperplasia with increased luteinizing hormone–dependent androgen production. In addition, acyclic follicle-stimulating hormone secretion results in an arrest of follicular genesis and inadequate granulosis cell aromatizing activity. The result is an increased concentration of androgens in the peripheral circulation in PCOS. Hyperinsulinemia is uniquely associated with PCOS. When total body insulin action is measured by the euglycemic glucose clamp technique, women with PCOS demonstrate peripheral insulin resistance similar to that found in persons with non–insulin-dependent diabetes mellitus (NIDDM).[46] Associated obesity has a synergistic deleterious impact on glucose tolerance in persons with PCOS. Twenty percent of obese women with PCOS have impaired glucose tolerance or NIDDM. In lean women with PCOS, β-cell function appears to be normal; however, the combination of PCOS and obesity results in β-cell dysfunction.[47,48] Other investigations have revealed

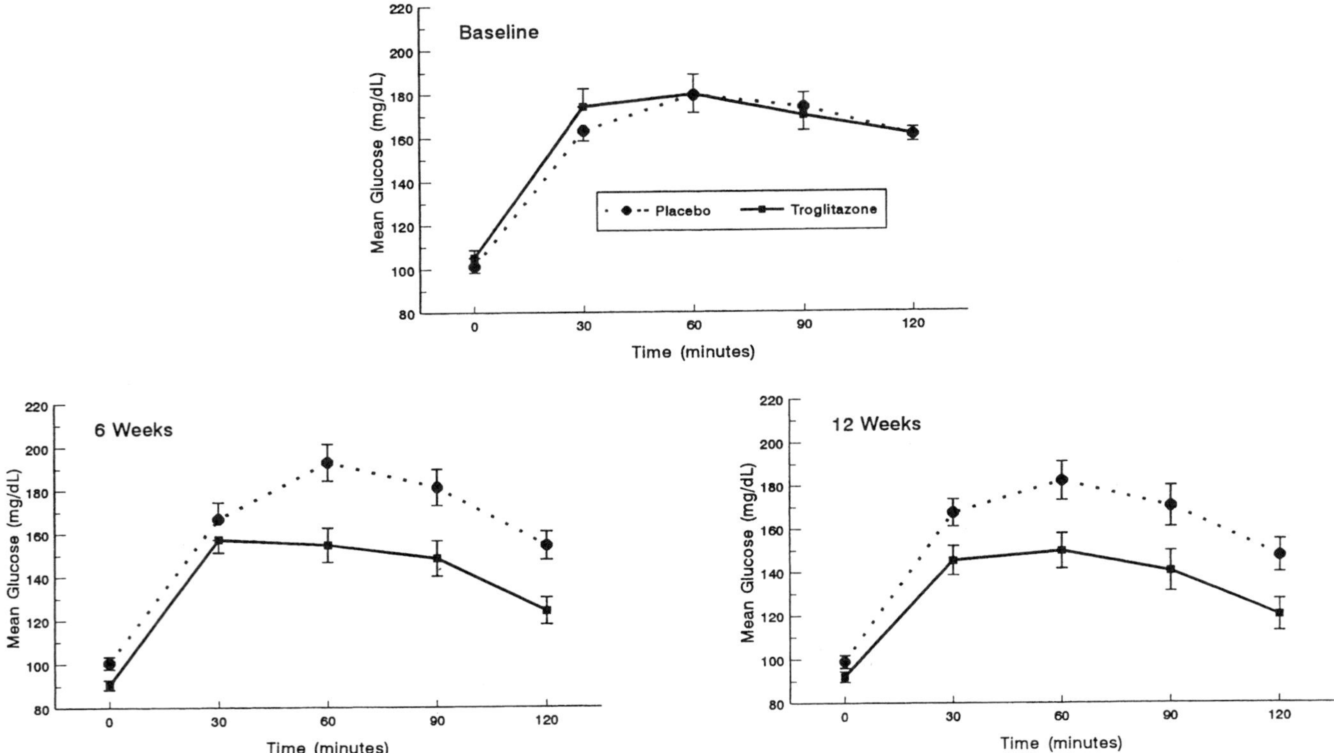

Figure 74-5. Mean ± standard error insulin response to a standard oral glucose tolerance test at baseline and after 6 and 12 weeks of treatment with troglitazone or placebo. The 120-minute values at 6 and 12 weeks are significantly lower ($p < 0.01$) for the troglitazone-treated group.

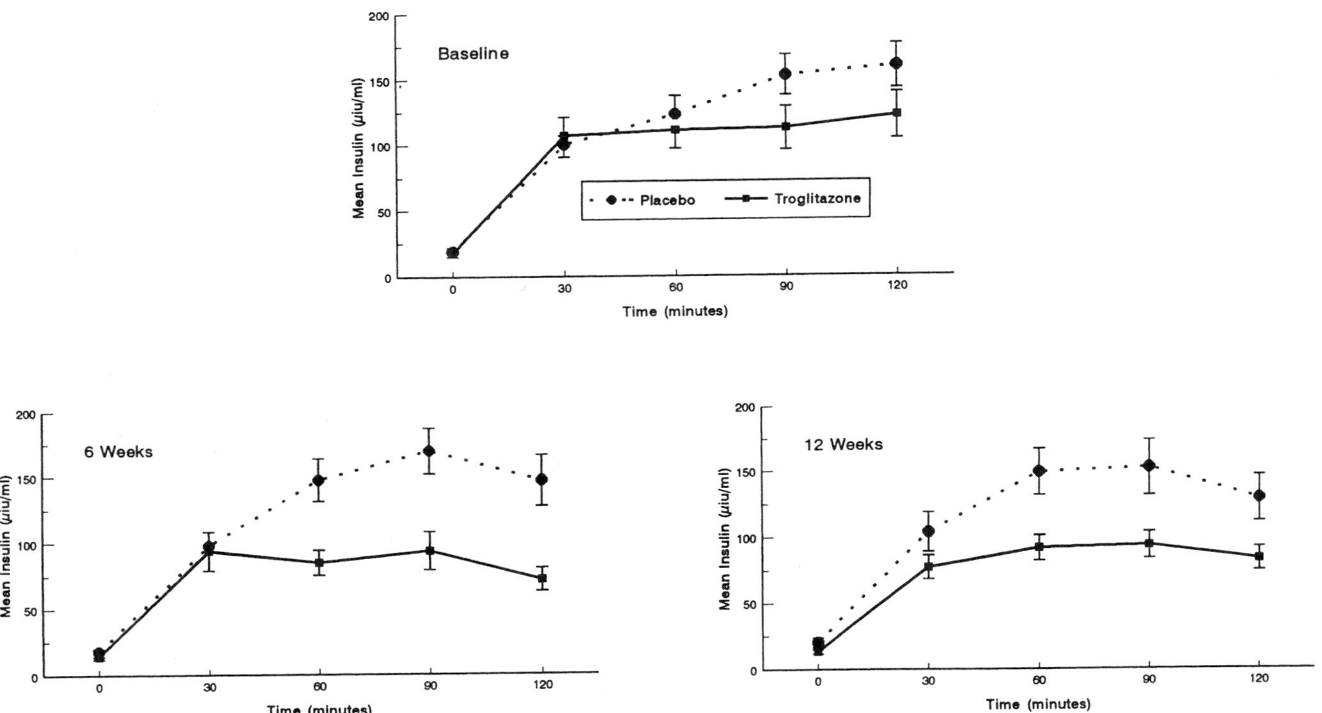

Figure 74-6. Mean ± standard error glucose response to a standard oral glucose tolerance test at baseline and after 6 and 12 weeks of treatment with troglitazone or placebo. The 120-minute values at 6 and 12 weeks are significantly lower ($p < 0.01$) for the troglitazone-treated group.

that patients with PCOS have a normal insulin receptor number but that there is a marked decrease in insulin receptor–mediated signal transduction. In addition, a modest decrease in GLUT-4 content has been noted.[49] It is of interest to note that insulin-like growth factor-1 receptors are present in the ovary and that insulin can exert an affect through these receptors.[45] In this setting, insulin can bond to the ligand-binding domain of the insulin-like growth factor-1 receptor and activate the tyrosine kinase activity of the β-subunit. Whether the increase under this influence is due to insulin or insulin-like growth factor-1 is not yet determined. It is not clear at present whether androgens enhance insulin resistance in patients with PCOS. Of interest is the observation that the insulin resistance in women with PCOS is not associated with hyperlipidemia or hypertension, which has been found to be prevalent in patients with insulin resistance due to NIDDM. Agents such as troglitazone, which directly increase insulin sensitivity, represent potentially important therapeutic modalities in the study of this disease state (i.e., the ability to separate insulin resistance from other endocrine disorders), as well as potentially therapeutic treatment for persons with these disorders.

Summary

Thiazolidinediones such as troglitazone represent a unique opportunity to study and treat insulin-resistant conditions such as non–insulin-dependent diabetes mellitus (NIDDM), impaired glucose tolerance, and polycystic ovarian syndrome (PCOS). Persons with other insulin-resistant states such as steroid-induced glucose intolerance and severe insulin resistance, as well as women with a history of gestational diabetes, are also populations in whom insulin-sensitizing agents would be valuable in both treating and potentially preventing hyperglycemic states.

References

1. Fujita T, Sugiyama Y, Taketomi S, et al. Reduction of insulin resistance in obese and/or diabetic animals by 3 [-4-(1 methylcyclohexylmethoxy) benzyl]-thiazolidine-2,4 dione (troglithazone), a new antidiabetic agent. Diabetes 1983;32:804
2. Fujiwara T, Yoshioka S, Yoshioka T, et al. Characterization of a new antidiabetic agent, CS-045. Studies in *KKA* and *ob/ob* mice and Zucker fatty rats. Diabetes 1988;37:1849
3. Lee MK, Miles PDG, Khoursheed M, et al. Metabolic effects of troglitazone on fructose-induced insulin resistance in the rat. Diabetes 1994;43:1435
4. Khoursheed M, Miles PDG, Gao KM, et al. Metabolic effects of troglitazone on fat induced insulin resistance in the rat. Metabolism 1995;in press
5. Tominaga M, Igarashi M, Daimon M, et al. Thiazolidinidiones (AD-4533 and CS-045) improve hepatic insulin resistance in streptozotocin-induced diabetic rats. Endocrine J 1993;40:343
6. Stevenson RW, McPherson RK, Genereux BE, et al. Antidiabetic agent englitazone enhances insulin action in nondiabetic rats without producing hypoglycemia. Metabolism 1991;40:1268
7. Bowen L, Steven PP, Stevenson R, Shulman CI. The effect of CP-68772, a thiazolidine derivative, on insulin sensitivity in lean and obese Zucker rats. Metabolism 1991;40:1025
8. Oakes ND, Kennedy CJ, Jenkins AB, et al. A new antidiabetic agent, BRL 49653, reduces lipid availability and improves insulin action and glucoregulation in the rat. Diabetes 1994;43:1203
9. Hofmann C, Lorenz K, Colca JR. Glucose transport deficiency in diabetic animals is corrected by treatment with the oral antihyperglycemic agent pioglitazone. Endocrinology 1991;129:1915
10. Sugiyama Y, Shimura Y, Ikeda H. Effects of pioglitazone on hepatic and peripheral insulin resistance in Wistar fatty rats. Arzneim Forsch 1990;40:436
11. Fujiwara T, Okuno A, Yoshioka S, Horikoshi H. Suppression of hepatic gluconeogenesis in chronic troglitazone (CS-045)-treated diabetic *KK* and C57BL/KSJ-*db/db* mice. Metabolism 1995;in press
12. Sugiyama Y, Teketomi S, Shimuoa V, et al. Effects of pioglitazone on glucose and lipid metabolism in Wistar fatty rats. Arzneim Forsch 1994;40:263
13. Kraegen E, James D, Jenkins AB, et al. A potent in vivo effect of ciglitazone on muscle insulin resistance induced by high fat feeding of rats. Metabolism 1989;38:1089
14. Castle CK, Colca JR, Melchior GW. Lipoprotein profile characterization of the KKA mouse, a rodent model of type II diabetes, before and after treatment with the insulin-sensitizing agent pioglitazone. Arterioscler Thromb 1992;13:307
15. Fujiwara T, Wade M, Fukuda K, et al. Characterization of CS-045, a new oral antidiabetic agent. II. Effects on glycemic control and pancreatic islet structure at a late stage of the diabetic syndrome in C57BL/KSJ-*db/db* mice. Metabolism 1991;40:1213
16. Reaven GM. Role of insulin resistance in human disease. Diabetes 1988;37:1595
17. Yoshioko J, Nishiyama H, Shiroki T, et al. Antihypertensive effects of CS-045 treatment in obese Zucker rats. Metabolism 1993;42:75
18. Zhang HY, Reddy SR, Kotchan TA. Antihypertensive effect of pioglitazone is not invariably associated with increased insulin sensitivity. Hypertension 1994;24:106
19. Kemnitz JW, Elson DF, Roecker EB, et al. Pioglitazone increases insulin sensitivity, reduces blood glucose, insulin and lipid levels, and lowers blood pressure in obese, insulin-resistant rhesus monkeys. Diabetes 1994;33:203
20. Saltiel AR. The paradoxical regulation of protein phosphorylation by insulin. FASEB J 1994;8:1034
21. Kletzien RF, Clark SD, Ulrich RG. Enhancement of adipocyte differentiation by an insulin-sensitizing agent. Mol Pharmacol 1992;41:393
22. Ohsumi J, Sakakibara S, Yamaguchi J, et al. Troglitazone prevents the inhibitory effects of inflammatory cytokines on insulin-induced adipocyte differentiation in 3T3-L1 cells. Endocrinology 1994;135:2279
23. Sandouk T, Reda D, Hofmann C. Antidiabetic agent pioglitazone enhances adipocyte differentiation of 3T3-F442A cells. Am J Physiol 1993;264:C1600
24. Tafuri S. Troglitazone stimulates glucose uptake in 3T3-L1 adipoyctes by enhancing expression of the GLUT1 and GLUT4 glucose transporters. Diabetes 1994;43:761A
25. Kreutter DK, Andrews KM, Gibbs EM, et al. Insulin-like activity of new antidiabetic agent CP68722 in 3T3-L1 adipocytes. Diabetes 1990;39:1414
26. Sandouk T, Reda D, Hofmann C. The antidiabetic agent pioglitazone increases expression of glucose transporters in 3T3-F442A cells by increasing messenger ribonucleic acid transcript stability. Endocrinology 1993;133:352
27. El-Kebbi IM, Roser S, Pollet RJ. Regulation of glucose transport by pioglitazone in cultured muscle cells. Metabolism 1994;43:953
28. Amri EZ, Bonino F, Ailhaud G, et al. Cloning of a protein that mediates transcriptional effects of fatty acids in preadipocytes. J Biol Chem 1995;270:2367
29. Ciraldi TP, Gilmore A, Olefsky JM, et al. In vitro studies on the action of CS-045, a new antidiabetic agent. Metabolism 1990;39:1056
30. Caro JF, Sinha MK, Raju JM, et al. Insulin receptor kinase in human skeletal muscle from obese subjects with and without noninsulin dependent diabetes. J Clin Invest 1987;79:1330
31. Muller HK, Kellerer M, Ermel B, et al. Prevention by protein kinase C inhibitors of glucose-induced insulin receptor tyrosine kinase resistance in rat fat cells. Diabetes 1991;40:1440
32. Baler S, Kiehn R, Haring HU. Effect of CS-045 on the activity of insulin receptor kinase in the skeletal muscle of insulin resistant Zucker rats. Diabetes Stoffweschel 1993;2:56
33. Kellerer M, Kroder G, Tippmer S, et al. Troglitazone prevents glucose-induced insulin resistance of insulin receptor in rat 1 fibroblasts. Diabetes 1994;43:447
34. Hofmann CA, Colca JR. New oral thiazolidinedione antidiabetic agents act as insulin sensitizers. Diabetes Care 1992;15:1075
35. Iwamoto Y, Kuzuya T, Matsuda A, et al. I. Effect of new oral antidiabetic agent CS-045 on glucose tolerance and insulin secretion in patients with NIDDM. Diabetes Care 1991;14:1083
36. Suter SL, Nolan JJ, Wallace P, et al. Metabolic effects of new oral hypoglycemic agent CS-045 in NIDDM subjects. Diabetes Care 1992;15:193
37. Valiquett TR, Balagtas CC, Whitcomb RW. Troglitazone dose-response study in patients with noninsulin dependent diabetes (abstract). Clin Res 1994;42:400A
38. Harris MI. Impaired glucose tolerance in the U.S. population. Diabetes Care 1989;12:464
39. Saad MF, Knowler WC, Pettit DJ, et al. Natural history of IGT in Pima Indians. N Engl J Med 1988;319:1500
40. Wingard DL, Scheidt-Nave C, Barrett-Connor EL, McPhillips JB. Prevalence of cardiovascular and renal complications in older adults with normal or impaired glucose tolerance or NIDDM. Diabetes Care 1993;12:1022
41. Nolan JJ, Ludvik B, Beerdsen P, et al. Improvement in glucose tolerance and insulin resistance in obese subjects treated with troglitazone. N Engl J Med 1994;331:1188
42. Antonucci T, Norris R, McClain R, Whitcomb R. An investigator-blinded, randomized, multicenter, placebo-controlled trial of the effect of troglitazone (CI-991) on impaired glucose tolerance (IGT) and insulin resistance. Diabetes 1994;43:253
43. Polson DW, Wadsworth J, Adams J, Franks S. Polycystic ovaries: A common finding in normal women. Lancet 1988;i:870
44. Gitsch E, Vytiska-Binstorfer E, Huber JC. Incidence of hyperandrogenemia. Gerburtshilfe Frauen 1987;47:796
45. Dunaif A, Givens JR, Haseltine FP, Merriam GR, eds. The Polycystic Ovary Syndrome. Cambridge, MA: Blackwell;1992
46. Dunaif A, Segal KR, Futterweit W, Dobrjansky A. Profound peripheral insulin

resistance, independent of obesity, in the polycystic ovary syndrome. Diabetes 1989;38:1165
47. Dunaif A, Graf M, Mandeli J, et al. Characterization of groups of hyperandrogenic women with acanthosis nigricans, impaired glucose tolerance and/or hyperinsulinemia. J Clin Endocrinol Metab 1987;65:499
48. Dunaif A, Green G, Finegood D. Pancreatic beta cell function is normal in insulin resistant women with the polycystic ovary syndrome. 74th Annual meeting of the Endocrine Society. 1992;280
49. Rosenbaum D, Haber R, Dunaif A. GLUT4 glucose transporter abundance correlates with decreased insulin responsiveness in adipocytes from polycystic ovary syndrome (PCOS) women, independent of obesity and glucose intolerance. Am J Physiol 1993;264:E197

Diabetes Mellitus, edited by Derek LeRoith, Simeon I. Taylor, and Jerrold M. Olefsky. Lippincott–Raven Publishers, Philadelphia © 1996.

CHAPTER 75
Fatty Acid Oxidation Inhibitors

JAMES E. FOLEY AND ROBERT ANDERSON

Introduction

Although fatty acid (FA) oxidation inhibitors are not currently available as drug therapy, their potential for the treatment of diabetes has been appreciated due to the association between the hypoglycemic effect of hypoglycin and its ability to inhibit FA oxidation (FAO).[1] In this chapter, the potential use of FAO inhibitors (FAOI) in the treatment of diabetes will be discussed. The role of FAO in both prandial glucose utilization and fasting glucose production will be examined. Finally, strategies for inhibiting FAO pharmacologically will be explored.

Role of Fatty Acid Oxidation in Prandial Glucose Utilization

The liver is the most important regulator of glycemia. After a meal, reduced hepatic gluconeogenesis and glycolysis, as well as increased hepatic glucose utilization by the liver, are major mechanisms by which peripheral glucose excursions are minimized.[2] Significant glucose does, however, escape regulation by the liver. This overflow of glucose is utilized via insulin-mediated peripheral glucose uptake, mainly by muscle.[3]

Although glucose and FA are competing sources of fuel by muscle (Fig. 75-1), FA are the preferred substrate. At the insulin concentrations prevalent during fasting, lipolysis rates are much higher than those after a meal. This leads to increased free FA (FFA) concentrations and increased fatty acid oxidation (FAO). The result is decreased glucose oxidation via feedback inhibition of pyruvate dehydrogenase and decreased glucose uptake via citrate feedback inhibition of phosphofructokinase. This, in turn, leads to feedback inhibition of hexokinase via accumulation of glucose-6-phosphate and to decreased net glucose transport by accumulation of glucose near the intracellular side of the glucose transporter. This FAO feedback mechanism was first demonstrated by Randle et al.[4] in rat heart over 30 years ago. Since that time, elevated free fatty acid (FFA) concentrations and the consequential elevated FAO rate have been implicated as a cause of insulin resistance.

The importance of this mechanism in the regulation of glucose uptake in human skeletal muscle, and thus as a cause of insulin resistance, is controversial. Most data from studies in humans in which FFA concentrations have either been raised or lowered suggest that the effect of fatty acid oxidation inhibitors (FAOI) on glucose oxidation via the inhibition of pyruvate dehydrogenase may well be a major factor in the generation of insulin resistance in the liver due to increased Cori cycling.[5] In such studies, however, the effect of FAO on glucose uptake via the Randle glucose uptake mechanism does not appear to be a major factor in the generation of insulin resistance in skeletal muscle.[6,7] Recent studies in which the role of intracellular fat depots in muscle has been evaluated suggest that these depots may sufficiently buffer any effect of modulating FFA.[8] The data suggest that if FAO is an important determinant of insulin resistance in skeletal muscle, then intervention is more likely to succeed by inhibiting FAO in muscle rather than decreasing FFA.

The same fatty acid (FA) and glucose oxidation mechanisms operating in skeletal muscle are operating in the heart. During ischemia, energy production is limited by availability of oxygen. Because FAO proceeds at a lower rate of ATP generated per unit

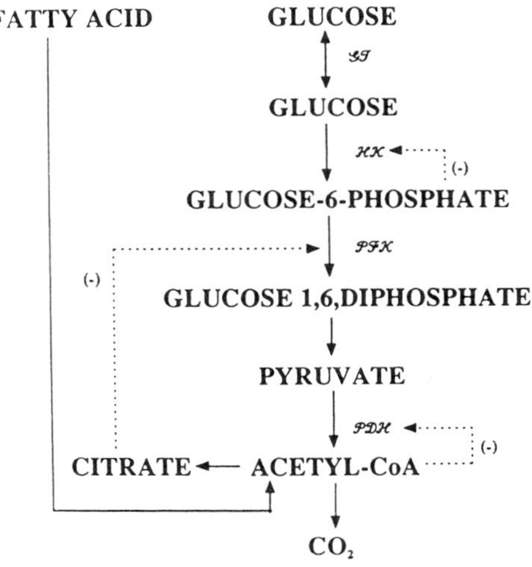

FIGURE 75-1. Regulation of glucose utilization in muscle by FAO. (Reproduced with permission from Foley JE. Rationale and application of fatty acid oxidation inhibitors in treatment of diabetes mellitus. Diabetes Care 1992;15:773.)

of oxygen utilized than does glucose oxidation, the heart maximizes ATP generation by switching from FAO to glucose oxidation.[9] This switch is associated with an increase in heart size. This change in heart size is reversible and appears to result from a compensatory increase in perfusion of heart muscle in response to perceived ischemia.[10] Increasing FAO would lead to decreased glucose oxidation and presumably less signal to increase cardiac perfusion. Thus, elevated FA concentrations are predicted to be deleterious in the ischemic heart.[11] Any agents that increase glucose oxidation, or decrease FAO and thus increase glucose oxidation, are predicted to increase heart size. No deleterious effects directly attributed to the increased heart weight have been seen. On the other hand, cardiac changes have been associated with heart weight changes after long-term administration of oxirane carboxylates such as Etomoxir and methyl 2-tetradecylglycidate.[12]

Role of Fatty Acid Oxidation in Fasting Glucose Production

It is clear that in non–insulin-dependent diabetes mellitus (NIDDM) patients whose hyperglycemia is more severe, there is increased hepatic glucose production (HGP) due to accelerated gluconeogenesis during the overnight fast.[6,13–17] It is also clear that at the insulin concentrations present during the overnight fast, the direct action of insulin on the liver does not determine the rate of gluconeogenesis.[18,19] It appears that the gluconeogenic rate is determined largely by the balance of energy production by the liver minus its nongluconeogenic utilization. Energy production from fatty acid oxidation (FAO) is preferred, but it can be supplemented by oxidation of gluconeogenic substrates such as lactate, glycerol, and alanine. Energy production is needed to supply the large energy requirements (ATP and reducing equivalents in the form of nicotinamide adenine denucleotide) of the liver, as well as for any gluconeogenesis (a much smaller component) (Fig. 75-2). From such a scheme, it is clear how an unusual energy demand on the liver could lead to hypoglycemia because energy production by the liver is an important determinant of gluconeogenesis. Fatty acids (FA) from triglyceride stores in the liver, as well as FA from free fatty acids (FFA) are a source of FA for hepatic FAO and hepatic energy production. Ultimately, it is the FFA concentrations that will determine hepatic energy production because hepatic triglyceride stores, in turn, are regulated by FFA concentrations.

To maintain normoglycemia during the overnight fast, FFA and gluconeogenic precursor fluxes to the liver are increased, leading to increased gluconeogenesis and HGP. In NIDDM, FFA concentrations may be twice as high as in normal persons,[20–23] leading presumably to a twofold elevation in FAO and resulting in inappropriate rates of gluconeogenesis during the overnight fast. A low dose of insulin at bedtime has been shown to be effective in controlling this glycemia.[24,25] The most likely explanation of this insulinotrophic effect is an antilipolytic effect in adipose tissue (see below) leading to decreased FFA concentrations and decreased hepatic FAO. Even after a meal, the major stimulus inhibiting gluconeogenesis may be the insulin-induced reduction in substrate fluxes to the liver rather than a direct effect of insulin on the liver by a change in the insulin:glucagon ratio.[26]

Most studies support the role of FAO in the control of gluconeogenesis. Changes in gluconeogenesis, however, are not always translated into changes in HGP.[7,27–30] The reason is that there are compensatory changes in glycogenolysis that can maintain constant HGP rates. This mechanism may in fact play a major role under experimental conditions. There are other potential levels of regulation, however, such as acute shifts to utilization of hepatic triglyceride versus FFA as precursors for FAO and in changes in the flux of gluconeogenic precursors to the liver. In addition, glycogenolysis rates depend on the replenishment of glycogen via gluconeogenesis. A major question is whether the liver will defend a hyperglycemic state by glycogenolysis. The fact that decreases in FFA concentrations or inhibition of FAO have been shown to decrease HGP (see below) indicates that, at least under some conditions, the liver will not defend hyperglycemia.

FAO also plays a role in the export, mobilization, and storage of triglyceride in the liver. When FFA concentrations are elevated in obesity, there is increased export of very low density lipoprotein-triglyceride and cholesterol from the liver. This export is decreased when FFA concentrations are normalized[31] and is reduced significantly in the presence of fatty acid oxidation inhibitors (FAOI).[32,33] This suggests that FAO and de novo FA synthesis are required for export of FA from the liver. It also predicts that some of the FA not oxidized will be stored as triglyceride in the liver and that the remaining FA not oxidized will lead to increased FFA concentrations. These situations occur chronically and acutely, respectively, as a consequence of FAOI.[32,34] Unexplained is a compensatory decrease in FFA to pre-FAOI levels within 24 hours even if FAO inhibition persists (unpublished observation). Because elevated FFA concentrations are not a persistent consequence of FAOI, the major concern is increased steady-state hepatic triglyceride concentrations. It is clear that a >90% inhibition of FAO 24 hours/day is predicted to cause increased steady-state hepatic triglyceride concentrations. The question is whether a 50% inhibition of FAO will lead to hepatic triglyceride concentrations that are greater than the already higher concentrations present in NIDDM. If they are higher, a further question is whether such an elevation is associated with any toxicity.

Regulation of Gluconeogenesis by Fatty Acid Oxidation

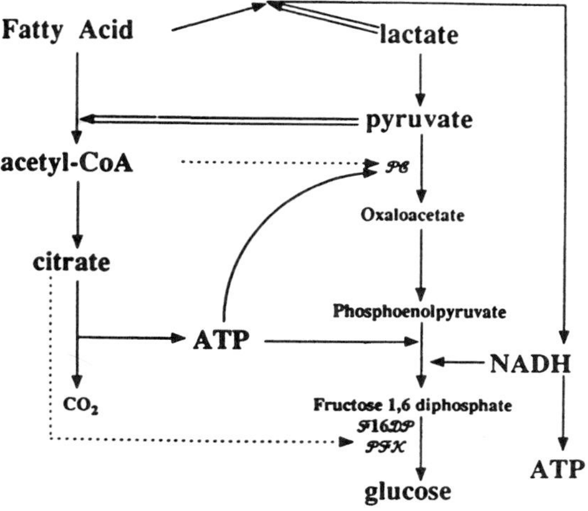

Figure 75-2. Regulation of gluconeogenesis by FAO. (Reproduced with permission from Foley JE. Rationale and application of fatty acid oxidation inhibitors in treatment of diabetes mellitus. Diabetes Care 1992;15:773.)

Inhibitors of Fatty Acid Oxidation

The major source of free fatty acids (FFA) is the fat cell (see "Fat Cell"). Long-chain fatty acids (FA) are the major chain length in most mammals, including primates and rodents. Although medium- and short-chain FA cross the mitochondrial membranes and are esterified to coenzyme A (CoA) esters within the mitochondria, long-chain FA must be esterified in the cytosol by CoA ligase (Fig. 75-3). Once esterified to CoA, the long-chain FA are transported across the mitochondrial membrane by the carnitine palmitoyltransferase system (see "Carnitine Palmitoyltransferase I" and

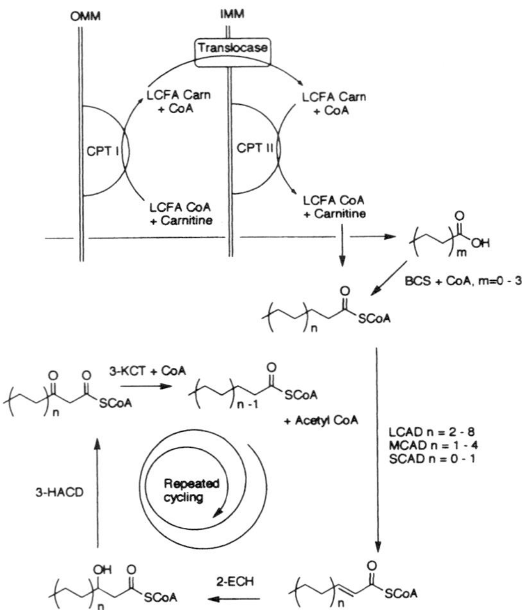

Figure 75-3. Schematic of the mitochondrial β-oxidation system. CPT I = carnitine palmitoyltransferase I; CPT II = carnitine palmitoyltransferase II; coA = coenzyme A; LCFA CoA = long-chain fatty acid coenzyme A ester; LCFA Carn = long-chain fatty acid carnitine ester; LCAD = long-chain acyl CoA dehydrongenase; MCAD = medium-chain acyl CoA dehydrogenase; SCAD = short-chain acyl CoA dehydrogenase; 2-ECH = 2-enoyl CoA hydratase; 3-HCAD = 3-hydroxyacyl CoA dehydrogenase; 3-KCT = 3-ketoacl CoA thiolase; BCS = butyryl-CoA synthetase; OMM = outer mitochondrial membrane; IMM = inner mitochondrial membrane.

"Carnitine Palmitoyltransferase II/Coenzyme A"). Once inside the mitochondria, FA undergo β-oxidation (see "Acyl Dehydrogenase Inhibitors").

Fat Cell

Fatty acid (FA) release from adipocytes is equally dependent on the rate of lipolysis and the rate of re-esterification of FA (Fig. 75-4). Lipolysis rates depend on the activities of hormone-sensitive lipase (HSL), and re-esterification depends on the rate of glucose transport. Inhibition of HSL and stimulation of glucose transport by insulin are the major mechanisms controlling FA release from adipocytes. This insulin action is much more sensitive than any other insulin action.

HSL and glucose transport are also regulated by a number of mediators, including catecholamines and adenosine, which bind to receptors coupled to G-proteins (see Fig. 75-4). Norepinephrine, released from sympathetic nerve endings, is the major stimulus to release FA from adipocytes.[35] Adenosine A1 receptor agonists have been shown to improve insulin sensitivity for both inhibition of HSL[36] and the stimulation of glucose transport,[37] and norepinephrine binding to the β-catecholamine receptor has been shown to decrease their sensitivity.[36,37] Nicotinic acid also binds to a putative receptor coupled to G-proteins in adipocytes. The action of nicotinic acid is similar to that of adenosine.[38]

Both glucose transport and HSL become insulin resistant in obesity and non–insulin-dependent diabetes mellitus (NIDDM),[39] but compensatory fasting hyperinsulinemia partially prevents free fatty acid (FFA) concentrations from rising. In NIDDM, however, this compensation diminishes during progression of the disease.[23] Potential solutions to the diminishing compensation by insulin are insulin therapy and the reversal of insulin resistance at the levels of HSL and glucose transport via drugs that bind to the putative nicotinic acid or the adenosine A1 receptor. Low-dose insulin therapy at bedtime has been used successfully for this purpose.[24, 25]

Nicotinic acid (Fig. 75-5) has been known for over 30 years to exert hypoglycemic effects under some conditions. Unfortunately, it has also been shown to cause insulin resistance and, in some cases, hyperglycemia. The latter effect is presumed to be due to a rebound in FFA concentrations.[40]

Recently, other compounds that bind to the putative nicotinic acid receptor and the adenosine A1 receptor have been evaluated as agents to improve insulin sensitivity in the adipocyte. Acipomox (see Fig. 75-5), which has less rebound than nicotinic acid,[41] has been tested extensively, with mixed results.[42–53]

Phenylisopropyladenosine has been shown to be effective in rats in increasing glucose uptake.[54] It is not orally active and has mixed A1 and A2 receptor activities. Although adipocytes do not appear to have A2 receptors, their presence in other tissues could contribute to insulin resistance. Using phenylisopropyladenosine as a starting point, several compounds have been evaluated for development that are orally active and are selective adenosine A1 agonists. Final evaluation of their utility in humans has not been reported.

Carnitine Palmitoyltransferase I

The carnitine palmitoyltransferase (CPT) system is a three-component system comprised of carnitine palmitoyltransferase I (CPT I), an acylcarnitine translocase, and carnitine palmitoyltransferase II (CPT II). CPT I, located on the inner surface of the outer mitochondrial membrane, catalyzes a reaction between long-chain fatty acid (FA) coenzyme A (CoA) esters and carnitine to give long-chain fatty acid (FA) carnitine esters and free CoA. CPT II, located on the inner surface of the inner mitochondrial membrane, catalyzes the reverse reaction. An acylcarnitine translocase is located in, and translocates long-chain FA carnitine esters across, the inner mitochondrial membrane—a membrane that forms an impermeable barrier to long-chain FA and their CoA esters. The CPT system is therefore a requisite shuttle system that allows long-chain FA access to the inner mitochondrial matrix and its fatty acid β-oxidation enzymes.[55]

CPT I and CPT II are highly homologous proteins with tissue-specific isoform distributions such that CPT II exists as the same isoform in liver, skeletal muscle, and heart muscle, whereas the predominant isoform of CPT I in heart and skeletal muscles is different from that in liver.[56] Relative to CPT II, CPT I's primary distinguishing characteristic is that it is potently inhibited by malonyl CoA. This regulation of CPT I by malonyl CoA explains the reciprocal relationship between lipogenesis and FA oxidation (malonyl CoA is the first committed intermediate in FA biosynthesis and concurrently plays a role in feedback regulation of fatty acid oxidation [FOA]), and is indicative of the key role that CPT I assumes as the rate-limiting step in FAO and thereby its ability to modulate gluconeogenesis.[55] The central role of the CPT system in ketogenesis and gluconeogenesis was initially exemplified with the aid of the CPT inhibitor decanoyl-D-carnitine, the decanoyl ester of the unnatural enantiomer of carnitine. These studies demonstrated the potential utility of such an inhibitor for the treatment of diabetes-related disorders.[57,58]

A number of other inhibitors of the CPT system have since been identified, the two most widely studied being tetradecylglycidic acid (TDGA) and ethyl 2-[6-(4-chlorophenoxy)hexyl]oxirane-2-carboxylate (Etomoxir)[32,59–67] (Fig. 75-6). After activation to their CoA esters, these agents are irreversible inhibitors of CPT I. Both TDGA and Etomoxir advanced to clinical trials, where they showed

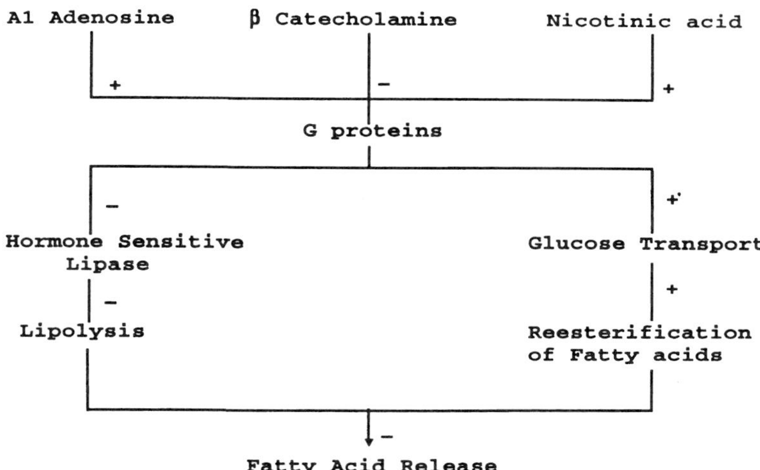

Figure 75-4. Receptor-mediated regulation of FA release from adipocytes.

promise as antidiabetic agents. For example, oral use of Etomoxir at doses of 12.5, 25, and 50 mg twice daily for 14 days in a multicenter, double-blind, parallel-group comparison against placebo with 48 patients with non–insulin-dependent diabetes mellitus (NIDDM) led to a 50% decrease in fasting β-hydroxybutyrate concentrations, a 20% decrease in glucose concentrations, a 30% decrease in triglyceride concentrations, and a 45% decrease in the ratio of low density lipoprotein to high density lipoprotein.[32] Neither of these agents, however, was fully developed as a clinically useful drug, probably due to concerns regarding drug-induced myocardial hypertrophy in animals. The heart is very dependent on FA oxidation as a primary fuel source, but when this fuel source becomes scarce, the heart will switch to oxidation of glucose. When this occurs, myocardial hypertrophy results. It is not known whether the myocardial hypertrophy is a direct effect of decreased FA oxidation, increased glucose oxidation, or both. The same type of hypertrophy can be created by fat-free diets, which also lead to decreased cardiac FA oxidation and increased carbohydrate utilization.[68] TDGA-induced hypertrophy has been directly linked to inhibition of heart muscle CPT I because, in the presence of octanoate, a medium-chain FA that bypasses the CPT system, TDGA-induced hypertrophy does not occur.[9] Thus, the additional complexity of myocardial hypertrophy is the result of the drug acting in an organ other than that intended. A more sophisticated approach would be one wherein the drug was selectively targeted to the liver.

At the enzyme level, this selectivity is not achievable with inhibitors of CPT II because the liver and muscle isoforms are the same. With CPT I, however, the liver and heart isoforms are different,[56] possibly with inhibitory isoenzyme selectivity, particularly if the drug also has appropriate pharmacokinetic properties that direct the drug to the liver and away from the heart. The problem with the glycidic acids TDGA and Etomoxir is that they are irreversible inhibitors and, time dependently, will completely inactivate both isoforms of CPT I, irrespective of any initial kinetic differences in enzyme binding. Furthermore, as demonstrated by their effects in the heart, they do not possess a pharmacokinetic profile beneficial to liver targeting. This is not unexpected. To achieve organ selectivity pharmacokinetically with an irreversible inhibitor would be very difficult because any quantity of the drug appearing in the organ would result in inactivation of the target enzyme, with overall inhibition of the enzyme depending on the rates of enzyme inactivation and turnover. Because, in general, the rate of enzyme inactivation will be much faster than the rate of enzyme turnover, essentially complete inactivation of the enzyme will occur over time. A reversible inhibitor, however, would display intrinsic, affinity-dependent isoenzyme selectivity. This intrinsic selectivity could be much more easily augmented by appropriate pharmacokinetic properties because small quantities of the drug could be allowed to enter unintended organs, with little effect on the target enzyme in those organs. None of the CPT inhibitors based on substrate analog structures, such as bromopalmitate, decanoyl-D-carnitine (Fig. 75-7), and *N*-palmitoylaminocarnitine, sufficiently meet the criteria to be considered for clinical development. By the application of a transition state analog design wherein the enzymatic reaction transition state is simulated sterically and electronically by a stable molecule, however, newer CPT inhibitors have been discovered that may prove useful in the treatment of diabetes.

SDZ CPI 975 (see Fig. 75-7) was designed with a stable tetrahedral phosphate anion to mimic the transient tetrahedral ester oxyanion hypothesized to exist in the reaction transition state. SDZ CPI 975 has been shown to be a reversible, competitive inhibitor of CPT I with respect to palmitoyl CoA and to selectively inhibit the liver isoform, with a dissociation constant (K_i) fourfold lower than that for the heart isoform. This intrinsic selectivity is enhanced pharmacokinetically by a 16:1 distribution of SDZ CPI 975 between liver and heart on oral dosing. SDZ CPI 975 is a potent inhibitor

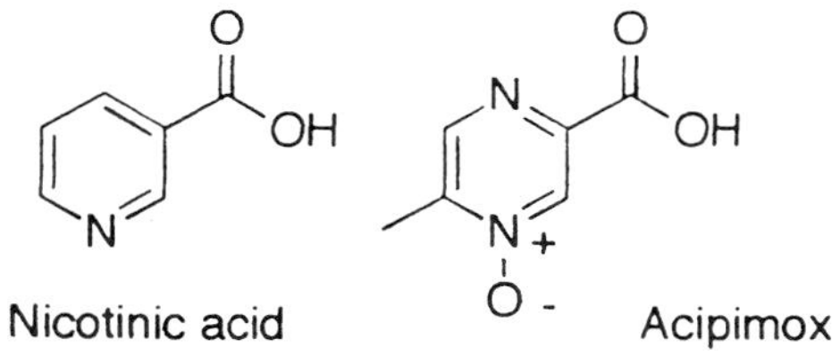

Figure 75-5. Chemical structures of nicotinic acid and Acipimox.

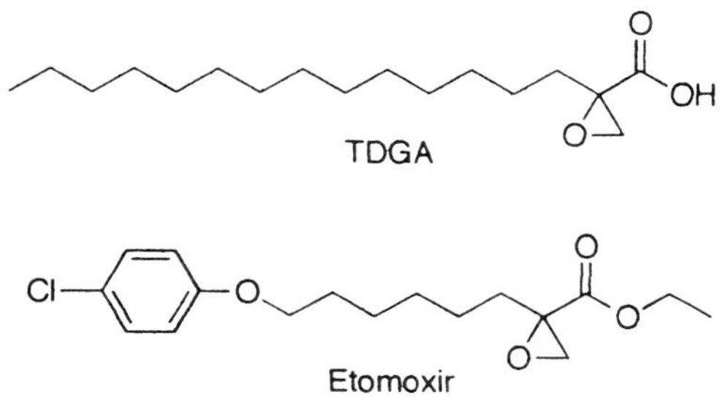

Figure 75-6. Chemical structures of TDGA and Etomoxir.

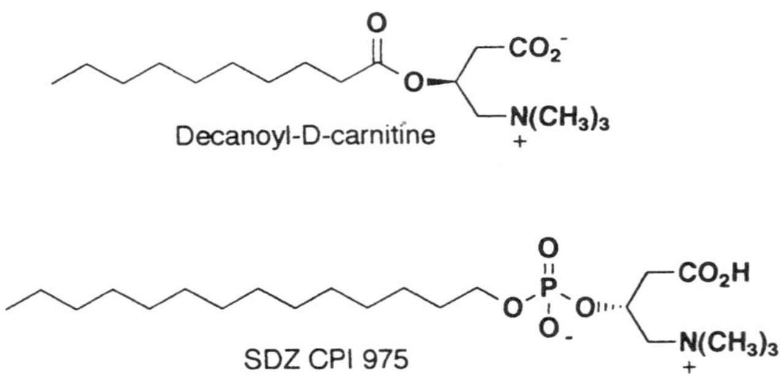

Figure 75-7. Examples of CPT inhibitors.

of ketogenesis in 18-hour fasted normal rats and is antihyperglycemic in a streptozotocin rat model of diabetes. Furthermore, SDZ CPI 975 lowers blood glucose concentrations in 18-hour fasted cynomolgus monkeys with a medium effective dose of 1.2 mg/kg. This hypoglycemic effect is limited by counter-regulation, which is consistent with the hypothesis that a fatty acid oxidation inhibitor (FAOI) per se leads to a counter-regulatable hypoglycemic effect. To ensure that the combined effects of the enzyme and pharmacokinetic selectivities were sufficient to circumvent myocardial hypertrophy, a 26-week study was conducted with SDZ CPI 975 in normal rats at oral doses of up to 100 mg/kg/day, with heart size and function being monitored by magnetic resonance imaging. Etomoxir was used as a positive control at a rate of 12.5 mg/kg/day. At the end of the study, Etomoxir had increased left ventricular mass by 10–15% with no effect on function, whereas SDZ CPI 975 had had no effect on either heart size or function. Thus, the concept of a reversible liver- versus heart-selective CPT I inhibitor is initially demonstrated and SDZ CPI 975 has entered into clinical trials, the results of which may clarify the overall utility of CPT inhibitors in the treatment of NIDDM.

Carnitine Palmyltransferase II/Coenzyme A

Intramitochondrial coenzymes A (CoAs) are a necessary cofactor by which carnitine palmyltransferase (CPT) II regenerates acyl-CoAs from acyl-carnitine. CPT II is predicted to be sensitive to these CoA levels.

Tert-butyl-benzoic acid is a good substrate for the medium-chain CoA ligase within mitochondria, leading to the formation of tert-butyl-benzoic acid CoA ester and depletion of intramitochondrial CoA (Fig. 75-8). This compound has been shown to be a potent hypoglycemic agent via this mechanism.[69,70] The compound is also associated with benzoic acid poisoning, however, due to nonspecific toxic effects of the tert-butyl-benzoic acid CoA esters, which accumulate to concentrations beyond those required to inhibit fatty acid oxidation (FAO).[71]

SDZ 51-641 has been shown to be an effective liver-selective fatty acid oxidation inhibitor (FAOI) in rats leading to decreased hepatic glucose production (HGP) and glycemia.[33] Subsequently, it was shown to be a prodrug of SDZ 53-450 (see Fig. 75-8), a compound that bears a striking resemblance to tert-butyl-benzoic acid, having only the addition of the hydroxymethyl group between the tert-butyl group and the benzoic acid. Remarkably, neither SDZ-51-641 nor any of several other prodrugs of SDZ 53-450 have shown any signs of benzoic acid poisoning. Apparently, there is a significant difference between the turnover of the CoA esters of SDZ 53-450 and tert-butyl benzoic acid, which may allow the use of SDZ 53-450 prodrugs in the treatment of non–insulin-dependent diabetes mellitus (NIDDM). A major question arises, however, as to whether the balance between formation and metabolism of SDZ 53-450 ester will be maintained across species. One prodrug, SDZ FOX 988, has been evaluated in humans, and it has been demonstrated that this balance is preserved, with enough turnover relative to formation, to prevent benzoic acid poisoning. At this time, however, no human data have been reported. Therefore, whether there is enough depletion of intramitochondrial CoA to reduce FAO sufficiently to decrease HGP remains to be established.

Acyl Dehydrogenase Inhibitors

In the β-oxidation of long-chain fatty acid coenzyme A (FA CoA) esters, the parent FA is consecutively oxidized to an α,β-unsaturated CoA ester, hydrated, oxidized to a β-keto ester, and then cleaved by CoA to give acetyl CoA and the parent FA CoA ester, now shortened by two carbon atoms. The initial step to form the α,β-unsaturated CoA ester is catalyzed by a family of flavin adenine dinucleotide coenzyme-dependent dehydrogenases that are physically distinct and identifiable by their discrete but overlapping chain-length selectivity. There are three dehydrogenases for the oxidation of unbranched FA CoA esters: long-chain acyl CoA dehydrogenase (LCAD); medium-chain acyl CoA dehydrogenase (MCAD); and short-chain acyl CoA dehydrogenase (SCAD).[72] (Recent evidence suggests a fourth dehydrogenase in mitochondria: very-long-chain acyl CoA dehydrogenase [VLCAD],[73] but other investigators claim that this enzyme is peroxisomal in origin.[74]) Thus, as a long-chain FA CoA ester is sequentially oxidized, physically different, FAD dependent, and chain-length selective, dehydrogenases are responsible for the initial step. Inhibition of any one of these enzymes would result in inhibition of FA oxidation at a chain-length specific site and lead to modulation of glycemia.

The first evidence for the relationship between acyl CoA dehydrogenase inhibition and hypoglycemic activity concerned Jamaican vomiting sickness. This condition results from eating the unripe fruit of the ackee tree. Hypoglycin, a component of this fruit, is metabolized to methylenecyclopropyl acetic acid CoA ester after ingestion, and MCPA is a potent and irreversible inhibitor of SCAD, MCAD, and a related branched chain acyl CoA dehydrogenase (BCAD) by covalently labeling the tightly bound FAD coenzyme. The resultant hypoglycemia and acidemia can lead to coma and death if not swiftly treated.[1,75] It has been suggested that if the hypoglycemic effects of hypoglycin could be controlled and separated from the concomitant toxic effects, regulation of FA oxidation at the level of the dehydrogenases could prove clinically useful.[76–78]

It has been suggested that the toxicity of hypoglycin is associated with its inhibition of SCAD and BCAD, causing accumulation of toxic short- and branched-chain acyl CoA esters, and that selective inhibition of MCAD or LCAD would give rise to a hypoglycemic effect without the accumulation of these toxic metabolites. Relative to SCAD, 3-mercaptopropionic acid is such a selective LCAD and MCAD inhibitor. Unfortunately, it causes convulsions in animals.[79] Recently, however, several MCPA analogs with appended alkyl side-chains (shown in Fig. 75-9) were synthesized and tested for their specificity against LCAD, MCAD, and SCAD. 12-Methylenecyclopropyl acetic acid CoA ester was found to be a reasonably selective inhibitor of LCAD and a potent hypoglycemic agent[78] devoid of drug-induced toxic acidemia. With increasing doses, however, non-counter-regulatable hypoglycemia results. It is hypothesized that an initial counter-regulatable hypoglycemic effect is brought about by a dose-dependent inhibition of LCAD

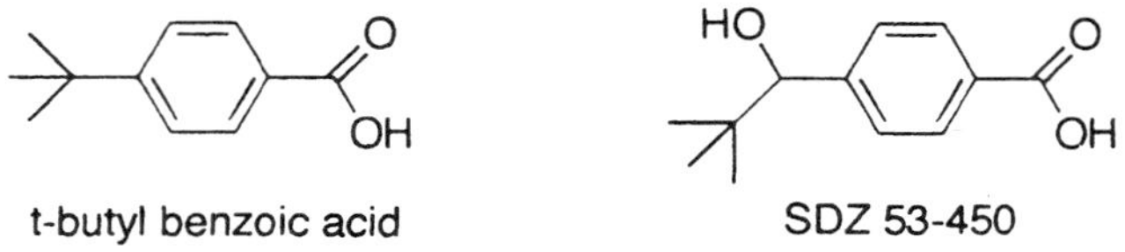

Figure 75-8. Chemical structures of tert-butyl-benzoic acid and SDZ 53-450.

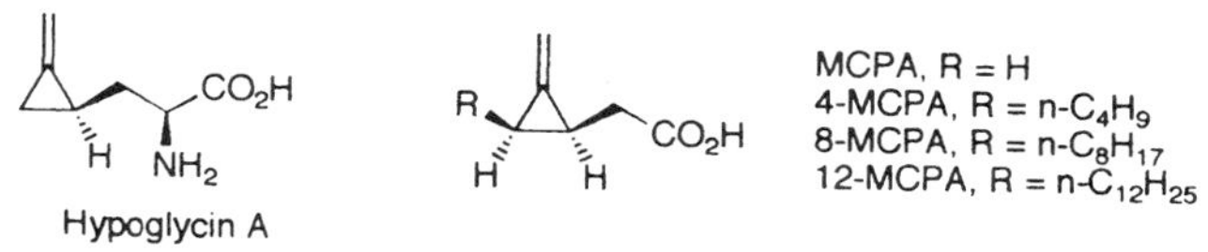

Hypoglycin A

MCPA, R = H
4-MCPA, R = n-C_4H_9
8-MCPA, R = n-C_8H_{17}
12-MCPA, R = n-$C_{12}H_{25}$

Figure 75-9. Examples of MCPA analogs with appended alkyl side chains.

but that, with increasing drug concentrations, further inhibition of gluconeogenesis is induced by accumulation of CoA esters of the drug substance. This results in CoA depletion, which presumably shuts down the Tricarboxylic acid (TCA) cycle.

Thus, there are no known dehydrogenase inhibitors (or inhibitors of the other enzymes in the long-chain FA β-oxidation pathway) that are of potential clinical utility.

Summary

Fatty acid oxidation inhibitors (FAOI) may be a feasible improvement on low-dose insulin therapy at bedtime for the treatment of excessive glucose production during the overnight fast. Liver-selective, reversible carnitine palmitoyltransferase (CPT) inhibitors that do not require activation to coenzyme A (CoA) esters may be the most desirable approach to inhibiting fatty acid oxidation.

References

1. Tanaka K, Ikeda Y. Hypoglycin and Jamaican vomiting sickness. In: Tanaka K, Coates PM, eds. Fatty Acid Oxidation: Clinical Biochemical and Molecular Aspects. New York: Alan R. Liss, Inc.; 1990:167
2. Mitrakou A, Kelly D, Venemen T, et al. Contribution of abnormal muscle and liver glucose metabolism to postprandial hyperglycemia in NIDDM. Diabetes 1990;39:1381
3. Groop LC, Bonadonna C, DelPrato S, et al. Glucose and free fatty acid metabolism in non–insulin-dependent diabetes mellitus: Evidence for multiple sites of insulin resistance. J Clin Invest 1989;84:205
4. Randle PJ, Hales CN, Garland PB, Newsholm EA. The glucose fatty-acid cycle: Its role in insulin sensitivity and the metabolic disturbances of diabetes mellitus. Lancet 1963;1:785
5. Kelley DE, Mokan M, Simoneau J-A, Mandarino LJ. Interaction between glucose and free fatty acid metabolism in human skeletal muscle. J Clin Invest 1993;92:91
6. Boden G, Jadali F. Effects of lipid on basal carbohydrate metabolism in normal men. Diabetes 1991;40:686
7. Yki-Jarvinen H, Puhakainen I, Koivisto VA. Effect of free fatty acids on glucose uptake and non-oxidative glycolysis across human forearm tissues in the basal state and during insulin stimulation. J Clin Endocrinol Metab 1991; 72:1268
8. Boden G, Jadali F, White J, et al. Effects of fat on insulin-stimulated carbohydrate metabolism in normal men. J Clin Invest 1991;88:960
9. Bressler R, Gay R, Copeland JG, et al. Chronic inhibition of fatty acid oxidation: New model of diastolic dysfunction. Life Sci 1989;44:1897
10. Burges RA, Gardiner DG, Higgins AJ. Protection of the ischaemic dog heart by oxfenicine. Life Sci 1981;29:1847
11. Shipp JC, Opie LH, Challoner D. Fatty acid and glucose metabolism in the perfused heart. Nature (Lond) 1961;189:1018
12. Lee SM, Bahl JJ, Bressler R. Prevention of the metabolic effects of 2-tetradecylglycidate by octanoic acid in the genetically diabetic mouse (*db/db*). Biochem Med 1985;33:104
13. Ferrannini E, Barrett EJ, Bevilacqua S, DeFronzo RA. Effect of fatty acids on glucose production and utilization in man. J Clin Invest 1983:1737
14. Campbell PJ, Mandarino LJ, Gerich JE. Quantification of the relative impairment in actions of insulin on hepatic glucose production and peripheral glucose uptake in non–insulin-dependent diabetes mellitus. Metabolism 1988;37:15
15. Hall SEH, Saunders J, Sonksen PH. Glucose and free fatty acid turnover in normal subjects and in diabetic patients before and after insulin treatment. Diabetologia 1979;16:297
16. Groop LC, Bonadonna C, DelPrato C, et al. Glucose and free fatty acid metabolism in non–insulin-dependent diabetes mellitus: Evidence for multiple sites of insulin resistance. J Clin Invest 1989;84:205
17. DeFronzo RA, Simonson D, Ferrannini E. Hepatic and peripheral insulin resistance: A common feature of type 2 (non–insulin-dependent) and type I (insulin-dependent) diabetes mellitus. Diabetologia 1982;23:313
18. Foley JE. Rationale and application of fatty acid oxidation inhibitors in the treatment of diabetes mellitus. Diabetes Care 1992;15:773
19. Prager R, Wallace P, Olefsky JM. Direct and indirect effects of insulin to inhibit hepatic glucose output in obese subjects. Diabetes 1987;36:607
20. Biermann E, Dole VP, Roberts TN. An abnormality of nonesterified fatty acid metabolism in diabetes mellitus. Diabetes 1957;6:475
21. Munkner C. Fasting concentrations of non-esterified fatty acids in diabetic and non-diabetic plasma and diurnal variations in normal subjects. Scand J Clin Lab Invest 1959;11:388
22. Fraze R, Donner CC, Swislocki ALM, et al. Ambient plasma free fatty acid concentrations in non–insulin-dependent diabetes mellitus: Evidence for insulin resistance. J Clin Endocrinol Metab 1985;61:807
23. Reaven GM, Chen Y-DI. Role of abnormal free fatty acid metabolism in the development of non–insulin-dependent diabetes mellitus. Am J Med 1988; 85:106
24. Taskinen MR, Sane T, Helve E, et al. Bedtime insulin for suppression of over-night free fatty acid, blood glucose, and glucose production in NIDDM. Diabetes 1989;38:580
25. Riddle MC. New tactics for type 2 diabetes: Regimens based on intermediate-acting insulin taken at bedtime. Lancet 1985;1:192
26. Bergman RN, Rebrin K, Steil GM. Free fatty acid as a link in the regulation of hepatic glucose output by peripheral insulin. Diabetes 1995;44:1038
27. Bonadonna RC, Groop LC, Zych K, et al. Dose-dependent effect of insulin on plasma free fatty acid turnover oxidation in humans. Am J Physiol 1990; 359:E736
28. Groop LC, Bonadonna RC, Shank M, et al. Role of free fatty acids and insulin in determining free fatty acid and lipid oxidation in man. J Clin Invest 1991;87:83
29. Saloranta C, Franssila-Kallunki, Ekstrand A. Modulation of hepatic glucose production by non-esterified fatty acids in type 2 (non–insulin-dependent) diabetes mellitus. Diabetologia 1991;34:409
30. Yki-Jarvinen H, Puhakainen I, Saloranta C, et al. Demonstration of novel feedback mechanism between FFA oxidation from intracellular and intravascular sources. Am J Physiol 1991;260:E680
31. Hoffman BB, Dall'Aglio E, Hollenbeck C, et al. Suppression of free fatty acids and triglycerides in normal and hypertriglyceridemic rats by the adenosine receptor agonist phenylisopropyladenosine. J Pharmacol Exp Ther 1986;239: 715
32. Wolf HPO. Acyl-substituted 2-oxirane carboxylic acids: A new group of antidiabetic drugs. In: Bailey CJ, Flatt PR, eds. New Antidiabetic Drugs. London: Smith Gorden; 1990:217
33. Young DA, Ho RS, Bell PA, et al. Inhibition of hepatic glucose production by SDZ 51641. Diabetes 1990;39:1408
34. Koundakjian PP, Turnbull DM, Bone AJ. Metabolic changes in fed rats caused by chronic administration of ethyl-2[5(4-chlorophenyl(pentyl]oxirane-2-carboxylate, a new hypoglycaemic compound. Biochem Pharmacol 1984;33:465
35. Wenke M. Effect of catecholamines on lipid metabolism. Adv Lipid Res 1966;4:69
36. Hoonor RC, Dhillon GS, Londos C. cAMP-dependent protein kinase and lipolysis in rat adipocytes. J Biol Chem 1985;260:15122
37. Kuroda M, Honnor RC, Cushman SW, et al. Regulation of insulin-stimulated glucose transport in the isolated rat adipocyte. J Biol Chem 1987;262:245
38. Ammon HPT, Estler CJ, Heim F, Okoronkwo B. Different effects of inhibition of lipolysis by nicotinic acid on the rate of glycolytic carbohydrate breakdown in brain skeletal muscle. Life Sci 1969;8:213
39. Foley JE. Mechanisms of impaired insulin action in isolated adipocytes from obese and diabetic subjects. Diabetes Metab Rev 1988;4:487
40. Molnar GD, Berge KG, Rosevear JW, et al. The effect of nicotinic acid in diabetes mellitus. Metabolism 1964;13:181
41. Fuccella LM, Goldaniga G, Lovisolo P, et al. Inhibition of lipolysis by nicotinic acid and by acipimox. Clin Pharmacol Ther 1980;28:790
42. Dulbecco A, Albenga C, Borretta G, et al. Effect of acipimox on plasma glucose levels in patients with non–insulin-dependent diabetes mellitus. Curr Ther Res Clin Exp 1989;46:478
43. Vaag AA, Skott P, Damsbo P, et al. Effect of the antilipolytic nicotinic acid analogue acipimox on whole-body and skeletal muscle glucose metabolism in patients with non–insulin-dependent diabetes mellitus. J Clin Invest 1991; 88:1282
44. Fulcher GR, Farrer M, Thow JC, et al. The glucose-fatty acid cycle in non–insulin-dependent diabetes mellitus: The acute effects of inhibition of lipolysis overnight with acipimox. Diab Nutr Metab 1990;4:285
45. Fulcher GR, Catalano C, Walker M, et al. A double blind study of the effect of acipimox on serum lipids, blood glucose control and insulin action in non-obese patients with type 2 diabetes mellitus. Diabetic Med 1992;9:908
46. Fulcher GR, Walker M, Catalano C, et al. Metabolic effects of suppression of non-esterified fatty acid levels with acipimox in obese NIDDM subjects. Diabetes 1992;41:1400
47. Fulcher GR, Walker M, Catalano C, et al. Acute metabolic and hormonal responses to the inhibition of lipolysis in non-obese patients with non–insulin-dependent (type 2) diabetes mellitus: Effects of acipimox. Clin Sci 1992;82:565
48. Fulcher GR, Walker M, Farrer M, et al. Acipimox increases glucose disposal in normal man independent of changes in plasma nonesterified fatty acid concentration and whole-body lipid oxidation rate. Metabolism 1993;42:308
49. Dean JD, McCarthy S, Betteridge DJ, et al. The effect of acipimox in patients with type 2 diabetes and persistent hyperlipidaemia. Diabetic Med 1992;9:611
50. Worm D, Henriksen JE, Vaag A, et al. Pronounced blood glucose–lowering effect of the antilipolytic drug acipimox in non–insulin-dependent diabetes

mellitus patients during a 3-day intensified treatment period. J Clin Endocrinol Metab 1994;78:717
51. Pulkakainen I, Yki-Jarvinen H. Inhibition of lipolysis decreases lipid oxidation and gluconeogenesis from lactate but not fasting hyperglycemia or total hepatic glucose production in NIDDM. Diabetes 1993;42:1694
52. Kumar S, Durrington PN, Bhatnagar D, Laing I. Suppression of non-esterified fatty acids to treat type A insulin resistance syndrome. Lancet 1994;343:1073
53. Saloranta C, Taskinen MR, Widen E, et al. Metabolic consequences of sustained suppression of free fatty acids by acipimox in patients with NIDDM. Diabetes 1993;42:1559
54. Reaven GM, Chang H, Hoffman BB. Additive hypoglycemic effects of drugs that modify free-fatty acid metabolism by different mechanisms in rats with streptozocin-induced diabetes. Diabetes 1988;37:28
55. McGarry JD, Woeltje KF, Kuwajima M, Foster DW. Regulation of ketogenesis and the renaissance of carnitine palmitoyltransferase. Diabetes Metab Rev 1989;5:271
56. Woeltje KF, Esser V, Weis BC, et al. Inter-tissue and inter-species characteristics of the mitochondrial carnitine palmitoyltransferase enzyme system. J Biol Chem 1990;265:10714
57. Williamson JR, Browning ET, Schloz R, et al. Inhibition of fatty acid stimulation of gluconeogenesis by (+)-decanoylcarnitine in perfused rat liver. Diabetes 1968;17:194
58. McGarry JD, Foser DW. Acute reversal of experimental diabetes ketoacidosis in the rat with (+)-decanoylcarnitine. J Clin Invest 1973;52:877
59. Declercq PE, Falcks JR, Kuwajima M, et al. Characterization of the mitochondrial carnitine palmitoyltransferase enzyme system. J Biol Chem 1987;262: 9812
60. Tutwiler GF, Kirsch T, Bridi G, Washington F. A pharmacologic profile of McN-3495 [N-(1-methyl-2-pyrrolidinylidene)-*N*′-phenyl-1-pyrrolidinecarboximidamide], a new orally effective hypoglycemic agent. Diabetes 1978;27:856
61. Tutwiler GF, Kirsch T, Mohrbacher RJ, Ho W. Pharmacologic profile of methyl 2-tetradecylglycidate (McN-3716)—an orally effective hypoglycemic agent. Metabolism 1978;27:1539
62. Tutwiler GF, Dellevigne P. Action of the oral hypoglycemic agent 2-tetradecylglycidic acid on hepatic fatty acid oxidation and gluconeogenesis. J Biol Chem 1979;254:2935
63. Tutwiler GF. Glucose fatty acid cycle—possible therapeutic implications for diabetes. Larkins R, Zimmet P, Chisholm D, eds. New York: Elsevier;1988: 175
64. Wolf HPO, Engel DW. Decrease of fatty acid oxidation, ketogenesis and gluconeogenesis in isolated perfused rat liver by phenylalkyl oxirane carboxylate (B807-27) due to inhibition of CPT 1 (EC 2.3.1.2.1). Eur J Biochem 1985;146:359
65. Koundakjian PP, Turnbull DM, Bone AJ. Metabolic changes in fed rats caused by chronic administration of ethyl-2[5(4-chlorophenyl)pentyl]oxirane-2-carboxylate, a new hypoglycaemic compound. Biochem Pharmacol 1984;33:465
66. Aigius L, Pillay D, Alberti KGMM, Sherratt HSM. Effects of 2[5(4-chlorophenyl)pentyl]oxirane-2-carboxylate on fatty acid synthesis and fatty acid oxidation in isolated rat hepatocytes. Biochem Pharmacol 1983;34:2651
67. Vaartjes WJ, DeHaas CGM, Haagsman HP. Effects of sodium 2-5(4-chlorophenyl)pentyl]oxirane-2-carboxylate (POCA) on intermediary metabolism in isolated rat liver cells. Biochem Pharmacol 1986;35:4267
68. Panos TC, Finerty JC. Effects of a fat-free diet on growing female rats, with special reference to the endocrine system. J Nutr 1953;49:397
69. McCune SA, Durant PJ, Flanders LE, Harris RA. Inhibition of hepatic gluconeogenesis and lipogenesis by benzoic acid, *p*-tert.-butylbenzoic acid, and a structurally related hypolipidemic agent SC-33459. Arch Biochem Biophys 1982;214:124
70. Swartzentruber MS, Harris RA. Inhibition of metabolic processes by coenzyme-A-sequestering aromatic acids. Prevention by para-chloro- and para-nitrobenzoic acids. Biochem Pharmacol 1987;36:3147
71. Gately SJ, Sherratt HSA. The synthesis of hippurate from benzoate and glycine by rat liver mitochondria. Submitochondrial localization and kinetics. Biochem J 1977;166:39
72. Schulz H. Mitochondrial β-oxidation. In: Tanaka K, Coates PM, eds. Fatty Acid Oxidation: Clinical, Biochemical, and Molecular Aspects. New York: Alan R Liss;1990:23
73. Hasimoto T. Peroxisomal and mitochondrial enzymes. In: Coates PM, Tanaka K, eds. New Developments in Fatty Acid Oxidation. New York: Wiley-Liss;1992:19
74. Jakobs BS, Wanders RJA. Resolution of the subcellular site of very long-chain fatty acid β-oxidation in human skin fibroblasts using a novel approach. In: Coates PM, Tanaka K, eds. New Developments in Fatty Acid Oxidation. New York: Wiley-Liss;1192:231
75. Billington D, Osmundsen H, Stanley H, Sherratt HSA. Mechanisms of the metabolic disturbances caused by hypoglycin and by pent-4-enoic acid in vitro studies. Biochem Pharmacol 1978;27:2879
76. Kean EA. Selective inhibition of acyl-CoA dehydrogenases by a metabolite of hypoglycin. Biochim Biophys Acta 1976;422:8
77. Melde K, Buettner H, Boschert W, et al. Mechanism of hypoglycaemic action of methylenecyclopropylglycine. Biochem J 1989;259:921
78. Bell P, Cheon SH, Fillers S, et al. Design of novel agents for the therapy of non-insulin dependent diabetes mellitus (NIDDM). Bioorganic Medicinal Chem Lett 1993;13:1007
79. Sabbach E, Cuebas D, Schulz H. 3-Mercaptopropionic acid, a potent inhibitor of fatty acid oxidation in rat mitochondria. J Biol Chem 1985;260:7337

Part VIII

Pregnancy

Diabetes Mellitus, edited by Derek LeRoith, Simeon I. Taylor, and Jerrold M. Olefsky. Lippincott–Raven Publishers, Philadelphia © 1996.

CHAPTER 76

Intermediary Metabolism During Pregnancy: Implications for Diabetes Mellitus

THOMAS A. BUCHANAN

Introduction

Human beings, along with many other higher animals, use energy continuously but ingest nutrients intermittently. As a result, humans alternate between periods of anabolism during feeding and catabolism during fasting. Pregnancy places considerable demands on mechanisms that normally regulate anabolism and catabolism because mothers must be able to store nutrients efficiently during feeding to provide for the ever-increasing nutrient demands of the developing fetus during fasting. There is considerable evidence that hormonal products of the fetoplacental unit modify maternal intermediary metabolism in ways that can benefit the mother and fetus, provided that maternal pancreatic β-cell function is normal. When maternal β-cell function is abnormal, as in diabetes mellitus, the impact of pregnancy on maternal metabolism can have serious consequences for both mother and fetus. The impact of pregnancy on maternal metabolism in normal and diabetic pregnancies will be the focus of the present chapter, and the implications of maternal diabetes for fetal development will be discussed in Chapter 78.

Intermediary Metabolism in Normal Pregnancy

Carbohydrate Metabolism

Insulin Resistance

One of the most prominent metabolic changes that occurs during pregnancy is resistance to the glucose-lowering effects of insulin. This resistance was demonstrated nearly four decades ago by Burt,[1] who noted that pregnant women experienced less hypoglycemia in response to exogenous insulin than did nonpregnant women. Subsequently, the development of methods to measure circulating insulin concentrations revealed that normal pregnant women had exaggerated insulin responses to ingested glucose, together with decreased glucose tolerance, compared to nonpregnant women.[2,3] The insulin resistance suggested by these early observations has been confirmed and quantified by more recent studies in which insulin sensitivity was measured directly by the euglycemic clamp technique[4,5] or by computer analysis of intravenous glucose tolerance test results.[6,7] With both techniques, whole body insulin sensitivity during the third trimester of pregnancy was found to be reduced 45–70% below nonpregnant values. Thus, late pregnancy is attended by some of the most marked physiologic insulin resistance that has been observed in humans[8] (Fig. 76-1).

At least four lines of evidence indicate that hormonal changes of pregnancy contribute to the development of insulin resistance. First, insulin resistance tends to increase during pregnancy,[5,7] in parallel with increasing concentrations of circulating maternal hormones such as human placental lactogen, progesterone, prolactin, and cortisol.[9] Second, administration of human placental lactogen,[10–12] progesterone,[13–15] or glucocorticoids[12] to nonpregnant individuals induces metabolic changes indicative of impaired insulin action. Third, in vitro exposure of adipose tissue[16] or skeletal muscle[17] to hormones that are elevated during pregnancy blunts insulin-mediated glucose uptake by those tissues, particularly when the exposure includes several hormones in combination.[16] Fourth, findings indicative of insulin resistance, such as increased insulin requirements in diabetic patients[18–20] and hyperinsulinemia with reduced glucose tolerance in normal women,[2,3,21] reverse very rapidly after delivery of the fetus and placenta,[20,21] suggesting that products of the conceptus mediate maternal insulin resistance. Thus, it is very likely that the fetoplacental unit, acting largely through hormonal products, plays an important role in the development of maternal insulin resistance during pregnancy. Moreover, animal studies in which suppression of maternal lipolysis partially reversed the insulin resistance of late pregnancy[22] suggest that hormonal stimulation of lipolysis and the resultant increased concentrations of free fatty acids (FFA) in the circulation (see "Lipid Metabolism") may be important for the development of insulin resistance in pregnancy, as has been proposed for other conditions of insulin resistance.[23,24] Increasing maternal adiposity[25] may contribute to the insulin resistance of pregnancy as well.

Considerable effort has been invested in the identification of tissues that contribute to the insulin resistance of pregnancy. Glucose clamp studies performed in vivo using labeled glucose have consistently revealed resistance to insulin-mediated glucose utilization in pregnant women[5] and in lower mammals.[22,26–30] Because skeletal muscle is the major site of glucose utilization during hyperinsulinemic clamp studies,[31] those studies provide strong evidence for insulin resistance in skeletal muscle during pregnancy. Hindlimb balance studies in rabbits[28,32] and measurements of labeled glucose uptake by individual tissues in rats[27] and rabbits[33] during glucose clamp studies have confirmed that insulin-mediated glucose utilization by skeletal muscle is reduced >40% in late pregnancy compared to nonpregnant animals. Insulin-mediated glucose uptake by cardiac muscle[33] and fat cells[17,27,34] from pregnant animals has also been reported to be reduced compared to nonpregnant animals, although the reductions appear to be less marked in fat than in muscle.[27,33]

In contrast to the well-documented reduction in sensitivity of peripheral tissues to insulin during pregnancy, the status of hepatic insulin sensitivity is not clear. Results of glucose clamp studies performed with labeled glucose in pregnant rats[26,30] and rabbits[22,30,32] have led investigators to conclude that endogenous glucose production is resistant to the suppressive effects of insulin in late gestation. The interpretation of all of those studies, however, is complicated by the fact that clamps were performed at lower ambient glucose concentrations in pregnant compared to nonpregnant animals. The lower glucose concentrations per se may have created some of the apparent hepatic insulin resistance because glucose has a suppressive effect on hepatic glucose production that is synergistic with the suppressive effects of insulin.[35] Nonetheless, two observations in rabbits suggest that there is true hepatic insulin resistance in late pregnancy, at least in that species. First, suppression of circulating FFA concentrations in late pregnancy caused a slight increase in hepatic sensitivity to insulin,[22] suggesting that hepatic

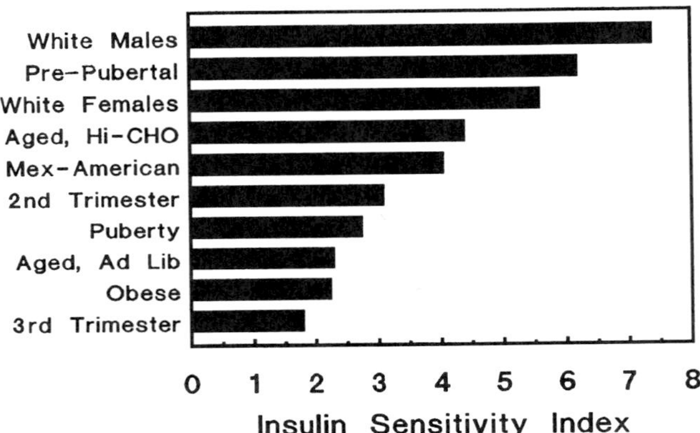

FIGURE 76-1. Range of insulin sensitivity in persons with normal glucose tolerance. Whole-body insulin sensitivity index (min^{-1}/ μU/mL) was measured with the Bergman minimal model technique[8] in 10 groups of persons with normal glucose tolerance. "Hi-CHO" denotes data collected after ingestion of a high carbohydrate diet. "Ad Lib" denotes data collected on an unrestricted diet. "Second Trimester" and "Third Trimester" denote results from pregnant women. (Adapted with permission from ref. 8.)

sensitivity was suppressed by the increased FFA concentrations that are characteristic of late gestation (see "Lipid Metabolism"). Second, Hauguel et al.[28] reported that hepatic insulin sensitivity was reduced in late pregnancy compared to midpregnancy despite similar ambient plasma glucose concentrations at the two stages, indicating a true decline in hepatic insulin sensitivity in late pregnancy. Studies of hepatic insulin sensitivity in human pregnancies have been limited to a small number of lean subjects studied serially from the preconception period.[36] Those studies did not reveal any reduction in hepatic insulin sensitivity during pregnancy, although the concentrations of insulin that were achieved during glucose clamps caused nearly complete suppression of glucose production before and during pregnancy. Thus, it remains unclear whether submaximal insulin concentrations will prove equally effective in suppressing endogenous glucose production in pregnant and nonpregnant humans.

The cellular mechanisms that underlie the insulin resistance of pregnancy have not been fully identified. Several groups have reported lower binding of insulin to adipocytes from pregnant compared to nonpregnant women.[37-39] Binding of insulin to hepatocytes[40,41] and to skeletal muscle,[42,43] quantitatively the most important tissue for insulin-mediated glucose uptake in vivo,[31] has been reported to be similar in pregnant and nonpregnant women. That finding suggests that postbinding events account for a large portion of the insulin resistance of pregnancy. Insulin-stimulated tyrosine kinase activity of hepatic insulin receptors has been reported to be decreased in rats during late pregnancy compared to nonpregnant control subjects.[41] By contrast, autophosphorylation of insulin receptors from human skeletal muscle has been reported to be unaffected by pregnancy,[42] as has the total content of GLUT-4 transporters in the same tissue in humans[44] and rats.[45] Thus, it appears that pregnancy induces peripheral insulin resistance by interfering with some aspect(s) of coupling between insulin receptor activation and glucose transport or metabolism in insulin target tissues such as skeletal muscle. A full definition of the intracellular events involved in that coupling in nonpregnant individuals may be required before the cellular mechanisms that mediate the insulin resistance of pregnancy are identified.

Hyperinsulinemia

It has been known for over three decades that circulating immunoreactive insulin concentrations are increased in late pregnancy compared to concentrations in women who are not pregnant.[2,3] Phelps et al.[46] and Kuhl[47] demonstrated that the increase was due to intact insulin rather than to other peptides with shared immunoreactivity, indicating true hyperinsulinemia in pregnancy. Burt and Davidson[48] and Bellman and Hartman[49] showed that the kinetics of insulin were similar in pregnant and nonpregnant women, indicating that enhanced pancreatic β-cell function must account for the hyperinsulinemia of pregnancy.

Longitudinal studies of insulin responses to glucose[2,5,50,51] have revealed a progressive increase in β-cell responsiveness that mirrors the progressive fall in insulin action during gestation.[5,7] This qualitatively inverse relationship between insulin action and pancreatic β-cell function during pregnancy is consistent with the proposal of Bergman and colleagues[8,52] that the normal relationship between insulin action and β-cell function is hyperbolic. The author's group[53] has demonstrated such a relationship in normal pregnant and nonpregnant women (Fig. 76-2), and Kahn et al.[54] have demonstrated a similar relationship in nonpregnant women and in men. Those findings, coupled with the fact that insulin resistance develops during pregnancy in the absence of endogenous β-cell function,[55] suggests that most of the hyperinsulinemia of normal pregnancy represents the pancreatic β-cell response to pregnancy-induced insulin resistance. That suggestion is supported by studies of pancreatic islets in vitro. Direct exposure of normal islets in vitro to conditions that mimic pregnancy had only a minor effect in enhancing β-cell responsiveness to insulin secretogogues.[56-58] Islets that were exposed in vivo to insulin resistance induced by pregnancy, or by administration of hormones such as progesterone and human placental lactogen exhibited much greater insulin secretory responses.[56,59-61]

The mechanisms that lead to enhanced insulin secretion in pregnancy are not known completely. A likely contributing factor is an increase in β-cell mass that appears, on the basis of animal studies,[62-64] to result from a combination of β-cell hypertrophy and hyperplasia. Hyperplasia of pancreatic islets has also been observed in human pregnancy.[65] The increased β-cell mass may contribute to the pattern of increased fasting insulin concentrations despite normal or lowered fasting glucose concentrations that has been observed in late pregnancy.[6,36] Increased β-cell mass may also contribute to an enhanced insulin response to secretogogues during pregnancy, although the magnitude of the enhanced β-cell responsiveness (i.e., two- to threefold above nonpregnant levels[6,36]) cannot

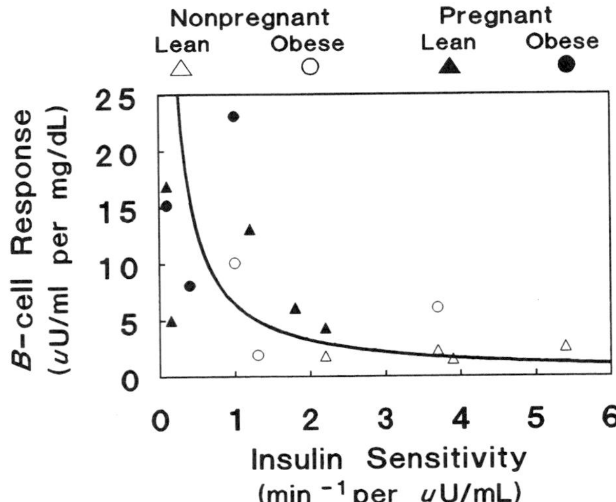

FIGURE 76-2. Relationship between insulin action and pancreatic β-cell function in pregnant and nonpregnant women with normal glucose tolerance. Measurements were made with the minimal model technique.[8] Symbols denote individual women; the line is a hyperbolic fit of the data, as originally proposed by Bergman et al.[52] (Adapted with permission from ref. 53.)

be explained on the basis of a 10–15% increase in β-cell mass.[65] Thus, the responsiveness of individual β-cells to nutrients must also be increased during pregnancy. The cellular mechanisms responsible for the increased responsiveness of β-cells have not been identified. Two groups of investigators[66,67] have reported evidence of increased activities of protein kinase A and/or protein kinase C in pancreatic tissue from pregnant compared to nonpregnant rats. Another recent report[68] indicated enhanced cell-to-cell communication in pancreatic islets from pregnant compared to nonpregnant animals. The relation of these phenomena to enhanced insulin secretion during pregnancy remains to be determined.

Lowered Fasting Glucose Concentrations

Fasting glucose concentrations tend to decline over the course of normal gestation. During the second trimester, the reduction is not apparent after a 12-hour overnight fast.[36,69] Extension of the fast by 72 hours, however, results in a significantly greater fall in circulating glucose concentrations compared to the result in nonpregnant women who fasted for the same period.[69] By the third trimester, plasma glucose concentrations after a 10-hour overnight fast are 10–20 mg/dL lower than in nonpregnant women,[6,36,70,71] and extension of the fast for as little as 4 additional hours results in a fall in plasma glucose concentrations in pregnant but not in nonpregnant women.[71]

The mechanisms responsible for the fasting hypoglycemia of pregnancy are only partly known. Endogenous glucose production rates during fasting have been measured in the third trimester, and most reports indicate that production rates are either the same or increased after an overnight fast compared to the rates in nonpregnant women.[36,70,72] The lowered fasting glucose concentrations in the face of increased glucose turnover rates are consistent with an expanded volume of distribution for glucose in late pregnancy.[70] The fact that the liver does not fully compensate for the reduced glucose concentrations suggests some restraint on glucose production compared to the nonpregnant condition. Indeed, the author's group[73] has shown that the fall in plasma glucose that occurs between 14 and 18 hours of fasting in the third trimester results from a fall in endogenous glucose production in the face of constant glucose clearance. Reduced availability of alanine as a substrate for gluconeogenesis, resulting both from impaired hepatic extraction of alanine[74] and from a reduced supply of alanine in the circulation[75,76] (see "Protein Metabolism"), has been implicated as a contributing factor to the fasting hypoglycemia of pregnancy. Enhanced β-cell function resulting in fasting insulin concentrations that are elevated relative to the ambient glucose concentrations[6,36,71] likely contributes to the fasting hypoglycemia as well.

Lipid Metabolism

Pregnancy is associated with two important alterations in lipid metabolism. The first is a stimulation of lipolysis and ketogenesis that is progressive over the course of gestation. In vitro data[77] indicate that the lipolysis results from the actions of placental hormones such as human placental lactogen, which directly stimulate free fatty acid (FFA) release from adipose tissue. The lipolytic effect normally is counterbalanced by the antilipolytic actions of insulin. Thus, the postprandial hyperinsulinemia of pregnancy maintains circulating FFA concentrations in a range that is only slightly higher than the range in nonpregnant women during the first 2–3 hours after eating[78] (Fig. 76-3). As circulating insulin concentrations fall in the postabsorptive period and during fasting, the lipolytic actions of placental hormones are unmasked, causing circulating FFA concentrations to rise. The FFA serve as a primary energy source for skeletal and cardiac muscles, and they provide the substrate for ketone production in the liver when insulin concentrations are low. The ketones can be used directly by the central nervous system as an energy source, providing an adaptive advantage by reducing the amount of glucose that must be produced from body protein stores. The magnitude of the accelerated fat catabolism increases during gestation, as can be seen from an examination of the duration of fasting required to generate exaggerated ketosis in pregnant compared to nonpregnant women. Felig and Lynch[69] observed exaggerated ketosis after 84 hours of fasting in the second trimester, and Metzger et al.[71] found a similar degree of exaggerated ketosis after only 14–18 hours of fasting in the third trimester.

The second major alteration of lipid metabolism that occurs during pregnancy is an increase in circulating triglyceride concentrations. Serum triglycerides in pregnant women are increased 1.5–2-fold above nonpregnant concentrations by the third trimes-

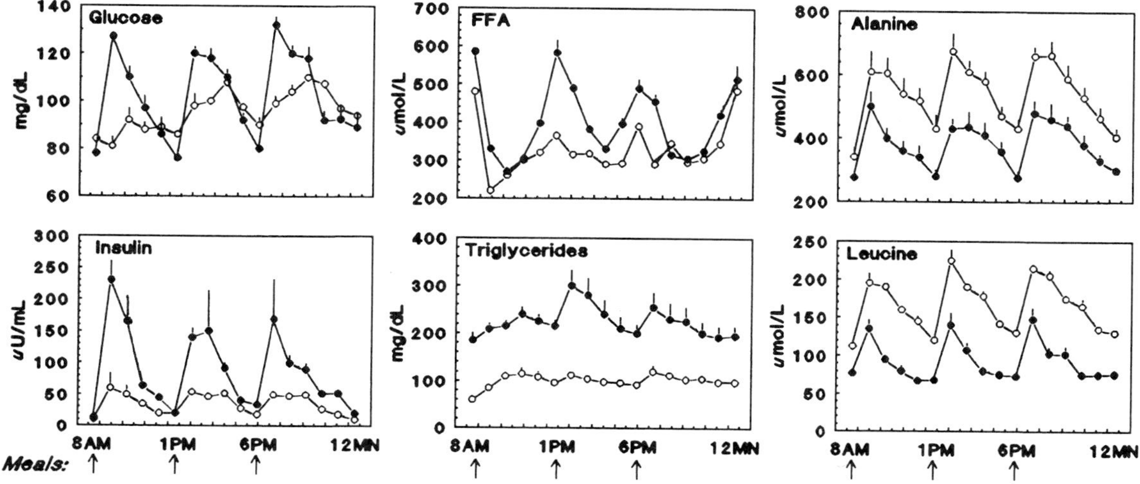

Figure 76-3. Profiles of plasma glucose, insulin, FFA, triglycerides, and two representative amino acids in eight nonpregnant women (open symbols) and eight pregnant women with normal glucose tolerance studied during the third trimester (closed symbols). Women were given liquid formula meals at arrows, and blood was collected hourly from indwelling venous catheters. (Adapted with permission from ref. 78.)

ter.[78] The hypertriglyceridemia appears to result from a combination of three factors[79]: (1) increased circulating FFA concentrations and hyperinsulinemia, which combine to promote triglyceride synthesis in the liver[80]; (2) increased food intake, resulting in increased appearance of chylomicrons from the gut; and (3) reduced activity of lipoprotein lipase in adipose tissue, resulting in reduced clearance of triglycerides from the circulation. The first factor can account for much of the increase in fasting triglyceride concentrations that occurs by late pregnancy, and all three factors are likely to contribute to hypertriglyceridemia in the fed state. As a result of these three factors, triglyceride concentrations are higher around the clock in third-trimester pregnant women compared to nonpregnant women.[78]

Protein Metabolism

Circulating concentrations of most amino acids are reduced in pregnant compared to nonpregnant women[78,81] (see Fig. 76-3). The mechanisms underlying the hypoaminoacidemia of pregnancy are not well understood.[73] The lowering of fasting amino acid concentrations may be due in part to an inhibition by placental hormones of amino acid release from skeletal muscle.[82,83] Mechanisms that may contribute to the postprandial hypoaminoacidemia of pregnancy include (1) accelerated maternal uptake of amino acids in response to postprandial hyperinsulinemia; (2) alterations in the distribution volume of amino acids as a result of intravascular and interstitial volume expansion during pregnancy; and (3) increased amino acid utilization by the fetus during late pregnancy. The last of these three factors may be important in polytocous species such as the rat, in which the fetal mass may comprise 20–30% of the total gravid body weight by the end of gestation. Data indicating that amino acid turnover is not increased in the third trimester of human pregnancies,[84] however, do not favor a role for fetal siphoning of maternal amino acids as a cause for hypoaminoacidemia in pregnant women.

Integrated Metabolism of Normal Pregnancy

As a result of the alterations in carbohydrate, lipid, and protein metabolism described above, intermediary metabolism in late pregnancy reflects an exaggeration of the normal swings between fed-state anabolism and fasting catabolism that occur in nonpregnant individuals (Fig. 76-4). During feeding, glucose and insulin concentrations rise rapidly as a result of the marked insulin resistance and compensatory hyperinsulinemia of late pregnancy. The hyperinsulinemia is sufficient to minimize, but not to eliminate, postprandial hyperglycemia. The hyperinsulinemia also counterbalances the lipolytic effects of placental hormones, thereby suppressing circulating free fatty acid (FFA) and ketone concentrations during feeding. Between meals, glucose concentrations fall more rapidly and to lower levels in pregnant compared to nonpregnant women. The fall in glucose is associated with a fall in circulating insulin concentrations, leaving unopposed the lipolytic effects of placental hormones. As a result, there is a brisk rise in circulating FFA concentrations between meals; ketone concentrations rise as well, especially during extended periods of fasting. Unlike the exaggerated cyclicity of glucose, insulin, and FFA, circulating triglycerides and amino acids exhibit more constant changes during late pregnancy. Triglyceride concentrations are higher and concentrations of nearly all amino acids are lower in pregnant than in nonpregnant women.

These metabolic changes of pregnancy appear to be mediated largely by the effects of placental hormones and thus represent the adaptive impact of the conceptus on maternal metabolism. That

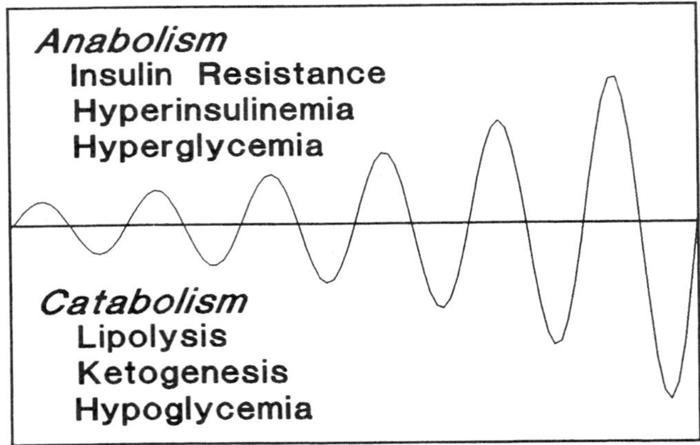

Figure 76-4. Schematic representation of maternal metabolic changes during gestation. Anabolism during feeding and catabolism during fasting are exaggerated in a progressive fashion, reflecting the combined effects of placental hormones and nutrient use by the fetus. (Reproduced with permission from Buchanan TA, Coustan DR. Diabetes Mellitus. In: Burrows GN, Ferris TF, eds. Medical Complications During Pregnancy. 4th ed. Philadelphia: WB Saunders;1994:29–61.)

impact increases in magnitude during pregnancy (see Fig. 76-4) and abates rapidly on delivery of the fetus and placenta. The adaptive significance of this impact on maternal metabolism may be threefold. First, the exaggerated excursions of maternal carbohydrate and lipid nutrients after feeding can be expected to promote transplacental passage of those nutrients, thereby providing energy substrates for fetal anabolism.[9,85] Second, to the extent that insulin resistance is more marked in skeletal muscle than in adipose tissue during pregnancy,[27,86,87] the compensatory hyperinsulinemia of pregnancy may promote a diversion of ingested nutrients toward storage in maternal adipose tissue, thereby enhancing maternal anabolism during feeding. Third, the accelerated fat catabolism and hypoglycemia that occur during fasting allow the mother to switch quickly from carbohydrate to fat as a predominant energy source for many tissues. That rapid switch, termed *accelerated starvation* by Freinkel,[88] allows the mother to utilize her fat stores for energy production, thereby minimizing the amount of her own muscle mass that must be consumed to meet maternal and fetal energy needs.

Implications for Diabetes in Pregnancy

The plasticity of pancreatic β-cell function plays a pivotal role in the normal maternal metabolic adaptations to pregnancy described thus far in this chapter. Women who lack that plasticity because of functional and/or structural abnormalities of their β-cells cannot respond appropriately to the adaptive impact of the conceptus on maternal metabolism. As a result, those women may exhibit abnormalities of carbohydrate, lipid, and protein metabolism that, in their mildest form, can alter fetal development and, in their most severe form, can threaten both maternal and fetal survival. The two normal metabolic changes of pregnancy that have the greatest potential impact on women with abnormal β-cell function are insulin resistance and accelerated fat catabolism. Those changes will be the focus of the remainder of this chapter, and their impact will be discussed in relation to women who are known to have diabetes before they become pregnant (i.e., women with pregestational diabetes) and women who are first discovered to have hyperglycemia during pregnancy (i.e., women with gestational diabetes).

Pregestational Diabetes

Insulin Resistance

Young women with diabetes may have insulin-dependent diabetes mellitus (IDDM), which generally is characterized by a complete lack of endogenous β-cell function, or non–insulin-dependent diabetes mellitus (NIDDM), which generally is characterized by impaired β-cell function. The absolute or relative insulin deficiency of these two conditions precludes normal pancreatic β-cell compensation for the insulin resistance of pregnancy. As a result, concentrations of glucose, triglycerides, and many amino acids may be elevated in the maternal circulation. Those metabolites, together with elevated concentrations of free fatty acids (FFA) and ketones that result from unregulated fat catabolism (see below), can alter embryonic and fetal development, leading to many of the perinatal complications of pregestational diabetes that are discussed in Chapter 78.

To minimize the impact of maternal diabetes on the fetus, exogenous insulin must be provided in a physiologic pattern and in sufficient amounts to normalize maternal intermediary metabolism. Because patients with IDDM generally have normal insulin sensitivity before pregnancy, the insulin resistance of pregnancy may lead to a substantial (i.e., 1.5–3-fold) increase in the amount of insulin required to maintain normoglycemia.[20,89] The majority of the increase occurs during the second half of gestation.[89] Patients with NIDDM also manifest an increase in exogenous insulin requirements during pregnancy, and their total insulin requirements are generally greater than those of patients with IDDM.[18,19] The insulin requirements of both groups of patients decrease markedly on delivery of the fetus and placenta.[20,21]

Accelerated Fat Catabolism

Patients with insulin-dependent diabetes mellitus (IDDM) are well known to be at risk for the development of ketoacidosis when rates of lipolysis and ketogenesis are not controlled by exogenous insulin. That risk is increased by the accelerated fat catabolism of pregnancy. Hormonal stimulation of lipolysis increases over the course of gestation, and increased insulin availability is needed to keep lipolysis and ketogenesis in check. As a result of these changes, pregnant women with IDDM may develop ketoacidosis rapidly (e.g., in 12–24 hours) and at relatively low circulating glucose concentrations (i.e., <400 mg/dL[91]) if they fail to take their insulin or if they develop an intercurrent illness. Intravenous administration of β-agonists (e.g., ritodrine) to arrest premature labor may add to the normal drive for lipolysis and ketosis in pregnancy and may also precipitate ketoacidosis in women with IDDM[92] unless they are managed aggressively.[93] Prevention and rapid treatment of ketoacidosis are important because of the high fetal mortality associated with that condition.[91]

Pregnant women with non–insulin-dependent diabetes mellitus (NIDDM) rarely develop diabetic ketoacidosis. The accelerated fat catabolism of pregnancy, however, has important implications for the dietary management of NIDDM during pregnancy. Caloric restriction, which has been shown to be effective in ameliorating hyperglycemia in nonpregnant people with NIDDM, may result in fasting ketosis during pregnancy.[71,94,95] Although the magnitude of the fasting ketosis is not sufficient to cause changes in maternal acid-base status, maternal ketonuria[96,97] and ketonemia[98] have been associated with impaired motor and intellectual development in offspring. Thus, the potential for ketosis during fasting limits the utility of hypocaloric diets in the management of overweight pregnant women with NIDDM.

Circulating Nutrient Concentrations

The concentrations of carbohydrate, lipid, and protein nutrients in the circulation of women with pregestational diabetes depend on the degree of metabolic regulation, which is usually assessed clinically by measuring circulating maternal glucose concentrations. Several groups[90,99–102] have shown that aggressive control of maternal glucose concentrations is associated with normalization of mean triglyceride, free fatty acid (FFA), ketone, and amino acid concentrations in the circulation of women with insulin-dependent diabetes mellitus (IDDM). Such normalization has generally been achieved with multiple daily insulin injections or continuous subcutaneous insulin infusions combined with frequent capillary glucose monitoring. Even when mean concentrations of maternal nutrients are normalized, however, daily variability may be increased, especially in the case of glucose and ketones.[99,100,102] Less successful management of circulating maternal glucose concentrations may be associated with elevations in ketone, FFA, triglyceride, and amino acid concentrations in the maternal circulation.

Gestational Diabetes

Insulin Resistance

In addition to people with overt diabetes, who generally have defective β-cell function under basal conditions, a subset of nondiabetic people appears to have a limitation of β-cell function that becomes manifest when these people encounter marked insulin resistance. Examples of nonpregnant people with such a limitation include individuals who develop diabetes mellitus in the face of the insulin resistance induced by Cushing's syndrome or acromegaly. A similar limitation in β-cell function appears to account for a majority of cases of gestational diabetes mellitus (GDM), defined as glucose intolerance that is first diagnosed during pregnancy.[103] Studies in which insulin sensitivity and insulin secretion have been measured in late pregnancy in women with mild to moderate GDM[5–7] have uniformly indicated that those women have the same degree of insulin resistance as normal women during late pregnancy. By contrast, the women with GDM exhibit impaired insulin secretory responses to glucose in late pregnancy compared to normal women.[5–7] Thus, it appears that a frequent pathogenesis for GDM is failure of β-cell compensation for the insulin resistance of late pregnancy. Women with GDM, especially those who are diagnosed early in pregnancy,[5,7] may have an additional component of insulin resistance that is not specifically related to pregnancy.[104,105] That additional insulin resistance may be similar to the chronic insulin resistance that has been noted in individuals at risk for non–insulin-dependent diabetes mellitus (NIDDM).[106–108] In fact, the combination of a β-cell defect and chronic insulin resistance may explain the relatively high rate of development of diabetes after pregnancy in women who have had GDM.[109,110]

Relatively few studies have investigated the mechanisms underlying the chronic insulin resistance of women who develop GDM. Garvey et al.[111] reported that the GLUT-4 content of rectus abdominus muscles was normal in women with GDM at term. By contrast, GLUT-4 content and subcellular trafficking in adipocytes were abnormal in women with GDM compared to nondiabetic pregnant women.[112] Ober et al.[113] have reported allele frequencies for restriction fragment length polymorphisms in the region of the insulin receptor gene and the insulin-like growth factor II gene that are different for white and African-American patients with GDM and race-matched, nondiabetic, pregnant women. The functional significance of these cellular defects and genetic associations in relation to insulin action in women with GDM remains to be determined.

The nature of the β-cell defect(s) in women with GDM is likely to be diverse. A minority of patients have evidence of autoimmunity directed against pancreatic islets.[114,115] Those women likely have evolving insulin-dependent diabetes mellitus (IDDM), and their limited β-cell capacity may be the result of immunologic damage to β-cells. The nature of the β-cell defects in other women with GDM is unclear, although a small minority of patients have mutations in the glucokinase gene that could be related to impaired β-cell function.[116]

Accelerated Fat Catabolism

The major implication of accelerated fat catabolism for women with gestational diabetes mellitus (GDM) is the risk of fasting ketosis (see "Pregestational Diabetes"). In the case of overweight patients with GDM, that risk has been shown to be equal to the risk in nondiabetic pregnant women.[94] Most overweight patients with GDM tolerate mild caloric restriction (e.g., to ~25 kcal per kilogram of actual body weight each day during the second half of gestation) without significant ketonuria.[95] More severe caloric restriction, however, may cause fasting ketosis, with the potential for long-term developmental problems in offspring.[96–98]

Circulating Nutrient Concentrations

As is true for pregestational diabetes, the imbalance between insulin resistance and pancreatic β-cell function that characterizes gestational diabetes mellitus (GDM) results in abnormal concentrations of carbohydrate, lipid, and protein nutrients in the maternal circulation. Metzger et al.[117] reported that concentrations of glucose, free fatty acids (FFA), triglycerides, and several branched-chain amino acids were increased in the circulation of women with GDM compared to normal pregnant women in the third trimester. Moreover, the magnitude of elevations of nonglucose nutrients paralleled the degree of hyperglycemia in the women with GDM. Normalization of circulating glucose concentrations in women with GDM has been reported to normalize circulating FFA and triglyceride concentrations as well.[118]

Summary

Metabolic changes, generated in large part by the effects of the feto-placental unit on maternal metabolism, allow mothers to store nutrients efficiently during feeding and utilize fat stores quickly during fasting while maintaining a supply of nutrients for fetal growth and development. The changes, which accentuate the normal fluctuations between anabolism during feeding and catabolism during fasting, increase in magnitude over the course of gestation. A normal response to these changes requires sufficient plasticity of pancreatic β-cell function to allow mothers to modulate the supply of insulin available to maternal tissues in response to the metabolic changes of pregnancy. Women with limited β-cell reserve cannot modulate their insulin secretion appropriately and incur significant metabolic abnormalities that may alter fetal development, as detailed in Chapter 77.

References

1. Burt RL. Peripheral utilization of glucose in pregnancy. III. Insulin tolerance. Obstet Gynecol 1956;2:558–664
2. Spellacy WN, Goetz FC. Plasma insulin in normal late pregnancy. N Engl J Med 1963;268:988–991
3. Bleicher SJ, O'Sullivan JB, Freinkel N. Carbohydrate metabolism in pregnancy. V. The interrelations of glucose, insulin and free fatty acids in later pregnancy and postpartum. N Engl J Med 1964;271:866–872
4. Ryan EA, O'Sullivan MJ, Skyler JS. Insulin action during pregnancy: Studies with the euglycemic glucose clamp technique. Diabetes 1985;34:380–389
5. Catalano PM, Tyzbir ED, Roman NM, et al. Longitudinal changes in insulin release and insulin resistance in nonobese pregnant women. Am J Obstet Gynecol 1991;165:1667–1672
6. Buchanan TA, Metzger BE, Freinkel N, Bergman RN. Insulin sensitivity and β-cell responsiveness to glucose during late pregnancy in lean and moderately obese women with normal glucose tolerance or mild gestational diabetes. Am J Obstet Gynecol 1990;162:1008–1014
7. Cousins L, Rea C, Crawford M. Longitudinal characterization of insulin sensitivity and body fat in normal and gestational diabetic pregnancies (abstract). Diabetes 1988;37(suppl 1):251A
8. Bergman RN. The Lilly Lecture 1989. Toward a physiological understanding of glucose tolerance: Minimal model approach. Diabetes 1989;38:1512–1528
9. Freinkel N. The Banting Lecture 1980. Of pregnancy and progeny. Diabetes 1980;29:1023–1035
10. Beck P, Daughaday WH. Human placental lactogen: Studies of its acute metabolic effects and disposition in normal man. J Clin Invest 1967;46:103
11. Samaan N, Yen SCC, Gonzalez D. Metabolic effects of placental lactogen in man. J Clin Endocrinol Metab 1968;28:485–491
12. Kalkhoff RK, Richardson BL, Beck P. Relative effects of pregnancy human placental lactogen and prednisolone on carbohydrate tolerance in normal and subclinical diabetic subjects. Diabetes 1969;18:153–175
13. Costrini NV, Kalkhoff RK. Relative effects of pregnancy, estradiol and progesterone on plasma insulin and pancreatic islet insulin secretion. J Clin Invest 1971;50:992–999
14. Beck P. Progestin enhancement of the plasma insulin response to glucose in rhesus monkeys. Diabetes 1969;18:146–152
15. Kalkhoff RK, Jacobson M, Lemper D. Progesterone, pregnancy and the augmented plasma insulin response. J Clin Endocrinol 1970;31:24–28
16. Ryan EA, Enns L. Role of gestational hormones in the induction of insulin resistance. J Clin Endocrinol Metab 1988;67:341–347
17. Leturque A, Haugel S, Sutter-Dub MT, Girard J. Effects of placental lactogen and progesterone on insulin stimulated glucose metabolism in rat muscles in vitro. Diabetes Metab 1989;15:176–181
18. Langer O, Anyaegbunam A, Brustman L, et al. Pregestational diabetes: Insulin requirements throughout pregnancy. Am J Obstet Gynecol 1988;159:616–621
19. Rudolf MC, Coustan DR, Sherwin RS, et al. Efficacy of the insulin pump in the home treatment of pregnant diabetics. Diabetes 1981;30:891–895
20. Jovanovic L, Peterson CM. Optimal insulin delivery for the pregnant diabetic patient. Diabetes Care 1982;5(suppl 1):24–37
21. Burt RL, Leake NH, Rhyne AL. Glucose tolerance during pregnancy and the puerperium. Obstet Gynecol 1969;33:634–641
22. Gilbert M, Basile S, Buadelin A, Pere MC. Lowering plasma free fatty acid levels improves insulin action in conscious pregnant rabbits. Am J Physiol 1993;264:E576–E582
23. Randle PJ, Garland PB, Hales CN, Newsholme EA. The glucose-fatty acid cycle: Its role in insulin sensitivity and the metabolic abnormalities of diabetes mellitus. Lancet 1963;1:785–789
24. Bonadonna RC, Groop LC, Simonson DC, DeFronzo RA. Free fatty acid and glucose metabolism in human aging: Evidence for operation of the Randle cycle. Am J Physiol 1994;266:501–509
25. Langhoff-Roos J, Wibell L, Gebre-Medhin M, Lindmark G. Placental hormones and maternal glucose metabolism: A study of fetal growth in normal pregnancy. Br J Obstet Gynaecol 1989;96:320–326
26. Leturque A, Burnol AF, Ferre P, Girard J. Pregnancy-induced insulin resistance in the rat: Assessment by glucose clamp technique. Am J Physiol 1984;246:E25–E31
27. Leturque A, Ferre P, Burnol AF, et al. Glucose utilization rates and insulin sensitivity in vivo in tissues of virgin and pregnant rats. Diabetes 1986;35:172–177
28. Hauguel S, Gilbert M, Girard J. Pregnancy-induced insulin resistance in liver and skeletal muscles of the conscious rabbit. Am J Physiol 1987;252: E165–E169
29. Gilbert M, Pere MC, Baudelin A, Battaglia FC. Role of free fatty acids in hepatic insulin resistance during late pregnancy in conscious rabbits. Am J Physiol 1991;260:E938–E945
30. Rossi G, Sherwin RS, Penzias AS, et al. Temporal changes in insulin resistance and secretion in 24-h-fasted conscious pregnant rats. Am J Physiol 1993;265:E845–E851
31. DeFronzo RA. Lilly Lecture 1987. The triumvirate: β-Cell, muscle, liver. A collusion responsible for NIDDM. Diabetes 1988;37:667–687
32. Bouisset M, Pere MC, Gilbert M. Net substrates balance across hindlimb in conscious rabbit during late pregnancy. Am J Physiol 1986;250:E42–E47
33. Hauguel S, Leturque A, Gilbert M, Girard J. Effects of pregnancy and fasting on muscle glucose utilization in the rabbit. Am J Obstet Gynecol 1988; 158:1215–1218
34. Toyoda N, Murata K, Sugiyama Y. Insulin binding, glucose oxidation, and methylglucose transport in isolated adipocytes from pregnant rats near term. Endocrinology 1985;116:998–1002
35. Ader M, and Bergman RN. Glucose synergizes insulin suppression of hepatic glucose output: Mechanism to avoid hyperglycemia (abstract). Diabetes 1988;37(suppl 1):77A

36. Catalano PM, Tyzbir ED, Wolfe RR, et al. Longitudinal changes in basal hepatic glucose production and suppression during insulin infusion in normal pregnant women. Am J Obstet Gynecol 1992;167:913–919
37. Pagano G, Cassader M, Massobrio M, et al. Insulin binding to human adipocytes during late pregnancy in healthy, obese and diabetic states. Horm Metab Res 1980;12:177–181
38. Hjolland E, Pedersen O, Espersen T, Klebe JG. Impaired insulin receptor binding and postbinding defects of adipocytes from normal and diabetic pregnant women. Diabetes 1986;35:598–603
39. Ciraldi TP, Kettel M, El-Roeiy A, et al. Mechanisms of cellular insulin resistance in human pregnancy. Am J Obstet Gynecol 1994;170:635–641
40. Davidson M. Insulin resistance of late pregnancy does not include the liver. Metabolism 1984;33:532–537
41. Martinez C, Ruiz P, Andres A, et al. Tyrosine kinase activity of liver insulin receptor is inhibited in rats at term gestation. Biochem J 1989;263:267–272
42. Damm P, Handberg A, Kuhl C, et al. Insulin receptor binding and tyrosine kinase activity in skeletal muscle from normal pregnant women and women with gestational diabetes. Obstet Gynecol 1993;82:251–259
43. Toyoda N, Deguchi T, Murata K, et al. Postbinding insulin resistance around parturition in the isolated rat epitrochlearis muscle. Am J Obstet Gynecol 1991;165:1475–1480
44. Garvey WT, Maianu L, Hancock JA, et al. Gene expression of GLUT4 in skeletal muscle from insulin-resistant patients with obesity, IGT, GDM, and NIDDM. Diabetes 1992;41:465–475
45. Okuno S, Maeda Y, Yamamguchi Y, et al. Expression of GLUT4 glucose transporter mRNA and protein in skeletal muscle and adipose tissue from rats in late pregnancy. Biochem Biophys Res Commun 1993;191:405–412
46. Phelps RL, Bergenstal R, Freinkel N. Carbohydrate metabolism in pregnancy. XII. Relationships between plasma insulin and proinsulin during late pregnancy in normal and diabetic subjects. J Clin Endocrinol Metab 1975;41: 1085–1091
47. Kuhl C. Serum proinsulin in normal and gestational diabetic pregnancy. Diabetologia 1976;12:295–300
48. Burt RL, Davidson IWF. Insulin half-life and utilization in normal pregnancy. Obstet Gynecol 1974;43:161–170
49. Bellman O, Hartman E. Influence of pregnancy on the kinetics of insulin. Am J Obstet Gynecol 1975;122:829–833
50. Spellacy WN, Goetz FC, Greenberg BZ. Plasma insulin in normal midpregnancy. Am J Obstet Gynecol 1965;92:11–15
51. Lind T, Billewicz WZ, Brown G. A serial study of changes occurring in the oral glucose tolerance test during pregnancy. J Obstet Gynaecol Br Commonw 1973;80:1033–1039
52. Bergman RN, Phillips LS, Cobelli C. Physiologic evaluation of factors controlling glucose tolerance in man. Measurement of insulin sensitivity and beta-cell sensitivity from the response to intravenous glucose. J Clin Invest 1981;68:1456–1467
53. Buchanan TA. Carbohydrate metabolism in pregnancy: Normal physiology and implications for diabetes mellitus. Isr J Med Sci 1991;27:432–441
54. Kahn SE, Prigeon RL, McCulloch DK, et al. Quantification of the relationship between insulin sensitivity and β-cell function in human subjects: Evidence for a hyperbolic function. Diabetes 1993;42:1663–1672
55. Schmitz O, Klebe J, Moller J, et al. In vivo insulin action in type I (insulin-dependent) diabetic pregnant women as assessed by the insulin clamp technique. J Clin Endocrinol Metab 1985;61:877–881
56. Costrini NV, Kalkhoff RK. Relative effects of pregnancy, estradiol and progesterone on plasma insulin and pancreatic islet insulin secretion. J Clin Invest 1971;50:992–999
57. Faure A, Suter-Dub MT. Insulin secretion from isolated pancreatic islets in the female rat. J Physiol (Paris) 1979;75:289–295
58. Howell SL, Tyhurst M, Green IC. Direct effects of progesterone on the islets of Langerhans in vivo and in tissue culture. Diabetologia 1977;13:579–583
59. Malaisse WJ, Malaisse-Lagae F, Picard C, Flament-Durand J. Effects of pregnancy and chorionic growth hormone upon insulin secretion. Endocrinology 1969;84:41–44
60. Hager D, Georg RH, Leitner JW, Beck P. Insulin secretion and content in isolated rat pancreatic islets following treatment with gestational hormones. Endocrinology 1972;91:977–981
61. Kalkhoff RK, Kim H-J. Effects of pregnancy on insulin and glucagon secretion by perfused rat pancreatic islets. Endocrinology 1978;102:623–631
62. Green IC, El Seifi S, Perrin D, Howell SL. Cell replication in the islets of Langerhans of adult rats: Effects of pregnancy, ovariectomy and treatment with steroid hormones. J Endocrinol 1981;88:219–224
63. Van Assche FA. Quantitative morphological and histoenzymatic study of the endocrine pancreas in non-pregnant and pregnant rats. Am J Obstet Gynecol 1974;118:39–41
64. Aerts L, Van Assche FA. Ultrastructural changes of the endocrine pancreas in pregnant rats. Diabetologia 1975;11:285–289
65. Van Assche FA, Aerts L, De Prins F. A morphological study of the endocrine pancreas in human pregnancy. Br J Obstet Gynaecol 1978;85:818–820
66. Hubinot CJ, Duframe SP, Malaisse WJ. Effect of pregnancy upon the activity of protein kinase A and C in rat pancreatic islets. Horm Metab Res 1985; 17:104–109
67. Tanigawa K, Tsuchiyama S, Kato Y. Differential sensitivity of pancreatic β-cells to phorbol ester TPA and C-kinase inhibitor H-7 in nonpregnant and pregnant rats. Endocrinol J 1990;37:883–891
68. Sheridan JD, Anaya PA, Parsons JA, Sorenson RL. Increased dye coupling in pancreatic islets from rats in later-term pregnancy. Diabetes 1988;37:908–911
69. Felig P, Lynch V. Starvation in human pregnancy: Hypoglycemia, hypoinsulinemia and hyperketonemia. Science 1970;170:990–992
70. Kalhan SC, D'Angelo LJ, Savin SM, Adam PAJ. Glucose production in pregnant women at term gestation. J Clin Invest 1979;63:388–394
71. Metzger BE, Ravnikar V, Vilesis R, Freinkel N. Accelerated starvation and the skipped breakfast in late normal pregnancy. Lancet 1982;1:588–592
72. Cowett RM. Hepatic and peripheral responsiveness to a glucose infusion in pregnancy. Am J Obstet Gynecol 1985;153:272–279
73. Bruschetta H, Buchanan TA, Steil GM, et al. Reduced glucose production accounts for the fall in plasma glucose during brief extension of an overnight fast in women with gestational diabetes (abstract). Clin Res 1994;42:27A
74. Kalhan SC, Gilfillian CA, Tserng KY, Savin SM. Glucose-alanine relationship in normal human pregnancy. Metabolism 1988;37:152–158
75. Felig P, Kim YJ, Lynch V, Hendler R. Amino acid metabolism during starvation in human pregnancy. J Clin Invest 1972;51:1195–1202
76. Metzger BE, Agnoli FS, Hare JW, Freinkel N. Carbohydrate metabolism in pregnancy. X. Metabolic disposition of alanine by the perfused liver of the fasting pregnant rat. Diabetes 1973;22:601–612
77. Turtle JR, Kipnis DM. The lipolytic action of human placental lactogen in isolated fat cells. Biochim Biophys Acta 1967;144:583–593
78. Phelps RL, Metzger BE, Freinkel N. Diurnal profiles of glucose, insulin, free fatty acids, triglycerides, cholesterol, and individual amino acids in late normal pregnancy. Am J Obstet Gynecol 1981;140:730–736
79. Herrera E, Gomez-Coronado D, Lasuncion MA. Lipid metabolism in pregnancy. Biol Neonate 1987;51:70–77
80. Topping DL, Mayes PA. The immediate effect of insulin and fructose on the metabolism of the perfused liver. Biochem J 1972;126:295–311
81. Kalhan SC, Assel BG. Protein metabolism in pregnancy. In: RM Cowett, ed. Principles of Perinatal-Neonatal Metabolism. New York: Springer Verlag; 1991:163–176
82. Morrow PG, Marshall WP, Kim H-J, Kalkhoff RK. Metabolic response to starvation I. Relative effects of pregnancy and sex steroid administration in the rat. Metabolism 1981;30:268–273
83. Morrow PG, Marshall WP, Kim H-J, Kalkhoff RK. Metabolic response to starvation II. Effects of sex steroid administration to pre- and post-menopausal women. Metabolism 1981;30:274–278
84. DeBenoist B, Jackson AA, Hall J. Whole-body protein turnover in Jamaican women during pregnancy. Hum Nutr Clin Nutr 1985;39:167–179
85. Freinkel N, Metzger BE, Nitzan M. Facilitated anabolism in late pregnancy: Some novel maternal compensations for accelerated starvation. In: Malaisse WJ, Pirart J, eds. Proceedings of the VIII Congress of the International Diabetes Federation. Excerpta Medica International Congress Series No. 312, Amsterdam: Excerpta Medica Co.; 1973:474
86. Andersen O, Kuhl C. Adipocyte insulin receptor binding and lipogenesis at term in normal pregnancy. Eur J Clin Invest 1988;18:575–581
87. Hauguel S, Leturque A, Gilbert M, Girard J. Effects of pregnancy and fasting on muscle glucose utilization in the rabbit. Am J Obstet Gynecol 1988; 158:1215–1218
88. Freinkel N. Effects of the conceptus on maternal metabolism during pregnancy. In: Leibel BS, Wrenshall GA, eds. On the Nature and Treatment of Diabetes. Amsterdam: Excerpta Medica; 1965:679–691
89. Rudolf MC, Coustan DR, Sherwin RS, et al. Efficacy of the insulin pump in the home treatment of pregnant diabetics. Diabetes 1981;30:891–895
90. Rigg L, Cousins L, Hollingsworth D, et al. Effects of exogenous insulin on excursions and diurnal rhythm of plasma glucose in pregnant patients with and without residual β-cell function. Am J Obstet Gynecol 1980;136:537–544
91. Montoro MN, Myers VP, Mestman JH, et al. Outcome of pregnancy in diabetic ketoacidosis. Am J Perinatol 1993;10:17–20
92. Mordes D, Kruetner K, Metzger W, Colwell JA. Dangers of intravenous ritrodrine in diabetic patients. JAMA 1982;248:973–975
93. Miodovnik M, Peros N, Holroyde JC, Siddiai TA. Treatment of premature labor in insulin-dependent diabetic women. Obstet Gynecol 1985;65:621–627
94. Buchanan TA, Metzger BE, Freinkel N. Accelerated starvation in late pregnancy: A comparison between obese normal pregnant women and women with gestational diabetes mellitus. Am J Obstet Gynecol 1990;162:1015–1020
95. Knopp RH, Magee MS, Raisys V, Benedetti T. Metabolic effects of hypocaloric diets in management of gestational diabetes. Diabetes 1991;40(suppl 2):165–171
96. Churchill JA, Berendez HW, Nemore J. Neuropsychological deficits in children of diabetic mothers. Am J Obstet Gynecol 1966;105:257–268
97. Stehbens JA, Baker GL, Kitchell M. Outcome at ages 1, 3, and 5 years of children born to diabetic women. Am J Obstet Gynecol 1977;127:408–413
98. Rizzo T, Metzger BE, Burns WJ, Burns K. Correlation between antepartum maternal metabolism and intelligence of offspring. N Engl J Med 1991; 325:911–916
99. Reece EA, Coustan DR, Sherwin RS, et al. Does intensive glycemic control in diabetic pregnancies result in normalization of other metabolic fuels? Am J Obstet Gynecol 1991;165:126–130
100. Potter JM, Reckless JPD, Cullen DR. The effect of continuous subcutaneous insulin infusion and conventional insulin regimes on 24-hour variations of blood glucose and intermediary metabolites in the third trimester of diabetic pregnancy. Diabetologia 1981;21:534–539
101. Hertz RH, King KC, Kalhan SC. Management of third-trimester diabetic

pregnancies with the use of continuous subcutaneous insulin infusion therapy: A pilot study. Am J Obstet Gynecol 1984;149:256–260
102. Jervell J, Stokke KT, Moe N, et al. Metabolic profiles in closely controlled diabetic pregnancies during the third trimester. Diabetologia 1979;16:229–233
103. Metzger BE and the Conference Organizing Committee. Summary and recommendations of the third international workshop-conference on gestational diabetes. Diabetes 1991;40(suppl 2):197–201
104. Ward WK, Johnston CLW, Beard JC, et al. Abnormalities of islet β-cell function, insulin action and fat distribution in women with a history of gestational diabetes: Relation to obesity. J Clin Endocrinol Metab 1985; 61:1039–1045
105. Ward WK, Johnston CLW, Beard JC, et al. Insulin resistance and impaired insulin secretion in subjects with a history of gestational diabetes mellitus. Diabetes 1985;34:861–869
106. Eriksson J, Franssila-Kallunki A, Ekstrand A, et al. Early metabolic defects in persons at increased risk for non–insulin-dependent diabetes mellitus. N Engl J Med 1989;231:337–343
107. Haffner SM, Stern MP, Mitchell BD, et al. Incidence of type II diabetes in Mexican Americans predicted by fasting insulin and glucose levels, obesity, and body-fat distribution. Diabetes 1990;39:283–288
108. Martin BC, Warram JH, Krolweski AS, et al. Role of glucose and insulin resistance in the development of type 2 diabetes mellitus: Results of a 25-year follow-up study. Lancet 1992;340:925–929
109. Kjos SL, Buchanan TA, Peters R, et al. Postpartum glucose tolerance testing identifies women with recent gestational diabetes who are at highest risk for developing diabetes within five years (abstract). Diabetes 1994;43(suppl 1):136A
110. Metzger BE, Cho NH, Roston SM, Radvany R. Prepregnancy weight and antepartum insulin secretion predict glucose tolerance five years after gestational diabetes mellitus. Diabetes Care 1994;16:1598–1605
111. Garvey WT, Maianu L, Hancock JA, et al. Gene expression of GLUT4 in skeletal muscle from insulin-resistant patients with obesity, IGT, GDM and NIDDM. Diabetes 1992;41:465–475
112. Garvey WT, Maianu L, Zhu J-H, et al. Multiple defects in the adipocyte glucose transport system cause cellular insulin resistance in gestational diabetes. Diabetes 1993;42:1773–1785
113. Ober C, Xiang K-S, Thisted RA, et al. Increased risk for gestational diabetes mellitus associated with insulin receptor and insulin-like growth factor II restriction fragment length polymorphisms. Gen Epidemiol 1989;6:559–569
114. Freinkel N, Metzger BE, Phelps RL, et al. Gestational diabetes mellitus: Heterogeneity of maternal age, weight, insulin secretion, HLA antigens, and islet cell antibodies and the impact of maternal metabolism on pancreatic β-cell function and somatic growth in the offspring. Diabetes 1985;34(suppl 2):1–7
115. Catalano PM, Tyzbir ED, Simms EAH. Incidence and significance of islet cell antibodies in women with previous gestational diabetes. Diabetes Care 1990;13:478–483
116. Stoffel M, Bell KL, Blackburn CL, et al. Identification of glucokinase mutations in subjects with gestational diabetes mellitus. Diabetes 1993;42: 937–940
117. Metzger BE, Phelps RL, Freinkel N, Navickas IA. Effects of gestational diabetes on diurnal profiles of plasma glucose, lipids, and individual amino acids. Diabetes Care 1980;3:402–409
118. Cowett RM, Carr SR, Ogburn PL. Lipid tolerance testing in pregnancy. Diabetes Care 1993;16:51–56

Diabetes Mellitus, edited by Derek LeRoith, Simeon I. Taylor, and Jerrold M. Olefsky. Lippincott–Raven Publishers, Philadelphia © 1996.

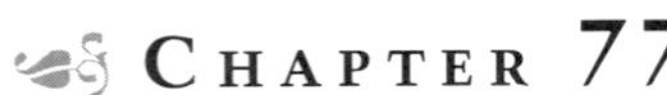

Chapter 77
Effects of Maternal Diabetes on Intrauterine Development

Thomas A. Buchanan

Introduction

Maternal diabetes can alter intrauterine development throughout gestation. The mechanisms by which diabetes alters development are incompletely understood, and they are likely to change over the course of pregnancy. At present, there is sufficient evidence to warrant separate discussions of two broad periods of development that can be altered by maternal diabetes: (1) the *first trimester,* during which maternal diabetes can lead to impaired growth, spontaneous abortions, and congenital anomalies through mechanisms that are not fully understood, and (2) the *second and third trimesters,* during which maternal diabetes can lead to fetal hyperinsulinism and excessive growth that appear to result from fetal overnutrition in the presence of an intact fetal pancreas. During each of these periods, the impact of maternal diabetes on the developing infant is determined by two factors: the intrauterine environment provided by the mother (see Chapter 76) and the fetal response to that environment.

Early Pregnancy: Effects on Embryogenesis

Normal Development and Maternal-Fetal Nutrient Transport

A review of normal human embryology reveals that the congenital malformations that have been reported in excess in diabetic pregnancies (Table 77-1; discussed below) occur during the first 6–7 weeks of intrauterine development.[1] The zygote spends the first 3 days of that period (development to the morula stage) in the fallopian tube and the next 2–3 days (development to the early blastocyst stage) in the uterus before initiating implantation on days 5–6 of development.[2] Implantation takes 5–6 days to complete, and the embryo establishes contact with the maternal blood via trophoblastic tissue near the end of implantation (days 11–12 of gestation; late blastocyst stage).

TABLE 77-1. Types and Timing of Malformations in Infants of Diabetic Mothers*

Type of Anomaly	Timing of Lesion (Weeks Postconception)
Skeletal	
Caudal regression	3
Spina bifida	6
Neural	
Anencephaly	4
Myelocele	4
Hydrocephalus	5
Cardiovascular	
Dextrocardia	4
Conus arteriosus defects	5
Ventricular septal defects	6
Renal	
Renal agenesis/hypoplasia	6

*The four major classes of malformations listed in italics have been reported in excess in diabetic pregnancies in five case-control studies.[40–42,45,46] Specific types of malformations have been reported in excess in three of those series.[40,41,46] Timing of malformations is based on normal events in human embryogenesis.[2]

Weeks 3–8 encompass organogenesis. The embryo develops into a trilaminar disc (endoderm, mesoderm, and ectoderm) with a primitive streak and notochord during week 3 (days 14–21). Neural tube formation and closure occur during weeks 3–4, an interval that is approximated by the in vitro studies of postimplantation rodent embryos discussed below (see ''Animal Models''). Formation of somites (precursors of the spinal cord) occurs from paraxial mesoderm during weeks 3–5. A single-chambered, beating heart with an embryonic circulation is established by the middle of week 4 (days 22–23). Cardiac septation occurs during weeks 4–5, and differentiation of the great vessels occurs during weeks 4–6. The ureteric bud begins to penetrate metanephric tissue to form the kidneys at the beginning of week 5; a primordial kidney is present by the end of week 6.

Embryos are exposed directly to fallopian and intrauterine fluid during their first 11–12 days of development (i.e., until implantation is complete and the implantation site is sealed off from the uterine cavity). Studies in rabbits[3] indicate that preimplantation embryos derive their energy supply from glucose as well as from nonglucose nutrients (probably lipids), and that they shift their pattern of glucose metabolism from aerobic to anaerobic glycolysis as they develop. Little is known about the nutrition and intermediary metabolism of human embryos after implantation. Studies in rodent embryos during that early postimplantation period, however, indicate that the embryo and its surrounding membranes are exposed to maternal plasma.[4,5] Small molecules such as glucose appear to be transported across the membranes, probably due to the presence of GLUT-1 transporter molecules in the membranes,[6] so that the embryos take up glucose in proportion to the surrounding glucose concentrations over a physiologic and pathologic range.[7] Larger molecules (e.g., peptides) may be processed by the membranes[8] and may not reach the embryo intact. Energy production from glucose during the early postimplantation period appears to occur predominantly through anaerobic glycolysis, so that relatively few high-energy phosphate molecules are produced per molecule of glucose metabolized when compared to later stages of development.[7,9–11] Early postimplantation embryos also metabolize glucose via the pentose phosphate pathway,[10,12,13] which is critical for production of ribose molecules for nucleic acid synthesis. Thus, the early postimplantation period when organogenesis begins can be characterized as a period when embryos need a constant supply of glucose to meet the energy[14–16] and synthetic[12,13] requirements of normal growth and development. At the same time, an oversupply of glucose during early organogenesis may lead to increased glucose uptake by embryos[7,17] and metabolism of glucose via deleterious pathways, resulting in severe developmental defects or death (see ''Animal Models''). Thus, there appears to be a relatively narrow range of glucose supply that is optimal for embryogenesis in the early postimplantation period. After establishment of the allantoic placenta and embryonic circulation at days 22–23 of development, rodent embryos shift to a greater predominance of aerobic metabolism[7,10–12,18] and thereby become less vulnerable to interruptions in their glucose supply.[19] Growth factors such as insulin[20,21] and insulin-like growth factors I and II[20] also appear to be important for normal embryo development at the early postimplantation stage. Maternal-fetal nutrient transport has not been well studied during this stage; the transport characteristics of the placenta during later stages of development are discussed below (see ''Later Pregnancy'').

Impact of Maternal Diabetes on Early Intrauterine Development

Three types of developmental abnormalities have been reported in association with maternal diabetes during the first trimester of human pregnancy: early growth delay, spontaneous abortions, and major congenital malformations. Because very little research has been conducted to elucidate the mechanisms underlying these three abnormalities in human pregnancies, this section will be limited to a description of the abnormalities and their relationship, when known, to maternal metabolic regulation in early human pregnancy. Potential mechanisms for the abnormalities will be discussed below (see ''Animal Models'').

Early Growth Delay

Early growth delay in diabetic pregnancies has been noted in two studies[22,23] in which women with insulin-dependent-diabetes (IDDM) and well-documented menstrual histories had ultrasound examinations to assess fetal size in the first and/or early second trimester of pregnancy. In both studies, the mean growth delay was mild (e.g., <5% reduction in crown-rump length compared to standard growth curves[23]), although infants who subsequently proved to have major congenital anomalies manifested more severe growth delay. Whether the apparent growth delay was due to a true slowing of embryonic growth in early pregnancy or to a change in the temporal relationship between menses and conception that produced an artifactually early estimated date of conception is unclear. Early growth retardation, however, has been a consistent feature in animal studies of diabetic pregnancies (see ''Animal Models''), suggesting that there may truly be early growth delay in human diabetic pregnancies as well. Although malformed human fetuses tended to have the greatest degree of early growth delay, the association was inconsistent. Thus, the phenomenon of early growth delay may be interesting from the standpoint of developmental biology, but it is not useful for the prediction of anomalies in individual patients.

Spontaneous Abortions

Some published reports have concluded that there is an increase in the spontaneous abortion rate in diabetic pregnancies.[24–26] Those studies, however, have lacked an appropriate control group to allow that conclusion to be drawn with certainty.[27] Two recent, well-controlled studies[28,29] have not revealed an overall increase in the spontaneous abortion rate in diabetic compared to nondiabetic

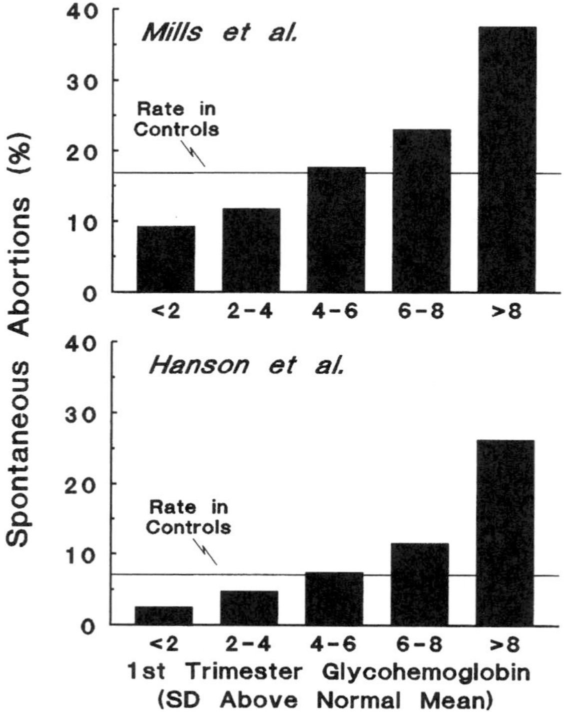

Figure 77-1. Relationship between spontaneous abortion rates and maternal first trimester glycohemoglobin concentrations in women with pregestational diabetes, as reported by Mills et al.[28] in the United States and Hanson et al.[29] in Sweden. Because techniques used to measure glycohemoglobin vary among laboratories, glycohemoglobin concentrations are expressed as standard deviations above the mean of persons without diabetes. A laboratory's normal range usually includes the normal mean plus or minus two standard deviations. Horizontal lines indicate the spontaneous abortion rates in nondiabetic subjects in each study.

women. In both of those studies and in two other reports,[30,31] however, there has been a clear increase in the spontaneous abortion rate in association with elevated maternal glycohemoglobin concentrations during the first or early second trimester, reflecting poor maternal glycemic control during very early pregnancy (Fig. 77-1). Thus, there can be little doubt that there is an increased risk of spontaneous abortion in diabetic pregnancies when maternal glycemic control is poor during early gestation. The temporal window of susceptibility for induction of spontaneous abortions by maternal diabetes is unknown.

Congenital Malformations

The best-known complication of maternal diabetes in early pregnancy is the generation of major congenital anomalies in infants, generally defined as anomalies that result in mortality, require surgical correction, or cause significant long-term morbidity. Studies spanning the period 1946–1988[32–39] indicate that, in the absence of special preconceptional diabetes care, 8–13% of infants born to mothers whose diabetes was present at conception are born with major malformations (Table 77-2). Those malformation rates are two to four times the rates reported for nondiabetic women in the general population or in prospectively recruited, nondiabetic control subjects.[32,37,38] Moreover, three population-based case-control studies[40–42] have reported risks of major malformations in diabetic pregnancies that are five to eight times the risks in nondiabetic pregnancies. Thus, there can be little doubt that the presence of maternal diabetes during early gestation can increase the risk of major malformations in infants. Prevalence rates of minor congenital anomalies (those not requiring surgical or medical intervention and not causing significant morbidity or mortality) do not appear to be increased by the presence of maternal diabetes.[38,43,44]

Several groups of investigators have examined the specific types of major malformations that occur in excess in diabetic pregnancies; most have taken a traditional organ system approach to the categorization of malformations. Results from five large case-control studies[40–42,45,46] indicate that maternal diabetes can increase the risk of malformations of the central nervous system,[40–42,46] heart and great vessels,[40–42,45] axial skeleton,[41,42,46] and urinary tract.[41,42,46] Cardiovascular and central nervous system defects appear to be the most common abnormalities associated with maternal diabetes. The skeletal abnormalities (particularly the caudal regression syndrome) are the most specific because of their rarity in offspring of nondiabetic mothers. Results from three large studies[42,46,47] indicate that rates of multiply-malformed infants are increased by maternal diabetes. That observation suggests that maternal diabetes may affect one or more developmental processes that lead to multiple defects rather than affecting any specific organ system. Indeed, Martinez-Frias[42,48] has presented evidence that maternal diabetes causes a group of defects that can be explained by disruption of specific developmental fields during blastogenesis, and Khoury et al.[47] have reported that a combination of vertebral and cardiovascu-

Table 77-2. Major Malformation Rates in Infants of Mothers with Pregestational Diabetes in the Absence of Special Preconceptional Diabetes Care*

Investigator	Years of Study	IDM with Anomalies	Control Infants with Anomalies
Pedersen[32]	1946–78	8%	3%
Karlsson and Kjellmer[33]	1961–70	11%	—
Gabbe et al.[34]	1971–75	7%	—
Miller et al.[35]	1977–80	13%	—
Fuhrman et al.[36]	1977–82	8%	—
Simpson et al.[37]	1977–81	8%	2%
Mills et al.[38]	1980–85	9%	2%
Kitzmiller et al.[39]	1982–88	11%	—

*Definitions of a major malformation vary among studies but usually require significant impact on the well-being of the infant (e.g., requiring surgery or causing mortality). IDM = infants of diabetic mothers. A control group of nondiabetic women was recruited prospectively in the studies of Simpson et al.[37] and Mills et al.[38] Malformation rates in the general population served as a control in the study by Pedersen.[32]

lar anomalies is characteristic of diabetic embryopathy in humans. The latter authors, however, also noted that the spectrum of anomalies associated with maternal diabetes could not be attributed to the disruption of any single developmental process, so that clinical diabetic embryopathy may represent the end result of more than one pathogenetic mechanism.

In theory, three specific components of maternal diabetes could contribute to the risk of malformations in infants of diabetic mothers: genetic transmission linked to genes for diabetes, long-term maternal vascular complications, and maternal metabolic abnormalities. Three observations suggest that the excess risk of malformations is not simply transmitted genetically along with susceptibility genes for diabetes: (1) malformations occur with increased frequency in offspring of women with insulin-dependent diabetes mellitus (IDDM) and non–insulin-dependent diabetes mellitus (NIDDM),[42,49] two diseases that are believed to be genetically distinct; (2) there is no excess risk of malformations in offspring of diabetic fathers[50]; and (3) the excess risk of malformations in women with IDDM can be reduced by careful preconceptional diabetes management.[36,39,51] Thus, although there is likely to be genetic variability in the susceptibility of embryos to the impact of maternal diabetes (see "Animal Models"), the overall excess risk cannot be attributed simply to genetic factors.

Studies in which malformation rates have been reported separately in offspring of diabetic women with and without diabetic microangiopathy[32–34,37,52,53] have consistently revealed higher rates in offspring of the women with microvascular disease. It is difficult to determine from most of those studies whether the increased anomaly rates were related specifically to the presence of microangiopathy because potential confounding factors such as maternal metabolic control were not provided. Miodovnik et al.[53] reported an association between maternal microangiopathy and congenital anomalies that was statistically independent of maternal glycemic control in early pregnancy, suggesting that the embryo derives a specific risk for malformations when the mother has diabetic retinopathy or nephropathy. That suggestion has not been confirmed in three other recent studies,[30,38,44] so that the impact of maternal microvascular disease on the risk of congenital anomalies remains controversial.

Most evidence from human pregnancies points to maternal metabolic abnormalities as the most important explanation for the increased risk of major malformations in diabetic pregnancies. The evidence comes from three general types of studies, all of which focus on maternal glucose as the index of metabolic control: (1) analysis of maternal blood glucose or glycohemoglobin concentrations in relation to malformation rates among unselected patients whose diabetes antedated conception; (2) comparison of malformation rates and measures of maternal glycemia between women who present for medical care when already pregnant and women who enroll in preconceptional diabetes care programs; and (3) comparison of malformation over time as overall diabetes control improves in a population. Results from the first type of study[29–31,35] indicate that the risk of malformations increases with increasing maternal glycemia, as assessed by maternal glycohemoglobin concentrations near the end of the first trimester (reflecting maternal glycemia during embryogenesis). Those studies reveal two important characteristics of the relationship between maternal glycemia and the risk of malformations (Fig. 77-2): (1) the risk increases in a nonlinear fashion with increasing maternal glycohemoglobin concentrations and (2) glycohemoglobin concentrations slightly above the normal range are not associated with an increased risk of malformations compared to the nondiabetic population. Results from at least five studies of preconceptional diabetes management programs[36,38,39,51,54] (Table 77-3) indicate that the risk of malformations is lower in women who attend those programs than in women who do not. Because all of the attenders were self-selected, it is possible that the lower malformation rates were the result of factors other than improved metabolic control. The observation that malformation rates are decreasing in the absence of special preconception clinics in parts of the world where diabetes care has improved in the population as a whole,[29,44,55] however, provides strong evidence that improved metabolic regulation can reduce the risk of congenital malformations in diabetic pregnancies. The metabolic factors that are reversed by improved glycemic control remain to be identified because maternal glucose has been the sole focus of the human studies cited above.

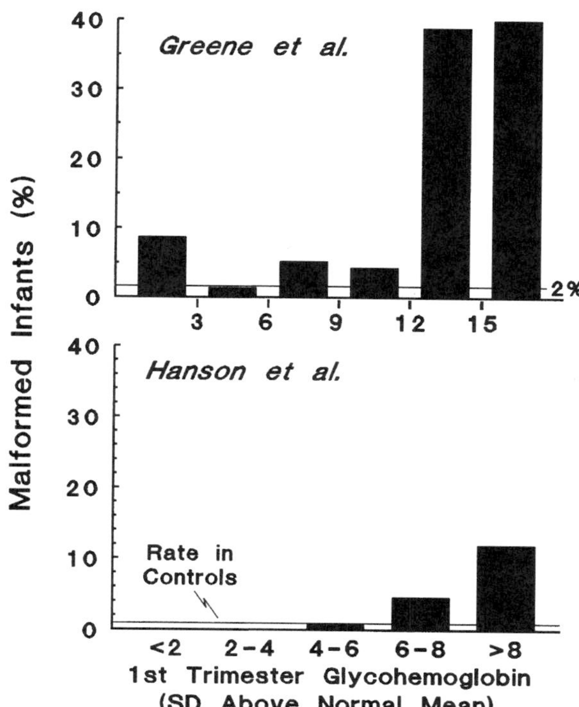

Figure 77-2. Relationship between rates of major malformations and maternal glycohemoglobin concentrations in women with pregestational diabetes, as reported by Greene et al.[30] in the United States and Hanson et al.[29] in Sweden. Glycohemoglobin concentrations are expressed relative to normal means, as in Figure 77-1. Note the difference in the range of the *x*-axis between figures.

Table 77-3. Rates of Major Congenital Malformations in Infants of Diabetic Women Who Participated in a Preconceptional Care Program and Those Who Did Not*

	Malformed Infants	
Investigators	Late Entrants	Early Entrants
Fuhrman et al.[36]	7.5%	0.8%
Goldman et al.[54]	9.6%	0.0%
Steel et al.[51]	10.4%	1.4%
Kitzmiller et al.[39]	10.9%	1.2%
Mills et al.[38]	9.0%	4.9%

*"Late entrants" received no special preconceptional care, and early entrants were enrolled in diabetes care programs before conception (or up to the third week postconception in the study of Mills et al.[38]). In the studies of Fuhrman, Goldman, Steel and Kitzmiller and their colleagues, attempts were made to maintain maternal glycemia as close to normal as possible before conception. No special glycemic goals were employed in the study of Mills et al. Malformation rates were significantly lower in the early entrants in each study.

Animal Models: Potential Mechanisms

Because practical and ethical issues limit the investigation of mechanisms underlying diabetic embryopathy in human pregnancies, a large number of investigators have turned to animal models in an attempt to identify teratogenic factors and mechanisms that may be operative in diabetic pregnancies. The investigations have been conducted in vivo, using genetic or induced models of diabetes, and in vitro, using culture techniques for preimplantation or early postimplantation embryos or embryonic tissues. Virtually all of the studies have been performed in rodent models of diabetes. These animal studies have yielded a wealth of important information regarding potential mechanisms for developmental anomalies induced by diabetes. The reader should keep in mind, however, that none of the currently available animal models is a perfect reflection of human diabetic embryopathy. For example, some of the rat strains that have been employed in whole-embryo culture studies in vitro do not develop congenital malformations when embryos are exposed to maternal diabetes in vivo.[56–58] Even the strains that do manifest anomalies in vivo may manifest only a particular type of anomaly (e.g., skeletal malformations[59]) in the presence of maternal diabetes. Mechanistic data from those strains cannot be extrapolated to anomalies of other organ systems or developmental fields in the absence of evidence to support such extrapolation. Finally, the technique for culture of whole postimplantation embryos[60] that has been employed by many investigators to study diabetic teratogenesis in vitro is very useful for detecting defects in development of the neural tube and the early axial skeleton. The technique, however, has limited utility in the study of defects in cardiac septation or development of the great vessels or kidneys. Despite these limitations, the information provided below may give important clues to the mechanisms that underlie diabetic embryopathy in humans.

Growth Retardation and Resorption

Growth retardation of early postimplantation embryos, manifested as a reduction in their size and content of protein and DNA, is a very frequent finding after exposure to maternal diabetes in utero[56] or to diabetic conditions in vitro.[61,62] The mechanisms that result in growth retardation under diabetic conditions are not known. In studies where exposure of embryos to diabetic conditions (e.g., high glucose concentrations) caused malformations in some embryos, however, growth retardation was often observed in the remaining, nonmalformed embryos. That observation suggests that growth retardation may be the mildest component of a spectrum of developmental abnormalities induced by diabetes during early development. Growth retardation induced by a brief metabolic insult to early postimplantation rat embryos in vivo[15] has been shown to persist until term,[63] suggesting that early growth retardation may contribute to the reduced birth weights that frequently occur in rodent models of diabetes in vivo.[57,59] Retardation of growth and development has also been reported in preimplantation rodent embryos that were exposed to a diabetic environment in vivo[64–66] or to diabetes-like conditions in vitro.[67–69] In at least one report,[70] the developmental delay affected the inner cell mass, that portion of the blastocyst that gives rise to embryonic tissues. Whether this very early developmental abnormality is related to the blastogenic developmental field defects reported by Martinez-Frias[48] in human diabetic pregnancies is unknown.

Resorption of embryos, the rodent analog of spontaneous abortions in humans, may comprise the most severe end of the spectrum of early developmental abnormalities induced by experimental maternal diabetes in vivo. Increased resorption rates have been reported at term in animal models of diabetes in which growth retardation and congenital malformations also occur.[59,71,72] The resorptions may reflect the loss of severely and/or multiply malformed embryos because delivery of a brief metabolic insult to early postimplantation rat embryos in vivo resulted in similar rates of severely malformed embryos at the end of organogenesis[15] and resorbed fetuses at term.[63] Mechanisms that lead to the resorption of embryos in diabetic pregnancies are not known.

Congenital Malformations

Most animal studies of diabetic embryopathy have focused on the pathogenesis of discrete congenital anomalies. Early studies revealed that it was possible to cause anomalies in offspring by the induction of diabetes in mothers with no genetic predisposition to diabetes,[73–75] supporting a metabolic rather than a genetic basis for the anomalies. The demonstration that insulin therapy administered throughout pregnancy[59,76] or during specific periods of embryogenesis[72] could reduce the rate of anomalies provided further support for mediation by some aspect of abnormal maternal metabolism. Maternal serum concentrations of glucose, ketones, triglycerides, and several amino acids correlated with the risk of skeletal anomalies and resorptions in one malformation-prone strain,[77] providing some candidate substances for the mediation of diabetic embryopathy in vivo.

Culture of whole rat or mouse embryos during the initial stages of neural tube development (analogous to days 18–28 of human embryogenesis[2]) has been used to study potential mediators of and mechanisms for diabetic embryopathy. The technique allows normal development of embryos during 24–48 hours of culture in normal serum.[60] Serum can be manipulated to test the effects of potential mediators and mechanisms of diabetic embryopathy on development, particularly of the neural tube and axial skeleton. Studies in which mouse embryos have been cultured in rat serum reveal that diabetic serum is teratogenic[78] and that the teratogenic effect can be reduced very rapidly (i.e., within 1–2 hours[79]) by insulin treatment of serum donors in vivo but not by addition of insulin to diabetic serum in vitro.[80] Studies in which potential teratogens have been added to normal serum before culture of rat or mouse embryos indicate that glucose[61,62,81–83] β hydroxybutyrate[61,62,83–85] and low molecular weight serum fractions containing an inhibitor of insulin-like growth factor I activity[61,62,86] are teratogenic in high concentrations and that those factors act synergistically (i.e., at lower concentrations than when added individually) to produce malformations.[61,62,83] Pyruvate and the amino acid analog α-ketoisocaproic acid have also been shown to enhance the teratogenic effects of glucose and β-hydroxybutyrate on cultured rat embryos from a strain that is prone to skeletal malformations when maternal diabetes is induced in vivo.[83]

At least four mechanisms have been suggested to explain the teratogenic effects of diabetes and diabetes-like conditions on early postimplantation-stage embryos: (1) disruption of normal function of the yolk sac,[87,88] which serves an important function in regulating nutrient transport from maternal plasma to the embryo during early neural tube development[87]; (2) depletion of intracellular myoinositol in embryos, with resultant disruption of arachidonic acid and prostaglandin metabolism[89–94]; (3) oxidative metabolism of the excess nutrients supplied by the mother, with resultant generation of free oxygen radicals that may be toxic to embryos, particularly if they are genetically predisposed to such toxicity[83,95]; and (4) glucose-induced mutations in embryonic DNA.[96,97] To date, these mechanisms have been identified in different rodent species or strains and under different experimental conditions. For example, disruption of myoinositol uptake and metabolism has been demonstrated in models of hyperglycemia alone, and the work on free oxygen radicals has been performed in a rat strain that is particularly prone to skeletal malformations. Therefore, it is not clear whether any of these four mechanisms can explain the wide spectrum of developmental abnormalities than are encompassed by diabetic embryopathy in rodents or whether any of the mechanisms contributes to diabetes-induced malformations in humans. Nonetheless, these mechanisms provide potential avenues for the investigation of diabetic embryopathy in human pregnancies.

Later Pregnancy: Effects on Fetal Development

Normal Fetal Development and Maternal-Fetal Nutrient Transport

Normal Development

A full discussion of fetal development during the second and third trimesters is beyond the scope of this chapter. Two events that are particularly relevant to fetal development in diabetic pregnancies, however, warrant mention. The first is the development by pancreatic β-cells of the capacity for nutrient-stimulated insulin secretion. Pancreatic islets of Langerhans differentiate during the 10th to 11th weeks of development, and according to studies performed with human fetal pancreatic tissue in vitro,[98,99] the islets begin to release insulin in response to nutrients as early as 11–15 weeks of development. Insulin responses to amino acids such as arginine and leucine have been reported to occur earlier than responses to glucose.[99] Insulin responses to glucose mature slowly in normal pregnancies[98,100,101] and remain poor relative to the adult situation throughout the early neonatal period.[99,102] Studies of rat fetal islets[103] indicate that immaturity of insulin stimulus-secretion coupling to glucose results from immaturity of glucose metabolism in the islets, precluding the normal generation of ATP that leads to insulin release when adult islets are stimulated by glucose.[104] Chronic exposure of rat fetal islets to glucose matures the stimulus-secretion coupling, and exposure to glucose or amino acids promotes proliferation of cultured fetal islets,[103] observations that may help to explain the enhancement of nutrient-stimulated insulin secretion by[98,102,105] and hyperplasia of[106–108] pancreatic islets in infants of diabetic mothers.

The other major event that is particularly relevant to pregnancies complicated by diabetes is the differentiation of adipose tissue and the storage of triglycerides therein. This process begins at approximately 26–28 weeks of gestation[109] and continues until term. The relatively late development of adipose tissue in the human fetus likely explains why factors that promote fat accumulation in infants (e.g., maternal diabetes and fetal hyperinsulinemia) have their greatest impact on rates and patterns of fetal growth during the last 2–3 months of intrauterine development.[110] Likewise, the virtual absence of fat in the rat fetus at term may explain in part why that species does not manifest excessive fetal growth in the presence of overt maternal diabetes.[57,59] Both of these patterns of growth reflect the importance of the interaction between the intrauterine environment and genetically programmed developmental events in determining the ultimate fetal outcome in diabetic pregnancies.

Maternal-Fetal Nutrient Transport

Once the allantoic placenta has developed, it serves as an important regulator of maternal-fetal nutrient transport (Fig. 77-3). Fetal glucose concentrations generally are 10–20 mg/dL lower than maternal concentrations, indicating that the placenta poses a barrier to free diffusion of glucose. The placenta, however, contains relatively high concentrations of insulin-independent glucose transport molecules (GLUT-1 and GLUT-3[111]), which are likely to be involved in the insulin-independent, facilitated transport of glucose from mother to fetus. The rate of transport by these glucose transporters is proportional to circulating glucose concentrations, so that the raising or lowering of maternal glucose concentrations causes parallel changes in glucose delivery to the fetus. Many amino acids are actively transported across the placenta.[112,113] Transport rates are concentration dependent for basic and neutral amino acids, so that elevated maternal amino acid concentrations result in increased maternal-fetal amino acid fluxes. Lipids vary in their maternal-fetal transport mechanisms. Ketones such as acetoacetate and 3-hydroxybutyrate are transferred by diffusion, so that fetal exposure parallels maternal plasma concentrations of those substances. Free

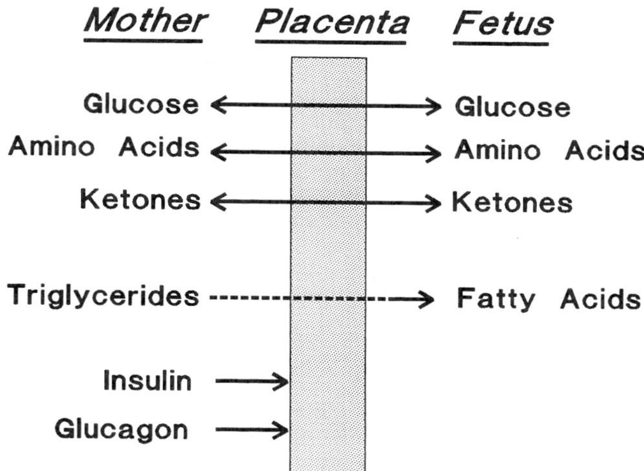

Figure 77-3. Schematic representation of maternal-fetal nutrient transport in humans. Glucose, ketones, and many amino acids are transported between the mother and fetus by concentration-dependent mechanisms, so that elevated maternal concentrations cause increased flux to the fetus. Maternal triglycerides are hydrolyzed in the placenta, and the component fatty acids may appear in the fetal circulation. Insulin and glucagon do not cross the human placenta but modify the fetal environment indirectly through their effects on maternal nutrient concentrations. (Adapted with permission from ref. 173.)

fatty acids are transported down a concentration gradient from mother to fetus, although the exact mechanism of transport remains unclear. Increased maternal concentrations of free fatty acids result in increased delivery to the fetus and an accumulation of fat in primates.[114,115] Intact triglycerides do not appear to cross the human placenta.[116] The placenta, however, contains enzymes capable of hydrolyzing triglycerides into their component fatty acids and glycerol.[117,118] Hummell et al.[119] reported that labeled fatty acids appeared in the circulation of fetal rats after administration of labeled triglycerides to their mothers, indicating transport of triglyceride-derived lipids from mother to fetus. Whether this process occurs in humans remains to be determined.

As a result of the transport processes described above, the nutrient mix contained in maternal plasma determines to a large extent the metabolic environment of the developing fetus (see Fig. 77-3). By contrast, the hormonal environment of the fetus is much less dependent on maternal hormone concentrations. Insulin and glucagon do not appear to cross the human placenta under normal conditions, although antibody-bound insulin may cross the placenta in insulin-treated diabetic patients.[120] The impact of maternal insulin on fetal development is mediated primarily through regulation of maternal nutrient levels. Insulin deficiency, whether absolute (as in insulin-dependent diabetes mellitus [IDDM]) or relative (as in non–insulin-dependent diabetes [NIDDM] or gestational diabetes [GDM]), results in increased levels of glucose, amino acids,[121] and lipids[122,123] in the maternal circulation and increased delivery of those nutrients to the fetus (see Chapter 76). The altered nutrient environment appears to play a major role in the genesis of fetal complications of diabetic pregnancies.

Impact of Maternal Diabetes on Fetal Development

Maternal diabetes during the second and third trimesters has been associated with a variety of fetal and neonatal morbidities related to abnormal fetal development, as well as to attempts by physicians to prevent some of the most serious fetal complications. The latter factor has led to confusion about the true impact of maternal diabetes on fetal development. To minimize that confusion, the reader should keep in mind the following historical framework when reading this section: (1) stillbirth rates in diabetic pregnancies were 20–30% in the five decades following the advent of insulin therapy[123]; (2) recognition of the timing of the stillbirths led to routine delivery at 36–37 weeks of gestation, a practice that reduced the stillbirth rate but increased complications related to prematurity (e.g., respiratory distress syndrome, jaundice, and hypocalcemia); (3) the parallel development in the last two decades of obstetric techniques to identify infants at greatest risk for fetal demise and medical techniques to improve maternal metabolic control now allows a majority of pregnancies to proceed to term with little, if any, excess risk of fetal demise unless congenital malformations are also present.[124] As a result, fetal hyperinsulinism and excessive growth have emerged as major developmental abnormalities in the second and third trimesters of well-managed diabetic pregnancies.

Stillbirth

A common outcome of pregnancy in women with diabetes in the middle of this century was unexpected fetal death during the last 3–6 weeks of gestation. The mechanisms responsible for this phenomenon have not been identified. It appears very likely that stillbirths are related to poor maternal metabolic control because programs to improve control have nearly eliminated the excess risk of stillbirths, an observation that cannot be explained simply by better obstetric surveillance in diabetic pregnancies. Data from fetal sheep[125,126] indicate that chronic hyperglycemia in late pregnancy leads to increased fetal glucose utilization, hypoxia, and acidosis, suggesting that hyperglycemia per se may be a link between maternal diabetes and the demise of anatomically normal fetuses. The observation that fetal pH in human diabetic pregnancies at term was inversely related to maternal and fetal glucose concentrations[127] is consistent with that suggestion.

Excessive Growth and Fetal Macrosomia

Infants of diabetic mothers tend to be heavy for a given gestational age compared to infants of nondiabetic mothers; one-fourth to one-third of infants born to mothers with pregestational[128–131] or gestational[132,133] diabetes weigh more than the 90th percentile for their age at birth. Assessment of neonatal adiposity by measurements of skinfold thickness have revealed that infants of diabetic mothers are fatter than infants of nondiabetic mothers of similar birth weight,[134] indicating a specific effect of maternal diabetes to increase fetal adipose tissue mass. The mass of other insulin-sensitive tissues such as liver and heart may be increased as well. The increased fetal size places infants at risk for birth trauma, cesarean delivery, and, as discussed below, obesity in later life.

Over four decades ago, Jorgen Pedersen proposed that the excessive growth of infants of diabetic mothers was due to increased maternal-fetal glucose transport, leading to stimulation of fetal insulin secretion and, in concert with an increased caloric supply, to accelerated fetal growth (Fig. 77-4). Four lines of clinical and experimental evidence supports Pedersen's *hyperglycemia-hyperinsulinemia* hypothesis. First, measures of maternal glycemia (especially postprandial glycemia[128,129]) in diabetic pregnancies have been correlated directly with fetal size corrected for gestational age. The excessive size and adiposity can be reduced by careful regulation of circulating maternal glucose concentrations starting as late as the third trimester.[135–137] Second, measures of pancreatic β-cell function in fetuses and neonates have been correlated directly with maternal glycemia during the second half of gestation in diabetic pregnancies.[138,139] Third, measures of fetal size have been correlated directly with measures of fetal insulin production during the third trimester.[138,139] Finally, chronic administration of insulin directly to normal fetal monkeys in utero caused excessive growth of fetal adipose tissue, heart, and liver in the absence of maternal hyperglycemia,[140] a finding that highlights the capacity of insulin to stimulate fetal growth. Observations of these four types have led to the widespread acceptance of the Pedersen hypothesis in explaining the excessive fetal growth and macrosomia that occur in many diabetic pregnancies. It also has become apparent, however, that the mediation of the excessive growth is more complex than was originally proposed by Pedersen.

One level of complexity results from the spectrum of maternal nutrients that may contribute to fetal macrosomia. Freinkel and Metzger[141] originally proposed that fetal macrosomia resulted from an overabundance not only of glucose, but also of amino acid and lipid nutrients in the presence of maternal diabetes. Indeed, concentrations of all three classes of nutrients are elevated in the circulation of pregnant women with diabetes,[121,142–144] and the concentrations have all been correlated with the birth weights of infants of diabetic mothers.[128,140,143,145,146] Thus, it is very likely that nonglucose nutrients, which are not routinely measured in diabetic pregnancies, contribute to the overgrowth of infants of diabetic mothers.

A second level of complexity is the efficiency of maternal-fetal nutrient transport, a phenomenon that has not been well studied in human diabetic pregnancies. It is clear, however, that maternal diabetes can induce anatomic[147] and functional[148] changes in the placenta that may alter the maternal-fetal nutrient transport depicted in Figure 77-3. The best example of this phenomenon may be the intrauterine growth retardation that has been observed in some diabetic pregnancies complicated by maternal microvascular disease.[43,149] Abnormalities of placental blood vessels and flow occur in the same pregnancies and may limit maternal-fetal nutrient delivery. In theory, very strict control of maternal glycemia could accen-

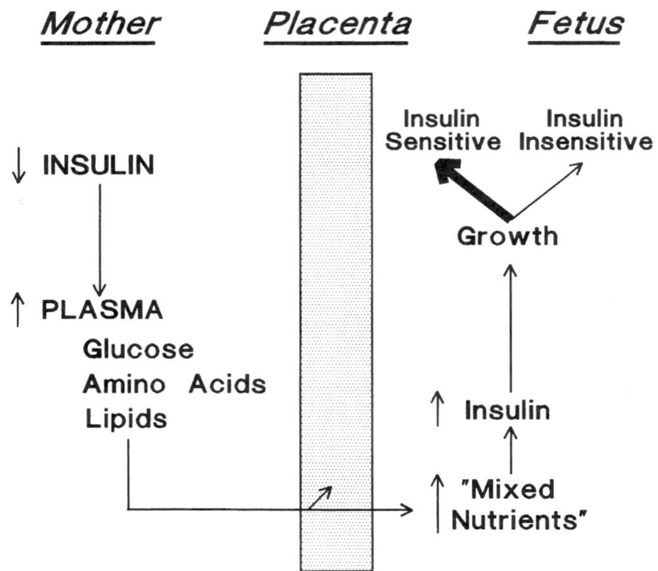

Figure 77-4. Schematic representation of the stimulation of fetal growth by maternal diabetes during the second and third trimesters of pregnancy. Absolute or relative insulin deficiency leads to increased concentrations of glucose, amino acids, and lipids in the maternal circulation. The increased nutrient concentrations increase the flux of nutrients to the fetus (see Fig. 77-3), stimulating maturation and secretion of insulin by the fetal pancreas. The combination of increased calories and hyperinsulinemia promote fetal growth, especially in insulin sensitive tissues (e.g., adipose tissue). (Adapted with permission from Freinkel N, Metzger BE, Potter J. Pregnancy in diabetes. In: Ellenberg M, Rifkin H, eds. Diabetes Mellitus: Theory and Practice. 3rd ed. New Hyde Park, N.Y.: Medical Examination;1983:698–714.)

tuate the growth retardation in such pregnancies. That theory remains to be tested.

A third level of complexity is the fetal response to maternal diabetes. Just as genetic factors appear to be important determinants of the risk of obesity in adults,[150,151] fetuses can be expected to vary in their susceptibility to excessive growth and macrosomia in the presence of the increased calories provided by maternal diabetes. This concept is supported by the observation that macrosomia rates differ among infants of white, black, and Hispanic mothers with gestational diabetes despite similar degrees of maternal metabolic dysregulation in the three groups.[152] Moreover, Gloria-Bottini et al.[153] have recently presented evidence of genetic variability in the region of the insulin-like growth factor I gene that alters the expression of macrosomia in offspring of mothers with pregestational diabetes. These observations, combined with the other two levels of complexity discussed above, indicate that macrosomia in diabetic pregnancies cannot be viewed simply in terms of maternal hyperglycemia and its impact on fetal development.

Neonatal Hypoglycemia

As discussed previously in this chapter, chronic exposure of fetal pancreatic β-cells to glucose in vitro results in maturation of fetal insulin secretion, and chronic exposure to glucose or amino acids leads to hyperplasia of the fetal islets. Similar changes in vivo are thought to account for the enhanced basal and glucose-stimulated insulin secretion that has been observed in infants of diabetic mothers.[102,154–156] The enhanced insulin release may lead to neonatal hypoglycemia, particularly during the first day of extrauterine life.[102,154,156] Indeed, prevalence rates of neonatal hypoglycemia (i.e., serum or plasma glucose <30 mg/dL for term infants or <20 mg/dL for preterm infants) have been reported to be in the range of 20–40% in infants of mothers with pregestational diabetes.[131,157,158] The hypoglycemia may result from reduced hepatic glucose production in the basal state[159] and from exaggerated disposition of glucose after a nutrient challenge.[102] Poor glucagon responses to lowered blood glucose concentrations[156,160] may add to the severity of hypoglycemia in infants of diabetic mothers.

The fact that measures of fetal insulin secretion and the risk of neonatal hypoglycemia are related to circulating maternal glucose[139,156,158,161–163] and amino acid[139] concentrations during mid-late pregnancy supports the concept that exposure to increased nutrient concentrations from the mother leads to fetal hyperinsulinemia and neonatal hypoglycemia. The programming of this process may begin early in the second trimester,[98,143] and the process can be mitigated by careful regulation of maternal blood glucose concentrations.[164] Even though fetal macrosomia and neonatal hypoglycemia appear to result from the same process of fetal overnutrition, the two phenomena do not necessarily occur together in diabetic pregnancies,[165] an observation that highlights the variability among fetuses in their responses to maternal diabetes.

Other Effects on the Fetus

Additional complications that have been reported in excess in infants of diabetic mothers include surfactant-deficient respiratory distress syndrome, hypocalcemia, jaundice, and polycythemia. The first three of these complications occur with increased frequency in premature infants, and early delivery of diabetic pregnancies likely accounted for a substantial portion of their excess in the past. These three complications are infrequent with modern management practices. Experimental data, however, suggest that exposure of fetuses to a diabetic environment may contribute to all four of these fetal complications. Exposure of type II pneumocytes to high concentrations of insulin in vitro decreases surfactant production by those cells,[166] an effect that could contribute to the delayed pulmonary maturation that has been reported in pregnancies with less than optimal maternal blood glucose control.[167] Poor maternal metabolic control has been associated with neonatal hypocalcemia and hypomagnesemia, an association that was independent of gestational age at delivery.[168] Maternal hyperglycemia[127,169,170] and fetal hyperinsulinemia[171] have been associated with increased fetal erythropoietin concentrations and polycythemia in infants of diabetic mothers. The increased erythrocyte mass and turnover may contribute to jaundice in some infants as well. Thus, poor maternal metabolic control may increase the risk of all four of these fetal complications of diabetic pregnancy.

Long-Term Impact on Offspring

Traditionally, the focus of investigation of fetal complications in diabetic pregnancies has been on the antenatal and perinatal complications detailed above. As proposed by Freinkel,[172] however, it is likely that the developmental abnormalities induced by maternal diabetes in utero will have a long-term impact on the phenotype expressed by infants of diabetic mothers. Certainly, the congenital malformations that may be induced by maternal diabetes will have a long-term impact on the health of the offspring. There is increasing evidence that exposure to maternal diabetes in utero can have a more subtle but important impact on the long-term health of the children of diabetic mothers. The evidence comes from studies in animal models of diabetes or hyperglycemia, as well as from long-term follow-up of infants of diabetic mothers.

Animal Models

Many of the animal data on the long-term impact of maternal diabetes come from studies of two types of exposure to hyperglycemia in utero: (1) hyperglycemia associated with maternal diabetes that is induced by chemical destruction of pancreatic β-cells and (2) hyperglycemia produced by a chronic infusion of glucose during the latter stages of gestation. All of the studies have been conducted in rats. Three different groups of investigators have reported that offspring of rats with overt[173,174] or mild[175] diabetes induced by streptozotocin administration before conception manifested reduced insulin sensitivity when studied as adults with the euglycemic clamp technique. Van Assche et al.[176] have reported that the adult offspring are not only insulin resistant but also glucose intolerant, indicating that vertical transmission of hyperglycemia may occur as a result of exposure to maternal diabetes in utero. Similar results have been reported from the chronic glucose infusion studies during pregnancy.[177] The long-term effects in this model must be interpreted with caution, however, because pregnant rats eat very little during high-dose glucose infusions, so that the model is characterized not only by hyperglycemia but also by reduced protein intake. Dahri et al.[178] have shown that maternal protein restriction during pregnancy can induce a long-lasting defect in the pancreatic β-cell function of offspring.

Human Studies

Two general types of abnormalities have been reported in children or young adult offspring of diabetic mothers: (1) impaired intellectual and motor development and (2) metabolic abnormalities including obesity, hyperinsulinemia, and hyperglycemia. Mild impairments of intellectual and motor development have been reported in young children, predominantly in association with maternal ketonuria[179,180] or ketonemia[181] during gestation. No cause-and-effect relationships can be inferred from the human data, although animal studies have revealed that exposure of fetal brain slices to β-hydroxybutyrate in vitro can inhibit the de novo synthesis of purines and pyrimidines needed for nucleic acid synthesis in the brain.[182,183]

Sells et al.[184] reported that verbal development was mildly impaired in young children of mothers who presented for diabetes care after conception and who did not maintain ideal glucose control thereafter, suggesting that poor maternal metabolic control during pregnancy may have a slightly adverse effect on brain development in humans.

At least three groups have reported that offspring of diabetic mothers are overweight during childhood compared to offspring of nondiabetic mothers.[185–187] Those findings could simply reflect a strong genetic association between diabetes and obesity. The observation that offspring of mothers with insulin-dependent diabetes mellitus (IDDM), who generally are not obese, demonstrated the same pattern of increased weight in childhood, however, suggests that intrauterine environmental factors may have contributed to the excessive weight. The fact that fetal[187] and neonatal[186] hyperinsulinism have been correlated with the risk of being overweight in childhood provides additional evidence that exposure to maternal diabetes in utero may increase the risk of obesity in later life. Pettitt et al.[188] have reported that offspring of Pima Indian mothers who were diabetic during pregnancy not only were overweight, but also had higher rates of diabetes in young adult life compared to offspring of control mothers who were not diabetic during pregnancy. That finding persisted when the control group consisted of offspring whose mothers eventually did develop diabetes (i.e., offspring with a genetic susceptibility to non–insulin-dependent diabetes mellitus [NIDDM] who were not exposed to diabetes in utero), a finding that highlights the importance of exposure to maternal diabetes in utero as a risk factor for future diabetes. Whether the risks of diabetes and obesity in offspring can be reduced by careful regulation of maternal metabolism during pregnancy remains to be tested.

Summary

During gestation, the human embryo and fetus are exposed to a metabolic environment that is determined largely by concentrations of nutrients in the maternal circulation. Maternal diabetes can alter circulating concentrations of a variety of maternal nutrients that, in turn, modify the metabolic environment for the developing embryo and fetus. Exposure to such an altered environment can disrupt normal intrauterine development, particularly when the maternal metabolic disturbance is severe. Disruptions during early pregnancy can result in growth retardation, congenital malformations, and/or demise of the developing embryo through mechanisms that are not fully identified. Disruptions of the fetal environment during the latter two-thirds of gestation lead to developmental abnormalities that are related predominantly to fetal overnutrition and hyperinsulinemia. The severity of the early and later developmental abnormalities induced by maternal diabetes appears to vary among offspring, perhaps on a genetic basis, and both types of abnormalities can have a significant long-term impact on the health of children of diabetic mothers. The impact of maternal diabetes on intrauterine development can be limited by careful regulation of maternal metabolism, which can greatly reduce the antenatal and perinatal morbidity and mortality in diabetic pregnancies. Whether that approach will also reduce the long-term impact of diabetes on the health of offspring remains to be determined.

References

1. Mills JL, Baker L, Goldman AS. Malformations in infants of diabetic mothers occur before the seventh gestational week: Implications for treatment. Diabetes 1979;28:292
2. Sadler TW. Langman's Medical Embryology, 5th ed. Baltimore: Williams & Wilkins;1985:19–78
3. Robinson DH, Benos DJ. Glucose metabolism in the trophectoderm and inner cell mass of the rabbit embryo. J Reprod Fertil 1991;91:493
4. Merker H-J, Villegas H. Elektronmikroskoposche untersuchngen zum problem des stoffaustausches zwischen mutter und keim bie rattenembtyonen des tages 7–10. Anat Entwicklungs-Geswch 1970;131:325
5. Unterman TG, Buchanan TA, Freinkel N. Access of maternal insulin to the rat conceptus prior to allantoic placentation. Diabetes Res 1989;10:115
6. Trocino RA, Akazawa S, Takino H, et al. Cellular-tissue localization and regulation of the GLUT-1 protein in both the embryo and the visceral yolk sac from normal and experimental diabetic rats during the early postimplantation period. Endocrinology 1994;134:869
7. Ellington SKL. In vitro analysis of glucose metabolism and embryonic growth in postimplantation rat embryos. Development 1987;100:431
8. Jollie WP. Ultrastructural studies of protein transfer across rodent yolk sac. Placenta 1986;7:263
9. Shepard TH, Tanimura T, Robkin MA. Energy metabolism in early mammalian embryos. Dev Biol 1970;4(suppl):42
10. Tanimura T, Shepard TH. Glucose metabolism by rat embryos in vitro. Proc Soc Exp Biol Med 1970;135:51
11. Nuebert D, Peters H, Tesks S, et al. Studies on the problem of "aerobic glycolysis" occurring in mammalian embryos. Naunyn-Schmiedebergs Arch Pharmak 1971;268:235
12. Clough JR, Whittingham DG. Metabolism of ^{14}C-glucose by postimplantation mouse embryos in vitro. J Embryol Exp Morphol 1983;74:133
13. Hunter ES, Sadler TW. Fuel-mediated teratogenesis: Biochemical effects of hypoglycemia during neurulation in mouse embryos in vitro. Am J Physiol 1989;257:E269
14. Freinkel N, Lewis NJ, Akazawa S, et al. The honeybee syndrome: Implications of the teratogenicity of mannose in rat embryo culture. N Engl J Med 1984;310:223
15. Buchanan T, Freinkel N, Lewis NJ, et al. Fuel-mediated teratogenesis: Use of D-mannose to modify organogenesis in the rat embryo in vivo. J Clin Invest 1984;75:1927
16. Buchanan TA, Freinkel N, Schemmer JK. Embryotoxic effects of brief maternal insulin-hypoglycemia during organogenesis in the rat. J Clin Invest 1986;78:643
17. Svensson AM, Borg LAH, Eriksson UJ. Glucose metabolism in embryos of normal and diabetic rats during organogenesis. Acta Endocrinol 1992;127:252
18. Mackler B, Grace R, Duncan HM. Studies of mitochondrial development during embryogenesis in the rat. Arch Biochem Biophys 1971;144:603
19. Buchanan TA, Sipos GF. Lack of a teratogenic effect of maternal insulin–induced hypoglycemia in the rat during late neurulation. Diabetes 1989; 38:1063
20. Travers JP, Exell L, Huang B, et al. Insulin and insulin-like growth factors in embryonic development. Diabetes 1992;41:318
21. Travers JP, Pratten MK, Beck F. Effects of low insulin levels on rat embryonic growth and development. Diabetes 1989;38:773
22. Pedersen JF, Molsted-Pedersen L. Early fetal growth delay detected by ultrasound marks increased risk of congenital malformation in diabetic pregnancy. Br Med J 1981;283:269
23. Brown ZA, Mills JL, Metzger BE, et al. Early sonographic evaluation for fetal growth delay and congenital malformations in pregnancies complicated by insulin-requiring diabetes. Diabetes Care 1992;15:613
24. Sutherland HW, Pritchard CW. Increased incidence of spontaneous abortion in pregnancies complicated by maternal diabetes. Am J Obstet Gynecol 1986; 155:135
25. Miodovnik M, Lavin JP, Knowles HC, et al. Spontaneous abortion among insulin-dependent diabetic women. Am J Obstet Gynecol 1984;150:372
26. Dicker D, Feldberg D, Samuel N, et al. Spontaneous abortion in patients with insulin-dependent diabetes mellitus: The effect of preconceptional diabetic control. Am J Obstet Gynecol 1988;158:1161
27. Kalter H. Diabetes and spontaneous abortion: A historical review. Am J Obstet Gynecol 1987;156:1243
28. Mills JL, Simpson JL, Driscoll SG, et al. Incidence of spontaneous abortion among normal women and insulin-dependent diabetic women whose pregnancies were identified within 21 days of conception. N Engl J Med 1988; 319:1617
29. Hanson U, Persson B, Thunell S. Relationship between hemoglobin A_{1c} in early type I (insulin-dependent) diabetic pregnancy and the occurrence of spontaneous abortion and fetal malformation in Sweden. Diabetologia 1990; 33:100
30. Greene MF, Hare JW, Cloherty JP, et al. First-trimester hemoglobin A_1 and risk for major malformation and spontaneous abortion in diabetic pregnancy. Teratology 1989;39:225
31. Rosenn B, Miodovnik M, Combs A, et al. Glycemic thresholds for spontaneous abortion and congenital malformations in insulin-dependent diabetes mellitus. Obstet Gynecol 1994;84:515
32. Pedersen J. The Pregnant Diabetic and Her Newborn: Problems and Management. 2nd ed. Baltimore: Williams & Wilkins;1977:191–197
33. Karlsson K, Kjellmer I. The outcome of diabetic pregnancies in relation to the mother's blood sugar level. Am J Obstet Gynecol 1972;112:213
34. Gabbe SG, Mestman JH, Freeman RK, et al. Management and outcome of pregnancy in diabetes mellitus, classes B to R. Am J Obstet Gynecol 1977;129:723
35. Miller E, Hare JS, Cloherty JP, et al. Elevated maternal hemoglobin A_{1c} in early pregnancy and major congenital anomalies in infants of diabetic mothers. N Engl J Med 1981;304:1331
36. Fuhrmann K, Reiher H, Semmler K, Glockner E. The effect of intensified

conventional insulin therapy before and during early pregnancy on the malformation rate in offspring of diabetic mothers. Exp Clin Endocrinol 1984; 83:173
37. Simpson JL, Elias S, Martin AO, et al. Prospective study of anomalies in offspring of mothers with diabetes mellitus. Am J Obstet Gynecol 1983; 146:263
38. Mills JL, Knopp RH, Simpson JL, et al. Lack of relation of increased malformation rates in infants of diabetic mothers to glycemic control during organogenesis. N Engl J Med 1988;318:671
39. Kitzmiller JL, Gavin LA, Gin GD, et al. Preconception care of diabetes. Glycemic control prevents congenital malformations. JAMA 1991;265:731
40. Becerra JE, Khoury MJ, Cordero JF, Erickson JD. Diabetes mellitus in pregnancy and the risk of specific birth defects: A population-based case-control study. Pediatrics 1990;85:1
41. Ramos-Arroyo MA, Rodriguez-Pinilla E, Cordero JF. Maternal diabetes: The risk for specific birth defects. Eur J Epidemiol 1992;8:503
42. Martinez-Frias ML. Epidemiological analysis of outcomes of pregnancy in diabetic mothers. Am J Med Genet 1994;51:108
43. Hod M, Merlob P, Friedman S, et al. Prevalence of minor congenital anomalies in newborns of diabetic mothers. Eur J Obstet Gynecol 1992;44:111
44. Damm P, Molsted-Pedersen L. Significant decrease in congenital malformations in newborn infants of an unselected population of diabetic women. Am J Obstet Gynecol 1989;161:1163
45. Pradat P. A case-control study of major congenital heart defects in Sweden: 1981–1986. Eur J Epidemiol 1992;8:789
46. McCarter RJ, Kessler II, Comstock GW. Is diabetes mellitus a teratogen or a coteratogen? Am J Epidemiol 1987;125:195
47. Khoury MJ, Becerra JE, Cordero JF, Erickson JD. Clinical-epidemiological assessment of patterns of birth defects associated with human teratogen: Application to diabetic embryopathy. Pediatrics 1989;84:658
48. Martinez-Frias ML. Developmental field defects and associations. Am J Med Genet 1994;49:45
49. Towner D, Kjos S, Leung B, et al. Congenital malformations in pregnancies complicated by NIDDM. Diabetes Care 1995;18:1446
50. Bennett PH, Webner C, Miller M. Congenital anomalies and the diabetic and prediabetic pregnancy. In: Pregnancy Metabolism, Diabetes and the Fetus. Ciba Foundation Symposium No. 63. Amsterdam: Excerpta Medica;1979: 207–225
51. Steel JM, Johnstone FD, Hepburn DA, Smith AF. Can prepregnancy care of diabetic women reduce the risk of anomalous babies? Br Med J 1990;301: 1070
52. Molsted-Pedersen L, Tygstrup I, Pedersen J. Congenital malformations in newborn infants of diabetic women. Correlation with maternal diabetic vascular complications. Lancet 1964;i:1124
53. Miodovnik M, Mimouni F, Dignan PSJ, et al. Major malformations in infants of IDDM women. Vasculopathy and early first-trimester poor glycemic control. Diabetes Care 1988;11:713
54. Goldman JA, Dicker D, Feldberg D. Pregnancy outcome in patients with insulin-dependent diabetes mellitus and preconceptional diabetes control: A comparative study. Am J Obstet Gynecol 1986;155:293
55. Gregory R, Tattesall RB. Are pre-pregnancy clinics worthwhile? Lancet 1992;340:656
56. Eriksson UJ, Lewis NJ, Freinkel N. Growth retardation during early organogenesis in embryos of experimentally diabetic rats. Diabetes 1984;33:281
57. Giavini E, Broccia ML, Prati M, et al. Effects of streptozotocin-induced diabetes on fetal development of the rat. Teratology 1986;34:81
58. Eriksson UJ. Importance of genetic predisposition and maternal environment for the occurrence of congenital malformations in offspring of diabetic rats. Teratology 1988;37:365
59. Eriksson U, Dahlstrom E, Larsson KS, Hellerstrom C. Increased incidence of congenital malformations in the offspring of diabetic rats and their prevention by maternal insulin therapy. Diabetes 1982;30:1
60. New DAT. Whole embryo culture and the study of mammalian embryos during organogenesis. Biol Rev 1978;53:81
61. Sadler TW, Hunter ES III, Wynn RE, Phillips LS. Evidence for multifactorial origin of diabetes-induced embryopathies. Diabetes 1989;38:70
62. Freinkel N, Cockroft DL, Lewis NJ, et al. Fuel-mediated teratogenesis during early organogenesis: The effects of increased concentrations of glucose, ketones, or somatomedin inhibitor during rat embryo culture. Am J Clin Nutr 1986;44:986
63. Buchanan TA, Freinkel N. Fuel-mediated teratogenesis: Symmetric growth retardation in the rat fetus at term after a circumscribed exposure to D-mannose during organogenesis. Am J Obstet Gynecol 1988;158:663
64. Vercheval M, De Hertogh R, Pampher S, et al. Experimental diabetes impairs rat embryo development during the preimplantation period. Diabetologia 1990;33:187
65. Diamond MP, Moley KH, Pellicer A, et al. Effects of streptozotocin- and alloxan-diabetes mellitus on mouse follicular and early embryo development. J Reprod Fert 1989;86:1
66. Beebe LFS, Kaye PL. Maternal diabetes and retarded preimplantation development of mice. Diabetes 1991;40:457
67. Gardner DK, Leese HJ. Concentrations of nutrients in mouse oviduct fluid and their effects on embryo development and metabolism in vitro. J Reprod Fert 1990;88:361
68. Ornoy A, Zusman I. Embryotoxic effect of diabetes on pre-implantation embryos. Isr J Med Sci 1991;27:487
69. Diamond MP, Pettway ZY, Logan J, et al. Dose-response effects of glucose, insulin, and glucagon on mouse pre-embryo development. Metabolism 1991; 40:566
70. Pampfer S, De Hertogh R, Vanderheyden I, et al. Decreased inner cell mass proportion in blastocysts from diabetic rats. Diabetes 1990;40:471
71. Giavani E, Broccia ML, Prati M, Roversi GD. Diet composition modifies the embryotoxic effects induced by experimental diabetes in rats. Biol Neonate 1991;59:278
72. Eriksson RSM, Thunberg L, Eriksson UJ. Effects of interrupted insulin treatment on fetal outcome of pregnant diabetic rats. Diabetes 1989;38: 764
73. Takano K, Nishimra H. Congenital malformations induced by alloxan diabetes in mice and rats. Anat Rec 1967;158:303
74. Endo A. Teratogenesis in diabetic mice treated with alloxan prior to conception. Arch Environ Health 1966;12:492
75. Deuchar EM. Embryonic malformations in rats resulting from maternal diabetes. J Embryol Exp Morphol 1977;41:93
76. Horii K, Watanabe G, Ingalls TH. Experimental diabetes in pregnant mice: Prevention of congenital malformations in offspring by insulin. Diabetes 1966;15:194
77. Styrud J, Thunberg L, Nybacka O, Eriksson UJ. Correlations between maternal metabolism and deranged development in the offspring of normal and diabetic rats. Pediatr Res 1995;37:343
78. Sadler TW. Effects of maternal diabetes on early embryogenesis. I. The teratogenic potential of diabetic serum. Teratology 1988;21:339
79. Buchanan TA, Denno K, Sipos GF, Sadler TW. Diabetic teratogenesis: Evidence for a multifactorial etiology with little contribution from glucose per se. Diabetes 1994;43:656
80. Sadler TW, Horton WE. Effects of maternal diabetes on early embryogenesis. The role of insulin and insulin therapy. Diabetes 1983;32:1070
81. Cockroft DL, Coppola PT. Teratogenic effects of excess glucose in head fold rat embryos in culture. Teratology 1977;16:141
82. Sadler TW. Effects of maternal diabetes on early embryogenesis: II. Hyperglycemia induced exencephaly. Teratology 1980;21:349
83. Eriksson UJ, Borg LAH. Diabetes and embryonic malformations. Role of substrate-induced free-oxygen radical production for dysmorphogenesis in cultured rat embryos. Diabetes 1993;42:411
84. Horton WE Jr, Sadler TW. Effects of maternal diabetes on early embryogenesis: Alterations in morphogenesis produced by the ketone body, β-hydroxybutyrate. Diabetes 1983;32:610
85. Hunter ES III, Sadler TW, Wynn RE. A potential mechanism of DL-β-hydroxybutyrate-induced malformations in mouse embryos. Am J Physiol 1987; 253:E72–E80
86. Sadler TW, Phillips LS, Balkan W, Goldstein S. Somatomedin inhibitors from diabetic rat serum alter growth and development of mouse embryos in culture. Diabetes 1986;35:861
87. Pinter E, Reece EA, Leranth CZ. Yolk sac failure in embryopathy due to hyperglycemia: Ultrastructural analysis of yolk sac differentiation associated with embryology in rat conceptuses under hyperglycemic conditions. Teratology 1986;33:73
88. Reece EA, Pinter E, Leranth C, et al. Yolk sac failure in embryopathy due to hyperglycemia: Horseradish peroxidase uptake in the assessment of yolk sac function. Obstet Gynecol 1989;74:755
89. Baker L, Piddington R, Goldman A, et al. Myo-inositol and prostaglandins reverse the glucose inhibition of neural tube fusion in cultured mouse embryos. Diabetologia 1990;33:593
90. Weigensberg MJ, Garcia-Palmer FJ, Freinkel N. Uptake of myo-inositol by early-somite rat conceptus. Diabetes 1990;39:575
91. Hod M, Star S, Passonneau J, et al. Glucose-induced dysmorphogenesis in the cultured rat conceptus: Prevention by supplementation with myo-inositol. Isr J Med Sci 1990;26:541
92. Hashimoto M, Akazawa S, Akazawa M, et al. Effects of hyperglycemia on sorbitol and myo-inositol contents of cultured embryos: Treatment with aldose reductase inhibitor and myo-inositol supplementation. Diabetologia 1990; 33:597
93. Sussman I, Matschinsky FM. Diabetes affects sorbitol and myo-inositol levels of neuroectodermal tissue during embryogenesis in rat. Diabetes 1988;37: 974
94. Goldman AS, Baker L, Piddington R, et al. Hyperglycemia-induced teratogenesis is mediated by a functional deficiency of arachidonic acid. Proc Natl Acad Sci USA 1985;82:8227
95. Eriksson UJ, Borg LAH. Protection by free oxygen radical scavenging enzymes against glucose-induced embryonic malformations in vitro. Diabetologia 1991;34:325
96. Endo A, Ingalls TH. Chromosomal anomalies in embryos of diabetic mice. Arch Environ Health 1968;16:316
97. Lee AT, Plump A, Desimone C, et al. A role for DNA mutations in diabetes associated teratogenesis in transgenic embryos. Diabetes 1994;44:20
98. Reiher H, Fuhrmann K, Noak S, et al. Age-dependent insulin secretion of the endocrine pancreas in vitro from fetuses of diabetic and nondiabetic patients. Diabetes Care 1983;6:446
99. Milner RDG, Ashworth MA, Barson AJ. Insulin release from human foetal pancreas in response to glucose, leucine, and arginine. J Endocrinol 1972; 52:497
100. Obershain SS, Adam PAJ, King KC, et al. Human fetal insulin response to sustained maternal hyperglycemia. N Engl J Med 1970;283:566

101. Otonkoski T, Andersson S, Knip M, Simell O. Maturation of insulin response to glucose during human fetal and neonatal development. Diabetes 1988; 37:286
102. Phelps RL, Freinkel N, Rubenstein AH, et al. Carbohydrate metabolism in pregnancy. XV. Plasma C-peptide during intravenous glucose tolerance in neonates from normal and insulin-treated diabetic mothers. J Clin Endocrinol Metab 1978;46:61
103. Hellerstrom C, Swenne I. Functional maturation and proliferation of fetal pancreatic β-cells. Diabetes 1991;40(suppl 2):89
104. Cook DL, Hales CN. Intracellular ATP directly blocks K^+-channels in pancreatic β-cells. Nature (Lond) 1984;311:271
105. Pildes RS, Hart RJ, Warrner R, Cornblath M. Plasma insulin response to oral glucose tolerance tests in newborns of normal and gestational diabetic mothers. Pediatrics 1969;44:76
106. Martin FIR, Dahlenburg GW, Russell J, Jeffrey P. Neonatal hypoglycemia in infants of insulin-dependent diabetic mothers. Arch Dis Child 1975;50:472
107. Milner RDG, Wirdnam PK, Tsanakas J. Quantitative morphology of B, A, D, and PP cells in infants of diabetic mothers. Diabetes 1981;30:271
108. Salzberger M, Liban E. Diabetes and fetal death. Isr J Med Sci 1975;11:623
109. Gellis SS, Hsia DYY. The infant of the diabetic mother. Am J Dis Child 1959;97:1
110. Ogata ES, Sabagha R, Metzger BE, et al. Serial ultrasonography to assess evolving fetal macrosomia. JAMA 1980;243:2405
111. Thorens B, Charron MJ, Lodish HF. Molecular physiology of glucose transporters. Diabetes Care 1990;13:209
112. Holzman IR, Lemons JA, Meschia G, Battaglia FC. Uterine uptake of amino acids and placental glutamine-glutamate balance in the pregnant ewe. J Dev Physiol 1979;1:137
113. Ghadimi H, Pecora P. Free amino acids of cord plasma as compared with maternal plasma during pregnancy. Clin Obstet Gynecol 1989;161:646
114. Portman OW, Behrman RE, Soltys P. Transfer of free fatty acids across the primate placenta. Am J Physiol 1696;216:143
115. Muller PS, Solomon F, Brown JR. Free fatty acid concentration in maternal plasma and fetal body fat content. Am J Obstet Gynecol 1964;88:196
116. Knopp RH, Magee MS, Bonet B, Gomez-Coronado D. Lipid metabolism in pregnancy. In: Cowett RM, ed. Principles of Perinatal-Neonatal Metabolism. New York: Springer-Verlag;1991:177–203
117. Malov S, Alousi AA. Lipoprotein lipase activity of rat and human placenta. Proc Soc Exp Biol Med 1965;119:301–306
118. Bonet B, Brunzell JD, Gown AM, Knopp RH. Metabolism of very-low-density lipoprotein triglyceride by human placental cells: The role of lipoprotein lipase. Metabolism 1992;41:596
119. Hummel L, Schwartze A, Schirrmeister W, Wagner H. Maternal plasma triglycerides as a source of fetal fatty acids. Acta Biol Med Ger 1976; 35:1635–1641
120. Menon RK, Cohen RM, Sperling MA, et al. Transplacental passage of insulin in pregnant women with insulin-dependent diabetes mellitus. N Engl J Med 1990;323:309
121. Metzger BE, Phelps RL, Freinkel N. Effects of gestational diabetes on diurnal profiles of plasma glucose, lipids and individual amino acids. Diabetes Care 1980;3:402
122. Hollingsworth DR. Alterations of maternal metabolism in normal and diabetic pregnancies: Differences in insulin-dependent, non–insulin-dependent, and gestational diabetes. Am J Obstet Gynecol 1983;146:417
123. Gabbe S. Medical complications of pregnancy. Management of diabetes in pregnancy: Six decades of experience. In: Pitkin RK, Zlatnik FJ, eds. Yearbook of Obstetrics and Gynecology. Part I: Obstetrics. Chicago: Year Book Medical Publishers;1980:37
124. Centers for Disease Control. Perinatal mortality and congenital malformations in infants born to women with insulin-dependent diabetes mellitus: United States, Canada and Europe, 1940–1988. MMWR 1190;39:363
125. Phillips AF, Porte PJ, Stabinsky S, et al. Effects of chronic fetal hyperglycemia upon oxygen consumption in the ovine uterus and conceptus. J Clin Invest 1984;74:279
126. Phillips AF, Dubin JW, Matty PJ, Raye J. Arterial hypoxemia and hyperinsulinemia in the chronically hyperglycemic fetal lamb. Pediatr Res 1982; 16:653
127. Salversen DR, Brudenell MJ, Nicolaides KH. Fetal polycythemia and thrombocythemia in pregnancies complicated by maternal diabetes mellitus. Am J Obstet Gynecol 1992;166:1287
128. Jovanovic-Peterson L, Peterson C, Reed GF, et al. Maternal postprandial glucose levels and infant birth weight: The Diabetes in Early Pregnancy Study. Am Obstet Gynecol 1991;164:103–111
129. Combs CA, Gundeson E, Kitzmiller JL, et al. Relationship of fetal macrosomia to maternal postprandial glucose control during pregnancy. Diabetes Care 1992;15:1251
130. Gregory R, Scott AR, Mohajar M, Tattersall RB. Diabetic pregnancy 1977–1990: Have we reached a plateau? J R Coll Phys 1992;26:162
131. Hanson U, Persson B. Outcome of pregnancies complicated by type I insulin dependent diabetes in Sweden: Acute pregnancy complications, neonatal mortality and morbidity. Am J Perinatol 1993;10:330
132. Langer O, Rodriguez DA, Xenakis MJX, et al. Intensified vs. conventional management of gestational diabetes. Am J Obstet Gynecol 1994;170:1036
133. Kjos SL, Henry OA, Montoro M, et al. Insulin-requiring diabetes in pregnancy: A randomized trial of active induction of labor and expectant management. Am J Obstet Gynecol 1993;169:611
134. Brans YW, Shannon DL, Hunter MA. Maternal diabetes and neonatal macrosomia. II. Neonatal anthropometric measurements. Early Hum Dev 1983; 8:297
135. Prophylactic insulin treatment of gestational diabetes reduces the incidence of macrosomia, operative delivery and birth trauma. Am J Obstet Gynecol 1984;150:836
136. Kalkhoff RK. Therapeutic results of insulin therapy in gestational diabetes mellitus. Diabetes 1985;34:(suppl 2):97
137. Buchanan TA, Kjos SL, Montoro MN, et al. Use of fetal ultrasound to select metabolic therapy for pregnancies complicated by mild gestational diabetes. Diabetes Care 1994;17:275
138. Weiss PAM, Hoffman HMH, Kainer F, Haas JG. Fetal outcome in gestational diabetes with elevated amniotic fluid insulin levels. Dietary vs. insulin treatment. Diabetes Res Clin Pract 1988;5:1
139. Metzger BE. Biphasic effects of maternal metabolism on fetal growth. Diabetes 1991;40(suppl 2):99
140. Susa JB, McCormick KL, Widness JA, et al. Chronic hyperinsulinemia in the fetal rhesus monkey: Effects on fetal growth and composition. Diabetes 1979;28:1058
141. Freinkel N, Metzger BE. Pregnancy as a tissue culture experience: The critical implications of maternal metabolism for fetal development. In: Pregnancy Metabolism, Diabetes and the Fetus. CIBA Foundation Symposium No. 65. Amsterdam: Excerpta Medica;1979:3–23
142. Persson B, Lunell NO. Metabolic control in diabetic pregnancy. Am J Obstet Gynecol 1975;122:737
143. Kalkhoff RK. Impact of maternal fuels and nutritional state on fetal growth. Diabetes 1991;40(suppl 2):61
144. Knopp RH, Magee MS, Walden CE, et al. Prediction of infant birth weight by GDM screening: Importance of plasma triglyceride. Diabetes Care 1992;15:1605
145. Freinkel N, Metzger BE, Phelps RL, et al. Gestational diabetes mellitus: Heterogeneity of maternal age, weight, insulin secretion, HLA antigens, and islet cell antibodies and the impact of maternal metabolism on pancreatic β-cell function and somatic growth in the offspring. Diabetes 1985;34(suppl 2):1
146. Knopp RH, Bergelin RO, Wahl PW, Walden CE. Relationship of infant birth size to maternal lipoproteins, apoproteins, fuels, hormones, clinical chemistries, and body weight at 36 weeks gestation. Diabetes 1985;34 (suppl 2):71
147. Bjork O. The fetal arterial vasculature in placentas of insulin-dependent diabetic mothers. Acta Pathol Microbiol Immunol Scand 1982;90:289
148. Thomas CR, Eriksson GL, Eriksson UJ. Effects of maternal diabetes on placental transfer of glucose in rats. Diabetes 1990;39:276
149. Kitzmiller JL, Brown ER, Phillippe M, et al. Diabetic nephropathy and perinatal outcome. Am J Obstet Gynecol 1981;141:741
150. Turula M, Kaprio J, Rissanen A, Koskenuo M. Body weight in the Finnish Twin Cohort. Diabetes Res Clin Pract 1990;10(suppl 1):S33
151. Bouchard C, Tremblay A, Despres JP, et al. The response to long-term overfeeding in identical twins. N Engl J Med 1990;322:1477
152. Dooley SL, Metzger BE, Cho N. Gestational diabetes: Influence of race on disease prevalence and perinatal outcome in a U.S. population. Diabetes 1991;40(suppl 2):25
153. Gloria-Bottini F, Gerlin G, Lucarini N, et al. Both maternal and foetal genetic factors contribute to macrosomia in diabetic pregnancy. Hum Hered 1994; 44:24
154. Knip M, Lautala P, Leppaluoto J, et al. Relation of enteroinsular hormones at birth to macrosomia and neonatal hypoglycemia in infants of diabetic mothers. J Pediatr 1983;103:603
155. Sosenko IR, Kitzmiller JL, Loo SW, et al. The infant of the diabetic mother: Correlation of increased cord C-peptide levels with macrosomia and neonatal hypoglycemia. N Engl J Med 1979;301:859
156. Kuhl C, Andersen GE, Hertel J, Molsted-Pedersen L. Metabolic events in infants of diabetic mothers during the first 24 hours after birth. Acta Pediatr Scand 1982;71:19
157. Hunter DJS, Burrows RF, Mohide PT, Whyte RK. Influence of maternal insulin-dependent diabetes mellitus on neonatal morbidity. Can Med Assoc J 1993;149:47
158. Anderson O, Hertel J, Schmolker L, Kuhl C. Influence of maternal plasma glucose concentration at delivery on the risk of hypoglycemia in infants of IDDM mothers. Acta Paediatr Scand 1985;74:268
159. Kalhan SC, Savin SM, Adams PAJ. Attenuated glucose production rate in newborn infants of insulin-dependent diabetic mothers. N Engl J Med 1977;296:375
160. Nurjhan N, Ktorza A, Ferre P, et al. Effects of gestational hyperglycemia on glucose metabolism and its hormonal control in the fasted, newborn rat during early postnatal life. Diabetes 1985;34:995
161. Light IJ, Keenan WJ, Sutherland JM. Maternal intravenous glucose administration a cause of hypoglycemic in the infant of the diabetic mother. Am J Obstet Gynecol 1972;113:345
162. Gillmer MDG, Berad RW, Oakley NW. Carbohydrate metabolism in pregnancy. Part II—relation between maternal glucose tolerance and glucose metabolism in the newborn. Br Med J 1975;3:402
163. Andersen O, Hertel J, Schmolker L, Kuhl C. Influence of the maternal plasma glucose concentrations at delivery on the risk of hypoglycemia in infants of insulin-dependent diabetic mothers. Acta Pediatr Scand 1985;74:268
164. Cowett RM, Susa JB, Giletti B, et al. Glucose kinetics in infants of diabetic mothers. Am J Obstet Gynecol 1983;146:781

165. Sosenko JM, Kitzmiller JL, Fluckiger R, et al. Umbilical cord glycosylated hemoglobin in infants of diabetic mothers: Relationships to neonatal hypoglycemia, macrosomia, and cord serum C-peptide. Diabetes Care 1982; 5:566
167. Stubbs WA, Stubbs SM. Hyperinsulinemia, diabetes mellitus and respiratory distress of the newborn: A common link? Lancet 1978;1:308
167. Piper JM, Langer O. Does maternal diabetes delay fetal pulmonary maturity? Am J Obstet Gynecol 1993;168:783
168. Demarini S, Mimouni F, Tsang R, et al. Impact of metabolic control of diabetes during pregnancy on neonatal hypocalcemia: A randomized study. Obstet Gynecol 1994;83:918
169. Green DW, Khoury J, Mimouni F. Neonatal hematocrit and maternal glycemic control in insulin-dependent diabetes. J Pediatr 1992;120:302
170. Salvesen DR, Brundell M, Snijders RJM, et al. Fetal plasma erythropoietin in pregnancies complicated by maternal diabetes mellitus. Am J Obstet Gynecol 1993;168:88
171. Widness JA, Susa JB, Garcia JF, et al. Increased erythropoiesis and elevated erythropoietin in infants born to diabetic mothers and in hyperinsulinemic rhesus fetuses. J Clin Invest 1981;67:637
172. Freinkel N. The Banting Lecture 1980. Of pregnancy and progeny. Diabetes 1980;29:1023
173. Holemans K, Aerts L, Van Assche FA. Evidence for an insulin resistance in the adult offspring of pregnant streptozotocin-diabetic rats. Diabetologia 1991;34:81
174. Grill V, Johansson B, Jalkanen P, Eriksson UJ. Influence of severe diabetes mellitus early in pregnancy in the rat: Effects on insulin sensitivity and insulin secretion in the offspring. Diabetologia 1991;34:373
175. Gelardi NL, Cha CM, Oh W. Evaluation of insulin sensitivity in obese offspring of diabetic rats by the hyperinsulinemic euglycemic clamps technique. Pediatr Res 1991;30:40
176. Van Assche FA, Aerts L, Holemans K. Metabolic alterations in adulthood after intrauterine development in mothers with mild diabetes. Diabetes 1991;40(suppl 2):106
177. Gauguier D, Bihoreau M-T, Picon L, Ktorza A. Insulin secretion in adult rats after intrauterine exposure to mild hyperglycemia during late gestation. Diabetes 1991;40(suppl 2):109
178. Dahri S, Snoeck A, Reusens-Billen B, et al. Islet function in offspring of mothers on low-protein diet during gestation. Diabetes 1991;40(suppl 2):115
179. Churchill JA, Berendez HW, Nemore J. Neuropsychological deficits in children of diabetic mothers. Am J Obstet Gynecol 1966;105:257
180. Stehbens JA, Baker GL, Kitchell M. Outcome at ages 1, 3, and 5 years of children born to diabetic women. Am J Obstet Gynecol 1977;127:408
181. Rizzo T, Metzger BE, Burns WJ, Burns K. Correlation between antepartum maternal metabolism and intelligence of offspring. N Engl J Med 1991; 325:911
182. Bhasin S, Shambaugh GE 3rd. Fetal fuels V. Ketone bodies inhibit pyrimidine biosynthesis in fetal rat brain. Am J Physiol 1982;243:E234
183. Shambaugh GE 3rd, Angulo MC, Koehler RR. Fetal fuels VII. Ketone bodies inhibit synthesis of purines in fetal rat brain. Am J Physiol 1984;247:E111
184. Sells CJ, Robinson NM, Brown Z, Knopp RH. Long-term developmental follow-up of infants of diabetic mothers. J Pediatr 1994;125:S9
185. Pettitt DJ, Baird HR, Aleck KA, et al. Excessive obesity in offspring of Pima Indian women with diabetes during pregnancy. N Engl J Med 1983;308:242
186. Kohlhoff R, Dorner G. Perinatal hyperinsulinism and perinatal obesity as risk factors for hyperinsulinaemia in later life. Exp Clin Endocrinol 1990; 96:105
187. Silverman BL, Rizzo T, Green OC, et al. Long-term prospective evaluation of offspring of diabetic mothers. Diabetes 1991;40(suppl 2):121
188. Pettitt DJ, Aleck KA, Baird HR, et al. Congenital susceptibility to NIDDM. Diabetes 1988;37:622

Diabetes Mellitus, edited by Derek LeRoith, Simeon I. Taylor, and Jerrold M. Olefsky. Lippincott–Raven Publishers, Philadelphia © 1996.

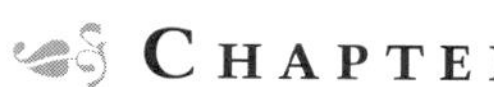

CHAPTER 78

Pregnancy and Complications of Type I Diabetes: Maternal and Fetal Implications

BARAK M. ROSENN AND MENACHEM MIODOVNIK

Introduction

Over the past two decades there has been a decrease in morbidity and mortality related to pregnancy in women with insulin-dependent diabetes mellitus (IDDM). These changes may be attributed to improved maternal glycemic control, advances in neonatal care, and close antepartum surveillance. Currently, the perinatal mortality rate for infants of mothers with IDDM approaches that of the population at large. Intrauterine fetal death in the last weeks of pregnancy, death due to the traumatic delivery of a macrosomic infant, and neonatal mortality arising from elective, physician-initiated premature delivery are presently unusual in women with IDDM who receive good prenatal care. Further, until recently, women with advanced diabetic disease were strongly advised not to conceive lest the pregnancy result in aggravation of the underlying disease, as well as a poor perinatal outcome. Many women with advanced IDDM can now gain access to specialized prenatal care and, in most instances, can expect a successful pregnancy without compromising their health or the well-being of their offspring. Nevertheless, even with the best care, maternal and perinatal complications in IDDM pregnancies are consistently more frequent than those in the general population. Indeed, diabetes and pregnancy may mutually affect each other over a range of interactions from conception to delivery, possibly with long-term ramifications for both the mother and her infant.

Since the introduction of insulin therapy, women with IDDM can conceive, carry a pregnancy to term, and expect to deliver a reasonably healthy, surviving infant. Many of these women, however, have been told that pregnancy may pose a long-term risk to their health. Specifically, physicians often warn these patients that pregnancy can accelerate the progression of retinopathy and nephropathy. As reviewed below, there are very few data available with which to counsel these women reliably.

Pregnancy and Diabetic Complications

Retinopathy

Several factors may contribute to the pathogenesis of diabetic retinopathy. Factors of particular concern during pregnancy include the role of glycemic control, angiogenic growth factors, and hypertension.

Strict glycemic control has become an accepted mode of management during pregnancy in women with IDDM that is expected to improve the outcome of pregnancy. Glycemic control, however, may be a two-edged sword in relation to the development and progression of retinopathy. Although most studies show that the presence and severity of retinopathy in nonpregnant subjects with IDDM are related to poor glycemic control,[1–5] several studies also show that rapid normalization of blood glucose can cause acute, albeit often transient, progression of retinopathy.[6–10]

The results of these studies may be relevant to the pregnant woman with IDDM because the goals of glycemic control used in the strictly controlled groups in these studies are similar to those often employed during pregnancy, and the period during which strict control was associated with progression rather than improvement is similar to the duration of pregnancy. One cannot necessarily extrapolate these findings to pregnancy, however, because of the physiologic, hemodynamic, and hormonal changes associated with the pregnant state.

It has been suggested that circulating and local factors may also contribute to the progression of retinopathy. These factors include growth hormone,[11–13] insulin-like growth factor 1,[14–16] and "angiogenic factors" isolated from the vitreous of patients with proliferative retinopathy that produce vessel proliferation in vitro.[17] The relevance of these findings to pregnancy is that the placenta also produces angiogenic factors that result in vessel proliferation in endothelial cell cultures in vitro.[18,19] Human placental lactogen circulates at high concentrations during pregnancy, with levels some 1000-fold greater than those of growth hormone,[20] and it is theoretically possible that its growth hormone–like actions could affect retinal tissue. Thus, the presence of placental factors could result in new-vessel formation during pregnancy, although it is unknown whether the systemic concentrations of these factors are high enough to affect other organs or whether they might act through intermediary substances to produce their effects.

Hypertension has also been consistently linked to the severity of retinopathy. The relation of hypertension to retinopathy may be particularly important during pregnancy because 10–20% of women with IDDM develop pregnancy-induced hypertension.[21] In a recent study,[22] pregnancy-induced hypertension and chronic hypertension were the most important factors associated with the progression of retinopathy during pregnancy.

Another concern is that the abrupt increases in blood pressure with maternal expulsive efforts during delivery may cause acute retinal hemorrhages in mothers with preproliferative changes. This concern has led some obstetricians to advocate cesarean delivery for these mothers. Others, however, argue that the vascular changes are predominantly postarteriolar and are unlikely to be affected by the Valsalva maneuver.[23] There are virtually no data with which to resolve this issue.

Because of the potential roles of glycemic control, growth factors, and hypertension in the pathogenesis of retinopathy, it is plausible to hypothesize that pregnancy may cause a worsening of the disease. This is especially important because most pregnant women with IDDM in whom retinopathy has been studied have had diabetes of 5 to 20 years' duration, so that the prevalence of background and preproliferative disease is relatively high. The possibility exists, then, that pregnancy may be a setting in which pathogenic mechanisms would accelerate retinal changes, creating a condition that could result in more pronounced changes years later.

Several recent studies have addressed the issue of progression of diabetic retinopathy during and after pregnancy (Table 78-1). In the only study that included nonpregnant controls,[24] Moloney and Drury[24] compared 53 pregnant women with diabetes and 39 nonpregnant control women with diabetes. Retinal examinations were performed in each trimester and at 6 months postpartum. During the 15-month period, there was no significant change in the nonpregnant patients, with only three patients developing streak or blob hemorrhages. Of the 53 pregnant patients, 24 showed progression during pregnancy. Changes in background retinopathy regressed in most patients 6 months after delivery, a finding that has also been demonstrated by others.[22,25,26] In this study, pregnant patients and nonpregnant controls did not undergo the same therapeutic intervention, that is, intensive insulin therapy. Furthermore, glycohemoglobin concentrations or other measures of glycemic control were not reported.

In a study by Dibble et al.,[27] 55 insulin-dependent pregnant women had fundus photography during each trimester and again at 8 weeks postpartum. Changes in retinopathy status were correlated with glycemic control, as calculated from the mean blood glucose concentrations from home monitoring records. Patients with hypertension and preeclampsia were excluded. Of the 55 patients studied, 23 had no eye disease, and none of these patients showed deterioration. Of 19 patients with background disease alone, 3 showed progression. Thirteen patients with proliferative disease were divided into two categories; seven patients had no photocoagulation therapy before pregnancy, and six had had prior treatment. Of the seven with no therapy, six showed progression of disease and required photocoagulation therapy. Only one patient with proliferative retinopathy that was treated before pregnancy showed progression requiring additional therapy during gestation. In this study, the presence and progression of retinopathy, excluding those in the proliferative group with antecedent therapy, correlated significantly with the duration of diabetes but not with glycemic control during gestation. The authors state that termination of pregnancy should be considered only in those patients with retinopathy that does not respond to photocoagulation therapy.

In contrast, data from Price et al.[28] on 23 pregnancies in women with diabetes showed that retinopathy did not appear in patients

Table 78-1. Progression of Diabetic Retinopathy in Pregnancy, Stratified by Initial Retinal Findings

		Number (%) with Progression Given Initial Findings		
Author	**Number of Pregnancies**	No Retinopathy	Background Retinopathy	Proliferative Retinopathy
Horvat et al.[25]	160	13/118 (11%)	11/35 (31%)	1/7 (14%)
Moloney and Drury[24]	53	8/20 (40%)	15/30 (50%)	1/3 (33%)
Dibble et al.[27]	55	0/23 (0%)	3/19 (16%)	7/13 (54%)
Price et al.[28]	31	0/14 (0%)	0/10 (0%)	5/7 (71%)
Ohrt[26]	100	4/50 (8%)	15/48 (31%)	1/2 (51%)
Phelps et al.[29]	38	3/13 (23%)	13/20 (65%)	5/5 (100%)
Serup[30]	45	6/19 (32%)	11/21 (52%)	0/5 (0%)
Rosenn et al.[22]	154	18/78 (23%)	28/68 (41%)	5/8 (63%)
Total	636	52/335 (16%)	96/251 (38%)	25/50 (50%)

who had normal eyes at the onset of pregnancy and that patients with pre-existing background retinopathy did not show disease progression during pregnancy or peripartum. In seven patients with pre-existing proliferative disease, five showed disease progress, with four of the five requiring laser photocoagulation during pregnancy or within 3 months postpartum. The small numbers in each group in this study, however, do not allow meaningful statistical conclusions.

In a prospective study by Ohrt,[26] 100 pregnancies in 75 women with diabetes were examined. Fifty patients had retinopathy at the time of examination, but proliferative retinopathy was present in only two patients. Four patients without retinopathy developed slight background changes during pregnancy, and proliferative changes developed in four more. Of 43 patients with background retinopathy, 15 showed only slight progression, the rest remaining unchanged. In 22 patients, background changes regressed during the postpartum period. In this study, there was no attempt to correlate changes with glycemic control.

Phelps et al.[29] studied the effects of intensive insulin therapy on eye changes during 38 pregnancies in 35 patients. Fundus photographs taken before 22 weeks' gestation were compared to those taken no later than 2 weeks postpartum. Background retinopathy worsened in 13 of 20 patients with pre-existing disease and was related to the abrupt, rapid institution of strict glycemic control. All five patients with pre-existing proliferative disease showed progression of retinopathy.

Serup[30] prospectively studied 145 women who were examined three times during pregnancy and three times postpartum, the last examination occurring 1 year after delivery. At the time of the report, 40 women had been followed for the entire period, with 73 followed to at least 2 months postpartum. Of the 40 women who completed the study, 19 had no retinopathy at entry. One of these 19 patients developed background changes that regressed postpartum. Of the 21 patients who had retinopathy at the initial examination, 11 had progression during pregnancy and none showed regression 1 year postpartum. Two patients developed proliferative disease; one required photocoagulation therapy 8 months after delivery, and the other had regression to background disease. Of the remaining 73 patients who were followed for 2 months postpartum, 5 developed proliferative retinopathy, 4 showing regression during the postpartum period. Five women entered the study with proliferative retinopathy, and none of these showed progression. The author recommended postponing photocoagulation therapy until 8–12 months postpartum.

Rosenn et al.[22] studied 154 women with IDDM who had eye examinations and fundus photography every trimester and again 6–12 weeks postpartum. Of 154 patients examined, 76 (49%) had retinopathy at the initial examination, 68 with background retinopathy and 8 with proliferative disease. The risk of progression was related to the degree of retinopathy at the initial examination. Of 78 patients without retinopathy early in gestation, 18 (23%) developed retinopathy during or after pregnancy. Of the 68 patients with background disease, 28 (41%) showed progression, with 7 requiring photocoagulation. Of the eight patients with proliferative disease, five (63%) showed deterioration that required photocoagulation. Progression was more likely to occur in patients with hypertensive disorders such as chronic or pregnancy-induced hypertension. Progression was also more likely to occur in those who initially had poor glycemic control and in those who had rapid institution of strict glycemic control in early pregnancy. Again, however, there was no nonpregnant control group, so it is premature to state whether the observed progression was related to pregnancy or whether it was simply a reflection of the progressive nature of the underlying disease.

The recent prospective, controlled study by Klein et al.[31] is not included in Table 78-1 because the results were not stratified by initial retinal findings. This study included 102 pregnant women with IDDM who had retinal examinations at an average of 11 weeks' gestation and again at an average of 9 weeks' postpartum. They were compared to 195 nonpregnant women with IDDM who had retinal examinations spanning a similar interval. The two groups had a similar distribution of baseline retinal findings, although the pregnancy group was younger, had a shorter duration of diabetes, lower baseline blood pressure, and better glycemic control at the first visit. At follow-up, 45 (43%) of the pregnant women and 77 (39%) of the nonpregnant controls had progression of retinopathy. Although this difference was obviously not significant, Klein et al. performed a logistic regression analysis to control for the confounding effect of the baseline difference in glycohemoglobin concentration between the pregnant and nonpregnant groups. On the basis of this analysis, pregnancy was associated with a higher risk of progression (odds ratio 1.8). Unfortunately, this study did not provide data on whether progression was related to the rapid institution of strict glycemic control in pregnancy. Further, the postpartum follow-up interval was rather short. It is therefore unclear to what extent the pregnancy-associated progression of retinopathy was only a transient phenomenon.

In summary, it is clear that retinopathy does progress with pregnancy and that the risk of progression is related to the severity of any baseline retinopathy: Women without baseline changes are at relatively low risk of progression, and women with proliferative retinopathy are at high risk. It is also clear that some women who show progression of retinopathy during pregnancy will show regression within 1 or 2 years postpartum. It is not clear, however, to what extent the irreversible progression observed during pregnancy is caused by pregnancy per se or simply reflects the natural history of a progressive disease. Also unclear is whether any changes attributable to pregnancy are caused primarily by the altered hormonal milieu of pregnancy, by the institution of strict glycemic control, by the occurrence of hypertensive complications of pregnancy, or by the hemodynamic stresses of pregnancy, labor, and delivery.

Nephropathy

Diabetic nephropathy is a progressive disease that affects 30–40% of patients with insulin-dependent diabetes mellitus (IDDM) and is the most common cause of end-stage renal disease in the United States (see Chapter 81). There appears to be a genetic basis for susceptibility to nephropathy.[32] In genetically susceptible persons, scattered sclerosis of glomeruli develops within a few years after the diagnosis of IDDM, and this can be demonstrated on renal biopsy even in the absence of clinical findings. Within 5–10 years, minute amounts of albumin and other anionic proteins can be detected in the urine. This is the phase of incipient nephropathy or so-called microalbuminuria. The phase of overt nephropathy is characterized by progressive, widespread glomerular sclerosis resulting in excretion of progressively larger amounts of protein. Ultimately, progressive renal insufficiency and end-stage renal disease occur, manifest as decreasing creatinine clearance, increasing serum creatinine, and uremia.

The precise cause of diabetic nephropathy is yet to be determined, but it is generally accepted that the primary insult is increased glomerular capillary pressure that leads to glomerular hyperfiltration.[33] These hemodynamic changes result in structural damage, which ultimately leads to renal functional deterioration. Several factors have been implicated in the development of nephropathy, such as glycemic control, dietary protein intake, and hypertension. Prospective trials have shown that modification of these factors can ameliorate the expected course of diabetic nephropathy.

Poor glycemic control has consistently been found to increase the glomerular filtration rate. Thus, the degree of glycemic control might theoretically influence the appearance of nephropathy or the rate of its progression. Indeed, several studies of the relationship of glycemic control to nephropathy have concluded that strict control results in improved renal function or a slower rate of progression of nephropathy.[4,10,34–42]

Diets with high protein content can result in hyperaminoacidemia and consequently in increased glomerular filtration rates.[43,44] Thus, reduction of dietary protein intake might theoretically delay the appearance of nephropathy or slow its progression. Several studies have shown that a low-protein diet has a beneficial effect on the course of incipient or overt diabetic nephropathy.[45–47]

Systemic arterial hypertension also appears to play a role in the rate of progression of nephropathy.[48–50] Hypertension is common in patients with overt diabetic nephropathy, as it is with many renal disorders. Strict control of blood pressure using angiotensin-converting enzyme (ACE) inhibitors or other antihypertensive agents appears to delay the progression from incipient to overt nephropathy and may also slow the progression from overt nephropathy to end-stage renal disease.[51,52]

Consideration of the foregoing factors makes it evident that pregnancy may have profound effects on the course of nephropathy. During normal pregnancy, there is a 40–60% increase in glomerular filtration rate and a moderate increase in the excretion of urinary protein. This physiologic hyperfiltration also occurs in some women with diabetic nephropathy.[53] To the extent that hyperfiltration causes injury to glomeruli, this pregnancy-related change might be expected to accelerate the progression of nephropathy. The increased dietary protein intake during pregnancy may also exacerbate glomerular hyperfiltration. In addition, pregnancy-induced hypertension affects 10–20% of all women with IDDM, and this rate is even higher among IDDM women with nephropathy.[21,54] Furthermore, Combs et al.[55] found a 40% rate of preeclampsia in women with incipient nephropathy and a 47% rate in women with overt nephropathy. To the extent that hypertensive disorders may damage glomeruli, an adverse effect on nephropathy could be expected.

It is possible that all of the above pregnancy-related changes may be too mild or too transient to have a permanent effect on diabetic nephropathy. Additionally, because pregnant women with IDDM are often managed with intensive insulin therapy, this factor might actually be expected to have a beneficial effect on renal function. Thus, the case can be made on theoretical grounds that pregnancy might worsen nephropathy, improve nephropathy, or have no effect. Unfortunately, only a few studies have examined the long-term effect of pregnancy on renal function, and have involved relatively few pregnant women and no nonpregnant controls. Most of these studies have appeared in the obstetric literature and emphasize the management and prognosis of patients with preexisting nephropathy, and most were done before the development of sensitive assays for microalbuminuria. To date, there are no published prospective studies dealing with glycemic control during pregnancy and the development or progression of nephropathy.

Kitzmiller et al.[56] obtained follow-up information on renal function in a group of 23 women with IDDM who had overt nephropathy at 9 to 35 months postpartum. They found that creatinine clearance decreased at an average rate of 10 mL/min/year, similar to the rate reported in nonpregnant subjects with diabetic nephropathy. Reece et al.[57] reported on 31 women with diabetes who had proteinuria during pregnancy, of whom 9 had preexisting overt nephropathy. From their tabulated data, Kitzmiller et al. calculated that the mean rate of fall in creatinine clearance averaged 10 mL/min/year over a 5–60-month postpartum follow-up period, which was no different than expected. Subsequently, Reece et al.[58] studied the change in serum creatinine concentrations in 11 women with diabetic nephropathy from prepregnancy up to 4 years postpartum. The observed decline in renal function through the end of the follow-up period appears to be consistent with the expected course of diabetic nephropathy in the absence of pregnancy. Thus, these studies concluded that renal function deteriorates after pregnancy in women with overt nephropathy, but the rate of deterioration is not different than would be expected without pregnancy. Kimmerle et al.[59] followed 29 women with diabetic nephropathy during pregnancy and for periods ranging from 4 months to 10 years after delivery. They concluded that the circumstantial evidence suggests that pregnancy does not accelerate the course of diabetic nephropathy. As expected, renal function declined more rapidly among those women who already had reduced renal function at the onset of pregnancy.

In contrast, Biesenbach et al.[60] studied five women with IDDM who had diabetic nephropathy with compromised renal function (creatinine clearance ≤75 mL/min) and hypertension. The mean rate of decline in creatinine clearance was greater than expected both during pregnancy (22 mL/min/year) and during the postpartum follow-up period (17 mL/min/year). Hypertension worsened in all 5 women during pregnancy, and all developed end-stage renal disease within 42 months postpartum (average, 29 months). The authors suggested that the accelerated decline in renal function may be related to increasing hypertension during pregnancy. Gordon et al.[61] reviewed the outcome of 29 patients with diabetic nephropathy (defined as ≥400 mg proteinuria per 24 hours) followed for a mean of 2.8 years postpartum. They found that creatinine clearance fell more than 10 mL/min/year in 12 patients. These authors concluded that pregnancy may accelerate loss of renal function in women with diabetic nephropathy.

None of the aforementioned studies included nonpregnant controls. Instead, they relied on literature reports on the rate of decline in renal function in patients with IDDM who had the diagnosis of nephropathy.

Grenfell et al.[61a] reported the outcome of pregnancy in 20 women with diabetic nephropathy, with follow-up on 15 of these patients for 6 months to 10 years (median, 2 years). They found that 11 women had normal creatinine levels, 3 had elevated serum creatinine levels, and 1 had died of renal failure. No conclusions could be drawn regarding the effect of pregnancy on progression of diabetic nephropathy. Carstensen et al.[61b] matched 22 pairs of women with IDDM by age and duration of disease. Each pair consisted of a woman who had never completed a pregnancy, matched with a woman who had completed one or two pregnancies. Their analysis showed no differences between the two groups with respect to the prevalence of microvascular complications up to 17.7 years after the birth of the oldest child and up to 24 years after the onset of diabetes.

Hemachandra et al.[61c] matched 80 nulliparous women with IDDM to 80 parous women with IDDM by age, duration of IDDM, race, and marital history. They found no differences between the groups regarding the prevalence of microvascular complications. They also followed a subgroup of 30 primiparous women for a period of 11.8 ± 7.7 months (mean ± standard deviation) following their pregnancy, matched to a group of 30 nulliparous women followed for the same period. There were no differences between the two groups in the incidence of diabetic nephropathy. They concluded that pregnancy does not appear to be a risk factor for complications of diabetes later in life.

Miodovnik et al.[61d] studied 182 women with IDDM, of whom 46 had overt diabetic nephropathy. These patients were treated with intensive insulin therapy throughout pregnancy, and followed for a period of 3–16 years (median, 9.1 years) after delivery. Of the 136 women without nephropathy at the time of pregnancy, only 13 (10%) eventually developed nephropathy later in life, within 10.1 ± 4.2 (mean ± standard deviation) years following the pregnancy. Proteinuria appearing during pregnancy and poor glycemic control during pregnancy were significantly associated with the subsequent development of nephropathy. Of the 46 women who had overt nephropathy prior to pregnancy, 12 (26%) progressed to end-stage renal disease after a median period of 6 years. Using life table analysis, the investigators found that the overall risk of developing nephropathy was 44% after 27 years of diabetes, and the risk of progressing to end-stage renal disease was 30% after 10 years of overt diabetic nephropathy. The risk of developing nephropathy de novo, and the risk of progressing from nephropathy to end stage renal disease were not associated with pregnancy or with increasing parity.

There are virtually no studies on whether pregnancy influences the rate of progression from the absence of nephropathy to incipient nephropathy or from incipient nephropathy to overt nephropathy.

In summary, pregnancy represents an altered physiologic state during which several hemodynamic, hormonal, dietary, and growth factors may potentially contribute to the microvascular changes of retinopathy and nephropathy in women with IDDM. Although there are many studies in the literature dealing with the issues of glycemic control and microvascular complications in subjects with IDDM, there are hardly any controlled, prospective studies addressing the effects of pregnancy on microvascular complications.

Data from independent prospective studies indicate that relatively intensive insulin therapy over a time span similar to that of pregnancy may contribute to acceleration of background retinopathy, although the long-term consequences have not yet been established. It is often stated that intensive insulin therapy to achieve near-euglycemia should be the goal for management of diabetes in pregnancy. Thus, it is possible that the retinal microvascular changes that occur during pregnancy and that have been reported in several uncontrolled studies may be a consequence of intensive insulin therapy rather than of pregnancy per se. The long-term effects of pregnancy on renal function in women with IDDM have never been studied in a prospective, controlled manner, and the few retrospective reports in the literature present conflicting data. Thus, at present, it is difficult to determine with certainty the long-term effects of pregnancy on the progression of microvascular complications in women with IDDM.

Coronary Heart Disease

Women with diabetes have a threefold risk of atherosclerosis and fatal myocardial infarction (see Chapter 86). The information in the medical literature concerning pregnancy in women with diabetes and coronary heart disease, however, is limited.[62–69] From these limited studies, it seems that the association of diabetes, pregnancy, and coronary heart disease poses significant risks to the mother and the fetus.

Maternal death occurred in 50% of the 16 cases reported: Four in women who suffered a myocardial infarction in the first trimester and four in women who suffered myocardial infarction in the third trimester or within 4 weeks postpartum. Of interest, two women who underwent coronary bypass surgery before pregnancy had a successful outcome.

These women are extremely vulnerable to myocardial damage and pulmonary edema in the immediate postpartum period. After a vaginal delivery, there is an immediate 60–80% increase in cardiac output[70] due to release of venocaval obstruction, autotransfusion of uteroplacental blood, and rapid mobilization of extravascular fluid, resulting in increased venus return and stroke volume. These fluid shifts are less pronounced after cesarean delivery using controlled analgesia.[71] An extended period of close postpartum follow-up is required for women with insulin-dependent diabetes mellitus (IDDM) who have ischemic heart disease because cardiovascular hemodynamics do not completely return to the pre-pregnancy state even by 12 weeks postpartum.[72]

Of particular concern in these patients are the consequences of hypoglycemia. Institution of strict glycemic control in pregnant women with IDDM is associated with a significant risk of hypoglycemia, primarily during the first half of pregnancy (see ''Pregnancy and Hypoglycemia''). Activation of the counter-regulatory responses to hypoglycemia will cause release of catecholamines, resulting in tachycardia, possible arrhythmia, and increased demands on the myocardium. These changes are particularly hazardous in a patient with underlying ischemic heart disease and may result in an acute myocardial infarction.

Because of the extremely high risk associated with pregnancy in women with diabetes and coronary heart disease, preconceptional consultation is of the utmost importance. It is prudent to make the patient aware of the serious maternal risk and to recommend a permanent method of sterilization. For the patient who has agreed to undertake these risks, a concerted effort must be made by the patient, the obstetrician, the diabetologist, and the cardiologist to obtain a thorough antenatal cardiac evaluation, attain strict glycemic control, maintain continuous surveillance of maternal and fetal status throughout pregnancy, and manage the delivery prudently.

Neuropathy

Little, if any, is known about the effects of diabetic neuropathy on pregnancy and the possible effects of pregnancy on neuropathy. Studies on the impact of pregnancy on diabetic neuropathy are basically limited to case reports, and any valid conclusions regarding such patients are difficult to make. The presence of gastroparesis is particularly relevant in that, with the hyperemesis of pregnancy, it results in exacerbation of nausea and vomiting. The result is irregular absorption of nutrients, inadequate nutrition, and aberrant glucose control.

From the few reported cases of pregnancy in women with autonomic neuropathy,[73–75] it may be concluded that although a successful outcome of the pregnancy is possible, significant maternal morbidity may be expected. Exacerbation of autonomic neuropathy during pregnancy has been reported by some authors,[73,74] whereas others have noticed transient improvement in symptoms during pregnancy.[75] Overall, it seems that pregnancy does not alter the natural course of diabetic autonomic neuropathy,[76] a complication associated with severe morbidity and mortality.[73]

Hypoglycemia

Hypoglycemia is a well-recognized complication of intensive insulin therapy in patients with insulin-dependent diabetes mellitus (IDDM) (see Chapter 13). Because pregnant women with IDDM are commonly treated with intensive insulin therapy, it is not surprising that hypoglycemia is a common complication in these patients. Indeed, several investigators have reported high rates of moderate and severe hypoglycemia in women with IDDM treated with intensive insulin therapy during pregnancy. Coustan et al.[77] reported a 72% rate of moderate hypoglycemia and a 46% rate of severe hypoglycemia among 22 pregnant women with IDDM. In a report by Kitzmiller et al.[78] on a group of 84 women who conceived after attending a preconception clinic, 58% had 1–17 hypoglycemic episodes per week during the first 7 weeks of pregnancy. Rayburn et al.[79] reported that 36% of pregnant women with IDDM had severe symptomatic hypoglycemia during pregnancy, with the peak incidence occurring during sleep between midnight and 8:00 A.M. Similar results were reported by Steel et al.[80] Kimmerle et al.[81] reported a 41% rate of severe hypoglycemia among their population of 77 women with IDDM, with the majority of episodes occurring during the first half of pregnancy. Rosenn et al.[82] studied 84 pregnant women with IDDM and found that significant hypoglycemia, requiring assistance from another person, occurred in 71%, with a peak incidence between 10 and 15 weeks. Thirty-four percent of the subjects had at least one episode of severe hypoglycemia, resulting in seizures, loss of consciousness, injury, emergency glucagon administration, or intravenous glucose treatment.

It is unclear why hypoglycemia occurs with such frequency in early pregnancy in women with IDDM. This phenomenon may be related to the institution of intensive insulin therapy. Such therapy results in diminished counter-regulatory hormonal responses to hypoglycemia[83] and an increased risk of hypoglycemia unawareness.[84] Consequently, the patient fails to recognize the impending hazards of hypoglycemia and may progress to a state of severe neuroglycopenia. Another possibility is that pregnancy itself independently increases the risk of hypoglycemia. This could be related to hormonal changes, or diminished counter-regulatory responses to hypoglycemia or to the nausea and vomiting of pregnancy. It is also possible that pregnancy and intensive insulin therapy produce an additive effect that increases the risk of hypoglycemia.

Some insight into the mechanisms underlying hypoglycemia during pregnancy have been provided by studies employing hypoglycemia-clamp techniques in pregnant women with IDDM. Diamond et al.[85] have demonstrated defective biochemical counter-regulatory responses to insulin-induced hypoglycemia in women with IDDM during pregnancy compared to nonpregnant, nondiabetic historic controls. Rosenn et al.[86] have shown that women with IDDM who have demonstrable defective counter-regulatory mechanisms in the nonpregnant state also have defective counter-regulation during pregnancy, that adrenegenic responses diminish further during pregnancy, and that growth hormone responses to hypoglycemia diminished progressively during pregnancy both in women with IDDM and in controls.

Diabetes and Obstetric Complications

Pregnancy-Induced Hypertension

Diabetes has long been considered a risk factor for the development of preeclampsia or pregnancy-induced hypertension (PIH). The rate of PIH in women with diabetes is generally accepted as being higher than the 7% rate in the general population.[87] There is lack of agreement, however, among reports in the literature concerning the incidence of PIH in diabetic pregnancies, and its correlation with the White class and glycemic control (Table 78-2). Analysis of data is confounded because there is a lack of unanimity among studies regarding inclusion and exclusion of different types of diabetes, definitions of preeclampsia and PIH, separate consideration of chronic hypertension, management of diabetes, management of labor and delivery, and study design.

In an early review published by Kyle in 1963,[88] the average rate of PIH in pregnant patients with diabetes was 25% (8–45%). Cousins[21] reviewed the English literature from 1965 to 1985 and reported an average rate of 11.7%, highly correlated with advanced White class, with a rate of 15.7% in classes B-RF. A similar correlation of PIH with White class was found by Jervell et al.[89] and by Diamond et al.[90] In a prospective study involving 491 women with insulin-dependent diabetes mellitus (IDDM), Hanson and Persson[91] found a 21% rate of preeclampsia or PIH, a fourfold increase compared to the general population in Sweden. The frequency of preeclampsia/PIH increased progressively with advanced White class. Other authors have reported different findings. Gabbe et al.[92] found no significant increase in the incidence of PIH among patients with diabetes (13% versus 10% in the general population in his report) and no increase of PIH in White classes D-R. In a small series reported by Coustan et al.,[93] the incidence of PIH was only 5.5%. Kitzmiller et al.[94] reported PIH in 5% of their patients with diabetes, not significantly different from the 3.8% rate of PIH in their general nondiabetic population.

Reference to glycemic control can be found in the study by Leveno et al.,[95] in which 24% of the patients with diabetes had PIH, which correlated with poor glycemic control during the patients' final hospitalization before delivery. On the other hand, Martin et al.[96] reported a 20% incidence of PIH in diabetes (twice that in the general population in their report) but found no correlation with glycemic control.

Siddiqi et al.[97] found that the rate of PIH in a study population of 175 women with IDDM was 15.4% and was significantly associated with nulliparity, poor glycemic control in the first and second trimesters, and advanced White class. The neonatal outcome was not significantly altered in the presence of PIH.

The etiology of preeclampsia/PIH has yet to be elucidated, but it seems to involve compromise of the normal process of adaptation of maternal vasculature in pregnancy. Furthermore, there is evidence that the vascular adaptation of the uteroplacental bed during the first half of pregnancy is restricted in pregnancies complicated by hypertensive disorders, including preeclampsia.[98] Poor glycemic control in women with IDDM during pregnancy may thus be associated with restriction of the normally occurring physiologic vascular changes and consequently with the development of preeclampsia/PIH. The association between preeclampsia/PIH and advanced White class may be related to the pathophysiologic process of microvascular disease. This process may involve autoregulative and adaptive mechanisms of the maternal vasculature in pregnancy, thus predisposing the mother to PIH.

Preterm Labor

Preterm labor leading to the delivery of a preterm low-birth-weight infant remains one of the foremost obstetric problems worldwide. Preterm delivery occurs in approximately 7% of all pregnancies in the United States, accounting for more than 75% of all perinatal morbidity and mortality.[99] Conflicting data exist regarding the incidence of spontaneous premature labor in insulin-dependent diabetic pregnancies; similar rates,[93] as well as increased[100] or decreased[101] rates, have been reported. Published studies are confounded by the high rate of iatrogenic prematurity in these pregnancies. Even as

Table 78-2. White Classification of Diabetes in Pregnancy

	Pregestational Diabetes				
Class	Age of Onset (year)		Duration (year)		Vascular Disease
A		Chemical diabetes			
B	≥20	and	<10		0
C	10–19	or	10–19		0
D	<10	or	≥20	or	Benign retinopathy
				or	Chronic hypertension
F	Any		Any		Nephropathy
R	Any		Any		Proliferative retinopathy
H	Any		Any		Ischemic heart disease
T	Any		Any		Renal transplant recipient

Source: Adapted with permission from White P. Classification of obstetric diabetes. Am J Obstet Gynecol 1978;130:228.

late as the 1970s, premature delivery was advocated for infants of mothers with diabetes because of the risk of intrauterine fetal death, especially after the 37th week of gestation.[102] Improved techniques for antepartum fetal surveillance, however, as well as meticulous glycemic control, have decreased the risk of intrauterine demise. Thus, the incidence of iatrogenic prematurity in insulin-dependent diabetes mellitus (IDDM) pregnancies has recently declined.

Greene et al.[103] found that 26.2% of women with IDDM delivered prior to 37 completed weeks of gestation compared to 9.7% of nondiabetic women. Preeclampsia was the most significant risk factor associated with premature delivery. Compared with the general population, most of the excess risk of prematurity in mothers with diabetes was confined to patients with hypertension or with advanced White class.

Mimouni et al.[104] found that the rate of spontaneous premature labor among 181 women with IDDM was 31.1%, significantly higher than that in their control population (20.2%). Premature labor was significantly associated with poor glycemic control and with the presence of urogenital infection. Rosenn et al.[54] found that 30% of women with IDDM delivered before 37 weeks' gestation, and 9.4% delivered prior to 34 weeks, compared to 12% and 5.3%, respectively, in the nondiabetic population. In this study, improved glycemic control was associated with a lower risk of premature delivery.

The association of preterm labor with poor glycemic control is an observation that eludes a straightforward rationale. Although the etiology of preterm labor has yet to be determined, it is possible that various pathophysiologic conditions may act independently toward a common mechanism, such as local release of prostaglandins in uterine muscle, that results in preterm labor. Prostaglandin production is increased in platelets from patients with diabetes,[105] but there are no data on uterine prostaglandin production in diabetic pregnancies. Furthermore, it is impossible to exclude the possibility that the patients with poor glycemic control are also those in whom behavioral and other factors may increase the risk of preterm labor.

Polyhydramnios

Polyhydramnios is considered a frequent complication of diabetic pregnancy. In a review by Cousins,[21] the overall incidence of polyhydramnios was 17.6% in patients with White classes B and C and 18.6% in patients with classes D, R, and F. High rates of polyhydramnios were reported by Lufkin et al.[106] (29% compared to 0.9% in controls) and by Kitzmiller et al.[94] (31%), but their study populations also included women with type II diabetes. Rosenn et al.[54] found that the rate of polyhydramnios was 26.4% among women with insulin-dependent diabetes mellitus (IDDM) compared to 0.6% in controls. Polyhydramnios was associated with poor glycemic control throughout the entire pregnancy, especially during the first two trimesters.

Although the diagnosis of polyhydramnios is subject to observer bias, the increasing use of the amniotic fluid index[107] in sonography may be expected to improve the objectivity of data on amniotic fluid volume in diabetic and nondiabetic pregnancies. Of note, the observed rate of polyhydramnios in control populations may be an underestimation of the true rate because women with uncomplicated pregnancies do not usually undergo sonographic examinations as frequently as pregnant women with diabetes. It is unclear why polyhydramnios is more common in women with diabetes and why it is associated with poor glycemic control. Although amniotic fluid volume is not related to the concentration of its solutes,[108] polyhydramnios in these circumstances may be related to an increased glucose content in the amniotic fluid, creating an osmotic pressure that equilibrates in the presence of an increased volume of amniotic fluid. In addition, if maternal hyperglycemia is associated with fetal hyperglycemia, this could be associated with fetal polyuria and, hence, cause polyhydramnios. Whether this is indeed the case remains to be studied because in one report, increased amniotic fluid volume was not associated with increased output of fetal urine measured sonographically.[109]

Morbidity Associated with Infection

Patients with insulin-dependent diabetes mellitus (IDDM) are at high risk for infection.[110] Several deficiencies in the immune mechanism involving defective leukocyte and lymphocyte activity[111–115] may explain their propensity to infection. These deficiencies appear to be linked to poor glycemic control.[113–115] Pregnancy is also generally thought to constitute a state of relative immune deficiency, specifically, impaired cell-mediated immunity.[116–118] Thus, pregnancy in the patient with IDDM is likely to represent an additional risk factor for infection.

There are few studies on the rate of specific infections in diabetic pregnancies. Vejlsgaards[119] reported an increased incidence of urinary tract infection in gravid women with diabetes compared with nondiabetic gravid women. In a study restricted to postpartum infections, Diamond et al.[120] also observed an increased rate of postpartum wound infection, endometritis, or both in pregnant women with diabetes. Cousins,[21] in his meta-analysis, found that pyelonephritis was reported in 2.2% of class B and C pregnant women with diabetes and in 4.9% of women with class D, F, and R diabetes. Pedersen and Mölsted-Pedersen[121] found that pyelonephritis was more common among class F women and stated that this condition is associated with increased perinatal mortality.

Glycemic control was not evaluated in the studies by Vejlsgaards[119] and Diamond et al.,[120] but Rayfield et al.[122] demonstrated a striking direct correlation between the overall prevalence of infection and the mean plasma glucose concentration. Stamler et al.[123] found that 83% of women with IDDM had at least one episode of antenatal infection compared to 26% of nondiabetic women. The rate of postpartum infection was five times higher in the women with IDDM, and they were susceptible to more kinds of infections. Glycohemoglobin values obtained before the infection were higher than during the infectious episode. Thus, infection appears to be associated with poor glycemic control, but the temporal relationships are not clear.

Effects of Diabetes on the Embryo, Fetus, and Neonate

Over the past 20 years, there has been a growing understanding of the pathophysiology of the diabetic pregnancy, development of specialized health care centers for pregnant women with diabetes, and remarkable improvements in neonatal care. All these have conjointly resulted in a markedly improved prognosis for the infant of the mother with diabetes. Despite these optimistic developments, however, it is prudent to bear in mind that these unborn infants developing in the sweet maternal environment are being set up for a bitter struggle against some rather unfavorable odds.

Conception

A variety of abnormalities in female reproductive function have been described in retrospective studies of women with diabetes mellitus. These include delayed menarche,[124] early menopause,[124] delayed ovulation,[125] and an increased incidence of menstrual cycle irregularities.[126] Kjaer et al.[127] reported that menstrual disturbances in women with diabetes occur with a frequency twice that of controls. In a retrospective analysis,[128] there was a positive correlation between increased duration of diabetes and later onset of menarche, even when the subject's maternal menarche was taken into account. There is a lack of data in the literature regarding the rate of conception in women with insulin-dependent diabetes mellitus (IDDM). A study from 1954 reported that the pregnancy rate in women with IDDM was 38% lower than in nondiabetic women.[124] Conversely, two recent reports found the same rates of spontaneous conception and sterility in women with or without diabetes.[127,129] From our own data, using life table analysis, we found that our population of women with diabetes had a lower cumulative pregnancy rate at each assessment time point over a 24-month period compared to nondiabetic women.[130] Additionally, the rate of conception was higher in women with good glycemic control, as assessed by glycohemoglobin concentrations (unpublished data).

The mechanisms underlying impaired fertility in women with IDDM are not entirely clear. They may be related to abnormal function of the hypothalamic-pituitary axis, such as a decreased luteinizing hormone response to gonadotropin-releasing hormone[131,132] or reductions in basal concentrations of luteinizing hormone and follicle-stimulating hormone,[126,133] low thyrotropin concentrations, leading to low circulating thyroxin and impaired prolactin synthesis or release,[133] or impaired synthesis of corticosterone.[134] IDDM may also modify female reproductive function through the direct effect on insulin-dependent mechanisms of cells within the ovary itself. Indeed, ovarian weights are reduced in rats with alloxan-induced diabetes, possibly due to decreased responsiveness of the ovaries to gonadotropins.[135] It has also been observed that granulosa cells isolated from women with IDDM demonstrate impaired insulin-stimulated synthesis of progesterone, even in cases of fair diabetic control.[136]

Diabetic Embryopathy

The developing embryo of the mother with diabetes is exposed to an altered milieu that may produce devastating toxic effects, resulting in a spectrum of time-specific pathologic consequences. In vitro animal studies and clinical data support the hypothesis that these insults are a result of "fuel-mediated teratogenesis,"[137] a process discussed in further detail in Chapter 77. An early insult after fertilization may result in a blighted ovum. Later, such an insult may result in spontaneous abortion or disruption of embryogenesis with the development of major congenital malformations.[138] Still later, insults may result in minor congenital malformations.[139] In addition to timing, the intensity of the insult may be important in determining its consequences.

Several clinical studies have demonstrated the association of poor glycemic control with an increased risk of spontaneous abortions and major congenital malformations. It is controversial, however, whether there is a threshold of poor glycemic control (glycohemoglobin or glucose concentration) below which the risks of diabetic embryopathy are low and above which these risks are high compared to those of the nondiabetic population. Alternatively, the risk of diabetic embryopathy could be directly correlated with the values of glycohemoglobin or glucose concentrations.

The specific toxic mediators and teratogenic mechanisms in diabetes have yet to be determined. Current data suggest that some aspect of glycemic control, or perhaps a related factor such as ketogenesis, is important. Animal studies have ascribed embryopathy to the effects of β-hydroxybutyrate,[140] free radicals,[140a] insulin,[141] disruption of arachidonic acid[142] and glycolytic metabolic pathways,[143] magnesium deficiency,[144] decreased fetal zinc uptake, increased fetal manganese uptake,[145] somatomedin inhibitors, hyperosmolarity, and biophysical modifications via nonenzymatic glycosylations.[137] Taken together, these studies indicate that no single parameter of the diabetic state can be viewed in isolation in an attempt to correlate diabetic embryopathy with maternal diabetic control.

Spontaneous Abortion

Whether or not women with insulin-dependent diabetes mellitus (IDDM) have an increased rate of spontaneous abortion (SAB) is a matter of controversy. A comprehensive review[146] of 58 studies spanning 37 years found an overall rate of 10%, which is probably not different from the rate of SAB in the general population. Most of these studies, however, suffer from methodologic shortcomings that cloud their interpretation. The rate of SAB in prospective, well-designed studies of IDDM pregnancies has ranged from 15% to 30%.[147–149] Several investigators have reported an association between SAB and poor glycemic control in the first trimester, as reflected by higher glycohemoglobin concentrations.[147,150–153] Further, SAB was related to glycemic control in the period close to conception rather than the period immediately before the abortion itself.[138] It has also been shown that patients who gain experience in a program specializing in diabetic pregnancies, and patients participating in a preconceptional program, have improved glycemic control early in pregnancy and have less SAB.[154–156] Furthermore, the association between SAB and poor glycemic control was demonstrated even in SAB occurring after ultrasonographically documented fetal cardiac activity.[144] The study on diabetes in early pregnancy (DIEP) demonstrated that increasingly higher first-trimester glycohemoglobin concentrations were associated with increasing rates of SAB, with no evidence of a threshold effect.[148] Conversely, a threshold effect was clearly demonstrated in two other studies.[152,157] This leads to the question: What is the mechanism of SAB in patients with diabetes? As mentioned previously, the increased risk in these pregnancies must be related to the toxic milieu to which the developing embryo is subjected (see Chapter 77). Most authors speculate that this may result in degeneration of the embryo and the appearance of a blighted ovum or in an increased rate of lethal malformations incompatible with intrauterine life. Other possible mechanisms underlying SAB in the face of poor glycemic control may be abnormal placentation[158] and vascularization,[159] and perhaps an increased incidence of chromosomal abnormalities. Whatever the mechanism, it appears that obtaining good glycemic control before conception and throughout the first trimester can reduce the risk of SAB in diabetic pregnancies.[154]

Congenital Malformations

Congenital malformations (CM) have emerged as the single most important cause of perinatal mortality among infants of mothers with diabetes, accounting for 50% of perinatal deaths compared to 20–30% in infants of nondiabetic mothers.[160] Women who are insulin-dependent at the time of conception are at high risk for having a malformed fetus, a fact that has been appreciated for decades.[161–168] For an in-depth discussion on the possible mechanisms underlying CM in infants of mothers with insulin-dependent diabetes mellitus (IDDM), see Chapter 77.

Several studies have established the relationship between CM and poor glycemic control in women with IDDM, demonstrating that higher first-trimester glycohemoglobin concentrations are associated with an increased risk of CM.[150–153,169–172] These observations support the aforementioned contention that the point in time and the time span during which diabetes is uncontrolled are major determinants of the embryopathic manifestations.[138] Two studies have also demonstrated a threshold effect of poor glycemic control with respect to the increased risk of CM.[152,157] The presence of diabetic vasculopathy in the mother was also associated with an increased risk of CM in some studies[169,170] but not in others.[152]

Thus, prevention of major CM in IDDM pregnancies should now focus on preconceptional and early postconceptional control of diabetes. Clearly, the patient with poor glycemic control and abnormally high blood glycohemoglobin concentrations (for which there are currently no standard definitions) is at increased risk for having an infant with CM.

Minor Malformations

In a recent study,[139] minor congenital malformations in infants of women with insulin-dependent diabetes mellitus (IDDM) were associated with poor glycemic control late in the first trimester and early in the second, corresponding to the late embryonic and early fetal development periods. These observations, however, were not confirmed in a retrospective analysis of diabetic pregnancies.[173]

Preconceptional Glycemic Control

Most pregnancies are not recognized clinically until 2 or more weeks after conception; thus, strict glycemic control is often started after the critical periods of embryogenesis and organogenesis have begun. Intensive blood glucose management initiated in early pregnancy may thus be inadequate to prevent adverse pregnancy outcomes. A few recent nonrandomized studies have reported improved outcomes of pregnancy in women with insulin-dependent diabetes mellitus (IDDM) who attended a preconception program for control of diabetes compared to women with IDDM who began care after conception.[78,154,174–177] Because these studies were not randomized, the possibility of selection bias cannot be ruled out.

The desired levels of glycemic control for women with IDDM during the preconceptional period and during pregnancy have not yet been determined. Most perinatologists recommend strict glycemic control or normalization of blood sugar concentrations for these women. There are no specifically defined targets of preconceptional glycemic control derived from a prospective, randomized clinical trial, however. Although strict glycemic control appears to be beneficial in terms of the pregnancy outcome, the potential benefits must be weighed against the increased burden on the patient and on the health care system and against the potential for increased morbidity associated with hypoglycemia.

Maternal Hypoglycemia and Fetal Development

Although concerns regarding the hazards of hypoglycemia are primarily related to the pregnant mother with diabetes, the potential effects of maternal hypoglycemia on the developing fetus need to be considered. In vivo and in vitro studies of rat and mice embryos have demonstrated an association between short- or long-term hypoglycemia and an increased rate of fetal malformations.[178–181] Brief exposure (1–4 hours) of mouse[178] and rat[179] embryos to hypoglycemic media during critical periods of embryonic development resulted in an increased rate of dysmorphogenic lesions and growth retardation. Furthermore, these effects were enhanced when the embryos exposed to hypoglycemia were subsequently cultured in hyperglycemic media.[179] In vivo studies in pregnant rats have shown that brief (1-hour) insulin-induced hypoglycemia at a critical time of embryonic development is associated with embryonic growth retardation and a small but significant incidence of gross developmental anomalies.[180]

The impact of maternal hypoglycemia on human fetal development and neonatal outcome has not been extensively studied. An early report on women undergoing psychiatric treatment with insulin shock therapy suggested an association between severe hypoglycemia induced during the first trimester and an adverse pregnancy outcome.[182] Since that report, however, not one of the studies involving pregnant women with insulin-dependent diabetes mellitus (IDDM) has found any association between maternal hypoglycemia and adverse fetal outcome.[77–82,151] In two separate reports, hypoglycemia in third-trimester women with IDDM was associated with changes in fetal baseline heart rate[183] and heart rate variability.[184] In clinical studies involving moderate hypoglycemia induced in pregnant women with IDDM, however, no changes were observed in fetal behavior or in fetal heart rate.[85]

Abnormal Fetal Growth

Macrosomia

Macrosomia has long been recognized as one of the hallmarks of diabetic fetopathy, found in 15–40% of diabetic pregnancies.[185–189] Macrosomia is most commonly defined as a gestational age-adjusted birth weight that exceeds the 90th percentile of a reference population or as a birth weight greater than 4000 g. Normal infants who are constitutionally large will obviously also be labeled macrosomic, but the macrosomia characteristic of the diabetic pregnancy is associated with altered body composition with increased body fat and may therefore be considered abnormal. Excessive fetal size is the principal factor contributing to the increased risk of birth trauma in infants of mothers with diabetes, with such mishaps as shoulder dystocia, asphyxia, brachial plexus injuries, and facial nerve palsies.[102,187] Macrosomia is also a major factor in the increased rate of cesarean delivery among women with diabetes.[21] Despite the prevailing trend in maintaining fairly strict glycemic control throughout pregnancy, it seems that the frequency of macrosomia has not decreased significantly over the past two decades.[190,191]

A biphasic intrauterine growth pattern has been observed in infants of mothers with diabetes.[192] An initial phase of early fetal growth delay in the first half of pregnancy,[193,194] affecting both head and abdominal growth, is followed by the typical accelerated abnormal fetal growth in the third trimester, with abnormal adipose deposition and distribution, visceral organ hypertrophy and hyperplasia, and acceleration of skeletal growth.[195]

Chapter 76 provides an in-depth discussion on the role of maternal nutrients in the development of macrosomia in infants of mothers with diabetes. Briefly, according to Pedersen's original hypothesis,[196] macrosomia in infants of mothers with diabetes is related to fetal pancreatic β-cell hypertrophy and hyperinsulinism secondary to maternal hyperglycemia. There is indeed evidence that β-cells in these infants undergo hypertrophy and hyperplasia and also demonstrate increased insulin content.[197] Insulin is a major anabolic growth hormone of the fetus[198] that increases cell size by stimulating protein synthesis[199] and increases glucose uptake and glycogenesis in peripheral tissues.[200] This intrauterine hyperinsulinemic state results in increased tissue fat, liver glycogen content, and total body size.[201] Salvesen et al.[202] found that the insulin:glucose ratio in umbilical venous blood samples obtained from diabetic pregnancies at 36–39 weeks' gestation is significantly correlated with the degree of fetal macrosomia. This implies that fetal pancreatic β-cell hyperplasia is central to the pathogenesis of macrosomia.

It is possible that an excess of maternal nutrients is not the sole etiologic stimulus for endogenous fetal hyperinsulinemia. The roles of insulinogenic amino acids and of insulin-like growth factors in this context have yet to be established.[203] Although it is generally believed that maternal insulin binds to placental receptors but does not cross the placenta, antibody-bound maternal insulin may be found in the fetal circulation and may, in theory, exert anabolic effects. Menon et al.[204] demonstrated the transfer of considerable amounts of antibody-bound insulin from mother to fetus in some women with insulin-dependent diabetes mellitus (IDDM) treated with animal insulin. Cord serum concentrations of animal insulin and anti-insulin antibodies correlated with the maternal concentrations of anti-insulin antibody. Concentrations of animal insulin in cord serum also correlated with fetal macrosomia, leading to the authors' conclusion that antibody-bound animal insulin transferred to the fetus has an etiologic role in fetal macrosomia. The incidence of macrosomia, however, has recently been studied by Rosenn et al.[205] in 209 pregnant patients with IDDM, 170 of whom were treated with animal insulin and 39 with human insulin. There were no differences between the two groups in infants' birth weights, ponderal indices, or rate of macrosomia.

Ballard et al.[206] studied the significance of disproportionate growth in infants of mothers with diabetes. The incidence of asymmetric macrosomia (macrosomia with a high ponderal index, reflecting excessive body weight relative to length) was 19% in diabetic pregnancies compared to 1% in controls. Furthermore, the incidence of neonatal metabolic complications (hypoglycemia, hyperbilirubinemia, and acidosis) was greatest among infants with asymmetric macrosomia, lower among infants with simple macrosomia, and least among nonmacrosomic infants. Thus, it appears that asymmetric macrosomia reflects the most pathologic manifestation of excessive fetal growth in diabetic pregnancy.

Whether strict glycemic control of the pregnant woman with IDDM can prevent macrosomia is a controversial issue. It appears that there is no excessive birth trauma in infants of mothers with well-controlled diabetes.[207] Although some investigators have found an association between glucose control and macrosomia,[185,208] others have failed to demonstrate such a relationship.[209–211] Thus, it appears that unless excellent glycemic control is maintained throughout pregnancy (and possibly even with it), approximately 20–30% of the infants of mothers with diabetes will be born with excessive weight and size.

Hypertrophic Cardiomyopathy

Infants of mothers with diabetes are at known risk for developing a hypertrophic type of cardiomyopathy[212,213] with a thickened interventricular septum and thickened ventricular walls. Myocardial changes include hypertrophy and hyperplasia of the myofibrils and a peculiar disruption of the normal myofibrillar pattern.[214,215] The hypertrophic muscle restricts filling and obstructs outflow, thus decreasing stoke volume and cardiac output.[216] The severity of cardiomyopathy can vary from incidental echocardiographic findings to severe heart failure. Several studies have noted that the risk of cardiomyopathy is associated with poor maternal glycemic control.[214,217,218] As noted previously, maternal hyperglycemia is associated with fetal hyperinsulinemia, macrosomia, and visceromegaly of the liver, heart, and placenta.[219,220] Cardiac hypertrophy was also found in fetal rhesus monkeys who were rendered hyperinsulinemic.[220]

The spectrum of cardiorespiratory symptoms in the newborn with cardiomyopathy includes cyanosis, tachypnea, tachycardia, and features of congestive heart failure. The majority of these infants need only supportive care because the cardiorespiratory symptoms usually resolve within the first weeks of life,[213,214,221] although the septal and wall hypertrophy may take many months to resolve.[222]

Neonatal Metabolic Aberrations

Hypocalcemia and Hypomagnesemia

The most significant clinical problem of calcium metabolism in the diabetic pregnancy is neonatal hypocalcemia, which may occur in 50% of the infants of mothers with diabetes during the first 3 days of life.[223] Furthermore, the rate and severity of hypocalcemia are directly related to the severity of maternal diabetes. Hypomagnesemia also occurs frequently in infants of mothers with diabetes, reported in up to 38% of newborns and associated with the severity of maternal diabetes and with prematurity.[224,225] The cause of hypomagnesemia and hypocalcemia in infants of mothers with diabetes is not fully understood. It has been suggested that hypomagnesemia in these infants may be due to maternal magnesium losses related to diabetes during pregnancy that result in reduced maternal and secondarily reduced fetal serum magnesium concentrations, which, in turn, causes decreased fetal urinary excretion of magnesium and decreased amniotic fluid magnesium concentrations.[226] Magnesium deficiency in the infant may cause a functional hypoparathyroidism that could result in neonatal hypocalcemia when the newborn is no longer provided with calcium of maternal origin through the placenta.[225–227]

Bone mineral content is also decreased in infants of mothers with diabetes, in correlation with maternal bone mineral content at delivery and poor glycemic control.[228] One possible explanation of this observation is that increased serum 1,25-$(OH)_2D$ concentrations in these infants[229] have a potent effect on bone resorption[230] and might be detrimental to bone mineralization. Decreased bone mineral content has not been correlated with neonatal hypocalcemia, possibly owing to the large bone reservoir of calcium relative to blood.

Hypoglycemia

Neonatal hypoglycemia is a frequent complication in infants of mothers with diabetes. The reported incidence of hypoglycemia occurring in the first 4 hours of life in these infants ranges from 10% to 50%,[231–233] with little change in this frequency observed over the last 20 years. The mechanism responsible for the occurrence of hypoglycemia has not been clearly established. Several hypotheses have been proposed, however. Pedersen's classic model states that maternal hyperglycemia causes fetal hyperglycemia and islet cell stimulation leading to fetal hyperinsulinemia.[196] At birth, interruption of the maternal glucose supply to the hyperinsulinemic neonate results in hypoglycemia. Alternatively, several authors have suggested that acute hyperglycemia in the mother with diabetes at the time of delivery may be the major etiologic determinant in the occurrence of neonatal hypoglycemia rather than chronic hyperglycemia.[234–238] This acute peripartum hyperglycemia results in an acute release of insulin by the fetal pancreas, and after the abrupt termination of the transplacental glucose supply, hypoglycemia occurs. Another plausible possibility relates to the fact that maternal exogenous insulin bound to IgG antibodies freely crosses the placenta and circulates in the fetal blood in concentrations very similar to those of the mother.[239,240] Withdrawal of maternal glucose at birth may then result in neonatal hypoglycemia. Whatever the cause, neonatal hypoglycemia tends to be less common and much milder in the infant whose mother has well-controlled diabetes throughout pregnancy and sustained euglycemia throughout labor and delivery.[188] Close monitoring of the infant's blood glucose concentration, and intravenous supplementation when necessary combined with early feeding within the first hours of life, further decrease the incidence of severe neonatal hypoglycemia.

The long-term prognosis of neonatal hypoglycemia is unknown. Low blood glucose values should be recognized and treated promptly because prolonged hypoglycemia is clearly associated with central nervous system abnormalities in children and adults.[188]

Polycythemia

Neonatal polycythemia, defined as a venous hematocrit of 65% or more, occurs in 3–5% of all newborns,[241,242] but it has been observed in up to 29% of infants of mothers with diabetes.[224,243] Neonatal polycythemia and its related increased viscosity may be associated with a spectrum of clinical sequelae, including cardiopulmonary failure, decreased renal function, renal vein thrombosis, necrotizing enterocolitis, and central nervous system damage.[244]

In the pregnant woman with insulin-dependent diabetes mellitus (IDDM), fetal hyperglycemia and hyperinsulinemia lead to reduced fetal arterial oxygen content.[245,246] Hyperketonemia in maternal and fetal sheep have the same effect.[247,248] Fetal hypoxemia may stimulate erythropoiesis, and elevated concentrations of erythropoietin have indeed been demonstrated in cord blood of infants of mothers with diabetes[249] and in hyperglycemic fetal lambs.[250] A direct correlation between fetal erythropoietin, fetal erythroblast count, fetal hemoglobin, and maternal glycohemoglobin concentration was demonstrated in fetal umbilical venous blood samples from diabetic pregnancies.[251] It has also been shown that acute maternal hypoxia in nondiabetic pregnancies results in acute fetal hypoxia and a significant shift of placental blood volume into the fetal compartment.[252] A similar pathophysiologic placental "transfusion" may occur under hyperglycemic and hypoxic conditions in the diabetic pregnancy. Although chronic hypoxia and placental transfusion may explain the increased incidence of polycythemia in infants of mothers with diabetes, it is quite possible that this phenomenon is related to additional factors such as decreased prostacyclin production, which may be associated with changes in fetal or placental vasculature[253] and body fluid volume shifts, such as transudation of fluid into the extravascular space after delivery.[242,254]

Hyperbilirubinemia

The risk of hyperbilirubinemia in infants of mothers with diabetes is higher than in normal infants[255] and has been associated with maternal glycemic control.[256,257] It is tempting to assume that hyperbilirubinemia is related to the increased incidence of polycythemia in these infants; however, this is not necessarily the case. In infants of nondiabetic mothers, the incidence of hyperbilirubinemia is comparable in polycythemic and control groups.[258–260] Furthermore, partial exchange transfusion for the treatment of polycythemia in newborns of mothers with diabetes does not prevent hyperbilirubinemia in these infants.[261]

There is an increased production rate of bilirubin in infants of mothers with diabetes compared to normal controls (up to 30% higher) that is unrelated to the hemoglobin concentration[255,262] and may be an important contributing factor to the propensity for severe hyperbilirubinemia. Infants of mothers with diabetes may also be subject to impairment of hepatocyte function, namely, uptake of bilirubin, its conjugation or excretion, resulting in delayed clearance of bilirubin.[263]

Chronically induced hyperinsulinemia in fetal rhesus monkeys results in increased concentrations of erythropoietin and increased erythropoiesis and reticulocytosis without polycythemia.[264] These findings suggest ineffective erythropoiesis or mild compensated hemolysis. As blood erythropoietin concentrations are elevated in as many as one-third of infants of mothers with diabetes,[264] and as an association between blood erythropoietin concentrations and bilirubin production has been observed in these infants,[265] ineffective erythropoiesis is a plausible explanation for the observed hyperbilirubinemia. Thus, it appears that there may be multiple causes of hyperbilirubinemia in infants of mothers with diabetes, and because these infants are often born prematurely, this too is often a contributing factor.[265]

Respiratory Decompensation

The reduced risk of intrauterine fetal death in infants of mothers with diabetes over the past decade has been associated with improvement in glycemic control during pregnancy, development of methods for fetal surveillance, and advances in neonatology. Even recent studies, however, have shown that 25–28% of these infants may have evidence of intrapartum asphyxia.[94,266]

Considerable experimental data have linked derangements in maternal and fetal carbohydrate metabolism with fetal asphyxia. Studies in fetal sheep have demonstrated that maternal hyperketonemia may lead to a significant reduction in fetal oxygenation.[267,268] Fetal hyperinsulinemia and hyperglycemia have been associated with decreased fetal oxygenation in sheep.[269,270] It has been suggested that increased concentrations of glycohemoglobin in women with diabetes result in increased oxygen affinity to hemoglobin,[271] leading to decreased availability of oxygen to the fetus. Another possibility is that diabetes-associated vasculopathy also affects placental vessels and their oxygen diffusion capacity. Additional pathophysiologic factors may be the increased proliferation of cytotrophoblastic cells and the enlargement of endothelial cells in villous capillaries.[272] Evidence that oxygen delivery to the fetus is related to maternal glucose control has also been obtained in human pregnancies. Fetal activity decreases during maternal hyperglycemia[273] and fetal acidemia,[274] and fetal heart rate variability is reduced during periods of maternal hyperglycemia.[275] Bradley et al.[276] studied umbilical blood samples obtained by cordocentesis in the late third trimester in 32 pregnancies complicated by maternal diabetes. They found a significant correlation between fetal plasma insulin immunoreactivity and fetal acidemia, suggesting that fetal pancreatic β-cell hyperplasia is involved in the pathogenesis of fetal acidemia in diabetic pregnancies.

Several investigators have reported that stricter glycemic control is associated with a decreased incidence of antepartum and intrapartum interventions prompted by suspected fetal jeopardy.[92,94,277] Such data support the contention that maintaining maternal normoglycemia reduces the risk of fetal hyperglycemia and hyperinsulinemia, and consequently reduces the risk of fetal hypoxemia and the need for elective intervention.

Maternal diabetes has been traditionally considered a predisposing factor for respiratory distress syndrome in neonates.[278] The high incidence of this syndrome in infants of mothers with diabetes may be due to a direct effect of maternal diabetes on fetal lung development, but the precise mechanism involved in delayed lung maturation remains to be elucidated. Animal studies addressing this issue have been conducted in sheep, rats, rabbits, and monkeys,[220,279–281] and all have virtually confirmed that fetal lung maturation is delayed in the presence of maternal diabetes. More recent studies have shown a decline in the incidence of respiratory distress syndrome in infants of mothers with diabetes[282,283] to a level no different than that of pair-matched control infants,[283] and some investigators have shown that the risk of this syndrome decreases with improved glycemic control of the mother.[284]

In summary, even though perinatal mortality of infants born to mothers with diabetes has decreased remarkably in recent years and now approaches that of the general population, these infants still face a multitude of potential complications, both in utero and postnatally, many of which are related to poor maternal glycemic control. Thus, the key to an improved pregnancy outcome lies in preconceptional counseling, specialized prenatal and postnatal care, and a commitment on the part of the mother to adhere to a regimen of meticulous glycemic control.

References

1. Alvarsson ML, Grill VE. Effect of long term glycemic control on the onset of retinopathy in IDDM subjects. A longitudinal and retrospective study. Diabetes Res 1989;10:75
2. Klein R, Klein BEK, Moss SE, et al. Glycosylated hemoglobin predicts the incidence and progression of diabetic retinopathy. JAMA 1988;260:2864
3. Brinchmann-Hansen O, Dahl-Jorgensen K, Sandvik L, Hanssen KF. Blood glucose concentrations and progression of diabetic retinopathy: The seven year results of the Oslo Study. Br Med J 1992;304:19
4. Reichard P, Britz A, Carlsson P, et al. Metabolic control and complications over 3 years in patients with insulin dependent diabetes (IDDM): The Stockholm Diabetes Intervention Study (SDIS). J Intern Med 1990;228:511
5. Singh R, Prakash V, Shukla PK, et al. Glycosylated hemoglobin and diabetic retinopathy. Ann Ophthalmol 1991;23:308
6. Kroc Collaborative Study Group. Blood glucose control and the evolution of diabetic retinopathy and albuminuria. N Engl J Med 1984;311:365
7. Lauritzen T, Larsen HW, Frost-Larensen K, Deckert T. The Steno Study Group: Effect of 1 year of near-normal glucose levels on retinopathy in insulin-dependent diabetics. Lancet 1983;1:200
8. Dahl-Jorgensen K, Brinchmann-Hansen O, Hanssen KF, et al. Rapid tightening of blood glucose leads to transient deterioration of retinopathy in insulin-dependent diabetes mellitus: The Oslo Study. Br Med J 1985;290:811
9. Helve E, Laatikainen L, Merenmies L, Kolvisto VA. Continuous insulin infusion therapy and retinopathy in patients with type 1 diabetes. Acta Endocrinol (Copenh) 1987;115:313

10. The Diabetes Control and Complications Trial Research Group. The effect of intensive treatment of diabetes on the development and progression of long-term complications in insulin-dependent diabetes mellitus. N Engl J Med 1993;329:977
11. Knopf RF, Fajans SS, Pek S, et al. Plasma levels of growth hormone and glucagon in diabetic patients and relatives of diabetic patients. Adv Metab Disord 1973;2:215
12. Sevin R. The correlation between human growth hormone (HGH) concentration in blood plasma and the evolution of diabetic retinopathy. Ophthalmologica 1972;165:71
13. Campbell J, Hausler HR, Munroe JS, Davidson IW. Effects of growth hormone in dogs. Endocrinology 1953;53:134
14. Grant M, Fitzgerald C, Merimee TJ. Insulin-like growth factors in vitreous: Studies in controls and diabetics with neovascularization. Diabetes 1986; 35:416
15. Arner P, Sjoberg S, Gjotterberg M, Skottner A. Circulating insulin-like growth factor I in type 1 (insulin-dependent) diabetic patients with retinopathy. Diabetologia 1989;32:753
16. Hyer SL, Sharp PS, Sleightholm M, et al. Progression of diabetic retinopathy and changes in serum insulin-like growth factor I (IGFI) during continuous subcutaneous insulin infusion (CSII). Horm Metab Res 1989;21:18
17. Hill CR, Kissun RD, Garner A. Angiogenic factor in vitreous from diabetic retinopathy. Experientia 1983;39:583
18. Frederick JL, Shimanuk T, DiZerega GS. Initiation of angiogenesis by human follicular fluid. Science 1984;224:389
19. Presta M, Mignatti P, Mullins DE, Moscatelli DA. Human placental tissue stimulates bovine capillary endothelial cell growth, migration and protease production. Biosci Rep 1985;5:783
20. Shafrir E, Bergman M, Felig P. The endocrine pancreas: Diabetes mellitus. In: Felig P, Baster JD, Broadus AE, Frohman LA, eds. Endocrinology and Metabolism. 2nd ed. New York: McGraw-Hill;1987:1157
21. Cousins L. Pregnancy complications among diabetic women: Review 1965–1985. Obstet Gynecol Surv 1987;42:140
22. Rosenn B, Miodovnik M, Kranias G, et al. Progression of diabetic retinopathy in pregnancy: Association with hypertension in pregnancy. Am J Obstet Gynecol 1992;166:1214
23. Elman KD, Welch RA, Frank RN, et al. Diabetic retinopathy in pregnancy: A review. Obstet Gynecol 1990;75:119
24. Moloney JBM, Drury MI. The effect of pregnancy on the natural course of diabetic retinopathy. Am J Ophthalmol 1982;93:745
25. Horvat M, Maclean H, Goldberg L, Crock GW. Diabetic retinopathy in pregnancy: A 12-year prospective survey. Br J Ophthalmol 1980;64:398
26. Ohrt V. The influence of pregnancy on diabetic retinopathy with special regard to the reversible changes shown in 100 pregnancies. Acta Ophthalmol 1984;62:603
27. Dibble CM, Kochenour NK, Worley RJ, et al. Effect of pregnancy on diabetic retinopathy. Obstet Gynecol 1982;59:699
28. Price JH, Hadden DR, Archer DB, Harley JM. Diabetic retinopathy in pregnancy. Br J Obstet Gynaecol 1984;91:11
29. Phelps RL, Sakol P, Metzger BE, et al. Changes in diabetic retinopathy during pregnancy. Arch Ophthalmol 1986;104:1806
30. Serup L. Influence of pregnancy on diabetic retinopathy. Acta Endocrinol 1986;277(suppl):122
31. Klein BEK, Moss SE, Klein R. Effect of pregnancy on progression of diabetic retinopathy. Diabetes Care 1990;13:34
32. Selby JV, FitzSimmons SC, Newman JM, et al. The natural history and epidemiology of diabetic nephropathy. Implications for prevention and control. JAMA 1990;263:1954
33. Hostetter TH. Pathogenesis of diabetic glomerulopathy: Hemodynamic considerations. Semin Nephrol 1990;10:219
34. Reichard P, Sule J, Rosenqvist U. Capillary loss and leakage after five years of intensified insulin treatment in patients with insulin-dependent diabetes mellitus. Ophthalmology 1991;98:1587
35. Chase HP, Jackson WE, Hoops SL, et al. Glucose control and the renal and retinal complications of insulin-dependent diabetes. JAMA 1988;261: 1155
36. Watts GF, Harris R, Shaw KM. The determinants of early nephropathy in insulin-dependent diabetes mellitus: A prospective study based on the urinary excretion of albumin. Q J Med New Series 1991;79:365
37. McCance DR, Hadden DR, Atkinson AB, et al. The relationship between long-term glycemic control and diabetic nephropathy. Q J Med New Series 1992;82:53
38. Kalk WJ, Osler C, Taylor D, Panz VR. Prior long term glycemic control and insulin therapy in insulin-dependent diabetic adolescents with microalbuminuria. Diabetes Res Clin Pract 1990;9:83
39. Reichard P, Rosenqvist U. Nephropathy is delayed by intensified insulin treatment in patients with insulin-dependent diabetes mellitus and retinopathy. J Intern Med 1989;226:81
40. Orchard TJ, Dorman JS, Maser RE, et al. Factors associated with avoidance of severe complications after 25 years of IDDM. Pittsburgh Epidemiology of Diabetes Complications Study I. Diabetes Care 1990;13:741
41. McNally GP, Burden AC, Swift PGF, et al. The prevalence and risk factors associated with the onset of diabetic nephropathy in juvenile-onset (insulin-dependent) diabetics diagnosed under the age of 17 years in Leicestershire 1930–1985. Q J Med New Series 1990;76:831
42. Feldt-Rasmussen B, Mathiesen ER, Jensen T, et al. Effect of improved metabolic control on loss of kidney function in type I (insulin-dependent) diabetic patients: An update of the Steno studies. Diabetologia 1991;34: 164
43. Castellino P, Shohat J, DeFronzo RA. Hyperfiltration and diabetic nephropathy: Is it the beginning? Or is it the end? Semin Nephrol 1990;10:228
44. Bank N. Mechanisms of diabetic hyperfiltration. Kidney Int 1991;40:792
45. Zeller KR. Low-protein diets in renal disease. Diabetes Care 1991;14:856
46. Dodds RA, Keen H. Low protein diet and conservation of renal function in diabetic nephropathy. Diabetes Metab 1990;16:464
47. Brouhard BH, LaGrone L. Effect of dietary protein restriction on functional renal reserve in diabetic nephropathy. Am J Med 1990;89:427
48. Nosadini R, Fioretto P, Trevisan R, Crepaldi G. Insulin-dependent diabetes mellitus and hypertension. Diabetes Care 1991;14:210
49. Mauer SM, Sutherland DER, Steffes MW. Relationship of systemic blood pressure to nephropathology in insulin-dependent diabetes mellitus. Kidney Int 1992;41:736
50. Mogensen CE, Hansen KW, Osterby R, Damsgaard EM. Blood pressure elevation versus abnormal albuminuria in the genesis and prediction of renal disease in diabetes. Diabetes Care 1992;15:1192
51. Parving H-H. Impact of blood pressure and antihypertensive treatment on incipient and overt nephropathy, retinopathy, and endothelial permeability in diabetes mellitus. Diabetes Care 1991;14:260
52. Jerums G, Allen TJ, Tsalamandris C, Cooper ME. The Melbourne Diabetic Nephropathy Study Group: Angiotensin converting enzyme inhibition and calcium channel blockade in incipient diabetic nephropathy. Kidney Int 1992;41:904
53. Davison JM, Dunlop W. Changes in renal hemodynamics and tubular function induced by normal human pregnancy. Semin Nephrol 1984;4:198
54. Rosenn B, Miodovnik M, Combs CA, et al. Poor glycemic control and antepartum obstetric complications in women with insulin-dependent diabetes. Int J Gynecol Obstet 1993;43:21
55. Combs CA, Rosenn B, Kitzmiller JL, et al. Early-pregnancy proteinuria in diabetes related to preeclampsia. Obstet Gynecol 1993;82:802
56. Kitzmiller JL, Brown ER, Phillippe M, et al. Diabetic nephropathy and perinatal outcome. Am J Obstet Gynecol 1981;141:741
57. Reece EA, Coustan DR, Hayslett JP, et al. Diabetic nephropathy: Pregnancy performance and fetomaternal outcome. Am J Obstet Gynecol 1988;159:56
58. Reece EA, Winn HN, Hayslett JP, et al. Does pregnancy alter the rate of progression of diabetic nephropathy? Am J Perinatol 1990;7:193
59. Kimmerle R, Zaß R-P, Cupisti S, et al. Pregnancies in women with diabetic nephropathy: Long-term outcome for mother and child. Diabetologia 1995; 38:227
60. Biesenbach G, Stoger H, Zazgornik J. Influence of pregnancy on progression of diabetic nephropathy and subsequent requirement of renal replacement therapy in female type I diabetic patients with impaired renal function. Nephrol Dial Transplant 1992;7:105
61. Gordon M, Landon MB, Samuels P, et al. Perinatal outcome and long-term follow-up associated with modern management of diabetic (DM) nephropathy (class F). Scientific Abstracts of the 15th Annual Meeting of the Society of Perinatal Obstetricians, Atlanta, GA, January 23–28, 1995. Am J Obstet Gynecol 1995;(Part 2)172(1):329. Abstract
61a. Grenfell A, Brudenell JM, Doddridge MC, Watkins PJ. Pregnancy in diabetic women who have proteinuria. QJM 1986;59(228):379
61b. Carstensen LL, Frost-Larsen K, Fugleberg S, Nerup J. Does pregnancy influence the prognosis of uncomplicated insulin-dependent diabetes mellitus? Diabetes Care 1982;5(1):1
61c. Hemachandra A, Ellis D, Lloyd CE, Orchard TJ. The influence of pregnancy on IDDM complications. Diabetes Care 1995;18(7):950
61d. Miodovnik M, Rosenn BM, Khoury J, et al. Does pregnancy increase the risk for development and progression of diabetic nephropathy? Am J Obstet Gynecol 1996 (in press)
62. Siegler AM, Hoffman J, Bloom O. Myocardial infarction complicating pregnancy. Obstet Gynecol 1956;7:306
63. Delaney JJ, Ptacek J. Three decades of experience with diabetic pregnancies. Am J Obstet Gynecol 1970;106:550
64. White P. Life cycle of diabetes in youth. 50th anniversary of the discovery of insulin (1921–1971). J Am Med Wom Assoc 1972;27:293
65. Hibbard LT. Maternal mortality due to cardiac disease. Clin Obstet Gynecol 1975;18:27
66. Hare JW, White P. Pregnancy in diabetes complicated by vascular disease. Diabetes 1977;26:953
67. Silfen SL, Wapner RJ, Gabbe SG. Maternal outcome in class H diabetes mellitus. Case reports. Obstet Gynecol 1980;55:749
68. Reece EA, Egan JFX, Coustan DR, et al. Coronary artery disease in diabetic pregnancies. Am J Obstet Gynecol 1986;154:150
69. Gast MJ, Rigg LA. Class H diabetes and pregnancy. Obstet Gynecol 1985;66:5S
70. Ueland K, Metcalfe J. Circulatory changes in pregnancy. Clin Obstet Gynecol 1975;18:41
71. Ueland K, Gills RE, Hansen JM, et al. Maternal cardiovascular dynamics. I. Cesarean section under subarachnoid block anesthesia. Am J Obstet Gynecol 1968;100:42
72. Capeless EL, Clapp JF. When do cardiovascular parameters return to their preconception values? Am J Obstet Gynecol 1991;165:883

73. Steel JM. Autonomic neuropathy in pregnancy. Letters and comments. Diabetes Care 1989;12:170
74. Macleod AF, Smith SA, Sönksen PH, Lowy C. The problem of autonomic neuropathy in diabetic pregnancy. Diabetic Med 1990;7:80
75. Scott AR, Tattersall RB, McPherson M. Improvement of postural hypotension and severe diabetic autonomic neuropathy during pregnancy. Letters and comments. Diabetes Care 1988;11:369
76. Airaksinen KEJ, Salmela PI. Pregnancy is not a risk factor for a deterioration of autonomic nervous function in diabetic women. Diabetic Med 1993;10:540
77. Coustan DR, Reece EA, Sherwin RS, et al. A randomized clinical trial of the insulin pump vs. intensive conventional therapy in diabetic pregnancies. JAMA 1986;255:631
78. Kitzmiller JL, Gavin LA, Gin GD, et al. Preconception care of diabetes: Glycemic control prevents congenital anomalies. JAMA 1991;265:731
79. Rayburn W, Piehl E, Jacober S, et al. Severe hypoglycemia during pregnancy: Its frequency and predisposing factors in diabetic women. Int J Gynaecol Obstet 1986;24:263
80. Steel JM, Johnstone FD, Hepburn DA, Smith AF. Can prepregnancy care of diabetic women reduce the risk of abnormal babies? BMJ 1990;301:1070
81. Kimmerle R, Heinemann L, Delecki A, Berger M. Severe hypoglycemia, incidence and predisposing factors in 85 pregnancies of type I diabetic women. Diabetes Care 1992;15:1034
82. Rosenn B, Miodovnik M, Holcberg G, et al. Hypoglycemia: The price of intensive insulin therapy in insulin-dependent diabetes mellitus pregnancies. Obstet Gynecol 1995;85:417
83. Simonson DC, Tamborlane WW, DeFronzo RA, Sherwin RS. Intensive insulin therapy reduces counterregulatory hormone responses to hypoglycemia in patients with type I diabetes. Ann Intern Med 1985;103:184
84. Cryer PE. Iatrogenic hypoglycemia as a cause of hypoglycemia-associated autonomic failure in IDDM: A vicious cycle. Diabetes 1992;41:2:55
85. Diamond MP, Reece EA, Caprio S, et al. Impairment of counterregulatory hormone responses to hypoglycemia in pregnant women with insulin-dependent diabetes mellitus. Am J Obstet Gynecol 1992;166:70
86. Rosenn B, Miodovnik M. Counterregulatory responses to hypoglycemia in pregnant women with insulin-dependent diabetes mellitus. Obstet Gynecol 1996 (in press)
87. Roberts JM. Pregnancy-related Hypertension. In: Creasy RK, Resnik R, eds. Maternal-Fetal Medicine: Principles and Practice. 3rd ed. Philadelphia: WB Saunders;1994:807
88. Kyle G. Diabetes and pregnancy. Ann Intern Med 1963;59(suppl 3):13
89. Jervell J, Moe N, Skjaeraasen J, et al. Diabetes mellitus in pregnancy: Management and results at Rikshospitalet, Oslo, 1970–1977. Diabetologia 1979; 16:151
90. Diamond MP, Shah DM, Hester RA, et al. Complication of insulin-dependent diabetic pregnancies by preeclampsia and/or chronic hypertension: Analysis of outcome. Am J Perinatol 1985;2:263
91. Hanson U, Persson B. Outcome of pregnancies complicated by type 1 insulin-dependent diabetes in Sweden: Acute pregnancy complications, neonatal mortality and morbidity. Am J Perinatol 1993;10:330
92. Gabbe S, Mestman J, Freeman R, et al. Management and outcome of pregnancy and diabetes mellitus, classes, B to R. Am J Obstet Gynecol 1977; 129:723
93. Coustan D, Berkowitz R, Hobbins J. Tight metabolic control of overt diabetes in pregnancy. Am J Med 1980;68:845
94. Kitzmiller J, Cloherty J, Younger M, et al. Diabetic pregnancy and perinatal morbidity. Am J Obstet Gynecol 1978;131:560
95. Leveno KJ, Hauth JC, Gilstrap LC, Whalley PJ. Appraisal of "rigid" blood glucose control during pregnancy in the overtly diabetic woman. Am J Obstet Gynecol 1979;135:853
96. Martin FIR, Heath P, Mountain KR. Pregnancy in women with diabetes mellitus: Fifteen years' experience: 1970–1985. Med J Aust 1987;146:187
97. Siddiqi T, Rosenn B, Mimouni F, et al. Hypertension during pregnancy in insulin-dependent diabetic women. Obstet Gynecol 1991;77:514
98. Brosens I, Robertson WB, Dixon HG. The physiological response of the vessels of the placental bed to normal pregnancy. J Pathol Bacteriol 1967; 93:569
99. Seigel DG, Stanley F. Statistics on perinatal morbidity and mortality. In: Quilligan EJ, ed. Fetal and Maternal Medicine. New York: Wiley;1980:3
100. Molsted-Pedersen L. Preterm labor and perinatal mortality in diabetic pregnancy. In: Sutherland HW, Stowers JM, eds. Obstetric Considerations, Carbohydrate Metabolism in Pregnancy and the Newborn. New York: Springer-Verlag;1979:392
101. Zalut J, Reed KL, Shenker L. Incidence of premature labor in diabetic patients. Am J Perinatol 1985;2:276
102. Tsang RC, Ballard JL, Braun C. The infant of the diabetic mother: Today and tomorrow. Clin Obstet Gynecol 1981;24:125
103. Greene MF, Hare JW, Krache M, et al. Prematurity among insulin-requiring diabetic gravid women. Am J Obstet Gynecol 1989;161:106
104. Mimouni F, Miodovnik M, Siddiqi TA, et al. High spontaneous premature labor rate in insulin dependent diabetic pregnant women: An association with poor glycemic control and urogenital infection. Obstet Gynecol 1988;72: 175
105. Halushka PV, Luric D, Colwell JA. Increased synthesis of prostaglandin-E-like material by platelets from patients with diabetes mellitus. N Engl J Med 1977;297:1306
106. Lufkin G, Nelson R, Hill L, et al. An analysis of diabetic pregnancies at Mayo Clinic, 1950–79. Diabetes Care 1984;7:539
107. Moore TR, Cayle JE. The amniotic fluid index in normal human pregnancy. Am J Obstet Gynecol 1990;162:1168
108. Cassady G. Amniocentesis. Clin Perinatol 1974;1:87
109. Van Otterlo L, Wladimiroff J, Wallenburg H. Relationship between fetal urine production and amniotic fluid volume in normal pregnancy and pregnancy complicated by diabetes. Br J Obstet Gynaecol 1977;84:205
110. Krall LP, ed. Joslin Diabetes Manual. 12th ed. Philadelphia: Lea & Febiger;1989:267
111. Mowat AG, Baum J. Chemotaxis of polymorphonuclear leukocytes from patients with diabetes mellitus. N Engl J Med 1971;284:621
112. MacCuish AC, Urbaniak SJ, Campbell CJ, et al. Phytohemagglutinin transformation and circulating lymphocyte subpopulations in insulin-dependent diabetic patients. Diabetes 1974;23:708
113. Bagdade JD, Stewart M, Walters E. Impaired granulocyte adherence: A reversible defect in host defense in patients with poorly controlled diabetes. Diabetes 1978;27:677
114. Bagdade JD, Root RK, Bulger RJ. Impaired leukocyte function in patients with poorly controlled diabetes. Diabetes 1974;23:9
115. Nolan CN, Beaty HN, Bagdade JD. Further characterization of the impaired bactericidal function of granulocytes in patients with poorly controlled diabetes. Diabetes 1978;27:889
116. Weinberg ED. Pregnancy associated depression of cell mediated immunity. Rev Infect Dis 1984;6:814
117. Falkoff R. Maternal immunologic changes in pregnancy: A critical appraisal. Clin Rev Allergy 1987;5:287
118. Sridama V, Pacini F, Yang SL, et al. Decreased levels of helper T cells: A possible cause of immunodeficiency in pregnancy. N Engl J Med 1982; 307:352
119. Vejlsgaards R. Studies on urinary infections in diabetes. Acta Med Scand 1973;193:33
120. Diamond MP, Entmann SS, Salyer SL, et al. Increased risk of endometritis and wound infection after cesarean section in insulin-dependent diabetic women. Am J Obstet Gynecol 1986;155:297
121. Pedersen J, Mölsted-Pedersen L. Prognosis of the outcome of pregnancy in diabetics. Acta Endocrinol 1965;50:70
122. Rayfield EJ, Ault MJ, Keusch GT, et al. Infection and diabetes: The case for glucose control. Am J Med 1982;72:439
123. Stamler EF, Cruz ML, Mimouni F, et al. High infectious morbidity in insulin-dependent diabetic pregnant women: An understated complication. Am J Obstet Gynecol 1990;163:1217
124. Bergqvist N. The gonadal function in female diabetics. Acta Endocrinol 1954;19:1
125. Steel JM, Johnstone SD, Corrie JET. Early assessment of gestation in diabetics (letter to the editor). Lancet 1984;2:975
126. Djursing H, Nyholm HC, Hagen C, et al. Clinical and hormonal characteristics in women with anovulation and insulin-treated diabetes mellitus. Am J Obstet Gynecol 1982;143:876
127. Kjaer K, Hagen C, Sando SH, Eshoj O. Infertility and pregnancy outcome in an unselected group of women with insulin-dependent diabetes mellitus. Am J Obstet Gynecol 1992;166:1412
128. Chitkara VK, Biro FM, Franklin A, Sperling MA. Duration of diabetes delays onset of menarche (abstract). Adolesc Med 1991;7:4a
129. Steel JM. Pregnancy counseling and contraception in the insulin-dependent diabetic patient. Clin Obstet Gynecol 1985;28:553
130. Guzick DS, Rock JA. Estimation of a model of cumulative pregnancy following infertility therapy. Am J Obstet Gynecol 1981;140:573
131. Kirchick HJ, Keyes PL, Frye BE. An explanation for anovulation in immature alloxan-diabetic rats treated with pregnant mare's serum gonadotropin: Reduced pituitary response to gonadotropin-releasing hormone. Endocrinology 1979;105:1343
132. Djursing H, Hagen C, Nyholm HC, et al. Gonadotropin responses to gonadotropin-releasing hormone and prolactin responses to thyrotropin-releasing hormone and metoclopramide in women with amenorrhea and insulin-treated diabetes mellitus. J Clin Endocrinol Metab 1983;56:1016
133. Djursing H, Nyholm HC, Hagen C, Pedersen LM. Depressed prolactin levels in diabetic women with anovulation. Acta Obstet Gynecol Scand 1982;61:403
134. Valdes CT, Elkind-Hirsch KE, Rogers DG. Diabetes-induced alterations of reproductive and adrenal function in the female rat. Neuroendocrinology 1990;51:406
135. Liu TYF, Lin HS, Johnson DC. Serum FSH, LH, and the ovarian response to exogenous gonadotropins in alloxan diabetic immature female rats. Endocrinology 1972;91:1172
136. Diamond MP, Lavy G, Polan ML. Progesterone production from granulosa cells of individual human follicles derived from diabetic and non-diabetic subjects. Int J Fertil 1989;34:204
137. Freinkel N. Diabetic embryopathy and fuel-mediated organ teratogenesis: Lessons from animal models. Horm Metab Res 1988;20:463
138. Mimouni F, Tsang RC. Pregnancy outcome in insulin-dependent diabetes: Temporal relationships with metabolic control during specific pregnancy periods. Am J Perinatol 1988;5:334
139. Rosenn B, Miodovnik M, Dignan PSJ, et al. Minor congenital malformations in infants of insulin-dependent diabetic women: Association with poor glycemic control. Obstet Gynecol 1990;76:745

140. Sheehan EA, Beck F, Clarke CA, Stanisstreet M. Effects of beta-hydroxybutyrate on rat embryos grown in cultures. Experientia 1985;41:273
140a. Sivan E, Wu YK, Homko C, Reece EA. Dietary vitamin E prophylaxis and diabetic embryopathy: Morphological, biochemical, and molecular analyses. Am J Obstet Gynecol 1995;171:303
141. Landaeur W. Is insulin a teratogen? Teratology 1972;5:129
142. Goldman AS, Baker L, Piddington R, et al. Hyperglycemia-induced teratogenesis is mediated by a functional deficiency of arachidonic acid. Proc Natl Acad Sci USA 1985;82:8227
143. Freinkel N, Lewis NJ, Akazawa S, et al. The honeybee syndrome—implications of the teratogenicity of mannose in rat-embryo culture. N Engl J Med 1984;310:223
144. Mimouni F, Miodovnik M, Tsang RC, et al. Decreased maternal serum magnesium concentration and adverse fetal outcome in insulin-dependent diabetic women. Obstet Gynecol 1987;70:85
145. Eriksson U. Diabetes in pregnancy: Retarded fetal growth, congenital malformations, and feto-maternal concentrations of zinc, copper, and manganese in the rat. J Nutr 1984;114:477
146. Kalter H. Diabetes and spontaneous abortion: A historical review. Am J Obstet Gynecol 1987;156:1243
147. Miodovnik M, Skillman C, Holroyde JC. Elevated maternal glycohemoglobin in early pregnancy and spontaneous abortion among insulin-dependent diabetic women. Am J Obstet Gynecol 1985;153:439
148. Mills JL, Simpson JL, Driscoll SG, et al. Incidence of spontaneous abortion among normal women and insulin-dependent diabetic women whose pregnancies were identified within 21 days of conception. N Engl J Med 1988; 319:1617
149. Miodovnik M, Mimouni F, Tsang RC, et al. Glycemic control and spontaneous abortion in insulin-dependent diabetic women. Obstet Gynecol 1986;68: 366
150. Key TC, Giuffrida R, Moore TR. Predictive value of early pregnancy glycohemoglobin in the insulin-treated diabetic patient. Am J Obstet Gynecol 1978;156:1096
151. Mills JL, Knopp RH, Simpson JL, et al. Lack of relation of increased malformation rates in infants of diabetic mothers to glycemic control during organogenesis. N Engl J Med 1988;318:671
152. Greene MF, Hare JW, Cloherty JP, et al. First-trimester hemoglobin A_1 and risk for major malformation and spontaneous abortion in diabetic pregnancy. Teratology 1989;39:225
153. Wright AD, Nicholson HO, Pollock A, et al. Spontaneous abortion and diabetes mellitus. Postgrad Med J 1983;59:295
154. Rosenn B, Miodovnik M, Combs CA, et al. Preconception management of insulin-dependent diabetes: Improvement of pregnancy outcome. Obstet Gynecol 1991;77:846
155. Dicker D, Feldberg D, Samuel N, et al. Spontaneous abortion in patients with insulin-dependent diabetes mellitus: The effect of preconceptional diabetic control. Am J Obstet Gynecol 1988;158:1161
156. Miodovnik M, Mimouni F, Siddiqi TA, et al. Spontaneous abortions in repeat diabetic pregnancies: A relationship with glycemic control. Obstet Gynecol 1990;75:75
157. Rosenn B, Miodovnik M, Combs CA, et al. Glycemic thresholds for spontaneous abortion and congenital malformations in insulin-dependent diabetes mellitus. Obstet Gynecol 1994;84:515
158. Kitzmiller JL, Watt N, Driscoll SG. Decidual arteriopathy in hypertension and diabetes in pregnancy: Immunofluorescent studies. Am J Obstet Gynecol 1981;141:773
159. Bendon RW, Mimouni F, Khoury J, Miodovnik M. Histopathology of spontaneous abortion in diabetic pregnancies. Am J Perinatol 1990;7:207
160. Kalter H. Perinatal mortality and congenital malformations in infants born to women with insulin-dependent diabetes mellitus: United States, Canada and Europe, 1940–1988. MMWR 1990;39:363
161. Bennett PH, Webner C, Miller M. Pregnancy, Metabolism, Diabetes and the Fetus. New York: Excerpta Medica;1979
162. Kucera J. Rate and type of congenital anomalies among offspring of diabetic women. J Reprod Med 1971;7:61
163. Becerra JE, Khoury MJ, Cordero JF, Erickson JD. Diabetes mellitus during pregnancy and the risks for specific birth defects: A population-based case-control study. Pediatrics 1990;85:1
164. Cousins L. Congenital anomalies among infants of diabetic mothers: Etiology, prevention, prenatal diagnosis. Am J Obstet Gynecol 1983;147:333
165. Gabbe SG. Congenital malformations in infants of diabetic mothers. Obstet Gynecol Surv 1977;32:125
166. Lowy C, Beard RW, Goldschmidt J. Congenital malformations in babies of diabetic mothers. Diabetic Med 1986;3:458
167. Reece EA, Hobbins JC. Diabetic embryopathy: Pathogenesis, prenatal diagnosis and prevention. Obstet Gynecol Surv 1986;41:325
168. Mills JL, Baker L, Goldman AS. Malformations in infants of diabetic mothers occur before the seventh gestational week: Implications for treatment. Diabetes 1979;28:292
169. Miodovnik M, Mimouni F, Dignan PSJ, et al. Major malformations in infants of IDDM women: Vasculopathy and early first-trimester poor glycemic control. Diabetes Care 1988;11:713
170. Miller E, Hare JW, Cloherty JP, et al. Elevated maternal hemoglobin A_{1c} in early pregnancy and major congenital anomalies in infants of diabetic mothers. N Engl J Med 1981;304:1331
171. Ylinen K, Aula P, Stenman UH, et al. Risk of minor and major fetal malformations in diabetics with high haemoglobin A_{1c} in early pregnancy. Br Med J 1984;289:345
172. Lucas MJ, Leveno KJ, Williams ML, et al. Early pregnancy glycosylated hemoglobin, severity of diabetes, and fetal malformations. Am J Obstet Gynecol 1989;161:426
173. Hod M, Merlob P, Friedman S, et al. Prevalence of minor congenital anomalies in newborns of diabetic mothers. Eur J Obstet Gynecol Reprod Biol 1992; 44:111
174. Steel JM, Johnstone SD, Smith AF, Duncan LJP. Five years' experience of a "prepregnancy" clinic for insulin-dependent diabetics. Br Med J 1982; 285:353
175. Fuhrmann K, Reiher H, Semmler K, Glockner E. The effect of intensified conventional insulin therapy before and during pregnancy on the malformation rate in offspring of diabetic mothers. Exp Clin Endocrinol 1984;83:173
176. Goldman JA, Dicker D, Feldberg D, et al. Pregnancy outcome in patients with insulin-dependent diabetes mellitus with preconceptional diabetic control: A comparative study. Am J Obstet Gynecol 1986;155:293
177. Damm P, Molsted-Pedersen L. Significant decrease in congenital malformations in newborn infants of an unselected population of diabetic women. Am J Obstet Gynecol 1989;161:1163
178. Smoak IW, Sadler TW. Embryopathic effects of short-term exposure to hypoglycemia in mouse embryos in vitro. Am J Obstet Gynecol 1990;163:619
179. Akazawa M, Akazawa S, Hashimoto M, et al. Effects of brief exposure to insulin-induced hypoglycemic serum during organogenesis in rat embryo culture. Diabetes 1989;38:1573
180. Buchanan TA, Schemmer JK, Freinkel N. Embryotoxic effects of brief maternal insulin-hypoglycemia during organogenesis in the rat. J Clin Invest 1986;78:643
181. Ellington SK. Development of rat embryos cultured in glucose-deficient media. Diabetes 1987;36:1372
182. Impastato DJ, Gabriel AR, Lardaro HH. Electric and insulin shock therapy during pregnancy. Dis Nerv Syst 1964;25:542
183. Langer O, Cohen WR. Persistent fetal bradycardia during maternal hypoglycemia. Am J Obstet Gynecol 1984;149:688
184. Stangenberg M, Persson B, Stange L, Carlström K. Insulin-induced hypoglycemia in pregnant diabetics. Acta Obstet Gynecol Scand 1983;62:249
185. Berk MA, Mimouni F, Miodovnik M, et al. Macrosomia in infants of insulin-dependent diabetic mothers. Pediatrics 1989;83:1029
186. Coustan DR, Berkowitz RL, Hobbins JC. Tight metabolic control of overt diabetes in pregnancy. Am J Med 1980;68:845
187. Gyves MT, Rodman HM, Little AB, et al. A modern approach to management of pregnant diabetics: A two-year analysis of perinatal outcomes. Am J Obstet Gynecol 1977;128:606
188. Hollingsworth DR, Moore TR. Diabetes and pregnancy. In: Creasy RK, Resnik R, eds. Maternal-Fetal Medicine: Principles and Practice. 2nd ed. Philadelphia, Pa: WB Saunders;1989:925
189. Lavin JP, Lovelace DR, Miodovnik M, et al. Clinical experience with one hundred seven diabetic pregnancies. Am J Obstet Gynecol 1983;147:742
190. Rosenn B, Miodovnik M, Holcberg G, et al. Why can't good glycemic control of diabetes in pregnancy eliminate the problem of macrosomia? Am J Obstet Gynecol 1994;170:293
191. Small M, Cameron A, Lunan CB, MacCuish AC. Macrosomia in pregnancy complicated by insulin-dependent diabetes mellitus. Diabetes Care 1987;10: 594
192. Siddiqi TA, Miodovnik M, Mimouni F, et al. Biphasic fetal intrauterine growth in insulin-dependent diabetic pregnancies. J Am Coll Nutr 1989;8:225
193. Eriksson UJ, Lewis NJ, Freinkel N. Growth retardation during early organogenesis in embryos of experimental diabetic rats. Diabetes 1984;33:281
194. Pedersen JF, Molsted-Pedersen L. Early growth retardation in diabetic pregnancy. Br Med J 1979;1:18
195. Ogata ES, Sabbagha R, Metzger BE, et al. Serial ultrasonography to assess evolving fetal macrosomia. Studies in 23 pregnant diabetic women. JAMA 1980;243:2405
196. Pedersen J. Weight and length at birth of infants of diabetic mothers. Acta Endocrinol 1954;16:330
197. Cardell BS. Hypertrophy and hyperplasia in the pancreatic islets in newborn infants. J Pathol Bacteriol 1953;66:335
198. Laron Z. Somatomedin, insulin, growth hormone, and growth. In: Chinmello G, Sperling M, eds. Recent Progress in Pediatric Endocrinology. New York: Raven Press;1983:67
199. Cheek DB, Greystone JE. The action of insulin, growth hormone, and epinephrine on cell growth in liver, muscle, and brain of the hypophysectomized rat. Pediatr Res 1969;3:77
200. Bocek RM, Young MK, Beatty CH. Effect of insulin and epinephrine on the carbohydrate metabolism and adenylate cyclase activity of rhesus fetal muscle. Pediatr Res 1973;7:787
201. Fee BA, Weil WB Jr. Body composition of infants of diabetic mothers by direct analysis. Ann NY Acad Sci 1963;110:869
202. Salvesen DR, Brudenell JM, Proudler AJ, et al. Fetal pancreatic beta-cell function in pregnancies complicated by maternal diabetes mellitus: Relationship to fetal acidemia and macrosomia. Am J Obstet Gynecol 1993;168:1363
203. Susa JB, Schwartz R. Effects of hyperinsulinemia in the primate fetus. Diabetes 1985;34:36
204. Menon RK, Cohen RM, Sperling MA, et al. Transplacental passage of insulin in pregnant women with insulin-dependent diabetes mellitus: Its role in fetal macrosomia. N Engl J Med 1990;323:309

205. Rosenn B, Miodovnik M, Combs CA, et al. Human versus animal insulin in the management of insulin dependent diabetes: Lack of effect on fetal growth. Obstet Gynecol 1991;78:590
206. Ballard JL, Rosenn B, Khoury JC, Miodovnik M. Diabetic fetal macrosomia: Significance of disproportionate growth. J Pediatr 1993;122:115
207. Mimouni F, Miodovnik M, Rosenn B, et al. Birth trauma in insulin-dependent diabetic pregnancies. Am J Perinatol 1992;3:205
208. Landon MB, Gabbe SG, Piana R, et al. Neonatal morbidity in pregnancy complicated by diabetes mellitus: Predictive value of maternal glycemic control. Am J Obstet Gynecol 1987;156:1089
209. Dandona P, Besterman HS, Freedman DB, et al. Macrosomia despite well-controlled diabetic pregnancy (letter). Lancet 1984;1:737
210. Knight G, Worth RC, Ward JD. Macrosomy despite a well-controlled diabetic pregnancy. Lancet 1983;2:1431
211. Diamond MP, Salyer SL, Vaughn WK, et al. Continuing neonatal morbidity in infants of women with class A diabetes. South Med J 1984;77:1386
212. Miller HC, Wilson HM. Macrosomia, cardiac hypertrophy, erythroblastosis, and hyperplasia of the islets of Langerhans in infants born to diabetic mothers. J Pediatr 1943;23:251
213. Gutgesell HP, Mullins CE, Gillette PG, et al. Transient hypertrophic subaortic stenosis in infants of diabetic mothers. J Pediatr 1976;89:120
214. Gutgesell HP, Speer ME, Rosenburg HS. Characterization of the cardiomyopathy in infants of diabetic mothers. Circulation 1980;61:441
215. Hurwitz D, Irving FC. Diabetes and pregnancy. Am J Med Sci 1937;194:85
216. Fanaroff AA, Sivakoff M, Veille JC. Cardiomyopathy in infants of diabetic mothers. In: Gabbe SG, Oh W, eds. Infant of the Diabetic Mother. Report of the Ninety-Third Ross Conference on Pediatric Research. Columbus, Ohio: Ross Laboratories;1987:117
217. Breitweser JA, Meyer RA, Sperling MA, et al. Cardiac septal hypertrophy in hyperinsulinemic infants. J Pediatr 1980;96:535
218. Mace S, Hirschfield SS, Riggs T, et al. Echocardiographic abnormalities in infants of diabetic mothers. J Pediatr 1979;95:1013
219. Cowett RM, Schwartz R. The infants of the diabetic mother: Symposium of the newborn. Pediatr Clin North Am 1982;29:1213
220. Susa JB, McCormick KL, Widness JA, et al. Chronic hyperinsulinemia in the fetal rhesus monkey: Effects of fetal growth and composition. Diabetes 1979;28:1058
221. Halliday HL. Hypertrophic cardiomyopathy in infants of poorly-controlled diabetic mothers. Arch Dis Child 1981;56:258
222. Way G, Wolfe R, Eshaghpour E, et al. The natural history of hypertrophic cardiomyopathy in infants of diabetic mothers. J Pediatr 1979;95:1020
223. Tsang RC, Kleinman LI, Sutherland JM, Light IJ. Hypocalcemia in infants of diabetic mothers. J Pediatr 1972;80:384
224. Mimouni F, Tsang RC, Hertzberg VS, Miodovnik M. Polycythemia, hypomagnesemia, and hypocalcemia in infants of diabetic mothers. Am J Dis Child 1986;140:798
225. Tsang RC, Strub R, Brown DR, et al. Hypomagnesemia in infants of diabetic mothers: Perinatal studies. J Pediatr 1976;89:115
226. Mimouni F, Miodovnik M, Tsang RC, et al. Decreased amniotic fluid magnesium concentration in diabetic pregnancy. Obstet Gynecol 1987;69:12
227. Tsang RC, Chen IW, Freidman MA, et al. Parathyroid function in infants of diabetic mothers. J Pediatr 1975;86:399
228. Mimouni F, Steichen JJ, Tsang RC, et al. Decreased bone mineral content in infants of diabetic mothers. Am J Perinatol 1988;5:339
229. Steichen JJ, Tsang RC, Ho M, Hug G. Perinatal magnesium, calcium and 1,25-$(OH)_2$D in relation to prospective randomized management of maternal diabetes. Calcif Tissue Int 1981;33:317
230. Raisz LG, Trummel CL, Holick MF, DeLuca HF. 1,25-Dihydroxycholecalciferol: A potent stimulator of bone resorption in tissue culture. Science 1972;175:178
231. Brans YW, Huff RW, Shannon DL, Hunter MA. Maternal diabetes and neonatal macrosomia—postpartum maternal hemoglobin Alc levels and neonatal hypoglycemia. Pediatrics 1982;70:576
232. Lemons JA, Vargas P, Delaney JJ. Infant of the diabetic mother: Review of 225 cases. Am J Obstet Gynecol 1981;57:187
233. Martin FIR, Dahlenburg GW, Russell J, Jeffery P. Neonatal hypoglycemia in infants of IDD mothers. Arch Dis Child 1975;50:472
234. Andersen O, Hertel JL, Schmolker L, Kuhl C. Influence of the maternal plasma glucose concentration at delivery on the risk of hypoglycemia in infants of insulin-dependent diabetic mothers. Acta Paediatr Scand 1985;74:268
235. Grylack LJ, Chu SS, Scanlon JW. Use of intravenous fluids before cesarean section: Effects on perinatal glucose before cesarean section. Obstet Gynecol 1984;63:654
236. Light IJ, Keenan WJ, Sutherland JM. Maternal intravenous glucose administration as a cause of hypoglycemia in the infant of the diabetic mother. Am J Obstet Gynecol 1972;113:345
237. Miodovnik M, Mimouni F, Tsang RC, et al. Management of the insulin-dependent diabetic during labor and delivery: Influences on neonatal outcome. Am J Perinatol 1987;4:106
238. West TET, Lowy C. Control of blood glucose during labor in diabetic women with controlled glucose and low dose insulin infusion. Br Med J 1977;1:1252
239. Fallucca F, Pachi A, Gerlini G, et al. Placental transfer of IgG insulin antibodies and metabolic and clinical complications in the IDMs. Diabetologia 1980;19:273
240. Mylvaganam R, Stowers JM, Steel JM, et al. Insulin immunogenicity in pregnancy: Maternal and fetal studies. Diabetologica 1983;24:19
241. Stevens K, Wirth FH. Incidence of neonatal hyperviscosity at sea level. J Pediatr 1980;97:118
242. Wirth FH, Goldberg KE, Lubchenco LO. Neonatal hyperviscosity: I. Incidence. Pediatrics 1979;63:833
243. Mimouni F, Miodovnik M, Siddiqi TA, et al. Neonatal polycythemia in infants of insulin-dependent diabetic mothers. Obstet Gynecol 1986;68:370
244. Black VD, Lubchenco LO, Luckey DW, et al. Developmental and neurologic sequelae of neonatal hyperviscosity syndrome. Pediatrics 1982;69:426
245. Phillips AF, Dubin JW, Matty PJ, Raye JR. Arterial hypoxemia and hyperinsulinemia in the chronically hyperglycemic fetal lamb. Pediatr Res 1982; 16:653
246. Stonestreet BS, Piasecki GJ, Oh W, Jackson BT. Cardiovascular responses to insulin infusions in the ovine fetus. Pediatr Res 1984;18:130A
247. Clark KE, Miodovnik M, Skillman CA, Mimouni F. Review of fetal cardiovascular and metabolic responses to diabetic insults in the pregnant ewe. Am J Perinatol 1988;5:312
248. Miodovnik M, Skillman CA, Hertzberg V, et al. Effect of maternal hyperketonemia in hyperglycemic pregnant ewes and their fetuses. Am J Obstet Gynecol 1986;154:394
249. Karlsson K, Kjellmer I. The outcome of diabetic pregnancies in relation to the mother's blood sugar level. Am J Obstet Gynecol 1972;122:213
250. Phillips AF, Widness JA, Garcia JF, et al. Erythropoietin elevation in the chronically hyperglycemic fetal lamb. Proc Soc Exp Biol Med 1982;170:42
251. Salvesen DR, Brudenell JM, Snijders RJ, et al. Fetal plasma erythropoietin in pregnancies complicated by maternal diabetes mellitus. Am J Obstet Gynecol 1993;168(1 pt 1):88
252. Oh W, Omori K, Emmanouilides GC, Phelps DL. Placenta to lamb fetus transfusion in utero during acute hypoxia. Am J Obstet Gynecol 1975;12:316
253. Stuart MJ, Sunderji SG, Allen JB. Decreased prostacyclin production in the infant of the diabetic mother. J Lab Clin Med 1981;98:412
254. Gross GP, Hathaway WE, McGaughey HR. Hyperviscosity in the neonate. J Pediatr 1973;82:1004
255. Peevy KJ, Landaw SA, Gross SJ. Hyperbilirubinemia in infants of diabetic mothers. Pediatrics 1980;66:417
256. Johnson JD, Trissel S, Angelus P, et al. Hyperbilirubinemia in human infants of diabetic mothers (IDM): Studies of bilirubin production and glycosylated hemoglobin. Pediatr Res 1986;20:412A
257. Ylinen K, Raivio K, Teramo K. Haemoglobin A_{1c} predicts the perinatal outcome in insulin-dependent diabetic pregnancies. Br J Obstet Gynaecol 1981;88:961
258. Black VD, Lubchenco LO. Neonatal polycythemia and hyperviscosity. Pediatr Clin North Am 1982;29:1137
259. Goldberg K, Wirth FH, Hathaway WE, et al. Neonatal hyperviscosity: II. Effect of partial plasma exchange transfusion. Pediatrics 1982;69:419
260. Ramamurthy RS, Brans YW. Neonatal polycythemia: I. Criteria for diagnosis and treatment. Pediatrics 1981;68:168
261. Gamsu HR. Neonatal morbidity in infants of diabetic mothers. J R Soc Med 1978;71:211
262. Stevenson DK, Bartoletti AL, Ostrander CR, Johnson JD. Pulmonary excretion of carbon monoxide in the human infant as an index of bilirubin production: II. Infants of diabetic mothers. J Pediatr 1979;94:956
263. Stevenson DK, Ostrander CR, Hopper AO, et al. Pulmonary excretion of carbon monoxide as an index of bilirubin production: IIa. Evidence for possible delayed clearance of bilirubin in infants of diabetic mothers. J Pediatr 1981;98:822
264. Stevenson DK. Bilirubin metabolism in the infant of the diabetic mother: An overview. In: Gabbe SG, Oh W, eds. Infant of the Diabetic Mother. Report of the Ninety-Third Ross Conference on Pediatric Research. Columbus, Ohio: Ross Laboratories;1987:109
265. Bucalo LR, Cohen RS, Ostrander CR, et al. Pulmonary excretion of carbon monoxide in the human infant as an index of bilirubin production: IIc. Evidence for the possible association of cord blood erythropoietin levels and postnatal bilirubin production in infants of mothers with abnormalities of gestational glucose metabolism. Am J Perinatol 1984;1:177
266. Mimouni F, Miodovnik M, Siddiqi TA, et al. Perinatal asphyxia in infants of insulin-dependent diabetic mothers. J Pediatr 1988;113:345
267. Miodovnik M, Lavin JP, Harrington DJ, et al. Effects of maternal ketoacidemia on the pregnant ewe and the fetus. Am J Obstet Gynecol 1982;144:585
268. Miodovnik M, Lavin JP, Harrington DJ, et al. Cardiovascular and biochemical effects of infusion of beta hydroxybutyrate into the fetal lamb. Am J Obstet Gynecol 1982;144:594
269. Carson BS, Philipps AF, Simmons MA, et al. Effects of a sustained insulin infusion upon glucose uptake and oxygenation of the ovine fetus. Pediatr Res 1980;14:147
270. Phillips AF, Rosenkrantz TS, Raye J. Consequences of perturbations of fetal fuels in ovine pregnancy. Diabetes 1985;34:32
271. Bunn HF, Briehl RW. The interaction of 2,3-diphosphoglycerate with various human hemoglobins. J Clin Invest 1970;49:1088
272. Jones CJP, Fox H. An ultrastructural and ultrahistochemical study of the placenta of the diabetic women. J Pathol 1976;119:91
273. Edelberg SC, Dierker L, Kalhan S, Rosen MG. Decreased fetal movements with sustained maternal hyperglycemia using the glucose clamp technique. Am J Obstet Gynecol 1987;156:1101
274. Patrick J, Campbell K, Carmichael L, et al. Patterns of gross fetal body movements over 24-hour observation intervals during the last 10 weeks of pregnancy. Am J Obstet Gynecol 1982;142:363

275. Kariniemi V, Forss M, Siegberg R. Reduced short-term variability of fetal heart rate in association with maternal hyperglycemia during pregnancy in insulin-dependent diabetic women. Am J Obstet Gynecol 1983;147:793
276. Bradley RJ, Brudenell JM, Nicolaides KH. Fetal acidosis and hyperlacticaemia diagnosed by cordocentesis in pregnancies complicated by maternal diabetes mellitus. Diabetic Med 1991;8:464
277. Jovanovic R, Jovanovic L. Obstetric management when normoglycemia is maintained in diabetic pregnant women with vascular compromise. Am J Obstet Gynecol 1984;149:617
278. Robert MF, Neff RK, Hubbell JP, et al. Association between maternal diabetes and the respiratory distress syndrome in the newborn. N Engl J Med 1976;294:357
279. Rhoades RA, Filler DA, Vannata B. Influence of maternal diabetes on lipid metabolism in neonatal rat lung. Biochem Biophys Acta 1979;572:132
280. Sosenko IR, Lawson EE, Demottay V, Frantz ID III. Functional delay in lung maturation in fetuses of diabetic rabbits. J Appl Physiol 1980;48:643
281. Warburton D. Chronic hyperglycemia reduces surface active material flux in tracheal fluid of fetal lambs. J Clin Invest 1983;71:550
282. Farrell PM, Engle MJ, Curet LB, et al. Saturated phospholipids in amniotic fluid of normal and diabetic pregnancies. Obstet Gynecol 1984;64:77
283. Mimouni F, Miodovnik M, Whitsett JA, et al. Respiratory distress syndrome in infants of diabetic mothers in the 1980s: No direct adverse effect of maternal diabetes with modern management. Obstet Gynecol 1987;69:191
284. Karlsson K, Kjellmer I. The outcome of diabetic pregnancies in relation to the mother's blood sugar level. Am J Obstet Gynecol 1972;112:213

Diabetes Mellitus, edited by Derek LeRoith, Simeon I. Taylor, and Jerrold M. Olefsky. Lippincott–Raven Publishers, Philadelphia © 1996.

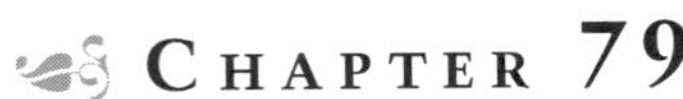

Chapter 79
Gestational Diabetes Mellitus

Robert E. Ratner

Gestational Diabetes Mellitus

Hyperglycemia first identified during pregnancy has been accepted as the arbitrary definition of gestational diabetes mellitus (GDM). The adverse effects of glycosuria and carbohydrate intolerance in pregnancy on fetal outcome were described nearly 100 years ago.[1] Subsequently, in 1917, Elliot P. Joslin described Case 309, which "showed sugar in 1897 during pregnancy, but following confinement, with resulting dead baby, it disappeared, but returned in 9 years in the form of moderate to severe diabetes. . . . [W]ith our present knowledge it is quite possible that such an outcome could be prevented by active treatment of the glycosuria from the very start."[2] Joslin's description emphasizes the importance that the identification of gestational diabetes has on perinatal morbidity and mortality, as well as subsequent development of diabetes in the mother. The differential effects on the mother and child have caused some dilemmas in both the ultimate diagnosis of the disorder and the aggressiveness with which it is sought and treated.

GDM may be viewed as

1. An unidentified pre-existing disease, or
2. The unmasking of a compensated metabolic abnormality by the added stress of pregnancy, or
3. A direct consequence of the altered maternal metabolism stemming from the changing hormonal milieu.

Based on a statistical analysis of the Second Health and Nutritional Examination and Survey, Harris[3] questioned the uniqueness of GDM. Glucose tolerance testing of 817 nonpregnant women of childbearing age with no previous history of diabetes found prevalence rates of carbohydrate intolerance virtually identical to those described in pregnancy. A substantial number of women identified as diabetic during pregnancy, therefore, could have been identified by the improved ascertainment arising from closer monitoring, as recommended during pregnancy. This is further suggested by the findings that those diagnosed with GDM before 24 weeks' gestation were significantly older and had a twofold greater incidence of required insulin therapy than did women diagnosed after 24 weeks' gestation.[4]

This controversial position can be refuted, at least partially, by the observation of the majority of subjects with GDM reverting to normal carbohydrate tolerance postpartum. Another limitation of the conclusion is the fact that Harris used glycemic parameters developed for the diagnosis of GDM, but in a nonpregnant population. Although the level of glycemia achieved by the two groups is comparable, neither the metabolic milieu nor the potential complications are the same. If traditional diagnostic criteria for diabetes in nonpregnant adults are applied to the population studied by the Second Health and Nutritional Examination and Survey, the prevalence of diabetes is considerably less. The critical point remains, however, that a substantial subset of women diagnosed with GDM, particularly those diagnosed early in pregnancy, may have had pre-existing disease that had gone undiagnosed. The apparent clinical correlate of this finding is the need to assess fasting glucose concentrations at the beginning of pregnancy in order to diagnose pre-existing carbohydrate intolerance.

A second possibility is that pregnancy creates a metabolic stress that simply pushes a woman with compensated insulin-dependent diabetes mellitus (IDDM) or non–insulin-dependent diabetes mellitus (NIDDM) into a decompensated hyperglycemic state. It is clear from the classic studies of Freinkel et al.[5] that insulin requirements rise substantially during normal pregnancy. If a woman has a limited β-cell response secondary to autoimmune β-cell destruction, as seen in IDDM, or has β-cell secretory reserve insufficient to meet the demands of pregnancy due to early NIDDM, she may decompensate from a normoglycemic state in the nonpregnant situation to a hyperglycemic state during pregnancy. Data supporting the hypothesis that pregnancy results in the decompensation of a prediabetic stage of IDDM include a twofold enrichment in the frequency of human leukocyte antigens DR3 and DR4 in women with GDM compared to that of a racially matched, carbohydrate-tolerant pregnant population[6] and the finding of islet cell antibodies in as many of 31% of women developing GDM.[7] In addition, 20% of women with previous GDM who subsequently develop diabetes develop traditional IDDM, as defined by a deficient C-peptide response to intravenous glucagon.[8] Others have been less successful in finding evidence of autoimmunity in women with GDM, suggesting that fewer than 10% may have incipient IDDM.[9]

It is far more likely that gestational diabetes results from decompensation of a prediabetic stage of NIDDM. Pathophysiologic observations of GDM are very similar to those seen in NIDDM and will be discussed in detail later in this chapter. Epidemiologically, however, the vast majority of persons who develop diabetes after a history of GDM have classic NIDDM. Review of 12 worldwide studies of diabetes among former patients with GDM indicates a wide range of incidence rates, from 19–87% for combined diabetes and impaired glucose tolerance to 6–62% for diabetes alone.[10] Depending on the ethnic group, conversion rates postpartum to nongestational diabetes may be as high as 9% within the first 6 weeks,[11] with 30% in the first year.[12] The initial observations of O'Sullivan and Mahan[13] in 752 unselected pregnant women in the 1960s demonstrated a 50% prevalence of diabetes after 28 years of follow-up in those in whom pregnancy was complicated by gestational diabetes. In addition, as will be shown subsequently, the prevalence of GDM parallels the prevalence of NIDDM in high-risk ethnic and racial groups.

How Is Gestational Diabetes Mellitus Defined?

The National Diabetes Data Group, together with all three International Gestational Diabetes Workshops, have accepted the modified criteria originally described by O'Sullivan and Mahan[13] in their classic study of 1964. A statistical analysis of glucose response over 3 hours to a 100-g oral glucose challenge in 752 healthy, pregnant women yielded values representing the mean plus or minus two standard deviations at baseline in the fasting state and at 1,2, and 3 hours. By arbitrarily declaring abnormal carbohydrate handling as that exceeding two standard deviations above the mean on two or more values, 2.5% of the population were defined as having gestational diabetes mellitus (GDM). This statistical means of defining disease is population specific, with a prevalence of GDM ranging from 0.5% in northern England to 12.3% in the inner-city (predominantly Hispanic and African-American) population.[14] With a mixed inner-city African-American and tertiary-care population, the George Washington University Medical Center has a 4% prevalence of GDM in its obstetric practice. In a review of an ethnically diverse cohort of 10,187 women undergoing standardized screening for glucose intolerance in New York City, the overall prevalence of GDM was 3.2%. The frequency of GDM was lowest for whites, followed by blacks, Hispanics, Orientals, and women classified as belonging to another "racial/ethnic group."[14] Thus, the purely statistical approach to the definition of GDM is inappropriate because it depends on the relative risk of the populations studied.

A more suitable method of defining disease is based on the morbidity associated with the condition. The O'Sullivan-Mahan criteria have stood the test of time as a predictor of subsequent diabetes in the mother, as previously mentioned. Perinatal maternal morbidity is likewise reflected in the significantly increased incidence of pregnancy-induced hypertension and preeclampsia.[15] With current aggressive glycemic management achieving postprandial euglycemia, the traditional maternal complications of polyhydramnios, preterm labor, abnormalities of labor, and birth trauma were not increased in this population with GDM. The predominant acute effects of GDM occur not to the mother but to the fetus.

Neonatal morbidity in the offspring of women with GDM has long been recognized. The occurrence of metabolic complications including hypoglycemia, hypocalcemia, macrosomia, and hyperbilirubinemia is excessive.[16] With improved neonatal care, it is difficult to demonstrate changes in fetal mortality. Older data, however, did report a fourfold increased mortality rate in infants of mothers with GDM.[17] The effects on the offspring are not limited, however, to the immediate perinatal period. As these offspring of mothers with GDM age, they are found to develop premature insulin resistance, obesity, and a high rate of carbohydrate intolerance.[18]

It would appear, therefore, that diagnosing GDM and instituting aggressive management of the mother are intended to reduce or eliminate the perinatal, neonatal, and long-term complications in the offspring. The current diagnostic criteria, however, in no way take the neonatal outcome into consideration. With this in mind, are the O'Sullivan-Mahan criteria too lax for the identification of persons at risk for perinatal morbidity associated with carbohydrate intolerance? The sanctity of these criteria have been seriously questioned.[19] The original criteria were based on whole blood determination of glucose by the Somogyi technique. This was subsequently modified by the National Diabetes Data Group by utilizing a conversion factor of 1.14 to represent plasma glucose determinations by the glucokinase technique.[20] Technical modifications of that conversion have been recommended by Carpenter and Coustan[21] as being more representative of the true plasma glucose determination. This modification results in a lowering of all glucose criteria in the 3-hour glucose tolerance test (Table 79-1). As such, a larger percentage of women undergoing glucose tolerance testing during pregnancy will be found to meet these modified criteria, thus increasing the sensitivity of the test; however, the effects of these more inclusive criteria on specificity remain in doubt.[22] By utilizing the lower modified criteria, the overall incidence of GDM increased by 56%. These excess cases were found to have perinatal morbidities similar to those of women diagnosed with GDM based on the more traditional criteria. Long-term maternal follow-up of this patient population is not yet available.

In addition to the debate concerning the appropriate glucose tolerance test criteria for utilization in the diagnosis of GDM, data are becoming increasingly available to suggest that a single abnormal value on glucose tolerance testing may better predict the occurrence of perinatal morbidity. Tallerigo et al.[23] examined the neonatal outcome in 249 women with normal glucose tolerance test results in the third trimester by the O'Sullivan-Mahan criteria.

Table 79-1. Historical Evolution of O'Sullivan-Mahan Criteria for the Diagnosis of Gestational Diabetes Mellitus

	O'Sullivan-Mahan Criteria (mM [mg%] Whole Blood)	National Diabetes Data Group Criteria (mM [mg%] Plasma)	Carpenter-Coustan Modification (mM [mg%] Plasma)
Fasting	5.0 (90)	5.83 (105)	5.28 (95)
1 hour	9.17 (165)	10.56 (190)	10.0 (180)
2 hours	8.06 (145)	9.17 (165)	8.61 (155)
3 hours	6.94 (125)	8.06 (145)	7.78 (140)

Adapted with permission from ref. 33.

They found that the 2-hour plasma glucose concentration after a 100-g oral glucose tolerance test significantly correlated with the infant's birth weight; the higher the 2-hour plasma glucose concentration, the greater the incidence of macrosomia, toxemia, and cesarean sections. A significant increase was noted as 2-hour plasma glucose concentrations exceeded 140 mg/dL compared to the 165 mg/dL cutoff noted in the traditional O'Sullivan-Mahan criteria. Others have correlated the rate of fall in plasma glucose concentration in the first hour after an IV glucose tolerance test with neonatal complications. Decreased glucose disposal, as manifested by a slower rate of decline in plasma glucose, correlated with increased infant birth weight, neonatal asphyxia, and congenital anomalies.[24] Validation of these findings has been provided by additional large-scale epidemiologic studies. Lindsay et al.[25] found both maternal and fetal morbidity increased in women with only a single abnormal value on glucose tolerance testing during pregnancy. Toxemia was increased in the affected group with an odds ration of 2.51, and macrosomia in the infants and subsequent shoulder dystocia were found to have odds ratios of 2.18 and 2.97, respectively. With only a single abnormal value on glucose tolerance testing, Berkus and Langer[26] found the incidence of infants who were large for gestational age to be twice that of mothers in whom the glucose tolerance test was entirely normal. Intervention to maintain normoglycemia during pregnancy reduced this adverse outcome to near-normal levels.

Finally, difficulties with the oral glucose tolerance test as a means of diagnosis have been raised, regardless of the criteria used. Poor reproducibility of glucose tolerance testing has been documented for 50 years.[27] This issue has been further examined during pregnancy, in which high-risk pregnant women underwent two sequential glucose tolerance tests 1 week apart; 24% were found to have discrepant test results on the two examinations.[28] Progression from normal to abnormal values stemming from progressive decompensation could not explain this inconsistency, as 80% of those discrepant tests reverted from abnormal to normal at the second examination.

Given the lack of reproducibility of the glucose tolerance test, together with the discrepancies in the number of abnormalities and the threshold for defining those abnormalities, much effort has gone into establishing simpler diagnostic criteria for GDM. Glycated proteins are extensively utilized to follow long-term levels of glycemic control. Many have hoped to adapt this simple blood test, which can be obtained without dietary preparation and at any time of day, as a diagnostic test for GDM. Unfortunately, neither glycated hemoglobin nor fructosamine is sufficiently sensitive for the identification of women with GDM.[29–31] Random glucose testing and use of reflectance meters lack the sensitivity for adequate identification of women at risk for GDM. The best screening test appears to be the 50-g 1-hour glucose challenge test. It is now recognized that a 50-g oral glucose load can be utilized in either the fasting or the fed state without reducing sensitivity or specificity.[32] Utilizing a screening threshold of 130 mg/dL provides a sensitivity approaching 100% while maintaining specificity at near 80%.[33] Alteration of this threshold for subsequent 3-hour 100-g glucose tolerance testing influences the sensitivity, specificity, and ultimate cost of universal screening. Universal screening of all pregnant women using a threshold value of 130 mg/dL results in an almost 100% sensitivity at a cost of $249 per case diagnosed. Limiting screening to women over the age of 25, or to younger women with the presence of risk factors, maintains the sensitivity at more than 95%, but with only a $35 reduction in cost per case diagnosed.

Glucose has traditionally been used as the marker for GDM because of its ease of measurement and test reproducibility among laboratories. It is now clear that alterations in insulin secretion, insulin sensitivity, and carbohydrate, fat, and amino acid metabolism are all intrinsic abnormalities in the state that we have come to accept as GDM. Developing more sensitive indices for the prediction of perinatal morbidity may require either intensification of glycemic criteria or the inclusion of more sophisticated metabolic measurements.

Currently accepted clinical management includes screening for GDM between gestational weeks 24 and 28 in all pregnant women who have not been previously identified as having glucose intolerance. A 1-hour plasma glucose determination in excess of 140 mg/dL (lower by Carpenter-Coustan criteria) constitutes a positive screen and requires the performance of a traditional 100-g oral glucose tolerance test for confirmation of GDM. Controversy over the amount and formulation of the oral glucose tolerance test, the criteria used for diagnosis, and the substitution of the more physiologic mixed-meal challenge have filled symposia and journals, but the modified O'Sullivan-Mahan criteria still stand firm for the diagnosis of GDM.

Etiology and Pathogenesis of Gestational Diabetes Mellitus

Epidemiologic evaluation of gestational diabetes mellitus (GDM) has much in common with the findings in non–insulin-dependent diabetes mellitus (NIDDM). Like NIDDM, the frequency of GDM increases with progressive age and body mass index and is seen more commonly in nonwhite populations. In various studies, the relative risk is increased by 1.6 to 3.5 in blacks, 1.8 in Hispanics, 8.5 in Southeast Asians, 10.9 in East Indians, and 15 in Native Americans.[35,36] These findings parallel those of NIDDM in these respective ethnic groups, as well as in relation to age and obesity. Metabolic assessment of women with previous histories of GDM further reveals findings consistent with NIDDM. In addition to the observation that over 90% of women developing nongestational diabetes after a history of GDM appear to have NIDDM,[37] metabolic studies suggest both β-cell defects and insulin resistance in women with a history of GDM.

It is useful, therefore, to examine the pathogenesis of GDM by examining the β-cell insulin response and subsequent insulin action in pregnant women both with and without GDM. Classic studies by Freinkel and others demonstrated a 1.5–2.5-fold augmentation in insulin secretion in response to either oral or intravenous glucose during pregnancy.[38] Clearly, limited β-cell reserve incapable of making this compensatory increase in insulin secretion would result in subsequent maternal carbohydrate intolerance. After an oral glucose challenge to women with GDM, significantly higher insulin levels are reached in pregnancy than are seen in the same individuals post-partum.[38]

In absolute terms, women with GDM have insulin responses almost identical to those of normal women during pregnancy.[39] Because the ambient glucose levels are higher in GDM, however, the insulin response per unit of glycemic stimulus (the insulinogenic index) is only half that seen in normal pregnancy.

Specific stimulation tests have revealed enhanced β-cell sensitivity to both glucose and amino acids in normal pregnancy. These responses, however, are significantly lower in women with GDM.[40] β-cell secretory dynamics may be assessed by IV glucose tolerance testing and analyzed by minimal modeling techniques.[41] First-phase insulin secretion was less than one-fourth that of the normal pregnant group.[42] In the second phase, insulin secretion was also found to be lower in the women with GDM, although not sufficient to reach statistical significance. In this group of 16 women with GDM, only 1, however, was found to have both normal first- and second-phase insulin secretion. These findings are entirely consistent with observations of β-cell response and dynamics in nongestational NIDDM.[43] It remains unclear whether this β-cell defect is present before conception. To date, no prospective studies before the occurrence of GDM have been published to demonstrate this proposed pre-existing β-cell defect. It is clear, however, that the β-cell defect persists after delivery. Oral glucose tolerance testing in women with previous GDM matched with women with a history of normal pregnancy demonstrates a 25–40% reduction in insulin responsiveness in both white and African-Caribbean patients. The insulin: glucose ratios are also reduced by 30–45% in these populations.[44]

As in NIDDM, it is not known whether the β-cell defect seen in GDM is a primary defect or occurs after insulin resistance. Nonetheless, insulin resistance is a well-described phenomenon in GDM. Utilizing techniques similar to those in NIDDM, insulin sensitivity is found to be markedly depressed in GDM and glucose disposal rates are markedly diminished. Utilizing a hyperinsulinemic-euglycemic clamp technique, Ryan et al.[45] demonstrated insulin resistance in women with normal pregnancies and GDM with decreasing glucose utilization of 18% and 58%, respectively, compared to normal nonpregnant women. Utilizing the minimal model technique, however, insulin sensitivity was reduced by two-thirds in both normal pregnant women and those with GDM compared to matched nonpregnant women. Thus, no differences were noted by this method in insulin action in GDM versus normal pregnancy.[42]

Examination of insulin action on peripheral tissues, specifically liver, adipocyte, and muscle, suggests normal insulin action in the two former sites and marked insulin resistance at the muscle. Phosphofructokinase and pyruvate kinase are significantly lower in muscle tissue from pregnant women compared to nonpregnant controls.[40] This results in decreased muscle glycolysis and glucose disposal.

These changes in insulin sensitivity are found inconsistently postpartum. Ryan et al.[45] found normal glucose disposal 3 days postpartum in two patients with a history of GDM. With larger samples, however, only 50% of women with previous GDM normalized their insulin sensitivity and glucose disposal.[46,47]

Like NIDDM, GDM is a genetically heterogeneous disorder. Ethnic differences in both phenotypic and genotypic features clearly exist. In both African-American and white subjects, the presence of genotypes 1,1 and 1,2 for the insulin receptor gene increase the relative risk of developing GDM.[48] These genotypic markers further interact with both body mass index (BMI) and a maternal history of diabetes. The presence of allele 1 of the insulin receptor gene confers an odds ratio of 3.72 when BMI equals 35. If a maternal history of diabetes is further factored in, the odds ratio rises to 62.84.[48]

In whites, the interaction between allele 1 positivity within the insulin receptor gene accounts for the entire increased odds ratio related to obesity. Thus, if BMI is 35 or greater, the odds ratio in allele 1–positive patients rises to 27.4, whereas it is not increased in women lacking the allele. A further interaction occurs between women with allele 1 positivity and insulin-like glucose factor 2 allele 2 positivity. This interaction further increases the odds ratio to 34. Hispanic patients in this analysis demonstrated none of the genetic risk factors found in either the white or African-American populations with GDM.

Despite these genetic observations, no definitive abnormalities in insulin receptor number, affinity, or activity have been noted. Available literature demonstrates a wide range of insulin receptor states in GDM. Thus, most investigators believe that the insulin resistance occurring in GDM stems from a postreceptor defect.

Examination of glucose transporter function has provided further evidence of the mechanism of insulin resistance. GLUT-4 content is entirely normal in skeletal muscle in both normal pregnancy and GDM.[49] GLUT-4 content in adipocytes, however, is abnormal in both absolute number and subcellular distribution.[50] Approximately 50% of patients with GDM have a profound cellular depletion of GLUT-4, whereas the other subgroup demonstrates normal total cellular GLUT-4 with an abnormal subcellular distribution. Insulin-stimulated translocation of GLUT-4 from microsomes into the plasma membrane was markedly deficient in all patients with GDM, with a subsequent 60% depression in glucose transport activity. It is unclear from these studies whether the defect in glucose transporter number, location, or activity is a primary defect present before gestation or if it persists postpartum. It is possible, however, that these defects are acquired as a result of either chronic hyperglycemia or hyperinsulinemia during the period of gestation. Further longitudinal studies of insulin action will be necessary before conclusive evidence is forthcoming.

Impact of Gestational Diabetes Mellitus on the Mother

The identification and treatment of women with gestational diabetes mellitus (GDM) are motivated as much by the desire to prevent obstetric complications as by the need to prevent fetal complications. A summary of observational studies revealed increased risks of polyhydramnios, pregnancy-induced hypertension, chronic hypertension, pyelonephritis, and the need for cesarean section delivery.[51] Improved obstetric care, and perhaps more intensive management of GDM, result in a reduction to control levels of most maternal complications.[52] Pregnancy-induced hypertension and preeclampsia, however, remain twice as common in women with GDM as in controls. This relationship persists even when matched for maternal BMI. In addition, both chronic hypertension/pregnancy-induced hypertension and preeclampsia are significantly more common (2.5% versus 1% and 19.8% versus 7.9%, respectively) in women with GDM compared to BMI-matched women with only a single abnormal value on glucose tolerance testing.[53]

Delivery by cesarean section occurs in 35% of mothers with GDM compared to controls.[54] Even when matched for body weight, women with GDM undergo cesarean section delivery twice as often as controls. Maternal BMI and nulliparity were the only maternal factors identified that predicted the need for cesarean section. Fetal factors associated with an increased risk of cesarean section included fetal presentation, percent body fat, and subscapular skinfold thickness. The single most common cause of cesarean section among women with GDM, however, remains repeat cesarean section.

GDM recurs in approximately 50% of subsequent pregnancies.[55] Additional predictors of recurrent GDM include absolute glucose tolerance test results, glucose response, the requirement of insulin, and the presence of macrosomia in the index pregnancy. Together with a BMI in excess of 35 in the subsequent pregnancy, these three additional risk factors in combination serve as excellent markers for recurrence. The presence of any two factors has an 82% positive predictive value, and the presence of any three carries with it a 100% positive predictive value.[56] Today the O'Sullivan and Mahan criteria remain the only long-term predictors of maternal carbohydrate tolerance. The incidence rates for diabetes among former patients with GDM varies from 6% to 62%, with the excess risk of diabetes among these women being as high as 31%.[10] Extensive efforts to identify factors predicting subsequent maternal nongestational diabetes have contributed extensively to the understanding of the pathophysiology of GDM. Pregnancy, despite its temporary diabetogenic state, is not associated with an increased risk of subsequent non–insulin-dependent diabetes mellitus (NIDDM).[57]

Pre-existing obesity and subsequent postpartum weight gain are strongly associated with the development of NIDDM.[58] Thus, the progression from GDM to NIDDM appears to be identical, though accelerated, to the course of NIDDM in the non-GDM population. Intensive examination of maternal and neonatal characteristics of a GDM population with postpartum follow-up confirms obesity (or BMI) and the fasting glucose value on the oral glucose tolerance test in pregnancy as the strongest predictors of subsequent development of NIDDM.[59–61] Interestingly, a family history of diabetes, maternal age, parity, and the need for therapeutic insulin during the index pregnancy were not consistently found to be significant predictors of the ultimate development of NIDDM.

GDM appears to be an early manifestation of NIDDM in populations at risk. Early identification allows longitudinal evaluation of metabolic parameters leading to the development of NIDDM and becomes an excellent model for prevention studies of nongestational diabetes mellitus.

Impact of Gestational Diabetes Mellitus on the Fetus

The fetus of the mother with gestational diabetes mellitus (GDM) is exposed to a metabolic milieu quite different from the normal one. Glucose, alanine, and free fatty acids are transferred from the maternal circulation to the fetus in excess quantity, resulting in an overfed fetus.[62] As a result, amniotic fluid insulin concentrations rise significantly as an indicator of fetal compensation for increased nutrient delivery.[63] Although glucose and glycated proteins, including hemoglobin, become the clearest parameters reflecting the maternal metabolic state, maternal triglyceride concentrations have been found to be the strongest predictor of birth weight.[64] Thus, the overall metabolic changes clearly affect fetal development and maturity, leading to a variety of morbid fetal outcomes. Improved maternal and neonatal care has reduced neonatal mortality to levels indistinguishable from those of control groups. The effects of maternal glucose and metabolic control tend to mask the incidence of neonatal complications but fail to ameliorate them entirely. Population-based studies of perinatal outcomes in patients with GDM reflect an increased prevalence of infants who are large for gestational age, macrosomia, hyperglycemia, hyperbilirubinemia, and polycythemia.[65,66] In these studies, triglycerides were not measured but maternal weight was significantly correlated with birth weight. Other neonatal morbidities, however, are unrelated to either maternal age or obesity but correlate to some degree with severity of maternal diabetes, as reflected by glycemic control.

Contemporary efforts to maintain normoglycemia during pregnancy with diet, exercise, and aggressive insulin therapy may result in normalization of glycated hemoglobin and near-normal glucose profiles throughout the day by self-monitoring of blood glucose concentrations. Despite this degree of near-normalization of glycemia, however, neonatal morbidities persist[16] (Table 79-2).

The in utero exposure to abnormal metabolic parameters has long-term consequences in addition to the short-term consequences seen in the perinatal period. Offspring of women with GDM are heavier for gestational age and heavier for height than offspring of nondiabetic women matched for age and BMI.[67] This neonatal obesity creates a problem that these children are apparently unable to overcome. As they age, within each age group, the offspring of diabetic women have a higher prevalence of obesity than their matched cohort. Similarly, these offspring have higher glucose concentrations after glucose tolerance tests and a higher prevalence of diabetes than their matched cohort. This study is particularly interesting in that the infants of women with GDM continued to have a significantly greater incidence of obesity and diabetes even when matched with infants of women with normal carbohydrate tolerance during the index pregnancy who subsequently developed NIDDM. Thus, the effects of the intrauterine environment may be separated from the effects of heredity, and can be demonstrated to have lasting effects on the anthropomorphic and metabolic development of the offspring.[67]

Conclusions

Discriminating the effects of maternal age, obesity, and degree of maternal glycemic control has complicated the assessment of fetal effects of gestational diabetes mellitus (GDM). Use of National Diabetes Data Group criteria for the diagnosis of GDM and differing thresholds for the initiation of insulin therapy, with resulting differences in maternal glycemic control, complicate our understanding of the impact of GDM on the fetus. Standardization of diagnostic criteria and therapeutic interventions, together with intensive examination of fetal and maternal metabolic parameters, will contribute significantly to our understanding of the impact of GDM. Nonetheless, GDM serves as an ideal model for examining the natural history of non–insulin-dependent diabetes mellitus (NIDDM) together with the effects of early intervention for prevention. Furthermore, infants of mothers with GDM provide a model for the effects of early nutrition, as well as an opportunity to reduce the occurrence of neonatal morbidities. New efforts are now underway to improve ascertainment of gestational diabetes, measurement of metabolic parameters, and examination of fetal outcomes in a controlled fashion.[68]

References

1. Williams JW. The clinical significance of glucosuria in pregnant women. Am J Med Sci 1909;137:1
2. Joslin EP. The Treatment of Diabetes Mellitus with Observation upon the Disease Based upon 1300 Cases. Philadelphia: Lea & Febiger;1917:448
3. Harris MI. Gestational diabetes may represent discovery of pre-existing glucose intolerance. Diabetes Care 1988;11:402
4. Berkowitz GS, Roman SH, Lapinski RH, Alvarez M. Maternal characteristics, neonatal outcome, and the time of diagnosis of gestational diabetes. Am J Obstet Gynecol 1991;167:976
5. Freinkel N, Metzger BE, Phelps RL, et al. Gestational diabetes mellitus: Heterogeneity of maternal age, weight, insulin secretion, HLA antigens, and islet antibodies and the impact of maternal metabolism on pancreatic beta cell and somatic development in the offspring. Diabetes 1985;34(suppl 2):1
6. McEvoy RC, Franklin B, Ginsberg-Fellner F. Gestational diabetes mellitus: Evidence for autoimmunity against the pancreatic beta cells. Diabetologia 1991;34:507
7. Damm P, Kuhl C, Bertelsen A, Molsted-Pedersen L. Predictive factors for the

Table 79-2. Neonatal Complications in Infants of Mothers with Gestational Diabetes Mellitus

Complication	GDM (n = 878)	Control (n = 380)	Relative Risk
Macrosomia	17.9%*	5.6%	3.2*
Hypoglycemia	5.1*	0.9	5.7*
Hyperbilirubinemia	16.5*	8.2	2.0*
Hypocalcemia	5.5*	2.7	2.0*
Polycythemia	13.3*	4.9	2.7*
Thrombocytopenia	0.6	0.9	0.7
Hyaline membrane disease	1.3	1.4	0.9
Major anomalies	3.0*	1.8	1.7*

*$p < 0.05$.
Adapted with permission from ref. 16.

development of diabetes in women with previous gestational diabetes mellitus. Am J Obstet Gynecol 1992;167:607
8. Catalano PM, Tyzbir ED, Simms EAH. Incidence and significance of islet cell antibodies in women with previous gestational diabetes. Diabetes Care 1990;13:478
9. O'Sullivan JB. Diabetes mellitus after GDM. Diabetes 1991;40(suppl 2):131
10. Hadden DR. Geographic, ethnic, and racial variations in the incidence of gestational diabetes mellitus. Diabetes 1985;34(suppl 2):8
11. Kjos SL, Buchanan TA, Greenspoon JS, et al. Gestational diabetes mellitus: The prevalence of glucose intolerance in diabetes mellitus in the first two months post-partum. Am J Obstet Gynecol 1990;163:93
12. Metzger BE, Bybee DE, Freinkel N, et al. Gestational diabetes mellitus: Correlations between the phenotypic and genotypic characteristics of the mother and abnormal glucose tolerance during the first year post-partum. Diabetes 1985;34(suppl 2):111
13. O'Sullivan JB, Mahan CM. Criteria for the oral glucose tolerance test in pregnancy. Diabetes 1964;13:278
14. Berkowitz GS, Lapinski RH, Wein R, Lee D. Racial/ethnicity and other risk factors for gestational diabetes. Am J Epidemiol 1992;135:965
15. Goldman M, Kitzmiller JL, Abrams B, et al. Obstetric complications with GDM: Effect of maternal weight. Diabetes 1991;40(suppl 2):79
16. Hod M, Merlob P, Friedman S, et al. Gestational Diabetes Mellitus a survey of perinatal complications in the 1980's. Diabetes 1991;40(suppl 2):74
17. O'Sullivan JB, Charles D, Mahan CM, et al. Gestational diabetes and perinatal mortality rate. Am J Obstet Gynecol 1973;116:901
18. Pettitt DJ, Bennett PH, Saad MF, et al. Abnormal glucose tolerance during pregnancy in Pima Indian women: Long-term effects on offspring. Diabetes 1991;40(suppl 2):126
19. Naylor CD. Diagnosing gestational diabetes mellitus: Is the gold standard valid? Diabetes Care 1989;12:565
20. National Diabetes Data Group. Classification and diagnosis of diabetes mellitus and other categories of glucose intolerance. Diabetes 1979;28:1039
21. Carpenter MW, Coustan DR. Criteria for screening tests for gestational diabetes. Am J Obstet Gynecol 1982;144:768
22. Magee MS, Walden CE, Benedetti TJ, Knopp RH. Influence of diagnostic criteria on the incidence of gestational diabetes and perinatal morbidity. JAMA 1993;269:609
23. Tallarigo L, Giampietro O, Penno G, et al. Relation of glucose tolerance test to complications of pregnancy in nondiabetic women. N Engl J Med 1986;315:989
24. Farmer G, Russell G, Hamilton-Nicol DR, et al. The influence of maternal glucose metabolism on fetal growth, development, and morbidity in 917 singleton pregnancies in nondiabetic women. Diabetologia 1988;31:134
25. Lindsay MK, Graves W, Klein L. The relationship of one abnormal glucose tolerance test value in pregnancy complications. Obstet Gynecol 1989;73:103
26. Berkus MD, Langer O. Glucose tolerance test: Degree of glucose abnormality correlates with neonatal outcome. Obstet Gynecol 1993;81:344
27. Freeman H, Looney JM, Hoskins RG. Spontaneous variability of oral glucose tolerance. J Clin Endocrinol 1942;2:431
28. Catalano PM, Avallone D, Drago NM, Amini SV. Reproducibility of the oral glucose tolerance test in pregnant women. Am J Obstet Gynecol 1993;169:874
29. Hod M, Orvieto R, Friedman S, et al. Glycated proteins in gestational diabetes mellitus. Isr J Med Sci 1990;26:638
30. Huter O, Drexel H, Brezinka C, et al. Low sensitivity of serum fructosamine as a screening parameter for gestational diabetes mellitus. Gynecol Obstet Invest 1992;34:20
31. Aziz NL, Abdelwahab S, Moussa M, Georgy M. Maternal fructosamine and glycosylated hemoglobin in the prediction of gestational glucose intolerance. Clin Exp Obstet Gynecol 1992;19:235
32. Coustan DR, Widness JA, Carpenter MW, et al. The breakfast tolerance test: Screening for gestational diabetes with a standard mixed nutrient meal. Am J Obstet Gynecol 1987;157:1113
33. Carpenter MW. Rationale and performance of tests for gestational diabetes. Clin Obstet Gynecol 1991;34:544
34. Second International Workshop Conference on Gestational Diabetes Mellitus: Summary and Recommendations. Diabetes 1985;34(suppl 2):123
35. Dornhorst A, Patterson CM, Nicholls JSD, et al. High prevalence of gestational diabetes in women from ethnic minority groups. Diabetic Med 1992;9:820
36. Benjamin E, Winters D, Mayfield J, Gohdes D. Diabetes in pregnancy in Zuni Indian women. Diabetes Care 1993;16:1231
37. Persson B, Hanson U, Hartling SG, Binder C. Follow-up of women with previous GDM: Insulin, C-peptide, and proinsulin responses to oral glucose load. Diabetes 1991;40(suppl 2):136
38. Freinkel N. Of Pregnancy and progeny. Diabetes 1980;29:1023
39. Hornnes PJ, Kuhl C, Lauritsen KB. Gastrointestinal insulinotropic hormones in normal and gestational diabetic pregnancy. Response to oral glucose. Diabetes 1981;30:504
40. Kuhl C. Aetiology of gestational diabetes. Bailliere's Clin Obstet Gynecol 1991;5:279
41. Bergman R, Finegood DT, Ader M. Assessment of insulin sensitivity in vivo. Endocrinol Rev 1985;6:45
42. Buchanan TA, Metzger BE, Freinkel N, Bergman RN. Insulin sensitivity and β cell responsiveness to glucose during late pregnancy in lean and moderately obese women with normal glucose tolerance or mild gestational diabetes. Am J Obstet Gynecol 1990;162:1008
43. Porte D. Beta cells in type II diabetes mellitus. Diabetes 1991;40:166
44. Dornhorst A, Chan SP, Gelding SV, et al. Ethnic differences in insulin secretion in women at risk of future diabetes. Diabetic Med 1992;9;258
45. Ryan EA, O'Sullivan MJ, Skyler JS. Insulin action during pregnancy. Studies with a euglycemic clamp technique. Diabetes 1985;34:380
46. Catalano PM, Bernstein IM, Wolfe RR, et al. Subclinical abnormalities of glucose metabolism in subjects with previous gestational diabetes. Am J Obstet Gynecol 1986;155:1255
47. Effendic S, Hanson U, Persson B, et al. Glucose tolerance, insulin release, and insulin sensitivity in normal weight women with previous gestational diabetes mellitus. Diabetes 1987;36:413
48. Ober C, Xiang K-S, Thisted RA, et al. Increased risk for gestational diabetes mellitus associated with insulin receptor and insulin-like growth factor 2 restriction fragment length polymorphisms. Genetic Epidemiol 1989;6:559
49. Garvey WT, Maianu L, Hancock JA, et al. Gene expression of GLUT 4 in skeletal muscle from insulin resistant patients with obesity, IGT, GDM, and NIDDM. Diabetes 1992;41:465
50. Garvey WT, Maianu L, Zhu J-H, et al. Multiple defects in the adipocyte glucose transport system cause cellular insulin resistance in gestational diabetes. Diabetes 1993;42:1773
51. Cousins L. Pregnancy complications among diabetic women: Review 1965–1985. Obstet Gynecol Surv 1987;42:140
52. Goldman M, Kitzmiller JL, Abrams B, et al. Obstetric complications with GDM: Effects of maternal weight. Diabetes 1991;40(suppl 2):79
53. Suhonen L, Teramo K. Hypertension and pre-eclampsia in women with gestational glucose intolerance. Acta Obstet Gynecol Scand 1993;72:269
54. Bernstein IM, Catalano PM. Examination of factors contributing to the risks of cesarean delivery in women with gestational diabetes. Obstet Gynecol 1994;83:462
55. Philipson EH, Super DM. Gestational diabetes mellitus: Does it recur in subsequent pregnancy? Am J Obstet Gynecol 1989;160:1324
56. Gaudier FL, Haugh JC, Poist M, et al. Recurrence of gestational diabetes mellitus. Obstet Gynecol 1992;80:755
57. Manson JE, Rimm EB, Colditz GA, et al. Parity and incidence of noninsulin dependent diabetes mellitus. Am J Med 1992;93:13
58. Dornhorst A, Bailey PC, Anyaoku V, et al. Abnormalities of glucose tolerance following gestational diabetes. Q J Med 1990;77:1219
59. Catalano PM, Vargo KM, Bernstein IM, Amini SB. Incidence and risk factors associated with abnormal postpartum glucose tolerance in women with gestational diabetes. Am J Obstet Gynecol 1991;165:914
60. Metzger BE, Cho NH, Roston SM, Radvany R. Prepregnancy weight and antepartum insulin secretion predict glucose tolerance five years after gestational diabetes mellitus. Diabetes Care 1993;16:1598
61. Coustan DR, Carpenter MW, O'Sullivan PS, Carr SR. Gestational diabetes: Predictors of subsequent disordered glucose metabolism. Am J Obstet Gynecol 1993;168:1139
62. Kalkoff RK. Impact of maternal fuels and nutritional state on fetal growth. Diabetes 1991;40(suppl 2):61
63. Weerasiri T, Riley SF, Sheedy MT, et al. Amniotic fluid insulin values in women with gestational diabetes as a predictor of emerging diabetes mellitus. Aust N Z J Obstet Gynecol 1993;33:358
64. Knopp RH, Magee MS, Waldon CE, et al. Prediction of infant birth weight by GDM screening tests. Diabetes Care 1992;15:1605
65. Jacobson JD, Cousins L. A population-based study of maternal and perinatal outcome of patients with gestational diabetes. Am J Obstet Gynecol 1989;161:981
66. Maresh M, Beard RW, Bray CS, et al. Factors predisposing to and outcome of gestational diabetes. Obstet Gynecol 1989;74:342
67. Pettitt DJ, Nelson RG, Saad MF, et al. Diabetes and obesity in the offspring of Pima Indian women with diabetes during pregnancy. Diabetes Care 1993;16:310
68. Blank A, Grave GD, Metzger BE. Effects of gestational diabetes on perinatal morbidity reassessed. Report of the International Workshop on Adverse Perinatal Outcomes of Gestational Diabetes Mellitus. Diabetes Care 1995; 18:127

Part IX

Complications: Descriptive and Clinical

Diabetes Mellitus, edited by Derek LeRoith, Simeon I. Taylor, and Jerrold M. Olefsky. Lippincott–Raven Publishers, Philadelphia © 1996.

CHAPTER 80
Pathophysiology of Diabetic Retinopathy

ZHEN Y. JIANG, HAMISH M.A. TOWLER, PHILIP LUTHERT, AND SUSAN LIGHTMAN

Introduction

Diabetic retinopathy is the most common cause of legal blindness in adults under the age of 65 in most Western countries.[1,2] It may occur with or without the other systemic complications of diabetes mellitus, and its incidence rises with increasing duration of disease. Although some of the clinical features of retinopathy respond to treatment, for example with laser photocoagulation, in the majority of patients the aim of treatment is to prevent or retard further visual loss rather than to improve vision. In addition, both laser therapy and surgical intervention have their own specific and potentially sight-threatening complications. A better understanding of the pathophysiology of diabetic retinopathy will hopefully allow prevention of visual loss or, failing that, more effective and earlier methods of treatment.

This chapter addresses the clinical features, pathology, and experimental evidence on which our understanding of the pathogenesis and treatment of diabetic retinopathy are based.

Clinical Features of Diabetic Retinopathy

Classically, diabetic retinopathy is divided into three stages: background, preproliferative, and proliferative retinopathy; a fourth type of retinopathy, namely, maculopathy, is also recognized. It may coexist with any of the other stages and is the most frequent single cause of diabetes-related blindness.

In type I diabetes, retinopathy is uncommon within the first 5 years, but the incidence rises rapidly thereafter to around 90% after 15 years.[3] Recent studies have shown that the onset and progression of retinopathy may be retarded by tight diabetic control,[4–6] although this may be associated with a transient worsening of retinopathy if improved control is rapidly imposed.[7] Because the exact onset of type II diabetes is more difficult to define, retinopathy appears to occur earlier and may even be present at diagnosis.

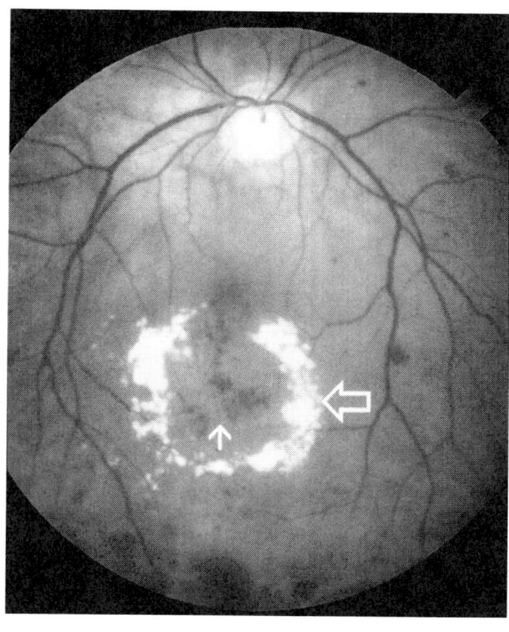

FIGURE 80-1. Fundus photograph showing a circinate hard exudate (↑) due to focal leakage from a cluster of microaneurysms (←). (See Color Fig. 80-1.)

Background Retinopathy

Microaneurysms are the earliest clinically visible structural manifestation of background diabetic retinopathy. When small, they may be evident only on fluorescein angiography, but as they enlarge, they appear as red dots. These represent focal saccular dilatations of retinal capillaries in the patent vascular bed adjacent to or surrounded by zones of capillary nonperfusion. Typically, microaneurysms gradually enlarge and then regress due to thickening of the vessel wall, followed by occlusion of the vascular lumen. Microaneurysms may bleed, causing small retinal hemorrhages ("blots"), or may allow focal leakage of lipoproteins, fibrinogen, and other proteins into the retina. These accumulate in the outer and inner plexiform layers of the retina as hard exudates (Fig. 80-1), often in a ring, or circinate, pattern.

There may also be a more generalized dilatation of the retinal vascular bed, in association with breakdown of the inner blood-retinal barrier, leading to retinal edema and thickening. This may involve the macula, resulting in diffuse macular edema, in contrast to the focal edema surrounding microaneurysms. Retinal capillary dilatation is inevitably associated with a variable amount of adjacent capillary closure and microaneurysm development, indicating that ischemia and edema always coexist to some degree.

Capillary nonperfusion is most easily demonstrated by fluorescein angiography (Fig. 80-2). The region surrounding the macula (the perifoveal capillary arcade) may be preferentially involved, but as there is considerable variation in the size of the foveal avascular zone in both normal persons and diabetic persons with normal vision, the assessment of macular ischemia can prove difficult.

Preproliferative Retinopathy

Increasing retinal ischemia due to capillary nonperfusion is responsible for the clinical features of this phase. Intraretinal microvascular abnormalities can result from significant vascular occlusion and may also leak, causing retinal edema. Retinal arteriolar occlusion leads to more severe retinal ischemia or infarction with impaired axoplasmic flow in retinal neurons, as manifested by cotton-wool spots, larger, dark-colored intraretinal hemorrhages, irregular or beaded veins (see Fig. 80-2), and venous "omega"

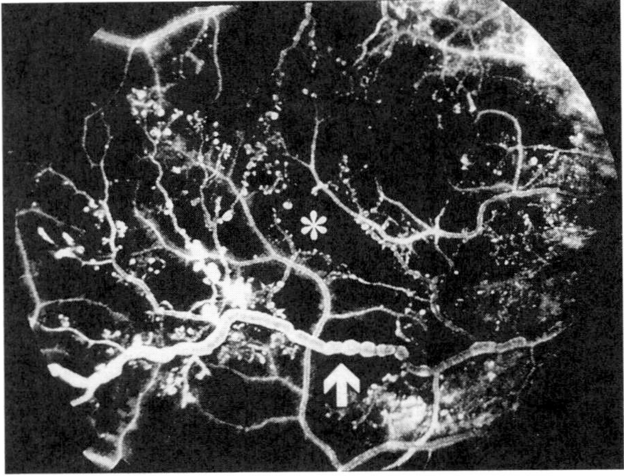

Figure 80-2. Fluorescein angiogram showing retinal capillary closure (*) and retinal venous beading (↑). (See Color Fig. 80-2.)

loop formation. This preproliferative phase of diabetic retinopathy will lead to proliferative disease within 15 months in about 50% of cases.

Proliferative Retinopathy

Proliferative diabetic retinopathy is defined as the presence of newly formed blood vessels and/or fibrous tissue arising from the retina or optic disc and extending along the inner surface or into the vitreous cavity. New vessels develop from retinal veins and may occur on the optic disc or elsewhere in the retina, but the majority occur within 45° of or on the optic disc. Early in their development, new vessels are very fine in diameter, but with growth their caliber increases and they frequently form networks resembling the spokes of a wheel (Fig. 80-3). The rate of growth of new vessels is extremely variable; the outgrowth of new vessels is usually accompanied by fibrous tissue that initially may be translucent but later appears white.

At first, the new blood vessels and fibrous tissue grow along the surface of the retina adhering to the posterior vitreous surface. When the vitreous detaches from the retina, hemorrhage may occur into or behind the vitreous (subhyaloid) due to traction on the new vessels. The subsequent reparative response and contraction of fibrovascular tissue can result in the retina's being pulled forward, causing traction retinal detachment.

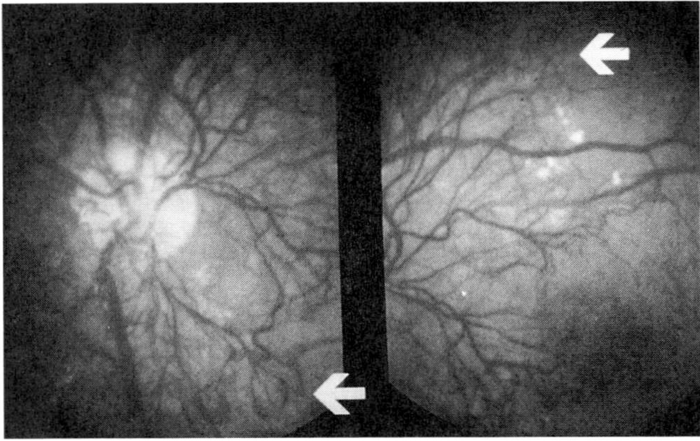

Figure 80-3. Fundus photograph showing extensive sheets of new vessels emanating from the optic disk (←). (See Color Fig. 80-3.)

Maculopathy

The classification of diabetic maculopathy into three types—focal edema, diffuse edema, and ischemic maculopathy—has enhanced our understanding of the natural history of maculopathy and helped determine the most appropriate treatment for each type.[8] The three groups are not mutually exclusive, however; they may occur together and contribute to visual impairment.

Treatment

Laser retinal photocoagulation[9–13] is the principal treatment for proliferative retinopathy and maculopathy. Localized leakage from microaneurysms threatening the macula can be treated by applying focal laser burns to and around the microaneurysm(s). Diffuse macular edema may respond to a wider application of low-intensity burns scattered over the macula, avoiding the fovea, a process known as *macular grid photocoagulation.* The exact mechanism by which this helps is unknown.

Proliferative retinopathy is treated by ablation of ischemic areas of the retina by more widespread laser therapy (*panretinal photocoagulation*). This will normally lead to regression of new vessels, although the amount of laser treatment required is quite variable. Unfortunately, the fibrous tissue associated with the new vessels may continue to contract and threaten vision. Vitreous hemorrhage may resolve spontaneously or may require surgical removal (*vitrectomy*). Traction retinal detachments or retinal surface membranes usually require an internal surgical approach for their removal to allow the retina to flatten.

Although laser photocoagulation is currently the mainstay of treatment for diabetic retinopathy, it is essentially a destructive tool that can lead to reduced retinal sensitivity and restriction of the visual field. As these changes in the retina are essentially irreversible, the primary goal in the management of diabetic retinopathy should be to prevent the occurrence of these devastating complications.

The Histopathology of Diabetic Retinopathy

The histopathology of diabetic retinopathy has been a subject of great interest and some controversy for over 30 years.[14,15] Three different stages are recognized according to the state of the retinal vasculature[14]: nonproliferative (background), preproliferative (advanced nonproliferative), and proliferative. Structural changes within the retinal microvessels are discernible clinically, and secondary functional pathology such as vessel occlusion, increased vessel permeability (leakiness), and rupture with hemorrhage lead to loss of vision. None of the abnormalities to be described below are entirely specific to diabetic retinopathy, similar changes being found in several conditions associated with retinal hypoxia. The pathologic abnormalities to be described, however, are often found in their most extreme form in patients with diabetes.

Nonproliferative and Preproliferative Diabetic Retinopathy

All levels of the vascular tree may ultimately become involved, but the earliest changes seem to take place in the capillary bed. Vascular basement membrane is a thin layer of proteinaceous mate-

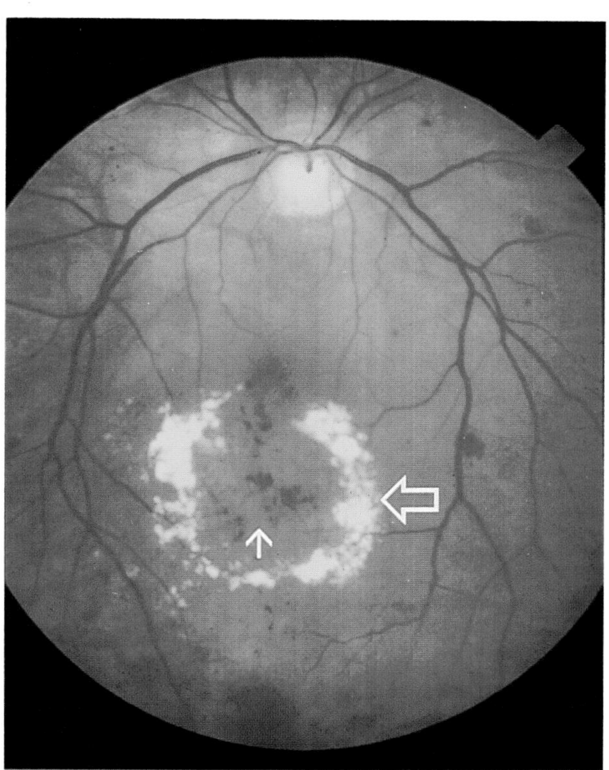

COLOR FIGURE **80-1.** Fundus photograph showing a circinate hard exudate (↑) due to focal leakage from a cluster of microaneurysms (←).

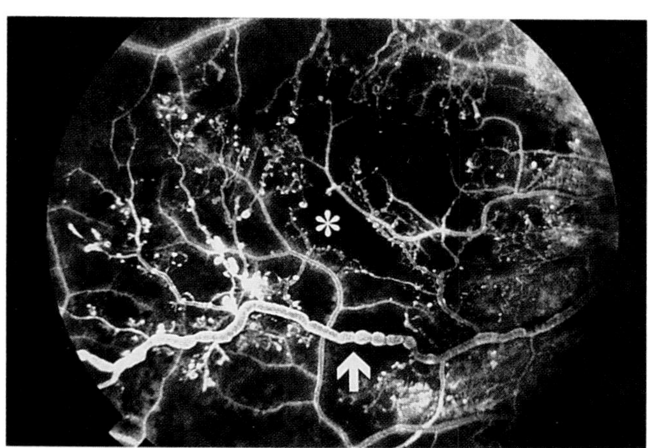

COLOR FIGURE **80-2.** Fluorescein angiogram showing retinal capillary closure (∗) and retinal venous beading (↑).

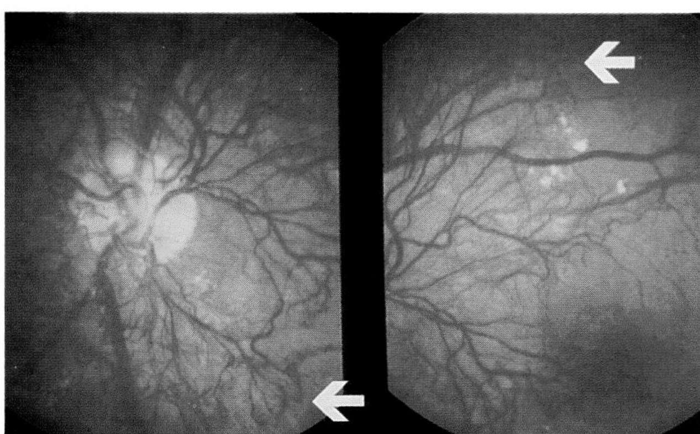

COLOR FIGURE **80-3.** Fundus photograph showing extensive sheets of new vessels emanating from the optic disk (←).

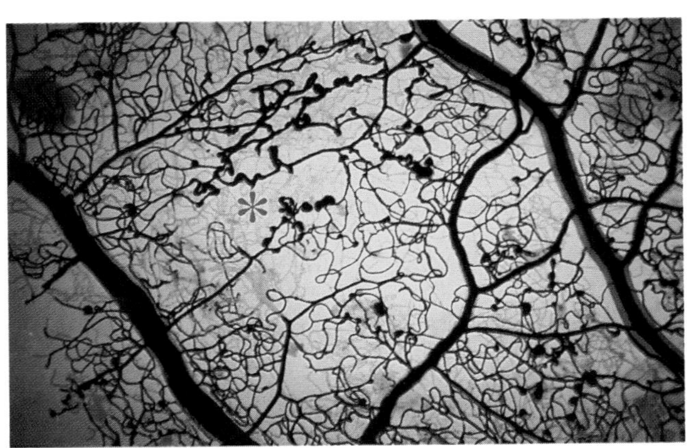

COLOR FIGURE 80-4. Low-power photomicrograph of a whole mount preparation of retina in which patent blood vessels are demonstrated by India ink injection. Note the area of nonperfusion (*), where the vessels are faint pink (not black), with nearby venous dilatation and microaneurysm formation. The microaneurysms are the small, round black swellings.

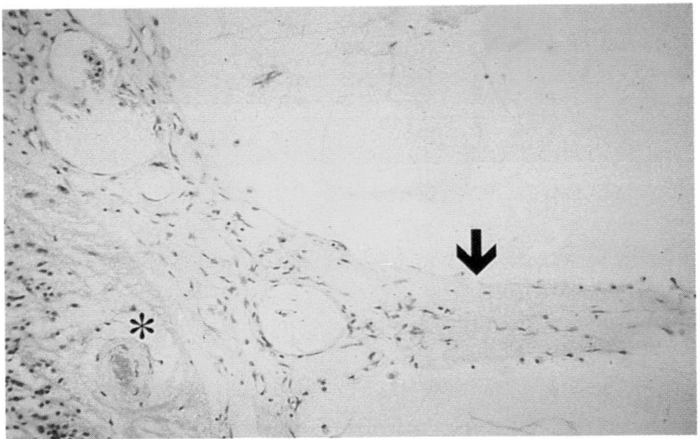

COLOR FIGURE 80-5. Medium-power photomicrograph showing the retina (bottom lefthand corner) with an arteriole with hyaline thickening of its wall (*). To the right of the retina is a fibrovascular membrane with large, thin-walled vessels that has a strand that has been pulled forward into the vitreous space (↓).

rial that separates the endothelial lining of blood vessels from the surrounding tissue and traps flattened cells known as *pericytes* that lie just external to the endothelium. Early in diabetic eye disease there is thickening of intraocular basement membranes at several sites, including around capillaries. The basement membrane may reach five times its normal thickness. Increased production of basement membrane proteins contributes to this increase in thickness, but accumulation of plasma proteins and alterations of protein turnover as a consequence of their nonenzymatic glycosylation are potentially also of importance. Another important change is the preferential loss of pericytes. Particularly in areas where there is pericyte loss, small focal dilatations of the capillaries (microaneurysms) form, either singly or in clusters. Pericytes are structurally similar to smooth muscle cells and lie in an analogous position in the smooth muscle of arterioles and venules. They may well have a structural role in resisting capillary intraluminal pressure, and their loss might be expected to lead to microaneurysm formation (Fig. 80-4). Other factors of potential importance in the development of microaneurysms are venous stasis and focal proliferation of endothelial cells leading to a focal bulge in the vessel wall. In some instances, microaneurysms appear to form from capillary loops that might be regarded as attempts at new-vessel formation.[15] Whether microaneurysms can truly resolve is unclear but apparent clinical resolution, at least in some instances, is a result of thrombosis of the aneurysmal lumen.[15]

There are two main complications of microaneurysms. The first is increased vessel permeability. This may also occur at other sites, particularly in the inner retina,[16] and is certainly a major feature of proliferative retinopathy (see below). The blood-retinal barriers normally keep plasma proteins out of the extracellular space of retinal tissue. Vessel leakage leads to the accumulation of protein/lipid-rich material (exudate) within the extracellular space that tends to follow the path of least resistance. The outer plexiform layer of the retina in the parafoveal region has a tangential arrangement of nerve fibers that are easily separated, and this is therefore a favored site of deposition. Thickening of this central portion of the retina is a major cause of visual loss in diabetic patients, and disturbed blood-retinal barrier function is likely to be a contributory factor. Swelling of Müller cells, one of the non-neuronal supporting cells of the retina, and their subsequent rupture to form cystic spaces, is an alternative or additional source of expanded extracellular space. Scavenging cells (macrophages) attempt, largely unsuccessfully, to clear this material back into the circulation.

The second complication of microaneurysm formation is hemorrhage due to rupture of the thinned vessel wall. The pattern of the hemorrhage depends on the organization of the extracellular space in the immediate vicinity. If blood extravasates in the innermost layer of the retina, which is composed mainly of nerve fibers running approximately parallel to one another, a flame- or splinter-shaped pattern results. In deeper layers (especially inner and outer plexiform layers and inner nuclear layers), more oval-shaped collections are formed. If they are large enough, hemorrhage from any layer can extend from the retina into the vitreous.

Occlusion of parts of the capillary bed is an important event, not only from the point of view of impaired local retinal function but also as a stimulant for other vascular changes. Microaneurysms often form around the edge of an area of poor perfusion, and retinal hypoxia secondary to any of several causes is a potent stimulus for new-vessel formation (Fig. 80-5). Small ischemic lesions of the nerve fiber layer of the retina interfere with the transport of proteins and organelles in both directions along the axons of the retinal ganglion cells that project, via the optic nerve, to the lateral geniculate nucleus of the brain. The resulting accumulation of intra-axonal material produces a cluster of axonal swellings that is clinically discernible as a cotton-wool spot. Each swollen axon resembles a cell, and somewhat confusingly, the term *cytoid bodies* has been applied to the histologic appearance of these lesions. There may be a transient associated disruption of the blood-retinal barrier, but the clinical term *soft exudate* is best avoided, as this is not the dominant pathologic process responsible for the appearances on fundoscopy.

Occlusive disease also affects terminal arterioles. In diabetes, hyalinization of arteriolar walls (see Fig. 80-5) occurs in many organs, and the retina is no exception. Associated narrowing of vessel lumina, especially at branch points, abnormalities of the endothelium, and a hypercoaguable state all predispose to thrombus formation. Areas of ischemic damage predominantly affect the inner retina and range in size from small focal lesions to extensive areas of atrophy.[17] Loss of ganglion cells may lead to areas of optic nerve atrophy.[17]

In advanced nonproliferative diabetic retinopathy (also known as *preproliferative retinopathy*), additional changes are present that are believed to be predictors of an increased likelihood of progression to proliferative disease. Vascular changes of significance include the formation of shunt vessels, dilated capillaries, venous beading, and intraretinal microvascular abnormalities, as

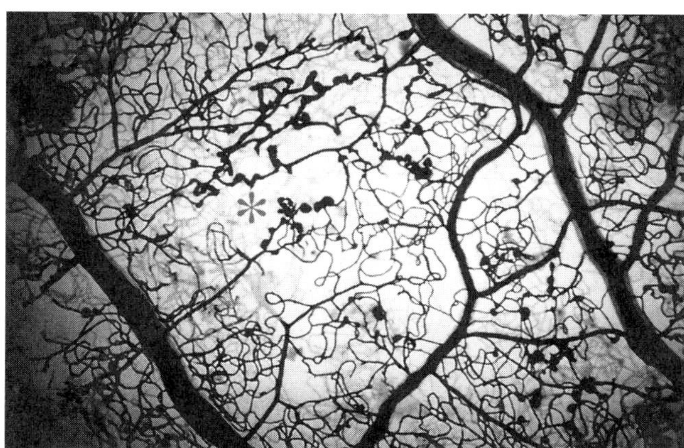

Figure 80-4. Low-power photomicrograph of a whole mount preparation of retina in which patent blood vessels are demonstrated by India ink injection. Note the area of nonperfusion (∗), where the vessels are faint pink (not black), with nearby venous dilatation and microaneurysm formation. The microaneurysms are the small, round black swellings. (See Color Fig. 80-4.)

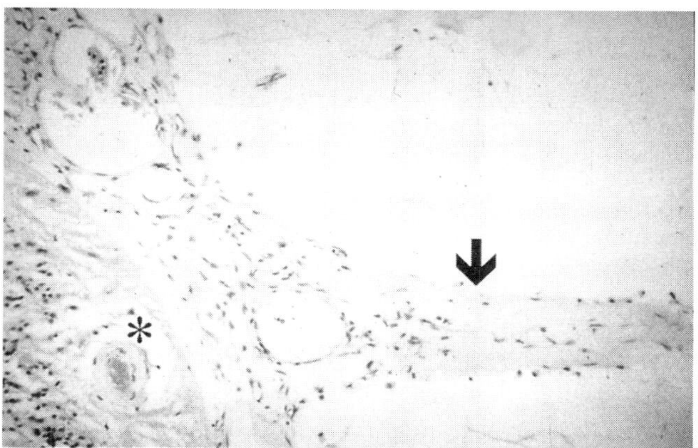

Figure 80-5. Medium-power photomicrograph showing the retina (bottom lefthand corner) with an arteriole with hyaline thickening of its wall (∗). To the right of the retina is a fibrovascular membrane with large, thin-walled vessels that has a strand that has been pulled forward into the vitreous space (↓). (See Color Fig. 80-5.)

well as abundant microaneurysms and extensive areas of impaired or lost perfusion. The appearances of some vessels in intraretinal microvascular abnormalities resemble those seen in surface proliferation and presumably have a similar pathogenesis. Unlike the former, however, these intraretinal vessels are not highly permeable.[18] This may be a consequence of the ability of glial components within the retina to induce a coherent system of tight junctions between adjacent endothelial cells. Pre-existing vessels become even more degenerate with loss of endothelial cells and pericytes and the formation of so-called ghost vessels.

Proliferative Diabetic Retinopathy

The critical event in proliferative retinopathy is the formation of new blood vessels anterior to the retina on its inner surface and within the vitreous (see Fig. 80-5). New vessels nearly always form from pre-existing veins, and the region of the optic disk is especially at risk, as there is no inner limiting membrane to act as a barrier to vessel growth, as there is elsewhere. Vessels then can grow over the retinal surface or into the substance of the vitreous. Traction on these fragile, newly formed vessels can lead to hemorrhage or can drag vessels farther forward. Tractional forces may be generated within the vitreous[19] or through contraction of the fibroglial tissue that becomes associated with the new blood vessels and forms epiretinal membranes. Diabetes is a predisposing factor for posterior vitreous detachment,[14] and it has been proposed that hyperglycemia-induced glycosylation changes in vitreous collagen may cause it to aggregate. Mild traction in the region of the macular may lead to distorted vision. Greater forces may lead to the formation of retinal cysts, slits between different layers (schisis), retinal detachment, and retinal tears.[14]

In conclusion, the histopathologic changes of diabetic retinopathy are primarily those of retinal hypoxia and its complications. Areas of poor or absent perfusion are often associated with microaneurysms and new-vessel formation, both of which may lead to sight-threatening hemorrhage. Macular edema and epiretinal membrane formation with possible retinal detachment also represent major causes of blindness in diabetic patients.

Experimental Evidence for Involvement of Biochemical Pathways

The cause of diabetic complications in humans is still an open question. Because hyperglycemia is the most common feature of diabetes, a number of studies have been conducted to investigate the possible relationship between hyperglycemia and the development of retinopathy. Pirart's pioneer study[20] reported that the annual prevalence and incidence of retinopathy in patients with type I and type II diabetes whose blood glucose concentrations were poorly controlled were much higher than those with good control over 25 years. The contributory effect of hyperglycemia to and the preventive effects of improved glycemic control on the onset and progression of retinopathy in type I diabetes have been confirmed by the well-designed 10-year multicenter Diabetes Control and Complications Trial study.[5] Over the past three decades, various biochemical mechanisms have been proposed to explain the adverse effects of hyperglycemia on the retina in patients with diabetes. These hypotheses are discussed separately in the following sections.

Polyol Pathway Metabolism

Aldose reductase (AR) and sorbitol dehydrogenase are the enzymes that constitute the polyol pathway. In this pathway, AR, utilizing reduced nicotinamide-adenine dinucleotide phosphate, reduces the aldehyde form of glucose or galactose to sorbitol or galactitol, respectively; galactose is a better substrate for AR than glucose. Sorbitol, but not galactitol, is metabolized to fructose by sorbitol dehydrogenase. When glucose concentrations are normal, intracellular sorbitol concentrations are very low due to the low affinity of AR for glucose. The polyol pathway, however, may play an important physiologic role in maintaining osmotic balance across the cellular membranes, particular in the kidney, as AR activity can also be regulated by osmotic pressure of the extracellular milieu.

Possible mechanisms that can cause cellular pathology in the eye by activating the polyol pathway were indicated in the studies of diabetic and galactosemic cataracts in animals. Van Heyningen[21] initially induced experimental cataracts in animals by raising the plasma concentration of aldose sugar, and demonstrated that the accumulation of polyol in the lens was directly related to the rapidity with which cataract develops. Kinoshita and coworkers[22] further proposed that the accumulation of polyols initiates the development of cataracts through an osmotic process. The osmotic hypothesis suggests that the activity of AR, which converts sugar to its polyol, is increased in hyperglycemic conditions. As the cell membranes are relatively impermeable to polyols, sorbitol or galactitol accumulates to high levels, resulting in a hypertonic intracellular state. This leads to an influx of water into the cell, with resultant cellular edema, changes of intracellular redox states, metabolic dysfunction such as depletion of intracellular myoinositol, and eventual cell death.

The role of the polyol pathway in the development of diabetic retinopathy has been studied intensively in recent years (see Chapter 89). Firstly, numerous studies have demonstrated that AR is expressed in the retina, particularly in retinal capillary pericytes, retinal pigment epithelium (RPE), and retinal endothelium in human, dogs, and rats. In vitro, AR is detectable in cultured human and bovine retinal pericytes, human RPE cells, and rat retinal endothelial cells.

Secondly, both AR expression and sorbitol concentrations are elevated and associated with retinal dysfunction and metabolic disorder in hyperglycemia. Vinores et al.[23] reported that AR was immunohistochemically undetectable in RPE of nondiabetic human eyes. AR, however, was detected in the RPE of 55% of diabetic patients with background retinopathy and 87.5% with proliferative retinopathy.[23] In diabetic BB rats, both AR activity and AR mRNA in retina and other tissues were increased. Intensive insulin treatment, which normalized blood glucose, significantly reversed these changes.[24] AR mRNA is upregulated under hyperglycemic conditions in cultured human RPE cells[25] and rat retinal endothelial cells (Jiang and Lightman, unpublished data). It has been reported that intracellular sorbitol concentrations were increased in these cells exposed to high concentrations of glucose. The increase in sorbitol concentrations was accompanied by a concomitant decrease in Na^+-K^+-ATPase activity but not by changes in intracellular levels of myoinositol, and these changes were prevented by inhibition of AR activity in cultured retinal endothelial cells exposed to high glucose concentrations.[26] In cultured RPE cells, depletion of myoinositol was associated with increased intracellular polyol levels and prevented by an AR inhibitor.[27]

Thirdly, histopathologic features of human diabetic retinopathy have been demonstrated in galactose-fed animals. Interestingly, these diabetic-like changes can be prevented by administration of AR inhibitors. It was reported that rats fed a diet high in galactose (50%) for 6 months developed retinal capillary basement membrane thickening, which was prevented by simultaneously feeding them the AR inhibitors Sorbinil or Tolrestat.[28] Early blood-retinal barrier breakdown has also been reported in rats fed galactose for 2.5 months. Inhibition of AR by Sorbinil also prevented the permeability changes in the blood-retinal barrier of galactosemic rats.[29] Long-term galactosemia (28 months) in rats induced retinal angiopathy identical to that occurring in patients with diabetes, including pericyte degeneration, endothelial cell proliferation, acellularity, capillary dilation, and microaneurysm formation. Inhibition of AR by

Tolrestat also prevented these retinal abnormalities.[30] Dogs fed galactose for up to 66 months developed diabetic-like preproliferative and proliferative retinal changes, including the appearance of broad areas of nonperfusion, cotton-wool spots, occluded arterioles, preretinal and intravitreal hemorrhages, and new-vessel growth.[31] In addition, the potential role of AR in the development of diabetic retinopathy has been further implicated by a recently reported study in which transgenic mice overexpressing AR developed occlusion of retinochoroidal vessels after fed a galactose diet for 1 week.[32]

Finally, there are a number of clinical studies supporting the view that activation of the polyol pathway may be associated with the development of diabetic retinopathy. For example, based on a 3-year study, epalrestat (an AR inhibitor) prevented the progression of diabetic retinopathy, including reduction or disappearance of microaneurysms, hemorrhage, and cotton-wool spots.[33]

Controversy remains, however, over the role of the polyol pathway in the development of diabetic retinopathy in humans. Although the polyol pathway may be responsible in part for diabetic cataract and possibly diabetic neuropathy, it is argued that the intracellular concentrations of sorbitol in other ocular tissues, such as retina, may not become high enough to produce significant changes in osmolarity. Activation of the polyol pathway in the diabetic retina, however, may result in other metabolic disorders, such as changes in redox states due to the consumption of nicotinamide-adenine dinucleotide phosphate, and thus may contribute in this way to retinal cell dysfunction. In contrast to the results reported by groups led by Robison[30] and Kador[31] in experimental diabetic or galactosemic animals, Engerman and Kern[34] found that Sorbinil, given for up to 5 years at a dose that prevented elevation of polyols in retina and erythrocytes, had no significant effect on the development of retinopathy in both diabetic and galactosemic dogs. The same group also reported that myoinositol concentrations in the retinas of diabetic and galactosemic dogs were higher, not lower, than those of the normal controls and were not altered by the administration of an AR inhibitor.[35] Furthermore, in a multicenter randomized clinical study involving 497 type I diabetic patients, treatment with Sorbinil for 41 months failed to show significant clinical improvement in retinopathy, although AR inhibition slightly slowed the rate of microaneurysm formation.[36] It is difficult to understand why some studies have demonstrated a beneficial effect of AR inhibition on diabetic and/or galactosemic retinopathy, whereas others have failed to do so. One possible explanation is that the degree of AR inhibition may be different with different AR inhibitors at different doses for different durations in those studies. Other pharmacologic activities (such as antioxidant activity) of some AR inhibitors may also contribute to the different results of those compounds on retinopathy in patients with diabetes and in animal models. Nevertheless, it is also possible that, based on those contradictory results referred to above, there may be other biochemical mechanisms contributing to the development of diabetic retinopathy.

Nonenzymatic Glycosylation

Nonenzymatic glycosylation (glycation) is a modification of macromolecules (proteins and DNA), occurring initially with the formation of a Schiff base intermediate between sugars in the open chain form and amine groups on protein or DNA, followed by the formation of the ketoamine (fructoselysine) by an Amadori rearrangement (see Chapter 90). The early glycated molecules (Amadori product) subsequently degrade into α-ketoaldehyde compounds such as 3-deoxyglucosone. These secondary compounds are more reactive than the parent monosaccharide and can react with proteins or DNA to form covalent adducts and cross-links called *advanced glycation end products* (*AGEs*).

The formation of AGEs in extracellular proteins may contribute to the capillary basement membrane thickening and vessel occlusion in diabetes. First, advanced protein glycation of matrix components alters their structure and functional properties.[37] For example, glucose-derived AGEs on collagen form heat-stable intermolecular cross-links and are resistant to proteolytic degradation. Advanced glycation of laminin causes decreased binding of heparin sulfate proteoglycan, a growth-regulating molecule. This may be responsible for the loss of immunoreactivity to heparin sulfate proteoglycan in diabetic retinas. Theoretically, the lack of heparin sulfate proteoglycan could stimulate the synthesis of other matrix components in diabetic retina. In addition, extensively glycated low density lipoproteins are poorly recognized by fibroblasts and preferentially accumulated by macrophages.[38]

AGEs could also alter cellular function by binding to AGE-specific receptors on macrophages and vascular endothelial cells.[37] Interaction between AGE protein and macrophages induces production of tumor necrosis factor, interleukin-1, and insulin-like growth factor 1 (IGF-1). These AGE-induced cytokines can promote growth responses in various cells and collagen synthesis. When AGE protein binds to its endothelial cell receptor, it enhances cellular oxidative stress, resulting in increased endothelial monolayer permeability and induction of procoagulatory activity on the endothelial cell surface. These findings indicate that AGE-receptor interactions could potentially contribute to the vascular lesions seen in chronic hyperglycemia.

Modification of intracellular macromolecules (proteins and DNA) by sugars may alter their physiologic functions. In vitro, AGEs induce DNA strand breakage, base modification, and transposition in plasmid DNA,[39] suggesting that AGEs may affect gene transcription. Glycated hemoglobin in erythrocytes has greater affinity for oxygen than normal, and it has been suggested that oxygen release to the tissues in diabetics may be reduced due to hemoglobin glycation.[40] Measurable AGE on hemoglobin in erythrocytes is increased in diabetic subjects. Glycated superoxide dismutase (SOD) in erythrocytes loses activity in vitro, and the increase in SOD glycation is strongly associated with the decreased activity in erythrocytes of patients with diabetes.[41]

In addition, a link between glycation and some diabetic-like vascular pathologic features has been demonstrated by injecting AGE-modified albumin into normal rats and rabbits.[42] These pathologic changes include an increase in vascular permeability, the activation of mononuclear cell migration across vascular walls, and impaired endothelium-dependent vasodilation.

Although most of the pathophysiologic role of glycation noted above is observed in studies using cells or tissues outside the retina, diabetic retinopathy changes in STZ-diabetic rats were also prevented by treatment with aminoguanidine,[43] an inhibitor of advanced glycosylation end product formation. After 26 weeks of treatment, aminoguanidine prevented endothelial cell proliferation and significantly decreased pericyte dropout in the retinas of diabetic rats. Aminoguanidine treatment for 75 weeks also significantly reduced the number of acellular capillaries and completely inhibited the formation of microaneurysms.

A number of clinical studies have focused on the relationship between AGE accumulation and diabetes, including patients with retinopathy. Sell et al.[44] reported that pentosidine concentrations were significantly elevated in skin collagen and serum from type I diabetics compared to control subjects, and collagen pentosidine concentrations correlated with the severity of diabetic retinopathy.[44] McCance et al.[45] measured collagen AGEs, including pentosidine and carboxymethyllysine, collagen-linked fluorescence, and fructoselysine (the initial glycation product) in the samples from type I diabetics and nondiabetic control subjects. The concentrations of these glycation products in collagen from diabetics increased progressively and significantly with the severity of retinopathy. Using anti-AGE-ribonuclease antisera to detect AGEs, it was found that the concentration of AGEs in serum from patients with diabetes was increased compared with those from normal subjects.[46]

Taken as a whole, the evidence suggests that glycation plays a role in some of the functional and structural changes observed in diabetic complications in general and in retinopathy in particular. Concerning the pathogenic role of glycation in diabetic retinopathy, however, some questions remain to be answered. Firstly, there is no evidence to date suggesting that AGEs concentrations are increased in the retinas of diabetic animals and that there is any correlation with the development of retinopathy. The direct effect of infusion of isolated AGEs on retinal vessels is unknown. Secondly, aminoguanidine is a compound with several different pharmacologic activities, including inhibition of advanced protein glycation, nitric oxide synthetase, and AR activities. It is possible that these different pharmacologic mechanisms may be involved in the inhibitory effect of aminoguanidine in the development of retinopathy in diabetic rats. Finally, clinical trials are needed to evaluate the potential of aminoguanidine in the treatment of diabetic retinopathy.

Oxidative Stress

Oxidative stress may be defined as increased reactive oxygen species in biologic systems, with consequent tissue damage. Glucose autoxidation and nonenzymatic protein glycation may be the source of reactive oxygen species that can initiate oxidative tissue damage in diabetes. Glucose is prone to transition metal–catalyzed autoxidation with the formation of O_2-., H_2O_2, and HO·.[47] Monosaccharides, such as glucose, can enolize and therefore reduce transition metal and molecular oxygen, yielding O_2-., whose dismutation forms H_2O_2 spontaneously. The latter can be further decomposed into HO·, a process catalyzed by transition metal ions such as copper and iron. Experiments in vitro show that glucose incubated with protein undergoes a similar process, with the formation of O_2-., H_2O_2, HO·, and dicarbonyls (α-ketoaldehyde). The latter is more reactive to protein, with the formation of ketoimine adducts. The on-site–formed HO· can attack protein attached to glucose and induce site-specific damage, including the oxidation of amino acids, the generation of flurophore (protein browning), and the fragmentation of protein. Thus, the term *autoxidative glycation* was introduced to describe the process of oxidative modification of protein by high glucose concentrations.

In addition, glycated proteins may serve as a source of oxygen radicals. It has been reported that the Amadori adduct of protein glycation is able to oxidize in the presence of oxygen and transition metals, leading to the formation of O_2-., the release of erythronic acid, and the products of oxidative cleavage of the glycated protein, that is, carboxymethylysine, carboxymethylhydroxylysine, and pentosidine. These compounds were termed *glycoxidation products* and were used as the biomarker of glucose-dependent protein damage.[48] It is interesting to note that the concentrations of carboxymethylysine and pentosidine were significantly elevated in patients with diabetic retinopathy, indicating an increase in oxidative protein damage by glycoxidation. Glycated protein or Amadori adducts also stimulate the peroxidation of lipids, causing oxidative damage to amine groups with subsequent fragmentation of protein.

Much of the evidence concerning a role for oxidative stress in the development of retinopathy comes from investigations comparing lipid peroxidation products in plasma and tissues from diabetics and age-matched controls. A possible association between diabetic retinopathy and oxidative activity is also suggested by studies of Uzel et al.,[49] which demonstrated significantly increased plasma lipid peroxide concentrations in type II diabetic patients with retinopathy compared to patients without retinopathy. More recently, Augustin et al.[50] reported that the concentration of malondialdehyde, the end product of lipid peroxidation, in the vitreous was elevated in patients with proliferative diabetic retinopathy (PDR) in comparison with patients with retinal detachment uncomplicated by proliferative vitreoretinopathy. The increase in lipid peroxidation in diabetic patients is also consistent with work on diabetic animals. In STZ-diabetic rats, the concentration of retinal and kidney lipid peroxides was increased about twofold,[51] was associated with a decrease in the concentration of lipid soluble antioxidants, and was inhibited by insulin treatment.

Oxidative tissue damage may also result from a decrease in antioxidant systems, including antioxidant enzymes and chemical antioxidants. Some evidence suggests alternations in the activity of tissue superoxide dismutase (SOD) in both experimental and clinical diabetes. It has been reported that Cu-Zn SOD activity is decreased in erythrocytes and retinas from STZ-diabetic rats.[52] Erythrocyte SOD activity was also reduced in both type I and type II patients with diabetes compared to normal controls.[53] It was reported that the percentage of the glycated form of Cu-Zn SOD, which has lower enzymatic activity, was significantly increased in erythrocytes of patients with diabetes compared to erythrocytes in normal subjects.[41] There have been a number of reports about the activity changes in other antioxidant enzymes, such as catalase and glutathione peroxidase, in experimental and clinical diabetes. The results to date are inconsistent and contradictory. Detailed discussion of these changes is beyond the scope of this chapter.

Chemical antioxidants such as glutathione, ascorbate, and vitamin E are also altered in experimental and human diabetes. Serum glutathione concentrations in type I and type II diabetic patients were lowered.[54] Erythrocyte concentrations of glutathione and glutathione peroxidase in erythrocyte membranes were also decreased 10–20% in type II diabetes, concomitant with a 40% increase in lipid peroxide; these changes were more significant in patients with retinopathy.[49] Plasma concentrations of ascorbic acid, a key aqueous-phase chain-breaking antioxidant, were decreased in both human and animal diabetes. At the same time, there was an increase in the dehydroascorbate : ascorbate ratio.[55] Likewise, the concentration of vitamin E, a lipophilic free radical scavenger, was significantly decreased in platelets of patients with type II diabetes, especially those with retinopathy, when compared to normal subjects.[56]

Diacylglycerol and Protein Kinase C

Protein kinase C (PKC) is a regulatory enzyme involved in a variety of cellular functions, including hormone and growth factor receptor turnover, DNA synthesis, vascular permeability, and vascular contractility. As noted above, polyol pathway activation may result in depletion of intracellular myoinositol and the consequent decrease of phosphoinositide-derived diacylglycerol (DAG), an endogenous activator of PKC. Therefore, it has been proposed that altered sorbitol and myoinositol metabolism are the biochemical basis for the decrease in PKC activity and the defective regulation of Na-K-ATPase observed in diabetic neuropathy.[57] It has been demonstrated, however, that membrane PKC activities are increased, rather than decreased, in retinal endothelial cells exposed to high-glucose or high-galactose conditions in vitro and in retinas of diabetic or galactosemic animals.[57,58] Interestingly, this increase in PKC activity is associated with the increase in intracellular concentrations of DAG,[58–60] a physiologic activator of PKC. Although the increase in sorbitol formation and the decrease in Na-K-ATPase activity in retinal endothelial cells exposed to high glucose concentrations are reversed by Sorbinil,[26] this AR inhibitor has no effect on the elevated concentrations of DAG and the increase in PKC activities in retinal endothelial cells when cultured in hyperglycemic conditions.[26,59] Thus, it is suggested that the increased PKC activity is induced by hyperglycemia via de novo synthesis of DAG, independent of polyol pathway activity. It has been shown recently that the glucose-induced activation of PKC leads to activation of cytosolic phospholipase A_2 ($cPLA_2$), which then mobilizes arachidonic acid, resulting in the inhibition of Na^+-K^+-ATPase in cultured vascular cells.[60] Activation of PKC by the vitreous injection of phorbol dibutyrate mimics the prolonged retinal blood circulation time observed in diabetic rats,[61] further implicating PKC activation in diabetic retinopathy. In addition, in diabetic animals,

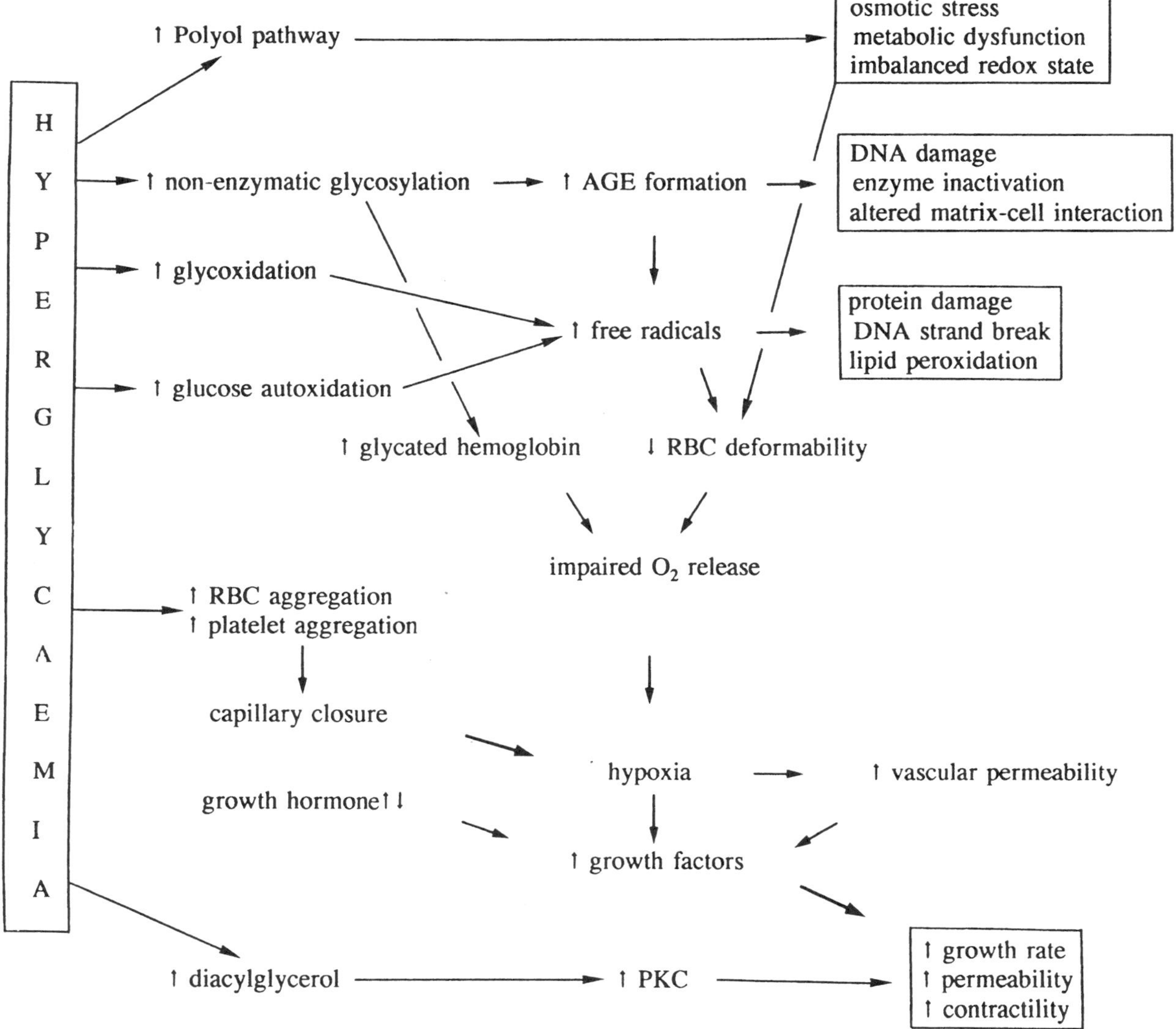

Figure 80-6. Biochemical mechanisms potentially involved in the development of diabetic retinopathy.

increased activity of the DAG-PKC pathway has been observed in many other vascular tissues such as aorta, heart, and renal glomeruli,[62,63] suggesting broad involvement of this pathway.

Hypoxia and Growth Factors

New-vessel formation on the surface of the retina, into the vitreous or at the optic disc, is found in PDR. Michaelson in 1948[64] first proposed that a diffusible "chemical factor" in retina stimulated retinal neovascularization. It is well known that preretinal neovascularization follows retinal capillary nonperfusion and inner retinal ischemia under diabetic conditions.[65] Later, it was proposed that retinal ischemia provides the stimulus for the release of an antigenic factor via an unknown mechanism.[66] In addition to retinal capillary nonperfusion resulting from capillary closure, impaired release of oxygen to the tissue from red blood cells in chronic hyperglycemia may lead to the development of retinal hypoxia, as glycated hemoglobin results in decreased dissociation of oxygen from the protein.[40] The deformability of red blood cells may also be reduced as the consequence of cellular membrane damage by glycation of membrane proteins or by free radical–induced lipid peroxidation and protein cross-linking.

In vitro studies have demonstrated that the proliferative ability of retinal endothelial cells and pericytes is upregulated by low oxygen tension in the culture medium.[67] Although the precise mechanism by which hypoxia regulates cell proliferation has yet to be elucidated, a number of studies have demonstrated the potential link between hypoxia and the expression of growth-regulating factors (see Chapters 92 and 94). Firstly, vascular endothelial growth factor (VGEF) mRNA concentrations are dramatically increased after exposing cultured cells to hypoxia.[68] Secondly, hypoxia induces the expression of growth factor receptors, such as those for VEGF and basic fibroblast growth factor (bFGF) and therefore may also activate cellular responsiveness to exogenous growth factors. Finally, hypoxia may induce venous dilatation and increase the permeability of the retinal vasculature, facilitating the release of growth factors, which, in turn, stimulate vasoproliferation in the diabetic retina.

A number of mitogenic and angiogenic factors in the eyes of diabetic patients and animal models have been studied. Both aFGF and bFGF (protein and mRNA) have been localized in various cells of the normal retina. The distribution of FGF is altered in the diabetic retina, however, and bFGF is present in the basement membrane of proliferative diabetic fronds and is increased in the vitreous of patients with PDR. It was proposed that ischemic tissue damage causes local release of FGFs, which bind to heparin in the basement matrix of retinal vessels. FGF may then act in a paracrine manner on neighboring retinal endothelial cells. The FGF receptor is also expressed in the inner retinal layer of the retina, and in vitro, bFGF stimulates the proliferation of endothelial cells. Recently, it was reported that intravitreal injection of bFGF affected retinal vessels in rabbits, causing rapid disruption of the blood-retinal barrier and neovascularization such as is seen in PDR.[69]

The insulin-like growth factors (IGFs) are thought to mediate the growth-stimulating effect of growth hormone. The latter is elevated in diabetics with poor metabolic control and may play a role in the development of diabetic retinopathy. It was reported that IGF-I, but not IGF-II, was increased in serum and vitreous from patients with PDR.[70] The vitreous concentrations of IGF-binding proteins, which regulate the bioavailability of these potent growth factors, were also increased in patients with diabetic retinopathy and diabetic animal models.[70] To our knowledge, the expression of IGFs in retinal cells has not been demonstrated. IGF receptors are found on retinal capillary endothelial cells and pericytes, however, and both types of cells respond to IGF-I with increased DNA synthesis. Intravitreal injection of IGF-1 also induced PDR-like vessel changes in the rabbit retina.[69] It has been suggested that IGFs produced systemically, rather than in the eye, may contribute to new-vessel formation in the diabetic retina.

VEGF is a secreted endothelial cell–specific angiogenic and vasopermeability factor. It is also present in normal human retina. In hypoxic conditions, VEGF mRNA is upregulated in retinal pericytes, retinal endothelial cells, and retinal pigment epithelial cells. Recently, two independent studies reported impressive evidence implicating elevated intraocular concentrations of VEGF with active neovascularization in PDR.[71,72] It is also interesting to note that vitreous samples from patients with active PDR stimulate the growth of retinal endothelial cells and that this in vitro stimulation is reduced by more than 65% by anti-VEGF antibody. This incomplete inhibition may suggest that there are simultaneous growth-stimulatory activity by other factors, such as bFGF and IGFs.

Conclusion

Retinopathy is a worldwide cause of blindness in the diabetic population, and new therapeutic agents are desperately needed for its prevention and treatment. Hyperglycemia is a major risk factor for its development, and it seems that multiple biochemical mechanisms could potentially be involved in its pathogenesis (Fig. 80-6). Further understanding of the mechanisms described above are necessary to aid the design of safe and effective pharmaceutical agents to prevent or interrupt these pathophysiologic changes, and it is possible that a polypharmacologic approach may be required.

References

1. The incidence and causes of blindness in England and Wales 1963–1968. In: Reports on Public Health and Medical Subjects, No. 28. London: Her Majesty's Stationary Office; 1972
2. National Diabetes Data Group. Diabetes in America: Diabetes data compiled 1984. (NIH Publication No. 85-1468). Bethesda, Md.: National Institutes of Health, 1985
3. Palmberg P, Smith M, Waltman S, et al. The natural history of retinopathy in insulin dependent juvenile onset diabetes. Ophthalmology 1981;88:613
4. Kroc Collaborative Study Group. Blood glucose control and the evolution of diabetic retinopathy and albuminuria: A preliminary multicenter trial. N Engl J Med 1984;311:365
5. The Diabetes Control and Complications Trial Research Group. The effect of intensive treatment of diabetes on the development and progression of long-term complications in insulin-dependent diabetes mellitus. N Engl J Med 1993;329:977
6. Reichard P, Nilsson B-Y, Rosenqvist U. The effect of long-term intensified insulin treatment on the development of microvascular complications of diabetes mellitus. N Engl J Med 1993;329:304
7. Dahl-Jorgensen K, Brinchmann-Hansen O, Hanssen KF, et al. Rapid tightening of blood glucose control leads to transient deterioration of retinopathy in insulin dependent diabetes mellitus. Br Med J 1985;290:811
8. Whitelocke RA, Kearns M, Blach RK, Hamilton AM. The diabetic maculopathies. Trans Ophthalmol Soc UK 1979;99:314
9. Meyer-Schwickerath GRE, Schott K. Diabetic retinopathy and photocoagulation. Am J Ophthalmol 1968;66:756
10. Cheng H. Multicentre trial of xenon-arc photocoagulation in the treatment of diabetic retinopathy: A randomised controlled clinical trial, interim report. Trans Ophthalmol Soc UK 1975;95:351
11. Diabetic Retinopathy Study Research Group. Photocoagulation treatment of proliferative diabetic retinopathy: The second report of Diabetic Retinopathy Study findings. Ophthalmology 1978;85:82
12. British Multicentre Study Group. Photocoagulation for proliferative diabetic retinopathy: A randomised controlled trial using the xenon arc. Diabetologia 1984;26:109
13. Diabetic Retinopathy Study Research Group. Photocoagulation treatment of proliferative diabetic retinopathy: Clinical application of Diabetic Retinopathy Study (DRS) findings, DRS report no. 8. Ophthalmology 1981;88:583
14. Green WR. Retina. In: Spencer WH, ed. Ophthalmic Pathology. Philadelphia: WB Saunders; 1985:589–1291
15. Garner A. Vascular diseases. In: Garner A, Klintworth GK, eds. Pathobiology of Ocular Disease. New York: Marcel Dekker; 1994:1625–1710
16. Vinores SA, Gadegbeku C, Campochiaro PA, Green WR. Immunohistochemical localisation of blood-retinal barrier breakdown in diabetics. Am J Pathol 1989;134:231
17. Kincaid MC, Green WR, Fine SL, et al. An ocular clinicopathologic correlative study of six patients from the diabetic retinopathy study. Retina 1983;3:218
18. Muraoka K, Shimizu K. Intraretinal neovascularization in diabetic retinopathy. Ophthalmology 1984;91:1440
19. Faulborn J, Bowald S. Microproliferations in proliferative diabetic retinopathy and their relationship to the vitreous: Corresponding light and electron microscopic studies (abstract). Graefes Arch Clin Exp Ophthalmol 1985;223:130
20. Pirart J. Diabetes mellitus and its degenerative complications: A prospective study of 4400 patients observed between 1947 and 1973. Part I. Diabetes Care 1978;1:168
21. Van Heyningen R. Formation of polyols by lens of the rat with sugar cataract. Nature 1959;184:194
22. Kinoshita JH, Merola LO, Dikmak E. Osmotic changes in experimental galactose cataract. Exp Eye Res 1962;1:405
23. Vinores SA, Campochiaro PA, Williams EH, et al. Aldose reductase expression in human diabetic retina and retinal pigment epithelium. Diabetes 1988; 37:1658
24. Ghahary A, Chakrabarti S, Sima AAF, Murphy LJ. Effect of insulin and Statil on aldose reductase expression in diabetic rats. Diabetes 1991;40:1391
25. Henry DN, Del Monte M, Greene DA, Killen PD. Altered aldose reductase gene regulation in cultured human retinal pigment epithelial cells. J Clin Invest 1993;92:617
26. Lee T-S, MacGregor LC, Fluharty ST, King GL. Differential regulation of protein kinase C and (Na,K)-adenosine triphosphatase activities by elevated glucose levels in retinal capillary endothelial cells. J Clin Invest 1989;83:90
27. Reddy VN, Lin L-R, Giblin FJ, et al. Study of polyol pathway and cell permeability changes in human lens and retinal pigment epithelium in tissue culture. Invest Ophthalmol Vis Sci 1992;33:2334
28. Robison WG Jr, Kador PF, Kinoshita JH. Retinal capillary: Basement membrane thickening by galactosemia prevented with aldose reductase inhibitor. Science 1983;221:1177
29. Vinores SA, Van Niel E, Swerdloff JL, Campochiaro PA. Electron microscopic immunocytochemical evidence for the mechanism of blood–retinal barrier breakdown in galactosemic rats and its association with aldose reductase expression and inhibition. Exp Eye Res 1993;57:723
30. Robison WG Jr, Tillis TN, Laver N, Kinoshita JH. Diabetes-like histopathologies of the rat retina prevented with an aldose reductase inhibitor. Exp Eye Res 1990;50:355
31. Takahashi Y, Wyman M, Ferris F, Kador PF. Diabetes-like preproliferative retinal changes in galactose-fed dogs. Arch Ophthalmol 1992;110:1295
32. Yamaoka T, Nishimura C, Yamashita K, et al. Acute onset of diabetic pathological changes in transgenic mice with human aldose reductase cDNA. Diabetologia 1995;38:255
33. Hotta N, Kakuta H, Ando F, Sakamoto N. Current progress in clinical trials of aldose reductase inhibitors in Japan. Exp Eye Res 1990;50:625
34. Engerman RL, Kern TS. Aldose reductase inhibition fails to prevent retinopathy in diabetic and galactosemic dogs. Diabetes 1993;42:820
35. Kern TS, Engerman RL. Retinal polyol and myoinositol in galactosemic dogs given an aldose reductase inhibitor. Invest Ophthalmol Vis Sci 1991;32:3175
36. Sorbinil Retinopathy Trial Research Group. A randomized trial of sorbinil, an aldose reductase inhibitor, in diabetic retinopathy. Arch Ophthalmol 1990; 108:1234
37. Brownlee M. Glycation and diabetic complications. Diabetes 1994;43:836
38. Steinbrecher UP, Witzum JL. Glycosylation of LDL to an extent comparable to that seen in diabetes slows their catabolism. Diabetes 1984;33:130

39. Mullokandov EA, Franklin WA, Brownlee M. DNA damage by glycation products of glyceraldehyde-3-phosphate and lysine. Diabetologia 1994;37: 145
40. Ditzel J. Affinity hypoxia as a pathogenetic factor of microangiopathy with particular reference to diabetic retinopathy. Acta Endocrinol 1980;94(suppl 238):39
41. Arai K, Iizuka S, Tada Y, et al. Increase in glucosylated form of erythrocyte Cu-Zn-superoxide dismutase in diabetes and close association of the non-enzymatic glucosylation with the enzyme activity. Biochem Biophys Acta 1987;924:192
42. Vlassara H, Fuh H, Makita Z, et al. Exogenous advanced glycosylation end products induce complex vascular dysfunction in normal animals: A model for diabetic and aging complications. Proc Natl Acad Sci USA 1992;89:12043
43. Hammes HP, Martin S, Federlin K, et al. Aminoguanidine treatment inhibits the development of experimental diabetic retinopathy. Proc Natl Acad Sci USA 1991;88:11555
44. Sell DR, Lapolla A, Odetti P, et al. Pentosidine formation in skin correlates with severity of complications in individuals with long-standing IDDM. Diabetes 1992;41:1286
45. McCance DR, Dyer DG, Dunn JA, et al. Maillard reaction products and their relation to complications in insulin-dependent diabetes mellitus. J Clin Invest 1993;91:2470
46. Mikita Z, Vlassara H, Cerami A, Bucala R. Immunochemical detection of advanced glycosylation end products in vivo. J Biol Chem 1992;267:5133
47. Wolff SP, Jiang ZY, Hunt JV. Protein glycation and oxidative stress in diabetes mellitus and ageing. Free Rad Biol Med 1991;10:339
48. Baynes J. Role of oxidative stress in development of complications of diabetes. Diabetes 1991;40:405
49. Uzel N, Sivas A, Uysal M, Oz H. Erythrocyte lipid peroxidation and glutathione peroxidase activities in patients with diabetes mellitus. Horm Metab Res 1987;19:89
50. Augustin AJ, Breipohl W, Boker T, et al. Increased lipid peroxide levels and myeloperoxidase activity in the vitreous of patients suffering from proliferative diabetic retinopathy. Graefe's Arch Clin Exp Ophthalmol 1993;231:647
51. Nishimura C, Kuriyama K. Alteration of lipid peroxide and endogenous antioxidant contents in retina of streptozotocin-induced diabetic rats: Effect of vitamin A administration. Jpn J Pharmacol 1985;37:365
52. Crouch R, Kimsey G, Priest DG, et al. Effect of streptozotocin on erythrocyte and retinal superoxide dismutase. Diabetologia 1978;15:53
53. Nath N, Chari SN, Rathi AB. Superoxide dismutase activity in diabetic polymorphonuclear leukocytes. Diabetes 1984;33:586
54. Awadallah R, El-Sessoukey EA, Doss H, Khalifa K. Blood reduced glutathione, pyruvic acid, citric acid, ceruloplasmin oxidase activity and certain mineral changes in diabetes mellitus before and after treatment. Z Ernahrungswiss 1978;17:72
55. Som S, Basu S, Mukherjee D, et al. Ascorbic acid metabolism in diabetes mellitus. Metabolism: Clin Exp 1981;30:572
56. Watanabe J, Umeda F, Wakasugi H, Ibayshi H. Effect of vitamin E on platelet aggregation in diabetes mellitus. Thromb Haemostas (Stuttgart) 1984;51:313
57. Greene DA, Lattimer SA, Sima AAF. Sorbitol, phosphoinositides, and sodium-potassium-ATPase in the pathogenesis of diabetic complications. N Engl J Med 1987;316:599
58. Lee T-S, Saltsman KA, Ohashi H, King GL. Activation of protein kinase C by elevation of glucose concentration: Proposal for a mechanism in the development of diabetic vascular complications. Proc Natl Acad Sci USA 1989;86:5141
59. Xia P, Inoguchi T, Kern TS, et al. Characterization of the mechanism for the chronic activation of diacylglycerol-protein kinase C pathway in diabetes and hypergalactosemia. Diabetes 1994;43:1122
60. Xia P, Kramer RM, King GL. Identification of the mechanism for the inhibition of Na^+-K^+-adenosine triphosphatase by hyperglycemia involving activation of protein kinase C and cytosolic phospholipase A_2. J Clin Invest 1995;96:733
61. Shiba T, Inoguchi T, Sportsman JR, et al. Correlation of diacylglycerol level and protein kinase C activity in rat retinal to retinal circulation. Am J Physiol 1993;265:E783
62. Inoguchi T, Battan R, Handler B, et al. Preferential elevation of protein kinase C isoform βII and diacylglycerol levels in the aorta and heart of diabetic rats: Differential reversibility to glycemic control by islet cell transplantation. Proc Natl Acad Sci USA 1992;89:11059
63. DeRubertis FR, Craven PA. Activation of protein kinase C in glomerular cells in diabetes: Mechanisms and potential links to the pathogenesis of diabetic glomerulopathy. Diabetes 1994;43:1
64. Michaelson IC. The mode of development of the vascular system of the retina, with some observations on its significance for certain retinal diseases. Trans Ophthalmol Soc UK 1948;68:137
65. Cogan DG, Toussaint D, Kuwabara T. Retinal vascular patterns: IV. Diabetic retinopathy. Arch Ophthalmol 1961;66:100
66. Ashton N. Studies of the retinal capillaries in relation to diabetic and other retinopathies. Br J Ophthalmol 1963;47:521
67. Rosen P, Boulton M, Moriarty P, et al. Effect of varying oxygen concentrations on the proliferation of retinal microvascular cells in vitro. Exp Eye Res 1991;53:597
68. Shweiki D, Itin A, Soffer D, Keshet E. Vascular endothelial growth factor induced by hypoxia may mediate hypoxia-initiated angiogenesis. Nature 1992;359:843
69. Grant MB, Mames RN, Fitzgerald C, et al. Insulin-like growth factor I acts as an angiogenic agent in rabbit cornea and retina: Comparative studies with basic fibroblast growth factor. Diabetologia 1993;36:282
70. Meyer-Schwickerath R, Pfeiffer A, Blnm WF, et al. Vitreous levels of the insulin-like growth factors I and II, and the insulin-like growth factor binding proteins 2 and 3, increased in neovascular eye disease. J Clin Invest 1993; 92:2620
71. Aiello LP, Avery RL, Arrigg PG, et al. Vascular endothelial growth factor in ocular fluid of patients with diabetic retinopathy and other retinal disorders. N Engl J Med 1994;331:1480
72. Adamis AP, Miller JW, Bernal MT, et al. Increased vascular endothelial growth factor levels in the vitreous of eyes with proliferative diabetic retinopathy. J Am Ophthalmol 1994;118:445

Diabetes Mellitus, edited by Derek LeRoith, Simeon I. Taylor, and Jerrold M. Olefsky. Lippincott–Raven Publishers, Philadelphia © 1996.

CHAPTER 81

Pathophysiology of Diabetic Nephropathy

ROBERTO TREVISAN AND GIANCARLO VIBERTI

Diabetic nephropathy is clinically defined as the presence of persistent proteinuria (total urinary protein excretion >0.5 g/24 h) in sterile urine of diabetic patients with concomitant retinopathy and elevated blood pressure, but without other renal disease or heart failure. Overt diabetic nephropathy is characterized by a progressive decline in renal function, resulting in end-stage renal disease.

Twenty-five to 50% of diabetic patients develop kidney disease and require dialysis or kidney transplantation. The mortality from all causes in diabetic patients with nephropathy is 20 to 40 times higher than that of patients without nephropathy.[1] Diabetic nephropathy is nowadays the single most common cause of renal failure in the Western world, and in some countries diabetic patients represent up to one-third of all patients entering renal replacement treatment programs. In the United States, the health-care cost for diabetic patients in renal failure exceeded $2 billion in 1993.

Natural History and Pathophysiology of Diabetic Nephropathy

Diabetic nephropathy evolves through several distinct but interconnected phases: an early phase of physiologic abnormalities of renal function, a "microalbuminuria phase," and a clinical phase with persistent clinical proteinuria progressing to end-stage renal failure.

Histologic changes of diabetic glomerulopathy are present in more than 96% of insulin-dependent diabetes mellitus (IDDM) patients with proteinuria and in approximately 85% of non–insulin-dependent diabetes mellitus (NIDDM) patients with proteinuria and concomitant retinopathy. A sizeable proportion (up to 30%) of NIDDM patients with proteinuria alone have a nondiabetic renal lesion.

Early Renal Abnormalities

Soon after the diagnosis of IDDM, several renal abnormalities may be observed. Supranormal values of renal plasma flow (RPF) and glomerular filtration rate (GFR; >135 mL/min/1.73 m^2) are found in approximately 20–40% of patients.[2] Hyperfiltration is partially related to the degree of metabolic control,[3] and intensified insulin therapy with improvement of blood glucose control reduces GFR toward normal values.[4] These hemodynamic abnormalities are associated with an increase in kidney size. Nephromegaly is a prerequisite for the occurrence of glomerular hyperfiltration. Whereas normal GFR can be found in patients with large kidneys, supranormal GFR is exceptional in patients with normal kidney size.[5] The prognostic significance of nephromegaly, however, remains unclear.

Elevated GFR has been implicated in the initiation and progression of renal disease. There is convincing evidence in animal diabetes models that hemodynamic factors, in particular intraglomerular pressure, play an important role in the development of glomerulopathy.[6–8] Still, the prognostic significance of glomerular hyperfiltration remains controversial in humans. In small groups of selected "hyperfiltering" patients, two retrospective studies have shown a correlation between the initially high GFR and the subsequent increase in urinary albumin excretion,[9,10] These findings were not confirmed in other reports. Two prospective studies of different designs, a case control and a cohort study, have failed to resolve the controversy after 8 years of observation.[11,12] No relationship between hyperfiltration and development of persistent proteinuria or hypertension was found in one study, whereas a positive association was claimed in the other. Both studies reported a faster rate of decline of GFR in diabetic patients with hyperfiltration, but the long-term significance of the phenomenon remains unclear at present.

The hemodynamic determinants of hyperfiltration have been investigated in animal diabetes models by direct measurements in single nephrons of glomerular plasma flow, transglomerular hydraulic pressure gradient, and systemic oncotic pressure and by calculation of ultrafiltration coefficient. RPF is on average 9–14% above normal values in diabetic patients, an elevation less than that of the GFR. There is a good correlation between GFR and RPF increases in diabetic patients, but increases in RPF can account only for approximately 60% of the increase in GFR.

Micropuncture studies in moderately hyperglycemic rats have shown a significant increase in transglomerular pressure gradient.[6,7] This resulted from a reduction of total glomerular vascular resistance, more marked at the afferent than at the efferent arteriole. The glomerular ultrafiltration coefficient, the product of the capillary hydraulic conductivity and the capillary surface area available to filtration, does not seem to be abnormal in diabetic animals. An increase in total glomerular capillary surface area was reported, however, in IDDM patients[13] and was significantly related to GFR.[14] In certain circumstances, therefore, an increase in the surface area available for filtration may contribute to the elevation of GFR. Systemic oncotic pressure is normal in diabetic patients.

Various metabolic and hormonal abnormalities of the diabetic state have been proposed as mediators of glomerular hyperfiltration (Table 81-1). Hyperglycemia per se increases GFR by 6–10%.[15] An increase in blood glucose concentration induces vasodilation in a number of tissues, including the glomerular capillaries.[16] Several mechanisms may account for this hemodynamic effect, such as an osmotic effect on endothelial cells,[17] an increase in formation of kallikrein and endothelium-derived–relaxing factor and modulation through renal prostaglandins.[18,19] High glucose concentration in the renal ultrafiltrate results in increased renal tubular reabsorption of glucose, a mechanism coupled with reabsortion of sodium. Increased sodium reabsorption may suppress the tubuloglomerular feedback system, thereby contributing to hyperfiltration.[20]

Ketone body infusion induces an increase in GFR of approximately 30%.[21] Glucagon and growth hormone, two counter-regulatory hormones often elevated in diabetic patients, are also capable of inducing a modest increase in GFR either acutely or in the long term.[22,23] Recent studies suggest that disturbances in prostaglandin production could play a role in the renal hemodynamic changes of diabetes.[24,25] An enhanced activity of vasodilatory prostaglandins with an imbalance between vasoconstrictive and vasodilatory eicosanoids has been proposed as a mechanism of hyperfiltration.[26] Findings that aspirin-induced inhibition of prostaglandin production reduces GFR in hyperfiltering diabetic patients would support this contention,[27] but other studies have failed to confirm these results.[28]

Several other mechanisms have been suggested as possible contributors to hyperfiltration,[1] such as decreased renin activity,[26] reduced numbers of glomerular angiotensin II (AII) receptors,[29] increased kinin production,[30] and hyporesponsiveness to vasoactive substances.[31] Atrial natriuretic peptide also has been implicated as one of the important determinants of glomerular hyperfiltration.[32] A consequence of hyperglycemia and peripheral hyperinsulinemia appears to be an increase in total exchangeable body sodium along with extracellular volume expansion.[33] This condition may induce hyperfiltration through a rise in atrial natriuretic peptide levels.

Protein intake also may play a role in diabetic hyperfiltration. The human kidney response to a meat meal is characterized by renal arteriolar vasodilation, increased GFR, and natriuresis.[34] Interestingly, restriction of dietary protein, a maneuver that affects glucagon and prostaglandin secretion, significant increases renal vascular resistance and reduces the elevated GFR independent of glycemic changes.[35] The type of protein ingested seems to be of importance to the magnitude of the GFR effect.[36]

Some of these perturbations increase GFR by elevating intraglomerular pressure, the factor implicated in the pathogenesis of glomerular histologic changes in animal models of diabetic renal disease.

TABLE 81-1. Potential Mediators of Diabetic Hyperfiltration

Hyperglycemia
Increased plasma concentrations of ketone body and other organic acids
Increased plasma levels of glucagon and growth hormone
Disturbances in renal prostaglandin production
Decreased renin activity
Increased atrial natriuretic peptide
Abnormalities of tubuloglomerular feedback mechanisms
Increased renal kallikrein production

Microalbuminuria

A proportion of diabetic patients exhibit elevated rates of urinary albumin excretion well before clinically persistent proteinuria develops. Microalbuminuria is defined as an increase in the albumin excretion rate to a range of 20 μg/min to 200 μg/min. Four longitudinal studies of cohorts of IDDM patients have demonstrated that microalbuminuria is a predictor for the development of clinical diabetic nephropathy,[37–40] and is associated with a 20-fold higher risk of progression to overt renal disease compared to normoalbuminuric patients. Albumin excretion rates in healthy individuals range from 1.5 to 20 μg/min (median, 6.5 μg/min). The average daily variation in albumin excretion rate is approximately 40% and is similar in both normal and diabetic subjects.[41] For this reason, an accurate classification of albumin excretion rate requires an average of multiple measurements (usually three urine collections) taken during a period of a few weeks.

Persistent microalbuminuria is found after 1 year of IDDM[42] and can be present at diagnosis in NIDDM patients.[43] The significance of microalbuminuria in patients with short-term diabetes is still unclear, but in patients with IDDM for 5 years or more, microalbuminuria is the consequence of definite, albeit early, renal damage.[44] Once microalbuminuria is established, the albumin excretion rate tends to increase with time at an average rate of approximately 15% per year.[45]

The filtration of proteins across the glomerular capillary barrier depends on four major determinants:

- The size and isoelectric point of the protein in question
- The size of the pores in the glomerular capillary glomerular barrier (*size-selectivity property*)
- The negative charge of the capillary wall (*charge-selectivity property*)
- The set of hemodynamic forces operating across the capillary wall.

The excess albumin excretion rate in diabetic patients with persistent microalbuminuria is most likely the result of an increased transglomerular flux, as suggested by normal tubular function in these subjects. The fractional clearance of albumin is increased at these early stages,[46] likely as a consequence of alterations in glomerular hemodynamics and, in particular, an increase in transglomerular pressure gradient. As microalbuminuria becomes persistent and increases in degree, the selectivity index (i.e., the ratio of immunoglobulin G clearance to albumin clearance) starts to decrease, reaching its lowest value when albumin excretion is approximately 90 μg/min. The decrease probably is due to a loss of the fixed negative electrical charge on the glomerular membrane.[46] Experiments measuring the clearance of neutral dextrans have shown that pore size is unchanged at this stage.[47] The transition to high-selectivity proteinuria signals the advent of heavier proteinuria, suggesting an important role for the loss of the charge barrier in the evolution of diabetic nephropathy.

Of particular interest is the consistent association of microalbuminuria with an increase in blood pressure. Several studies have confirmed a positive linear correlation between blood pressure and albumin excretion rate that is independent of age, sex, duration of diabetes, body mass index, and blood glucose control.[48] The magnitude of this increase in blood pressure is approximately 10–15%, compared to the blood pressure of diabetic patients with normal albumin excretion.[48,49] This phenomenon has been elegantly documented in a number of recent studies using 24-hour blood pressure monitoring.[50] This blood pressure increase, which occurs most often within the so-called normal blood pressure range, documents clearly that patients with microalbuminuria are not "normotensive" relative to their counterparts with normoalbuminuria. Often at this stage of microalbuminuria, there is no hint of renal failure, and GFR can even be supranormal.[48] Therefore, it is difficult to ascribe hypertension to renal functional impairment. Studies of transition from normoalbuminuria to microalbuminuria have documented that the diabetic patients who progress to microalbuminuria already exhibit a blood pressure increase as the albumin excretion rate rises within the normal range.[50,51] In some ethnic groups of NIDDM patients, there is evidence that blood pressures recorded before NIDDM onset positively relate to the development of proteinuria after NIDDM onset.[52,53] This raises the possibility that elevated blood pressure may be one factor contributing to renal damage or, alternatively, that high blood pressure and an increase in albumin excretion may represent concomitant manifestations of a common process responsible for the development of diabetic nephropathy.

Morphologic studies have shown that structural lesions, as evidenced by increased mesangial fractional volume and decreased filtration surface density, are more advanced, on average, when albumin excretion rate exceeds 45 mg/24 h,[44] confirming that microalbuminuria is a sign of early glomerulopathy. These findings underlie the importance of searching for other earlier markers to identify patients at risk for diabetic nephropathy.

Associations between microalbuminuria and the enhanced risk of renal and cardiovascular complications are of particular interest in IDDM patients. Higher levels of plasma lipids,[54] abnormalities of coagulation factors[54] and endothelial function,[55] echocardiographic evidence of left ventricular hypertrophy,[56] enhanced sodium retention,[56] and increased transcapillary escape rate of albumin[57] have all been reported in patients with microalbuminuria and may have potentially important prognostic implications. Table 81-2 lists the concomitants of microalbuminuria (the "microalbuminuria syndrome").

With the euglycemic insulin clamp technique, diabetic patients with microalbuminuria have been found to be more insulin resistant than normoalbuminuric patients.[58] This altered insulin sensitivity may explain the reason why microalbuminuric patients tend to have a poorer metabolic control in comparison with normoalbuminuric patients. It is of particular interest that insulin resistance is an independent risk factor for coronary artery disease in the nondiabetic population.

Thus, risk factors for both renal and cardiovascular complications cluster in IDDM and NIDDM patients with microalbuminuria. In a 23-year follow-up study of 63 IDDM patients, cardiovascular mortality was found to be more than twice as high in microalbuminuric IDDM patients than in normoalbuminuric IDDM patients, independent of patient age and duration of diabetes.[59] In NIDDM patients, microalbuminuria is the strongest predictor for risk of cardiovascular disease.[60]

The importance of identifying and detecting microalbuminuric diabetic patients at an early stage is twofold. They may respond

Table 81-2. Concomitants of Microalbuminuria: The Microalbuminuria Syndrome

Elevated blood pressure
Atherogenic lipid profile (increased VLDL-tryglicerides, decreased HDL-cholesterol, increased Lpa)
Elevated plasma fibrinogen levels
Decreased insulin sensitivity
Increased total body exchangeable sodium
Increased transcapillary escape of albumin
Impaired basal endothelium-dependent vasorelaxation
Increased left ventricular volume
High sodium-lithium countertransport activity
Diabetic retinopathy
Increased prevalence of diabetic neuropathy
Increased prevalence of peripheral vascular disease
"Silent" ischemic heart disease

HDL = high-density lipoprotein; VLDL = very-low-density lipoprotein.

to preventive treatment, and their study may provide insights into the pathogenesis of diabetic nephropathy before the clinical phase of the disease sets in.

Overt Nephropathy

In diabetic patients who progress to overt, persistent albuminuria (albumin excretion rate >300 mg/24 h), GFR gradually declines in a linear fashion at a rate ranging from 0.1 to 2.4 mL/min/month.[61] The reason for the differences in the rates of progression are not known, but blood pressure control could be important. Before the introduction of early, intensive treatment for hypertension in diabetic patients, end-stage renal failure occurred an average of 7 years after the onset of proteinuria. Today, period between onset of overt proteinuria and renal replacement therapy is more than double what it once was. Overt nephropathy is characterized by progressive mesangial and interstitial expansion and capillary occlusion. These histologic lesions of diabetic glomerulopathy restrict filtration surface area and consequently reduce the ultrafiltration coefficient, contributing to the observed decline in GFR. As the GFR decreases, the degree of proteinuria increases and there is a change from high- to low-selectivity proteinuria.[46] Studies of neutral dextran sieving curves reveal the appearance of a size-selectivity defect.[62] The fractional clearance of molecules with radii >4.6 nm is elevated, and analysis of membrane permeability using a theoretic model suggests that this abnormality is related to the appearance of a small population of large, unselective pores (*shunt pathway*) within the glomerular capillary wall. These large pores would explain the heavy proteinuria of advanced diabetic nephropathy. Although the precise morphologic counterpart of this shunt pathway still is unclear, detachment of epithelial cells from the basement membrane and defects within the glomerular membrane itself could contribute to the loss of size selectivity. It also is likely that a defect in charge selectivity contributes to clinical proteinuria. In diabetic patients with established nephropathy, sialic acid and heparan sulfate proteoglycans content in the glomerular barrier is reduced,[63,64] leading to rarefaction of the fixed negative charge of the glomerular capillary wall.

Elevation of blood pressure is a feature of approximately 85% of patients, with proteinuria and blood pressure increases of approximately 7% per year in association with progressive renal failure. The excess of arterial hypertension in IDDM seems to be largely accounted for by overt clinical nephropathy; however, long-term uncomplicated diabetic patients tend to have lower blood pressures than those of age-matched normal controls. The degree of proteinuria is related to the extent of renal damage. The appearance of the nephrotic syndrome is predictive of a poor renal outcome.

Diabetic retinopathy and hyperlipidemia (characterized by increased levels of cholesterol, low-density lipoprotein [LDL] cholesterol, and triglycerides; and by decreased levels of high-density lipoprotein [HDL] cholesterol) are present in most patients with nephropathy. At this stage, the course of renal failure does not seem to be reversible, and available treatment modalities can only slow the rate of decline in renal function and delay the need for renal replacement therapy.

Pathogenesis of Diabetic Kidney Disease

An understanding of the pathogenesis and pathophysiology of diabetic kidney disease is crucial to design strategies to prevent or arrest the development of such a devastating long-term complication of diabetes.

There is no doubt that the diabetic milieu is necessary for diabetic glomerular lesions to develop. Microangiopathic lesions can be observed in chemically induced diabetes in the animal model, and these lesions can be prevented or greatly reduced by near-normalization of blood glucose levels, depending on the time of the start of intensified insulin treatment after the induction of diabetes. Moreover in the kidney, the morphologic lesions typical of the diabetic state, such as mesangial expansion, are reversed by the transplantation of the diabetic kidney into a normal animal.

Renal lesions also can be seen in humans with chronic hyperglycemia secondary to pancreatitis and without any evidence of a genetic predisposition to diabetes. Both retrospective and prospective studies have suggested a relationship between blood glucose control and risk of diabetic nephropathy. The recently reported Diabetes Control and Complication Trial (DCCT study) has now precisely documented that the rate of development and progression of diabetic nephropathy is closely associated with glycemic control.[65] Nevertheless in many patients, despite several years of poor diabetes control, no renal disease develops, as assessed by levels of urinary albumin excretion rate. It thus appears that in humans hyperglycemia is necessary, but not sufficient, to cause renal damage and that other factors are needed for the manifestation of the clinical syndrome.

Several biochemical mechanisms have been advocated to explain the deleterious effects of high glucose concentrations in the kidney (Table 81-3).

Nonenzymatic Glycosylation

A possible link between elevated glucose level and diabetic nephropathy resides in nonenzymatic glycosylation of cellular proteins.[66] The exposure of lysine amino terminal groups of circulating or structural protein to an increasing amount of glucose would lead, by basic chemical stoichiometry, to increasing covalent binding of glucose to protein. These covalent products can then participate in cross-linking between or within proteins, producing *advanced glycosylation end products* (AGEPs). The new combination may impair the original function of either protein and may affect normal processes of turnover and clearance, so that AGEPs accumulate in tissues. The extent of glycosylation is dependent on protein half-life and the mean glucose level.[66] Direct proof that these AGEPs cause tissue injury in human diabetes is still lacking, although correlative studies have been performed. The amount of glycosylated products is related to the extent and severity of advanced complications of diabetes.[67] Recent studies have shown that the AGEPs lead to synthesis and secretion of cytokines when bound to a specific AGEP receptor identified in macrophages.[68] AGEPs can induce an excess cross-linking of collagen molecules in the glomerular plasma membrane affecting the assembly and architecture of the glomerular basement membrane and mesangial matrix,

Table 81-3. Biochemical Basis for the Effect of Hyperglycemia on the Pathogenesis of Diabetic Nephropathy

Glucose toxicity
Nonenzymatic glycosylation of protein
Abnormal polyol metabolism
Glucose-induced growth factor gene expression
Increased sodium reabsorption
Increased protein kinase C activity
Increased cytokine production
Alteration of extracellular matrix
Disturbances in cell cycle and proliferation rate
Decreased anionic charge of cell membranes
Abnormal lipid metabolism
Abnormal cation transport

and can potentially act on mesangial cells via platelet-derived growth factor, causing cells to synthesize more extracellular matrix.[66] All these processes may lead to enhanced deposition of extracellular matrix proteins in the mesangium, interfere with the mesangial clearance of macromolecules, and alter macrophage function, therefore contributing to mesangial expansion and glomerular occlusion.

Aminoguanidine, a hydrazine derivative that binds irreversibly to early glycosylation products, prevents AGEP formation and AGEP-induced protein crosslinking. The efficacy of this new drug in preventing some of the complications of diabetes in animal models supports the role of AGEPs in the pathogenesis of diabetic complications.

The Polyol Pathway

Another possible mechanism of tissue injury involves excessive intracellular production of sorbitol from glucose, a reaction catalyzed by aldose reductase. Chronic hyperglycemia may lead to sorbitol accumulation in a variety of tissues, including renal tubuli and glomeruli. Sorbitol accumulation causes tissue damage via a disruption of cellular osmoregulation along with a depletion of *myo*-inositol.[69]

Some beneficial effect of aldose reductase inhibition has been reported in diabetic animals. The increased GFR and proteinuria in rats with streptozotocin-induced diabetes was reduced by inhibitors of aldose reductase[70] or by supplementation of *myo*-inositol.[71] Recent studies showed that cells may counter-regulate inositol depletion and that the histologic lesions of glomerular disease were unaffected by the administration of an aldose reductase inhibitor in the rat made diabetic with streptozotocin.[72] Renal damage in the diabetic kidney therefore is unlikely to occur through a mechanism involving the polyol pathway.

Glucotoxicity

A further possibility is that glucose itself has a direct toxic effect on the cells. Lorenzi[73] demonstrated that cultured human endothelial cells chronically exposed to high glucose concentrations exhibit important abnormalities in cell function that could not be ascribed to alteration of the polyol pathway. High glucose levels determine alterations in cell cycle and proliferation and lead to increased synthesis and gene expression of collagen, fibrinonectin, and laminin, which may explain the increase in extracellular matrix production observed in the diabetic kidney. Mesangial cells exposed to elevated glucose concentrations synthesize less heparan sulfate, and theoretically this could contribute to a reduction of the electronegative charge that physiologically restricts the transcapillary flux of circulating albumin, thus giving rise to proteinuria. Moreover in mesangial cells high glucose levels induce the transcription and secretion of transforming growth factor (TGF-β), unique among the cytokines in stimulating matrix synthesis and inhibiting matrix degradation.

Hemodynamic and Hypertrophic Pathways

Glomerular hemodynamic disturbances with elevations of blood flow and filtration rate occur early in the course of diabetes. These alterations have been suggested to be directly responsible for the development of glomerulosclerosis and its attendant proteinuria.[74] Several observations give support to the notion that renal hyperfusion and hyperfiltration contribute to renal damage (Fig. 81-1). In several animal models with spontaneous or induced diabetes, both single-nephron GFR and glomerular plasma flow are increased

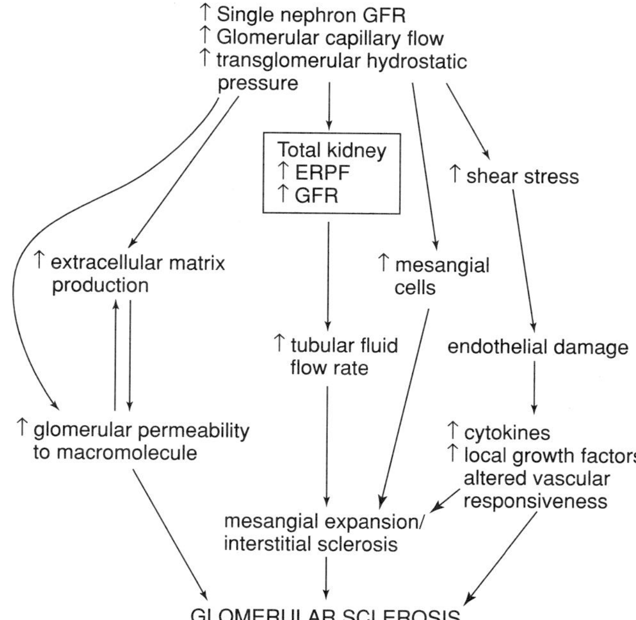

Figure 81-1. Possible sequence of events from intrarenal hemodynamic abnormalities to onset of diabetic nephropathy. ERPF = effective renal plasma flow.

whereas intrarenal vascular resistances is reduced. Despite normal systemic blood pressures, transmission of systemic pressures to the glomerular capillaries is facilitated by a proportionally greater reduction in afferent versus efferent arteriolar resistance. Consequently, the glomerular capillary hydraulic pressure rises. Elevated intraglomerular pressure via increased mechanical stress and shear forces may damage the endothelial surface and disrupt the normal structure of the glomerular barrier, eventually leading to mesangial proliferation, increase in extracellular matrix production, and thickening of the glomerular basement membrane. Evidence that these glomerular hemodynamic abnormalities contribute to the development and progression of diabetic nephropathy has been provided by studies involving maneuvers that aggravate or ameliorate glomerular hyperperfusion and hyperfiltration without affecting metabolic control. For example, both a low-protein diet and inhibition of angiotensin converting enzyme have been shown to prevent not only the disturbed hemodynamics but also the glomerular histologic lesions that are found in untreated diabetic control animals.

In other studies, a dissociation between the hemodynamic perturbations and subsequent sclerosis has been reported. In different strains of diabetic rats, no relationship was found between level of glomerular hyperfiltration and pressure and subsequent degree of glomerular sclerosis.[75]

The hemodynamic abnormalities so far described usually are associated with hypertrophic changes in the glomerulus. Marked renal hypertrophy is a very early event in diabetes, and it has been argued that hyperplastic and hypertrophic changes in the diabetic kidney may precede the hemodynamic abnormalities. Although the exact role of growth factors in the development of diabetic kidney disease is not yet fully understood, growth hormone, insulin-like growth factors (IGFs), transforming growth factor (TGFβ), platelet derived growth factor (PDGF), and other growth promoters may be of importance in the long-term renal changes of diabetes. They may activate mesangial cell proliferation and increase mesangial matrix synthesis or decrease matrix degradation, giving rise to the histologic alterations that are pathognomonic of diabetic glomerulopathy.

Familial and Genetic Aspects

The annual incidence of diabetic nephropathy rises rapidly during the first 15–20 years of diabetes and then declines sharply afterward. This leads to a cumulative incidence that, after approximately 20 years of diabetes, plateaus at approximately 30–35%.[76,77] This pattern of risk is compatible with an individual susceptibility to renal damage partly independent of the environmental perturbations caused by diabetes, and makes it necessary to identify contributing factors other than glycemic control.

That there is an individual predisposition to diabetic nephropathy is supported by the observation that this complication clusters in families. Seaquist et al.[78] reported that 83% of IDDM siblings of probands with diabetic nephropathy have evidence of renal disease, compared to only 17% of IDDM siblings of probands without diabetic nephropathy. This striking familial aggregation of diabetic kidney disease was also confirmed in a Danish population.[79] A similar familial influence on development of nephropathy has been described in Pima Indians with NIDDM.[80] Overt proteinuria occurred in 14% of the diabetic offspring of diabetic parents without proteinuria, in 23% if one parent had proteinuria, and in 46% if both parents had proteinuria. Although these studies are consistent with the possibility that genetic factors play an important role in the susceptibility to diabetic nephropathy, they cannot entirely exclude shared environmental influences and do not provide insight into the nature of these factors. Further information has come from other family studies of risk factors for nephropathy.

Earle et al.[81] demonstrated that a family history of cardiovascular disease greatly increases the risk of nephropathy in diabetic patients compared to that of patients without family history for cardiovascular disease (odds ratio, 3.2) and enhances the likelihood of cardiovascular disease in diabetic patients who have nephropathy (odds ratio, 6.2). This observation has been confirmed by recent studies, which also have revealed that first-degree nondiabetic relatives of IDDM patients with albuminuria have reduced insulin sensitivity and abnormal lipid profiles.[82,83] This familial aggregation of renal and cardiovascular disease and their risk factors has led to the suggestion that these disorders may share a common pathogenetic basis.

Family studies of blood pressure have provided further insights. Higher arterial pressure was measured in parents of diabetic patients with proteinuria than in parents of patients without proteinuria.[84] A higher prevalence of arterial hypertension among the parents of IDDM patients with nephropathy was also found by a subsequent study.[85] A relative risk for developing overt nephropathy of approximately 3.3 was found if at least one of the parents had hypertension. That the hypertension associated with diabetic nephropathy is not merely a consequence of the renal disease is confirmed by several studies indicating that elevations of arterial pressure develop at very early stages in both IDDM and NIDDM patients with normoalbuminuria, who subsequently progress to microalbuminuria,[51–53] and persist at the microalbuminuria stage.[86,87] All these studies suggest that hypertension or a predisposition to it may be important components in determining the susceptibility to renal disease in diabetes.

The suggestion that hereditary causes are involved in the development of diabetic nephropathy has stimulated the search for cell and genetic markers that would allow early diagnosis and identification of patients at risk as well as help clarify the molecular mechanisms of this complication.

Sodium-Lithium Countertransport

An increase in red blood cell sodium-lithium countertransport, a cell membrane cation transport system, is consistently associated with essential hypertension and its vascular complications.[88] Up to 80% of the interindividual variability of the activity of this transport system is explained by genetic influence representing the sum of a major gene with polygene effects.[89]

Increased rates of sodium-lithium countertransport activity have been reported by several, though not all, authors both in IDDM and NIDDM patients with microalbuminuria or macroalbuminuria.[90–92] A significant correlation in the activity of this transport system found between diabetic probands with nephropathy and their parents strongly suggests heritability of elevated activities in diabetic nephropathy.[93] The importance of genetic factors was confirmed by the close association of sodium-lithium countertransport activities found in diabetic identical twins.[94] That elevated sodium-lithium countertransport activity may confer an increased risk for nephropathy and its vascular complications is supported by a clustering of metabolic, hemodynamic, and morphologic abnormalities (e.g., poorer metabolic control, reduced insulin sensitivity, a more atherogenic lipid profile, greater proximal tubular reabsorption of sodium, higher GFRs, increased left ventricular thickness, larger kidney size) in patients with high sodium-lithium countertransport activities, but without overt proteinuria.[56]

Sodium-Hydrogen Antiporter

Sodium-lithium countertransport activity is determined by measuring sodium-driven lithium efflux from red blood cells loaded with lithium in an in vitro artifactual system. Because this system does not operate in vivo, the relevance of this abnormality to the pathogenesis of diabetic renal disease remains uncertain. The close similarities between sodium-lithium countertransport and a physiologic cell membrane exchanger, the sodium-hydrogen antiporter, has prompted the search for abnormalities in this latter system in diabetic nephropathy.

Sodium-hydrogen antiport is an integral plasma membrane protein that catalyzes the electroneutral exchange of extracellular sodium for intracellular hydrogen with a stoichiometry of 1:1. Molecular cloning studies have so far revealed the presence of five subtypes of sodium-hydrogen exchangers. These isoforms share a similar structure, but exhibit differences with respect to amiloride sensitivity, cellular localization, kinetic parameters, regulation by various stimuli, and plasma membrane targeting. They define a new gene family of vertebrate transporters.[95]

The most widely studied sodium-hydrogen isoform, referred to as *NHE1*, is ubiquitously expressed and involved in a variety of cellular functions by virtue of its ability to control intracellular pH. It is inhibited by the diuretic compound amiloride and its five amino-substituted derivatives. The *NHE1* gene is located on the short arm of chromosome 1. It encodes a protein of 815 amino acids with two distinct domains. The N-terminal domain contains 10–12 transmembrane segments, whereas the C-terminal domain is cytoplasmic. Sodium-hydrogen antiport is involved in three important cellular functions: (1) intracellular pH regulation; (2) cell volume control; and (3) stimulus-response coupling and cell proliferation. In the kidney, the isoform *NHE2,* expressed on the apical membrane of polarized epithelia, is directly involved in sodium reabsorption.

An essential feature of this transport system is its allosteric activation by intracellular protons, which are presumed to interact at a "modifier" site that is separate from the sites involved in sodium and hydrogen transport. The activity and expression level of this antiport can be modulated by a large variety of stimuli, including growth factors, tumor promoters, and hormones, as well as physical factors such as changes in cell volume, extracellular acidification, and degree of cell spreading (Fig. 81-2).

Protein kinases appear to play an important role in the regulation of the antiport, but the molecular mechanisms of activation are not yet fully elucidated. It has been reported that growth factors activate the antiporter by shifting the pH dependence of the modifier site, adjusting the set point upward by 0.15–0.30 pH units. The

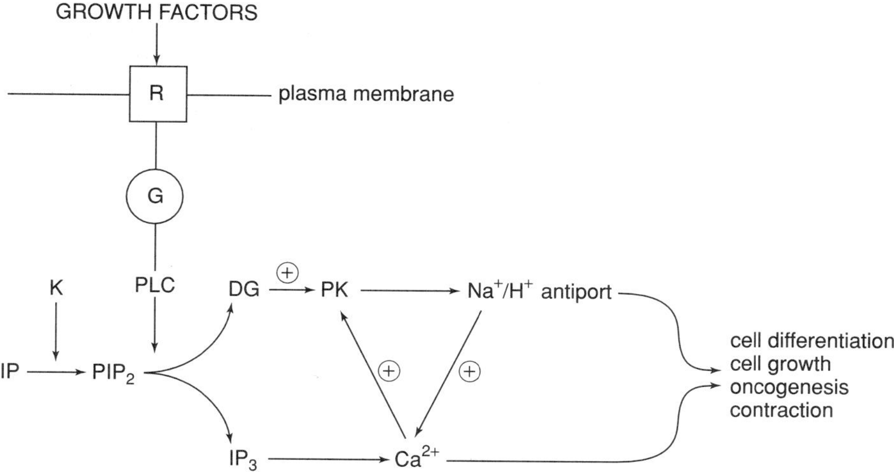

FIGURE 81-2. Schematic representation of interaction between growth factors and the sodium-hydrogen antiport and calcium-dependent cell activities. R = receptor; G = regulatory protein; PLC = phospholipase C; K = kinases; IP = inositol phosphate; PIP_2 = phosphatidylinositol-4,5 biphosphate; DG = 1,2-diacylglycerol; IP_3 = inositol-1,4-5-triphosphate; PK = protein kinase C.

alteration in the set point probably is mediated by phosphorylation of the antiporter itself or of an ancillary protein.

Increased sodium-hydrogen antiport activity has been reported in leukocytes of IDDM patients with nephropathy[96] as well as in patients with essential hypertension.[97] A higher activity also has been found in red blood cells from IDDM patients with microalbuminuria.[98] In these studies, however, measurements were performed soon after blood sampling, and potential confounding effects of the disturbed diabetic environment on circulating cells could not be excluded. Skin fibroblasts, which can be cultured for several passages in well-defined conditions, were used by Trevisan et al.[99] to measure sodium-hydrogen antiport activity from IDDM patients with and without nephropathy. The kinetic parameters of sodium-hydrogen antiporter were determined by measuring the initial velocity of amiloride-sensitive net sodium uptake under pH gradient conditions. There was significantly increased sodium-hydrogen antiport activity in the cells of IDDM patients with nephropathy compared to that found in cells of IDDM patients without nephropathy, which was comparable to the activity found in cells of the nondiabetic controls (Fig. 81-3). The increased activity was found to be caused by an increased maximal velocity for extracellular sodium, whereas the Km for extracellular sodium was similar in all patients. The intracellular pH, measured using the distribution of 7-^{14}C-benzoic acid, was also higher in fibroblasts exposed to serum from IDDM patients with nephropathy than in those of IDDM patients without nephropathy. These findings in long-term cultured cells are consistent with an intrinsic overactivity of sodium-hydrogen exchange in patients with nephropathy.

These results were confirmed by another study, in which sodium-hydrogen antiport activity was determined by a different technique, using the pH-sensitive dye 2′-7′-bis(carboxyethyl)-5,6-carboxyfluorescein (BCECF).[100] Resting intracellular pH was more alkaline in growing fibroblasts from IDDM patients with nephropathy than in those of IDDM patients without nephropathy. This was associated with increased sodium-hydrogen antiport activity when intracellular pH was clamped at pH 6.5, but not when pH was clamped at 6.2. It was suggested that the abnormal activity of the exchanger in patients with nephropathy was accounted for by an increased apparent affinity of the antiporter for hydrogen ions at the internal hydrogen modifier site.

A recent study established that this abnormal phenotype is conserved in Epstein–Barr-immortalized lymphoblasts.[101] The maximal velocity was significantly elevated, and the Hill coefficient for internal hydrogen binding was lower in lymphoblasts of IDDM patients with nephropathy than in those of both normal controls and normoalbuminuric diabetic patients. By means of specific polyclonal antisera to the C-terminus of *NHE1*, it was shown that the elevated maximal velocity of sodium-hydrogen exchange was not due to an increased *NHE1* density, which was similar in IDDM patients with and without nephropathy, but to an increased turnover rate per site.

Although the enhanced sodium-hydrogen exchange activity could be caused theoretically by a reduced intracellular buffer capacity for hydrogen ions in nephropathic patients, this possibility has been excluded in all the above-reported studies, which found intracellular buffer capacity to be similar in all subjects.

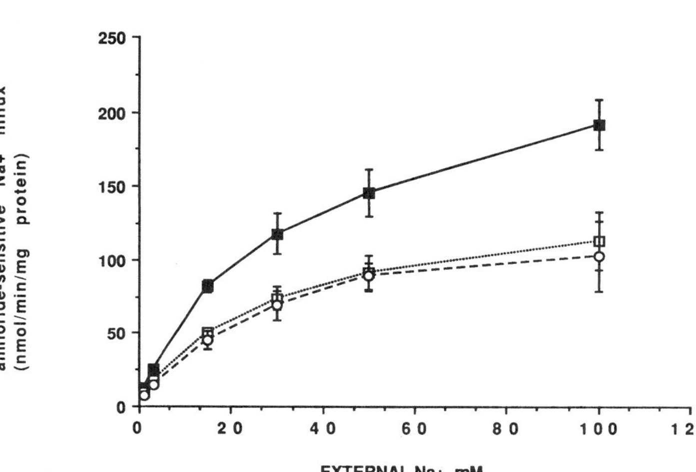

FIGURE 81-3. Amiloride-sensitive $^{22}Na^{+}$ influx as a function of external Na^{+} concentration in acid-loaded fibroblasts from IDDM patients with (■) and without (□) nephropathy, and normal subjects (○).

Potential Involvement of the Sodium-Hydrogen Antiporter in the Pathogenesis of Diabetic Nephropathy

The kinetic abnormalities of sodium-hydrogen antiport described in cells from IDDM patients with nephropathy are similar to those reported in cells from patients with essential hypertension and may be determined by genetic factors. This supports the contention that an inherited predisposition to essential hypertension increases the risk of diabetic nephropathy.

A critical question arises from these studies: Is this altered cation transport system implicated in the pathogenesis of diabetic nephropathy, and if so, how?

The abnormalities of sodium-hydrogen antiport seem unlikely to reflect modifications in a sodium-hydrogen antiport gene (or genes). Genetic linkage analysis has yielded no evidence for *NHE1* as a candidate gene in hypertension.[102] The possibility that the increased maximal velocity could be due to an increased gene expression of *NHE1* was excluded both in patients with essential hypertension and in diabetic patients with nephropathy.

It seems more likely that some of the regulatory pathways of the sodium-hydrogen exchange may be important for its overactivity in diabetic nephropathy. Inhibition of protein kinase C in lymphocytes of IDDM patients with albuminuria was found to normalize the elevated activity of the antiporter.[103] These preliminary findings suggest that a more extensive degree of phosphorylation may determine a more active antiport.

Several other phenotypic abnormalities have been described in cultured cells from IDDM patients with nephropathy. Increased sodium-hydrogen antiport activity is closely associated with abnormal cell proliferation in several cell types in patients with both essential hypertension and diabetic nephropathy. Enhanced DNA synthesis after stimulation of quiescent fibroblasts with serum has been described in skin fibroblasts from patients with diabetic nephropathy, suggesting a difference in the ability of these cells to enter the synthetic S phase after mitogen stimulation.[99] These preliminary data have been confirmed by the finding of abnormalities in the cell cycle and cell life span of these fibroblasts. Extracellular matrix synthesis, in particular collagen production, also has been found to be significantly enhanced in fibroblasts from patients with nephropathy.[104] Because sodium-hydrogen antiport may be activated by extracellular matrix protein,[105] this coexistence of an altered matrix synthesis with an overactive cation transport system may help to understand the reason for the excessive matrix deposition that leads to glomerular sclerosis in diabetic nephropathy.

Whether the enhanced activity of sodium-hydrogen antiporter reflects the appropriate response to an abnormal growth tendency or constitutes a primary permissive factor leading to cell function disturbances remains to be clarified. In any case, it is clear that in diabetic nephropathy the reason for an increased susceptibility is likely to reside in the host cell response to the dysregulation brought about by diabetes.

Many growth factors and vasoactive compounds are elevated in diabetes both in the circulation and at the tissue level. In glomeruli from rats made diabetic with streptozocin, an increased and sustained mRNA expression of a variety of growth factors have been found.[106]

More insight into the relationship between the disturbed milieu of diabetes and the sodium-hydrogen antiport activity has come from a recent study by Williams and Howard[107] that demonstrated that elevated glucose concentrations significantly increased sodium-hydrogen antiport activity in cultured vascular smooth muscle cells via a glucose-induced protein kinase C (PCK)-dependent mechanism, thereby providing a biochemical basis for a further increase in the activity of the antiport in the vascular tissues of patients with IDDM.

It is possible to speculate that increased concentrations of growth factors and plasma glucose may exert a more profound effect in the subset of diabetic patients who are characterized by an intrinsic overactivity of sodium-hydrogen antiport or who are predisposed to overreact to any hypertrophic or hyperplastic stimulus.

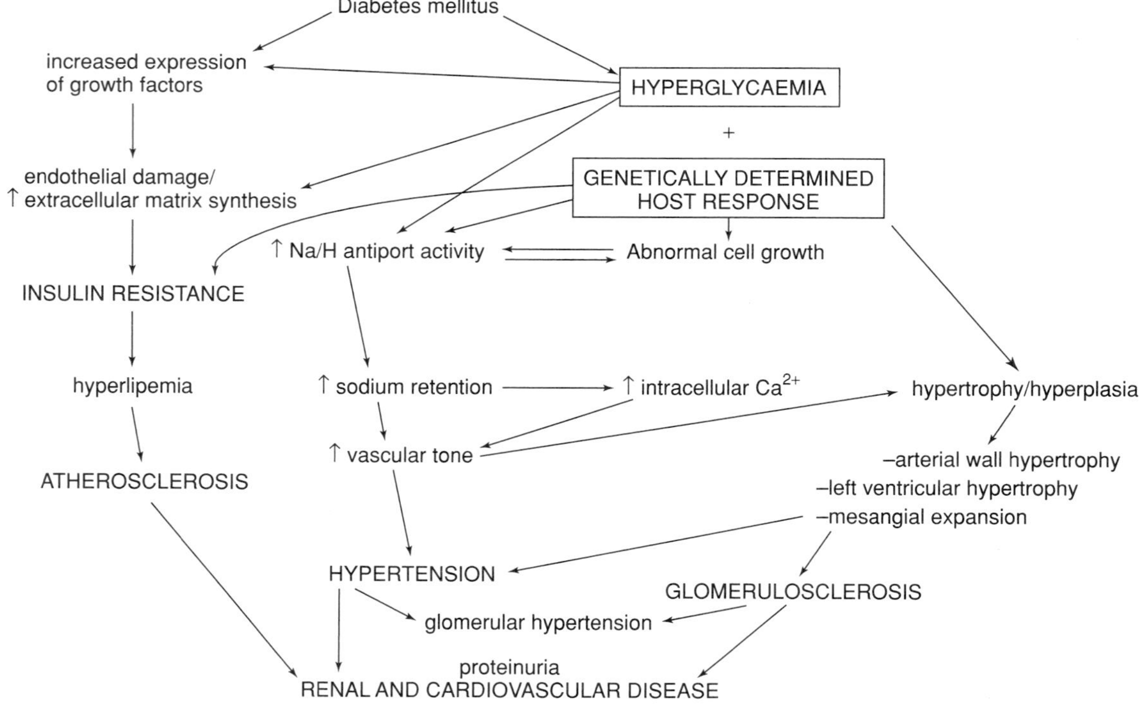

Figure 81-4. Hypothetic representation of a sequence of events leading to the development of renal and cardiovascular disease in a subset of susceptible diabetic patients.

A possible sequence of events leading to diabetic nephropathy are represented in Figure 81-4. Diabetic subjects exhibiting an overactivity of this membrane ion transporter could have increased tubular sodium reabsorption, which would increase renal plasma flow and lead to glomerular hyperfiltration in order to maintain sodium balance. The hypertrophic/hyperplastic processes of smooth muscle cells in arteries and arterioles associated with raised Na^+/H^+ antiport activity could lead to increased vascular tone and an increase in systemic and intraglomerular pressure. The same process could cause mesangial expansion. An alteration of extracellular matrix synthesis associated with sodium-hydrogen antiport overactivity may contribute to excessive matrix deposition in the mesangium and interstitium. These abnormalities would trigger a cycle of events producing systemic and glomerular hypertension, more severe glomerulosclerosis, and finally, glomerular occlusion and renal failure.

Candidate Genes for Diabetic Nephropathy

The search for polymorphism in genes potentially involved in susceptibility to the development of diabetic nephropathy recently has generated intensive research activity and contrasting reports. Significant associations between DNA sequence differences at the locus of angiotensin I-converting enzyme (ACE) and diabetic nephropathy have been reported by some groups. DNA from 151 IDDM patients was genotyped at the ACE locus by a three-allele restriction fragment-melting polymorphism (*DdeI*) and a two-allele insertion/deletion recognized as a restriction fragment-length polymorphism (*XbaI*). Carriers of *XbaI/DdeI* "+ =" haplotype had a fourfold risk of having diabetic nephropathy.[108] In another study, an imbalance of ACE genotype distribution, with a low proportion of subjects homozygotic for insertion II (XbaI "−"), was observed in IDDM patients with nephropathy compared to their control subjects. Higher plasma ACE levels also were found in IDDM patients with nephropathy. The authors concluded that this genotype of *ACE* gene (XbaI "−") is a marker for reduced risk for diabetic nephropathy.[109] More recent data in larger series, however, have been unable to confirm an association between *ACE*-polymorphism and nephropathy, but do show a relationship with the cardiovascular complications of diabetic nephropathy.[110]

The presence of allele 2 of the anti-inflammatory interleukin-1 receptor antagonist gene (*IL1*) has been reported to confer a fourfold increased risk for diabetic nephropathy in both IDDM and NIDDM patients. Moreover, strong association has been described between allele frequency of the rarer allele of *IL1β* gene and diabetic nephropathy in NIDDM patients.[111] Whether these proinflammatory genes contribute to the pathogenesis or are a simple chromosomal marker remains to be established.

The candidate gene approach may not represent the best strategy to identify susceptibility genes for diabetic renal disease. Other techniques, including differential display of mRNA by polymerase chain reaction (PCR) or genome search by microsatellite in multiplex diabetic nephropathy families, must be explored.

Conclusions

In the past few years new evidence has been accumulating on the complex interaction among metabolic, hemodynamic, and cellular factors involved in the pathophysiology of diabetic nephropathy. Preliminary data support a genetic basis for each of these factors. A better understanding of the genetic factors conferring susceptibility to diabetic nephropathy, and of its pathophysiology, will help those patients at risk of developing this complication of diabetes to be identified earlier and treated more successfully.

References

1. Viberti GC, Walker JD, Pinto J. Diabetic nephropathy. In: Alberti KGMM, De Fronzo RA, Keen H, Pinto J, eds. International Textbook of Diabetes Mellitus. New York, NY: John Wiley & Sons;1992:1267–1328
2. Mogensen CE. Glomerular filtration rate and renal plasma flow in short-term and long-term juvenile diabetes mellitus. Scand J Clin Lab Invest 1971;28:91
3. Wiseman MJ, Viberti GC, Keen H. Threshold effect of plasma glucose in the glomerular hyperfiltration in diabetics. Nephron 1984;48:257
4. Wiseman MJ, Saunders AJ, Keen H, Viberti GC. Effect of blood glucose on increased glomerular filtration rate and kidney size in insulin-dependent diabetes. N Engl J Med 1985;312:617
5. Wiseman MJ, Viberti GC. Kidney size and GFR in type 1 insulin-dependent diabetes mellitus revisited. Diabetologia 1983;25:530
6. Zatz R, Meyer TM, Rennke HG, Brenner BM. Predominance of hemodynamic rather than metabolic factors in the pathogenesis of diabetic glomerulopathy. Proc Natl Acad Sci U S A 1985;82:5963
7. Hostetter TH, Troy JC, Brenner BM. Glomerular hemodynamics in experimental diabetes mellitus. Kidney Int 1981;19:410
8. Berkman J, Rifkin H. Unilateral nodular diabetic glomerulosclerosis (Kimmelstiel-Wilson): Report of a case. Metabolism 1973;22:715
9. Mogensen CE. Early glomerular hyperfiltration in insulin-dependent diabetics and late nephropathy. Scand J Clin Lab Invest 1984;46:201
10. Mogensen CE, Christensen CK. Predicting diabetic nephropathy in insulin-dependent diabetic patients. N Engl J Med 1984;311:89
11. Rudberg S, Persson B, Dalquist G. Increased glomerular filtration rate as a predictor of diabetic nephropathy: An 8 year prospective study. Kidney Int 1992;41:822
12. Messent J, Jones SL, Wiseman M, Viberti CC. Glomerular hyperfiltration and albuminuria—an 8 year prospective study [abstract]. Diabetologia 1991; 34 (suppl 2):A1
13. Kroustrup JP, Gundersen HJG, Osterby R. Glomerular size and structure in diabetes mellitus: III. Early enlargement of the capillary surface. Diabetologia 1977;13:207
14. Hirose K, Tsuchida H, Osterby R, Gundersen HJG. A strong correlation between glomerular filtration rate and filtration surface area in diabetic kidney hyperfiltration. Lab Invest 1980;43:434
15. Christiansen JS, Frandsen M, Parving HH. Effect of intravenous glucose infusion on renal function in normal man and in insulin-dependent diabetics. Diabetologia 1981;21:368
16. Mathiesen ER, Hilsted J, Feldt-Rasmussen B, et al. The effect of metabolic control on hemodynamics in short-term insulin-dependent diabetic patients. Diabetes 1985;34:1301
17. Gray SD. Effect of hypertonicity on vascular dimensions in skeletal muscle. Microvasc Res 1971;3:117
18. Harvey JN, Edmundson AW, Jaffa AA, et al. Renal excretion of kallikrein and eicosanoids in patients with type 1 (insulin-dependent) diabetes mellitus: Relationship to glomerular and tubular function. Diabetologia 1992;35:857
19. Perico N, Benigni A, Gabanelli M, et al. Atrial natriuretic peptide and prostacyclin synergistically mediate hyperfiltration and hyperperfusion of diabetic rats. Diabetes 1992;41:533
20. Blantz RC, Peterson OW, Gushwa L, Tucker BJ. Effect of modest hyperglycemia on tubuloglomerular feedback activity. Kidney Int 1982;22:S206
21. Trevisan R, Nosadini R, Fioretto P, et al. Ketone bodies increase glomerular filtration rate in normal man and in patients with type 1 (insulin-dependent) diabetes. Diabetologia 1987;30:214
22. Parving HH, Christiansen JS, Noer I, et al. The effect of glucagon infusion on kidney function in short term insulin-dependent juvenile diabetics. Diabetologia 1980;10:350
23. Christiansen JS, Gammelgaard J, Frandsen M, et al. Kidney function and size in normal subjects before and during growth hormone administration for one week. Eur J Clin Invest 1981;11:487
24. Kasiske BL, O'Donnell MP, Keane WF. Glucose induced increase in renal hemodynamic function: Possible modulation by renal prostaglandins. Diabetes 1985;34:360
25. Schambelan M, Blake S, Sraer J, et al. Increased prostaglandin production by glomeruli isolated from rats with streptozotocin-induced diabetes mellitus. J Clin Invest 1985;75:404
26. Viberti GC, Benigni A, Bognetti E, et al. Glomerular hyperfiltration and urinary prostaglandins in type 1 diabetes mellitus. Diabet Med 1989;6:219
27. Esmatjes E, Fernandez MR, Halperin I, et al. Renal hemodynamic abnormalities in patients with short-term insulin-dependent diabetes mellitus: Role of renal prostaglandins. J Clin Endocrinol Metab 1985;60:1231
28. Christiansen JS, Feldt-Rasmussen B, Parving HH. Short-term inhibition of prostaglandin synthesis has no effect on the elevated glomerular filtration rate of early insulin-dependent diabetes. Diabetic Med 1985;2:17
29. Ballerman BJ, Skorecki KL, Brenner BM. Reduced glomerular angiotensin II receptor density in early untreated diabetes mellitus in the rat. Am J Physiol 1984;247:F110
30. Mayfield RK, Margolius HS, Levine JH, et al. Urinary kallikrein excretion in insulin-dependent diabetes mellitus and its relationship to glycemic control. J Clin Endocrinol Metab 1984;59:278
31. Christlieb AR. Renin, angiotensin and norepinephrine in alloxan diabetes. Diabetes 1974;23:962

32. Ortola FV, Ballerman BJ, Anderson S, et al. Elevated plasma natriuretic peptide levels in diabetic rats. J Clin Invest 1987;80:670
33. Skott P, Hother-Nielsen O, Bruun NE, et al. Effects of insulin on kidney function and sodium excretion in healthy subjects. Diabetologia 1989;32:694
34. Hostetter TH. Human renal response to a meat meal. Am J Physiol 1986; 250:F13
35. Wiseman MJ, Bognetti E, Dodds R, et al. Changes in renal function in response to protein restricted diet in type 1 insulin-dependent diabetic patients. Diabetologia 1987;30:154
36. Kontessis P, Jones SL, Dodds RA, et al. Renal, metabolic and hormonal responses to ingestion of animal and vegetable proteins. Kidney Int 1990; 38:136
37. Viberti CC, Jarrett RJ, Mahmud U, et al. Microalbuminuria as a predictor of clinical nephropathy in insulin-dependent diabetes mellitus. Lancet 1982;1:1430
38. Parving H-H, Oxenboll B, Svendsen PA, et al. Early detection of patients at risk of developing diabetic nephropathy: A longitudinal study of urinary albumin excretion. Acta Endocrinol 1982;100:550
39. Mathiesen ER, Oxenboll B, Johansen K, et al. Incipient nephropathy in type 1 (insulin-dependent) diabetes. Diabetologia 1984;26:406
40. Mogensen CE, Christensen CK. Predicting diabetic nephropathy in insulin-dependent diabetic patients. N Engl J Med 1984;311:89
41. Cohen DL, Close CF, Viberti GC. The variability of overnight urinary albumin excretion in insulin-dependent diabetic and normal subjects. Diabet Med 1987;4:427
42. EURODIAB IDDM Complications Study Group. Microvascular and acute complications in IDDM patients: The EURODIAB IDDM Complications Study. Diabetologia 1994;37:278
43. Uusitupa M, Siitonen O, Penttila I, et al. Proteinuria in newly diagnosed type II diabetic patients. Diabetes Care 1987;10:191
44. Fioretto P, Steffes MW, Mauer M. Glomerular structure in nonproteinuric IDDM patients with various levels of albuminuria. Diabetes 1994;48:1358
45. Feldt-Rasmussen B, Mathiesen E, Deckert T. Effect of two years of strict metabolic control on the progression of incipient nephropathy in insulin-dependent diabetes. Lancet 1986;2:1300
46. Viberti GC, Keen H. The patterns of proteinuria in diabetes mellitus: Relevance to pathogenesis and prevention of diabetic nephropathy. Diabetes 1984;33:686
47. Deckert T, Kofoed-Enevoldsen A, Vidal P, et al. Size- and charge-selectivity of glomerular filtration in IDDM patients with and without albuminuria. Diabetologia 1993;36:244
48. Wiseman M, Viberti GC, Mackintosh D, et al. Glycaemia, arterial pressure and microalbuminuria in type I (insulin-dependent) diabetes mellitus. Diabetologia 1984;26:401
49. Mogensen CE, Christensen CK. Blood pressure changes and renal function changes in incipient and overt diabetic nephropathy. Hypertension 1985; 7:II64
50. Poulsen L, Hansen KW, Mogensen CE. Ambulatory blood pressure in the transition from normo- to microalbuminuria. Diabetes 1994;43:1248
51. Microalbuminuria Collaborative Study Group. Risk factors for the development of microalbuminuria in insulin-dependent diabetic patients: A cohort study. BMJ 1993;306:1235
52. Nelson RG, Pettitt DJ, Baird HR, et al. Prediabetic blood pressure predicts urinary albumin excretion after the onset of type 2 (non-insulin-dependent) diabetes mellitus in Pima Indians. Diabetologia 1993;36:998
53. Haneda M, Kikkawa R, Togawa M, et al. High blood pressure is a risk factor for the development of microalbuminuria in Japanese subjects with non-insulin-dependent diabetes mellitus. J Diabetes Complications 1992;6:181
54. Jones SL, Close CE, Mattock MB, et al. Plasma lipid and coagulation factor concentrations in insulin-dependent diabetics with microalbuminuria. BMJ 1988;29:487
55. Jensen T. Increased plasma level of von Willebrand factor in type 1 (insulin-dependent) diabetic patients with incipient nephropathy. BMJ 1989;298:27
56. Trevisan R, Nosadini R, Fioretto P, et al. Clustering of risk factors in hypertensive insulin-dependent diabetics with high sodium-lithium countertransport. Kidney Int 1992;41:855
57. Feldt-Rasmussen B. Increased transcapillary escape rate of albumin in type 1 (insulin-dependent) diabetic patients with microalbuminuria. Diabetologia 1986;29:282
58. Yip J, Mattock M, Sethi M, et al. Insulin resistance in insulin-dependent diabetic patients with microalbuminuria. Lancet 1993;342:883
59. Messent J, Elliott T, Hill R, et al. Prognostic significance of microalbuminuria in insulin-dependent diabetes mellitus: A twenty-three year follow-up study. Kidney Int 1992;41:836
60. Mattock MB, Morrish NJ, Viberti GC, et al. Prospective study of microalbuminuria as predictor of mortality in NIDDM. Diabetes 1992;41:736
61. Viberti GC, Bilous RW, Mackintosh D, Keen H. Monitoring glomerular function in diabetic nephropathy. Am J Med 1983;74:256
62. Myers BD, Winetz JA, Chui F, Michaels AS. Mechanisms of proteinuria in diabetic nephropathy: A study of glomerular barrier function. Kidney Int 1982;21:633
63. Wahl P, Deppermann D, Hasslacher C. Biochemistry of glomerular basement membrane of the normal and diabetic human. Kidney Int 1982;21:744
64. Shimomura H, Spiro RG. Studies on the macromolecular components of human glomerular basement membrane and alterations in diabetes: Decreased levels of heparan sulfate proteoglycan and laminin. Diabetes 1987;36: 374
65. The Diabetes Control and Complications Trial Research Group. The effect of intensive treatment of diabetes on the development and progression of long-term complications in insulin-dependent diabetes mellitus. N Engl J Med 1993;329:977
66. Brownlee M, Cerami A, Vlassara H. Advanced glycosylation end products in tissue and the biochemical basis of diabetic complications. N Engl J Med 1988;318:1315
67. Vogt BW, Schleicher E, Wieland OH. Aminolysine bound glucose in human tissues obtained at autopsy: Increase in diabetes mellitus. Diabetes 1982; 31:1123
68. Vlassara H, Brownlee M, Cerami A. Novel macrophage receptor for glucose-modified proteins is distinct from previously described scavenger receptors. J Exp Med 1986;164:1301
69. Greene D. The pathogenesis and its prevention of diabetic neuropathy and nephropathy. Metabolism 1988;37(suppl 1):25
70. Tilton RG, Chang K, Pugliese G, et al. Prevention of hemodynamic and vascular albumin filtration changes in diabetic rats by aldose reductase inhibitors. Diabetes 1989;38:1258
71. Pugliese G, Tilton RG, Speedy A, et al. Modulation of hemodynamics and vascular filtration changes in diabetic rats by dietary myoinositol. Diabetes 1990;39:312
72. Rasch R, Osterby R. Lack of influence of aldose reductase inhibitor treatment for 6 months on the glycogen nephrosis in streptozotocin diabetic rats. Diabetologia 1990;32:532A
73. Lorenzi M. Glucose toxicity in the vascular complications of diabetes: The cellular perspective. Diabetes Metab Rev 1992;8:85
74. Vora JP, Anderson S, Brenner BM. Pathogenesis of diabetic glomerulopathy: The role of glomerular hemodynamic factors. In: Mogensen CE, ed. The Kidney and Hypertension in Diabetes Mellitus. 2nd ed. Norwell, MA: Kluwer Academic Publishers; 1994:223–232
75. Bank N, Klose R, Aynedjian AS, et al. Evidence against increased glomerular pressure initiating diabetic nephropathy. Kidney Int 1987;31:898
76. Andersen AR, Christiansen JS, Andersen JK, et al. Diabetic nephropathy in type I (insulin-dependent) diabetes: An epidemiological study. Diabetologia 1983;25:496
77. Krolewski AS, Warram JH, Christlieb AR, et al. The changing natural history of nephropathy in type I diabetes. Am J Med 1985;78:785
78. Seaquist ER, Goetz FC, Rich S, Barbosa J. Familial clustering of diabetic kidney disease: Evidence for genetic susceptibility to diabetic nephropathy. N Engl J Med 1989;320:1161
79. Borch-Johnsen K, Norgaard K, Hommel E, et al. Is diabetic nephropathy an inherited complication? Kidney Int 1992;41:719
80. Pettitt DJ, Saad MF, Bennett PH, et al. Familial predisposition to renal disease in two generations of Pima Indians with type 2 (non-insulin-dependent) diabetes mellitus. Diabetologia 1990;33:438
81. Earle K, Walker J, Hill C, Viberti GC. Familial clustering of cardiovascular disease in patients with insulin-dependent diabetes and nephropathy. N Engl J Med 1992;326:673
82. Yip J, Mattock M, Sethi M, et al. Insulin resistance in family members of insulin-dependent diabetic patients with microalbuminuria. Lancet 1993; 341:369
83. De Cosmo S, Bacci S, De Cicco ML, et al. Increased prevalence of cardiovascular disease, reduced insulin sensitivity in parents of IDDM patients with elevated albumin excretion rate. Diabetologia 1994;37(suppl 1):A23
84. Viberti GC, Keen H, Wiseman MJ. Raised arterial pressure in parents of proteinuric insulin-dependent diabetic. BMJ 1987;295:515
85. Krolewski AS, Canessa M, Warram J, et al. Predisposition to hypertension and susceptibility to renal disease in insulin-dependent diabetes mellitus. N Engl J Med 1988;318:140
86. Poulsen PL, Hansen KW, Mogensen CE. Ambulatory blood pressure in the transition from normo- to microalbuminuria: A longitudinal study in IDDM patients. Diabetes 1994;43:1248
87. Hansen KW, Christensen CK, Andersen PH, et al. Ambulatory blood pressure in microalbuminuric type 1 diabetic patients. Kidney Int 1992;41:847
88. Morgan DB, Steward AD, Davidson C. Relations between erythrocyte lithium efflux, blood pressure and family history of hypertension and cardiovascular disease: Studies in a factory workforce and hypertension clinic. J Hypertens 1986;4:609
89. Hasstedt SJ, Wu LL, Ash KO, et al. Hypertension and sodium-lithium countertransport in Utah pedigrees: Evidence for major locus inheritance. Am J Hum Genet 1988;43:14
90. Mangili R, Bending JJ, Scott G, et al. Increased sodium-lithium countertransport activity in red cells of patients with insulin-dependent diabetes and nephropathy. N Engl J Med 1988;318:146
91. Jones SL, Trevisan R, Tariq T, et al. Sodium-lithium countertransport in microalbuminuric insulin-dependent diabetic patients. Hypertension 1990; 15:570
92. Morocutti A, Barzon I, Solini A, et al. Poor metabolic control and predisposition to hypertension, rather than hypertension itself, are risk factors for nephropathy in type 2 diabetes. Acta Diabet 1992;29:123
93. Walker JD, Tariq T, Viberti GC. Sodium-lithium countertransport activity in red cells of patients with insulin-dependent diabetes and nephropathy and their parents. BMJ 1990;301:635

94. Hardman TC, Dubrey SW, Leslie RDG, et al. Erythrocyte sodium-lithium countertransport and blood pressure in identical twin pairs discordant for insulin-dependent diabetes. BMJ 1992;305:215
95. Rosskopf D, Dusing R, Siffert W. Membrane sodium-proton exchange and primary hypertension. Hypertension 1993;21:607
96. Ng LL, Simmons D, Frighi V, et al. Leukocyte sodium-hydrogen antiport activity in type 1 (insulin-dependent) diabetic patients with nephropathy. Diabetologia 1990;33:371
97. Ng LL, Dudley C, Bomford J, Hawley D. Leukocyte intracellular pH and sodium-hydrogen antiport activity in human hypertension. J Hypertens 1989; 7:471
98. Semplicini A, Mozzato MG, Sama B, et al. Sodium-hydrogen and lithium-sodium exchange in red cells of normotensive and hypertensive patients with insulin-dependent diabetes mellitus. Am J Hypertens 1989;2:174
99. Trevisan R, Li LK, Messent J, et al. Na H antiport activity and cell growth in cultured skin fibroblasts of IDDM patients with nephropathy. Diabetes 1992;41:1239
100. Davies JE, Ng LL, Kofoed-Enevoldsen A, et al. Intracellular pH and sodium-hydrogen antiport activity of cultured skin fibroblasts from diabetics. Kidney Int 1992;42:1184
101. Ng LL, Davies JE, Siczkowski M, et al. Abnormal sodium-hydrogen antiporter phenotype and turnover of immortalized lymphoblasts from type 1 diabetic patients with nephropathy. J Clin Invest 1994;93:2750
102. Lifton RP, Hunt SC, Williams RR, et al. Exclusion of the sodium-hydrogen antiporter as a candidate gene in human essential hypertension. Hypertension 1991;17:8
103. Ng LL, Simmons D, Frighi V, et al. Effect of protein kinase C modulators on the leukocyte sodium-hydrogen antiport in type 1 diabetic subjects with albuminuria. Diabetologia 1990;33:278
104. Yip J, Trevisan R, Li LK, Viberti GC. Enhanced collagen synthesis in cultured skin fibroblasts from insulin-dependent diabetic patients with nephropathy. Diabetologia 1993;36(suppl 1):A11
105. Schwartz MA, Lechene C, Ingber DE. Insoluble fibronectin activates the sodium-hydrogen antiporter by clustering and immobilizing integrin, independent of cell shape. Proc Natl Acad Sci U S A 1991;88:7849
106. Nakamura T, Fukui M, Ebihara I, et al. mRNA expression of growth factors in glomeruli from diabetic rats. Diabetes 1993;42:450
107. Williams B, Howard RL. Glucose-induced changes in Na/H antiport activity and gene expression in cultured vascular muscle cells. J Clin Invest 1994; 93:2623
108. Doria A, Warram JH, Krowlewski AS. Genetic predisposition to diabetic nephropathy: Evidence for a role of the angiotensin I-converting enzyme gene. Diabetes 1994;43:690
109. Marre M, Bernadet P, Gallois Y, et al. Relationships between angiotensin I converting enzyme gene polymorphism, plasma levels, and diabetic retinal and renal complications. Diabetes 1994;43:384
110. Tarnow L, Cambien F, Rossing P, et al. Angiotensin-converting enzyme gene polymorphism, diabetic nephropathy and coronary heart disease in IDDM patients. Diabetologia 1994;37(suppl 1):A126
111. Gonzalez AM, di Giovine F, Cox A, et al. Diabetic nephropathy in type 2 diabetes is associated with an allele of the IL-1 beta gene. Diabet Med 1994;8(suppl 1):S13

Diabetes Mellitus, edited by Derek LeRoith, Simeon I. Taylor, and Jerrold M. Olefsky. Lippincott–Raven Publishers, Philadelphia © 1996.

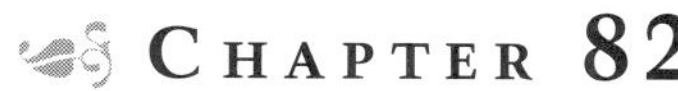

Chapter 82

Diabetic Neuropathies: An Overview of Clinical Aspects

Aaron I. Vinik, Pauline Newlon, Zvonko Milicevic, Patricia McNitt, and Kevin B. Stansberry

Diabetic neuropathy is a heterogeneous condition that encompasses a wide range of dysfunction and, whose development might be attributable to diabetes per se or to factors associated with the disease. The most common form of diabetic neuropathy is *distal symmetric polyneuropathy,* which can afflict somatic sensory or motor nerves and the autonomic nervous system. In general it is an insidious disorder with slow progression and a predilection for early involvement of the longest axons. Thus, symptoms often begin in the feet and progress proximally to involve the hands. Similarly, damage to the long vagal nerve fibers precedes that of the shorter sympathetic nervous system fibers. Focal or multifocal forms are asymmetric and affect cranial, trunk, or limb innervation. The most striking feature seen histopathologically is the loss of nerve fibers affecting the most remote nerve trunks first. The loss of sensation is what predisposes diabetic patients to ulceration, infection, and ultimately limb loss, accounting for the high morbidity. Once the autonomic nervous system is involved, mortality may be as high as 50% within 5 years, pointing to the serious consequences of this complication. The disorder can be manifested, by obvious symptoms, or it can be subclinically apparent, with abnormalities detectable only with careful testing. Frequently, the diagnosis of diabetic neuropathy is difficult to make because the manifestations are nonspecific and may occur in a number of other conditions. Neuropathy is not confined to a single type of diabetes, but can occur in insulin-dependent and non–insulin-dependent diabetes mellitus (IDDM and NIDDM) and in various forms of acquired diabetes.[1–3] Although there is considerable uncertainty as to the prevalence of neuropathy in the diabetic population, it is generally accepted that neuropathy is the most common, and often the most troublesome, of the major complications afflicting this group. In this chapter, we present an overview of current thinking on the etiology, pathogenesis, clinical presentations, diagnostic tests, and various forms of specific and general therapies for diabetic neuropathies.

Classification

Table 82-1 is offered as a current classification of diabetic neuropathy; this clearly will be modified as our understanding of the disease process improves. The signs, symptoms, and neurologic deficits vary depending on the classes of nerve fibers involved. Neuropathies may be either sensory or motor[4–6] and may involve primarily small or large nerve fibers.[7] Small nerve fiber damage usually (although not always) precedes large nerve fiber damage and is manifested first in the lower limbs, with pain and hyperalgesia, followed by a loss of thermal sensitivity and reduced light touch and

Table 82-1. Classification of Diabetic Neuropathies

Type	Description
Distal Sensorimotor peripheral polyneuropathy	Pain and dysesthesias Glove and stocking sensory loss Loss of reflexes Muscle weakness and wasting
Autonomic	Tachycardia, ventricular dysfunction, cardiac denervation, orthostatic hypotension, impaired cutaneous blood flow Gastroparesis, diarrhea Urogenital dysfunction, impotence, atonic bladder Gustatory sweating, pupillary abnormalities, anhidrosis, hypoglycemia unresponsiveness/unawareness
Mononeuropathy	Cranial nerve palsy Carpal tunnel and tarsal tunnel syndromes Ulnar, peroneal, and femoral nerve palsies
Amyotrophy (proximal neuropathy)	Acute anterior thigh pain Weakness of hip flexion and fasciculation, wasting
Radiculopathy	Pain and sensory loss in dermatomal distribution

pinprick sensation.[8] When pain occurs, nerve conduction velocity (NCV) is often normal or only minimally reduced.[9] Large fiber neuropathies are manifested by reduced vibration and position sense, weakness, muscle wasting, and depressed tendon reflexes. Most diabetic peripheral neuropathy is of the ''mixed'' variety—a combination of both large and small nerve fiber involvement. In our own outpatient population, only 15.0% of patients with symptoms of confirmed neuropathy had no objective signs, and 63.7% of patients with signs had no symptoms.[8] A very small proportion show ''pure'' small nerve or large nerve fiber deficit.[7,8] Involvement of the autonomic nervous system can occur as early as the first year after diagnosis[10–12] and may involve any system in the body. Subclinical abnormalities in cardiovascular[13] and gastrointestinal function[14] may be found at diagnosis,[15] or even in teenage diabetic persons.[16] The clinical features, however, often are unsuspected and without careful scrutiny may go undetected. These features include the following: resting tachycardia with exercise intolerance, orthostatic hypotension, impaired sweating and cutaneous blood flow regulation, hypoglycemic unawareness, delayed gastric emptying, diarrhea alternating with constipation, bladder atony, and impotence in male patients.

Prevalence of Neuropathy

Prevalence data for diabetic neuropathy are sparse. Few population-based studies have been undertaken, and because the prevalence of undiagnosed diabetes in the general population is estimated to be at least as great as the prevalence of diagnosed diabetes,[17] there must be a significant number of undisclosed cases. Furthermore, most published studies entail substantial selection biases because they are limited to that portion of the diabetic population with access to medical care. In addition, lack of consensus as to the appropriate diagnostic criteria for diabetic neuropathy has resulted in a wide range of prevalence estimates reported in the literature, ranging from 0% to 93%![18] When neuropathy is defined as loss of Achilles reflexes with symptoms or objective signs of polyneuropathy, then prevalence is 7% for persons within 1 year of being diagnosed with diabetes, rising to 50% for those who have had diabetes for >25 years.[19] In a cohort of 278 healthy IDDM subjects enrolled in the feasibility phase of the Diabetes Control and Complication Trial (DCCT), subclinical polyneuropathy was detectable in 39% of the asymptomatic subjects on careful examination.[20] Evidence of autonomic neuropathy[21] and reduction in motor nerve conduction velocities have been documented, even among diabetic children,[22,23] as have reductions in vibratory sensation.[21]

There are few published estimates of the prevalence of other syndromes of somatic neuropathy, mainly because these conditions occur so infrequently. In a sample of 351 patients attending our diabetes clinic, we observed prevalence rates for mononeuropathy, radiculopathy, and amyotrophy to be 3.0%, 3.5%, and 2.1%, respectively.[19,24]

Estimates of the prevalence of autonomic neuropathy based on the presence of abnormalities of cardiovascular autonomic reflexes have ranged in the literature from 14% to nearly 50%.[25–29] The prevalence is associated both with duration of diabetes[28] and with age,[25] and is equal or higher in NIDDM than in IDDM,[30] although these correlations may not hold for all indices of autonomic function. A striking association has been found among autonomic neuropathy and hypertension, elevation of low-density lipoprotein (LDL) cholesterol, and reduced high-density lipoprotein (HDL) cholesterol.[31] In addition, an increased prevalence of autonomic neuropathy has been found among female patients and patients with a relatively high body mass index.[32]

Natural History

Slowing of NCVs is one of the earliest neuropathic abnormalities that occur in diabetes and often is present even at diagnosis,[15,33–35] especially in NIDDM cases. After diagnosis, slowing of NCV generally progresses at a steady rate by approximately 1 m/sec/year, and level of impairment is positively correlated with duration of diabetes.[36] The large initial decline seen in NIDDM is possibly responsible for the difficulty in obtaining significant reversibility when intervention is made late in the disease process. Sensory fibers are usually affected first, followed by motor fibers, testifying to the need for sophisticated measures of sensory function if early intervention is to be possible.[37] Although slowing of NCV is common in diabetes and often occurs early in the course of the disease, there is considerable uncertainty as to the relevance of these abnormalities to the future development of either subclinical manifestations or clinically apparent diabetic neuropathy. Although most studies have documented that symptomatic patients are more likely to have slower nerve conduction velocities than patients without symptoms,[37–42] NCV does not appear to be related to the severity of symptoms.[43] Symptoms referable to one fiber tract may not relate to those of other tracts. For example, progressive reduction of vibratory sensation and loss of tendon reflexes has been observed in patients who at the same time reported an improvement in pain symptoms.[44,45]

Much remains to be learned of the natural history of diabetic autonomic neuropathy. Testing of cardiovascular reflexes has revealed that signs of autonomic neuropathy may occur relatively early in the course of diabetes.[25,28,46] Both sympathetic and parasympathetic nerve fibers may be affected, with parasympathetic dysfunction preceding sympathetic dysfunction.[28,46,47] Improvements in the methods to measure sympathetic function have now shown, though, that sympathetic damage may occur earlier than previously thought.[48] For example, using infrared pupillometry, Ziegler et al. demonstrated that the speed of pupillary dilation may be slowed even at diagnosis of IDDM.[35]

Although symptomatic somatomotor neuropathy usually precedes the development of symptomatic autonomic neuropathy,[5,49] signs of parasympathetic neuropathy sometimes appear prior to other signs of neuropathy.[50] In contrast, sympathetic nerve abnormalities are rarely found in the absence of signs of somatomotor neuropathy.[50] The mortality for diabetic autonomic neuropathy has been estimated to be of the order of 44% within 2.5 years of diagnosis of symptomatic autonomic neuropathy,[46] but based even on asymptomatic subjects with only abnormalities in autonomic function tests, the overall mortality rate may be as high as 25–40% over 10 years.[51]

Pathogenesis

Figure 82-1 summarizes current theories of pathogenesis of diabetic neuropathy. More detailed discussions of the various theoretic aspects of the pathogenesis are to be found in Chapters 83, 84, and 85 and are not presented here. Most persons with diabetes will develop subclinical or clinical neuropathy given sufficient time. The condition can be exacerbated by a genetic predisposition, excessive consumption of alcohol, or smoking. Height plays a role inasmuch as the longer the nerve fiber the greater its vulnerability to injury. Prevailing concepts of injury invoke metabolic, autoimmune, and vascular pathogenesis. Favored metabolic theories for nerve damage embrace persistent hyperglycemia (or glucose toxicity) causing increased polyol flux; accumulation of sorbitol and fructose; deficiencies in myo-inositol, formation of dihomogamma linolenic acid from linoleic acid, and N-acetyl-L-carnitine; and impairment of the Na^+ pump. Autoimmune mechanisms of nerve destruction are predominantly humoral and may be directed at antigens within nerves, or at the supporting lectins, growth factors, and their receptors. Microvascular insufficiency, either functional or organic, may cause ischemia or failure to deliver appropriate growth factors to the site of need. Glycation of proteins may alter their immunogenicity and enhance autoimmunity, or may contribute to the loss of elasticity of vasa nervorum and promote ischemia. Once structural damage occurs, growth factors become necessary if appropriate repair is to be achieved. Failure to do so results in imperfect repair and perpetuates loss of function.

Clinical Manifestations

From a clinical perspective, it is useful to classify diabetic neuropathy into the two broad categories of somatic and autonomic neuropathies, each with its own further subdivisions. The somatic neuropathies tend to fall into three major subdivisions: symmetric distal polyneuropathies, proximal motor neuropathies, and focal neuropathies. Although it is convenient to consider these separately, in practice observed patterns often overlap, and involvement of sensory, motor, and autonomic nerves usually coexists.[7,52,53]

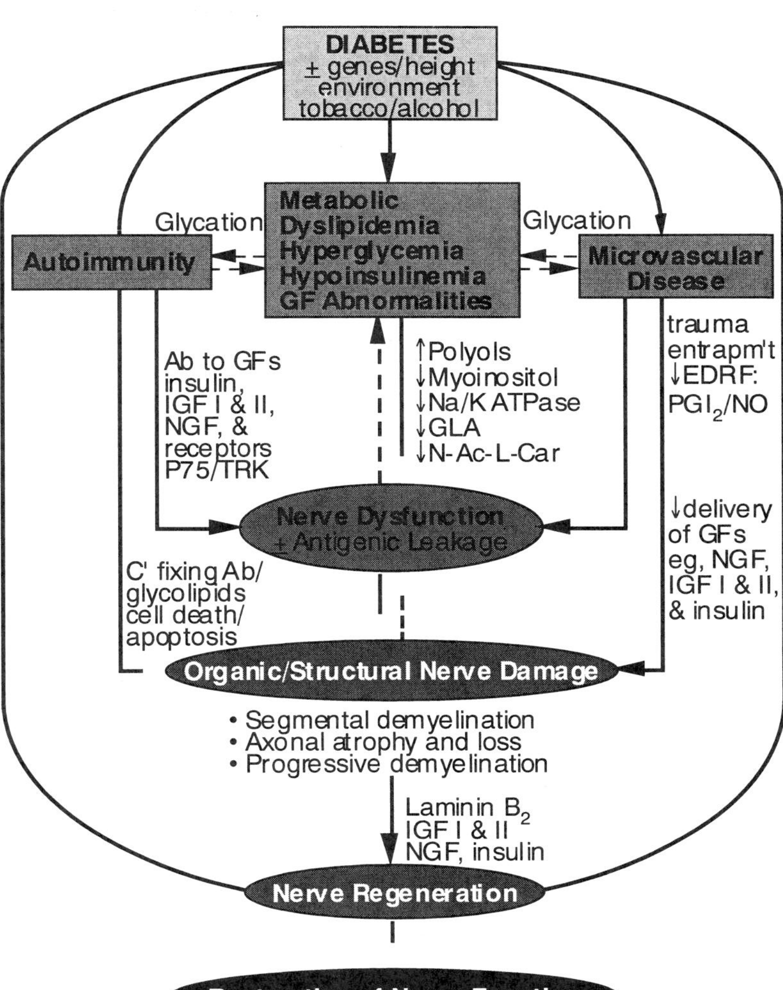

FIGURE 82-1. Theoretic framework for the pathogenesis of diabetic neuropathy.

Somatic Neuropathies

Symmetric Distal Polyneuropathy

Symmetric distal polyneuropathy is the most common and widely recognized form of diabetic neuropathy. The onset is usually insidious but occasionally acute following stress or initiation of therapy for diabetes. The deficit is predominantly sensory, with lesser involvement of motor fibers. Signs include depression or loss of ankle jerks and vibratory sensation, with calf tenderness and hyperalgesia in some patients. The neurologic deficit is peripheral, involving the distal sensorimotor nerves in a "glove and stocking" distribution of the hands, arms, legs, and feet. The lower extremities receive the major brunt of the affliction. The stocking is not a single line of loss of one modality of sensation; rather, there are multiple gloves and stockings, one for each modality. In general, the long fibers that are most severely affected, such as those for position sense and touch, have the highest stocking and the short pain fibers the lowest stocking. The type of neuropathy varies with the type of nerve fiber involved. *Large fibers* are associated with loss of position and vibration sense, some light touch, and sensory ataxia with loss of ankle reflexes. The symptoms may be minimal: sensations of walking on cotton, floors feeling "strange," inability to turn the pages of a book, or inability to discriminate among coins. In contrast, *small fiber* involvement is associated with pain initially, followed by a loss of pain sensation and temperature discrimination.

Generalized motor weakness may occur in *peripheral symmetric neuropathy,* but wasting of the small muscles of the hands and feet is a very characteristic finding. This usually occurs in very advanced cases and may resemble motor neuron disease, although the latter has no sensory component. Loss of the deep tendon reflexes is a hallmark of peripheral symmetric neuropathy, and when pure motor neuropathy is found, causes other than diabetes must be considered.

Acute Painful Neuropathy

Some patients develop a predominantly *small-fiber neuropathy,* which is manifested by pain and paresthesia. Symptoms often are exacerbated at night and are manifested in the feet more than the hands. Spontaneous episodes of pain can be severely disabling. The pain varies in intensity and character. In some patients, the pain has been variably described as burning, lancinating, stabbing, tearing, aching, or like a dog gnawing at the bones. In others, it has been described as dull, like a tooth ache in the bones of the feet, or even crushing or cramp-like. Pain often is accompanied by paresthesia or episodes of distorted sensation, such as pins and needles, tingling, coldness, numbness, or burning.[54] The lower legs may be exquisitely tender to touch, with any disturbance of the hair follicles resulting in excruciating pain. Because pain can be aggravated by repeated contact of the lower limbs with foreign objects, even basic daily activities such as sitting at a desk may be disrupted. Pain often occurs at the onset of the disease[9] and is often worsened by initiation of therapy with insulin or sulfonylureas.[55–57] In this early form of the painful syndrome, the condition often remits spontaneously and the management entails supportive therapy. It may be associated with profound weight loss and severe depression that has been termed *diabetic neuropathic cachexia*.[58] The syndrome occurs predominantly in male patients and may occur at any time in the course of both IDDM and NIDDM.

There is another variety of painful polyneuropathy with onset occurring later in the course of the diabetes, often years later, in which the pain persists and becomes quite debilitating. This condition may lead to tolerance to narcotics and analgesics, and finally to addiction. Although this variety is relatively rare, it is inordinately resistant to all forms of intervention, and most trying to the patient and his or her physician.

The mechanism for acute pain in small-fiber neuropathy is not well understood. In some patients the heralding features of their diabetes may be the onset of acute painful neuropathy[58]; in others the condition may appear soon after initiation of therapy.[57] Hyperglycemia may be a factor in lowering the pain threshold[59]; however, in some patients there is a striking amelioration of symptoms with the intravenous administration of insulin.[9,56] Pain frequently occurs when objective measures suggest recovery from the neuropathy, implying that regrowth of small fibers may be an important constituent of this syndrome. Indeed, loss of pain with evidence of progression of the disease may be indicative of nerve death and thus may not be a welcome occurrence.

Neuropathic (Perforating) Ulcer

Foot ulcer constitutes a major source of morbidity among individuals with diabetes. Loss of protective sensation and repetitive trauma (e.g., walking) are the major causes. Ulceration occurs most frequently over the metatarsal heads, but also appears at other areas of increased pressure. Loss of tone in the small muscles of the feet leads to an imbalance between the flexors and extensors, ultimately resulting in the classic hammer-claw toe. The altered architecture of the foot is associated with increased pressure over the ball of the foot corresponding to the heads of the metatarsals. Also, the normal person constantly shifts the area of pressure in the foot while walking or running, whereas the diabetic with neuropathy is unable to do so because of lack of the sensory input from the soles of the feet. This constant pressure causes calluses with increase in pressure and ultimately ulceration in the high-pressure areas. The hyperhidrosis, cracked and dry skin, and increased small blood vessel flow due to autonomic dysfunction create an excellent milieu for infection to take hold and proliferate.[60] Infection develops after the skin breaks down and, combined with ischemia, can eventually lead to gangrene.

Neuropathic Arthropathy (Charcot's Joints)

Neuropathic arthropathy, or Charcot's joints, occurs in the presence of impaired sensations of pain and proprioception, intact motor power, and repeated minor trauma and usually is found in feet with normal pulses and warmth. The clinical course may be one of acute, painful joint destruction, but usually is painless, characterized by nonedematous enlargement of the foot so that the foot becomes shorter, wider, everted, and externally rotated with a flattening of the arch. The gait becomes abnormal, and clubfoot develops. It is generally limited to the ankle and tarsal joints in diabetes. Pathologic radiographic features include osteopenia, bone lysis, fragmentation, and eburnation. There is disarticulation and dissolution of the joints with bony overgrowth followed by calcification in and around the joints. Eventually pressure ulcers, infection, and osteomyelitis develop. The feet of diabetics often have bounding pulses that suggest an adequate large blood vessel supply. The impression is erroneous, however, and these pulses are now thought to be due to the shunting of blood through the small arteriovenous fistulae normally regulated by the sympathetic nervous system. The enhanced blood flow may be conducive to excessive bone resorption, fractures, and osteoarthropathy.[12,61]

Proximal Motor Neuropathies

Diabetic Amyotrophy (Proximal Neuropathy)

This syndrome is recognized by the triad of pain, severe muscle atrophy in the limb girdle distribution, and fasciculation of the muscles. The onset is usually acute,[62] but it may be subacute and evolve gradually during a period of weeks.[63] Patients also experience generalized weight loss and diabetic cachexia. Asymmetric proximal muscle weakness and wasting of lower extremity muscles, predominantly the iliopsoas, quadriceps, and adductor muscles, occurs. Patients often cannot stand unsupported, climb stairs, or rise from the kneeling or sitting position. The differential diagnosis is Cushing's syndrome, thyrotoxicosis, or a neoplasm, all of which produce proximal myopathy without evidence of nerve lesions and are characterized by intact reflexes. Other differential diagnoses include the proximal neuropathies in which there is no pain or fasciculation, such as Guillain–Barré syndrome. Diabetic amyotrophy is often accompanied by pain in the thigh muscles and sometimes lumbar or perineal regions. The knee jerks are depressed, but little or no sensory involvement is found. The anterolateral muscle group in the lower legs may also be involved, producing the *anterior compartment syndrome*. Occasionally, the upper limb girdle also is affected, and wasting of the deltoids is seen. This syndrome occurs primarily in older patients with NIDDM who frequently have only mild diabetes. It has been postulated that the acute and chronic varieties of the syndrome derive from different pathogenic mechanisms, the acute variety being due to multiple infarcts in the proximal nerve trunks and the lumbosacral plexus and the slowly evolving variety being due to metabolic or autoimmune factors.[64,65] The condition resolves spontaneously, but it can last 1–3 years. New evidence suggests that the course can be modified by immune therapy and resolution of symptoms can occur within 3 weeks.[66]

Truncal Mononeuropathy (Radiculopathy)

This syndrome is primarily a sensory neuropathy affecting the nerve root, which is almost always unilateral and asymmetric. The gender distribution is equal, and older patients are affected primarily. Occasionally, young patients with IDDM of long duration are affected. It usually is associated with peripheral neuropathy and can resemble diabetic cachexia. Hyperesthesia often is found in the root distribution, and the clinical presentation may mimic acute abdominal or thoracic crisis, resulting in unnecessary invasive procedures. Denervation of muscles in the root segment may also occur.[67–71] This syndrome sometimes resembles herpes zoster infection in the prevesicular phase and, occasionally, spinal cord compression from neoplasms or other causes. Nocturnal exacerbation of pain is troublesome, but there is spontaneous remission, usually within 3 months of the onset, dictating a need for supportive therapy during the painful phase.

Focal Neuropathies

Focal and multifocal diabetic neuropathies cause neurologic deficits confined to the distribution of a single nerve (*mononeuropathy*) or multiple individual nerves (*mononeuropathy multiplex*). The onset is typically acute, often heralded by severe pain, and the differential diagnosis must exclude a vascular catastrophe. There is no clear relationship with the age or sex of the patient nor is there a relationship with the type of diabetes, its duration, the degree of diabetes control, or treatment. For common mononeuropathies in diabetes see Chapter 84.

Cranial Nerve Lesions

Lesions in the cranial nerves are manifested as isolated or multiple palsies that occur primarily in the older population, sometimes in the absence of other evidence of neuropathy. The onset is generally abrupt, and although painless in 50% of patients, may be extremely painful in others for reasons that are not understood.[72] The 3rd nerve lesion is most common. It characteristically presents as sudden onset, with a severe ipsilateral headache often preceding the neurologic deficit by several days. Ptosis and ophthalmoplegia are found, but in contrast with the posterior communicating aneurysm rupture, the pupils usually are spared.[73] Of the other extraocular ophthalmoplegias, the 6th nerve is less commonly involved and the 4th nerve seldom involved. The 7th nerve may also be affected, resulting in an isolated Bell's palsy. All other cranial nerves have been reported to be involved, but much less commonly.

Recovery is generally complete within 6–8 weeks and does not appear to be a function of diabetes control.

Isolated Peripheral Nerve Lesions

Isolated peripheral neuropathies involve particularly the ulnar, median, radial, femoral, and lateral cutaneous nerves of the thigh. *Carpal tunnel syndrome* occurs twice as frequently in the diabetic population compared to the normal healthy population. This may be related to repeated, undetected trauma; metabolic changes; or edema within the confined space of the carpal tunnel. The nerves involved usually are mixed or motor, but pure sensory lesions occasionally occur. Nerves at risk for compression are the peroneal nerve at the head of the fibula, the ulnar nerve at the elbow, the median nerve at the wrist, and the lateral cutaneous nerve of the thigh (affected patients may present with unexplained pain and hyperesthesia in the upper, outer quadrant of the thigh) and the peroneal nerves.[74,75] Again, these lesions are self-limiting but may take somewhat longer to resolve than the cranial nerve lesions. For common nerve entrapments and their distinction from mononeuropathies see Chapter 84.

Autonomic Neuropathies

Diabetic autonomic neuropathy may involve any system in the body. Its manifestations are protean, and the onset often is insidious. Using cardiovascular reflex tests, the prevalence is reported to be 17–40%.[16,76–79] Of teenagers with IDDM, 31% have abnormal tests.[16] The relationship with sensorimotor neuropathy is variable, but in general autonomic and sensory motor abnormalities coexist. In people with peripheral neuropathy, 50% have asymptomatic autonomic neuropathy. When symptoms of autonomic neuropathy are present, the anticipated mortality is 15–40% within 5 years.[51,80–82] With gastroparesis, 35% die within 3 years, usually of aspiration pneumonia. Reduced exercise tolerance, edema, paradoxic supine or nocturnal hypertension,[83] and intolerance to heat due to defective thermoregulation are a consequence of autonomic neuropathy. Silent myocardial infarction, respiratory failure and sudden death are hazards for the diabetic with cardiac autonomic neuropathy.[84–87] It is therefore vitally important to make this diagnosis early so that appropriate intervention can be instituted. For a complete discussion of the clinical and biochemical features of autonomic neuropathy and its management, the reader is referred to our recent extensive review.[88] Table 82-2 lists the common manifestations of autonomic neuropathy.

Table 82-2. Common Manifestations of Autonomic Neuropathy

I. Pupillary abnormalities
II. Cardiorespiratory dysfunction
  A. Impaired systolic and diastolic function
  B. Cardiac denervation; silent myocardial infarction
  C. Orthostatic hypotension without compensatory tachycardia
  D. Impaired cutaneous blood flow
  E. Respiratory dysfunction; impaired hypoxia-induced respiratory drive
III. Motor disturbances of gastrointestinal tract
  A. Esophageal enteropathy
  B. Gastroparesis diabeticorum
  C. Diabetic enteropathy
  D. Gut neuroendocrine abnormalities
IV. Genitourinary tract disturbances
  A. Neurogenic vesical dysfunction
  B. Impotence
  C. Retrograde ejaculation
V. Sweating disturbances
VI. Hypoglycemia unawareness and unresponsiveness
VII. Hypoglycemia associated autonomic failure
VIII. Lowered glycemic thresholds

Diagnosis of Diabetic Neuropathies

The American Diabetes Association and the American Academy of Neurology recommend that at least one parameter from each of the following five categories be measured to establish the presence of diabetic neuropathy: symptoms profiles, neurologic examination, quantitative sensory testing (QST), nerve conduction studies, and quantitative autonomic function testing (QAFT).[89] The panel recommended that the neurologic examination be a systematic assessment "of neuropathic signs and symptoms, including sensory, motor and reflex measures in upper and lower extremities, cranial nerves and autonomic function." Suggested motor and sensory nerve conduction studies included amplitudes and conduction velocities from both an arm and a leg.

Clinical Evaluation

A thorough clinical examination is essential in the evaluation of patients suspected of neuropathy—with special attention to the feet, examining for (1) dryness, shiny skin, cracking of the skin, (2) ulceration; (3) loss of hair; (4) levels of loss of sensory modalities, with particular emphasis on vibratory and thermal sensation, (5) reflexes, and (6) motor power. Diabetic neuropathy is diagnosed by exclusion of a variety of other causes of neuropathy (Table 82-3).

Systematic questioning, including a family history of nondiabetic peripheral nerve disease and the presence of toxic, metabolic, mechanical, and vascular causes of nerve disease, should be carried out. If any other potentially neuropathic factors are present, other diagnostic methods should be used to determine the etiology of nerve disease. Appropriate laboratory screening for the differential diagnoses (listed in Table 82-3) should be performed.

To aid in the assessment of neuropathy during a clinical examination, coded scores of neurologic function have been developed that allow assignment of broad categories of functional abnormalities based on the clinical examination (e.g., 1 = normal, 2 = mild abnormality, 3 = moderate abnormality, 4 = severe abnormality, and 5 = total loss of function). Both signs and symptoms can be scored, and the nerve symptom score can be maintained as a record of the patient's response to treatment. Equally important, and neglected in the routine physical examination, are the functional correlates of nerve impairment. The nerve disability score is a useful instrument, and an activity of daily living instrument to measure the functional impact of neuropathy has been developed by us, which ascertains the degree of restriction associated with tasks of living (e.g., the ability to put on a shirt, button a shirt, squeeze toothpaste, use a fork, turn the pages of a book). We also routinely have the patient fill out a neuropathy quality-of-life questionnaire, which, in these days of outcomes consciousness, is often the primary interest of the patient and the health-care providers. These tests have not been applied widely in the evaluation of diabetic neuropathy, but they offer a means of evaluating the degree of restriction of activities that are of vital importance to the patient as well as monitoring progress of the neuropathy.

TABLE 82-3. Differential Diagnosis of Distal Symmetric Polyneuropathy

Congenital/Familial: Charcot Marie tooth
Traumatic: Entrapment syndromes
Inflammatory: AIDS, sarcoidosis, leprosy, lyme disease
Neoplastic: Carcinoma—paraneoplastic syndromes, myeloma, monoclonal gammopathies, amyloid reticuloses, leukemias, lymphomas
Metabolic/Endocrine: Diabetes mellitus, uremia, pernicious anemia (B12 and B6 deficiency), hypothyroidism, malnutrition, porphyria (acute intermittent)
Vascular: Diabetes mellitus, vasculitides
Toxic: Alcohol, heavy metals (lead, mercury, arsenic), hydrocarbons, chemotherapeutic agents, phenytoin (Dilantin), nitrofurantoin, Taxol, vincristine, amiodarone, metronidazole, cisplatin
Autoimmune: Diabetes, collagen vascular disorders, chronic inflammatory demyelinating neuropathy, Multifocal motor neuropathy, Guillain-Barré syndrome

Quantitative Testing in Diabetic Neuropathy

More objective indices are found in the QST[90] and QAFT.[91] Combined, these tests cover vibratory, proprioceptive, tactile, pain, thermal, and autonomic function.[92–94] QST provides standardized procedures for evaluating neuropathy that are sensitive, specific, and reproducible in detecting dysfunction before symptoms appear.[90] We use standardized equipment to determine levels of cutaneous sensitivity. This equipment provides (1) interval data, (2) more precise methods of stimulus presentation, and (3) minimal subject and operator bias.

The QAFT consists of a series of simple, noninvasive tests for detecting cardiovascular autonomic neuropathy. Developed by Ewing and Clarke,[95] they have been successfully applied by many.[96–99] These tests can be done at the bedside and provide an index of the neuropathy that correlates roughly with the vibration threshold and certain other measures of somatic and gut neuropathy.[95,100] The precise relationship between autonomic and somatic neuropathy remains unclear. Positive correlations of various degrees using different indices of somatic function have been reported,[89,95,100–102] but further study of the relationship between autonomic and somatic large and small fiber involvement in diabetic neuropathy is required.

Laser Doppler measurement of cutaneous blood flow in the pulp of the fingers and toes may be the most sensitive measurement of sympathetic autonomic dysfunction in the extremities.[103] Flow autoregulation in these areas is modulated by sympathetic input and hence depends on the integrity of those fibers, providing us another measure of autonomic function.

Quantification of Cutaneous Sensitivity

Quantitative sensory testing is the determination of the sensory threshold, defined as the minimal energy reliably detected for a particular modality. It is a logical extension of the sensory portion of the clinical neurologic examination and has the principal advantage of assigning a numeric value. In recent years we have witnessed the development of a number of relatively inexpensive devices that allow suitable assessment of somatosensory function, including vibration, thermal energy, and light touch.

QST can be used to document subtle sensory loss, to characterize patients at the onset of a clinical trial, and to monitor a modality known to be associated with a specific complication of diabetic neuropathy.[104–106] The evaluation contributes to the differentiation of the relative deficit in small (e.g., temperature) versus large (e.g., vibration) diameter axons, as well as polyneuropathy versus mononeuropathy.

Calibration and units of measure should be expressed in standard terminology, such as μm (vibration), °C (temperature), and dyne/cm^2 (light touch), and the physical dimensions of stimulation (e.g., waveform, frequency, rise-time) should be reported.

Two testing procedures are emerging as the "standards" in the field: (1) modified "up-down" stimulation with two alternative forced choice responses; and (2) ramping of stimulus intensity (method of limits) combined with "yes-no" paradigm.[107] With the first procedure, the most common definition of threshold is the stimulus intensity corresponding to the 75% correct response point. With the second procedure, threshold usually is defined as the stimulus intensity corresponding to 50% correct detection. To be acceptable, the two alternative procedures must allow sufficient reversals to converge on a true threshold. The yes-no paradigm must include "catch trials" (where stimulus is not delivered) in sufficient numbers and variable ramps to minimize guessing. More details concerning the different psychophysical methods, response paradigms, and their critical evaluation can be found in Maurissen's study.[108]

Sensory Modalities

Vibration Perception Testing. This measure is the most widely studied QST procedure and has produced the most extensive normal and neuropathy data bases. If frequencies of 120–200 Hz are used, it principally assesses function in Meissner and Pacinian corpuscles and their associated large-diameter fibers. Typical sites of assessment are the glabrous skin of the fingers and toes.

Thermal Perception Testing. This measure assesses function in free-nerve endings and their associated unmyelinated and thinly myelinated fibers. The value and reliability of this measure is enhanced by separately assessing warm and cold perception. Although thermal thresholds have proven to be especially variable, they uniquely index small-fiber dysfunction.[109]

Light Touch. Quantitative esthesiometry techniques require a relatively sophisticated stimulus delivery system. This measure tests the integrity of Merkel touch domes and Meissner corpuscles and their associated large-diameter fibers. The expanded use of this technique in assessing diabetic neuropathy will be a function of the anticipated increased availability of devices specific for this modality.

In addition to the above modalities, QST procedures are available for *pain thresholds* and *cutaneous current perception.*[110] Pain thresholds test nociceptors and C-fibers. Although they may be important for selected studies, the *Consensus Statement*[89] rejected their inclusion in a general assessment of diabetic neuropathy because of subject discomfort and the limited experience in multicenter trials. Current perception assesses the detection threshold for electrical sine wave stimuli produced by a constant current generator and delivered to the skin through surface electrodes. There are no known receptors for electrical current, and this form of stimulation appears to excite the cutaneous axons directly. Multiple frequencies have been reported to excite different axonal subgroups, but this claim awaits validation. Studies in persons with diabetes suggest strong correlations with other QST measures.[105,111] Additional studies are required, however, to explore the specificity and sensitivity of current perception for the assessment of diabetic neuropathy.

Nerve conduction indices and sensory symptom status are highly correlated with QST.[112–114] Utilizing electrophysiologic findings and symptoms to identify neuropathic patients, an elevated vibration threshold was associated with a sensitivity of 73% and a false-positive rate of 7%.[112] Furthermore, asymptomatic diabetic patients have significantly higher thresholds than nondiabetic individuals, suggesting that QST may be useful in detecting subclinical neuropathy.

Average intrasubject coefficients of variation for normal subjects have been reported as low as 7–10% for vibration thresholds. In diabetic subjects, coefficients of variation for vibration thresholds are on the order of 10–20%, whereas levels >20% have been observed for thermal thresholds. We have shown that the greatest sensitivity for detection of neuropathy is obtained by using a combination of thermal and vibration perception tests.[90]

Thorough assessment of the neurologic status of patients presenting with clinical signs or symptoms of a peripheral sensory neuropathy requires an evaluation of neural afferent function in the peripheral skin. Recent technologic advancements have provided more sophisticated measures of some dimensions of sensory function. A variety of instruments are now available for the detection of impairment in thermal sensitivity and vibration perception, as well as electrical current, pressure, and pain perception. These types of instruments allow for cutaneous sensory functions to be assessed noninvasively, and their measurements are, by definition, correlates of specific nerve fiber function. The proper application of these instruments will lead to advances in descriptions of cutaneous sensitivity, with a level of detail regarding the magnitude of impairment of different cutaneous sensory modalities that is useful to both the researcher and the clinician. Information concerning fiber-specificity and progression of sensory neuropathies cannot be assessed fully until advances in the quantification of cutaneous sensory function are put to use in both research and clinical assessments of sensory neuropathies. The use of standardizable equipment to determine levels of cutaneous sensitivity provides distinct advantages over otherwise-derived assessments, primarily through its allowance for (1) improvements in scaling techniques, and (2) more exacting and standardized methods of stimulus presentation and response.

Electrophysiological Testing in Diabetic Neuropathy

Electrodiagnostic nerve conduction studies yield values of amplitude and velocity that can be related to numbers of viable axons, extent of demyelination, axonal resistance, and conduction block.[115,116] Electrophysiologic testing is not specific for diabetic neuropathy, but plays an important role in detecting, characterizing, and measuring progress of the different forms of diabetic neuropathies.[89] Sensory conduction delays and absence of response commonly are found in patients with neuropathic symptoms, and as many as 20% of asymptomatic patients have positive electrophysiologic findings.[116] Nerve conduction velocity (NCV) provides a measure of transmission time in the largest myelinated fibers. Transmission time may be influenced by a number of factors, including fiber size, degree of myelination, nodal and internodal length, axonal resistance and temperature.[115,116] In diffuse neuropathies, slowing of conduction velocity may become more apparent if measurement is obtained over long nerve segments. F-response latency measurement, which includes conduction over the entire motor nerve, is thus a sensitive method for detecting neuropathy.[117] F-wave latencies also provide a means of assessing proximal motor nerve function which may be useful in conditions such as diabetic amyotrophy or proximal neuropathies.[106] Conduction studies also help to identify and localize focal lesions within a nerve by demonstrating localized slowing or conduction block, both of which can occur in diabetic neuropathy. This is helpful especially when there is coincident carpal tunnel or tarsal tunnel entrapment, to which diabetics are susceptible.

Electrophysiologic tests correlate with nerve biopsy results,[118,119] and they serve well as a surrogate for histology in longitudinal studies. There are limitations, however, in the prognostic relevance of these abnormalities. The demonstration of a conduction delay in an asymptomatic patient does not provide specific information about what pattern of neuropathy may subsequently develop, nor does the NCV disclose dysfunction in the various fiber subtypes within a nerve. For example, even though small fibers that mediate pain and autonomic function are often the first to demonstrate dysfunction, these fibers are essentially silent in the routine NCV study. Another potential limitation of the standard electrophysiologic techniques is in detecting therapeutic benefit. Clinical studies have failed to show large or rapid improvements in conduction velocity with treatments that have beneficial behavioral effects.[120]

Needle electromyography (EMG) in conjunction with nerve conduction studies may reveal fibrillation, a sensitive indicator of axonal degeneration that precedes other clinical or electrophysiologic evidence of neuropathy.[121] The needle examination is also helpful in determining the distribution of nerve involvement. EMG, for instance, is the electrodiagnostic study of choice in the evaluation of diabetic polyradiculopathy[122,123] and provides important information in the assessment of both proximal motor neuropathy[124,125] and plexopathy.

Additional quantitative testing can be done with single-fiber EMG, which allows measurement of muscle fiber density and evaluation of neuromuscular transmission.[117] Muscle fiber density is increased in cases of axonal loss with subsequent reinnervation by collateral sprouting. Ongoing collateral sprouting also may be assessed quantitatively by the jitter, which reflects neuromuscular transmission.

Other modalities useful in the evaluation of diabetic neuropathy, but which may not be available at all centers, include near-nerve recording, somatosensory evoked potentials, or repetitive stimulation with measurement of refractory periods. Sensory evoked potentials have been shown to be very useful diagnostic and prognostic tools in neurologic disease and trauma. A number of investigators have described evoked potential (EP) abnormalities in diabetic patients.[126–137] Most reports have concentrated on the somatosensory pathways,[127,128,130,132,133,137] although visual and auditory modalities have received some attention.[126,129,131,134,136] Consistent with nerve conduction studies, EPs show upper- and lower-extremity peripheral conduction delays in diabetic patients[127,128,130,131,132–135,137] that may be related to the duration of disease[130,133,135]; however, the evidence for central conduction abnormalities is equivocal. Several authors have reported an incidence of central nervous system abnormalities ranging from 20% to 50%.[128,129,131,134,138] Many of these studies were of patients with minimal or no signs of peripheral neuropathy. Other investigators, however, have failed to demonstrate significant evidence of central[127] or supraspinal dysfunction[130,131] in somatosensory pathways. Ziegler et al.[137] used tibial nerve sensory EPs to evaluate 100 IDDM patients grouped into Dyck's stages 0, 1, and 2.[139] They found that the latency, interpeak latencies, and amplitude of scalp-recorded components of tibial nerve potentials correlated with small-fiber dysfunction, as indicated by heart rate variation and thermal perception threshold. Despite inconsistencies and gaps in the literature, there are enough data available to suggest that EPs are very sensitive to subtle levels of neural dysfunction and may be able to detect subclinical or occult lesions of prognostic significance. This has yet to be demonstrated conclusively, particularly with regard to central dysfunction. Further study of large, well-defined populations would be desirable to address this question. Multi-modality EPs are capable of disclosing a variety of patterns of abnormality in diabetic patients quite early in the disease, and there is a trend over time toward progression of EP abnormalities to include new areas of the nervous system.[135]

The peripheral autonomic surface potential (also known as the sympathetic skin response) is an electrodermal potential that has been utilized for many years as an indicator of autonomic integrity.[140–144] This response is mediated by muscarinic mechanisms, and a few studies in diabetic patients have shown that the response is very diminished or absent in patients with autonomic dysfunction.[141–143]

The utility of electrophysiologic testing lies in its reliability and reproducibility. These measurements are largely independent of patient cooperation and are reproducible among different examiners in different centers. They have also been shown to play an important role in studies evaluating disease progression or regression and the response to medical treatment.[118,145]

It is important when performing these tests to control for sources of error.[89] One factor of particular importance is *limb temperature*. Amplitude, latency, and conduction velocity all vary with limb temperature.[115] As the limb cools, there is less dispersion of the evoked response, and the amplitude subsequently increases. At the same time, decreases in conduction velocity and increases in distal latencies are seen. It is generally recommended, therefore, that limb temperatures be kept at 32–36°C,[121] with warming of limbs occasionally necessary to maintain them in the ideal range. It may be difficult in some patients to maintain proper temperature due to ischemia or denervation, in which case corrections can be made as outlined in other texts.[121]

Quantification of Autonomic Function

Cardiovascular Tests. There are a series of simple noninvasive tests that are capable of detecting cardiovascular autonomic neuropathy. These were developed by Ewing and colleagues[46] and have been successfully applied by others and ourselves.[146–152] The following is a list of the measures and the normal values:

1. **Resting heart rate:** >100 beats per minute is abnormal.
2. **Beat-to-beat heart rate variation:** With the patient at rest and supine, breathing 6 breaths per minute with heart rate monitored by electrocardiography (ECG), a difference (maximal-minimal) in heart rate of >15 beats per minute is normal; a difference of 10 beats per minute or less is abnormal.
3. **Valsalva maneuver:** The subject blows into mouthpiece of manometer to 40 mmHg for 15 seconds with continuous ECG monitoring before, during, and after the procedure. Healthy subjects normally develop tachycardia and peripheral vasoconstriction during strain, and an overshoot rise in blood pressure and bradycardia on release. The Valsalva ratio is longest *R-R*/shortest R-R; the normal value is ≥ 1.21.
4. **Heart rate response to standing:** The subject stands with continuous ECG monitoring, and one measures the R-R interval at beats 15 and 30. The 30/15 ratio is normally >1.03. Tachycardia at beat 15 and bradycardia at beat 30 is normal.
5. **Systolic blood pressure response to standing:** The response is abnormal if the blood pressure falls >30 mmHg within 2 minutes of standing.
6. **Diastolic blood pressure rise with sustained exercise:** A hand-grip dynamometer is squeezed to 30% of maximum (predetermined in the subject) for 5 minutes. The normal response is a rise of diastolic blood pressure >16 mmHg.
7. **QT interval on ECG:** The QT interval corrected for the cardiac cycle length (QTc) is = QT/square root of longest-shortest R-R interval. Normal is a QTc ≤440 msec.

Gastrointestinal Tests. A number of imaging studies and laboratory tests have been developed to investigate gastrointestinal neuropathy. These include the following:

- Technetium resin and chicken liver gastric emptying studies[153]: A positive test is retention of more than one half of the radioactivity in the stomach for >100 minutes.
- Pressure/motility studies of intestinal function.[153]
- Insulin hypoglycemia test of pancreatic polypeptide and catecholamine responses.[154–158]

Special Tests of Bladder Function. In suspect cases of a vesical dysfunction there may be a need to do the following tests:

- Cystometry
- Sphincter electromyography
- Uroflometry
- Urethral pressure profile
- Electrophysiologic test of bladder innervation.

Special Tests of Penile Function. A variety of tests have been developed to quantitate erectile impotence. These are designed to distinguish psychogenic from organic, and vascular from neuropathic impotence and include the following:

- Doppler ultrasound measurement of brachial and penile systolic blood pressure
- Nocturnal penile tumescence and rigidity measurement by strain gauge
- Penile responses to intracavernosal injection of vasodilators
- Bulbocavernosus reflex response latency and sensory tests.

Sudomotor Sympathetic Function. Sudomotor function can be evaluated with the thermoregulatory sweat test, quantitative sudomotor axon reflex test, skin potentials, or sweat imprint quantitation.

Peripheral Skin Blood Flow Reactions. Microvascular skin blood flow may be accurately measured noninvasively using laser Doppler flowmetry.[159] Smooth-muscle microvasculature in the periphery reacts sympathetically and parasympathetically to a number of stressor tasks.

Hypoglycemia Unawareness/Unresponsiveness

Testing for the presence of these syndromes requires elaborate and expensive equipment and is best done in a research environment with the stepped hypoglycemic clamp technique.[160] The insulin infusion test, applied to normal subjects and patients with IDDM, also has been described in detail.[161] The test must be performed by two persons, one of whom must be a physician (because a medical judgment must be made as to whether or not an endpoint is reached and insulin infusion should be stopped). It also requires accurate glucose measurement at the bedside.

Biopsy

Biopsy of nerve tissue may be helpful for excluding other causes of neuropathy, such as the familial hypertrophic forms, amyloid, sarcoid, and other granulomata, but the pathology of diabetic neuropathy is not unique. The pathology of the early sensorimotor neuropathy is not known, but in established neuropathy, the characteristic picture is that of distal fiber loss and degeneration. Histologic data have been reexamined recently in light of the subtle asymmetries and focal nature of the clinical presentation; findings have supported the hypothesis that there are differences in the types of neuropathies occurring in IDDM versus NIDDM. Unlike IDDM, in NIDDM the major observation is *Wallerian degeneration,* which may be patchy and irregular, supporting the notion of a vascular origin of the disease[13,162–167] in this form of diabetes. While these findings cannot be distinguished clearly from other causes of neuropathy, a microvascular occlusive picture in the absence of known vasculitides may, however, be pathognomonic of diabetes.

Management

Management of diabetic neuropathy may be divided into general and specific measures. The specific measures include diabetes control and drug therapies directed at the underlying cause of the symptom complex. The general measures include symptomatic, palliative, and supportive treatment directed at the symptom complex present.

Specific Measures

Diabetes Control. The outcome of the multicenter Diabetes Control and Complications Trial[168] has clearly shown that, with the elimination of persons with symptomatic neuropathy, rigorous diabetes control can decrease the prevalence of symptomatic, electrophysiologic, and autonomic indicators of neuropathy by 38–59%. The respective roles of insulin administration per se and the many other variables that were altered in this trial in the amelioration of neuropathy are not yet apparent, nor is it clear why so many did not respond, and the degree of response in any given individual was small.[168] Nonetheless, it would be prudent to normalize diabetes control as much as possible, especially in those patients who have evidence of early neuropathy.

Nutritional Factors. A variety of nutritional factors have been implicated in the pathogenesis of neuropathy, including deficiencies in vitamin B12, vitamin A, and pyridoxine (B6), as well as a host of macronutrients and micronutrients. There are data to suggest that supplementing the diet with 3.2 g of inositol and 500 mg of dihomo-γ-linolenic acid (evening primrose oil) or N-acetyl L-carnitine may have some beneficial effects; however, studies have not been well controlled, and the present recommendation is to maintain adequate and healthy nutrition and to give only supplements that are innocuous. Excessive intake of pyridoxine, for example, results in a severe form of sensory neuropathy.

Aldose Reductase Inhibitors. Aldose reductase inhibitors trials are still very much in the research arena, and although there are some promising reports on improvement in symptoms and in some objective measures of neuropathy, the degree of benefit obtained has not been outstanding. At the present it is too early to evaluate the place of aldose reductase inhibitors in the management of diabetic neuropathy.[145,169–179]

None of the aldose reductase inhibitors are currently approved for clinical use in the United States; all patients receiving treatment are participants of trials conducted by various centers. A major problem related to the interpretation of the data generated in the early studies has been a lack of standardized approaches to the following: (1) determination of clinical symptomatic responsiveness; (2) measurement of subtle changes in thermal and vibratory perception; (3) electrophysiologic quantification of improvement; and (4) use of surrogate data as supportive evidence of nerve regeneration. Furthermore, variability in the measurements carried out by different centers in control studies have been considerable, thus highlighting the need for minimizing both intercenter and intracenter variability. Thus, for trials of this nature to be successful and for meaningful results to be achieved, it will be necessary to standardize carefully the clinical measurements of symptoms and physical findings, as well as those for quantitative physiologic testing, and to identify prospectively the histologic endpoints to be used as primary goals of therapy.

As alluded to earlier, patient selection is also an important consideration, with ideal candidates afflicted with only mild or very modest neuropathy. Because many of these patients will experience predominantly small-fiber neuropathy, which is not detected by electrophysiologic measures, quantitation of neural deficits are based predominantly on subjective responses. Therefore these studies should be blinded and placebo-controlled.

***myo*-Inositol.** *myo*-Inositol deficiency has been reported in animal models and intolerance to *myo*-inositol has been reported in diabetic humans. There are several studies suggesting that *myo*-inositol supplements of the normal diet will improve neuropathy,[43,180–182] but the treatment may have to be prolonged for at least 6 months for a significant effect to be achieved.[43] In desperate situations, however, persons whose normal *myo*-inositol intake is 800 mg per day may increase this to 3200 mg per day. This is easily obtainable by purchasing Brewer's yeast (or inositol) from a health food store, where it comes in two forms, one containing 400 mg and one containing 800 mg of inositol, with the appropriate number of tablets prescribed per day.

Gangliosides. Gangliosides are sialoglycolipids found in nerve cell membranes and nerve growth cones. A series of studies reported from Europe[118,183–187] and one from the United States[188] have shown some improvement in lower extremity sensation, following ganglioside administration in small groups of patients, but without changes in the electrophysiologic measures of nerve function. Although these studies held promise, the development of Guillain Barré syndrome in many of the recipients of the brain extracts has led to a moratorium on further therapeutic trials or research.

Evening Primrose Oil. Diabetic subjects have an inability to convert linoleic acid to γ-linolenic acid, a necessary precursor for membrane phospholipids, and thus have a deficient substrate for the synthesis of certain prostaglandin derivatives. In a Dutch study, and in a multicenter British and European study, diabetic subjects were treated for one year or longer with γ-linolenic acid, which bypasses the enzyme block, and these patients showed improved nerve function compared with a placebo-treated group.[189,190] The results generated by these small trials are exciting because γ-linolenic acid also has an important effect in reducing lipid concentrations and thus could be useful in the general management of diabetes. Further exploration in this area is needed.

Aminoguanidine. New studies in rats have shown that aminoguanidine may be of value in reversing the glycation of proteins implicated in the pathogenesis of diabetic complications[191] Studies are being carried out on a research basis, and the product is not yet available for human use.

Symptomatic Therapy

Pain Control

Control of pain in diabetic neuropathy may present one of the most trying problems for both physician and patient. Often patients are depressed, and the depression does not appear to be a function of the extent or severity of the neuropathy, but rather of a sense of hopelessness. An accompanying sense of "weakness" may also be present, and this often is due not to a muscle deficit, but again to a feeling of hopelessness. Enrollment of some patients into various drug trials for neuropathy has yielded improvement in approximately 50% of subjects even before institution of the drug therapy or with the administration of placebo. This trial effect highlights the need for physicians to treat these patients with compassion, sympathy, understanding, and with a sense of hope. Simple maneuvers, such as wearing body stockings to decrease movement of hair follicles, can be very helpful.

There are generally two types of pain in neuropathy. The first type is marked by hyperesthesia and a burning, lancinating dysesthetic component. This subgroup may respond to topical application of capsaicin.[192] The second type is dull and gnawing, like a toothache, and generally does not respond well to topical therapy. Figure 82-2 outlines treatment paths for these two types of neuropathic pain.

Analgesics. Various analgesic drugs have been used for the management of pain in diabetic neuropathy, including aspirin, paracetamol, the nonsteroidal anti-inflammatory drugs, and meperidine (Demerol). Care must be exercised in the use of more potent analgesics for fear of addiction.

Phenytoin (Dilantin). Long advocated in the treatment of pain, phenytoin is generally not thought to be of value in diabetic neuropathy.[193,194] One problem is that it tends to yield toxicity (e.g., macrocytic anemia, hypertrophic gums, ataxia) before a therapeutic effect is observed.

Carbamazepine. Carbamazepine is very useful in the management of epilepsy in children, and it has been shown to be of some benefit in cases of diabetic neuropathy in double-blind placebo-controlled studies.[195–197] In general, however, this drug is too toxic to be considered as the first-line drug.

Clonidine. Interest in clonidine in the management of painful diabetic neuropathy has been motivated by the considerable success achieved by this drug in the management of patients who have been withdrawn from alcohol and other drugs. It also seems to work reasonably well in many causalgic situations. One should start with a small dose of 75–100 μg given at night to avoid hypotension and sleepiness and then increase the dose gradually until a desired effect is achieved. About one-third of patients will respond in this manner.

Amitriptyline. Several studies have examined the effects of various tricyclic drugs in combination with phenothiazines, and have reported a beneficial effect that is unrelated to the relief of depression.[198–200] The usual treatment is amitriptyline 50–150 mg in divided doses plus fluphenazine 1–2 mg orally at night. Unfortunately, however, the dysautonomia, dry mouth, and visual disturbances caused by tricyclics may be limiting and the tardive dyskinesia caused by phenothiazines troublesome. A benefit of treatment with tricyclics alone in double-blind placebo-controlled studies has been reported, indicating greater effectiveness of the drug compared with placebo.[201,202] As mentioned earlier, many of these patients are very depressed, and a trial of imipramine alone or amitriptyline given together with fluphenazine may be of benefit in a number of patients.

Transcutaneous Nerve Stimulation. Transcutaneous nerve stimulation must be considered if only for the reason that it represents one of the most benign approaches to management. Often this approach is abandoned prematurely when the practitioner fails to move the electrodes around sufficiently to identify sensitive areas. Salutary results usually are obtained only when the electrodes are moved to multiple areas, including those not in the distribution of the nerves involved.

Nerve Blocking. The administration of lidocaine by slow infusion of 5 mg/kg in a period of 30 minutes has been shown recently to provide relief of intractable pain for a period of 3–21 days.[203] When the pain is localized to a nerve root distribution, the temporary pain relief provided by the local nerve blockers may constitute sufficient management because such pain is self-limiting. If a positive response to lidocaine is found, then therapy can be continued with oral mexilitene in divided doses totalling ≤10 mg/kg/day.

Rheologic Agents. Pentoxifylline is a rheologic agent that increases the deformability of red blood cells and increases blood flow with enhanced oxygenation of tissues. Use of this agent has been reported sporadically in diabetic neuropathy but results of the completed six-center clinical investigation of its safety and efficacy in painful diabetic neuropathy were negative.

Neuropathic Ulcers

It must be stressed that neuropathic ulcers constitute the greatest hazard to loss of limbs in patients with diabetes, and it is the responsibility of the physician to ensure that the patient understands the importance of foot care.

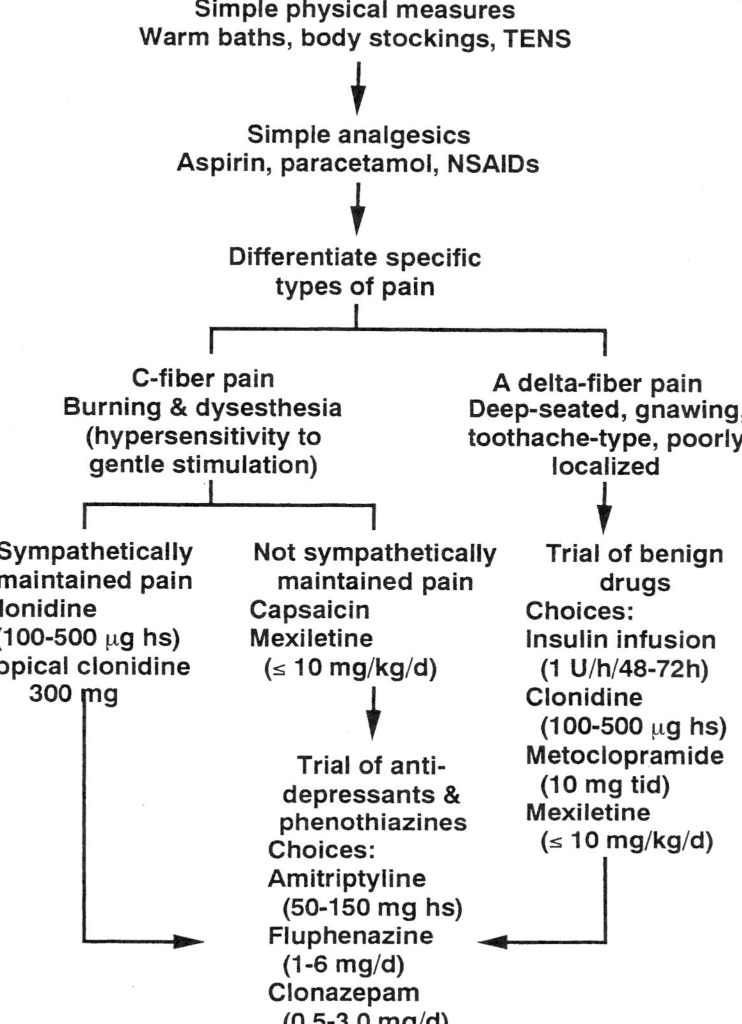

Figure 82-2. Pain management in diabetic neuropathy. (Modified from Vinik AI, Holland MT, LeBeau JM, et al. Diabetic neuropathies. Diabetes Care 1992;15:1926.)

Meticulous Foot Care. Drying between the toes after bathing and application of drying powder (e.g., talcum, cornstarch) and softening creams (e.g., lanolin) are critical measures for the prevention of foot ulcers. Daily inspection of the feet is paramount, and patients must be taught proper toenail-cutting techniques.

Orthotic Devices. If a patient presents with marked loss of sensation with the development of ulcers in the pressure areas of the foot (discussed above), the purchase of a shoe one size larger than regular with an insert of plastozet or alzet, which will mold to the foot and distribute the pressure, can result in healing of ulcers within several months. A simple, yet effective measure is to wear padded socks, e.g. Thotlo, a maneuver shown to reduce the likelihood of foot ulceration.

Ulcer Care. Ulcer care requires debridement of necrotic tissue, repeated sterile dressings, removal from further pressure with supportive devices, or even bed rest or a plaster cast! Infection must be treated aggressively, with appropriate antibiotics often prescribed for at least 3 weeks and an underlying osteomyelitis excluded by x-ray. Trials of topical platelet-derived growth factor as a means of accelerating wound healing are being undertaken in several U.S. cities. This area probably constitutes the single greatest cause of mismanagement of patients with diabetes giving rise to medical lawsuits.

Charcot's Joints: Orthotic Devices

Once destruction of a Charcot's joint is complete and there is total loss of joint pain and perception, the only means of treatment is with orthotic devices.

Mononeuropathies

Physiotherapy is important to prevent contractures, and the joints should be protected until spontaneous recovery occurs.

Autonomic Neuropathies

The management of the wide variety of disorders found in association with autonomic neuropathy is beyond the scope of this chapter; the reader is referred to several excellent reviews.[83,88,204]

Prognosis

The tendency for neuropathy, nephropathy, and retinopathy to cluster together in the same patient has long been recognized[205] and is now referred to as a *triopathy*. This clustering is independent of age and duration of diabetes.[206–208] Neuropathy is often the first of these complications to become manifest and thus may serve as a marker for those at high risk for future development of retinopathy, as suggested by Knowler et al.[209] and perhaps for other diabetic complications.

Peripheral and possibly autonomic neuropathy is also an important contribution to the development of neuropathic foot ulceration, which can be a devastating complication for some patients. It has been estimated that >50% of all nontraumatic amputations in this country occur in diabetic patients and that one-half of these are potentially preventable.[210] These statistics highlight the need for careful attention to foot care in diabetic patients.

The presence of autonomic neuropathy may also lead to accelerated development of other morbid conditions. Among women with diabetes, for example, it is reported that those with cardiovascular autonomic neuropathy have a higher prevalence rate of bacteriuria than women of similar age, duration of diabetes, and glycosylated hemoglobin but without cardiovascular autonomic neuropathy.[211] The increased mortality risk associated with diabetic autonomic neuropathy is well established, and is in the range of 25–50% within 5–10 years of diagnosis.[10,80,212] Patients who die prematurely are, however, more likely to present with postural hypotension, gastric symptoms, and hypoglycemic unawareness at baseline examination. Possible mechanisms for the increased risk associated with diabetic autonomic neuropathy have been discussed earlier.

Prospects for the Future

It is now abundantly clear that neuropathy is heterogeneous and that hyperglycemia and its metabolic consequences can account only for a proportion of the susceptibility to this complication. With the recognition that autoimmunity, vascular insufficiency, and growth factor deficiency may also contribute to this complication, either in conjunction with the metabolic imbalance or as independent culprits, newer therapies directed toward these mechanisms might achieve a greater degree of success than that currently enjoyed by clinicians handling these patients. Indeed, there are now early trials of growth factor therapy for growth factor–deprived patients, and soon there will be attempts to address the autoimmune and vascular pathology as well. When considered in the light of the types of nerve fibers involved and the dependence of the specific fibers on particular growth factors, it seems reasonable to predict that before long targeted "cocktails" of growth factors directed toward the specific lesion in a given individual will make their way into our therapeutic armamentarium.

Summary

Diabetic neuropathy is a common complication of diabetes that often is associated both with considerable morbidity (e.g., painful polyneuropathy, neuropathic ulceration) and mortality (e.g., autonomic neuropathy). The epidemiology and natural history of diabetic neuropathy is clouded with uncertainty, largely due to confusion regarding the definition and measurement of this disorder.

We have reviewed a variety of the clinical manifestations associated with somatic and autonomic neuropathy and have discussed current views related to the management of the different abnormalities. Although unproved, the best evidence suggests that near-normal control of blood glucose in the early years after onset of diabetes may help delay the development of clinically significant nerve impairment. Intensive therapy to achieve normalization of blood glucose also may lead to reversibility of early diabetic neuropathy, but again this has not been proved.

Our ability to manage successfully the many different manifestations of diabetic neuropathy depends ultimately on our success in uncovering the pathogenic processes underlying this disorder. The recent resurgence of interest in the vascular hypothesis, for example, and the possibility that autoimmunity may play a role has opened up new avenues of investigation for therapeutic intervention. Paralleling our increased understanding of the pathogenesis of diabetic neuropathy, there must be refinements in our ability to measure quantitatively the different types of defects that occur in this disorder, so that appropriate therapies of growth factors can be targeted to specific fiber types. These tests must be validated and standardized to allow comparability between studies and a more meaningful interpretation of study results.

References

1. Deckert T. Late diabetic manifestations in "pancreatogenic" diabetes mellitus. Acta Med Scand 1960;168:439
2. Galton D. Diabetic retinopathy and haemochromatosis. Br Med J 1965;1:1169
3. Bank S, Marks I, Vinik A. Clinical and hormonal aspects of pancreatic diabetes. Am J Gastroenterol 1975;64:13
4. Thomas PK, Eliasson SG. Diabetic neuropathy. In: Peripheral Neuropathy. Dyck PJ, Thomas PK, Lambert EH, Bunge R, eds. Philadelphia, Pa: W.B. Saunders;1984:1773
5. Ellenberg M. Diabetic neuropathy. In: Diabetes Mellitus: Theory and Practice. Ellenberg M, Rifkin H, eds. New York, New York: McGraw-Hill;1982:777
6. Greene DA, Pfeifer MA. Diabetic neuropathy. In: Diabetes Mellitus: Management and Complications. Olefsky JM, Sherwin RS, eds. New York, New York: Churchill Livingston;1985:223
7. Brown M, Asbury A. Diabetic neuropathy. Ann Neurol 1984;15:2
8. Vinik AI, Holland MT, LeBeau JM, et al. Diabetic neuropathies. Diabetes Care 1992;15:1
9. Archer A, Watkins P, Thomas P, et al. The natural history of acute painful neuropathy in diabetes mellitus. J Neurol Neurosurg Psychiatry 1983;46:491
10. Ewing DJ, Campbell IW, Clarke BF. The natural history of diabetic autonomic neuropathy. Quart J Med 1980;49:95
11. Pfeifer MA, Weinberg CR, Cook DL, et al. Autonomic neural dysfunction in recently diagnosed diabetic subjects. Diabetes Care 1984;7:447
12. O'Brien AI, O'Hare JP, Lewin IG, Corrall RJ. The prevalence of autonomic neuropathy in insulin-dependent diabetes mellitus: A controlled study based on heart rate variability. Quart J Med 1986;61:957
13. Ewing D, Bellavere G, Espi F, et al. Correlation of cardiovascular and neuroendocrine tests of autonomic function in diabetes. Metabolism 1986;35:349
14. Feldman M, Schiller L. Disorders of gastrointestinal motility associated with diabetes mellitus. Ann Intern Med 1983;98:378
15. Fraser D, Campbell I, Ewing D, et al. Peripheral and autonomic nerve function in newly diagnosed diabetes mellitus. Diabetes 1977;26:546
16. Young R, Ewing D, Clarke B. Nerve function and metabolic control in teenage diabetics. Diabetes 1983;32:142
17. Orchard T, Dorman J, LaPorte R, et al. Host and environmental interactions in diabetes mellitus. J Chron Dis 1986;39:979
18. Bruyn GW, Garland H. Neuropathies of endocrine origin. In: Vinkin PJ, Bruyan GW, eds. Handbook of Clinical Neurology. Amsterdam: North-Holland Publishing Company;1970:29–71
19. Vinik AI, Mitchell BD, Leichter SB, et al. Epidemiology of the complications of diabetes. In: Leslie RDG, Robbins DC, eds. Diabetes: Clinical Science in Practice. Cambridge: Cambridge Univ Press;1995:221–287
20. The DCCT Research Group. Factors in development of diabetic neuropathy. Baseline analysis of neuropathy in feasibility phase of Diabetes Control and Complications Trial (DCCT). Diabetes 1988;37:476
21. Sosenko J, Boulton A, Kubrusly D, et al. The vibratory perception threshold in young diabetic patients: Associations with glycemia and puberty. Diabetes Care 1985;8:605
22. Marcus J, Ehrlich R, Kelly M, et al. Nerve conduction in childhood diabetes. Can Med Assoc J 1973;108:116
23. Kruger M, Brunko E, Dorchy H, et al. Femoral versus peroneal neuropathy in diabetic children and adolescents—relationships to clinical status, metabolic control and retinopathy. Diabete Metab 1987;13:110
24. Mitchell BD, Hawthorne BD, Hawthorne VM, Vinik AI. Cigarette smoking and neuropathy in diabetic patients. Diabetes Care 1990;13:434
25. Jeyarajah R, Samarawickrama P, Jameel M. Autonomic function tests in non-insulin dependent patients and apparently healthy volunteers. J Chron Dis 1986;39:479
26. Sharpey-Schafer E, Taylor P. Absent circulatory reflexes in diabetic neuritis. Lancet 1960;1:559
27. Ewing D, Irving J, Wildsmith J, et al. Cardiovascular response to sustained handgrip in normal subjects and in patients with diabetes mellitus: A test of autonomic function. Clin Sci Mol Med 1974;46:295
28. Dryberg T, Benn J, Christiansen JS, et al. Prevalence of diabetic autonomic neuropathy measured by simple bedside tests. Diabetologia 1981;20:190
29. Burke C, O'Doherty A, Flanagan A, et al. Autonomic neuropathy in a diabetic clinic. Irish Med J 1984;77:202
30. Veglio M, Carpano-Maglioli P, Tonda L. Autonomic neuropathy in non-

insulin-dependent diabetic patients: Correlation with age, sex, duration and metabolic control of diabetes. Diabete Metab 1990;16:200
31. Maser R, Pfeifer M, Dorman J. Diabetic autonomic neuropathy and cardiovascular risk. Arch Intern Med 1990;150:1218
32. Bergstrom B, Lilja B, Osterlin S. Autonomic neuropathy in non-insulin dependent (type II) diabetes mellitus. J Intern Med 1990;227:57
33. Ward J, Bowes C, Fisher D, et al. Improvement in nerve conduction following treatment in newly diagnosed diabetics. Lancet 1971;1:428
34. Christensen NJ. Diabetic macroangiopathy blood flow and radiological studies. In: Camerini-Davalos RA, Cole HS, eds. Vascular and Neurological Changes in Early Diabetes. New York: Academic Press;1973:129–134
35. Ziegler D, Cicmir I, Wiefels K, et al. Peripheral and autonomic nerve dysfunction in newly diagnosed insulin-dependent diabetics (IDDM) [abstract]. Diabetes 1986;35:102A
36. Gregersen G. Diabetic neuropathy: Influence of age, sex, metabolic control and duration of diabetes on motor conduction velocity. Neurology 1967;17:972
37. Lamontagne A, Buchthal F. Electrophysiological studies in diabetic neuropathy. J Neurol Neurosurg Psychiatry 1970;33:442
38. Boulton A, Knight G, Drury J, Ward J. The prevalence of symptomatic, diabetic neuropathy in an insulin-treated population. Diabetes Care 1985;8:125
39. Haimanot R, Abdulkadir J. Neuropathy in Ethiopian diabetics: A correlation of clinical and nerve conduction studies. Trop Geogr Med 1985;37:62
40. Osuntokun B, Akinkugbe F, Francis T, et al. Diabetes mellitus in Nigerians: A study of 832 patients. West Afr Med J 1971;20:925
41. Mulder D, Lambert E, Bastron J, et al. The neuropathies associated with diabetes mellitus: A clinical and electromyographic study of 103 unselected diabetic patients. Neurology 1961;11:275
42. Skillman T, Johnson E, Hamwi G, et al. Motor nerve conduction velocity in diabetes mellitus. Diabetes 1961;10:46
43. Greene DA, Brown MJ, Braunstein SN, et al. Comparison of clinical course and sequential electrophysiological tests in diabetes with symptomatic polyneuropathy and its implications for clinical trials. Diabetes 1981;30:139
44. Bischoff A. The natural course of diabetic neuropathy: A follow-up. Horm Metab Res 1980;9:98
45. Mayne N. The short-term prognosis in diabetic neuropathy. Diabetes 1968;17:270
46. Ewing D, Clarke B. Diagnosis and management of diabetic autonomic neuropathy. Br Med J 1982;285:916
47. Bellavere F, Bosello G, Cadone C, et al. Evidence of early impairment of parasympathetic reflexes in insulin dependent diabetics without autonomic symptoms. Diabete Metab 1985;11:152
48. Watkins P, Edmonds M. Sympathetic nerve failure in diabetes. Diabetologia 1983;25:73
49. Thomas PK, Ward JD, Watkins PJ. Diabetic Neuropathy. London: Edward Arnold Publishing Company;1982:1–109
50. Sundkvist G. Autonomic nervous function in asymptomatic diabetic patients with signs of peripheral neuropathy. Diabetes Care 1981;4:529
51. O'Brien IA, Lewin I, O'Hare J, et al. Abnormal circadian rhythm of melatonin in diabetic autonomic neuropathy. Clin Endocrinol 1986;24:359
52. Evans R, Harati Y. Review of clinical presentations, pathophysiology and treatment of diabetic neuropathies. Tex Med 1983;79:50
53. Dyck PJ, Karnes J, O'Brien PC. Diagnosis, staging and classification of diabetic neuropathy and association with other complications. Philadelphia, Pa: WB Saunders;1987:36–44
54. Said G, Slama G, Selva J. Progressive centripetal degeneration of axons in small fiber type diabetic polyneuropathy: A clinical and pathological study. Brain 1983;106:791
55. Llewelyn J, Thomas P, Fonseca V, et al. Acute painful diabetic neuropathy precipitated by strict glycemic control. Acta Neuropathol (Berl) 1986;72:157
56. Boulton A, Drury J, Clarke B, Ward J. Continuous subcutaneous insulin infusion in the management of painful diabetic neuropathy. Diabetes Care 1982;5:386
57. Ellenberg M. Diabetic neuropathy precipitating after institution of diabetic control. Am J Med Sci 1958;236:466
58. Ellenberg M. Diabetic neuropathic cachexia. Diabetes 1974;23:418
59. Morley G, Mooradian A, Levine A, Morley J. Mechanisms of pain in diabetic peripheral neuropathy: Effect of glucose on pain perception in humans. Am J Med 1984;77:79
60. Ahmed M, LeQuesne P. Quantitative sweat test in diabetics with neuropathic foot lesions. J Neurol Neurosurg Psychiatry 1986;49:1059
61. Archer A, Roberts V, Watkins P. Blood flow patterns in painful diabetic neuropathy. Diabetologia 1984;27:563
62. Raff M, Sangalang V, Asbury A. Ischemic mononeuropathy multiplex associated with diabetes mellitus. Arch Neurol 1968;18:487
63. Chokroverty S, Reyes M, Rubino F, Tonaki H. The syndrome of diabetic amyotrophy. Ann Neurol 1977;2:181
64. Asbury A. Proximal diabetic neuropathy. Ann Neurol 1977;2:179
65. Said G, Goulon-Goeau C, Lacroix C, Moulonguet A. Nerve biopsy findings in different patterns of proximal diabetic neuropathy. Ann Neurol 1994;35:559
66. Krendel DA, Costigan DA, Hopkins LC. Successful treatment of neuropathies in patients with diabetes mellitus. Arch Neurol 1995;52:1053
67. Ellenberg M. Diabetic truncal mononeuropathy—a new clinical syndrome. Diabetes Care 1978;1:10
68. Longstreth G, Newcomer A. Abdominal pain caused by diabetic radiculopathy. Ann Intern Med 1977;86:166
69. Boulton AJ, Angus E, Ayyar DR, Weiss DR. Diabetic thoracic polyradiculopathy presenting as abdominal swelling. Br Med J (Clin Res Ed) 1984;289:798
70. Streib E, Sun S, Paustian F, et al. Diabetic thoracic radiculopathy: Electrodiagnostic study. Muscle Nerve 1986;9:548
71. Harati Y, Niakan E. Diabetic thoracoabdominal neuropathy: A cause for chest and abdominal pain. Arch Intern Med 1986;146:1493
72. Edvinsson L, Ekman R, Jansen I, et al. Peptide-containing nerve fibers in human cerebral arteries: Immunocytochemistry, radioimmunoassay, and in vitro pharmacology. Ann Neurol 1987;21:431
73. Zorilla E, Kozak J. Opthalmophegia in diabetes mellitus. Ann Intern Med 1967;67:968
74. Fraser D, Campbell I, Ewing D, Clarke B. Mononeuropathy in diabetes mellitus. Diabetes 1979;28:96
75. Calverley J, Mulder D. Femoral neuropathy. Neurology 1960;10:963
76. Niakan E, Harati Y, Comstock J. Diabetic autonomic neuropathy. Metabolism 1986;35:224
77. McLeod J, Tuck R. Disorders of the autonomic nervous system: I. Pathophysiology and clinical features. Ann Neurol 1987;21:419
78. McLeod J, Tuck R. Disorders of the autonomic nervous system: II. Investigation and treatment. Ann Neurol 1987;21:519
79. Ewing D, Clarke B. Diabetic autonomic neuropathy: Present insights and future prospects. Diabetes Care 1986;9:648
80. Ewing D, Campbell I, Clarke B. Mortality in diabetic autonomic neuropathy. Lancet 1976;1:601
81. Kahn J, Sisson J, Vinik A. QT interval prolongation and sudden cardiac death in diabetic autonomic neuropathy. J Clin Endocrinol Metab 1987;64:751
82. Sampson M, Wilson S, Karaginnnis P. Progression of diabetic autonomic neuropathy over a decade in insulin-dependent diabetics. Q J Med 1990;278:635
83. Zola BE, Vinik AI. Effects of autonomic neuropathy associated with diabetes mellitus on cardiovascular function. Curr Sci 1992;3:33
84. Hosking D, Bennett T, Hamptom J. Diabetic autonomic neuropathy. Diabetes 1978;22:1043
85. Faerman I, Faccio E, Milei R. Autonomic neuropathy and painless myocardial infarction in diabetic patients: Histologic evidence of their relationship. Diabetes 1977;26:1147
86. Campbell I, Ewing D, Clarke B. Painful myocardial infarction in severe diabetic autonomic neuropathy. Acta Diabetol Lat 1978;15:201
87. Hreidarsson A, Gunderson H. The pupillary response to light in type I (insulin-dependent) diabetes. Diabetologia 1985;28:815
88. Vinik AI, Suwanwalaikorn S, Holland MT, et al. Diagnosis and management of diabetic autonomic neuropathy. In: deFronzo R, ed. Current Management of Diabetes Mellitus. Mosby-Year Book, Inc., St. Louis, in press
89. American Diabetes Association and American Academy of Neurology. Consensus statement: Report and recommendations of the San Antonio conference on diabetic neuropathy. Diabetes Care 1988;11:592
90. Vinik AI, Suwanwalaikorn S, Stansberry KB, et al. Quantitative measurement of cutaneous perception in diabetic neuropathy. Muscle Nerve 1995;18:574
91. Zola BE, Vinik AI. Effects of autonomic neuropathy associated with diabetes mellitus on cardiovascular function. Coron Artery Dis 1992;3:33
92. Boulton AJM, Knight G, Drury J, Ward JD. The prevalence of symptomatic diabetic neuropathy in an insulin-treated population. Diabetes Care 1985;8:125
93. Thomson FJ, Masson EA, Boulton AJ. Quantitative vibration perception testing in elderly people: An assessment of variability. Age Ageing 1992;21:171
94. Wetherill GB, Chen H, Vasudeva RB. Sequential estimation of quantal response curves: A new method of estimation. Biometrika 1966;53:439
95. Ewing DJ, Martyn CN, Young RJ, Clarke BF. The value of cardiovascular autonomic function tests: 10 years experience in diabetes. Diabetes Care 1985;8:491
96. Abrahm DR, Hollingsworth PJ, Smith CB, et al. Decreased alpha 2-adrenergic receptors on platelet membranes from diabetic patients with autonomic neuropathy and orthostatic hypotension. J Clin Endocrinol Metab 1986;63:906
97. Kahn JK, Zola BE, Juni JE, Vinik AI. Decreased exercise heart rate and blood pressure response in diabetic subjects with cardiac autonomic neuropathy. Diabetes Care 1986;9:389
98. Nesto R, Phillips R. Asymptomatic myocardial ischemia in diabetic patients. Am J Med 1992;80:40
99. Levitt N, Vinik A, Sive P, et al. The effect of dietary fiber on glucose and hormone responses to mixed meal in normal subjects and in diabetic subjects with and without autonomic neuropathy. Diabetes Care 1980;3:515
100. Pfeifer M, Weinberg C, Cook D. Correlation among autonomic, sensory and motor neural function tests in untreated non-insulin-dependent diabetic individuals. Diabetes Care 1985;8:576
101. Goodman JI, Baumoel S, Frankel L. The Diabetic Neuropathies. Springfield, Ill.: Charles C. Thomas;1953:1–138
102. Shenfield GM, McCann VJ, Tjokresetio R. Acetylator status and diabetic neuropathy. Diabetologia 1982;22:441
103. McDaid EA, Monaghan B, Parker AI, et al. Peripheral autonomic impairment in patients newly diagnosed with type II diabetes. Diabetes Care 1994;17:1422
104. Arrezzo J, Laudadio C, Schaumburg H. The optacon tactile tester and the Pfizer thermal tester: New devices for the detection of diabetic neuropathy [abstract]. Diabetes 1984;33(suppl 1):185A
105. Masson EA, Veves A, Fernando D, Boulton AJ. Current perception thresholds: A new, quick, and reproducible method for the assessment of peripheral neuropathy in diabetes mellitus. Diabetologia 1989;32:724

106. Sosenko JM, Kato M, Soto R, Bild DE. Comparison of quantitative sensory-threshold measures for their association with foot ulceration in diabetic patients. Diabetes Care 1990;13:1057
107. Wetherill GB, Chen H, Vasudeva RB. Sequential estimation of quantal response curves: A new method of estimation. Biometrika 1966;53:439
108. Maurissen JP. Quantitative sensory assessment in toxicology and occupational medicine: Applications, theory and critical appraisal. Toxicol Lett 1988;43: 321
109. Sosenko JM, Kato M, Soto RA, et al. Specific assessments of warm and cool sensitivities in adult diabetic patients. Diabetes Care 1988;11:481
110. Katims JJ, Naviasky EH, Rendell MS, et al. Constant current sine wave transcutaneous nerve stimulation for the evaluation of peripheral neuropathy. Arch Phys Med Rehabil 1987;68:210
111. Rendell MS, Dovgan DJ, Bergman TF, et al. Mapping diabetic sensory neuropathy by current perception threshold testing. Diabetes Care 1989;12: 636
112. Sosenko JM, Gadia MT, Natori N, et al. Neurofunctional testing for the detection of diabetic peripheral neuropathy. Arch Intern Med 1987;147:1741
113. Rendell MS, Katims JJ, Richter R, Rowland F. A comparison of nerve conduction velocities and current perception thresholds as correlates of clinical severity of diabetic sensory neuropathy. J Neurol Neurosurg Psychiatry 1989;52:502
114. Masson EA, Boulton AJ. The neurometer: Validation and comparison with conventional tests for diabetic neuropathy. Diabetic Med 1991;8:563
115. Kimura J. Electrodiagnosis in disease of nerve and muscle: Principles and practice. Philadelphia, Pa: FA Davis;1989:709
116. Daube JR. Electrophysiologic Testing in Diabetic Neuropathy. Philadelphia, Pa: W.B. Saunders;1987:1–162
117. Argyropoulos CJ, Panayiotopolus CP, Scarpalezos S, Nastas PE. F-wave and M-response conduction velocity in diabetes mellitus. Electromyogr Clin Neurophysiol 1979;19:443
118. Bassi S, Albizati M, Calloni E, Frattola L. Electromyographic study of diabetic and alcoholic polyneuropathy patients treated with gangliosides. Muscle Nerve 1981;5:351
119. Fagius J. Effects of aldose reductase inhibitor treatment in diabetic polyneuropathy: a clinical and neurophysiological study. J Neurol Neurosurg Psychiatry 1981;44:991
120. Greene D. American Diabetes Association Symposium, New Orleans. DCCT: One year later, 1994
121. Greene DA, Sima AA, Albers JW, Pfeifer MA. Diabetic Neuropathy. New York, NY: Elsevier Science Publishing;1990:1–710
122. Kitka DG, Breuer AC, Wilbourn AJ. Thoracic root pain in diabetes: The spectrum of clinical and electromyographic findings. Ann Neurol 1982;11:80
123. Sun SF, Streib WE. Diabetic thoracoabdominal neuropathy: Clinical and electrodiagnostic features. Ann Neurol 1981;9:75
124. Chokroverty S. Proximal nerve dysfunction in diabetic proximal amyotrophy. Electrophysiology and electron microscopy. Arch Neurol 1982;39:403
125. Williams IR, Mayer RF. Subacute proximal diabetic neuropathy. Neurology 1976;26:108
126. Cirillo D, Gonfiantini E, DeGrandis D, et al. Visual evoked potentials in diabetic children and adolescents. Diabetes Care 1984;7:273
127. Collier A, Reid W, McInnes A, et al. Somatosensory and visual evoked potentials in insulin-dependent diabetics with mild peripheral neuropathy. Diabetes Res Clin Pract 1988;5:171
128. Cracco J, Castells S, Mark E. Spinal somatosensory evoked potentials in juvenile diabetes. Neurol 1984;15:55
129. Donald MW, Bird CE, Lawson JS, et al. Delayed auditory brain stem responses in diabetes mellitus. J Neurol Neurosurg Psychiatry 1981;44:641
130. Gupta PR, Dorfman LJ. Spinal somatosensory conduction in diabetes. Neurology 1981;31:841
131. Harkin SW, Gardner DF, Anderson RA. Auditory and somatosensory far-field evoked potentials in diabetes mellitus. Int J Neurosci 1985;28:41
132. Nakamura R, Noritake M, Hosoda Y, et al. Somatosensory conduction delay in central and peripheral nervous system of diabetic patients. Diabetes Care 1992;15:532
133. Nakamura Y, Takahashi M, Kitaguchi M, et al. Clinical utility of somatosensory evoked potentials in diabetes mellitus. Diabetes Res Clin Pract 1989;7:17
134. Pozzessere G, Rozzo PA, Valle E, et al. Early detection of neurological involvement in IDDM and NIDDM. Multimodal evoked potentials versus metabolic control. Diabetes Care 1988;11:473
135. Pozzessere G, Rizzo PA, Valle E, et al. A longitudinal study of multimodal evoked potentials in diabetes mellitus. Diabetes Res 1989;10:17
136. Pozzessere G, Valle E, DeCrignis S, et al. Abnormalities of cognitive function in IDDM revealed by P300 event-related potential analysis. Diabetes 1991;40:952
137. Ziegler D, Muhlen H, Dannehl K, Gries FA. Tibial nerve somatosensory evoked potentials at various stages of peripheral neuropathy in insulin dependent diabetic patients. J Neurol Neurosurg Psychiatry 1993;56:58
138. Fedele D, Martini A, Cardonne C, et al. Impaired auditory brainstem-evoked responses in insulin-dependent diabetic subjects. 1984;33:1085
139. Dyck PJ. Detection, characterization and staging of polyneuropathy: Assessed in diabetes. 1988;11:21
140. Shahani B, Halperin J, Boulu P, Cohen J. Sympathetic skin response. A method of assessing unmyelinated axon dysfunction in peripheral neuropathies. J Neurol Neurosurg Psychiatry 1984;47:536
141. Hoeldtke RD, Davis KM, Hshieh PB, et al. Autonomic surface potential analysis: Assessment of reproducibility and sensitivity. Muscle Nerve 1992;15:926
142. Soliven B, Maselli R, Jaspan J, et al. Sympathetic skin response in diabetic neuropathy. Muscle Nerve 1987;10:711
143. Knezevic W, Bajada S. Peripheral autonomic surface potential. A quantitative technique for recording sympathetic conduction in man. J Neurol Sci 1985;67: 239
144. Shahani BT, Day TJ, Cros D, et al. RR interval variation and the sympathetic skin response in the assessment of autonomic function in peripheral neuropathy. Arch Neurol 1990;47:659
145. Fagius J. Effects of aldose reductase inhibitor treatment in diabetic polyneuropathy: A clinical and neurophysiological study. J Neurol Neurosurg Psychiatry 1981;44:991
146. Nesto R, Phillips R. Asymptomatic myocardial ischemia in diabetic patients. Am J Med 1992;80:40
147. Abrahm DR, Hollingsworth PJ, Smith CB, et al. Decreased alpha 2-adrenergic receptors on platelet membranes from diabetic patients with autonomic neuropathy and orthostatic hypotension. J Clin Endocrinol Metab 1986;63:906
148. Vinik AI, Abrahams D, Jim L, Smith CB. Platelet alpha-2 receptors and in vivo blood pressure (BP) regulation [Abstract]. Diabetes 1985;34(suppl 1):12A
149. Zola B, Kahn J, Juni J, Vinik A. Abnormal cardiac function in diabetics with autonomic neuropathy in the absence of ischemic heart disease. J Clin Endocrinol Metab 1986;63:208
150. Kahn J, Zola B, Juni J. Radionuclide assessment of left ventricular diastolic filling in diabetes mellitus. J Am Coll Cardiol 1985;7:1303
151. Kahn JK, Zola B, Juni JE, Vinik AI. Decreased exercise heart rate and blood pressure response in diabetic subjects with cardiac autonomic neuropathy. Diabetes Care 1986;9:389
152. Levitt N, Vinik A, Sive A, et al. The effect of dietary fiber on glucose and hormone responses to mixed meal in normal subjects and in diabetic subjects with and without autonomic neuropathy. Diabetes Care 1980;3:515
153. Achem-Karem S, Funakoshi A, Vinik A, Owyang C. Plasma motilin concentration and interdigestive migrating motor complex in diabetic gastroparesis: Effect of metaclopramide. Gastroenterology 1985;88:492
154. Levitt N, Vinik A, Sive A, et al. Impaired pancreatic polypeptide responses to insulin-induced hypoglycemia in diabetic autonomic neuropathy. J Clin Endocrinol Metab 1980;50:445
155. Krarup T, Schwartz T, Hilsted J, et al. Impaired response of pancreatic polypeptide to hypoglycaemia: An early sign of autonomic neuropathy in diabetics. Br Med J 1979;2:1544
156. Hilsted J, Madsbad S, Krarup T, et al. No response of pancreatic hormones to hypoglycemia in diabetic autonomic neuropathy. J Clin Endocrinol Metab 1982;54:815
157. White N, Gingerich R, Levandoski L, et al. Plasma pancreatic polypeptide response to insulin-induced hypoglycemia as a marker for defective glucose counterregulation in insulin-dependent diabetes mellitus. Diabetes 1985; 34:870
158. Hoeldtke R, Boden G, Shuman C, Owen O. Reduced epinephrine secretion and hypoglycemia unawareness in diabetic autonomic neuropathy. Ann Intern Med 1982;96:459
159. Rendell M, Bergman T, O'Donnell G, et al. Microvascular blood flow, volume, and velocity measured by laser doppler techniques in IDDM. Diabetes 1989;38:819
160. Boyle PJ, Schwartz NS, Shah SD, et al. Plasma glucose concentrations at the onset of hypoglycemic symptoms in patients with poorly controlled diabetes and in nondiabetics. N Engl J Med 1988;318:1487
161. White N, Skor D, Cryer P, et al. Identification of type I diabetic patients at increased risk from hypoglycemia during intensive therapy. N Engl J Med 1983;308:485
162. Yasuda H, Dyck P. Abnormalities of endoneurial microvessels and sural nerve pathology in diabetic neuropathy. Neurology 1987;37:20
163. Johnson P, Doll S, Cromey D. Pathogenesis of diabetic neuropathy. Ann Neurol 1986;19:450
164. Dyck P, Hansen S, Karnes J. Capillary number and percentage closed in human diabetic sural nerve. Proc Natl Acad Sci U S A 1985;82:2513
165. Dyck P, Karnes J, O'Brien P, et al. The spatial distribution of fiber loss in diabetic polyneuropathy suggests ischemia. Ann Neurol 1986;19:440
166. Dyck P, Lais A, Karnes J, et al. Fiber loss is primary and multifocal in sural nerves in diabetic polyneuropathy. Ann Neurol 1986;19:425
167. Williams E, Timperley W, Ward J, Duckworth T. Electron microscopical studies of vessels in diabetic peripheral neuropathy. J Clin Pathol 1980;33:462
168. The Diabetes Control and Complication trial (DCCT): Design and methodologic considerations for the feasibility phase. Diabetes 1986;35:530
169. Christensen J, Varnek L, Gregersen G. The effect of an aldose reductase inhibitor (Sorbinil) on diabetic neuropathy and neural function of the retina: A double-blind study. Acta Neurol Scand 1985;71:164
170. Judzewitsch R, Jaspan J, Polonsky J. Aldose reductase inhibition improves nerve conduction velocity in diabetic patients. N Engl J Med 1983;308:119
171. Handelsman D, Turtle J. Clinical trial of an aldose reductase inhibitor in diabetic neuropathy. Diabetes 1981;30:459
172. Culebras A, Alio J, Herrera J-L, Lopez-Fraile IP. Effect of an aldose reductase inhibitor on diabetic peripheral neuropathy: Preliminary report. Arch Neurol 1981;38:133
173. Gabbay K, Spack N, Loo S, et al. Aldose reductase inhibition: Studies with alrestatin. Metabolism 1979;28:471

174. Jaspan J, Towle L, Maselli R, Herold K. Clinical studies with an aldose reductase inhibitor in the autonomic and somatic neuropathies of diabetes. Metabolism 1986;35:83
175. Young R, Ewing D, Clarke B. A controlled trial of sorbinil, an aldose reductase inhibitor, in chronic painful diabetic neuropathy. Diabetes 1983;32:938
176. Fagius J, Brattberg A, Jameson S, Berne C. Limited benefit of treatment of diabetic polyneuropathy with an aldose reductase inhibitor: A 24-week controlled trial. Diabetologia 1985;28:323
177. Lewin I, O'Brien I, Morgan M, Corrall R. Clinical and neurophysiological studies with the aldose reductase inhibitor, sorbinil, in symptomatic diabetic neuropathy. Diabetologia 1984;26:445
178. Boulton A. Effects of tolrestat, a new aldose reductase inhibitor, on nerve conduction and paresthetic symptoms in diabetic neuropathy [abstract]. Diabetologia 1986;29:521A
179. Harati Y, Niakan E, Comstock J, Logan C. Aldose reductase inhibitor (tolrestat) therapy in patients with diabetic peripheral neuropathy [abstract]. Ann Neurol 1987;22:129
180. Salway J, Whitehead L, Finnegan J, et al. Effect of myo-inositol on peripheral-nerve function in diabetes. Lancet 1978;2:1282
181. Clements R Jr, Vourganti B, Kuba T. Dietary myo-inositol intake and peripheral nerve function in diabetic neuropathy. Metabolism 1979;28:477
182. Gregersen G, Borsting H, Theil P, Servo C. Myoinositol and function of peripheral nerve in human diabetics: A controlled clinical trial. Acta Neurol Scand 1978;58:241
183. Pozza G, Saibene V, Comi G. The effect of ganglioside administration in human diabetic peripheral neuropathy. In: Gangliosides in Neurological and Neuromuscular Function, Development and Repair. Rapport MM, Gorio A, eds. New York: Raven Press;1981:253–257
184. Abraham R, Wynn V. A double-blind placebo-controlled trial of mixed gangliosides in diabetic peripheral and autonomic neuropathy. Adv Exp Med Biol 1984;174:607
185. Bradley W, Tandan R, Fillyaw M. Double-blind controlled trials of cronassial in chronic peripheral neuropathies [abstract]. Neurology 1987;37:254
186. Naarden A, Davidson J, Harris L, et al. Treatment of painful diabetic polyneuropathy with mixed gangliosides. Adv Exp Med Biol 1983;174:581
187. Crepaldi G, Fedele D, Tiengo A. Ganglioside treatment in diabetic peripheral neuropathy: A multicenter trial. Acta Diabetol Lat 1983;10:265
188. Horowitz S. Ganglioside therapy in diabetic neuropathy. Muscle Nerve 1986;9:531
189. Jamal GA, Carmichael H. The effect of gamma-linolenic acid on human diabetic peripheral neuropathy: A double-blind placebo-controlled trial. Diabetic Med 1990;7:319
190. Keen H, Payan J, Allawi J, et al. Treatment of diabetic neuropathy with γ-linolenic acid. Diabetes Care 1993;16:8
191. Brownlee M. Glycation products and the pathogenesis of diabetic complications. Diabetes Care 1992;15:1835
192. Vinik AI. Management of painful syndromes in diabetes mellitus. Clin Diabetes 1991;9:57
193. Ellenberg M. Treatment of diabetic neuropathy with diphenylhydantoin. N Y State J Med 1968;68:2653
194. Saudek C, Werns S, Reidenberg M. Phenytoin in the treatment of diabetic symmetrical polyneuropathy. Clin Pharmacol Ther 1977;22:196
195. Rull J, Quibrera R, Gonsalez-Millan H, Lozano-Castaneda O. Symptomatic treatment of peripheral diabetic neuropathy with carbamazepine (Tegretol): Double-blind crossover study. Diabetologia 1969;5:215
196. Wilton T. Tegretol in the treatment of diabetic neuropathy. S Afr Med J 1974;48:869
197. Chakrabarti A, Samantaray S. Diabetic peripheral neuropathy: Nerve conduction studies before, during and after carbamazepine therapy. Aust N Z J Med 1976;6:565
198. Davis J, Lewis S, Gerich J, et al. Peripheral diabetic neuropathy treated with amitriptyline and fluphenazine. JAMA 1977;238:2291
199. Mendel C, Klein R, Chappell D. A trial of amitriptyline and fluphenazine in the treatment of painful diabetic neuropathy. JAMA 1986;255:637
200. Gomez-Perez F, Rull J, Dies H, et al. Nortriptyline and fluphenazine in the symptomatic treatment of diabetic neuropathy: A double-blind cross-over study. Pain 1985;23:395
201. Young R, Clarke B. Pain relief in diabetic neuropathy: The effectiveness of imipramine and related drugs. Diabetic Med 1985;2:363
202. Max M, Culnane M, Schafer S. Amitriptyline relieves diabetic neuropathy pain in patients with normal or depressed mood. Neurology 1987;37:589
203. Kastrup J, Petersen P, Dejgard A, et al. Intravenous lidocaine infusion—a new treatment of chronic painful diabetic neuropathy? Pain 1987;28:69
204. Vinik AI, Milicevic Z. Preventive measures and treatment options for diabetic neuropathy. Contemp Int Med 1994;6:41
205. Root H, Pote W, Frehner H. Triopathy of diabetes: Sequence of diabetes, retinopathy and nephropathy in one hundred and fifty-five patients. Arch Intern Med 1954;94:931
206. Pirart J. [Diabetes mellitus and its degenerative complications: A prospective study of 4,400 patients observed between 1947 and 1973 (author's transl)]. Diabete Metab 1977;3:97
207. Pirart J. [Diabetes mellitus and its degenerative complications: A prospective study of 4,400 patients observed between 1947 and 1973 (2nd part) (author's transl)]. Diabete Metab 1977;3:173
208. Pirart J. [Diabetes mellitus and its degenerative complications: A prospective study of 4,400 patients observed between 1947 and 1973 (3rd and last part) (author's transl)]. Diabete Metab 1977;3:245
209. Knowler W, Bennett P, Ballintine E. Increased incidence of retinopathy in diabetics with elevated blood pressure: A six-year follow-up study in Pima Indians. N Engl J Med 1980;302:645
210. American Diabetes Association Staff. The physician's guide to non–insulin-dependent (Type II) diabetes: Diagnosis and treatment. New York, NY: American Diabetes Association;1988:1–98
211. Sawyers J, Todd W, Kellett H. Bacteriuria and autonomic nerve function in diabetic women. Diabetes Care 1986;9:460
212. Clarke B, Campbell I, Ewing D. Prognosis in diabetic autonomic neuropathy. Horm Metab Res 1980;9:101

Diabetes Mellitus, edited by Derek LeRoith, Simeon I. Taylor, and Jerrold M. Olefsky. Lippincott–Raven Publishers, Philadelphia

Chapter 83

Autoimmune Mechanisms of Diabetic Neuropathy

Gary L. Pittenger, Zvonko Milicevic, and Aaron I. Vinik

There has been growing evidence since the early 1980s that autoimmunity plays a role in the development of diabetic neuropathy, especially in insulin-dependent diabetes mellitus (IDDM), with studies regarding the involvement of the immune system in the development of IDDM having been performed by a number of investigators. In IDDM, disease pathogenesis is characterized by the autoimmune destruction of β-cells of the endocrine pancreas and subsequent insulinopenia, hyperglycemia, and development of chronic neurologic, ophthalmologic, and renal complications. Investigators have confirmed the appearance of autoantibodies before β-cell failure and clinical manifestation of diabetes, with progressive target-cell destruction developing during a period of several years.[1,2] It has been speculated that an autoimmune reaction resulting in diabetic complications could be induced by shared antigens between β-cells and other tissues, or as a part of larger defect in self-tolerance. If the defects occur because of a predisposition to autoimmunity, one might expect to find a genetic component. Immunogenetic studies in diabetic patients support the concept of an autoimmune origin of both IDDM and its complications.[3] Investigators have reported that 60% of the inheritance of IDDM can be accounted for by genes within the major histocompatibility complex (MHC), in particular the class II region, and 95% of white individuals with IDDM express either human leukocyte antigen (HLA)-DR3 or DR4 MHC antigens.[4] It is believed that the role of MHC class II molecules in antigen presentation underlies their importance in disease expression.

There are many similarities between β-cells and neurons. Studies by Teitelman et al.[5–7] suggest that islet cells and pancreatic cholinergic neurons may arise from a common precursor cell. In addition, neurons release neurotransmitters in much the same manner as pancreatic islets release hormone in response to stimuli, even exhibiting a membrane depolarization. There also is evidence that nerve growth factor (NGF) may play a role in the development of β-cells. RINm5F cells, representative of a pancreatic β-cell early in development, express both low- and high-affinity NGF receptors and can be induced by NGF to extend neurite-like (neurofilament-containing) processes.[8] In addition, some cell-surface markers for neurons (e.g., gangliosides) also are present on pancreatic islets.[9,10] Because neuropathy is a common complication of IDDM, an autoimmune disease, if neurons were to share some related antigenic characteristics, that would imply that the same immunoglobulins may play a role in attacking β-cells in the neuronal dysfunction. Supporting this idea, monoclonal antiganglioside antibody produced by immunization with fetal rat brain was shown to react specifically with the cell surfaces of all cell types in pancreatic islets of human, rat, and mouse subjects.[11]

A growing body of evidence suggests that antibodies generated in the autoimmune response to β-cells can lead to deficits in tissues other than β-cells, resulting in some of the complications associated with diabetes. The first suggestion of the connection between autoimmunity and diabetic neuropathy arose in the early 1980s, when Guy et al.[12] described the correlation between autoimmune iritis and diabetic autonomic neuropathy. The increased frequency of other organ-specific autoimmune diseases (including Addison's disease, autoimmune thyroiditis [Graves' disease, Hashimoto's thyroiditis], myasthenia gravis, pernicious anemia, and polyglandular syndromes) in patients with IDDM (~10%) suggests that there is likely to be an underlying susceptibility to autoimmune disease in a certain population of patients that will contribute to multiple organ failure.

It is generally thought that in organ-specific autoimmune disease, the autoantibodies are specific for each organ and do not cross-react.[13] Some diabetes-related autoantigens (e.g., gangliosides), however, are present in greater amounts in certain organs, such as pancreatic islets, neurons, kidney glomeruli, and adrenal medulla, and thus it is feasible that the same or similar antigens may participate in multiple organ damage, resulting in the complications associated with diabetes. Further work must be done to examine the primary defect resulting in autoimmune complications of diabetes, whether it be autoantibodies to single antigens affecting several organs, or an underlying susceptibility to autoimmunity.

Nondiabetic Autoimmune Neuropathies

A number of observations during the last 20 years suggest a primary or contributing role of immunologic system effectors in the pathogenesis of a large group of peripheral neurologic disorders. Multiple sclerosis and myasthenia gravis are examples of MHC class II– and probably TcR Vβ gene–related disorders. Both conditions have a well-defined role for the immune system in their pathogenesis, including the identification of autoantibodies to specific antigens recognized during disease initiation and T-cell activation. Chronic inflammatory demyelinating polyneuropathy (CIDP), Guillain–Barré syndrome (GBS), multifocal motor polyneuropathy (MMP), and polyneuropathies associated with monoclonal gammopathies of undetermined significance (MGUS) are a group of peripheral neuropathies with no clearly established genetic background.[14–16]

The clinical presentations of these autoimmune neuropathies suggest a specificity of antigens for clinical manifestations. For example, in MMP, GBS, and CIDP, there is predominantly a motor loss, with reduced nerve conduction velocity on electromyography concomitant with demyelination and axonal degeneration involving mainly large Aα-fibers. The time courses, however, are varied for these syndromes, and only GBS has been reported to involve significant sensory and autonomic deficit, reflecting dysfunction of small, unmyelinated C-fibers. This is in contrast to the neural deficits seen in the majority of patients with diabetic neuropathy, where the predominant abnormalities are loss of sensory and autonomic function, reflecting C-fiber and sensory Aδ fiber loss, and where there is little motor fiber loss. Examination of the antigens associated with the syndromes helps explain the differences in the clinical characteristics of these conditions. MMP, GBS, and CIDP have all been associated with anti-GM1 autoantibody production; however, only GBS has been associated with significant disialoganglioside and trisialoganglioside autoantibodies. CIDP has been associated with myelin glycoprotein autoantibodies. The potential autoantigens in diabetes are very different from the mainly motor neuropathies addressed thus far. Thus, patients with peripheral neuropathies present with variations in clinical features, and these variations can be associated with specific sets of autoantigens.

In most patients with CIDP and GBS, and in some with MMP, immune cell infiltration in peripheral nerves is observed during postmortem examination.[14,16–19] The production of specific humoral effectors resulting in nerve destruction, and signs and symptoms of peripheral sensory or motor polyneuropathy, or both, are a generally accepted mechanism for the pathogenesis of this group of neurologic diseases. GBS is closely associated with anti-GM1 and anti-GD1b antibodies, and antibodies against the membrane glycolipids P0 and P2 also have been described.[20,21] Typical serologic findings in CIDP patients were autoantibodies specific for glycolipids P0 and P2 and beta-tubulin.[21,22] Autoantibodies against ganglioside GM1 were found in patients with MMP.[23,24] In more than 50% of patients with MGUS, monoclonal antibodies specific for myelin-associated glycoprotein (MAG) have been found.[25–27] Thus it seems that specific neurologic deficits can be related to autoantibodies recognizing specific neuronal antigens.

One difficulty in ascribing cause and effect to autoimmunity in neuropathies is the lack of correlation of antibody titer with neuropathic symptoms. Closer examination of the literature, however, allows an explanation of this observation (Fig. 83-1). It is reasonable to assume that the antibody titer will be highest at the time of the first neuropathic damage, when the severity of symptoms is low. With longer duration of disease, the severity of the symptoms will increase, while the antigen level and subsequently antibody titer eventually will begin to diminish. Thus, a simple correlation analysis may not reflect the true relationship between autoantibody and development of neuropathic syndromes. In many patients autoantibodies have been found without signs or symptoms of neuropathy. Studies by Rabinowe et al.[28] have supported this hypothesis, demonstrating the presence of complement-fixing antiadrenal medullary antibodies in 19% of patients with IDDM for ≤16 years, but in only 3% of those with IDDM for ≥16 years. It has been speculated that autoantibodies recognizing nerve growth factor (NGF) might also contribute to diabetic neuropathy[12]; however, a recent study by Zanone et al.[29] found no such correlation. The subjects for this study had a mean duration of diabetes of >20 years, and the authors suggested that studies of subjects with a shorter duration of disease might be more revealing. Thus, prospective studies examining the development of neuropathy in those patients with autoantibodies are needed to establish a cause-and-effect relationship between autoantibodies and the development of diabetic neuropathy.

Lending further support to the observation of the pathogenetic potential of autoantibodies described in patients with peripheral neuropathies are immunotherapies allowing for removal or neutral-

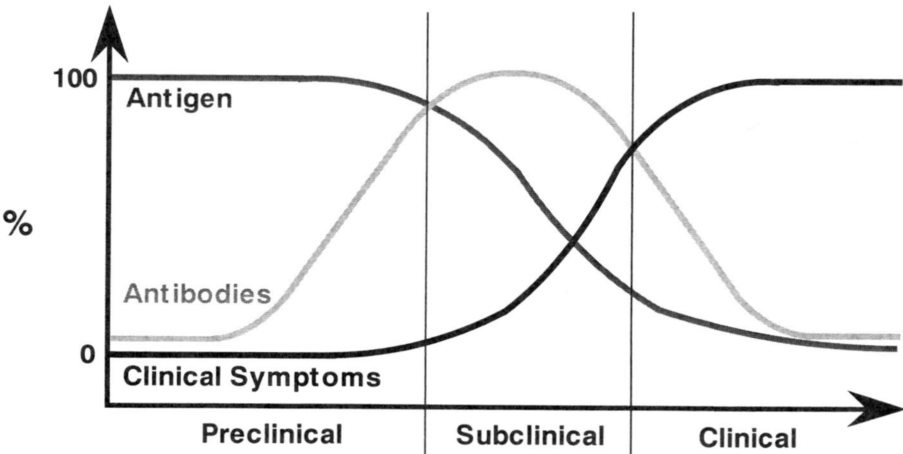

Figure 83-1. The interrelationships among severity of neuropathic symptoms, autoantibody titers, and antigen presentation in IDDM patients with neuropathy.

ization of the offending immunoglobulins (e.g., plasmapheresis,[30,31] administration of high IV doses of pooled, polyspecific human IG [IVIg][32]). The application of IVIg appears to have substantial short- and long-term therapeutic potential. Investigations during different stages of the natural course of disease have shown the presence of suppressive activity against antineural cell autoantibodies in sera from patients who have spontaneously recovered from GBS or CIDP.[33,34] The F(ab′)2 fragments have been found to mediate the inhibitory effect, suggesting idiotype–anti-idiotype interaction as a basic mechanism in disease remission. Anti-idiotypic autoantibodies are present in IVIg preparations, and in studies in vitro, inhibition of the activity of specific pathogenic autoantibodies has been induced exclusively by IVIg fractions containing F(ab′)2 fragments.[33] The appearance of anti-idiotypic antibodies was found to correlate with subsequent remission of the syndrome in patients with spontaneously acquired factor VIII:C inhibitors, recurrent spontaneous abortions associated with antiphospholipid antibodies, and myasthenia gravis.[35–37] It seems that this mechanism of tolerance induction by anti-idiotypic antibodies also is involved in the induction of graft tolerance in polytransfused patients.[38] A recent report also has determined that IVIg treatment significantly affects cytokine levels in the blood.[39] The role of cytokines in the regulation of autoimmune processes leading to neuropathy remains to be determined. Finally, plasmapheresis, which removes the primary antibody, was particularly effective for improving neuropathy in patients with IgA and IgG gammopathies.[30] Furthermore, plasmapheresis and IVIg appear to be complementary,[40] suggesting that removing the primary antibody and employing anti-idiotypic antibody may improve the chance of success in clinical efforts to reverse neuropathy.

The most well characterized antigens associated with peripheral neuropathy are the *glycolipids*. Several different autoantibodies in human sera that can react with epitopes in neuronal cells have been reported. For example, the gangliosides GM1, GD1b, and asialo-GM1 are bound by IgM recognizing the epitope Gal(β1-3)GalNAc in patients with lower motor neuron disease, multifocal motor polyneuropathy, and acute axonal neuropathies.[41–44] The three-sulfated glucuronic acid (SO_4-3-GlcA), an epitope designated HNK-1, is recognized by antimyelin-associated IgM in patients with demyelinating peripheral neuropathy associated with plasma cell dyscrasia.[45] Both antigens can be demonstrated on the surface of human neuroblastoma cells using immunohistochemistry. Gangliosides are overexpressed in many neuroblastoma cell lines[46] and play a regulating role in the proliferation and differentiation of neuroblastoma cells. A murine monoclonal antibody specifically recognizing disialoganglioside GD2 lyses a number of human neuroblastoma cell lines by antibody- and complement-dependent cytotoxicity.[47] Other studies indicate that IDDM serum IgG specifically binds to neuronal type cell surfaces. The property of the surface binding pattern is similar to the antibody binding pattern reported with the use of antiganglioside antibody. Gangliosides have been successfully used in functional recovery after central nervous system damage[48] and offer partial protection in experimental allergic neuritis. Studies are under way to determine whether gangliosides could rescue neuronal cells in IDDM, either by autoantibody neutralization or by direct neurotrophic effects.

The pathogenetic potential of antibodies associated with peripheral neuropathies has been shown in vitro by studies of their specificity and in vivo by immunoglobulin transfer in experimental models. For example, IgM the sera of MGUS patients contain IgM that binds MAG and is apparently specific, because it can be completely inhibited by MAG isolated from human myelin.[25] In addition, anti-MAG IgM has been shown to bind with complement to peripheral nerve myelin.[49,50] Levels of anti-MAG antibodies have been found to correlate with severity of neurologic signs and symptoms.[51] Sural nerve biopsies examining IgA, IgG, and IgM monoclonal proteins have shown their association with a mixed fiber involvement, including fiber loss, segmental demyelination, and axonal degeneration.[52] A number of transfer studies also have been performed. Injection of sera from patients with monoclonal gammopathy into the sciatic nerves of cats in one study resulted in demyelination and conduction block.[53] Injection of serum from patients with MMP exhibiting anti-GM1 activity into rat tibial nerves yielded similar results in another study.[54] Thus, it is clear that immunoglobulins, probably via a complement-mediated mechanism, are capable of inducing neuropathic conditions.

Evidence for Autoimmune Mechanisms in the Pathogenesis of Diabetic Neuropathy

It has been recognized for many years that IDDM is a chronic inflammatory disease with a long prodromal phase,[55] involving both CD4+ and CD8+ T-cell infiltration, and is often associated with production of antibodies that react with islet cells.[56–59] Islet cell antibody (ICA), directed to unknown islet cell cytoplasmic antigens, was the first specific immune marker detected in IDDM patients.[13,57,60] Although a pathogenic role for ICA has not been confirmed, there is a strong correlation between ICA and the development of IDDM. Several other antigens possibly involved in immune system sensitization have been described, but there has been no definitive identification of those antigens that are responsible for causing IDDM in humans. A recent study has established a strong correlation between glutamic acid decarboxylase (GAD) autoantibodies and IDDM; loss of tolerance to GAD has been shown to correlate with the development of diabetes in the autoimmune nonobese diabetic (NOD) mouse model.[61] Anti-GAD activity as a cause of IDDM, however, has not been established, and some investigators find GAD to be insufficient to cause diabetes by itself.

An interesting study by Björk et al.[62] has presented evidence that the epitope of GAD identified by autoantibodies in IDDM is different from that identified in patients with autoimmune polyendocrine syndrome type I (APS I) and stiff man syndrome (SMS),[62] a neuropathic condition often associated with diabetes. Whereas both APS I and SMS sera were able to block the enzymatic activity of GAD in vitro, IDDM serum was not able to block GAD activity, and in some cases even enhanced activity. Thus, the role for the autoantibodies to islet cell antigens in the development of diabetic neuropathy remains unknown.

There is fairly strong evidence to support both tissue and humoral immune mechanisms in the pathogenesis of diabetic autonomic neuropathy. The most important pathologic change in diabetic polyneuropathy is a loss of myelinated and unmyelinated nerve axons. *Segmental demyelination* in diabetes may be primary, from loss of individual Schwann cells, or secondary, the result of responses to a change in axonal caliber. No clear infiltration has been described in patients with typical distal sensorimotor diabetic polyneuropathy. In 1983 Segal et al.[63] demonstrated an association between diabetic neuropathy and sensitization of lymphocytes to basic encephalitogenic protein and P_2, antigens from the central nervous system and peripheral nerve tissue, respectively. Other investigators have described lymphoplasmocytic infiltrates in sympathetic ganglia of IDDM subjects studied at autopsy.[64,65] Brown et al. also reported on the high frequency of adrenal medullary fibrosis in patients with long-standing IDDM.[66] In another retrospective autopsy study, using formalin-fixed tissue and monoclonal antibodies specific for anti-HLA, anti–B-lymphocyte antigen, and anti-CD45 antigen, signs of moderate to severe adrenal medullary infiltration were detected in 20% of IDDM patients and mild to severe fibrosis in another 52%.[65] Accordingly, one can argue that inflammatory infiltration is present in certain autonomic nervous system structures of IDDM patients, but not elsewhere in the system. Vagal nerve examination showed loss of myelinated axons and marked excess of collagen, with no clear infiltration.[64] The sympathetic postganglionic myelinated fibers in the splanchnic nerves are also severely damaged in diabetic neuropathy,[67] but no inflammation was reported. It is not clear whether all these changes in the autonomic nervous system are of the same origin, or whether different pathogenetic mechanisms could be involved in the development of lesions in different parts of the autonomic nervous system. The differences in histopathologic findings between the different parts of the autonomic nervous system, or between autonomic and peripheral sensorimotor nervous systems, may be the result of different pathogenetic mechanisms for certain chronic neurologic complications of the disease. An important issue is the possible antigenic differences between sympathetic and parasympathetic structures, which could result in differences in the susceptibility to immune destruction. The histopathologic differences that have been described support this concept. Accordingly, it is possible that the parasympathetic lesion in IDDM is mediated by humoral immune effectors, or not mediated immunologically at all.

Organ-specific, complement-fixing autoantibodies against unknown antigens from adrenal medulla (CF-ADM) and sympathetic ganglia (CF-SG) have been demonstrated in IDDM patients.[28,68–72] With a duration of diabetes of >5 years, CF-ADM was found to occur in both ICA-positive and ICA-negative patients, suggesting that the antigenic targets in adrenal medulla and pancreatic islets are different. Because these were cross-sectional studies, it is unknown whether the generation of antibody preceded neuronal destruction. Observations by Zanone et al.[70] on the prevalence of CF-SG antibodies or at least one of the autoantibodies directed to autonomic nervous system structures (CF-SG, CF-ADM, or complement-fixing vagal [CF-V] autoantibody) in patients with diabetic autonomic neuropathy strongly support the relationship between autoantibodies to autonomic structures and autonomic neuropathy in IDDM. Recent studies have demonstrated that there is an immunoglobulin, probably IgG, in the serum of patients with IDDM and clinical neuropathy that is able to inhibit the growth, and in some cases induce death, of an adrenergic neuroblastoma cell clone, which is an in vitro model for sympathetic neurons.[73,74] In patients with IDDM but with no signs of clinical neuropathy, there is no consistent effect, although some of these sera also inhibit cell proliferation, suggesting that these patients might be preneuropathic. In contrast, the sera of NIDDM patients with neuropathy exhibited little effect on cell proliferation, suggesting that the development of neuropathy in IDDM and NIDDM might occur via different mechanisms.

The differences in the presentation of neuropathy observed by various investigators may simply reflect a different pathogenesis of chronic neurologic complications of IDDM, perhaps generated by different antigen-antibody complexes. A number of autoantigens have been described in IDDM patients that might induce immune system responses resulting in nerve damage, including phospholipids, glycolipids, and GAD. Rabinowe et al.[75] reported the finding of an antiganglioside GT1b IgG antibody in IDDM patients, and they correlated this antibody to changes in orthostatic blood pressure,[75] suggesting a role in autonomic neuropathy. Anti-GT1b autoantibody recognizes sympathetic ganglia and adrenal medullary antigens. There are probably other, as yet unrecognized, antigens associated with IDDM that may participate in neuronal recognition. Immunogenetic analyses of IDDM patients have shown a significantly higher frequency of the heterozygous genetic constellation HLA-DR3/DR4 in those with mild and severe autonomic diabetic neuropathy of the cardiovascular system, compared with those who did not have any signs of autonomic nervous system disturbances.[3] This observation suggests a relationship between diabetic autonomic neuropathy and immune response genes within the MHC, which is in accordance with other evidence of autoimmunity generated against sympathetic nervous system structures in IDDM patients.

In recent studies of *antiphospholipid antibodies* (anti-PLAs), a family of closely related immunoglobulins that interact with one or more negatively charged phospholipids (constituents of nervous tissues), we have found their increased prevalence in IDDM patients, with a further increase in those who had concomitant neuropathy. There does not appear to be a direct correlation between autonomic neuropathy and PLAs, but we have found that sera with high titers of IgG PLA inhibit cell growth and differentiation in a neuroblastoma cell line.[76] PLAs have been described in a number of autoimmune, neurologic, and hematologic disorders. In these disorders, PLA appearance increases the risk of arteriovenous thrombosis, thrombocytopenia, hemolytic anemia, and fetal loss. These features, occurring by themselves or commonly together, have been described as the *antiphospholipid syndrome,* found in PLA-positive persons without clinical or serologic signs of any other disease. Thus, the possibility that PLA might contribute to diabetic neuropathy, either by direct neuronal toxicity or by compromise of the neuronal vessels, must be considered. In one study PLAs were found in 88% of a diabetic population with neuropathy, compared to 32% of diabetic patients without neurologic complications and 2% in the general population. Most of the PLA-positive patients were positive for the IgG fraction.[76] Correlation between PLA level and warm perception threshold suggests that small, unmyelinated C-fibers contain a specific antigen recognized by PLAs. Results obtained from experimental investigations in humans as well as other species demonstrate that autoimmunity may be caused not only by functional immunocyte disorders, but also by the changed antigenicity of target cells. It is reported that there is a change in the phospholipid composition of the extracellular leaflet of the plasma membrane of erythrocytes, with an increase in phosphatidylserine, in response to hyperglycemia in diabetes.[77] It is as yet unclear whether this "phospholipid asymmetry" is a common cellular effect of diabetes. In light of the increased prevalence of PLAs in patients with diabetic neuropathy, it must be considered that these events acting in combination may be important in neuronal destruction.

It has been argued that PLAs are of no pathologic consequence, but are an epiphenomenon resulting from tissue damage and the subsequent generation of an immune response. Considerable circumstantial evidence supports the notion that PLAs may indeed be capable of inflicting injury, and that the damage may be selective for specific parts of the nervous system as well as other tissues.[78,79] In addition, concurrent vascular changes may lead to significant interaction between the two pathogenetic mechanisms. Future studies should help resolve questions about the role of PLAs in the development of neuropathic syndromes.

Glycolipid autoantibodies may also play a significant role in diabetic neuropathy. Autoantibodies to the gangliosides sialo- and asialo-GM1 have been described in diabetic patients.[80] Pestronk et al.[81] have characterized GM-1 autoantibodies to be regulated by T-cell independent B-cells; however, Bansal et al.[82] reported that although they found anti-GM1 IgM to be clearly associated with multifocal motor neuropathy, they found no correlation with anti-GM1 titer in patients with diabetic peripheral neuropathy. The latter group, however, did not divide the diabetic patient population according to type of neuropathy (e.g., motor, sensorimotor, autonomic) and therefore may have oversimplified their analysis. As described previously, anti-GM1 is most often associated with lower motor neuropathies, and therefore may not play a major role in diabetic neuropathies, which for the most part do not have a large motor component.

The 67-kD form of GAD, which is a product of a different gene than GAD-65, is the predominant form in neurons.[83] Antibodies to GAD are found in patients with the neurologic disorder SMS,[84–86] in whom there is a high prevalence of IDDM. Harrison et al.[87] reported the presence of GAD antibodies in IDDM patients, with a progressive decline in anti-GAD titer with increasing duration of diabetes.[87] In nine patients with autonomic neuropathy these antibody levels persisted, suggesting a role in the pathogenesis of neuropathy. This has, however, been contested[88,89] and is not compatible with observations by other investigators.[76,89] Furthermore, GAD is a cytoplasmic enzyme in neurons, and access of the autoantibody to the protein in live cells is problematic. Thus, the role of anti-GAD antibodies in diabetic neuropathy remains to be determined.

Other target antigens associated with diabetes or neuropathy, or both, such as growth factors, also must be considered. *Insulin autoantibodies* are a common feature of both IDDM and NIDDM. There are structural and biochemical similarities between the insulin family of peptides and NGF.[90,91] NGF was discovered nearly 50 years ago. Since the pioneering work of Levi-Montalcini and Booker,[92] it has been known that neural crest–derived cells, sympathetic neurons, and dorsal root ganglion (DRG) neurons are developmentally dependent on NGF. More recently, it has been shown that adult DRG and sympathetic neurons, both of which are affected in diabetic neuropathy, are dependent on NGF either for their maintenance[93] or survival.[94] It has been suggested that antibodies to insulin may cross-react with NGF and contribute to an effective reduction in NGF available to nerves, thereby contributing to the development of neuropathy.[95] This is significant because transgenic mice that have an inactive low-affinity NGF receptor, p75, present a similar neuropathic condition to that seen in diabetic neuropathy, with loss of sensory (especially temperature perception) and autonomic innervation.[96] Thus, autoimmunity may play a role in the NGF deficiency reported in diabetes by mechanisms related to immune neutralization of available NGF.

In 1991, Anand et al.[97] described a 30-year-old woman with long-standing dizziness who was found to have severe orthostasis and a reduced skin-flare response. Autonomic tests indicated a selective impairment of adrenergic nerve function. Plasma levels of norepinephrine, epinephrine, dopamine, and dopamine β-hydroxylase were undetectable. Skin biopsy showed loss of tyrosine hydroxylase and neuropeptide Y, markers of adrenergic sympathetic fibers, and loss of the sensory neuropeptides, substance P and calcitonin gene-related peptide (CGRP). Sural nerve biopsy showed depletion of small, unmyelinated C-fibers, and assay showed reduced NGF content. Because NGF selectively induces tyrosine hydroxylase and dopamine β-hydroxylase, is necessary for the survival of sympathetic nerve fibers, and is required for the expression of substance P and CGRP in adult sensory neurons, immune neutralization of NGF could possibly generate a clinical syndrome similar to that found in diabetic neuropathy. Guy et al.[12] found an association between diabetic autonomic neuropathy and iritis, suggesting an immunologic background. Because iritis itself is an immunologically mediated disorder with circulating immune complexes, they speculated that the associated small-fiber damage that results in autonomic neuropathy might be due to autoimmunity. Furthermore, the iris has a high NGF content and it must be considered that, because of the homology between NGF and the insulin family of proteins, insulin autoantibodies might recognize epitopes on NGF in the iris, resulting in iritis. Thus, insulin autoantibody formation, which is universal in IDDM patients and also can occur as a primary phenomenon, may contribute not only to diabetic neuropathy, but also to other autoimmune conditions (e.g., iritis) through interaction with NGF.

Studies have demonstrated that the *insulin-like growth factors* (IGFs) are widely distributed throughout the nervous system and exert profound effects on developing neurons (see Chapter 85). To summarize briefly, whether acting via paracrine, autocrine, or endocrine mechanisms, the rationale for implicating IGFs in the pathogenesis of diabetic neuropathy is as follows: (1) IGFs in nervous tissue are regulated by insulin; (2) IGF receptors are present in the appropriate tissues (e.g., neurons, Schwann cells, ganglia) involved in diabetes-associated nerve disorders; (3) IGFs exert numerous effects on nerve tissue growth and function, including indirect effects such as those mediated through NGF; and (4) IGF-binding proteins are present in the nervous system, are regulated by insulin and the glycemic state, and have been shown to modulate IGF action in nervous tissue. As yet, however, there are no data to support a role for autoimmune processes acting on IGFs in the neuronal deficits of diabetic neuropathy.

Neuropathy developing in NIDDM patients is likewise difficult to attribute to autoimmune processes. As yet there is no known autoimmune mechanism in the pathogenesis of the disease. It has recently been determined, however, that a subgroup of NIDDM patients are more accurately classified as latent autoimmune diabetes of aging (LADA).[98] These patients are determined actually to have a slower time course of autoimmune disease than the typical IDDM patient, yet autoimmune processes are responsible for the ensuing diabetes. In a study by Zimmet et al.[98] it was found that both GAD antibody titer and anti-GAD positivity was significantly higher in LADA patients compared to NIDDM patients. Thus, the consideration of LADA patients as a distinct group may help elucidate the contribution of autoimmunity in the development of diabetic neuropathy in what is likely to be a heterogeneous group of patients previously classified as having NIDDM.

Summary

Diabetic neuropathy has a complex mechanism of pathogenesis that may be multifactorial, with contributions from not only autoimmune but also metabolic, growth factor, and vascular dysfunctions. Table 83-1 presents a comparison of the clinical profiles for several autoimmune neuropathies with the typical clinical profile for diabetic neuropathy. Candidate antigens for autoantibodies related to diabetic neuropathy include insulin, phospholipids, nerve growth factor or its receptors, gangliosides, and GAD. In addition, there may be an underlying genetic predisposition to autoimmunity in IDDM patients that may contribute to the process. Further studies of the interplay between the various physiologic defects in these patients should provide information that can lead to better therapeutic approaches to prevent and reverse the development of neuropa-

TABLE 83-1. Autoimmune Peripheral Neuropathies: Pathologic, Clinical and Immunologic Characteristics

	Diabetic Neuropathy	Guillain-Barré Syndrome	Chronic Inflammatory Demyelinating Polyneuropathy	Multifocal Motor Neuropathy	Polyneuropathy Associated with MGUS
Pathology	Demyelination Axonal degeneration Multifocal[80]	Demyelination Axonal degeneration Inflammation ++ APC, T- and B-cells, Ig + complement Multifocal[17,18,99]	Demyelination Axonal degeneration Inflammation +[14,19]	Demyelination Axonal degeneration Inflammation ±[16,100]	Demyelination Axonal degeneration[50,101,102]
Time course	Chronic[80]	Acute Relapsing[103]	Subacute Chronic Relapsing[104,105]	Chronic[16,24,100]	Chronic[101]
Lesion distribution NDS NSS	Motor +* Sensory +++ NDS ↓, NSS ↓[80]	Motor +++ Sensory + NDS →↓, NSS ↓[103]	Motor +++ Sensory + NDS (MRS) ↓, NSS (done, no specific data)[104,105]	Motor +++ Sensory ± NDS (MRS, MRCS) ↓ NSS →[16,24,100]	Motor ++ Sensory +++ NDS ↓ NSS ↓[101]
Electromyographic findings	Sensory ↓+++ Motor ↓+[80]	Motor ↓+++ Sensory ↓++[106]	Motor ↓+++ Sensory ↓+[105,107]	Motor ↓+++ Sensory ±[24,107,108]	Motor ↓++ Sensory ↓ +++[102,105]
Antigen-derived antibodies	GM1 Ab Asialo-GM1-Ab GT1b Ab[74,80]	GM1 Ab (IgG>IgM) GD1a (IgG>IgM) GD1b Ab (IgG) GT1b (IgM) Anti-glycolipids P0 and P2 and anti-MAG Ab[20,21,103]	MAG Ab (IgM) Antiglycolipids P0 and P2 Ab Antitubulin Ab[21,103,104,109]	GM1 Ab (IgM) GD1b Ab (IgM)[24,42,110]	MAG Ab (IgM>IgG>IgA) Anti-GM1 Ab (IgM) Anti-GD1b Ab (IgM)[105,111]
Natural antibody	PLA (IgG>IgM>IgA)[75,76]	PLA (IgM>IgG)[112]	PLA[113]		
Associated autonomic neuropathy	Myelinating fibers Sympathetic (postgang. ADM, SG) Parasympathetic[28,66–69,114]	Small fibers Sympathetic (pregang.) Parasympathetic No inflammation[109,115,116]	Mild, rarely[117]	No data	No data
Quantitative sensory testing	Vibratory sen. ↓+++ Pinprick sen. ↓+++ Light touch sen. ↓+++ Position sen. ↓+++[80]	No data in recent studies	Vibratory sen. ↓ Pinprick sen. ↓[105]	Preserved (no specific data)[24]	Vibratory sen. ↓+++ Position sen. ↓+ Pain sen. ↓+ Light touch ↓+[101]
Autonomic function tests	Sympath. tests ↓ Parasympath. tests ↓[80,118]	No data in recent studies	No data in recent studies	No data	No data
Sensory evoked potentials	Prolonged or nonevokable[119]	Proximal conduction block Reduced amplitude Generalized slowing[120]	Refractory period increase Pronounced slowing[120]	No data	Median nerve + Ulnar nerve + Tibial nerve ± Peroneal nerve ±[101]
Immunotherapy	None	Immunosuppressive drugs Plasma exchange IVIg[14,106,121]	Immunosuppressive drugs Plasma exchange IVIg[14,122,123]	Immunosuppressive drugs Plasma exchange IVIg[16,51,124]	Immunosuppressive drugs Plasma exchange IVIg[30,32,125,126]

*Frequency of disturbances: ± = rarely; + = infrequently; ++ = moderately; +++ = frequently.
MAG = myelin-associated glycoprotein; MGUS = monoclonal gammopathies of undetermined significance; ADM = adrenal medulla; SG = sympathetic ganglia; MRCS = Medical Research Council score; MRS = modified Rankin score; NDS = neuropathy disability score; NSS = neuropathy sensory score; sen. = sensation.

thy, thus allowing physicians to determine those patients at highest risk for developing neuropathic complications before the onset of symptomatic neuropathy.

References

1. Herold KC, Rubenstein AH. New directions in the immunology of autoimmune diabetes. Ann Intern Med 1992;117:436
2. Boitard C. The differentiation of the immune system towards anti-islet autoimmunity. Clin Prospects 1992;35:1101
3. Barzilay J, Warram JH, Rand LI, et al. Risk for cardiovascular autonomic neuropathy is associated with the HLA-DR3/4 phenotype in type I diabetes mellitus. Ann Intern Med 1992;116:544
4. Todd JA. Genetic control of autoimmunity in type I diabetes. Immunol Today 1990;11:122
5. Teitelman G. Cellular and molecular analysis of pancreatic islet cell lineage and differentiation. Recent Prog Horm Res 1991;47:259
6. Teitelman G, Joh TH, Reis DJ. Linkage of the brain-skin-gut axis: Islet cells originate from dopaminergic precursors. Peptides 1981;2(suppl 2):157
7. Teitelman G, Lee JK. Cell lineage analysis of pancreatic islet development: Glucagon and insulin cells arise from catecholaminergic precursors present in the pancreatic duct. Dev Biol 1987;121:454
8. Polak M, Scharfmann R, Seilheimer B, et al. Nerve growth factor induces neuron-like differentiation of an insulin-secreting pancreatic beta cell line. Proc Natl Acad Sci U S A 1993;90:5781
9. Srinivasan J, Hays AP, Thomas FP. Autoantigens in human neuroblastoma cells. J Neuroimmunol 1990;26:43
10. Pearse AGE. Islet cell precursors are neurons. Nature 1982;295:96
11. Ariga T, Kohriyama T, Freddo L. Characterization of sulfated glucuronic acid containing glycolipids reacting with IgM M-proteins in patients with neuropathy. J Biol Chem 1987;262:848
12. Guy RJC, Richards F, Edmonds ME, Watkins PJ. Diabetic autonomic neuropathy and iritis: An association suggesting an immunological cause. Br Med J 1984;289:343
13. Bottazzo GF, Todd I, Mirakian R, et al. Organ-specific autoimmunity: A 1986 overview. Immunol Rev 1986;94:137
14. Feasby TE. Inflammatory-demyelinating polyneuropathies. Neurologic Clin 1992;10:651
15. Davidson DLW, O'Sullivan AF, Morley KD. HLA antigens in familial Guillain-Barré syndrome. J Neurol Neurosurg Psychol 1992;1282:7684
16. Parry GJ, Sumner AJ. Multifocal motor neuropathy. Neurologic Clin 1992;10:671
17. Al-Hakim M, Cohen M, Daroff RB. Postmortem examination of relapsing acute Guillain-Barré syndrome. Muscle Nerve 1993;16:173
18. Honavar M, Tharakan JKJ, Hughes RAC, et al. A clinicopathological study of the Guillain-Barré syndrome. Brain 1992;114:1245
19. Dyck PJ, Lais A, Ohta M, et al. Chronic inflammatory polyradiculoneuropathy. Mayo Clin Proc 1975;50:621
20. Yuki N, Yamada M, Sato S, et al. Association of IgG anti-GD1 antibody with severe Guillain-Barré syndrome. Muscle Nerve 1993;16:642
21. Khalili-Shirazi A, Atkinson P, Gregson N, Hughes RA. Antibody response to P0 and P2 myelin proteins in Guillain-Barré syndrome and chronic idiopathic demyelinating polyradiculopathy. J Neuroimmunol 1993;46:245
22. Connolly AM, Pestronk A, Trotter JL, et al. High titer selective serum anti-beta-tubulin antibodies in chronic inflammatory demyelinating polyneuropathy. Neurology 1993;43:557
23. Pestronk A, Cornblath DR, Ilyas AA, et al. A treatable multifocal motor neuropathy with antibodies to GM1 ganglioside. Ann Neurol 1988;24:73
24. Pestronk A, Chaudhury V, Feldman EL, et al. Lower motor neuron syndromes detected by patterns of weakness, nerve conduction abnormalities, and high titers of antiglycolipid antibodies. Ann Neurol 1990;27:316
25. Steck AJ, Murray N, Meier C, et al. Demyelinating neuropathy and monoclonal IgM antibody to myelin-associated glycoprotein. Neurology 1983;33:19
26. Hafler DA, Johnson D, Kelly JJ, et al. Monoclonal gammopathy and neuropathy: Myelin-associated glycoprotein reactivity and clinical characteristics. Neurology 1986;36:75
27. Melmed C, Frail D, Duncan I, et al. Peripheral neuropathy with IgM kappa monoclonal immunoglobulin directed against myelin-associated glycoprotein. Neurology 1983;33:1397
28. Rabinowe SL, Brown FM, Watts M, et al. Anti-sympathetic ganglia antibodies and postural blood pressure in IDDM subjects of varying duration and patients at high risk of developing IDDM. Diabetes Care 1989;12:1
29. Zanone MM, Banga JP, Peakman M, et al. An investigation of antibodies to nerve growth factor in diabetic autonomic neuropathy. Diabet Med 1994;11:378
30. Dyck PJ, Low PA, Windebank AJ, et al. Plasma exchange in polyneuropathy associated with monoclonal gammopathy of undetermined significance. N Engl J Med 1991;325:1482
31. Haas DC, Tatum AH. Plasmapheresis alleviates neuropathy accompanying IgM anti-myelin associated glycoprotein paraproteinemia. Ann Neurol 1988;23:394
32. Cook D, Dalakas M, Galdi A, et al. High-dose intravenous immunoglobulin in the treatment of demyelinating neuropathy associated with monoclonal gammopathy. Neurology 1990;40:212
33. Lundkvist I, Van Doorn PA, Vermeulen M, Brand A. Spontaneous recovery from the Guillain-Barré syndrome is associated with anti-idiotypic antibodies recognizing a cross-reactive idiotype on anti-neuroblastoma cell line antibodies. Clin Immunol Immunopathol 1993;67:192
34. Van Doorn PA, Rossi F, Brand A, et al. On the mechanism of high-dose intravenous immunoglobulin treatment of patients with chronic inflammatory demyelinating polyneuropathy. J Neuroimmunol 1990;29:57
35. Sultan Y, Kazatchkime MD, Nydegger U, et al. Intravenous immunoglobulin in the treatment of spontaneously acquired factor VIII:C inhibitors. Am J Med 1991;91(suppl 5A):35S
36. Orvieto R, Achiron A, Ben-Rafael Z, Achiron R. Intravenous immunoglobulin treatment for recurrent abortions causes by antiphospholipid antibodies. Fertil Steril 1991;56:1013
37. Ferrero B, Durelli L, Cavallo R, et al. Therapies for exacerbation of myasthenia gravis: The mechanism of action of intravenous high-dose immunoglobulin G. Ann N Y Acad Sci 1993;681:563
38. Nishimura M, Sakai K, Akaza T, et al. Anti-idiotypic antibody to T-cell receptor in multiply transfused patients may play a role in resistance to graft-versus-host disease. Transfusion 1992;32:719
39. Aukrust P, Fröland SS, Liabakk N-B, et al. Release of cytokines, soluble cytokine receptors, and interleukin-1 receptor antagonist after intravenous immunoglobulin administration in vivo. Blood 1994;7:2136
40. Herson S, Cherin P, Coutellier A. The association of plasma exchange synchronized with intravenous gamma globulin therapy in severe intractable polymyositis. J Rheumatol 1992;19:828
41. Freddo L, Yu RK, Latov N. Gangliosides GM1 and GD1b are antigens for IgM M-protein in a patient with motor neuron disease. Neurology 1986;36:454
42. Latov N. Neuropathy and anti-GM1 antibodies. Ann Neurol 1990;27:S41
43. Quarles RH, Ilyas AA, Willison HJ. Serum antibodies to gangliosides in Guillain-Barre syndrome. Ann Neurol 1990;27:S48
44. Weng NP, Yu-lee L, Sanz I. Structure and specificities of anti-ganglioside autoantibodies associated with motor neuropathies. J Immunol 1992;149:2518
45. Freddo L, Ariga T, Latov N. The neuropathy of plasma cell dyscrasia: Binding of IgM M-proteins to peripheral nerve glycolipids. Neurology 1985;35:1420
46. Wu G, Hua Z, Ledeen RW. Correlation of gangliotetraose gangliosides with neurite forming potential of neuroblastoma cells. Dev Brain Res 1991;61:217
47. Mujoo K, Cheresh DA, Yang HM, Reisfeld RA. Disialoganglioside GD2 on human neuroblastoma cells: Target antigen for monoclonal antibody-mediated cytolysis and suppression of tumor growth. Cancer Res 1984;47:1098
48. Geisler FH, Dorsey FC, Coleman WP. Recovery of motor function after spinal cord injury—A randomized, placebo-controlled trial with GM-1 ganglioside. N Engl J Med 1991;324:1829
49. Monaco S, Bonetti B, Ferrari S, et al. Complement-mediated demyelination in patients with IgM monoclonal gammopathy and polyneuropathy. N Engl J Med 1990;322:649
50. Takatsu M, Hays AP, Latov N, et al. Immunofluorescence study of patients with neuropathy and IgM M proteins. Ann Neurol 1985;18:173
51. Nobile-Orazio E, Francomano E, Daverio R, et al. Anti-myelin-associated glycoprotein IgM antibody titers in neuropathy associated with macroglobulinemia. Ann Neurol 1989;26:543
52. Yeung KB, Thomas PK, King RH, et al. The clinical spectrum of peripheral neuropathies associated with benign monoclonal IgM, IgG and IgA paraproteinemia. J Neurol 1991;238:383
53. Hays AP, Latov N, Takatsu M, Sherman WH. Experimental demyelination of nerve induced by serum of patients with neuropathy and an anti-MAG IgM M-protein. Neurology 1987;37:242
54. Uncini A, Santoro M, Corbo M, et al. Conduction abnormalities induced by sera of patients with multifocal motor neuropathy and anti-GM1 antibodies. Muscle Nerve 1993;16:610
55. Gorsuch AN, Spencer KM, Lister J, et al. The natural history of type I (insulin-dependent) diabetes mellitus: Evidence for a long pre-diabetic period. Lancet 1981;2:363
56. Vives M, Somoza N, Soldevilla G. Reevaluation of autoantibodies to islet cell membrane in IDDM. Diabetes 1992;41:1624
57. Bottazzo GF, Florin-Christensen AF, Doniach D. Islet cell antibodies in diabetes mellitus with autoimmune polyendocrine deficiencies. Lancet 1974;2:1279
58. Baekkeskov S, Nielsen JH, Marner B, et al. Autoantibodies in newly diagnosed diabetic children immunoprecipitate human pancreatic islet cell proteins. Nature 1982;298:167
59. Lernmark Å. Islet cell antibodies. Diabet Med 1987;4:285
60. Atkinson MA, Maclaren NK. Islet cell autoantigens in insulin-dependent diabetes. J Clin Invest 1993;92:1608
61. Tisch R, Yang XD, Singer SM, et al. Immune response to glutamic acid decarboxylase correlates with insulitis in non-obese diabetic mice. Nature 1993;366:15
62. Björk E, Velloso LA, Kämpe O, Karlsson FA. GAD autoantibodies in IDDM, stiff-man syndrome, and autoimmune polyendocrine syndrome type I recognize different epitopes. Diabetes 1994;43:161
63. Segal P, Teitelbaum D, Ohry A. Cell-mediated immunity to nervous system antigens in diabetic patients with neuropathy. Isr J Med Sci 1983;19:7

64. Duchen LW, Anjorin NA, Watkins PJ, Mackay JD. Pathology of autonomic neuropathy in diabetes mellitus. Ann Intern Med 1980;92:301
65. Brown FM, Smith AM, Longway S, Rabinowe SL. Adrenal medullitis in type I diabetes. J Clin Endocrinol Metabol 1990;71:1491
66. Brown FM, Zuckerman M, Longway S, Rabinowe SL. Adrenal medullary fibrosis in IDDM of long duration. Diabetes Care 1989;12:494
67. Low PA, Walsh JC, Huang CY, McLeod JG. The sympathetic nervous system in diabetic neuropathy—a clinical and pathological study. Brain 1975;98:341
68. Brown FM, Kamalesh M, Adri MNS, Rabinowe SL. Anti-adrenal medullary antibodies in IDDM subjects and subjects at high risk for developing IDDM. Diabetes Care 1988;11:30
69. Brown FM, Brink SJ, Freeman R, Rabinowe SL. Anti-sympathetic nervous system autoantibodies: Diminished catecholamines with orthostasis. Diabetes 1989;38:938
70. Zanone MM, Peakman M, Purewal T, et al. Autoantibodies to nervous tissue structures are associated with autonomic neuropathy in type 1 (insulin-dependent) diabetes mellitus. Diabetologia 1993;36:564
71. Brown FM, Vinik AI, Ganda OP. Different effects of duration on prevalence of anti-adrenal medullary and pancreatic islet cell antibodies in type I diabetes mellitus. Horm Metabol Res 1988;21:434
72. Sundkvist G, Lind P, Bergstrom B, et al. Autonomic nerve antibodies and autonomic nerve function in type 1 and type 2 diabetic patients. J Intern Med 1991;229:505
73. Pittenger GL, Liu D, Vinik AI. The toxic effects of serum from patients with type I diabetes mellitus on mouse neuroblastoma cells: A new mechanism for development of autonomic neuropathy. Diabet Med 1993;10:925
74. Pittenger GL, Liu D, Vinik AI. The neuronal toxic factor in serum of type 1 diabetic patients is a complement-fixing autoantibody. Diabet Med 1995;12:380
75. Rabinowe SL, Myerov A, Brown F. Anti-ganglioside GT1b IgG antibodies in type I diabetes: Orthostatic blood pressure and autonomic antibodies [Abstract]. Clin Res 1991;39:364A
76. Vinik AI, Pittenger GL, Stansberry KB, Powers A. Antiphospholipid and glutamic acid decarboxylase antibodies in diabetic neuropathy. Diabetes Care 1995;18:1225
77. Wilson MJ, Richter Lowney K, Daleke DL. Hyperglycemia induces a loss of phospholipid asymmetry in human erythrocytes. Biochemistry 1993;32:11302
78. Lockshin MD, Druzin ML, Goei S, et al. Antibody to cardiolipin as a predictor of fetal distress or death in pregnant patients with systemic lupus erythematosus. N Engl J Med 1985;313:152
79. Lockshin MD, Qamar T, Druzin ML, Goei S. Antibody to cardiolipin, lupus anticoagulant, and fetal death. J Rheumatol 1987;14:259
80. Vinik AI, Holland MT, LeBeau JM, et al. Diabetic neuropathies. Diabetes Care 1992;15:1926
81. Pestronk A, Adams RN, Kuncl RW, et al. Differential effects of prednisone and cyclophosphamide on autoantibodies in human neuromuscular disorders. Neurology 1989;39:628
82. Bansal AS, Abdul-Karim B, Malik RA, et al. IgM ganglioside GM1 antibodies in patients with autoimmune disease or neuropathy, and controls. J Clin Pathol 1994;47:300
83. Kaufman DL, Houser CR, Tobin AJ. Two forms of the gamma-aminobutyric acid synthetic enzyme glutamate decarboxylase have distinct intraneuronal distributions and cofactor interactions. J Neurochem 1991;56:720
84. Solimena M, Folli F, Denis-Donini S, et al. Autoantibodies to glutamic acid decarboxylase in a patient with stiff-man syndrome, epilepsy, and type 1 diabetes mellitus. N Engl J Med 1988;318:1012
85. Solimena M, Folli F, Aparisi A, et al. Autoantibodies to GABA-ergic neurons and pancreatic beta cells in stiff-man syndrome. N Engl J Med 1990;322:1555
86. Baekkeskov S, Aanstoot HJ, Christgau S, et al. Identification of the 64K autoantigen in insulin-dependent diabetes as the GABA-synthesizing enzyme glutamic acid decarboxylase. Nature 1990;347:151
87. Harrison LC, Honeyman MC, DeAizpurua HJ, et al. Inverse relation between humoral and cellular immunity to glutamic acid decarboxylase in subjects at risk of insulin-dependent diabetes. Lancet 1993;341:1365
88. Tuomi T, Zimmet PZ, Rowley MJ, et al. Persisting antibodies to glutamic acid decarboxylase in type 1 (insulin-dependent) diabetes mellitus are not associated with neuropathy [Letter]. Diabetologia 1993;36:685
89. Zanone MM, Petersen JS, Peakman M, et al. High prevalence of autoantibodies to glutamic acid decarboxylase in long-standing IDDM is not a marker of symptomatic autonomic neuropathy. Diabetes 1994;43:1146
90. Frazier WA, Hogue-Angeletti R, Bradshaw RA. Nerve growth factor and insulin, structural similarities indicate an evolutionary relationship reflected by physiological action. Science 1972;176:482
91. Mobley WC. Nerve growth factor, 2nd of 3 parts. N Engl J Med 1977;297:1149
92. Levi-Montalcini R, Booker B. Destruction of the sympathetic ganglia in mammals by an antiserum to the nerve-growth promoting factor. Proc Natl Acad Sci U S A 1960;42:384
93. Matheson SF, Gold B, Mobley WC. Somatofugal axonal atrophy in intact adult sensory neurons following injection of nerve growth factor (NGF) antiserum. Soc Neurosci Abst 1989;15:707
94. Rich KM, Luszczynski JR, Osborne PA, Johnson EM Jr. Nerve growth factor protects adult sensory neurons from cell death and atrophy caused by nerve injury. J Neurocytol 1987;16:261
95. Bennett T. Physiological investigation of diabetic autonomic failure. In: Bannister R, ed. Autonomic Failure: A Textbook of Clinical Disorders of the Autonomic Nervous System. Oxford: Oxford University Press;1983:406–436
96. Smeyne RJ, Klein R, Schnapp A, et al. Severe sensory and sympathetic neuropathies in mice carrying a disrupted Trk/NGF receptor gene. Nature 1994;368:246
97. Anand P, Rudge P, Mathias CJ, et al. New autonomic and sensory neuropathy with loss of adrenergic sympathetic function and sensory neuropeptides. Lancet 1991;337:1253
98. Zimmet PZ, Tuomi T, Mackay IR, et al. Latent autoimmune diabetes mellitus in adults (LADA): The role of antibodies to glutamic acid decarboxylase in diagnosis and prediction of insulin dependency. Diabet Med 1994;11:299
99. Brown F. Sural nerve biopsies in Guillain-Barre syndrome: Axonal degeneration and macrophage-associated demyelination and absence of cytomegalovirus genome. Muscle Nerve 1993;16:112
100. Kaji R, Oka N, Tsuji T, et al. Pathological findings at the site of conduction block in multifocal motor neuropathy. Ann Neurol 1993;33:152
101. Suarez GA, Kelly JJ Jr. Polyneuropathy associated with monoclonal gammopathy of undetermined significance: Further evidence that IgM-MGUS neuropathies are different than IgG-MGUS. Neurology 1993;43:1304
102. Kelly JJ, Adelman LS, Berkman E, Bhan I. Polyneuropathies associated with IgM monoclonal gammopathies. Arch Neurol 1988;45:1355
103. Yu RK, Ariga T, Kohriyama T, et al. Autoimmune mechanisms in peripheral neuropathies. Ann Neurol 1990;27(suppl):30
104. Dalakas MC, Engel WK. Chronic relapsing (dysimmune) polyneuropathy: Pathogenesis and treatment. Ann Neurol 1981;9(suppl):134
105. Simmons Z, Albers JW, Bromberg MB, Feldman EL. Presentation and initial clinical course in patients with chronic inflammatory demyelinating polyradiculopathy: Comparison of patients without and with monoclonal gammopathy. Neurology 1993;43:2202
106. van der Meche FGA, Schmitz PIM, Dutch Guillain–Barre Study Group. A randomized trial comparing intravenous immune globulin and plasma exchange in Guillain-Barre syndrome. N Engl J Med 1992;326:1123
107. Bromberg MB, Feldman EL, Albers JW. Chronic inflammatory demyelinating polyradiculoneuropathy: Comparison of patients with and without an associated monoclonal gammopathy. Neurology 1992;42:1157
108. Krarup C, Stewart JD, Sumner AJ, et al. A syndrome of asymmetrical limb weakness with motor conduction block. Neurology 1990;40:118
109. McLeod JG. Invited review: Autonomic dysfunction in peripheral nerve disease. Muscle Nerve 1992;15:3
110. Baba H, Daune GC, Ilyas AA, et al. Anti-G_{M1} ganglioside antibodies with differing fine specificities in patients with multifocal motor neuropathy. J Neuroimmunol 1989;25:143
111. Latov N, Hays AP, Donofrio PD, et al. Monoclonal IgM with unique specificity to gangliosides GM1 and GD1b and to lacto-N-tetraose associated with human motor neuron disease. Neurology 1988;38:763
112. Harris EN, Englert H, Derue G, et al. Antiphospholipid antibodies in acute Guillain-Barré syndrome. Lancet 1983;2:1361
113. Korn-Lubetzki I, Abramsky O. Acute and chronic demyelinating inflammatory polyradiculoneuropathy: Association with autoimmune disease and lymphocyte response to human neuritogenic protein. Arch Neurol 1986;43:604
114. Brown FM, Brink SJ, Freeman R, Rabinowe SL. Different effects of duration on prevalence of anti-adrenal medullary and pancreatic islet cell antibodies in type 1 diabetes mellitus. Horm Metabol Res 1989;21:434
115. Matsuyama H, Haymaker W. Distribution of lesions in the Guillain-Barre syndrome with emphasis on involvement of the sympathetic system. Acta Neuropathol (Berl) 1967;8:203
116. Tuck RR, McLeod JG. Autonomic dysfunction in Guillain-Barre syndrome. J Neurol Neurosurg Psychiatry 1981;44:983
117. Ingall TJ, McLeod JG, Tamura N. Autonomic function and unmyelinated fibers in chronic inflammatory polyradiculopathy. Muscle Nerve 1990;13:70
118. Ewing D, Martyn C, Young R. The value of cardiovascular function tests: 10 years experience in diabetes. Diabetes Care 1985;8:491
119. Ziegler D, Mühlen H, Dannehl K, Gries FA. Tibial nerve somatosensory evoked potentials at various stages of peripheral neuropathy in insulin dependent diabetic patients [Abstract]. J Neurol Neurosurg Psychiatry 1993;56:58
120. Daube JR. Electrodiagnosis in Clinical Neurology. New York: Churchill Livingstone;1992:280–283
121. Soueidan SA, Dalakas MC. Treatment of autoimmune neuromuscular diseases with high-dose intravenous immune globulin. Pediatr Res 1992;33(suppl 1):S95
122. Van Doorn PA, Brand A, Strengers PWF, et al. High dose immunoglobulin (IVIg) treatment in chronic inflammatory demyelinating polyneuropathy: A double-blind placebo-controlled study. Neurology 1990;40:209
123. Vermeulen M, Van Doorn PA, Brand A, et al. Intravenous immunoglobulin treatment in patients with chronic inflammatory demyelinating polyneuropathy: A double blind, placebo controlled study. J Neurol Neurosurg Psychiatry 1993;56:36
124. Feldman EL, Bromberg MB, Albers JW, Pestronk A. Immunosuppressive treatment in multifocal motor neuropathy. Ann Neurol 1991;30:397
125. Siciliano G, Moriconi L, Gianni G, et al. Selective techniques of apheresis in polyneuropathy associated with monoclonal gammopathy of undetermined significance. Acta Neurol Scand 1994;89:117
126. Kyle RA. Monoclonal proteins in neuropathy. Neurol Clin 1992;10:713

Diabetes Mellitus, edited by Derek LeRoith, Simeon I. Taylor, and Jerrold M. Olefsky. Lippincott–Raven Publishers, Philadelphia © 1996.

CHAPTER 84

Microvascular and Compression Mechanisms in the Etiology of Diabetic Neuropathy

MICHAEL A. HILL, LAWRENCE B. COLEN, AND AARON I. VINIK

Although considerable progress has been made in the treatment and monitoring of the metabolic disturbances that are characteristic of diabetes mellitus, neuropathy remains a major long-term cause of the increased morbidity and mortality. Clinically, the most common form of neural dysfunction in diabetes is sensorimotor polyneuropathy co-existing with autonomic neuropathy which results in abnormal sensory perception and function of the cardiovascular, respiratory, sudomotor, digestive, and urogenital systems. More detailed descriptions of the clinical manifestations of diabetic neuropathy can be found in Chapter 82 by Vinik et al. Despite the extent of neural dysfunction, the exact etiology of this disorder is uncertain. In particular, controversy exists as to whether diabetic neuropathy represents a primary neural disturbance, occurs secondarily to microangiopathy, or results from a combination of neural and microvascular events. This controversy results, at least in part, from the fact that both neural tissue and vascular cells (smooth muscle and endothelial cells) are subject to the biochemical consequences of hyperglycemia (e.g., polyol accumulation, nonenzymatic glycosylation, and de novo synthesis of diglyceride).[1,2]

Although the exact relationship between microvascular dysfunction and the development of diabetic neuropathy remains uncertain, the possibility of a vascular component to the neural disorder has been considered for some 100 years. For example, in 1929 Woltman and Wilder[3] wrote the following in the introduction of their article: "That it owes its origin to a primary disturbance of the nervous system is possibly an open question; it may result from a defective blood supply." They concluded from histologic studies that "the marked thickening of the walls of the intraneural vessels are consistent with the idea that arteriosclerosis and resulting ischemia were factors of significance." In the late 1950s Fagerberg[4] attributed the neural degeneration of diabetic neuropathy to vascular lesions as well as including hyalinosis, increased wall thickness, and a narrowing of the vessel lumen. He documented the increase in vessel wall thickness by demonstrating an accumulation of Periodic–acid-Schiff staining material. After Fagerberg's studies implicating a vascular component, for a period of time it generally was accepted that a vascular mechanism would be limited to asymmetric focal neuropathies.[5] Substantial evidence exists for a vascular component to mononeuropathies such as third cranial nerve palsy.[6] The mononeuropathies are characteristically acute in development consistent with a vascular etiology. Patients with this disorder present with sudden loss of nerve function accompanied by severe pain; spontaneous recovery generally occurs within 6–8 weeks.[7] This contrasts with distal symmetric polyneuropathy, which is slow in development and does not exhibit significant recovery.[7] More recently, however, there has been a resurgence of interest as to the possibility that microangiopathy contributes to the more common diffuse symmetric neuropathies associated with diabetes. Such interest has arisen principally from studies demonstrating diabetes-induced structural and functional abnormalities of neural microvasculature (described below). Functional abnormalities, in particular, may lead to a generalized state of absolute or relative neural hypoxia, which in turn leads to functional and structural abnormalities in the nerves themselves.

With respect to the epidemiology of diabetic neuropathy, factors concomitant with neural dysfunction are aging, increased blood pressure, body mass index, and existence of generalized cardiovascular disease. This seems to suggest that macrovascular disease plays a role in diabetic neuropathy, but this has not been supported by studies of nerve pathology.[8] Neuropathy shows an apparent relationship with HLA DR3/4 phenotype[9] and is associated with the presence of microvascular complications.[10] Therefore the possibility exists that microvascular insufficiency could underlie the development of diabetic neuropathy.

Difficulty in understanding the exact relationship between neural and microvascular components, particularly at the cellular level, stems from the fact that any of the following pathogenetic scenarios is feasible:

1. Similar mechanisms underlie both neural and microvascular dysfunction with no interaction between the tissues occurring.
2. The microvascular derangements directly lead to neural dysfunction and ultimately degeneration.
3. A primary neural dysfunction (e.g., arteriovenous shunts), leads to impaired regulation of specific microvascular segments.
4. There is an interdependence between neural and vascular tissue that, when impaired, leads to neural dysfunction and degeneration.

The material described below briefly considers evidence relevant to the latter three possibilities. For additional material, see the recent reviews by Dyck,[8] Tooke,[11] and Tesfaye et al.[12]

Evidence for Involvement of Ischemia in Diabetic Neuropathy

In support of a role for ischemia in the development of neuropathy, a number of human and experimental animal studies have demonstrated decreased endoneurial blood flow as well as decreased neural Po_2. For example, Tuck et al.,[13] using a H_2 clearance technique, found sciatic nerve blood flow to be significantly decreased by approximately 35%, compared to that measured in control animals, after 4 months of streptozocin-induced diabetes in the rat. Using platinum microelectrodes, these authors further demonstrated that impaired blood flow was associated with a decrease in endoneurial Po_2.

These results have since been confirmed by a number of investigators, using tracer (H_2 clearance[14] and [^{14}C] butanol distribution[15]) and laser Doppler techniques,[16] and have been extended to examine the time course for development of impaired blood flow. Several studies have reported neural blood flow to be significantly decreased after only 1 week of experimental diabetes, and thereafter exhibiting a duration-dependent decline.[16,17] In contrast, Cameron et al.[18] found neural blood flow to be markedly decreased after 1 week (approximately 60% of that of control animals), after which flow remained relatively unchanged. The reasons underlying the apparent difference in time course are uncertain, but may relate to severity of diabetes or to the acute effects of dehydration and contraction of plasma volume caused by the diabetes onset.

Several lines of evidence suggest that the decrease in neural blood flow in experimental diabetes is causally related to impairment of neural function. In particular, it has been shown that treatment of streptozocin-induced diabetic rats with a variety of pharmacologic agents that cause smooth muscle relaxation, and hence vasodilatation, improve neural function as assessed by conduction velocity.[16,19–23] Such treatments, including calcium-channel antagonists,[16,21] adrenergic antagonists,[22] and angiotensin-converting enzyme inhibitors,[23] improve neural function in the absence of improved diabetic control. In human diabetic subjects, administration of either the prostacyclin analog iloprost[24] or a prostaglandin E_1 derivative[25] (potent vasodilators) improves peripheral nerve function and decreases pain and hyperesthesia. These agents, rather than having a specific inhibitory effect on mechanisms leading to the development of neuropathy, may normalize blood flow by inhibiting the level of basal vascular tone. Further indirect support for the role of blood flow is provided by the observation that neural function in diabetic animals can be improved by maintaining the animals in a high-oxygen environment.[26]

Studies of neural blood flow in human diabetic subjects are limited to the recent report from Tesfaye et al.[27] These authors used a fluorescein angiographic method, under local anesthesia, to measure epineural blood flow in sural nerves of control subjects and diabetic subjects with and without clinically apparent neuropathy. Blood flow was estimated by fluorescein appearance time and intensity. Both flow indices were significantly altered in the neuropathic subjects compared to both non-neuropathic and control groups. A calculated vascular pathology score correlated significantly with indices of neuropathic impairment (nerve conduction velocity, vibration, and thermal perception), in addition to showing a strong correlation with clinically detectable microangiopathy, as evidenced by retinopathy. These studies confirmed earlier measurements of sural nerve oxygen tension, which were taken to be indicative of decreased nerve blood flow.[28] Direct studies of human sural nerve blood flow have been limited in extent because of the invasive nature of the procedure. It is hoped that future studies can be conducted to address the natural history of neuropathy and to determine whether blood flow changes predate abnormal neural function in diabetic subjects. At present this question is being studied indirectly by examination of the relationships between skin blood flow (measured with laser Doppler techniques) and indices of early neural dysfunction.[29,30]

Not all studies, however, have demonstrated decreased neural blood flow in experimental models of diabetes. Zochodne and Ho[31,32] have consistently reported unchanged sciatic nerve blood flow in streptozocin-induced diabetic rats, despite using the H_2 clearance method referred to above. Similarly, Sutera et al.[33] and Williamson et al.,[34] from the same institution, used the method of radioactive microspheres; both studies suggested that in the streptozocin-induced diabetic rat there is an early phase of normal or increased perfusion.

The latter data have been used to support the hypothesis of a *hemodynamic process,* whereby an early stage of hyperperfusion initiates a process of vascular damage that ultimately leads to vascular sclerosis, vessel closure, and hypoperfusion. Although this is an attractive hypothesis, which has been applied to microangiopathy in general, it is uncertain whether the discordant neural blood flow results represent stages of a pathologic process or are a function of methodologic differences. In particular, the use of microspheres can be criticized for the following reasons: 1. Only a small number of microspheres would be expected to accumulate in a nerve sample. 2. Diabetes-induced alterations in arteriolar diameter could conceivably affect the entrapment rate of the microspheres. In favor of the use of microspheres, however, is the fact that the technique does not require the surgical isolation of the nerve, which is required for H_2 clearance and laser Doppler methods.[34] Recent studies in normal animals have suggested that this surgical preparation leads to a prolonged period of hyperemia.[35] Such a response may well be impaired in diabetic animals: There have been a number of reports suggesting that experimental diabetes leads to a generalized impairment in vasodilatory capacity. This being the case, "base-line" blood flow may appear low in diabetic animals, while the vasodilatation evident in control arterioles may obscure local blood flow regulatory mechanisms. It is unlikely that the apparent discrepancies in blood flow data can be explained by the various methods of measuring different indices of neural perfusion (e.g., epineural, endoneural, or combined blood flow).

An additional complicating factor may be the severity of diabetes induced in the animal models. It has been shown by several investigators that renal hyperperfusion is evident only in so-called moderately hyperglycemic rats, whereas severely hyperglycemic rats exhibit increased renal vascular resistance.[36,37] Thus it is possible that similar results may be obtained for the effects of diabetes on neural blood flow depending on the severity of the disorder. There is currently a lack of nerve blood flow data in experimental models of diabetes in which animals have been treated with a low dose of insulin to prevent the initial dehydration, and to provide adequate body weight gain while maintaining hyperglycemia. Such future studies may provide insight into the developmental stages of functional neural impairment in an experimental animal model in which the metabolic derangement more closely resembles poorly controlled human diabetes.

Possible Factors Contributing to Neural Ischemia

If it is accepted that diabetes, both human and experimental, is associated with decreased neural blood flow, what then is the basis of the increased vascular resistance? Possible factors include functional abnormalities resulting in vasoconstriction; structural reduction of vessel diameter or vessel number, or both; and hemorrheologic disturbances. The possible contribution of each mechanism to diabetic neuropathy is discussed briefly in the following sections.

The finding that a variety of pharmacologic interventions, which would favor vasodilatation, reverse the impairment in nerve conduction velocity found in early experimental diabetes,[19–21] suggests that at least the initial phases of the development of neuropathy may involve a functional disturbance that impacts on microvascular reactivity. Neural blood supply consists of epineural and endoneural vessels connected by perineural arterioles. Increased reactivity of arteriolar smooth muscle at the level of epineural or perineural vessels would be expected to have an impact on endoneurial capillary blood flow. Such an increase in local resistance could result from alterations of endothelial or vascular smooth muscle function or from increased adrenergic stimulation via innervation of the vasa nervorum. Diabetes-induced abnormalities in microvascular reactivity have been demonstrated in a variety of vascular beds both in vivo and in vitro.[38–41] Consistent with the possibility of increased vascular resistance in neural vessels, there have been reports of increased responsiveness to vasoconstrictors (e.g., adrenergic agonists,[39] angiotensin II[40]) and a decreased ability to respond to a variety of vasodilators (e.g., acetylcholine,[42] prostacyclin,[40] ATP-sensitive K+-channel openers[43]). Altered responsiveness to vasoactive agents may reflect abnormalities in receptor interactions, calcium handling, production of second messengers, or alterations to the mechanical properties of the arteriolar wall.

In addition to altered microvascular responsiveness, there is evidence of decreased neural synthesis of endothelium-derived vasodilators (e.g., nitric oxide,[20] prostacyclin[44]) and increased production of vasoconstrictors such as endothelin.[45] That a decreased capacity to vasodilate could be of relevance to the pathogenesis of diabetic neuropathy is shown by the observation that nerve conduction velocity can be impaired in normal animals chronically treated with inhibitors of nitric oxide synthase and cyclo-oxygenase.[20]

A number of histologic studies have indicated an increased frequency of endoneurial blood vessel plugging with material containing fibrin, platelets, and red blood cells.[46–48] Consistent with these observations, there have been numerous reports of a generalized increase in platelet reactivity and impaired fibrinolysis in diabetes (see Chapter 93 by Nolan and Vinik). Although accumulation of material in endoneurial blood vessels may be a reflection of such increased clotting or decreased fibrinolytic activity, it also may occur as a result of preexisting microvascular disease. Regardless of the mechanism underlying the accumulation of such material in the vessel lumen, if such a phenomenon were sufficiently widespread, it could conceivably increase vascular resistance and contribute to ischemia. If intravascular deposition of fibrin-like material is an early event in the development of neuropathy, then evidence of vessel plugging should occur before the development of clinically evident neuropathy. There is a dearth of detailed data examining nerve morphology in diabetic subjects before clinical and neurophysiologic evidence of neuropathy, but such studies are in progress.[49]

Diabetes-induced alterations in the hemorheologic properties of blood could provide an additional impediment to effective microvascular blood flow.[50] In particular, decreased erythrocyte deformability and increased whole blood and plasma viscosity, resulting from increased acute-phase plasma proteins[51] and circulating immune complexes,[52] could conceivably compromise blood flow in the endoneurial microvasculature. Numerous studies have demonstrated altered blood rheology in diabetic subjects,[53,54] and such changes are evident before neural disturbances are clinically apparent.[55] As with the coagulation data described above, it is uncertain whether altered hemorrheology (e.g., red cell aggregation resulting from increased plasma fibrinogen levels) is a primary factor in the development of diabetic complications or a response to preexisting injury. It is of interest to note, however, that alterations in red cell deformability and blood viscosity are present in diabetic children, before the onset of overt microangiopathy or neuropathy.[55]

In a recent study that examined morphologic characteristics of endoneurial microvessels in sural nerve biopsies, Giannini and Dyck[56] concluded that diabetic neuropathy is associated with alterations in the structure of the vessel wall, rather than factors decreasing the effective patency of the lumen. In particular, these authors described reduplication of basement membranes, pericyte degeneration, and endothelial cell hypertrophy/hyperplasia. These diabetes-induced changes in vessel wall structure did not appear to be a function of age, as had been suggested previously.[57] Giannini and Dyck further concluded that the data did not directly support an ischemia/hypoxia basis for polyneuropathy because changes in vessel number, intercapillary distance, or vessel lumen area were not evident. In contrast, studies of sural nerve perineural vessels by Malik et al.[58] reported that the endothelial cell hypertrophy/hyperplasia contributes to narrowing of the vessel lumen and is thus consistent with an ischemic component to diabetic neuropathy. This group has also reported that the degree of endoneurial vessel pathology (e.g., endothelial cell number, basement membrane thickening) is related to the severity of nerve fiber abnormalities and overt neuropathy.[10] These histologic observations do not, however, preclude the possibility that under in vivo conditions, impaired blood flow results from a functional increase in arteriolar resistance. This situation is evident in experimental models of early diabetes, in which decreased nerve blood flow and conduction velocity occurs in the presence of a normal complement of microvessels, yet nerve function can be improved by administration of vasodilators.[19–21]

As modeled by Myers et al.,[59] compression of endoneurial blood vessels could theoretically occur as a result of local swelling or edema because of polyol accumulation in the presence of a relatively rigid perineurium. Transperineural arterioles, in particular, have been suggested to be prone to constriction, due to entrapment, during edema. Galactosemic rats exhibit marked galactitol accumulation and endoneurial swelling, yet in some studies blood flow has been reported to be relatively normal.[13] Similarly, 5 years of galactose feeding in dogs did not result in decreased nerve conduction velocity.[60] In a recent study, a sorbitol dehydrogenase inhibitor was administered to streptozocin-induced diabetic rats to prevent the formation of fructose from sorbitol.[61] As a result of inhibiting oxidation of the polyol, accumulation of intracellular sorbitol occurs. Despite the increase in sorbitol levels (and presumably osmotic stress) the inhibitor was reported to improve nerve conduction velocity.[61] As a final consideration on this point, it appears unlikely that sufficient accumulation of osmotically active substances (e.g., sorbitol, fructose) occurs as early as 1 week after the induction of experimental diabetes, which is when nerve blood flow has been reported to be decreased.[18]

In addition to an overt decrease in neural blood flow with resulting ischemia, local impairment of nutritional blood flow (i.e., capillary or near-capillary level) may result from abnormal arteriovenous shunting. Arteriovenous shunts provide a potential low-resistance pathway by which blood flow can be diverted from the arteriolar to venular circulations, bypassing the capillary bed. The suggestion of increased shunting of blood flow in diabetes and its possible relationship to the development of neuropathic ulcers was provided by the studies of Boulton Ward et al.[62,63] and Edmonds et al.[64] These authors demonstrated increased venular oxygen levels, apparent ischemic lesions despite the presence of palpable pulses, and raised skin temperatures in the distal extremities—observations suggested to be consistent with arteriovenous shunting. Because control of arteriovenous shunt vessel diameter is mediated by sympathetic nerves,[65] these data were taken to be consistent with a primary neural impairment. Arteriovenous shunt vessels also have been demonstrated in the epineural circulation and, using fluorescein angiography, have been shown to be more evident in sural nerves of diabetic subjects with established neuropathy.[27] Consistent with these observations Beggs et al.,[66] using a histologic approach, demonstrated decreased perivascular innervation in sural nerve biopsies taken from diabetic subjects. Thus, denervation of the epineural shunt vessels may lead to partitioning of blood flow, causing decreased perfusion and ischemia at the level of the endoneurial capillaries.

Is the Level of Ischemia Observed in the Diabetic Nerve Pathophysiologically Significant?

An important question in regard to the ischemia hypothesis is whether Po_2 decreases to levels that would be expected to impair nerve function. To protect against ischemia, the vasculature of nerves contains an extensive network of arterio-arterio shunts (*arcades*), perineural and epineural autoregulation (albeit weakly), and peripheral nerve itself exhibits relatively low metabolic activity. With respect to local microvascular control mechanisms, it has been reported that the endoneurial microcirculation is relatively ineffective in autoregulating blood flow, resulting in a situation where flow varies with changes in perfusion pressure.[67] This may, however, be a result of the necessary surgical preparation to perform such studies: Arterioles from most tissues can be shown to develop a level of spontaneous basal tone and to exhibit myogenic reactivity.

An additional consideration is whether blood flow in the diabetic nerve is appropriate to the metabolic state of the tissue. Primary nerve fiber loss could conceivably reduce the metabolic requirements of a given nerve. Under normal conditions, microvascular blood flow is generally closely coupled to metabolic demand. In this regard it is of interest to note that energy metabolism has been reported to be significantly decreased in diabetic nerves.[68,69] If blood flow were matched with demand, however, a decreased neural Po_2 in diabetics (relative to that in controls) might not be expected, nor would the apparent effectiveness of vasodilators on nerve function as assessed by conduction velocity.

Decrease in neural blood flow found in ischemic conditions, as may occur in experimental diabetes, has been demonstrated to be sufficient to cause functional or structural alterations in peripheral nerves with the use of normal animal models, in which specific vascular beds have been rendered ischemic by the infusion of microspheres.[70,71] Nerve conduction velocity has been shown to decrease with increasing numbers of infused *microspheres*, suggesting a relationship between nerve function and the level of ischemia.[71] Because of the extensive collateral circulation supplying peripheral nerves, large quantities of microspheres are required to induce structural damage (i.e., fiber degeneration). Nukada[72] further demonstrated that infusion of a quantity of microspheres, which was subthreshold with respect to nerve pathology in control animals, caused marked structural alterations in the nerves of rats with streptozocin-induced diabetes. It was suggested that the mild ischemia caused by the microsphere infusion, in combination with diabetes-related alterations in hemorrheologic factors and microvascular function, was sufficient to result in structural nerve damage. An additional approach to examine the effects of ischemia on nerve function was taken by Smith et al.,[73] who studied animals chronically maintained in a *hypoxic environment*. Chronic (i.e., 5 weeks') hypoxia resulted in a 30% reduction in nerve conduction velocity and a decrease in sciatic nerve substance P immunoreactivity. Because these changes occurred in the absence of hyperglycemia, and because there were no resultant disturbances of nerve Na^+K^+-ATPase and *myo*-inositol depletion, a more complex situation may exist in the in vivo diabetic condition in humans.

An apparent paradox with respect to the relationship between ischemia and nerve function has been described in both human subjects and experimental animal models. It has been reported consistently that, after an acute occlusion of the blood supply, nerve conduction velocity is maintained for a longer period in diabetic nerves compared to control nerves.[74,75] This phenomenon has been termed *resistance to ischemic conduction failure*. Although the mechanism underlying this acute resistance to ischemia is uncertain, it has been suggested that protection may be afforded by the metabolic state of the diabetic nerve in terms of increased available energy stores, decreased metabolic requirements, and increased dependence on anaerobic metabolism.[74] It is interesting that this phenomenon is observed in subjects who have become hypoxic as a result of chronic obstructive pulmonary disease[76] and that it can be induced in experimental animals[77]; in both cases nerve glucose levels would be expected to be normal. It appears that the resistance to ischemia is not directly related to indices of impaired nerve function in diabetes because several pharmacologic treatments have been shown to normalize conduction velocity while being relatively ineffective in reversing ischemic resistance.[20,21] In addition, it has been suggested that resistance to ischemia occurs earlier in the history of diabetes than does a reduction in absolute nerve conduction velocity,[74] although early changes in electrophysiologic activity may go undetected. Although the exact physiologic significance of this phenomenon is unclear, it may act as a protective mechanism in the diabetic nerve during acute short-term ischemic episodes[78]; however, during chronic ischemia the nerve remains more susceptible to structural damage.[74]

Interactions Between Neural and Vascular Tissue in the Development of Neuropathy

An additional possibility for an underlying vascular component to neuropathy is that diabetes induces a disturbance in the normal relationship between vascular smooth muscle and neural tissue. In particular, it has been suggested that vascular smooth muscle may be a source of *growth factors* (e.g., nerve growth factor) that are necessary for neuronal growth and maintenance,[79,80] and thus may contribute to the maintenance of a functional microvascular-nerve unit (additional material relating to growth factors and neuropathy can be found in Chapter 85 by Liuzzi and Depto). A decreased production of such growth factors by the highly innervated arteriovenous shunt vessels, for example, could lead to neural degeneration with loss of sympathetic tone and shunting of blood away from nutritional capillary circuits. That vascular smooth muscle can augment neuronal growth via release of *nerve growth factor* (NGF) has been demonstrated in co-culture experiments. Creedon and Tuttle[79] and Ueyama et al.[80] have shown that whereas growth of cells from sympathetic ganglia is impaired under serum-free conditions, co-culture with vascular smooth muscle prolongs neuronal cell survival and promotes cell growth, as evidenced by neurite extension. These investigators further showed that an anti-NGF antibody negated the vascular smooth muscle effect and that the smooth muscle cells both contained the mRNA for NGF and secreted the protein.[79] The possibility that a decrease in growth factor availability contributes to diabetic neuropathy is supported by the observation that NGF levels are decreased both in sympathetically innervated target organs of rats with streptozocin-induced diabetes[81] and mice with genetic diabetes[82] and in the plasma of diabetic human subjects.[83] The role of vascular elements as a source of required neural growth and maintenance factors in diabetes, however, has not been examined.

Histologic studies have shown that diabetes is associated with decreased innervation of the vasa nervorum,[66] which would be expected to impair control of microvascular blood flow in the nerve itself, conceivably making it susceptible to hemodynamic and ischemic damage. As described above, regression of the normal innervation to arteriovenous shunt vessels, secondary to an impaired growth factor axis, could result in loss of a tonic constrictor influence and the opening of low-resistance vascular pathways that bypass the nutritional circulation.

Involvement of the microcirculation in the maintenance of neuronal integrity may not be limited to the direct supply of growth factors. Zochodne and Ho[32] suggested that diabetes-induced impairment of dilator responses to agents such as substance P and calcitonin gene–related peptide (CGRP) may impair local hyperemia during the axon response to injury. The decreased ability to exhibit a hyperemic response would be further impaired by a diabetes-induced reduction in such paracrine factors, as has been reported in several experimental studies.[84,85] Impairment of dilator responses, after injury may hinder the delivery of factors necessary for effective neuronal repair.

A disturbance in the normal relationship between neurons and their associated microvasculature could conceivably result from alterations in the permeability barrier between the tissues. Altered vascular permeability is a characteristic of a number of non-neural tissues in both human diabetic subjects and experimental animal models.[86–88] Similarly, there have been a number of reports of increased permeability of the blood-nerve barrier to small (e.g., mannitol[89]) and large (e.g., albumin[90,91]) molecules in diabetes, although several studies have failed to confirm the finding of increased permeability.[92,93] Changes in the effective permeability barrier may result from physical damage or alterations to its character (e.g., changes in ion selectivity, nonenzymatic glycosylation of constituent proteins), or they may occur secondary to alterations in the structure of transported molecules, as has been reported

Table 84-1. Common Nerve Entrapment Sites in Diabetes

Site	Nerve	Clinical Presentation
Carpal tunnel	Median	Pain; numbness; tingling; weakness of thumb, index, and middle fingers
Elbow	Ulnar	Pain and weakness in small and ring fingers and in medial aspects of forearm
Posterior humerus	Radial	Sensory loss at dorsum of thumb and hand
Hip	Femoral	Weak knee extension and loss of knee jerk
Inguinal canal	Lateral cutaneous	Pain and sensory loss, upper lateral aspect of the thigh
Upper fibula	Peroneal	Footdrop, sensory loss at outer foot
Posterior tibia	Medial/lateral plantar	Pain and sensory loss, medial or lateral plantar region, weakness of plantar extensor muscles
Posterior calf	Sural	Sensory loss of lateral foot
Buttock	Sciatic	Lateral thigh pain, ankle jerk absent, footdrop

for nonenzymatically glycosylated proteins.[94,95] The relationship, if any, between the development of diabetic neuropathy and the altered chemical environment that follows the increase in permeability is uncertain.

Compression Mechanisms Contributing to Diabetic Neuropathy

Peripheral nerves are vulnerable to injury from compressive forces transmitted from surrounding structures such as bone and soft tissue. Studies in experimental animal models[96] have shown that the histopathologic changes associated with chronic nerve compression, or entrapment, progress from endoneurial edema to extrafasicular and interfasicular epineural fibrosis and perineural thickening, followed by incremental thinning of myelin and segmental demyelination. The extent of damage is found to be greater in the peripheral fascicles, with decreasing severity observed toward the center of the nerve. Few human nerves have been available for detailed study of compression injury, but the available data are consistent with those described in experimental animal models.[97]

In an effort to explain the higher-than-expected incidence of combined nerve entrapment syndromes (e.g., cervical disk disease, carpal tunnel syndrome), the *double crush hypothesis* was formulated by Upton and McComas in 1973.[98] This hypothesis states that serial constrictions affecting axoplasmic flow may combine to cause nerve dysfunction (i.e., dysfunction would not have occurred after a single constriction). It was further suggested that a systemic disease that impairs axoplasmic flow, such as diabetes, may represent one of the serial constrictions. Support for this hypothesis has been provided by both human studies and experimental animal models. Placement of a mildly constricting band around the sciatic nerve of rats was shown in one study to predispose the nerve to a second distally placed band, which then caused significant impairment of nerve conduction velocity and amplitude.[99] Chronic sciatic nerve banding in rats with streptozocin-induced diabetes was shown in another study to result in a greater impairment in indices of nerve function than is seen in comparably treated control animals, suggesting that the diabetic nerve may be more susceptible to nerve compression.[100] These results are similar to those reported by Nukada,[72] referred to earlier, who reported that local infusion of a dose of microspheres, subthreshold for damage in control animals, resulted in significant nerve pathology in diabetic animals.

Clinical observations suggest that diabetic subjects exhibit increased susceptibility to compression injury compared to the nondiabetic population; for example, carpal tunnel syndrome has been reported to be twice as common in the diabetic population.[7] A list of common sites of neural entrapment and clinical presentation is shown in Table 84-1. These can be distinguished from the mononeuropathies (Table 84-2) by certain distinctive clinical features (Table 84-3). It is conceivable that in certain diabetic subjects the susceptibility toward compression injury, combined with the diabetes-related alterations in nerve blood flow and metabolism, combine to produce a degree of neural impairment that would not be expected for either insult alone. Given the above hypotheses, and the finding that there are similarities in nerve pathology between nerve compression and diabetic neuropathies, it is important for the clinician to exclude nerve compression when treating diabetic patients for symptoms of peripheral neuropathy. Effective medical and surgical treatment is available for nerve compression in diabetic patients.

Conclusions

There is considerable evidence for a vascular component in the etiology of the diffuse symmetrical neuropathies characteristic of long-term diabetes mellitus. The major question to be resolved is

Table 84-2. Common Mononeuropathies in Diabetes

Site	Nerve
Cranial	3rd, 4th, 6th, 7th
Thoracic	Mononeuritis multiplex
Peripheral	Peroneal, sural, sciatic, femoral, ulnar, median

Table 84-3. Comparison of Features of Mononeuritis and Entrapment

	Mononeuritis	Entrapment
Onset	Sudden	Gradual
Pain	Acute	Chronic
Multiplex	Occurs	Rare
Course	Resolves	Persists without intervention
Treatment	Physical therapy	Rest/splints/surgery

whether the vascular dysfunction provides a primary neural insult, plays a supporting role to biochemical disturbances occurring within the nerve itself, or is a manifestation of neuronal damage and breakdown. There is also a strong possibility that several independent vascular mechanisms contribute to nerve damage in diabetes, such as alterations in vascular reactivity, vessel wall structure, and supply of required neural growth and maintenance factors. A brief summary of the possible relationships between the metabolic disturbances of diabetes and vascular factors in the development of neuropathy is provided in Figure 84-1. If a vascular component is a contributing factor to the development of diabetic neuropathy, then the following questions remain to be answered: (1) Do the changes in microvascular function precede the appearance of structural vascular changes? and (2) Is microvascular dysfunction a generalized process, or does it affect specific vascular segments, such as arteriovenous shunt vessels? An understanding of such relationships should prompt the development of more effective pharmacologic therapies for preventing diabetic neuropathy that would supplement the standard treatment for the metabolic disturbances in diabetes mellitus.

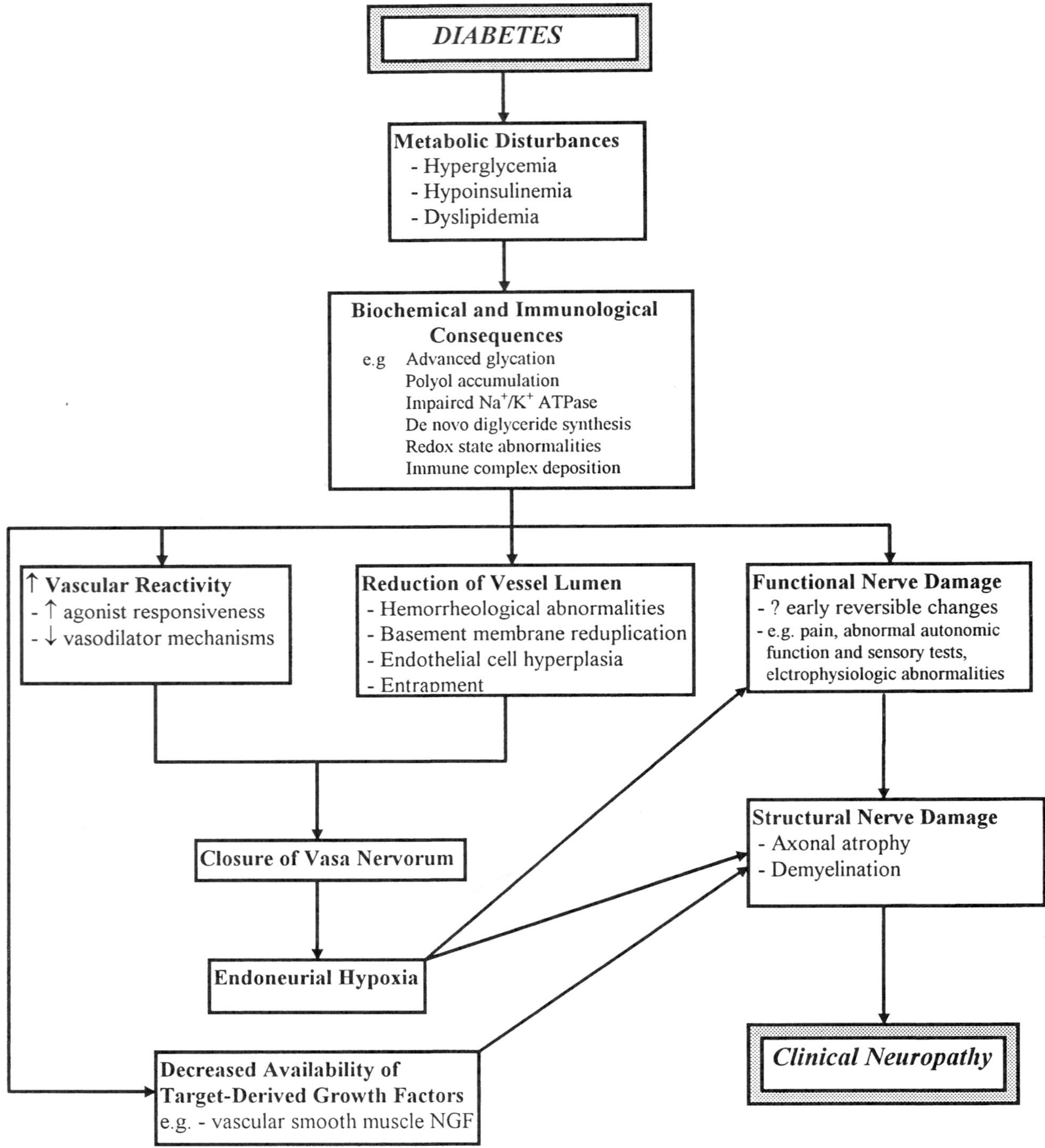

FIGURE 84-1. Interrelationships between metabolic and vascular factors in the development of diabetic neuropathy.

References

1. Ruderman NB, Williamson JR, Brownlee M. Glucose and diabetic vascular disease FASEB J 1992;6:2905
2. Brownlee M. Glycation products and the pathogenesis of diabetic complications. Diabetes Care 1992;15:1835
3. Woltman HW, Wilder RM. Diabetes mellitus: Pathological changes in the spinal cord and peripheral nerve. Arch Intern Med 1929;44:576
4. Fagerberg SE. Diabetic neuropathy, a clinical and histological study on the significance of vascular affections. Acta Med Scand 1959;345(suppl 164):1
5. Raff MC, Sangalang V, Asbury AK. Ischemic mononeuropathy multiplex associated with diabetes mellitus. Arch Neurol 1968;18:487
6. Asbury AK, Aldredge H, Hershberg R, Fisher CM. Oculomotor palsy in diabetes mellitus: A clinico-pathological study. Brain 1970;93:555
7. Vinik AI, Milecevic Z. Preventive measures and treatment options for diabetic neuropathy. Contemp Int Med 1994;6:41
8. Dyck PJ. Hypoxic neuropathy: Does hypoxia play a role in diabetic neuropathy? Neurology 1989;39:111
9. Barzilay J, Warram JH, Rand LI, et al. Risk for cardiovascular autonomic neuropathy is associated with the HLA-DR3/4 phenotype in type 1 diabetes mellitus. Annals Intern Med 1992;116:544
10. Malik RA, Newrick PG, Sharma AK, et al. Microangiopathy in human diabetic neuropathy: Relationship between capillary abnormalities and severity of neuropathy. Diabetologia 1989;32:92
11. Tooke JE. Microcirculation and diabetes. Br Med Bull 1989;45:206
12. Tesfaye S, Malik R, Ward JD. Vascular factors in diabetic neuropathy. Diabetologia 1994;37:847
13. Tuck RR, Schmelzer JD, Low PA. Endoneurial blood flow and oxygen tension in the sciatic nerves of rats with experimental diabetic neuropathy. Brain 1984;107:935
14. Hotta N, Kakuta H, Fukasawa H, et al. Effect of niceritrol on streptozocin-induced diabetic neuropathy in rats. Diabetes 1992;41:587
15. Monafo WW, Eliasson SG, Shimazaki S, Sugimoto H. Regional blood flow in resting and stimulated sciatic nerve of diabetic rats. Exp Neurol 1988;99:607
16. Kappelle AC, Biessels GJ, Van Buren T, et al. Effects of nimodipine on sciatic nerve blood flow and vasa nervorum responsiveness in the diabetic rat. Eur J Pharmacol 1993;250:43
17. Stevens EJ, Carrington AL, Tomlinson DR. Nerve ischemia in diabetic rats: Time-course of development, effect of insulin treatment plus comparison of streptozotocin and BB models. Diabetologia 1994;37:43
18. Cameron NE, Cotter MA, Low PA. Nerve blood flow in early experimental diabetes in rats: Relation to conduction deficits. Am J Phsiol 1991;261:E1
19. Cameron NE, Cotter MA, Robertson S. Essential fatty acid diet supplementation: Effects on peripheral nerve and skeletal muscle function and capillarization in streptozotocin-induced diabetic rats. Diabetes 1991;40:532
20. Cameron NE, Cotter MA, Dines KC, Maxfield EK. Pharmacological manipulation of vascular endothelium function in non-diabetic and streptozotocin-diabetic rats: Effects on nerve conduction, hypoxic resistance and endoneurial capillarization. Diabetologia 1993;36:516
21. Robertson S, Cameron NE, Cotter MA. The effect of the calcium channel antagonist nifedipine on peripheral nerve function in streptozotocin-diabetic rats. Diabetologia 1992;35:1113
22. Cameron NE, Cotter MA, Ferguson K, et al. Effects of chronic alpha-adrenergic receptor blockade on peripheral nerve conduction, hypoxic resistance, polyols, Na^+-K^+-ATPase activity and vascular supply in STZ-D rats. Diabetes 1991;40:52
23. Cameron NE, Cotter MA, Robertson S. Angiotensin converting enzyme inhibition prevents the development of muscle and nerve dysfunction and stimulates angiogenesis in streptozotocin-diabetic rats. Diabetologia 1992;35:12
24. Shindo H, Tawata M, Aida K, Onaya T. Clinical efficacy of a stable prostacyclin analog, iloprost, in diabetic neuropathy. Prostaglandins 1991;41:85
25. Shindo H, Tawata M, Inoue M, et al. The effect of prostaglandin E1.aCD on vibratory threshold determined with the SMV-5 vibrometer in patients with diabetic neuropathy. Diabetes Res Clin Pract 1994;24:173
26. Low PA, Tuck RR, Dyck PJ, et al. Prevention of some electrophysiologic and biochemical abnormalities with oxygen supplementation in experimental diabetic neuropathy. Proc Natl Acad Sci USA 1984;81:6894
27. Tesfaye S, Harris N, Jakubowski JJ, et al. Impaired blood flow and arterio-venous shunting in human diabetic neuropathy: A novel technique of nerve photography and fluorescein angiography. Diabetologia 1993;36:1226
28. Newrick PG, Wilson AJ, Jakubowski J, et al. Sural nerve oxygen tension in diabetes. Br Med J 1986;293:1053
29. Stansberry KB, Hill MA, McNitt PM, Bhatt BA. Cutaneous blood flow reactivity and neuropathy. Diabetes 1994;43:A107
30. Stansberry KB, Hill MA, McNitt PM, et al. Peripheral vasomotion in diabetes. Diabetes 1995;44:172A
31. Zochodne DW, Ho LT. Normal blood flow but lower oxygen tension in diabetes of young rats: microenvironment and the influence of sympathectomy. Can J Physiol Pharmacol 1992;70:651
32. Zochodne DW, Ho LT. Diabetes mellitus prevents capsaicin from inducing hyperaemia in the rat sciatic nerve. Diabetologia 1993;36:493
33. Sutera SP, Chang K, Marvel J, Williamson JR. Concurrent increases in regional hematocrit and blood flow in diabetic rats: Prevention by sorbinil. Am J Physiol 1992;263:H945
34. Williamson J, Chang K, Allison W, Kilo C. Endoneurial blood flow changes in diabetic rats. Diabet Med 1993;10(suppl 2):49S
35. Kinoshita Y, Monafo WW. Effect of surgical trauma on regional blood flow in rat sciatic nerve. Exp Neurol 1994;125:296
36. Jensen PK, Christiansen JS, Steven K, Parving H-H. Renal function in streptozotocin diabetic rats. Diabetologia 1981;21:409
37. Hill MA, Larkins RG. Alterations in distribution of cardiac output in experimental diabetes in rats. Am J Physiol 1989;257:H571
38. Brody MJ, Dixon RL. Vascular reactivity in experimental diabetes mellitus. Circ Res 1964;14:494
39. Morff RJ. Microvascular reactivity to norepinephrine at different arteriolar levels and durations of streptozotocin-induced diabetes. Diabetes 1990;39:354
40. Hill MA, Larkins RG. Altered microvascular reactivity in streptozotocin-induced diabetes in rats. Am J Physiol 1989;257:H1438
41. Hill MA, Meininger GA. Impaired arteriolar myogenic reactivity in early experimental diabetes. Diabetes 1993;42:1226
42. Hill MA, Ege EA. Active and passive mechanical properties of isolated arterioles from STZ-induced diabetic rats: Effect of aminoguanidine treatment. Diabetes 1994;43:1450
43. Mayhan WG, Faraci FM. Responses of cerebral arterioles in diabetic rats to activation of ATP-sensitive potassium channels. Am J Physiol 1993;265:H152
44. Ward KK, Low PA, Schmelzer JD, Zochodne DW. Prostacyclin and noradrenaline in peripheral nerve of chronic experimental diabetes in rats. Brain 1989;112:197
45. Takahashi K, Ghatei MA, Lam H-C, et al. Elevated plasma endothelin in patients with diabetes mellitus. Diabetologia 1990;33:306
46. Timperley WR, Ward JD, Preston FE, et al. Clinical and histological studies in diabetic neuropathy: A reassessment of vascular factors in relation to intravascular coagulation. Diabetologia 1976;12:237
47. Dyck PJ, Hansen S, Karnes J, et al. Capillary number and percentage closed in human diabetic sural nerve. Proc Natl Acad Sci U S A 1985;82:2513
48. Ford I, Malik RA, Newrick PG, et al. Relationship between hemostatic factors and capillary morphology in human diabetic neuropathy. Thromb Haemost 1992;69:628
49. Malik RA, Tesfaye S, Ward JD, Boulton AJM. Nerve fiber damage in diabetic patients before clinical and neurophysiologic evidence of neuropathy. Diabetes 1994;43:16A
50. McMillan DE. The effect of diabetes on blood flow properties. Diabetes 1983;32(suppl 2):56
51. McMillan DE. Plasma protein changes, blood viscosity and diabetic microangiopathy. Diabetes 1976;25(suppl 2):858
52. Gisinger C, Lopes-Virella MF. Lipoprotein-immune complexes and diabetic vascular complications. Diabetes 1992;41(suppl 2):92
53. Schmid-Schonbien H, Volger E. Red cell aggregation and red cell deformability. Diabetes 1976;25(suppl 2):897
54. Juhan I, Vague Ph, Buonocore M, et al. Abnormalities of erythrocyte deformability and platelet aggregation in insulin dependent diabetics corrected by insulin in vivo and in vitro. Lancet 1982;1:535
55. Hill MA, Court JM, Mitchell GM. Blood rheology and microalbuminuria in type 1 diabetes mellitus. Lancet 1982;2:985
56. Giannini C, Dyck PJ. Ultrastructural morphometric abnormalities of sural nerve endoneurial microvessels in diabetes mellitus. Ann Neurol 1994;36:408
57. Sima AAF, Nathaniel V, Prashar A, et al. Endoneurial microvessels in human diabetic neuropathy: Endothelial cell disjunction and lack of a treatment effect by an aldose reductase inhibitor. Diabetes 1991;40:1090
58. Malik RA, Tesfaye S, Thompson SD, et al. Transperineural capillary abnormalities in the sural nerve of patients with diabetic neuropathy. Microvasc Res 1994;48:236
59. Myers R, Murakami H, Powell HC. Reduced nerve blood flow in edematous neuropathies: A biomechanical mechanism. Microvasc Res 1986;32:145
60. Engerman RL, Kern TS, Larson ME. Nerve conduction and aldose reductase inhibition during 5 years of diabetes or galactosaemia in dogs. Diabetologia 1994;37:141
61. Tilton RG, Chang K, Nyengaard JR, et al. Inhibition of sorbitol dehydrogenase: Effects on vascular and neural dysfunction in streptozotocin-induced diabetic rats. Diabetes 1995;44:234
62. Boulton AJM, Scarpello JHB, Ward JD. Venous oxygenation in the diabetic neuropathic foot: Evidence for arterio-venous shunting? Diabetologia 1982;22:6
63. Ward JD, Simms JM, Knight G, et al. Venous distension in the diabetic neuropathic foot (physical sign of arteriovenous shunting). J Roy Soc Med 1983;76:1011
64. Edmonds ME, Roberts VC, Watkins PJ. Blood flow in the diabetic neuropathic foot. Diabetologia 1982;22:9
65. Hales JRS, Iriki M, Tsuchiya K, Kozawa E. Thermally induced cutaneous sympathetic activity related to blood flow through capillaries and arteriovenous anastomoses. Pflugers Arch 1978;375:17
66. Beggs J, Johnson PC, Olafsen A, Watkins CJ. Innervation of the vasa nervorum: Changes in human diabetics. J Neuropathol Exp Neurol 1992;51:612
67. Low PA, Tuck RR. Effects of changes in blood pressure, respiratory acidosis and hypoxia on blood flow in the sciatic nerve of the rat. J Physiol 1984;347:513
68. Greene DA, Lattimer SA. Impaired energy utilization and Na-K-ATPase in diabetic peripheral nerve. Am J Physiol 1984;246:E311
69. Thurston JH, McDougal DB, Hauhart RE, Schulz DW. Effects of acute,

subacute, and chronic diabetes on carbohydrate and energy metabolism in rat sciatic nerve: Relation to mechanisms of peripheral neuropathy. Diabetes 1995;44:190
70. Nukada H, Dyck PJ. Microsphere embolization of nerve capillaries and fiber degeneration. Am J Pathol 1984;115:275
71. Kihara M, Zollman PJ, Schmelzer JD, Low PA. The influence of dose of microspheres on nerve blood flow, electrophysiology, and fiber degeneration of rat peripheral nerve. Muscle Nerve 1993;16:1383
72. Nukada H. Mild ischemia causes severe pathological changes in experimental diabetic nerve. Muscle Nerve 1992;15:1116
73. Smith WJ, Diemel LT, Leach RM, Tomlinson DR. Central hypoxaemia in rats provokes neurological defects similar to those seen in experimental diabetes mellitus: Evidence for a partial role of endoneurial hypoxia in diabetic neuropathy. Neuroscience 1991;45:255
74. Nukada H. The susceptibility of rat diabetic nerve to ischemia: Increased or decreased? J Neurol Sci 1993;119:162
75. Newrick PG, Boulton AJM, Ward JD. Nerve ischemia-resistance: An early abnormality in diabetes. Diabetic Med 1987;4:517
76. Masson EA, Church SE, Woodcock AA, et al. Is resistance to ischemic conduction failure induced by hypoxia? Diabetologia 1988;31:762
77. Low PA, Schmelzer JD, Ward KK, Yao JK. Experimental chronic hypoxic neuropathy: Relevance to diabetic neuropathy. Am J Physiol 1986;250:E94
78. Dyck PJ, Englestad JK, Giannini C, et al. Resistance to axonal degeneration after nerve compression in experimental diabetes. Proc Natl Acad Sci U S A 1989;86:2103
79. Creedon D, Tuttle JB. Nerve growth factor synthesis in vascular smooth muscle. Hypertension 1991;18:730
80. Ueyama T, Hamada M, Hano T, et al. Release of nerve growth factor from cultured aortic smooth muscle cells. Blood Vessels 1991;28:532
81. Fernyhough P, Diemel LT, Brewster WJ, Tomlinson DR. Deficits in sciatic nerve neuropeptide content coincide with a reduction in target tissue nerve growth factor mRNA in streptozotocin-diabetic rats: Effects of insulin treatment. Neurosci 1994;62:337
82. Kasayama S, Oka T. Impaired production of nerve growth factor in the submandibular gland of diabetic mice. Am J Physiol 1989;257:E400
83. Faradji V, Sotelo J. Low serum levels of nerve growth factor in diabetic neuropathy. Acta Neurol Scand 1990;81:402
84. Diemel LT, Stevens EJ, Willars GB, Tomlinson DR. Depletion of substance P and calcitonin gene-related peptide in sciatic nerve of rats with experimental diabetes: Effects of insulin and aldose reductase inhibition. Neurosci Lett 1992;137:253
85. Sango K, Verdes JM, Hikawa N, et al. Nerve growth factor (NGF) restores depletion of calcitonin gene-related peptide and substance P in sensory neurons from diabetic mice in vitro. J Neurol Sci 1994;126:1
86. Parving HH. Increased microvascular permeability to plasma proteins in short- and long-term juvenile diabetics. Diabetes 1976;25(suppl 2):884
87. Joyner WL, Mayhan WG, Johnson RL, Phares K. Microvascular alterations develop in Syrian hamsters after the induction of diabetes mellitus by streptozotocin. Diabetes 1981;30:93
88. Viberti G, MacKintosh D, Keen H. Determinants of the penetration of proteins through the glomerular barrier in insulin-dependent diabetes mellitus. Diabetes 1983;32(suppl 2):92
89. Rechthand E, Smith QR, Latker CH, Rapoport SI. Altered blood-nerve permeability to small molecules in experimental diabetes mellitus. J Neuropathol Exp Neurol 1987;46:302
90. Ohi T, Poduslo JF, Dyck PJ. Increased endoneurial albumin in diabetic polyneuropathy. Neurology 1985;35:1790
91. Williamson JR, Chang K, Tilton RG, et al. Increased vascular permeability in spontaneously diabetic BB/W rats and in rats with mild versus severe streptozocin-induced diabetes: Prevention by aldose reductase inhibitors and castration. Diabetes 1987;36:813
92. Sima AAF, Robertson DM. The perineural and blood-nerve barriers in experimental diabetes. Acta Neuropathol 1978;44:189
93. Kihara M, Schmelzer JD, Poduslo JF, et al. Aminoguanidine effects on nerve blood flow, vascular permeability, electrophysiology, and oxygen free radicals. Proc Natl Acad Sci U S A 1991;88:6107
94. Patel NJ, Misra VP, Dandona P, Thomas PK. The effect of non-enzymatic glycation of serum proteins on their permeation into peripheral nerve in normal and streptozotocin-diabetic rats. Diabetologia 1991;34:78
95. Poduslo JF, Curran GL. Glycation increases the permeability of proteins across the blood-nerve and blood-brain barriers. Mol Brain Res 1994;23:157
96. O'Brien JP, Mackinnon SE, MacLean AR, et al. A model of chronic nerve compression in the rat. Ann Plast Surg 1987;19:430
97. Neary D, Ochoa J, Gilliatt RW. Subclinical entrapment neuropathy in man. J Neurol Sci 1975;24:283
98. Upton AR, McComas AJ. The double crush in nerve entrapment syndromes. Lancet 1973;2:359
99. Dellon AL, Mackinnon SE. Chronic nerve compression model for the double crush hypothesis. Ann Plast Surg 1991;26:259
100. Dellon AL, MacKinnon SE, Seiler WA. Susceptibility of the diabetic nerve to chronic compression. Ann Plast Surg 1988;20:117

Diabetes Mellitus, edited by Derek LeRoith, Simeon I. Taylor, and Jerrold M. Olefsky. Lippincott–Raven Publishers, Philadelphia © 1996.

Chapter 85

Neuropathy: Growth Factors and Nerve Regeneration

Francis J. Liuzzi and Alison S. Depto

Throughout life neurons are dependent on neurotrophic factors. During development, the birth, migration, and survival of neurons is regulated by neurotrophic factors within their environment. Classic experiments by Viktor Hamburger, Rita Levi-Montalcini, and others (see Oppenheim for a review[1]) have shown that competition for growth factors at critical stages in nervous system development determines whether a neuron will live or die.

Although in adulthood many neurons become more independent of neurotrophic factors, at least for survival, much of neuronal gene expression and consequent function continues to be regulated by neurotrophic factors. These factors include circulating peptides in serum, retrogradely transported target-derived trophic factors, and paracrine products of non-neuronal supporting cells, such as the satellite cells of the spinal and sympathetic ganglia and Schwann cells in peripheral nerve. Any disturbance of neurotrophic factor availability from any of these sources can severely affect neuronal gene expression and function and axonal regeneration, and in some instances can result in neuronal death. Clearly, disease processes that affect neurotrophic factor availability manifest themselves in these ways.

Substantial evidence indicates that diabetes mellitus causes decreased synthesis of neurotrophic factors and possibly decreased neurotrophic factor receptor binding, uptake, and retrograde axonal transport. The contribution that these changes make to the etiology of diabetic neuropathy is the focus of ongoing research in a number of laboratories. Numerous studies have shown that diabetes mellitus is associated with a decline in neurotrophic factor availability, and the data from these studies support the idea that this decline contributes to the development of diabetic neuropathy. The pathologic features of diabetic neuropathy only need to be compared to those of diminished neurotrophic support seen in experimental animals and in human disease processes to begin to understand how a decline in such support might play an important role in the pathogenesis of neuropathy.

Further evidence for a "neurotrophic factor hypothesis" of diabetic neuropathy comes from observations of impaired peripheral nerve regeneration in diabetic rats[2,3] and patients.[4] The profound importance of neurotrophic factors in peripheral nerve regeneration is well established (see Liuzzi and Tedeschi for a review[5]). Therefore, any study of the mechanisms underlying impaired nerve regeneration must consider the likelihood of disturbances in the availability of the various neurotrophic factors that are necessary to mount an effective regenerative response in injured neurons and their environment.

Few proponents of the "neurotrophic factor hypothesis" of diabetic neuropathy believe that a decline in the availability of neuronal trophic support is the single cause of diabetic neuropathy. Indeed, the etiology of diabetic neuropathy is complex and likely to involve a number of interacting pathogenic mechanisms. Hyperglycemia, the major consequence of insulinopenia, for example, causes nonenzymatic glycosylation,[6] myoinositol deficiency, inhibition of Na^+/K^+ ATPase, and increased flux in the polyol pathway within peripheral nervous tissue.[7] The relationship between hyperglycemia and nerve damage is well documented.

It is important to consider, however, that neurotrophic factors not only are essential for normal neuronal maintenance and function but also are neuroprotective.[8,9] For example, guanethidine, when chronically administered, causes an immune-mediated destruction of sympathetic neurons in rats.[8] Nerve growth factor (NGF), which is essential for sympathetic neuron development and survival, prevents that destruction. Similarly, NGF, basic fibroblast growth factor (bFGF), and epidermal growth factor (EGF) enhanced PC12 cell survival in an in vitro model of ischemia.[9] It could be speculated that a decline of neurotrophic, neuroprotective factors in diabetes might increase nervous tissue susceptibility to glucose toxicity, ischemia, and autoimmune destruction, all potential factors in the development of diabetic neuropathy.

In addition, in a consideration of the pathogenesis of diabetic neuropathy it is important to examine the direct effects of insulinopenia and its potential consequences on neuronal maintenance and function. Increasing evidence indicates that insulin has effects beyond glucose regulation and is itself a neurotrophic factor. Moreover, insulin directly affects the availability of other neurotrophic factors that are essential for neuronal maintenance and function. Insulin influences NGF synthesis[10] as well as NGF receptor binding.[11] Insulin also has been implicated in the regulation of serum and tissue levels of the insulin-like growth factors (IGFs) and their binding proteins (IGFBPs).[12,13]

Insulin as a Neurotrophic Factor

The neurotrophic factor most obviously affected by pancreatic β-cell destruction in diabetes is insulin. Researchers who culture neurons have long been aware that insulin is an essential component of the culture medium. It supports the survival of primary cultures of peripheral[14] and central neurons[15] in serum-free media. Its receptors are present in central[16] and peripheral nervous system tissues.[17]

Llewelyn and colleagues[18] examined insulin binding in dorsal root ganglia, sciatic nerve, and superior cervical ganglion and found that all three bind insulin.[17] Sensory neurons in dorsal root ganglia and possibly non-neuronal cells, and satellite and Schwann cells abundantly express insulin receptors.[18] An in vitro analysis of glucose and amino acid uptake by whole dorsal root ganglia showed that insulin had no effect on either glucose or amino acid uptake,[17] suggesting that insulin may not be involved in acute neuronal metabolic processes. By contrast, Recio-Pinto and Ishii[11] showed that insulin increased the uptake of leucine and uridine, stimulated protein synthesis, and enhanced neurite extension in human neuroblastoma cells.

Insulin has been implicated in the regulation of neuronal maturation in the central nervous system.[19] Ishii and colleagues, in a number of related studies, have shown that insulin acts as a neurotrophic factor for cultured neuroblastoma, sympathetic ganglion, and dorsal root ganglia neurons.[14] Moreover, insulin, although less effective than the IGFs (IGF-1 and IGF-2), regulates tubulin expression in cultured neurons.[14]

In cultures of adult rat primary sensory neurons, insulin had no effect on neuronal survival.[20] However, insulin alone, added to defined medium, increased the rate of neurite outgrowth (regeneration) by 3.5 times over controls.[20]

Effects of Insulin on Other Neurotrophic Factors

Although the evidence indicates that insulin itself is a neurotrophic factor, the effect of diabetic insulinopenia on neuronal trophic support may be mediated via insulin's effects on the availability of other neurotrophic factors. For example, insulin acts in synergy with NGF. In serum-free media, human SH-SY5Y neuroblastoma cells lose their ability to bind NGF, whereas addition of insulin to the media dramatically increases specific NGF receptor binding.[11] Similarly, Fernyhough and colleagues[20] observed an additive effect of insulin and NGF on neurite outgrowth from cultured adult dorsal root ganglia neurons. These data suggest that diabetic insulinopenia acts on NGF availability by decreasing NGF receptor binding. Such a decrease in NGF receptor binding by sensory and sympathetic neurons might contribute to the decrease in retrograde transport of NGF that characterizes diabetes. In addition, insulinopenia may directly affect NGF synthesis by neuronal target tissues.[10]

Diabetic insulinopenia also affects the availability of IGF-1 and IGF-2. The relationship of insulin and IGF-1 is more direct than that between insulin and NGF. IGF-1 mRNA is most abundant in the liver,[21] and there is evidence that insulin regulates serum IGF-1 levels by direct action on the liver such that low insulin levels result in low serum IGF-1 levels.[13] Like insulin, but more potent, IGF-1 has neurotrophic activity.[14] It has been shown to enhance neurite outgrowth from cultured neurons and has been implicated as an important factor in sciatic nerve regeneration.[14] IGF-1, which is growth hormone–dependent, is decreased in the sera of diabetic animals and insulin-dependent patients.[3,13,22–25] In diabetic swine, IGF-1 mRNA levels are decreased in heart, liver, and muscle, and this decreased gene expression is correlated with decreased serum levels.[24]

The relationship of insulin and IGF-2 is less clear than that between insulin and IGF-1. IGF-2 mRNA is most abundant in the brain,[21] particularly in the choroid plexus. Like the other members of the insulin gene family, IGF-2 is a neurotrophic factor, it is produced by non-neuronal cells in regenerating nerve, and it enhances axonal regeneration in vivo.[14] There is, however, some controversy regarding the effects of diabetes mellitus on serum IGF-2 levels. Some investigators report that IGF-2 serum levels are diminished,[25] others say they remain unchanged,[24] whereas still others say that they are elevated[23] in diabetics.

The IGFs, but not insulin, are bound to carrier proteins, IGFBPs, in the serum.[12] The role of IGFBPs in diabetes is as yet unclear. However, it has been shown that the low-molecular-weight (30–34 kd) IGFBP, which is insulin-dependent, is elevated in patients with insulin-dependent diabetes mellitus (IDDM).[22,23,26] This binding protein binds IGF-1 with five times greater affinity than the IGF type I receptor.[22] Elevated binding proteins in diabetic sera or tissues could decrease the availability of the IGFs to sensory, motor, and sympathetic neurons.

Nerve Growth Factor in Development, Peripheral Nerve Regeneration, and Neuropathy

Nerve growth factor (NGF) was the first discovered neurotrophic factor. It is the most well characterized of a growing list of neurotrophic factors. NGF is a member of the neurotrophin family which includes brain-derived neurotrophic factor (BDNF), neurotrophin-3 (NT-3), and NT-4/5 (see Lindsay and colleagues for a review[27]). The pioneering work of Levi-Montalcini and her colleagues showed that NGF is essential for the differentiation and survival of neural crest–derived neurons during development.[1] Administration of exogenous NGF decreases naturally occurring cell death in developing sympathetic ganglia, whereas antiserum to NGF increases that cell loss.[1]

NGF is produced by target organs, such as the skin, heart, and salivary glands, taken up by sensory[28,29] and sympathetic[28] axons, and retrogradely transported to their cell bodies. NGF binds to receptors on the axon terminals; the receptor-ligand complex is internalized and retrogradely transported.[30]

NGF and the other neurotrophins bind two types of receptors, a low-affinity, 75 kd (p75) receptor and a high-affinity trk (tyrosine kinase) receptors that are believed to subserve signal transduction by activation of second messenger pathways. The neurotrophins all bind the low-affinity receptor with similar avidity. Binding to the trk receptors exhibits more specificity, with NGF binding to trkA, whereas BDNF and NT-4 bind to trkB and NT-3 binds to trkB and trkC.[27,31] Recent data show that different subpopulations of dorsal root ganglia neurons are dependent upon different neurotrophins for their normal development and maintenance.[27,31]

In adulthood, all autonomic neurons remain dependent on NGF for their survival.[1] However, only a subpopulation of dorsal root ganglia sensory neurons remain dependent on the factor for their survival. In adult rats, this set of dependent neurons dies following axotomy of their peripheral processes, whereas local administration of exogenous NGF rescues 100% of these cells.[5]

Another feature of axotomy of dorsal root ganglia neuronal peripheral processes is somal and axonal atrophy. Administration of exogenous NGF to the cut proximal end of the sciatic nerve prevents, in part, this axotomy-induced atrophy of sensory neurons. Conversely, injections of NGF antisera cause atrophy of uninjured axons and an approximate 2.5-fold increase in the number of dorsal root ganglia neurons displaying eccentric nuclei.[5] The NGF antisera-induced atrophy might be explained by the relationship between neurofilament synthesis and axon diameter[32] and the observation by Verge and colleagues[33] that NGF restores neurofilament (NF) gene expression in NGF-receptive dorsal root ganglia neurons following axotomy.

NGF may be important in peripheral nerve regeneration. In adult peripheral nerve, under normal conditions, Schwann cells produce very little NGF.[34] However, nerve injury causes a biphasic increase in NGF expression within the nerve.[35] Within 2–6 hours after injury, there is an upregulation of NGF within the endoneurium of the proximal and distal nerve stumps. The second phase begins at 2 days after injury and is confined to the injury site and distal nerve.[35] This latter phase corresponds to the immigration of macrophages and may be stimulated by macrophage-derived interleukin-1.[35] Moreover, Schwann cell low-affinity NGF receptor binding[36] and receptor mRNA expression increase distal to the injury site.[34] When regenerating axons arrive within an area of regenerating nerve, Schwann cell NGF receptor expression within that area is downregulated.[36] These data suggest that Schwann cell upregulation of NGF and the NGF receptor plays an important role in peripheral nerve regeneration.

Rich and colleagues[37] examined the role of NGF in peripheral nerve regeneration using a tube model in which a 6-mm nerve gap is bridged by an impermeable silicone tube. In the experimental animals, the tubes were filled with NGF. In the controls, the tubes were filled with saline. After 4 weeks, the rats were sacrificed and the tubes containing the regenerating nerves were removed. In the NGF-treated nerves, there were more than twice as many myelinated axons in the distal 2-mm segment of the tube as in control nerves. Interestingly, the total number of axons, myelinated and unmyelinated together, were approximately equal in the two conditions. The greater number of large, myelinated axons in the NGF-treated condition might not reflect an effect on the rate of axonal regeneration. Rather, it may be attributable to the effect of NGF on neurofilament gene expression[33] and axon diameter. In this experiment, NGF might also have had local effects on Schwann cells and endoneurial fibroblasts. As the authors pointed out, such effects might explain the advanced maturation of the NGF-treated nerve.[37]

Diamond and colleagues [38] have challenged the idea that NGF plays a role in axonal regeneration. They crushed cutaneous nerves and examined the effect of anti-NGF treatment on regeneration. Interestingly, they found that regeneration-related recovery of nociception, mediated by unmyelinated c-fibers and small myelinated Aδ fibers, was not impaired by anti-NGF treatment. By contrast, collateral sprouting of uninjured C and Aδ fibers into denervated regions of skin was impaired by anti-NGF treatments. These findings indicate that collateral sprouting is a very different process than axonal regeneration. It is difficult, however, to reconcile the anti-NGF regeneration data from Diamond and colleagues' study with previous data suggesting an important role for NGF in sensory neuronal survival, gene expression, and regeneration. It is important, however, to note that after axotomy, sensory neurons downregulate both the high (trk) and low-affinity (p75) NGF receptors.[39] This results in a threefold decrease in the retrograde transport of NGF.[35]

The observations of impaired retrograde axonal transport of NGF in diabetic rat nerves were the seminal findings leading to the formulation of the neurotrophic hypothesis of diabetic neuropathy. The finding by Lindsay and Hamar[40] that NGF regulates substance P synthesis combined with the observations of reduced substance P transport in sciatic nerves of diabetic rats further galvanized the idea that decreased NGF availability contributes to the pathogenesis of diabetic neuropathy.

Diemel and colleagues[41] have shown a decrease in preprotachykinin (PPT) mRNA and substance P in diabetic rat dorsal root ganglia. The PPT gene encodes for a protein that is post-translationally cleaved to produce substance P.[40] Substance P is a putative nociceptive transmitter, and its depletion results in thermal analgesia.[42]

It has already been stated that substance P synthesis in sensory ganglion neurons is regulated by NGF.[40,43] Retrograde axonal transport of NGF is impaired in diabetic rats,[44,45] and serum NGF levels are reduced in diabetic patients.[46] Both NGF transport and synthesis, as previously discussed, may be influenced by serum insulin levels.

The interaction of insulin and NGF availability is illustrated by the findings of Diemel and colleagues,[47] which show that insulin treatment restores substance P levels in diabetic nerve. Originally, the restoration was attributed by the authors to "tight glycemic" control. Interestingly, though, their later experiments showed that tight glycemic control was not necessary for the restoration of substance P levels in sciatic nerve and PPT mRNA levels in the dorsal root ganglia of diabetic rats.[41,47] NGF infusions restored those levels despite the fact that blood glucose levels in the NGF-treated diabetic rats were no different from those of vehicle-treated diabetic rats that showed no change.[41] Diemel and colleagues' work supports the idea that serum insulin level, rather than glucose level, may be important to the regulation of substance P (PPT) gene expression via its effect on NGF availability. Their work also provides compelling evidence that some neuropathic changes in diabetes are independent of glycemic state.

In addition to the regulation of PPT gene expression in dorsal root ganglia neurons, NGF regulates neurofilament gene expression in those dorsal root ganglia neurons that are NGF-receptive, that is, those that express the trkA receptor.[33] Neurofilaments have been implicated as important in the maintenance of axon diameter.[32]

Axon diameter affects both axon conduction velocity and degree of myelinization. Interestingly, axonal atrophy characterizes diabetic neuropathy and a reduction in neurofilament numbers correlates with this atrophy.[48] Preliminary in situ hybridization studies in our laboratory using a cRNA probe for the low molecular weight (68 kd) neurofilament subunit suggest that diabetes causes a downregulation of neurofilament gene expression in dorsal root ganglia of streptozotocin-induced diabetic rats. This is similar to what occurs following axotomy of dorsal root ganglia neuronal peripheral processes, which separates the neurons from target-derived growth factors.

Exactly how diabetes mellitus affects NGF availability is not fully understood. As stated above, serum NGF levels are reduced in diabetic patients.[46] By contrast, Hellweg and Hartung[44] have shown an initial decrease in autonomic neuronal target tissue NGF levels in diabetic rats, followed by a later increase in NGF levels in these tissues. The increased target tissue NGF levels, however, may be the result of decreased NGF receptor-binding, axonal uptake, and retrograde transport.

More recently, Fernyhough and colleagues[10] found a direct link between insulin treatment and NGF mRNA levels in diabetic skin. In their study, streptozocin-induced diabetic rats maintained on low-dose insulin had a nearly 50% decrease in NGF mRNA in footpad skin. By contrast, diabetic rats treated with intensive insulin had essentially the same levels of NGF mRNA in footpad skin as nondiabetic controls. Although intensive insulin treatment reduced blood glucose levels in the diabetic rats, their blood glucose levels remained more than twice as high as controls. These latter observations suggest that insulin rather than glucose regulates tissue NGF expression in diabetic rats.

Changes in NGF levels, uptake, and receptor binding in diabetes and the amelioration of some of the sensory neuronal perturbations by exogenous NGF suggest that NGF might be useful in the clinical treatment of some diabetic sensory neuropathies. Moreover, the continued dependence of sympathetic neurons on NGF in adulthood suggests that autonomic neuropathies might especially be effectively treated with exogenous NGF. A multicenter clinical trial using NGF as a treatment for diabetic neuropathy is about to commence in this country.

Insulin-like Growth Factors in Development, Peripheral Nerve Regeneration, and Neuropathy

The IGFs share structural homology with insulin, and like insulin, both IGF-1 and IGF-2 have neurotrophic activity.[14] Just as NGF has been shown to promote neurite extension from culture neurons, IGF-1 and IGF-2 have been shown to enhance neurite outgrowth from neurons in vitro.[14] The IGFs, like NGF, have also been shown to regulate neuronal gene expression, particularly tubulin and neurofilament expression.[14] Moreover, like NGF, the IGFs have been shown to be produced by neuronal target organs, such as muscle, and to be retrogradely transported within axons.[49]

Although the role of IGFs in nervous system development has not been as clearly elucidated as that of NGF, there is evidence that the IGFs may be involved in central nervous system as well as peripheral nervous system development. The IGFs are differentially distributed throughout the nervous system, central and peripheral, and are abundantly expressed in regions of the developing nervous system.[50]

As described above, many fetal neurons, particularly those of neural crest origin, are dependent upon NGF for survival and differentiation. Similarly, there is evidence that the IGFs may be important for fetal neuronal survival and for the promotion of neurite outgrowth from these cells. Svrzic and Schubert[51] have shown that fetal cortical neuronal survival in culture is enhanced by IGF-1. Similarly, the survival of cultured chick dorsal root ganglion neurons in the absence of NGF is significantly enhanced by the presence of IGF-2 in media.[52] Moreover, neurite extension from these cultured neurons was increased by IGF-2 in the media by nearly the same extent as it was by NGF in the media.[52]

Ralphs and colleagues[53] used an antibody to human IGF-1 to examine the distribution of this peptide in developing chicks and concluded from their observations that the IGFs were involved in the differentiation of nervous tissue cells. Unfortunately, since the antibody used in their study bound strongly to IGF-1 and weakly to IGF-2 under their conditions,[53] the differential distribution of these peptides during development could not be determined. However, in the case of nervous tissues, IGF-positive immunostaining was observed in developing peripheral nerves and within the developing neuraxis.

Interestingly, in nerves, IGF immunostaining was associated with axons, whereas Schwann cells were unlabeled.[53] These observations might suggest that developing Schwann cells are not synthesizing IGFs. However, in regenerating adult nerves, IGF synthesis is upregulated in Schwann cells.[14] Moreover, axonal staining with the antibody might suggest either neuronal synthesis and transport of the peptides or uptake of the peptides from surrounding tissues. In the developing central nervous system, IGF-positive immunostaining was associated with axonal tracts and was present in the mantel zone, a region of neuronal differentiation.[53]

A more precise understanding of the role of IGFs in neural development may come from studies like that of Bondy and colleagues[50] using in situ hybridization with probes to IGF-1, IGF-2, and IGF-1 receptor to study the differential distribution of these mRNAs in fetal rats. They found that IGF-1 mRNA, but not IGF-2 mRNA, was particularly abundant in the mesenchyme associated with developing nerves and dorsal root ganglia. By contrast, IGF-2 mRNA was most abundant in the central nervous system-vascular interfaces of the choroid plexus and organum vasculosum of the lamina terminalis.[50] In the central nervous system, IGF-1 receptor mRNA was widely distributed but was most abundant in the ventral floorplate of the hindbrain. In the peripheral nervous system, IGF-1 receptor mRNA was present in dorsal root ganglia.

In the adult, IGF-1 has been implicated in central nervous system remyelinization following experimental demyelinization.[54] However, more important for diabetic neuropathy, the IGFs have been implicated in peripheral nerve regeneration and nerve-muscle targeting (see Ishii and colleagues for a review[14]). IGF-1, like NGF, is retrogradely transported in sciatic nerves of normal adult rats[49] and therefore local production of IGF-1 may influence axonal regeneration at the level of the neuronal cell bodies. Indeed, infusions of IGF-1 or IGF-2 at the site of nerve injury enhanced the rate of sciatic nerve regeneration following nerve injury in rats.[14]

In diabetes mellitus, IGF-1, which is growth hormone–dependent, is decreased in the sera of diabetic animals and insulin-dependent patients.[3,13,22–25] In diabetic swine, IGF-1 mRNA levels are decreased in heart, liver, and muscle, and this decreased gene expression is correlated with decreased serum levels.[24] There is evidence that insulin regulates serum IGF-1 levels by direct action on the liver such that low insulin levels result in low serum IGF-1 levels.[13]

As mentioned earlier, the issue of IGF-2 and its role in diabetic neuropathy is less clear than that of IGF-1. At present, some controversy remains over whether serum IGF-2 levels are diminished,[25] remain unchanged,[24] or are increased[23] in diabetes.

Sciatic nerve regeneration in diabetic rats is severely impaired.[2,3] Changes in the availability of IGFs to sensory and motor axons might contribute to the impaired nerve regeneration observed in diabetics. Ekström and colleagues[3] linked low serum IGF-1 levels in streptozotocin-induced diabetic rats to diminished sciatic nerve regeneration and reported that elevation of IGF-1 levels was linked to improved regeneration. However, the method used to elevate IGF-1 levels in their rats was insulin infusion. Considering the neurotrophic effects of insulin and the effects of the hormone on hyperglycemia and consequently its effects on the diabetic nerve, it is difficult to accept the conclusion that IGF acted alone to improve regeneration. However, in very recent studies, Ishii and colleagues reported that a downregulation of IGF gene expression in sciatic nerves in streptozotocin-treated rats precedes neuropathy,[55] whereas local IGF infusions improve sciatic nerve regeneration in those diabetic rats.[56] The improved regeneration was in the presence of hyperglycemia,[56] suggesting that hyperglycemia may not contribute significantly to impaired peripheral nerve regeneration in diabetics.

As in the case of NGF, the data suggest that a decreased availability of the IGFs may contribute to the pathogenesis of diabetic neuropathy. Clinical trials of IGF-1 for the treatment of amyotrophic lateral sclerosis are currently under way. Considering the mounting evidence that IGFs are important in the maintenance of the peripheral nervous system and that their expression may be disturbed by diabetes, clinical trial using IGFs for diabetic neuropathy are not far off.

Laminin in Development, Peripheral Nerve Regeneration, and Neuropathy

Laminin is not traditionally included in a discussion of neurotrophic factors. However, the available data suggest that the large, heterotrimeric, cruciform glycoprotein plays an important role in nervous system development and repair.

Laminin, the major component of all basal lamina, is composed of three subunits, a large A chain and two smaller B chains, B1 and B2.[57] In peripheral nervous tissue, the A chain is replaced by the A chain variant, the merosin, or M chain.[58] There, basal laminar components are synthesized by Schwann cells and form continuous basal laminar tubes within the endoneurium.

Laminin appears to play an important role in the developing nervous system, guiding neuronal migration and neurite extension in the peripheral and central nervous systems. It has been shown to enhance neurite extension from cultured neurons.[59] Moreover, studies of peripheral nerve injury have implicated Schwann cell basal laminar tubes as the mechanical guides along which regenerating axons grow.[60]

A recent study by Federoff and colleagues[61] showed that nonenzymatic glycosylation of laminin and the laminin peptide IKVAV inhibit neuritic outgrowth by cultured neuroblastoma cells. Interestingly, however, the normal carbohydrate moieties of laminin appear to be essential for neurite outgrowth and cell migration.[62] Indeed, Dean and colleagues[62] report that unglycosylated laminin inhibits neurite outgrowth and that glycosylation is necessary for cell migration and neurite outgrowth but not for cell adhesion. Advanced glycosylation of laminin, however, causes aberrant cross-links that alter the cruciform shape of the molecule and impair self-assembly of the molecule.[63] These changes might inhibit laminin receptor binding as well as laminin interactions with heparan sulfate and type IV collagen within basal laminae. Furthermore, impairment of laminin self-assembly may affect the normal turnover of Schwann cell basal laminae within the nerve and contribute to their thickening.

Advanced glycosylation of Schwann cell basal laminar components is likely to occur in the high glucose environment of diabetic nerves. Examination of streptozotocin-treated diabetic rat nerves indicates the presence of advanced glycosylation end products.[64] However, whether Schwann cell basal laminae are specifically subjected to advanced glycosylation in diabetic nerves remains to be shown. An inhibitor of advanced glycosylation, aminoguanidine has been shown to improve motor nerve conduction velocities and affect myelinated fiber size and axon diameter in streptozotocin-treated diabetic rat peripheral nerves.[64] However, no hypothesis of how advanced glycosylation might influence those functional and morphologic parameters has been proposed. More important, since advanced glycosylation of laminin inhibits neurite outgrowth in culture, it will be important to determine whether aminoguanidine treatment improves axonal regeneration in diabetic rat nerves.

Our laboratory has been interested in laminin not as an extracellular matrix component but as a neurotrophic factor. We have shown, using in situ hybridization, that all normal adult dorsal root ganglia neurons express the laminin B2 chain gene,[65] and we believe that this expression may be essential to neuronal maintenance. Additionally, a subpopulation of smaller dorsal root ganglia neurons express the B1 laminin subunit gene.[65] This more restricted neuronal gene expression could have implications for the specificity of neuron-target interactions in the periphery as well as within the spinal cord. Primary sensory neurons do not appear to express the A chain gene or the merosin, M chain gene.[65] However, the merosin M chain gene is expressed by satellite and Schwann cells within the ganglia.[65]

During sciatic nerve regeneration in nondiabetic rats, laminin B2 gene expression is upregulated by axotomized dorsal root ganglia neurons.[66] This upregulation of laminin B2 in neurons during regeneration suggests that neuronal B2 laminin plays a role in the regenerative response of those cells. Neuronal laminin may act locally, within the ganglion, in a paracrine or possibly autocrine fashion. Alternatively, it may be anterogradely transported to the growth cone region where it might affect local cellular events within the regenerating nerve.

Studies of laminin gene expression in peripheral nervous tissue are currently under way in our laboratory. It is important to determine whether B2 laminin gene expression is disturbed in diabetic dorsal root ganglia neurons. Moreover, since upregulation of laminin B2 message appears to be a part of the normal regenerative response of dorsal root ganglia neurons, it is important to determine whether that regenerative response is impaired by diabetes.

Schwann cell laminin gene expression, which appears to be important in nerve regeneration, might also be impaired by diabetes. It might be postulated that advanced glycosylation of laminin and its effects on laminin assembly and its interactions with other extracellular matrix components in diabetes might affect laminin's expression by Schwann cells and ultimately the environment through which regenerating axons must grow.

In light of all the unanswered questions about neuronal and Schwann cell laminin gene expression in diabetes, it is likely that the clinical use of laminin as a treatment for diabetic neuropathy is years away. Many questions need to be addressed. It is important to determine first how neuronal laminin gene expression is regulated and what role it plays in normal neuronal maintenance and regeneration. Additionally, it is important to determine whether therapeutic treatments of diabetic rats with insulin or other neurotrophic factors affect laminin gene expression and restore the regenerative response of dorsal root ganglia neurons.

Future Perspectives for the Treatment of Diabetic Neuropathy With Neurotrophic Factors

In the nearly half-century since the earliest studies of neurotrophism, a growing list of neurotrophic factors has been compiled. Relatives of NGF, members of the neurotrophin family, have been identified. Many of their actions have been studied and their receptors have been characterized. New information about the neurotrophins is available on a nearly daily basis. Similarly, there has been an explosion of information available about insulin's relatives, the IGFs.

Many diseases of the nervous system, from Alzheimer's disease to ALS, have been linked to disturbances in growth factor availability. Clinical trials for neurotrophic factor treatment of these diseases either have been proposed or are now under way.

It is increasingly obvious that perturbations of growth factor availability may play a major role in the pathogenesis of diabetic neuropathy. Clinical trials using NGF for the treatment of diabetic neuropathy are currently under way. IGF-1 is being used in clinical trials to treat amyotrophic lateral sclerosis, and trials to test the efficacy of IGFs in the treatment of diabetic neuropathy cannot be far off. As more information is garnered about laminin and the many other growth factors, such as ciliary neurotrophic factor, which is currently being used in clinical trials for the treatment of amyotrophic lateral sclerosis,[27] new treatments for diabetic neuropathy may evolve. Indeed, as more information becomes available about neurotrophic factors and their specific actions and interactions, carefully formulated combinations may become available for the treatment or prevention of diabetic neuropathy.

References

1. Oppenheim RW. Cell death during development of the nervous system. Annu Rev Neurosci 1991;14:453
2. Longo FM, Powell HC, LeBeau JM, et al. Delayed nerve regeneration in streptozotocin diabetic rats. Muscle Nerve 1986;9:385
3. Ekström PAR, Kanje M, Skottner A. Nerve regeneration and serum levels of insulin-like growth factor-I in rats with streptozotocin-induced insulin deficiency. Brain Res 1989;496:141
4. Britland ST, Young RJ, Sharma AK, Clarke BF. Association of painful and painless diabetic neuropathy with different patterns of nerve fiber degeneration and regeneration. Diabetes 1990;39:898
5. Liuzzi FJ, Tedeschi B. Peripheral nerve regeneration. In: Burchiel KM, ed. Surgical Management of Peripheral Nerve Injury and Entrapment. Philadelphia: WB Saunders Co; 1991:31
6. Brownlee MA, Cerami A, Vlassara H. Advanced glycosylation end products in tissue and the biochemical basis of diabetic complications. N Engl J Med 1988;318:1315
7. Greene DA, Lattimer SA, Sima AA. Are disturbances of sorbitol, phosphoinositide, and Na^+-K^+-ATPase involved in the pathogenesis of diabetic neuropathy? Diabetes 1988;37:688
8. Manning PT, Russell JH, Simmons B, Johnson EM Jr. Protection from guanethidine-induced neuronal destruction by nerve growth factor: Effect of NGF on immune function. Brain Res 1985;340:61
9. Boniece IR, Wagner JA. Growth factors protect PC12 cells against ischemia by a mechanism that is independent of PKA, PKC, and protein synthesis. J Neurosci 1993;13:4220
10. Fernyhough P, Carrington AL, Tomlinson DR. Reduced nerve growth factor mRNA in skin of diabetic rats: Effects of insulin (abstract). Br J Pharmacol 1992;107:426P
11. Recio-Pinto E, Ishii DN. Effects of insulin, insulin-like growth factor-II and nerve growth factor on neurite outgrowth in cultured neuroblastoma cells. Brain Res 1984;302:323
12. Cohick WS, Clemmons DR. The insulin-like growth factors. Ann Rev Physiol 1993;55:131
13. Griffein SC, Russell SM, Katz LS, Nicoll CS. Insulin exerts metabolic and growth-promoting effects by direct action on the liver in vitro: Clarification of the functional significance of the portal vascular link between the beta cells of the pancreatic islets and the liver. Proc Natl Acad Sci USA 1987;84: 7300
14. Ishii DN, Glazner GW, Pu S-F. Role of insulin-like growth factors in peripheral nerve regeneration. Pharmacol Ther 1994;62:125
15. Aizenman Y, de Vellis J. Brain neurons develop in a serum and glial free environment: Effects of transferrin, insulin, insulin-like growth factor I and thyroid hormone on neuronal survival, growth and differentiation. Brain Res 1987;406:32
16. Heidenreich KA, Brandenburg D. Oligosaccharide heterogeneity of insulin receptors. Comparison of N-linked glycosylation of insulin receptors in adipocytes and brain. Endocrinology 1986;118:1835
17. Patel NJ, Llewelyn JG, Wright DW, Thomas PK. Glucose and leucine uptake by rat dorsal root ganglia is not insulin sensitive. J Neurol Sci 1994;121:159
18. Llewelyn JG, Patel NJ, Thomas PK, et al. Autoradiographic localization of (^{125}I) insulin binding in peripheral nerve tissue. In: Scarpini E, Fiori MG, Pleasure G, Scarlato G, eds. Peripheral Nerve Development and Regeneration: Recent Advances in Clinical Application. Padova, Italy: Liviana Press; 1989:149
19. Puro DG, Agardh E. Insulin-mediated regulation of neuronal maturation. Science 1984;225:1170
20. Fernyhough P, Willars GB, Lindsay RM, Tomlinson DR. Insulin and insulin-like growth factor I enhance regeneration in cultured adult rat sensory neurones. Brain Res 1993;607:117
21. Murphy LJ, Bell GI, Friesen HG. Tissue distribution of insulin-like growth factor I and II messenger ribonucleic acid in the adult rat. Endocrinology 1987;120:1279
22. Crosby SR, Tsigos C, Anderton CD, et al. Elevated plasma insulin-like growth factor binding protein-1 levels in type 1 (insulin-dependent) diabetic patients with peripheral neuropathy. Diabetologia 1992;35:868
23. Hall K, Johansson BL, Povoa G, Thalme B. Serum levels of insulin-like growth factor (IGF) I, II and IGF binding protein in diabetic adolescents treated with continuous subcutaneous insulin infusion. J Int Med 1989;225:273
24. Leaman DW, Simmen FA, Ramsay TG, White ME. Insulin-like growth factor-I and -II messenger RNA expression in muscle, heart and liver of streptozotocin-diabetic swine. Endocrinology 1990;126:2850
25. Yang H, Scheff AJ, Schalch DS. Effects of streptozotocin-induced diabetes mellitus on growth and hepatic insulin-like growth factor I gene expression in the rat. Metabolism 1990;39:295
26. Suikkari A-M, Koivisto VA, Rutanen E-M, et al. Insulin regulates the serum levels of low molecular weight insulin-like growth factor-binding protein. J Clin Endocrinol 1988;66:266
27. Lindsay RM, Wiegand SJ, Altar CA, DiStefano PS. Neurotrophic factors: From molecule to man. Trends Neurosci 1994;17:182
28. Stoeckel K, Schwab M, Thoenen H. Specificity of retrograde transport of nerve growth factor (NGF) in sensory neurons: A biochemical and morphological study. Brain Res 1975;89:1
29. Richardson PM, Riopelle RJ. Uptake of nerve growth factor along peripheral and spinal axons of primary sensory neurons. J Neurosci 1984;4:1683
30. Johnson EM, Taniuchi M, Clark HB, et al. Demonstration of retrograde transport of nerve growth factor receptor in the peripheral and central nervous system. J Neurosci 1987;7:923
31. Snider WD. Functions of the neurotrophins during nervous system development: What the knockouts are teaching us. Cell 1994;77:627
32. Hoffman PN, Cleveland DW, Griffin JW, et al. Neurofilament gene expression: A major determinant of axonal caliber. Proc Natl Acad Sci USA 1987;84: 3472
33. Verge VMK, Tetzlaff W, Bisby MA, Richardson PM. Influence of nerve growth factor on neurofilament gene expression in mature primary sensory neurons. J Neurosci 1990;10:2018
34. Heumann R, Lindholm D, Bandtlow C, et al. Differential regulation of mRNA encoding nerve growth factor and its receptor in rat sciatic nerve during development, degeneration and regeneration: Role of macrophages. Proc Natl Acad Sci USA 1987;84:8735
35. Raivich G, Kreutzberg GW. Nerve growth factor and regeneration of peripheral nervous system. Clin Neurol Neurosurg 1993;95(suppl):S84
36. Tanuichi M, Clark HB, Schweitzer JB, Johnson EM Jr. Expression of nerve growth factor receptors by Schwann cells of axotomized peripheral nerve: Ultrastructural location, suppression by axon contact, and binding properties. J Neurosci 1988;8:664
37. Rich KM, Alexander TD, Pryor JC, Hollowell JP. Nerve growth factor enhances regeneration across gaps within silicone chambers. Exp Neurol 1989;105:45
38. Diamond J, Foester A, Holmes M, Coughlin M. Sensory nerves in adult rats regenerate and restore sensory function to the skin independently of exogenous NGF. J Neurosci 1992;12:1467
39. Verge VMK, Merlio JP, Grandin J, et al. Colocalization of NGF binding sites, trk mRNA, and low-affinity NGF receptor mRNA in primary sensory neurons: Response to injury and infusion of NGF. J Neurosci 1992;12:4011
40. Lindsay RM, Hamar AJ. Nerve growth factor regulates expression of neuropeptide genes in adult sensory neurons. Nature 1989;337:362
41. Diemel LT, Brewster WJ, Fernyhough P, Tomlinson DR. Expression of neuropeptides in experimental diabetes; effects of treatment with nerve growth factor or brain-derived neurotrophic factor. Mol Brain Res 1994;21:171
42. Yaksh TL, Farb DH, Leeman SE, Jessell TM. Intrathecal capsaicin depletes substance P in the rat spinal cord and produces prolonged thermal analgesia. Science 1979;206:481
43. Wong J, Oblinger MM. NGF rescues substance P expression but not neurofilament or tubulin gene expression in axotomized sensory neurons. J Neurosci 1991;11:543
44. Hellweg R, Hartung HD. Endogenous levels of nerve growth factor (NGF) are altered in experimental diabetes mellitus: A possible role for NGF in the pathogenesis of diabetic neuropathy. J Neurosci Res 1990;26:258
45. Schmidt RE, Grabau GC, Yip HK. Retrograde transport of (^{125}I) nerve growth factor in ileal mesenteric nerves in vitro: Effect of streptozotocin diabetes. Brain Res 1986;378:325
46. Faradji V, Sotelo J. Low serum levels of nerve growth factor in diabetic neuropathy. Acta Neurol Scand 1990;81:402
47. Diemel LT, Stevens EJ, Willars GB, Tomlinson DR. Depletion of substance P and calcitonin gene-related peptide in sciatic nerve of rats with experimental diabetes; effects of insulin and aldose reductase inhibition. Neurosci Lett 1992;137:253
48. Yagihashi S, Kamijo M, Watanabe K. Reduced myelinated fiber size correlates with loss of axonal neurofilaments in peripheral nerve of chronically streptozotocin diabetic rats. Am J Pathol 1990;136:1365
49. Hansson HA, Rozell B, Skottner A. Rapid axonal transport of insulin-like growth factor I in the sciatic nerve of adult rats. Cell Tissue Res 1987;247: 241
50. Bondy CA, Werner H, Roberts CT, LeRoith D. Cellular pattern of IGF I and type II IGF receptor gene expression in early organogenesis: Comparison with IGFII gene expression. Molec Endocrinol 1990;4:1386
51. Svrzic D, Schubert D. Insulin-like growth factor 1 supports embryonic nerve cell survival. Biochem Biophys Res Commun 1990;172:54
52. Bothwell M. Insulin and somatomedin MSA promote nerve growth factor-independent neurite formation by cultured chick dorsal root ganglionic sensory neurons. J Neurosci Res 1982;8:225

53. Ralphs JR, Wylie L, Hill DJ. Distribution of insulin-like growth factor peptides in the developing chick embryo. Development 1990;109:51
54. Komoly S, Hudson LD, Webster HD, Bondy CA. Insulin-like growth factor I gene expression is induced in astrocytes during experimental demyelinization. Proc Natl Acad Sci USA 1992;89:1894
55. Wuarin L, Guertin DM, Ishii DN. Reduction of insulin-like growth factor (IGF) gene expression in nerves precedes the onset of diabetic neuropathy (abstract). Soc Neurosci Abst 1993;20:415
56. Zhuang HX, Pu S-F, Ishii DN. Insulin-like growth factors (IGFs) prevent diabetic neuropathy (impaired regeneration and hyperalgesia) in rats despite hyperglycemia (abstract). Soc Neurosci Abst 1993;20:415
57. Timple R. Structure and biological activity of basement membrane proteins. Eur J Biochem 1989;180:487
58. Ehrig K, Leivo I, Argraves WS, et al. Merosin, a tissue-specific basement membrane protein, is a laminin-like protein. Proc Natl Acad Sci USA 1990; 87:3264
59. Manthrorpe M, Engvall E, Ruoslahti E, et al. Laminin promotes neuritic regeneration from cultured peripheral and central neurons. J Cell Biol 1983; 97:1882
60. Ide C, Tohyama K, Yokata R, et al. Schwann cell basal lamina and nerve regeneration. Brain Res 1983;288:61
61. Federoff HJ, Lawrence D, Brownlee M. Nonenzymatic glycosylation of laminin and the laminin peptide CIKVAVS inhibits neurite outgrowth. Diabetes 1993;42:509
62. Dean JW III, Chandrasekaran S, Tanzer ML. A biological role for carbohydrate moieties of laminin. J Biol Chem 1990;265:12553
63. Charonis AS, Reger LA, Dege JE, et al. Laminin alterations after in vitro nonenzymatic glycosylation. Diabetes 1990;39:807
64. Yagahashi S, Kamijo M, Baba M, et al. Effect of aminoguanidine on functional and structural abnormalities in peripheral nerve of STZ-induced diabetic rats. Diabetes 1992;41:47
65. Le Beau JM, Liuzzi FJ, Depto AS, Vinik AI. Differential laminin gene expression in dorsal root ganglion neurons and non-neuronal cells. Exp Neurol 1994;127:1
66. Le Beau JM, Liuzzi FJ, Vinik AI. Differential expression of laminin genes in dorsal root ganglia during sciatic nerve regeneration (abstract). Soc Neurosci Abst 1993;19:679

Diabetes Mellitus, edited by Derek LeRoith, Simeon I. Taylor, and Jerrold M. Olefsky. Lippincott–Raven Publishers, Philadelphia © 1996.

CHAPTER 86
Diabetes, Lipids, and Atherosclerosis

ALAN CHAIT AND JOHN D. BRUNZELL

Diabetes and Atherosclerosis

Atherosclerotic cardiovascular disease remains the most important cause of morbidity and mortality in both insulin-dependent diabetes mellitus (IDDM) and non–insulin-dependent diabetes mellitus (NIDDM) today.[1,2] Despite years of study, the mechanisms by which diabetes so dramatically increases atherosclerosis risk remains poorly understood. The onset of diabetic renal disease markedly increases the risk of atherosclerosis.[1,3] Nonetheless, risk is increased in IDDM, and especially in NIDDM, even when renal function is unimpaired.[1,3] Therefore, factors common to both IDDM and NIDDM are likely to play an important role in the pathogenesis of atherosclerosis in diabetes and should provide clues to pathogenetic mechanisms.

Abnormalities of plasma lipid and lipoprotein metabolism are very common in diabetes[4] and have long been thought to play a role in atherogenesis in diabetes, much as they do in the nondiabetic state. However, the nature and mechanism of the dyslipidemia differ between the two types of diabetes, and disturbances of plasma lipids and lipoproteins alone are not likely to account for all the increased atherosclerotic risk associated with diabetes.

The mechanisms by which lipids and lipoproteins are involved in the atherogenic process has received considerable recent attention. Lipids and lipoproteins are involved in the initiation and progression of atherosclerosis and also are likely to be involved in the thrombotic events that herald the onset of acute myocardial infarction. It is now appreciated that several modified forms of lipoproteins, especially oxidized lipoproteins, are involved in many of the biologic events associated with atherogenesis. Therefore, the effect of the diabetic state on lipoprotein modification might be an important cause of the increased atherosclerotic risk associated with diabetes. This chapter reviews potentially atherogenic changes in lipid and lipoproteins in diabetes and describes how their interaction with the artery wall might account for the increased atherosclerotic risk associated with this disorder. It also reviews currently available therapeutic approaches that might interfere with these atherogenic processes and outlines directions for future research that are likely to provide additional insights into the pathogenesis and management of the accelerated atherosclerosis associated with diabetes.

Lipids and Atherosclerosis

Epidemiologic studies have demonstrated a consistent and strong association between plasma cholesterol levels and atherosclerosis risk[5,6] that presumably is due to low-density lipoprotein (LDL), which is the major determinant of plasma cholesterol levels. Conversely, high-density lipoprotein (HDL) cholesterol levels are inversely associated with cardiovascular risk.[7] Some forms of hypertriglyceridemia, especially when associated with small, dense very low-density lipoproteins (VLDLs), are associated with increased cardiovascular risk, whereas hypertriglyceridemia associated with larger VLDL particles is not.[8,9] Thus, hypertriglyceridemia seen in familial combined hyperlipidemia, IDDM, NIDDM, and the insulin resistance syndrome, and chronic renal disease may be associated with increased cardiovascular risk, whereas hypertriglyceridemia caused by some forms of familial hypertriglyceridemia, ethanol, bile acid binding therapy, high carbohydrate diets, and estrogen may not be associated with increased risk. In those disorders associated with increased atherosclerotic risk, the hypertriglyceridemia is probably a marker of other lipoprotein abnormalities, such as the presence of increased levels of LDL, small, dense LDL, low HDL levels, or accumulation of remnant lipoproteins. Remnants of the triglyceride-rich lipoproteins have themselves been implicated as cardiovascular risk factors,[10] although the mechanism by which they exert their atherogenic effect is not known. Although some recent studies have suggested that Lp(a) is not an independent cardiovascular risk factor,[11,12] most studies in which the plasma has been correctly stored have shown it to be an important indicator of increased premature cardiovascular disease risk.[13–15]

Mechanisms by Which Lipids Are Involved in Atherogenesis

Lipids and lipoproteins appear to be involved at all phases of atherogenesis. The earliest lesion of atherosclerosis is the *fatty streak,* which consists of macrophages loaded with cholesterol derived from lipoproteins that have entered the subendothelial space by transcytosis. Macrophages in culture do not accumulate cholesterol after exposure to unmodified LDL because of down-regulation of the LDL receptor under conditions of cholesterol excess. However, macrophages accumulate cholesterol after uptake of modified forms of LDL via the scavenger receptor, which is not regulated by cell cholesterol content.[16] The most likely contender for a naturally occurring lipoprotein that results in delivery of cholesterol to macrophages via the scavenger receptor is oxidized LDL[17] (see later on), although VLDL[18] and Lp(a)[19] also can undergo oxidative modification. Oxidized LDL also affects several other processes involved in the recruitment, activation, and maturation of macrophages (see later on), thereby playing a major role in the early phases of atherogenesis. β-VLDL, a lipoprotein formed in response to a diet high in fat and cholesterol,[20] also is taken up by and leads to cholesterol accumulation in macrophages.[21]

During the progression from a fatty streak to a *fibrofatty plaque,* smooth muscle cells migrate from the media to the intima, where they undergo proliferation in response to a number of cytokines and growth factors.[22] Lipoproteins modulate the expression of several growth factors and therefore influence this stage of atherogenesis as well. Lipoprotein-derived cholesterol also accumulates in arterial smooth muscle cells by mechanisms that are not well understood. Smooth muscle cells usually do not express scavenger receptors[23] but can accumulate lipid in the absence of functional LDL receptors (e.g., in homozygous familial hypercholesterolemia). Uptake may be mediated by interaction with cell surface proteoglycans,[24] by selective uptake from lipoprotein,[25] or by direct translocation of unesterified cholesterol from lipoproteins to the surface of arterial smooth muscle cells.[26] Lipoproteins also accumulate extracellularly in association with matrix molecules to which apo B- and E-containing lipoproteins and Lp(a) bind with high affinity.[27] The accumulation of a large mass of extracellular matrix and fibrous tissue is another hallmark of the fibrofatty lesion. It, too, may be influenced by lipids and lipoproteins, since the secretion of proteoglycans by arterial smooth muscle cells can be modulated by their exposure to lipoproteins.[28] Thus, lipoproteins containing apo B and E can be involved in the pathogenesis of many of the features of the atherosclerotic plaque.

The accumulation of cholesterol represents the net balance between uptake and removal of cholesterol, a process that involves HDL. Binding of HDL to cell surface-binding sites triggers the translocation of cholesterol from intracellular pools to the cell surface, from where it can be removed by acceptor particles such as HDL itself.[29] HDL-binding sites on the cell surface increase in response to accumulation of cholesterol,[30] providing a mechanism for the cell to rid itself of excess cholesterol. The cholesterol then is esterified, transferred to lower density lipoproteins, and transported to the liver from where it can be excreted, in a process known as reverse cholesterol transport. Thus HDL particles can facilitate the removal of excess cholesterol from cells of the artery wall, thereby exerting an antiatherogenic effect.

Lp(a) is a lipoprotein that consists of an LDL particle in disulfide linkage with apo (a), a protein that has considerable sequence homology with plasminogen without its protease function.[31] Lp(a) can undergo oxidative modification,[19] bind to extracellular matrix,[32] and be taken up by macrophages, although the receptor involved in the mechanism of uptake is not clear.[33] Therefore, Lp(a) can deliver cholesterol to the artery wall and be atherogenic. Because it competes with plasminogen for binding sites but does not cause thrombolysis, Lp(a) is thrombogenic as well,[34] which probably accounts for the markedly increased atherosclerotic risk associated with elevated levels of this lipoprotein. In addition to Lp(a), an increased tendency to thrombosis has been demonstrated in association with hypertriglyceridemia.[35]

Plaques tend to undergo necrosis and fissure, followed by hemorrhage into the plaque.[36] These events can lead to plaque rupture and intravascular thrombosis, which is the event that immediately precedes a myocardial infarction. Features of the unstable plaque, which is prone to rupture and thrombosis, include the presence of a large lipid core, lipid-filled macrophages at the shoulder of the lesion, and a thin fibrous cap.[37]

Oxidized Low-Density Lipoproteins and Other Modified Lipoproteins

As alluded to earlier, it is believed that lipoproteins often undergo modification prior to their interacting adversely with arterial wall cells and matrix. Alterations such as oxidative modification are likely to occur in the milieu of the artery wall rather than in the plasma and therefore are difficult to detect. LDL can be oxidized by endothelial cells, smooth muscle cells, and macrophages[38,39] by several mechanisms that require the presence of transitional metals,[40] including the generation of superoxide[41,42] and via lipoxygenases.[43] Monocyte-macrophages also can oxidatively modify LDL by myeloperoxidase, which does not require transition metals.[44] Oxidized LDL can affect many biologic processes involved in atherogenesis,[38,39] including the adhesion and chemotaxis of monocytes to endothelial cells, activation and differentiation of monocyte-macrophages by colony-stimulating factors, modulation of cytokine and growth factor expression, uptake by macrophage scavenger receptors leading to foam cell formation, cytotoxicity, vasoreactivity, thrombosis by stimulating the expression of tissue factor and plasminogen activator inhibitor-1, and metalloprotease expression.

Epitopes, using antibodies generated against oxidized LDL, have been demonstrated in atherosclerotic lesions from experimental animals and humans.[45,46] Lipoproteins with many properties of oxidized LDL have been eluted from the artery wall,[47] and circulating autoantibodies against oxidized LDL have been found.[47] These observations suggest that oxidatively modified forms of lipoproteins exist in vivo and play a role in atherogenesis. Perhaps the most compelling evidence that oxidized lipoproteins are atherogenic is from studies that demonstrate that both lipoprotein oxidation and atherosclerosis can be inhibited by a number of antioxidants in several animal species.[48] Thus, a role for oxidized LDL in atherogenesis is plausible, likely, and amenable to therapy. However, because lipoprotein oxidation occurs in the interstitial space rather than in the vascular compartment, detection of oxidized forms of lipoproteins must be achieved by indirect measures,[49] such as evaluation of the susceptibility of LDL to oxidation mediated by a controlled oxidative stress ex vivo.[50]

Lipids and Diabetes

Epidemiology

Hyperlipidemia, especially hypertriglyceridemia, occurs frequently in diabetes mellitus, although the prevalence varies in different studies, in part because of the criteria used to define hyperlipidemia and in part because of differences in selection criteria. Population-based studies that obviate selection biases have shown that hypertriglyceridemia is commonly observed, independent of age and relative body weight,[51] whereas total plasma cholesterol levels are not elevated. However, despite normal LDL cholesterol levels in NIDDM, VLDL cholesterol levels are elevated and HDL cholesterol levels are decreased.[52] Elevated LDL has been noted occasionally, although most studies still report LDL as d=1.006–1.063 g/mL, which includes intermediate density lipoproteins (IDL) composed largely of remnants of triglyceride-rich lipoprotein catabolism. When ILD (d=1.006–1.019 g/mL) has been separated from LDL (d=1.019–1.063 g/mL), most of the elevation in "LDL" in NIDDM is caused by an increase in IDL.[53] HDL cholesterol levels tend to be normal or even increased in treated patients with IDDM[54] and are low in patients with NIDDM.[55]

Hypertriglyceridemia appears to be associated with an increased cadiovascular risk in diabetes. In the large WHO Multinational Study of Vascular Disease in Diabetes, ischemic heart disease was more strongly associated with plasma triglyceride levels than with cholesterol.[2] Similar results have been obtained in other studies.[56–59]

Insulin-Dependent Diabetes Mellitus

Hypertriglyceridemia caused by increased levels of VLDL occurs commonly in untreated IDDM.[60–62] Persistent hypertriglyceridemia[62,63] and low HDL levels also are associated with poor glycemic control.[62,64] Triglyceride levels fall with improved glycemic control, especially when blood glucose levels are normalized by the use of continuous subcutaneous insulin injections or with multiple insulin injections.[65–70] HDL cholesterol levels also improve with treatment[67,71] and are normal[71] or even elevated[54] in treated IDDM patients. They did not change in the Diabetes Control and Complications Trial (DCCT), possibly because most subjects gained weight during intensive therapy[72] and weight gain leads to a reduction in HDL cholesterol.[73] Although LDL cholesterol levels usually are in the normal range in IDDM,[74] they nonetheless fall in response to intensive insulinization.[66,67,72] Studies in children who embarked on a multistage program of intensification of insulin therapy suggest that greater metabolic improvement occurs after early routine therapeutic measures than after intensification of therapy.[75] Recent detailed evaluation of the lipids and lipoproteins in subjects participating in the DCCT showed that the decrease in "LDL" levels was due to a reduction in Lp(a), a decrease in IDL, and a shift from dense LDL to more buoyant particles.[76] Thus, subtle compositional changes that are likely to be beneficial are obscured by the simple measurement of "LDL cholesterol."

The hypertriglyceridemia seen with the initial presentation of IDDM is caused by decreased adipose tissue lipoprotein lipase activity,[77–79] which is restored to normal within 3 months of the onset of therapy.[77,79] Lipoprotein lipase activity also is reduced in IDDM patients with ketonuria without ketoacidosis[80] but is normal in most chronically treated IDDM patients and is not related to the degree of glycemic control.[79] The improvement in triglyceride levels seen with intensive insulin therapy is attributable to decreased secretion of VLDL[71,82] rather than to improved removal of triglycerides from plasma. Similarly, the reduction in LDL levels seen with intensive therapy is caused by decreased production of LDL.[83] The reduced HDL cholesterol in untreated IDDM is in part because of replacement of cholesterol in the core of HDL by triglycerides and in part because of increased catabolism of HDL associated with impaired lipoprotein lipase activity.[84] These abnormalities normalize with therapy. The increased levels of HDL cholesterol observed in some studies may be related to relatively low body weights in some IDDM subjects.[85] In summary, in IDDM, the major abnormality of plasma lipoproteins is an increased level of VLDL, and all lipoprotein abnormalities improve with good glycemic control.

Non–Insulin-Dependent Diabetes Mellitus

The effect of NIDDM on lipids and lipoproteins is more difficult to ascertain because of the heterogeneity of therapy for diabetes, the impact of glycemic control, the confounding effect of obesity, the use of other medications for associated disorders, and the effect of complications (see later on), which often are present in this disorder.

Patients with NIDDM who have never received insulin or oral sulfonylureas frequently are hypertriglyceridemic and have low levels of HDL cholesterol.[55,86,87] Their plasma triglyceride levels are inversely related to the extent of glycemic control,[88,89] especially when the effects of relative body weight are considered. Commencement of therapy with either insulin or oral sulfonylureas leads to a reduction in VLDL levels and an increase in HDL cholesterol despite the weight gain that often accompanies the initiation of therapy.[55,87] The effect of initiation of therapy is far greater than improving glycemic control in previously treated patients.[55,87]

Hypertriglyceridemia and decreased HDL levels often persist in NIDDM despite treatment[90–92] and appear to be independent of the degree of glycemic control.[93] These residual abnormalities have been termed "diabetic dyslipidemia" and include the presence of small, dense LDL particles,[94] accumulation of remnants of the triglyceride-rich lipoproteins, and abnormalities in the composition of HDL.[95]

The hypertriglyceridemia seen in mild to moderately hyperglycemic NIDDM subjects not receiving insulin or oral agents is mainly the result of an increase in VLDL secretion,[96–99] although, VLDL catabolism may be impaired simultaneously[100] despite normal levels of lipoprotein lipase.[101] Lipoprotein lipase activity is decreased, however, in the more severely hyperglycemic untreated patient with NIDDM,[77–79,89] in whom greater relative insulin deficiency accompanies the insulin resistance. However, VLDL oversecretion may occur concomitantly. Therapy, whether with insulin or oral hyperglycemic agents, leads to a correction of the lipoprotein lipase defect after several weeks to months,[79,89,92] with a parallel reduction in plasma triglyceride levels. Chronically treated patients with NIDDM have normal lipoprotein lipase levels, which are unrelated to the extent of glycemic control.[79] Residual hypertriglyceridemia appears to be the result of VLDL oversecretion.[79]

Remnants of the triglyceride-rich lipoproteins also are increased in NIDDM. In studies in which IDL (d=1.006–1.019 g/mL) has been measured separately from LDL (d=1.019–1.063 g/mL), the remnant-rich IDL levels are increased, whereas true LDL levels are normal.[53,102–104] VLDL also are enriched in the ratio of cholesterol/triglycerides,[105–107] suggesting that they, too, are enriched in remnant lipoproteins, which are believed to impart an increased risk of atherosclerosis.[9,10]

LDL metabolism also is disturbed in NIDDM. With mild untreated NIDDM, LDL synthesis and removal rates are increased concomitantly, resulting in normal LDL cholesterol levels.[108] In untreated or poorly controlled moderately hyperglycemic patients, impaired LDL catabolism can lead to mildly elevated LDL levels.[108,109]

HDL cholesterol levels are decreased in NIDDM[55,86,110] and increase with weight loss,[111,112] and administration of insulin [55,113] and oral sulfonylureas.[78,114] As with IDDM, this can in part be accounted for by a replacement of cholesterol in the core of HDL by triglycerides from hypertriglyceridemia that is present. HDL cholesterol levels rise if triglycerides levels fall during treatment owing to a reversal of this effect. HDL levels also may increase during therapy as a result of improved catabolism of VLDL, with transfer of surface components of VLDL catabolism to HDL.[110]

Insulin Resistance Syndrome and Dyslipidemia in the Treated NIDDM Patient

Insulin resistance is a feature of NIDDM but also occurs in individuals with normal blood glucose levels. In both situations there is a clustering of cardiovascular risk factors and a markedly increased risk of cardiovascular disease.[115,116] These risk factors include dyslipidemia (consisting of hypertriglyceridemia, low HDL, accumulation of remnant lipoproteins, and the presence of small, dense, cholesterol-depleted LDL particles), hypertension, impaired glucose tolerance, increased levels of fibrinogen, and decreased levels of plasminogen-activator inhibitor-1.[117] This constellation of findings has been termed syndrome X.[117] The hallmark of this syndrome is the presence of a central, especially visceral, distribution of body fat,[118,119] which can be detected by computed tomography of the abdomen.[120]

The cause of this syndrome is under intense investigation. One hypothesis is that the primary defect is insulin resistance, although the cause and nature of the defect are unknown. Alternatively, the hyperinsulinemia may be secondary to the visceral adiposity. The compensatory hyperinsulinemia that results in either case is believed to lead to all the other features of the syndrome, including the dyslipidemia. The increased secretion of VLDL apo B is believed to be related to an increased portal flux of free fatty acids, which also stimulates hepatic lipase activity.[121] This, in turn, leads to the formation of small, dense LDL particles.[122]

Lp(a)

There has been considerable recent interest in the effect of diabetes on Lp(a) levels because of the potential importance of Lp(a) as a cardiovascular risk factor.[13–15] Lp(a) levels have been reported to be increased in IDDM and to improve with improved glycemic control.[123] In the DCCT, Lp(a) levels were slightly higher in the conventional therapy than in the intensively treated group,[76] suggesting that levels may in part be influenced by glycemic control. Opinions differ as to whether Lp(a) levels are increased in uncomplicated NIDDM,[123] although the onset of diabetic nephropathy or even microalbuminuria[123,124] has been reported to be associated with increased levels of this lipoprotein. Clearly, further studies are required to ascertain the effect of diabetes and its complications on Lp(a) levels and the role of Lp(a) in the macrovascular disease associated with diabetes.

Effect of Complications

The major complication of diabetes that affects lipoproteins is renal disease. Microalbuminuric diabetic subjects with normal renal function have higher triglyceride and apo B levels than do subjects without microalbuminuria.[125] Intermediate levels of albuminuria are associated with further increases in apo B levels and a markedly increased risk of cardiovascular disease in IDDM.[126] With the development of marked proteinuria and the nephrotic syndrome, both VLDL and LDL levels become markedly increased,[127,128] similar to what is seen in nephrotic patients without diabetes. Similarly, hypertriglyceridemia and low HDL cholesterol levels are typical of both diabetic and nondiabetic patients with end-stage renal disease.[127–129] Dialysis is associated with elevations in VLDL and IDL levels and with a decrease in true LDL (d=1.1019–1.063 g/mL) and HDL levels. After renal transplantation, the increase in both VLDL and LDL levels appears to be related to the use of cyclosporine and prednisone for immunosuppression.[127,130]

Patients with IDDM have an increased incidence of autoimmune thyroid disease. Untreated hypothyroidism can lead to increases in both LDL and VLDL and their remnants,[127,131] which return to normal with thyroid replacement therapy.[131] There is an increased prevalence of hypertension in both IDDM and NIDDM. Some drugs used to treat hypertension, especially diuretic and β-adrenergic blocking agents, can adversely affect plasma lipids and lipoproteins.[132,133]

The Chylomicronemia Syndrome

The chylomicronemia syndrome occurs when plasma triglyceride levels exceed 2000 mg/dL[134] and is characterized by a constellation of signs and symptoms that includes eruptive xanthomata, abdominal pain and pancreatitis, lipemia retinalis, reversible memory loss, and dysesthesias.[134] The most common cause of severe hypertriglyceridemia of this magnitude is the coexistence of undiagnosed or untreated NIDDM with a genetic form of hypertriglyceridemia such as familial combined hyperlipidemia or familial hypertriglyceridemia.[127,134] Although marked hypertriglyceridemia has been described in IDDM,[135] it is likely also to represent the interaction of diabetes with a genetic form of hypertriglyceridemia and is much less commonly seen than in NIDDM, probably because of the different approach to treatment in the two disorders. Very high triglyceride levels are the result of saturation of lipoprotein lipase-mediated triglyceride removal by the combined genetic disorder and oversecretion of VLDL as a result of NIDDM.[136] Impaired lipoprotein lipase activity secondary to severe insulin deficiency, either relative in NIDDM or absolute in IDDM (see earlier NIDDM section), can further reduce triglyceride removal from plasma. As a result of saturation of triglyceride removal systems, chylomicrons accumulate in addition to VLDL.

Modified Lipoproteins and Diabetes

Diabetes can lead to several modifications of lipoproteins that can affect their interactions with cells of the artery wall and thereby contribute to the increased risk of atherosclerosis associated with diabetes. The two lipoprotein modifications that are likely to be common in both IDDM and NIDDM are oxidation and glycation. Formation of lipoprotein immune complexes and compositional changes that alter cell interactions also may occur in both types of diabetes.

Oxidized Lipoproteins

Evidence is accruing that oxidative stress, that is, an imbalance between the generation of free radicals and antioxidant defenses, is increased in diabetes.[137,138] Glucose autoxidation[139] and glycation of proteins[140] lead to the generation of oxygen-free radicals that can enhance the oxidation of LDL.[141–143] Antioxidant defenses also are reduced in both IDDM[143] and NIDDM.[144] These include reduced levels of vitamin C[145,146] and uric acid,[143] which play a role in protecting lipoproteins from oxidative modification. Since the oxidation of lipoproteins is believed to occur in the interstitial space rather than in the circulation, indirect measures have been used to evaluate this process in diabetes. Thus, LDL isolated from subjects with poorly controlled IDDM[143] and NIDDM[144] is more susceptible to oxidative modification than LDL from control subjects without diabetes. Further, the small, dense LDL that is characteristic of NIDDM and the insulin-resistant state (see earlier) also undergoes oxidation more readily than does more buoyant LDL.[147] Even though lipoprotein oxidation is believed to occur extravascularly, some studies in diabetic animal models[148] and humans with diabetes[149,150] suggest that circulating lipoproteins show evidence of increased oxidation, although the methods used for these studies are rather nonspecific. Further evidence for the occurrence of lipoprotein oxidation in vivo is the finding of circulating autoantibodies against oxidized LDL[47] (see later on). The postulated role of oxidized lipoproteins in atherogenesis was described earlier.

Glycated Lipoproteins, Including the Formation of LDL with Advanced Glycosylation End-Products

Another modification of lipoproteins that is common to both IDDM and NIDDM and that is related to the extent of chronic glycemic control is nonenzymatic glycation. Glycation of the apolipoproteins in all classes of circulating lipoproteins has been found in diabetes.[151] Approximately 2–5% of apo B in the plasma of subjects with diabetes is glycated compared with about 1% in plasma from nondiabetic control subjects.[152] Increased glycation of the circulating C apolipoproteins probably is a reflection of their increased residence time in plasma relative to VLDL and HDL, between which they shuttle. Advanced glycation end-products (AGE) have recently been reported to be associated with LDL[153] with modification of amino groups on both proteins and phospholipids.[154] This observation suggests that the formation of AGE may occur more rapidly than previously believed, or that AGE-LDL can enter plasma from extravascular tissues such as the artery wall. As with oxidized LDL, circulating autoantibodies that react with glycated LDL have been demonstrated in some patients with diabetes.[155]

Glycated LDL interacts poorly with the LDL receptor,[152] thereby increasing its residence time in plasma[156] and presumably the extracellular space of the artery wall where oxidative modification can occur. Some studies also suggest that glycated LDL has increased susceptibility to oxidative modification.[157] Glycated HDL has impaired ability to stimulate cholesterol efflux from cells.[158] AGE proteins bind to specific receptors on macrophages and other cell types[159] and can stimulate the release of cytokines and growth factors,[160] which may play a role in atherogenesis.

Immune Complexes and Aggregates

Phagocytosis of aggregated lipoproteins by an LDL receptor-mediated mechanism can lead to massive lipid accumulation and foam cell formation in macrophages.[161] Oxidation of LDL increases the propensity of this lipoprotein to aggregate.[162,163] Lipoprotein immune complexes, for example with antibodies against oxidized or glycated LDL, also can lead to the formation of foam cells after phagocytosis by Fc receptors on macrophages.[164,165] Both of these processes could be increased in diabetes. Both lipoprotein aggregates[166] and lipoprotein immune complexes[167] have been observed in atherosclerotic lesions.

Compositional Changes, Including Small, Dense Low-Density Lipoprotein and Surface Cholesterol Enrichment

Several changes in the composition of lipoproteins that might alter their interactions with cells have been described in diabetes. Diabetes is associated with a relative increase in the ratio of unesterified cholesterol to phospholipid in all lipoprotein classes,[168] which improves but nonetheless persists with intensive insulin therapy.[169,170] These changes in the surface of the lipoprotein particle favor a net flux of cholesterol from lipoproteins to cells rather than in the opposite direction.[171] As discussed earlier, NIDDM and insulin-resistant states are characterized by the presence of small, dense LDL, which are susceptible to oxidative modification[147] and its consequences. Small, dense LDL also binds more avidly to proteoglycans than does more buoyant LDL.[172] This may increase its retention on extracellular matrix, where it can undergo oxidation and glycation. Finally, the triglyceride-rich lipoproteins may become enriched with apo E in diabetes.[173] This may in part account for increased uptake of the triglyceride-rich lipoproteins and their remnants in diabetes, which would favor foam cell formation. Thus, several subtle changes in lipoprotein composition can occur in diabetes, all of which can interfere with the interaction of these lipoproteins with cells and which may be factors in increasing the propensity to atherosclerosis in diabetics.

Approach to Management

Although our understanding of the relationship of lipoproteins to atherosclerosis is not complete, several things can be done at present that are likely to reduce the risk of atherosclerosis in diabetes. These include giving attention to all known cardiovascular risk factors, including lipids. Patients with diabetes should not smoke, and hypertension should be treated early, especially with angiotensin-converting enzyme inhibitors.[174] The guidelines of the Adult Treatment Panel of the National Cholesterol Education Program[175] can be applied to patients with both IDDM and NIDDM who often require both diet and drug treatment of their hyperlipidemia because of borderline high levels of LDL in the presence of two or more net other risk factors or because of the presence of established atherosclerotic disease.

The low saturated fat and low cholesterol diet recommended for treatment of hyperlipidemic patients without diabetes is appropriate for most diabetic patients. Triglyceride levels can increase in some patients when carbohydrates replace fat in the diet.[176] This carbohydrate induction of hypertriglyceridemia often is transient[177] and may be reduced by a gradual change in the diet.[178] When central obesity accompanies diabetes, as it so often does in NIDDM, therapy should include a decrease in calories from fat and an exercise program aimed at weight control. Triglyceride levels tend to fall with weight reduction.

Lipid-lowering drug therapy for the patient with diabetes is similar to that in the nondiabetic patient. However, the presence of hypertriglyceridemia is a relative contraindication to the use of bile acid-binding resins. Also, nicotinic acid increases insulin resistance and therefore is difficult to use in diabetes. Its use in patients with IDDM often requires an increase in the dose of insulin. Worsening glycemic control in NIDDM often precludes its use. The initial drug of choice usually is a reductase inhibitor or a fibric acid derivative, depending on whether the major abnormality is an increase in cholesterol or triglycerides. Triglyceride levels often do not return to normal with a reductase inhibitor,[179] and LDL levels often increase when triglyceride levels fall during treatment with a fibric acid derivative.[180] Therefore, the combination of a reductase inhibitor with a fibrate may be required. This combination should be used with caution because of the increased risk of myopathy, especially in the presence of renal disease.

Management of the chylomicronemia syndrome is undertaken mainly to prevent pancreatitis. Therapy includes treatment of the diabetes by whatever means is otherwise indicated but usually also requires the use of a specific lipid-lowering agent such as a fibric acid derivative (gemfibrozil, clofibrate, fenofibrate, or bezofibrate) to control the markedly elevated plasma triglyceride levels.[134] Secondary forms of hypertriglyceridemia other than diabetes that may be contributing to the marked hypertriglyceridemia should be sought and treated in their own right. Drugs that increase triglycerides, especially β-blocking agents, diuretics, estrogens, and glucocorticoids should be avoided, as should the use of ethanol.[127] Although triglyceride levels fall with weight loss, the loss of more than a few pounds of weight is discouraged in this disorder, since triglyceride levels increase, sometimes dramatically, when weight is regained, as is usually the case.

Future Directions

A better understanding of the mechanisms whereby the dyslipidemia associated with diabetes so dramatically increases atherosclerosis risk should ultimately lead to a more rational approach to therapy. Several lines of investigation should provide additional therapeutic insights in the near future. For example, the question of whether tight glycemic control results in a reduction of atherosclerosis risk, as suggested by the DCCT study,[72] needs to be carefully addressed, especially in NIDDM. The weight gain that is likely to accompany tight glycemic control[181] in this disorder may increase central obesity and the risk factors associated with it, such as dyslipidemia and hypertension, which may offset any potentially beneficial effects of reduced blood glucose levels and glycated proteins, including lipoproteins. Studies that use multiple approaches, including lipid-lowering therapy, to intervene in the multiple risk factors present in NIDDM and the insulin resistance syndrome need to be performed. The role of antioxidants, both dietary and pharmacologic, in the prevention of atherosclerosis needs to be formally evaluated by placebo-controlled clinical trials. Because of the increased oxidant stress that occurs in diabetes, it is an ideal situation to test the effect of antioxidants on atherosclerosis prevention. Finally, the effect on atherosclerosis of aminoguanidine, which inhibits the formation of advanced glycation endproducts,[182] needs to be tested. The effect of reduced glycation of the extracellular matrix of the artery wall might alter the interaction of lipoproteins with the matrix, thereby reducing their retention in the artery wall where they are able to exert their atherogenic damage. Although the significance of AGE-LDL is not yet known, aminoguanidine should reduce the amount of this modified form of lipoproteins as well. Thus, advances in the foreseeable future should provide further valuable information about (1) the mechanism by which abnormalities of lipoprotein composition and metabolism lead to increased atherosclerosis in diabetes, and (2) therapeutic approaches to prevent the very high incidence of macrovascular complications in diabetes.

References

1. Krolewski AS, Kosinski EJ, Warram JH, et al. Magnitude and determinants of coronary artery disease in juvenile-onset, insulin-dependent diabetes mellitus. Am J Cardiol 1987;59:750
2. West KM, Ahuja MMS, Bennett PH, et al. The role of circulating glucose and triglyceride concentrations and their interactions with other ''risk factors'' as determinants of arterial disease in nine diabetic population samples from the WHO multinational study. Diabetes Care 1983;6:361
3. Jarrett RJ. Risk factors for coronary heart disease in diabetes mellitus. Diabetes 1992;41:1
4. Brunzell JD, Chait A. Diabetic dyslipidemia—pathology and treatment. In: Rifkin H and Porte D Jr, eds. Ellenberg and Rifkin's Diabetes Mellitus, 5th ed. New York: Elsevier; in press
5. Tyroler HA. Serum lipoproteins as risk factors: Recent epidemiological studies in individuals with and without cardiovascular disease. Eur Heart J 1990;11:21
6. Kannel WB, Neaton JD, Wentworth D, et al. Overall and coronary heart disease mortality rates in relation to major risk factors in 325,348 men screened for the MRFIT. Multiple Risk Factor Intervention Trial. Am Heart J 1986;112:825
7. Jacobs DR Jr, Mebane IL, Bangdiwala SI, et al. High density lipoprotein cholesterol as a predictor of cardiovascular disease mortality in men and women: The follow-up study of the Lipid Research Clinics Prevalence Study. Am J Epidemiol 1990;131:32
8. Brunzell JD, Albers JJ, Chait A, et al. Plasma lipoproteins in familial combined hyperlipidemia and monogenic familial hypertriglyceridemia. J Lipid Res 1983;24:147
9. Brunzell JD, Schrott HG, Motulsky AG, Bierman EL. Myocardial infarction in the familial forms of hypertriglyceridemia. Metabolism 1976;25:313
10. Zilversmit DB. Atherogenic nature of triglycerides, postprandial lipidemia, and triglyceride-rich remnant lipoproteins. Clin Chem 1995;41:153
11. Ridker PM, Hennekens CH, Stampfer MJ. A prospective study of lipoprotein (a) and the risk of myocardial infarction. JAMA 1993;270:2195
12. Jauhiainen M, Koskinen P, Ehnholm C, et al. Lipoprotein (a) and coronary heart disease risk: A nested case-control study of the Helsinki Heart Study participants. Atherosclerosis 1991;89:59
13. Rosengren A, Wilhelmsen L, Ericksson E, et al. Lipoprotein (a) and coronary heart disease: A prospective case-control study in a general population of middle aged men. Br Med J 1990;301:1248
14. Schaefer EJ, Lamon-Fava S, Jenner JL, et al. Lipoprotein(a) levels and risk of coronary heart disease in men. The Lipid Research Clinics Coronary Primary Prevention Trial. JAMA 1994;271:999
15. Sigurdsson G, Baldursdottir A, Sigvaldason H, et al. Predictive value of apolipoproteins in a prospective survey of coronary artery disease in men. Am J Cardiol 1992;69:1251
16. Brown MS, Goldstein JL. Lipoprotein metabolism in the macrophage: Implications for cholesterol deposition in atherosclerosis. Annu Rev Biochem 1983;52:223
17. Henriksen T, Mahoney EM, Steinberg D. Enhanced macrophage degradation of low density lipoprotein previously incubated with cultured endothelial cells. Recognition by receptors for acetylated low density lipoproteins. Proc Natl Acad Sci USA 1981;78:6499
18. Morh D, Stocker R. Radical-mediated oxidation of isolated human very-low-density lipoprotein. Arterioscler Thromb 1994;4:1186
19. Naruszewicz M, Selinger E, Davignon J. Oxidative modification of lipoprotein(a) and the effect of beta-carotene. Metabolism 1992;41:1215
20. Mahley RW. Atherogenic hyperlipoproteinemia. The cellular and molecular biology of plasma lipoproteins altered by dietary fat and cholesterol. Med Clin North Am 1982;66:375
21. Mahley RW, Innerarity TL, Brown MS, et al. Cholesteryl ester synthesis in macrophages: Stimulation of beta–very low density lipoproteins from cholesterol-fed animals of several species. J Lipid Res 1980;21:970
22. Ross R. The pathogenesis of atherosclerosis: A perspective for the 1990s. Nature 1993;362:801
23. Pitas RE. Expression of the acetyl low density lipoprotein receptor by rabbit fibroblast and smooth muscle cells. Up-regulation by phorbol esters. J Biol Chem 1990;265:12722
24. Saxena U, Klein MG, Goldberg IJ. Metabolism of endothelial cell-bound lipoprotein lipase. Evidence for heparan sulfate proteoglycan-mediated internalization and recycling. J Biol Chem 1990;265:12880
25. Rinninger F, Jaeckle S, Pittman RC. A pool of reversibly cell-associated cholesteryl esters involved in the selective uptake of cholesteryl esters from high-density lipoproteins by Hep G2 hepatoma cells. Biochim Biophys Acta 1993;1166:275
26. Slotte JP, Chait A, Bierman EL. Cholesterol accumulation in aortic smooth muscle cells exposed to low density lipoproteins: Contribution of free cholesterol transfer. Arteriosclerosis 1988;8:750
27. Camejo G, Camejo EH, Olsson U, Bondjers G. Proteoglycans and lipoproteins in atherosclerosis. Curr Opin Lipidol 1993;4:385
28. McManus BM, Malcom G, Kendall TJ, et al. Lipid overload and proteoglycan expression in chronic rejection of the human transplanted heart. Clin Transplant 1994;8:336
29. Oram JF, Mendez AJ, Slotte JP, Johnson TF. High density lipoprotein apolipoproteins mediate removal of sterol from intracellular pools but not from plasma membranes of cholesterol-loaded fibroblasts. Arterioscler Thromb 1991;11:403
30. Oram JF, Brinton EA, Bierman EL. Regulation of HDL receptor activity in cultured human skin fibroblasts and human arterial smooth muscle cells. J Clin Invest 1983;72:1611
31. Scanu AM. Lipoprotein (a): A potential bridge between the fields of atherosclerosis and thrombosis. Arch Pathol Lab Med 1988;112:1045
32. Kostner GM, Bihari-Varga M. Is the atherogenicity of Lp(a) caused by its reactivity with proteoglycans? Eur Heart J 1990;11:184
33. Bottalico LA, Keesler GA, Fless GM, Tabas I. Cholesterol loading of macrophages leads to marked enhancement of native lipoprotein (a) and apoprotein (a) internalization and degradation. J Biol Chem 1993;268:8569
34. Loscalzo J. Lipoprotein (a): A unique risk factor for atherothrombotic disease. Arteriosclerosis 1990;10:672
35. Miller GJ. Lipoproteins and the haemostatic system in atherothrombotic disorders. Baillières Clin Haematol 1994;7:713
36. Davies MJ, Woolf N, Katz DR. The role of endothelial denudation injury, plaque fissuring, and thrombosis in the progression of human atherosclerosis. Atherosclerosis Rev 1991;23:105
37. Davies MJ, Richardson PD, Woolf N, et al. Risk of thrombosis in human atherosclerotic plaques: Role of extracellular lipid, macrophage, and smooth muscle cell content. Br Heart J 1993;69:377
38. Witztum JL, Steinberg D. Role of oxidized low density lipoprotein in atherogenesis. J Clin Invest 1991;88:1785
39. Chait A, Heinecke JW. Lipoprotein modification: Cellular mechanisms. Curr Opin Lipidol 1994;5:365
40. Heinecke JW, Rosen H, Chait A. Iron and copper promote modification of low density lipoprotein by human arterial smooth muscle cells. J Clin Invest 1984;74:1890
41. Heinecke JW, Baker L, Rosen H, Chait A. Superoxide-mediated free radical modification of low density lipoprotein by arterial smooth muscle cells. J Clin Invest 1986;77:757

42. Steinbrecher UP. Role of superoxide in endothelial-cell modification of low density lipoproteins. Biochim Biophys Acta 1988;959:20
43. Sparrow CP, Parthasarathy S, Steinberg D. Enzymatic modification of low density lipoprotein by purified lipoxygenase plus phospholipase A2 mimics cell-mediated oxidative modification. J Lipid Res 1988;29:745
44. Heinecke JW, Li W, Francis GA, Goldstein JA. Tyrosyl radical generated by myeloperoxidase catalyzes the oxidative crosslinking of proteins. J Clin Invest 1993;91:2866
45. Boyd HC, Gown AM, Wolfbauer G, Chait A. Direct evidence for a protein recognized by a monoclonal antibody against oxidatively-modified low density lipoprotein in atherosclerotic lesions from a Watanabe heritable hyperlipidemic rabbit. Am J Pathol 1989;35:815
46. Rosenfeld ME, Palinski W, Ylä-Herttuala S, et al. Distribution of oxidation specific lipid-protein adducts and apolipoprotein B in atherosclerotic lesions of varying severity from WHHL rabbits. Arteriosclerosis 1990;10:336
47. Palinski W, Rosenfeld ME, Ylä-Herttuala S, et al. Low density lipoprotein undergoes oxidative modification in vivo. Proc Natl Acad Sci USA 1989; 86:1372
48. Steinberg D. Antioxidants in the prevention of human atherosclerosis. Summary of the Proceedings of a National Heart, Lung, and Blood Institute Workshop: September 5–6, 1991, Bethesda, MD. Circulation 1992;85:2337
49. Chait A. Methods for assessing lipid and lipoprotein oxidation. Curr Opin Lipidol 1992;3:389
50. Esterbauer H, Striegl G, Puhl H, Rotheneder M. Continuous monitoring of in vitro oxidation of human low density lipoprotein. Free Radic Res Commun 1989;6:67
51. Barrett-Connor E, Grundy SM, Holdbrook MJ. Plasma lipids and diabetes mellitus in an adult community. Am J Epidemiol 1982;115:657
52. Barrett-Connor E, Witztum JL, Holdbrook M. A community study of high density lipoproteins in adult noninsulin-dependent diabetics. Am J Epidemiol 1983;117:186
53. Gabor J, Spain M, Kalant N. Composition of serum very-low-density and high-density lipoproteins in diabetes. Clin Chem 1980;26:1261
54. Eckel RH, Albers JJ, Cheung MC, et al. High density lipoprotein composition in insulin-dependent diabetes mellitus. Diabetes 1981;30:132
55. Rabkin SW, Boyko E, Streja DA. Changes in high density lipoprotein cholesterol after initiation of insulin therapy in non-insulin dependent diabetes mellitus: Relationship to changes in body weight. Am J Med Sci 1983;285: 14
56. Solerte SB, Carnevale-Schiana GP, Adamo S. Lipid and lipoprotein changes in diabetes mellitus in relation to metabolic control and vascular degenerative complications. Med Biol Environ 1985;13:755
57. Fontbonne A. Relationship between diabetic dyslipoproteinaemia and coronary heart disease risk in subjects with non-insulin-dependent diabetes mellitus. Diabetes Metab Rev 1991;7:179
58. Stern MP, Haffner SM. Dyslipidemia in type II diabetes. Implications for therapeutic intervention. Diabetes Care 1991;14:1144
59. Shaten BJ, Smith GD, Kuller LH, Neaton JD. Risk factors for the development of type II diabetes among men enrolled in the Usual Care group of the Multiple Risk Factor Intervention Trial. Diabetes Care 1993;16:1331
60. Kobbah M, Vessby B, Tuvemo T. Serum lipids and apolipoproteins in children with type 1 (insulin-dependent) diabetes during the first two years of the disease. Diabetologia 1988;31:195
61. Sosenko JM, Breslow JL, Miettinen OS, Gabbay KH. Hyperglycemia and plasma lipid levels: A prospective study of young insulin-dependent diabetic patients. N Engl J Med 1980;302:650
62. Lopes-Virella MF, Wohltmann HJ, Loadholt CB, Buse MG. Plasma lipids and lipoproteins in young insulin-dependent diabetic patients: Relationship with control. Diabetologia 1981;21:216
63. Andersen GE, Christiansen JS, Mortensen HB, et al. Serum lipids and lipoproteins in 157 insulin dependent diabetic children and adolescents in relation to metabolic regulation obesity and genetic hyperlipoproteinemia. Acta Paediat Scand 1983;72:361
64. Carvajal F, Quesada X, Gonzalez P. High density lipoprotein cholesterol in insulin-dependent diabetic children. Acta Diabetica Lat 1983;20:289
65. Tamborlane WV, Sherwin RS, Genel M, Felig P. Restoration of normal lipid and amino acid metabolism in diabetic patients treated with a portable insulin-infusion pump. Lancet 1979;1:1258
66. Pietri A, Dunn FL, Raskin P. The effect of improved diabetic control on plasma lipid and lipoprotein levels: A comparison of conventional therapy and continuous subcutaneous insulin infusion. Diabetes 1980;29:1001
67. Dunn FL, Pietri A, Raskin P. Plasma lipid and lipoprotein levels with continuous subcutaneous insulin infusion in type I diabetes mellitus. Ann Int Med 1981;95:426
68. Hershcopf R, Plotnick LP, Kaya K, et al. Short term improvement in glycemic control utilizing continuous subcutaneous insulin infusion: The effect on 24-hour integrated concentrations of counterregulatory hormones and plasma lipids in insulin-dependent diabetes mellitus. J Clin Endocrinol Metab 1982; 54:504
69. Lopes-Virella MF, Wohltmann HJ, Mayfield RK, et al. Effect of metabolic control on lipid, lipoprotein, and apolipoprotein levels in 55 insulin-dependent diabetic patients. A longitudinal study. Diabetes 1983;32:20
70. Vlachokosta FV, Asmal AC, Ganda OP, Aoki TT. The effect of strict control with the artificial beta-cell on plasma lipid levels in insulin-dependent diabetes. Diabetes Care 1983;6:351
71. Falko JM, O'Dorisio TM, Cataland S. Improvement of high-density lipoprotein-cholesterol levels. Ambulatory type I diabetics treated with the subcutaneous insulin pump. JAMA 1982;247:37
72. The Diabetes Control and Complications Trial Research Group. The effect of intensive treatment of diabetes on the development and progression of long-term complications in insulin-dependent diabetes mellitus. N Engl J Med 1993;329:977
73. Katzel LI, Busby-Whitehead MJ, Goldberg AP. Adverse effects of abdominal obesity on lipoprotein lipids in healthy older men. Exp Gerontol 1993;28:411
74. Kern PA. Lipid disorders in diabetes mellitus. Mt Sinai J Med 1987;54:245
75. Daneman D, Epstein LH, Siminerio L, et al. Effects of enhanced conventional therapy on metabolic control in children with insulin-dependent diabetes mellitus. Diabetes Care 1982;5:472
76. Purnell JQ, Marcovina SM, Kennedy H, et al. Lp(a) levels in IDDM: Effect of intensive diabetes therapy in the DCCT. Diabetes 1994;43:75A
77. Pykalisto OJ, Smith PH, Brunzell JD. Determinants of human adipose tissue lipoprotein lipase. Effect of diabetes and obesity on basal- and diet-induced activity. J Clin Invest 1975;56:1108
78. Taskinen MR, Beltz WF, Harper I, et al. Effects of NIDDM on very-low-density lipoprotein triglyceride and apolipoprotein B metabolism. Studies before and after sulfonylurea therapy. Diabetes 1986;35:1268
79. Brunzell JD, Porte D Jr, Bierman EL. Abnormal lipoprotein-lipase-mediated plasma triglyceride removal in untreated diabetes mellitus associated with hypertriglyceridemia. Metabolism 1979;28:897
80. Rubba P, Capaldo B, Falanga A, et al. Plasma lipoproteins and lipoprotein lipase in young diabetics with and without ketonuria. J Endocrinol Invest 1985;8:433
81. Pietri AO, Dunn FL, Grundy SM, Raskin P. The effect of continuous subcutaneous insulin infusion on very-low-density lipoprotein triglyceride metabolism in type I diabetes mellitus. Diabetes 1983;32:75
82. Dunn FL, Carroll PB, Beltz WF. Treatment with artificial beta-cell decreases very-low-density lipoprotein triglyceride synthesis in type I diabetes. Diabetes 1987;36:661
83. Rosenstock J, Vega GL, Raskin P. Effect of intensive diabetes treatment on low-density lipoprotein apolipoprotein B kinetics in type I diabetes. Diabetes 1988;37:393
84. Magill P, Rao SN, Miller NE, et al. Relationships between the metabolism of high-density and very-low-density lipoproteins in man: Studies of apolipoprotein kinetics and adipose tissue lipoprotein lipase activity. Eur J Clin Invest 1982;12:113
85. Brunzell JD. Obesity and coronary heart disease. A targeted approach. Arteriosclerosis 1984;4:180
86. Taskinen M-R, Nikkila EA, Kuusi T, Harno K. Lipoprotein lipase activity and serum lipoproteins in untreated type 2 (insulin-dependent) diabetes associated with obesity. Diabetologia 1982;22:46
87. Abbate SL, Brunzell JD. Pathophysiology of hyperlipidemia in diabetes mellitus. J Cardiovasc Pharmacol 1990;16:S1
88. Schmitt JK, Poole JR, Lewis SB, et al. Hemoglobin A1 correlates with the ratio of low-to-high-density-lipoprotein cholesterol in normal weight type II diabetics. Metabolism 1982;31:1084
89. Pfeifer MA, Brunzell JD, Best JD, et al. The response of plasma triglyceride, cholesterol, and lipoprotein lipase to treatment in non-insulin-dependent diabetic subjects without familial hypertriglyceridemia. Diabetes 1983;32:525
90. Briones ER, Mao SJT, Palumbo PJ, et al. Analysis of plasma lipids and apolipoproteins in insulin-dependent and non-insulin-dependent diabetics. Metabolism 1984;33:42
91. Biesbroeck RC, Albers JJ, Wahl PW, et al. Abnormal composition of high density lipoproteins in non-insulin-dependent diabetics. Diabetes 1982; 31:126
92. Jialal I, Joubert SM, Asmal AC. Cholesterol, triglyceride and high-density lipoprotein cholesterol levels in non-insulin-dependent diabetes in the young. S Afr Med J 1982;61:393
93. Stern MP, Mitchell BD, Haffner SM, Hazuda HP. Does glycemic control of type II diabetes suffice to control diabetic dyslipidemia? Diabetes Care 1992;15:638
94. Barakat HA, Carpenter JW, McLendon VD, et al. Influence of obesity, impaired glucose tolerance, and noninsulin dependent diabetes on low density lipoprotein structure and composition: Possible link between hyperinsulinemia and atherosclerosis. Diabetes 1990;39:1527
95. Barakat HA, McLendon VD, Marks R, et al. Influence of morbid obesity and non-insulin-dependent diabetes mellitus on high-density lipoprotein composition and subpopulation distribution. Metabolism 1992;41:37
96. Kissebah AH, Alfarsi S, Evans DJ, Adams PW. Integrated regulation of very low density lipoprotein triglyceride and apolipoprotein-B kinetics in non-insulin-dependent diabetes mellitus. Diabetes 1982;31:217
97. Greenfield M, Kolterman O, Olefsky J, Reaven GM. Mechanism of hypertriglyceridaemia in diabetic patients with fasting hyperglycaemia. Diabetologia 1980;18:441
98. Ginsberg H, Grundy SM. Very low density lipoprotein metabolism in non-ketotic diabetes mellitus: Effect of dietary restriction. Diabetologia 1982; 23:421
99. Abrams JJ, Ginsberg H, Grundy SM. Metabolism of cholesterol and plasma triglycerides in nonketotic diabetes mellitus. Diabetes 1982;31:903
100. Dunn FL, Raskin P, Bilheimer DW, Grundy SM. The effect of diabetic control on very low-density lipoprotein—triglyceride metabolism in patients with type II diabetes mellitus and marked hypertriglyceridemia. Metabolism 1984;33:117

101. Taskinen MR. Lipoprotein lipase in diabetes. Diabetes Metab Rev 1987;3:551
102. Kasama T, Yoshino G, Iwatani I, et al. Increased cholesterol concentration in intermediate density lipoprotein fraction of normolipidemic non-insulin-dependent diabetes. Atherosclerosis 1987;63:263
103. Hughes TA, Clements RS, Fairclough PK, et al. Effects of insulin therapy on lipoproteins in non-insulin-dependent diabetes mellitus (NIDDM). Atherosclerosis 1987;67:105
104. Lisch HJ, Sailer S. Lipoprotein patterns in diet, sulphonylurea, and insulin treated diabetics. Diabetologia 1981;20:118
105. Weisweiler P, Drosner M, Schwandt P. Dietary effects on very low-density lipoproteins in type 2 (non-insulin-dependent) diabetes mellitus. Diabetologia 1982;23:101
106. Fielding CJ, Reaven GM, Fielding PE. Human noninsulin-dependent diabetes: Identification of a defect in plasma cholesterol transport normalized in vivo by insulin and in vitro by selective immuno-absorption of apolipoprotein E. Proc Natl Acad Sci USA 1982;79:6365
107. Fielding CJ, Reaven GM, Liu G, Fielding PE. Increased free cholesterol in plasma low and very low density lipoproteins in non-insulin-dependent diabetes mellitus: Its role in the inhibition of cholesteryl ester transfer. Proc Natl Acad Sci USA 1984;81:2512
108. Kissebah AH, Alfarsi S, Evans DJ, Adams PW. Plasma low density lipoprotein transport kinetics in non-insulin-dependent diabetes mellitus. J Clin Invest 1983;71:655
109. Howard BV, Abbott WGH, Beltz WF, et al. Integrated study of low density lipoprotein metabolism and very low density lipoprotein metabolism in non-insulin-dependent diabetes. Metabolism 1987;36:870
110. Nikkila EA. High density lipoproteins in diabetes. Diabetes 1981;30:82
111. Kennedy L, Walshe K, Hadden DR, et al. The effect of intensive dietary therapy on serum high density lipoprotein cholesterol in patients with type 2 (non-insulin-dependent) diabetes mellitus: A prospective study. Diabetologia 1982;23:24
112. Wolf RN, Grundy SM. Influence of weight reduction on plasma lipoproteins in obese patients. Arteriosclerosis 1983;3:160
113. Agardh C-D, Nilsson-Ehle P, Schersten B. Improvement of the plasma lipoprotein pattern after institution of insulin treatment in diabetes mellitus. Diabetes Care 1982;5:322
114. Paisey R, Elkeles RS, Hambley J, Magill P. The effects of chlorpropamide and insulin on serum lipids, lipoproteins and fractional triglyceride removal. Diabetologia 1978;15:81
115. Wingard DL, Barrett-Connor E, Criqui MH, Suarez L. Clustering of heart disease risk factors in diabetic compared to nondiabetic adults. Am J Epidemiol 1983;117:19
116. Haffner SM, Valdez RA, Hazuda HP, et al. Prospective analysis of the insulin-resistance syndrome (syndrome X). Diabetes 1992;41:715
117. Reaven GM. Syndrome X: 6 years later. J Intern Med Suppl 1994;736:13
118. Bjorntorp P. Abdominal fat distribution and the metabolic syndrome. J Cardiovasc Pharmacol 1992;20:S26
119. Desprès JP. Abdominal obesity as important component of insulin-resistant syndrome. Nutrition 1993;9:452
120. Fujimoto WY, Leonetti DL, Newell Morris L, et al. Relationship of absence or presence of a family history of diabetes to body weight and body fat distribution in type 2 diabetes. Int J Obes 1991;15:111
121. Brunzell JD, Austin MA, Deeb SS, et al. Familial combined hyperlipidemia and genetic risk for atherosclerosis. In: Woodruff FP, Davignon J, Sniderman A, eds. Atherosclerosis X. Amsterdam: Elsevier;1995:624–627
122. Zambon A, Austin MA, Brown BG, et al. Effect of hepatic lipase on LDL in normal men and those with coronary artery disease. Arterioscler Thromb 1993;13:427
123. Haffner SM. Lipoprotein(a) and diabetes. An update. Diabetes Care 1993; 16:835
124. Jenkins AJ, Steele JS, Janus ED, Best JD. Increased plasma apolipoprotein (a) levels in IDDM patients with microalbuminuria. Diabetes 1991;40:787
125. Vannini P, Ciavarella A, Flammini M, et al. Lipid abnormalities in insulin-dependent diabetic patients with albuminuria. Diabetes Care 1984;7:151
126. Borch-Johnson K, Kreiner S. Proteinuria: Value as predictor of cardiovascular mortality in insulin dependent diabetes mellitus. Br Med J 1987;294:1651
127. Chait A, Brunzell JD. Acquired hyperlipidemia (secondary dyslipoproteinemias). Endocrinol Metab Clin North Am 1990;19:259
128. Joven J, Villabona C, Vilella E. Pattern of hyperlipoproteinemia in human nephrotic syndrome: Influence of renal failure and diabetes mellitus. Nephron 1993;64:565
129. Attman PO, Nyberg G, William-Olsson T, et al. Dyslipoproteinemia in diabetic renal failure. Kidney Int 1992;42:1381
130. Cassader M, Ruiu G, Gambino R, et al. Lipoprotein-apolipoprotein changes in renal transplant recipients: A 2-year-follow-up. Metabolism 1991;40: 922
131. Lithell H, Boberg J, Hellsing K, et al. Serum lipoprotein and apolipoprotein concentrations and tissue lipoprotein lipase activity in overt and subclinical hypothyroidism: The effects of substitution therapy. Eur J Clin Invest 1981;11:3
132. Rohlfing JJ, Brunzell JD. Effects of diuretics and adrenergic blocking agents on plasma lipids. West J Med 1986;145:210
133. Weinberger MH. Antihypertensive therapy and lipids. Paradoxical influences on cardiovascular disease risk. Am J Med 1986;80:64
134. Chait A, Brunzell JD. Chylomicronemia syndrome. Adv Intern Med 1992;37:249
135. Bagdade JD, Porte D Jr, Bierman EL. Diabetic lipemia. A form of acquired fat-induced lipemia. N Engl J Med 1967;276:427
136. Brunzell JD, Hazzard WR, Porte D Jr, Bierman El. Evidence for a common, saturable, triglyceride removal mechanism for chylomicrons and very low density lipoproteins in man. J Clin Invest 1973;52:1578
137. Baynes JW. Role of oxidative stress in development of complications in diabetes. Diabetes 1991;40:405
138. Wolff SP, Jiang ZY, Hunt JV. Protein glycation and oxidative stress in diabetes mellitus and ageing. Free Radic Biol Med 1991;10:339
139. Thornalley PJ. Monosaccharide auto-oxidation in health and disease. Environ Health Perspect 1985;64:297
140. Gillery P, Monboisse JC, Maquart FX, Borel JP. Glycation of proteins as a source of superoxide. Diabete Metab 1988;14:25
141. Kawamura M, Heinecke JW, Chait A. Pathophysiological concentrations of glucose promote oxidative modification of low density lipoprotein by a superoxide-dependent pathway. J Clin Invest 1994;94:155
142. Hunt JV, Smith CC, Wolff SP. Autoxidative glycosylation and possible involvement of peroxides and free radicals in LDL modification by glucose. Diabetes 1990;39:1420
143. Tsai EC, Hirsch IB, Brunzell JD, Chait A. Reduced plasma peroxyl radical trapping capacity and increased susceptibility of LDL to oxidation in poorly controlled IDDM. Diabetes 1994;43:1010
144. Sinclair AJ, Lunec J, Girling AJ, Barnett AH. Modulators of free radical activity in diabetes mellitus: Role of ascorbic acid. EXS 1992;62:342
145. Stankova L, Riddle M, Larned J, et al. Plasma ascorbate concentrations and blood cell dehydroascorbate transport in patients with diabetes mellitus. Metabolism 1984;33:347
146. Sinclair AJ, Taylor PB, Lunec J, et al. Low plasma ascorbate levels in patients with type 2 diabetes mellitus consuming adequate dietary vitamin C. Diabet Med 1994;11:893
147. Chait A, Brazg RL, Tribble DL, Krauss RM. Susceptibility of small, dense low density lipoproteins to oxidative modification in subjects with the atherogenic lipoprotein phenotype, pattern B. Am J Med 1993;94:350
148. Morel DW, Chisolm GM. Antioxidant treatment of diabetic rats inhibits lipoprotein oxidation and cytotoxicity. J Lipid Res 1989;30:1827
149. Nishigaki I, Hagihara M, Tsunekawa H, et al. Lipid peroxide levels of serum lipoprotein fractions of diabetic patients. Biochem Med 1981;25:373
150. Faure P, Corticelli P, Richard MJ, et al. Lipid peroxidation and trace element status in diabetic ketotic patients: Influence of insulin therapy. Clin Chem 1993;39:789
151. Curtiss LK, Witztum JL. Plasma apolipoproteins AI, AII, B, CI, and E are glycosylated in hyperglycemic diabetic subjects. Diabetes 1985;34:452
152. Steinbrecher UP, Witztum JL. Glucosylation of low-density lipoproteins to an extent comparable to that seen in diabetes slows their catabolism. Diabetes 1984;33:130
153. Bucala R, Makita Z, Vega G, et al. Modification of low density lipoprotein by advanced glycation end products contributes to the dyslipidemia of diabetes and renal insufficiency. Proc Natl Acad Sci USA 1994;91:9441
154. Bucala R, Makita Z, Koschinsky T, et al. Lipid advanced glycosylation: Pathway for lipid oxidation in vivo. Proc Natl Acad Sci USA 1993;90:6434
155. Witztum JL, Steinbrecher UP, Kesaniemi YA, Fisher M. Autoantibodies to glucosylated proteins in the plasma of patients with diabetes mellitus. Proc Natl Acad Sci USA 1984;81:3204
156. Witztum JL, Mahoney EM, Branks MJ, et al. Nonenzymatic glucosylation of low-density lipoprotein alters its biologic activity. Diabetes 1982;31:283
157. Bowie A, Owens D, Collins P, et al. Glycosylated low density lipoprotein is more sensitive to oxidation: Implications for the diabetic patient? Atherosclerosis 1993;102:63
158. Duell PB, Oram JF, Bierman EL. Nonenzymatic glycosylation of HDL and impaired HDL receptor-mediated cholesterol efflux. Diabetes 1991;40:377
159. Schmidt AM, Hori O, Brett J, et al. Cellular receptors for advanced glycation end products. Implications for induction of oxidant stress and cellular dysfunction in the pathogenesis of vascular lesions. Arterioscler Thromb 1994; 14:1521
160. Vlassara H, Brownlee M, Manogue KR, et al. Cachectin/TNF and IL-1 induced by glucose-modified proteins: Role in normal tissue remodeling. Science 1988;240:1546
161. Heinecke JW, Suits AG, Aviram M, Chait A. Phagocytosis of lipase-aggregated low density lipoprotein promotes macrophage foam cell formation. Sequential morphological and biochemical events. Arterioscler Thromb 1991;11:1643
162. Hazell LJ, van den Berg JJ, Stocker R. Oxidation of low-density lipoprotein by hypochlorite causes aggregation that is mediated by modification of lysine residues rather than lipid oxidation. Biochem J 1994;302:297
163. Kawabe Y, Cynshi O, Takashima Y, et al. Oxidation-induced aggregation of rabbit low-density lipoprotein by azo initiator. Arch Biochem Biophys 1994;310:489
164. Griffith RL, Virella GT, Stevenson HC, Lopes-Virella MF. Low density lipoprotein metabolism by human macrophages activated with low density lipoprotein immune complexes. A possible mechanism of foam cell formation. J Exp Med 1988;168:1041
165. Khoo JC, Miller E, Po F, et al. Monoclonal antibodies against LDL further enhance macrophage uptake of LDL aggregates. Arterioscler Thromb 1992;12:1258
166. Nievelstein PF, Fogelman AM, Mottino G, Frank JS. Lipid accumulation in rabbit aortic intima 2 hours after bolus infusion of low density lipoprotein.

A deep-etch and immunolocalization study of ultrarapidly frozen tissue. Arterioscler Thromb 1991;11:1795
167. Ylä-Herttuala S, Palinski W, Butler SW, et al. Rabbit and human atherosclerotic lesions contain IgG that recognizes epitopes of oxidized LDL. Arterioscler Thromb 1994;14:32
168. Lane JT, Subbaiah PV, Otto ME, Bagdade JD. Lipoprotein composition and HDL particle size distribution in women with non-insulin-dependent diabetes mellitus and the effects of probucol treatment. J Lab Clin Med 1991;118:120
169. Bagdade JD, Helve E, Taskinen MR. Effects of continuous insulin infusion therapy on lipoprotein surface and core lipid composition in insulin-dependent diabetes mellitus. Metabolism 1991;40:445
170. Bagdade JD, Buchanan WE, Kuusi T, Taskinen MR. Persistent abnormalities in lipoprotein composition in noninsulin-dependent diabetes after intensive insulin therapy. Arteriosclerosis 1990;10:232
171. Fielding CJ, Reaven GM, Fielding PE. Human noninsulin-dependent diabetes: Identification of a defect in plasma cholesterol transport normalized in vivo by insulin and in vitro by selective immuno-absorption of apolipoprotein E. Proc Natl Acad Sci USA 1982;79:6365
172. Parks JS, Gebre AK, Edwards IJ, Wagner WD. Role of LDL subfraction heterogeneity in the reduced binding of low density lipoproteins to arterial proteoglycans in cynomolgus monkeys fed a fish oil diet. J Lipid Res 1991;32:2001
173. Syvanne M, Rosseneu M, Labeur C, et al. Enrichment with apolipoprotein E characterizes postprandial TG-rich lipoproteins in patients with non-insulin-dependent diabetes mellitus and coronary artery disease: A preliminary report. Atherosclerosis 1994;105:25
174. Sano T, Kawamura T, Matsumae H, et al. Effects of long-term enalapril treatment on persistent micro-albuminuria in well-controlled hypertensive and normotensive NIDDM patients. Diabetes Care 1994;17:420
175. Adult Treatment Panel II. Summary of the second report of the National Cholesterol Education Program (NCEP) Expert Panel on Detection, Evaluation, and Treatment of High Blood Cholesterol in Adults. JAMA 1993; 269:3015
176. Garg A, Bantle JP, Henry RR, et al. Effects of varying carbohydrate content of diet in patients with non-insulin-dependent diabetes mellitus. JAMA 1994;271:1421
177. Milne RM, Mann JI, Chisholm AW, Williams SM. Long-term comparison of three dietary prescriptions in the treatment of NIDDM. Diabetes Care 1994;17:74
178. Ullmann D, Connor WE, Hatcher LF, et al. Will a high-carbohydrate, low-fat diet lower plasma lipids and lipoproteins without producing hypertriglyceridemia? Arterioscler Thromb 1991;11:1059
179. Garg A, Grundy SM. Treatment of dyslipidemia in non-insulin-dependent diabetes mellitus with lovastatin. Am J Cardiol 1988;62:44J
180. Garg A, Grundy SM. Gemfibrozil alone and in combination with lovastatin for treatment of hypertriglyceridemia in NIDDM. Diabetes 1989;38:364
181. Henry RR, Gumbiner B, Ditzler T, et al. Intensive conventional insulin therapy for type II diabetes. Metabolic effects during a 6-month outpatient trial. Diabetes Care 1993;16:21
182. Brownlee M. Glycation products and the pathogenesis of diabetic complications. Diabetes Care 1992;15:1835

Diabetes Mellitus, edited by Derek LeRoith, Simeon I. Taylor, and Jerrold M. Olefsky. Lippincott–Raven Publishers, Philadelphia © 1996.

CHAPTER 87

Pathogenesis of Hypertension in Diabetes

NAFTALI STERN AND MICHAEL L. TUCK

Arterial hypertension is more common in both insulin-dependent (IDDM) and non–insulin-dependent diabetes mellitus (NIDDM) than in the general population.[1] Traditionally, hypertension in IDDM was attributed to chronic renal failure, whereas in NIDDM it was thought to reflect concurrence of two common conditions: essential hypertension and NIDDM. Recent observations concerning interrelationships among glucose, insulin, body mass, sodium homeostasis, renal function, and the systemic vasculature in blood pressure regulation offer new insights into the mechanisms underlying high blood pressure in diabetes mellitus.

Sodium and Volume in Diabetic Hypertension

Almost all studies evaluating total body exchangeable sodium in diabetic patients have found increased sodium content, 10% higher than in nondiabetic subjects.[2,3,4] The increase in exchangeable sodium is explained partially by active reabsorption of glucose and ketones in the kidney as sodium salts.[5] Increased extracellular fluid osmolarity caused by hyperglycemia can also lead to water retention in the vascular space.[6,7] Hypervolemia in diabetes can be further aggravated by abnormalities in several sodium- and volume-regulating systems such as the renin-angiotensin-aldosterone system, insulin, atrial natriuretic peptide, sodium transport pathways, vessel compliance, and renal function, resulting in an enhanced propensity to hypertension.

The Renin-Angiotensin-Aldosterone System

Most studies show normal to suppressed aldosterone activity and low to normal renin levels in patients with uncomplicated and complicated diabetes mellitus.[2,7,8,9] In experimentally induced diabetes, plasma renin activity (PRA) declines within several days to weeks.[10,11] Even normal renin and aldosterone levels, however, may be inappropriately elevated for the increased exchangeable sodium and increased intravascular volume in diabetes mellitus. Low PRA levels are noted in diabetic subjects with autonomic neuropathy,[12,13] probably reflecting defective neural control of renin release.[14] Hyporeninemic hypoaldosteronism, which is most often seen in diabetic patients with nephropathy,[2,7,15] is associated with elevated arterial pressure and hyperkalemia.

The microvascular complications affect renin release, as both diabetic nephropathy and retinopathy are associated with reduced PRA levels.[2,7] However, diabetes itself, independent of microvascular complications, alters renin release as PRA levels are decreased with control high- and low-sodium diets in uncomplicated normotensive and hypertensive NIDDM.[16] Impaired β-adrenergic regulation of renin secretion[13,14,17] and decreased prostacyclin secretion[18] contribute to the low PRA levels in diabetes mellitus. Microvascular disease is also associated with increased levels of inactive renin,[19,20] which can serve as an early indicator of complications. Increased inactive renin may represent altered post-translational processing of inactive renin to active renin.[21]

The suppression of circulating PRA in diabetes suggests that this axis is unrelated to the evolution of high blood pressure. However, the protective effect on renal function of blocking this system with angiotensin-converting enzyme (ACE) inhibitors in diabetes[22–24] suggests that renin is important in the etiology of hypertension. Increased activity of the tissue renin-angiotensin system, especially vascular renin with local generation of angiotensin II and enhanced arterial sensitivity, has been proposed in diabetes. Indeed, during streptozocin-induced diabetes in rats, circulating PRA declines while aortic and adrenal renin increase[10,11] and renal renin mRNA remains unchanged.[11] Increased plasma ACE has been reported in IDDM subjects with nephropathy[26] and retinopathy,[27] and ACE genotypes conferring either protection from[26] or enhanced susceptibility[28] to nephropathy may exist. ACE is increased in the serum and mesenteric arteries of animals with experimentally induced diabetes.[29,30] Increased ACE could lead to increased tissue generation of angiotensin.

Atrial Natriuretic Peptide

Basal atrial natriuretic peptide (ANP) levels are increased in experimental diabetes[31] and in diabetic subjects.[32] Because ANP directly increases glomerular filtration rate, high circulating ANP levels may promote the glomerular hyperfiltration found in diabetes.[31] However, ANP action and secretion can be blunted in diabetes. When challenged with saline infusion, diabetics have a smaller rise in ANP along with a blunted natriuretic response[32,33]; this could promote sodium retention and hypertension.

Digitalis-like Substance

Streptozocin-induced diabetes in the rat is associated with hypertension when renal mass is reduced by 25%.[34] In this model, circulating digitalis-like substance, a factor often associated with hypervolemic states, is elevated. Further, digitalis-like substance is positively related to arterial pressure and inversely related to heart microsomal Na^+, K^+ ATPase activity. Thus, enhanced digitalis-like substance activity leading to inhibition of cardiovascular Na^+, K^+ ATPase may contribute to hypertension in diabetes in association with hypervolemia. In humans, this factor appears to be related to body mass index and is increased in individuals with impaired glucose tolerance.[35]

Sodium-Lithium Countertransport and Proximal Tubule Handling of Sodium

Abnormal sodium transport could contribute to sodium retention and hypervolemia in diabetes. Measurement of the erythrocyte sodium-lithium countertransport system may be an index of sodium reabsorption in the proximal tubule.[36] The activity of this system is increased in erythrocytes from patients with essential hypertension[37] as well as in patients with IDDM and nephropathy.[38,39] A strong family history of hypertension is found in the 30–40% of IDDM patients who develop diabetic nephropathy. Because increased erythrocyte sodium-lithium countertransport activity is observed both in patients with essential hypertension and in IDDM patients with nephropathy, a possible association may exist between abnormal renal sodium handling, hypertension, and renal failure in genetically susceptible IDDM patients. However, one study found no difference in renal sodium and lithium handling in diabetics with a genetic predisposition to essential hypertension.[40] In NIDDM subjects, erythrocyte countertransport is high in most patients regardless of renal function.[33,41]

Insulin and Diabetic Hypertension

Hypertension is associated with hyperinsulinemia in obese diabetic subjects, nondiabetic obese subjects, and in patients with essential hypertension.[42] In essential hypertension, hyperinsulinemia can occur independent of body weight or glucose intolerance.[43–48] Although decreased metabolic clearance of insulin may be present in patients with essential hypertension,[48] it appears that reduced tissue response to insulin is the key factor leading to hyperinsulinemia. Insulin-mediated glucose disposal (insulin sensitivity) is decreased in both nonobese and obese hypertensive patients, and there is a negative correlation of insulin sensitivity to systolic blood pressure.[45] The presence of hypertension in diabetics aggravates insulin resistance. Recently, impairment in insulin-induced glucose uptake by extrahepatic tissue was observed not only in diabetic hypertensive individuals but also in nonobese normotensive NIDDM subjects who, in the course of a 6-year follow-up period, developed hypertension and microalbuminuria.[49] Thus, impaired nonhepatic glucose utilization, presumably independent of obesity, may precede the onset of hypertension in subjects with NIDDM.

The link between insulin and blood pressure, although apparently consistent in whites, is by no means ubiquitous. In normotensive, nondiabetic Pima Indians and African-Americans, blood pressure is not related to insulin sensitivity.[50] In the San Antonio Heart Study, Mexican-Americans were found to be hyperinsulinemic relative to nonHispanic whites, but they displayed a lower prevalence of hypertension.[51] However, fasting insulin level may be a determinant of future hypertension in the nonobese participants in this study.[51] In a mixed population composed of Afro-Caribbeans, Gujerati Indians, and white Europeans, no relation between indices of insulin secretion and hypertension was found.[52] Data from the Mauritius Non-Communicable Disease Study Group also show that insulin and blood pressure are not independently related in three different ethnic groups cohabiting this country.[53] Collectively, these studies underscore the complexity of the relationship between insulin and blood pressure.

Experimental Models of Insulin and Hypertension

Experimental induction of abnormal carbohydrate metabolism may lead to increases in blood pressure. Sprague-Dawley rats fed a fructose-enriched diet develop insulin resistance, hyperinsulinemia, and hypertriglyceridemia and show significant increments in systolic blood pressure.[54] Exercise or somatostatin, which reduces insulin resistance, also reduces blood pressure in these animals.[54,55] In the spontaneously hypertensive rat, insulin resistance and hyperinsulinemia have been described,[56] but enhanced insulin sensitivity has also been demonstrated in this genetic model of hypertension.[57] In the two-kidney, one-clip model of renovascular hypertension,[58] insulin sensitivity is normal, suggesting that induction of hypertension does not impair insulin action. Insulin infusion in dogs does not alter blood pressure even after uninephrectomy, high salt intake, and simultaneous infusion of pressor agents.[59] In glucose-fed rats, however, chronic insulin infusion increases systolic and diastolic blood pressures beyond the increments induced by glucose feeding itself.[60] In the Zucker fatty rat, which is considered a genetic model of insulin resistance and hyperinsulinemia, blood pressure has been found to be either normal or high.[61] Therefore, experimental models have offered some insight into the relationship between insulin and blood pressure, but variation in responses among species has been a problem.

Patterns of Insulin Resistance

Ferrannini and coworkers[43] and DeFronzo and Ferrannini[46] have characterized the pattern of insulin resistance in different hypertensive conditions, including essential hypertension, hypertension in NIDDM, and hypertension in obesity. These conditions share diminished insulin-mediated whole-body glucose uptake but differ in degree of sensitivity to other actions of insulin (Table 87-1). Essential hypertensive subjects show reduced insulin sensitivity only through the nonoxidative pathway for glucose disposal, whereas obese and NIDDM patients also have reduced glucose uptake through the oxidative pathway and reduced effects of insulin to suppress hepatic glucose output. In essential hypertension, insulin resistance appears to be present mainly in skeletal muscles involving reduced glycogen synthesis.[62] This type of insulin resistance may be related to a decreased number of the insulin-sensitive slow-twitch, type I muscle fibers observed in hypertensive individuals or to restriction of the muscular microcirculation.[47,62] Insulin sensitivity is related to skeletal blood flow (capillary density) and fiber type. Slow-twitch fibers demonstrate high insulin binding, sensitivity, and glucose uptake compared with fast-twitch fibers.[63]

Upper body adiposity, even without marked increase in body mass index, is strongly linked to both hypertension and hyperinsulinemia.[64] Intra-abdominal adipocytes readily release free fatty acids in response to adrenergic stimulation.[65] The combination of excessive adrenergic tone and increased abdominal adipocyte response to adrenergic stimulation in obese subjects facilitates excess release of free fatty acids in this condition. Increased free fatty acids in turn impair both hepatic insulin clearance and muscle glucose uptake.

The coexistence of hypertension and NIDDM may be associated with a unique form of insulin resistance. Laakso and coworkers[66] noted that insulin resistance in extrahepatic tissues is more pronounced in hypertensive than in normotensive NIDDM subjects. In support of this finding, impairment in insulin-induced glucose uptake by extrahepatic tissues was observed only in NIDDM patients exhibiting hypertension or microalbuminuria.[49]

The mechanisms involved in insulin's cellular uptake of glucose also appear to be related to vascular function and have been implicated in insulin resistance. In lean individuals, insulin stimulates muscle blood flow by a vasodilatory effect, and this may be a determinant of insulin-mediated glucose uptake.[67] In obese, insulin-resistant subjects[67–69] and in NIDDM, insulin fails to enhance muscle blood flow possibly because of a specific impairment of sympathetic neural responsiveness in skeletal muscle.[69] Insulin reduces the pressor response to norepinephrine and increases the metabolic clearance rate of norepinephrine in lean but not in obese subjects.[70] Additionally, norepinephrine induces a larger fall in leg vascular resistance in lean compared with obese men.[70] These abnormal vascular responses to insulin may diminish peripheral blood flow and glucose delivery and could also contribute to hypertension in NIDDM. Insulin-mediated amino acid uptake may also modulate arterial blood pressure through central nervous system control mechanisms, regulating both sympathetic activity and feeding behavior.[71,72]

Insulin and the Renin-Angiotensin System

Insulin resistance is not found in renovascular hypertension,[58] and the interaction between angiotensin II and insulin on blood pressure has been thought to be minimal.[73] However, angiotensin II may affect insulin-mediated glucose utilization, as studies show that angiotensin II increases peripheral glucose uptake.[74,75] Another report indicated that angiotensin II precipitated insulin resistance in rats.[76] ACE inhibitors improve insulin action in nondiabetic and type II diabetics with or without hypertension, perhaps by reducing angiotensin II.[77–81] Additionally, angiotensin II has been shown to directly inhibit glycogen synthesis and stimulate phosphorylase activity in hepatocytes in vitro.[82] Some have been unable to demonstrate improved glucose metabolism or insulin sensitivity during ACE therapy.[83–85]

Insulin and Sympathetic Nervous System Activity

Nutrient intake can modulate sympathetic nervous system activity.[72,86] Restricted caloric intake leads to a reduction in plasma catecholamines in humans and to diminished tissue norepinephrine turnover in rats.[72,86] Conversely, sucrose overfeeding enhances tissue norepinephrine turnover in normal rats and increases blood pressure in hypertensive animals.[72,86] In a study using insulin and a euglycemic clamp technique, high doses of insulin increased plasma norepinephrine and blood pressure levels in normal subjects.[87] Thus both glucose and insulin may act as signals that couple a dietary load to enhancement in sympathetic flow.

Using microneurography to evaluate regional sympathetic discharge, obese individuals were noted to exhibit greater basal activity. However, insulin increased the number of sympathetic bursts only in normal individuals and not in obese or diabetic (NIDDM) subjects.[69,88] Insulin also fails to normally enhance skeletal muscle flow, a neurally mediated effect, in IDDM[89] and NIDDM subjects.[68] Increased circulating norepinephrine has been observed in obese individuals,[90,91] and there is a close relationship between reduction in plasma norepinephrine levels and blood pressure during weight loss.[91,92]

Table 87-1. Patterns of Insulin Resistance in Subjects with Obesity, Non–Insulin-Dependent Diabetes Mellitus, and in Elderly and Essential Hypertensive Subjects

	Obesity	NIDDM	Elderly	Hypertension
Whole-body glucose uptake	↓↓↓	↓↓↓	↓↓	↓↓
Glucose oxidation	↓↓	↓↓	↓	0
Nonoxidative glucose disposal	↓↓	↓↓↓	↓↓	↓↓
Suppression of hepatic glucose production	↓	↓	0	0

(Modified from references 26 and 29, with permission.)
Downward arrows indicate reduced insulin action; 0 indicates normal effect.

Insulin and the Vascular Bed

Human Studies. Epidemiologic and clinical studies reinforce the relationship between insulin and vascular disease. Atherosclerotic conditions such as macrovascular disease, coronary artery disease, cerebrovascular disease, and hypertension all show a strong, independent correlation with hyperinsulinemia.[93,94] Hyperinsulinemia could actually enhance atherosclerosis in diabetes mellitus.[95,96] Early changes in vascular structure are crucial to the development of hypertension,[97] and the atherosclerotic process facilitates these effects via reduction in vessel compliance and vasodilatory mechanisms.

Effects of Insulin on Vascular Smooth Muscle Cells

The growth-promoting effect of insulin may induce structural and functional changes in the arterial bed. Insulin stimulates the proliferation of vascular smooth-muscle cells[98] and increases DNA synthesis in the rat aorta.[99] Insulin also augments the expression of insulin-like growth factor 1 (IGF 1) in rat aortic cultured smooth muscle cells.[100] This provides a potential amplification mechanism, since the proliferative effects of insulin may be exerted via the IGF 1 receptor.[101,102] Since these effects are not necessarily impaired in states of insulin resistance, a grossly exaggerated proliferative response may take place due to hyperinsulinemia.[103] Supernatants obtained from platelets of insulin-treated patients are 83% more active in promoting growth of rat vascular smooth muscle cells than those obtained from normals.[104] Vascular smooth-muscle cell migration from the media to the intima is a key step in the atherogenesis process. Insulin pretreatment enhances the migration of smooth muscle cells induced by 12-hydroxyeicosatetraenoic acid, a product of lipoxygenase metabolism of arachidonic acid.[105]

Effects of Insulin on Endothelial Cells

Although insulin has no proliferative effect on large vessel endothelial cells,[106–108] it enhances the expression of the endothelin-I gene in cultured endothelial cells.[107,108] This may have both paracrine and endocrine vasopressor effects, since increased circulating endothelin levels have been reported in diabetes mellitus.[109] Insulin also increases endothelin receptor density and endothelin-mediated DNA synthesis in vascular smooth muscle cells.[110] Proinsulin, the concentration of which is increased in NIDDM, increases mRNA expression and the release of plasminogen activator-inhibitor type I in cultured endothelial cells.[111] Because this endothelial cell–derived factor acts to enhance coagulation and since plasminogen activator-inhibitor type I circulating levels are increased in NIDDM, this effect could provide an additional mechanism by which islet β-cell products promote vasculopathy.

Effects of Insulin on Vascular Lipid Metabolism

Hyperinsulinemia promotes fat deposition into the vasculature via the lipogenic effect of insulin.[96] Insulin increases low-density lipoprotein binding to smooth-muscle cells, fibroblasts, and monocytes.[112] In monocytes, which are the precursors of the foam cells of the atheromatous lesion, insulin stimulates the activity of 3-hydroxy-3-methylglutaryl-coenzyme A reductase, the rate-limiting enzyme of cholesterol synthesis.[113]

Insulin and Vascular Tone

Insulin exerts multiple effects on vascular tone, and these effects vary among different vascular compartments and species.[2,6] Insulin stimulates muscle blood flow and reduces leg vascular resistance, presumably via activation of sympathetic pathways that induce local vasodilation.[66–68] In humans, the effects of insulin on adrenergic pressor responses may vary with the experimental setting. Insulin has been reported to augment the cardiovascular response to norepinephrine[114] but to reduce the rise in forearm vascular resistance in response to phenylephrine.[115] In vitro, insulin attenuates the vasoconstrictive response to norepinephrine and angiotensin II in rabbit vessels[116] and diminishes vasopressin- and angiotensin II-induced calcium transients in cultured vascular smooth muscle cells.[117–120] This effect partly depends on reduced mobilization of intracellular calcium stores owing to reduced sensitivity of inositol-triphosphate–mediated release of calcium.[118] Insulin also reduces arginine vasopressin-induced inward calcium currents in vascular cells.[117] Enhancement of isoproterenol-induced relaxation may represent an additional mechanism by which insulin diminishes arterial wall tension.[121] Insulin increases regional blood flow, and this vasodilatory effect is inhibited by beta blockers.[122]

Collectively, these studies support the role of insulin as a potential vasodilator. Just how important these effects are for normal vascular function and whether or not the derangement of these vasodilatory mechanisms would have effects on systemic blood pressure are unknown.

Insulin and Ion Transport

Several membrane ion transport systems are altered by insulin, including the Na, K-ATPase pump, the Ca^{++}-ATPase pump, and the sodium-hydrogen (Na/H) antiporter system. Insulin stimulates Na/H antiport activity in vitro in several tissues.[123] Increased renal Na/H antiport activity increases Na reabsorption, and high antiport activity in vascular smooth muscle has been linked to increased intracellular sodium and calcium. Augmented Na/H antiport would raise intracellular pH, facilitating growth of vascular smooth-muscle cells.[124] Aviv and Livne[124] have proposed that elevated cytosolic calcium stimulates the Na/H antiport. Insulin has been shown to cause elevations in cytosolic calcium in isolated adipocytes[125] but not in vascular cells.[118]

Insulin stimulates Ca^{++}-ATPase activity, blocks Ca^{++} currents, and attenuates calcium-driven action potentials.[126] Vascular smooth-muscle cells resistant to these effects of insulin could result in elevation of cytosolic calcium. The genetically obese, insulin-resistant Zucker rat exhibits both reduced membrane Ca^{++}-ATPase activity and increased cellular calcium levels.

Recent research has linked hypertension and diabetes to common defects in calcium and magnesium metabolism. Hypercalciuria is found in insulin-deficient streptozocin-induced diabetic rats[127] as a result of a specific defect in renal tubular calcium reabsorption. In humans, a hypercalciuric response to induced hyperinsulinemia also has been demonstrated.[127] Hypercalciuria in diabetes mellitus is associated with low to normal serum ionized calcium levels and with decreased duodenal calcium transport.[127] Reduced Ca^{++}-ATPase activity is found in cells of diabetic animals and of diabetic patients.[7] Magnesium may also provide a nexus between hypertension, peripheral insulin resistance, and diabetes mellitus. Total red blood cell magnesium levels increase in normal subjects after an oral glucose load and with elevated insulin levels.[127] These insulin effects on cellular magnesium uptake are impaired both in hypertensive patients and in NIDDM subjects. Because magnesium regulates the activity of rate-limiting glycolytic enzymes as well as Na, K-ATPase activity, hyperinsulinemia and hypertension may be influenced by decreased intracellular free magnesium.

Insulin and Sodium Homeostasis

As recently reviewed,[128,129] there are now substantial data documenting abnormal sodium metabolism in diabetes mellitus. Acute insulin administration to normal subjects significantly reduces sodium excretion. The antinatriuretic effect of insulin is not impaired in hypertensive patients[130,131] or in insulin-resistant obese individuals.[132] A reduction in insulin dosage in IDDM patients leads to natriuresis, weight loss, and lower blood pressure.[133] Increased sodium reabsorption in IDDM subjects is accompanied by increased glomerular filtration rate (GFR) but normal renal plasma clearance of lithium.[134] In these studies, both the fractional and absolute sodium reabsorption rates in the proximal tubules were significantly elevated in diabetic subjects. Variations in plasma insulin may result in changes in renal Na handling, as glucose reabsorption is coupled in Na transport in the proximal tubules. Impaired sodium excretion has been demonstrated in IDDM during water immersion, which induces central volume expansion.[135]

The effect of insulin on sodium reabsorption is direct, as shown by insulin infusion to the renal artery or to the isolated perfused kidney,[2] acting on the proximal and distal segments of the tubule to enhance sodium reabsorption and decrease free water clearance. The effect of insulin could be via direct stimulation of the Na/H antiport system or on the Na, K-ATPase pump in the renal tubule.[136,137] Studies with micropipettes in proximal convoluted tubules suggest that this site is where insulin enhances volume absorption.[138,139] In a recent study, insulin was shown to blunt the natriuretic effect of atrial natriuretic peptide in hypertensive men.[130] Mogensen and coworkers[140] reported a decrease in glomerular filtration rate and in renal blood flow in IDDM patients after they received an intravenous injection of insulin at doses to normalize serum glucose levels. Christiansen and associates[141] also observed reductions in glomerular filtration rate and renal blood flow with insulin administration, but the effect of insulin could be abolished by preventing the glucose changes, suggesting that glucose was more important than insulin in these effects on renal hemodynamics.

Can Insulin Cause Hypertension? An Overview

Hyperinsulinemia and/or insulin resistance is present in at least three clinical settings that are not necessarily associated with hypertension. First, in patients with insulinoma, hypertension is not a recognized complication. Second, women with polycystic ovarian syndrome are frequently insulin-resistant but are usually normotensive. Finally, in some individuals with marked obesity, insulin resistance and hyperinsulinemia are present for years, although they have entirely normotensive levels of blood pressure. Although these observations argue against the possibility that hyperinsulinemia leads to hypertension, sufficient clinical and experimental evidence exists to suggest a link, especially in individuals who have other factors that make them susceptible to hypertension.

There are two potential pathways by which abnormalities in insulin could elicit arterial hypertension (Fig. 87-1). According to one proposal, the primary defect resides in insulin's effect on glucose utilization, whereas tissue responses to all other biologic effects of insulin are preserved. The compensatory hyperinsulinemia leads to enhanced insulin effects in target tissues not affected by insulin resistance. Candidate effects of insulin excess include sodium retention, upper body adiposity, stimulation of vascular smooth muscle cell growth and cytosolic calcium, induction of endothelin secretion, and enhancement of vascular lipid deposition (see Fig. 87-1). An alternative hypothesis emphasizes a role for the vasodilatory effects of insulin in the maintenance of arterial tone (see Fig. 87-1). Impaired insulin-dependent arterial vasodilation could occur in conditions associated with hypertension and hyperinsulinemia. Thus, defective insulin-mediated attenuation of vasoconstriction would lead to increased vascular tone

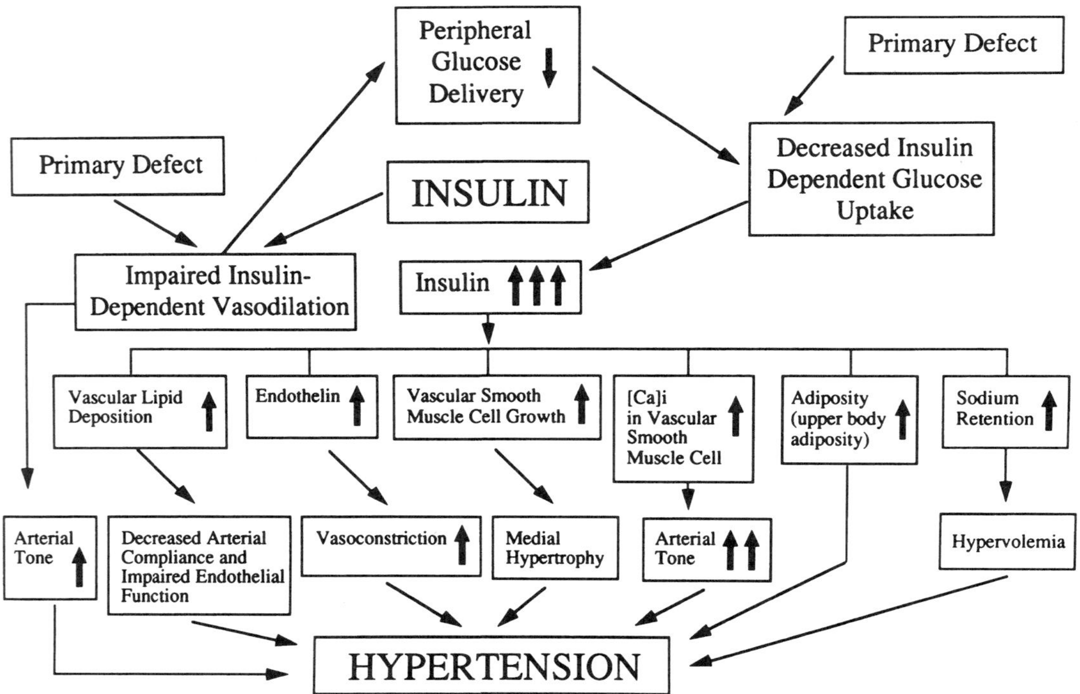

Figure 87-1. Mechanisms of insulin effect on blood pressure. One potential mechanism is a primary defect in insulin-dependent glucose uptake leading to hyperinsulinemia and activation of several pressor factors. Another hypothesis is that impaired insulin-dependent vasodilation causes decreased peripheral glucose delivery and increased arterial tone.

and hypertension. The two hypothetical pathways are not mutually exclusive.

Glucose and Diabetic Hypertension

The demonstration by the Diabetes Control and Complications Trial (DCCT) that improved glycemic control reduces microvascular complications in IDDM[142] indicates a role for glucose in diabetic vasculopathy. Many surveys have shown a positive correlation between blood pressure and plasma glucose level.[2] Reduction in blood pressure has been shown to occur with better glucose control in diabetic subjects despite increases in plasma volume and exchangeable sodium.[143] In contrast, during controlled insulin withdrawal, blood pressure increases with worsening of metabolic control.[144] Experimental agents that directly reverse insulin resistance and improve metabolic control can lower blood pressure.[145] These studies imply that abnormalities in both glucose and insulin can modulate blood pressure.

Cellular Actions of Glucose

Elevated glucose levels have been shown to impair endothelium-dependent relaxation via activation of protein kinase C and a decrease in nitric oxide formation in endothelial cells.[146] Glucose directly increases the secretion of endothelin-I from cultured endothelial cells,[147] which may account for the increased circulating endothelin levels in diabetics.[109] Hyperglycemia also diminishes Na^+, K^+ ATPase in the aorta,[148] and this effect may also depend on reduced endothelium-derived nitric oxide formation.[149] Low vascular smooth-muscle cell Na^+, K^+ ATPase, in turn, leads to increased vascular tone as a result of an increase in cytosolic calcium. Decreased nitric oxide generation in human[149] and experimental[150] diabetes may reflect direct effects of glucose and contribute to hypertension in patients with chronic hyperglycemia. Increased glucose concentration may also have a direct toxic effect on endothelial cells resulting in delayed cell replication and accelerated cell death.[151] Possibly, hyperglycemia is also responsible for the increased ACE activity in diabetic individuals.[152] In porcine vascular smooth muscle cells, glucose enhances angiotensin II–induced 12-hydroxyeicosatetraenoic acid formation,[153,154] an intercellular metabolite that participates in angiotensin II-dependent calcium signal[154] and stimulates vascular smooth-muscle cell migration.[105] Finally, glucose has been shown to directly enhance low-density lipoprotein oxidation in vitro.[155] Since oxidized low-density lipoprotein has been implicated in the acceleration of multiple events along the atherogenic cascade, including monocyte chemotaxis, cytotoxicity, cytokine, and growth factor synthesis, inhibition of nitric oxide effects, and foam cell formation, a possibility exists that chronic hyperglycemia might augment these effects by facilitation of low-density lipoprotein oxidation.[155]

Glucose and Glycosylated Proteins

Circulating glucose reacts nonenzymatically with proteins, leading to the formation of highly reactive, late addition products termed advanced glycosylation end-products (AGEs). AGEs remain irreversibly bound to proteins at multiple sites, particularly to subendothelial basement-membrane proteins, and their deposition takes place at an accelerated rate in diabetes. AGEs elicit multiple effects that could promote vasculopathy and elevation of arterial pressure. Following binding to specific receptors on monocytes, AGEs induce the secretion of growth-promoting cytokines such as interleukin I and insulin-like growth factor 1 by these cells.[156,157] AGEs also promote the transendothelial migration of monocytes toward the subendothelial space and subsequently enhance the expression of platelet-derived growth factor by these cells.[158] Finally AGEs inhibit the antiproliferative effects of nitric oxide,[159] which may be important in attenuating the progression of medial hypertrophy in hypertension.

Vascular Reactivity and Diabetic Hypertension

Blood pressure sensitivity to pressor factors is markedly exaggerated in diabetes[4,6,7]; this effect is seen early in the disease in both normotensive and hypertensive patients with IDDM and NIDDM. In experimental diabetes, there is also an early exaggeration in blood pressure response to stimuli.[7] The abnormality in vascular reactivity is completely corrected by diuretic drugs in diabetics, indicating an effect of sodium on blood pressure.[4] There may be an abnormal interaction between sodium, angiotensin II, and blood pressure in diabetes. In obese NIDDM, the blood pressure response to angiotensin II is not normally diminished by sodium restriction, and this may explain the high incidence of salt-sensitive hypertension in diabetes.[6]

This enhanced blood pressure reactivity in diabetes could be attributed to alterations in the physical properties of the resistance arteries or to abnormal paracrine regulation of vascular tone. Indeed, there is an early decrease in the passive distensibility of the vascular bed in diabetes.[160] The production of prostacyclin, an endothelial cell-derived vasodilator and antiaggregant, is diminished, whereas thromboxane, which promotes aggregation and vasoconstriction, is increased in experimental diabetes.[161] Observations in animal and human tissues that endothelial nitric oxide–mediated dilation is impaired in diabetes[162–165] could account for enhanced vascular reactivity. It is well documented that systemic inhibition of nitric acid synthesis in animals results in increased arterial pressure.[165] Advanced glycosylation products may account for defective nitric acid–dependent vasodilation in diabetes, since AGEs can quench nitric oxide activity.[167] Insulin can prevent the development of impaired vascular relaxation owing to abnormal nitric acid levels in mesenteric resistance arteries from streptozocin-induced diabetic rats.[168]

Nephropathy and Diabetic Hypertension

Epidemiologic and Clinical Studies

Hypertension is a hallmark of overt diabetic nephropathy and is present in more than 90% of diabetics with impaired renal function.[7,169] Hypertension and nephropathy develop in parallel as suggested by the inverse correlation between creatinine clearance and arterial pressure as well as by the direct relation between protein excretion and blood pressure.[169,170] Hypertension itself accelerates the deterioration in renal function in diabetic subjects,[171] and antihypertensive therapy retards the decline in glomerular filtration rate and reduces proteinuria.[172] Contrary to earlier beliefs, hypertension is clearly not a late complication of diabetic nephropathy. Rather, elevations in arterial pressure can occur at the very early stages of renal dysfunction in diabetes.[169,170] Although often still within the normal range, blood pressure levels are higher in IDDM patients with microalbuminuria compared with those in controls. In normoalbuminuric diabetic subjects, the appearance of microalbuminuria seems to precede increases in blood pressure,[173,174] although the reverse sequence has also been documented.[175] Very subtle changes in blood pressure such as diminished day-to-night variation may herald the evolution of hypertension in IDDM patients.[176] Although microalbuminuria may also be present in essential hypertension,[177,178] albumin excretion is 100-fold greater in diabetics compared with essential hypertensive subjects for a given level of blood pressure.[7,173] However, microalbuminuria can be detected in offspring of nondiabetic essential hypertensive individuals, suggesting that alterations in glomerular function precede hypertension.[179] The association between microalbuminuria and hypertension is more consistent in IDDM than in NIDDM, although in a report of 510 NIDDM subjects, diastolic pressure was higher in patients with proteinuria.[180]

Genetics of Diabetic Nephropathy

Nephropathy in IDDM is related to a genetic predisposition to essential hypertension.[39,181] Indicators of genetic susceptibility to hypertension in diabetic nephropathy include parental hypertension and increased erythrocyte sodium-lithium countertransport. Nondiabetic parents of patients with IDDM and nephropathy have higher blood pressures than do parents of IDDM patients who are free of renal involvement.[181] Previous reports that some patients with uncomplicated, longstanding IDDM have relatively low blood pressures[182] lend additional support to the notion of susceptibility to nephropathy in certain patients. Red blood cell sodium-lithium countertransport cannot be considered a genetic marker for nephropathy or hypertension in NIDDM: It was reported to be normal in one study of patients with NIDDM, regardless of the presence of hypertension[183] and was elevated in NIDDM patients regardless of level of renal function in another report.[41]

Structural-Functional Relationships in Diabetes

Mauer and coworkers[184] reported that no structural glomerular parameter precisely predicted albumin excretion among 45 IDDM patients. They found, however, that mesangial expansion was highly predictive of hypertension, and in these patients filtration was distinctly decreased. Identical structural lesions have been reported in markedly obese patients with overt proteinuria in the absence of hypertension or decreased glomerular filtration rate. Obese patients can have nephrotic range proteinuria and supranormal creatinine clearance.[185] In renal biopsy, obese subjects show focal glomerulosclerosis, diabetic nephropathy, and minimal change disease.[186] There may be a relationship between insulin resistance, blood pressure, and renal functional and structural changes in obesity, essential hypertension, aging, NIDDM, and IDDM[187] (Table 87-2). Aging is associated with progressive loss of renal function and glomerular basement membrane thickening, increased glomerular mesangium, and reduced effective filtering area.[188] Similar renal changes can be found in essential hypertension and obesity. These abnormal renal functional and anatomic changes may be linked to the syndromes of insulin resistance.[187]

Functional Renal Alterations in Diabetes

A state of generalized hyperperfusion of the peripheral vessels is described in diabetes as best documented in the glomerular capillary circulation.[189] Morphologic studies of diabetic vessels from humans and animal models demonstrate capillary dilatation, congestion, or tortuosity in several vascular beds.[190] Increased renal nitric oxide synthesis is noted in experimental diabetes,[191] and inhibition of nitric oxide eliminates hyperfiltration in the streptozocin-induced diabetic rat.[192] Enhanced efferent arteriolar wall sensitivity to angiotensin II has been advocated as one of the major mechanisms to raise intraglomerular pressure in diabetes. The intrarenal renin-angiotensin system also accelerates glomerular growth and sclerosis via mechanisms independent of its effects on glomerular hemodynamics.[193,194] Glomerulosclerosis can evolve in the absence of glomerular hypertension and is attenuated by ACE inhibitors independent of changes in intraglomerular pressure.[193–195] Direct studies of cultured mesangial cells showed that angiotensin II stimulates the synthesis of matrix protein and that this effect is mediated via induction of transforming growth factor-β expression.[196] Hyperglycemia activates protein kinase C in the glomerulus, increasing endothelial cell permeability to albumin and enhancing matrix protein synthesis in mesangial cells.[197]

Hypertension in Non–Insulin-Dependent Diabetes Mellitus

Using the World Health Organization guidelines for the diagnosis of high blood pressure (>160/95 mm Hg), the incidence of hypertension in NIDDM may be as high as 40% in men and 53% in women. This high incidence is partly explained by associated obesity, older age, and essential hypertension. Kelleher and coworkers[198] compared the prevalence of hypertension among subjects

TABLE 87-2. Physiologic and Morphologic Characteristics of Subjects with Various Insulin-Resistant States

	IDDM	NIDDM	Obesity	Age	Essential Hypertension
Insulin resistance	+	+++	+++	++	++
Prevalence of hypertension	20% to 30%	40% to 50%	40% to 50%	45% to 55%	100%
Na, Li CTT	↑	↑	+/−	nl	↑
Kidney Function					
Mean kidney volume	↑	↑	↑	↓	nl
Glomerular filtration rate	↑	↑	↑	↓	nl
RPF	↑	↑	↑	↓	↓
Na excretion	↓	↓	↓	↑/↓	↑
Renin	↑/↓	↓	↓	↓	↑/↓
Microalbuminuria	+	+	+/−	+/−	+
Microscopic Anatomy					
Mesangial volume	↑↑	↑↑	↑↑	↑	↑
Filtration area	↓	↓	↓	↓	↓
Glomerulosclerosis	↑	↑	↑	↑	↑

Na, Li CTT = Sodium-lithium countertransport in red blood cells.

with IDDM and NIDDM and nondiabetic subjects, noting an increase with both age and body mass index in the three groups. Although the increased prevalence among NIDDM subjects compared with nondiabetic subjects persisted when controlled for age and body mass index, the difference between IDDM and NIDDM was not seen when these variables were controlled for. The incidence of nephropathy in NIDDM may be equal to or less frequent (20–30%) than that in IDDM (30–40%). Fabre and coworkers[180] found only an 8.4% incidence of compromised GFR in 510 NIDDM hypertensive subjects. Tiernay and colleagues,[199] however, reported a 30% incidence of renal insufficiency in 2965 subjects with NIDDM and hypertension. Racial differences may account for this widely discrepant outcome, since the ethnic composition of these studies appears grossly distinct. In 10 otherwise healthy NIDDM patients, Schmitz and coworkers[200] studied glomerular filtration rate, kidney volume, and albumin excretion at the time of diagnosis and 3 months after initiation of treatment. They found a significant reduction in glomerular filtration rate, total kidney volume, and albumin excretion after metabolic control. Their study suggests that renal hypertrophy and hyperfiltration, which are characteristic of patients with IDDM, are shared features with NIDDM.

Hypertension often precedes diabetes in NIDDM,[187] which possibly reflects a familial clustering of essential hypertension in NIDDM and mechanisms related to obesity. Reubi and associates[201] reported that in the absence of nephropathy, few differences existed in the overall pattern of blood pressure and renal function between NIDDM patients in whom hypertension was diagnosed either before or after the emergence of diabetes. Whether hypertension emerges in parallel to nephropathy in NIDDM individuals in the same way as that seen in IDDM patients is not known. Baba and coworkers[202] have shown in a 10-year follow-up of normotensive NIDDM patients that 38% of normotensive NIDDM patients who developed hypertension had proteinuria on entry into the study. Although this finding suggests that nephropathy precedes hypertension in most NIDDM, a recent study assessing the prevalence of hypertension in NIDDM using the Joint National Committee on Detection, Evaluation and Treatment of Hypertension (JNC-V) criteria (that is, >140/90 mm Hg) found that hypertension is present in 71% of normoalbuminuric type II diabetic patients.[203]

Treatment of Hypertension in Diabetes

In 1994, the National High Blood Pressure Education Program (NHBPEP) Working Group on Hypertension in Diabetes issued its second consensus statement advocating an algorithmic approach to treatment of hypertension in diabetes[204] (Fig. 87-2). The report

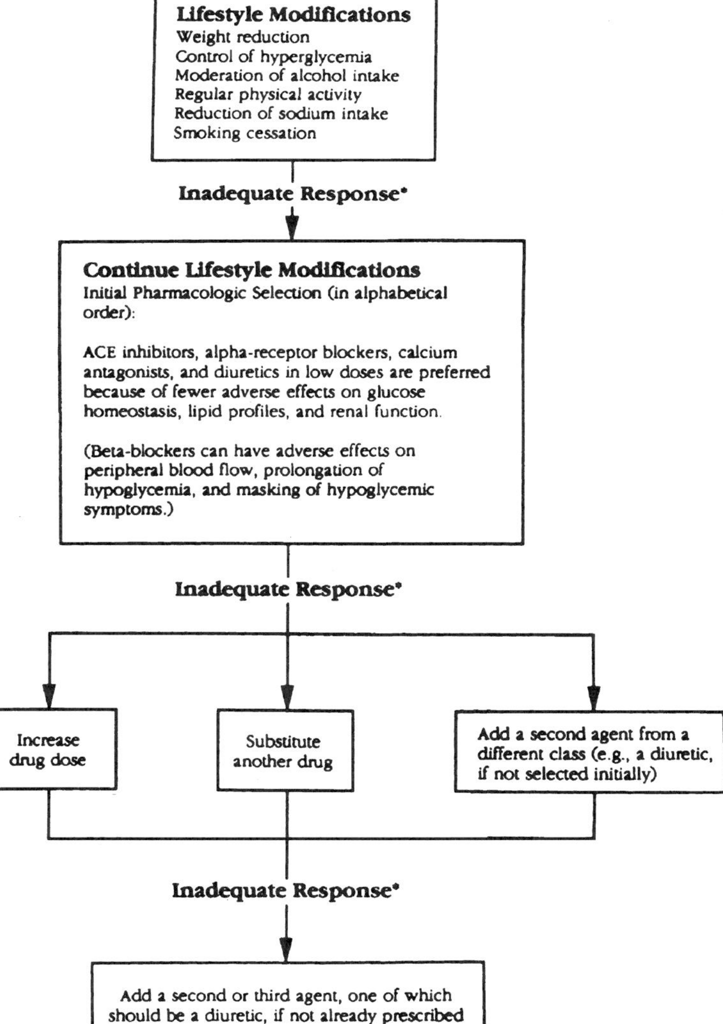

FIGURE 87-2. Hypertension treatment algorithm for diabetic patients. (Reproduced with permission from the National High Blood Pressure Education Program Working Group Report on Hypertension in Diabetes. Hypertension 1994;23:145.)

emphasized the need to start with lifestyle changes and if these are not sufficient, to begin drug monotherapy but not using the traditional stepped-care approach. Initial recommendations for monotherapy might include thiazide diuretics, converting-enzyme inhibitors (CEIs), calcium channel blockers, or α_1-adrenergic blockers. There was a caution noted for the role of β-blockers in treatment of hypertension in diabetes because of their metabolic and other side effects.[204] Other expert reports, including the American Diabetes Association Consensus Statement on the Treatment of Hypertension in Diabetes[205] and the Report of the Canadian Hypertension Consensus Conference on Hypertension in Diabetes,[206] also cautioned about using diuretics and β-blockers in diabetics except in certain circumstances. The NHBPEP Working Group defined goal blood pressure as 135/85 mm Hg or less for the treatment of hypertension in diabetes.

Lifestyle Modifications

The NHBPEP Working Group advocated lifestyle modification as the initial treatment for hypertension in subjects with diabetes mellitus. Control of body weight was recognized as most important in NIDDM, as a relatively small amount of weight loss can produce substantial reductions in blood pressure.[207] This mode of therapy also helps correct the metabolic abnormalities in NIDDM subjects. As a high proportion of hypertensive diabetics retain sodium and have salt-sensitive hypertension,[2,6] sodium restriction should be effective in blood pressure control. Indeed, one recent study has documented that sodium restriction is effective to control blood pressure in most hypertensive NIDDM.[208] A diet moderately restricting sodium chloride to 100 mM/day (2.3 g sodium/day, 6 g sodium chloride/day) is recommended. Moderation in alcohol intake, daily exercise, and smoking cessation are also very important in the diabetic.

Antihypertensive Agents

Converting-Enzyme Inhibitors

CEIs are considered by many to be the most effective in the treatment of hypertension in diabetes. As vasodilators, these agents lower total peripheral resistance and have a positive effect on cardiac performance. They do not cause sodium retention as do the direct-acting vasodilators. CEIs favorably affect intermediary metabolism and insulin-mediated glucose disposal[209] and are either lipid-neutral or reduce cholesterol.[210] Their well-documented capacity to lower urine protein excretion[23,211] and slow the progression of renal failure[24] is a very attractive feature in either normotensive or hypertensive diabetic subjects with nephropathy. They also reduce left ventricular hypertrophy.[212] The side-effect profile of CEIs is quite good, and they have less unfavorable effects on sexual function compared to diuretics, β-blockers and other sympatholytic antihypertensive agents. Borderline hyperkalemia during CEI therapy may occur especially in those diabetics with type IV renal tubular acidosis. CEI therapy can accelerate renal insufficiency in subjects with bilateral renal artery stenosis.

Calcium Channel Blockers

Calcium channel blockers are highly effective in control of hypertension in diabetes and have the advantage of exerting neutral effects on lipid metabolism.[213] In subjects without heart failure, these agents do not adversely affect cardiac function and have been shown to reverse cardiac hypertrophy. The effect of calcium channel blockers on protein excretion in diabetic nephropathy has been controversial. In general, the nondihydropyridine agents (diltiazem, verapamil) reduce proteinuria in hypertensive IDDM, whereas the dihydropyridines have less beneficial effects on proteinuria.[214,215] The calcium channel blockers can potentially impair insulin secretion and insulin-mediated glucose disposal, but the clinical significance of these effects is minimal.[216]

α_1-Adrenergic Blockers

The α_1-adrenergic blocking agents prazosin, terazosin, and doxazosin have been shown to effectively lower blood pressure in diabetics with hypertension.[207,213] These agents have a very good side-effect profile for glucose and lipid metabolism.[207,217,218] Although orthostatic hypotension is considered a first-dose phenomenon with prazosin, it may persist in diabetics with autonomic neuropathy. Additionally, prazosin can have diminished antihypertensive efficacy over time related to reactive salt and water retention.

Diuretic Agents

Diabetic subjects have a 10% increase in total body exchangeable sodium and exaggerated blood pressure responses to vasopressors.[2] These abnormalities are normalized by diuretic therapy, suggesting a selectivity of action in diabetes. Because of their adverse side-effect profile, these agents may not be considered the first choice in patients with hypertension and high-risk metabolic disorders. Diuretics are frequently used, however, in combination therapy, as when they are added in low doses to patients on either CEIs or beta blockers. Hypokalemia worsens glycemic control and increases susceptibility to complex ventricular ectopy; these complications can be minimized by potassium supplements or potassium-sparing diuretics. Diuretics adversely affect lipid profiles, increasing total and low-density lipoprotein cholesterol and to a lesser extent increasing very low-density lipoprotein triglycerides and lowering high-density lipoprotein cholesterol.[218] It has been argued that the glucose and lipid changes do not persist over time and that diuretics are safe to use in hypertensive subjects.[219] Indeed, a retrospective study of prescription patterns in hypertensive patients shows that diuretics do not require more orders for hypoglycemic drugs than any other class of antihypertensives.[220] Diuretics activate the renin angiotensin system, which may offset their hypotensive effect. The ability of diuretics to reverse left ventricular hypertrophy has been variable, most trials showing no effect but a few showing reductions.[212] Long-term thiazide diuretic therapy produces sexual dysfunction in a number of individuals.

β-Adrenergic Blocking Agents

Most β-adrenergic blocking agents have proven efficacy in control of hypertension in diabetes.[213,221] β-Blockers are especially indicated in younger diabetics who may have active coronary heart disease, tachyarrhythmias, recent myocardial infarction, or concentric ventricular hypertrophy. In overt diabetic nephropathy and hypertension, these agents can reduce protein excretion and the rate of progression of renal disease.[222] The adverse effects of β-blockers in diabetes are numerous. They markedly worsen insulin resistance[221] and glucose control in NIDDM. Both cardioselective and nonselective β-blockers increase serum triglycerides and decrease high-density lipoprotein cholesterol levels.[218,223] There is evidence that these agents may increase the incidence of diabetes in hypertensive individuals,[224] but they may be safer to use when combined with lifestyle modifications.[225] β-Blockers mask the warning signs of hypoglycemia in IDDM patients receiving insulin and delay recovery. Peripheral vascular resistance is increased during β-blockade, exacerbating intermittent claudication and Raynaud's phenomenon. In diabetic cardiomyopathy, the negative inotropic effects of β-blockade may worsen cardiac performance.

References

1. Major SG. Blood pressure in diabetes mellitus: A statistical study. Arch Intern Med 1989;44:797
2. Stern N, Tuck ML. Mechanisms of hypertension in diabetes mellitus. In: Laragh JH, Brenner BM, eds. Hypertension: Pathophysiology, Diagnosis, and Management. New York: Raven Press; 1995:2301–2314
3. Feldt-Rasmussen B, Mathiesen ER, Deckert T, et al. Central role for sodium in the pathogenesis of blood pressure changes independent of angiotensin, aldosterone and catecholamines in type I (insulin-dependent) diabetes mellitus. Diabetologia 1987;30:610
4. Weidmann P. Pathogenesis of hypertension accompanying diabetes mellitus. Contrib Nephrol 1988;73:73
5. Ditzel J, Brochner-Mortesen J. Tubular reabsorption rates as related to elevated glomerular filtration in diabetic children. Diabetes 1983;32(suppl 2):28
6. Tuck ML, Corry D, Trujillo A. Salt-sensitive blood pressure and exaggerated vascular reactivity in the hypertension of diabetes mellitus. Am J Med 1990;88:210
7. Sower JR, Epstein M. Diabetes mellitus and associated hypertension, vascular disease and nephropathy. An update. Hypertension 1995;26(pt 1):869
8. Ritz E, Fliser D, Nowicki M. Hypertension and vascular disease as complications of diabetes. In: Laragh JH, Brenner BM, eds. Hypertension: Pathophysiology, Diagnosis and Management. New York: Raven Press; 1995:2321–2334
9. Drury PL. Diabetes and arterial hypertension. Diabetologia 1983;24:1
10. Ubeda M, Hernandez I, Fenoy F, Quesada T. Vascular and adrenal renin-like activity in chronically diabetic rats. Hypertension 1988;11:339
11. Corrila-Rotter R, Hostetter TH, Rosenberg ME. Renin and angiotensin gene expression in experimental diabetes mellitus. Kidney Int 1992;41:796
12. Christlieb AR, Munichoodappa K, Braaten JT. Decreased response of plasma renin activity to orthostasis in diabetic patients with orthostatic hypotension. Diabetes 1973;23:835
13. Fernandez Cruz A Jr, Noth RH, Lassman MN, et al. Low plasma renin activity in normotensive patients with diabetes mellitus: Relationship to neuropathy. Hypertension 1981;3:87
14. Tuck ML, Sambhi MP, Levin L. Hyporeninemic hypoaldosteronism in diabetes mellitus: Studies of the autonomic nervous system control of renin release. Diabetes 1979;28:237
15. Baretta-Piccoli C, Weidmann P, Fraser R. Responsiveness of plasma 18-hydroxycorticosterone and aldosterone to angiotensin II or corticotropin in nonazotemic diabetes mellitus. Diabetes 1983;32:1
16. Trujillo A, Eggena P, Barrett J, Tuck M. Renin regulation in type II diabetes mellitus: Influence of dietary sodium. Hypertension 1989;13:200
17. Veldhuis JD, Melby J. Isolated aldosterone deficiency in man: Acquired and inborn errors in the biosynthesis or action of aldosterone. Endocrine Rev 1981;4:495
18. Nadler JL, Lee FO, Hsueh W, Horton R. Evidence of prostacyclin deficiency in the syndrome of hyporeninemic hypoaldosteronism. N Engl J Med 1986;314:1015
19. Hsueh WA, Carlson EZ, Luetscher JA, Grislis G. Activation and characterization of inactive big renin in plasma of patients with diabetic nephropathy and unusual active renin. J Clin Endocrinol Metab 1980;51:535
20. Luetscher JA, Kraemer FB, Wilson DM, et al. Increased plasma inactive renin in diabetes mellitus: A marker of microvascular complications. N Engl J Med 1985;312:1412
21. Hseuh WA. Effect of renin-angiotensin system in the vascular disease of type II diabetes mellitus. Am J Med 1992;92(suppl):13s
22. Anderson S, Rennkle HG, Garcia OL, Brenner BM. Short and long term effects of antihypertensive therapy in the diabetic rat. Kidney Int 1989;36:523
23. Ravid M, Savin H, Jutrin I, et al. Long-term stabilizing effect of angiotensin-converting enzyme inhibition on plasma creatinine and on proteinuria in normotensive type II diabetic patients. Ann Intern Med 1993;118:577
24. Lewis EJ, Hunsicker LG, Bain RP, Rhode RD. The effect of angiotensin-converting enzyme inhibition on diabetic nephropathy. N Engl J Med 1993;329:1456
25. Dzau VJ. Circulating versus local renin-angiotensin system in cardiovascular homeostasis. Circulation 1988;77(suppl I):I-I
26. Marre M, Bernadet P, Gallois Y, et al. Relationship between angiotensin I converting enzyme gene polymorphism, plasma levels and diabetic retinal and renal complications. Diabetes 1994;43:384
27. Feman SS, Mericle RA, Reed GW, et al. Serum angiotensin converting enzyme in diabetic patients. Am J Med Sci 1993;305:280
28. Doria M, Warram JH, Krolewski AS. Genetic predisposition to diabetic nephropathy. Evidence for a role of angiotensin I converting enzyme gene. Diabetes 1994;43:690
29. Erman A, Van Dyk DJ, Chen-Gal B, et al. Angiotensin converting enzyme activity in the serum, lung, and kidney of diabetic rats. Eur J Clin Invest 1993;23:615
30. Jandeleit K, Rumble J, Jackson R, Cooper ME. Mesenteric vascular angiotensin converting enzyme is increased in experimental diabetes mellitus. Clin Exp Pharmacol Physiol 1992;19:343
31. Ortola FV, Ballermann BJ, Anderson S, et al. Elevated plasma atrial natriuretic peptide levels in diabetic rats: Potential mediator of hyperfiltration. J Clin Invest 1987;80:670
32. DeChatel R, Toth M, Barra I. Exchangeable body sodium: Its relationship with blood pressure and atrial natriuretic factor in patients with diabetes mellitus. J Hypertens 1986;4:S256
33. Nosadini R, Floretto P, Trevisan R, Crepaldi G. Insulin-dependent diabetes mellitus and hypertension. Diabetes Care 1991;14:210
34. Chen S, Yeen C, Clough D, et al. Role of digitalis-like substance in the hypertension of reduced renal mass rats. Am J Hypertens 1994;6(5 Pt 1): 397
35. Takahashi H, Matsusawa M, Nishimura M, et al. Digoxin-like immunoreactivity may contribute to hyperinsulinemia-associated hypertension in patients with glucose intolerance. J Cardiovasc Pharmacol 1993;22(suppl 2):S22
36. Weder AB. Red cell lithium-sodium countertransport and renal lithium clearance in hypertension. N Engl J Med 1986;314:198
37. Canessa M, Adragna N, Solomon HS, et al. Increased sodium-lithium countertransport in red cells of patients with essential hypertension. N Engl J Med 1980;302:772
38. Mangili R, Bending JJ, Scoot G, et al. Increased sodium-lithium countertransport activity in red cells of patients with insulin-dependent diabetes and nephropathy. N Engl J Med 1988;318:146
39. Krowlewski AS, Canessa M, Warram J, et al. Predisposition to hypertension and susceptibility to renal disease in insulin-dependent diabetes mellitus. N Engl J Med 1988;381:140
40. Hannedouche TP, Marques LP, Guicheney P, et al. Predisposition to essential hypertension and renal hemodynamics in recent onset insulin-dependent diabetic patients. J Am Soc Nephrol 1992;3(suppl 4):S34
41. Gall MA, Rossing P, Jensen JS, et al. Red cell Na+, Li+ countertransport in non-insulin-dependent diabetics with diabetic nephropathy. Kidney Int 1991;39:135
42. Modan M, Halkin H, Almog S, et al. Hyperinsulinemia: A link between hypertension, obesity and glucose intolerance. J Clin Invest 1985;75:809
43. Ferrannini E, Buzzigoli G, Bonadonna R, et al. Insulin resistance in essential hypertension. N Engl J Med 1987;317:350
44. Reaven GM, Hoffman BB. Hypertension as a disease of carbohydrate and lipoprotein metabolism. Am J Med 1989;87(suppl 6A):2S
45. Pollare T, Lithell H, Berne C. Insulin resistance is a characteristic feature of primary hypertension independent of obesity. Metabolism 1990;39:167
46. DeFronzo RA, Ferrannini E. Insulin resistance: A multifaceted syndrome responsible for NIDDM, obesity and hypertension, dyslipidemia and atherosclerotic cardiovascular disease. Diabetes Care 1991;14:173
47. Julius S, Gundrandsson T, Jamerson K, et al. The hemodynamic link between insulin resistance and hypertension. J Hypertens 1991;9:983
48. Salvatore T, Cozzolino D, Giunta R, et al. Decreased insulin clearance as a feature of essential hypertension. J Clin Endocrinol Metab 1992;74:144
49. Nosadini R, Solini A, Velussi M, et al. Impaired insulin-induced glucose uptake by extrahepatic tissue is a hallmark of NIDDM patients who have or will develop hypertension and microalbuminuria. Diabetes 1994;43:491
50. Saad MF, Lillioja S, Nyomba BL, et al. Racial differences in the relation between blood pressure and insulin resistance. N Engl J Med 1991;324:733
51. Bennet PH, Stern PH. Patient population and genetics: Role in diabetes. Am J Med 1991;90(suppl A):76S
52. Cruickshank JK, Cooper J, Burnett M, et al. Ethnic differences in fasting plasma C-peptide and insulin in relation to glucose tolerance and blood pressure. Lancet 1991;338:842
53. Dowse GK, Collins VR, Alberti KG, et al. Insulin and blood pressure are not independently related in Mauritians of Asian Indian, Creole or Chinese origin. The Mauritius Non-Communicative Disease Study Group. J Hypertens 1991;15:297
54. Reaven G, Ho H, Hoffman BB. Attenuation of fructose-induced hypertension in rats by exercise training. Metabolism 1988;12:129
55. Reaven G, Ho H, Hoffman BB. Somatostatin inhibition of fructose-induced hypertension. Hypertension 1989;14:117
56. Mondon CE, Reaven GM. Evidence of abnormalities of insulin metabolism in rats with spontaneous hypertension. Metabolism 1988;37:303
57. Buchanan T, Sipos G, Liu C, Campese V. Hyperinsulinemia in spontaneously hypertensive rats. Clin Res 1990;38:109A
58. Buchanan TA, Sipos GF, Gadalah S, et al. Glucose tolerance and insulin action in rats with renovascular hypertension. Hypertension 1991;18:341
59. Hall JE, Coleman TG, Mizelle HL, Smith MJ. Chronic hyperinsulinemia and blood pressure regulation. Am J Physiol 1990;258:F722
60. Meehan WP, Buchanan TA, Hsueh W. Chronic insulin administration elevates blood pressure in rats. Hypertension 1994;23(part 2):1012
61. Kurtz TW, Morris RC, Pershadsingh HA. The Zucker fatty rat as a genetic model of obesity and hypertension. Hypertension 1989;13:896
62. Natali A, Santoro O, Palombo C, et al. Impaired insulin action on skeletal muscle metabolism in essential hypertension. Hypertension 1991;17:170
63. Lillioja S, Young AA, Culter CL. Skeletal muscle capillary density and fiber

type are possible determinants of in vivo insulin resistance in man. J Clin Invest 1988;80:415
64. Peiris AN, Sothman MS, Hoffman FG, et al. Adiposity, fat distribution and cardiovascular risk. Ann Intern Med 1989;110:867
65. Peiris AN, Mueller RA, Smith GA, et al. Splanchnic insulin metabolism in obesity. J Clin Invest 1986;78:1642
66. Laakso M, Sarlund H, Mykkanen L. Essential hypertension and insulin resistance in non-insulin dependent diabetes mellitus. Eur J Clin Invest 1989;19:518
67. Laakso M, Edelman SV, Brechtel G, Baron D. Decreased effect of insulin to stimulate muscle blood flow in obese men. A novel mechanism for insulin resistance. J Clin Invest 1990;85:1844
68. Laakso M, Edelman SV, Brectel G, Baron D. Impaired insulin-mediated skeletal muscle flow in patients with NIDDM. Diabetes 1990;41:1076
69. Vollenweider P, Randin D, Tappy L, et al. Impaired insulin-induced sympathetic neural activation and vasodilation in skeletal muscle in obese humans. J Clin Invest 1994;93:2365
70. Baron AD, Brechtel G, Johnson A, et al. Interactions between insulin and norepinephrine on blood pressure and insulin sensitivity: Studies in lean and obese men. J Clin Invest 1994;93:2453
71. Fukagawa NK, Minaker KL, Young VR, Rowe JW. Insulin dose-dependent reductions in plasma amino acids in man. Am J Physiol 1986;250:E13
72. Kreiger DR, Landsberg L. Mechanisms in obesity-related hypertension: Role of insulin and catecholamines. Am J Hypertens 1988;1:84
73. Vierhapper H. Effect of exogenous insulin on blood pressure regulation in healthy and diabetic subjects. Hypertension 1975;7(suppl II):II49
74. Buchanan TA, Thawani H, Kades W, et al. Angiotensin II increases glucose utilization during acute hyperinsulinemia via a hemodynamic mechanism. J Clin Invest 1993;92:720
75. Townsend RR, DiPette DJ. Pressor doses of angiotensin II increase insulin-mediated glucose uptake in normotensive men. Am J Physiol 1993;265:E362
76. Rao RH. Effects of angiotensin II on insulin sensitivity and fasting glucose metabolism in rats. Am J Hypertens 1994;7:655
77. Torlone E, Britta M, Rambotti AM, et al. Improved glycemic control after long term angiotensin-converting enzyme inhibition in subjects with arterial hypertension and type II diabetes. Diabetes Care 1993;16:1347
78. Gans ROB, Bilo HJG, Nauta JJP, et al. The effect of angiotensin I converting enzyme inhibition on insulin action in healthy volunteers. Eur J Clin Invest 1991;21:527
79. Pollare T, Lithell H, Berne C. A comparison of the effects of hydrochlorothiazide and captopril on glucose and lipid metabolism in patients with hypertension. N Engl J Med 1989;321:866
80. Paolisso G, Gambardella A, Verza M, et al. ACE inhibition improves insulin sensitivity in aged insulin-resistant hypertensive patients. J Hum Hypertens 1992;6:175
81. Vuorinen-Markkola H, Ykj-Jarvinen H. Antihypertensive therapy with enalapril improves glucose storage and insulin sensitivity in hypertensive type II diabetic patients (Abstract). Diabetologia 1992;35(suppl 1):A93
82. Garrison JO, Borland MK, Florio VA, et al. The role of calcium ion as mediator of the effect of angiotensin, catecholamines and vasopressin on the phosphorylation and activity of enzymes in isolated hepatocytes. J Biol Chem 1979;254:7147
83. Seefeldt T, Orskov L, Rasmussen O, et al. Lack of effects of angiotensin converting enzyme inhibitors on glucose metabolism in insulin-dependent diabetes mellitus. Diabetic Med 1990;7:700
84. Santoro D, Natali A, Palombo C, et al. Effects of chronic angiotensin-converting enzyme inhibition on glucose tolerance and insulin sensitivity in essential hypertension. Hypertension 1992;20:181
85. Seghieri G, Yin W, Boni C, et al. Effect of chronic ACE inhibition on glucose tolerance and insulin sensitivity in hypertensive type II diabetic patients. Diabetic Med 1992;9:732
86. Landsberg L. Hyperinsulinemia: Possible role in obesity-induced hypertension. Hypertension 1992;19(suppl 1):I–61
87. Rowe JW, Young JB, Minaker KL, et al. Effect of insulin and glucose infusions on sympathetic nervous system activity in normal man. Diabetes 1981;30:219
88. Anderson EA, Hoffman RP, Balon TW, et al. Hyperinsulinemia produces both sympathetic neural activation and vasodilation in normal humans. J Clin Invest 1991;87:2246
89. Baron AO, Laakso M, Brechtel G, Edelman SW. Mechanism of insulin resistance in insulin dependent diabetes mellitus: A major role for reduced skeletal muscle blood flow. J Clin Endocrinol Metab 1991;73:637
90. Sowers JR, Whitfield LA, Catania RA, et al. Role of the sympathetic nervous system in blood pressure maintenance in obesity. J Clin Endocrinol Metab 1982;54:1181
91. Tuck ML. Obesity, the sympathetic nervous system and essential hypertension. Hypertension 1992;19(suppl 1):I-67
92. Tuck ML, Sowers JR. Dornfield L, et al. Reductions in plasma catecholamines and blood pressure during weight loss in obese subjects. Acta Endocrinol (Copenh) 1983;102:252
93. Fontbonne AM, Eschwege EM. Insulin and cardiovascular disease: Paris Prospective Study. Diabetes Care 1991;14:461
94. Reaven GM. Banting lecture 1988: Role of insulin resistance in human disease. Diabetes 1988;37:1595
95. Stolar MW. Atherosclerosis in diabetes: The role of hyperinsulinemia. Metabolism 1988;37(suppl 1):1
96. Stout RW. Insulin and atheroma: 20-year perspective. Diabetes Care 1990; 13:631
97. Folkow B. Cardiovascular structural adaptation: Its role in the initiation and maintenance of primary hypertension: The fourth Volhard lecture. Clin Sci Mol Med 1978;55(suppl):3s
98. King GL, Goodman AM, Buzngy S, et al. Receptors and growth promoting effects of insulin and insulin-like growth factors on cells from bovine retinal capillaries and aorta. J Clin Invest 1985;75:1028
99. Capron L, Jamet J, Kazandjian S, Housset E. Growth-promoting effects of diabetes and insulin on arteries. Diabetes 1986;35:973
100. Murphy LJ, Ghahary A, Chakrabart S. Insulin regulation of IGF-I expression in rat aorta. Diabetes 1990;39:657
101. King GL, Kahn CR, Rechler MM, Nissley SR. Direct demonstration of separate receptors for growth and metabolic activities of insulin and multiplication-stimulating activity (an insulin-like growth factor). J Clin Invest 1980;66:120
102. Bornfeldt KE, Arnquist HJ, Capron L. In vivo proliferation of rat vascular smooth muscle in relation to diabetes mellitus, insulin-like growth factor-I and insulin. Diabetologia 1992;35:104
103. Stout RW. Insulin and atherogenesis. Eur J Epidemiol 1992;8(suppl 1):134
104. Hamet P, Sugimoto H, Umeda I, et al. Abnormalities of platelet-derived growth factors in insulin-dependent diabetes. Metabolism 1985;34(suppl 1):25
105. Nakoo J, Ito H, Kanayasu T, Murota SI. Stimulatory effect of insulin on aortic smooth muscle cell migration induced by 12-hydroxy-5,8,10,14-eicosatetraenoic acid and its modulation by elevated extracellular glucose levels. Diabetes 1985;34:185
106. Taggart H, Stout RW. Control of DNA synthesis in cultured vascular endothelial and smooth muscle cells. Atherosclerosis. 1980;37:549
107. Oliver FJ, de La-Rubia G, Fenner EP, et al. Stimulation of endothelin-I gene expression by insulin in endothelial cells. J Biol Chem 1991;266:23251
108. Hattori Y, Kasai K, Nakamura T, et al. Effects of glucose and insulin on immunoreactive endothelin-I released from cultured porcine aortic endothelial cells. Metabolism 1991;40:165
109. Takahashi K, Ghatei MA, Lam HC, et al. Elevated plasma endothelin in patients with diabetes mellitus. Diabetologia 1990;33:306
110. Frank HJ, Levin ER, Hu RM, Pedram A. Insulin stimulates endothelin binding and action in cultured vascular smooth muscle cells. Endocrinology 1993;133:1092
111. Schneider DJ, Nordt TK, Sobel BE. Stimulation by proinsulin of expression of plasminogen activator inhibitor type I in endothelial cells. Diabetes 1992;41:890
112. Oppenheimer MJ, Sundquist K, Bierman EL. Downregulation of high density lipoprotein receptor in human fibroblasts by insulin and IGF-I. Diabetes 1989;38:117
113. Krone W, Naegle H, Belinki B, Greten H. Opposite effects of insulin and catecholamines on LDL-receptor activity in human mononuclear leukocytes. Diabetes 1988;37:1386
114. Gans ROB, Bilo HJG, Maarschalkerweerd Heine RJ, et al. Exogenous insulin augments in healthy volunteers the cardiovascular reactivity to noradrenaline but not to angiotensin II. J Clin Invest 1991;88:512
115. Saki K, Imaizumi T, Masaki H, Takeshita A. Intraarterial infusion of insulin attenuates vasoreactivity in human forearm. Hypertension 1993;22:67
116. Yagi S, Takata S, Kiyokawa H, et al. Effects of insulin on vasoconstrictive responses to norepinephrine in rabbit femoral artery and vein. Diabetes 1988;37:1064
117. Standley PR, Zhang F, Ram JL, et al. Insulin attenuates vasopressin-induced calcium transients and a voltage dependent calcium response to rat vascular smooth muscle cells. J Clin Invest 1991;88:1230
118. Saito F, Hori MT, Fittingoff M, et al. Insulin attenuates agonist-mediated calcium mobilization in cultured rat vascular smooth muscle cells. J Clin Invest 1993;92:1161
119. Touyz RM, Tolleczko B, Schiffrin EL. Insulin attenuates agonist-evoked calcium transients in vascular smooth muscle cells. Hypertension 1994;23 (suppl I):I-25
120. Kahn AM, Seidel CL, Allen JC, et al. Insulin reduces contraction and intracellular calcium concentration in vascular smooth muscle. Hypertension 1993;22:735
121. Gros R, Borkowski KR, Feldman RD. Human insulin-mediated enhancement of vascular beta-adrenergic responsiveness. Hypertension 1994;23:551
122. Creager MA, Liang CS, Coffman JD. Beta-adrenergic-mediated vasodilator response to insulin in the human forearm. J Pharmacol Exp Ther 1985;235: 709
123. Huot SJ, Aronson PS. Na-H exchanger and its role in essential hypertension and diabetes mellitus. Diabetes Care 1991;14:521
124. Aviv A, Livne A. The Na+/H+ antiport, cytosolic free Ca2+, and hypertension: A hypothesis. Am J Hypertens 1988;1:410
125. Drazin B, Kao M, Sussman KE. Insulin and glyburide increase cytosolic free calcium concentrations in isolated rat adipocytes. Diabetes 1987;36:174
126. Sowers JR, Khoury S, Standley P, et al. Mechanisms of hypertension in diabetes mellitus. Am J Hypertens 1991;4(2 pt 1):177
127. Resnick LM. Calcium metabolism in hypertension and allied metabolic disorders. Diabetes Care 1991;14:505
128. Beretta-Piccoli C, Weidmann P. Body sodium and renin activity in diabetes mellitus. Diabete Metab 1989;15:296

129. Nosadini R, Fioretto P, Giorato C, et al. Sodium metabolism in insulin-dependent patients: Role of insulin and atrial natriuretic peptide. Diabete Metab 1989;15:301
130. Abonchacra S, Baines AD, Zinman B, et al. Insulin blunts the natriuretic action of atrial natriuretic peptide in hypertension. Hypertension 1994;23 (part 2):1054
131. Natali A, Quinones Galvan A, Santoro D, et al. Relationship between insulin release, antinatriuresis and hypokalemia after glucose ingestion in normal and hypertensive men. Clin Sci 1993;85:327
132. Rocchini AP, Katch V, Kveselis D, et al. Insulin and renal sodium retention in obese adolescents. Hypertension 1989;14:367
133. Tedde R, Sachi LA, Marigliano A, et al. Antihypertensive effect of insulin reduction in diabetic hypertensive patients. Am J Hypertens 1989;2:163
134. Ditzel J, Lervang H-H, Brochner-Mortensen J. Renal sodium metabolism in relation to hypertension in diabetes. Diabete Metab 1989;15:292
135. O'Hare JA, Roland JM, Walters G, Corrall RJM. Impaired sodium excretion in response to volume expansion induced by water immersion in insulin-dependent diabetes mellitus. Clin Sci 1986;71:403
136. Moore RD. Effects of insulin on ion transport. Biochim Biophys Acta 1983;737:1
137. Fidelman ML, May JM, Biber TUL, Watlington CO. Insulin stimulation of Na+ transport and glucose metabolism in cultured kidney cells. Am J Physiol 1982;242:C121
138. Baum M. Insulin stimulates volume absorption in the proximal convoluted tubules. J Clin Invest 1987;79:1104
139. Skott P, Hothe-Nielsen G, Bruun NE, et al. Effects of insulin on kidney function and sodium excretion in healthy subjects. Diabetologia 1989;32:694
140. Mogensen CE, Christensen NJ, Gunderson HJG. The acute effect of insulin on renal hemodynamics and protein excretion in diabetics. Diabetologia 1978;15:153
141. Christiansen JS, Frandsen M, Parving HH. The effect of intravenous insulin infusion on kidney function in insulin-dependent diabetes mellitus. Diabetologia 1981;20:199
142. The Diabetes Control and Complication Trial Research Group. The effect of intensive treatment of diabetes on the development and progression of long term complications in insulin dependent diabetes mellitus. N Engl J Med 1993;329:977
143. Ferris JB, O'Hare JA, Kelleher CCM, et al. Diabetic control and the renin angiotensin system, catecholamines and blood pressure. Hypertension 1985; 7(suppl 2):II58
144. Randeree HA, Omar MAK, Motala AA, Seedat MA. Effect of insulin therapy on blood pressure in NIDDM patients with secondary failure. Diabetes Care 1992;15:1258
145. Anderson EA, Mark AL. The vasodilator action of insulin. Implications for the insulin hypothesis of hypertension. Hypertension 1993;21:136
146. Tesfamariam B, Brown ML, Cohen RA. Elevated glucose impairs endothelium dependent relaxation by activation of protein kinase C. J Clin Invest 1991;87:1643
147. Yamauchi T, Ohnaka K, Takayanagi R, et al. Enhanced secretion of endothelin-I by elevated glucose levels from cultured bovine aortic endothelial cells. FEBS Lett 1990;267:16
148. Gupta S, Sussman I, McArthur CVS, et al. Endothelium-dependent inhibition of Na^+, K^+ ATPase activity in rabbit aorta by hyperglycemia. Possible role of endothelium-derived nitric oxide. J Clin Invest 1992;90:727
149. McVeigh CE, Brennan GM, Johnston GD, et al. Dietary fish oil augments nitric oxide production or release in patients with type 2 diabetes mellitus. Diabetologia 1993;36:33
150. Thompson ABR, Kappagoda T. Endothelium-dependent relaxation in aorta from diabetic rats. Diabetes 1987;36:979
151. Lorenzi M, Cagliero E, Toledo S. Glucose toxicity for human endothelial cells in culture: Delayed replication, disturbed cell cycle and accelerated death. Diabetes 1985;34:621
152. Scurnthuner G, Schwarzer C, Kuzmito R, et al. Increased angiotensin-converting enzyme activities in diabetes mellitus: Analysis of diabetes type, state of metabolic control and occurrence of diabetic vascular disease. J Clin Pathol 1984;37:307
153. Natarajan R, Gu JL, Rossi J, et al. Elevated glucose and angiotensin II increase 12-lipoxygenase activity and expression in porcine aortic smooth muscle cells. Proc Natl Acad Sci (USA) 1993;90:4947
154. Saito F, Hori M, Ideguchi Y, et al. 12-Lipoxygenase products modulate calcium signals in vascular smooth muscle cells. Hypertension 1992;20: 268
155. Kawamura M, Heinecke JW, Chait A. Pathophysiological concentrations of glucose promote oxidative modification of low density lipoprotein by a superoxide-dependent pathway. J Clin Invest 1994;94:771
156. Vlassara H, Brownlee M, Monague KR, et al. Cachectin/TNF and IL-I induced by glucose modified proteins: Role in normal tissue remodelling. Science 1988;240:1546
157. Kirstein M, Aston C, Hintz R, et al. Receptor-specific induction of insulin-like growth factor I in human monocytes by advanced glycosylation and product-modified proteins. J Clin Invest 1992;90:439
158. Kirstein M, Brett J, Radoff S, et al. Advanced protein glycosylation induces transendothelial human monocyte chemotaxis and secretion of platelet-derived growth factor: Role in vascular disease of diabetes and aging. Proc Natl Acad Sci USA 1991;87:9010
159. Hogan M, Cerami A, Bucala R. Advanced glycosylation end products block the antiproliferative effect of nitric oxide: Role in the vascular and renal complications of diabetes mellitus. J Clin Invest 1992;90:1110
160. Faris I, Agerskov K, Henrikenson O. Decreased distensibility of a passive vascular bed in diabetes mellitus; an indicator of microangiopathy. Diabetologia 1982;23:411
161. Halushka PV, Mayfield R, Colwell JA. Insulin and arachidonic acid metabolism in diabetes mellitus. Metabolism 1985;34(suppl 1):32
162. Durante W, Sen AK, Sunahara FA. Impairment of endothelium-dependent relaxation of aortae from spontaneously diabetic rats. Br J Pharmacol 1980;94:463
163. Saenez de Tejada I, Goldstein I, Azadzoi K, et al. Impaired neurogenic and endothelial-mediated relaxation of penile smooth muscle from diabetic men with impotence. N Engl J Med 1989;320:1025
164. Calver A, Collier J, Vallace P. Inhibition and stimulation of nitric oxide synthesis in the human forearm arterial bed of patients with diabetes mellitus. J Clin Invest 1992;90:2548
165. Rees DD, Palmer RMJ, Moncada S. Role of endothelium-derived nitric oxide in the regulation of blood pressure. Proc Natl Acad Sci USA 1988;86:3375
166. Monnies VM, Kohn RR, Cerami A. Accelerated age-related browning of human collagen in diabetes mellitus. Proc Natl Acad Sci USA 1984;81:583
167. Bucola R, Tracey KJ, Cerami A. Advanced glycosylation products quench nitric oxide and mediate defective endothelium-dependent vasodilation in experimental diabetes. J Clin Invest 1991;87:432
168. Taylor PD, Oon BB, Thomas CR, Poston L. Prevention by insulin treatment of endothelial dysfunction but not enhanced noradrenaline-induced contractility in mesenteric resistance arteries from streptozotocin diabetic rats. Br J Pharmacol 1994;111:35
169. Ritz E, Hasslacher C, Guo J-Z, Mann JFE. Role of hypertension in diabetic nephropathy. In: Heidland A, Koch KM, Heidborder E, eds. Diabetes and the Kidney. Basel, Switzerland: Karger;1989:91–101
170. Mogensen CE, Christensen CK. Blood pressure changes and renal function in incipient and overt diabetic nephropathy. Hypertension 1985;7(suppl II):II64
171. Standl E, Stiegler H, Roth R, et al. On the impact of hypertension on the prognosis of NIDDM: Results of the Schwabing GP-program. Diabete Metab 1989;15:352
172. Bakris GL. The effects of calcium antagonists on renal hemodynamics, urinary protein excretion, and glomerular morphology in diabetic states. J Am Soc Nephrol 1991;2:S21
173. Feldt-Rasmussen B, Borch-Johnson K, Mathiesen ER. Hypertension in diabetes as related to nephropathy: Early blood pressure changes. Hypertension 1985;7(suppl II):II18
174. Mathiesen ER, Ronn B, Jensen T, et al. Relationship between blood pressure and urinary albumin excretion in development of microalbuminuria. Diabetes 1990;39:245
175. Chase HP, Sarg SK, Harris S, et al. High-normal blood pressure and early diabetic nephropathy. Arch Intern Med 1990;150:639
176. Poulsen PL, Hansen KW, Mogensen CE. Ambulatory blood pressure in transition from normo- to microalbuminuria: A longitudinal study in IDDM patients. Diabetes 1994;43:1248
177. Christensen CK, Krusell LR, Mogensen CE. Increased blood pressure in diabetes: Essential hypertension or diabetic nephropathy. Scand J Clin Lab Invest 1987;47:363
178. Ljungman S, Granerus G. The evaluation of kidney function in hypertensive patients. In: Laragh JH, Brenner BM, eds. Hypertension, Pathophysiology, Diagnosis and Management. New York: Raven Press;1995:1987–2004
179. Grunfeld B, Perelstein E, Simsolo R, et al. Renal function and microalbuminuria in offspring of hypertensive parents. Hypertension 1990;15:257
180. Fabre J, Balant LP, Dayer PG, et al. The kidney in maturity-onset diabetes mellitus: A clinical study of 510 patients. Kidney Int 1982;21:730
181. Viberti GC, Keen H, Wiseman MJ. Raised arterial pressure in parents of proteinuric insulin-dependent diabetics. Br Med J 1982;295:515
182. Borch-Johnsen K, Nissen H, Nerup J. Blood pressure after 40 years of insulin-dependent diabetes. Diabetic Nephrol 1985;4:11
183. Trevisan M, Vaccaro O, Laurenzi M, et al. Hypertension, non-insulin-dependent diabetes and intracellular sodium metabolism. Hypertension 1988;11:264
184. Mauer SM, Steffes MW, Ellis EN, et al. Structural-functional relationships in diabetic nephropathy. J Clin Invest 1984;74:1143
185. Wesson DE, Kurtzman NA, Frommer JP. Massive obesity and nephrotic proteinuria with a normal renal biopsy. Nephron 1985;40:235
186. Kasiske BL, Crosson JT. Renal disease in patients with massive obesity. Arch Intern Med 1986;146:1105
187. Corry D, Tuck ML. Hypertension and diabetes. Semin Nephrol 1991;11:561
188. Kaplan C, Pasternack B, Shah H, et al. Age-related incidence of sclerotic glomeruli in human kidneys. Am J Pathol 1975;80:227
189. Zatz R, Brenner BM. Pathogenesis of diabetic microangiopathy: The hemodynamic view. Am J Med 1986;80:443
190. Bohlen HG, Hankins KD. Early arteriolar and capillary changes in streptozotocin-induced diabetic rats and in intraperitoneal hyperglycemic rats. Diabetologia 1982;22:344
191. Bank N, Aynedjian HS. Role of EDRF (nitric oxide) in diabetic renal hyperfiltration. Kidney Int 1993;43:1306
192. Tolins JP, Shultz PJ, Raij L, et al. Abnormal renal hemodynamic response to reduced renal perfusion pressure in diabetic rats; role of NO. Am J Physiol 1993;165(6 pt 2):F886

193. Ichikawa I, Harris RC. Angiotensin II actions in the kidney: Renewed insight into the old hormone. Kidney Int 1991;40:583
194. Wolf G, Neilson EG. Angiotensin II as a renal growth factor. J Am Soc Nephrol 1993;3:1531
195. Kakinuma Y, Kawamura T, Bills T, et al. Blood pressure-independent effects of angiotensin-converting enzyme inhibition on vascular lesions of chronic renal failure. Kidney Int 1993;42:46
196. Kagami S, Border WA, Miller DE, Noble NA. Angiotensin II stimulates extracellular matrix protein synthesis through induction of transforming growth factor-B expression in rat glomerular mesangial cells. J Clin Invest 1994;93:2431
197. Derubertis PR, Craven PA. Activation of protein kinase C in glomerular cells in diabetes: Mechanisms and potential links to the pathogenesis of diabetic glomerulopathy. Diabetes 1994;43:1
198. Kelleher C, Kingston S, Barry SM, et al. Hypertension in diabetic clinic patients and their siblings. Diabetologia 1988;31:76
199. Tierney WM, McDonald CJ, Luft FC. Renal disease in hypertensive adults: Effect of race and type II diabetes mellitus. J Kidney Dis 1989;6:485
200. Schmitz A, Hansen HH, Christensen T. Kidney function in newly diagnosed type 2 (non-insulin-dependent) diabetic patients before and during treatment. Diabetologia 1989;32:434
201. Reubi F, Franz KA, Horber F. Hypertension as related to renal function in diabetes mellitus. Hypertension 1985;7(suppl 2):II21
202. Baba T, Murabyashi S, Aoyagi K, et al. Prevalence of hypertension in diabetes mellitus; its relation to diabetic nephropathy. Tohoku J Exp Med 1985; 145:167
203. Tarnow L, Rossing P, Gali MA, et al. Prevalence of arterial hypertension in diabetic patients before and after the JNC-V. Diabetes Care 1994;17: 1247
204. The National High Blood Pressure Education Program Working Group. National High Blood Pressure Education Program Working Group Report on Hypertension in Diabetes. Hypertension 1994;23:145
205. American Diabetes Association. Consensus statement on the treatment of hypertension in diabetes. Diabetes Care 1993;16:1394
206. Dawson KG, McKenzie JK, Ross SA, et al. Report of the Canadian Hypertension Consensus Conference: 5, Hypertension and diabetes. Can Med Assoc J 1993;149:821
207. Stern N, Tuck M. Drug therapy of hypertension in diabetic patients. J Hum Hypertens 1991;5:295
208. Dodson PM, Beevers M, Hallworth R, et al. Sodium restriction and blood pressure in hypertensive type II diabetics: Randomized blind controlled and crossover studies of moderate sodium restriction and sodium supplementation. Br Med J 1989;298:227
209. Pollare T, Lithell H, Berne C. A comparison of the effects of hydrochlorothiazide and captopril on glucose and lipid metabolism in patients with hypertension. N Engl J Med 1989;321:868
210. Costa EV, Borghi C, Mussi A, et al. Use of captopril to reduce serum lipids in hypertensive patients with hyperlipidemia. Am J Hypertens 1988;1: 221S
211. Kasiske BL, Kalil RSN, Ma JZ, et al. Effect of antihypertensive therapy on the kidney in patients with diabetes: A meta-regression analysis. Ann Intern Med 1993;118:129
212. Hachamivitz S, Sonnenblick EH, Storm JA, et al. Left ventricular hypertrophy in hypertension and the effects of antihypertensive drug therapy. Curr Prob Cardiol 1988;13:369
213. Stein P, Black H. Drug treatment of hypertension in patients with diabetes mellitus. Diabetes Care 1991;14:425
214. Bakris GL, Barnhill BW, Sadler R. Treatment of arterial hypertension in diabetic humans: Importance of therapeutic selection. Kidney Int 1992;141: 912
215. Mogensen CE. Management of the diabetic patient with elevated blood pressure or renal disease. In: Laragh JH, Brenner BM, eds. Hypertension: Pathophysiology, Diagnosis and Management. New York: Raven Press;1995: 2335–2365
216. Tuck ML, Bravo EL, Krakoff LR, Friedman CP, and the Modern Approach to the Treatment of Hypertension Study Group: Endocrine and renal effects of nifedipine gastrointestinal therapeutic system in patients with essential hypertension: Results of a multicenter trial. Am J Hypertens 1990;3: 333S
217. Lund L, Pollare T, Berne C, et al. Long-term metabolic effects of antihypertensive drugs. Am Heart J 1994;128:1177
218. Kassike BL, Ma JZ, Kalil RSN, Louis TA. Effects of antihypertensive therapy on serum lipids. Ann Intern Med 1995;122:133
219. Freis E. The efficacy and safety of diuretics in treating hypertension. Ann Intern Med 1995;122:223
220. Gurwitz JH, Bohn RL, Glynn RJ, et al. Antihypertensive drug therapy and the initiation of treatment for diabetes mellitus. Ann Intern Med 1992;118: 273
221. Pollare T, Lithell H, Morlin C, et al. Metabolic effects of diltiazem and atenolol: Results from a randomized, double-blind study with parallel groups. J Hypertens 1989;7:551
222. Parving HH, Andersen AR, Smidt UM, et al. Early aggressive antihypertensive treatment reduces rate of decline in kidney function in diabetic nephropathy. Lancet 1983;1:1176
223. Pollare T, Lithell H, Selinus I, et al. Sensitivity to insulin during treatment with atenolol and metoprolol: A randomized double blind study of effects on carbohydrate and lipoprotein metabolism in hypertensive patients. Br Med J 1989;298:1152
224. Mykkanen L, Haffner SM, Kuusisto V, et al. Hypertensives with beta blocker or diuretic therapy have an increased risk of developing type II diabetes. Diabetologia 1993;36:A212
225. Neaton JD, Grimm RH, Prineas RJ, et al. for the Treatment of Mild Hypertension Study Research Group. Treatment of Mild Hypertension Study: Final results. JAMA 1993;270:713

Diabetes Mellitus, edited by Derek LeRoith, Simeon I. Taylor, and Jerrold M. Olefsky. Lippincott–Raven Publishers, Philadelphia © 1996.

CHAPTER 88
Macrovascular Complications of Diabetes Mellitus

BARBARA V. HOWARD

Macrovascular complications, such as atherosclerosis in the coronary arteries, cerebral arteries, and large arteries of the lower extremities, are the major causes of morbidity and mortality in individuals with diabetes mellitus.[1] The occurrence of these complications and their relationship to known risk factors for arteriosclerosis are the subjects of this chapter. Also explored are mechanisms for the increased incidence of cardiovascular disease among individuals with diabetes.

Epidemiology

Mortality from coronary heart disease (CHD) among individuals with insulin-dependent diabetes mellitus (IDDM) is significantly higher than that for the general population, some studies showing rates as much as 9 times higher for men and 14 times higher for women.[2] In the non–insulin-dependent diabetes mellitus (NIDDM)

Table 88-1. Gender and Risk of Coronary Heart Disease in Non–Insulin-Dependent Diabetes Mellitus

Study	Method of Diagnosis of NIDDM	Age Range (yr)	Relative Risk (Women/Men)
Framingham[3]	Medical history	45–74	3.3/1.7
Rancho Bernardo[4]	Self report or fasting glucose	40–79	3.5/2.4
Chicago Workers[5]	GTT	35–64	4.7/3.8
Rochester, MN[6]	GTT	>30	3.2/2.7
NHANES I[7]	Self report	40–77	2.2/2.6
Strong Heart[8]	GTT	45–74	4.6/1.8

GTT = glucose tolerance test.

population, the literature uniformly shows a 1.5–3-fold increase in CHD mortality compared with the general population. Many of these studies reveal a disproportionate impact of CHD on diabetic women (Table 88-1).

Mortality rates from stroke also are higher among diabetic individuals.[9,10] In one study, age- and sex-standardized stroke mortality among diabetic subjects was 4.1 (IDDM patients[2]) and 2.0 (NIDDM patients) times higher than in the general public. Data from the First National Health and Nutrition Examination Survey (NHANES I)[11] indicated 2.5-fold higher rates of stroke among diabetic men and women, both white and African-American. The prevalence of peripheral vascular disease among those of both sexes, as judged by ankle/arm blood pressure ratios or velocimetry, is 22–34% among those with IDDM[12,13] and 22% among NIDDM subjects.[14]

Atherosclerosis has been evaluated directly in diabetic subjects through autopsy studies. In 1968, an examination of 23,000 sets of coronary arteries from autopsies performed in 14 countries showed an increase in the extent of lesions in diabetic subjects.[15] More recently, diabetic patients were shown to have greater occlusion of the left main artery and a greater prevalence of multivessel disease.[1]

Risk Factors for Atherosclerosis in Diabetic Individuals

The increased prevalence of atherosclerotic vascular disease among diabetic individuals appears to be due, in part, to diabetes-induced increases in hypertension, dyslipidemia, and hyperinsulinemia (Table 88-2).

Table 88-2. Summary of Risk Factors for Atherosclerosis Often Exacerbated in Diabetes

Hypertension
Dyslipidemia
- Elevated total and VLDL cholesterol
- Decreased HDL
- Increased total and LDL cholesterol

Hyperinsulinemia and insulin resistance
Obesity

HDL = high-density lipoprotein; LDL = low-density lipoprotein; VLDL = very low-density lipoprotein.

Hypertension

Elevated blood pressure levels have been observed consistently in those with diabetes, independent of age or the presence of obesity or renal disease.[16–19] The prevalence of hypertension increases with the duration of diabetes[20] and is greatly exacerbated in the presence of diabetic nephropathy.[21–24] In IDDM, the prevalence of hypertension rises to nearly 50% among patients more than 50 years old.[25] NHANES II data showed that hypertension is more than twice as prevalent among NIDDM patients than among those with normal glucose tolerance.[26] The mechanisms of increased hypertension in diabetic individuals without nephropathy is not well understood. One possible cause is the increase in exchangeable sodium and enhanced cardiovascular reactivity, which occur in both IDDM and NIDDM. Alternatively, increased intracellular calcium and decreased magnesium have been reported among diabetic hypertensive patients. Further, the insulin resistance syndrome, with accompanying hyperinsulinemia (see below), may contribute to hypertension in individuals with NIDDM.[27,28]

Several studies have demonstrated that hypertension is a significant risk factor for the development of vascular disease in individuals with diabetes. Mortality rates among diabetics have been shown to be four times greater in those with elevated blood pressures,[29] and the Whitehall study revealed an increased relative risk of death among diabetic individuals with systolic hypertension.[30] When it accompanies diabetes, hypertension is a primary risk factor for the development of cerebral vascular disease. In a 1985 study, diabetic patients with hypertension were twice as likely as normotensive patients to develop this disease.[31] There also is a close relationship between systolic hypertension and peripheral vascular disease among individuals with diabetes.[32]

Altered Lipoprotein Concentrations

Lipoprotein alterations occur in and are associated with atherogenesis, both in IDDM and NIDDM. Foremost among these are hypertriglyceridemia, low circulating levels of high-density lipoprotein (HDL), and increased total and low-density lipoprotein (LDL) cholesterol (see Table 88-2).

Hypertriglyceridemia

Hypertriglyceridemia, which is represented by increased levels of very low-density lipoprotein (VLDL) and remnants of VLDL and chylomicron metabolism, is very common among individuals with IDDM and NIDDM.[33–35] The elevations in VLDL in diabetic subjects have several possible mechanisms:

1. Increased free fatty acid and glucose availability to the hepatocyte lead to overproduction of VLDL.
2. Abnormalities of lipoprotein lipase result in decreased clearance both of chylomicrons and VLDL.
3. Prolonged postprandial hypertriglyceridemia leads to accumulation of chylomicron remnants.

Although there has been conflicting evidence concerning the relationship between hypertriglyceridemia and atherosclerotic cardiovascular disease in the nondiabetic population,[36] several studies have demonstrated that elevated triglycerides are a risk factor for atherosclerotic disease among diabetics, even after adjustment for other risk factors.[37–40] Other studies have highlighted the causative role of hypertriglyceridemia in diabetes-associated peripheral vascular disease.[41,42] Although it is not clear why hypertriglyceridemia predisposes diabetic patients to atherosclerosis, hypertriglyceridemia is associated with increased concentrations of chylomicron remnants[43] and smaller VLDL remnant-like particles.[44] This increase in remnants, which contain a higher proportion of cholesterol than does LDL[45] and are known to be atherogenic,[46] may impart the increased risk via remnant uptake by macrophages and subsequent lipid accumulation in the vessel wall.

Decreased High-Density Lipoprotein Concentrations

Decreased concentrations of HDL cholesterol are observed uniformly in NIDDM patients and in IDDM patients with poor glycemic control. There are several possible mechanisms for this HDL decrease. In diabetic patients, the impaired metabolism of triglyceride-rich lipoproteins, with decreased activity of lipoprotein lipase, impairs transfer of materials to the HDL compartment.[47] In addition, levels of hepatic lipase are higher among diabetic patients.[48] Finally, insulin resistance may be a direct cause of decreased HDL concentrations.[8]

HDL is a strong inverse risk factor for vascular disease, and a strong association has been made between low HDL levels and CHD in both NIDDM and IDDM.[49,50] Although it is not clear how low HDL predisposes diabetic individuals to atherosclerosis, it is likely that, as in nondiabetic persons, HDL mediates critical steps in lipoprotein transport that influence the flux of cholesterol to and from the arterial wall.[51,52] HDL is thought to interact with a cell surface receptor; free cholesterol is transferred from the cell to the core of HDL, and then exchanged with triglycerides during the metabolism of triglyceride-rich lipoproteins. This creates a cholesterol transport process that theoretically results in removal of cholesterol from the vessel wall and excretion through the liver. Another possibility is that the HDL decrease reflects the impaired catabolism of triglyceride-rich lipoproteins and the presence of their atherogenic remnants.

Increased Levels of Total and Low-Density Lipoprotein Cholesterol

Levels of LDL are sometimes elevated among diabetic subjects.[53] The NHANES survey has shown that among whites with diabetes, total and LDL cholesterol levels are significantly higher than levels among nondiabetic persons.[54] This was not observed, however, among African Americans or Latinos with NIDDM. Elevation of total or LDL cholesterol is a strong risk factor for coronary artery disease in both nondiabetic and diabetic persons.[55] LDL is also thought to facilitate atherosclerosis in both diabetic and nondiabetic persons; that is, it binds to the LDL receptor in vascular cells and is incorporated into the atherosclerotic plaque. This process may be greatly enhanced by the *alterations* in LDL composition that occur in conjunction with diabetes (see below).

Hyperinsulinemia and the Insulin Resistance Syndrome

In three prospective population-based studies, hyperinsulinemia was shown to be a precursor of CHD, independent of other risk factors.[56–58] In diabetes, the role of high insulin levels in the pathogenesis of atherosclerosis is suggested by the following:

1. IDDM patients treated with exogenous insulin have elevated circulating free insulin levels.
2. NIDDM patients frequently have endogenous hyperinsulinemia in association with insulin resistance.[45]

It is not clear, however, whether it is the elevated insulin concentrations or the insulin resistance that contributes to atherosclerosis. Recent results from the Diabetes Control and Complications Trial indicate that increased insulin administration is not associated with increased CHD among IDDM patients.[59] It is thus likely that insulin level predicts atherosclerosis because hyperinsulinemia is a component of the insulin resistance syndrome. This syndrome is associated with central intra-abdominal adiposity and dyslipidemia and may also be associated with hypertension,[60,61] a constellation of metabolic disorders accelerating the progression of atherosclerosis.

Factors Unique to Diabetes

Multivariate analyses of several prospective population studies[1] suggest that the increased CHD risk among diabetics cannot be explained fully by increases in the known CHD risk factors (i.e., hypertension, changes in lipoprotein and insulin concentrations). Thus, the diabetic state itself appears to increase the risk for atherosclerosis, in addition to its potentiating effect on known risk factors (see Table 88-2). This was clearly demonstrated in both the Multiple Risk Factor Intervention Trial[61a] and the Framingham study,[3] in which, for varying levels of each major risk factor analyzed, diabetics had a higher risk than nondiabetics at the same level of each risk factor.

Alterations in Lipoprotein Composition

Diabetes not only changes lipoprotein concentrations, but it induces a number of alterations in lipoprotein composition that may influence the atherosclerotic process (Table 88-3). Many of these changes involve LDL—the most important lipoprotein in the atherogenic process. In diabetes, the single apoprotein in LDL, apo

TABLE 88-3. Summary of Possible Mechanisms of Diabetes-Associated Vascular Disease

Abnormalities of lipoprotein composition
• Proliferation of cholesterol-bearing VLDL remnants
• Small dense LDL
• Glycated LDL
• Oxidized LDL
• Decreased proportion of HDL_2
• Glycated HDL
Glycated connective tissue proteins
Endothelial dysfunction
Clotting abnormalities
Cardiomyopathy

HDL = high-density lipoprotein; LDL = low-density lipoprotein; VLDL = very low-density lipoprotein.

B, is *glycated*.[62] Glycated LDL has been shown to interact abnormally with macrophages.[63] Recognition of the glycated LDL by the classic LDL receptor is impaired; however, it is recognized by the receptor on macrophages and other scavenger cells that recognize modified LDL.[64] The glycated LDL is recognized by a high-capacity, low-affinity pathway on monocyte-derived macrophages, which accelerates its uptake by these cells and thus enhances foam cell formation. A second modification observed in diabetic LDL is increased extent of *oxidation*. Oxidatively modified LDL is believed to play an important role in atherogenesis because it (1) stimulates the production of foam cells by macrophages,[65,66] (2) induces adhesion of monocytes to endothelial cells,[67] (3) stimulates monocyte chemotaxis,[68] and (4) can be cytotoxic to endothelial cells.[69] Further, it has been shown that glycated LDL is more susceptible to oxidation.[45,70] Thus, the processes of glycation and oxidation are closely interwoven and may produce a vicious circle of vascular injury.

Glycated[71] and oxidized[72] LDL also may stimulate the production of circulating antibodies, which suggests that these modified lipoprotein species can be *immunogenetic*.[45] Circulating lipoprotein immune complexes may accelerate atherosclerosis[73,74] via stimulation of (1) macrophage foam cell formation by immune complex uptake, or (2) atherogenetic immune mechanisms in arterial wall cells.

Another primary alteration in LDL composition is the presence of small, dense LDL particles. This shift in distribution of LDL particle size toward the sub-type B pattern defined by Austin and colleagues[75] has been associated with several markers of cardiovascular disease in studies of nondiabetic patients. A greater proportion of small, dense LDL particles has been demonstrated to be associated with the insulin resistance syndrome[61] and to be more prevalent among diabetic patients.[76,77] In addition, these particles have been shown to be more susceptible to oxidation, thus enhancing the vicious circle of oxidation and glycation referred to above.

Alterations in HDL composition also are associated with diabetes. Diabetics have a smaller proportion of the larger HDL_2 subfraction and a greater proportion of HDL_3, a distribution known to be associated with atherosclerosis. Additionally, glycation of HDL also has been reported in diabetic subjects, which could interfere further with the metabolic actions of HDL. Glycation hastens HDL clearance from plasma[78] and impairs stimulation of cholesterol efflux from arterial cells.[79,80]

Glycated Proteins

In addition to the effects of glycation on lipoproteins, the process of glycation may influence other macromolecules that play a role in atherogenesis. Increased glycation of antithrombin III has been shown to impair its inhibition of the coagulation cascade.[81] In diabetes, longer-lived proteins are increasingly likely to undergo excessive glycation.[45] Collagen, for example, has been shown to have an increased rate of glycation in diabetics,[55] which may facilitate atherogenesis by trapping lipoproteins in the extracellular matrix. Glycated collagen also stimulates platelet aggregation.[82] The initial glycation process leads to further chemical changes and subsequent formation of advanced glycation end products,[83] which serve as a catalyst for the transendothelial migration of monocytes and the expression of growth factors by macrophages—mechanisms that could stimulate the atherogenetic process.[84]

Disturbed Cellular Function

The diabetic state also may produce abnormalities in arterial wall and circulating blood cell metabolism, which may play a role in atherogenesis. A low-molecular-weight growth factor has been described in plasma from NIDDM subjects.[85] Cells in the vessel walls, such as smooth muscle cells, have been shown to produce mitogens (e.g., colony-stimulating factors) and cytokines (e.g., IL-1, TNF-α).[86] Elevated glucose concentrations also have been shown to cause abnormalities in endothelial cells, enhanced vascular permeability,[87–89] and abnormalities in contractility.[90] Cellular proliferation and loss also are prominent features of the diabetic endothelium.[90] Several of these anomalies may be caused by abnormalities in growth factors, as described above.

The mechanisms of the adverse effects of hyperglycemia on endothelial function are not clear. The production of *sorbitol* and its possible toxicity have been well studied.[91–93] Another hypothesis is that nonenzymatic glycation of cell proteins could lead to endothelial injury. Further, hyperglycemia has been shown to result in increased diacylglycerol levels and protein kinase C activity. Finally, elevations in glucose may change the membrane potential of the cells, thus serving as a source of toxicity. Elevations in glucose levels, then, may affect many important pathways in the cell and vascular function, causing cellular dysfunction and acceleration of the atherosclerotic process.

Thrombosis

Diabetes is associated with an increased propensity for thrombosis, as indicated by in vitro measures.[94] Abnormalities of platelet adherence and aggregation in diabetes have been reported, as have increased levels of several clotting factors and the plasminogen activation inhibitor (PAI-1), which may lead to a procoagulant state.[95] Fibrinogen levels also are elevated.[96] Platelets can contribute to vascular disease by releasing factors that can modify the vessel wall and by forming thrombi.

There is evidence for enhanced platelet adhesion in diabetic subjects.[97] Hypersensitivity to aggregating agents, and subsequent increased sensitivity to the release of their granular contents, is associated with IDDM and NIDDM.[98] This is thought to be caused by (1) increased arachidonate mobilization, (2) fibrinogen binding to platelets, (3) alterations in nonarachidonate pathways, or (4) alterations in the platelet membrane lipid fluidity.[98]

Diabetic Cardiomyopathy

In addition to the enhanced atherosclerotic process, it has been proposed that additional cardiac dysfunction is associated with diabetes. The small and medium vessels that penetrate the ventricular wall may be altered in individuals with diabetes, perhaps because of the presence of microangiopathy.[99] This appears to be associated with left ventricular dysfunction, diffuse subendocardial fibrosis, and glycoprotein deposits.[100]

The *autonomic nervous system* also seems to be involved in diabetic cardiomyopathy. Diabetics have altered autonomic dysfunction resulting in tachycardia, postural hypertension, and silent ischemia. This may involve destruction of the cardiac sympathetic fibers[101] and hence cardiac dysfunction. Parasympathetic nerve dysfunction, which influences heart rate, has been demonstrated in diabetic patients.[102–103] In addition, sympathetic nerve dysfunction also can cause dysfunction in the peripheral circulation, thus exacerbating peripheral arterial disease.

Summary and Conclusions

Increased atherosclerotic vascular disease involving vessels of the heart, brain, and periphery has been well established in the diabetic population and is responsible for a large proportion of the morbidity and mortality. Part of the increased propensity for atherosclerosis appears to be related to the effect of diabetes-induced increases of known risk factors: hypertension, dyslipidemia, and hyperinsulinemia. Diabetes also, however, appears to be associated with increased risk for atherosclerosis, even when the classic risk factors are taken into account. There are multiple possible explanations for the *independent effect* of diabetes on enhancing atherosclerosis. Many alterations in lipoprotein composition, especially glycation and oxidation, are known to accelerate the atherosclerotic process. In addition, the vessel wall cells of diabetic patients appear to have altered function. These alterations may be induced as a result of the glycation process or through the secretion or alteration of mitogen and cytokine activity. There is ample evidence for increased rates of thrombosis among diabetics. Finally, diabetes appears to be associated with specific cardiomyopathy.

Even though our knowledge of the mechanism of macrovascular disease in diabetes is not complete, there is much information to guide atherosclerosis-prevention strategies. These strategies must be aimed toward reducing the presence of all possible risk factors. Thus, blood pressure should be carefully controlled, dyslipidemia appropriately treated, and smoking cessation required. Efforts to increase weight loss and physical activity will contribute to reducing these risk factors by reducing plasma insulin concentrations and reducing insulin resistance. Aggressive control of plasma glucose will decrease the rate of glycation, thus potentially reversing many of the abnormalities of lipoprotein composition and cellular dysfunction. Maintenance of normoglycemia also should reduce the adverse effects of diabetes that can cause thrombosis and impaired cardiac function. Further work must be done to improve our understanding of the mechanisms of diabetic vascular disease so that we can design more specific and successful strategies for its prevention and control.

References

1. Pyörälä K, Laakso M, Uusitupa M. Diabetes and atherosclerosis: An epidemiologic view. Diabetes Metab Rev 1987;3:463
2. Moss SE, Klein R, Klein BEK. Cause-specific mortality in a population-based study of diabetes. Am J Public Health 1991;81:1158
3. Kannel WB, McGee DL. Diabetes and glucose tolerance as risk factors for cardiovascular disease: The Framingham study. Diabetes Care 1979;2:120
4. Barrett-Connor E, Wingard DL. Sex differential in ischemic heart disease mortality in diabetics: A prospective population-based study. Am J Epidemiol 1983;118:489
5. Pan WH, Cedres LB, Liu K, et al. Relationship of clinical diabetes and asymptomatic hyperglycemia to risk of coronary heart disease mortality in men and women. Am J Epidemiol 1986;123:504
6. Elveback LR, Connolly DC, Melton LJ 3d. Coronary heart disease in residents of Rochester, Minnesota: VII. Incidence 1950 through 1982. Mayo Clin Proc 1986;61:896
7. Kleinman JC, Donahue RP, Harris MI, et al. Mortality among diabetics in a national sample. Am J Epidemiol 1988;128:389
8. Howard BV. Insulin action in vivo: Insulin and lipoprotein metabolism. In: Alberti KGMM, DeFronzo RA, Zimmet P, eds. International Textbook of Diabetes Mellitus. 2nd ed. Sussex: John Wiley & Sons;1996.
9. Jarrett RJ. Cardiovascular disease and hypertension in diabetes mellitus. Diabetes Metab Rev 1989;5:547
10. Haffner SM, Stern MP, Rewers M. Diabetes and atherosclerosis: Epidemiological considerations. In: Draznin R, Eckel RH, eds. Diabetes and Atherosclerosis: Molecular Basis and Clinical Aspects. New York, NY: Elsevier;1993:229
11. Kittner SJ, White LR, Losonczy KG, et al. Black-white difference in stroke incidence in a national sample: The contribution of hypertension and diabetes mellitus. JAMA 1990;264:1267
12. Beach KW, Brunzell JD, Conquest LL, Strandness DE. The correlation of arteriosclerosis obliterans with lipoproteins in insulin-dependent and non-insulin-dependent diabetes. Diabetes 1979;28:836
13. Orchard TJ, Dorman JS, Maser RE, et al. Prevalence of complications in IDDM by sex and duration: Pittsburgh Epidemiology of Diabetes Complications Study II. Diabetes 1990;39:1116
14. Beach KW, Bedford GR, Bergelin RO, et al. Progression of lower-extremity arterial occlusive disease in type II diabetes mellitus. Diabetes Care 1988;11:464
15. Robertson WB, Strong JP. Atherosclerosis in persons with hypertension and diabetes mellitus. Lab Invest 1968;18:538
16. Christlieb AR, Warram JH, Krolewski AS, et al. Hypertension, the major risk in juvenile-onset insulin-dependent diabetics. Diabetes 1981;30:90
17. Barrett-Connor E, Criqui MH, Klauber MR, Holdbrook M. Diabetes and hypertension in a community of older adults. Am J Epidemiol 1981;113:276
18. Keen H, Chlouverakis C, Fuller J, Jarrett RJ. The concomitants of raised blood sugar: Studies in newly detected hyperglycaemics: II. Urinary albumin excretion, blood pressure and their relation to blood sugar levels. Guys Hosp Rep 1969;118:247
19. Modan M, Halkin H, Almog S, et al. Hyperinsulinemia: A link between hypertension, obesity and glucose intolerance. J Clin Invest 1985;75:809
20. Krolewski AS, Warram JH, Christlieb AR, et al. The changing natural history of nephropathy in type I diabetes. Am J Med 1985;78:785
21. Wiseman M, Viberti GC, Mackintosh D, et al. Glycaemia, arterial pressure and micro-albuminuria in type 1 (insulin-dependent) diabetes mellitus. Diabetologia 1984;26:401
22. Feldt-Rasmussen B, Borch-Johnson K, Mathiesen ER. Hypertension in diabetes as related to nephropathy: Early blood pressure changes. Hypertension 1985;7(suppl 2):18
23. Berglund J, Lins PE, Adamson U, Lins LE. Microalbuminuria in long-term insulin-dependent diabetes mellitus: Prevalence and clinical characteristics in a normotensive population. Acta Med Scand 1987;222:333
24. Gall M, Skott P, Damsbo P, et al. The prevalence of micro- and macroalbuminuria, retinopathy, arterial hypertension and large vessel disease in type 2 (non-insulin dependent) diabetes mellitus [Abstract]. Diabetologia 1988;31:492A
25. Keen H, Track NS, Sowry GCS. Arterial pressure in clinically apparent diabetics. Diabet Metab 1975;1:159
26. Harris MI. Impaired glucose tolerance in the U.S. population. Diabetes Care 1989;12:464
27. Rossetti L, Frontoni S. Mechanisms of hypertension in diabetes mellitus. In: Draznin R, Eckel RH, eds. Diabetes and Atherosclerosis: Molecular Basis and Clinical Aspects. New York, NY: Elsevier;1993:277
28. Ferrannini E, Buzzigoli G, Bonadonna R, et al. Insulin resistance in essential hypertension. N Engl J Med 1987;317:350
29. Dupree EA, Meyer MB. Role of risk factors in the complications of diabetes mellitus. Am J Epidemiol 1980;112:100
30. Janka HU, Dirschedl P. Systolic blood pressure as a predictor for cardiovascular disease in diabetes: A 5-year longitudinal study. Hypertension 1985;7:II90
31. Kuller LH, Dorman JS, Wolf PA. Cerebrovascular disease and diabetes. In Diabetes in America. Washington, DC: US Department of Health and Human Services;1985:1–18. Publication 85-1468.
32. Tuck ML. Diabetes and hypertension. Postgrad Med J 1988;64(suppl 3):76
33. Barrett-Connor E, Grundy SM, Holdbrook MJ. Plasma lipids and diabetes mellitus in an adult community. Am J Epidemiol 1982;115:657
34. Laakso M, Voutilainen E, Sarlund H, et al. Serum lipids and lipoproteins in middle-aged non-insulin-dependent diabetics. Atherosclerosis 1985;56:271
35. Howard BV, Howard WJ. Dyslipidemia in non-insulin dependent diabetes mellitus. Endocr Rev 1994;15:263
36. Assmann G, Gotto AM Jr, Paoletti R. The hypertriglyceridemias: Risk and management. Am J Cardiol 1991;68:1A
37. West KM, Ahuja MMS, Bennett PH, et al. The role of circulating glucose and triglyceride concentrations and their interactions with other risk factors as determinants of arterial disease in nine diabetic population samples from the WHO multinational study. Diabetes Care 1983;6:361
38. Janka HU. Five-year incidence of major macrovascular complications in diabetes mellitus. Horm Metab Res Suppl 1985;15:15
39. Fontbonne A, Eschwege E, Cambien F, et al. Hypertriglyceridemia as a risk factor for coronary heart disease mortality in subjects with impaired glucose tolerance or diabetes: Results from the 11-year follow-up of the Paris Prospective study. Diabetologia 1989;32:300
40. Santen RJ, Willis PW, Fajans SS. Atherosclerosis in diabetes mellitus: Correlations with serum lipid levels, adiposity and serum insulin levels. Arch Intern Med 1972;130:833
41. Laakso M, Pyörälä K. Lipid and lipoprotein abnormalities in diabetic patients with peripheral vascular disease. Atherosclerosis 1988;74:55
42. Uusitupa MI, Niskanen LK, Siitonen O, et al. 5-year incidence of atherosclerotic vascular disease in relation to general risk factors, insulin level, and abnormalities in lipoprotein composition in non-insulin-dependent diabetic and nondiabetic subjects. Circulation 1990;82:27
43. Ochiai S, Onuma T, Boku A, et al. Change of chylomicron remnant in non-insulin-dependent diabetes mellitus [Abstract]. In: Proceedings of the Eighth International Symposium on Atherosclerosis. Amsterdam: Excerpta Medica;1989:677
44. Rivellese A, Riccardi G, Romano G, et al. Presence of very low density lipoprotein compositional abnormalities in type 1 (insulin-dependent) diabetic patients: Effects of blood glucose optimisation. Diabetologia 1988;31:884
45. Chait A, Bierman EL. Pathogenesis of macrovascular disease in diabetes. In: Kahn CR, Weir GC, eds. Joslin's Diabetes Mellitus. 13th ed. Philadelphia, PA: Lea & Febiger;1994:648
46. Zilversmit DB. Relative atherogenicity of different plasma lipoproteins. Adv Exp Med Biol 1978;109:45
47. Eisenberg S. High density lipoprotein metabolism. J Lipid Res 1984;25:1017
48. Taskinen M-R, Kuusi T, Helve E, et al. Insulin therapy induces antiatherogenic changes of serum lipoproteins in noninsulin-dependent diabetes. Arteriosclerosis 1988;8:168

49. Laakso M, Pyörälä K, Sarlund H, Voutilainen E. Lipid and lipoprotein abnormalities associated with coronary heart disease in patients with insulin-dependent diabetes mellitus. Arteriosclerosis 1986;6:679
50. Laakso M, Voutilainen E, Pyörälä K, Sarlund H. Association of low HDL and HDL_2 cholesterol with coronary heart disease in noninsulin-dependent diabetics. Arteriosclerosis 1985;5:653
51. Bagdade JD, Subbaiah PV. Whole-plasma and high-density lipoprotein subfraction surface lipid composition in IDDM men. Diabetes 1989;38:1226
52. Fielding CJ, Reaven GM, Fielding PE. Human noninsulin-dependent diabetes: Identification of a defect in plasma cholesterol transport normalized in vivo by insulin and in vitro by selective immunoadsorption of apolipoprotein E. Proc Natl Acad Sci U S A 1982;79:6365
53. Reavan PD, Picard S, Witztum JL. Low density lipoprotein metabolism in diabetes. In: Draznin R, Eckel RH, eds. Diabetes and Atherosclerosis: Molecular Basis and Clinical Aspects. New York, NY: Elsevier; 1993:17
54. Cowie CC, Howard BV, Harris MI. Serum lipoproteins in African Americans and Whites with non-insulin-dependent diabetes in the US population. Circulation 1994;90:1185
55. Stamler J. Epidemiology, established major risk factors, and the primary prevention of coronary heart disease. In: Parmley WW, Chatterjee K, eds. Cardiology. Vol 2. Philadelphia, PA: JB Lippincott; 1989:1
56. Pyörälä K, Savolainen E, Kaukola S, Haapakoski J. Plasma insulin as coronary heart disease risk factor: Relationship to other risk factors and predictive value during 9 1/2-year follow-up of the Helsinki Policemen Study Population. Acta Med Scand Suppl 1985;701:38
57. Welborn TA, Wearne K. Coronary heart disease incidence and cardiovascular mortality in Busselton with reference to glucose and insulin concentrations. Diabetes Care 1979;2:154
58. Fontbonne A, Charles MA, Thibult N, et al. Hyperinsulinaemia as a predictor of coronary heart disease mortality in a healthy population: The Paris Prospective Study, 15-year follow-up. Diabetologia 1991;34:356
59. The Diabetes Control and Complications Trial. N Engl J Med 1993;329:683
60. DeFronzo RA, Ferrannini E. Insulin resistance: A multifaceted syndrome responsible for NIDDM, obesity, hypertension, dyslipidemia, and atherosclerotic cardiovascular disease. Diabetes Care 1991;14:173
61. Reaven GM, Chen YDI, Jeppesen J, et al. Insulin resistance and hyperinsulinemia in individuals with small, dense low density lipoprotein particles. J Clin Invest 1993;92:141
61a. Stamler J, Vaccaro O, Neaton JD, Wentworth D. Diabetes, other risk factors, and 12-year cardiovascular mortality for men screened in the Multiple Risk Factor Intervention Trial. Diabetes Care 1993;16(2):434
62. Witztum JL, Mahony EM, Branks MJ, et al. Nonenzymatic glycosylation of low-density lipoprotein alters its biologic activity. Diabetes 1982;31:283
63. Lopes-Virella MF, Klein RL, Lyons TJ, et al. Glycosylation of low-density lipoprotein enhances cholesteryl ester synthesis in human monocyte-derived macrophages. Diabetes 1988;37:550
64. Lyons TJ, Klein RL, Baynes JW, et al. Stimulation of cholesteryl ester synthesis in human monocyte-derived macrophages by low-density lipoproteins from type 1 (insulin-dependent) diabetic patients: The influence of nonenzymatic glycosylation of low-density lipoprotein. Diabetologia 1987; 30:916
65. Lyons TJ. Oxidized low density lipoproteins—a role in the pathogenesis of atherosclerosis in diabetes? Diabetic Med 1991;8:411
66. Lyons TJ, Lopes-Virella MF. Glycosylation-related mechanisms. In: Draznin R, Eckel RH, eds. Diabetes and Atherosclerosis: Molecular Basis and Clinical Aspects. New York, NY: Elsevier; 1993:169
67. Berliner JA, Territo MC, Sevanian A, et al. Minimally modified low density lipoprotein stimulates monocyte endothelial interactions. J Clin Invest 1990; 85:1260
68. Cushing SD, Berliner JA, Valente AJ, et al. Minimally modified low density lipoprotein induces monocyte chemotactic protein 1 in human endothelial cells and smooth muscle cells. Proc Natl Acad Sci U S A 1990;87: 5134
69. Morel DW, Hessler JR, Chisolm GM. Low density lipoprotein cytotoxicity induced by free radical peroxidation of lipid. J Lipid Res 1983;24:1070
70. Hunt JV, Smith CCT, Wolff SP. Autoxidative glycosylation and possible involvement of peroxides and free radicals in LDL modification by glucose. Diabetes 1990;39:1420
71. Witztum JL, Koschinsky T. Metabolic and immunological consequences of glycation of low density lipoproteins. Prog Clin Biol Res 1989;304:219
72. Palinski W, Rosenfeld ME, Ylä-Herttuala S, et al. Low density lipoprotein undergoes oxidative modification in vivo. Proc Natl Acad Sci U S A 1989;86:1372
73. Wissler RW. Update on the pathogenesis of atherosclerosis. Am J Med 1991;91:35
74. Orekhov AN. Lipoprotein immune complexes and their role in atherogenesis. Curr Opin Lipidol 1991;2:329
75. Austin MA, Breslow JL, Hennekens CH, et al. Low density lipoprotein subclass patterns and risk of myocardial infarction. JAMA 1988;260: 1917
76. Selby JV, Austin MA, Newman B, et al. LDL subclass pattern and the insulin resistance syndrome in women. Circulation 1993;88:381
77. Haffner SM, Mykkänen L, Valdez RA, et al. LDL size and subclass pattern in a biethnic population. Arterioscler Thromb 1993;13:1623
78. Witztum JL, Fisher M, Pietro T, et al. Nonenzymatic glycosylation of high-density lipoproteins accelerates its catabolism in guinea pigs. Diabetes 1982;31:1029
79. Duell PB, Oram JF, Bierman EL. Nonenzymatic glycosylation of HDL resulting in inhibition of high-affinity binding to cultured human fibroblasts. Diabetes 1990;39:1257
80. Duell PB, Bierman EL. Nonenzymatic glycosylation of HDL inhibits HDL receptor-mediated cholesterol efflux [Abstract]. Arteriosclerosis 1989; 9:716A
81. Brownlee M, Vlassara H, Cerami A. Inhibition of heparin-catalyzed antithrombin III activity by non-enzymatic glycosylation: Possible role in fibrin deposition in diabetes. Diabetes 1984;33:532
82. Le Pape A, Guitton JD, Gutman N, et al. Nonenzymatic glycosylation of collagen in diabetes: Incidence on increased normal platelet aggregation. Haemostasis 1983;13:36
83. Brownlee M, Cerami A, Vlassara H. Advanced glycosylation end products in tissue and the biochemical basis of diabetic complications. N Engl J Med 1988;318:1315
84. Kirstein M, Brett J, Radoff S, et al. Advanced protein glycosylation induces transendothelial human monocyte chemotaxis and secretion of platelet-derived growth factor: Role in vascular disease of diabetes and aging. Proc Natl Acad Sci U S A 1990;87:9010
85. Koschinsky T, Bünting CE, Rütter R, Gries FA. Vascular growth factors and the development of macrovascular disease in diabetes mellitus. Diabetes Metab 1987;13:318
86. Filonzi EL, Zoellner H, Stanton H, Hamilton JA. Cytokine regulation of granulocyte-macrophage colony stimulating factor and macrophage colony-stimulating factor production in human arterial smooth muscle cells. Atherosclerosis 1993;99:241
87. Wallow IHL, Engerman RL. Permeability and patency of retinal blood vessels in experimental diabetes. Invest Ophthalmol Vis Sci 1977;16:447
88. Williamson JR, Chang K, Rowold E, et al. Sorbinil prevents diabetes-induced increases in vascular permeability but does not alter collagen cross-linking. Diabetes 1985;34:703
89. Cunha-Vaz J, De Abrew JRF, Campose AJ. Early breakdown of the retinal barrier in diabetes. Br J Ophthalmol 1975;59:649
90. King GL, Banskota NK, Shiba T, et al. Endothelial cell abnormalities in diabetes. In: Draznin R, Eckel RH, eds. Diabetes and Atherosclerosis: Molecular Basis and Clinical Aspects. New York, NY: Elsevier; 1993:191
91. Greene DA, Lattimer SA, Sima AA. Sorbitol, phosphoinositides, and sodium-potassium ATPase in the pathogenesis of diabetic complications. N Engl J Med 1987;316:599
92. MacGregor LC, Matschinsky FM. Treatment with aldose reductase inhibitor of myoinositol arrests deterioration of the electroretinogram of diabetic rats. J Clin Invest 1985;24:1250
93. Gabbay KH. The sorbitol pathway and the complications of diabetes. N Engl J Med 1973;288:831
94. Banga JD, Sixma JJ. Diabetes mellitus, vascular disease and thrombosis. Clin Haematol 1986;15:465
95. Bierman EL. Atherogenesis in diabetes. Arter Thromb 1992;12:647
96. Jones RL, Peterson CM. Hematologic alterations in diabetes mellitus. Am J Med 1981;70:339
97. Colwell JA, Winocour PD, Lopes-Virella MF. Platelet function and platelet-plasma interactions in atherosclerosis and diabetes mellitus. In: Rifkin H, Porte D, eds. Ellenberg and Rifkin's Diabetes Mellitus, Theory and Practice. 4th ed. Amsterdam: Elsevier; 1990:249
98. Winocour PD, Richardson M. Thrombosis and atherogenesis in diabetes. In: Draznin R, Eckel RH, eds. Diabetes and Atherosclerosis: Molecular Basis and Clinical Aspects. New York, NY: Elsevier; 1993:213
99. Sniderman A, Michel C, Racine N. Heart disease in patients with diabetes mellitus. In: Draznin R, Eckel RH, eds. Diabetes and Atherosclerosis: Molecular Basis and Clinical Aspects. New York, NY: Elsevier; 1993:255
100. Regan TJ, Lyons MM, Ahmed SS, et al. Evidence for cardiomyopathy in familial diabetes mellitus. J Clin Invest 1977;60:884
101. Faerman I, Faccio E, Milei J, et al. Autonomic neuropathy and painless myocardial infarction in diabetic patients: Histologic evidence of their relationship. Diabetes 1977;26:1147
102. Ewing DJ, Campbell IW, Clarke BF. Assessment of cardiovascular effects in diabetic autonomic neuropathy and prognostic implications. Ann Intern Med 1980;92:308
103. Ewing DJ. Cardiovascular reflexes and autonomic neuropathy. Clin Sci Mol Med 1978;55:321

Part X

Complications: Mechanisms

Diabetes Mellitus, edited by Derek LeRoith, Simeon I. Taylor, and Jerrold M. Olefsky. Lippincott–Raven Publishers, Philadelphia © 1996.

CHAPTER 89
The Sorbitol-Osmotic and Sorbitol-Redox Hypotheses

DOUGLAS A. GREENE AND MARTIN J. STEVENS

The pathogenesis of the complications associated with chronic diabetes, including neuropathy, is thought to be complex and multifactorial. Yet the consistent parallelism between glycemic exposure and the onset and progression of the neuropathic and vascular complications of diabetes, as well as the proven efficacy of improved metabolic control in their prevention, strongly implicates hyperglycemia or other metabolic abnormalities intrinsic to the diabetic state as overriding pathogenetic elements.[1–5] However, the precise mechanisms by which the effects of prevailing hyperglycemia or insulin deficiency, or both, precipitate metabolic and vascular defects in nerve and other complication-prone tissues, and their precise cellular localization, remain highly speculative.[4,6–11]

The most commonly cited metabolic defects include activation of the polyol or sorbitol pathway, abnormalities in lipid metabolism, advanced glycosylated end product formation, and increased oxidative damage.[4,6–17] These metabolic defects may directly damage specific critical cellular components of complications-prone tissue (e.g., peripheral nerve axons or Schwann cells), or they may contribute to end-organ dysfunction and cause damage indirectly through functional or structural defects involving supporting mesenchymal elements, such as the extracellular matrix or microvasculature.[18,19]

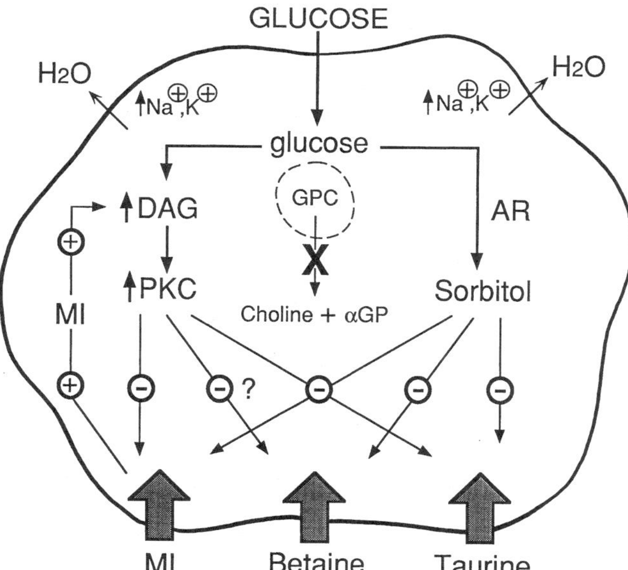

FIGURE 89-1. Aldose reductase–mediated osmotic dysregulation in isotonic hyperglycemia. Isotonic hyperglycemia may perturb the intracellular milieu by promoting sorbitol accumulation through the provision of excess substrate for the high-Km aldose reductase (AR). In the absence of an osmotic stress, intracellular sorbitol accumulation and changes in protein kinase activity produce a compensatory downregulation of other alternative osmolytes, causing their intracellular depletion, which may become rate-limiting for their normal metabolic functions. Intracellular *myo*-inositol (MI) accumulation may inhibit its own uptake by activation of PKC. *GPC,* Glycerophosphorylcholine; *αGP*, α-glycerophosphate.

Alternatively, metabolic defects can induce systemic or localized rheologic abnormalities,[20,21] or defects in vasoactive (e.g., nitric oxide[16,17] or eicosanoids[13]) or growth-promoting agents which, in turn, alter target-organ structure or function, or both.

Despite these uncertainties, considerable evidence has implicated activation of the sorbitol pathway by glucose as an early component in these various pathogenetic cascades, with special emphasis on those thought to underlie diabetic peripheral neuropathy.[4,6,7] The sorbitol pathway is activated by hyperglycemia in numerous cells and tissues expressing the enzymes aldose reductase and sorbitol dehydrogenase and in which transport is not rate-limiting for overall glucose metabolism.[7] In these tissues, excess glucose is metabolized to sorbitol and fructose by these adenine-nucleotide–linked oxoreductases,[4,22] resulting in an accumulation of the intracellular organic osmolyte sorbitol, as well as shifts in the $NADP^+/NADPH$ and $NAD^+/NADH$ redox couples. Sorbitol accumulation is associated with reciprocal depletion of alternative organic intracellular physiologic osmolytes, such as *myo*-inositol (also a precursor for phosphoinositide synthesis)[4,6,7] and taurine (a β-amino acid).[23] As will be discussed later, in certain cell types, depletion of these alternative osmolytes is thought to limit their metabolism, thereby perturbing phosphoinositide- and calcium-mediated signal transduction and other cellular and metabolic functions that they subserve. Moreover, shifts in the redox potential of the adenine-nucleotide cofactors, induced by exaggerated flux through the sorbitol pathway, are thought to alter a wide range of adenine-nucleotide–linked cellular and metabolic processes.

The Sorbitol-Osmotic ("Compatible Osmolyte") Hypothesis and Altered *Myo*-Inositol and Taurine Metabolism in Diabetes

For more than two decades, activation of aldose reductase by mass action has been viewed as a critical link between hyperglycemia, cellular osmotic dysregulation, and tissue damage in diabetes.[24–26] In the renal medulla, aldose reductase is now recognized to play a physiologic role in intracellular osmoregulation during antidiuresis.[26] Indeed, the observation that the expression of the aldose reductase gene is strongly and specifically induced by extracellular hyperosmolality[27] has led to a "compatible osmolyte hypothesis," which argues that certain nonionic and, therefore, "nonperturbing"[28] osmotically active compounds, such as sorbitol, *myo*-inositol, and taurine, function as alternative organic intracellular osmolytes that respond coordinately to changes in external osmolality, thereby buffering otherwise injurious shifts in the intracellular electrolyte and water composition.[27–29] Osmotic stress produces a compensatory increase or decrease in the intracellular concentration of one or more of these alternative osmolytes by induction or suppression of the relevant synthetic or degradative enzymes (aldose reductase in the case of sorbitol[27]) or membrane transporters (the sodium-*myo*-inositol and taurine transporters[29,30]), thus accumulating or disposing of these osmolytes in a coordinated fashion (Fig. 89-1). Isotonic hyperglycemia perturbs this osmoregulatory system by promoting sorbitol accumulation through the provision of excess substrate for high-Km aldose reductase, rather than through osmotic induction of its gene.[28] In the absence of osmotic stress, intracellular sorbitol accumulation produces a compensatory down-regulation of other alternative osmolytes, causing their intracellular depletion. Although initially regarded as metabolically inert, these alternative organic osmolytes are now thought to have important metabolic, as well as osmoregulatory, roles.[31-33] Thus, as detailed later, *myo*-inositol may become limiting for phosphoinositide signaling,[33] and taurine depletion may exacerbate oxidative stress[32] and lead to disruption of intracellular calcium homeostasis.[31] Taurine has been implicated as a modulator of neuronal hyperexcitability,[34] and it has also been implicated in the regulation of neurotransmitter release and ion conductance.[35,36] Given the osmoregulatory and metabolic importance of taurine and *myo*-inositol under isosmolar as well as hypertonic conditions, abnormal expression of the osmoresponsive genes that modulate compatible osmolyte metabolism might exaggerate the deleterious effects of otherwise trivial osmolar or metabolic stress (such as might occur in diabetes mellitus), thereby predisposing that individual to the development of diabetic neuropathy. Indeed, provocative, fragmentary, but conflicting data suggest a possible association between increased aldose reductase enzymatic activity or protein, or both, and the presence of late diabetic complications.[37,38]

Sorbitol and the *Myo*-Inositol Depletion Hypothesis, Protein Kinase C, and (Na,K)-ATPase Activity

The two-decade-old "*myo*-inositol depletion hypothesis"[39,40] is now regarded as a subset of the sorbitol-osmotic hypothesis[4] because the major (but not the sole[41]) cause of tissue *myo*-inositol depletion in diabetes appears to be compensatory to sorbitol accumulation.[42,43] Nerve *myo*-inositol depletion has been presented as an important mediator of the effect of sorbitol pathway activation on nerve conduction slowing in acute experimental diabetes,[4,6,39-43] although this view has now been challenged.[8-10,12,44-46] *myo*-Inositol supplementation or aldose reductase inhibitors (ARIs) normalize nerve *myo*-inositol content and nerve conduction velocity in streptozotocin-induced and spontaneously diabetic rats.[40,42,43,47,48] Thus, the action of ARIs on the acute and rapidly reversible slowing of nerve conduction in experimental diabetes is thought to be mediated, in part, by correction of sorbitol-pathway–induced *myo*-inositol depletion.[49] Depletion of intracellular *myo*-inositol has been thought to render it rate-limiting for membrane phosphoinositide synthesis and turnover,[4,6] which are necessary for phospholipase-C–mediated, G-protein–associated signal transduction. This has been speculated to lead to diminished phosphoinositide-derived diacylglycerol (DAG) and impaired activation of protein kinase C (PKC), which may link altered *myo*-inositol metabolism to defective (Na,K)-ATPase regulation[50] in diabetic nerve. This assertion is based on the observations that (Na,K)-ATPase activity,[39,47,50,51] arachidonyl-DAG levels,[52] and PKC activation[53] are diminished in diabetic nerve, and that dietary *myo*-inositol supplementation in vivo,[51,54] or exogenous PKC agonists in vitro,[54] correct impaired nerve (Na,K)-ATPase activity.

Antiparallel Effects of Glucose on Protein Kinase C

The relationship between ambient glucose and PKC activity is now suspected to be considerably more heterogeneous and cell-specific than was previously supposed. Indeed, physiologic hyperglycemia has now been speculated to alter phosphoinositide signal transduction by two separate mass-action mechanisms with antiparallel effects.[55] In peripheral nerve, as outlined earlier, glucose-induced, aldose reductase–catalyzed sorbitol accumulation and reciprocal *myo*-inositol depletion diminish phosphoinositide synthesis and turnover, as well as the subsequent release of phosphoinositide-derived arachidonyl-DAGs.[4] Elements of this pattern of metabolic glucotoxicity have recently been studied in tissue culture[55,56] using retinal pigment epithelial cells[55] and retinal microvascular pericytes[56] expressing high levels of aldose reductase.[57,58] In these cells, basal and/or agonist-stimulated phosphoinositide turnover and release of inositol phosphates and/or DAG was diminished after exposure to 20–25 mM of glucose. In retinal pigment epithelial cells expressing low aldose reductase activity,[55] as well as in other incubated cells and tissues with relatively low aldose reductase expression[57,58] (such as retinal microvascular endothelial cells[59] and isolated renal glomeruli[60,61]), a different pattern of metabolic glucotoxicity is observed. In such cells and tissues, exposure to elevated glucose levels increases DAG precursors, such as α-glycerophosphate and phosphatidic acid, which are thought to increase de novo synthesis of DAG in an aldose reductase–independent fashion. These studies thus suggest the existence of two distinct metabolic responses that appear to reflect the level of aldose reductase gene expression and activity, and the presence or absence of *myo*-inositol depletion (Fig. 89-2).

As recently discussed,[55] the intriguing possibility that glucose could have opposite effects on DAG in cells with high or low aldose reductase activity warrants further investigation, especially in view of the cell-specific localization of aldose reductase in cellularly heterogeneous tissues, such as the retina,[57] renal glomerulus,[62] arterial wall,[58] and peripheral nerve,[63] all of which exhibit diabetic complications. For example, discordant effects of glucose on DAG levels and molecular species in retinal pericytes[56] and endothelial cells[59] could produce simultaneous, but diametrically opposite (or at least divergent)[64] effects on growth factor responsiveness and the cell cycle, promoting the simultaneous pericyte loss and endothelial cell replication characteristic of early diabetic

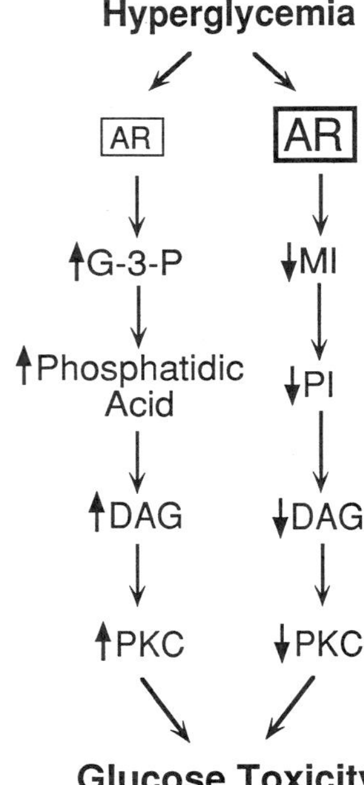

Figure 89-2. Antiparallel effects of glucose on protein kinase C activity. Tissue-specific differences in the level of aldose reductase (AR) gene expression and activity, and the presence or absence of *myo*-inositol (MI) depletion may determine the cellular metabolic response to hyperglycemia and the ultimate change in PKC activity implicated in glucose toxicity. *PI*, phosphoinositides; *G-3-P*, glycerol-3-phosphate.

retinopathy. Similarly, aldose reductase–related reductions in arachidonyl-DAG and related molecular species in diabetic nerve could also explain some of the reported beneficial effects of dietary essential fatty acid supplementation[12,65] or prostaglandin analogues[66] on nerve function in the streptozotocin-induced diabetic rat. Variations in aldose reductase gene expression or activity over time and between species, which produce antiparallel effects on *myo*-inositol and DAG, could also partially explain the socalled "*myo*-inositol paradox" described by Matchinsky and coworkers.[67] Finally, the use of ARIs may convert the biochemical response to hyperglycemia from one pattern to another in a tissue-specific manner, depending upon the intrinsic level of aldose reductase activity, the degree and site of ARI, and the propensity for increasing de novo synthesis of phosphoinositide-related compounds from glucose.

Potentially just as paradoxical is the fact that PKC *activation* has been associated with *diminished* (Na,K)-ATPase activity in peripheral nerve in at least one animal model—the chronically diabetic mouse—with *low* aldose reductase levels.[59] Therefore, it is possible that PKC activation may itself have bidirectional effects on (Na,K)-ATPase activity or, alternatively, that chronic stimulation of PKC could potentially lead to compensatory upregulation or downregulation of its action in this animal model. This is of physiologic relevance because a reduced level of nerve (Na,K)-ATPase has emerged as a possible mechanism for impaired nerve conduction based on detailed electrophysiologic studies in acutely and chronically diabetic rats.[68] Moreover, pharmacologic manipulation of nondiabetic rats with agents that decrease nerve (Na,K)-ATPase levels has permitted researchers to reproduce diabetic nerve conduction slowing.[69] Thus, the relationship between nerve (Na,K)-ATPase activity and nerve conduction velocity in acutely diabetic rodents remains a cornerstone of the explanation for early and reversible slowing of nerve conduction in diabetic animal models,[39,47,50,51] even though a full and precise understanding of this relationship and the details of the underlying metabolic cause(s) remains elusive. Finally, the application of the sorbitol-*myo*-inositol-(Na,K)-ATPase hypothesis to chronic human diabetes remains problematic. For example, ARIs are known to diminish sorbitol accumulation and increase nerve conduction in human diabetic neuropathy, but whether the *myo*-inositol level (or that of other, alternative intracellular osmolytes) is reduced in human diabetic nerve remains controversial,[70,71] and (Na,K)-ATPase activity has not yet been reported.

Sorbitol, Taurine Depletion, and Altered Calcium Homeostasis in Diabetes

The β-amino acid taurine (2-aminoethanesulfonic acid) may also be important in the pathogenesis of diabetic complications. It is found in the highest concentrations in tissues prone to diabetic complications.[72] Our current knowledge of the function of taurine in these diverse tissues, its interactions with phosphoinositide (PI) metabolism, and its depletion in diabetes[23,32] suggests that alterations in taurine metabolism may significantly disrupt the intracellular milieu in the diabetic state.

Taurine is an antioxidant[32,73,74] that may help scavenge the increased free radical production in diabetic tissues.[75] High concentrations of taurine have been identified in tissues that produce oxidants, such as the lung, where taurine has been shown to protect against bronchiolar damage induced by NO_2,[73] ozone, and amiodarone.[76] Taurine has neurotrophic actions[77] and may serve to promote neuronal regeneration, which is depressed in diabetes.[6] In the eye, taurine depletion has been implicated in cataract formation[32] and in structural and functional retinal abnormalities.[78] In the kidney, taurine has been shown to prevent glucose-induced lipid peroxidation and excess collagen production.[79] As discussed later, many of taurine's wide-ranging effects may result from regulation of intracellular Ca^{++} levels.[31,80,81]

Taurine, like *myo*-inositol, behaves as an osmolyte in complications-prone diabetic tissues, reciprocally depleting as sorbitol accumulates, thereby maintaining the intracellular milieu.[23,28,32] Intracellular taurine levels are maintained by endogenous synthesis and active uptake.[82] Taurine uptake occurs by two different transport processes: one that is carrier-mediated and one that is diffusion-limited.[83,84] The gradient-dependent uptake component is thought to be the same Na-independent mechanism that mediates efflux.[84] Like *myo*-inositol, taurine is accumulated by an Na-dependent transporter,[82–89] which requires Cl^-.[85] The human taurine transporter (HTT) has an Na^+/Cl^-/taurine stoichiometry of 2:1:1.[88] The cDNAs for the dog,[89] rat,[90] mouse,[91] and, recently, HTTs[92] have been cloned and shown to be regulated by both hypertonicity[89] and extracellular taurine levels.[93] Cellular taurine release occurs in response to depolarizing agents, including K^+ and excitatory amino acids (EAAs),[94] as well as cell swelling.[95] Acute hypotonicity-induced cell swelling is followed by cellular osmolyte efflux by an Na-independent, but Cl-dependent, route,[96] which may be the taurine efflux pathway.[97] This efflux route has a broad specificity, allowing both taurine and inositol efflux,[97] as well as mannitol and sorbitol, to enter the cell by this mechanism. This efflux route can be inhibited by anion transport blockers,[98] removal of extracellular Cl^-,[99] Cl^- transport blockers,[100] and arachidonic acid.[101]

Organic osmolyte fluxes may principally be regulated by fluctuations in osmotic stress, together with alterations in transmembrane transport induced by kinase activation and inhibition. PKC may regulate osmolyte fluxes; in cell culture, for example, stimulation of PKC by active phorbol esters inhibits taurine uptake and stimulates efflux.[93,102] Activation of the polyol pathway in diabetes may regulate intracellular taurine metabolism by two competing mechanisms: (1) osmotically induced taurine depletion may be compensatory to sorbitol accumulation; and (2) impaired PKC activity resulting from osmotically induced *myo*-inositol (MI) depletion (inhibiting phosphoinositol [PI] turnover) may stimulate taurine uptake. In tissues with low levels of polyol pathway activity, however, glucose-induced PKC activation may be the predominant mechanism producing taurine depletion. Thus, tissue-specific differences in these regulatory factors may predict tissue susceptibility to diabetic complications.

Both taurine[72] and *myo*-inositol[22] are found in high concentrations in the retina.[72,82,103] Moreover, sorbitol accumulates in diabetic retina,[104] and ARIs, which restore tissue taurine and *myo*-inositol levels, have been found to prevent some diabetes- or galactosemia-induced complications.[104,105] Taurine inhibits phosphorylation of specific retinal proteins[106] and may limit the detrimental effects of glucose-induced activation of PKC in tissues (such as retinal capillary endothelium) with low levels of AR expression. In the nervous system, taurine is localized in both glial and neuronal fractions.[107] It is thought to act as an osmoregulator, neuromodulator, or inhibitory neurotransmitter.[108] Taurine may modulate neuronal hyperexcitability[34] by stimulating hyperpolarization[109] and by inhibiting calcium/calmodulin-dependent protein kinases.[34] Taurine may also modulate the growth and differentiation of nervous tissue as it stimulates differentiation of retinal sensory neurons and binds to the insulin receptor.[110]

Many of the protective effects of taurine may be mediated by its effect on intracellular Ca^{++} levels.[31,81] Taurine does not chelate calcium, but modifies its binding to biologic membranes.[81] Taurine can decrease cytosolic Ca^{++} by stimulating mitochondrial Ca^{++} uptake,[111] inhibiting the turnover of phosphoinositides,[111] and decreasing internal flux of Ca^{++}.[112] Moreover, taurine has been shown to protect the cell from excess internal flux of Ca^{++} when the external concentration is high, as it decreases intracellular ionization after ionophore activation or depolarization.[112] These actions also serve to inhibit Ca^{++}-dependent PKC-catalyzed phosphorylation.[111] Indeed, taurine has been shown to block phorbol ester–activated phosphorylation of proteins in rat cortical tissue.[113] These inhibitory effects of taurine may play a vital role in cellular protection after EAA-mediated neuroexcitotoxicity (e.g., during hypoglycemia or ischemia[114]) that is caused by excess Ca^{++} influx stimulating increased protein phosphorylation.[115] Thus, intracellular taurine may play a vital role in intracellular Ca^{++} homeostasis and may serve as a ''counter-regulatory osmolyte,'' helping to modulate the potentially deleterious effects of widespread, uncontrolled activation of protein kinases.

The Sorbitol-Redox Hypothesis

Flux of glucose through AR and sorbitol dehydrogenase stochiometrically oxidizes nicotinamide-adenine dinucleotide phosphate (reduced form) (NADPH)/$NADP^+$ (oxidized form) and reduces NADH/NAD^+ ratios, respectively. Activation of the sorbitol pathway in diabetes could produce redox disturbances if the redox buffering reserve of the cell is otherwise compromised or is overwhelmed (Fig. 89-3). Although direct supportive evidence is lacking,[116] increased oxidative tissue damage in diabetes has been proposed to result from the oxidation of NADPH/$NADP^+$ and the resulting depletion of reduced glutathione. Depletion of NADPH may also limit NADPH-dependent synthase reactions, such as that responsible for the synthesis of nitric oxide (NO), a potent vasodilator and neuromodulator. This could lead to NO depletion, with secondary effects on nerve blood flow and energy reserve, which could further impair redox buffering capacity and other energy-requiring processes [e.g., (Na,K)-ATPase, as discussed later]. The reduction of the NADH/NAD^+ couple by the metabolic oxidation of glucose-derived sorbitol to fructose by sorbitol dehydrogenase is viewed as reproducing the redox effects of hypoxia,[117] a state described as ''metabolic pseudohypoxia.''[46] This has also been identified as the major putative defect contributing to the pathogenesis of diabetic neuropathy.[46] It is thought that the resulting shifts in cytoplasmic NADH/NAD^+ divert glycolytic intermediates to the synthesis of phospholipid precursors, such as α-glycerophosphate, phosphatidic acid, DAG, and cytidine-diphospho-diglyceride (CDP-DG), while simultaneously interfering with β-oxidation of long-chain fatty acids,[46] which are known to accumulate in diabetic nerve. By this construct, the beneficial effects of *myo*-inositol administration on nerve conduction velocity in diabetic rodents could be explained by the accelerated disposal of excess DAG and CDP-DG through stimulation of phosphoinositide synthesis.[46] It seems reasonable to assume that this metabolic model would be most damaging in tissues that limit oxidative capacity, such as the erythrocyte or renal medulla, or in tissues in which oxygen delivery is compromised in diabetes. These relationships are currently being assessed in both cell culture and animal models. Interestingly, one of the cornerstones of the ''metabolic pseudohypoxia hypothesis'' is the ability of millimolar concentrations of pyruvate, which should oxidize the NADH/NAD^+ redox couple, to counteract the effect of glucose on tissue function.[46] A recent study in cultured retinal pigment epithelial cells suggests that pyruvate, rather than correcting a putative alteration in cytoplasmic redox, may enhance sodium-dependent *myo*-inositol transport, thereby counteracting glucose-induced AR-dependent *myo*-inositol depletion and providing an alternative explanation for the beneficial effects of pyruvate.[118] This observation suggests that the sodium-dependent *myo*-inositol transporter is regulated by metabolic as well as osmotic factors, and opens the possibility that ischemic hypoxia, by reducing pyruvate levels, may exacerbate *myo*-inositol depletion under some circumstances.

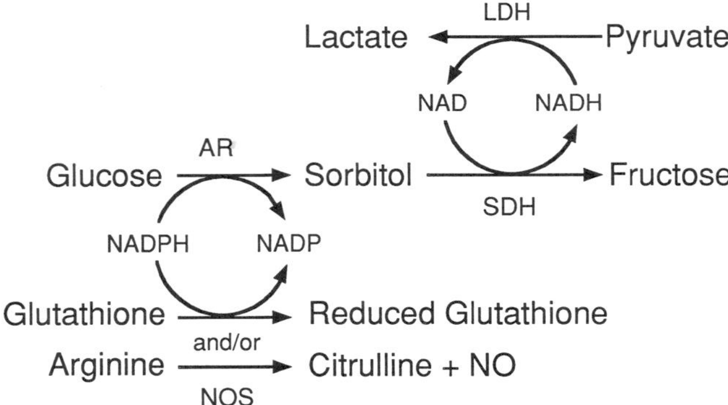

Figure 89-3. Redox relationships in the sorbitol pathway. High glucose flux through aldose reductase (AR) and sorbitol dehydrogenase (SDH) oxidizes the NADPH/$NADP^+$ and reduces the NADH/NAD^+ redox couples, respectively, thereby perturbing other adenine nucleotide–linked reactions. Oxidation of the NADPH/$NADP^+$ couple may increase susceptibility to oxidative tissue damage in diabetes through depletion of reduced glutathione, and to increased superoxide radical–mediated tissue injury. NADPH depletion may also become rate-limiting for nitric oxide (NO) synthesis. Alternatively, a "metabolic pseudoischemia" has been described in which the reduction of NADH/NAD^+ couples by the oxidation of glucose-derived sorbitol to fructose generates phospholipid precursors that may interfere with β-oxidation of long-chain fatty acids that accumulate in diabetic nerve. (Modified with permission from Greene DA, Sima AAF, Stevens MJ, et al. Aldose reductase inhibitors: An approach to the treatment of diabetic nerve damage. Diabetes Metab Rev 1993;9:206.)

This is particularly important given the increasing evidence that nerve ischemia plays a central role in the pathogenesis of diabetic neuropathy, and that nerve blood flow is corrected by ARIs. Hemodynamic and oximetric measurements in anesthetized rats have demonstrated reduced endoneurial blood flow and oxygen tension in chronically diabetic rats,[8,9] which may occur as early as 1 week after the induction of diabetes[9] (although this contention is disputed by some[119]). A wide variety of vasodilatory agents have been shown to partially or completely correct nerve conduction slowing in diabetic rats.[10,66] Fragmentary clinical evidence in support of the role of nerve hypoxia in the development of neuropathy has been derived from the finding of reduced endoneurial oxygen in the sural nerves of diabetic patients with advanced polyneuropathy,[120] and the observation of some abnormalities of neural conduction in nondiabetic hypoxic patients with chronic obstructive airway disease.[121] Nondiabetic animals exposed to chronic hypoxia show some impairment of nerve conduction velocity and resistance to ischemic conduction block, which abnormalities are reversible when the hypoxia is corrected.[122] Finally, an experimentally induced reduction in caudal nerve action potential in diabetic rats can be normalized by hyperbaric oxygenation, but nerve conduction velocity has not been found to improve.[123] Thus, although hypoxia may play a role in the development of diabetic neuropathy, it may not be the sole mechanism; sorbitol pathway and *myo*-inositol depletion may be potential causes and consequences of ischemia in diabetes.

The Impact of the Sorbitol-Osmotic and Sorbitol-Redox Hypotheses on Vasoactive Agents in Diabetes

Theoretical and empirical considerations suggest that sorbitol pathway activation and the resultant alterations in compatible osmolytes and cellular redox could alter the secretion and action of a variety of important vasomodulatory agents. For example, glucose-induced impairment of phosphoinositide signal transduction in retinal pericytes could diminish their responsiveness to endothelin-1, one of the most potent known vasoconstrictors, thereby contributing to increased retinal blood flow in early diabetes.[56] Similarly, the decrease in nerve blood flow observed in early experimental diabetic neuropathy has been ascribed to depletion of nitric oxide[69] or an imbalance in the thromboxane:prostacyclin ratio,[13] both of which, as discussed in the following section, are potentially related to the sorbitol-osmotic and sorbitol-redox hypotheses.

The Sorbitol-Osmotic and Sorbitol-Redox Hypotheses and Nitric Oxide in Diabetes

Over the last few years, the once obscure endothelium-derived relaxing factor NO has been identified as a potent mediator of vasodilatation, macrophage cytotoxicity, and neurotransmission,[124,125] and may be of critical importance to the pathogenesis of diabetic complications, including diabetic neuropathy. Endothelial cells, vascular smooth muscle cells, and sympathetic ganglia are potential sites of action of NO synthase (NOS), the enzyme catalyzing the conversion of L-arginine to citrulline and NO at the expense of NADPH.[125] So-called ''constitutively expressed'' forms of NOS (cNOS) are, indeed, constitutively expressed in endothelial (eNOS) and neuronal (nNOS) cells at the mRNA and protein level, but the activity of the gene product is dependent on post-translational modification by calcium/calmodulin-dependent, and perhaps, other protein kinases, including PKC.[16,124,125] Because sorbitol pathway activation appears to alter NADPH via the redox hypothesis, and protein kinases and calcium via the osmotic hypothesis, it is not unreasonable to speculate that sorbitol metabolism in diabetes could interfere with NO metabolism and action. Locally released NO in the endoneurial microvasculature, along with locally derived prostacyclins, would presumably modulate regional blood flow. Moreover, elevated plasma levels of the immunoreactive vasoconstrictor endothelin have been found in diabetic subjects,[126] and this may further exaggerate the effects of abnormal NO metabolism and action on vascular tone in diabetes. Endothelium-dependent relaxation of smooth muscle has been shown to be impaired in both human diabetics[128] and animals with experimentally induced diabetes.[128,129] The mechanisms underlying this deficit are unclear, but may involve depletion of NO[16,128–130] or an altered smooth muscle sensitivity to NO.[131] Impaired local synthesis of NO may alter basal vascular tone, either by reduced activation of soluble guanylate cyclase in vascular smooth muscle[69,129,132] or by decreased Na/K-ATPase,[133] potentially resulting in decreased blood flow in the endoneurium of peripheral nerves. The impaired endoneurial vasodilatory responses to acetylcholine[128,129] and attendant preserved endothelium-independent vasodilatory responses to, for example, sodium nitroprusside,[129] nitroglycerin,[16] and other agents that release NO directly, suggest a defect or defects in endoneurial NO synthesis or release as the cause of impaired vascular responses in diabetes.

Recently, NO has emerged not only as an important local direct vasoactive substance, but also as an important neurotransmitter, with both central and peripheral effects.[134] In the sympathetic autonomic nervous system, NO may function as an inhibitory neurotransmitter that is released by postsynaptic sympathetic neurons, thereby inhibiting the presynaptic release of acetylcholine and reducing sympathetic tone[69] (Fig. 89-4). Thus, NADPH depletion or alterations in PK or calcium regulation of nNOS in postsynaptic sympathetic neurons could increase sympathetic vascular tone,[4] possibly explaining the observation that inhibition of basal sympathetic vascular tone by guanethidine restores both nerve blood flow and nerve conduction to normal levels in acute experimental diabetes.[9] Thus, for example, in diabetes, if NO depletion at the level of the sympathetic ganglia is an early event, increased vasoconstricting sympathetic tone to the nerve vasculature may result, precipitating nerve ischemia and acute nerve conduction slowing.

Altered NO metabolism (together with prostaglandin metabolism) in diabetes may be the means by which the divergent metabolic and vascular hypotheses evoked in the pathogenesis of diabetic neuropathy are linked.[4,135] Metabolic competition for NADPH by AR and NOS has been proposed as a possible mechanism linking these hypotheses[4,135] (see Fig. 89-3). Evidence is also accumulating that PKC, the activity of which is altered in diabetic tissues, may also regulate NOS by direct phosphorylation.[136] The effect of PKC on NOS is controversial, however, as PKC activation has been reported to both increase[136] and decrease[137] NOS activity. Moreover, the bidirectional effects of hyperglycemia on DAG levels and PKC activation, which may reflect cell-specific variations in AR expression and activity in different tissues (see Fig. 89-2), suggest that tissue-specific differences in these regulatory factors may determine the predominant response of NOS to hyperglycemia. Finally, AR-mediated consumption of NADPH may not only directly impair the activity of NOS, but may also lead to increased levels of superoxide radicals (which may chemically quench NO[17]), as NADPH is also required for the production of reduced glutathione[7] (see Fig. 89-4). In diabetes, the endothelium is abnormally sensitive to damage mediated by both increased production of superoxide radicals and increased formation of advanced glycosylation end products by glucose[7] and fructose, which may quench NO. Evidence of metabolic competition between NOS and AR, and/or AR-mediated abnormalities in PKC is provided by the fact that ARIs not only restore osmolyte and redox balance in the nerve,[6,23] but also

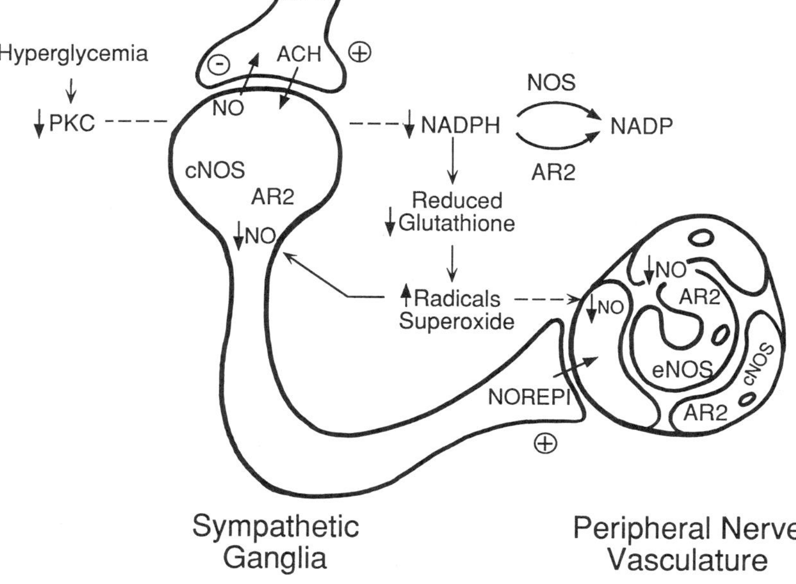

Figure 89-4. Alterations in nitric oxide (NO) metabolism in sympathetic ganglia, vascular smooth muscle cell, and an endothelial cell. Reduced endoneurial blood flow in diabetes may result from depletion of NO at the level of the autonomic ganglia or within the endoneurial vasculature. *AR2*, aldose reductase; *ACH*, acetylcholine; *NOREPI*, norepinephrine. (Modified with permission from Greene DA, Sima AAF, Stevens MJ, et al. Aldose reductase inhibitors: An approach to the treatment of diabetic nerve damage. Diabetes Metab Rev 1993;9:206.)

improve nerve blood flow.[66] AR protein is found within the endoneurium as well as the perineurium[63] and, presumably, the sympathetic ganglia, which would make such metabolic interactions possible at any of these sites. Moreover, in a 3-month experiment involving a streptozotocin-diabetic (STZ-D) rat model, ARI treatment was demonstrated to restore endothelium-dependent relaxation to within normal limits.[135] Recently, a NO synthase inhibitor—L-nitro-N-methyl arginine ester (L-NAME)—was found to reverse the effects of ARI in acute experimental diabetic neuropathy, despite the ability of ARI to decrease nerve sorbitol significantly and increase nerve *myo*-inositol in the L-NAME–treated rats.[69] L-NAME appeared to have little acute effect on nerve conduction velocity in untreated diabetic animals.[69] Short-term (3-week) treatment of nondiabetic control animals with L-NAME only insignificantly reduced nerve conduction, but did slow nerve conduction and reduce Na/K-ATP-ase activity.[69] These data support a role for NO in mediating, at least partially, the beneficial effects of ARIs on nerve blood flow and nerve conduction in diabetic rats, as well as in maintaining nerve Na/K-ATPase levels.

Therefore, decreased production of NO in diabetics, resulting from sorbitol pathway–related osmolyte depletion or redox imbalance, could contribute to slowing of nerve conduction through a decrease in endoneurial blood flow produced both by an acute increase in vascular sympathetic tone[4] and by localized vascular endothelial and smooth muscle depletion. Alternatively, NO depletion may exert more distal effects on nerve function, independently of nerve blood flow, via direct effects on nerve Na/K-ATPase activity, as suggested earlier.

The Sorbitol-Osmotic and Sorbitol-Redox Hypotheses and Eicosanoid Metabolism in Diabetes

Altered eicosanoid metabolism has been implicated in the pathogenesis of diabetic complications. The possible interactions are potentially quite complex between sorbitol pathway activity, its effect on osmolyte composition and redox balance, and the secondary effects of these disturbances on overall tissue metabolism. Arachidonic acid, which can become rate-limiting for eicosanoid metabolism, is released from membrane phosphoinositides and is dependent upon cytoplasmic redox for synthesis and metabolism. Altered prostaglandin production and hypersensitivity in diabetes may predispose an individual to either tissue hyperemia or ischemia, depending on the balance between vasoconstrictive and vasodilatory eicosanoids. Microvascular tone is dependent on the opposing actions of prostacyclin (which is located within the endothelial cells and which, together with NO, elicits vasodilatation) and thromboxane A2, which is found mainly in blood platelets (but also in endothelium) and produces vasoconstriction.[138] Increases in vasoconstricting thromboxanes prostaglandin H_2 (PGH_2),[139] thromboxane A_2 (TXA_2),[138] and PGF_{2a}, as well as reductions in vasodilating prostacyclin, have been described in isolated diabetic vascular tissue.[140] An increase in the thromboxane:prostacyclin ratio[13] may contribute to a reduction of blood flow and, possibly, Na/K-ATPase activity in diabetic nerve. Ischemia in the nerve may activate phospholipase A_2,[141] which disrupts membrane phospholipids and generates prostaglandins from activated arachidonic acid[142] (Fig. 89-5). A hypoxic insult may also be one of the triggers for the production of the superoxide radical via the breakdown of ATP and the generation of reducing equivalents, such as NADPH, in the xanthine-xanthine oxidase reaction.[13] The generation of lipid hydroperoxides by the action of free radicals may result in increased cyclo-oxygenase activity and reduced prostacyclin synthase activity, thereby increasing the thromboxane:prostacyclin ratio, with resultant vasoconstriction and platelet aggregation. Phospholipase activation may also generate leukotrienes, which may further compound the damage to the endothelial cell. Superoxide dismutase, which has an important role in neutralizing superoxide radicals, may be reduced in diabetic peripheral nerve. Eicosanoids may also serve to limit the detrimental effects of ischemia, however, by inhibiting superoxide anion production.[143]

There is compelling evidence in the diabetic rat model of a role for disruption of prostaglandin metabolism in experimental nerve conduction slowing. As prostacyclin levels are typically not depleted early in experimental neuropathy, however, they probably

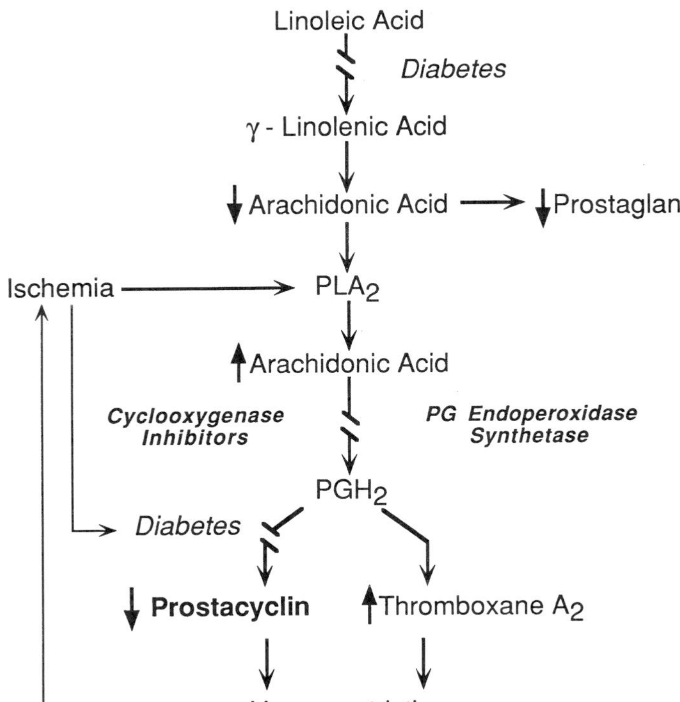

FIGURE 89-5. Prostaglandin synthesis in diabetic nerve. In diabetes, defects in desaturation of linoleic acid and ischemia-induced activation of phospholipase A_2 (***PLA_2***), together with inhibition of prostacyclin synthetase by free radical–generated lipid hydroperoxides, may lead to overproduction of vasoconstricting thromboxane A_2 with a depletion in prostacyclin, favoring vasoconstriction of the endoneurial vasculature and reduced nerve blood flow.

do not precipitate the early decrease in endoneurial blood flow that is observed (although eicosanoids may modulate autonomic tone as both PGE_1 and PGE_2 inhibit sympathetic neurotransmission, mainly by reducing the release of norepinephrine from adrenergic nerve terminals[144]). Reduced nerve prostacyclin has been found in chronic (4-month) experimental diabetes,[13] and PGE_1 analogue administration has been shown to restore nerve conduction velocity to normal in diabetic rats.[66] cAMP levels are reduced in experimental diabetic neuropathy,[145] and nerve prostacyclin levels, cAMP,[146] and Na/K-ATPase activity[45] have been found to correlate with each other and to be corrected by PGE_1 administration. It is thus possible that prostaglandin metabolism may be a key modulator of both endoneurial blood flow and nerve Na/K-ATPase activity in experimental diabetic neuropathy. Moreover, therapeutic manipulations that have been shown to correct nerve conduction slowing, such as MI supplementation or gamma-linolenic acid (GLA, from evening primrose oil),[12,40,51,146] may, in fact, exert their effect, at least in part, by increasing prostacyclin production, as both may increase arachidonic acid, which is rate-limiting for prostaglandin synthesis.

Summary

In summary, the potential mechanisms by which glucose metabolism, through the two simple reactions of the sorbitol pathway, influences the biochemistry, function, and structure of tissues prone to diabetic complications form a complex web of interactions at the molecular, biochemical, and microvascular level. Two proximal metabolic consequences of sorbitol pathway activation include perturbations of the metabolism of intracellular nonionic osmolytes and adenine-nucleotide–linked chemical reactions. They proceed to involve cellular fuel metabolism, redox potential, and signal transduction in a profound way. It is likely that these effects vary from cell to cell in complex heterogeneous tissues, and differentially affect different vascular beds in diverse ways. Although we are just beginning to appreciate the full impact of these diverse molecular, metabolic, and physiologic perturbations in a tissue-specific fashion, clinical trials are examining the beneficial effects of inhibition of the initial inciting event, namely the metabolism of glucose through AR using both specific enzymatic inhibitors and tight blood glucose control. As the full web of consequences of sorbitol pathway activation become understood more fully, tissue-specific interventions tailored to the predominant impact of the sorbitol pathway will likely be developed, thereby adding to the therapeutic armamentarium available to treat or prevent diabetic complications resulting from sorbitol pathway activation.

References

1. DCCT Research Group: Factors in the development of diabetic neuropathy: Baseline analysis of neuropathy in the feasibility phase of the Diabetes Control and Complications Trial (DCCT). Diabetes 1988;37:476
2. Pirart J. Diabetes mellitus and its degenerative complications: A prospective study of 4,400 patients observed between 1947 and 1973. Diabetes Care 1978;1:168
3. Young MJ, Boulton AJM, Macleod AF, et al. A multi-centre study of the prevalence of diabetic peripheral neuropathy in the United Kingdom hospital clinic population. Diabetologia 1993;36:150
4. Greene DA, Sima AAF, Stevens MJ, et al. Complications: Neuropathy, pathogenetic considerations. Diabetes Care 1992;15:1902
5. DCCT Research Group: The effect of intensive treatment of diabetes on the development and progression of long-term complications in insulin-dependent diabetes mellitus. N Engl J Med 1993;329:977
6. Greene DA, Lattimer SA, Sima AAF. Sorbitol, phosphoinositides and sodium-potassium-ATPase in the pathogenesis of diabetic complications. N Engl J Med 1987;316:599
7. Dvornik D. Hyperglycemia in the pathogenesis of diabetic complications. In: Porte D, ed. Aldose Reductase Inhibition: An Approach to the Prevention of Diabetic Complications. New York: McGraw-Hill;1987:69
8. Tuck RR, Schmelzer JD, Low PA. Endoneurial blood flow and oxygen tension in the sciatic nerves of rats with experimental diabetic neuropathy. Brain 1984;107:935
9. Cameron NE, Cotter MA, Low PA. Nerve blood flow in early experimental diabetes in rats: Relation to conduction deficits. Am J Physiol 1991;261:E1
10. Cameron NE, Cotter MA, Ferguson K, et al. Effects of chronic alpha-adrenergic receptor blockade on peripheral nerve conduction, hypoxic resistance, polyols, Na/K-ATPase activity, and vascular supply in STZ-D rats. Diabetes 1991;40:1652
11. Horrobin DF. Gamma linolenic acid. Rev Contemp Pharmacother 1990;1:1
12. Cameron NE, Cotter MA, Robertson S. Effects of essential fatty acid dietary supplementation on peripheral nerve and skeletal muscle function and capillarisation in streptozotocin diabetic rats. Diabetes 1991;40:532
13. Ward KK, Low PA, Schmelzer JD, Zochodne DW. Prostacyclin and noradrenaline in peripheral nerve of chronic experimental diabetic in rats. Brain 1989;112:197
14. Brownlee M. Glycation products and the pathogenesis of diabetic complications. Diabetes Care 1992;15:1835
15. Richard S, Tamas C, Sell DR, Monnier VM. Tissue-specific effects of aldose reductase inhibition on fluorescence and cross-linking of extracellular matrix in chronic galactosemia. Relationship to pentosidine cross-links. Diabetes 1991;40:1049
16. Moncada S, Palmer RMJ, Higgs EA. Nitric oxide: Physiology, pathophysiology and pharmacology. Pharmacol Rev 1991;43:109
17. Gryglewski RJ, Palmer RMJ, Moncada S. Superoxide anion is involved in the breakdown of endothelium-derived vascular relaxing factor. Nature 1986;320:454
18. Dyck PJ, Karnes JL, O'Brien P, et al. The spatial distribution of fiber loss in diabetic polyneuropathy suggests ischemia. Ann Neurol 1986;19:440
19. Vracko R. A comparison of the microvascular lesions in diabetic mellitus with those of normal aging. J Am Geriatr Soc 1982;30:201
20. Lowe GDO, Lowe JM, Drummond MM, et al. Blood viscosity in young male diabetics with or without retinopathy. Diabetologia 1980;18:359
21. Bauersachs RM, Shaw SJ, Ziedler A, Meiselman HJ. Red blood cell aggregation and blood viscosity in poorly controlled type 2 diabetes mellitus. Clin Hemorheol 1989;9:935
22. Marano CW, Matchinsky FM. Biochemical aspects of diabetes mellitus in microscopic layers of the cornea and retina. Diabetes Metab Rev 1989;5:1
23. Stevens MJ, Lattimer SA, Kamijo M, et al. Osmotically induced nerve taurine depletion and the compatible osmolyte hypothesis in experimental diabetic neuropathy in the rat. Diabetologia 1993;36:608
24. Dvornik D. In: Porte D, ed. Aldose Reductase Inhibition: An Approach to the Prevention of Diabetic Complications. New York: McGraw-Hill;1987:222
25. Kinoshita JH. Mechanism initiating cataract formation. Invest Ophthalmol 1974;13:713
26. Moriyama T, Garcia-Perez A, Burg MB. Factors affecting the ratio of different organic osmolytes in renal medullary cells. Am J Physiol 1990;259:F847
27. Moriyama T, Garcia-Perez A, Burg MB. High extracellular NaCl stimulates synthesis of aldose reductase, an osmoregulatory protein, in renal medullary cells. Kidney Int 1989;35:499
28. Burg MB, Kador PF. Sorbitol, osmoregulation, and the complications of diabetes. J Clin Invest 1988;81:635
29. Moo Kwon H, Yamauchi A, Uchida S, et al. Renal Na-*myo*-inositol cotransporter mRNA expression in Xenopus oocytes: Regulation by hypertonicity. Am J Physiol 1991;260:F258
30. Uchida S, Nakanishi T, Kwon HM, et al. Taurine behaves as an osmolyte in Madin-Darby canine kidney cells. J Clin Invest 1991;88:656
31. Huxtable RJ. From heart to hypothesis: A mechanism for the calcium modulatory effects actions of taurine. In: Huxtable RJ, Franconi F, Giotti A, eds. The Biology of Taurine: Methods and Mechanisms. New York: Plenum Press;1987:371
32. Malone JI, Lowitt S, Cook WR. Nonosmotic diabetic cataracts. Pediatr Res 1990;27:293
33. Nakamura J, Del Monte MA, Shewach D, et al. Inhibition of phosphatidylinositol synthase by glucose in human retinal pigment epithelial cells. Am J Physiol 1992;262:E417
34. Lombardi JB. Effects of taurine on calcium ion uptake and protein phosphorylation in rat retinal membrane preparations. J Neurochem 1985;45:268
35. Cheung WY. Calmodulin plays a pivotal role in cellular regulation. Science 1980;207:17
36. Nestler EJ, Greengard P. Protein phosphorylation in the brain. Nature 1983;305:583
37. Dent MT, Tebbs SE, Gonzales AM, et al. Neutrophil aldose reductase activity and its association with established diabetic microvascular complications. Diabetes Med 1991;8:439
38. Vinores SA, Campochiaro PA, Williams EH, et al. Aldose reductase expression in human diabetic retina and retinal pigment epithelium. Diabetes 1988;37:1658
39. Greene DA, Lattimer SA. Impaired energy utilization and Na-K-ATPase in diabetic peripheral nerve. Am J Physiol 1984;246:E311
40. Greene DA, DeJesus PV, Wingrad AI. Effects of insulin and dietary *myo*-inositol on impaired motor nerve conduction velocity in acute streptozotocin diabetes. J Clin Invest 1975;55:1326
41. Greene DA, Lattimer SA. Sodium- and energy-dependent uptake of *myo*-inositol by rabbit peripheral nerve: Competitive inhibition by glucose and lack of an insulin effect. J Clin Invest 1982;70:1009

42. Tomlinson DR, Sidenius P, Larsen JR. Slow component-a of axonal transport, nerve *myo*-inositol and aldose reductase inhibition in streptozotocin-diabetic rats. Diabetes 1986;34:398
43. Finegold D, Lattimer S, Nolle S, et al. Polyol pathway activity and *myo*-inositol metabolism. Diabetes 1983;32:988
44. Hermenegildo C, Felipo V, Minana M-D, et al. Sustained recovery of Na^+-K^+-ATPase activity in sciatic nerve of diabetic mice by administration of H7 or calphostin C, inhibitors of PKC. Diabetes 1993;42:257
45. Sonobe M, Yasuda H, Hisanaga T, et al. Amelioration of nerve Na/K-ATPase activity independently of *myo*-inositol level by PGE1 analogue OP-1206.a-CD in streptozotocin-induced diabetic rats. Diabetes 1991;40:726
46. Williamson JR, Chang K, Frangos M, et al. Hyperglycemic "pseudohypoxia" and diabetic complications. Diabetes 1993;42:801
47. Greene DA, Lattimer SA. Action or sorbinil in diabetic peripheral nerve. Relationship of polyol (sorbitol) pathway inhibition to a *myo*-inositol-mediated defect in sodium-potassium ATPase activity. Diabetes 1984;33:712
48. Tomlinson DR, Mayer JH. Reversal of deficits in axonal transport and nerve conduction velocity by treatment of streptozotocin diabetic rats with *myo*-inositol. Exp Neurol 1985;89:420
49. Greene DA, Lattimer S, Ulbrecht J, Carroll P. Glucose-induced alterations in nerve metabolism: Current perspective on the pathogenesis of diabetic neuropathy and future directions for research and therapy. Diabetes Care 1985;8:290
50. Das PK, Bray GM, Aguayo AJ, Rasminsky M. Diminished ouabain sensitive, sodium potassium ATPase activity in sciatic nerves of rats with streptozotocin induced diabetes. Exp Neurol 1976;53:285
51. Greene DA, Lattimer SA. Impaired rat sciatic nerve sodium-potassium adenosine trisphosphatase in acute streptozotocin diabetes and its correction by dietary *myo*-inositol supplementation. J Clin Invest 1983;72:1058
52. Zhu X, Eichberg J. 1,2-Diacylglycerol content and its arachidonyl-containing molecular species are reduced in sciatic nerve from streptozotocin-induced diabetic rats. J Neurochem 1990;55:1087
53. Kim J, Rushovich EA, Thomas TA, et al. Diminished specific activity of cytosolic protein kinase C in sciatic nerve of streptozotocin-diabetic rats, and its correction by dietary *myo*-inositol. Diabetes 1991;40:1545
54. Kim J, Kyriazi H, Greene DA. Normalization of Na,K-ATPase activity in isolated membrane fraction from sciatic nerves of streptozotocin-induced diabetic rats by dietary *myo*-inositol supplementation in vivo or protein kinase C agonists in vitro. Diabetes 1990;40:558
55. Thomas TP, Feldman EL, Nakamura J, et al. Ambient glucose and aldose reductase-induced *myo*-inositol depletion modulate basal and carbachol-stimulated inositol phospholipid metabolism and diacylglycerol accumulation in human retinal pigment epithelial cells in culture. Proc Natl Acad Sci USA 1993;90:9712
56. De La Rubia G, Oliver FJ, Inoguchi T, King GL. Induction of resistance of endothelin-1's biochemical actions by elevated glucose levels in retinal pericytes. Diabetes 1992;41:1533
57. Akagi Y, Yajima PF, Kador PF, et al. Localization of aldose reductase in the human eye. Diabetes 1984;33:562
58. Ludwigson MA, Sorenson RL. Immunohistochemical localization of aldose reductase. I. Enzyme purification and antibody preparation-localization in peripheral nerve, artery and testis. Diabetes 1980;29:438
59. Lee T-S, Slatsman KA, Ohashi H, King GL. Activation of protein kinase C by elevation of glucose concentration: Proposal for a mechanism in the development of diabetic vascular complications. Proc Natl Acad Sci USA 1989;86:5141
60. Craven PA, DeRubertis FR. Protein kinase C is activated in glomeruli from streptozotocin diabetic rats: Possible mediation by glucose. J Clin Invest 1989;83:1667
61. Kunisaki M, Bursell S-E, Umeda F, et al. Normalization of diacyglycerol-protein kinase C activation by vitamin E in aorta of diabetic rats and cultured rat smooth muscle cells exposed to elevated glucose levels. Diabetes 1994; 43:1372
62. Ludwigson MA, Sorenson RL. Immunohistochemical localization of aldose reductase. 2. In rat eye and kidney. Diabetes 1980;29:450
63. Chakrabarti S, Sima AAF, Nakajima T, et al. Aldose reductase in the BB rat: Isolation, immunological identification and localization in the retina and peripheral nerve. Diabetologia 1987;30:244
64. Leach KL, Ruff VA, Wright TM, et al. Dissociation of protein kinase C activation and sn-1,2-diacylglycerol formation. Comparison of phosphatidylinositol- and phosphatidylcholine-derived diglycerides in thrombin-stimulated fibroblasts. J Biol Chem 1991;266:3215
65. Tomlinson DR, Robinson JP, Compton A, Keen P. Essential fatty acid treatment—Effects on nerve conduction, polyol pathway and axonal transport in streptozotocin diabetic rats. Diabetologia 1989;32:655
66. Yasuda HS, Masanobu M, Yamashita M, et al. Effect of prostaglandin E, analogue TFC612 on diabetic neuropathy in streptozotocin-induced diabetic rats. Comparison with aldose reductase inhibitor ONO2235. Diabetes 1989; 38:832
67. Loy A, Kurie KG, Ghosh A, et al. Diabetes and the *myo*-inositol paradox. Diabetes 1990;39:1305
68. Brismar T, Sima AAF, Greene DA. Reversible and irreversible nodal dysfunction in diabetic neuropathy. Ann Neurol 1987;21:504
69. Stevens MJ, Dananberg J, Feldman EL, et al. The linked roles of nitric oxide, aldose reductase and (Na^+,K^+)-ATPase in the slowing of nerve conduction in the streptozotocin diabetic rat. J Clin Invest 1994;94:853
70. Sima AAF, Bril V, Nathaniel V, et al. Regeneration and repair of myelinated fibers in sural nerve biopsies from patients with diabetic neuropathy treated with an ARI. N Engl J Med 1988;319:548
71. Dyck PJ, Zimmerman BR, Vilen TH, et al. Nerve glucose, fructose, sorbitol, *myo*-inositol and fiber degeneration and regeneration in diabetic neuropathy. N Engl J Med 1988;319:542
72. Jacobsen JG, Smith LH. Biochemistry and physiology of taurine and taurine derivatives. Physiol Rev 1968;48:424
73. Gould RE, Shaked AA, Solano DF. Taurine protects hamster bronchioles from acute NO_2-induced alteration. Am J Pathol 1986;125:585
74. Pasantes-Morales H, Cruz C. Taurine and hypotaurine inhibit light-induced lipid peroxidation and protect rod outer segment structure. Brain Res 1985;330:154
75. Low PA, Nickander KK. Oxygen free radical effects in sciatic nerve in experimental diabetes. Diabetes 1991;40:873
76. Wang QJ, Hollinger MA, Giri SN. Attenuation of amiodarone-induced lung fibrosis and phospholipidosis in hamsters by taurine and/or niacin treatment. J Pharmacol Exp Ther 1992;262:127
77. Oja SS, Kontro P. Neuromodulatory and trophic actions of taurine. In: Taurine: Functional Neurochemistry, Physiology and Cardiology. Pasantes Morales H, Martin DL, Shain W, Martin del Río, eds. New York, NY: Wiley-Liss;1990:1
78. Nakagawa M. Homeostatic and protective effects of taurine. In: Taurine: Functional Neurochemistry, Physiology, and Cardiology. New York, NY: Wiley-Liss;1990:447
79. Trachtman H, Futterweit S, Bienkowski RS. Taurine prevents glucose-induced lipid peroxidation and increased collagen production in cultured rat mesangial cells. Biochem Biophys Res Commun 1993;191:759
80. Li Y-P, Lombardini JB. Inhibition by taurine of the phosphorylation of specific synaptosomal proteins in the rat cortex: Effects of taurine on the stimulation of calcium uptake in the mitochondria and inhibition of phosphoinositide turnover. Brain Res 1991;553:89
81. Huxtable RJ. The interaction between taurine, calcium and phospholipids: Further investigations of a trinitarian hypothesis. In: Taurine: Functional Neurochemistry, Physiology, and Cardiology. Pasantes Morales H, Martin DL, Shain W, Martin del Río, eds. New York, NY: Wiley-Liss;1990:185
82. Miyamoto Y, Palaniappan K, Leibach FH, Ganapathy V. Taurine uptake in apical membrane vesicles from the bovine retinal pigment epithelium. Invest Ophthalmol Visual Sci 1991;32:2542
83. Sanchez-Olea R, Moran J, Schousboe A, Pasantes-Morales H. Changes in taurine transport evoked by hyperosmolarity in cultured astrocytes. J Neurosci Res 1992;32:86
84. Beetsch JW, Olson JE. Taurine transport in rat astrocytes adapted to hyperosmotic conditions. Brain Res 1993;613:10
85. Karl PI, Fisher SE. Taurine transport by microvillous membrane vesicles and the perfused cotyledon of the human placenta. Am J Physiol 1990;258: C443
86. Wolf NA, Kinne R. Taurine transport by rabbit brush-border membranes: Coupling to sodium, chloride, and membrane potential. J Membr Biol 1988; 102:131
87. Turner RJ. B-Amino acid transporter across the renal brush-border membrane is coupled to both Na and Cl. J Biol Chem 1988;261:16060
88. Ramamoorthy S, Leibach FH, Mahesh VB, et al. Functional characterization and chromosomal localization of a cloned taurine transporter from human placenta. Biochem J 1994;300:893
89. Uchida S, Moo Kwon H, Yamauchi A, et al. Molecular cloning of the cDNA for an MDCK cell Na^+- and Cl^--dependent taurine transporter that is regulated by hypertonicity. Proc Natl Acad Sci USA 1992;89:8230
90. Smith KE, Borden LA, Wang C-HD, et al. Cloning and expression of a high-affinity taurine transporter from rat brain. Mol Pharmacol 1992;42:563
91. Liu Q-R, Lopez-Corcuera B, Nelson H, et al. Cloning and expression of a cDNA encoding the transporter of taurine and B-alanine in mouse brain. Proc Natl Acad Sci USA 1992;89:12145
92. Jhaing SM, Fithian L, Smanik P, et al. Cloning of the human taurine transporter and characterization of taurine uptake in thyroid cells. FEBS Lett 1993;318:139
93. Jones DP, Miller LA, Dowling C, Chesney RW. Regulation of taurine transporter activity in LLC-PK1 cells: Role of protein synthesis and protein kinase C activation. J Am Soc Nephrol 1991;2:1021
94. Oja SS, Kontro P. Taurine. In: Lajtha A, ed. Handbook of Neurochemistry. Vol. 3. 2nd ed. New York: Plenum Press;1983:510
95. Martin DL, Madelian V, Seligmann B, Shain W. The role of osmotic pressure and membrane potential in the K^+-stimulated taurine release from cultured astrocytes and LRM55 cells. J Neurosci 1990;10:571
96. Strange K, Morrison R. Volume regulation during recovery from chronic hypertonicity in brain glial cells. Am J Physiol 1992;263(Cell Physiol. 32):C412
97. Banderalli U, Roy G. Anion channels for amino acids in MDCK cells. Am Physiol Soc 1992;263:1200
98. Kirk K, Ellory JC, Young JD. Transport of organic substrates via a volume-activated channel. J Biol Chem 1992;267:23475
99. Faff-Michalak L, Reichenbach A, Dettmer D, et al. K^+-hypoosmolality, and $NH4^+$-induced taurine release from cultured rabbit Muller cells: Role of Na^+ and Cl^- ions and relation to cell volume changes. Glia 1994;10: 114
100. Sanchez-Olea R, Pena C, Moran J, Pasantes-Morales H. Inhibition of volume

regulation and efflux of osmoregulatory amino acids by blockers of Cl- transport in cultured astrocytes. Neurosci Lett 1993;156:141
101. Jackson PS, Strange K. Volume-sensitive anion channels mediate swelling-activated inositol and taurine efflux. Am J Physiol 1993;265(Cell Physiol. 34):C1489
102. Brandsch M, Miyamoto Y, Ganapathy V, Leibach FH. Regulation of taurine transport in human colon carcinoma cell lines (HT-29 and Caco-2) by protein kinase C. Am J Physiol 1993;264(Gastrointest. Liver Physiol. 27):G939
103. Voaden MJ, Lake N, Marshall J, Morjaria B. Studies on the distribution of taurine and other neuroactive amino acids in the retina. Exp Eye Res 1977;25:249
104. Robison WG Jr, Kador PF, Kinoshita JH. Retinal capillaries: Basement membrane thickening by galactosemia prevented with aldose reductase inhibitor. Science 1983;221:1177
105. Cunha-Vaz JG, Mota CC, Leite EC, et al. Effect of sulindac on the permeability of the blood retinal barrier in early diabetic retinopathy. Arch Ophthalmol 1985;103:1307
106. Lombardini JB. Effects of taurine on protein phosphorylation in mammalian tissues. In: Lombardini JB, Schaffer SW, Azuma J, eds. Advances in Experimental Medicine and Biology. Taurine: Nutritional Value and Mechanisms of Action. New York: Plenum Press;1992:309
107. Sellstrom A, Sjoberg L-B, Hamberger A. Neuronal and glial systems for gamma aminobutyric acid metabolism. J Neurochem 1975;25:393
108. Davidson AN, Kaczmarek LN. Taurine—A possible neurotransmitter? Nature 1971;234:107
109. Lerma J, Herranz AS, Herreras O, et al. Gamma-aminobutyric acid increases the in vivo extracellular taurine in the rat hippocampus. J Neurochem 1985;44:983
110. Maturo J, Kulakowski EC. Taurine binding to the purified insulin receptor. Biochem Pharmacol 1988;37:3755
111. Li Y-P, Lombardini JB. Inhibition by taurine of the phosphorylation of specific synaptosomal proteins in the rat cortex: Effects of taurine on the stimulation of calcium uptake in the mitochondria and inhibition of phosphoinositide turnover. Brain Res 1991;553:89
112. Whitton PS, Nicholson RA, Strong HC. Effect of taurine on calcium accumulation in resting and repolarized insect synaptosomes. J Neurochem 1988a; 50:1743
113. Lombardini JB. Regional and subcellular studies on taurine in the rat central nervous system. In: Huxtable R, Barbeau A, eds. Taurine. New York: Raven Press;1976:311
114. Choi DW. Calcium-mediated neurotoxicity: Relationship to specific channel types and role in ischemic damage. Trends Neurosci 1988;11:465
115. Woolf CJ. Excitatory amino acids increase glycogen phosphorylase activity in the rat spinal cord. Neurosci Lett 1987;73:209
116. Carroll PB, Thornton BM, Greene DA. Glutathione redox state is not the link between polyol pathway activity and diminished (Na,K)-ATPase activity in experimental diabetic neuropathy. Diabetes 1986;35:1282
117. Williamson JR, Arrigoni-Martelli E. The roles of glucose-induced metabolic hypoxia and imbalances in carnitine metabolism in mediating diabetes-induced vascular dysfunction. Int J Clin Pharmacol Res 1992;12:247
118. Thomas TP, Porcellati F, Kato K, et al. Effects of glucose on sorbitol pathway activation, cellular redox and metabolism of *myo*-inositol, phosphoinositide and diacylglycerol in cultured human retinal pigment epithelial cells. J Clin Invest 1994;93:2718
119. Tilton RG, Pugliese G, Eades DM, et al. Prevention of hemodynamic and vascular albumin filtration changes in diabetic rats by ARIs. Diabetes 1989; 38:1258
120. Newrick PG, Wilson AJ, Jakubowski J, et al. Sural nerve oxygen tension in diabetes. Br Med J 1986;293:1053
121. Appenzeller O, Parks RD, MacGee J. Peripheral neuropathy in chronic disease of the respiratory tract. Am J Med 1968;44:873
122. Low PA, Schmelzer JD, Ward KK. Experimental hypoxic neuropathy: Relevance to diabetic neuropathy. Am J Physiol 1986b;250:E94
123. Low PA, Schmelzer JD, Ward KK, et al. Effect of hyperbaric oxygenation on normal and chronic streptozotocin diabetic peripheral nerves. Exp Neurol 1988;99:201
124. Garthwaite J, Charles S, Chess-Willaims R. Endothelium-derived relaxing factor release on activation of NMDA receptors suggests role as intercellular messenger in the brain. Nature 1988;336:385
125. Moncada S, Palmer RMJ, Higgs EA. Biosynthesis of nitric oxide from L-arginine: A pathway for the regulation of cell function and communication. Biochem Pharmacol 1989;38:1709
126. Takahashi K, Ghatei MA, Lam HC, et al. Elevated plasma endothelin in patients with diabetes mellitus. Diabetologia 1990;33:306
127. Saenz de Tejada I, Goldstein I, Azadzoi K, et al. Impaired neurogenic and endothelium-mediated relaxation of the penile smooth muscle from diabetic men with impotence. N Engl J Med 1989;320:1025
128. Durant W, Amar K, Sen Sunahara FA. Impairment of endothelium-dependent relaxation in aorta from spontaneously diabetic rats. Br J Pharmacol 1988;94: 463
129. Kamata K, Miyata N, Kasuya Y. Impairment of endothelium-dependent relaxation and changes in levels of cyclic GMP in aorta from streptozotocin-induced diabetic rats. Br J Pharmacol 1989;97:614
130. Vallence P, Collier J, Moncada S. Effects of endothelium-derived nitric oxide on peripheral arterial tone in man. Lancet 1989;2:997
131. Calver A, Collier J, Vallance P. Inhibition and stimulation of nitric oxide synthesis in the human forearm arterial bed of patients with insulin-dependent diabetes. J Clin Invest 1992;90:2548
132. Rapoport RM, Murad F. Agonist-induced endothelium-dependent relaxation in rat thoracic aorta may be mediated through cGMP. Circ Res 1983;52:352
133. Gupta S, Sussman I, McArthur CS, et al. Endothelium-dependent inhibition of Na/K-ATPase activity in rabbit aorta by hyperglycemia. J Clin Invest 1992;90:727
134. Bult H, Boeckxstaens GE, Pelckmans PA, et al. Nitric oxide as an inhibitory nonadrenergic noncholinergic neurotransmitter. Nature (Lond) 1990a;345:346
135. Cameron NE, Cotter MA. Impaired contraction and relaxation in aorta from streptozotocin-diabetic rats: Role of polyol pathway. Diabetologia 1992;35: 1011
136. Nakane M, Mitchel L, Forstermann U, Murad F. Phosphorylation by calcium calmodulin-dependent protein kinase II and protein kinase C modulates the activity of nitric oxide synthetase. Biochem Biophys Res Commun 1991;180: 1396
137. Bredt DS, Ferris CD, Snyder SH. Nitric oxide synthetase regulatory sites. J Biol Chem 1992;267:10976
138. Subbiah MTR, Deitemeyer D. Altered synthesis of prostaglandins in platelet and aorta from spontaneously diabetic Wistar rats. Biochem Med 1980;23: 231
139. Shimizu K, Muramatsu M, Kakegawa Y, et al. Role of prostaglandin H2 as an endothelium-derived contracting factor in diabetic state. Diabetes 1993;42: 1246
140. Harrison HE, Reece AH, Johnson M. Decreased vascular prostacyclin in experimental diabetes. Life Sci 1978;23:354
141. Bazan NG. Effects of ischemia and electroconvulsive shock on free fatty acid pool in the brain. Biochim Biophys Acta 1970;218:1
142. Wolfe LS. Eicosanoids, prostaglandins, thromboxanes, leukotrienes, and other derivatives of carbon-2 unsaturated fatty acids. J Neurochem 1982;38:1
143. Simpson PJ, Mickelson J, Fantone JC, et al. Reduction of experimental canine infarct size with prostaglandin E1: Inhibition of neutrophil migration and activation. J Pharmacol Exp Therapeut 1988;244:619
144. Hedqvist P, Wennmalm A. Comparison of the effects of prostaglandins E1, E2 and F2 alpha on the sympathetically stimulated rabbit heart. Acta Physiol Scand 1971;83:156
145. Shindo H, Tawata M, Aida K, Onaya T. The role of cyclic adenosine 3′, 5′-monophosphate and polyol metabolism in diabetic neuropathy. J Clin Endocrinol Metab 1992;74:393
146. Houtsmiller AJ, van Hal-Ferwerda J, Zahn KJ, Henkes HE. Favourable influences of linoleic acid on the progression of diabetic macro- and microangiopathy in adult onset diabetes mellitus. Prog Lipid Res 1982;20:377

Diabetes Mellitus, edited by Derek LeRoith, Simeon I. Taylor, and Jerrold M. Olefsky. Lippincott–Raven Publishers, Philadelphia © 1996.

CHAPTER 90
Advanced Glycation End Products and the Pathogenesis of Diabetic Complications

HANS-PETER HAMMES AND MICHAEL BROWNLEE

Hyperglycemia Causes Complications by Both Intracellular and Extracellular Mechanisms

A causal relationship between chronic hyperglycemia and diabetic microvascular disease, long inferred from a variety of animal and clinical studies,[1] has now been definitely established by data from the Diabetes Control and Complications Trial (DCCT), a multicenter, randomized, prospective controlled clinical study.[2] A relationship between chronic hyperglycemia and diabetic macrovascular disease in patients with non–insulin-dependent diabetes mellitus (NIDDM) is also supported by recent literature.[3]

The mechanisms by which hyperglycemia causes tissue damage and the resultant clinical complication syndromes can be conceptually divided into two categories. The first of these involves rapid changes in intracellular metabolites in response to diabetic hyperglycemia. These changes can revert to normal when hyperglycemia is abolished, but their cumulative effect leads to irreversible tissue damage. Examples of such intracellular mechanisms include increased polyol pathway flux, increased de novo diacylglycerol synthesis, altered intracellular redox state, and formation of advanced glycation end products (AGEs).[4–8] The second type of mechanism by which hyperglycemia causes tissue damage involves slow changes in extracellular molecules as a result of hyperglycemia-induced covalent modification. These changes are irreversible for the life of the extracellular molecule. Examples of such extracellular mechanisms include covalent modification by lipid peroxidation products and by advanced glycation end products.[9,10] This chapter focuses on the role of AGEs in the pathogenesis of diabetic complications. Following an overview of AGE biochemistry, both intracellular and extracellular mechanisms are reviewed. The effects of AGE inhibitors on diabetic complications in animal models are summarized in the final section.

Advanced Glycation End Products Form Nonenzymatically from Sugar-Derived Intermediates

Advanced glycation end products may arise by two mechanisms (Fig. 90-1). It has long been recognized that AGEs can be produced by oxidation of the so-called Amadori product, a 1-amino-1-deoxyketose produced by the reaction of reducing sugars with protein amino groups.[2] This occurs via reactive dicarbonyl intermediates, such as 3-deoxyglucosone.[11–20] Recently, it has been shown that dicarbonyl AGE intermediates may also form from metal-catalyzed auto-oxidation of sugars.[21] Moreover, glucose has recently been found to have the slowest rate of glycosylation product formation of any naturally occurring sugar. Thus, the rate of AGE formation by such intracellular sugars as fructose, glucose-6-phosphate, and glyceraldehyde-3-phosphate is considerably faster than the rate for glucose.[22] In in vitro studies, the level of fructose-derived AGEs after 5 days was found to be 10 times greater than the level of glucose-derived AGEs.[23] For this reason, the rate of intracellular

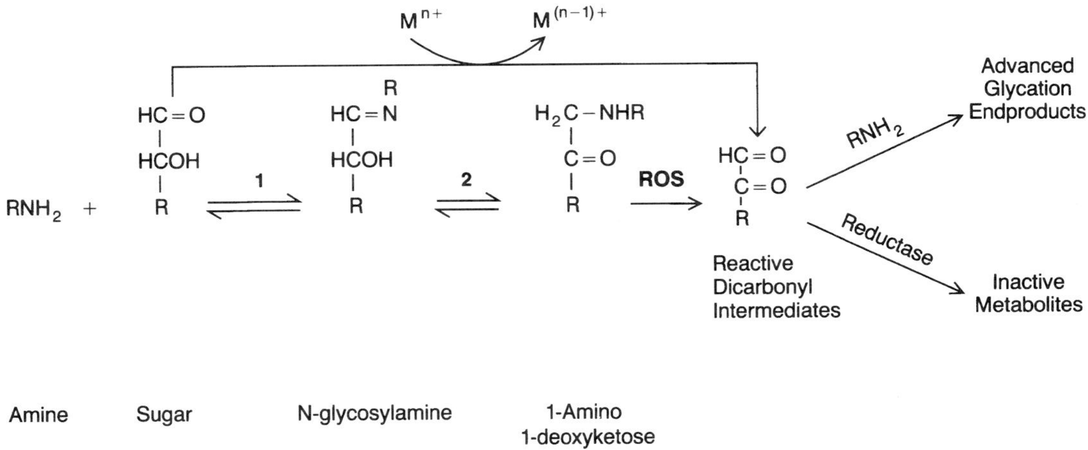

FIGURE 90-1. Advanced glycation end products form nonenzymatically from reactive dicarbonyl intermediates that arise from both oxidation of the 1-amino-1-deoxyketose Amadori product and from metal-catalyzed auto-oxidation of sugars. Specific reductases can detoxify reactive dicarbonyl intermediates to inactive metabolites. ROS = reactive oxygen species; M^n = transition metal. (Adapted from Brownlee M. Lilly lecture, 1993: Glycation and diabetic complications. Diabetes 1994;43:836.)

AGE formation is much more rapid than the rate of AGE formation in the extracellular compartment. The reactive dicarbonyl intermediates formed from Amadori products and from sugars react with protein amino groups to form a variety of AGEs. Studies with antibodies to AGEs suggest that immunologically similar structures form from the reaction of a number of different sugars with proteins.[24–27]

3-Deoxyglucosone is reduced to a relatively inactive product, deoxyfructose. In order to ascertain whether the AGE-intermediate 3-deoxyglucosone is actually produced in significant quantities in normal humans, levels of 3-deoxyfructose levels have been measured in plasma and urine.[28] Calculations based on the results obtained indicate that several milligrams of 3-deoxyglucosone are formed in the nondiabetic body per day, and are detoxified by reduction to 3-deoxyfructose. In diabetic rats, plasma levels of 3-deoxyglucosone are elevated several-fold compared to those in nondiabetics.[29] The quantity of 3-deoxyfructose in plasma and urine strongly suggests that specific reductase enzymes in the body detoxify AGE precursors and prevent AGE formation. For example, 2-oxoaldehyde dehydrogenase oxidizes 3-deoxyglucosone to 2-keto-3-deoxyglyconic acid,[30] and methylglyoxal reductase appears to reduce deoxyglucosone to 3-deoxyglucose.[31] A 2-oxoaldehyde reductase that reduces 3-deoxyglucosone to 3-deoxyfructose has been isolated and cloned. This enzyme appears to be identical to aldehyde reductase.[32] The nature and efficiency of such enzymes could be an important determinant of the amount of AGEs that form at any given level of blood glucose in both diabetic and nondiabetic patients. In the aggregate, patients with higher levels of mean blood glucose, like diabetic animals, have a higher prevalence of diabetic complications. Among individual patients, however, there are some with poor glucose control who escape complications and others with excellent control who develop severe complications. Inherited differences in the ability to detoxify AGE intermediates, such as 3-deoxyglucosone, by enzymatic means may be one of the genetic factors responsible for determining the impact of a given level of glycemia on diabetic complications.

The qualitative relationship between blood glucose level, tissue accumulation of AGEs, and extent of tissue pathology has been most extensively studied in animals. In retinal vessel preparations from nondiabetic and diabetic rats, AGE-specific fluorescence increased 2.6 fold after 26 weeks of diabetes.[33] A similar magnitude of change in AGE-specific fluorescence has been observed in diabetic lens proteins[34] and renal cortex.[35] These increases in AGE accumulation preceded and were accompanied by histologic evidence of diabetic tissue damage. Recently, enzyme-linked immunosorbent assays (ELISA) using AGE-specific antibodies have shown that these same diabetic samples have 10–45 times more AGEs than nondiabetic samples after 5–20 weeks of diabetes. These results suggest that nonfluorescent AGEs predominate over fluorescent AGEs in diabetic tissues, and show that AGE formation increases at a much greater rate than the increase in blood glucose. This relationship suggests that even modest elevations in diabetic blood glucose levels result in substantial increases in AGE accumulation.

There are three general mechanisms by which AGE formation may cause pathologic changes (Fig. 90-2). First, rapid intracellular AGE formation by glucose, fructose, and more highly reactive, metabolic pathway-derived intermediates can directly alter protein function in target tissues. Second, AGEs alter signal transduction pathways involving ligands on extracellular matrix. Third, AGEs alter the level of soluble signals, such as cytokines, hormones, and free radicals, through interactions with AGE-specific cellular receptors. These three mechanisms are discussed individually in the following sections.

AGEs Increase Much More Rapidly Inside Cells than Outside, Altering Protein Function

Advanced glycation end products have been thought to form only on long-lived extracellular macromolecules because the rate of AGE formation from glucose is so slow that intracellular proteins that are more rapidly turned over would not exist long enough to accumulate them. Recently, however, it has been demonstrated that AGEs do, in fact, form on proteins in vivo. In erythrocytes, AGE

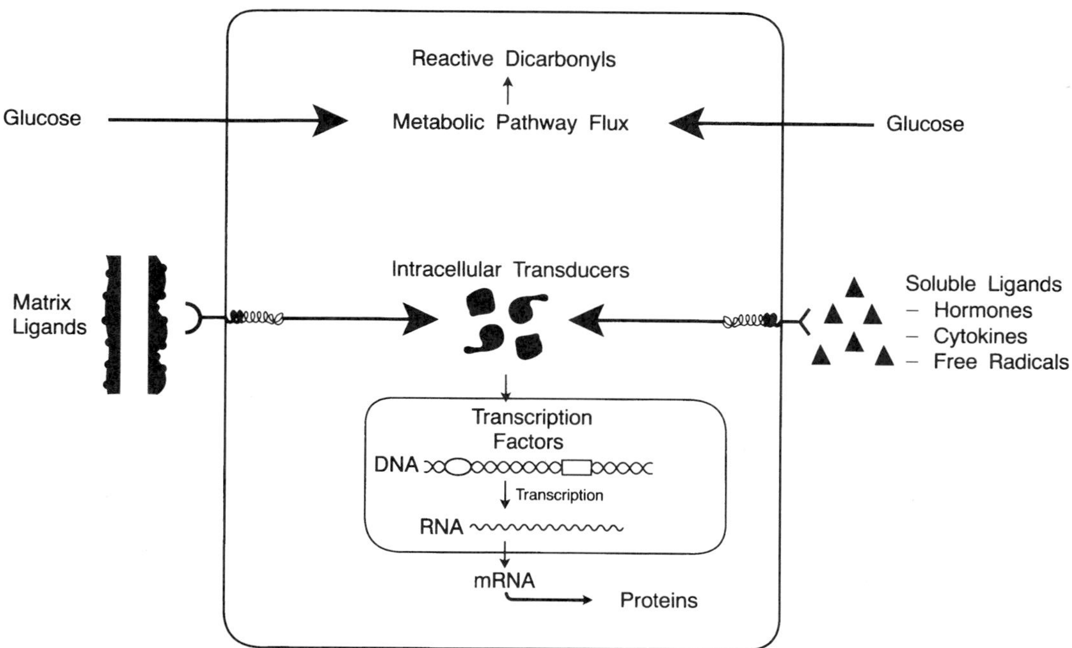

FIGURE 90-2. There are three general mechanisms by which AGEs may cause pathologic changes: (1) intracellular formation of AGEs can alter protein function; (2) extracellular AGEs can interfere with normal matrix function; and (3) extracellular AGEs can induce receptor-mediated soluble ligand production. (Adapted from Brownlee M. Lilly lecture, 1993: Glycation and diabetic complications. Diabetes 1994;43:836.)

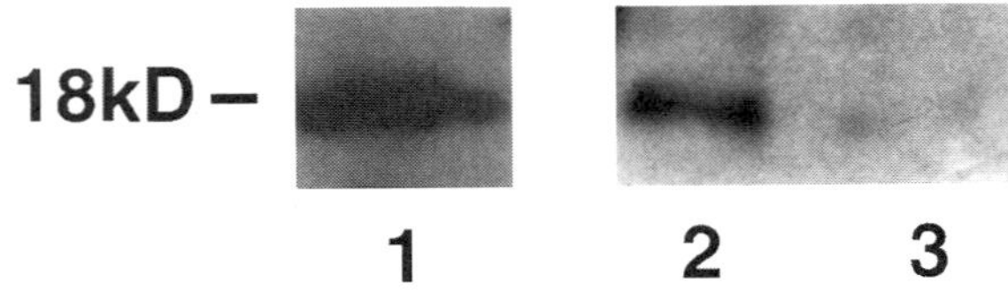

Figure 90-3. Immunoblot of AGE-bFGF from endothelial cell cytosol after cell culture in different glucose concentrations. Lane 1 shows 100 pg of recombinant bFGF, lanes 2 and 3 show 50 μg of cytosolic preparations obtained from cells pre-exposed to either 5mM of glucose (lane 3) or 30 mM of glucose (lane 2) for 168 hours. (Reproduced with permission from Giardino I, Edelstein D, Brownlee M. Nonenzymatic glycosylation in vitro and in bovine endothelial cells alters basic fibroblast growth factor activity. A model for intracellular glycosylation in diabetes. Clin Invest 1994;94:110, and by copyright permission of The American Society for Clinical Investigation.)

hemoglobin accounts for 0.42% of circulating hemoglobin in normal subjects and 0.75% in diabetics.[36] In endothelial cells, a primary site for hyperglycemia-induced damage, increased AGE formation is even more pronounced. After only 1 week, AGE content increased 13.8 fold in endothelial cells cultured in media containing high levels of glucose.[8] This extremely rapid rate of AGE formation most likely reflects hyperglycemia-induced increases in intracellular sugars that are much more reactive than glucose, such as fructose, glucose-6-phosphate, and glyceraldehyde-3-phosphate.[22] Both in vitro and in vivo, antioxidants profoundly inhibit hyperglycemia-induced intracellular AGE formation (I. Giardino and M. Brownlee, unpublished data, 1995).

Basic fibroblast growth factor (bFGF) is the major AGE-modified protein in endothelial cells, but other proteins are also modified (Fig. 90-3). Endothelial cell cytosol mitogenic activity is reduced 70% by AGE formation when cytosolic AGE-bFGF is increased 6.1 fold. These data support the hypothesis that AGE modification of intracellular proteins can alter vascular cell function. Intracellular AGE formation occurs in retinal pericytes and Muller cells as well (I. Giardino, unpublished data, 1995).

Intracellular AGE formation may also affect DNA function. AGEs form on prokaryotic DNA in vitro and cause mutations and DNA transposition in bacteria and mammalian cells.[37–41] If AGEs also form on DNA in vivo, deleterious effects on gene expression may occur.

Increased intracellular AGE formation may underlie the development of a diabetic nephropathy-like syndrome in normoglycemic patients with glycogen storage disease type I.[42,43]

AGEs Interfere with Normal Matrix-Matrix and Matrix-Cell Interactions

AGE formation alters the functional properties of several important matrix molecules. Collagen was the first matrix protein used to demonstrate that glucose-derived AGEs form covalent, intermolecular bonds.[44,45] On type I collagen, this cross-linking induces an expansion of the molecular packing.[46] Soluble plasma proteins, such as low-density lipoprotein (LDL) and immunoglobulin G (IgG), are also covalently cross-linked by AGEs on collagen.[47–49] The luminal narrowing that characterizes diabetic vessels may arise, in part, from accumulation of subendothelial AGE-linked plasma proteins. AGE formation on type IV collagen from basement membrane inhibits lateral association of these molecules into a normal network-like structure by interfering with binding of the noncollagenous NC1 domain to the helix-rich domain.[50]

AGE formation on laminin causes decreased polymer self-assembly, decreased binding to type IV collagen, and decreased binding of heparan sulfate proteoglycan.[51] AGE formation on the adhesive matrix molecule vitronectin decreases site-specific binding of heparin and collagen (H.P. Hammes, K. Preissner, M. Eppinger-Albrecht, et al., unpublished data, 1995). Diabetes-induced loss of matrix-bound heparan sulfate proteoglycan (HSPG) secondary to AGE modification of vitronectin and laminin could explain the observed decrease in binding of HSPG to diabetic basement membrane,[52] which is thought to stimulate a compensatory overproduction of other matrix components in the vessel wall.[53,54]

AGE formation on extracellular matrix not only interferes with matrix-matrix interactions, it interferes with matrix-cell interactions as well. For example, AGE modification of type IV collagen's cell-binding domains decreases endothelial cell adhesion,[55] and AGE modification of a six–amino acid growth-promoting sequence in the A chain of the laminin molecule markedly reduces neurite outgrowth.[56]

These AGE-induced abnormalities in extracellular matrix function alter the structure and function of intact vessels. For example, AGEs are known to decrease elasticity in large vessels from diabetic rats, even after vascular tone is abolished, and to increase fluid filtration across the carotid artery.[57] Defects in the vasodilatory response to nitric oxide correlate with the level of accumulated AGEs in diabetic animals owing to dose-dependent quenching by AGEs. These defects are prevented by inhibition of AGE formation.[58] AGEs also block the cytostatic effect of nitric oxide on aortic smooth muscle cells,[59] suggesting that extracellular AGE accumulation may contribute to accelerated atherosclerosis in diabetes.

AGE Receptors Mediate Pathologic Changes in Gene Expression

Specific receptors for AGEs were first identified on monocytes and macrophages. These cells have a binding affinity for AGE-modified proteins of $1.75 \times 10^{-7}M^{-1}$, similar to that of the Fc receptor. There are 1.5×10^{-5} AGE receptors per cell.[60] Two AGE-binding proteins isolated from rat liver are both present on monocyte/macrophages. Antisera to either the 60-kd or 90-kd protein blocks AGE binding.[61] AGE protein binding to this receptor stimulates macrophage production of interleukin-1, insulin-like growth factor I, tumor necrosis factor α, and granulocyte/macrophage colony-stimulating factor at levels that have been shown to increase glomerular synthesis of type IV collagen and to stimulate proliferation of both arterial smooth muscle cells and macrophages.[62–64]

AGE receptors have also been identified on glomerular mesangial cells. In vitro, AGE protein binding to its receptor on mesangial cells stimulates platelet-derived growth factor secretion, which, in turn, mediates production of type IV collagen, laminin, and HSPG.[65,66] In vivo, chronic administration of AGEs to otherwise healthy rats leads to focal glomerulosclerosis, mesangial expansion, and albuminuria.[67] A 4-week course of AGE administration in mice has been found to induce an increase in mRNAs for glomerular type α1 IV collagen, laminin B1, and transforming growth factor β_1.[68]

Vascular endothelial cells also express AGE-specific receptors. A 35-kd and a 46-kd AGE-binding protein have been purified to homogeneity from endothelial cells (Fig. 90-4).[69–71] The N-terminal sequence of the 35-kd protein was identical to lactoferrin, whereas the 46-kd protein was novel. A full-length, 1.5-kb cDNA for the 46-kd protein was cloned and sequenced. This novel AGE-binding protein appears to be a member of the immunoglobulin superfamily, with three disulfide-bonded immunoglobulin homology units. Cross-linking studies with endothelial cells show formation of a new, higher-molecular-weight band that reacts with antibodies to both proteins.

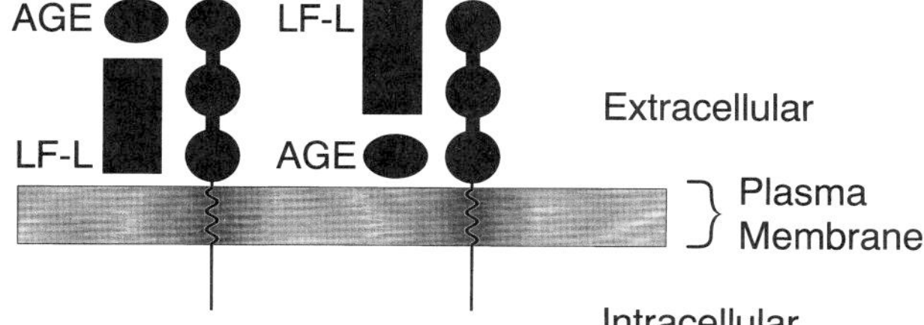

Figure 90-4. Model of AGE binding to a receptor composed of an integral membrane protein and its noncovalently associated lactoferrin-like (LF-L) polypeptide. (Reprinted with permission from Brownlee M. Lilly lecture, 1993: Glycation and diabetic complications. Diabetes 1994;43:836.)

The two purified proteins bind together in vitro with high affinity (k_d = 100 pM). AGE binding to endothelial cells is blocked by antibodies to either protein, suggesting that the two proteins are closely associated on the cell surface. Two AGE-binding proteins that are immunochemically related to the endothelial cell receptor are found on human monocytes.[72] Antibodies to either protein block monocyte chemotaxis.

The AGE receptor appears to mediate signal transduction through the generation of oxygen free radicals. Reactive oxygen species are generated by AGE binding to endothelial cells. These reactive oxygen species activate the free radical–sensitive transcription factor NFκB, a pleiotropic regulator of many "response-to-injury" genes. This signal transduction cascade can be blocked by antibodies to either of the AGE receptor components, as well as by antibodies to AGEs themselves.[73]

In endothelial cells, such AGE-induced changes in gene expression include alterations in thrombomodulin and tissue factor.[74] These changes induce two additive procoagulatory changes in the endothelial surface. One procoagulatory change is a rapid reduction in thrombomodulin activity. This prevents activation of the anticoagulant protein C pathway. The other procoagulatory change induced by AGE receptor binding is an increase in tissue factor activity. This increase activates coagulation factors IX and X through factor VIIa binding. Together, these AGE-induced changes in endothelial cell function favor thrombus formation at sites of extracellular AGE accumulation.

AGE Inhibitors Prevent Diabetic Complications in Animal Models

Pharmacologic agents that specifically inhibit AGE formation have made it possible to investigate the role of AGEs in the development of diabetic complications in animal models. The hydrazine compound aminoguanidine was the first AGE inhibitor discovered,[44] and it has been by far the most extensively studied. Aminoguanidine reacts mainly with non–protein-bound dicarbonyl intermediates, such as 3-deoxyglucosone,[75] rather than with Amadori products on proteins. More detailed studies of the underlying mechanisms using nuclear magnetic resonance imaging (NMR), mass spectroscopy, and x-ray diffraction have shown that aminoguanidine reacts with the AGE precursor 3-deoxyglucosone to form 3-amino-5- and 3-amino-6-substituted triazines.[76] These triazines are produced as a result of initial hydrazone formation at either C-1 or C-2. Similarly, aminoguanidine reacts with methylglyoxal to form 3-amino-5-methyl-1,2,4- and 3-amino-6-methyl-1,2,4-triazines.[77] In addition to inhibiting AGE formation, aminoguanidine has been shown to inhibit the inducible form of nitric oxide synthase in vitro.[78] In vivo, however, 8–16 times the dosage used to inhibit AGEs is necessary to affect nitric oxide levels significantly.[79]

The effects of aminoguanidine on diabetic pathology have been investigated in retina, kidney, nerve, and artery (Table 90-1). In the rat retina, diabetes causes a 19-fold increase in the number of acellular capillaries. Aminoguanidine treatment of diabetics was found to prevent excess AGE accumulation and to reduce the number of acellular capillaries by 80%. Aminoguanidine treatment had a similar effect on the number of diabetic eyes positive for microaneurysms. Diabetes-induced pericyte dropout was also markedly reduced by aminoguanidine treatment.[33] Aminoguanidine treatment also inhibited the development of accelerated diabetic retinopathy in the spontaneously hypertensive rate model, suggesting that hypertension-induced deposition of AGEs in the retinal vasculature plays an important role in the acceleration of diabetic retinopathy by hypertension.[80]

Similar results have been obtained in animal models of diabetic kidney disease.[81–83] Diabetes increased AGEs in the renal glomerulus, and aminoguanidine treatment prevented this diabetes-induced increase. Within 32 weeks, untreated diabetic animals developed albuminuria that averaged 30 mg/24 h. This was more than a 10-fold increase above control levels. In aminoguanidine-treated diabetics, the level of albumin excretion was reduced nearly 90%.[81] In hypertensive diabetic rats, aminoguanidine treatment also prevented albuminuria without affecting blood pressure.[83] Untreated diabetic animals also developed the characteristic structural feature of human diabetic nephropathy; increased fractional mesangial volume. When diabetic animals were treated with aminoguanidine, this increase in fractional mesangial volume was completely prevented.

In peripheral nerve of diabetic rats, both motor nerve and sensory nerve conduction velocity were found to be decreased after 8 weeks of diabetes.[84] Nerve action potential amplitude was decreased by 37%, and peripheral nerve blood flow was reduced by 57% after 24 weeks of diabetes.[85] Aminoguanidine treatment was found to prevent these abnormalities of diabetic peripheral nerve function.[84,85]

Inhibition of AGE formation by aminoguanidine treatment also ameliorates the effects of diabetes on the large arteries. In

Table 90-1. Effects of Aminoguanidine Treatment on Diabetic Target Tissues*

	Nondiabetic	Diabetic	Diabetic Treatment
Retinal acellular capillaries (mm^2)[33]	9 ± 2	167 ± 27	33 ± 11
Retinal microaneurysms (% positive)[33]	0	37.5	0
Urinary albumin excretion (mg/24 h)[81]	2.4 ± 1.3	38.9 ± 1.4	5.1 ± 1.5
Mesangial volume fraction (%)[81]	12.5 ± 2.5	18.8 ± 2.5	13.7 ± 0.6
Motor nerve conduction velocity (m/s)[84]	65.5 ± 2	52.4 ± 3	64 ± 2
Nerve action potential amplitude[85]	100%	63%	97%
Arterial elasticity (nL/mmHg/mm)[57]	—	7.5 ± 1.5	10.8 ± 3
Arterial fluid filtration (nL/sec/mm)[57]	—	0.9	0.45

*Reprinted with permission from Brownlee M. Lilly lecture, 1993: Glycation and diabetic complications. Diabetes 1994;43:836.

animal models, aminoguanidine treatment increased vessel elasticity, as measured by static compliance, aortic input impedance, and left ventricular power output. Abnormal increases in fluid filtration across the carotid wall were also significantly reduced.[57]

Clinical Trials Will Define the Role of AGE Inhibitors in Patients

It is now known that AGEs accumulate as a function of the level of chronic hyperglycemia via generation of reactive dicarbonyl intermediates. Inside cells, AGEs accumulate rapidly and cause altered function of intracellular proteins. Outside cells, AGEs accumulate over longer periods of time, interfering with normal extracellular matrix interactions and causing AGE-receptor–mediated pathologic changes in gene expression. In animal models, pharmacologic inhibition of AGE formation prevents diabetic complications in the retina, glomerulus, peripheral nerve, and artery. Will AGE inhibitors also prevent diabetic complications in humans? At what point in the natural history of the disease would treatment be most effective? To answer these questions a multicentered, randomized, double-blind study is currently being conducted to examine the effects of aminoguanidine on various end points in both overt and end-stage diabetic nephropathy. Other clinical studies will be necessary in order to define the place of AGE inhibitors in the prevention and treatment of diabetic retinopathy, neuropathy, and accelerated atherosclerosis.

References

1. Nathan D. Relationship between metabolic control and long-term complications of diabetes. In: Kahn CR, Weir G, eds. Joslin's Diabetes. Philadelphia: Lea & Febiger; 1994
2. The Diabetes Control and Complications Trial Research Group. The effect of intensive treatment of diabetes and progression of long term complications in insulin dependent diabetes mellitus. N Engl J Med 1993;329:977
3. Kuusisto J, Mykkanen L, Pyorala K, et al. NIDDM and its metabolic control predict heart disease in elderly subjects. Diabetes 1994;43:7
4. Kinoshita JH. A thirty-year journey in the polyol pathway. Exp Eye Res 1990;50:567
5. DeRubertis FR, Craven PA. Activation of protein kinase C in glomerular cells in diabetes. Mechanisms and potential links to the pathogenesis of diabetic glomerulopathy. Diabetes 1994;43:1
6. King GL, Shiba T, Oliver J, et al. Cellular and molecular abnormalities in the vascular endothelium of diabetes mellitus. Annu Rev Med 1994;45:179
7. Williamson JR, Chang K, Frangos M, et al. Hyperglycemic pseudohypoxia and diabetic complications. Diabetes 1993;42:801
8. Giardino I, Edelstein D, Brownlee M. Nonenzymatic glycosylation in vitro and in bovine endothelial cells alters basic fibroblast growth factor activity. A model for intracellular glycosylation in diabetes. J Clin Invest 1994;94:110
9. Bucala R, Makita Z, Koschinsky T, et al. Lipid advanced glycosylation: Pathway for lipid oxidation in vivo. Proc Natl Acad Sci USA 1993;90:6434
10. Brownlee M, Vlassar H, Cerami A. Advanced glycosylation endproducts in tissue and the biochemical basis of complications. (Beth Israel Seminar in Medicine). N Engl J Med 1988;318:1315
11. Fu M-X, Wells-Knecht KJ, Blackledge JA, et al. Glycation, glycoxidation, and cross-linking of collagen by glucose: Kinetics, mechanisms and inhibition of late stages of the Mailliard reaction. Diabetes 1994;43:676
12. Giardino I, Horiuchi S, Brownlee M. Accelerated formation of extracellular advanced glycation end products (AGEs) detected by a specific monoclonal antibody. Diabetes 1994;43:320
13. Brownlee M. Advanced products of non-enzymatic glycosylation and the pathogenesis of diabetic complications. In: Rifkin H, Porte D Jr, eds. Diabetes Mellitus: Theory and Practice. New York: Elsevier; 1990:279
14. Monnier V. Toward a Maillard reaction theory of aging. In: Baynes JW, Monnier VM, eds. The Maillard Reaction in Aging, Diabetes and Nutrition: An NIH Conference. New York: Alan R. Liss; 1989:1–22
15. Baynes JW, Thorpe SR, Murtiashaw MH. Nonenzymatic glucosylation of lysine residues in albumin. In: Wold F, Moldave K, eds. Methods in Enzymology: Postranslational Modifications. Vol. 106. New York: Academic Press; 1984:88
16. Higgins PJ, Bunn HF. Kinetic analysis of the nonenzymatic glucosylation of hemoglobin. J Biol Chem 1981;256:5204
17. Mortensen HB, Christophersen C. Glucosylation of human haemoglobin A in red blood cells studied in vitro. Kinetics of the formation and dissociation of haemoglobin A_{1c}. Clin Chim Acta 1983;134:317
18. Kato H, Hayase F, Shin DB, et al. 3-Deoxyglucasone, an intermediate product of the Maillard reaction. In: Baynes JW, Monnier VM, eds. The Maillard Reaction in Aging, Diabetes, and Nutrition: An NIH Conference. New York: Alan R. Liss; 1989:69–84
19. Kato H, Shin DB, Hayase F. 3, Deoxyglucosone cross links proteins under physiological conditions. Agric Biol Chem 1987;51:2009
20. Kato H, Cho RK, Okitani A, Hayase F. Responsibility of 3 deoxyglucosone for the glucose-induced polymerization of proteins. Agric Biol Chem 1987;51:683
21. Wolff SP, Dean RT. Glucose autooxidation and protein modification. The potential role of 'autoxidative glycosylation' in diabetes. Biochem J 1987;245:243
22. Monnier V. Toward a Malliard Reaction theory of aging. In: Baynes JW, Monnier VM, eds. The Malliard Reaction in Aging, Diabetes and Nutrition: An NIH Conference. New York: Alan R. Liss; 1988:1–69
23. McPherson JD, Shelton BH, Walton DJ. Role of fructose in glycation and crosslinking of proteins. Biochemistry 1988;27:1901
24. Araki N, Ueno N, Chakrabarti B, et al. Immunochemical evidence for the presence of advanced glycation end products in human lens protein and its positive correlation with aging. J Biol Chem 1992;267:10211
25. Dyer DG, Blackledge JA, Thorpe SR, Baynes JW. Formation of pentosidine during nonenzymatic browning of proteins by glucose: Identification of glucose and other carbohydrates as possible precursors of pentosidine in vivo. J Biol Chem 1991;266:11654
26. Horiuchi S, Araki N, Morino Y. Immunochemical approach to characterize advanced glycation end products of the Maillard reaction: Evidence for the presence of a common structure. J Biol Chem 1991;266:7329
27. Makita Z, Vlassara H, Cerami A, Bucala R. Immunochemical detection of advanced glycosylation end products in vivo. J Biol Chem 1992;267:5133
28. Knecht KG, Feather MS, Baynes JW. Detection of 3 deoxyfructose and 3 deoxyglucosone in human urine and plasma: Evidence for intermediate stages of the Maillard reaction in vivo. Arch Biochem Biophys 1992;294:130
29. Yamada H, Miyata S, Igaki N, et al. Increase in 3-deoxyglucasone levels in diabetic rat plasma. Specific in vivo determination of intermediate in advanced Maillard reaction. J Biol Chem 1994;269:20275
30. Jellum E. Metabolism of the ketoaldehyde 2-keto-3-deoxyglucose. Biochim Biophys Acta 1968;165:357
31. Kato H, Miyauchi Y, Nishimura T, Liang ZQ. Purification and partial characterization of NADH-dependent methylglyoxal-reducing enzyme from porcine liver. Agric Biol Chem 1988;52:2641
32. Takahashi M, Fujii J, Teshima T, et al. Identity of a major 3 deoxyglucosone reducing enzyme with aldehyde reductase in rat liver established by amino acid sequencing and cDNA expression. Gene 1993;127:249
33. Hammes H-P, Martin S, Federlin K, et al. Aminoguanidine treatment inhibits the development of experimental diabetic retinopathy. Proc Natl Acad Sci USA 1991;88:11555
34. Nakayama H, Mitsuhashi T, Kuwajima S, et al. Immunochemical detection of advanced glycation end products in lens cystallins from streptozotocin-induced diabetic rats. Diabetes 1993;42:345
35. Mitsuhashi T, Nakayama H, Itch S, et al. Immunochemical detection of advanced glycation end products in renal cortex from STZ induced diabetic rat. Diabetes 1993;42:826
36. Makita Z, Vlassara H, Rayfield E, Cartwright K, et al. Hemoglobin-AGE: A circulating marker of advanced glycosylation. Science 1992;258:651
37. Bucala R, Model P, Cerami A. Modification of DNA by reduced sugars: A possible mechanism for nucleic acid aging and age-related dysfunction in gene expression. Proc Natl Acad Sci USA 1984;81:105
38. Bucala R, Model R, Russl M, Cerami A. Modification of DNA by glucose-6-phosphate induces DNA rearrangements in an *E. coli* plasmid. Proc Natl Acad Sci USA 1985;82:8439
39. Lee AT, Cerami A. Elevated glucose 6-phosphate levels are associated with plasmid mutations in vivo. Proc Natl Acad Sci USA 1987;84:8311
40. Mullokandov EA, Franklin WA, Brownlee M. DNA damage by the glycation products of glyceraldehyde-3-phosphate and lysine. Diabetologia 1994;37:145
41. Bucala R, Lee AT, Rourke L, Cerami A. Transposition of an Alu-containing element induced by DNA-advanced glycosylation endproducts. Proc Natl Acad Sci USA 1993;90:2666
42. Baker L, Dahlem S, Goldfarb S, et al. Hyperfiltration and renal disease in glycogen storage disease, type I. Kidney Int 1989;35:1345
43. Chen YT, Coleman RA, Scheinman JI, et al. Renal disease in type I glycogen storage disease. N Engl J Med 1988;318:7
44. Brownlee M, Vlassara H, Kooney T, et al. Aminoguanidine prevents diabetes-induced arterial wall protein cross-linking. Science 1986;232:1629
45. Kent MJC, Light ND, Bailey AJ. Evidence for glucose-mediated covalent cross-linking of collagen after glycosylation in vitro. Biochem J 1985;225:745
46. Tanaka S, Avigad G, Brodsky B, Eikenberry EF. Glycation induces expansion of the molecular packing of collagen. J Mol Biol 1988;203:495
47. Brownlee M, Pongor S, Cerami A. Covalent attachment of soluble protein by nonenzymatically glycosylated collagen: Role in the in situ formation of immune complexes. J Exp Med 1983;158:1739
48. Sensi M, Tanzi P, Bruno RM, et al. Human glomerular basement membrane: Altered binding characteristics following in vitro non-enzymatic glycosylation. Ann NY Acad Sci 1986;488:549
49. Brownlee M, Vlassara H, Cerami A. Non-enzymatic glycosylation products on collagen covalently trap low-density lipoprotein. Diabetes 1985;34:938
50. Tsilbary EC, Charonis AS, Reger LA, et al. The effect of nonenzymatic glucosylation on the binding of the main noncollagenous NC1 domain to type IV collagen. J Biol Chem 1990;263:4302

51. Charonis AS, Reger LA, Dege JE, et al. Laminin alterations after in vitro nonenzymatic glucosylation. Diabetes 1988;39:807
52. Klein DJK, Oegema TR, Brown DM. Release of glomerular heparan-$^{35}SO_4$ proteoglycan by heparin from glomeruli of streptozocin-induced diabetic rats. Diabetes 1989;38:130
53. Rohrbach DH, Hassel JR, Kleinman HK, Martin GR. Alterations in basement membrane (heparin sulfate) proteoglycan in diabetic mice. Diabetes 1982;31: 185
54. Ruoslahti E, Yamaguchi Y. Proteoglycans as modulators of growth factor activities. Cell 1991;64:867
55. Haitoglou CS, Tsilibary EC, Brownlee M, Charonis AS. Altered cellular interactions between endothelial cells and nonenzymatically glucosylated laminin/type IV collagen. J Biol Chem 1992;267:12404
56. Federoff HJ, Lawrence D, Brownlee M. Nonenzymatic glycosylation of laminin and the laminin peptide CIKVAVS inhibits neurite outgrowth. Diabetes 1993;42:509
57. Huijberts MSP, Wolffenbuttel BRH, Struijker Boudier HAJ, et al. Aminoguanidine treatment increases elasticity and decreases fluid filtration of large arteries from diabetic rats. J Clin Invest 1993;92:1407
58. Bucala R, Tracey KJ, Cerami A. Advanced glycosylation products quench nitric oxide and mediate defective endothelium-dependent vasodilation in experimental diabetes. J Clin Invest 1991;87:432
59. Hogan M, Cerami A, Bucala R. Advanced glycosylation end products block the antiproliferative effect of nitric oxide. J Clin Invest 1992;90:1110
60. Vlassara H, Brownlee M, Cerami A. High-affinity receptor-mediated uptake and degradation of glucose-modified proteins: A potential mechanism for the removal of senescent macromolecules. Proc Natl Acad Sci USA 1985;82:5588
61. Yang Z, Makita Z, Horii Y, et al. Two novel rat liver membrane proteins that bind advanced glycosylation endproducts: Relationship to macrophage receptor for glucose-modified proteins. J Exp Med 1991;174:515
62. Vlassara H, Brownlee M, Monogue K, et al. Cachectin/TNF and IL-1 induced by glucose-modified proteins: Role in normal tissue remodeling. Science 1988;240:1546
63. Kirstein M, Aston C, Hintz R, Vlassara H. Receptor-specific induction of insulin-like growth factor I in human monocytes by advanced glycosylation end product-modified proteins. J Clin Invest 1992;90:439
64. Yui S, Sasaki T, Araki N, et al. Induction of macrophage growth by advanced glycation end products of the Maillard reaction. J Immunol 1994;152:1943
65. Skolnik EY, Yang Z, Makita Z, et al. Human and rat mesangial cell receptors for glucose-modified proteins: Potential role in kidney tissue remodelling and diabetic nephropathy. J Exp Med 1991;174:931
66. Doi T, Vlassara H, Kirstein M, et al. Receptor specific increase in extracellular matrix productions in mouse mesangial cells by advanced glycosylation end products is mediated via platelet derived growth factor. Proc Natl Acad Sci USA 1992;89:2873
67. Vlassara H, Striker LJ, Teichberg S, et al. Advanced glycation end products induce glomerular sclerosis and albuminuria in normal rats. Proc Natl Acad Sci USA 1994;91:11704
68. Yang CW, Vlassara H, Peten E, et al. Advanced glycation end products upregulate gene expression found in diabetic glomerular disease. Proc Natl Acad Sci USA 1994;91:9436
69. Schmidt AM, Vianna M, Gerlach M, et al. Isolation and characterization of two binding proteins for advanced glycosylation end products from bovine lung which are present on the endothelial cell surface. J Biol Chem 1992;267:14987
70. Neeper M, Schmidt AM, Brett J, et al. Cloning and expression of RAGE: A cell surface receptor for advanced glycosylation end products of proteins. J Biol Chem 1992;267:14998
71. Schmidt AM, Mora R, Cao K, et al. The endothelial cell binding site for advanced glycation endproducts consists of A complex: An integral membrane protein and a lactoferrin-like polypeptide. J Biol Chem 1994;269:9882
72. Schmidt AM, Yan SD, Brett J, et al. Regulation of human mononuclear phagocyte migration by cell surface-binding proteins for advanced glycation end products. J Clin Invest 1993;91:2155
73. Yan SD, Schmidt AM, Anderson GM, et al. Enhanced cellular oxidant stress by the interaction of advanced glycation end products with their receptors/binding proteins. J Biol Chem 1994;269:9889
74. Esposito C, Gerlach H, Brett J, et al. Endothelial receptor-mediated binding of glucose modified albumin is associated with increased monolayer permeability and modulation of cell surface coagulant properties. J Exp Med 1992;170: 1387
75. Edelstein D, Brownlee M. Mechanistic studies of advanced glycosylation end product inhibition by aminoguanidine. Diabetes 1992;41:26
76. Hirsch J, Baines CL, Feather MS. X-ray structures of a 3-amino-5- and a 3-amino-6-substituted triazine, produced as a result of a reaction of 3-deoxy-D-erythro-hexos-2-ulose (3-Deoxyglucosone) with aminoguanidine. J Carbohydrate Chem 1992;11:891
77. Lo TW, Selwood T, Thornalley PJ. The reaction of methylglyoxal with aminoguanidine under physiological conditions and prevention of methylglyoxal binding to plasma proteins. Biochem Pharmacol 1994;48:1865
78. Corbett JA, Tilton RG, Chang K, et al. Aminoguanidine, a novel inhibitor of nitric oxide formation, prevents diabetic vascular dysfunction. Diabetes 1992; 41:552
79. Cross AH, Misko TP, Lin RF, et al. Aminoguanidine, an inhibitor of inducible nitric oxide synthase, ameliorates experimental autoimmune encephalomyelitis in SJL mice. J Clin Invest 1994;93:2684
80. Hammes H-P, Brownlee M, Edelstein D, et al. Aminoguanidine inhibits the development of accelerated diabetic retinopathy in the spontaneous hypertensive rat. Diabetologia 1994;37:32
81. Soules-Liparota T, Cooper M, Papazoglou D, et al. Retardation by aminoguanidine of development of albuminuria, mesangial expansion, and tissue fluorescence in streptozocin-induced diabetic rat. Diabetes 1991;40:1328
82. Edelstein D, Brownlee M. Aminoguanidine ameliorates albuminuria in diabetic hypertensive rats. Diabetologia 1992;35:96
83. Ellis EN, Good BH. Prevention of glomerular basement membrane thickening by aminoguanidine in experimental diabetes mellitus. Metabolism 1991;40: 1016
84. Cameron NE, Cotter MA, Dines K, Love A. Effects of aminoguanidine on peripheral nerve function and polyol pathway metabolites in streptozotocin-diabetic rats. Diabetologia 1992;35:946
85. Kihara M, Schmelzer JD, Poduslo JF, et al. Aminoguanidine effects on nerve blood flow, vascular permeability, electrophysiology and oxygen free radicals. Proc Natl Acad Sci USA 1991;88:6107

Diabetes Mellitus, edited by Derek LeRoith, Simeon I. Taylor, and Jerrold M. Olefsky. Lippincott–Raven Publishers, Philadelphia © 1996.

CHAPTER 91
Hyperinsulinemia

ELE FERRANNINI

Insulin stands out among hormones on account of the following properties:

1. It is a phylogenetically ancient peptide, which, during evolution has accumulated both acute effects on intermediary metabolism and chronic actions on tissue growth and differentiation.
2. It is potentially lethal by virtue of its tight and rapid control of plasma glucose concentration, and therefore, brain function.
3. It is not known to be directly regulated by any ad hoc pituitary or hypothalamic hormone; that is, it lacks central integration.
4. Its action is antagonized by a host of other hormones (growth hormone, cortisol, glucagon, catecholamines, thyroid hormones, sex steroids), which collectively constitute the redundant countersystem that is typical of vital functions.

Absolute insulin deficiency causes insulin-dependent diabetes (IDDM), whereas variable degrees of insulin deficiency are associated with non–insulin-dependent diabetes (NIDDM). However, unlike all other classical hormones for which both deficiency and excess produce distinct clinical syndromes, we still do not understand what disease is caused by insulin excess. Because persistent insulin excess is incompatible with life, insulin resistance can be thought to have evolved as a means to blunt the effects of hyperinsulinism. The cost of such adaptation is, however, hidden. This chapter attempts to bring some aspects of it to light.

Circulating Insulin

Insulin circulates in plasma at a concentration that is a simultaneous function of its secretion, distribution, and degradation. Although secretion rate rapidly responds to metabolic and neural signals, neither the apparent total volume of distribution nor the clearance rate of insulin is a major regulatory or regulatable step of in vivo insulin action.[1] Insulin is distributed into a space that includes the intravascular volume, the interstitial fluid, and the plasma membrane insulin receptors.[2] Insulin clearance from peripheral plasma averages 13 $mLmin^{-1}kg^{-1}$ ($\pm 20\%$) under normal circumstances, whereas hepatic insulin uptake is at least twice as high as peripheral removal because of the large portosystemic insulin concentration gradient.[3] Saturation of insulin clearance is readily detectable within the physiologic concentration range,[4] but is most evident when plasma insulin levels exceed 150–200 μU/mL.[3,4] Changes in insulin distribution affect circulating insulin levels only in those rare conditions in which the density of membrane insulin receptors is profoundly reduced. In these cases, insulin clearance is also impaired, and circulating insulin levels rise because insulin degradation may be largely receptor-mediated.[5] Hepatic or renal parenchymal insufficiency causes hyperinsulinemia by depressing insulin degradation.[3]

In the absence of organ failure, and except for rare insulin resistance syndromes, the cause of hyperinsulinemia is an increased secretory rate. In addition, when β-cell activity is persistently stimulated, the hepatic capacity for insulin degradation may be exceeded, and the pancreatic insulin overflowing into the general circulation contributes to the systemic hyperinsulinemia. This typically is the case in massive obesity.[6]

In the process of insulin synthesis, proinsulin is enzymatically cleaved at both the A-chain/C-peptide (at amino acid residues 65–66) and the B-chain/C-peptide (residues 32–33) junction to yield insulin and C-peptide in equimolar proportions. Incomplete cleavage at either junction gives rise to split proinsulins, and removal of a pair of basic amino acids from these precursors generates des 64,65 split and des 31,32 split proinsulin. Small amounts of proinsulin and its split products (particularly, the des forms) are released from β-cells into the portal circulation (at a rate of ~3 $pmolmin^{-1}$ in the case of proinsulin), escaping hepatic uptake and accumulating in peripheral plasma because of their slow, mostly renal, clearance (~3.5 $mLmin^{-1}kg^{-1}$ in the case of proinsulin). Most polyclonal antisera raised against insulin recognize several epitopes common to proinsulin, split, and des split proinsulins. Thus, using ordinary radioimmunoassay kits, cross-reactivity of proinsulin with insulin ranges between 35% and 100%.[7] Monoclonal antibodies and two-site immunometric assays improve the specificity of the insulin assay. The availability of biosynthetic human proinsulin has made it possible to raise both polyclonal and monoclonal antibodies with less cross-reactivity with partially processed proinsulin molecules.

Fasting serum proinsulin, which comprises 5–20% of total immunoreactive insulin in normal subjects, is increased in subjects with impaired glucose tolerance (IGT) or NIDDM, roughly in proportion to the degree of fasting hyperglycemia.[8] In these conditions, therefore, the use of nonspecific insulin assays overestimates true insulin levels and may mask insulin deficiency.[9] Under normal circumstances, however, this confounding effect has been shown to be modest.[10] At a simplistic level, increased circulating proinsulin levels are considered to be an index of β-cell secretory dysfunction. These precursor peptides may carry their own message as markers for cardiovascular risk factors, as has recently been suggested.[11]

In summary, keeping in mind the above caveats, a persistent increase in plasma insulin concentration, or hyperinsulinemia, is the expression of exaggerated β-cell secretory activity, whether primary (i.e., true hypersecretion) or adaptive (to resistance to insulin action).

Hyperinsulinemia

Epidemiology

Plasma insulin concentration has been measured in multiple population-based studies. For example, in the San Antonio Heart Study, a survey involving ~3000 subjects stratified by age and socioeconomic condition, fasting insulin levels were typically in the range of 1–50 μU/mL (6 and 300 pM), whereas postglucose plasma insulin concentrations (2 hours after a standard oral load) were in the range of 1–700 μU/mL (6 and 4200 pM). Both sets of insulin measurements are distributed with a clear rightward skew, similar to those of serum cholesterol and blood pressure. Logarithmic transformation of plasma insulin values yields a distribution that does not appreciably deviate from a normal distribution. If obese subjects (i.e., those with a body mass index [BMI] of > 27 kg/m^2) and individuals with IGT or NIDDM are excluded, the distribution is still skewed (Fig. 91-1). Logarithmic transformation of fasting insulin levels in this nonobese, nondiabetic segment of the whole population yields a normal distribution. If one defines hyperinsulinemia as a value 2 SDs above the mean (or the top 2.5%) of this group, the cut-off is 31 μU/mL (see Fig. 91-1). In the whole population, ~8% of those screened have fasting insulin values exceeding 31 μU/mL. Thus, by this purely statistical criterion, roughly 1 in 10 subjects between 20–65 years of age are hyperinsulinemic in the Southwestern United States. Clearly, however, the prevalence of hyperinsulinemia may be different in different populations, depending on a number of factors. Different cut-off values may be chosen depending on the ratio of sensitivity to specificity that is needed for the particular purpose of such an analysis.

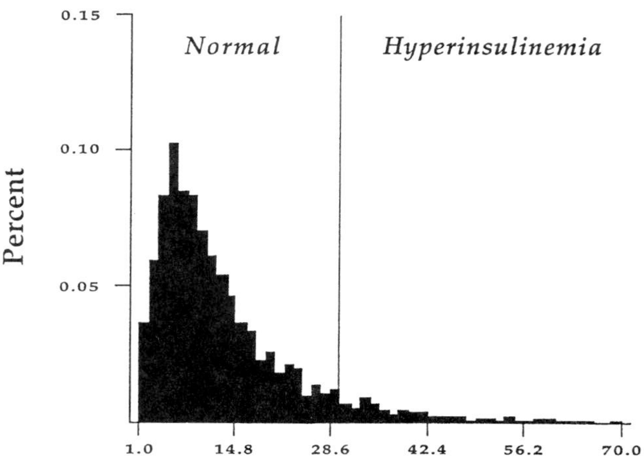

FIGURE 91-1. Frequency distribution plot of fasting plasma insulin concentrations in a population-based survey of 2930 individuals (the San Antonio Heart Study). The cut-off point for hyperinsulinemia is set at 31 μU/mL (see text for explanation).

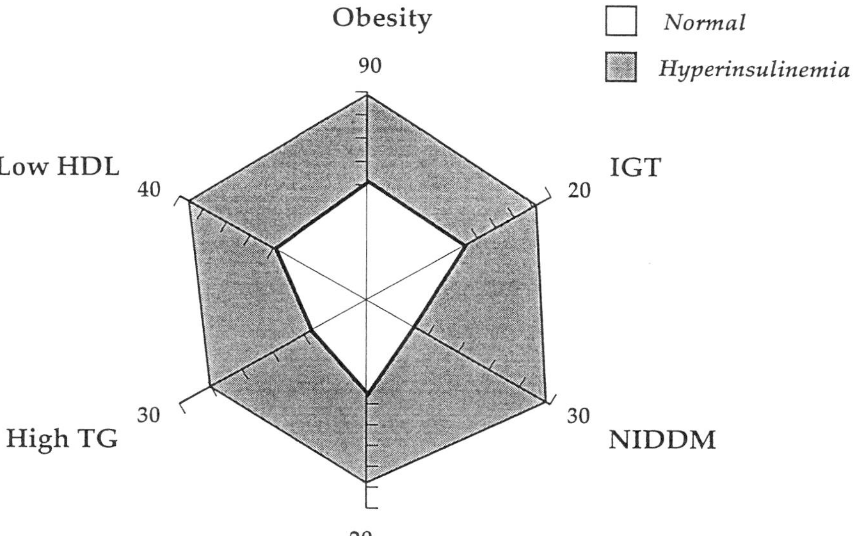

Figure 91-2. Prevalence rates (expressed in %) of obesity, IGT, NIDDM, hypertension, hypertriglyceridemia, and low HDL cholesterol levels in the normoinsulinemic (n = 2700) and hyperinsulinemic (n = 239) segment of the general population (from the San Antonio Heart Study). *TG*, triglyceride.

Clinical Definition

A quantitative definition of hyperinsulinemia may be useful if a clinically relevant end point is identified. In the San Antonio Heart Study, the clinical impact of hyperinsulinemia is significant. As shown in Figure 91-2, obesity, IGT, NIDDM, hypertension, hypertriglyceridemia (arbitrarily defined as a serum triglyceride concentration > 250 mg/dL [2.9 mM]), and low concentrations of high-density lipoprotein (HDL) cholesterol (<35 mg/dL [0.94 mM]) were found to be 2–3 times more prevalent in the 239 individuals with fasting insulin levels of greater than 31 μU/mL than in the 2700 subjects with fasting insulins below that level. Thus, in this population, hyperinsulinemia segregates not only with obesity, but also with the components of a metabolic/hemodynamic syndrome, which Reaven has termed "syndrome X."[12] In addition, in a population in which plasma insulin levels are an independent predictor of cardiovascular morbidity, it would be logical to set the boundary of hyperinsulinemia at the lowest insulin concentration associated with a statistical increase in the probability of cardiovascular disease. This would be analogous to what has been done with arterial blood pressure or serum cholesterol values, and, like the latter, is subject to change as more information is gained from longitudinal studies and/or intervention trials.

Obesity

The strongest acquired factor that impacts on the circulating concentration of insulin is obesity. As shown in Figure 91-3, fasting plasma insulin concentration increases with body mass, in men as well as in women, by roughly 4 pmol/L for each BMI unit. Excess weight comprises both fat tissue and lean mass, in an approximate ratio of 2:1. In a series of observations in which fat mass was directly quantitated (by electrical bioimpedance) in nondiabetic subjects, the relationship between fat mass and BMI was found to be depicted in Figure 91-4. Among lean individuals, women have a greater percentage of fat mass (~30% of body weight) than do men (~20%). With increasing degrees of obesity, both men and women reach the same proportion of body weight as fat. This means that men accrue relatively more fat than women as they

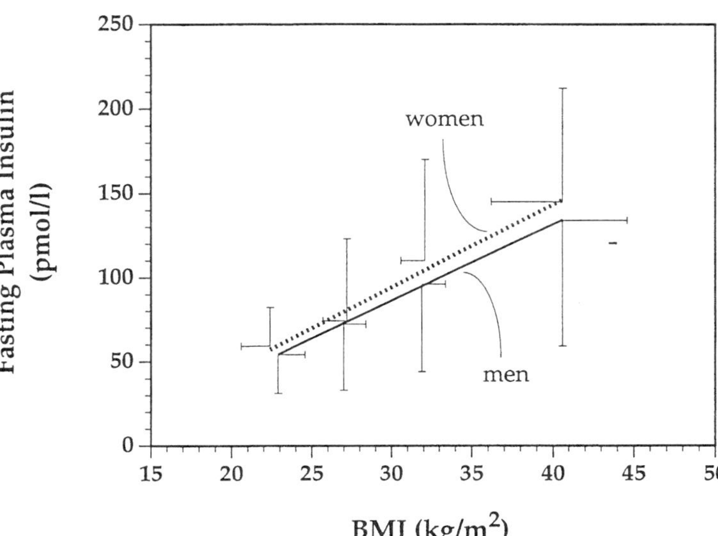

Figure 91-3. Relationship between fasting plasma insulin concentrations and BMI in 760 nondiabetic subjects (unpublished data). Vertical and horizontal bars denote 1 SD.

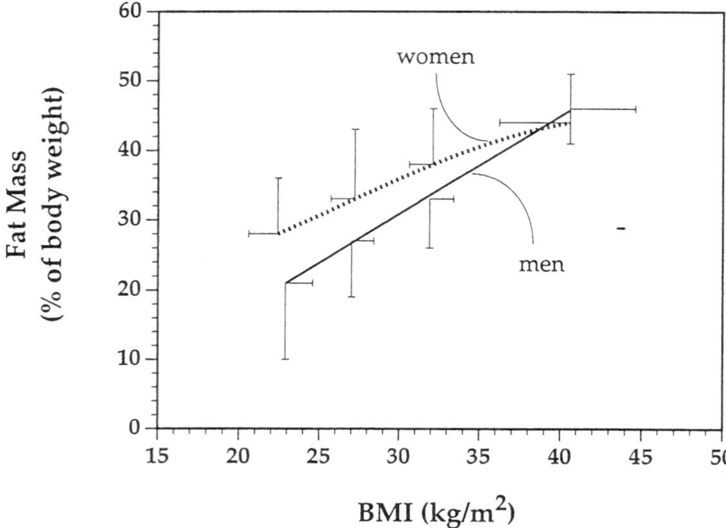

Figure 91-4. Relationship between fat mass (expressed as % of body weight) and BMI in the same subjects as in Figure 91-3.

gain weight. In support of this interpretation are the longitudinal data from the San Antonio Heart Study. In 1485 subjects who underwent follow-up studies for 8 years, fasting plasma insulin concentrations were significantly related to the weight change occurring over 8 years (Fig. 91-5), and the same weight gain was associated with a significantly larger increment in fasting insulin in men than in women. This gender difference was canceled when adjusting for skinfold (subscapular and triceps) thickness, a measure of adiposity. Thus, fat deposition leads to hyperinsulinemia, and men appear to be more susceptible than women to obesity-induced hyperinsulinemia, at least in part because they accumulate relatively more fat mass with gain weight than do women.

Upper body (or android) rather than lower body (or gynoid) accumulation of fat has been shown to be independently associated with hyperinsulinemia.[13] The relative proportion of adipose mass that is found on the trunk rather than in the extremities is most commonly expressed as the waist-to-hip circumference ratio (WHR). In the nondiabetic segment of the San Antonio Heart Study cohort, fasting plasma insulin concentrations are modestly correlated with the WHR ($r^2 < 3\%$ in both nonobese and obese individuals). These relationships are still statistically significant when simultaneously accounting for BMI, suggesting that there is an additive effect of obesity and body fat distribution on plasma insulin levels. The WHR is a constitutive characteristic, with marked sexual dimorphism. In smaller-scale investigations, direct quantitation of visceral fat mass is far superior to the WHR in predicting hyperinsulinemia.[14] The hormonal background against which fat is preferentially routed to the abdominal region is not fully characterized, although steroid hormones (cortisol, androgens, estrogen) seem to play a dominant role.[15] The extent to which homing of adipose mass to the subcutaneous and visceral depots is also affected by other environmental factors, such as stress, diet, and physical activity, has yet to be studied in detail.[16]

In summary, accumulation of adipose mass, particularly in the visceral area, is associated with hyperinsulinemia in a very consistent manner, both cross-sectionally and longitudinally. For this reason, in unselected population samples, hyperinsulinemia should be evaluated after adjusting for adipose mass and, possibly, its relative body distribution. Two considerations are of special importance in this regard. First, hyperinsulinemia, however defined, can be found in individuals with normal body weight, in whom it shows the same pattern of associations (described later) found in obese subjects or in the population at large. To classify such hyperinsulinemic lean subjects as "metabolically obese" is just

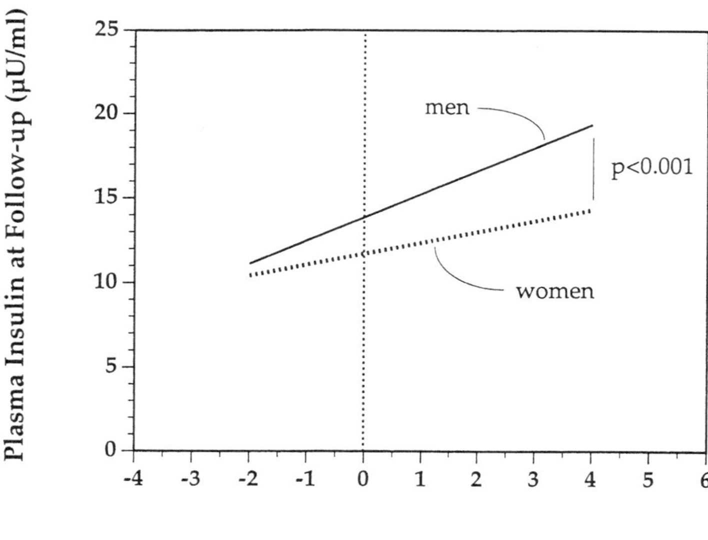

Figure 91-5. Fasting plasma insulin concentrations at follow-up examination as a function of the body weight change occurring during an 8-year period in 1485 subjects studied in the San Antonio Heart Study. Regressions are adjusted for age and baseline BMI. The slope of the regression is significantly steeper in men than in women.

another way of describing the same phenomenon. Second, and conversely, being overweight can be associated with apparently normal plasma insulin concentrations. In the San Antonio Heart Study data base, roughly 20% of the healthy (nondiabetic, normotensive, normolipidemic) subjects with a BMI > 27 kg/m^2 (n=850) had both fasting (~4 μU/mL) and postglucose (~40 μU/mL) insulin values that were superimposable on those of their lean counterparts. Nevertheless, this subset of normoinsulinemic obese subjects still showed changes characteristically associated with obesity—that is, increased arterial blood pressure levels, increased serum triglyceride and decreased serum HDL cholesterol concentrations. It is not known whether, in these individuals, plasma insulin level is unrelated to the other metabolic/hemodynamic abnormalities, or would be even lower if the subjects were not obese.

Obesity results from a chronically positive energy balance, usually attributable to overeating. In particular, a diet rich in carbohydrates increases plasma insulin concentrations in humans.[17] In addition, it has been determined that physical training reduces plasma insulin levels,[18] whereas smoking, a sympathoexcitatory stimulus, raises plasma insulin.[19]

In summary, the circulating plasma insulin concentration in any given individual is the integrated result of environmental influences, including (1) current or past overeating, (2) a hormonal mode favoring accumulation of excess fat in the trunk, (3) a sedentary lifestyle, and (4) chronic stress.

Inheritance

Despite powerful environmental effects, growing evidence indicates that the fasting plasma insulin concentration is, to some extent, controlled by genetic factors. Hyperinsulinemia has been described in nondiabetic Mexican Americans in the San Antonio Heart Study, a population at high risk for NIDDM,[20] and in the nondiabetic offspring of parents with NIDDM.[21] In more than 200 family members of patients with NIDDM,[22] fasting insulin levels segregate as an autosomal recessive allele, with a frequency of 0.25. Although such estimates depend on the number and quality of pedigrees available for analysis (and ultimately represent only the best statistical fit of the data from a range of compatible models), they do suggest that the fasting insulin concentration is a moderately inheritable trait, subject to modulation by a relatively small number of quantifiable external factors.

Metabolic Correlates

Plasma Glucose Levels

Increased glucose levels are invariably coupled with increased insulin concentrations except in severely diabetic individuals (i.e., in only a small percentage of the population). For example, in nondiabetics in the San Antonio Heart Study, fasting and postglucose plasma insulin and glucose levels were found to be interrelated, as shown in Table 91-1. Thus, both the glucose and the insulin response to the test (oral glucose) are strongly predicted by the respective fasting level (with insulin being better correlated than glucose). Within each state, glucose and insulin are directly related to one another (stimulated state better than fasting). Other cross-associations are weaker. This pattern of associations is the expression of the glucose-insulin homeostatic system. Whereas acute increases in insulin lower plasma glucose, chronic increments in insulin (e.g., from hyperalimentation or tissue insulin resistance) downregulate insulin action via an effect on hormone binding to membrane receptors.[23] Chronically increased plasma glucose levels, however, are believed to downregulate glucose-induced insulin secretion, one of the manifestations of the glucose toxicity phenomenon.[24] The overall result of this homeostatic system and its loops is such that the two variables—plasma insulin and plasma glucose level—will always vary in direct proportion to one another (unless insulin secretion fails).

Lipids

In the San Antonio Heart Study population, both fasting and postglucose insulin concentrations were found to be directly related to serum triglyceride levels (r=0.21 and r=0.20, respectively) and inversely related to serum HDL cholesterol concentrations (r=−0.17 and r=−0.11, respectively). These associations are the result of another homeostatic system involving plasma free fatty acid (FFA) levels, hepatic secretion of very low-density lipoprotein (VLDL) triglycerides and VLDL cholesterol, delipidation, and removal of lipoproteins. Recent population data (Haffner SM, et al. unpublished observations, 1996) show that, in nondiabetics, fasting FFA levels rise with female gender, age, BMI, and WHR. Following glucose ingestion, FFA levels promptly decline because of insulin inhibition of triglyceride hydrolysis. As in the case of glucose, however, insulin acutely lowers FFA, but under steady-state conditions, increased insulin is associated with increased levels of FFA. Impaired suppression of circulating FFA by insulin is accompanied by increased triglyceride and glucose levels. In patients with NIDDM, both fasting and postglucose FFA levels are increased, and FFA suppression is compromised, in comparison with the values measured in subjects with normal glucose tolerance. Hepatic secretion of VLDL triglycerides is a simultaneous function of FFA supply to the liver and plasma insulin concentrations. Furthermore, removal of circulating VLDL is delayed, and the rate of clearance of HDL is increased, in hyperinsulinemic individuals.[25] Finally, recent evidence has shown that hyperinsulinemia is coupled with a relative abundance of small, dense, LDL cholesterol particles in nondiabetic subjects.[26] There is no independent association of LDL cholesterol and plasma insulin in the general population, however, and no evidence of hyperinsulinemia in patients with type IIA familial hypercholesterolemia.[27] Thus, the associations between insulin and serum lipids are the expression of insulin regulation of triglyceride removal (through stimulation of lipoprotein lipase), triglyceride hydrolysis (via inhibition of hormone-sensitive tissue

Table 91-1. Univariate Correlation Coefficients Between Plasma Glucose and Insulin Levels in the General Population*

	Fasting Glucose Level	Fasting Insulin Level	2-Hour Glucose Level	2-Hour Insulin Level
Fasting glucose	—	0.30	0.35	0.18
Fasting insulin	—	—	0.28	0.55
2-Hour glucose	—	—	—	0.64

*Data from 2650 nondiabetic subjects screened in the San Antonio Heart Study.

lipase), de novo hepatic synthesis of FFA and apolipoproteins, and, possibly, the pattern of transfer of lipid moieties among apolipoproteins.

Uric Acid

Hyperuricemia is often found in association with glucose intolerance, obesity, diabetes, and hypertension. In healthy subjects, serum uric acid concentrations are directly related to insulin levels, whereas uric acid clearance, a determinant of uricemia, is inversely related to plasma insulin.[28] Acute insulin infusion causes a coupled reduction in the urinary excretion of uric acid and sodium.[29]

Nonmetabolic Correlates

Blood Pressure

A direct relationship between plasma insulin and blood pressure is clearly evident in the San Antonio Heart Study data base. Indeed, this relationship was noted in the whole population sample, as well as in the healthy (nonobese, nondiabetic, normotensive, normolipidemic) segment of the population, and persisted after adjustment for age, gender, BMI, and WHR.[30] In several other epidemiologic studies, a similar relationship between some measure of arterial blood pressure (systolic, diastolic, mean, or pulse pressure) and some measure of plasma insulin (fasting, single postglucose value, or sum of postglucose values) has been reported, often with adjustment for age, gender, or BMI. The association, however, has generally been rather weak, and this may explain why some surveys have yielded negative results. Interethnic variability, which was evident in the San Antonio Heart Study,[31] contributes to this relative inconsistency. The physiologic structure of the link between insulin and blood pressure is still imperfectly understood. It seems established that high blood pressure per se does not give rise to hyperinsulinemia, as secondary forms of hypertension are not conspicuously associated with elevated plasma insulin levels. Hyperinsulinemia, however, has the potential of raising blood pressure through a variety of mechanisms (stimulation of renal sodium reabsorption, activation of the adrenergic nervous system, stimulation of smooth muscle cell growth, alteration of transmembrane ion traffic).[32]

Ion Abnormalities

A high rate of sodium/lithium countertransport (Na/Li CT) activity, a marker related to hypertension heritability as a monogenic trait,[33] is associated with insulin resistance and hyperinsulinemia in nondiabetic hypertensive patients.[34] Furthermore, high Na/Li CT activity identifies a subgroup of patients with IDDM who are prone to hypertension and diabetic nephropathy,[35] and segregates with insulin resistance, lipid disturbances, and microalbuminuria in hypertensive patients with NIDDM.[36] In red blood cells, insulin increases both the Km and the Vmax of Na/Li CT,[37] and by this change may promote cell growth.[38]

High intracellular calcium concentrations have been described in adipocytes of obese, insulin-resistant subjects.[39] Acute insulin administration causes a paradoxical rise in intracellular calcium levels in platelets of insulin-resistant individuals, whereas no such effect is seen in insulin-sensitive subjects.[40] Low intracellular magnesium levels have been found in circulating cells of patients with insulin resistance and hyperinsulinemia.[41] These findings have led to the concept that opposite changes in the free cytosolic levels of calcium and magnesium are possible mediators of insulin action in insulin-resistant states.[42]

Microalbuminuria

Microalbuminuria has recently been found to be associated with hyperinsulinemia and increased serum triglyceride levels in nondiabetic subjects, both with and without hypertension.[43] In NIDDM, microalbuminuria clusters with insulin resistance and dyslipidemia.[36] An increased rate of urinary albumin excretion is found more often in patients with essential hypertension than in the normotensive population,[44] and those with microalbuminuria and hypertension are hyperinsulinemic in comparison with normoalbuminuric hypertensives.[45] The nature of the link between hyperinsulinemia and albumin excretion is obscure.

Fibrinolysis

Increased plasma concentrations of plasminogen activator inhibitor 1 (PAI-1) have been associated with obesity (particularly, central obesity), NIDDM, essential hypertension, hypertriglyceridemia, and coronary heart disease[46]—that is, in conditions of hyperinsulinemia and insulin resistance. Although in vitro insulin stimulates PAI-1 secretion by cultured liver cells,[47] in vivo acute insulin administration does not change circulating PAI-1 levels. Defective fibrinolysis caused by excess PAI-1 has been hypothesized to mediate the putative atherogenic effects of insulin.

Birth Weight

A low birth weight has been linked with development of hypertension[48] and glucose intolerance[49] in adult life, both in Caucasians[50] and in the biethnic population of the San Antonio Heart Study.[51] Reduced fetal growth has, therefore, been proposed as a general antecedent of adult hyperinsulinemia and its correlates. Hyperinsulinemia is physiologic during pregnancy. In healthy mothers, a higher degree of hyperinsulinemia during the third trimester of pregnancy is associated with a lower weight of the neonate.[52] Thus, in addition to genetic factors, hyperinsulinemia may also be inheritable through intrauterine influences.

Summary

As mentioned previously, the hyperinsulinemic segment of the population includes subjects who are obese, glucose-intolerant, overtly diabetic, hypertensive, or dyslipidemic (or combinations thereof). Analysis of the pattern of association of plasma insulin concentrations with the physiologic variables that define these disorders (body fat, plasma glucose level, blood pressure, and the lipid couple triglyceride/HDL cholesterol) confirms that the presence of hyperinsulinemia in these disorders is merely an extension into the pathologic domain of connections that exist throughout the physiologic range. In addition, hyperinsulinemia is associated with a number of other changes (elevated intracellular calcium/magnesium ratio, raised PAI-1, microalbuminuria, hyperuricemia, maternal hyperinsulinemia) that do not identify distinct diseases. According to available evidence, these associations often have a sound physiologic substrate. Admittedly, this is an ''insulinocentric'' view insofar as many significant relations also exist between other variables of the set (e.g., between BMI and triglycerides, WHR and HDL cholesterol, and BMI and blood pressure). It could, therefore, be argued that placing insulin—rather than BMI or WHR or lipids or blood pressure—at the core of the set reflects the investigator's bias rather than a necessary key to interpreting the whole.

Hyperinsulinemia and Insulin Resistance

General Observations

Insulin action modulates insulin secretion by setting the demand for insulin by the body tissues. Accordingly, when both insulin secretion (as reflected by the circulating insulin concentration) and insulin sensitivity (measured as whole-body glucose disposal under conditions of stable euglycemic hyperinsulinemia, such as that achieved using an insulin clamp) have been determined in a given population, an inverse relationship has been observed. As depicted in Figure 91-6, however, the scatter around the regression line is wide, and the explained variance (8%) is small. Thus, at any level of insulin sensitivity, insulin concentrations can vary over a wide range; conversely, any level of plasma insulin can be associated with very different degrees of sensitivity. Clearly, this depends on the precision of the two measurements (and on the kinetics of plasma insulin removal), as well as on individual set-points of the homeostatic couple. Furthermore, when insulin secretion is deficient (as in the case of IDDM and severe NIDDM) but insulin action is impaired, the set-points will decline to the left and below the regression line. Thus, although hyperinsulinemia is customarily viewed as an adaptation to insulin resistance, the underlying physiologic state may range from one in which normal insulin sensitivity is associated with true insulin hypersecretion to one in which normal or low insulin levels coexist with insulin insensitivity. This implies that other, unknown factors contribute to the control of insulin sensitivity, as well as to insulin secretion. Furthermore, in any given hyperinsulinemic/insulin-resistant individual, it is impossible to determine whether hypersecretion is the primary event with insulin resistance developing secondarily, or the other way around.

An important concept to keep in mind is that the primary target of insulin action is glucose homeostasis. When glucose metabolism is impeded in refractory tissues, the plasma glucose level itself signals back to the β-cell to increase insulin secretion. For all we know, insulin sensitivity is geared to maintaining circulating glucose levels and preserving glycogen stores. Although protein or lipid depots also depend on insulin and can interfere with insulin action on glucose (e.g., by substrate competition[53]), their own regulation does not feed back through insulin sensitivity. It follows that insulin resistance can be restricted to glucose metabolism, in which case the nonresistant pathways will be exposed to compensatory hyperinsulinemia. A crucial issue in the interpretation of hyperinsulinemia is whether its associated changes (in terms of metabolic and nonmetabolic functions, as discussed in the previous sections) result from the high insulin concentrations per se or the underlying insulin resistance.

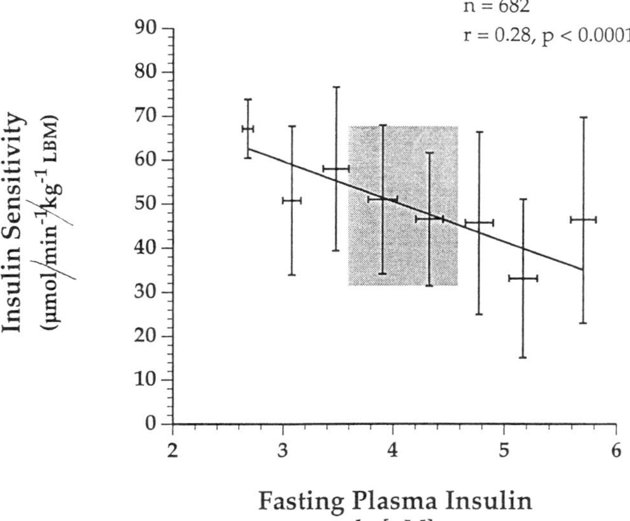

FIGURE 91-6. Relationship between insulin sensitivity (as measured during a euglycemic insulin clamp) and fasting plasma insulin concentrations in nondiabetic individuals. Vertical and horizontal bars denote 1 SD. The shaded area includes the mean x and y values ± 1 SD. *LBM,* lean body mass.

Specific Situations

Insulin resistance is present in most patients with NIDDM or IGT, whether lean or obese.[54] Insulin resistance (or weight-adjusted hyperinsulinemia) has also been noted in the nonobese offspring of diabetic parents,[55,56] in whom the full spectrum of metabolic changes associated with NIDDM is already present at a time when their glucose metabolism is still within normal limits.[57] In longitudinal studies, both insulin resistance and hyperinsulinemia have been shown to precede and predict the appearance of diagnostic hyperglycemia in nondiabetic subjects[58–60] and in the normoglycemic offspring of parents with NIDDM.[61]

A significant proportion of patients with essential hypertension are insulin-resistant.[62] Interestingly, this finding, unlike the results obtained with plasma insulin measurements, has been entirely consistent.[63] As with plasma insulin levels,[31] the relationship between insulin sensitivity and blood pressure shows distinct ethnic variability.[64] Altered insulin sensitivity is found in young black men with borderline hypertension (a frequent antecedent of established hypertension)[65] and in normotensive, lean, young subjects with a hypertensive parent.[66] In follow-up investigations, a high baseline insulin concentration is a significant predictor of the subsequent development of hypertension in both nondiabetic[67] and diabetic subjects.[68,69]

Insulin sensitivity is reduced in hypercholesterolemia with high triglycerides (familial combined hyperlipoproteinemia), but is fully preserved in true familial hypercholesterolemia.[27] Plasma insulin has also been found to be a predictor of both hypertriglyceridemia and low HDL cholesterol in nondiabetic subjects included in the San Antonio Heart Study.[70]

With regard to disease associations, patients having NIDDM and essential hypertension[71] or hypertriglyceridemia[72] are more insulin-resistant than diabetic patients without either. In familial dyslipidemic hypertension,[73] a condition in which high blood pressure and dyslipidemia are associated in multiple members of the family, plasma insulin levels are elevated more than can be accounted for by obesity, and the condition is concordant in male twins.[74] A parental history of diabetes is associated with higher triglyceride levels, lower HDL cholesterol, higher blood pressure, and higher plasma glucose levels in offspring.[75] Even in children, plasma glucose and insulin concentrations, as well as blood pressure levels, are significantly associated with one another.[76]

In longitudinal observations of lean, prehypertensive subjects, the association of insulin levels with future hypertension was found to cluster with increased triglyceride and total cholesterol levels and decreased HDL cholesterol concentrations.[67] Furthermore, subjects with NIDDM at baseline were found to have an increased incidence of hypertension at follow-up compared to subjects with normal glucose tolerance (17% versus 8%).[67] Fasting hyperinsulinemia simultaneously predicted NIDDM, hypertension, and dyslipidemia in the San Antonio Heart Study.[70] In the general population, increased blood pressure values and serum cholesterol levels have been found to be significant predictors of NIDDM.[77] Conversely, in nondiabetic subjects, an increased plasma glucose response to oral glucose predicts development of hypertension over a period of 18 years.[78]

Summary

In summary, then, the following points may be made:

1. Insulin sensitivity, like the plasma insulin level, is controlled by genetic factors.
2. Insulin resistance is present in NIDDM, essential hypertension, and dyslipidemia, independent of obesity.
3. Insulin insensitivity is consistently found in groups of healthy individuals who are at risk for NIDDM or hypertension.
4. Insulin resistance (or weight-adjusted hyperinsulinemia) precedes and predicts the development of NIDDM, dyslipidemia, and (albeit more weakly) hypertension.
5. The presence (in probands or their families) of one condition—NIDDM or hypertension—predicts the subsequent appearance of the other.

Thus, across individual diseases and their combinations, hyperinsulinemia and insulin resistance remain parallel. On the grounds of independence (of obesity), antecedence (of the actual diseases), and cross-predictivity, hyperinsulinemia/insulin resistance is the substrate from which the clinical triad of disordered glucose, lipid, and blood pressure homeostasis evolves later in life. It is important to recognize that insulin resistance is often, but not always, found in patients with diabetes, hypertension, or dyslipidemia, all of which are heterogeneous conditions. Furthermore, even when insulin resistance is present, it appears to anticipate or precipitate, but is insufficient to directly cause, full-blown diabetes, hypertension, or dyslipidemia.

Clinical Significance

Hyperinsulinemia is potentially related to atherosclerotic cardiovascular diseases (CVDs). Several correlates of hyperinsulinemia have been shown to be (in isolation) risk factors for CVD: namely, increased glucose and blood pressure values, as well as high triglyceride/low HDL cholesterol levels, high PAI-1 levels, high WHR, hyperuricemia, microalbuminuria, and low birth weight. For example, microalbuminuria has emerged as an independent predictor of CVD in both nondiabetic[79] and diabetic individuals,[80,81] and Barker and colleagues[82] have established a correlation between low birth weight and CVD mortality.[82] In a large prospective survey conducted in Sweden (the Malmö Study), several of the independent risk factors for the development of overt NIDDM (or IGT) in normoglycemic individuals during a 6-year period were also found to be established risk factors for CVD (i.e., obesity, sedentary lifestyle, increased fasting and 2-hour plasma glucose concentrations, a family history of diabetes, and treatment for hypertension).[83] This provides a logical explanation for the finding[84] that, in a 24-year follow-up study, cardiovascular mortality in men and women with NIDDM was higher than that in the nondiabetic population, even just 3 years after diagnosis. Similar conclusions have been drawn from an analysis of cardiovascular risk factors in confirmed prediabetic individuals,[85] which supports the concept that the "clock" for CVD starts "ticking" long before the onset of clinical diabetes. Plasma insulin concentration itself has emerged as an independent risk factor for CVD in three longitudinal studies,[86–88] although more recent findings have failed to confirm this association. Patients with coronary heart disease are hyperinsulinemic and insulin-resistant, even when accounting for cardiovascular risk factors that are themselves associated with insulin resistance (BMI, WHR, plasma glucose and lipid levels, blood pressure).[89] In vitro, insulin promotes the growth of smooth muscle cells.[90] In animal models, chronic insulin administration induces atherosclerotic lesions[91] and aortic smooth muscle cell proliferation following endothelial injury.[92]

In conclusion, hyperinsulinemia/insulin resistance stands for an ensemble of metabolic and nonmetabolic changes that are more or less tightly interconnected through cause-and-effect relationships. The pathogenic potential of hyperinsulinemia/insulin resistance is suggested from disparate, mostly circumstantial evidence; its exact expression is under active investigation. Whether a marker or a mechanism, hyperinsulinism of any origin is likely to take a sizeable toll in terms of cardiovascular morbidity.

References

1. Navalesi R, Pilo A, Ferrannini E. Kinetic analysis of plasma insulin disappearance in nonketotic diabetic patients and in normal subjects. A tracer study with ^{125}I-insulin. J Clin Invest 1978;61:197
2. Ferrannini E, Cobelli C. The kinetics of insulin in man. I. General aspects. Diabetes Metab Rev 1987;3:335
3. Ferrannini E, Cobelli C. The kinetics of insulin in man. I. Role of the liver. Diabetes Metab Rev 1987;3:365
4. Morishima T, Bradshaw C, Radziuk J. Measurement using tracers of steady-state turnover and metabolic clearance of insulin in dogs. Am J Physiol 1985; 248:E203
5. Flier JS, Minaker KL, Landsberg L, et al. Impaired in vivo insulin clearance in patients with severe target cell resistance to insulin. Diabetes 1982;31:132
6. Polonski KS, Given BD, Hirsch L, et al. Quantitative study of insulin secretion and clearance in normal and obese subjects. J Clin Invest 1988;81:435
7. Clark PMS, Hales CN. How to measure plasma insulin. Diabetes Metab Rev 1994;10:79
8. Yoshioka N, Kuzuya T, Matsuda A, et al. Serum proinsulin levels of fasting and after oral glucose load in patients with type 2 (non–insulin-dependent) diabetes mellitus. Diabetologia 1988;31:355
9. Temple RC, Carrington CA, Luzio SD, et al. Insulin deficiency in non–insulin dependent diabetes. Lancet 1989;1:293
10. Reaven GM, Chen YD-I, Hollenbeck CB, et al. Plasma insulin, C-peptide and proinsulin concentrations in obese and non-obese individuals with varying degrees of glucose intolerance. J Clin Endocrinol Metab 1993;76:44
11. Nagi DK, Hendra TJ, Ryle AJ, et al. The relationships of concentrations of insulin, intact proinsulin and 32-33 split proinsulin with cardiovascular risk factors in Type II (non–insulin-dependent) diabetic subjects. Diabetologia 1990;33:532
12. Reaven GM. Role of insulin resistance in human disease. Diabetes 1988; 37:1595
13. Kissebah AH, Vydelingum N, Murray R, et al. Relation of body fat distribution to metabolic complications of obesity. J Clin Endocrinol Metab 1982; 54:254
14. Lemieux S, Després JP, Nadeau A, et al. Heterogeneous glycaemic and insulinaemic responses to oral glucose in non-diabetic men: Interactions between duration of obesity, body fat distribution and family history of diabetes mellitus. Diabetologia 1992;35:653
15. Kissebah AH, Evans DJ, Peiris A, Wilson CR. Endocrine characteristics in regional obesities: Role of sex steroids. In: Vague J, Björntorp P, Guy-Grand B, et al., eds. Metabolic Complications of Human Obesities. Amsterdam: Elsevier Science;1985:115
16. Björntorp P. Visceral fat accumulation: The missing link between psychosocial factors and cardiovascular disease? J Intern Med 1991;230:195
17. Adamo M, LeRoith D, Simon J, Roth J. Effect of altered nutritional states on insulin receptors. Annu Rev Nutr 1988;8:149
18. Rodnick KJ, Haskell WL, Solomon R, et al. Improved insulin action in muscle, liver, and adipose tissue in physically trained human subjects. Am J Physiol 1987;253:E489
19. Facchini F, Hollenbeck CB, Jeppesen J, et al. Insulin resistance and cigarette smoking. Lancet 1992;339:1128
20. Haffner SM, Stern MP, Hazuda HP, et al. Hyperinsulinemia in a population at high risk for non-insulin-dependent diabetes mellitus. N Engl J Med 1986;315:220
21. Haffner SM, Stern MP, Hazuda HP. Increased insulin concentrations in non-diabetic offspring of diabetic parents. N Engl J Med 1988;319:1297
22. Schumacher MC, Hasstedt SJ, Hunt SC, et al. Major gene effect for insulin levels in familial NIDDM pedigrees. Diabetes 1992;41:416
23. Roth J, Kahn CR, Lesniak MA, et al. Receptors for insulin, NSILA-s and growth hormone: Applications to disease states in man. Rec Progr Horm Res 1975;31:95
24. Unger RH, Grundy S. Hyperglycaemia as an inducer as well as a consequence of impaired islet cell function and insulin resistance: Implications for the management of diabetes. Diabetologia 1985;28:119
25. Reaven GM. A syndrome of resistance to insulin-stimulated glucose uptake (Syndrome X): Definition and implications. Cardiovasc Risk Factors 1993;3:2
26. Reaven GM, Chen Y-DI, Jeppesen J, et al. Insulin resistance and hyperinsulinemia in individuals with small, dense, low density lipoprotein particles. J Clin Invest 1993;92:141
27. Quiñones-Galvan A, Santoro D, Natali A, et al. Insulin sensitivity in familial hypercholesterolemia. Metabolism 1993;42:1359
28. Facchini F, Chen Y-DI, Hollenbeck CB, Reaven GM. Relationship between resistance to insulin-mediated glucose uptake, urinary uric acid clearance, and plasma uric acid concentration. JAMA 1991;226:3008

29. Quiñones-Galvan A, Natali A, Baldi S, et al. Effect of insulin on uric acid excretion in humans. Am J Physiol 1995;268:E1
30. Ferrannini E, Haffner SM, Stern MP. Essential hypertension: An insulin-resistant state. J Cardiovasc Pharmacol 1990;15(Suppl 5):S18
31. Ferrannini E, Haffner SM, Stern MP, et al. High blood pressure and insulin resistance: Influence of genetic background. Eur J Clin Invest 1991;21:280
32. Ferrannini E, DeFronzo RA. The association of hypertension, diabetes and obesity: A review. J Nephrol 1989;1:3
33. Williams RR, Hasstedt SJ, Hunt SC, et al. Genetic traits related to hypertension and electrolyte metabolism. Hypertension 1991;17(Suppl 1):169
34. Doria A, Fioretto P, Avogaro A, et al. Insulin resistance is associated with high sodium-lithium countertransport in essential hypertension. Am J Physiol 1991;261:E694
35. Mangili R, Bending JJ, Scott G, et al. Increased sodium-lithium countertransport activity in red cells of patients with insulin-dependent diabetes and nephropathy. N Engl J Med 1988;318:146
36. Groop L, Ekstrand A, Forsblom C, et al. Insulin resistance, hypertension and microalbuminuria in patients with Type 2 (non–insulin-dependent) diabetes mellitus. Diabetologia 1993;36:642
37. Canessa M, Zerbini P. Insulin modulation of Na^+/Li^+ countertransport: Impact on hypertension and diabetes. Acta Diabetol 1992;29:186
38. Mahnensmith RL, Aronson PL. The plasma membrane sodium-hydrogen exchanger and its role in physiological and pathophysiological process. Circ Res 1985;56:443
39. Draznin B, Sussman KE, Eckel RH, et al. Possible role of cytosolic free calcium concentrations in mediating insulin resistance of obesity and hyperinsulinemia. J Clin Invest 1988;82:1848
40. Baldi S, Natali A, Buzzigoli G, et al. In vivo effect of insulin on intracellular calcium concentrations: Relation to insulin resistance. Metabolism; in press.
41. Paolisso G, Scheen A, D'Onofrio F, Lefebvre PJ. Magnesium and glucose homeostasis. Diabetologia 1990;33:511
42. Ram JL, Standley PR, Sowers JR. Hypertension, insulin function, and calcium. In: Draznin B, Eckel RH, eds. Diabetes and Atherosclerosis. Molecular Basis and Clinical Aspects. Amsterdam: Elsevier;1993:291
43. Haffner SM, Stern MP, Koslowski-Gruber MK, et al. Microalbuminuria. Potential marker for increased cardiovascular risk factors in nondiabetic subjects? Arteriosclerosis 1990;10:727
44. Parving HH, Mogensen CE, Jensen HAE, Ervin PE. Increased urinary albumin excretion rate in benign essential hypertension. Lancet 1974;1:1190
45. Bianchi S, Bigazzi R, Valtriani C, et al. Elevated serum insulin levels in patients with essential hypertension and microalbuminuria. Hypertension 1994;23:681
46. Juhan-Vague I, Alessi MC, Vague P. Increased plasminogen activator inhibitor 1 levels. A possible link between insulin resistance and atherothrombosis. Diabetologia 1991;34:457
47. Alessi MC, Juhan-Vague I, Kooistra T, et al. Insulin stimulates the synthesis of plasminogen activator inhibitor 1 by the human hepatocellular line HepG2. Thromb Haemost 1988;60:491
48. Barker DJP, Bull AR, Osmond C, Simmonds SJ. Fetal and placental size and risk of hypertension in adult life. BMJ 1990;301:259
49. Hales CN, Barker DJP, Clark PMS, et al. Fetal and infant growth and impaired glucose tolerance at age 64. Br Med J 1991;303:1019
50. Barker DJP, Hales CN, Fall CHD, et al. Type 2 (non-insulin-dependent) diabetes mellitus, hypertension and hyperlipidaemia (syndrome X): Relation to reduced fetal growth. Diabetologia 1993;36:62
51. Athens M, Valdez R, Stern M. Effect of birthweight on future development of "Syndrome X" in adult life. Diabetes 1993;42(Suppl 1):61A
52. Breschi MC, Seghieri G, Bartolomei G, et al. Relation of birthweight to maternal plasma glucose and insulin concentrations during normal pregnancy. Diabetologia 1993;36:1315
53. Groop LC, Ferrannini E. Insulin action and substrate competition. In: Ferrannini E, ed. Insulin Resistance and Disease. Baillière's Clinical Endocrinology & Metabolism. Vol. 7. 1993:1007
54. DeFronzo RA. The triumvirate: Beta cell, muscle, liver. A collusion responsible for NIDDM. Diabetes 1988;37:667
55. Martin BC, Warram JH, Rosner B, et al. Familial clustering of insulin sensitivity. Diabetes 1992;41:850
56. Eriksson J, Franssila-Kallunki A, Ekstrand A, et al. Early metabolic defects in persons at increased risk for non–insulin-dependent diabetes mellitus. N Engl J Med 1989;321:337
57. Gulli G, Ferrannini E, Stern MP, et al. The metabolic profile of non–insulin-dependent diabetes mellitus is fully established in glucose tolerant offspring of two non-insulin dependent diabetic parents. Diabetes 1992;41:1575
58. Sicree RA, Zimmet PZ, King HOM, Coventry JS. Plasma insulin response among Nauruans (1987). Prediction of deterioration in glucose tolerance over six years. Diabetes 1987;36:179
59. Lillioja S, Mott DM, Howard BV, et al. Impaired glucose tolerance as a disorder of insulin action: Longitudinal and cross-sectional studies in Pima Indians. N Engl J Med 1988;318:1217
60. Haffner SM, Stern MP, Mitchell BD, et al. Incidence of type II diabetes in Mexican Americans predicted by fasting insulin and glucose levels, obesity, and body-fat distribution. Diabetes 1990;39:283
61. Warram JH, Martin BC, Krolewski AS, et al. Slow glucose removal rate and hyperinsulinemia precede the development of type II diabetes in the offspring of diabetic parents. Ann Intern Med 1990;113:909
62. Ferrannini E, Buzzigoli G, Bonadonna R, et al. Insulin resistance in essential hypertension. N Engl J Med 1987;317:350
63. Pollare T, Lithell H, Berne C. Insulin resistance is a characteristic feature of primary hypertension independent of obesity. Metabolism 1990;39:167
64. Saad MF, Lillioja S, Nyomba BL, et al. Racial differences in the relation between blood pressure and insulin resistance. N Engl J Med 1991;324:733
65. Falkner B, Hulman S, Tannenbaum J, Kushner H. Insulin resistance and blood pressure in young black men. Hypertension 1990;16:708
66. Ferrari P, Weidmann P, Shaw S, et al. Altered insulin sensitivity, hyperinsulinemia, and dyslipidemia in individuals with a hypertensive parent. Am J Med 1991;91:589
67. Haffner SM, Ferrannini E, Hazuda HP, Stern MP. Clustering of cardiovascular risk factors in confirmed prehypertensive individuals. Hypertension 1992;20:38
68. Skarfors ET, Lithell HO, Selinus I. Risk factors for the development of hypertension: A 10-year longitudinal study in middle-aged men. J Hypertens 1991; 9:217
69. Niskanen LK, Uusitupa MI, Pyörälä K. The relationship of hyperinsulinemia to the development of hypertension in type 2 diabetic patients and in non-diabetic subjects. J Hum Hypertens 1991;5:155
70. Haffner SM, Valdez RA, Hazuda HP, et al. Prospective analysis of the insulin resistance syndrome (Syndrome X). Diabetes 1992;41:715
71. Laakso M, Sarlund H, Mykkänen I. Essential hypertension and insulin resistance in non–insulin-dependent diabetes. Eur J Clin Invest 1989;19:518
72. Widen E, Ekstrand A, Saloranta C, et al. Localization of insulin resistance in type 2 (non–insulin-dependent) diabetic patients with hypertriglyceridemia. Diabetologia 1992;35:1140
73. Hunt SC, Wu LL, Hopkins PN, et al. Apolipoprotein, low density lipoprotein subfraction and insulin associations with familial combined hyperlipidemia: Study of Utah patients with familial dyslipidemic hypertension. Arteriosclerosis 1989;9:335
74. Selby JV, Newman B, Quiroga J, et al. Concordance for dyslipidemic hypertension in male twins. JAMA 1991;265:2079
75. Haffner SM, Stern MP, Hazuda HP, et al. Parental history of diabetes is associated with increased cardiovascular risk factors. Arteriosclerosis 1989;9: 928
76. Florey C du V, Uppal S, Lowy C. Relation between blood pressure, weight, and plasma sugar and serum insulin levels in schoolchildren aged 9–12 years in Westland, Holland. Br Med J 1976;1:1368
77. Medalie JH, Papier CM, Goldbourt H, Herman JB. Major factors in the development of NIDDM in 10,000 men. Arch Intern Med 1975;135:811
78. Salomaa VV, Strandberg TE, Vanhanen H, et al. Glucose tolerance and blood pressure: Long-term follow-up in middle aged men. Br Med J 1991;302:493
79. Yudkin JS, Forrest RD, Jackson CA. Microalbuminuria as predictor of vascular disease in nondiabetic subjects. Lancet 1988;2:530
80. Fuller JH, Head J. Blood pressure, proteinuria and their relationship with circulatory mortality: The WHO multinational study of vascular disease in diabetics. Diabetes Metab 1989;15:273
81. Mattock MB, Morrish NJ, Viberti G, et al. Prospective study of microalbuminuria as predictor of mortality in NIDDM. Diabetes 1992;41:736
82. Barker DJP, Winter PD, Osmond C, et al. Weight in infancy and death from ischemic heart disease. Lancet 1989;2:577
83. Eriksson K-F. Prevention of non–insulin-dependent diabetes mellitus. A population study with special reference to insulin secretion, skeletal muscle morphology and metabolic capacity. Lund, Sweden: University of Lund;1992. Doctoral Thesis.
84. Krolewski AS, Warram JH, Valsania P, et al. Evolving natural history of coronary artery disease in diabetes mellitus. Am J Med 1991;90(Suppl 2A):56S
85. Haffner SM, Stern MP, Hazuda HP, et al. Cardiovascular risk factors in confirmed prediabetic individuals: Does the clock for coronary heart disease start ticking before the onset of clinical diabetes? JAMA 1990;263:2893
86. Welborn TA, Wearne K. Coronary disease incidence and cardiovascular mortality in Busselton with reference to glucose and insulin concentrations. Diabetes Care 1979;2:154
87. Pyörälä K. Relationship of glucose tolerance and plasma insulin to the incidence of coronary heart disease: Results from two population studies in Finland. Diabetes Care 1979;2:131
88. Ducimetiere P, Eschwege E, Papoz L, et al. Relationship of plasma insulin levels to the incidence of myocardial infarction and coronary heart disease mortality in a middle-aged population. Diabetologia 1980;19:205
89. Paolisso G, Gambardella A, Galzerano D, et al. Metabolic features of patients with and without coronary heart disease but with a superimposable cluster of cardiovascular risk factors. Coronary Artery Dis 1993;4:1085
90. Stout RW. Insulin and atheroma: 20-year perspective. Diabetes Care 1990; 13:631
91. Sato Y, Shiraishi S, Oshida T, et al. Experimental atherosclerosis-like lesions induced by hyperinsulinism in Wistar rats. Diabetes 1989;38:91
92. Ridray S, Heudes D, Michel O, et al. Increased SMC proliferation after endothelial injury in hyperinsulinemic obese Zucker rats. Am J Physiol 1994; 267:H1976

Diabetes Mellitus, edited by Derek LeRoith, Simeon I. Taylor, and Jerrold M. Olefsky. Lippincott–Raven Publishers, Philadelphia © 1996.

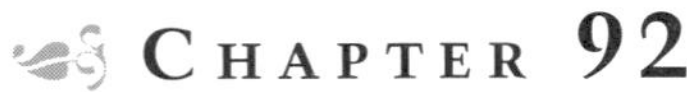

Chapter 92

The Role of Growth Factors in the Pathogenesis of Diabetic Vascular Complications

Vicky A. Blakesley and Derek LeRoith

The complications of diabetes mellitus have been well described clinically for many years. The specific mechanisms that perturb normal cellular and organ function, however, are not yet completely understood. In recent years, there have been many advances in our knowledge of the interactions of growth factors and their target cells in the eye, kidney, and peripheral vascular system. The following is a discussion of the current knowledge of the best characterized growth factors associated with the common complications of diabetes mellitus. Given the rapid accumulation of information concerning new growth factors, it is likely that the list of growth factors involved in this common disease will continue to expand.

Diabetic Retinopathy

Proliferative diabetic retinopathy is the result of a sequence of events. Microvascular ischemia, by stimulating release of angiogenic factors, is thought to play a crucial role in the pathogenesis of retinopathy. The specific mechanisms by which these angiogenic factors, now known to include several growth factors, modulate the events resulting in diabetic retinopathy have not been elucidated fully. Morphologically, the earliest identified steps in diabetic retinopathy are loss of capillary pericytes and degradation of the basement membranes of small capillaries within the retina.[1–3] Vascular endothelial cells then migrate through these defects in the basement membranes and proliferate, forming a new endothelial capillary sprout protruding from the retina into the vitreal space. Proliferation of endothelial cells extends the capillary sprout. Alignment of endothelial cells to form tubes results in a new vascular network extending from the retina. Retinal microvascular pericytes migrate along the vascular network. These aberrant capillary networks lack functional tight junctions between endothelial cells and have a scant basement membrane and a paucity of pericytes. These networks are prone to leakage with minimal provocation, and the resulting hemorrhage induces further neovascularization. The process of neovascularization is a perturbation in the balance between proteinases and proteinase inhibitors. Disruption of the basement membrane requires synthesis of several proteinases, including, but not limited to, plasminogen activators (PAs). These enzymes catalyze the conversion of plasminogen to the serine proteinase plasmin. Plasmin is partially responsible for the proteolysis of many extracellular matrix components, including laminin, fibronectin, type V collagen, and proteoglycans.[4] Plasmin can also activate procollagenase.[5] A naturally occurring inhibitor of PAs is plasminogen activator inhibitor-1 (PAI-1). Matrix metalloproteinase (MMP-2), which degrades type IV collagen, may also be involved in the disruption of the basement membrane. The proteinases and proteinase inhibitors are thought to be regulated by circulating and locally produced growth factors.[4,6–8] These growth factors also modulate endothelial cell migration and proliferation. Many investigators now believe that the endothelial cell alone is capable of producing all of the information required to orchestrate neovascularization.[7]

The concept that chemical reagents might control the development of retinal neovascularization was first postulated by Michaelson in 1948.[9] Ashton et al. extended this hypothesis to the release of a "vasoformative factor" from the retina in response to hypoxia.[9a] Since that time, investigators have searched for "factor X," the presumed growth factor hypothesized by Michaelson to be the trigger in the initiation of diabetic retinopathy. Numerous studies have documented the presence of several growth factors and their receptors within structures of the eye. Investigators recently have begun to elucidate the specific growth factors involved in diabetic retinopathy and the mechanisms by which the growth factors mediate their angiopathic effects. Until recently, however, none of the growth factors studied satisfied two criteria thought to be essential for identification of a specific growth factor as "factor X:" (1) the growth factor must be found consistently in the eyes of patients or animals with retinopathy, and (2) retinal vessel occlusion with retinal ischemia must result in accumulation of the growth factor within the eye.

The role of insulin-like growth factor-I (IGF-I) or somatomedin-C in the pathogenesis of diabetic retinopathy has been extensively studied. Using the dog as a model system, hypophysectomy was shown to improve the diabetic state, whereas injection of either pituitary extracts or purified growth hormone was found to convert normoglycemic dogs to diabetic dogs.[10] In 1969 and 1970, it was found that some patients with diabetes had increased circulating levels of growth hormone (GH).[11,12] In a controlled clinical trial, retinopathy regressed following pituitary ablation, and the degree of regression correlated with the degree of GH deficiency.[13] Subsequently, with the knowledge that most of the metabolic effects of GH are mediated by IGF-I, the role of IGF-I in the pathogenesis of diabetic retinopathy was investigated. The development or worsening of diabetic retinopathy has been observed in several cases when serum IGF-I levels have increased. In the prepubertal state, when serum IGF-I levels are low, the development of retinopathy is rare.[14–17] During puberty, with a rise in growth hormone and circulating IGF-I, diabetic retinopathy develops. Conversely, the progression of retinopathy is slowed in diabetic patients with hypopituitarism who have low serum IGF-I levels.[18,19] Further speculation that IGF-I is involved in the pathogenesis of diabetic retinopathy is based on observations that diabetic retinopathy worsens immediately following improved glycemic control, at a time when serum IGF-I levels increase as a result of improved metabolic status.[20–22] Although there are conflicting data concerning circulating serum levels of IGF-I in diabetic patients,[23,24] some investigators have documented a transient rise in serum IGF-I levels in the early phase of retinal neovascularization.[25,26] However, several cross-sectional studies of diabetic patients with and without retinopathy reveal no consistent correlation between serum IGF-I levels and retinopathy.[24,27–31] Only a few cohorts of diabetic patients have been studied longitudinally with respect to serum IGF-I levels and incidence and progression of retinopathy. One study reported a significant correlation between elevated serum IGF-I levels and progression of retinopathy.[26] Two other studies supported the conclusion that serum IGF-I was not a predictor of diabetic retinopathy.[25,32] With the knowledge that IGF-I is produced locally in tissues and may serve in a paracrine/autocrine fashion, rather than being limited to an endocrine role where it is synthesized and released from the liver following simulation by growth hormone, many investigators have begun to examine the location of IGF-I production and its actions on structures and specific cell types of the eye.[33] Vitreal levels of IGF-I were threefold higher in diabetic patients undergoing therapeutic vitrectomy than in nondiabetic patients.[23] Those patients with more rapid progression of their retinopathy had the highest levels of IGF-I in the vitreous.[26] IGF-I receptors have been localized to the retinal pigment epithelial cells and the neural retina of humans, cattle, and rodents.[23,34–38] In the retina of diabetic rats, IGF-I synthesis was not increased, but IGF-I receptors were found in all layers of the retina, and were more abundant than receptors in nondiabetic rat retina.[39] In in vivo models, active capillary proliferation was documented after implantation of intracorneal pellets containing IFG-I.[40] Results from in vitro studies support the role of IGF-I in neovascularization. IGF-I receptors are present on bovine retinal endothelial cells and microvascular pericytes grown in culture, and there is a fivefold increase in thymidine incorporation into DNA when these cells are stimulated with IGF-I.[41] IGF-I has been shown to stimulate the proliferation of human retinal pigment epithelial cells (HRECs) and to potentiate the proliferation by the more potent growth factors fibroblast growth factor (FGF) and epidermal growth factor (EGF).[42] IGF-I significantly modulates the chemotaxis of human and bovine retinal endothelial cells in a dose-dependent fashion.[8,43] The understanding of the chain of events by which IGF-I may modulate neovascularization is far from fully understood. Returning to the postulated mechanism that PA is involved in the pathogenesis of proliferative retinopathy, investigators have found that IGF-I stimulates the release of PA from HRECs of diabetic patients, but not from HRECs isolated from nondiabetic patients.[44] Thus, the evolving scenario suggests that IGF-I modulates several important processes in the pathogenesis of diabetic retinopathy, including endothelial cell proliferation, cellular migration, and release of proteinases capable of disrupting the basement membrane of the retina. Despite the body of evidence that IGF-I is involved in the progression of diabetic retinopathy, it is now considered unlikely that IGF-I is "factor X," the presumed initiation growth factor. Although IGF-I can stimulate endothelial cells in culture, IGF-I is not consistently found in the eyes of diabetic patients with retinopathy. This latter criterion is thought to be essential for the factor that initiates the pathologic effects following oxygen depletion of the retina.

Basic FGF (b-FGF) has been identified in the retina.[45,46] b-FGF binding to heparan sulfate residues in the basement membrane results in an accumulation of glycosaminoglycans, which most likely are major determinants in stabilizing the basement membrane.[47–49] It has been shown that vascular endothelial cells cultured on intact basement membrane matrices undergo decreased proliferation and have increased anatomic evidence of differentiation as compared with cells cultured on other substrates.[50–52] b-FGF has been shown to modulate several of the events thought to be crucial to the development of proliferative retinopathy. b-FGF is synthesized and released from microvascular endothelial cells[53,54] and retinal pigment epithelial cells.[55] It induces endothelial cell proliferation[45,46] and functions as a chemoattractant for endothelial cell migration in culture.[56–58] The mitogenic effect of b-FGF was synergistic with IGF-I when both were tested on HRECs, in culture.[57] In in vivo assays, such as the corneal implant assay, b-FGF stimulated neovascularization.[59] Injection of b-FGF into the vitreous cavity of cats resulted in increased uptake of radioactive thymidine into the nuclei of retinal cells as compared to that in retinal cells of control cats.[60] This result is supported by the finding of increased thymidine incorporation in cell culture after HRECs were stimulated with b-FGF.[57] The release of PA was shown to be stimulated by b-FGF,[61] and stimulation of tissue-type PA (t-PA) mRNA was seen following treatment of HRECs with b-FGF.[57] This latter effect was stimulated further by the addition of IGF-I.[57] Clinical studies also support a crucial role for b-FGF in the pathogenesis of retinopathy. Elevated levels of b-FGF were found in vitrectomy samples of diabetic patients with proliferative retinopathy, and those with active disease (hemorrhage) had higher levels of b-FGF than did patients with inactive proliferative retinopathy.[62] This growth factor is thought by some authors[63] to be a more potent mitogen and, thus, a more likely candidate for stimulation of neovascularization in the diabetic eye, than IGF-I. There is now evidence that the effects of IGF-I and b-FGF are synergistic in the steps leading to proliferative retinopathy.[57] Because b-FGF appears not to be actively secreted from intact endothelial cells, it has been postulated that the pathologic events mediated by b-FGF are triggered only when the endothelial cell is injured, thus releasing b-FGF into the vascular space. Thus, while in both in vivo and in vitro models, b-FGF accounts for most of the mitogenic activity, its angiogenic potential appears to be synergistic with the action of IGF-I on neovascularization. Like IGF-I, however, b-FGF is not consistently found in the eyes of patients with diabetic retinopathy. It is, thus, considered to be a growth factor that participates in the progression of diabetic retinopathy, but is not the initiation growth factor, "factor X."

A closely related form of fibroblast growth factor, known as acidic fibroblast growth factor (a-FGF), shares similar biologic functions with b-FGF, interacts with the same receptor, and has a similarly high binding affinity to heparin.[64] a-FGF has been shown to stimulate migration and proliferation of vascular endothelial cells, fibroblasts, glial cells, and retinal pigment epithelial cells, but has been shown to be less potent than b-FGF in these actions.[64] Investigators utilizing immunohistochemical techniques have identified a-FGF within normal human ocular structures[65] and preretinal structures (conjunctival and corneal epithelia, subcapsular epithelium of the lens, and ciliary processes) and within the retina from patients with proliferative diabetic retinopathy.[33] Stimulation by a-FGF induces vascular endothelial cells to synthesize PA, thereby implicating a-FGF as a growth factor in the progression of neovascular sprouts and development of proliferative diabetic retinopathy.[66]

EGF has been found in the preretinal membranes of patients with proliferative diabetic retinopathy[33] and, when implanted in corneal pockets in rabbits, it has been noted to stimulate neovascularization.[59] EGF receptors have also been detected in bovine retinal vessels.[67] Although EGF is known to stimulate endothelial cell growth in vitro,[68] it is less angiogenic than b-FGF.[47] The angiogenic effect of EGF is potentiated by thrombin.[68] EGF has potent mitogenic activity on HRECs, and this effect has been shown to be synergistic with that of b-FGF.[42] Because EGF has been shown to be present in plasma and platelets,[69] some investigators have postulated that retinal capillary ischemia results in thrombin release, which acts in concert with EGF from platelets and plasma to stimulate proliferation of endothelial cells. Further, synergistic action of FGF and EGF may stimulate pigment epithelial cell migration and proliferation, resulting in preretinal membrane formation.[33] To date, it has not been firmly established that EGF directly mediates any of the essential actions that lead to proliferative diabetic retinopathy. A structurally related growth factor—transforming growth factor α (TGFα)—has been shown to stimulate neovascularization in model systems other than the retina, but there is little experimental evidence to suggest its role in diabetic retinopathy. The TGFα receptor has been detected in bovine retinal vessels.[67] Once again, these growth factors do not fulfill both of the criteria thought to be essential for the growth factor that can initiate the events of neovascularization following ischemic injury in the diabetic eye.

Within the past few years, mounting evidence has led investigators to hypothesize that a growth factor that is apparently specific for the vascular epithelium is the postulated "factor X." Vascular endothelial growth factor (VEGF) was originally described from tumors and shown to make blood vessels leaky.[70,71] VEGF can induce proliferation and migration of vascular endothelial cells in culture and appears to be specific to these cells.[72–77] The VEGF receptor has been characterized from vascular endothelial cells.[70,78,79] VEGF has been shown to be produced by retinal epithelial cells, and the synthesis and release of VEGF is increased when the cells are grown under conditions of reduced oxygen tension. In animal models, the correlation between elevated levels of VEGF and the development of a disordered vascular network, which is a hallmark of diabetic retinopathy, has been studied by several groups. Following laser ablation of retinal veins in a monkey model, VEGF concentrations rose in the eye just as neovascularization was occurring on the irides.[80] As vitreal levels of VEGF declined, vascular growth stopped. In a mouse model of retinal blood vessel occlusion, VEGF levels in the eye rose just before neovascularization.[81] Furthermore, the cells producing VEGF appear to be at the leading edge of the newly vascularized retina in both mouse and kitten models.[81] Two small cross-sectional studies of patients with retinopathy showed increased vitreal VEGF levels in patients with diabetic retinopathy.[82,83] Vitreal VEGF levels were significantly elevated in patients with active blood vessel growth, whether they had proliferative diabetic retinopathy or occluded retinal veins. VEGF levels dropped an average of 75% in those patients who underwent successful laser therapy of the neovascular network.[84] In support of the hypothesis that VEGF is a vascular growth factor, vitreal fluid from patients with active retinopathy has been shown to stimulate endothelial cells in culture.[84] This stimulated proliferation could be reduced if the vitreal fluids were treated with antibodies to VEGF.[84] Of all of the growth factors yet studied, VEGF possesses the most characteristics thought to be essential for the pathologic function of "factor X." To date, VEGF has been consistently found in the eyes of patients and animals suffering from ischemia-produced proliferative retinopathy. There is a close temporal relationship between elevated vitreal VEGF levels and the appearance of new vessels. Truly convincing evidence of the role of VEGF as the initiation growth factor will be forthcoming as several investigating groups search for an inhibitor of the neovascular action of VEGF in animal models. Once a growth factor has been established as a vascular-specific initiation growth factor, therapeutic inhibitors will likely be developed and tested.

Other growth factors, such as growth hormone and platelet-derived growth factor, may be involved in the development and progression of diabetic retinopathy; however, little experimental work has been done to elucidate their roles. It is of interest to note that there may be at least one growth factor that has an inhibitory effect on the development of retinopathy. b-FGF-induced proliferation and migration of cultured fetal bovine heart endothelial cells have been found to be strongly inhibited by transforming growth factor β (TGFβ). Co-culture of retinal endothelial cells and retinal microvascular pericytes has been observed to result in decreased proliferation of the endothelial cells.[85] In one study, TGFβ was released by pericytes, provided the pericytes were contacting, or in close proximity to, retinal endothelial cells.[86] Consideration of the proposed function of TGFβ may explain the functional importance of one of the earliest morphologic changes seen in diabetic retinopathy, that is, loss of retinal capillary pericytes. The loss of pericytes would likely reduce the amount of TGFβ that could be released following appropriate stimuli. Furthermore, thickening of the basement membrane, which is a pathologic hallmark of diabetic angiopathy, would prevent the pericyte processes from contacting the endothelial cells, thereby releasing the endothelial cells from the inhibitory influence of TGFβ.[63] Both loss of pericytes and a reduction in pericyte-endothelial cell contact could result in increased endothelial cell production. Further study of the regulation of TGFβ will be needed before its role in maintenance of normal retinal vascular architecture and function can be completely understood. Further investigations will need to be done before possible therapeutic manipulations enhancing the normal inhibitory growth factors of the retinal vessels can be proposed and tested.

Diabetic Nephropathy

An increased glomerular filtration rate (GFR) has been recognized as an early manifestation of diabetes mellitus for many years.[87–91] Renal hypertrophy, however, has only been recognized clinically as a manifestation of early diabetic nephropathy for the past 20 years.[92–97] Histologically, the early changes include increased glomerular volume, increased capillary lumen area per glomerulus, and significant mesangial expansion.[98–102] In one study, intensive blood glucose control in subjects newly diagnosed with type I diabetes mellitus reduced GFR, but did not affect the renal hypertrophy.[96] A portion of diabetic patients will develop microalbuminuria within 10–20 years of diagnosis. These patients go on to develop overt diabetic nephropathy.[102a] Similar to the lack of diabetic retinopathy prior to puberty, microalbuminuria is seen in juvenile diabetics only after the age of 15 years.[103,104] This observation has led to the suggestion that GH and IGF-I are involved in the pathogenesis of diabetic nephropathy. Octreotide was found to decrease kidney volume in insulin-dependent diabetic patients as compared to patients given a placebo, without affecting glucose control.[105] Although this finding also suggests a role for GH and IGF-I in renal hypertrophy, it should be noted that somatostatin analogues are not specific GH inhibitors, and these findings do not conclusively prove that the mechanism of octreotide inhibition involves the reduction of circulating IGF-I.

Animal studies and studies of kidney cells grown in culture have implicated IGF-I in the development of diabetic nephropathy. IGF-I synthesized by the kidney does increase in hypophysectomized rats treated with growth hormone.[106,107] IGF-I mRNA has been isolated from rat and human kidneys.[106,108–112] The IGF-I protein has been found to be released from principal cells of the collecting duct and glomerular mesangial cells in culture.[108,113–115] The suggestion that locally synthesized IGF-I is involved in renal function in an autocrine or paracrine fashion is supported by the finding of IGF-I receptors throughout the kidney.[116–125] Moreover, IGF-I receptors have been identified in mesangial cells in culture.[27,117,126] Endothelial cells and epithelial cells do not produce IGF-I in culture, but have high-affinity receptors for IGF-I.[115,120] Studies to distinguish the specific roles of IGF-I produced by the liver following stimulation by growth hormone or IGF-I synthesized locally in the kidney suggest that circulating IGF-I causes glomerular enlargement, but that mesangial proliferation is not directly correlated with circulating IGF-I.[127] IGF-I synthesis in the kidney is regulated by GH[107,128–131] and GH-independent factors.[118] Streptozotocin (STZ)-diabetic rats were found to have a transient increase in renal tissue IGF-I protein just prior to the development of the initial renal hypertrophy, with levels declining to basal values in a few days.[109,123,132–136] STZ-diabetic rats rendered euglycemic by the administration of insulin did not develop renal hypertrophy, and there was no increase in IGF-I.[132,134,135] Although it did not affect blood glucose when administered to STZ-diabetic rats, octreotide did prevent an increase in kidney size and the transient rise in serum IGF-I.[133] If an IGF-I infusion is administered after the initial renal hypertrophy but when IGF-I levels have returned to basal levels, kidney tissue levels of IGF-I are again elevated and the renal hypertrophy is reaccelerated.[137] These results support the hypothesis that IGF-I is the growth factor responsible for kidney growth in early experimental diabetes mellitus. The mechanism by which IGF-I is elevated in the kidney is somewhat unclear. Although an early short-term study indicated a transient increase in kidney tissue mRNA,[138] another short-term study showed no increase in renal IGF-I mRNA.[109] More recently, a long-term study revealed that kidney tissue IGF-I mRNA was decreased from the induction of diabetes and throughout the study period.[139] Investigators have postulated either sequestration of renal IGF-I by IGF-I receptors or IGF binding proteins as the mechanism by which elevated IGF-I levels are maintained in the diabetic kidney. Increased numbers of IGF-I receptors have been observed in the kidneys of STZ-diabetic rats at later time points as compared to control rats.[122,140] IGF binding proteins are transiently increased in STZ-diabetic rats.[122,141] Also, there is a significant shift in the amounts of specific IGF binding proteins within the medulla and cortex of the kidney in experimental diabetic rats.[139] Given that some IGF binding proteins are known to potentiate the effects of IGF-I, this or the increase in IGF-I receptors may result in chronic IGF-I stimulatory effects on the kidney, despite the return of IGF-I to normal levels. The increase in kidney size may also include the expansion of extracellular material. IGF-I stimulates protein synthesis by mesangial cells in culture,[142] and in the diabetic rat model, GH administration results in increased glomerular basement membrane collagen synthesis.[143] In glomerulosclerosis, mesangial expansion is associated with increased fibronectin deposition by mesangial cells.[144] In STZ-diabetic rats, the synthesis and processing of fibronectin in fibroblasts are altered.[145] Additionally, IGF-I increases fibronectin levels in rat mesangial cells.[146] In nonobese diabetic (NOD) mice, which spontaneously develop immune-mediated insulin-dependent diabetes mellitus (IDDM) and nephropathy, laminin b1 mRNA and protein levels were increased when compared to age-matched control mice.[147] This protein is a major component of the peripheral basement membrane and glomerular mesangium. This increase of laminin b1 has also been noted in the STZ-diabetic rat model.[148–150]

The role of IGF-I on increased GFR and the subsequent development of nephropathy in the diabetic patient is less clear than the role of IGF-I in the development of renal hypertrophy. The hypothesis that IGF-I is involved in the control of GFR is supported by the finding that GH-deficient patients have low renal plasma flow (RPF) and GFR, both of which normalize after administration of GH.[151] Serum IGF-I levels rise in parallel with the increases in GFR and RPF.[152] Infusion of IGF-I into humans or rats has been found to result in increases in GFR;[152–154] however, because circulating levels of IGF-I do not strictly correlate with renal hypertrophy, some caution must be exercised in interpreting the impact of IGF-I infusions on renal function. Also of interest is the lack of correlation between kidney size and the progressive decline in GFR seen in diabetic patients as they develop diabetic nephropathy,[155,156] which suggests that those factors important for growth are not necessarily involved in renal hemodynamics. Micropuncture studies in rats receiving IGF-I by infusion show a decline in efferent and afferent arteriolar resistance, coupled with an increase in the glomerular ultrafiltration coefficient.[157] Further IGF-I infusion studies in rats have suggested that the IGF-I vasodilatory effect is mediated by kinins,[158] which are known to increase RPF.[159] Kinins generate potent stimuli for nitric oxide production, and inhibition of nitric oxide synthesis ablates the vasodilatory effect of IGF-I.[160] Thus, there is evidence that IGF-I has a direct effect on known vasodilators in the kidney, and that the concentration of IGF-I in the renal tissue or circulation may account for the hyperfiltration seen in early diabetic nephropathy.

In the STZ-diabetic rat, the early increase in kidney size is paralleled by an increase in GFR;[161,162] however, the rise in GFR persists much longer than the local increase in IGF-I levels.[162] Here again, then, mechanisms other than increased circulating IGF-I levels must be responsible for the prolonged perturbation in renal hemodynamics.

Diabetic nephropathy is considered to be a low renin state which, in some diabetic patients, may be associated with hyporeninemic hypoaldosteronism.[163–165] Renin-secreting cells are derived from vascular smooth muscle, which is known to express the IGF-I gene and to secrete IGF-I.[166,167] Renin activity in STZ-diabetic renal tissue has been found to be reduced after stimulation with IGF-I as compared to renin activity in control rats,[168] suggesting a resistant state in the diabetic rat.

EGF has been postulated to have a role in diabetic nephropathy because the urinary excretion of EGF is reduced during the development of diabetic nephropathy,[169,170] although transient increases in urinary EGF excretion can be seen early in the disease. The kidney is one of the major sites for EGF production. EGF increases IGF-I mRNA and protein in isolated rat renal collecting duct,[171] suggesting synergistic action between these two growth factors. Receptors for EGF have been identified in several segments of the nephron.[172,173] Functionally, urinary excretion of EGF has been found to correlate positively with GFR.[169]

TGF-β1 has been postulated to have a role in the pathogenesis of glomerulosclerosis. TGF-β1 is thought to be involved in the regulation of extracellular matrix deposition and has been shown to be increased in glomerosclerotic diseases in which there is an accumulation of extracellular matrix.[174] In culture, TGF-β1 has been found to stimulate extracellular matrix synthesis by glomerular epithelial cells[175] and to increase production of tenascin, an extracellular matrix protein, by fibroblasts.[176] Rat mesangial cells increase in size in response to chronic TGF-β1 treatment.[177] In animal models, the accumulation of extracellular matrix was found to be blocked by inhibition of TGF-β1 action.[178] Increased glomerular TGF-β1 mRNA levels were found 4 weeks after induction of diabetes in STZ-diabetic rats.[179] In NOD mice, increased expression of TGF-β1 mRNA correlated with increased levels of tenascin and laminin early in the development of IDDM.[147] Hyperglycemia induces nonenzymatic glycosylation of proteins and specifically leads to accumulation of kidney advance glycosylation end products (AGEs) in diabetic patients. The accumulation of AGEs has been implicated in the pathogenesis of diabetic nephropathy.[180] In cultured mesangial cells, AGEs stimulate expression of several extracellular matrix genes.[181] mRNA levels of TGF-β1 and several extracellular matrix genes were found to be increased in normal mice injected with AGEs.[182] In NOD mice, AGEs were increased concomitantly with increased TGF-β1 mRNA.[147] These observations suggest that TGF-β1 may have a role in the initiation and/or progression of renal hypertrophy in the diabetic animal. The increased expression of TGF-β1 may be in response to the accumulation of AGEs in the hyperglycemic diabetic animal.

To date, the most extensively studied growth factor involved in the pathogenesis of diabetic nephropathy has been IGF-I; however, it is obvious from the observations cited earlier that other mechanisms and, presumably, other growth factors are involved in this particular complication of diabetes mellitus. In the diabetic patient, nephropathy may also be affected by hypertension. Clinically, it has been established that reduction of blood pressure in the hypertensive diabetic patient slows the progression of renal insufficiency. Growth factors are likely mediators of the detrimental changes within the kidney in the setting of hypertension. In cultured glomerular mesangial cells of hypertensive rats, cellular mitogenesis is enhanced in the presence of IGF-I and PDGF. PDGF also stimulates cell-associated fibronectin accumulation and incorporation of proline in collagenous protein in these same cells.[183] These growth factor-stimulated increases in cellular proliferation and matrix accumulation likely contribute to glomerulosclerosis secondary to hypertension. In one study, the administration of an inhibitory antibody to PDGF to rats with mesangioproliferative glomerulonephritis prevented mesangial cell proliferation and matrix accumulation.[184] Thus, in the setting of the hypertensive diabetic patient, growth factors released in response to elevated blood pressure may mediate additional morphologic and physiologic changes in the kidney.

Diabetic Macrovascular Disease

The macrovascular complications of diabetes mellitus—stroke and coronary artery disease—are also mediated, to some degree, by growth factors. Macrovascular disease associated with diabetes mellitus shares many features with artherosclerosis seen in the absence of diabetes. The natural history includes the early "fatty streak" consisting of lipid-rich macrophages and T-lymphocytes, the intermediate atherosclerotic lesions composed of macrophages and smooth muscle cells, and finally, the fibrous plaques seen in advanced vascular occlusive disease. The development of these lesions involves the complex interaction of vascular endothelium with several growth factors produced by platelets, macrophages, T lymphocytes, and smooth muscle cells. These growth factors stimulate migration, proliferation, proteolytic activity, and organizational behavior of endothelial cells.[185] In culture, cells of various origins produce several growth factors. For example, platelets produce and, when aggregated, release PDGF, EGF/TGFα, and TGFβ; macrophages release VEGF, bFGF, and EGF/TGFα; endothelial cells release bFGF and PDGF; and smooth muscle cells release bFGF and VEGF.[186] The interaction between cell types has been studied using isolated rat aortic explants. Vascular outgrowth consisting of microvessels has been noted upon exposure of the aortic explants to VEGF.[187] PDGF and IGF-I stimulate outgrowths consisting mostly of fibroblast-like cells. By contrast, both TGF-β1 and IL-1α inhibit neovascularization. These inhibitory actions of TGF-β1 and IL-1α have also been demonstrated in cells in culture.[188,189]

In cultured cells, VEGF stimulates endothelial proliferation and migration.[75] VEGF acts synergistically with bFGF in stimulating angiogenesis.[186,190–192] Microvascular endothelial cells also proliferate in response to PDGF-BB.[193–195] In large vessels, the endothelial cells may also respond to PDGF because there is transient expression of PDGF receptors during wound healing.[196] However, it may be just as likely that the effect of PDGF on large blood vessel walls is indirect. PDGF is known to activate the expression of growth factors in other cells. The release of these factors may, in turn, stimulate angiogenesis in vivo. Likewise, in in vitro systems, IGF-I has been shown to stimulate endothelial cell proliferation.[197,198]

Conclusion

Since the postulation by Michaelson[9] in 1948 of a chemical factor released from the retina in diabetic patients in the initiation and progression of vascular changes in retina, several growth factors have been implicated in the pathogenesis of diabetic retinopathy. Although there is to date no conclusive evidence of the exact growth factor that would satisfy the criteria of an initiator molecule, it has become increasingly clear that growth factors working by both autocrine and paracrine pathways are involved in the pathogenesis of diabetic retinopathy. By analogy, and with a growing body of scientific evidence, the initiation and progression of diabetic nephropathy and macrovascular diseases are also thought to be mediated by specific growth factors. The exact inciting events that lead to activation of the growth factor-mediated pathologic events remain to be fully elucidated. In the case of diabetic glomerulosclerosis, the accumulation of AGEs appears to have a distinct role. Retinal hypoxia may be one of the initial events in the development of diabetic retinopathy. No matter the initial signal, it now appears certain that one or more growth factors are responsible for the subsequent changes in the retina and kidney characteristic of diabetes mellitus. Elucidation of the growth factors involved and their specific actions will lead not only to a better understanding of the pathogenesis of the detrimental complications of diabetes, but will also allow intervention at more specific sites to prevent or slow the progression of these complications.

References

1. Cogan DG, Toussaint D, Kuwabara T. Retinal vascular patterns. IV. Diabetic retinopathy. Arch Ophthalmol 1961;66:366
2. Kalebic T, Garbisa S, Glaser B, Liotta LA. Basement membrane collagen: Degradation by migrating endothelial cells. Science 1983;221:281
3. Ausprunk DH, Folkman J. Migration and proliferation of endothelial cells in preformed and newly formed blood vessels during tumor angiogenesis. Microvasc Res 1977;14:53
4. Gross JL, Moscatelli D, Rifkin DB. Increased capillary endothelial cell protease activity in response to angiogenic stimuli. Proc Natl Acad Sci U S A 1983;80:2623
5. Bauer PI, Machovich R, Buki KG, et al. Interaction of plasmin with endothelial cells. Biochem J 1984;218:119
6. Moscatelli D, Jagge E, Rifkin DB. Teredecanoyl phorbol acetate stimulates latent collagenase production by cultured human endothelial cells. Cell 1980;20:343
7. Sholley MM, Ferguson GP, Seibel HR, et al. Mechanisms of neovascularization. Vascular sprouting can occur without proliferation of endothelial cells. Lab Invest 1984;51:624
8. Grant M, Jerdan J, Merimee TJ. Insulin-like growth factor-I modulates endothelial cell chemotaxis. J Clin Endocrinol Metab 1987;65:370
9. Michaelson IC. The mode of development of the vascular system of the retina, with some observations on its significance for certain retinal diseases. Trans Opthalmol Soc UK 1948;68:137

9a. Ashton N, Ward B, Serpell G. Effect of oxygen on developing retinal vessels with particular reference to the problems of retrolental fibroplasia. Br J Ophthalmol 1954;38:397

10. Campbell J, Davidson IWF, Lei HP. The production of permanent diabetes by highly purified growth hormone. Endocrinology 1950;46:588
11. Yde H. Abnormal growth hormone response to ingestion of glucose in juvenile diabetics. Acta Med Scand 1969;186:499
12. Hansen AaP, Johansen K. Diurnal pattern of blood glucose, serum FFA, insulin, glucagon and growth hormone in normals and juvenile diabetics. Diabetologia 1970;6:27
13. Lundbaek K, Malmros R, Andersen HC, et al. Hypophysectomy for diabetic angiopathy: A controlled clinical trial. In: Symposium on the Treatment of Diabetic Retinopathy. Washington, DC: Public Health Service;1989:291
14. Frank RN, Hoffman WH, Podgor MJ, et al. Retinopathy in juvenile-onset diabetes of short duration. Ophthalmology 1980;87:1
15. Klein R, Klein BEK, Moss SE, et al. Retinopathy in young-onset diabetic patients. Diabetes Care 1985;8:311
16. Murphy RP, Nanda M, Plotnick L, et al. The relationship of puberty to diabetic retinopathy. Arch Opthalmol 1990;108:215
17. Kostraba JN, Dorman JS, Orchard TJ, et al. Contribution of diabetes duration before puberty to development of microvascular complications in IDDM subjects. Diabetes Care 1989;12:686
18. Merimee TJ, Fineberg SE, McKusick VA, Hall J. Diabetes mellitus and sexual ateliotic dwarfism: A comparative study. J Clin Invest 1970;49:1096
19. Merimee TJ. A follow up study of vascular disease in growth hormone deficient dwarfs with diabetes. N Engl J Med 1978;298:1217
20. The Kroc Collaborative Study Group. Blood glucose control and the evolution of diabetic retinopathy and albuminuria. A preliminary multicenter trial. N Engl J Med 1984;311:365
21. Lauritzen T, Frost-Larsen K, Larsen H-W, Deckert T, The Steno Study Group. Two years experience with continuous subcutaneous insulin infusion in relation to retinopathy and nephropathy. Diabetes 1985;34(Suppl 3):74
22. Hanssen KF, Dahl-Jorgensen K, Lauritzen T, et al. Diabetic control and microvascular complications: The near normoglycaemic experience. Diabetologia 1986;29:677
23. Grant M, Russell B, Fitzgerald C, Merimee TJ. Insulin-like growth factors in vitreous: Studies in control and diabetic subjects with neovascularization. Diabetes 1986;35:416
24. Arner P, Sjoberg S, Gjotterberg M, Skottner A. Circulating insulin-like growth factor I in type I (insulin-dependent) diabetic patients with retinopathy. Diabetologia 1989;32:753
25. Hyer SL, Sharp PS, Brooks RA, et al. A two-year follow-up study of serum insulin-like growth factor-I in diabetics with retinopathy. Metabolism 1989;38:586
26. Merimee TJ, Zapf J, Froesch ER. Insulin-like growth factors: Studies in diabetics with and without retinopathy. N Engl J Med 1983;309:527
27. Cohen MP, Jasti K, Rye DL. Somatomedin in insulin-dependent diabetes mellitus. J Clin Endocrinol Metab 1977;45:236
28. Tan K, Baxter RC. Serum insulin-like growth factor levels in adult diabetic patients: The effect of age. J Clin Endocrinol Metab 1986;63:651
29. Hyer SL, Sharp PS, Brooks RA, et al. Serum IGF-I concentration in diabetic retinopathy. Diabetes Med 1988;5:356
30. Hyer SL, Sharp PS, Sleightholm M, et al. Progression of diabetic retinopathy and change in serum insulin-like growth factor I (IGF-I) during continuous subcutaneous insulin infusion (CSII). Horm Metab Res 1989;21:18
31. Nardelli GM, Guastamacchia E, Paolo SD, et al. Somatomedin-C (SM-C). Study in diabetic patients with and without retinopathy. Acta Diabetol Lat 1989;26:217
32. Wang Q, Dills DG, Klein R, et al. Does insulin-like growth factor I predict incidence and progression of diabetic retinopathy? Diabetes 1995;44:161

33. Fredj-Reygrobellet D, Baudouin Ch, Negre F, et al. Acidic FGF and other growth factors in preretinal membranes from patients with diabetic retinopathy and proliferative vitreoretinopathy. Ophthalmic Res 1991;23:154
34. Ocrant I, Valentino KL, King MC, et al. Localization and structural characterization of insulin-like growth factor receptors in mammalian retina. Endocrinology 1989;125:2407
35. Das A, Pansky B, Budd G, Kollaritis C. Immunocytochemistry of mouse and human retina with antisera to insulin and S-100 protein. Curr Eye Res 1984;3:1397
36. Das A, Pansky B, Budd G. Demonstration of insulin-specific mRNA in cultured rat retinal glial cells. Invest Ophthalmol Vis Sci 1987;28:1800
37. Waldbillig RJ, Fletcher RT, Sommers RL, Chader GF. IGF-I receptor in the bovine neural retina: Structure, kinase activity and comparison with retinal insulin receptors. Exp Eye Res 1988;47:587
38. Martin DM, Yee D, Feldman EL. Gene expression of the insulin-like growth factors and their receptors in cultured human retinal pigment epithelial cells. Mol Brain Res 1992;12:181
39. Charkrabarti S, Ghahary A, Murphy LJ, Sima AAF. Insulin-like growth factor-I expression is not increased in the retina of diabetic BB/W-rats. Diabetes Res Clin Pract 1991;14:91
40. Fitzgerald C, Grant M, Guay C. Stimulation of in vivo neovascularization by insulin-like growth factor-I. Invest Ophthalmol Vis Sci 1990;31:195
41. King GL, Goodman AD, Buzney S, et al. Receptors and growth-promoting effects of insulin and insulin-like growth factors on cells from bovine retinal capillaries and aorta. J Clin Invest 1985;75:1028
42. Leschey KH, Hackett SF, Singer JH, Campochiaro PA. Growth factor responsiveness of human retinal pigment epithelial cells. Invest Ophthalmol Vis Sci 1990;31:839
43. Grant MB, Guay C, Marsh R. Insulin-like growth factor I stimulates proliferation, migration, and plasminogen activator release by human retinal pigment epithelial cells. Curr Eye Res 1990;9:323
44. Grant MB, Guay C. Plasminogen activator production by human retina endothelial cells of nondiabetic and diabetic origin. Invest Ophthalmol Vis Sci 1991;32:53
45. Baird A, Esch F, Gospodarowicz D, Guillemin L. Retina- and eye-derived endothelial cell growth factors: Partial molecular characterization and identity with acidic and basic fibroblast growth factors. Biochemistry 1985;24:7855
46. Gospodarowicz D, Massoglia S, Cheng J, Fujii DK. Effect of retina-derived basic and acidic fibroblast growth factor and lipoproteins on the proliferation of retina-derived capillary endothelial cells. Exp Eye Res 1986;43:450
47. Folkman J, Klagsbrun M, Sasse J, et al. A heparin-binding angiogenic protein—basic fibroblast growth factor—is stored within basement membrane. Am J Pathol 1988;130:393
48. Vigny M, Ollier-Hartmann MP, Lavigne M, et al. Specific binding of basic fibroblast growth factor to basement membrane-like structures and to purified heparan sulfate proteoglycan of the EHS tumor. J Cell Physiol 1988; 137:321
49. Gonzalez A-M, Buscaglia M, Ong M, Baird A. Distribution of basic fibroblast growth factor in the 18-day rat fetus: Localization in the basement membranes of diverse tissues. J Cell Biol 1990;110:753
50. Madri JA, Williams SK, Capillary endothelial cell cultures: Phenotypic modulation by matrix components. J Cell Biol 1983;97:153
51. Kubota Y, Kleinman HK, Martin GR, Lawley TJ. Role of laminin and basement membrane in the morphological differentiation of human endothelial cells into capillary-like structures. J Cell Biol 1988;107:1589
52. Kennedy A, Frank RN, Sotolongo LB, et al. Proliferative response and macromolecular synthesis by ocular cells cultured on extracellular matrix materials. Curr Eye Res 1990;9:307
53. Schweigerer L, Neufeld G, Friedman J, et al. Capillary endothelial cells express basic fibroblast growth factor, a mitogen that promotes their own growth. Nature 1987;325:257
54. McNeil PL, Muthukrishnan L, Warder E, D'Armore PA. Growth factors are released by mechanically wounded endothelial cells. J Biol Chem 1989; 109:811
55. Schweigerer L, Malerstein B, Neufeld G, Gospodarowicz D. Basic fibroblast growth factor is synthesized in cultured retinal pigment epithelial cells. Biochem Biophys Res Commun 1987;143:934
56. Gospodarowicz D. Localisation of a fibroblast growth factor and its effect alone and with hydrocortisone on 3T3 cell growth. Nature 1974;249:123
57. Grant MB, Caballero S, Millard WJ. Inhibition of IGF-I and b-FGF stimulated growth of human retinal endothelial cells by the somatostatin analogue, octreotide: A potential treatment for ocular neovascularization. Regul Pept 1993;48:267
58. Herman IM, D'Amore PA. Capillary endothelial cell migration. Loss of stress fibers in response to retina-derived growth factor. J Muscle Res Cell Motil 1984;5:697
59. Gospodarowicz D, Bialecki H, Thakral T. The angiogenic activity of the fibroblast and epidermal growth factor. Exp Eye Res 1979;28:501
60. de Juan E, Strefansson E, Ohiro A. Basic fibroblast growth factor stimulates ^{3}H-thymidine uptake in retinal venular and capillary endothelial cells in vivo. Invest Ophthalmol Vis Sci 1990;31:1238
61. Presta M, Moscatelli D, Joseph-Silverstein J, Rifkin DB. Purification from a human hepatoma cell line of a basic fibroblast growth factor-like molecule that stimulates capillary endothelial cell plasminogen activator production, DNA synthesis, and migration. Mol Cell Biol 1986;6:4060
62. Sivalingam A, Kenney J, Brown GC, et al. Basic fibroblast growth factor levels in the vitreous of patients with proliferative diabetic retinopathy. Arch Ophthalmol 1990;108:869
63. Frank RN. On the pathogenesis of diabetic retinopathy: A 1990 update. Ophthalmology 1991;98:586
64. Gospodarowicz D, Ferrara N, Schweigerer L, Neufeld G. Structural characterization and biological functions of fibroblast growth factor. Endocr Rev 1987;8:95
65. Baudouin Ch. Fredj-Reygrobellet D, Caruelle JP. Acidic fibroblast growth factor distribution in normal human eye and possible implications in ocular pathogenesis. Ophthalmic Res 1990;22:73
66. Montesano R, Vassali JD, Baird A, et al. Basic growth factor induces angiogenesis in vitro. Proc Natl Acad Sci U S A 1986;83:7297
67. Fassio JB, Brockman EB, Jumblatt M, et al. Transforming growth factor alpha and its receptor in neural retina. Invest Ophthalmol Vis Sci 1989;30:1916
68. Gospodarowicz D, Brown KD, Birdwell CR, Zetter BR. Control of proliferation of human vascular endothelial cells. Characterization of the response of human umbilical vein endothelial cells to fibroblast growth factor, epidermal growth factor and thrombin. J Cell Biol 1978;77:774
69. Byyny RL, Orth DN, Cohen S. Epidermal growth factor: Effects of androgens and adrenergic agents. Endocrinology 1974;95:776
70. Houck KA, Leung DW, Rowland AM, et al. Dual regulation of vascular endothelial growth factor bioavailability by genetic and proteolytic mechanisms. J Biol Chem 1992;267:26031
71. Senger DR, Van de Water L, Brown LF, et al. Vascular permeability factor (VPF, VEGF) in tumor biology. Cancer Metastasis Rev 1993;12:303
72. Connolly DT, Heuvelman DM, Nelson R, et al. Tumor vascular permeability factor stimulates endothelial cell growth and angiogenesis. J Clin Invest 1989;84:1470
73. Gospodarowicz D, Abraham JA, Schilling J. Isolation and characterization of a vascular endothelial cell mitogen produced by pituitary-derived folliculo stellate cells. Proc Natl Acad Sci U S A 1989;86:7311
74. Keck PJ, Hauser SD, Krivi G, et al. Vascular permeability factor, an endothelial cell mitogen related to PDGF. Science 1989;246:1309
75. Leung DW, Cachianes G, Kuang WJ, et al. Vascular endothelial growth factor is a secreted angiogenic mitogen. Science 1989;246:1306
76. Plouet D, Gitay-Goren H, Safran M, et al. Isolation and characterization of a newly identified endothelial cell mitogen produced by AtT-20 cells. EMBO J 1989;8:3801
77. Tischer E, Gospodarowicz D, Mitchell R, et al. Vascular endothelial growth factor: A new member of the platelet-derived growth factor gene family. Biochem Biophys Res Commun 1989;165:1198
78. Plouet J, Moukadiri H. Characterization of the receptor to vasculotropin on bovine adrenal cortex-derived capillary endothelial cells. J Biol Chem 1990; 265:22071
79. Olander JV, Connolly DT, DeLarco JE. Specific binding of vascular permeability factor to endothelial cells. Biochem Biophys Res Commun 1991; 175:68
80. Miller JW, Adamis AP, Shima DT, D'Amore PA. Vascular endothelial growth factor/vascular permeability factor is temporally and spatially correlated with ocular angiogenesis in a primate model. Am J Pathol 1994;145:574
81. Pierce EA, Avery RL, Foley ED, et al. Vascular endothelial growth factor/ vascular permeability factor expression in a mouse model of retinal neovascularization. Proc Natl Acad Sci U S A 1995;92:905
82. Adamis AP, Miller JW, Bernal M-T, C'Amico DJ. Increased vascular endothelial growth factor levels in the vitreous of eyes with proliferative diabetic retinopathy. Am J Ophthalmol 1994;118:445
83. Malecaze F, Clamens S, Simorre-Pinatel V, et al. Detection of vascular endothelial growth factor messenger RNA and vascular endothelial growth factor-like activity in proliferative diabetic retinopathy. Arch Ophthalmol 1994;112:1476
84. Aiello LP, Avery RL, Arrigg PG, et al. Vascular endothelial growth factor in ocular fluid of patients with diabetic retinopathy and other retinal disorders. N Engl J Med 1994;331:1480
85. Orlidge A, D'Amore PA. Inhibition of capillary endothelial cell growth by pericytes and smooth muscle cells. J Cell Biol 1987;105:1455
86. Antonelli-Orlidge A, Saunders KB, Smith SR, D'Amore PA. An activated form of transforming growth factor β is produced by cocultures of endothelial cells and pericytes. Proc Natl Acad Sci U S A 1989;86:4544
87. Stadler G, Schmid R. Severe functional disorders of glomerular capillaries and renal hemodynamics in treated diabetes mellitus during childhood. Ann Pediatr 1959;193:129
88. Mogensen CE. Kidney function and glomerular permeability to macromolecules in early juvenile diabetes. Scand J Clin Lab Invest 1971;28:79
89. Mogensen CE. Glomerular filtration rate and renal plasma flow in short-term and long-term juvenile diabetes. Scand J Clin Lab Invest 1971;28:91
90. Ditzel J, Junker K. Abnormal glomerular filtration rate, renal plasma flow and renal protein excretion in recent short-term diabetics. Br Med J 1972;2:13
91. Mogensen CE. Glomerular filtration rate and renal plasma flow in long-term juvenile diabetics without proteinuria. Br Med J 1972;4:257
92. Mogensen CE, Andersen MJF. Increased kidney size and glomerular filtration rate in early juvenile diabetes. Diabetes 1973;22:706
93. Mogensen CE. Renal function changes in diabetes. Diabetes 1976;25:872
94. Garcia-Puig J, Anton FM, Grande C, et al. Relation of kidney size to kidney function in early insulin-dependent diabetes. Diabetologia 1981;21:363
95. Christiansen JS, Gammelgaard J, Frandsen M, Parving H-H. Increased kidney size, glomerular filtration rate and renal plasma flow in short-term insulin-dependent diabetics. Diabetologia 1981;20:451

96. Christiansen JS, Gammelgaard J, Tronier B, et al. Kidney function and size in diabetics before and during initial insulin treatment. Kidney Int 1982;21:683
97. Schweiger J, Fine LG. Renal hypertrophy, growth factors, and nephropathy in diabetes mellitus. Semin Nephrol 1990;10:242
98. Kroustrup JP, Gundersen HJG, Osterby R. Glomerular size and structure in diabetes mellitus. III. Early enlargement of the capillary surface. Diabetologia 1977;13:207
99. Hirose K, Tsuchida H, Osterby R, Gundersen HJG. A strong correlation between glomerular filtration rate and filtration surface area in diabetic kidney hyperfunction. Lab Invest 1980;43:434
100. Gundersen HJG, Gotzsche O, Hirose K, et al. Early structural changes in glomerular capillaries. Acta Endocrinol 1981;242(Suppl.):19
101. Osterby R, Gundersen HJG. Glomerular size and structure in diabetes mellitus. Late abnormalities. Diabetologia 1975;11:225
102. Mauer SM, Steffes MW, Ellis EN, et al. Structural-functional relationships in diabetic nephropathy. J Clin Invest 1984;74:1143
102a. Mogensen CE, Christensen CK. Predicting diabetic nephropathy in insulin-dependent diabetic patients. N Engl J Med 1984;311:89
103. Dahlquist G, Rudberg S. Microalbuminuria in diabetic children and adolescents and its relationship to puberty. Pediatr Adolesc Endocrinol 1988;17:153
104. Mathiesen ER, Saurbrey N, Hommel D, Parving H-H. Microalbuminuria in children with insulin-dependent diabetes mellitus. Pediatr Adolesc Endocrinol 1988;17:162
105. Serri O, Beauregard H, Brazeau P, et al. Somatostatin analogue, octreotide, reduces increased glomerular filtration rate and kidney size in insulin-dependent diabetes. JAMA 1991;264:888
106. D'Ercole AJ, Stiles AD, Underwood LE. Tissue concentrations of somatomedin C: Further evidence for multiple sites of synthesis and paracrine or autocrine mechanisms of action. Proc Natl Acad Sci U S A 1984;81:935
107. Lajara R, Rotwein P, Bortz JD, et al. Dual regulation of insulin-like growth factor I expression during renal hypertrophy. Am J Physiol 1989;257:F252
108. Bortz JD, Rotwein P, DeVol D, et al. Focal expression of insulin-like growth factor 1 in rat kidney collecting duct. J Cell Biol 1988;107:811
109. Flyvbjerg A, Bornfeldt KE, Marshall SM, et al. Kidney IGF-I mRNA in initial renal hypertrophy in experimental diabetes in the rat. Diabetologia 1990;33:334
110. Murphy LJ, Bell GI, Freisen HG. Tissue distribution of insulin-like growth factor I and II ribonucleic acid in the adult rat. Endocrinology 1987;120:1279
111. Hammerman MR, Miller SB. The growth hormone insulin-like growth factor axis in kidney revisited. Am J Physiol 1993;265:F1
112. Flyvbjerg A, Marshall SM, Fystyk J, et al. Insulin-like growth factor I in initial renal hypertrophy in potassium depleted rats. Am J Physiol 1992;262:F1023
113. Andersson I, Billig H, Fryklund L, et al. Localization of IGF-I in adult rats: Immunohistochemical studies. Acta Physiol Scand 1986;126:311
114. Hansson HA, Nilsson A, Isgard J, et al. Immunohistochemical localisation of insulin-like growth factor I in the adult rat. Histochemie 1988;89:403
115. Conti FG, Striker LJ, Elliot SJ, et al. Synthesis and release of insulin-like growth factor I by mesangial cells in culture. Am J Physiol 1988;255:F1214
116. Hammerman MR, Rogers S. Distribution of IGF receptors in the plasma membrane of proximal tubular cells. Am J Physiol 1987;253:F841
117. Arnqvist HJ, Ballerman BJ, King GL. Receptors for and effects of insulin and IGF-I in rat glomerular mesangial cells. Am J Physiol 1988;254:C411
118. Conti FG, Striker LJ, Lesniak MA, et al. Studies on binding and mitogenic effect of insulin and insulin-like growth factor 1 in glomerular mesangial cells. Endocrinology 1988;122:2788
119. Pillion DJ, Haskell JF, Meezan E. Distinct receptors for insulin-like growth factor I in rat renal glomeruli and tubules. Am J Physiol 1988;255:E504
120. Aron DC, Rosenzweig JL, Abboud HE. Synthesis and binding of insulin-like growth factor 1 by human glomerular mesangial cells. J Clin Endocrinol Metab 1989;68:585
121. Conti FG, Elliot SJ, Striker LJ, Striker GE. Binding of insulin-like growth factor-I by glomerular endothelial and epithelial cells: Further evidence for IGF-I action in the renal glomerulus. Biochem Biophys Res Commun 1989;163:952
122. Werner H, Shen-Orr Z, Stannard B, et al. Experimental diabetes increases insulin-like growth factor I and II receptor concentration and gene expression in kidney. Diabetes 1990;39:1490
123. Bach LA, Cox AJ, Mendelsohn FAO, et al. Focal induction of IGF binding proteins in proximal tubules of diabetic rat kidney. Diabetes 1992;41:499
124. Chin E, Bondy C. Insulin-like growth factor system gene expression in the human kidney. J Clin Endocrinol Metab 1992;75:962
125. Flyvbjerg A, Nielsen S, Sheikh MI, et al. Luminal and basolateral uptake and receptor binding of IGF-I in rabbit renal proximal tubules. Am J Physiol 1993;43:797
126. Norman JT, Kleinman KS, Bacay A, Fine LG. Renal tubular epithelial cells release factors which modulate fibroblast function: Implications for pathogenesis of interstitial nephritis (Abstract). Kidney Int 1989;35:179
127. Doi T, Striker LJ, Quaife C, et al. Progressive glomerulosclerosis develops in transgenic mice chronically expressing growth hormone and growth hormone releasing factor but not in those expressing insulin-like growth factor 1. Am J Pathol 1988;131:398
128. D'Ercole AJ, Underwood LE. Estimation of tissue concentrations of somatomedin C/insulin-like growth factor I. Methods Enzymol 1988;146:227
129. Murphy LJ, Bell GI, Friesen HG. Growth hormone stimulates sequential induction of c-myc and insulin-like growth factor I expression in vivo. Endocrinology 1987;120:1806
130. Rogers SA, Miller SB, Hammerman MR. Growth hormone stimulates IGF-I gene expression in isolated rat renal collecting duct. Am J Physiol 1990;259:F474
131. Miller SB, Rotwein P, Bortz JD, et al. Renal expression of IGF-I in hypersomatrotropic states. Am J Physiol 1990;259:F251
132. Flyvbjerg A, Thorlacius-Ussing O, Nearaa R, et al. Kidney tissue somatomedin C and initial renal growth in diabetic and uninephrectomized rats. Diabetologia 1988;31:310
133. Flyvbjerg A, Fyrstyk J, Thorlacius-Ussing O, Orskov H. Somatostatin analogue administration prevents increase in kidney somatomedin C and initial renal growth in diabetic and uninephrectomized rats. Diabetologia 1989; 32:261
134. Flyvbjerg A, Frystyk J, Osterby R, Orskov H. Kidney IGF-I and renal hypertrophy in GH deficient dwarf rats. Am J Physiol 1992;262:E956
135. Flyvbjerg A. The role of insulin-like growth factor I in initial renal hypertrophy in experimental diabetes. In: Flyvbjerg A, Orskov H, Alberti KBMM, eds. Growth Hormone and Insulin-Like Growth Factor I in Human and Experimental Diabetes. Chichester: Wiley;1993:271
136. Bach LA, Jerums G. Effect of puberty on initial kidney growth and rise in kidney IGF-I in diabetic rats. Diabetes 1990;39:557
137. Flyvbjerg A, Bornfeldt KE, Orskov H, Arnqvist HJ. Effect of insulin-like growth factor I infusion on renal hypertrophy in experimental diabetes mellitus in rats. Diabetologia 1991;34:715
138. Bach LA, Stevenson JL, Allen TJ, et al. Kidney insulin-like growth factor I mRNA levels are increased in postpubertal diabetic rats. J Endocrinol 1991; 129:5
139. Landau D, Chin E, Bondy C, et al. Expression of insulin-like growth factor binding proteins in the rat kidney: Effects of long-term diabetes. Endocrinology 1995;136:1835
140. Oemar BS, Foellmer HG, Hodgdon-Anandant L, Rosenzweig SA. Regulation of insulin-like growth factor I receptors in diabetic mesangial cells. J Biol Chem 1991;266:2369
141. Flyvbjerg A, Kessler U, Dorka B, et al. Transient increase in renal IGF binding proteins during initial kidney hypertrophy in experimental diabetes in rats. Diabetologia 1992;35:589
142. Moran A, Brown DM, Kim Y, Klein DJ. Effects of IGF-I and glucose on protein and proteoglycan synthesis by human fetal mesangial cells in culture. Diabetes 1991;40:1346
143. Reddi AS. Metabolism of glomerular basement membrane in normal, hypophysectomized, and growth-hormone-treated diabetic rats. Exp Mol Pathol 1985;43
144. Bergijk EC, Munaut C, Baelde JJ, et al. A histologic study of the extracellular matrix during the development of glomerulosclerosis in murine chronic graft-versus-host disease. Am J Pathol 1992;140:1147
145. Phan-Thanh I, Robert L, Derouette JC, Labat-Robert J. Increased biosynthesis and processing of fibronectin in fibroblasts from diabetic mice. Proc Natl Acad Sci U S A 1987;84:1911
146. Tamaroglio TA, Lo CS. Regulation of fibronectin by insulin-like growth factor-I in cultured rat thoracic aortic smooth muscle cells and glomerular mesangial cells. Exp Cell Res 1994;215:338
147. Yang C-W, Hattori M, Vlassara H, et al. Overexpression of TGF-β1 mRNA is associated with upregulation of glomerular tenascin and laminin gene expression in diabetic NOD mice. J Am Soc Nephrol 1995;5:1610
148. Killen PD, Ebihara I, Martin GR, et al. mRNA levels for laminin and collagen IV chains in diabetic kidneys (Abstract). Kidney Int 1987;31:171
149. Poulsom R, Kurkinen M, Prockop DJ, Boot-Handford RP. Increased steady-state levels of laminin B1 mRNA in kidneys of long-term streptozotocin-diabetic rats. No effect of an aldose reductase inhibitor. J Biol Chem 1988; 263:10072
150. Fukui M, Nakamura R, Ebihara I, et al. ECM gene expression and its modulation by insulin in diabetic rats. Diabetes 1992;41:1520
151. Christiansen JS, Gammelgaard J, Orskov H, et al. Kidney function and size in normal subjects before and during growth hormone administration for one week. Eur J Clin Invest 1981;11:487
152. Hirschberg R, Kopple JD. Evidence that insulin-like growth factor 1 increases renal plasma flow and glomerular filtration rate in fasted rats. J Clin Invest 1989;83:326
153. Guler H-P, Eckardt K-U, Zapf J, et al. Insulin-like growth factor 1 increases glomerular filtration rate and renal plasma flow in man. Acta Endocrinol 1989;121:101
154. Hirschberg R, Brunori G, Kopple JD, Guler H-P. Effects of insulin-like growth factor I on renal function in normal men. Kidney Int 1993;43:387
155. Wiseman MJ, Saunders AJ, Keen H, Viberti GC. Effect of blood glucose control on increased glomerular filtration rate and kidney size in insulin-dependent diabetes. N Engl J Med 1985;312:617
156. Christensen CK, Christiansen JS, Christensen T, et al. The effect of six months continuous subcutaneous insulin infusion on kidney function and size in insulin-dependent diabetes. Diabetes Med 1986;3:29
157. Hirschberg R, Kopple JD, Blantz RC, Tucker BJ. Effects of recombinant human insulin-like growth factor 1 on glomerular dynamics in the rat. J Clin Invest 1991;87:1200
158. Jaffa AA, LeRoith D, Roberts CT Jr, et al. Insulin-like growth factor I produces renal hyperfiltration by a kinin-mediated mechanism. Am J Physiol 1994;266:F102
159. Baylis C, Deen WM, Myers D, Brenner BM. Effects of some vasodilator drugs on transcapillary fluid exchange in renal cortex. Am J Physiol 1976; 230:1148

160. Haylor J, Singh I, El Nahas MA. Nitric oxide synthesis inhibitor prevents vasodilation by insulin like growth factor 1. Kidney Int 1991;39:333
161. Cortes P, Levin NW, Dumler F, et al. Uridine triphosphate and RNA synthesis during diabetes-induced renal growth. Am J Physiol 1980;238:E349
162. Allen TJ, Cooper ME, O'Brien RC, et al. Glomerular filtration rate in streptozocin-induced rats: Role of exchangeable sodium, vasoactive hormones and insulin therapy. Diabetes 1990;39:1182
163. Christlieb AR. Diabetes and hypertensive vascular disease. Mechanisms and treatment. Am J Cardiol 1973;32:592
164. Christlieb AR. Angiotensin-aldosterone system in diabetes mellitus. Diabetes 1976;25:820
165. Cohen A, McCarthy D, Rosset R. Renin secretion by the spontaneously diabetic rat. Diabetes 1986;35:341
166. Barajas L. Anatomy of the juxtaglomerular apparatus. Am J Physiol 1979; 249:F175
167. Delafontaine P, Bernstein K, Alexander R. Insulin-like growth factor I gene expression in vascular cells. Hypertension 1991;17:693
168. Jost-Vu E, Horton R, Antonipillai I. Altered regulation of renin secretion by insulinlike growth factors and angiotensin II in diabetic rats. Diabetes 1992;41:1100
169. Mathiesen ER, Nexo E, Hommel E, Parving H-H. Reduced urinary excretion of epidermal growth factor in incipient and overt diabetic nephropathy. Diabetes Med 1989;6:121
170. Dagogo-Jack S, Marshall SM, Kendall-Taylor P, Alberti KGMM. Urinary excretion of human epidermal growth factor in the various stages of diabetic nephropathy. Clin Endocrinol (Oxf) 1989;31:167
171. Rogers SA, Miller SB, Hammerman MR. Insulin-like growth factor I gene expression in isolated rat renal collecting duct is stimulated by epidermal growth factor. J Clin Invest 1991;87:347
172. Breyer J, Harris R. EGF binds to specific EGF receptors and stimulates mitogenesis in renal medullary interstitial cells (Abstract). Kidney Int 1988; 33:255
173. Gustavson B, Cowley G, Smith JA, Ozanne B. Cellular localization of human epidermal growth factor receptor. Cell Biol Int Rep 1984;8:649
174. Sharma K, Ziyadeh FN. The transforming growth factor-β system and the kidney. Semin Nephrol 1993;13:116
175. Nakamura T, Miller D, Ruoslahti E, Border WA. Production of extracellular matrix by glomerular epithelial cells is regulated by transforming growth factor-β1. Kidney Int 1992;41:1213
176. Pearson CA, Pearson D, Shibahara S, et al. Tenascin: cDNA cloning and induction of TGF-β. EMBO J 1988;7:2977
177. Choi ME, Kim EG, Huang Q, Ballermann BJ. Rat mesangial cell hypertrophy in response to transforming growth factor-β1. Kidney Int 1993;44:948
178. Border WA, Noble NA, Yamamoto T, et al. Natural inhibitor of transforming growth factor-β protects against scarring in experimental kidney disease. Nature 1992;360:361
179. Nakamura T, Fukui M, Ebihara I, et al. mRNA expression of growth factors in glomeruli from diabetic rats. Diabetes 1993;42:450
180. Brownlee M, Cerami A, Vlassara H. Advanced glycosylation end products in tissue and the biochemical basis of diabetic complications. N Engl J Med 1988;318:1315
181. Doi T, Vlassara H, Kirstein M, et al. Receptor-specific increase in extracellular matrix production in mouse mesangial cells by advanced glycosylation end products is mediated via platelet-derived growth factor. Proc Natl Acad Sci U S A 1992;89:2873
182. Yang C-W, Vlassara H, Peten EP, et al. Advanced glycation endproducts up-regulate gene expression found in diabetic glomerular disease. Proc Natl Acad Sci U S A 1994;91:9436
183. Heidenreich S, Tepel M, Lang D, et al. Differential effects of insulin-like growth factor I and platelet-derived growth factor on growth response, matrix formation, and cytosolic free calcium of glomerular mesangial cells of spontaneously hypertensive and normotensive rats. Nephron 1994;68:481
184. Iida H, Seifert R, Alpers CE, et al. Platelet-derived growth factor (PDGF) and PDGF receptor are induced in mesangial proliferative nephritis in the rat. Proc Natl Acad Sci U S A 1991;88:6560
185. Folkman J, Shing Y. Angiogenesis. J Biol Chem 1992;267:10931
186. Ferrara N, Winer J, Burton T. Aortic smooth muscle cells express and secrete vascular endothelial growth factor. Growth Factors 1991;5:141
187. Nicosia RF, Nicosia SV, Smith M. Vascular endothelial growth factor, platelet-derived growth factor, and insulin-like growth factor-1 promote rat aortic angiogenesis *in vitro*. Am J Pathol 1994;145:1023
188. RayChaudhury A, D'Amore PA. Endothelial cell regulation by transforming growth factor β. J Cell Biochem 1991;47:224
189. Cozzolino F, Torcia M, Aldinucci D, et al. Interleukin 1 as autocrine regulator of human endothelial cell growth. Proc Natl Acad Sci U S A 1990;87: 6487
190. Finkenzeller G, Marme D, Weich HA, Hug H. Platelet-derived growth factor–induced transcription of the vascular endothelial growth-factor gene is mediated by protein kinase C. Cancer Res 1992;52:4821
191. Pepper MS, Ferrara N, Orci L, Montesano R. Potent synergism between vascular endothelial growth factor and basic fibroblast growth factor in the induction of angiogenesis *in vitro*. Biochem Biophys Res Commun 1992; 189:824
192. Bobik A, Campbell JH. Vascular derived growth factors: Cell biology, pathophysiology, and pharmacology. Pharmacol Rev 1993;45:1
193. Bar RS, Boes M, Booth BA, et al. The effects of platelet-derived growth factor in cultured microvessel endothelial cells. Endocrinology 1989; 124:1841
194. Beitz JG, Kim IS, Calabresi P, Frackelton AR Jr. Receptors for platelet-derived growth factor on microvascular endothelial cells. EXS 1992;61:85
195. Marx M, Perlmutter RA, Madri JA. Modulation of platelet-derived growth factor expression in microvascular endothelial cells during in vitro angiogenesis. J Clin Invest 1994;93:131
196. Antoniades HN, Galanopoulos T, Neville-Golden J, et al. Injury induces *in vivo* expression of platelet-derived growth factor (PDGF) and PDGF receptor mRNAs in skin epithelial cells and PDGF mRNA in connective tissue fibroblasts. Proc Natl Acad Sci U S A 1991;88:565
197. Nakao-Hayashi J, Ito H, Kanayasu T, et al. Stimulatory effects of insulin and insulin-like growth factor I on migration and tube formation by vascular endothelial cells. Atherosclerosis 1992;92:141
198. Grant MB, Mames RN, Fitzgerald C, et al. Insulin-like growth factor I as an angiogenic agent. *In vivo* and *in vitro* studies. Ann NY Acad Sci 1993;692:230

Diabetes Mellitus, edited by Derek LeRoith, Simeon I. Taylor, and Jerrold M. Olefsky. Lippincott–Raven Publishers, Philadelphia © 1996.

CHAPTER 93
Pathogenesis of Platelet Dysfunction in Diabetes

ROGER D. NOLAN AND AARON I. VINIK

Platelets are small, anucleate, discoid cells that circulate in the bloodstream and participate in hemostasis. Their main function is to plug holes in blood vessel walls, and they do this by undergoing a change in shape, adhering to subendothelial surfaces, secreting the contents of intracellular organelles, and aggregating to form a thrombus in response to stimuli present in the area surrounding a damaged site in a blood vessel. Such stimuli are proaggregatory and include thrombin, collagen, and epinephrine, which are exogenous to the platelet; and agents, such as ADP (which is secreted from platelet storage granules) and thromboxane A_2 (TxA_2, which is synthesized by the platelets during activation) (see review in refs. 1 and 2).

During aggregation, platelets secrete components of the blood coagulation pathway and growth factors necessary for healing the wound in the vessel. Activation of platelets also results in changes in the level of expression of surface glycoproteins (GP) (both integrins and nonintegrins), which act as receptors for platelet agonists and for adhesive proteins involved in platelet aggregation (Fig. 93-1). P-selectin (also known as GMP-140) is translocated from the membrane of α-granules to the plasma membrane after thrombin activation of platelets,[3] the GPIIb-IIIa complex on the plasma membrane undergoes a conformational change that exposes a fibrinogen binding site,[4] thrombospondin binding to GPIV is increased by platelet activation,[5] and the von Willebrand factor–binding site on the GPIb-IX complex is downregulated by thrombin.[6] Detection of these activation-dependent platelet surface changes by specific antibodies has been utilized as a sensitive assay of platelet activation in whole blood.[7]

Antiaggregatory agents also contribute to platelet function. They are released by intact vascular endothelium and antagonize the effects of proaggregants so that thrombi do not form in healthy segments of blood vessels. Two of the most-studied antiaggregants are the eicosanoid prostacyclin (PGI_2) and the endothelium-derived relaxing factor nitric oxide (NO) (reviewed in refs. 8 and 9).

Both proaggregants and antiaggregants exert their effects by binding to specific receptors on the platelet surface; a notable exception is NO, which traverses the membrane and directly activates guanylate cyclase. The signals emitted by the activated receptors are transmitted to the interior of the platelet via a distinct number of signal transduction mechanisms, each involving GTP-binding proteins (G-proteins).[1,2] The effect of stimulation of the proaggregatory signal transduction mechanisms is the activation of effector systems, such as phospholipase C (PLC)–induced hydrolysis of inositol phospholipids and opening of ion channels. The effector system of the antiaggregatory mechanisms is the activation of adenylate cyclase and guanylate cyclase. Activation of all these effector systems leads to various physiologic responses by inducing changes in phosphorylation state, enzymatic activity, and structural properties of key platelet proteins.

There are multiple interactions between these molecular pathways such that amplification, inhibition, or synergism can occur in response to agonists. Amplification is seen when TxA_2 and ADP are released from activated platelets and act as local hormones, binding to their receptors on the same and neighboring platelets to trigger a chain reaction. Epinephrine synergizes with other proaggregants, probably by inhibiting platelet adenylate cyclase and inhibiting the breakdown of active second messengers induced by the other agonists. Likewise, the antiaggregants PGI_2 and NO synergize in inhibiting platelet aggregation (reviewed in refs. 8 and 9).

There are various congenital defects in platelets that cause reduced platelet activity and lead to bleeding disorders. For example, congenital deficiencies in platelet membrane glycoproteins cause impaired platelet adhesion to damaged vessel walls and impaired platelet aggregation, and are associated with bleeding disorders and hemorrhage. Some conditions, however, may result in increased platelet activity and an increased tendency for thrombus formation. Such cases occur in atherosclerosis, heart disease, hypertension, and diabetes. Abnormalities may occur in potentially all the mechanisms regulating platelet function (discussed earlier) involving platelet-agonist interaction, platelet–vessel wall interaction, platelet-platelet interaction, platelet secretion, and platelet-

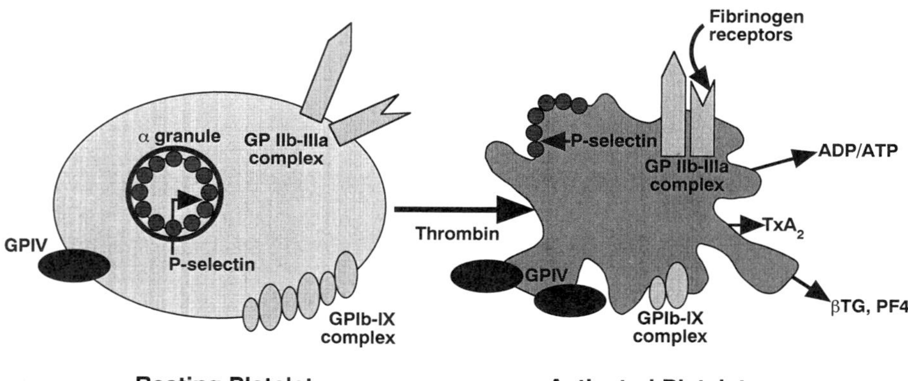

FIGURE 93-1. Surface markers of platelet activation. Changes in the number of glycoprotein (GP) receptors on the platelet surface occur after activation. Expression on the external platelet surface of GPIIb-IIIa, GPIV and P-selectin increases with activation, whereas that of GPIb-IX decreases. Detection of these glycoproteins with specific antibodies allows for a sensitive measurement of platelet activation. *βTG*, beta-thromboglobulin; *PF4*, platelet factor-4. (Adapted from Kestin AS, Ellis PA, Barnard MR, et al. Effect of strenuous exercise on platelet activation state and reactivity. Circulation 1993;88:1502.)

coagulant protein interaction. The transcellular regulatory mechanisms involving endothelial cells and platelets are, therefore, vital in vascular disorders, and this chapter focuses on abnormalities in this transcellular communication, as well as on intrinsic platelet abnormalities, in diabetes.

Diabetes and Platelets

Vascular diseases and related complications represent the main causes of morbidity and mortality in subjects with diabetes. The complications of neuropathy, nephropathy, retinopathy, and reduced tissue perfusion result from reduced capillary microcirculation and are diabetes-dependent; diabetic subjects are 17 times more prone to develop renal failure and 25 times more prone to develop blindness than normal subjects.[10,11] This trend in microangiopathy is more evident in insulin-dependent diabetes mellitus (IDDM) and proceeds as a function of the duration of the diabetes.[12] Macroangiopathy leads, in particular, to accelerated coronary arterial disease, but also to cerebral and peripheral arterial disease, and is increased in diabetes. The incidence of mortality from cardiovascular diseases is 2–4 times higher in diabetic persons than in nondiabetic persons.[10] Cardiovascular mortality is responsible for a higher proportion of deaths in non–insulin-dependent diabetes mellitus (NIDDM) than in IDDM.[13] Studies also show that, in diabetes, the prevalence of cardiovascular disease is the same in both men and women,[14,15] indicating that the relative resistance of premenopausal women to cardiovascular disease in the nondiabetic population is lost in diabetes, so that the impact of diabetes on cardiovascular disease is greater in women than in men.

Coronary heart disease in diabetes is associated with advanced atherosclerosis because of the increased incidence of atherosclerosis in the coronary arteries of diabetic persons relative to nondiabetic persons.[16,17] In contrast to microvascular disease, macrovascular disease is not strongly correlated with either the duration of diabetes or the level of glycemic control; in only some of the studies performed were glucose levels significantly associated with cardiovascular deaths,[18] and there is a lack of correlation between duration of diabetes and presence of heart disease.[16,19]

Besides diabetes itself, other cardiovascular risk factors, including high blood pressure, high triglyceride levels, and low high-density lipoprotein (HDL) cholesterol levels, are present in diabetic patients.[20] Of these, elevated triglyceride level has been shown to be a stronger predictor of coronary heart disease mortality in subjects with abnormal glucose tolerance than cholesterol, glucose, insulin, or obesity.[21] There is evidence, however, that insulin may promote atherosclerosis directly,[22] in addition to inducing adverse changes in other cardiovascular risk factors.[23]

In addition to coronary heart disease, cerebrovascular and peripheral vascular disease occur twofold to threefold and twofold to fivefold, more frequently, respectively, in diabetic persons than in nondiabetic persons.[24–27] The incidence of peripheral gangrene, a disease of both the large and small vessels, is increased fivefold by diabetes.[10]

The pathogenesis of atherosclerosis in diabetes has several potential contributors, including increased intravascular thrombin generation and reduced fibrinolytic potential.[28–30] Fibrinogen levels may also be elevated in diabetes,[31] which would contribute to fibrin clot formation and platelet aggregation (Fig. 93-2). Fibrinolytic activity has been reported to be low in type II diabetes,[32,33] and is thought to be attributable to high levels of plasminogen-activator inhibitor 1 (PAI-1), which inhibits the formation of fibrinolytic plasmin from plasminogen (see Fig. 93-2). PAI-1 levels have been found to be strongly correlated with body mass index and fasting plasma insulin levels in NIDDM,[33] and also with triglyceride levels in nondiabetic obese subjects.[34] Furthermore, PAI-1 levels decrease and fibrinolysis improves when insulin resistance and hyperinsulinemia are reduced by weight loss.[35] The elevated PAI-1 levels

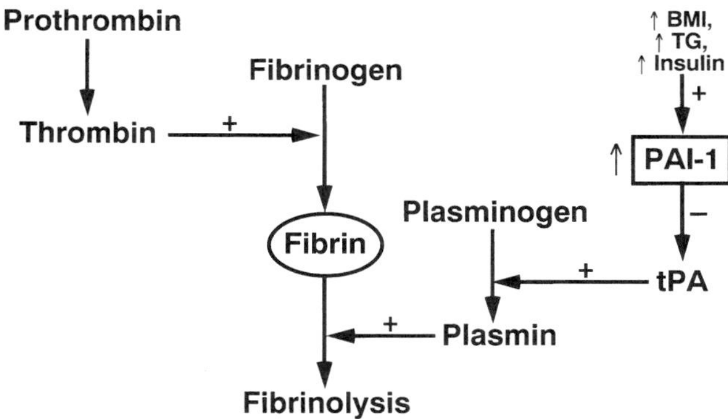

Figure 93-2. Changes in the fibrinolytic system in diabetes. The diagram shows the steps involved in regulating formation and dissolution of a fibrin clot in hemostasis. Activation (+) and inhibition (−) of various steps by the respective regulators are indicated. Changes secondary to diabetes are indicated with small arrows. *BMI*, body mass index; *TG*, triglycerides.

in subjects with NIDDM may, therefore, be explained by the insulin resistance of these individuals, and may explain why vascular complications are more common in obese than in nonobese patients with NIDDM.

Atherosclerosis is also accompanied by dyslipidemia, as is diabetes. NIDDM is associated with elevated triglyceride levels, reduced HDL cholesterol levels, and, less commonly, elevated low-density lipoprotein (LDL) cholesterol levels.[36,37] These lipoprotein abnormalities are strongly correlated with increased coronary risk. Their possible mechanisms of action in diabetic atherosclerosis are discussed later in this chapter.

Endothelial injury may be the initial event in atherogenesis, followed by platelet adhesion and aggregation at the site of injury, and resulting in release of growth factors by platelets, which provokes smooth muscle proliferation. However, in diabetes with or without vascular disease, there appears to be enhanced adhesiveness and response of platelets to several aggregating agents.[38–40] Platelets may, therefore, assume an important role in the initiation of atherosclerosis in diabetes. This thesis is substantiated by the results of studies in which antiplatelet drugs, such as aspirin and dipyridamole, provided protection against stroke and myocardial infarction in both diabetic and nondiabetic individuals, as well as against diabetic retinopathy.[41] This effect was generally not seen in studies that included subjects with advanced diabetic macroangiopathy or microangiopathy. The evidence is strong, however, that aspirin therapy is very beneficial for patients with less advanced microvascular disease, for survivors of myocardial infarction and stroke, and in subjects with unstable angina or transient ischemic attacks.

The involvement of platelet activation in cardiovascular disease[42] and the evidence of in vitro platelet hyperaggregability in diabetes have, therefore, combined to implicate the platelet in the high incidence of cardiovascular disease in diabetes. Work is ongoing to determine the potential contributions to enhanced platelet sensitivity of other concomitant factors associated with diabetes (e.g., hyperlipidemia, hypertension, smoking, obesity, and lack of exercise). However, the platelet is central to thrombus formation, and its interaction with other cells, including endothelium, in the microenvironment of the platelet aggregate is important in the regulation of thrombus formation and dissolution and vascular response.

Platelet-Endothelial Cell Interactions

There are two potential main causes of platelet hyperaggregability in diabetes: altered responses of platelets to extrinsic factors and altered levels of these extrinsic factors themselves. Extrinsic factors among the proaggregants are thrombin, epinephrine, and fibrinogen, whereas platelet modulators are represented by PGI_2 and NO released by the endothelium.

In healthy vessels, PGI_2 and NO combine to prevent platelet adherence to endothelium and aggregation (reviewed in refs. 8 and 9). These antiaggregants are released continually by healthy endothelium, but their synthesis is increased in the vicinity of aggregating platelets in response to plasma thrombin and bradykinin, and to platelet-released serotonin, platelet-derived growth factor, interleukin-1, and ADP (Fig. 93-3). This negative feedback mechanism is thought to limit the growth of the platelet plug to the area of vessel damage and de-endothelialization.

PGI_2 binds to a specific platelet receptor of the classic seven-transmembrane domain structure linked to a G-protein that is stimulatory (G_s) for adenylate cyclase. A G-protein that is inhibitory (G_i) for adenylate cyclase is linked to the α_2-adrenergic receptor that binds epinephrine.[43,44] NO, a much smaller, shorter-lived molecule, diffuses across the platelet membrane and directly activates guanylate cyclase. These inhibitory pathways culminate in phosphorylation by cAMP- and cGMP-dependent protein kinases, respectively, and inactivation of platelet proteins crucial for aggregation.[9,45–47]

Clearly, any condition that compromises the ability of the vascular endothelial cells to synthesize and release PGI_2 and NO will result in increased platelet activation. Such a situation is thought to occur in diabetes. There have been several reports in the literature of decreased vascular synthesis of PGI_2 in different models of diabetes,[48,49] including humans,[50,51] and of decreased synthesis and release of NO in diabetes.[52–56] Studies in animals have indicated that metabolic control with insulin or pancreatic islet transplantation returns vascular PGI_2 synthesis to normal.[48,49] Clearly, impaired synthesis and release of antiaggregants would result in increased platelet activity and response to proaggregants, but the same effect would result if platelets were less sensitive to antiaggregants in diabetes.

There have been several reports in which platelets have been shown to respond to PGI_2 and NO to a lesser degree in vascular disease caused by diabetes or other factors. Reports from the laboratories of the author and others have indicated that platelets from diabetic subjects have diminished sensitivity to PGI_2[57,58] and NO.[59] Reduced sensitivity of coronary vascular smooth muscle to NO has been suggested in acute ischemic heart disease,[60] indicating that insensitivity to NO may be a defect common to vascular diseases.

A variety of mechanisms may be responsible for an observed decrease in sensitivity to PGI_2 and NO. First, PGI_2 receptor activity could be impaired. A decrease in receptor number has not been described in diabetes, but has been described in heart disease,[61] a condition in which receptor number was returned to normal by insulin.[62–64]

It is interesting to speculate that platelet PGI_2 receptor levels are decreased in diabetes also when the effects of insulin are blunted; however, there is no confirmation of this hypothesis in the literature and, in fact, Modesti et al.[65] report that platelets from both type I and II diabetic patients have normal numbers of PGI_2 receptors. Altered responses to PGI_2 may also be manifested through G-protein malfunction, downstream of the receptor. Livingstone et al.[66] have found that there is a decrease in the level of G_i in the membranes of platelets from patients with NIDDM. This decrease correlates with a decreased stimulation of adenylate cyclase in response to activation of the PGI_2 receptor by prostaglandin E_1 (PGE_1). The mechanism of this impaired cAMP response remains to be determined, but the facts that G-protein function may be altered in diabetes, and that this defect may affect adenylate cyclase activity, are well noted.

The notion that diabetes affects the activity and expression of G-proteins is not novel. There are other reports in the literature that suggest changes in G-proteins in diabetes. Vinik and colleagues have demonstrated that GTP-stimulated, but not basal, platelet PLC activity is decreased in IDDM,[67] and that alterations in the subcellular distribution of small-molecular-weight G-proteins in IDDM are correlated with increased aggregation in response to thrombin.[68] Reynet and Kahn[69] have reported that there is overexpression of a ras-related G-protein, rad, in skeletal muscle in NIDDM. Work from our laboratory indicates that there is a 10-fold increase in the translocation of rap1B to the cytoskeleton in activated platelets from patients with NIDDM, in the absence of a concomitant increase in the expression of rap1B.[70]

It has yet to be determined what the differences in expression, activity, and cellular localization of G-proteins in diabetes mean. In NIDDM, at least, it appears that there may be genetic anomalies in the activity of G-proteins, caused by differences in either level of expression or sequence of genes. Mutations in the G-protein genes themselves may account for the changes in cellular distribution or, alternatively, these changes may be brought about by malfunction of the machinery that carries out post-translational processing of G-proteins in diabetes.[71] The latter possibility is discussed by Bastyr et al.[68] It is quite possible that, in a disease with a genetic basis, such as diabetes, there is defective post-translational processing of proteins, which leads to inappropriate activity or subcellular localization of the proteins. The mutant gene in human choroideremia encodes a protein component of rab geranylgeranyl transferase which results in impairment in isoprenylation of the ras-related G-protein rab3A and expression of the choroidemia phenotype characterized by retinitis pigmentosa and blindness.[72]

Apart from the work of Livingstone et al.,[66] little is known about the activities of adenylate and guanylate cyclases in diabetes.

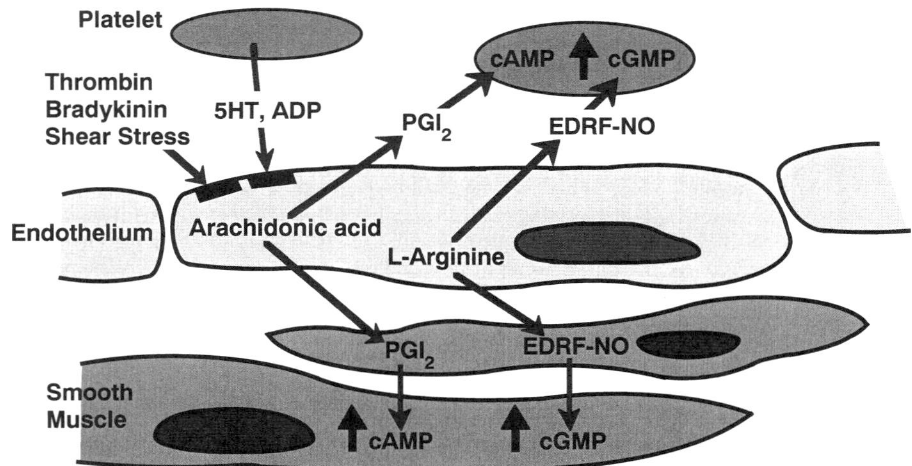

Figure 93-3. Synthesis and actions of PGI_2 and NO in blood vessels. Stimulation of endothelial cell receptors by platelet-derived 5-HT (serotonin) or ADP, or by thrombin, bradykinin, or shear stress, leads to release of the vasodilators/antiaggregants. PGI_2 relaxes smooth muscle and inhibits platelet aggregation via the cAMP pathway. Endothelium-derived relaxing factor (EDRF)-NO also relaxes smooth muscle and inhibits platelet aggregation and adhesion via the cGMP pathway. (Adapted from Vane JR, Änggård EE, Botting RM. Mechanisms of disease: Regulatory functions of the vascular endothelium. N Engl J Med 1990;323:27.)

There is evidence, however, of increased cGMP-phosphodiesterase activity in experimental and human diabetes; this is discussed by Hamet et al.,[73] and may explain abnormalities in sensitivity to antiaggregants in the absence of other defects. Further work needs to be done to elucidate whether there are inherent abnormalities in the specific cyclic nucleotide–dependent protein kinase enzymes, because altered activity of these proteins would clearly affect the way platelets respond to antiaggregants.

It has been apparent for two decades that the endothelium may also contribute to platelet activation in diabetes by releasing von Willebrand factor, a glycoprotein constituent of the factor VIII complex, which promotes platelet clumping by binding to the platelet GPIb-IX and IIb-IIIa complexes. A number of studies have been published showing elevated levels of von Willebrand factor activity and antigen in the plasma of diabetic subjects (reviewed in ref. 74). It is thought that the increased release of von Willebrand factor in diabetes is an indicator of endothelial damage. There is evidence that insulin therapy can reduce the elevated von Willebrand factor level in experimental diabetes,[75] which may provide an explanation for the beneficial effect of insulin in reducing platelet activity.

Intrinsic Abnormalities in the Platelet

Not only may platelets come into contact with an increased number of proaggregatory agents in the diabetic milieu, but there is an ever-expanding body of literature on enhanced platelet sensitivity to a variety of aggregating agents in vitro, including epinephrine, ADP, thrombin, and collagen.[74] A summary of the many tests used to measure platelet activation is shown in Table 93-1. It is not yet clear whether the platelet abnormalities are intrinsic to the platelet or are a consequence of circulating factors that affect platelet function, as has been demonstrated for insulin immunocomplexes.[76] It has been reported that the response to epinephrine, ADP, and thrombin are enhanced in human diabetes,[77–81] although it has been difficult to consistently demonstrate hyperaggregatory responses in patients with NIDDM whose disease is moderately well-controlled.[82,83]

The hyperaggregability of diabetic platelets, which appears to be independent of the ADP and arachidonate pathways,[77–83] is not diminished after insulinization of diabetic patients for 7 days, which normalizes blood glucose levels but does not return the lipid profile to normal.[84] Colwell et al.[85] hypothesized that, "in diabetes a vicious cycle may be set up in which vascular disease may lead to platelet damage and altered platelet function may contribute to vascular disease." It seems, therefore, that perturbations in the extensive network of cross-talk between tissues may be a factor in the pathogenesis of diabetic vascular complications, although there is evidence of an intrinsic abnormality in platelets in diabetes.

Much of the early work concentrated on the role of the arachidonic acid pathway in the enhanced aggregation of platelets in diabetes. Sagel and coworkers found that inhibition of cyclo-oxygenase significantly decreased the effect of diabetes on platelets.[77] This was attributed to the increased synthesis of PGE_2 and TxA_2 in activated platelets obtained from diabetic subjects.[86–90] Although platelets from diabetic subjects were less sensitive to inhibition of the synthesis and action of TxA_2,[86] TxA_2 synthesis is not necessarily correlated with platelet aggregation.[91–93] This is consistent with the evidence that the enhanced platelet aggregation is multifactorial. Moreover, in the multicenter Veterans Administration study, aspirin did not reduce the likelihood of loss of the surviving limb after gangrene of one limb.[94]

As discussed earlier, the increase in platelet aggregability may not be caused solely by the onset of vascular disease. In an animal model of diabetes, enhanced platelet aggregation and TxA_2 synthesis was detected within days of making rats diabetic with streptozotocin,[49,95] before vascular disease was evident. Also, vascular disease is promoted by platelet activation and the release of mitogens, which stimulate vascular smooth muscle cell proliferation, suggesting a role for platelets in the etiology of atherosclerosis. Data such as these highlight the difficulties in relating in vitro findings with the situation in vivo. It is, therefore, important to investigate platelet behavior in vivo in the various models of diabetes; previous studies set up along those lines have indicated that there is increased platelet turnover in vivo in diabetes,[96,97] which is suggestive of increased platelet aggregation in the circulation.

After the burst of interest in platelet TxA_2 production in the late 1970s and early 1980s had waned, researchers began to focus on possible alternative mechanisms to explain the enhanced platelet sensitivity to agonists in diabetes. The discovery that inositol phospholipid turnover and calcium release were early events in the platelet response,[98] preceding secretion and eicosanoid synthesis, focused attention in that area. Most proaggregants, including thrombin, collagen, ADP, and TxA_2, initiate platelet aggregation by binding to specific G-protein–linked receptors and activating PLC-mediated hydrolysis of phosphoinositide (4,5)P_2, which results in release of the calcium-elevating messenger inositol triphosphate and the protein kinase C stimulator diacylglycerol (reviewed in refs. 1 and 2).

Although efforts have been made to establish an effect of diabetes on platelet phosphoinositide (PI) turnover, a uniform trend has not appeared. For example, PI turnover was shown to be elevated in hyperaggregating platelets in NIDDM,[99,100] but decreased in IDDM.[101] It would seem that enhanced sensitivity to primary agonists of platelet aggregation would be accompanied by an increase in PI turnover but, because of the multifactorial nature of diabetic platelet hyperaggregability, decreased activity of the PI cycle in IDDM may represent a compensatory response of platelets to increased activity of another pathway. Alternatively, much of the discrepancy in these studies could be attributable to case selection and definition of hyperaggregability. To compound the issue, the increase in platelet activity observed with aging has been associated with increased PI turnover[102]; this is compatible with the hypothesis that increased platelet activity is associated with increased PI turnover.

Studies on calcium homeostasis in platelets from subjects with diabetes may shed some light on the involvement of the PI cycle in platelet hyperfunction. It has been shown that resting platelets from patients with IDDM who have poor metabolic control (HbA_{1c}>8%) have higher calcium content than those from controls, whereas thrombin-induced calcium levels are augmented only in patients with good metabolic control who are free from complications.[103] These data are consistent with the report of decreased

Table 93-1. Assays for Increased Platelet Activity

Marker of Activation	Test
Aggregability	Spontaneous platelet aggregation
	Agonist-induced platelet aggregability
Formation of "circulating" platelet aggregates	Platelet count ratio
	Flow cytometry (monoclonal antibody against glycoprotein Ib)
Activation of surface marker	Flow cytometry (monoclonal antibody against glycoprotein IIb/IIIa)
	Flow cytometry (monoclonal antibody against P-selectin)
Release of platelet activation products	β-thromboglobulin (enzyme immunoassay)
	Platelet factor-4 (enzyme immunoassay)
	Urinary 2,3-dinor-thromboxane B_2 (TxB_2) (gas chromatography-mass spectrometry)
	Urinary 11-dehydro-TxB_2 (radioimmunoassay)

thrombin-induced PI pathway activity in hyperaggregating platelets in IDDM (mentioned earlier),[101] and fit in with the compensatory response theory. Higher basal and collagen-stimulated calcium levels have been reported in platelets of subjects with NIDDM than in those of controls,[104] which is consistent with the PI data in experiments with NIDDM platelets discussed earlier. Interestingly, the IDDM-dependent changes in platelet calcium and aggregation are not affected by acute alterations in in vitro glucose concentration, indicating that glucose does not affect platelet aggregation directly.

Products of advanced glycosylation, the terminal adducts of the nonenzymatic reaction between glucose and the amino groups of protein, accumulate in tissues at an accelerated rate in diabetes.[105] The increased extent of glycosylation of platelet membrane proteins in diabetes appears to be related to reduced membrane fluidity,[106] which modulates cell function, possibly through alterations in receptor availability. The reduced membrane fluidity of platelets in diabetes may contribute to platelet hyperfunction. Also, enhanced glycosylation of subendothelial proteins may quench NO produced by the endothelium,[53] contributing to reduced platelet inhibition. Platelet membrane fluidity can also be affected by the plasma lipoprotein profile, which is altered in diabetes.[107] Moreover, the increased glycosylation of LDLs in IDDM has been shown to be responsible for enhanced platelet sensitivity to the aggregating agents thrombin, collagen, and ADP. Watanabe et al.[108] reported that LDL isolated from patients with IDDM was taken up by platelets to a greater extent, and enhanced aggregation to a greater extent, that LDL isolated from matched controls. These properties of LDL from subjects with IDDM were correlated with the degree of glycosylation only; there was no difference in lipid composition of LDL isolated from diabetic and control subjects, and no change in platelet lipid composition. These results suggest a mechanism for the altered membrane fluidity and platelet hyperaggregability in diabetes.

There is also evidence for increased glycoprotein expression on the platelet surface in diabetes. Increased numbers of GPIb and GPIIb-IIIa complex are present on platelets in both IDDM and NIDDM.[109] GPIb acts as a receptor for von Willebrand factor, to which platelets are exposed at injury sites, and as a substrate for thrombin, and GPIIb-IIIa acts as a receptor for several adhesive proteins, including fibrinogen, which are involved in aggregation. Increases in GP expression on platelets may, therefore, contribute to platelet hypersensitivity of diabetes.

It is quite possible and very probable that the etiology of platelet hyperaggregability is different in the two major forms of diabetes and in other instances of vascular complications. It remains to be seen whether the relatively novel PI 3-kinase pathway, which appears to be involved in platelet secretion and aggregation,[110–112] is altered in diabetes. Even if it is, the challenge will be to demonstrate whether it is the cause or an effect of the underlying tendency to hyperaggregate.

Insulin May Have Direct and Indirect Actions on Platelets

The hypothesis that platelets behave differently in IDDM and NIDDM raises the discussion of the role insulin plays in diabetic platelet hyperaggregability. Platelets have been shown to be targets of insulin action because they retain a functional insulin receptor capable of insulin-binding and autophosphorylation.[113] Insulin is generally thought to reduce platelet responses to the agonists ADP, collagen, thrombin, arachidonate, and platelet-activating factor.[114,115] A clue to this action of insulin is the finding that insulin downregulates the number of α_2-adrenergic receptors on platelets.[116] Note, however, that although platelet α_2-adrenergic receptor numbers are low in diabetes, they are even lower in diabetic persons with autonomic neuropathy.[117] Because epinephrine potentiates the effects of other aggregating agents[118] and stimulates G_i-mediated inhibition of adenylate cyclase,[119,120] it is clear that insulin's modifying effect on the action of epinephrine would tone down platelet responses to the other aggregants.

The picture may not be that clear, however. The complication in this case is the evidence that platelet activity may be enhanced by the action of insulin. Lopez-Aparicio and colleagues[121] have reported that insulin phosphorylates and activates cGMP-inhibited cAMP phosphodiesterase in human platelets. This meshes with the reported effect of insulin in decreasing platelet cAMP,[122] and would be expected to result in a decreased effect of PGI_2. Also, insulin infusion has been reported to make human platelets more sensitive to ADP,[93] and intravenous bolus injection enhances platelet TxA_2 in diabetes.[123] Murer et al.[124] investigated this further, demonstrating that insulin decreased the threshold for induction by ADP of aggregation of human platelets in vitro.

The relevance of all these data to diabetes is not clear. It is important, however, to consider the effects of insulin, as presented, in light of the insulin concentrations and sensitivity in all forms of diabetes. There is scant reference in the literature to the sensitivity of platelets to insulin in diabetes. It may be expected that patients with IDDM, however responsive they are to the effects of insulin on platelets, suffer from a prolonged deficiency of insulin, whereas subjects with NIDDM have insulin-insensitive platelets. Of interest is the isolated report of Udvardy et al.,[125] who reported

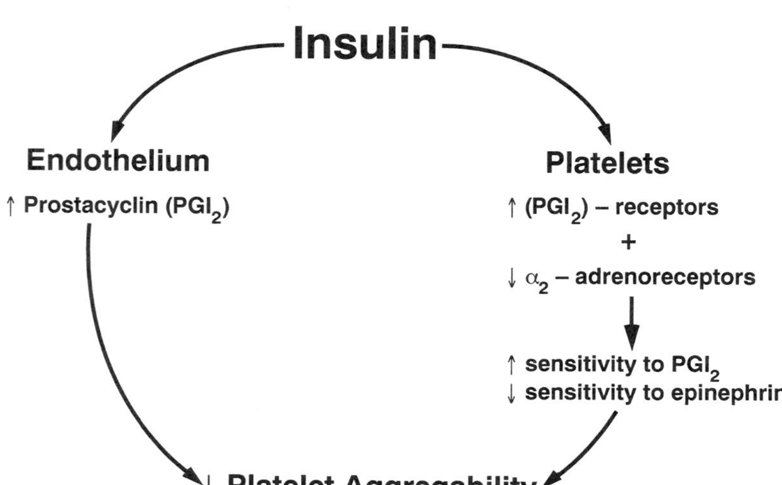

FIGURE 93-4. Effects of insulin on platelet aggregability. The effects of insulin on platelet and endothelial parameters involved in the regulation of platelet activation are indicated with small arrows.

decreased platelet insulin receptor number and affinity in subjects with NIDDM.

An interesting analogy may be the effects of insulin on platelets in coronary heart disease. Work from Kahn, et al.[126] has shown that, in nondiabetic patients with acute ischemic heart disease, there is decreased binding of insulin and PGI_2 to platelets and decreased plasma insulin level. These deficiencies are transient and improve after recuperation. The same researchers showed, in other studies, that the impaired responses of platelets to PGI_2 in coronary heart disease are normalized by physiologic quantities of insulin administered both in vitro[62] and in vivo.[63] The effect of insulin was to increase the number of PGI_2 binding sites on platelets, which increased the cAMP response to PGI_2. This effect was observed in platelets from patients with acute ischemic heart disease and from normal controls,[62,127] and the increase was more than twofold.

These studies indicate the potential importance of insulin in maintaining normal platelet sensitivity to PGI_2, and suggest a possible mechanism whereby platelets are more active in diabetes. There appear to be no data in the literature on the effects of insulin on PGI_2 responsiveness of platelets from subjects with diabetes, although this is clearly an important issue. The authors' laboratory is investigating this question. The effects of insulin, which are known to influence platelet activity, are summarized in Figure 93-4.

Insulin is known to have other effects on the cardiovascular system, and it is generally assumed that these are important in the pathogenesis of diabetic vascular disease. Insulin's role as a growth factor may be important in arterial smooth muscle[128] and megakaryocyte[129] proliferation. Both these functions, along with the finding that it also upregulates GPIIb-IIIa expression in megakaryocytes of experimentally-diabetic rats,[129] incriminate insulin as potentially atherogenic. The number of known actions of insulin underscores how difficult it is to determine the role of insulin in atherogenesis. Clearly, it is important to isolate the individual effects of insulin by continuing with in vitro studies. Only after such studies and long-term in vivo studies, taking into account all the other risk factors, will the question be able to be resolved.

Table 93-2. Reported Alterations in Diabetes that May Affect Platelet Function

Endothelium-related
Release of PGI_2
Release of NO
Release of fibrinolytic activity
Release of plasminogen-activator inhibitor
Platelet-related
Platelet survival
Surface glycoprotein activity/number
Proaggregant and antiaggregant receptor activity/number
Activity/expression of G-proteins
Arachidonate pathway
Phosphoinositide pathway
Activity of cyclic nucleotide phosphodiesterases
Lipid uptake
Insulin-related
Hyperinsulinemia
Hypoinsulinemia
Platelet insulin receptor number
Platelet PGI_2 receptor number
Platelet α_2-receptor number
Circulation-related
Plasma glucose
Plasma lipid profile
Glycation of lipoproteins

Summary

Platelets are essential for hemostasis, and knowledge of their function is basic to an understanding of the pathophysiology of vascular disease in diabetes. Moreover, platelets are an easily accessible tissue from the human subject and, because they share many functional mechanisms with other cells, they mirror the anormalies that occur in other tissues, such as vascular smooth muscle, in diabetes. These are the reasons why platelets have been so well studied in an attempt to understand the mechanisms of atherogenesis.

The mechanisms of atherosclerosis in diabetes are believed to be similar to those in the nondiabetic population. Anomalies in a number of mechanisms involved in platelet action can be seen in diabetic platelets in vitro. These anomalies account for hypersensitivity of platelets to aggregants and hyposensitivity to antiaggregants, and are thought to contribute to enhanced atherosclerosis via increased platelet activity at sites of vessel injury. The changes in platelets in diabetes include enhanced glycoprotein receptor binding of agonists and adhesive proteins; decreased membrane fluidity; enhanced activation of the arachidonic acid pathway, resulting in increased TxA_2 formation; altered PI turnover, leading to changes in diacylglycerol and inositol triphosphate production, calcium mobilization and protein phosphorylation; impaired responses to antiaggregants, resulting in decreased PGI_2 receptor binding, cyclic nucleotide production, and cyclic nucleotide–dependent protein phosphorylation; and altered sensitivity to insulin. A summary of the alterations that are known to occur in diabetes and that may contribute to platelet hyperfunction is presented in Table 93-2.

It is generally accepted from in vitro studies that platelets from diabetic patients behave differently from those of normal subjects. There is also evidence of increased platelet activity in vivo in diabetes, but whether this reflects platelet hyperfunction or increased activation of platelets by already diseased vasculature remains to be shown. Whatever the cause, platelet activity is augmented in diabetes, and this contributes to the enhanced atherosclerosis and the resulting complications in the diabetic population. The origin of the platelet abnormalities and the extent to which they contribute to the pathogenesis of cardiovascular disease require further investigation.

References

1. Siess W. Molecular mechanisms of platelet activation. Physiol Rev 1989; 69:58
2. Ashby B, Daniel JL, Smith JB. Mechanisms of platelet activation and inhibition. Hematol Oncol Clin North Am 1990;4:1
3. Stenberg PE, McEver RP, Shuman MA, et al. A platelet alpha-granule membrane protein (GMP-140) is expressed on the plasma membrane after activation. J Cell Biol 1985;101:880
4. Shattil SJ, Hoxie JA, Cunningham M, Brass LF. Changes in the platelet membrane glycoprotein IIb-IIIa complex during platelet activation. J Biol Chem 1985;260:11107
5. Michelson AD, Barnard MR. The thrombospondin receptor on platelet membrane glycoprotein IV: Surface expression on resting platelets and modulation by thrombin. Blood 1988;72:332
6. Coller BS, Peerschke EI, Scudder LE, Sullivan CA. Studies with a murine monoclonal antibody that abolishes ristocetin-induced binding of von Willebrand factor to platelets: Additional evidence in support of GPIb as a platelet receptor for von Willebrand factor. Blood 1983;61:99
7. Kestin AS, Ellis PA, Barnard MR, et al. Effect of strenuous exercise on platelet activation state and reactivity. Circulation 1993;88:1502
8. Vane JR, Anggard EE, Botting RM. Regulatory functions of the vascular endothelium. N Engl J Med 1990;323:27
9. Gryglewski RJ, Botting RM, Vane JR. Mediators produced by the endothelial cell. Hypertension 1988;12:530
10. Crofford OB, Boshell BR, Cahill GF Jr. Report of the National Commission on Diabetes. The long-range plan to combat diabetes Vol. 1. Bethesda, MD: 1976. DHEW publication (NIH)76-1018
11. Tchobroutsky G. Relation of diabetic control to development of microvascular complications. Diabetologia 1978;15:143
12. McMillan DE. Deterioration of the microcirculation in diabetes. Diabetes 1975;24:944

13. Moss SE, Klein R, Klein BE. Cause-specific mortality in a population-based study of diabetes. Am J Public Health 1991;81:1158
14. West KM, Ahuja MM, Bennett PH, et al. The role of circulating glucose and triglyceride concentrations and their interactions with other 'risk factors' as determinants of arterial disease in nine diabetic population samples from the WHO multinational study. Diabetes Care 1983;6:361
15. Morrish NJ, Stevens LK, Fuller JH, et al. Incidence of macrovascular disease in diabetes mellitus: The London cohort of the WHO Multinational Study of Vascular Disease in Diabetics. Diabetologia 1991;34:584
16. Waller BF, Palumbo PJ, Lie JT, Roberts WC. Status of the coronary arteries at necropsy in diabetes mellitus with onset after age 30 years: Analysis of 229 diabetic patients with and without clinical evidence of coronary heart disease and comparison to 183 control subjects. Am J Med 1980;69:498
17. Robertson WB, Strong JB. Atherosclerosis in persons with hypertension and diabetes mellitus. Lab Invest 1968;18:538
18. International Collaborative Group. Joint discussion. J Chronic Dis 1979; 32:829
19. Vigorita VJ, Moore GW, Hutchins GM. Absence of correlation between coronary arterial atherosclerosis and severity or duration of diabetes mellitus of adult onset. Am J Cardiol 1980;46:535
20. Steiner G. Diabetes and atherosclerosis: An overview. Diabetes 1981;30 (Suppl 2):1
21. Fontbonne A, Eschwege E, Cambien F, et al. Hypertriglyceridaemia as a risk factor of coronary heart disease mortality in subjects with impaired glucose tolerance of diabetes: Results from the 11-year follow-up of the Paris Prospective Study. Diabetologia 1989;32:300
22. Stout RW. Insulin and atheroma: 20-Year perspective. Diabetes Care 1990; 13:631
23. Donahue RP, Orchard TJ, Becker DJ, et al. Sex differences in the coronary heart disease risk profile: A possible role for insulin. The Beaver County Study. Am J Epidemiol 1987;125:650
24. Kannel WB, McGee DL. Diabetes and cardiovascular risk factors: The Framingham Study. Circulation 1979;59:8
25. Kannel WB, McGee DL. Diabetes and cardiovascular disease: The Framingham Study. JAMA 1979;241:2035
26. Brand FN, Abbott RD, Kannel WB. Diabetes, intermittent claudication and risk of cardiovascular events. The Framingham Study. Diabetes 1989;38:504
27. Palumbo PJ, Melton LJ. Peripheral vascular disease and diabetes. In: Diabetes in America. Diabetes Data Compiled 1984, National Diabetes Data Group. NIH publication 1985;85:1486
28. Fearnley GR, Chakraborti R, Avis PRD. Blood fibrinolytic activity in diabetes mellitus and its bearing on ischemic heart disease and obesity. Br Med J 1963;1:921
29. Almer L, Nilsson IM. On fibrinolysis in diabetes mellitus. Acta Med Scand 1975;198:101
30. Almer L, Pandolfi M. Fibrinolysis and diabetic retinopathy. Diabetes 1976; 25(Suppl 2):807
31. Banga JD, Sixma JJ. Diabetes mellitus, vascular disease and thrombosis. Clin Haematol 1986;15:465
32. Auwerx J, Bouillon R, Collen D, Geboers J. Tissue-type plasminogen activator antigen and plasminogen activator inhibitor in diabetes mellitus. Arteriosclerosis 1988;8:68
33. Juhan-Vague I, Roul C, Alessi MC, et al. Increased plasminogen activator inhibitor activity in non–insulin-dependent diabetic patients. Relationship with plasma insulin. Thromb Haemost 1989;61:370
34. Vague P, Juhan-Vague I, Chabert V, et al. Fat distribution and plasminogen activator inhibitor activity in nondiabetic obese women. Metabolism 1989; 38:913
35. Folsom AR, Qamhieh HT, Wing RR, et al. Impact of weight loss on plasminogen activator inhibitor (PAI-1), factor VII, and other hemostatic factors in moderately overweight adults. Arterioscler Thromb 1993;13:162
36. Ginsberg HN. Lipoprotein physiology in nondiabetic and diabetic states: Relationship to atherogenesis. Diabetes Care 1991;14:839
37. Howard BV. Lipoprotein metabolism in diabetes mellitus. J Lipid Res 1987; 28:613
38. Bern MM. Platelet functions in diabetes mellitus. Diabetes 1978;27:342
39. Peterson CM, Jones RL, Koenig RJ, et al. Reversible hematologic sequelae of diabetes mellitus. Ann Intern Med 1977;86:425
40. Colwell JA, Halushka PV, Sarji KE, et al. Vascular disease in diabetes: Pathophysiological mechanisms and therapy. Arch Intern Med 1979;139:225
41. Colwell JA. Antiplatelet drugs and prevention of macrovascular disease in diabetes mellitus. Metabolism 1994;41(Suppl 1):7
42. Ross R. The pathogenesis of atherosclerosis—An update. N Engl J Med 1986; 314:488
43. Haslam RJ, Davison MM. Guanine nucleotides decrease the free [Ca2+] required for secretion of serotonin from permeabilized blood platelets. Evidence of a role for a GTP-binding protein in platelet activation. FEBS Lett 1984;174:90
44. Jakobs KH, Aktories K, Minuth M, Schultz G. Inhibition of adenylate cyclase. Adv Cyclic Nucleotide Protein Phosphorylation Res 1985;19:137
45. Lapetina EG, Lacal JC, Reep BR, Molina y Vedia L. A ras-related protein is phosphorylated and translocated by agonists that increase cAMP levels in human platelets. Proc Natl Acad Sci U S A 1989;86:3131
46. Lazarowski ER, Winegar DA, Nolan RD, et al. Effect of protein kinase A on inositide metabolism and rap 1 G-protein in human erythroleukemia cells. J Biol Chem 1990;265:13118
47. Walter U, Waldmann R, Nieberding M. Intracellular mechanism of action of vasodilators. Eur Heart J 1988;9(Suppl H):1
48. Harrison HE, Reece AH, Johnson M. Effect of insulin treatment on prostacyclin in experimental diabetes. Diabetologia 1980;18:65
49. Gerrard JM, Stuart MJ, Rao GHR, et al. Alteration in the balance of prostaglandin and thromboxane synthesis in diabetic rats. J Lab Clin Med 1980; 95:950
50. Johnson M, Harrison HE, Raftery AT, Elder JB. Vascular prostacyclin may be reduced in diabetes in man [Letter]. Lancet 1979;1:325
51. Silberbauer K, Schernthaner G, Sinzinger H, et al. Decreased vascular prostacyclin in juvenile-onset diabetes [Letter]. N Engl J Med 1979;300:366
52. Saenz de Tajada I, Goldstein I, Azadzoi K, et al. Impaired neurogenic and endothelium-mediated relaxation of penile smooth muscle from diabetic men with impotence. N Engl J Med 1989;320:1025
53. Bucala R, Tracey KJ, Cerami A. Advanced glycosylation products quench nitric oxide and mediate defective endothelium-dependent vasodilation in experimental diabetes. J Clin Invest 1991;87:432
54. Chin JH, Azhar S, Hoffman BB. Inactivation of endothelial-derived relaxing factor by oxidized lipoproteins. J Clin Invest 1992;89:10
55. Kamata K, Miyata N, Kasuya Y. Impairment of endothelium-dependent relaxation and changes in levels of cyclic GMP in aorta from streptozotozin-induced diabetic rats. Br J Pharmacol 1989;97:614
56. Harris KH, MacLeod KM. Influence of the endothelium on contractile responses of arteries from diabetic rats. Eur J Pharmacol 1988;153:55
57. Betteridge DJ, El Tahir KE, Reckless JP, Williams KI. Platelets from diabetic subjects show diminished sensitivity to prostacyclin. Eur J Clin Invest 1982;12:395
58. Akai T, Naka K, Okuda K, et al. Decreased sensitivity of platelets to prostacyclin in patients with diabetes mellitus. Horm Metab Res 1983;15:523
59. Nolan RD, Platt KH, Loose PG. The resistance to nitric oxide inhibition of platelet aggregation is due to decreased phosphorylation of rap1B in platelets of NIDDM compared with control subjects [Abstract]. Diabetes 1994; 43(Suppl 1):101A
60. Forstermann U, Mugge A, Alheid U, et al. Selective attenuation of endothelium-mediated vasodilation in atherosclerotic human coronary arteries. Circ Res 1988;62:185
61. Kahn NN, Mueller HS, Sinha AK. Impaired prostaglandin E1/I2 receptor activity of human blood platelets in acute ischemic heart disease. Circ Res 1990;66:932
62. Kahn NN, Mueller HS, Sinha AK. Restoration by insulin of impaired prostaglandin E1/I2 receptor activity of platelets in acute ischemic heart disease. Circ Res 1991;68:245
63. Kahn NN, Najeeb MA, Ishaq M, et al. Normalization of impaired response of platelets to prostaglandin E1/I2 and synthesis of prostacyclin by insulin in unstable angina pectoris and in acute myocardial infarction. Am J Cardiol 1992;70:582
64. Kahn NN, Bauman WA, Hatcher VB, Sinha AK. Inhibition of platelet aggregation and the stimulation of prostacyclin synthesis by insulin in humans. Am J Physiol 1993;265:H2160
65. Modesti PA, Fortini A, Gensini GF, et al. Human prostacyclin platelet receptors in diabetes mellitus. Thromb Res 1991;63:541
66. Livingstone C, McLellan AR, McGregor M, et al. Altered G-protein expression and adenylate cyclase activity in platelets of non-insulin-dependent diabetic (NIDDM) male subjects. Biochim Biophys Acta 1991;1096:127
67. Bastyr EJ III, Vinik AI. Reduced guanine nucleotide-stimulated polyphosphoinositide specific phospholipase C in platelet hyperaggregation in IDDM. Thromb Res 1992;65:241
68. Bastyr EJ III, Lu J, Stowe R, et al. Low molecular weight GTP-binding proteins are altered in platelet hyperaggregation in IDDM. Oncogene 1993; 8:515
69. Reynet C, Kahn CR. Rad: A member of the Ras family overexpressed in muscle of type II diabetic humans. Science 1993;262:1441
70. Nolan RD, Burch MG, Salter LM, Platt KH. Abnormalities in the distribution of rap1B in platelets of NIDDM [Abstract]. Diabetes 1993;42(Suppl 1): 72A
71. Hancock JF, Magee AI, Childs JE, Marshall CJ. All ras proteins are polyisoprenylated but only some are palmitoylated. Cell 1989;57:1167
72. Seabra MC, Brown MS, Goldstein JL. Retinal degeneration in choroideremia: Deficiency of Rab geranylgeranyl transferase. Science 1993;259:377
73. Hamet P, Skuherska R, Pang SC, Tremblay J. Abnormalities of platelet function in hypertension and diabetes. Hypertension 1985;7:II 135
74. Colwell JA, Lopes-Virella M, Halushka PV. Pathogenesis of atherosclerosis in diabetes mellitus. Diabetes Care 1981;4:121
75. Winocour PD, Lopes-Virella M, Laimins M, Colwell JA. Effect of insulin treatment in streptozocin-induced diabetic rats on in vitro platelet function and plasma von Willebrand factor activity and factor VIII-related antigen. J Lab Clin Med 1985;106:319
76. Van Zile J, Kilpatrick M, Laimins M, et al. Platelet aggregation and release of ATP after incubation with soluble immune complexes purified from the serum of diabetic patients. Diabetes 1981;30:575
77. Sagel J, Colwell JA, Crook L, Laimins M. Increased platelet aggregation in early diabetes mellitus. Ann Intern Med 1975;82:733
78. Kutti J, Wadenvik H, Henestam B, Stenstrom G. Evaluation of platelet reactivity in diabetes mellitus. Acta Med Scand 1986;219:195
79. Colwell JA, Halushka PV, Sarji K, et al. Altered platelet function in diabetes mellitius. Diabetes 1976;25(Suppl 2):826

80. Kobbah M, Ewald U, Tuvemo T. Platelet aggregation during the first year of diabetes in childhood. Acta Paediatr Scand 1985;320(Suppl):50
81. Bastyr EJ III, Kadrofske MM, Vinik AI. Hyperaggregatory function of platelets in type I diabetic subjects (IDDM) occurs in receptor-specific first phase [Abstract]. Diabetes 1987;36(Suppl 1):208A
82. DiMinno G, Silver MJ, Cerbone AM, et al. Platelet fibrinogen binding in diabetes mellitus. Differences between binding to platelets from non-retinopathic and retinopathic diabetic patients. Diabetes 1986;35:182
83. Bensoussan D, Levy-Toledano S, Passa P, et al. Platelet hyperaggregation and increased plasma level of von Willebrand factor in diabetics with retinopathy. Diabetologia 1975;11:307
84. Winocour PD, Halushka PV, Colwell JA. Platelet involvement in diabetes mellitus. In: Longenecker GL, ed. The Platelets: Physiology and Pharmacology. New York: Academic Press;1985:341
85. Colwell JA, Gisinger C, Klein R. Altered platelet function in diabetes mellitus: Effect of glycemic regulation and antiplatelet agents. In: Ruderman N, Williamson J, Brownlee M, eds. Hyperglycemia, Diabetes, and Vascular Diseases. Oxford, U.K.: Oxford University Press;1992:30
86. Halushka PV, Rogers RC, Loadholt CB, Colwell JA. Increased platelet thromboxane synthesis in diabetes mellitus. J Lab Clin Med 1981;97:87
87. Halushka PV, Lurie D, Colwell JA. Increased synthesis of prostaglandin E-like material by platelets from patients with diabetes mellitus. N Engl J Med 1977;297:1306
88. Ziboh VA, Maruta H, Lord J, et al. Increased biosynthesis of thromboxane A2 by diabetic platelets. Eur J Clin Invest 1979;9:223
89. Lagarde M, Burtin M, Berciaud P, et al. Increase of platelet thromboxane A2 formation and of its plasmatic half-life in diabetes mellitus. Thromb Res 1980;19:823
90. Brunner D, Klinger J, Weisbort J, et al. Thromboxane, prostacyclin, beta-thromboglobulin, and diabetes mellitus. Clin Ther 1984;6:636
91. de Gaetano G, Cerletti C, Bertele V. Pharmacology of antiplatelet drugs and clinical trials on thrombosis prevention: A difficult link. Lancet 1982;2: 974
92. Bertele V, Tomasiak M, Falanga A, et al. Aspirin inhibits platelet aggregation but not because it prevents thromboxane synthesis [Letter]. Lancet 1982;2: 775
93. Mayfield RK, Halushka PV, Wohltmann HJ, et al. Platelet function during continuous insulin infusion treatment in insulin-dependent diabetic patients. Diabetes 1985;34:1127
94. Colwell JA, Bingham SF, Abraira C, et al. Veterans Administration Cooperative Study on antiplatelet agents in diabetic patients after amputation for gangrene. II. Effects of aspirin and dipyridamole on atherosclerotic vascular disease rates. Diabetes Care 1986;9:140
95. Honour AJ, Hockaday TD, Mann JI. The synergistic effect of aspirin and dipyridamole upon platelet thrombi in living blood vessels. Br J Exp Pathol 1977;58:268
96. Colwell JA, Sagel J, Crook L, et al. Correlation of platelet aggregation, plasma factor activity, and megathrombocytes in diabetic subjects with and without vascular diseases. Metabolism 1977;26:279
97. Garg SK, Lackner H, Karpatkin S. The increased percentage of megathrombocytes in various clinical disorders. Ann Intern Med 1972;77:361
98. Kaibuchi K, Sano K, Hoshijima M, et al. Phosphatidylinositol turnover in platelet activation: Calcium mobilization and protein phosphorylation. Cell Calcium 1982;3:323
99. Ishii H, Umeda F, Hashimoto T, Nawata H. Changes in phosphoinositide turnover, Ca2+ mobilization, and protein phosphorylation in platelets from NIDDM patients. Diabetes 1990;39:1561
100. Ishii H, Umeda F, Hashimoto T, Nawata H. Increased inositol phosphate accumulation in platelets from patients with NIDDM. Diabetes Res Clin Pract 1991;14:21
101. Bastyr EJ III, Kadrofski MM, Dershimer RC, Vinik AI. Decreased platelet phosphoinositide turnover and enhanced platelet activation in IDDM. Diabetes 1989;38:1097
102. Bastyr EJ III, Kadrofske MM, Vinik AI. Platelet activity and phosphoinositide turnover increase with advancing age. Am J Med 1990;88:601
103. Pellegatta F, Folli F, Ronchi P, et al. Deranged platelet calcium homeostasis in poorly controlled IDDM patients. Diabetes Care 1993;16:178
104. Tschope D, Rosen P, Gries FA. Increase in the cytosolic concentration of calcium in platelets of diabetics type II. Thromb Res 1991;62:421
105. Brownlee M. Advanced products of nonenzymatic glycosylation and the pathogenesis of diabetic complications. In: Rifkin H, Porte D Jr, eds. Diabetes Mellitus, Theory and Practice. New York: Elsevier;1990:277
106. Winocour PD, Watala C, Kinlough-Rathbone RL. Membrane fluidity is related to the extent of glycation of proteins, but not to alterations in the cholesterol to phospholipid molar ratio in isolated platelet membranes from diabetic and control subjects. Thromb Haemost 1992;67:567
107. Winocour PD, Bryszewska M, Watala C, et al. Reduced membrane fluidity in platelets from diabetic patients. Diabetes 1990;39:241
108. Watanabe J, Wohltmann HJ, Klein RL, et al. Enhancement of platelet aggregation by low-density lipoproteins from IDDM patients. Diabetes 1988;37:1652
109. Tschoepe D, Roesen P, Kaufmann L, et al. Evidence for abnormal glycoprotein receptor expression on diabetes mellitus. Eur J Clin Invest 1990;20:166
110. Nolan RD, Lapetina EG. Thrombin stimulates the production of a novel polyphosphoinositide in human platelets. J Biol Chem 1990;265:2441
111. Kucera GL, Rittenhouse SE. Human platelets form 3-phosphorylated phosphoinositides in response to alpha-thrombin, U46619, or GTP gamma S. J Biol Chem 1990;265:5345
112. Zhang J, Fry MJ, Waterfield MD, et al. Activated phosphoinositide 3-kinase associates with membrane skeleton in thrombin-exposed platelets. J Biol Chem 1992;267:4686
113. Falcon C, Pfliegler G, Deckmyn H, Vermylen J. The platelet insulin receptor: Detection, partial characterization, and search for a function. Biochem Biophys Res Commun 1988;157:1190
114. Hiramatsu K, Nozaki H, Arimori A. Reduction of platelet aggregation induced by euglycaemic insulin clamp. Diabetologia 1987;30:310
115. Trovati M, Anfossi G, Cavalot F, et al. Insulin directly reduces platelet sensitivity to aggregating agents: Studies in vitro and in vivo. Diabetes 1988; 37:780
116. Kahn NN, Sinha AK. Down regulation of alpha-2 adrenergic receptor numbers in platelets by insulin. Biochim Biophys Acta 1992;1134:292
117. Abrahm DR, Hollingsworth PJ, Smith CB, et al. Decreased alpha 2-adrenergic receptors on platelet membranes from diabetic patients with autonomic neuropathy and orthostatic hypotension. J Clin Endocrinol Metab 1986;63:906
118. Lanza F, Beretz A, Stierle A, et al. Epinephrine potentiates human platelet activation but is not an aggregating agent. Am J Physiol 1988;255:H1276
119. Jakobs KH, Saur W, Schultz G. Reduction of adenylate cyclase activity in lysates of human platelets by the alpha-adrenergic component of epinephrine. J Cyclic Nucleotide Res 1976;2:381
120. Atlas D, Steer ML. Clonidine p-isothiocyanate, an affinity label for alpha 2-adrenergic receptors on human platelets. Proc Natl Acad Sci U S A 1982; 79:1378
121. Lopez-Aparicio P, Rascon A, Manganiello VC, et al. Insulin-induced phosphorylation and activation of the cGMP-inhibited cAMP phosphodiesterase in human platelets. Biochem Biophys Res Commun 1992;186:517
122. Trovati M, Anfossi G, Mularoni E, et al. Insulin reduces platelet sensitivity to platelet activating factor in washed human platelets resuspended in a calcium-free medium. Diabetes Metab Nutr 1989;2:151
123. McDonald JW, Dupre J, Rodger NW, et al. Comparison of platelet thromboxane synthesis in diabetic patients on conventional insulin therapy and continuous insulin infusions. Thromb Res 1982;28:705
124. Murer EH, Gyda MA, Martinez NJ. Insulin increases the aggregation response of human platelets to ADP. Thromb Res 1994;73:69
125. Udvardy M, Pfliegler G, Rak K. Platelet insulin receptor determination in non-insulin dependent diabetes mellitus. Experientia 1985;41:422
126. Kahn NN, Bauman WA, Sinha AK. Transient decrease of binding of insulin to platelets in acute ischemic heart disease. Am J Med Sci 1994;307:21
127. Kahn NN, Sinha AK. Stimulation of prostaglandin E1 binding to human blood platelet membrane by insulin and the activation of adenylate cyclase. J Biol Chem 1990;265:4976
128. Stout RW. Diabetes and atherosclerosis—The role of insulin. Diabetologia 1979;16:141
129. Tschope D, Schwippert B, Schettler B, et al. Increased GPIIB/IIIA expression and altered DNA-ploidy pattern in megakaryocytes of diabetic BB-rats. Eur J Clin Invest 1992;22:591

Diabetes Mellitus, edited by Derek LeRoith, Simeon I. Taylor, and Jerrold M. Olefsky. Lippincott–Raven Publishers, Philadelphia © 1996.

Chapter 94
Free Radicals, Nitric Oxide, and Diabetic Complications

Jerry L. Nadler and Lori Winer

Increasing evidence suggests that increased oxidative stress and changes in nitric oxide (NO) formation or activity play major roles in the complications of diabetes. In this chapter, an overview of free radical and nitric oxide pathways is presented. Subsequently, the potential mechanisms underlying diabetes-induced alterations of the activity of these pathways are reviewed in the context of the relevance of these changes to the development of vascular complications of diabetes. Finally, the practical application of this information and future considerations for prevention of diabetes complications are discussed.

Overview of Free Radicals

Free radicals are highly reactive molecules with unpaired electrons in the outer orbital. Free radicals perform beneficial tasks, such as aiding in the destruction of microorganisms and cancer cells. Excessive production of free radicals or inadequate antioxidant defense mechanisms, however, can lead to damage of cellular structures and enzymes.[1] Damage to entire tissues can result from free radical–mediated oxidative alteration of fatty acids, also known as lipid peroxidation.[2] There are well-characterized reactions that lead to the formation of the superoxide anion, hydrogen peroxide, and the highly toxic hydroxyl radical.[1] The cytotoxic potential of the superoxide anion is derived mainly from its ability to be converted to the hydroxyl radical directly or via interaction with hydrogen peroxide. The superoxide anion can also interact with NO to form peroxynitrite, which can degrade to form the hydroxyl radical.[3] Peroxy radicals can remove hydrogen from lipids, such as polyunsaturated fatty acids, resulting in the formation of lipid hydroperoxides and further propagation of the radical pathways by regeneration of alkyl radicals.[4]

Hydroperoxides have direct toxic effects for endothelial cells and can also degrade to form the hydroxyl radical.[1] Hydroperoxides may also react with transition metals to form stable aldehydes, such as malondialdehyde (MDA), which damages membranes by facilitating the formation of protein cross-links and other end products.[5] Rao and Berk have shown that active oxygen species can stimulate vascular smooth muscle cell (VSMC) growth and proto-oncogene expression.[6] These authors suggest that arterial injury, active oxygen species production, and VSMC proliferation are strongly related. In support of this hypothesis is genetic evidence for a common pathway mediating oxidative stress, inflammatory gene induction, and aortic fatty streak formation in mice.[7]

New evidence suggests that certain enzymatic pathways of arachidonic or linoleic acid metabolism can participate in the formation of free radicals and lipid peroxides in the vascular and renal systems. It has been suggested that certain lipoxygenase (LO) enzymes that react with arachidonic or linoleic acids play an important role in atherosclerosis by inducing the oxidation of low-density lipoprotein (LDL).[8] Data suggest that a 15-LO is co-localized in macrophage-rich areas of human atherosclerotic lesions.[9] Furthermore, there is evidence that a leukocyte type of 12-LO is expressed in human vascular and mononuclear cells.[10] In addition, the leukocyte type of 12-LO is an important mediator of the effects of angiotensin II.[11–13] The hydroperoxyeicosatetraenoic acids (HPETEs) and more stable hydroxyeicosatetraenoic acids (HETEs) can lead to VSMC migration.[14] Also, 12-HPETE and 12-HETE are potent direct inhibitors of renin secretion in isolated kidney preparations.[15] These LO products also activate many of the pathways linked to increased vascular and renal disease, including protein kinase C (PKC), oncogene activation, and increased matrix production.[16–18] In particular, these LO enzymes can generate superoxide radicals via oxidation of pyridine nucleotides.[19] Furthermore, new evidence indicates that one product of the 12-LO enzyme has potent angiogenic properties at subnanomolar concentrations.[20] Table 94-1 summarizes several potential actions of these LO products that are relevant to vascular complications of diabetes.

Morrow and coworkers[21] have reported that a series of free radical–catalyzed peroxidation products of arachidonic acid, called isoprostanes, can be formed in vivo in models of oxidative stress. These prostanoids are formed in a cyclo-oxygenase–independent manner and remain associated with membrane phospholipids until they are released by phospholipases. One isoprostane—8 epi-$PGF_2\alpha$—is potentially relevant to diabetic vascular disease based on its potent vascular and renal vasoconstrictive properties and its growth-promoting actions for vascular smooth muscle.[22] There is new evidence that 8 epi-$PGF_2\alpha$ concentration is increased in VSMCs cultured in elevated (25 mM) glucose.[23]

Antioxidant defense mechanisms are critically important for the ultimate effects of oxidative stress and free radicals on cells and tissues. Antioxidants may interrupt lipid peroxidation and inorganic free radical reactions or scavenge the reactive intermediates formed. Nonenzymatic antioxidants that affect lipid peroxidation (LPO) include vitamin E, which inhibits the initiation step; vitamin C, which, along with vitamin E, inhibits hydroperoxide formation; thiol-containing compounds, such as glutathione, cysteine, methio-

Table 94-1. Potential Roles of the 12- and 15-Lipoxygenase Pathway in Cardiovascular Disorders

Inhibition of renal renin release (particularly the 12-lipoxygenase pathway)
Inhibition of prostacyclin synthesis
Direct vasoconstriction of certain vascular beds
Mediator of angiotensin II action in blood vessels and adrenal glomerulosa (particularly the 12-lipoxygenase pathway)
Growth-promoting effect on endothelial and VSMCs
Possible involvement in oxidative modification of LDL

nine, ubiquinone, and urate, which degrade hydroperoxides into nonradical metabolites; chelators, such as penicillamine, which bind transition metals necessary for some reactions involved in LPO; and vitamins A and E, which scavenge free radicals to produce a less reactive species.[24] Glutathione peroxidase (GPx) is an enzymatic antioxidant that degrades hydroperoxides to less reactive products.[24]

Nonenzymatic antioxidants involved in inorganic free radical reactions include metal chelators that inhibit the Fenton and Haber-Weiss-type reactions; scavengers of free radicals, such as vitamin A, vitamin E, and urate;[4,5,25–26] and inactivators of inorganic reactions, such as glutathione (GSH). Enzymatic antioxidants that promote inactivation of inorganically derived free radicals include superoxide dismutase (SOD), catalase (CAT), GPx, and gluthione reductase (GR), which replenishes the intracellular supply of GSH.[27]

Overview of Nitric Oxide

Nitric oxide (NO) has emerged as one of the most important molecules released from the endothelium and a variety of other tissues. Several recent excellent reviews have detailed aspects of NO synthesis and function.[28–33] NO is a free radical that can act as a neurotransmitter or in a paracrine or autocrine manner to produce diverse cellular responses, both beneficial and detrimental.

Many cells and tissues contain specific isoforms of NO synthase (NOS), which oxidize the guanidino nitrogen of arginine to form citrulline and NO. The enzymes utilize reduced nicotinamide adenine dinucleotide phosphate, flavin adenine dinucleotide, flavin mononucleotide, and tetrahydrobiopterin as cofactors. The human NOSs have been isolated and cloned, and can generally be divided into three major categories (Table 94-2): endothelial NOS (ecNOS or type III NOS), inducible NOS (iNOS or type II NOS) and neuronal NOS (ncNOS or type I NOS). nc and ecNOS are constitutive, calcium/calmodulin-dependent enzymes that synthesize small basal quantities of NO.[28,30] New evidence suggests, however, that ecNOS activity can be regulated by certain cytokines and sex hormones.[34,35] In addition, new evidence suggests that insulin may lead to vasodilation by activating NOS.[36] Furthermore, we have shown that nerve stimulation can directly increase the release of NO from isolated rat skeletal muscle.[37] In contrast to the constitutive forms, the activity and expression of iNOS is low or absent in resting cells. In an increasing number of cell types, iNOS expression and activity can be induced rapidly by the action of certain cytokines and lipopolysaccharide.[29] The activity of iNOS appears to be largely independent of intracellular calcium concentrations.[29] iNOS can be expressed in many cells, including pancreatic β-cells, macrophages, fibroblasts, vascular endothelial and smooth muscle cells, mesangial cells, and cardiac myocytes.[29] iNOS can produce large bursts of NO, which can be cytotoxic or can inhibit pathogens.

In most cases, NO binds to and activates the soluble form of guanylate cyclase to generate cyclic guanosine monophosphate (cGMP), resulting in biologic effects.[32,33] However, NO may also exert its effects by a mechanism that does not involve cGMP, such as through the promotion of ADP ribosylation.[33,38]

NO produces many desirable effects that act to maintain the normal vascular tone and reduce the rate of atherosclerosis (Table 94-3). NO was originally identified as a potent endothelial-derived relaxing factor for vascular smooth muscle. New evidence indicates that NO can antagonize the actions of the pressor peptides, such as angiotensin II.[39] NO also inhibits platelet aggregation and adhesion through a cGMP mechanism.[40] Upon activation, platelets release NO, resulting in a negative feedback loop to inhibit further activation. NO can inhibit leukocyte adhesion to activated endothelium,[41] thus blocking a critical step in the atherosclerotic process. Furthermore, NO can inhibit VSMC growth and migration,[32,40,42] and can reduce the oxidation of LDL by macrophages.[3] Very recent studies also indicate that NO can reduce expression of endothelin and platelet-derived growth factor in normal or hypoxic endothelium.[43] Cooke and coworkers[43] have shown that supplementation of L-arginine, the precursor for NO, can reduce the rate of atherosclerosis in the hypercholesterolemic rabbit model.[44]

A wide variety of studies, therefore, have demonstrated the beneficial actions of NO in the prevention of cardiovascular disease. In specific circumstances, however, NO, when generated in large quantities for long periods of time, can be cytostatic or cytotoxic for organisms or cells.

The oxidative state profoundly affects NO function.[31] Superoxide generating systems can inhibit constitutive NOS activity.[45] The superoxide anion can also react with NO to yield peroxynitrite which, in turn, decomposes to the toxic hydroxyl radical.[3] The hydroxyl radical subsequently can lead to substantial vessel injury.[46] Peroxynitrite is also a mediator of lipoprotein oxidation.[47] A very recent study has shown that, under certain circumstances, derivatives of NO can lead to biologically active oxidized LDL, which could accelerate atherosclerosis.[48] Therefore, under states of oxidative stress, as in diabetes, it is possible that a lack of NO formation or NO conversion to toxic radicals could contribute to the development and progression of cardiovascular disease. Clearly, hypertension and atherosclerosis, in general, have been characterized as states showing reduced ecNOS activity.[38]

Table 94-3. Beneficial Vascular Actions of Nitric Oxide

Potent vasodilation of smooth muscle
Inhibition of platelet aggregation and adhesion
Inhibition of leukocyte adhesion to activated endothelium
Inhibition of VSMC migration and proliferation
Reduction of macrophage-dependent oxidation of LDL
Inhibition of expression of endothelin and platelet-derived growth factor by the vascular endothelium

Table 94-2. Various Forms of Nitric Oxide Synthase (NOS) in Humans

Type	Calcium/Calmodulin Dependence	Constitutive	Chromosomal Location
ecNOS (also known as type II NOS)	Yes	Yes	7q35–36
iNOS (also known as type II NOS)	No	No	17cen–q12
ncNOS (also known as type I NOS)	Yes	Yes	12q 24.2

ecNOS = endothelial nitric oxide synthase; iNOS = inducible nitric oxide synthase; ncNOS = neuronal nitric oxide synthase; Ca = calcium; CaM = calmodulin

Table 94-4. Potential Mechanisms by Which Hyperglycemia Can Lead to Free Radicals and Lipid Peroxidation

Through direct autooxidation of glucose
Induction and activation of various lipoxygenase enzymes
Activation of glycation pathways
Promotion of the interaction of nitric oxide with superoxide anions to produce peroxynitrite and hydroxyl radicals
Reduction of the activity of the antioxidant defense mechanisms

Mechanisms by Which Elevated Glucose Could Lead to Increased Oxidative Stress

In order for increased oxidative stress to be a plausible factor in the development of diabetic complications, the diabetic milieu must encourage an enhanced oxidative state. Table 94-4 describes several possible mechanisms by which hyperglycemia could increase the formation of free radicals and lipid peroxides. Glucose autoxidation, as described in cell-free systems, is a means by which glucose itself initiates free radical production.[49] Glucose, in its enediol form, may be autoxidized in a transition metal-dependent reaction to an enediol radical anion, which is then converted to ketoaldehyde, which can yield the superoxide anion. Superoxide anion then undergoes conversion to hydrogen peroxide and, ultimately, to the hydroxyl radical.[50–52] The hydroxyl radical produced specifically by glucose autoxidation has been shown to damage proteins.[53] In addition, glucose catalyzes LPO reactions.[54]

Elevated glucose has also been shown to increase the activity and expression of the LO enzymes. Endothelial cells cultured in elevated glucose have been found to produce more 15-HETE than cells maintained in normal glucose concentrations.[55] We have found that elevated glucose concentrations increase the rate of porcine VSMC growth.[56] Elevated glucose markedly increases basal 12-LO RNA expression[57] using a specific reverse transcriptase polymerase chain reaction (RT-PCR) technique (Fig. 94-1). Furthermore, elevated glucose conditions markedly enhance the effects of angiotensin II to increase 12-LO expression (see Fig. 94-1) and to stimulate fibronectin concentration in VSMCs.[18]

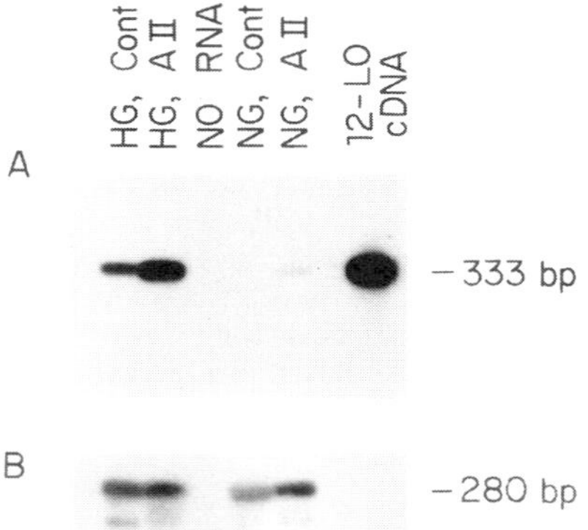

Figure 94-1. Regulation of porcine leukocyte-type 12-LO mRNA by angiotensin II (100 nM) treatment for 24 hours in porcine VSMCs cultured in normal glucose (NG) or high glucose (HG) concentrations. mRNA samples (0.5 μg each) were amplified for 25 cycles with porcine leukocyte 12-LO primers. Similar results were obtained in two separate experiments involving hybridization with 12-LO oligonucleotide (***A***) and GAPDH probes (***B***), respectively. (Reproduced with permission from Natarajan R, Gu JL, Rossi J, et al. Elevated glucose and angiotensin II increase 12-lipoxygenase activity and expression in porcine aortic smooth muscle cells. Proc Natl Acad Sci USA 1993;90:4947.)

Association of Free Radicals and Advanced Glycated End Products

Nonenzymatic glycosylation of proteins, or the Maillard reaction, begins with the interaction of glucose with protein to form early glycosylation products, known as Schiff bases and Amadori products. Amadori products may be degraded oxidatively to form carboxymethyllsine (CML),[58] or they may form glucose-derived protein cross-links, known as advanced glycosylation end products (AGEs) (as reviewed in Chapter 90). Protein and glucose mixtures in cell-free systems generate nanomolar quantities of H_2O_2,[51] and glucose can increase H_2O_2 levels in endothelial cells,[59] whereas Schiff bases and Amadori products are sources of the superoxide radical.[60] In addition, superoxide anion production by glycated polylysine, a glycated protein, is suppressed by SOD.[61] Glycosylated proteins drive other free radical reactions, as evidenced by the catalysis of LPO by glycated collagen[54] and glucose-treated LDL.[62] Vitamin E was found to inhibit completely, and SOD only partially to inhibit LPO catalyzed by glycated polylysine. However, catalase was found to have no effect, which demonstrates the nonuniformity of antioxidant effects on LPO induced by this process. CML and pentosidine, which are sugar-derived autoxidation products known as glycoxidation products, may initiate and propagate free radical reactions.[63] Another means by which AGE formation plays a role in diabetes-related oxidative stress is through glycation of antioxidant enzymes, such as copper, zinc (Cu-Zn) SOD,[64] resulting in inhibition of its activity.

Mailliard intermediates are capable of promoting free radical production. However, free radical reactions may also promote AGE formation. Glucose autoxidation, for example, enhances the covalent attachment of glucose to protein.[65] MDA, an end product of LPO, facilitates protein cross-linking, a destructive and final step in AGE formation. Conversely, the antioxidants vitamin E and lipoic acid prevent protein glycosylation.[66,67] Therefore, blockade of free radical formation could provide a mechanism for preventing AGE formation or blocking AGE action.

Antioxidant defense mechanisms may also be reduced in diabetes. In one study, endothelial cells of untreated diabetic rabbits showed reduced activity of Cu-Zn SOD and GPX.[68] Insulin either completely or partially restored these activities. Endothelial cell growth is inhibited by elevated glucose,[69] but these effects are reversed by GSH, SOD, and CAT,[70] suggesting that oxidative stress is an important mechanism for the glucose-induced decline in endothelial cell growth. In platelets from diabetic patients, the reduced GSH levels may be associated with increased platelet reactivity.[71]

It remains unclear whether circulatory or tissue levels of vitamin E are altered in diabetes given the marked heterogeneity of patients with diabetes. Unlike the mixed results with vitamin E,[72–74] most evidence suggests that ascorbic acid levels in plasma are low in people with diabetes.[75] Additional clarification of the levels of organic or inorganic antioxidant status in well-defined larger groups of diabetic patients will be required, however, before any general conclusions about this area can be made.

Evidence for an Enhanced Oxidative State in People with Diabetes

A state of enhanced oxidative stress in diabetes is suggested by a number of studies in which a variety of free radical measurements have been performed on the plasma or serum of patients with

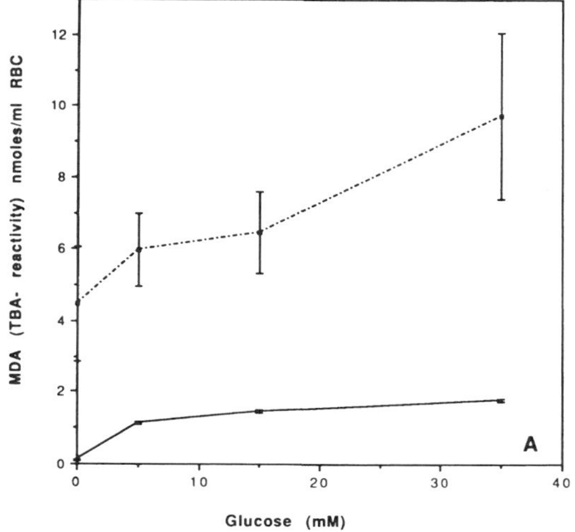

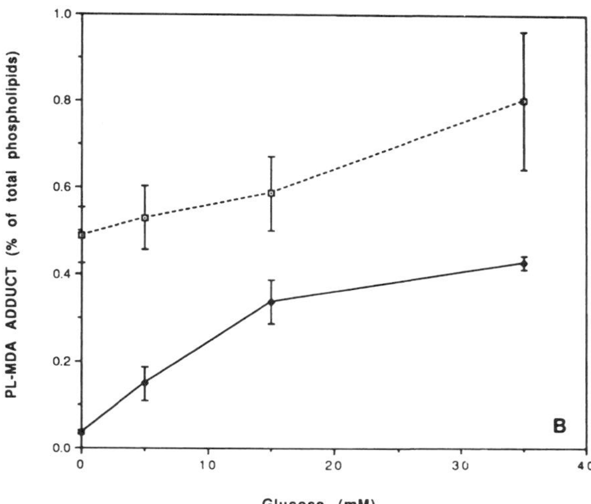

Figure 94-2. Effect of glucose on (*A*) malonyldialdehyde (MDA) and (*B*) phospholipid-MDA (PL-MDA) adduct formation in erythrocytes of diabetic (---■---) and normal healthy controls (——■—■——). Erythrocytes (45% hematocrit) in phosphate-buffered saline (PBS) with a pH of 7.4 were incubated with glucose (0–35 mM) for 24 hours at 37°C. At the end of incubation, erythrocytes were washed three times in PBS, and from the aliquots, the formation of MDA and phospholipid-MDA adduct was determined (as described in materials and methods). Each value represents mean ± S.D. (n = 25 for type II diabetics; n = 10 for normal healthy controls). *TBA*, thiobarbituric acid. (Reproduced with permission from Rajeswari P, Natarajan R, Nadler JL, et al. Glucose induces lipid peroxidation and inactivation of membrane-associated ion-transport enzymes in human erythrocytes in vivo and in vitro. J Cell Physiol 1991;149:100. © 1991. Reprinted by permission of John Wiley & Sons, Inc.)

IDDM and NIDDM. Plasma 2,3-dihydroxybenzoate levels, formed by direct hydroxyl radical attack on preadministered salicylate, are higher in well-controlled diabetic patients than in control subjects.[76] Superoxide anion production, as determined by the ferricytochrome C method, is greater in the serum of patients with IDDM than in that of normal subjects, and it correlates with glycemic control.[77] Plasma thiobarbituric acid (TBAR) levels, a measure of MDA that is an indirect index of LPO, are significantly higher in patients with poorly controlled NIDDM than in patients with well-controlled disease or in controls,[78] and urinary MDA levels are five times greater in poorly controlled diabetic rats compared to nondiabetic controls.[79] Levels of methylguanidine, a metabolic product of guanidine regulated by free radicals, are significantly higher in children with poorly controlled IDDM compared to those whose disease is well-controlled or control subjects.[80] Many of these studies support an association between blood glucose level and free radical load, which is consistent with the pathways outlined in Table 94-4.

Jain et al.[81] have demonstrated increased LPO in erythrocyte membranes of patients with IDDM. In more recent studies,[82] it has been found that erythrocytes from patients with NIDDM show an 8- to 10-fold increase in lipid MDA, and 13-fold higher levels of phospholipid MDA adduct (Fig. 94-2) when compared to healthy controls. Furthermore, as shown in Figure 94-2, glucose further increases MDA and phospholipid MDA adduct. In this same report, it was found that LO inhibitors, but not cyclo-oxygenase inhibitors, could reduce LPO induced by glucose.

Not all studies, however, demonstrate an increased free radical load in the diabetic state. Plasma TBAR levels in well-controlled diabetic patients were not significantly different than in control subjects.[76] Level of blood glucose control may be one factor responsible for these findings. Despite the heterogeneity of methodology, the bulk of the experimental data favors enhanced free radicals in diabetes, especially in the poorly-controlled state. Further studies will be required to evaluate fully whether oxidative stress in patients with diabetes varies with the presence of complications. These analyses will need to take into account the possible role of genetic variation in antioxidant activity or expression, which could modulate the effects of glucose on free radical formation.

NO: Effects of Diabetes

Emerging evidence suggests that diabetes mellitus can produce major changes in NO production or action. There are several likely mechanisms that explain how diabetes can alter NO pathways (Table 94-5).

In the diabetic rat and rabbit aorta, high glucose conditions result in impaired relaxation response to acetylcholine, implying a reduced release or action of NO.[83,84] This impaired dilation response is reversed by SOD, again suggesting an important role of free radicals in NO pathway dysfunction in diabetes.[84] Blockade of PKC has been found to reverse the high glucose–induced impairment of endothelium-dependent relaxation.[85] Furthermore, reduced NO-mediated increases in cGMP in glomeruli from diabetic rats are mediated, in part, by PKC activation,[86] suggesting that glucose-induced increases in PKC could be a factor in reduced NO action in diabetes.

It has been suggested that inhibition of Na^+-K^+ ATPase activity by elevated glucose could be a factor contributing to both microvascular and macrovascular disease.[87] It has been shown that

Table 94-5. Mechanisms by Which Diabetes Can Alter Nitric Oxide (NO) Pathways

Reduction of NO production
Reduction of NO action by interaction with AGEs
Reaction of NO with superoxide anions to produce peroxynitrite, which can promote oxidation of LDL and lead to LPO
Increased renal production or sensitivity of NO in early diabetic nephropathy

the glucose-induced reduction of Na^+-K^+ ATPase activity can be completely reversed by L-arginine or sodium nitroprusside (Fig. 94-3), implying that glucose effects are secondary to inhibition of NO formation.[87]

In a very recent preliminary report,[88] glucose was demonstrated to reduce NOS activity in endothelial cells. Studies in porcine aortic endothelial cells exposed to high glucose conditions, however, actually demonstrated a net increase in NO formation owing to an enhanced free calcium concentration.[89] Furthermore, spontaneous NO release was greater in diabetic rat aorta than in controls, although NO activity was reduced.[90] The results of these in vitro studies indicate that diabetes can reduce NO action. However, additional carefully controlled studies in appropriate models evaluating NO expression, enzyme activity, and NO release will be required to clarify the effects of diabetes on NO production.

There have been several important human studies indicating that diabetes may alter NO action. In a study of 15 patients with IDDM,[91] it was found that forearm vasodilatory responses to methacholine were reduced in this population compared to controls (Fig. 94-4). In another study of patients with IDDM, it was found that blockade of NO with an NO inhibitor or exogenous NO administration with nitroprusside produced less of a forearm flow response in the diabetic patients than in controls.[92] In this and another study in patients with IDDM without complications,[93] no difference in stimulated NO action was demonstrated between the diabetics and controls, suggesting that abnormalities in NO may not directly occur in diabetes unless another factor, such as enhanced AGEs or free radicals, is also present.

It is likely that NO action is reduced in NIDDM. This interesting premise will require further investigation, however, particularly taking into account the role of hyperlipidemia, insulin resistance, hypertension, and altered ions, such as calcium and magnesium, in NO production and action.

Diabetes can also have a profound influence on NO action and metabolism through effects of free radicals and AGEs on NO. In an earlier section, evidence was reviewed showing that NO can react with superoxide anions to produce peroxynitrite, which can lead to membrane damage and LPO. AGEs also exert substantial effects on NO. AGEs have been shown to quench NO in vitro and in rat models.[94] Highly glycosylated hemoglobin inhibits acetylcholine-induced, endothelium-dependent relaxation in rat aorta, whereas nonglycosylated and low-glycosylated hemoglobin have no inhibitory effects.[95] The time course of NO quenching, which occurs after formation of Amadori products, is similar to the time course of free radical production by AGEs.[94] This temporal relationship provides support for NO quenching by an enhanced free radical load induced by glucose. AGEs also have been shown to block the antiproliferative effect of NO in rat aortic smooth muscle and murine glomerular mesangial cells.[96] In some studies, aminoguanidine has been found to be an inhibitor of NO, thus confounding the relationship between NO and AGEs. Bucala et al.[94] demonstrated that when aminoguanidine was administered to rats that were diabetic for less than 1 month the vasodilatory impairment otherwise observed in these diabetic animals was ameliorated, suggesting that aminoguanidine, presumably by blocking AGE formation, increased NO. Aminoguanidine treatment at later time points, however, had no effect. Other studies have found that aminoguanidine exerts its beneficial effects by inhibiting the formation of NO. Aminoguanidine administration exerts effects similar to those of an NO inhibitor in rat insulinoma cells.[97] Aminoguanidine also has been found to be equipotent to an NO inhibitor in its ability to inhibit glucose-induced increases in vascular albumin clearance in a skin chamber granulation model. The similarities between the NO inhibitor and aminoguanidine action provide indirect evidence for aminoguanidine functioning as an NO inhibitor.

In support of this hypothesis, Tilton et al.[98] have demonstrated that aminoguanidine inhibits NOS, as measured by L-arginine conversion to L-citrulline. Methylguanidine, which is equipotent to aminoguanidine as an inhibitor of NOS, but which has limited ability to prevent AGE formation, was found to reduce regional vascular albumin hyperpermeation induced by diabetes to levels comparable to those of aminoguanidine. These data suggest that, in some instances, the mechanism by which aminoguanidine normalizes diabetes-induced vascular dysfunction is related to its ability to inhibit NO production instead of its action to prevent AGE formation. Therefore, further studies using analogues of aminoguanidine that do not alter NO action may be needed to clarify the relative effects of AGEs versus altered NO metabolism in this agent's ability to reduce diabetic complications.

There also may be a situation in which excess production or action of NO could participate in the development of diabetic complications. Early states of diabetic nephropathy are associated with an increase in glomerular filtration rate (GFR). This increase in GFR may be a risk factor for the development of overt diabetic nephropathy.[99] The mechanisms responsible for increases in GFR remain poorly understood. Experiments using L-arginine analogues

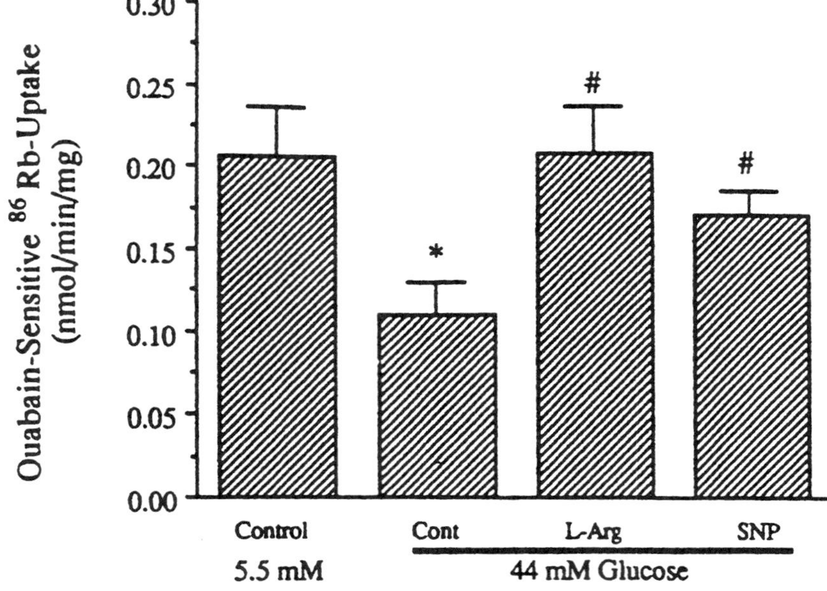

Figure 94-3. Reversal of hyperglycemia-induced inhibition of ouabain-sensitive (OS) ^{86}Rb-uptake by L-arginine and sodium nitroprusside (SNP) in endothelium-intact aorta. L-arginine (0.3 mM) and SNP (10 μM) were added to the incubation media during the final 30 and 10 minutes, respectively, of the 3-hour incubation; hyperglycemia failed to decrease OS ^{86}Rb-uptake. Results are means ± SE of five experiments. The asterisk (*) denotes values that are significantly different from those in aorta incubated in 5.5 or 44 mM glucose ($P < 0.05$). Cont = control (Reproduced with permission from Gupta S, Sussman I, McArthur CS, et al. Endothelium-dependent inhibition of Na^+-K^+ ATPase activity in rabbit aorta by hyperglycemia: Possible role of endothelium-derived nitric oxide. J Clin Invest 1992;90:727.)

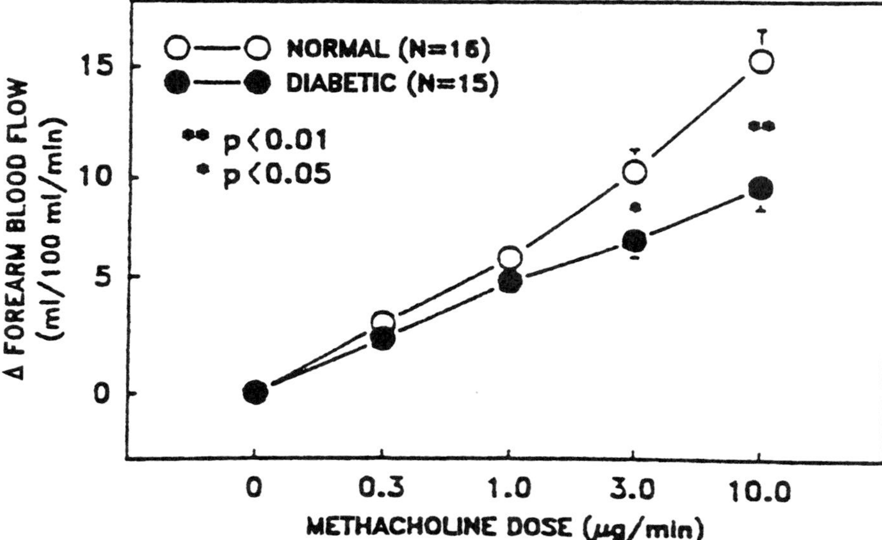

Figure 94-4. Plot of forearm blood flow response to intra-arterial infusion of methacholine chloride in normal and diabetic subjects. Cholinergic vasodilation was less in the diabetic group than in the normal group. The difference between groups was significant at the 3 and 10 μg/min doses. (Reproduced with permission from Johnstone MT, Creager SJ, Scales KM, et al. Impaired endothelium-dependent vasodilation in patients with insulin-dependent diabetes mellitus. Circulation 1993;88:2510.)

to inhibit NO, such as N-monomethyl-2-arginine (L-NMMA) or nitro-L-arginine methylester (L-NAME), have shown that NO is a potent renal vasodilator.[100] Recent evidence using these NO inhibitors or NO donors in experimental animal models suggests that increases in NO release or action may, in part, be responsible for diabetic renal hyperfiltration.[101,102] The trigger for increased NO production in early diabetes is not clear, but evidence suggests that increases in diacylglycerol by elevated glucose could result in increased NO production.[86,98]

Conclusions and Future Prospects for New Methods to Prevent Diabetic Vascular Complications

The weight of experimental and human evidence supports a clear role for increased oxidant stress in many of the proposed biochemical pathways linked to the microvascular and macrovascular complications of diabetes. In particular, very recent evidence has underscored the particular role elevated glucose plays in oxidative modification of LDL by a superoxide-dependent pathway,[103] and has demonstrated that, in people with poorly controlled IDDM, there is increased LDL oxidation associated with reduced antioxidant defenses.[104]

Most of the studies in the literature have focused on the role of oxidative stress as it relates to the effects of hyperglycemia on diabetic complications. It has been established, however, that insulin resistance and hyperinsulinemia are important factors linked to hypertension and atherosclerotic cardiovascular disease (reviewed in other chapters). Several lines of evidence now support the concept that NO activation may be an important mechanism in insulin-induced vasodilatory effects. Two recent independent studies using inhibitors of NOS have demonstrated a reduction in insulin's vasodilatory actions.[36,105] The source of NO in response to insulin, however, was not fully evaluated in these studies. It is now clear, though, that skeletal muscle can synthesize NO,[37] suggesting that blood vessels and skeletal muscle may be potential sources of NO release in response to insulin.

One area for future investigation will be to determine whether altered NO release or action could be involved in altered vascular function and hypertension in insulin-resistant states. The results of these types of studies could provide a rationale for modulation of the NO system to reduce diabetic complications associated with hyperinsulinemia.

The particular role of NO in insulin's metabolic functions remains to be evaluated. There are several intriguing human studies, however, that show that administration of antioxidants improves insulin action in humans with NIDDM.[106,107] It is possible, therefore, that increased oxidative stress plays a role in the reduced metabolic effects of insulin.

One obvious question that arises from the information available is whether supplementation with antioxidants, such as vitamins C and E, is warranted to prevent diabetic complications. A recent study by Kunisaki et al.[108] highlights this issue by showing that vitamin E and another antioxidant, probucol, normalize the changes in diacylglycerol and PKC activation in diabetic rats. Despite additional studies in nondiabetics supporting the potential benefit of vitamin E to reduce vascular disease,[109–111] one must use caution in recommending antioxidant supplements to people with diabetes without appropriate controlled trials in these subjects. One basis for this caution is that, under certain circumstances, vitamin E or C can actually act as a pro-oxidant.[112,113] Also, vitamin C shares several cellular transport mechanisms with glucose,[114] and it can increase the rate of absorption of iron, which is a pro-oxidant. The American Diabetes Association has recently published a consensus statement on this issue, which states that supplementation with antioxidant vitamins cannot be recommended for all diabetics at this time.[115] Clearly, a large-scale clinical trial in patients with diabetes evaluating the role of antioxidants on parameters linked to glucose control, as well as insulin and NO action, will be needed to fully address this important issue.

The role of nutrition should be considered as a factor related to increased oxidative stress in diabetes. Evidence in diabetic animals shows that oxidized lipids in the diet make a major contribution to the levels of oxidized lipids in lipoproteins, and that diabetes increases the rate of oxidized lipid absorption.[116] Furthermore, magnesium deficiency, which is a common problem in patients with NIDDM,[117,118] has been associated with increased free radical damage, insulin resistance, and increased vasomotor tone.[119,120] One study in diabetics from St. Louis,[121] and our data in 50 nonselected patients with NIDDM in Duarte (unpublished observations, 1995), indicate that more than 50% of diabetics consume less than the recommended dietary allowance of Mg. Thus, studies are warranted that would address the effect on diabetic complications of modified dietary intake of factors that reduce oxidant stress.

In conclusion, it is likely that, in the near future, new pharmacologic or nutritional approaches for reducing diabetic complications will become available as we gain knowledge of the mechanisms by which diabetes may lead to oxidative stress and altered function or synthesis of NO.

Acknowledgments

The authors would like to thank Elizabeth Rees for preparing the manuscript and Rachmiel Levine, M.D. for his inspiration and support. J. Nadler's research is supported in part by grants from the NIH DK 39721, HL 41295 and PO1 HL55798 and the Juvenile Diabetes Foundation.

References

1. Southorn PA. Free radicals in medicine. 1. Chemical nature and biologic reactions. Mayo Clin Proc 1988;63:381
2. Halliwell B, Gutteridge JMC. Free Radicals in Biology and Medicine. New York: Oxford University Press;1985:139
3. Hogg N, Kalyanaraman B, Joseph J, et al. Inhibition of low-density lipoprotein oxidation by nitric oxide: Potential role in atherogenesis. FEBS Lett 1993; 334:170
4. Halliwell B, Gutteridge JM. Role of free radicals and catalytic metal ions in human diseases: An overview. In: Packer L, Glazer AN, eds. Oxygen Radicals in Biological Systems. (Part B: Oxygen Radicals and Antioxidants). Methods Enzymol 1990;186:1
5. Freeman BA, Crapo JD. Biology of disease: Free radicals and tissue injury. Lab Invest 1982;47:412
6. Rao GN, Berk BC. Active oxygen species stimulate vascular smooth muscle cell growth and proto-oncogene expression. Circ Res 1992;70:593
7. Feng L, Andalibi A, Qiao JH, et al. Genetic evidence for a common pathway mediating oxidative stress, inflammatory gene induction, and aortic fatty streak formation in mice. J Clin Invest 1994;94:877
8. Kuhn H, Belkner J, Suzuki H, Yamamoto S. Oxidative modification of human lipoproteins by lipoxygenases of different positional specificities. J Lipid Res 1994;35:1749
9. Ylä-Hertuala S, Rosenfeld ME, Parthasarathy S, et al. Colocalization of 15-lipoxygenase mRNA and protein with epitopes of oxidized low density lipoprotein in macrophage-rich areas of atherosclerotic lesions. Proc Natl Acad Sci USA 1990;87:6959
10. Kim J, Gu J, Natarajan R, et al. A leukocyte type of 12-lipoxygenase is expressed in human vascular and mononuclear cells. Arterioscler Thromb Vasc Biol 1995;15:942
11. Nadler JL, Natarajan R, Stern N. Specific action of the lipoxygenase pathway in mediating angiotensin II-induced aldosterone synthesis in isolated adrenal glomerulosa cells. J Clin Invest 1987;80:1763
12. Gu J, Natarajan R, Ben-Ezra J, et al. Evidence that a leukocyte type of 12-lipoxygenase is expressed and regulated by angiotensin II in human adrenal glomerulosa cells. Endocrinology 1994;134:70
13. Nozawa K, Tuck M, Golub M, et al. Inhibition of the lipoxygenase pathway reduces blood pressure in renovascular hypertensive rats. Am J Physiol 1990;259:H174
14. Nakao J, Ooyama T, Ito H, et al. Comparative effect of lipoxygenase products of arachidonic acid on rat aortic smooth muscle cell migration. Atherosclerosis 1982;44:339
15. Antonipillai I, Nadler JL, Robin EC, Horton R. The inhibitory role of 12- and 15-lipoxygenase products on renin release. Hypertension 1987;10:61
16. Natarajan R, Lanting L, Xu L, Nadler J. Role of specific isoforms of protein kinase C in angiotensin II and lipoxygenase action in rat adrenal glomerulosa cells. Mol Cell Endocrinol 1994;101:59
17. Haliday E, Ramesha C, Ringold G. TNF induces c-fos via a novel pathway requiring conversion of arachidonic acid to a lipoxygenase metabolite. EMBO J 1991;10:109
18. Natarajan R, Gonzales N, Lanting L, Nadler J. Role of the lipoxygenase pathway in angiotensin II-induced vascular smooth muscle cell hypertrophy. Hypertension 1994;23:142
19. Roy P, Roy SK, Mitra A, Kulkarni AP. Superoxide generation by lipoxygenase in the presence of NADH and NADPH. Biochim Biophys Acta 1994;1214:171
20. Laniado-Schwartzman M, Lavrovsky Y, Stoltz R, et al. Activation of nuclear factor kB and oncogene expression by 12(R)-hydroxyeicosatrienoic acid, and angiogenic factor in microvessel endothelial cells. J Biol Chem 1994;269: 24321
21. Morrow JD, Awad JA, Hollis JB, et al. Non–cyclooxygenase-derived prostanoids (F_2-isoprostanes) are formed *in situ* on phospholipids. Proc Natl Acad Sci USA 1992;89:10721
22. Fukunaga M, Makita N, Roberts JL, et al. Evidence for the existence of F_2-isoprostane receptors on rat vascular smooth muscle cells. Am J Physiol 1993;264:1619
23. Natarajan R, Lanting L, Nadler J. Formation of a F_2-isoprostane, 8-epi-prostaglandin $F_2\alpha$ in vascular smooth muscle cells (VSMC) by elevated glucose and growth factors. Am J Physiol (In press, 1996)
24. Feher J, Csomos G, Vereckei A. Free Radical Reactions in Medicine. 1st ed. Germany: Springer-Verlag;1987:11
25. Moser U, Bendich A. Vitamin C. In: Machlin LJ, ed. Handbook of Vitamins. 2nd ed. New York: Marcel Dekker, Inc.;1991:195
26. Machlin LJ. Vitamin E. In: Machlin LJ, ed. Handbook of Vitamins. 2nd ed. New York: Marcel Dekker;1991:99
27. Frank L, Massaro D. Oxygen toxicity. Am J Med 1980;69:117
28. Knowles R, Moncada S. Nitric oxide synthases in mammals. Biochem J 1994;298:249
29. Xie O, Nathan C. The high output nitric oxide pathway: Role and regulation. J Leukoc Biol 1994;56:576
30. Nathan C, Xie Z. Nitric oxide synthases: Roles, tolls and controls. Cell 1994;78:915
31. Stamler JS. Redox signalling: Nitrosylation and related target interactions of nitric oxide. Cell 1994;78:931
32. Schmidt HH, Walter U. NO at work. Cell 1994;78:919
33. Schmidt HH, Lohmann S, Walter U. The nitric oxide and cGMP signal transduction system. Biochim Biophys Acta 1993;1178:153
34. Weiss P, Sessa W, Milstein S, et al. Regulation of nitric oxide synthesis by proinflammatory cytokines in human umbilical vein endothelial cells. J Clin Invest 1994;93:2236
35. Weiner C, Lizasoain I, Baylis S, et al. Induction of calcium-dependent nitric oxide by sex hormones. Proc Natl Acad Sci USA 1994;91:5212
36. Steinberg H, Brechtel G, Johnson A, et al. Insulin-mediated skeletal muscle vasodilation is nitric oxide dependent: A novel action of insulin to increase nitric oxide release. J Clin Invest 1994;94:1172
37. Balon TW, Nadler JL. Nitric oxide release is present in skeletal muscle. J Appl Physiol 1994;77:2519
38. Dinerman JL, Lowenstein CJ, Snyder SH. Molecular mechanisms of nitric oxide regulation: Potential relevance to cardiovascular disease. Circ Res 1993;73:217
39. Ito S, Johnson CS, Carretero OA. Modulation of angiotensin II-induced vasoconstriction by endothelium-derived relaxing factor in the isolated microperfused rabbit afferent arteriole. J Clin Invest 1991;87:1656
40. Moncada S, Higgs A. The L-arginine-nitric oxide pathway. N Engl J Med 1993;329:2002
41. Kubes P, Suzuki M, Granger DN. Nitric oxide: An endogenous modulator of leukocyte adhesion. Proc Natl Acad Sci USA 1991;88:4651
42. Garg UC, Hassid A. Nitric oxide-generating vasodilators and 8-bromo-cyclic guanosine monophosphate inhibit mitogenesis and proliferation of cultured rat vascular smooth muscle cells. J Clin Invest 1989;83:1774
43. Kourembanas S, McQuillan LP, Leung GK, Faller DV. Nitric oxide regulates the expression of vasoconstrictors and growth factors by vascular endothelium under both normoxia and hypoxia. J Clin Invest 1993;92:99
44. Cooke JP, Singer AH, Tsao P, et al. Antiatherogenic effects of L-arginine in the hypercholesterolemic rabbit. J Clin Invest 1992;90:1168
45. Rengasamy A, Johns RA. Inhibition of nitric oxide synthase by a superoxide generating system. J Pharm Exp Ther 1993;267:1024
46. Beckman JS, Beckman TW, Chen J, et al. Apparent hydroxyl radical production by peroxynitrite: Implications for endothelial injury from nitric oxide and superoxide. Proc Natl Acad Sci USA 1990;87:1620
47. White CR, Brock TA, Chang L-Y, et al. Superoxide and peroxynitrite in atherosclerosis. Proc Natl Acad Sci USA 1994;91:1044
48. Chang GJ, Woo P, Honda HM, et al. Oxidation of LDL to a biologically active form by derivatives of nitric oxide and nitrite in the absence of superoxide. Arterioscler Thromb 1994;14:1808
49. Wolff SP, Crabbe MJC, Thornalley PJ. The autoxidation of glyceraldehyde and other simple monosaccharides. Experientia 1984;40:244
50. Wolff SP, Jiang Z-Y, Hunt JV. Protein glycation and oxidative stress in diabetes mellitus and aging. Free Radic Biol Med 1991;10:339
51. Jiang Z-Y, Woolard ACS, Wolff SP. Hydrogen peroxide production during experimental protein glycation. FEBS Lett 1990;268:69
52. Thornalley P, Wolff S, Crabbe M, Stern A. The autoxidation of glyceraldehyde and other simple monosaccharides under physiological conditions catalysed by buffer ions. Biochim Biophys Acta 1984;797:276
53. Hunt JV, Dean RT, Wolff SP. Hydroxyl radical production and autoxidative glycosylation: Glucose autoxidation as the cause of protein damage in the experimental glycation model of diabetes mellitus and aging. Biochem J 1988;256:205
54. Hicks M, Delbridge L, Yue DK, Reeve TS. Catalysis of lipid peroxidation by glucose and glycosylated collagen. Biochem Biophys Res Comm 1988;151:649
55. Brown ML, Jakubowski JA, Leventis JJ, Deykin D. Elevated glucose alters eicosanoid release from procine aortic endothelial cells. J Clin Invest 1988;82: 2136
56. Natarajan R, Gonzales N, Xu L, Nadler J. Vascular smooth muscle cells exhibit increased growth in response to elevated glucose. Biochem Biophys Res Commun 1992;187:552
57. Natarajan R, Gu JL, Rossi J, et al. Elevated glucose and angiotensin II increase 12-lipoxygenase activity and expression in porcine aortic smooth muscle cells. Proc Natl Acad Sci USA 1993;90:4947
58. Ahmed MU, Thorpe SR, Baynes JW. Identification of N^E-carboxymethyllysine as a degradation product of fructoselysine in glycated protein. J Biol Chem 1986;261:4889

59. Kashiwagi A, Asahina T, Ikebuchi M, et al. Abnormal glutathione metabolism and increased cytotoxicity caused by H_2O_2 in human umbilical vein endothelial cells cultured in high glucose medium. Diabetologia 1994;37:264
60. Mullarley CJ, Edelstein D, Brownlee M. Free radical generation by early glycation products: A mechanism for accelerated atherogenesis in diabetes. Biochem Biophys Res Comm 1990;173:932
61. Sakurai T, Sugioka K, Nakano M. 0_2-generation and lipid peroxidation during the oxidation of a glycated polypeptide, glycated polylysine, in the presence of iron-ADP. Biochim Biophys Acta 1990;1043:27
62. Hunt JV, Smith CCT, Wolff SP. Autoxidative glycosylation and possible involvement of peroxides and free radicals in LDL modification by glucose. Diabetes 1990;39:1420
63. Baynes JW. Role of oxidative stress in development of complications in diabetes. Diabetes 1991;40:405
64. Arai K, Maguchi S, Fujii S, et al. Glycation and inactivation of human Cu-Zn-superoxide dismutase: Identification of the in vitro glycated sites. J Biol Chem 1987;262:16969
65. Wolff SP, Dean RT. Glucose autoxidation and protein modification: The potential role of autoxidative glycosylation in diabetes. Biochem J 1987;245: 243
66. Ceriello A, Giugliano D, Quatraro A, et al. Vitamin E reduction of protein glycosylation in diabetes: New prospect for prevention of diabetic complications? Diabetes Care 1991;14:68
67. Kawabata T, Packer L. α-Lipoate can protect against glycation of serum albumin, but not low density lipoprotein. Biochem Biophys Res Comm 1994; 203:99
68. Tagami S, Yoshida K, Shimada M, et al. Antioxidant enzyme status of aortic endothelial cells in alloxan-induced diabetic rabbits (Abstract). Diabetes 1991;40(Suppl 1):221A
69. Nakao-Hayashi J, Ito H, Kawashima S. An oxidative mechanism is involved in high glucose-induced serum protein modification causing inhibition of endothelial cell proliferation. Atherosclerosis 1992;97:89
70. Curcio F, Ceriello A. Decreased cultured endothelial cell proliferation in high glucose medium is reversed by antioxidants: New insights on the pathophysiological mechanisms of diabetic vascular complications. In Vitro Cell Dev Biol 1992;28A:787
71. Thomas G, Skrinska V, Lucas FV, Schumacher OP. Platelet glutathione and thromboxane synthesis in diabetes. Diabetes 1985;34:951
72. Asayama K, Uchida N, Nakane T, et al. Antioxidants in the serum of children with insulin-dependent diabetes mellitus. Free Radic Biol Med 1993;15:597
73. Caye-Vaugien C, Krempf M, Lamarche P, et al. Determination of alpha-tocopherol in plasma, platelets, and erythrocytes of type I and type II diabetic patients by high-performance liquid chromatography. Int J Vitamin Nutr Res 1990;60:324
74. Jain SK, Levine SN, Duett J, Hollier B. Reduced vitamin E and increased lipofuscin products in erythrocytes of diabetic rats. Diabetes 1991;40:1241
75. Yue DK, McLenna S, Fisher E, et al. Ascorbic acid metabolism and polyol pathway in diabetes. Diabetes 1989;38:257
76. Ghiselli A, Laurenti O, De Mattie G, et al. Salicylate hydroxylation as an early marker of in vivo oxidative stress in diabetic patients. Free Radic Biol Med 1992;13:621
77. Ceriello A, Giugliano D, Quatraro A, et al. Metabolic control may influence the increased superoxide generation in diabetic serum. Diabetic Med 1991;8: 541
78. Altomare E, Vendemiale G, Chicco D, et al. Increased lipid peroxidation in type 2 poorly controlled diabetic patients. Diabetes Metab 1992;18:264
79. Galliaher DP, Cassalany AS, Shoeman DW, Olson JM. Diabetes increases excretion of urinary malonaldehyde conjugates in rats. Lipids 1993;28:663
80. Nagashima K, Yagi H, Yutani S, et al. Relationship between serum levels of methylguanadine and glycemic control in IDDM children. Diabetes Care 1993;16:1196
81. Jain SK, McVie R, Duett J, Herbst JJ. Erythrocyte membrane lipid peroxidation and glycosylated hemoglobin in diabetes. Diabetes 1989;38:1539
82. Rajeswari P, Natarajan R, Nadler JL, et al. Glucose induces lipid peroxidation and inactivation of membrane-associated ion-transport enzymes in human erythrocytes in vivo and in vitro. J Cell Physiol 1991;149:100
83. Tesfamariam B. Free radicals in diabetic endothelial cell dysfunction. Free Radic Biol Med 1994;16:383
84. Pieper GM, Mei DA, Langenstroer P, O'Rourke ST. Bioassay of endothelium-derived relaxing factor in diabetic rat aorta. Am J Physiol 1992;263:H676
85. Tesfamariam B, Brown JL, Cohen RA. Elevated glucose impairs endothelium-dependent relaxation by activating protein kinase C. J Clin Invest 1991; 86:1643
86. Craven PA, Studer RK, DeRubertis FR. Impaired nitric oxide–dependent cyclic guanosine monophosphate generation in glomeruli from diabetic rats: Evidence for protein kinase C–mediated suppression of the cholinergic response. J Clin Invest 1994;93:311
87. Gupta S, Sussman I, McArthur CS, et al. Endothelium-dependent inhibition of Na^+-K^+ ATPase activity in rabbit aorta by hyperglycemia: Possible role of endothelium-derived nitric oxide. J Clin Invest 1992;90:727
88. Gupta S, Tieken K, Ruderman N. Inhibition of nitric oxide synthase activity by hyperglycemia in endothelial cells (Abstract). Diabetes 1994;43(Suppl 1):100A
89. Graier WF, Wascher TC, Lackner L, et al. Exposure to elevated d-glucose concentrations modulates vascular endothelial cell vasodilatatory response. Diabetes 1993;42:1497
90. Langenstroer P, Pieper GM. Regulation of spontaneous EDRF release in diabetic rat aorta by oxygen free radicals. Am J Physiol 1992;263:H257
91. Johnstone MT, Creager SJ, Scales KM, et al. Impaired endothelium-dependent vasodilation in patients with insulin-dependent diabetes mellitus. Circulation 1993;88:2510
92. Calver A, Collier J, Vallance P. Inhibition and stimulation of nitric oxide synthesis in the human forearm arterial bed of patients with insulin-dependent diabetes. J Clin Invest 1992;90:2548
93. Smits P, Kapma J-A, Jacobs M-C, et al. Endothelium-dependent vascular relaxation in patients with type 1 diabetes. Diabetes 1993;42:148
94. Bucala R, Tracey KJ, Cerami A. Advanced glycosylation products quench nitric oxide and mediate defective endothelium-dependent vasodilatation in experimental diabetes. J Clin Invest 1991;87:432
95. Rodriguez-Manas L, Arribas S, Giron C, et al. Interference of glycosylated human hemoglobin with endothelium-dependent responses. Circulation 1993; 88:2111
96. Hogan M, Cerami A, Bucala R. Advanced glycosylation end products block the antiproliferative effect of nitric oxide: Role in the vascular and renal complications of diabetes mellitus. J Clin Invest 1992;90:1110
97. Corbett JA, Tilton RG, Chang K, et al. Aminoguanidine, a novel inhibitor of nitric oxide formation, prevents diabetic vascular dysfunction. Diabetes 1992;41:552
98. Tilton RG, Chang K, Hasan KS, et al. Prevention of diabetic vascular dysfunction by guanidines: Inhibition of nitric oxide synthase versus advanced glycation end-product formation. Diabetes 1993;42:221
99. Mogensen CE, Christensen CK. Predicting diabetic nephropathy in insulin-dependent patients. N Engl J Med 1984;311:89
100. Tolins JP, Palmer RM, Moncada S, Raij L. Role of endothelium-derived relaxing factor in regulation of renal hemodynamic responses. Am J Physiol 1990;258:655
101. Komers R, Allen TJ, Cooper ME. Role of endothelium-derived nitric oxide in the pathogenesis of the renal hemodynamic changes of experimental diabetes. Diabetes 1994;43:1190
102. Tolin JP, Schultz PJ, Raij L, et al. Abnormal renal hemodynamic response to reduced renal perfusion pressure in diabetic rats: Role of NO. Am J Physiol 1993;265:886
103. Kawamura M, Heinecke JW, Chait A. Pathophysiological concentrations of glucose promote oxidative modification of low density lipoprotein by a superoxide-dependent pathway. J Clin Invest 1994;94:771
104. Tsai EC, Hirsch IB, Brunzell JD, Chait A. Reduced plasma peroxyl radical trapping capacity and increased susceptibility of LDL to oxidation in poorly controlled IDDM. Diabetes 1994;43:1010
105. Scherrer U, Randin D, Vollenweider P, et al. Nitric oxide release accounts for insulin's vascular effects in humans. J Clin Invest 1994;94:2511
106. Paolisso G, Di Maro G, Pizza G, et al. Plasma GSH/GSSG affects glucose homeostasis in healthy subjects and non–insulin-dependent diabetics. Am J Physiol 1992;263:235
107. Paolisso G, D'amore A, Balbi V, et al. Plasma vitamin C affects glucose homeostasis in healthy subjects and in non–insulin-dependent diabetics. Endocrinol Metab 1994;266:251
108. Kunisaki M, Bursell S-E, Umeda F, et al. Normalization of diacylglycerol-protein kinase C activation by vitamin E in aorta of diabetic rats and cultured rat smooth muscle cells exposed to elevated glucose levels. Diabetes 1994;43:1372
109. Rimm EB, Stampfer MJ, Ascherio A, et al. Vitamin E consumption and the risk of coronary heart disease in men. N Engl J Med 1993;328:1450
110. Stampfer MJ, Hennekens CH, Manson JE, et al. Vitamin E consumption and the risk of coronary disease in women. N Engl J Med 1993;328:1444
111. Steinberg D. Antioxidant vitamins and coronary heart disease. N Engl J Med 1993;328:1487
112. Bowry VW, Ingold KU, Stocker R. Vitamin E in human low-density lipoprotein: When and how this antioxidant became a pro-oxidant. Biochem J 1992;288:341
113. Hunt JV, Bottoms MA, Mitchinson MJ. Ascorbic acid oxidation: A potential cause of the elevated severity of atherosclerosis in diabetes mellitus? FEBS Lett 1992;311:161
114. Mooradian AD. The effect of ascorbate and dehydroascorbate on tissue uptake of glucose. Diabetes 1987;36:1001
115. Mooradian AD, Failla M, Hoogwerf B, et al. Selected vitamins and minerals in diabetes. Diabetes Care 1994;17:464
116. Staprans I, Rapp JH, Pan X-M, Feingold KR. The effect of oxidized lipids in the diet on serum lipoprotein peroxides in control and diabetic rats. J Clin Invest 1993;92:638
117. Nadler JL, Malayan S, Luong E, et al. Intracellular free magnesium plays a key role in increased platelet reactivity in type II diabetes. Diabetes Care 1992;15:835
118. Resnick LM, Gupta RK, Bhargava KK, et al. Cellular ions in hypertension, diabetes and obesity. Hypertension 1991;17:951
119. Weglicki WB, Phillips TM. Pathobiology of magnesium deficiency: A cytokine/neurogenic inflammation hypothesis. Am J Physiol 1992;263:734
120. Nadler JL, Buchanan T, Natarajan R, et al. Magnesium deficiency produces insulin resistance and increased thromboxane synthesis. Hypertension 1993;21:1024
121. Schmidt LE, Arfken CL, Heins JM. Evaluation of nutrient intake in subjects with non–insulin-dependent diabetes mellitus. J Am Dietetic Assoc 1994; 94:773

Index

Page numbers followed by *t* and *f* indicate tables and figures, respectively.